ANTIMICROBIAL AGENTS
AND
CHEMOTHERAPY

VOLUME 10

WASHINGTON, D.C. 20006

1976

ANTIMICROBIAL AGENTS AND CHEMOTHERAPY

VOLUME 10 • 1976

EDITORIAL BOARD

EX OFFICIO

Antimicrobial Agents and Chemotherapy, an interdisciplinary publication of the American Society for Microbiology, 1913 I St., N.W., Washington, D.C. 20006, is devoted to the dissemination of knowledge relating to all aspects of antimicrobial agents and chemotherapy, including cancer chemotherapy. *Antimicrobial Agents and Chemotherapy* is published monthly, and the twelve numbers are divided into two volumes per year. The nonmember subscription price is $50 per year. The member subscription price is $13 per year. Single copies are $5. Correspondence relating to subscriptions, reprints, defective copies, availability of back issues, lost or late proofs, disposition of submitted manuscripts, and general editorial matters should be directed to the ASM Publications Office, 1913 I St., N.W., Washington, D.C. 20006 (area 202 833-9680).

Second class postage paid at Washington, D.C. 20006, and at additional mailing offices.
Made in the United States of America.

Volume 10

Contents for July

Number 1

Biosynthesis; Chemistry; Mechanisms of Action and Resistance

Specific Inactivation of Herpes Simplex Virus by Silver Nitrate at Low Concentrations and Biological Activities of the Inactivated Virus. FUMIO SHIMIZU,* YOSHINOBU SHIMIZU, AND KATSUO KUMAGAI 57

Antiviral Activity of Arabinosyladenine and Arabinosylhypoxanthine in Herpes Simplex Virus-Infected KB Cells: Selective Inhibition of Viral Deoxyribonucleic Acid Synthesis in the Presence of an Adenosine Deaminase Inhibitor. PAULINE M. SCHWARTZ, CHARLES SHIPMAN, JR., AND JOHN C. DRACH* 64

Inactivation of the Enveloped Bacteriophage $\phi 6$ by Butylated Hydroxytoluene and Butylated Hydroxyanisole. PAUL WANDA, JAMES CUPP, WALLACE SNIPES,* ALEC KEITH, TOM RUCINSKY, LOUIS POLISH, AND JEFFREY SANDS 96

Beta-Lactamase Activity in Anaerobic Bacteria. A. ELISE WEINRICH AND VICTOR E. DEL BENE* 106

Antiviral Action and Cellular Toxicity of Four Thymidine Analogues: 5-Ethyl-, 5-Vinyl-, 5-Propyl-, and 5-Allyl-2′-Deoxyuridine. YUNG-CHI CHENG,* BARBARA A. DOMIN, RAM A. SHARMA, AND MIROSLAV BOBEK 119

Phleomycin-Induced Solubilization of Deoxyribonucleic Acid in Uninfected and T Bacteriophage-Infected *Escherichia coli* B. KAREN SHIVE AND C. F. EARHART* 150

Photoinactivation of Venezuelan Equine Encephalitis Virus Mediated by Tetracyclines. JOSE ESPARZA,* CARMEN I. PIÑA, AND ERNESTO NOVO 176

Absence of Penicillin-Degrading Enzymes in Penicillin-Resistant Strains of *Neisseria gonorrhoeae*. J. L. BEEBE,* P. LIGETI, AND T. J. WLODKOWSKI ... 179

Nalidixic Acid Inhibition of Post-Ultraviolet Recovery in *Escherichia coli* K-12: Requirement for *recBC* Function. MICHAEL A. PURDY* AND K. LEMONE YIELDING 182

Physiological Effects and Microbial Susceptibility

In Vitro Activity of Gentamicin and Minocycline Alone and in Combination Against Bacteria Associated with Intra-Abdominal Sepsis. ROBERT J. FASS,* DANIEL E. RUIZ, RICHARD B. PRIOR, AND ROBERT L. PERKINS 34

Susceptibility of *Prototheca* Species to Antifungal Agents. ESTER SEGAL, ARVIND A. PADHYE,* AND LIBERO AJELLO 75

Short-Term Storage of Six Penicillins and Cephalothin in Microdilution Trays for Antimicrobial Susceptibility Tests. A. L. BARRY,* L. J. EFFINGER, AND R. E. BADAL 83

Susceptibility of *Acinetobacter calcoaceticus* var. *anitratus* (*Herellea vaginicola*) to Minocycline. J. Z. MONTGOMERIE,* M. J. PICKETT, R. N. YOSHIMORI, A. W. CHOW, AND L. B. GUZE 102

Susceptibility Testing of Anaerobic Bacteria with 100-μg Carbenicillin Disks. W. W. LASLIE* AND D. W. LAMBE, JR. 112

R Factor-Mediated Antibiotic Resistance in *Serratia marcescens*. ROBERT C. COOKSEY, GRACE M. THORNE, AND W. EDMUND FARRAR, JR.* 123

Antimicrobial Susceptibility of Group B Streptococci Isolated from a Variety of Clinical Sources. CAROL J. BAKER,* BETTE J. WEBB, AND FRED F. BARRETT 128

In Vitro Comparison of Netilmicin, a Semisynthetic Derivative of Sisomicin, and Four Other Aminoglycoside Antibiotics. S. A. KABINS,* C. NATHAN, AND S. COHEN 139

In Vitro Antimicrobial Activity of Cinoxacin Against 2,968 Clinical Bacterial Isolates. R. N. JONES* AND P. C. FUCHS 146

* Asterisk refers to person to whom inquiries regarding the paper should be addressed.

Synergism of Cefazolin-Gentamicin Against Enterococci. MICHAEL BOURQUE, RICHARD QUINTILIANI,* AND RICHARD C. TILTON 157

Inhibition of L5178Y Cells in Culture by Methotrexate and Antibiotics. P. L. CHELLO* AND H. W. BRUCKNER 185

In Vitro Activity of Josamycin and Rosamicin Against *Bacteroides fragilis* Compared with Clindamycin, Erythromycin, and Metronidazole. JEROME SANTORO, DONALD KAYE, AND MATTHEW E. LEVISON* 188

Pharmacology and Therapeutics

In Vitro and In Vivo Evaluation of Ceftezole, a New Cephalosporin Derivative. MINORU NISHIDA,* TAKEO MURAKAWA, TOSHIAKI KAMIMURA, NAOHIKO OKADA, HIROSHI SAKAMOTO, SHIGEMI FUKADA, SHOJI NAKAMOTO, YOSHIKO YOKOTA, AND KAZUYO MIKI 1

Antiviral and Interferon-Inducing Activity of a New Glutarimide Antibiotic, 9-Methylstreptimidone. NORIYUKI SAITO, FUJIO SUZUKI, KENJI SASAKI, AND NAKAO ISHIDA* 14

Bioevaluation of the Antibacterial Flumequine for Urinary Tract Use. S. R. ROHLFING,* J. F. GERSTER, AND D. C. KVAM 20

Pharmacokinetic Parameters of Sisomicin. BURT R. MEYERS, SHALOM Z. HIRSCHMAN,* STANLEY YANCOVITZ, AND BRUCE RIBNER 25

Antiviral Effect of Pyran Against Systemic Infection of Mice with Herpes Simplex Virus Type 2. RONALD S. MCCORD, MARY K. BREINIG, AND PAGE S. MORAHAN* 28

Characterization and Quantitation of Experimental Surgical-Wound Infections Used to Evaluate Topical Antibacterial Agents. R. J. MCRIPLEY* AND R. R. WHITNEY 38

Responsiveness of Experimental Surgical-Wound Infections to Topical Chemotherapy. R. J. MCRIPLEY* AND R. R. WHITNEY 45

Cefazolin in the Treatment of Acute Enteric Fever. MARWAN UWAYDAH 52

Gentamicin- and Cephalothin-Associated Rises in Blood Urea Nitrogen. W. LEE FANNING, DIETER GUMP, AND HERSHEL JICK* 80

Influence of Subtherapeutic Levels of a Combination of Neomycin and Oxytetracycline on *Salmonella typhimurium* in Swine, Calves, and Chickens. A. E. GIRARD,* A. R. ENGLISH, D. G. EVANGELISTI, J. E. LYNCH, AND I. A. SOLOMONS 89

Laboratory Evaluation of 3-(5-Tetrazolyl)Penam, a New Semisynthetic Beta-Lactam Antibacterial Agent with Extended Broad-Spectrum Activity. ARTHUR R. ENGLISH,* JAMES A. RETSEMA, AND JOHN E. LYNCH 132

Acute Diffuse Interstitial Nephritis Related to Chemotherapy of Tuberculosis. WILLIAM J. STONE,* JAMES A. WALDRON, JOHN H. DIXON, JR., R. KIRBY PRIMM, AND ROBERT G. HORN 164

Triple Crossover Study on Absorption and Excretion of Ampicillin, Talampicillin, and Amoxycillin. L. VERBIST 173

Volume 10

Contents for August

Number 2

Biosynthesis; Chemistry; Mechanisms of Action and Resistance

Inducible Oxacillin-Hydrolyzing Penicillinase in *Aeromonas hydrophila* Isolated from Fish. TETSUO SAWAI,* KAYOKO MORIOKA, MAYUMI OGAWA, AND SABURO YAMAGISHI 191

Indirect Method for Assessing the Penetration of Beta-Lactamase-Nonsusceptible

Penicillins and Cephalosporins in *Escherichia coli* Strains. M. H. RICHMOND,* D. C. CLARK, AND SANDRA WOTTON 215

Comparative Study of Seven Cephalosporins: Susceptibility to Beta-Lactamases and Ability to Penetrate the Surface Layers of *Escherichia coli*. M. H. RICHMOND* AND SANDRA WOTTON 219

Comparison of Tetracycline Action on *Staphylococcus aureus* and *Escherichia coli* by Microbial Kinetics. SAMUEL M. HEMAN-ACKAH 223

Photoinactivation of Latent Herpes Simplex Virus in Rabbit Kidney Cells. J. J. KELLEHER* AND J. VARANI 229

Hydroxyquinolines Inhibit Ribonucleic Acid-Dependent Deoxyribonucleic Acid Polymerase and Inactivate Rous Sarcoma Virus and Herpes Simplex Virus. WOLFGANG ROHDE, PETER MIKELENS, JEAN JACKSON, JANE BLACKMAN, JACK WHITCHER, AND WARREN LEVINSON* 234

A New Cephalosporin with a Dual Mode of Action. CYNTHIA H. O'CALLAGHAN,* R. B. SYKES, AND SUSAN E. STANIFORTH 245

Dual-Action Cephalosporin Utilizing a Novel Therapeutic Principle. D. GREENWOOD* AND F. O'GRADY 249

New Plasmid-Mediated Nucleotidylation of Aminoglycoside Antibiotics in *Staphylococcus aureus*. F. LE GOFFIC,* A. MARTEL, M. L. CAPMAU, B. BACA, P. GOEBEL, H. CHARDON, C. J. SOUSSY, J. DUVAL, AND D. H. BOUANCHAUD ... 258

Nutrition of *Bacillus brevis* ATCC 9999, the Producer of Gramicidin S. E. J. VANDAMME AND A. L. DEMAIN* 265

Mode of Action of a Purified Antitumor Protein from the Proteinaceous Crystal of *Bacillus thuringiensis* subsp. *thuringiensis* on Yoshida Ascites Sarcoma Cells. S. S. S. V. PRASAD* AND Y. I. SHETHNA 293

Genetic Basis of Streptococcin A-FF22 Production. J. R. TAGG AND L. W. WANNAMAKER* 299

Specific Action of 4-Nitropyridine 1-Oxide on *Escherichia coli* K-12 Pro^+ Strains Leading to the Isolation of Proline-Requiring Mutants: Isolation and Characterization of Pro^- Mutants. MANABU INUZUKA,* HIROSHI MIYANO, AND MUNEMITSU TOMOEDA 325

Specific Action of 4-Nitropyridine 1-Oxide on *Escherichia coli* K-12 Pro^+ Strains Leading to the Isolation of Proline-Requiring Mutants: Mechanism of Action of 4-Nitropyridine 1-Oxide. MANABU INUZUKA,* HIROMI TOYAMA, HIROSHI MIYANO, AND MUNEMITSU TOMOEDA 333

Formation of Methylated and Phosphorylated Metabolites During the Fermentation Process of Verdamicin. B. K. LEE,* R. G. CONDON, G. H. WAGMAN, AND M. J. WEINSTEIN 363

Physiological Effects and Microbial Susceptibility

Comparison of Direct and Standardized Antimicrobial Susceptibility Testing of Positive Blood Cultures. JAMES E. JOHNSON AND JOHN A. WASHINGTON II* .. 211

Comparative Activity In Vitro of Ticarcillin, BL-P1654, and Carbenicillin. THEODORE E. EICKHOFF* AND JOSEPHINE M. EHRET 241

In Vitro Susceptibility of Common Clinical Anaerobic and Aerobic Isolates Against Josamycin. RICHARD E. REESE, ROBERT F. BETTS,* LOLA W. GOEDDE, AND R. GORDON DOUGLAS, JR. 253

Susceptibility of *Streptococcus mutans* to Antimicrobial Agents. JOSEPH F. FERRETTI* AND MARGIE WARD 274

In Vitro Evaluation of the New Oral Cephalosporin Cefatrizine: Comparison with Other Cephalosporins. C. CAROLINE BLACKWELL,* EARL H. FREIMER, AND GREGORY C. TUKE 288

Susceptibility of *Haemophilus influenzae* Type b to Cefatrizine, Ampicillin, and Chloramphenicol. THOMAS BROTHERTON, TRACY LEES, AND RALPH D. FEIGIN* 322

Chloramphenicol: an Enzymological Microassay. PAUL S. LIETMAN,* THOMAS J. WHITE, AND WILLIAM V. SHAW 347

Inhibition of *Neisseria gonorrhoeae* by a Bacteriocin from *Pseudomonas aeruginosa*. STEPHEN A. MORSE,* PATRICK VAUGHAN, DEANNE JOHNSON, AND BARBARA H. IGLEWSKI 354

In Vitro Susceptibility of Pathogenic *Naegleria* and *Acanthamoeba* Species to a Variety of Therapeutic Agents. RICHARD J. DUMA* AND RUTH FINLEY 370

Genotypic Stability of Methicillin Resistance in *Staphylococcus aureus* at Supraoptimal Temperature. FERENC ROZGONYI 377

Comparative In Vitro Activity of Sch 20656, Netilmicin, Gentamicin, and Tobramycin. CHATRCHAI WATANAKUNAKORN 382

Pharmacology and Therapeutics

In Vitro Effects of Low Concentrations of Penicillin and Sulfadiazine on *Streptococcus mutans*. H. G. WELD AND H. J. SANDHAM* 196

Effect of Long-Term Therapies with Penicillin and Sulfadiazine on *Streptococcus mutans* and Lactobacilli in Dental Plaque. H. G. WELD AND H. J. SANDHAM* 200

Amikacin in Newborn Infants: Comparative Pharmacology with Kanamycin and Clinical Efficacy in 45 Neonates with Bacterial Diseases. JORGE B. HOWARD, GEORGE H. MCCRACKEN, JR.,* HUGO TRUJILLO, AND EDGAR MOHS 205

Renal Extraction of Gentamicin in Anesthetized Dogs. PETER J. S. CHIU,* ARTHUR BROWN, GEORGE MILLER, AND JAMES F. LONG 277

Pharmacokinetic Interpretation of Cephradine Levels in Serum After Intravenous and Extravascular Administration in Humans. ELISABETH S. RATTIE, PETER D. BERNARDO, AND LOUIS J. RAVIN* 283

Comparative Pharmacokinetics and Metabolism of Cephapirin in Laboratory Animals and Humans. B. E. CABANA, D. R. VAN HARKEN,* AND G. H. HOTTENDORF 307

Treatment of Murine Coccidioidomycosis with Polymyxin B. M. S. COLLINS* AND D. PAPPAGIANIS 318

Effect of Gentamicin on Growth of Viral, Chlamydial, and Rickettsial Agents in Mice and Embryonated Eggs. LENDELL A. WHITE,* HENRIETTA E. HALL, T. TZIANABOS, AND W. ADRIAN CHAPPELL 344

Change in Susceptibility of Group B Streptococci to Penicillin G from 1968 Through 1975. M. J. SEVERIN* AND J. L. WILEY 380

Comparison of Activity of Sisomicin and Gentamicin in Mouse Protection Tests with Gram-Negative Bacilli. BURT R. MEYERS AND SHALOM Z. HIRSCHMAN* 384

Volume 10 # Contents for September **Number 3**

Biosynthesis; Chemistry; Mechanisms of Action and Resistance

Inhibition of the Apparent Rate of Synthesis of the Vacuolar Glycoprotein Carboxypeptidase Y and Its Protein Antigen by Tunicamycin in *Saccharomyces cerevisiae*. ANDREJ HASILIK AND WIDMAR TANNER* 402

Substrate Inhibition of Beta-Lactamases, a Method for Predicting Enzymatic Stability of Cephalosporins. DAVID F. MAHONEY, G. A. KOPPEL, AND J. R. TURNER* 470

Antitrichomonad Action, Mutagenicity, and Reduction of Metronidazole and Other Nitroimidazoles. DONALD G. LINDMARK* AND MIKLÓS MÜLLER 476

Basis for the Design of Anticandidal Agents from Studies of Peptide Utilization in *Candida albicans*. WAYNE D. LICHLITER, FRED NAIDER, AND JEFFREY M. BECKER* 483

Chemical Nature of Agrocin 84 and Its Effect on a Virulent Strain of *Agrobacterium tumefaciens*. BARBARA A. MCCARDELL AND C. F. POOTJES* 498

Evolution of Transferable Antibiotic Resistance in Coliform Bacteria from Remote Environments. SHARON J. BURT AND D. R. WOODS* 567

Physiological Effects and Microbial Susceptibility

Antimicrobial Susceptibility of *Propionibacterium acnes* and Related Microbial Species. U. HOEFFLER, H. L. KO, AND G. PULVERER* 387

Activity of Newer Aminoglycosides and Carbenicillin, Alone and in Combination, Against Gentamicin-Resistant *Pseudomonas aeruginosa*. M. I. MARKS,* S. HAMMERBERG, G. GREENSTONE, AND BARRY SILVER 399

Mutants of *Pseudomonas aeruginosa* That Show Specific Hypersensitivity to Aminoglycosides. B. J. MILLS AND B. W. HOLLOWAY* 411

Bacteriocin Production by *Neisseria gonorrhoeae*. WILLIAM D. LAWTON,* MARY ANN BELLINGER, MARION SCHLING, AND HASSAN A. GAAFAR 417

Laboratory Evaluation of BL-S786, a Cephalosporin with Broad-Spectrum Antibacterial Activity. F. LEITNER,* M. MISIEK, T. A. PURSIANO, R. E. BUCK, D. R. CHISHOLM, R. G. DEREGIS, Y. H. TSAI, AND K. E. PRICE 426

Reproducibility of Control Strains for Antibiotic Susceptibility Testing. MARIE B. COYLE,* MARY F. LAMPE, CONNIE L. AITKEN, POLLY FEIGL, AND JOHN C. SHERRIS 436

Comparison of the In Vitro Activity of Several Cephalosporin Antibiotics Against Gram-Negative and Gram-Positive Bacteria Resistant to Cephaloridine. ALEXANDER L. KISCH* AND LUANNA BARTHOLOMEW 507

In Vitro Synergistic Effect of Netilmicin, a New Aminoglycoside Antibiotic. KWUNG P. FU AND HAROLD C. NEU* 511

Selection and Characterization of Strains of *Staphylococcus aureus* Displaying Unusual Resistance to Aminoglycosides. STEPHEN G. WILSON* AND CHRISTINE C. SANDERS 519

In Vitro Study of Netilmicin Compared with Other Aminoglycosides. KWUNG P. FU AND HAROLD C. NEU* 526

Synergy of Mecillinam, a Beta-Amidinopenicillanic Acid Derivative, Combined with Beta-Lactam Antibiotics. HAROLD C. NEU 535

New Method for Detecting In Vitro Inactivation of Penicillins by *Haemophilus influenzae* and *Staphylococcus aureus*. WIE-SHING LEE* AND LOUIS KOMARMY 564

Inhibition of Antibiotic Activity In Vitro by Synthetic Melanin. MICHAEL BARZA,* JULES BAUM, AND ANNE KANE 569

Pharmacology and Therapeutics

Pharmacological Study of Cefazolin During Intermittent and Continuous Infusion: a Crossover Investigation in Humans. J. P. THYS,* B. VANDERKELEN, AND J. KLASTERSKY 395

Comparative Pharmacokinetics of Cefamandole, Cephapirin, and Cephalothin in Healthy Subjects and Effect of Repeated Dosing. MICHAEL BARZA,* SRIKUMARAN MELETHIL, STEPHEN BERGER, AND E. CHAIM ERNST 421

Active Metabolites of Isoxazolylpenicillins in Humans. H. H. W. THIJSSEN* AND H. MATTIE 441

Reversible Thrombocytosis and Anemia Due to Miconazole Therapy. LEROY C. MARMION, KENNETH B. DESSER,* RALPH B. LILLY, AND DAVID A. STEVENS .. 447

Comparative Pharmacology of Josamycin and Erythromycin Stearate. LARRY J. STRAUSBAUGH, W. KLINE BOLTON, JOHN A. DILWORTH, RICHARD L. GUERRANT, AND MERLE A. SANDE* 450

Pharmacokinetics of Cefamandole in Patients Undergoing Hemodialysis and Peritoneal Dialysis. MARY JEAN AHERN, FREDERIC O. FINKELSTEIN, AND VINCENT T. ANDRIOLE* 457

Concentrations of Trimethoprim-Sulfamethoxazole in Blood After a Single, Large Oral Dose. THOMAS T. YOSHIKAWA* AND LUCIEN B. GUZE 462

Effect of Renal Failure and Dialysis on the Serum Concentration of the Aminoglycoside Amikacin. T. MADHAVAN,* K. YAREMCHUK, N. LEVIN, D. POHLOD, K. BURCH, E. FISHER, F. COX, AND E. L. QUINN 464

Comparison of Thrombophlebitis Associated with Three Cephalosporin Antibiotics. W. T. SIEBERT,* E. L. WESTERMAN, J. D. SMILACK, M. W. BRADSHAW, AND T. W. WILLIAMS, JR 467

Pirbenicillin: Pharmacokinetic Parameters in Mice. ARTHUR R. ENGLISH,* DENNIS GIRARD, AND JAMES A. RETSEMA 491

Effect of Organic Mercurials and Sulfhydryl Compounds on the Urease Activity of *Proteus*: Inhibition by Urine and Ascorbic Acid. CALVIN M. KUNIN 503

5″-Amino-5″-Deoxybutirosin, a Semisynthetic Analogue of Butirosin A: Antibacterial Activity In Vitro and in Mice. C. L. HEIFETZ,* C. A. FREY, I. A. PEARSON, AND J. C. SESNIE 543

Therapeutic Effects of Ribavirin Given by the Intraperitoneal or Aerosol Route Against Influenza Virus Infections in Mice. E. L. STEPHEN,* J. W. DOMINIK, J. B. MOE, AND J. S. WALKER 549

Can Mannitol Reduce Amphotericin B Nephrotoxicity? Double-Blind Study and Description of a New Vascular Lesion in Kidneys. WARD E. BULLOCK,* ROBERT G. LUKE, CHARLES E. NUTTALL, AND DINYAR BHATHENA 555

Antiviral Effects of Virazole in Chronic Hepatitis B Surface Antigen-Seropositive Chimpanzees. ALEXANDER E. DENES,* JAMES W. EBERT, KENNETH R. BERQUIST, BERT L. MURPHY, AND JAMES E. MAYNARD 571

Volume 10

Contents for October

Number 4

Biosynthesis; Chemistry; Mechanisms of Action and Resistance

Mode of Action of Penicillins In Vivo and In Vitro in *Bacillus megaterium*. TETSUO OKA 579

Kinetics of the Actions of Tetracyclines on *Escherichia coli* as Studied by Microcalorimetry. PER-ANDERS MÅRDH,* TORVALD RIPA, KARL-ERIK ANDERSSON, AND INGEMAR WADSÖ 604

Growth of *Physarum gyrosum* on Agar Plates and in Liquid Culture. RICHARD L. TAYLOR AND M. F. MALLETTE* 613

Tirandamycin, an Inhibitor of Bacterial Ribonucleic Acid Polymerase. FRITZ REUSSER 618

Differential Effects of 5-Methylmercapto-2′-Deoxyuridine on the Replication of Herpes Simplex Virus Type 1 in Two Cell Systems. ROBERT HARDI, R. G. HUGHES, JR.,* Y. K. HO, K. C. CHADHA, AND T. J. BARDOS 682

Suppression of the Lytic and Bactericidal Effects of Cell Wall-Inhibitory Antibiotics. RUBEN LOPEZ, CONCHITA RONDA-LAIN, ALFONSO TAPIA, SUSAN B. WAKS, AND ALEXANDER TOMASZ* 697

Correlation of Resistance to Proflavine and Penicillin in *Escherichia coli*. ROBIN C. MCKELLAR, COLIN N. MCKENZIE, AND DONN J. KUSHNER* 765

Physiological Effects and Microbial Susceptibility

Classification of R Plasmids by Incompatability in *Pseudomonas aeruginosa*. H. SAGAI,* K. HASUDA, S. IYOBE, L. E. BRYAN, B. W. HOLLOWAY, AND S. MITSUHASHI 573

Comparative Activity of Netilmicin, Gentamicin, Amikacin, and Tobramycin Against *Pseudomonas aeruginosa* and *Enterobacteriaceae*. DALIUS J. BRIEDIS AND HUGH G. ROBSON* 592

Antibiotic Resistance of Bacteria in Water Containing Ornamental Fishes. T. J. TRUST* AND J. L. WHITBY 598

Multiple Antibiotic Resistance in Clinical Strains of *Neisseria gonorrhoeae* Isolated in South Carolina. JAMES T. POWELL AND JOHN H. BOND* 639

Comparison of the Antibacterial Activity of Nine Cephalosporins Against *Enterobacteriaceae* and Nonfermentative Gram-Negative Bacilli. LUDO VERBIST 657

Enzymatic Adenylylation by Aminoglycoside 4′-Adenylyltransferase and 2″-Adenylyltransferase as a Means of Determining Concentrations of Aminoglycoside Antibiotics in Serum. P. SANTANAM AND F. H. KAYSER* 664

In Vitro Susceptibility of Gentamicin-Resistant *Enterobacteriaceae* and *Pseudomonas aeruginosa* to Netilmicin and Selected Aminoglycoside Antibiotics. RICHARD D. MEYER,* LINDA L. KRAUS, AND KAREN A. PASIECZNIK 677

Variation in the Susceptibility of Strains of *Staphylococcus aureus* to Oxacillin, Cephalothin, and Gentamicin. C. G. MAYHALL, G. MEDOFF,* AND J. J. MARR 707

Susceptibility of Respiratory Tract Anaerobes to Orally Administered Penicillins and Cephalosporins. DAVID F. BUSCH, LUBNA AFZAL KURESHI, VERA L. SUTTER, AND SYDNEY M. FINEGOLD* 713

Antimicrobial Susceptibility Testing of Yeasts: a Turbidimetric Technique Inpendent of Inoculum Size. JOHN N. GALGIANI* AND DAVID A. STEVENS 721

Aerobically Incubated Thioglycolate Broth Disk Method for Antibiotic Susceptibility Testing of Anaerobes. TERRENCE A. KURZYNSKI,* JOHN W. YRIOS, ARLAN G. HELSTAD, AND CHARLES R. FIELD 727

Susceptibility of Anaerobic Bacteria to 23 Antimicrobial Agents. VERA L. SUTTER* AND SYDNEY M. FINEGOLD 736

R-Plasmid Transfer In Vivo in the Absence of Antibiotic Selection Pressure. V. PETROCHEILOU, J. GRINSTED, AND M. H. RICHMOND* 753

Inhibition of Bacteriophage Lambda, T1, and T7 Development by R Plasmids of the H Incompatibility Group. DIANE E. TAYLOR* AND ROBERT B. GRANT 762

In Vitro Comparison of Gentamicin, Tobramycin, Sisomicin, and Netilmicin. K. N. BROWN,* J. BENEDICTSON, AND S. SWANBY 768

Josamycin and Rosamicin: In Vitro Comparisons with Erythromycin and Clindamycin. SMITH SHADOMY,* MARGARET TIPPLE, AND LARRY PAXTON 773

New Medium for In Vitro Susceptibility Studies with Amphotericin B. C. J. UTZ, S. WHITE, AND S. SHADOMY* 776

Pharmacology and Therapeutics

Effects of Doxycycline in Actively Purging Cholera Patients: a Double-Blind Clinical Trial. M. Mujibur Rahaman,* M. A. Majid, A. K. M. Jamiul Alam, and M. Rafiqul Islam 610

Pharmacokinetics of Cefamandole in the Presence of Renal Failure and in Patients Undergoing Hemodialysis. Gerald B. Appel, Harold C. Neu,* Michael F. Parry, Mark J. Goldberger, and Ginette B. Jacob 623

Nosocomial Infection with Gentamicin-Carbenicillin-Resistant *Pseudomonas aeruginosa*. Ian M. Baird,* Jerry M. Slepack, Carol A. Kauffman, and John P. Phair 626

Metabolism of [^{14}C]Cefaclor, a Cephalosporin Antibiotic, in Three Species of Laboratory Animals. Hugh R. Sullivan,* Susan L. Due, Donald L. K. Kau, John F. Quay, and Warren M. Miller 630

Synergistic Activity of Carbenicillin and Gentamicin in Experimental *Pseudomonas* Bacteremia in Neutropenic Rats. Rita E. Scott and Hugh G. Robson* 646

Radioimmunoassay of Iodinated Tobramycin. Alan Broughton,* James E. Strong, Larry K. Pickering, and Gerald P. Bodey 652

Effect of Treatment with Exogenous Interferon, Polyinosinic Acid-Polycytidylic Acid, or Polyinosinic Acid-Polycytidylic Acid–Poly-L-Lysine Complex on Encephalomyocarditis Virus Infections in Mice. Gregg A. Olsen,* Earl R. Kern, Lowell A. Glasgow, and James C. Overall, Jr. 668

Comparative Toxicological Studies of Amphotericin B Methyl Ester and Amphotericin B in Mice, Rats, and Dogs. G. R. Keim, Jr.,* P. L. Sibley, Y. H. Yoon, J. S. Kulesza, I. H. Zaidi, M. M. Miller, and J. W. Poutsiaka 687

Antiviral Activity of BL-3849A, a Low-Molecular-Weight Oral Interferon Inducer. Earl R. Kern,* John R. Hamilton, James C. Overall, Jr., and Lowell A. Glasgow 691

Concentration of Cefamandole in Serum Interstitial Fluid, Bile, and Urine. N. G. Waterman,* H. U. Eickenberg, and L. Scharfenberger 733

Therapeutic Effects of Small-Particle Aerosols of Ribavirin on Parainfluenza (Sendai) Virus Infections of Mice. E. W. Larson,* E. L. Stephen, and J. S. Walker 770

Errata

Acute Diffuse Interstitial Nephritis Related to Chemotherapy of Tuberculosis. William J. Stone,* James A. Waldron, John H. Dixon, Jr., R. Kirby Primm, and Robert G. Horn 778

Gentamicin- and Cephalothin-Associated Rises in Blood Urea Nitrogen. W. Lee Fanning, Dieter Gump, and Hershel Jick* 778

Volume 10 Contents for November Number 5

Biosynthesis; Chemistry; Mechanisms of Action and Resistance

Inhibition of Conjugal Transfer of R Plasmids by Pipemidic Acid and Related Compounds. Shinichi Nakamura,* Satoru Inoue, Masanao Shimizu, Shizuko Iyobe, and Susumu Mitsuhashi 779

Effects of Antibiotics on Metabolism of Peptidoglycan, Protein, and Lipids in *Bifidobacterium bifidum* subsp. *pennsylvanicus*. G. C. Molenkamp and J. H. Veerkamp* 786

R Plasmids in *Streptococcus agalactiae* (Group B). THEA HORODNICEANU,* D. H. BOUANCHAUD, G. BIETH, AND Y. A. CHABBERT 795

Effect of Osmolality on the Response of *Escherichia coli* to Mecillinam. DAVID GREENWOOD 824

Preparation of Isolated Intestinal Villi Useful for Studying Hydrolysis Rates of Penicillin and Cephalosporin Esters. WALTER E. WRIGHT* AND VERLE D. LINE 861

Physiological Effects and Microbial Susceptibility

Combination of Bacteriostatic and Bactericidal Drugs: Lack of Significant In Vitro Antagonism Between Penicillin, Cephalothin, and Rolitetracycline. FRANZ D. DASCHNER 802

Biological Activity of Netilmicin, a Broad-Spectrum Semisynthetic Aminoglycoside Antibiotic. GEORGE H. MILLER,* GEORGE ARCIERI, MARVIN J. WEINSTEIN, AND J. ALLAN WAITZ 827

Antifungal Properties of Electrically Generated Metallic Ions. T. J. BERGER,* J. A. SPADARO, RICHARD BIERMAN, S. E. CHAPIN, AND R. O. BECKER 856

Sisomicin Versus Netilmicin: In Vitro Susceptibility Testing. D. J. FLOURNOY . 864

Stability of Gentamicin in Serum. SUE M. JONES, DONNA J. BLAZEVIC, AND HENRY H. BALFOUR, JR.* 866

Pharmacology and Therapeutics

Effect of Ribavirin on Murine Cytomegalovirus Infection. JOHN N. DOWLING,* BOSKO POSTIC, AND LUCILLE O. GUEVARRA 809

Cefamandole: In Vitro and Clinical Pharmacokinetics. R. S. GRIFFITH,* H. R. BLACK, G. L. BRIER, AND J. D. WOLNY 814

Ticarcillin in Combination with Cephalothin or Gentamicin as Empiric Antibiotic Therapy in Granulocytopenic Cancer Patients. STEPHEN C. SCHIMPFF,* SHELDON LANDESMAN, DAVIS M. HAHN, HAROLD C. STANDIFORD, CLARENCE L. FORTNER, VIOLA MAE YOUNG, AND PETER H. WIERNIK 837

Comparative Nephrotoxicities of Netilmicin and Gentamicin in Rats. FRIEDRICH C. LUFT,* MOO NAHM YUM, AND STUART A. KLEIT 845

Antibiotic Penetrance of Ascitic Fluid in Dogs. DALE N. GERDING,* JAMES P. KROMHOUT, JOHN J. SULLIVAN, AND WENDELL H. HALL 850

Volume 10 — Contents for December — Number 6

Biosynthesis; Chemistry; Mechanisms of Action and Resistance

Bacteriocin Production by Group A Streptococcal L-Forms. WALERIA HRYNIEWICZ* AND JOHN R. TAGG 912

Physiological Effects and Microbial Susceptibility

Reevaluation of the Disk Diffusion Method for Sulfonamide Susceptibility Testing of *Neisseria meningitidis*. SUSAN HAMMERBERG, MELVIN I. MARKS,* AND GERRY WEINMASTER 869

In Vitro Activity of Gentamicin, Amikacin, and Netilmicin Alone and in Combination with Carbenicillin Against *Serratia marcescens*. STEVEN M. POGWIZD AND STEPHEN A. LERNER* 878

Antibiotic Synergy and Antagonism Against Clinical Isolates of *Klebsiella* Species. ROBERT M. D'ALESSANDRI, DAVID J. MCNEELY, AND RONICA M. KLUGE* 889

Cultivation of *Staphylococcus auerus* in a Synthetic Medium of Low Ultraviolet Absorptivity. B. G. CHARLES AND B. D. RAWAL* 915

Comparative In Vitro Studies of Cinoxacin, Nalidixic Acid, and Oxolinic Acid. RALPH C. GORDON,* LYNNE I. STEVENS, CHARLES E. EDMISTON, JR., AND KANWAL MOHAN 918

Procedure for Expediting Determinations of Antibiotic Susceptibility of Gram-Negative, Urinary Tract Pathogens. DENNIS L. WEGNER* AND THOMAS R. NEBLETT 921

Chemically Defined Medium for Susceptibility Testing of Antimicrobial Agents. PAULA F. DOUGHERTY,* DAVID W. YOTTER, AND THOMAS R. MATTHEWS 923

Medium for Use in Antibiotic Susceptibility Testing of Anaerobic Bacteria. TRACY D. WILKINS* AND SARAH CHALGREN 926

Pharmacology and Therapeutics

Comparison of the Epidemiology of Bacterial Resistance to Mecillinam and Ampicillin. J. D. ANDERSON,* MONICA A. ADAMS, JANE C. BARRINGTON, W. N. SPENCE, AND C. A. SHEPHERD 872

Effect of 9-β-D-Arabinofuranosyladenine 5′-Monophosphate and 9-β-D-Arabinofuranosylhypoxanthine 5′-Monophosphate on Experimental Herpes Simplex Keratitis. HERBERT E. KAUFMAN AND EMILY D. VARNELL* 885

Effect of Clindamycin on Aminoglycoside Activity in a Murine Model of Invasive *Escherichia coli* Infection. EDEM EKWO AND GEORGES PETER* 893

Comparison of Josamycin and Erythromycin in the Therapy of *Mycoplasma pneumoniae* Pneumonia. RICHARD P. WENZEL,* J. OWEN HENDLEY, WENDELL K. DODD, AND JACK M. GWALTNEY, JR. 899

Cephalosporin and Aminoglycoside Concentrations in Peritoneal Capsular Fluid in Rabbits. DALE N. GERDING,* WENDELL H. HALL, ELIZABETH A. SCHIERL, AND ROBERT E. MANION 902

Erratum

Mutanolysin, Bacteriolytic Agent for Cariogenic Streptococci: Partial Purification and Properties. KANAE YOKOGAWA, SHIGEO KAWATA, SHINZO NISHIMURA, YASUHIKO IKEDA, AND YOSHIO YOSHIMURA 929

ANTIMICROBIAL AGENTS AND CHEMOTHERAPY, July 1976, p. 1-13

Vol. 10, No. 1
Printed in U.S.A.

In Vitro and In Vivo Evaluation of Ceftezole, a New Cephalosporin Derivative

MINORU NISHIDA,* TAKEO MURAKAWA, TOSHIAKI KAMIMURA, NAOHIKO OKADA, HIROSHI SAKAMOTO, SHIGEMI FUKADA, SHOJI NAKAMOTO, YOSHIKO YOKOTA, AND KAZUYO MIKI

Research Laboratories, Fujisawa Pharmaceutical Co., Ltd., Osaka, Japan

Received for publication 24 November 1975

Ceftezole, a new cephalosporin derivative, was compared with cefazolin, cephaloridine, and cephalothin. Data obtained indicate that it is a broad-spectrum antibiotic, with almost identical antimicrobial activity against pathogenic organisms isolated from patients. The therapeutic effect of ceftezole on experimental infections in mice was similar to that of cefazolin and was superior to that of cephalothin. The binding of ceftezole to serum proteins was somewhat less than that of cefazolin. The concentrations of ceftezole in the sera of test animals and human volunteers were determined after intramuscular injection of 20 mg/kg and after a single dose of 500 mg, respectively. The concentration of ceftezole in the serum of volunteers peaked at 24.9 μg/ml 15 min after injection and remained effective (about 2.6 μg/ml) at 4 h. The half-life in serum under the same conditions was 56 min, i.e., about one-half that of cefazolin. The 24-h urinary recovery rate was 87.5%. Most of the administered ceftezole was excreted unchanged mainly through the urinary tract. The biliary excretion rate in SD strain rats after intramuscular injection of 20 mg/kg was about 4.4%. As compared with commercially available cephalosporins, ceftezole was second only to cefazolin in biliary excretion rate. Various tissue levels of ceftezole in animals were higher than cephalothin but, with the exception of renal levels in the early stage after administration, were lower than cefazolin.

During the screening of new cephalosporin derivatives in Fujisawa Research Laboratories, cefazolin was identified as an agent of outstanding potential. It has since been proved to have excellent antimicrobial activity and tolerance (4) and has been widely tested in clinical situations (1–3).

In subsequent screening, some potentially more useful derivatives were found among those closely related to cefazolin in chemical structure. Of these, ceftezole (Fig. 1) has recently been developed and is reported here.

In the present study, the in vitro and in vivo antimicrobial activity, absorption, excretion, and tissue distribution of ceftezole were investigated and compared with those of related cephalosporins.

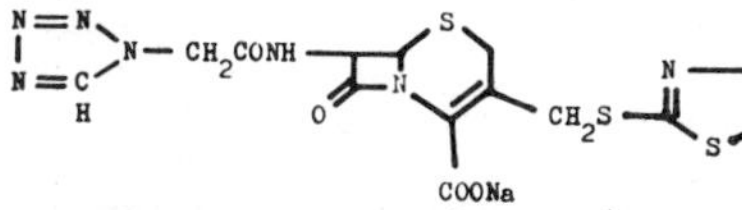

FIG. 1. *Chemical structure of ceftezole. Sodium (6R, 7R)-3-[(1,3,4-thiadiazol-2-yl)-thiomethyl]-8-oxo-7-[2-(1H-tetrazol-1-yl) acetamido]-5-thia-1-azabicyclo-[4,2,0] oct-2-ene-2-carboxylate. ($C_{13}H_{11}N_8O_4S_3Na$: molecular weight, 462.47).*

MATERIALS AND METHODS

Test antibiotics. Ceftezole and cephalosporin C were provided by Fujisawa Research Laboratories, cefazolin was provided by Fujisawa Pharmaceutical Co., Ltd., and cephaloridine and cephalothin were provided by Eli Lilly & Co.

Subjects. The following subjects were included: male ICR strain mice, each weighing 17 to 23 g, 4 weeks of age; male SD strain rats, each weighing 170 to 245 g, 6 weeks of age; male beagle dogs, each weighing 9.5 to 12.5 kg; male rhesus monkeys, each weighing 6.4 to 9.9 kg; and healthy male adult volunteers, each weighing 55 to 75 kg.

Measurement of in vitro antimicrobial activity. The in vitro antimicrobial activity of the test antibiotics was determined by the agar dilution method. An overnight broth culture and decimal dilutions thereof were spot-inoculated, using a multiple inoculator onto heart infusion agar (Difco) containing graded concentrations of the test drugs. The minimum inhibitory concentration (MIC) was estimated after incubation at 37 C for 20 h. For testing of activity against three species of *Streptococcus* and against *Corynebacterium diphtheriae*, 10% rabbit blood was added to the above media.

Bactericidal activity. Heart infusion broth containing one-fourth the MIC, the MIC, and four times the MIC of each test drug was inoculated with *Escherichia coli* NIHJ JC-2 in a quantity sufficient to yield a final concentration of 10^6 cells/ml. The cultures were then incubated at 37 C with shaking for an initial 8 h and without shaking for a subsequent 16-h period. The number of viable cells was measured at regular intervals throughout the incubation period.

Protein binding. (i) Ultrafiltration method. To 4.5 ml of human serum (Consera) or of fresh serum from each animal, 0.5 ml of antibiotic solution (300 μg/ml) in M/15 phosphate buffer (pH 7.0) was added and incubated at 37 C for 1 h. The mixture was poured into a Visking tube (8/32 in size) hung in a 15-ml polypropylene tube and centrifuged at 1,000 $\times$ *g* for 30 min. The concentration-free antibiotic in the ultrafiltrate was determined by the disk method. When these values are expressed as X and the values obtained in the reference experiment with buffer in place of serum are expressed as Y, the binding rate (B) of the antibiotics was determined as follows:

$$B\ (\%) = \frac{Y - X}{Y} \times 100$$

(ii) Effect of buffer dilution on antibiotic-protein binding. The antibiotic solution (500 μg/ml) was mixed with ninefold volumes of human serum (Consera). The mixture was allowed to stand at room temperature for 1 h, and then was diluted two-, four-, and eightfold with M/15 phosphate buffer (pH 7.0). The concentration of antibiotic in each dilution was determined by the disk method. When M/15 phosphate buffer was used instead of serum, the concentration of antibiotic was expressed in terms of relative value as 100.

Protective effect on infections in mice. Male ICR white mice, 4 weeks of age and each weighing 17 to 23 g, were used in groups of 10 mice each. The organisms were cultivated overnight at 37 C on brain heart infusion agar and were then suspended in 2 or 5% mucin solution to obtain microbial cell concentrations of 1×10^6 to 4×10^6/ml. Mice were inoculated intraperitoneally with 0.5 ml of the suspension. Each of the test antibiotics was administered subcutaneously in varying dosages to a group of 10 mice, 1 h after challenge. The mean effective dose (ED_{50}) values were found by the probit method from the number of surviving animals after 2 weeks of observation.

Microbiological assay. Each 10 ml of agar medium (1% sodium citrate, 0.5% polypeptone, 0.3% meat extract, and 1% agar) was inoculated with 10^5 spores of *Bacillus subtilis* ATCC 6633 per ml and placed in petri dishes. Test disks (6 or 8 mm in diameter were immersed in the standard solutions or test solutions containing the antibiotics under study. After removing excess water, the disks were placed on the above media. After standing at 37 C for 20 h, the diameters of the inhibitory zones were measured.

Absorption and excretion. (i) Drug concentrations in serum. The test drugs were given intramuscularly in a dose of 20 mg/kg to experimental animals and in a dose of 500 mg to healthy human volunteers. Groups of 10 rats each were anesthetized with chloroform, and blood was collected from the heart at 0.25, 0.5, 1, 1.5, and 2 h. The blood was collected from dogs, monkeys, and human volunteers from the foreleg veins at 0.5, 1, 2, 4, and 6 h. The concentrations of antibiotic in each serum sample was determined by the disk method, using standard solutions prepared with sera of respective animals and volunteers.

(ii) Urinary excretion. Urine of rats was collected with a urine collector at 0 to 3, 3 to 6, and 6 to 24 h after intramuscular injection of 20 mg of the test drugs per kg. Urine was collected from dogs and monkeys with a catheter at specified intervals after intramuscular injection. The concentration of antibiotic in each urine sample was bioassayed with the standard buffer at pH 7.0, and the urinary recovery rate was calculated.

(iii) Identification of active substances excreted into urine. Ceftezole was given intramuscularly to experimental animals (20 mg/kg) and human volunteers (500 mg). The urine was collected over a period of 6 h after administration and examined by thin-layer chromatography and bioautography. The standard ceftezole solution (1 mg/ml) and urine samples were examined chromatographically by the use of Eastman Chromagram sheet no. 6061. The sheet was then dried and developed with the solvent system *n*-butanol-acetic acid-water (4:1:5, top layer). The dried sheet was then placed on an agar plate that had been seeded with 0.2% of the spore suspension (2×10^8 spores/ml) of *B. subtilis* ATCC-6633.

(iv) Biliary excretion. Rats anesthetized with pentobarbital were fixed in a supine position, and a polyethylene cannula was inserted into the bile duct. Bile samples were collected at 0 to 3, 3 to 6, and 6 to 24 h after intramuscular injection of 20 mg of the test drugs per kg. The antibiotic levels in the bile samples were assayed with the standard solutions prepared with M/15 phosphate buffer (pH 7.0).

(v) Tissue distribution. Groups of three rats each received intramuscularly 20 mg of each of the test antibiotics per kg and were sacrificed at 30, 60, and 90 min after drug administration. Liver, kidneys, lungs, heart, and spleen were removed and after light washing in saline solution, the organs from each group of animals were pooled, mixed with ethanol, and homogenized in a polytron homogenizer. The concentrations of antibiotic in the supernatants obtained by centrifuging the tissue homogenates at 10,000 rpm for 10 min were bioassayed with the standard solutions prepared with M/15 phosphate buffer (pH 7.0) containing 66% ethanol. Each experiment was repeated three times in the same manner, and the values were averaged.

(vi) Antibiotic concentrations in pouch exudates. After subcutaneous injection of 20 ml of air into the backs of rats, 1 ml of 1% olive oil containing croton oil was injected into the pouch of each animal to obtain aseptic inflammation. A 20-mg amount of each antibiotic per kg was given intramuscularly on day 6 or 7 after formation of the pouch, and the exudates were collected at 0.5, 1, 2, 3, and 4 h. The antibiotic concentrations in the exudates were bioassayed with the standard solutions diluted with the exudates.

RESULTS

Antimicrobial activity. In the experiments conducted as a part of this study, ceftezole showed a broad spectrum of antimicrobial activity against gram-positive and gram-negative bacteria, as did cefazolin and the other two cephalosporins tested (Table 1). Ceftezole was inactive against *Proteus vulgaris* IAM-1025 and *Pseudomonas aeruginosa* IAM-1095.

The susceptibilities of 354 strains isolated from patients to ceftezole are shown in Table 2. *Staphylococcus aureus, E. coli, Klebsiella pneumoniae,* and *P. mirabilis* were tested, using an inoculum of 10^8 microbial cell units/ml. The MICs of ceftezole against 40 strains of *S. aureus* ranged from 0.2 to 3.13 μg/ml. The MIC of ceftezole for 21 (52.5%) of the 40 strains was 0.39 μg/ml. All strains tested were susceptible to ceftezole and to the other cephalosporins examined. The susceptibility of the strains was greatest for cephaloridine; cephalothin was the next most active. The susceptibility of these strains to ceftezole was almost the same as to cefazolin. The susceptibility of *S. aureus* to cephalosporins was greater than that of the gram-negative organisms tested. The susceptibility of 40 strains of *E. coli* to ceftezole was almost the same as that of cefazolin. The MICs ranged from 1.56 to >400 μg/ml and were most frequently 6.25 μg/ml (20 [50%] of the 40 strains). Four (10%) of the 40 test strains were highly resistant, the MICs being 100 μg/ml or greater. The antimicrobial activity of ceftezole against *E. coli* was almost the same as that of cefazolin and was markedly superior to that of cephalothin. The susceptibility of 60 strains of *K. pneumoniae* to ceftezole was almost the same as that of cefazolin. The MICs ranged from 1.56 to 400 μg/ml and were 3.13 μg/ml for 37 (61.7%) of the 60 strains. Five (8.3%) of the 60 strains were highly resistant, the MICs being 100 μg/ml or more. From these data, it can be assumed that the antimicrobial activity of cef-

TABLE 1. *Antimicrobial spectra of ceftezole and other cephalosporins*[a]

Strain	MIC (μg/ml) of:			
	Ceftezole	Cefazolin	Cephaloridine	Cephalothin
Staphylococcus aureus 209P JC-1	0.2	0.39	0.1	0.39
S. aureus Newman	0.39	0.78	0.1	0.39
S. aureus Terashima	0.78	1.56	0.1	0.39
S. aureus Smith	0.2	0.39	0.025	0.2
S. aureus ATCC-6538 P	0.39	0.39	0.05	0.2
Bacillus subtilis ATCC-6633	0.2	0.39	0.05	0.05
B. subtilis PCI-219	0.2	0.39	0.05	0.05
Micrococcus luteus PCI-1001	0.39	0.39	0.025	0.1
Streptococcus pneumoniae III[b]	0.2	0.39	0.1	0.2
S. pyogenes S-23[b]	0.2	0.2	0.05	0.1
S. pyogenes A-S-8[b]	0.2	0.2	0.05	0.1
S. faecalis 6733[b]	25	50	25	25
Corynebacterium diphtheriae PW-8[b]	0.05	0.1	0.05	1.56
C. diphtheriae A-7[b]	0.39	0.78	0.2	1.56
C. diphtheriae M 406 MGL[b]	0.39	0.78	0.2	0.39
Escherichia coli NIHJ JC-2	6.25	3.13	6.25	25
E. coli Yukitoshi	6.25	3.13	6.25	12.5
E. coli K-12	0.78	1.56	1.56	25
Klebsiella pneumoniae NCTC-418	3.13	3.13	12.5	25
Proteus vulgaris IAM-1025	>100	>100	100	100
Pseudomonas aeruginosa IAM-1095	>100	>100	>100	>100
Salmonella typhi T-287	0.78	1.56	3.13	1.56
S. typhi O-901	1.56	1.56	3.13	3.13
S. paratyphi A 1015	1.56	3.13	3.13	3.13
S. schottmuelleri 8006	1.56	3.13	3.13	12.5
S. typhimurium 1406	1.56	3.13	3.13	3.13
S. enteritidis 1891	3.13	3.13	3.13	3.13
Shigella dysenteriae A1 Shiga	3.13	3.13	6.25	12.5
S. flexneri 1a EW-8	3.13	6.25	6.25	6.25
S. flexneri 1b Showa 15	6.25	3.13	3.13	12.5
S. flexneri 2a Komagome B III	3.13	3.13	3.13	12.5
S. flexneri 3a EW-14	3.13	3.13	6.25	25
S. flexneri 4a Saigon-Arai	1.56	1.56	3.13	12.5
S. sonnei I EW-33	1.56	0.78	1.56	6.25
S. sonnei II EW-34	3.13	3.13	3.13	25

[a] Inoculum size, 10^8 microbial cell units/ml.
[b] Supplemented with 10% rabbit blood.

TABLE 2. *Susceptibility of clinical isolates to ceftezole and other cephalosporins*

Organism	Antibiotic	No. of organisms with an MIC (μg/ml) of:														
		≦0.05	0.1	0.2	0.39	0.78	1.56	3.13	6.25	12.5	25	50	100	200	400	>400
Staphylococcus aureus[a] (40 strains)	Ceftezole			9	21	3	5	2								
	Cefazolin			6	19	9	4	2								
	Cephaloridine	10	14	3	6	2	3	2								
	Cephalothin			14	19	7										
Escherichia coli[a] (40 strains)	Ceftezole						2	5	20	3	4	2		1	2	1
	Cefazolin						5	5	18	2	3	2		3	1	1
	Cephaloridine							5	18	3	4	2	2	4		2
	Cephalothin								2	3	10	16	4		1	4
Klebsiella pneumoniae[a] (60 strains)	Ceftezole						5	37	4	2	5	2	3	1	1	
	Cefazolin						4	31	9	7	4	1	3		1	
	Cephaloridine							4	19	27	2	1	3	1	2	1
	Cephalothin						1	1	12	30	8	2	4	2		
Proteus mirabilis[a] (41 strains)	Ceftezole							1	11	23	6					
	Cefazolin							3	5	17	11	5				
	Cephalordine								1	9	25	6				
	Cephalothin							2	8	18	11	2				
P. vulgaris[b] (21 strains)	Ceftezole												7	2	10	2
	Cefazolin												2	4	6	9
	Cephaloridine													2	5	14
	Cephalothin												2		3	16
P. morganii[b] (20 strains)	Ceftezole											2	8	7	1	2
	Cefazolin												3	10	3	4
	Cephaloridine													1	8	11
	Cephalothin															20
P. rettgeri[b] (20 strains)	Ceftezole					1	1			2	2	1	3	10		
	Cefazolin					1	1	1		1	2	1		6	7	
	Cephaloridine									2	1		1	16		
	Cephalothin									1	1	1	1	1	2	13
P. inconstans B[b] (20 strains)	Ceftezole						1		3	4	6	3	3			
	Cefazolin							1	2	8	2	4	3			
	Cephaloridine										3	2	8	4	3	
	Cephalothin									1	1	7	5	3	3	
Citrobacter[b] (20 strains)	Ceftezole					1				1	6	4	4			4
	Cefazolin						1				5	2	4	3	1	4
	Cephaloridine							1				2	4	7	3	3
	Cephalothin								1	2		8	2	2	1	4
Enterobacter aerogenes[b] (19 strains)	Ceftezole						1	4	4	1		3	3	1	2	
	Cefazolin						2	4	3	1	1	1	3	2	2	
	Cephaloridine								2	1	2	2	5	4	3	
	Cephalothin									3	4	3		4		5
E. cloacae[b] (20 strains)	Ceftezole						1		1						6	12
	Cefazolin						1		1						4	14
	Cephaloridine								1		1			1	4	13
	Cephalothin										1	1				18
Serratia marcescens[b] (18 strains)	Ceftezole															18
	Cefazolin															18
	Cephaloridine														6	12
	Cephalothin															18
Acinetobacter[b] (15 strains)	Ceftezole				1	1				1		1	1	2	1	7
	Cefazolin				1		1			1			2	2	2	6
	Cephaloridine					1		1	1		2	1	3	1	2	3
	Cephalothin				1			1		1		1		2	4	5

[a] Inoculum size, 10^8 microbial cell units/ml.
[b] Inoculum size, 10^6 microbial cell units/ml.

tezole against *K. pneumoniae* may be very similar to that of cefazolin and greater than that of other cephalosporins.

The MICs of ceftezole against 41 strains of *P. mirabilis* ranged from 3.13 to 25 μg/ml. The MICs of ceftezole were 12.5 μg/ml for 23 (57.5%) of the 41 strains. No strains resistant to more than 50 μg/ml (MIC) were found. Ceftezole was the most active of the cephalosporin derivatives.

Indole-positive *Proteus, Citrobacter, Enterobacter aerogenes, E. cloacae, Serratia marcescens,* and *Acinetobacter* were tested using inocula of 10^6 microbial cell units/ml. The MICs of ceftezole against 21 strains of *P. vulgaris* ranged from 100 to >400 μg/ml, and those against 20 strains of *P. morganii* ranged from 50 to >400 μg/ml. Most of the strains were resistant to ceftezole and to the other cephalosporins tested. The MICs to ceftezole against 20 strains of *P. rettgeri* and 20 strains of *P. inconstans* B ranged from 0.78 to 200 μg/ml and from 1.56 to 100 μg/ml, respectively. The MICs of ceftezole against *Citrobacter* ranged from 0.78 to >400 μg/ml, and those against *E. aerogenes* (19 strains) ranged from 1.56 to 400 μg/ml. The susceptibility of these organisms was distributed widely. Two of the 20 strains of *E. cloacae* were susceptible to ceftezole (MIC, 1.56 and 6.25 μg/ml), but other strains were highly resistant (MIC, ≥400 μg/ml). The 18 strains of *S. marcescens* were all resistant to cephalosporins. Two or 3 out of 15 strains of *Acinetobacter* were susceptible to cephalosporins, but the remaining strains were resistant to cephalosporins.

To evaluate the effect of various test conditions on antimicrobial activity, the antimicrobial activity of ceftezole was compared by using five conventional agar media. As shown in Table 3, no abnormal fluctuations in antimicrobial activity of ceftezole and cefazolin against four test strains were noted in any of the five different media.

The effect of pH on the MIC of ceftezole was very similar to that of cefazolin (Table 3). *K. pneumoniae* 4106 was greatly influenced by the pH, i.e., an eightfold difference in MIC. *S. faecalis* 1215 was the least influenced.

Generally, the MICs of ceftezole against various test strains became correspondingly smaller when the inoculum size was reduced. Ceftezole closely resembled cefazolin in this respect.

When 10, 25, and 50% serum was added to each medium, there was little change in antimicrobial activity against most strains. The effect of serum on the antimicrobial activity of ceftezole was slightly less than that on the activity of cefazolin.

The bactericidal activity of ceftezole against *E. coli* NIHJ JC-2 in heart infusion broth was compared with that of cefazolin (Fig. 2).

Viable cell counts of *E. coli* NIHJ JC-2 decreased for 4 h after the start of incubation in broth containing one-fourth the MIC of ceftezole and, as in the case with cefazolin, increased 6 h after incubation. Under the same conditions, an increase of viable cell counts was more rapid for cephalothin than for ceftezole and cefazolin. At the MIC and four times the MIC, bactericidal activity of ceftezole was nearly the same as that of cefazolin and cephalothin, and viable cell counts did not increase even after prolonged incubation.

The hydrolysis of ceftezole and other cephalosporins by penicillinase type or cephalosporinase type β-lactamases isolated from various bacterial strains was investigated. The results were expressed as the relative hydrolysis rate of ceftezole and related cephalosporins in comparison with the hydrolysis rate of cefazolin under the same experimental conditions (Table 4). Under the conditions of these experiments, the hydrolysis rate of ceftezole was higher than that of cefazolin by penicillinase type β-lactamases isolated from *E. coli* 40 and two strains of *K. pneumoniae*. Among the five cephalosporinase type β-lactamases, the hydrolysis of ceftezole differed; two showed lower and three showed higher rates than did cefazolin. The results show that ceftezole is hydrolyzed slightly more easily than cefazolin.

Binding of ceftezole to human and animal serum protein was determined by the ultrafiltration method. Table 5 shows that there were differences in binding rates among different animal species. The binding of ceftezole to human serum protein was 86%, as was the case with cephalothin, higher than that of cephaloridine but lower than that of cefazolin. The binding of ceftezole to rat and rabbit serum protein was approximately 90%, i.e., almost the same as that of cefazolin, but the binding of ceftezole to mouse and dog serum protein was 27% and 19%, respectively, i.e., lower than that of cefazolin.

To determine the liberation of free drug from a protein-drug complex, antibiotic-serum solutions were diluted twofold with M/15 phosphate buffer (pH 7.0), and their antimicrobial potencies were compared.

As shown in Fig. 3, when ceftezole-serum solution was diluted fourfold with the phosphate buffer, the potency of ceftezole was completely recovered. When the cefazolin-serum so-

TABLE 3. *Influence of various factors on the antimicrobial activity of ceftezole and cefazolin*

Factor	Antibiotic	MIC (μg/ml) of organism:			
		A[a]	B	C	D
Medium					
HI[b] agar (Difco)	Ceftezole	0.2	12.5	3.13	1.56
Nutrient agar (Difco)		0.1	3.13	3.13	1.56
BHI[b] agar (Difco)		0.1	3.13	6.25	3.13
Trypticase soy agar (BBL)		0.1	3.13	6.25	3.13
Mueller-Hinton agar (Difco)		0.1	3.13	6.25	3.13
HI agar (Difco)	Cefazolin	0.2	12.5	1.56	1.56
Nutrient agar (Difco)		0.1	6.25	1.56	1.56
BHI agar (Difco)		0.2	6.25	1.56	1.56
Trypticase soy agar (BBL)		0.2	6.25	1.56	3.13
Mueller-Hinton agar (Difco)		0.2	6.25	1.56	1.56
pH					
6.0	Ceftezole	≦0.05	6.25	1.56	1.56
7.0		0.1	12.5	1.56	0.78
8.0		0.2	12.5	1.56	1.56
9.0		0.2	12.5	6.25	6.25
6.0	Cefazolin	0.1	6.25	1.56	3.13
7.0		0.2	12.5	1.56	1.56
8.0		0.2	12.5	1.56	1.56
9.0		0.2	12.5	6.25	12.5
Inoculum size					
10^8	Ceftezole	0.39	25	3.13	3.13
10^6		0.2	12.5	3.13	1.56
10^4		0.1	6.25	1.56	0.78
10^8	Cefazolin	0.39	25	3.13	3.13
10^6		0.2	12.5	1.56	1.56
10^4		0.1	6.25	1.56	1.56
Serum[c]					
0	Ceftezole	0.2	12.5	1.56	0.78
10%		0.2	25	3.13	1.56
25		0.39	25	1.56	3.13
50		0.39	50	1.56	3.13
0	Cefazolin	0.2	12.5	3.13	0.78
10%		0.2	25	3.13	1.56
25		0.39	50	1.56	3.13
50		0.39	50	1.56	6.25

[a] Organism A, *S. aureus* 209-P JC-1; B, *S. faecalis* 1215; C, *E. coli* NIHJ JC-2; D, *K. pneumoniae* 4106.
[b] HI, Heart infusion; BHI, brain heart infusion.
[c] Serum, rabbit.

lution was diluted fourfold with the phosphate buffer, approximately 80% of its potency was recovered, but when diluted eightfold complete potency was recovered. The results obtained from cephalothin-serum solution diluted with the phosphate buffer in the same manner show that the liberation of cephalothin is less than that of ceftezole. The liberation of dicloxacillin was the least of the test antibiotics. From the above results, the binding of ceftezole in the protein-drug complex is thought to be comparatively loose.

The protective effect of ceftezole in experimental infection was studied in mice according to the procedures outlined in the experimental method. As shown in Table 6, the ED_{50} of subcutaneously administered ceftezole against infections due to *E. coli* 362 was 0.92 mg/mouse, a protective effect which corresponded to that of cefazolin. The protective effect of ceftezole against infection produced by *E. coli* 362 was superior to that of cephalothin but inferior to that of cephaloridine. The ED_{50} of subcutaneously administered ceftezole on infections produced by *K. pneumoniae* 410 was 0.05 mg/mouse, the effect being almost the same as that of cephaloridine. The protective effect against infection due to these organisms was superior to cephalothin and inferior to cefazolin. The ED_{50} of ceftezole in infections produced by *P. mirabilis*

504 was 0.37 mg/mouse, the effect being nearly equal to that of cefazolin and cephaloridine and superior to that of cephalothin. The ED_{50} of ceftezole in infections produced by *Citrobacter* 821 was 3.60 mg/mouse, which was nearly equal to that of cefazolin. The effect of ceftezole in infections produced by *Citrobacter* 821 was superior to that of cephaloridine and cephalothin.

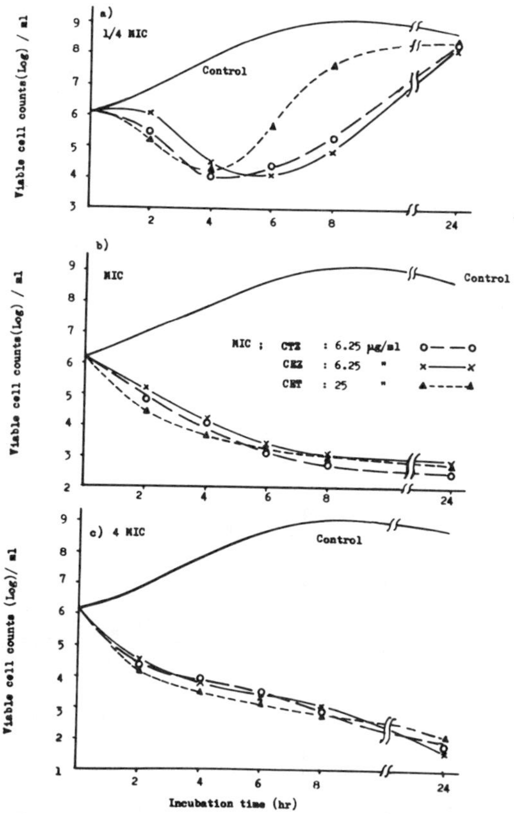

FIG. 2. *Bactericidal activity of ceftezole (CTZ), cefazolin (CEZ), and cephalothin (CET) against E. coli NIHJ JC-2.*

Absorption and excretion. (i) Serum levels. The concentrations of ceftezole in serum of SD strain rats after intramuscular injection of 20 mg/kg are shown in Fig. 4. The mean drug concentrations peaked at 33.8 μg/ml 15 min after injection and fell to 10.5 μg/ml within 1 h and to 0.9 μg/ml by 2 h. The peak concentrations and the concentrations at 30 min after ceftezole administration were about one-half those of cefazolin. The concentrations of ceftezole in serum were higher than those of the other cephalosporin derivatives tested, i.e., cephaloridine and cephalothin.

The mean concentrations of ceftezole in serum of beagle dogs after intramuscular injection of 20 mg/kg peaked at 49.7 μg/ml at 30 min and were 1.1 μg/ml at 6 h (Fig. 5). The concentrations of ceftezole in serum of dogs at the intervals specified in Fig. 5 (except 30 min) did not differ greatly from those of cefazolin and cephaloridine. The concentrations of cephalothin in serum however, were lower than those of ceftezole, cefazolin, and cephaloridine.

The concentrations of ceftezole in serum of monkeys after intramuscular injection of 20 mg/kg were compared with those of cefazolin, cephaloridine, and cephalothin. As shown in Fig. 6, the concentrations of ceftezole in serum were 40.0 μg/ml 30 min after injection, 1.3 μg/ml at 4 h, and not detectable at 6 h. After intramuscular injection of an equal dose of cephaloridine, the values were nearly the same. The concentrations of ceftezole in serum of monkeys were about one-half the levels of cefazolin in the early stage after administration but were higher than those of cephalothin, as was the case with rats.

TABLE 4. *Hydrolysis of ceftezole and other cephalosporins by different types of β-lactamases*[a]

Substrate	Penicillinase type			Cephalosporinase type					
	Escherichia coli 40	*Klebsiella pneumoniae*[b] 118	*K. pneumoniae*[c] 164	*E. coli* 36	*Enterobacter aerogenes* 3	*Citrobacter freundii* 15	*Pseudomonas aeruginosa* 79	*Proteus rettgeri* 8
Cefazolin	100[d]	100	100	100	100	100	100	100
Ceftezole	129	171	128	204	157	79	162	98
Cephaloridine	487	549	78	133	159	97	83	74
Cephalothin	200	147	82	710	479	95	404	120
Cephalosporin C	1,133	32	8	1,170	468	216	175	205

[a] β-lactamase was partially purified by gel filtration on Sephadex G-200. β-lactamase activity; initial hydrolysis velocity at the concentration of 50 μg/ml at 37 C by ultraviolet method.

[b] Indole-negative *K. pneumoniae*.

[c] Indole-positive *K. pneumoniae*.

[d] Relative activity (velocity of cefazolin = 100).

TABLE 5. *Extent of protein binding of ceftezole and other cephalosporins by centrifugal ultrafiltration technique*

Antibiotic	Extent of protein bindings (%) in serum of:				
	Humans	Dogs	Rabbits	Rats	Mice
Ceftezole	86	19	97	90	27
Cefazolin	93	54	92	94	49
Cephaloridine	55	22	55	67	32
Cephalothin	86	44	86	87	57
Dicloxacillin	96	92	96	94	60

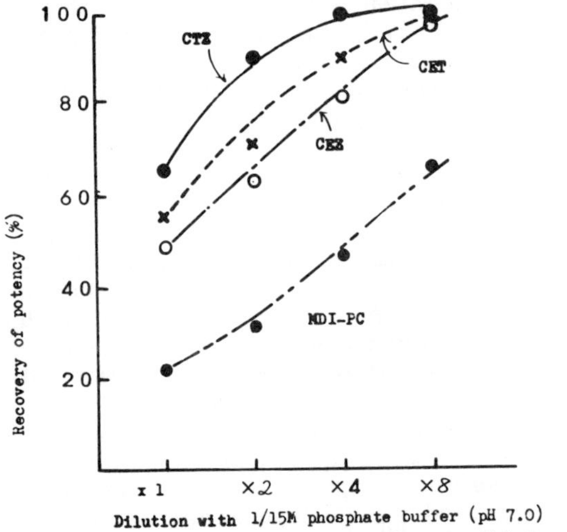

FIG. 3. *Release of free antibiotics from antibiotic-protein complex by buffer dilution. See legend to Fig. 2 for abbreviations.*

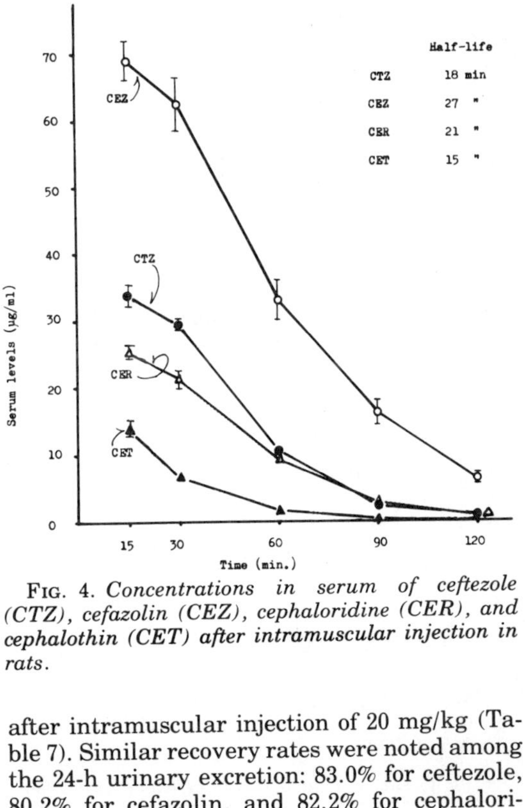

FIG. 4. *Concentrations in serum of ceftezole (CTZ), cefazolin (CEZ), cephaloridine (CER), and cephalothin (CET) after intramuscular injection in rats.*

As shown in Fig. 7, the concentrations of ceftezole in serum of seven healthy male volunteers after intramuscular injection of 500 mg peaked at a mean of 24.9 μg/ml at 15 min and were 17.5 μg/ml at 1 h, 10.0 μg/ml at 2 h, 2.6 μg/ml at 4 h, and not detectable in six subjects at 6 h. The half-life of ceftezole in serum of men was 56 min.

(ii) Urinary excretion. The urinary excretion of ceftezole in rats was determined at 24 h after intramuscular injection of 20 mg/kg (Table 7). Similar recovery rates were noted among the 24-h urinary excretion: 83.0% for ceftezole, 80.2% for cefazolin, and 82.2% for cephaloridine. This high recovery in urine shows that ceftezole is less readily metabolized than cepha-

TABLE 6. *Protective effect of ceftezole and other cephalosporins against experimental infections in mice*[a]

Organism		ED$_{50}$ (mg/mouse) of:			
		Ceftezole	Cefazolin	Cephaloridine	Cephalothin
Escherichia coli	362	0.92 (0.451–2.004)[b]	0.63 (0.317–1.289)	0.19 (0.087–0.447)	7.03 (7.014–7.055)
Klebsiella pneumoniae	410	0.05 (0.033–0.073)	0.03 (0.010–0.039)	0.06 (0.038–0.087)	0.90 (0.591–1.339)
Proteus mirabilis	504	0.37 (0.23–0.71)	0.51 (0.35–0.78)	0.45 (0.23–0.96)	1.53 (0.79–3.08)
Citrobacter	821	3.60 (2.365–5.357)	4.19 (2.787–6.409)	5.00 (3.31–7.68)	>20

[a] All animals were challenged by the intraperitoneal route; drugs were administered subcutaneously.
[b] Numbers in parentheses = 95% confidence limit.

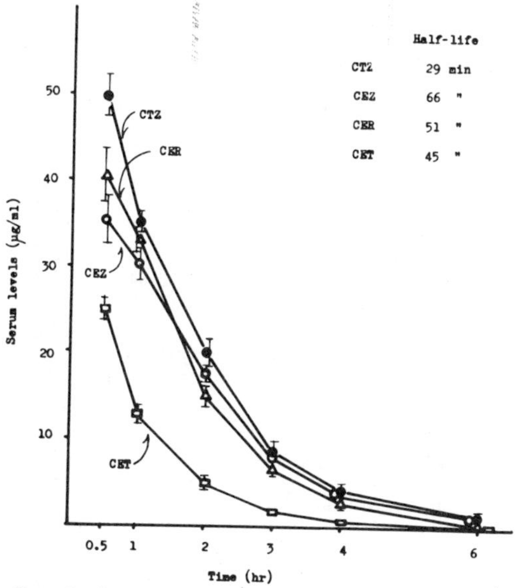

FIG. 5. *Concentrations in serum of ceftezole (CTZ), cefazolin (CEZ), cephaloridine (CER), and cephalothin (CET) after intramuscular injection in dogs.*

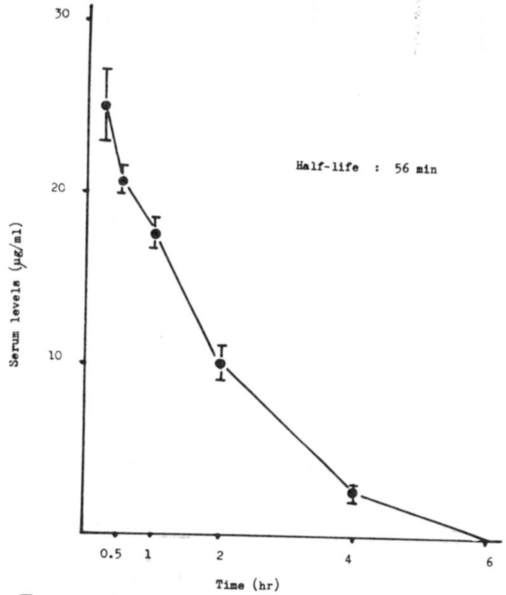

FIG. 7. *Concentrations in serum of ceftezole after intramuscular injection in seven healthy human volunteers.*

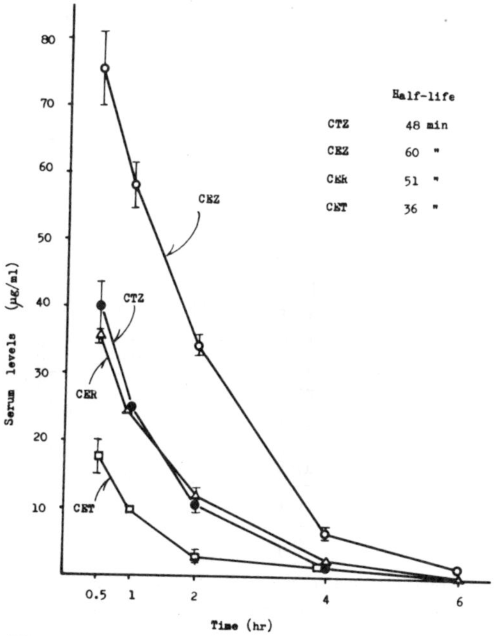

FIG. 6. *Concentrations in serum of ceftezole (CTZ), cefazolin (CEZ), cephaloridine (CER), and cephalothin (CET) after intramuscular injection in monkeys.*

lothin (22.1%).

The urinary excretion in beagle dogs for 24 h after intramuscular injection of 20 mg/kg averaged 73.5% of the administered dose for ceftezole, 80.1% for cefazolin, and 78.9% for cephaloridine (Table 8). These cephalosporin derivatives show high recovery in urine. No statistically significant differences were noted among these antibiotics. The urinary excretion of cephalothin, however, was 35.1%, significantly lower than that of ceftezole.

The urinary excretion of ceftezole in monkeys for 24 h after intramuscular injection of 20 mg/kg was compared with those of cefazolin, cephaloridine, and cephalothin (Table 9). The urinary excretion was 72.7% for ceftezole, 80.3% for cefazolin, and 74.4% for cephaloridine. No significant differences in urinary excretion were observed among these antibiotics, as was the case with other test animals. The urinary excretion of cephalothin was lower (49.4%).

The 24-h urinary excretion of ceftezole in seven healthy male volunteers after a single intramuscular injection of 500 mg averaged 86.6% (Table 10). The results show that ceftezole is stable in the human body. About 87.5% of the total excretion was recovered within 3 h after intramuscular injection. The urinary excretion of ceftezole was rapid. The urinary levels of ceftezole peaked at a mean of 2,390 µg/ml at 1 h and averaged 244 µg/ml (80 to 440 µg/ml) at 3 to 6 h. These levels were high enough to inhibit the growth of susceptible organisms.

An investigation was done by the thin-layer

TABLE 7. *Urinary excretion of ceftezole and other cephalosporins after intramuscular injection in rats*

Antibiotic	Urinary excretion at:							
	0–3 h		3–6 h		6–24 h		Total	
	μg/ml	%	μg/ml	%	μg/ml	%	mg	%
Ceftezole (n = 10)	1,900 (368)[a]	72.0 (2.7)	168 (32.0)	5.80 (1.20)	4.50 (1.50)	0.53 (0.15)	3.41 (0.10)	83.0 (1.9)
Cefazolin (n = 10)	1,580 (195)	75.7 (1.9)	171 (24.7)	4.05 (0.50)	4.04 (0.90)	0.44 (0.09)	3.59 (0.06)	80.2 (1.7)
Cephaloridine (n = 10)	1,430 (125)	79.7 (2.1)	83.6 (12.6)	2.2 (0.30)	2.02 (0.35)	0.31 (0.05)	3.54 (0.12)	82.2 (2.2)
Cephalothin (n = 10)	391 (60.4)	21.8 (1.5)	12.2 (3.2)	0.3 (0.07)	0.25 (0.15)	0.02 (0.01)	0.95 (0.06)	22.1 (1.5)

[a] Numbers in parentheses = standard error.

TABLE 8. *Urinary excretion of ceftezole and other cephalosporins after intramuscular injection in dogs*

Antibiotic	Urinary excretion at:							
	0–3 h		3–6 h		6–24 h		Total	
	μg/ml	%	μg/ml	%	μg/ml	%	mg	%
Ceftezole (n = 6)	2,480 (447)[a]	54.1 (3.5)	896 (215)	15.9 (2.8)	119 (48.1)	3.6 (1.3)	170 (6.7)	73.5 (2.1)
Cefazolin (n = 5)	3,030 (743)	64.5 (2.8)	718 (95)	14.2 (0.6)	29.1 (4.8)	1.4 (0.1)	175 (8.4)	80.1 (2.9)
Cephaloridine (n = 5)	2,040 (344)	70.1 (4.7)	388 (30)	7.8 (0.6)	19.6 (3.2)	1.0 (0.1)	177 (8.6)	78.9 (4.8)
Cephalothin (n = 5)	622 (54)	33.1 (2.3)	71 (25)	1.5 (0.3)	6.7 (3.9)	0.4 (0.2)	76.3 (6.0)	35.1 (2.0)

[a] Numbers in parentheses = standard error.

TABLE 9. *Urinary excretion of ceftezole and other cephalosporins after intramuscular injection in monkeys*

Antibiotic	Urinary excretion at:									
	0–2 h		2–4 h		4–6 h		6–24 h		Total	
	μg/ml	%	μg/ml	%	μg/ml	%	μg/ml	%	mg	%
Ceftezole (n = 6)	2,020 (859)[a]	52.7 (2.8)	1,020 (132)	15.8 (0.8)	354 (121)	4.0 (1.4)	3.0 (0.9)	0.2 (0.04)	108 (4.8)	72.7 (1.4)
Cefazolin (n = 3)	1,410 (139)	45.0 (8.3)	1,240 (441)	28.6 (6.8)	139 (38)	4.6 (0.7)	48.6 (17.5)	2.2 (0.7)	120 (10)	80.3 (0.5)
Cephaloridine (n = 3)	764 (37)	58.6 (2.9)	780 (234)	15.8 (3.2)	218 (75)	2.2 (0.6)	6.3 (2.0)	0.3 (0.1)	115 (10)	74.4 (1.5)
Cephalothin (n = 3)	602 (92)	38.8 (4.7)	405 (63.3)	9.8 (4.1)	25.4 (9.1)	0.83 (0.27)	0.25 (0.03)	0.02 (0.01)	77.2 (8.2)	49.4 (2.7)

[a] Numbers in parentheses = standard error.

chromatographic and bioautographic methods to confirm whether active substances in the urine of animals and human volunteers after intramuscular injection of ceftezole included unchanged ceftezole. Figure 8 shows the bioautograms. Only one active substance was found in urine samples, the R_f value of which corresponded to intact ceftezole.

(iii) Biliary excretion. The biliary excretion of ceftezole in rats for 24 h after intramuscular injection of 20 mg/kg was compared with that of the other cephalosporin derivatives (Table 11). The biliary excretion was 4.4% of the administered dose for ceftezole and 9.9% for cefazolin. The excretion of ceftezole was lower than that of cefazolin but was higher than that of cephaloridine and cephalothin.

(iv) Tissue distribution. The tissue distribution of ceftezole after intramuscular injection of 20 mg/kg was determined (Table 12). Ceftezole

TABLE 10. *Urinary excretion of ceftezole after intramuscular injection in healthy human volunteers*

Volunteer		Urinary excretion at:											
		0–1 h		1–2 h		2–3 h		3–6 h		6–24 h		Total	
No.	Wt (kg)	μg/ml	%	μg/ml	%	μg/ml	%	μg/ml	%	μg/ml	%	mg	%
A	75	887	24.0	887	26.2	730	17.7	395	20.0	11.7	3.86	459	91.8
B	69	1,150	39.8	897	31.6	540	13.8	144	7.34	3.40	0.86	467	93.4
C	60	1,440	41.4	835	25.0	690	12.3	185	5.00	2.74	1.06	424	84.8
D	60	8,000	38.4	4,630	33.4	1,380	8.0	440	7.66	4.30	0.82	441	88.3
E	56	1,370	29.0	1,170	30.0	780	12.3	358	17.2	3.00	0.83	447	89.3
F	55	1,710	30.4	960	27.2	290	12.4	80.0	7.64	2.50	0.91	393	78.6
G	69	2,170	41.6	670	24.6	305	11.7	105	1.55	1.48	0.29	399	79.7
Mean		2,390	34.9	1,440	28.3	674	12.6	244	9.48	4.16	1.23	433	86.6
		(948)[a]	(2.7)	(535)	(1.3)	(139)	(1.1)	(56.5)	(2.50)	(1.29)	(0.44)	(10.8)	(2.17)

[a] Numbers in parentheses = standard error.

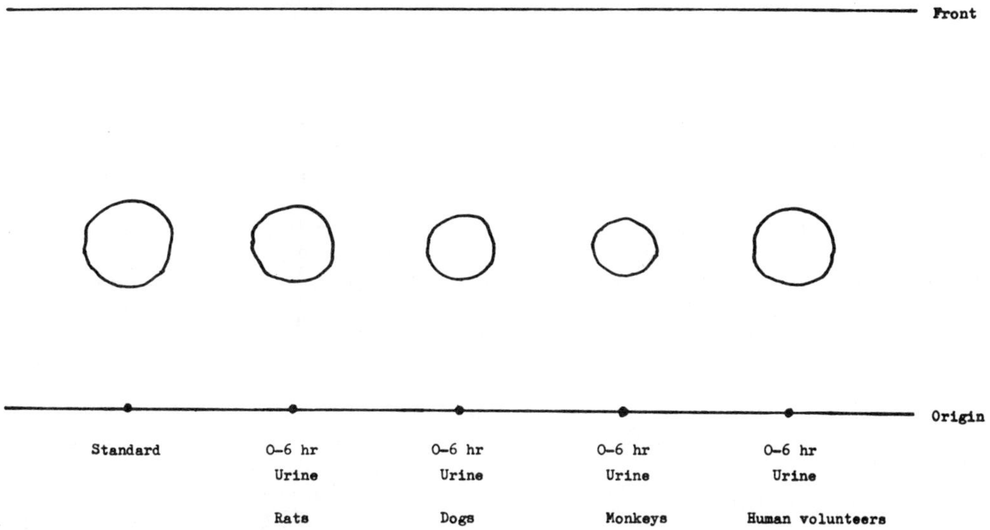

FIG. 8. *Bioautograms of urine of rats, dogs, monkeys (20 mg/kg), and healthy human volunteers (500 mg) after intramuscular injection of ceftezole.*

TABLE 11. *Biliary excretion of ceftezole and other cephalosporins after intramuscular injection in rats*

Antibiotic	Biliary excretion at:							
	0–3 h		3–6 h		6–24 h		Total	
	μg/ml	%	μg/ml	%	μg/ml	%	mg	%
Ceftezole	67.4	4.3	1.6	0.08	ND[a]	ND	0.194	4.4
(n = 10)	(10.2)[b]	(0.6)	(0.4)	(0.02)			(0.029)	(0.6)
Cefazolin	141	9.4	12.3	0.5	0.05	0.01	0.430	9.9
(n = 10)	(17.1)	(1.3)	(1.3)	(0.05)	(0.02)	(0.00)	(0.06)	(1.3)
Cephaloridine	6.0	0.37	1.23	0.05	0.05	0.01	0.017	0.44
(n = 10)	(0.72)	(0.05)	(0.14)	(0.01)	(0.02)	(0.00)	(0.002)	(0.06)
Cephalothin	12.0	0.90	0.05	0.0	0.05	0.01	0.041	0.91
(n = 10)	(1.8)	(0.14)	(0.02)	(0.00)	(0.02)	(0.00)	(0.007)	(0.14)

[a] ND, Not detected.
[b] Numbers in parentheses = standard error.

was detected in all the tissue samples. The peak tissue levels at 15 to 30 min were 71.3 μg/g in the kidney, 9.8 μg/g in the liver, 8.7 μg/g in the lung, 5.1 μg/g in the heart, and 2.3 μg/g in the spleen. When these tissue levels were compared with those of cefazolin, all were lower

TABLE 12. *Tissue distribution of ceftezole and other cephalosporins after intramuscular injection in rats*

Antibiotic	Time (min)	Tissue levels (μg/g) in:					Concn in serum (μg/ml)
		Liver	Kidneys	Lungs	Heart	Spleen	
Ceftezole	15	9.2	71.3	8.7	5.1	2.3	33.1
(*n* = 6)	30	9.8	48.0	6.4	4.8	1.9	29.0
	60	4.8	22.8	3.5	2.2	0.6	13.5
	90	1.4	6.9	0.9	0.5	ND[a]	3.8
Cefazolin	15	11.0	53.4	13.2	8.3	3.2	63.8
(*n* = 9)	30	16.3	45.4	10.9	5.8	2.7	50.0
	60	9.5	33.4	6.6	4.7	1.8	30.8
	90	5.0	13.6	3.5	2.1	1.0	12.5
Cephaloridine	30	8.6	70.3	6.8	3.0	2.1	19.6
(*n* = 9)	60	6.8	27.9	3.3	1.4	1.1	7.8
	90	4.9	8.7	1.3	0.7	1.0	2.7
Cephalothin	30	2.4	8.5	0.6	0.3	ND	5.5
(*n* = 9)	60	0.4	1.6	0.1	ND	ND	1.4
	90	ND	ND	ND	ND	ND	0.3

[a] ND, Not detected.

except renal levels at 15 to 30 min after injection. All the tissue levels of ceftezole were higher than those of cephalothin.

(v) Levels in rat pouch exudate. Ceftezole levels in the exudate of pouches with aseptic inflammation after intramuscular injection of 20 mg/kg to SD strain rats were compared with cefazolin levels (Fig. 9a and b). Ceftezole and cefazolin levels on day 6 and 7 after formation of pouches differed, and these levels decreased with the lapse of time. The levels of ceftezole in the exudate were slightly lower than those of cefazolin under all conditions.

DISCUSSION

No significant differences in antimicrobial activity of ceftezole and cefazolin against the clinical isolates tested were noted. The antimicrobial activity of ceftezole against most often encountered gram-negative bacilli, *E. coli*, *P. mirabilis*, and *K. pneumoniae* was higher than any of the other known cephalosporins. Among gram-negative bacilli considered to be resistant to cephalosporin derivatives, such as *P. rettgeri*, *P. inconstans* B, *Citrobacter*, and *E. aerogenes*, susceptibility to ceftezole and cefazolin was considerably higher with small sizes of inocula.

Apparent differences in serum-protein binding were observed between ceftezole and cefazolin. These differences were not great, but the protein binding of ceftezole was estimated to be looser than that of cefazolin on the basis of the dissociation rate of the active substance from

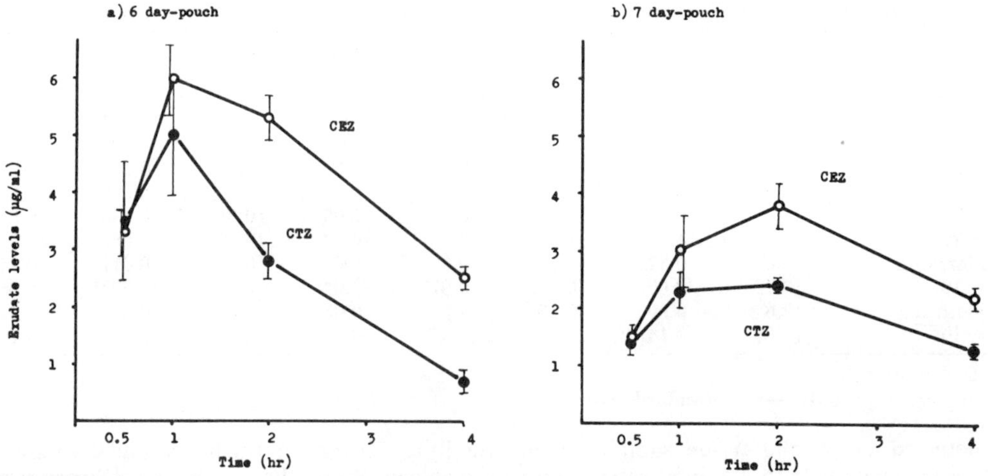

FIG. 9. *Exudate levels of ceftezole (CTZ) and cefazolin (CEZ) after intramuscular injection in rats with granuloma pouch.*

the binding conjugation by the buffer dilution (5). The influence of protein binding of antibiotics on clinical effect has been discussed but still remains controversial. The clinical trials of both drugs, which are similar in in vitro antimicrobial activity but different in protein binding, may be useful to elucidate the influence of serum-protein binding on clinical effect.

In rats, renal levels of ceftezole were markedly higher than those of cefazolin in the early stage after administration.

The ratio of renal levels to concentrations in serum of ceftezole was 2.15 at 15 min, 1.65 at 30 min, and 1.69 at 60 min. The renal levels of ceftezole at each time were 1.6 to 2 times the concentrations in serum. High levels of ceftezole in the kidneys were maintained, whereas the renal levels of cefazolin at each interval were nearly the same as concentrations in serum: 0.84 times at 15 min, 0.91 times at 30 min, and 1.08 times at 60 min. The ratios of all the tissue levels to concentrations in serum, except kidneys, were higher than those of cefazolin. These results indicate that the diffusion rates of ceftezole into the tissues from the blood is higher than that of cefazolin and may be explained by the weaker serum-protein binding of ceftezole. Furthermore, the extremely high renal levels of ceftezole in the early stage after administration may suggest that renal excretion of ceftezole is faster than that of cefazolin. The half-life of concentrations of ceftezole in serum of healthy volunteers after intramuscular injection was about 1 h, one-half that of cefazolin.

This new antibiotic, which equals cefazolin in antimicrobial activity and exceeds cefazolin in speed of renal clearance, may be useful in treating patients with renal dysfunction, when accumulation of an antibiotic is an important consideration.

LITERATURE CITED

1. **Ishiyama, S. (ed.).** 1970. Cefazolin. Chemotherapy (Japan) **18**:481–843.
2. **Kass, H. (ed.).** 1973. Clinical symposium on cefazolin. J. Infect. Dis. **128**(Suppl.):S307–424.
3. **Knothe, H., W. Marget, and R. Timmler (ed.).** 1974. Cefazolin; ein neues Cephalosporin. Infection **2** (Suppl. 1):S1–106.
4. **Nishida, M., T. Matsubara, T. Murakawa, Y. Mine, Y. Yokota, S. Kuwahara, and S. Goto.** 1970. In vitro and in vivo evaluation of cefazolin, a new cephalosporin C derivative, p. 236–243. Antimicrob. Agents Chemother. 1969.
5. **Shimizu, T.** 1974. Studies on protein binding of cefazolin and other antibiotics. Jpn. J. Antibiot. **27**:296–301.

ANTIMICROBIAL AGENTS AND CHEMOTHERAPY, July 1976, p. 14-19
Vol. 10, No. 1

Antiviral and Interferon-Inducing Activity of a New Glutarimide Antibiotic, 9-Methylstreptimidone

NORIYUKI SAITO, FUJIO SUZUKI, KENJI SASAKI, AND NAKAO ISHIDA*

Department of Bacteriology, Tohoku University School of Medicine, Sendai, Japan

Received for publication 17 December 1975

The antiviral effect of 9-methylstreptimidone (9-MS) was examined in mice infected with mouse-adapted influenza A_2 (H_2N_2) virus. Both a single and continuous prophylactic administration of 9-MS protected mice from virus infection, and comparison between the minimal effective and the 50% lethal dose gave a therapeutic index of 60. When the treatment was started after infection, however, no antiviral effect was demonstrated. After a single intraperitoneal administration of 9-MS, a highly potent virus-inhibitory factor was detected in the lungs (10 h later) and the sera (16 h later) of uninfected mice, which was assumed to be an interferon on the basis of the biological characteristics. These results suggest that the protective activity of the antibiotic is due to interferon induction in mice.

An approach to the control of virus diseases is to find a nontoxic inducer of interferon. The inducers studied most frequently are large anionic polymers (6, 25), highly base-paired ribonucleic acids (5, 9), and polycarboxylates (4, 8), which are difficult to characterize because of their polydispersity and because they caused toxic side effects (2, 7, 16, 19). Some low-molecular-weight inducers, such as tilorone hydrochloride (18), quinacrine (10), BL-20803 (24), CP-20961 (12), and cycloheximide (30), were also examined for their antiviral effects, with unencouraging results. Tilorone hydrochloride (18), an orally active inducer in mice, and CP-20961, which has a high therapeutic index (300) in the infection model of vesicular stomatitis virus, showed little, if any, protective activity against influenza virus infection in mice (12). Cycloheximide induced circulating interferon only at the level at which it coincidentally inhibited protein synthesis in animals (30). The rest have not been examined in influenza infection in mice.

The present report describes the effect of 9-methylstreptimidone (9-MS), a new glutarimide antibiotic having low acute and subacute toxicity (23), on influenza A_2 virus infection in mice. This compound evoked interferon, which was apparently responsible for the antiviral activity.

MATERIALS AND METHODS

Drug preparation. 9-MS used in this study was purified from culture filtrate of *Streptomyces* sp. S-885 (23). The final product, pale yellowish viscous oil, was dissolved in sterile phosphate-buffered saline (PBS), pH 7.2, containing 0.1% ethanol and 0.001% Tween 80 and used for animal experiments.

Amantadine hydrochloride was kindly provided by Daiichi Pharmaceutical Co. Ltd. and *Escherichia coli* endotoxin was prepared in our laboratory by Westphal's method. Both were dissolved in sterile PBS.

Mice. The ddI strain of mice of both sexes, weighing 14 to 16 g, was used throughout. They were obtained from the Central Breeding Farm of Tohoku University, where care was taken to prevent infections with Sendai virus and *Mycoplasma*.

Cell cultures. Monolayer cultures of the thymidine-kinaseless mutant strain of mouse fibroblasts, L-1D cells (14), were grown in Roux bottles in Eagle minimal essential medium supplemented with 10% calf serum. RK-13 cells grown in Eagle minimal essential medium supplemented with 10% bovine serum and primary chicken embryo cells in Hanks solution containing 0.5% lactalbumin hydrolysate and supplemented with 10% bovine serum were used to examine the host species specificity of the mouse interferon.

Viruses. The mouse-adapted Kumamoto strain of influenza A_2 (H_2N_2) virus (27) was propagated once in the allantoic cavity of embryonated eggs, and 48-h allantoic fluid was used as the inoculum after light centrifugation. The 50% egg infectious dose of the fluid was $10^{9.4}$/ml.

The Indiana strain of vesicular stomatitis virus, propagated in L-1D cell cultures and stored at −80 C, was used as the challenge virus to assay interferon. The 50% tissue culture infectious dose of the virus was $10^{7.5}$/ml.

In vivo infections. To infect mice with influenza virus, 10 ml of allantoic fluid diluted with nutrient broth was sprayed within 30 min with a vaponephrine-type nebulizer connected to a compressor. This procedure resulted in an inoculation of 0.002 ml of the fluid per mouse (13). The 50% lethal dose

(LD_{50}) was determined according to the Reed and Muench procedure (22), and the dose per mouse was specified in each experiment.

Drug evaluation. According to the schedules, the drug dissolved in PBS was administered intraperitoneally (i.p.) on a milligram per kilogram basis. The criteria of anti-influenza activity were increase in the mean survival time of mice succumbing to infection during the 30-day observation period and increase in the number of survivors on day 30. They were evaluated statistically by means of Student's *t* and chi-square tests, respectively. If the *P* value obtained in each test was below 0.05, the drug dose was considered to have statistically significant antiviral activity.

Virus titration in mouse lungs. The lungs of infected mice were disrupted in sea sand with a mortar and pestle to make a 10% suspension in PBS, followed by centrifugation at 1,580 × *g* for 10 min. The supernatant was serially diluted twofold with PBS, and the hemagglutinin titers were determined with 0.5% chicken erythrocytes, as described previously (13).

Interferon. Interferon was titrated in an L-1D cell-vesicular stomatitis virus system (28). Serum and lung specimens were taken at appropriate time intervals from the mice injected with 9-MS. Samples diluted with Eagle minimal essential medium supplemented with 2% heated calf serum (maintenance medium) were added to 3-day-old monolayer cultures in tubes. After 12 to 18 h of incubation at 37 C, cells were washed with Hanks balanced salt solution and challenged with 500 50% tissue culture infective doses of vesicular stomatitis virus in new maintenance medium. Mouse serum interferon induced by *E. coli* endotoxin served as a positive control. The maximal cytopathic effect was evident in control cultures within 18 to 25 h. Interferon units were expressed as the reciprocal of the maximal sample dilution giving 50% protection against cytopathic effect.

RESULTS

Protective effect of 9-MS against influenza infection in mice. Three groups of 10 mice and one group of 20 mice were simultaneously infected intranasally with 5 LD_{50} of influenza virus. The first two groups received, respectively, i.p. injection of 20 and 10 mg of 9-MS per kg three times, 24, 3, and 1 h, before and twice, 1 and 3 h, after infection and once daily for 4 consecutive days. The third and fourth groups were given, respectively, 15 mg of amantadine hydrochloride per kg and 0.5 ml of PBS according to the same schedule; these served as positive and negative controls. Whereas 95% of the mice receiving PBS died within 20 days, 70% of the mice treated with 20 mg of 9-MS per kg survived for the observation period of 30 days (Table 1). Both 10 mg of 9-MS and 10 mg of amantadine hydrochloride per kg gave a survival rate of 30%. The mean survival time of 9-MS-treated mice dying before day 30 was also significantly increased.

The pulmonary virus contents were then assayed in the mice infected with the same dose of the virus. In the mice treated with 9-MS according to the above-mentioned schedule, it was not until 4 days after infection that the virus was detected, and the hemagglutinin titer reached a peak ($10^{2.7}$) 2 days thereafter. But, in the untreated mice, the virus was already detectable 2 days after infection and the titer reached the maximum ($10^{3.1}$) on day 4. Thus, 9-MS was shown to inhibit virus growth in lungs.

The administration of 9-MS also improved the status of the mice infected with as high as 10 LD_{50} of the virus. The treatments with 20

TABLE 1. *Effect of 9-MS on influenza A_2 (H_2N_2) virus infection in mice*

Drug[a]	Single dose (mg/kg)	No. of mice[b]	Survival		Mean survival	
			%[c]	Significance[d] (*P*)	Time (days)	Significance[e] (*P*)
Challenge with 5 LD_{50}						
9-MS	20	10	70	<0.01	23.9	<0.005
9-MS	10	10	30	0.04	17.2	0.01
Amantadine	15	10	30	0.04	13.3	0.1
PBS	0.5 ml	20	5		11.8	
Challenge with 10 LD_{50}						
9-MS	20	10	50	<0.01	20.0	<0.001
9-MS	10	10	30	<0.01	15.7	<0.005
PBS	0.5 ml	30	0		9.7	

[a] Treatment schedule: the drug was administered i.p. 24, 3, and 1 h before and 1 and 3 h after infection and once daily for 4 consecutive days.

[b] Mice were infected in an aerosol chamber.

[c] Percentage of survival on day 30 postinfection.

[d] Probability value obtained by use of chi-square analysis.

[e] Probability value obtained by use of the Student *t* test.

and 10 mg of 9-MS per kg following the above schedule produced survival rates of 50 and 30%, respectively, along with a significant increase in the mean survival time (Table 1). With such a high dose challenge, all the control mice receiving PBS died within 15 days.

Dose-dependent protective effect of 9-MS against influenza infection. Groups of 10 mice were infected with 10 LD_{50} of influenza virus and treated with 1.2 to 22 mg of 9-MS per kg according to the schedule described above. The protective effect was dose related and was demonstrated with all doses higher than 1.2 mg/kg (Fig. 1). The data show that the minimal protective dose of 9-MS administered according to the above-mentioned schedule was 2 mg/kg in mice infected with 10 LD_{50} of influenza virus, which corresponded to 1/50 of the minimal subacute toxic dose (100 mg/kg per day) (23).

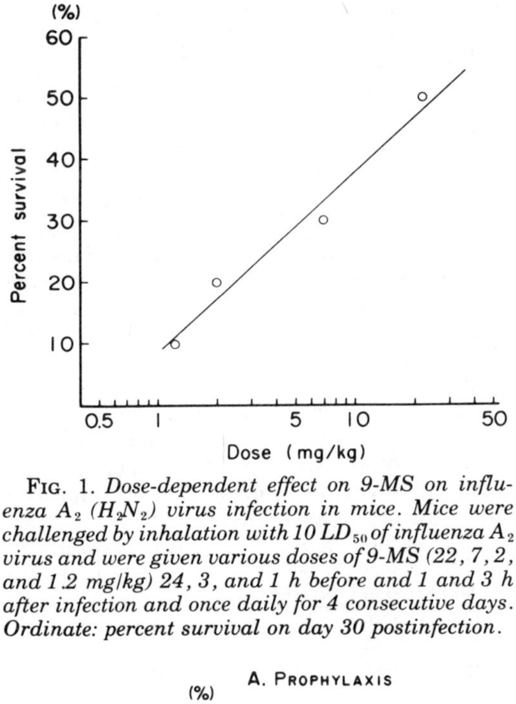

FIG. 1. *Dose-dependent effect on 9-MS on influenza A_2 (H_2N_2) virus infection in mice. Mice were challenged by inhalation with 10 LD_{50} of influenza A_2 virus and were given various doses of 9-MS (22, 7, 2, and 1.2 mg/kg) 24, 3, and 1 h before and 1 and 3 h after infection and once daily for 4 consecutive days. Ordinate: percent survival on day 30 postinfection.*

Dependence of the antiviral action of 9-MS on the treatment schedule. The effect of time of administration on the antiviral action of 9-MS was investigated. Half of the mice given 30 mg of 9-MS per kg i.p. three times, 24, 3, and 1 h, before infection with 10 LD_{50} of the virus survived for more than 30 days (Fig. 2A), whereas all the control mice receiving PBS died within 13 days. However, all the mice treated with the same dose of 9-MS three times, 24, 48, and 72 h, after infection died within 12 days, as did the untreated controls (Fig. 2B). Thus, it was only the prophylactic administration of the antibiotic that demonstrated the antiviral activity against influenza infection in mice.

In the next experiment, mice were given an almost toxic dose (260 mg/kg) of 9-MS i.p. as a single administration 2 to 72 h before infection. No treatments, except one performed 2 h before infection, conferred statistically significant protection (Table 2). In addition, a nontoxic single dose (5 mg/kg) of the antibiotic administered 2 h before infection significantly increased the survival rate (by 20%) as well as the mean survival time (Table 2). The therapeutic index was computed, therefore, at 60 by comparison between the minimal effective dose (5 mg/kg) and LD_{50} (300 mg/kg).

Mechanism of the antiviral effect. The infectivity of $10^{7.5}$ 50% egg infectious doses of influenza virus was not reduced by incubation with 1 mg of 9-MS per ml in serum-free Eagle minimal essential medium at 37 C for 12 h. Besides, the antibiotic was shown not to exercise any inhibitory activity against influenza

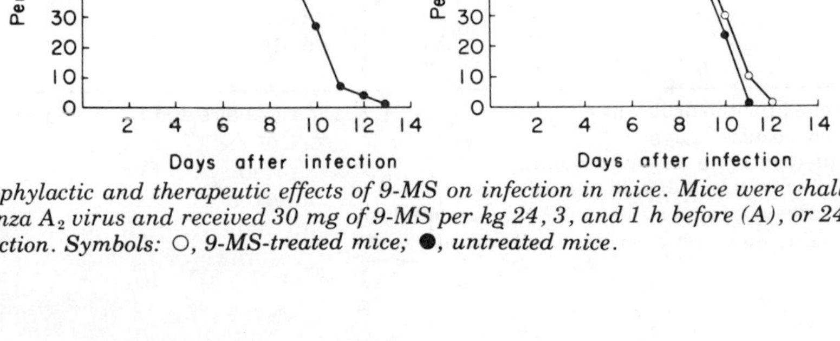

FIG. 2. *Prophylactic and therapeutic effects of 9-MS on infection in mice. Mice were challenged with 10 LD_{50} of influenza A_2 virus and received 30 mg of 9-MS per kg 24, 3, and 1 h before (A), or 24, 48, and 72 h after (B), infection. Symbols: ○, 9-MS-treated mice; ●, untreated mice.*

TABLE 2. *Dependence of the activity of 9-MS on time of treatment*

Single dose (mg/kg)	Time of treatment before virus injection[a] (h)	No. of mice[b]	Survival		Mean survival	
			%[c]	Significance[d] (*P*)	Time (days)	Significance[e] (*P*)
Almost toxic						
260	72	10	0		7.6	
260	48	10	0		8.0	
260	24	10	0		8.0	
260	2	10	40	<0.01	17.5	<0.001
0		27	0		8.2	
Nontoxic						
5	2	10	20	0.027	14.5	<0.001
0		28	0		7.4	

[a] 9-MS was given i.p. at each time before virus challenge.
[b] Ten LD_{50} of influenza A_2 virus were given by inhalation.
[c] Percentage of survival on day 30.
[d] Probability value obtained by use of chi-square analysis.
[e] Probability value obtained by use of the Student *t* test.

virus proliferation in chicken embryo fibroblasts at a concentration lower than 12.5 μg/ml, whereas it was observed to inhibit the growth of the cells at a concentration of 10μg/ml. The compound proved, therefore, to possess neither virocidal nor virostatic activity in vitro.

The lack of virocidal or virostatic activity in vitro and the requirement of prophylactic treatment mentioned above suggested that the antibiotic brought about the protective effect through mediation by interferon. Therefore, evidence for an interferon activity was sought in the serum and lung samples taken from the treated mice. Figure 3 shows the kinetics of viral inhibitors in the serum and lung after i.p. injection of 30 mg of 9-MS per kg. The inhibitor was found in the serum 12 h later. The titer subsequently reached a peak 4 h thereafter and steadily declined to undetectable levels within the following 16 h. On the other hand, the activity was detected much earlier in the lung and reached a peak 10 h after the injection. It then fell linearly, as did that in the serum. In addition, the administration of 5 to 260 mg of 9-MS per kg similarly induced inhibitors in the lung and serum.

The activity in the serum was characterized for species specificity, trypsin susceptibility, heat stability, and pH stability, in comparison with the mouse serum interferon induced 2 h after the intravenous injection of endotoxin. The inhibitory activities in both serum specimens were not detectable in the primary cultures of chicken embryo fibroblasts or in rabbit RK-13 cell cultures challenged with vesicular stomatitis virus, and they were completely destroyed by trypsin treatment (Table 3). The inhibitory activity stimulated with 9-MS treatment was abolished after incubation at 56 C for

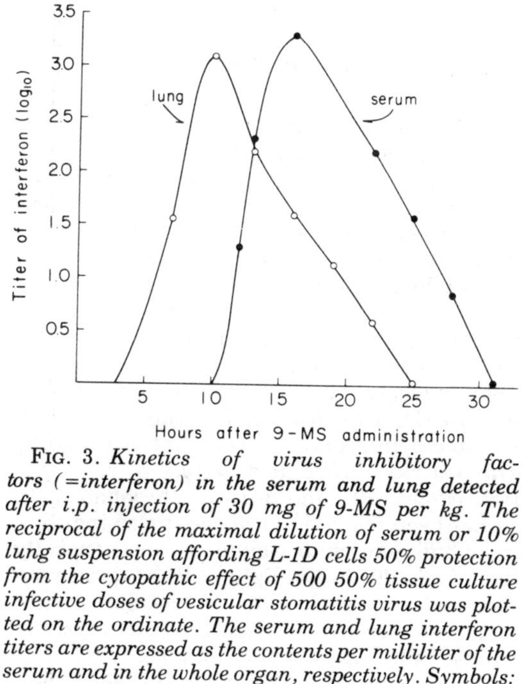

FIG. 3. *Kinetics of virus inhibitory factors (=interferon) in the serum and lung detected after i.p. injection of 30 mg of 9-MS per kg. The reciprocal of the maximal dilution of serum or 10% lung suspension affording L-1D cells 50% protection from the cytopathic effect of 500 50% tissue culture infective doses of vesicular stomatitis virus was plotted on the ordinate. The serum and lung interferon titers are expressed as the contents per milliliter of the serum and in the whole organ, respectively. Symbols:* ○, *lung;* ●, *serum.*

30 min and after dialysis against glycine-HCl buffer (pH 2.0) for 24 h at 4 C. On the other hand, the mouse serum interferon induced by endotoxin was relatively resistant to heat and acid treatments. Both of them, however, were not dialyzable at neutral pH. The inhibitor detected in the mouse lung after 9-MS administration showed almost the same characteristics as that detected in the serum. Taken together, these data indicate that the serum and lung inhibitors stimulated by 9-MS were interferon.

TABLE 3. *Characterization of mouse serum inhibitors[a] obtained after injection of 9-MS and endotoxin*

Test procedures	Titer[b] of the inhibitor induced with:	
	9-MS	Endotoxin
Species specificity		
Mouse L-fibroblasts (L-1D)	200	640
Chicken embryo fibroblasts	<12	<10
Rabbit RK-13 cells	<12	<10
Trypsin sensitivity (100 μg/ml, pH 7.4, 3 h, 37 C)	<12	<20
Thermoresistance (56 C, 30 min)	<12	80
pH resistance[c] (pH 2.0, 24 h, 4 C)	<12	80
Effect of dialysis (24 h, 4 C)[d]	200	640
Stock preparation[e]	200	640

[a] The serum specimens were obtained 16 h after i.p. administration of 30 mg of 9-MS per kg or 2 h after the intravenous injection of 0.5 mg of *E. coli* endotoxin per kg.

[b] Titers are expressed as the reciprocal of the serum dilution that gave 50% protection against a challenge of 500 50% tissue culture infective doses of vesicular stomatitis virus.

[c] Dialysis against 0.1 M glycine-HCl buffer, pH 2.0, was conducted at 4 C for 24 h, followed by dialysis against PBS (pH 7.2) for 24 h.

[d] Mouse serum was dialyzed against distilled water.

[e] Stored at −20 C as a control.

DISCUSSION

Influenza virus has generally been regarded as more sensitive to the action of interferon (17, 20) than herpes simplex and other viruses (3). It has generally been reported that the prophylactic administration of such interferon inducers as polyinosinic:polycytidylic acid (injected i.p.; 21), bacterial endotoxin (26), CP-20961 (12), and tilorone hydrochloride (15) does not exert any protective effect against influenza infection in mice. On the other hand, a small but significant protective effect has been exhibited by other inducers, such as chlorite-oxidized oxyamylose (1), polyinosinic:polycytidylic acid (administered intranasally) (11), natural double-stranded ribonucleic acid extracted from *Lentinus edotes* (29), and dextran phosphate (26). As has been pointed out above, these inducers are of high molecular weight and are generally toxic (7, 6, 19). In the light of these data, nontoxic inducers with a low molecular weight have been screened for their protective activity against influenza infection in mice.

9-MS, a unique glutarimide antibiotic, was found to improve the course of influenza infection and to stimulate interferon production in mouse lung and serum. The prophylactic administration of 9-MS displayed a reproducible protective effect (Table 1). Given in a therapeutic manner, however, the antibiotic was no longer effective (Fig. 2). A high dose of 9-MS exerted protection only when administered 2 h before infection (Table 2). A completely nontoxic dose of the antibotic injected 2 h before infection also increased significantly both the survivor number and the mean survival time. These data suggest that the antiviral effect of 9-MS is brought about by host-mediated, rather than direct, antiviral activity, such as interferon induction.

Fifteen minutes after the administration of an almost toxic dose (260 mg/kg) of 9-MS, 0.3 mg of the antibiotic was recovered in the lung by means of bioassay with *Saccharomyces sake* (data not shown); however, the pulmonary content fell to undetectable levels within 1 h. In addition, it has been reported that it is not until 2 days after infection with 5 to 20 LD_{50} of mouse-adapted influenza virus that the virus is seen to proliferate in the mouse lung (13, 26, 27), and our present data also sustain this observation. In addition, the antibiotic was shown to possess no virocidal activity, as mentioned above. Taken together, these results rule out direct interactions of 9-MS with influenza virus in the lung. Although direct evidence is still lacking to show that induced interferon inhibited virus growth, these data suggest that 9-MS exerts its protective effect against influenza infection through interferon induction or, alternatively, through other as yet unestablished host-mediated defense mechanisms. The low toxicity of the antibiotic (23) should warrant further detailed evaluation of the activity against various infections in vivo. Positive prophylactic but negative therapeutic effects should be examined in these various infectious systems.

ACKNOWLEDGMENTS

This work was supported by grants from the Ministry of Education, Science and Culture and from the Science and Technology Agency of Japan.

We wish to thank the staff of the Fermentation Division of Mitsubishi Chemicals Co. Ltd., Tokyo, for the supply of 9-MS.

LITERATURE CITED

1. **Billiau, A., J. Desmyter, and P. De Somer.** 1970. Antiviral activity of chlorite-oxidized oxyamylose, a polyacetal carboxylic acid. J. Virol. 5:321–328.
2. **Black, D. R., F. Eckstein, E. De Clercq, and T. C. Merigan.** 1973. Studies on the toxicity and antiviral activity of various polynucleotides. Antimicrob. Agents Chemother. 3:198–206.
3. **Catalano, L. W., Jr., and S. Baron.** 1970. Protection against herpes virus and encephalomyocarditis virus encephalitis with a double-stranded RNA inducer of interferon. Proc. Soc. Exp. Biol. Med. 133:684–687.
4. **Claes, P., A. Billiau, E. De Clercq, J. Desmyter, E. Schonne, H. Vanderhaeghe, and P. De Somer.** 1970. Polyacetal carboxylic acid: a new group of antiviral polyanions. J. Virol. 5:313–320.
5. **De Clercq, E., F. Eckstein, and T. C. Merigan.** 1970. Structural requirement for synthetic polyanions to act as interferon inducers. Ann. N.Y. Acad. Sci. 173:444–461.
6. **De Clercq, E., and T. C. Merigan.** 1969. An active interferon inducer obtained from *Hemophilus influenzae* type B. J. Immunol. 103:899–906.
7. **De Clercq, E., W. E. Stewart II, and P. De Somer.** 1972. Interferon production linked to toxicity of polyriboinosinic acid-polyribocytidylic acid. Infect. Immun. 6:344–347.
8. **De Somer, P., E. De Clercq, A. Billiau, E. Schonne, and M. Claesen.** 1968. Antiviral activity of polyacrylic and polymethacrylic acids. II. Mode of action in vivo. J. Virol. 2:886–893.
9. **Field, A. K., A. A. Tytell, G. P. Lampson, and M. R. Hilleman.** 1967. Inducers of interferon and host resistance. II. Multistranded synthetic polynucleotide complexes. Proc. Natl. Acad. Sci. U.S.A. 58:1004–1010.
10. **Glaz, E. T., E. Szolgay, I. Stoger, and M. Talas.** 1973. Antiviral activity and induction of interferon-like substance by quinacrine and acranil. Antimicrob. Agents Chemother. 3:537–541.
11. **Hill, D. A., S. Baron, and R. M. Chanock.** 1969. The effect of an interferon inducer on influenza virus. Bull. W.H.O. 41:689–693.
12. **Hoffman, W. W., J. J. Korst, J. D. Niblack, and T. H. Cronin.** 1973. *N,N*-dioctadecyl-*N′,N′*-bis (2-hydroxyethyl)propanediamine: antiviral activity and interferon stimulation in mice. Antimicrob. Agents Chemother. 3:498–502.
13. **Ishida, N., Y. Kosaka, and Y. Sasaki.** 1959. Studies on experimental influenza in mice. II. Absolute amount of virus introduced into the respiratory tract of mice by standard inhalation procedure. Tohoku J. Exp. Med. 71:151–161.
14. **Kits, S., D. R. Dubbs, L. J. Piekrski, and T. C. Hsu.** 1963. Deletion of thymidine kinase activity from L cells resistant to bromodeoxyuridine. Exp. Cell Res. 31:297–312.
15. **Kruger, R. F., and G. D. Mayer.** 1970. Tilorone hydrochloride: an orally active antiviral agent. Science 169:1213–1214.
16. **Leonard, B. J., E. Eccleston, and D. Jones.** 1969. Toxicity of interferon inducers of double-stranded RNA type. Nature (London) 224:1023–1024.
17. **McLaren, C., and C. W. Potter.** 1973. The relationship between interferon and virus virulence in influenza virus infections of the mouse. J. Med. Microbiol. 6:21–32.
18. **Mayer, G. D., and R. F. Kruger.** 1970. Tilorone hydrochloride: mode of action. Science 169:1214–1215.
19. **Merigan, T. C., E. De Clercq, and G. H. Bausek.** 1970. Nonviral interferon inducers. J. Gen. Physiol. 56:57s–75s.
20. **Murphy, B. R., S. Baron, E. G. Chalhub, C. P. Uhlendorf, and R. M. Chanock.** 1973. Temperature-sensitive mutants of influenza virus. IV. Induction of interferon in the nasopharynx by wild-type and a temperature-sensitive recombinant virus. J. Infect. Dis. 128:488–492.
21. **Nemes, M. M., A. A. Tytell, G. P. Lampson, A. K. Field, and M. R. Hilleman.** 1969. Inducers of interferon and host resistance. IV. Antiviral efficacy of poly I:C in animal models. Proc. Soc. Exp. Biol. Med. 132:776–783.
22. **Reed, L J., and H. Muench.** 1938. A simple method of estimating fifty percent end points. Am. J. Hyg. 27:493–497.
23. **Saito, N., F. Ktame, M. Kikuchi, and N. Ishida.** 1974. Studies on a new antiviral antibiotic, 9-methylstreptimidone. I. Physicochemical and biological properties. J. Antibiot. 27:206–214.
24. **Siminoff, P., A. M. Bernard, V. S. Hursky, and K. E. Price.** 1973. BL-20803, a new, low-molecular-weight interferon inducer. Antimicrob. Agents Chemother. 3:742–743.
25. **Stinebring, W. R., and J. S. Youngner.** 1964. Pattern of interferon appearance in mice injected with bacteria and bacterial endotoxin. Nature (London) 204:217.
26. **Suzuki, F., N. Ishida, M. Suzuki, T. Sato, and S. Suzuki.** 1975. Effect of interferon inducer, dextran phosphate, on influenza virus infection in mice. Proc. Soc. Exp. Biol. Med. 149:847–853.
27. **Suzuki, F., J. Ohya, and N. Ishida.** 1974. Effect of antilymphocyte serum on influenza virus infection in mice. Proc. Soc. Exp. Biol. Med. 146:78–84.
28. **Suzuki, F., T. Suganuma, and N. Ishida.** 1974. Interferon induction by an antitumor antibiotic, lymphomycin. J. Antibiot. 27:346–348.
29. **Tsunoda, A., and N. Ishida.** 1970. A mushroom extract as an interferon inducer. Ann. N.Y. Acad. Sci. 173:719–726.
30. **Youngner, J. S., W. R. Stinebring, and S. E. Taube.** 1965. Influence of inhibitors of protein synthesis on interferon formation in mice. Virology 27:541–550.

ANTIMICROBIAL AGENTS AND CHEMOTHERAPY, July 1976, p. 20-24 Vol. 10, No. 1

Bioevaluation of the Antibacterial Flumequine for Urinary Tract Use

S. R. ROHLFING,* J. F. GERSTER, AND D. C. KVAM

Riker Laboratories, Inc., St. Paul, Minnesota 55101

Received for publication 17 February 1976

The antimicrobial activity of flumequine (R-802) was characterized by in vitro and in vivo procedures. Assay of the minimal inhibitory concentrations for 321 recent clinical isolates revealed that 88% of the gram-negative bacteria were inhibited by an R-802 concentration of 6.2 μg/ml or less. Cross-resistance in laboratory-derived mutants of *Proteus vulgaris* was essentially complete for R-802, nalidixic acid, and oxolinic acid, although quantitative differences were evident. R-802 was more effective than either of these quinolone antibacterials in preventing the development of experimental murine pyelonephritis (*P. vulgaris*). R-802 and trimethoprim/sulfamethoxazole (1:5) were equally effective in resolving a *P. mirabilis*-induced prostatitis of rats.

Flumequine (R-802) is a synthetic antibacterial, selected from a series of tricyclic quinolines prepared in Riker Laboratories. The compound is 6,7-dihydro-9-fluoro-5-methyl-1-oxo-1H,5H (ij) quinolizine-2-carboxylic acid (Fig. 1). This report describes the bioevaluation of R-802 and its comparison with several antimicrobials in clinical use.

(This work was reported in part at the Annual Meeting of the Federation of American Societies for Experimental Biology, 1974, Atlantic City, N.J.)

MATERIALS AND METHODS

Bacteria. Laboratory stock cultures were used. Susceptibility testing of clinical isolates was accomplished with cultures from urine specimens taken at the St. Paul Veterans Administration Hospital, St. Paul, Minn. These isolates were identified using conventional microbiological methods (1). Wound isolates of *Staphylococcus aureus* were obtained from the St. Louis Park Clinic, Minneapolis.

Antimicrobials. Flumequine (R-802) was synthesized in Riker Research Laboratories. Stock solutions of R-802 (1%) for in vitro use were prepared with 0.1 N sodium hydroxide. Nalidixic acid and oxolinic acid were provided by Winthrop Laboratories and Warner-Lambert Research Institute, respectively. Bactrim (sulfamethoxazole and trimethoprim, 5:1), Erythrocin (erythromycin stearate), and Terramycin (oxytetracyline-hydrochloride) were obtained in commercial form.

Susceptibility. The antimicrobial spectrum of R-802 was surveyed on tryptone soy agar (TSA) plates with a $\log_{10}$ dilution series. Microliter aliquots of stock solution were mixed with molten TSA in individual screw-cap vials and dispensed into petri dishes. These preparations were allowed to harden and were surface inoculated with stock culture suspensions. The conditions of incubation were overnight at 37 C in a humidified atmosphere enriched with 10% carbon dioxide. Growth inhibition of those strains that appeared to be most susceptible to R-802 was further examined by a $\log_2$ dilution tube technique in nutrient broth (5). Nalidixic acid and oxolinic acid were included in this titration as reference quinolone antibacterials. *Bacillus subtilis* was deleted in this comparison because of pellicle formation in static broth culture; *Proteus vulgaris*, which was not tested on TSA because of the "swarming" phenomenon, was included here. The minimal inhibitory concentrations (MICs) of R-802 for clinical isolates of urinary tract infection were similarly determined; the influence of culture medium pH was examined in selected strains at 0.2-unit intervals over the range 6.0 to 8.0.

Cross-resistance of mutant clones selected by growth on oxolinic acid, nalidixic acid, and R-802 was assessed by the replica plating technique (6). Approximately 10^9 cells were spread over the surface of drug plates containing TSA plus 0.15% bile salts to inhibit swarming of *P. vulgaris* 210. The levels of drug permitting development of approximately 10 colonies/plate were as follows: R-802 and oxolinic acid, 10 μg/ml; nalidixic acid, 50 μg/ml. No colonies were observed on plates containing 25 μg of R-802 or oxolinic acid per ml. An imprint of the colonies developing on each original plate was transferred to sterile velveteen templates. These in turn were used to reproduce the patterns on several test plates containing the individual drugs. All plates were scored after 2 days of incubation at 37 C.

Efficacy. Preclinical evaluation of R-802 for treatment of urinary tract infection used a rat model, which mimics the development of bacterial pyelonephritis in humans (8). One-tenth milliliter of an overnight shake culture of *P. vulgaris* 210 was injected into the partially ligated bladder of female Simonsen rats. Tryptone soy broth was used as the growth medium and diluent. The temperature of

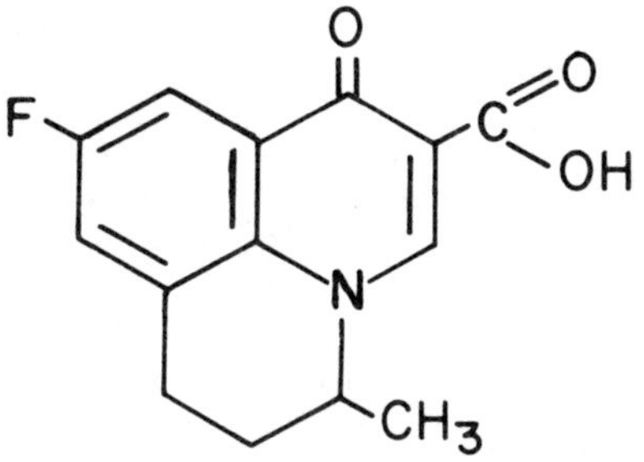

FIG. 1. *Structure of flumequine (R-802).*

incubation was 35 to 37 C with rotary agitation at 200 rpm. The highest dilution (usually 1:10) producing uniform bladder infections, which persisted for at least 10 days, was used. Antimicrobials were suspended in 4% aqueous acacia and homogenized with a ground-glass tissue mill. Treated animals were dosed daily by oral gavage beginning 24 h postinfection for a period of 3 weeks. Treatment periods of only 10 days at elevated doses (namely, 100 mg of R-802/kg per day) were inadequate based on culture of excised tissue. Infection control animals received no treatment. Water was supplied ad libitum. Animals were sacrificed 24 h post-treatment to culture both kidneys and the urinary bladder. Kidney slices and bladder fragments were placed on TSA agar to reveal the characteristic swarming outgrowth in positive cultures. No antibacterial activity could be demonstrated in excised tissues by using sensitive indicator bacteria. Infection relapse was assessed by retaining animals for a period of 2 weeks post-treatment prior to sacrifice and culture.

An experimental prostatitis was induced in male Simonsen rats according to the method of Friedlander and Braude (4). The growth conditions for *P. mirabilis* 120 were the same as those described for *P. vulgaris* 210. The undiluted culture in a nonrefluxing volume (0.05 ml) was injected into the unrestricted bladder of surgically prepared animals. Antimicrobials were suspended in 4% aqueous acacia and homogenized with a ground-glass tissue mill. Treated animals were dosed daily by oral gavage beginning 5 days postinfection for a period of 3 weeks. Infection control animals received no treatment. Water was supplied ad libitum. Animals were sacrificed after a total of 25 days to culture the ventral prostate, the urinary bladder, and both kidneys on TSA plates; the dorsolateral prostate is less frequently involved and was not monitored for evidence of infection.

Urinary levels of active drug were estimated by agar diffusion assay using *Klebsiella pneumoniae* 113 as the indicator bacterium. In lieu of cylinders, a stainless-steel template containing six wells (bioassay plate no. 1310, Labline Instruments, Inc.) was placed on the surface of seeded TSA plates. R-802 standards and pooled urine samples were diluted in tryptone soy broth. Each rat (three per group) received a single dose of 10 or 25 mg of R-802 per kg prior to 24-h urine collection.

RESULTS

In vitro. The susceptibility to R-802 of selected strains of microorganisms is presented in Table 1. The concentrations of R-802 inhibiting growth of bacteria ranged from 1 to 100 μg/ml, whereas no antifungal activity was evident at 100 μg of R-802 per ml. Antibacterial activity was unchanged by the addition of 10% (vol/vol) horse serum to the TSA growth medium.

The MICs of quinolone antibacterials presented in Table 2 suggested that a study of the response of recent clinical isolates from urinary tract infection to R-802 should be pursued. No "skip-tube" end points indicating rapid selection of resistant progeny were evident in this experiment.

Assay of the R-802 MICs for 321 recent clinical isolates (Table 3) revealed that 88% of the gram-negative bacteria were inhibited at a concentration of 6.2 μg/ml or less. The majority of gram-positive strains exhibited an MIC of 12.5 μg/ml or more. A different response to R-802 by these two groups of bacteria was also suggested by the influence of growth medium pH on antimicrobial activity in broth culture. The MIC values for *Escherichia coli* VA-1, *P. vulgaris*

TABLE 1. *Antimicrobial activity of R-802*[a]

Microorganism	MIC (μg/ml)	
	Serum free	10% Horse serum
Streptococcus pyogenes 114	100	100
Staphylococcus aureus 1	10	10
Bacillus subtilis 6	1	1
Escherichia coli 22	1	1
Pseudomonas aeruginosa 12	100	100
Streptococcus faecalis 196	100	100
Klebsiella pneumoniae 197	10	10
Aspergillus niger 18	>100	>100
Candida albicans 20	>100	>100

[a] Growth inhibition of laboratory stock cultures determined by TSA plate dilution.

TABLE 2. *MICs of quinolone antibacterials*[a]

Bacterium	MIC (μg/ml)		
	Nalidixic acid	Oxolinic acid	R-802
Proteus vulgaris 210	12.5	0.8	0.8
Klebsiella pneumoniae 197	0.8	0.4	0.4
Escherichia coli 22	3.1	0.4	0.8
Staphylococcus aureus 1	12.5	1.6	1.6

[a] Growth inhibition of laboratory stock cultures determined by the serial dilution tube technique in nutrient broth.

TABLE 3. *Cumulative percentage of clinical isolates inhibited at various R-802 concentrations*[a]

Bacterium	MIC (μg/ml):							Total isolates
	0.8	1.6	3.1	6.2	12.5	25.0	>25	
Escherichia coli	26	48	84	100	—[b]	—	—	58
Proteus vulgaris	—	14	43	71	100	—	—	7
Proteus mirabilis	8	28	58	80	100	—	—	40
Proteus rettgeri	14	29	43	71	100	—	—	7
Proteus morganii	35	57	78	87	100	—	—	23
Klebsiella pneumoniae	2	9	39	78	100	—	—	64
Enterobacter aerogenes	—	7	46	96	100	—	—	28
Pseudomonas aeruginosa	—	4	17	79	88	100	—	24
Serratia marcescens	12	44	75	100	—	—	—	32
Providence	17	50	50	83	100	—	—	6
Streptococcus faecalis	—	—	—	4	62	85	100	26
Staphylococcus aureus[c]	—	—	—	—	100	—	—	6

[a] Growth inhibition determined by the serial dilution tube technique in nutrient broth.
[b] —, Zero incidence.
[c] Wound isolates.

VA-1, and *P. mirabilis* VA-3 were invariant in the pH range 6.0 to 8.0; the MIC for *S. aureus* 148 increased 10-fold to a maximum of 25.0 μg/ml at pH 8.0.

Cross-resistance in laboratory-derived mutants of *P. vulgaris* was essentially complete for R-802, nalidixic acid, and oxolinic acid (Table 4). Although discrete colonies were evident on nalidixic acid selection plates containing 10 μg of drug per ml, a background lawn of additional mutants was confirmed on replica plates. Multistep mutants selected by serial transfers in increasing concentrations of each drug confirmed these observations: cross-resistance was demonstrated for *P. vulgaris* clones capable of growing on TSA containing 100 μg of R-802, 100 μg of oxolinic acid, or 500 μg of nalidixic acid per ml.

In vivo. the R-802 dose response obtained in an ascending rat urinary tract infection model is presented in Table 5. The median effective dose based on several titrations in this model was approximately 10 mg/kg per day. The data were not cumulatively scored as the sum of all positive cultures for each dose level, because upon cessation of treatment animals with infected bladders would surely develop infected kidneys in due course. A variable number of animals succumbed to fatal infections prior to terminating the experiment, as indicated in the column of survivors.

The comparative efficacy of R-802 and two urinary tract antimicrobials is presented in Table 6. The performance of nalidixic acid was comparable to that of oxolinic acid, whereas R-802 was clearly more effective in preventing the development of pyelonephritis as defined in this model. Bladder isolates from the two R-802 treatment failures were indistinguishable from the infecting culture in terms of antimicrobial susceptibility.

The absence of infection relapse in a short-term follow-up experiment is evident in Table 7. Bladder isolates from the four rats treated

TABLE 4. *Cross-resistance of P. vulgaris clones isolated in the presence of certain quinolone antibacterials*

Original selection plate			Cross-resistant clones on test replica plate			
Quinolone	Concn (μg/ml)	No. of colonies	Oxolinic acid (10 μg/ml)	Nalidixic acid 10 μg/ml	Nalidixic acid 50 μg/ml	R-802 (10 μg/ml)
Oxolinic acid	10	12	16	16	16	13
	10	11	12	12	12	11
Nalidixic acid	10	~44	10	TNTC[a]	TNTC	4
	50	9	4	TNTC	9	4
R-802	10	13	12	12	12	9
	10	7	7	7	7	2
	10	9	5	6	5	6

[a] TNTC, Too numerous to count.

TABLE 5. *Ascending rat urinary tract infection model: titration of R-802*[a]

Group	Survivors (21 days)	Left kidney	Right kidney	Bladder
Infection controls (*P. vulgaris*)	8/10	6/8	6/8	7/8
Infected and treated with R-802 (mg/kg per day)				
100	10/10	0/10	0/10	1/10
75	10/10	0/10	0/10	0/10
50	10/10	0/10	0/10	0/10
25	10/10	0/10	0/10	0/10
10	9/10	2/9	1/9	4/9

[a] Each group consisted of 10 animals; the last three columns indicate the ratio of positive cultures to survivors.

TABLE 6. *Ascending rat urinary tract infection model: comparison of R-802 with reference quinolones*[a]

Group	Survivors (21 days)	Left kidney	Right kidney	Bladder
Infection controls (*P. vulgaris*)	8/10	7/8	7/8	7/8
Infected and treated with:				
R-802, 25 mg/kg per day	10/10	0/10	0/10	2/10
Nalidixic acid, 25 mg/kg per day	9/10	2/9	4/9	4/9
Oxolinic acid, 25 mg/kg per day	9/10	3/9	4/9	6/9

[a] Each group consisted of 10 animals; the last three columns indicate the ratio of positive cultures to survivors.

with 25 mg of R-802/kg per day were again unchanged in terms of R-802 susceptibility.

The therapeutic response to R-802 and three reference antimicrobials in a *P. mirabilis*-induced prostatitis is presented in Table 8. In three experiments, the incidence of positive prostate cultures from infection control groups of 10 animals each ranged from 0.72 to 0.86; positive cultures from both kidneys of each animal closely paralleled the incidence of prostate infection. The incidence of bladder infection was slightly higher, as indicated. R-802 was essentially ineffective in this model at a dose of 25 mg/kg per day. A dose of 50 mg/kg per day resulted in a 65% reduction in the incidence of prostatitis and pyelonephritis, as measured by in vitro culture of excised tissue. Oral administration of erythromycin and trimethoprim/sulfamethoxazole significantly reduced the incidence of positive prostate cultures at 50 and 100 mg/kg per day. These reductions were not closely paralleled by results obtained from tissues of the urinary tract per se. Oxytetracycline was poorly effective in this model by comparison with the other antimicrobials examined.

Based on the in vitro activity of R-802, the levels of active drug achieved in a 24-h urine collection from rats receiving a single oral dose were 15 μg/ml at 10 mg of R-802 per kg of body weight and 41 μg/ml at 25 mg of R-802 per kg of body weight.

TABLE 7. *Ascending rat urinary tract infection model: infection incidence 14 days post-treatment*[a]

Group	Time (days)	Survivors	Left kidney	Right kidney	Bladder
Infection controls (*P. vulgaris*)	21	5/10	4/5	4/5	4/5
Infected and treated with R-802 (mg/kg per day)					
50	21	7/7	0/7	0/7	0/7
50	21 (+14)	7/8	0/7	0/7	0/7
25	21	6/8	2/6	1/6	3/6
25	21 (+14)	6/7	1/6	0/6	1/6

[a] The infection control group consisted of 10 animals; 15 animals were treated in each dosage group as indicated. The last three columns indicate the ratio of positive cultures to survivors.

DISCUSSION

Quinolone antimicrobials are broad-spectrum agents reserved primarily for urinary tract use. Therapeutic advantages for *Proteus* sp. infections, in particular, were suggested in a comparative study of 2,081 clinical isolates which used Neg-gram sensitivity disks (9). In one study of urinary tract infections, nalidixic acid performed significantly better than sulfadimidine, producing cure rates of 93.7 and 81.4%, respectively; this result led the authors to regard nalidixic acid as a drug of choice when bacteriological facilities are not available (2). It is also clear that development of resistant organisms after administration of existing quinolones is a frequent problem (3,7). There is an

TABLE 8. *Efficacy of R-802 and reference antimicrobials in P. mirabilis-induced prostatitis*[a]

Treatment	Survivors	Prostate	Bladder	Right kidney	Left kidney
Infection controls	24/30	19/24 (0.79)	22/24 (0.92)	20/24 (0.83)	20/24 (0.83)
Infected and treated with					
R-802 (mg/kg per day)					
25	10/10	7/10 (0.70)	8/10 (0.80)	8/10 (0.80)	8/10 (0.80)
50	29/30	8/29 (0.28)	16/29 (0.55)	9/29 (0.31)	9/29 (0.31)
100	10/10	0/10	0/10	0/10	0/10
Erythromycin (mg/kg per day)					
50	7/10	1/7 (0.14)	6/7 (0.86)	6/7 (0.86)	6/7 (0.86)
100	8/10	2/8 (0.25)	6/8 (0.75)	4/8 (0.50)	2/8 (0.25)
Oxytetracycline (mg/kg per day)					
50	10/10	5/10 (0.50)	6/10 (0.60)	6/10 (0.60)	6/10 (0.60)
100	9/10	4/9 (0.44)	7/9 (0.78)	6/9 (0.67)	6/9 (0.67)
Trimethoprim/sulfamethoxazole (mg/kg per day)					
50	8/10	3/8 (0.38)	8/8 (1.00)	7/8 (0.88)	6/8 (0.75)
100	10/10	1/10 (0.10)	6/10 (0.60)	2/10 (0.20)	4/10 (0.40)

[a] Survival ratios indicate the number of animals that succumbed to infection between day 5, when treatment was initiated, and day 25, when specimens were taken. The last four columns indicate the ratio of positive cultures to survivors; the incidence of infection calculated from this ratio is shown in parentheses.

apparent absence of transferable drug resistance with these compounds, due in part to the prescribed indications. Laboratory-induced mutations to quinolone resistance occur in stepwise fashion, and the synthesis of oxolinic acid that enhanced in vitro activity improved the potential therapeutic value of these compounds. The results obtained in the present study utilizing appropriate rodent models demonstrate the added potential of R-802.

In vitro testing of R-802 demonstrated significant antibacterial activity for the principal pathogens in urinary tract infection. In addition to *E. coli*, *Proteus* sp., and the *Klebsiella-Enterobacter* group, the clinical isolates examined in this study also included 32 *Serratia marcescens*; *S. marcescens* is usually regarded as an index of nosocomial infection and appeared to resemble *E. coli* in terms of R-802 susceptibility. The pronounced influence of pH on antibacterial activity versus *S. aureus* has been observed with other quinolones and is unexplained at present.

In vivo testing of R-802 was aimed at determining efficacy for intended use. The *Proteus* sp.-induced pyelonephritis is a good model for comparing quinolone antibacterials for reasons previously cited. It is less useful for antibiotics, e.g., ampicillin, but attempts to substitute other infecting bacteria have met with limited success. Prostatitis can be a significant treatment problem and source of chronic bacteruria (10). The rodent model used to challenge R-802 for this indication is idealized in terms of the infecting agent; nevertheless, the method provides a measure of antimicrobial efficacy rather than antimicrobial activity partitioned into prostatic secretions. The reference antimicrobials in this experiment were selected largely on the basis of clinical interest. Oxytetracycline hydrochloride would be a poor choice based on in vitro susceptibility of most strains of *P. mirabilis* (9). The in vitro activity of erythromycin stearate is favored by slightly alkaline conditions, and the pH of mammalian prostatic fluid is usually less than 7.0. Nevertheless, erythromycin was effective in eliminating bacteria from the prostate. The therapeutic responses to R-802 and trimethoprim/sulfamethoxazole were dose related and comparable for prostatitis. Additional indications for R-802 have been investigated in this laboratory and will be reported in a separate communication.

ACKNOWLEDGMENTS

We express our appreciation to J. Chernay, St. Paul Veterans Administration Hospital, who collected and identified clinical isolates used in this study. Technical assistance was provided by P. L. Betterman, G. K. Hill, and R. M. Winandy. Chemical technology was provided by S. Pecore and R. Stern.

LITERATURE CITED

1. **Blair, J. E., E. H. Lennette, and J. P. Truant (ed.).** 1970. Manual of clinical microbiology, p. 151–198. American Society for Microbiology, Bethesda, Md.
2. **Brown, P. C. C., M. C. Donaghy, P. H. Dootson, D. H. M. Titcombe, and D. M. MacLaren.** 1971. Sulphadimidine and nalidixic acid therapy in urinary-tract infections in general practice. Practitioner **207:**819–826.
3. **Clark, H., N. K. Brown, J. F. Wallace, and M. Turck.** 1971. Emergence of resistant organisms as a function of dose in oxolinic acid therapy. Am. J. Med. Sci. **261:**145–148.
4. **Friedlander, A. M., and A. I. Braude.** 1972. Experimental prostatitis-relationship to pyelonephritis. J. Infect. Dis. **125:**645–651.
5. **Grove, D. C., and W. A. Randall.** 1955. Assay methods of antibiotics, a laboratory manual, p. 190–192. Medical Encyclopedia, Inc., New York.
6. **Lederberg, J., and E. M. Lederberg.** 1952. Replica plating and indirect selection of bacterial mutants. J. Bacteriol. **63:**399–406.
7. **Madsen, P. O., and P. R. Rhodes.** 1971. Oxolinic acid, a new chemotherapeutic agent in the treatment of urinary tract infection. J. Urol. **105:**870–872.
8. **Miraglia, G. J.** 1970. Model infections in the evaluation of antimicrobial agents. Trans. N.Y. Acad. Sci. **32:**338–344.
9. **Roupas, A., and J. D. Piguet.** 1968. Sensibilité aux antibiotiques de 2081 souches bactériennes, isolées d'infections urinaires. Schweiz. Med. Wochenschr. **98:**2008–2016.
10. **Stamey, T. A.** 1971. Part II: the clinical aspects of urinary tract infections – observations on the clinical use of nalidixic acid. Postgrad. Med. J. **47:**21–26.

ANTIMICROBIAL AGENTS AND CHEMOTHERAPY, July 1976, p. 25-27
Vol. 10, No. 1

Pharmacokinetic Parameters of Sisomicin

BURT R. MEYERS, SHALOM Z. HIRSCHMAN,* STANLEY YANCOVITZ, AND BRUCE RIBNER

Department of Medicine, The Mount Sinai School of Medicine of the City University of New York, New York, New York 10029

Received for publication 10 February 1976

Sisomicin in doses of 1 mg/kg was administered intramuscularly to 10 healthy volunteers, and 1 week later the same volunteers received sisomicin at the same dose intravenously. A peak serum concentration of sisomicin of 3.08 μg/ml was obtained 1 h after intramuscular injection, and a peak serum concentration of 7.12 μg/ml was achieved 30 min after a 30-min intravenous infusion. The sisomicin elimination data were analyzed according to a two-compartment model. Pharmacokinetic parameters derived from the intramuscular and intravenous studies were quite similar.

Aminoglycoside antibiotics, such as gentamicin, have become increasingly important in the therapy of infections due to gram-negative bacteria (1, 5). Sisomicin is a new aminoglycoside antibiotic isolated from the fermentation broth of *Micromonospora inyoensis* and closely resembles gentamicin C_{1a}, a component of the gentamicin complex (11). Since aminoglycoside antibiotics can be both nephro- and ototoxic, careful investigation of the pharmacological properties of these antibiotics is mandatory. We report results of pharmacokinetic studies with sisomicin in 10 healthy human volunteers.

MATERIALS AND METHODS

Ten healthy volunteers, aged 19 to 34 years, five male and five female, were the subjects of these studies. The volunteers ranged in weight from 49.9 to 107.3 kg, with a mean weight of 64.92 ± 17 (standard deviation) kg. Informed consent was obtained from all volunteers, in accord with institutional policies.

In the first phase of the study, the 10 volunteers were given 1-mg/kg doses of sisomicin intramuscularly (i.m.). The volunteers voided before injection of the drug, were in the fasting state, and remained sedentary during the study period. Blood samples were obtained just before injection and then at 0.5, 1, 2, 4, 6, 8, and 24 h after injection. Urine was collected for the first 8 h and then during 8 to 24 h after drug administration.

One week later, the same volunteers were used for study with intravenous (i.v.) infusion. Doses of 1 mg of sisomicin per kg were dissolved in 250 ml of 5% dextrose and water and administered i.v. over a 30-min period. Blood samples were collected just before injection and at 0.25, 0.5, 1, 1.5, 2, 4, 6, and 24 h after the end of the infusion. Urine was collected for the first 8 h and then for the following 8 to 24 h.

Serum and urine concentrations of sisomicin were determined by the cup plate assay method, using *Bacillus subtilis* as the test organism by methods previously described (7).

The following laboratory studies were determined before and after administration of both i.m. and i.v. doses of sisomicin: hemogram, urine analysis, blood urea nitrogen, serum creatinine, glutamic oxaloacetic transaminase, glutamic pyruvic transaminase, alkaline phosphatase, bilirubin, phosphorus, sodium, potassium, chloride, calcium, albumin, and globulin.

Pharmacokinetic parameters were determined by means of a program written for a Wang 700B programmable calculator. The data were fitted to two regression lines, and the following pharmacokinetic parameters, based on a two-compartment model (2), were calculated: elimination constant, K_e (per hour); transfer rate constants between the central (V_1) and peripheral (V_2) compartments, K_{12} and K_{21} (per hour); "concentration times time" area below the curve, A (micrograms per milliliter per hour); the total apparent volume of distribution (by the area method [2]), V_d (liters per 100 kg); plasma clearance, C (milliliters per minute); and the half-life of the beta elimination phase, $t_{1/2\beta}$ (hours). The corrections developed by Loo and Riegelman (4) were used for the calculation of pharmacokinetic parameters after i.v. infusion.

RESULTS

The average serum concentrations obtained after i.m. injection of sisomicin are listed in Table 1. The highest serum concentration of sisomicin, 3.08 μg/ml, was found 1 h after injection. Serum concentrations decreased during the ensuing 8 h, and no drug was detectable at 24 h. Of the total injected dose of sisomicin, 33.5% was excreted in the urine during the first 8 h, followed by only 6.3% during the next 16 h. The average urine concentration of sisomicin during the first 8 h was 87 μg/ml, and that during the 8- to 24-h period was 10 μg/ml.

After i.v. administration of 1-mg/kg doses of sisomicin, an average peak serum level of 7.12 μg/ml was obtained 30 min after infusion (Table 1). Serum levels decreased over the next 5.5 h, and no drug was detected in the serum at 24 h (Table 1). The average urine concentration of sisomicin during the first 8 h after infusion was 64 μg/ml, and that during the next 16-h period was 5.1 μg/ml. Of the total dose administered, 29.5% was excreted during the first 8 h and only 3.7% was excreted during the following 16 h.

The volunteers tolerated the administration of sisomicin without mishap. There were no complaints of prolonged or excessive pain after i.m. injection. The laboratory tests examined remained normal after administration of sisomicin.

The pharmacokinetic parameters derived for sisomicin from the i.m. and i.v. studies with these 10 volunteers were quite similar (Table 2). The elimination constants (K_e) after i.m. and i.v. administration of sisomicin were 0.449 and 0.51/h, respectively. The transfer constants, K_{21} and K_{12}, also were quite similar for the two studies. The $t_{1/2\beta}$ was 158 min after i.m. injection and 153 min after i.v. injection. The total apparent volume of distribution (V_d) derived from the study with i.m. doses of sisomicin was 25 liters/100 kg, and a very similar value of 24 liters/100 kg was obtained from the i.v. study (Table 2). A plasma clearance value of 72 ml/min was derived from both studies.

DISCUSSION

The serum concentrations after parenteral administration of sisomicin were comparable to those reported previously from this laboratory (6) for two other aminoglycoside antibiotics, gentamicin and tobramycin, except that the serum concentrations of gentamicin and tobramycin were slightly higher from the 1st to 4th h after i.v. infusion (6). However, greater percentages of the administered doses of both gentamicin (59%) and tobramycin (79%) were excreted during the first 24 h than were found with sisomicin. The average concentration of these antibiotics in the urine (6) also was greater than that found with sisomicin.

TABLE 1. *Serum concentrations after 1-mg/kg parenteral doses of sisomicin*

Time after dose (h)	Serum concn (μg/ml)	
	i.m.	i.v.
0.25		2.7 ± 0.68
0.5	2.58 ± 0.3[a]	7.12 ± 1.56
1	3.08 ± 0.39	3.1 ± 0.91
1.5		2.5 ± 0.54
2	1.4 ± 0.3	1.6 ± 0.48
4	0.95 ± 0.3	1.02 ± 0.39
6	0.61 ± 0.16	0.54 ± 0.17
8	0.28 ± 0.14	
24	0	0

[a] Mean ± standard deviation.

TABLE 2. *Pharmacokinetic parameters of sisomicin after parenteral administration of 1-mg/kg doses*

Route	Parameter						
	K_e (per h)	K_{21} (per h)	K_{12} (per h)	A (μg/ml per h)	$t_{1/2\beta}$ (h)	V_d (liters/ 100 kg)	Clearance (ml/ min)
i.m.	0.449	0.463	0.141	15.11	2.63	25	72
i.v.	0.51	0.499	0.2	15.21	2.55	24	72

In our previous studies with tobramycin and gentamicin (6), we found that the regression lines constructed for the drug elimination data could be fitted to a one-compartment model; other investigators reported similar findings (8, 10). However, the elimination data we obtained after parenteral administration of sisomicin were clearly best resolved into two regression lines. Indeed, the alpha distribution phase (2) was much more prolonged with sisomicin than what we previously found for both tobramycin and gentamicin. The pharmacokinetic parameters we derived in this study for sisomicin are different from those reported by both Rodriguez et al. (9) and Lode et al. (3). Rodriguez et al. (9) appear to have analyzed their data by a one-compartment model. Curiously, these authors stated that the serum half-life of sisomicin after i.m. doses of 20 mg of sisomicin per m^2 was 120 min, whereas the serum half-life determined after a 30-min i.v. infusion of sisomicin at a dose of 30 mg/m^2 was 160 min. It is difficult to resolve these differences in the half-life. These data were obtained in hospitalized patients with neoplasms. Indeed, close perusal of the data presented by Rodriguez et al. (9) shows a prolonged alpha elimination phase. We cannot directly compare our study with that presented by Lode and co-workers (3). These authors determined pharmacokinetic parameters for gentamicin, tobramycin, and sisomicin after 1-h infusions of 1-mg/kg doses of the three aminoglycoside antibiotics; the antibiotics were dissolved in 50 ml of saline and, to achieve a steady-state serum concentration, 70% of the dose was infused during the first 10 min and the remainder was infused over 50 min. The half-life derived for sisomicin was 122 ± 27 min. However, if we calculate the pharmacokinetic parameters of our i.v. data according to a one-compartment model, then a half-life of 130 min is obtained approximating that given by Lode et al. (3); the apparent volume of distribution derived from our i.m. data according to a one-compartment analysis was 22 liters, a value similar to those given by Regamey et al. (8) for gentamicin (21 liters) and tobramycin (23 liters), also calculated from i.m. studies according to a one-compartment system. Clearly, tobramycin and gentamicin yield almost identical pharmacokinetic parameters, yet the elimination data we found with sisomicin definitely showed two phases. Furthermore, one of the basic assumptions of the two-compartment model (2) is that the pharmacokinetic data derived from i.v. and i.m. studies should be the same. Our results after i.m. and i.v. administration of sisomicin in the volunteers yielded similar pharmacokinetic parameters.

ACKNOWLEDGMENTS

This work was supported by grants from the Public Health Service (T01AI00410 from the National Institute of Allergy and Infectious Diseases) and Schering Corp., Bloomfield, N.J.

LITERATURE CITED

1. **Cox, C., and L. L. Harrison.** 1971. Comparison of gentamicin and polymyxin B-kanamycin in therapy of bacteremia due to gram-negative bacilli. J. Infect. Dis. **124S**:156–163.
2. **Greenblatt, D. J., and J. Koch-Weser.** 1975. Clinical pharmacokinetics. N. Engl. J. Med. **293**:702–705.
3. **Lode, H., B. Kemmerich, and P. Koeppe.** 1975. Comparative clinical pharmacology of gentamicin, sisomicin and tobramycin. Antimicrob. Agents Chemother. 8:396–401.
4. **Loo, J. C. K., and S. Riegelman.** 1970. Assessment of pharmacokinetic constants from postinfusion blood curves obtained after i.v. infusion. J. Pharm. Sci. **59**:53–55.
5. **Martin, C. M. A., A. J. Cuomo, M. J. Geraghty, J. R. Zager, and T. C. Mandes.** 1969. Gram-negative rod bacteremia. J. Infect. Dis. **119**:506–517.
6. **Meyers, B. R., and S. Z. Hirschman.** 1972. Pharmacologic studies on tobramycin and comparison with gentamicin. J. Clin. Pharmacol. **12**:321–324.
7. **Meyers, B. R., B. Leng, and S. Z. Hirschman.** 1975. Comparison of the anti-bacterial activities of sisomicin and gentamicin against gram-negative bacteria. Antimicrob. Agents Chemother. **8**:757–758.
8. **Regamey, C., R. C. Gordon, and W. M. M. Kirby.** 1973. Comparative pharmacokinetics of tobramycin and gentamicin. Clin. Pharmacol. Ther. **14**:396–403.
9. **Rodriguez, V., G. P. Bodey, M. Valdivieso, and R. Feld.** 1975. Clinical pharmacology of sisomicin. Antimicrob. Agents Chemother. **7**:38–41.
10. **Siber, G. R., P. Echeverria, A. L. Smith, J. W. Paisley, and D. H. Smith.** 1975. Pharmacokinetics of gentamicin in children and adults. J. Infect. Dis. **132**:637–651.
11. **Weinstein, M. J., J. A. Marquez, R. T. Testa, G. H. Wagman, E. M. Oden, and J. A. Waitz.** 1970. Antibiotic 6640, a new micromonospora-produced aminoglycoside antibiotic. J. Antibiot. **23**:551–554.

ANTIMICROBIAL AGENTS AND CHEMOTHERAPY, July 1976, p. 28-33 Vol. 10, No. 1

Antiviral Effect of Pyran Against Systemic Infection of Mice with Herpes Simplex Virus Type 2

RONALD S. McCORD, MARY K. BREINIG, AND PAGE S. MORAHAN*

Department of Microbiology, Medical College of Virginia, Virginia Commonwealth University, Richmond, Virginia 23298

Received for publication 9 February 1976

The immunomodulator pyran markedly protected 5-week-old mice from lethal intravenous infection with herpes simplex virus type 2. The 50% lethal dose was increased almost 100-fold in pyran-treated mice as compared with controls. Although the protection was not as marked in older mice (10 and 16 weeks old), there was a significant increase in mean survival time. When the pathogenesis of herpesvirus disease was monitored in control and drug-treated mice, the effect of pyran was most evident in the spinal cord, where virus was recovered from 20 of 25 control mice and from only 6 of 25 pyran-treated mice. There was also a significant reduction in the titer of virus present, and virus appeared later in the spinal cord of pyran-treated mice than in control mice. The protective effect of pyran was observed only when the drug was administered 24 h before viral challenge, was seen after both intraperitoneal and intravenous injection, and was not due to direct inactivation of the virus.

Adequate antiviral chemotherapy is not available for herpesvirus infections such as herpes encephalitis, herpes zoster, or herpes labialis or genitalis. The results of recent clinical investigations with adenine arabinoside and phosphonoacetic acid have been equivocal (T. C. Merigan [ed.], J. Infect. Dis., in press). In certain clinical situations, treatment with related antiviral chemotherapeutic agents such as iododeoxyuridine (8), cytosine arabinoside (31), or neutral red (26) has produced adverse effects in terms of unacceptable toxicity or exacerbation of the viral disease itself. An alternate or adjuvant approach to the control of herpesvirus infections might be the use of immunomodulators. Therapy with immunomodulators as adjuvants with surgery or chemotherapy has proven more effective than either alone in inhibiting tumor growth (13). Treatment with the biological immunomodulator BCG has been reported to ameliorate recurrent herpes vaginalis in women (1). Prophylactic treatment of rabbits and mice with BCG resulted in some protection against systemic herpesvirus infection (3, 19). Protection could also be produced by the synthetic polyanions polyriboinosinic-cytidylic acid (9, 14) and chlorite-oxidized oxyamylose (4, 5). Another synthetic polyanion, pyran, a copolymer of maleic anhydride and divinyl ether, profoundly alters the reticuloendothelial system (25) and various immunological responses (2, 24) and induces interferon (21). Pyran has been shown to be an effective antiviral agent against several ribonucleic acid viruses, including vesicular stomatitis virus (12), foot-and-mouth disease virus (30), encephalomyocarditis (24) and mengovirus (20), ribonucleic acid leukemia viruses (10, 22, 29), and one deoxyribonucleic acid virus, vaccinia (11). We have previously demonstrated that pyran is protective against intravenous or intravaginal infection of mice with herpes simplex virus type 2 (HSV-2) (23). In the present study, we examined the effect of varying the route and the time of administration of the drug and monitored the effect of pyran on the pathogenesis of systemic herpesvirus disease.

(This paper was presented in part at the 75th Annual Meeting of the American Society for Microbiology, New York, 27 April to 2 May 1975.)

MATERIALS AND METHODS

Mice. Female BALB/c mice (Flow Research Animals, Inc., Dublin, Va., and Laboratory Supply, Indianapolis, Ind.) were received at 4 to 5 weeks of age and usually were used for experiments at 5 to 6 weeks of age.

Cells. HEp-2 cells (Microbiological Associates, Bethesda, Md.) and Vero cells (courtesy of Byron Murray) were grown in Eagle minimal essential medium with Hanks balanced salt solution (HMEM), 10% heat-inactivated fetal calf serum, and no antibiotics. For virus titrations, HMEM with 2% fetal calf serum, 1% methyl cellulose, 200 U of penicillin per ml, 100 μg of streptomycin per ml, and 1 μg of amphotericin B (Fungizone) per ml was used.

Virus. The virus used in this study was a recent human isolate identified as HSV-2 by the indirect hemagglutinin test (courtesy of John Stewart, Center for Disease Control, Atlanta Ga.). Virus was propagated in HEp-2 cells and had a titer of 5×10^6 plaque-forming units (PFU)/ml.

Virus titrations. Virus was titrated for PFU on cells grown in 24-well tissue culture plates (Linbro Chemical Co., New Haven, Conn.). The virus-infected cells were incubated for 2 days, and cells were stained with crystal violet to visualize plaques. Virus titrations were performed on HEp-2 cells, except where indicated.

Drugs. Pyran, a polyanionic copolymer of maleic anhydride and divinyl ether, lot XA 124-177, was obtained from David Breslow, Hercules, Inc., Wilmington, Del. The drug was solubilized in 0.15 N NaCl brought up to pH 7.0 with NaOH.

Animal experiments. Groups of 10 mice were injected with pyran intravenously (i.v.) (0.5 mg/mouse) or intraperitoneally (i.p.) (1.5 mg/mouse) and infected with virus 24 h later. These doses are similar to those reported effective against other viruses (20, 24) and are not toxic. The acute mean lethal dose (LD_{50}) is approximately 1.5 mg/mouse by i.v. injection. Mice were checked daily for mortality and the percent mortality was calculated. The majority of deaths occurred within 14 days after infection, and all had occurred by 25 days.

The mean survival time was calculated using 25 days as the day of death for the surviving mice. Statistical analysis of mortality data was performed using the chi-square test with Yates' correction factor, and mean survival time was evaluated by the Student's *t* test. For some experiments, groups of 10 animals were infected with several 10-fold dilutions of virus, and the PFU required for the LD_{50} was calculated by the method of Reed and Muench (28).

Pathogenesis studies. Mice were treated with 0.15 N NaCl or drug and infected as described. Groups of five control or drug-treated mice were sacrificed on various days after infection, organs were removed, and the individual samples were triturated in mortars. Blood, kidney, spleen, liver, spinal cord, cerebellum and brain stem, and cerebrum were collected from each animal, and the clinical status of the animal (well, hunched with ruffled fur, paralyzed, moribund) was noted. Ten percent (wt/vol) suspensions of all organs, except spinal cord and blood, were prepared in viral diluent containing Hanks balanced salt solution, 0.5% gelatin, 0.25% lactalbumin hydrolysate, and antibiotics. Spinal cord was prepared as a 5% suspension, and clotted blood was prepared as a 33% suspension. Specimens were centrifuged at $1,000 \times g$, and the supernatant fluids were frozen at -70 C until the separate specimens from individual mice were assayed for virus by plaque formation on Vero cells.

RESULTS

Antiviral action of pyran in mice of various ages. A marked age-related resistance to systemic infection with HSV has been noted to occur in mice between birth and 4 weeks of age (15, 16). Experiments were performed to determine whether this age-related resistance continued to increase in early adulthood and to follow the antiviral effects of pyran during this period. The LD_{50} of HSV-2 increased 50-fold between 5 and 10 weeks of age and remained relatively constant thereafter (Table 1). Prophylactic treatment with pyran markedly protected 5-week-old mice from HSV-2 lethality; the LD_{50} was increased 80-fold, from $10^{1.4}$ PFU in control animals to $10^{3.3}$ PFU in pyran-treated animals. Although the protective effects of pyran were not as marked in the 10- and 16-week-old mice, the LD_{50} was increased four- to eightfold, and the mean survival time of mice was significantly increased over controls. Although the older mice were larger, the milligrams per kilogram dose ranged from only 25 to 33 mg/kg, both dosages which we have shown to be effective in older mice.

Effect of pyran on HSV-2 pathogenesis. To follow quantitatively the course of HSV-2 infection in control and drug-treated 5-week-old animals, organs from individual mice whose clinical status was noted were collected at various times during infection and assayed individually for virus. Groups of 10 control and drug-treated mice were followed for mortality. In this experiment prophylactic i.v. treatment with pyran reduced the mortality from $^8/_{10}$ in control mice to $^1/_{10}$ in pyran-treated mice.

No virus was detected in any samples of blood, spleen, or liver assayed between days 1 and 13 after i.v. virus infection. However, low levels of virus (less than 10^3 PFU/g) were sporadically detected in the kidney in 2 of 25 samples from control mice and in 6 of 25 samples from pyran-treated mice harvested on days 6 to 13 after infection. Amounts of virus in the cerebellum-brain stem reached peak mean titers of less than 10^2 PFU/g between days 8 and 11 in both control and drug-treated groups. A titer of 10 PFU/g of cerebral tissue was observed in only one drug-treated mouse on day 11 after infection.

The effect of pyran treatment on the pathogenesis of HSV-2 was most evident in the spinal cord. The geometric mean titers of virus present in the spinal cord were significantly reduced in drug-treated as compared with control mice on days 6 through 10 after infection (Fig. 1). Furthermore, virus was recovered from the spinal cord in 20 of 25 control mice and from only 6 of 25 pyran-treated mice that were sacrificed between days 6 and 13 after virus infection. Virus also appeared later in the drug-treated mice. A level of 3×10^3 PFU/g of tissue was observed on day 6 in control animals,

TABLE 1. *Antiviral action of pyran in mice of various ages*

Treatment	5-week-old mice		10-week-old mice		16-week-old mice	
	LD_{50}[a]	MST ± SE[b]	LD_{50}	MST ± SE	LD_{50}	MST ± SE
Control	1.4	9.8 ± 1.0	3.1	13.4 ± 1.7	3.5	20.5 ± 1.5
Pyran[c]	3.3	20.6 ± 2.1[d]	4.0	24.5 ± 2.3[d]	4.1	>25.0[d]

[a] LD_{50} expressed as $\log_{10}$ PFU per 0.2 ml of inoculum per mouse.
[b] Mean survival time ± standard error in mice inoculated with $10^{3.3}$ or $10^{3.6}$ PFU/mouse.
[c] Pyran (0.5 mg/mouse, i.v.) was inoculated 24 h before i.v. HSV-2 challenge.
[d] $P < 0.05$.

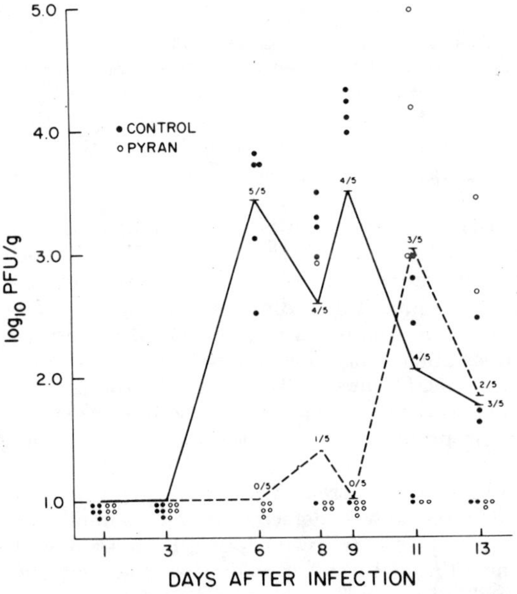

FIG. 1. *Effect of pyran on growth of HSV-2 in spinal cord. Mice were treated with 0.15 N NaCl or pyran and infected i.v. with HSV-2 24 h later; five mice in each group were sacrificed on the days indicated, and virus present in the spinal cord was determined by plaque formation on Vero cells. Symbols: ●, control mice; ○, pyran-treated mice. The bars represent the geometric mean virus titer of all five mice, with the number of positive mice indicated.*

whereas a similar level was not obtained until day 11 in drug-treated mice. The inhibitory effect of pyran was even greater than the data indicate. Because we wanted to evaluate the ability to correlate clinical illness with HSV-2 present in the central nervous system, a particular effort was made to include both sick and apparently well mice in each group when organs were harvested. In general, the presence of HSV-2 in the spinal cord correlated well with the clinical status of the animal. Except on day 6, when all control animals appeared well but exhibited virus in the central nervous system, virus was only recovered from mice with clinical illness.

Lack of direct inactivation of HSV-2 by pyran. Inhibition of HSV-2 could occur by direct inactivation of the virus. Pyran has been reported to inactivate certain viruses (20). However, when HSV-2 was mixed with varying concentrations of pyran in vitro for 1 h at 36 C, there was little loss in infectivity (Table 2). Concentrations of 12.5 mg of pyran per ml were required to reduce the virus titer one $\log_{10}$. Since mice were treated with 0.5 mg, it seemed unlikely that direct inactivation of the virus could account for the antiviral effect of the drug. However, it was possible that pyran could be altered in vivo to an active inhibitory form. Serum and 10% spleen homogenates were prepared from mice 24 h after i.v. injection with pyran, at the time when mice were protected in vivo against i.v. challenge with virus. These serum and spleen homogenates did not directly inactivate HSV-2 in vitro (data not shown).

Effect of varying the route of administration of pyran. The antiviral effect of polyanions has been reported to be a primarily local effect (20). Mice were treated with pyran either i.v. (0.5 mg) or i.p. (1.5 mg) and infected 24 h later

TABLE 2. *Effect of incubation of pyran and HSV-2 in vitro*[a]

Final concn of pyran (mg/ml)	HSV-2 titer (PFU/ml)
Expt 1	
None	4.8×10^6
1.25	2.5×10^6
2.5	4.8×10^6
Expt 2	
None	5.5×10^5
1.55	3.1×10^5
3.12	1.9×10^5
6.25	3.2×10^5
12.5	4.6×10^4
25.0	1.1×10^3

[a] Varying concentrations of pyran were mixed with a constant amount of HSV-2, the mixture was incubated for 1 h at 36 C, and the titer of residual virus was determined. Virus was incubated alone in diluent for the control.

with HSV-2 i.p. Administration of the drug by either route was effective in reducing mortality from HSV-2 infection (Table 3) and in increasing the mean survival time of mice (data not shown).

Effect of varying the time of administration of pyran. The protective effect of pyran was limited with respect to the time of drug administration relative to viral inoculation. Marked protection against virus lethality was observed only when pyran was administered 24 h before viral challenge (Table 4).

Effect of pinworm infestation on HSV-2 infection and pyran protection. Evidences of either pinworm infestation or *Pasteurella pneumotropica* infection of the brain were observed in certain shipments of mice. To determine whether pinworm infestation affected experiments, pinworm-infested and pinworm-free mice were treated with pyran and infected with HSV-2. Half of one shipment of mice was treated orally with piperazine (11 mg of piperazine citrate per ml of drinking water) for 2 weeks until they were found to be completely pinworm free, whereas the pinworm-infested mice were housed normally but kept isolated from other mice. Pinworm infestation did not markedly affect the HSV-2 infection (Table 5). Although pyran appeared to be equally effective in pinworm-free and -infested mice at day 17 after virus infection, subsequent late deaths occurred in the pyran-treated, pinworm-infested mice. The effects of *Pasteurella* infection could not be directly ascertained since the organism could not readily be passed serially in mice. However, this experience emphasizes the role intercurrent infections may play in modifying drug-virus-host interactions.

DISCUSSION

Several studies have investigated the antiviral activity of the immunomodulator pyran against ribonucleic acid viruses (12, 20, 30). The mode of antiviral action of pyran has not been completely elucidated. Prophylactic administration was essential for activity against HSV-2 infection, as has been previously reported for activity against mengovirus infection (20). Merigan and Finkelstein (20) showed that 1 to 5 mg/ml reduced plaque formation by mengovirus, vesicular stomatitis virus, and vaccinia virus; the authors concluded that direct virus inactivation was unlikely to account for the in vivo protection. With the HSV-2 used in the present studies, a dose of 10 mg/ml was required to reduce virus titer by one $\log_{10}$. These results are consistent with the previous data. The slight difference in amount of drug required for direct inactivation may reflect differences in viruses or the source of drug. Pyran has been demonstrated to be a potent inhibitor of ribonucleic acid-dependent deoxyribonucleic acid polymerase in vitro and to slightly inhibit alpha- and beta-mammalian polymerases (27). The necessity for prophylactic drug treatment is inconsistent with a mode of action involving

TABLE 3. *Effect of route of pyran administration on protection against HSV-2 infection*[a]

Route of pyran	No. of dead mice/total in expt: 1	2	3	Total	P value
None	8/10	7/10	10/10	25/30	
i.p.	2/10	1/10	NT	3/20	<0.001
i.v.	NT	3/10	5/10	8/20	<0.005

[a] Pyran (1.5 mg i.p. or 0.5 mg i.v.) was inoculated 24 h before i.p. challenge of 5-week-old mice with $10^{2.3}$ PFU of HSV-2. NT, Not tested.

TABLE 4. *Effect of varying the time of administration of pyran on protection against HSV-2*

Time of pyran treatment (h)[a]	No. of dead/total	MST ± SE[b]
None	20/20	9.0 ± 0.6
−168	10/10	8.4 ± 0.6
−96	9/10	12.2 ± 1.1 (<0.025)[c]
−48	10/10	9.2 ± 0.9
−36	10/10	11.3 ± 1.0 (<0.05)
−24	5/10 (<0.005)	16.0 ± 1.3 (<0.005)
−12	7/7	10.9 ± 0.6 (<0.05)
−2	10/10	9.3 ± 0.6
+24	8/10	12.2 ± 1.4 (<0.05)

[a] Pyran (0.5 mg/mouse) was inoculated i.v. at varying times between −168 to +24 h with respect to the time of i.v. challenge of 5-week-old mice with $10^{2.8}$ PFU of HSV-2.

[b] Mean survival time ± standard error.

[c] Numbers in parentheses represent *P* values.

TABLE 5. *Effect of pinworm infestation on HSV-2 infection and pyran protection*[a]

Pinworm infestation	Pyran treatment	No. of dead/total on: Day 17	Day 20	MST ± SE[b]
−	−	14/15	14/15	9.6 ± 0.8
−	+	8/15[c]	8/15[c]	15.0 ± 1.2[c]
+	−	14/15	14/15	9.9 ± 0.8
+	+	7/14[c]	10/14	15.9 ± 1.0[c]

[a] Pinworm-free and -infested 6-week-old mice were treated i.v. with pyran (0.5 mg/mouse) 24 h before i.v. challenge with HSV-2 ($10^{3.0}$ PFU).

[b] Mean survival time ± standard error.

[c] $P < 0.05$.

either direct virus inactivation or inhibition of virus replication. Furthermore, the systemic as well as local action of the drug argues against local drug effects.

In view of the known immunomodulating activity of the compound, enhancement of host resistance responses against the virus appears likely. The pathogenesis data indicated that pyran inhibited spread of the virus into the central nervous system. Similar to reports by Kern et al. (18), we have been unable to define completely the early pathogenesis of HSV-2 in the visceral organs in adult mice. However, pyran appears to reduce this early virus production, since mice treated with pyran who survive infection with HSV are often less resistant to rechallenge than are untreated mice (M. C. Breinig, P. F. Cline, and P. S. Morahan, Abstr. Annu. Meet. Am. Soc. Microbiol. 1976, E88, p. 78).

It would be tempting to suggest interferon involvement in this early antiviral effect. However, there is no compelling evidence for a significant role for interferon in the antiviral effects of pyran. We have previously demonstrated that the antiviral effect of pyran against encephalomyocarditis virus was not correlated with induction of interferon (24). Similar conclusions were reached by Billiau et al. concerning the antiviral action of another polyanion, chlorite-oxidized oxyamylose, against mengovirus infection (5). The authors postulated that the antiviral effect might be related to macrophage activation in the peritoneal cavity. The fact that herpesviruses are generally among the most resistant to the antiviral effects of interferon also argues against an important role for interferon.

Pyran is an immunoadjuvant for certain humoral immune responses (2). However, we have seen no evidence for increased neutralizing antibody production in pyran-treated as compared with untreated mice (Breinig et al., Abstr. Annu. Meet. Am. Soc. Microbiol. 1976, E88, p. 78). Cell-mediated immunity has been implicated as important in recovery of animals from primary herpesvirus infections (7, 32), but we have shown that pyran was effective against HSV-2 in mice depleted of thymus-derived lymphocytes by adult thymectomy, lethal irradiation, and bone marrow reconstitution (23). These data suggest that pyran may exert its antiviral activity not through modulation of specific immunological responses toward HSV-2 but by activating macrophages for enhanced nonspecific antiviral activity. The increased efficacy of the drug in 5-week as compared with 15-week-old mice may have some bearing on this point. Hirsch et al. (15) have demonstrated that macrophages from young mice are immature in regard to resistance to HSV replication in vitro. Blaese (6) has demonstrated that a variety of immunomodulating agents such as BCG and polyriboadenylic-uridylic acid can cause immature macrophages to develop competence for immunological helper function. Pyran treatment, therefore, may enable immature macrophages to express antiviral resistance. Other evidence for a role for activated macrophages comes from observations that pyran-activated peritoneal cells exhibit cytotoxicity for tumor cells (17) and inhibit HSV-2 and vaccinia virus growth in vitro (unpublished data). However, a definitive role for macrophages activated by pyran in the inhibition of HSV-2 replication in vivo remains to be established.

ACKNOWLEDGMENTS

This work was supported by Public Health Service research grant CA 16193 from the National Cancer Institute, grant IN-105A from the American Cancer Society, and Public Health Service training grant AI 00382 from the National Institute of Allergy and Infectious Diseases. PSM is a recipient of Public Health Service research career development award AI 70863 from the National Institute of Allergy and Infectious Diseases.

The technical assistance of Paul F. Cline is greatly appreciated.

LITERATURE CITED

1. **Anderson, F. D., R. N. Ushijima, and C. L. Larson.** 1974. Recurrent herpes genitalis. Treatment with *Mycobacterium bovis* (BCG). Obstet. Gynecol. **43:**797–805.
2. **Baird, L. G., and A. M. Kaplan.** 1975. Immunoadjuvant activity of pyran copolymer. I. Evidence for direct stimulation of T-lymphocytes and macrophages. Cell. Immunol. **20:**167–176.
3. **Baker, M. B., C. L. Larson, R. N. Ushijima, and F. D. Anderson.** 1974. Resistance of female mice to vaginal infection induced by *Herpesvirus hominis* type 2: effects of immunization with *Mycobacterium bovis*, intravenous injection of a specific *Herpesvirus hominis* type 2 antiserum, and a combination of these procedures. Infect. Immun. **10:**1230–1234.
4. **Billiau, A., J. DeSmyter, and P. DeSomer.** 1970. Antiviral activity of chlorite-oxidized oxyamylose, a polyacetal carboxylic acid. J. Virol. **5:**321–328.
5. **Billiau, A., J. J. Muyembe, and P. DeSomer.** 1971. Mechanism of antiviral activity of polycarboxylates which induce interferon. Nature (London) **232:**183–186.
6. **Blaese, R. M.** 1975. Macrophages and the development of immunocompetence, p. 309–317. *In* J. A. Bellanti and D. H. Dayton (ed.), Phagocytic cell in host resistance. Raven Press, New York.
7. **Blanden, R. J.** 1974. T-cell response to viral and bacterial infections. Transplant. Rev. **19:**56–88.
8. **Boston Interhospital Virus Study Group and the NIAID-sponsored Cooperative Antiviral Clinical Study.** 1975. Failure of high dose 5-iodo-2′-deoxyuridine in the therapy of herpes simplex virus encephalitis. N. Engl. J. Med. **292:**599–603.
9. **Catalano, L. W., Jr., and S. Baron.** 1970. Protection against herpes virus and encephalomyocarditis virus encephalitis with a double-stranded RNA inducer of interferon. Proc. Soc. Exp. Biol. Med. **133:**684–687.

10. **Chirigos, M. A., W. Turner, J. Pearson, and W. Griffin.** 1969. Effective antiviral therapy of two murine leukemias with an interferon-inducing synthetic carboxylate copolymer. Int. J. Cancer 4:267–278.
11. **DeClercq, E., and P. DeSomer.** 1969. Prolonged antiviral protection by interferon inducers. Proc. Soc. Exp. Biol. Med. 132:699–703.
12. **DeClercq, E., and T. C. Merigan.** 1969. Local and systemic polyanionic interferon inducers in mice against intranasal vesicular stomatitis virus. J. Gen. Virol. 5:359–368.
13. **Gutterman, J. U., G. Mavligit, J. A. Gottlieb, M. A. Burgess, C. E. McBride, L. Einhorn, E. J. Freireich, and E. M. Hersh.** 1974. Chemoimmunotherapy of disseminated malignant melanoma with dimethyl triazeno imidazole carboxamide and Bacillus Calmette-Guerin. N. Engl. J. Med. 291:592–597.
14. **Hamilton, L. D., V. I. Babcock, and C. M. Southan.** 1969. Inhibition of herpes simplex virus by synthetic double-stranded RNA (polyriboadenylic and polyribouridylic acids and polyriboinosinic and polyribocytidylic acids). Proc. Natl. Acad. Sci. U.S.A. 64:878–883.
15. **Hirsch, M. S., B. Zisman, and A. C. Allison.** 1970. Macrophages and age-dependent resistance to herpes simplex virus in mice. J. Immunol. 104:1160–1165.
16. **Johnson, R. T.** 1964. The pathogenesis of herpesvirus encephalitis. II. A cellular basis for the development of resistance with age. J. Exp. Med. 120:359–374.
17. **Kaplan, A. M., P. S. Morahan, and W. Regelson.** 1974. Induction of macrophage mediated tumor cell cytotoxicity by pyran copolymer. J. Natl. Cancer Inst. 52:1919–1923.
18. **Kern, E. R., J. C. Overall, Jr., and L. A. Glasgow.** 1975. *Herpesvirus hominis* infection in newborn mice: treatment with interferon inducer polyinosinic-polycytidylic acid. Antimicrob. Agents Chemother. 7:793–800.
19. **Larson, C. L., R. N. Ushijima, R. Karin, M. B. Baker, and R. E. Baker.** 1972. *Herpesvirus hominis* type 2 infections in rabbits. Effect of prior immunization with attenuated *Mycobacterium bovis* (BCG) cells. Infect. Immun. 6:465–468.
20. **Merigan, T. C., and M. S. Finkelstein.** 1968. Interferon-stimulating and *in vivo* antiviral effects of various synthetic anionic polymers. Virology 35:363–374.
21. **Merigan, T. C., and W. Regelson.** 1967. Interferon induction in man by a polyanion of defined composition. N. Engl. J. Med. 277:1283–1287.
22. **Mohr, S. J., M. A. Chirigos, F. S. Fuhrman, and J. W. Pryor.** 1975. Pyran copolymer as an effective adjuvant to chemotherapy against a murine leukemia and solid tumor. Cancer Res. 35:3750–3754.
23. **Morahan, P. S., and R. S. McCord.** 1975. Resistance to herpes simplex type 2 virus induced by an immunopotentiator (pyran) in immunosuppressed mice. J. Immunol. 115:311–313.
24. **Morahan, P. S., W. Regelson, and A. F. Munson.** 1972. Pyran and polyribonucleotides: differences in biological activities. Antimicrob. Agents Chemother. 2:16–22.
25. **Munson, A. E., W. Regelson, W. Lawrence, Jr., and W. R. Wooles.** 1970. Biphasic response of the reticuloendothelial system (RES) induced by pyran copolymer. J. Reticuloendothel. Soc. 1:375–385.
26. **Myers, M. G., M. N. Oxman, J. E. Clark, and K. A. Arndt.** 1975. Failure of neutral-red photodynamic inactivation in recurrent herpes simplex virus infections. N. Engl. J. Med. 293:945–949.
27. **Papas, T. S., T. W. Pry, and M. A. Chirigos.** 1974. Inhibition of RNA-dependent DNA polymerase of avian myeloblastosis virus by pyran copolymer. Proc. Natl. Acad. Sci. U.S.A. 71:367–370.
28. **Reed, L. S., and H. Muench.** 1938. A simple method for estimating fifty percent end points. Am. J. Hyg. 27:493–500.
29. **Regelson, W.** 1967. Prevention and treatment of Friend leukemia virus (FLV) infection by interferon-inducing synthetic polyanions. Adv. Exp. Med. Biol. 1:315–332.
30. **Richmond, J. Y., and C. H. Campbell.** 1972. Influence of divinyl ether-maleic anhydride (pyran) on foot-and-mouth disease virus infection: effect on adsorption and multiplication in mouse tissues. Arch. Gesamte Virusforsch. 36:232–239.
31. **Stevens, D. A., G. W. Jordan, T. F. Waddell, and T. C. Merigan.** 1973. Adverse effect of cytosine arabinoside on disseminated zoster in a controlled trial. N. Engl. J. Med. 289:873–878.
32. **Zisman, B., M. S. Hirsch, and A. C. Allison.** 1970. Selective effects of anti-macrophage serum, silica and anti-lymphocyte serum on pathogenesis of herpes virus infection of young adult mice. J. Immunol. 104:1155–1159.

Antimicrobial Agents and Chemotherapy, July 1976, p. 34-37
Vol. 10, No. 1

In Vitro Activity of Gentamicin and Minocycline Alone and in Combination Against Bacteria Associated with Intra-Abdominal Sepsis

ROBERT J. FASS,* DANIEL E. RUIZ, RICHARD B. PRIOR, AND ROBERT L. PERKINS

Division of Infectious Diseases, Department of Medicine, The Ohio State University College of Medicine, Columbus, Ohio 43210

Received for publication 20 February 1976

The minimal inhibitory concentrations of gentamicin and minocycline alone and in combination were determined by a broth microdilution method for 100 aerobic, facultative, and anaerobic isolates representative of pathogens recovered from patients with intra-abdominal sepsis. Gentamicin inhibited all strains of *Klebsiella, Enterobacter,* and *Pseudomonas aeruginosa* in concentrations of 0.4 to 3.1 μg/ml and all strains of *Escherichia coli* and *Proteus mirabilis* in concentrations of 0.8 to 12.5 μg/ml. Whereas minocycline did not consistently inhibit these organisms in concentrations of 1.6 μg or less/ml, it did act synergistically with gentamicin against 43% of the *Enterobacteriaceae* tested in clinically achievable concentrations; significant synergy was most common with *E. coli* (60%). Minocycline inhibited 62% of *Bacteroides fragilis,* 71% of *Clostridium,* 40% of anaerobic cocci, and 40% of enterococci tested in concentrations of 1.6 μg or less/ml. Whereas gentamicin rarely inhibited these organisms in concentrations of 6.2 μg or less/ml, it did act synergistically with minocycline against 20% of *B. fragilis,* 67% of *Clostridium,* 22% of anaerobic cocci, and 22% of enterococci (which had minimal inhibitory concentrations of minocycline within the range tested) at clinically achievable concentrations. Although only four (13%) of the 30 isolates resistant to both gentamicin and minocycline alone were inhibited by clinically achievable concentrations of the combination, the observed synergy, particularly against strains of *E. coli,* was considered to be of potential clinical usefulness. Antagonism between gentamicin and minocycline was not observed at the concentrations tested.

Intra-abdominal sepsis associated with gastrointestinal or gynecological disease is usually mixed in etiology. The most frequently isolated organisms include gram-negative aerobic and facultative bacilli, enterococci, and anaerobes (3). Gentamicin has a broad spectrum of activity against gram-negative aerobic and facultative bacilli. Minocycline is active against some of the same organisms, some strains of enterococci, and many anaerobic bacteria (R. J. Fass, D. E. Ruiz, W. G. Gardner, and C. A. Rotilie, Arch. Intern. Med., in press). Because the two antibiotics have complementary spectrums of activity, which together include many of the bacterial species associated with intra-abdominal sepsis, they might be used in combination to treat such mixed infections.

The present study was designed to determine the in vitro activity of gentamicin and minocycline alone and in combination against a variety of aerobic, facultative, and anaerobic bacterial pathogens commonly associated with mixed intra-abdominal sepsis.

MATERIALS AND METHODS

Bacteria. One hundred clinical isolates from patients in University Hospitals, Columbus, Ohio, were studied. They included: 20 strains of *Escherichia coli,* 5 strains of *Klebsiella,* 5 strains of *Enterobacter,* 5 strains of *Proteus mirabilis,* 5 strains of *Pseudomonas aeruginosa,* 10 strains of enterococcus, 26 strains of *Bacteroides fragilis,* 14 strains of *Clostridium* (including 6 strains of *C. perfringens* and 8 strains of other *Clostridium* species), and 10 strains of anaerobic cocci (including 4 strains of *Peptococcus,* 4 strains of *Peptostreptococcus,* and 2 strains of *Veillonella).* The isolates tested had known susceptibility patterns prior to their selection, and a disproportionate number of minocycline-resistant strains were included to obtain sufficient data on this group of organisms (Table 1).

Antibiotics. Commercially available laboratory standards were dissolved in sterile distilled water. Working solutions with concentrations of 100 and 50 μg of gentamicin and 50 and 25 μg of minocycline per ml were stored at −20 C until used.

Susceptibility tests. Minimal inhibitory concentrations (MICs) of gentamicin and minocycline alone and in combinations were determined using a broth microdilution method (2). Serial twofold dilutions of each antibiotic were made in duplicate to test each antibiotic alone and in a checkerboard fashion so that 121 different combinations of concentrations ranging from 25 to 0.02 μg/ml for gentamicin and 12.5 to 0.01 μg/ml for minocycline were tested. For gentamicin, MICs of 6.2 μg or less/ml were considered to signify susceptibility. For minocycline, MICs of 1.6 μg or less/ml were considered to signify susceptibility. The combined action of gentamicin and minocycline was considered synergistic when the MIC of each drug in combination was one-fourth or less of the MIC of each respective drug when tested alone. Synergy was considered to be of potential clinical significance only if the MICs of gentamicin and minocycline in combination were 6.2 μg or less and 1.6 μg or less/ml, respectively. The combination was considered antagonistic when the MIC of each drug in combination was four or more times the MIC of each respective drug when tested alone. When MICs of each drug in combination were not both at least fourfold different from MICs when tested alone, the combination was considered to be indifferent, since twofold (one concentration) variations of MICs are commonly observed with serial dilution tests.

TABLE 1. *Percentage of clinical isolates from University Hospitals[a] and of isolates selected for the present study that were susceptible to gentamicin (MIC, 6.2 μg or less/ml) and minocycline (MIC, 1.6 μg or less/ml)*

Organisms	Gentamicin		Minocycline	
	University Hospitals	Present study	University Hospitals	Present study
E. coli	87	85	73	50
Klebsiella	100	100	71	20
Enterobacter	100	100	42	0
P. mirabilis	89	60	0	0
P. aeruginosa	100	100	0	0
Enterococci	0	0	17	40
B. fragilis	1	0	78	62
Clostridium	6	7	92	71
Anaerobic cocci	24	20	65	40

[a] Fass et al., in press.

RESULTS

The in vitro susceptibilities of the 100 clinical isolates tested to gentamicin and minocycline alone and in combinations are shown in Fig. 1 and 2. Gentamicin inhibited all strains of *Klebsiella*, *Enterobacter*, and *P. aeruginosa* in concentrations of 3.1 μg or less/ml and 80% of *E.*

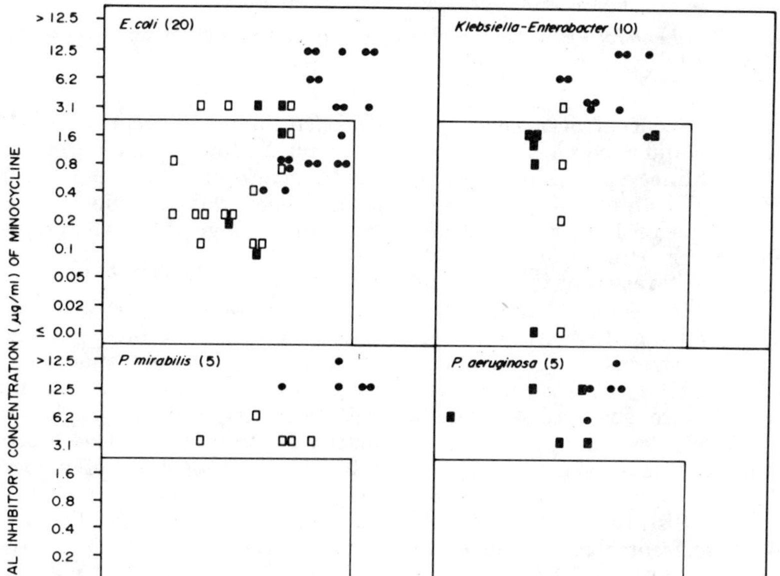

FIG. 1. *Susceptibility of Enterobacteriaceae and P. aeruginosa to gentamicin and minocycline alone and in combinations. Symbols:* ●, *gentamicin and minocycline alone;* ■, *nonsynergistic combinations;* □, *synergistic combinations. MICs of gentamicin that were 6.2 μg or less/ml and MICs of minocycline that were 1.6 μg or less/ml were considered to indicate susceptibility.*

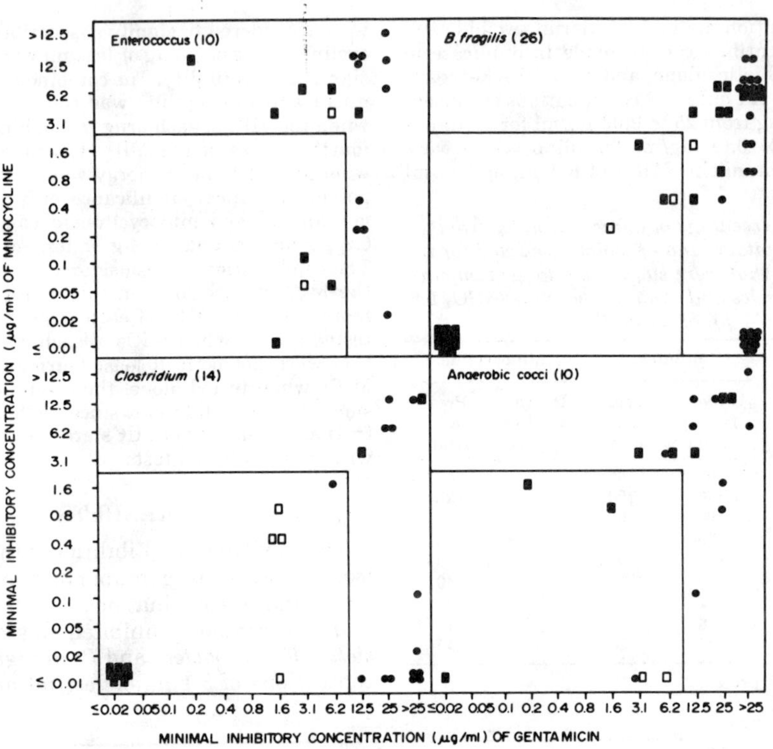

FIG. 2. *Susceptibility of enterococci and anaerobes to gentamicin and minocycline alone and in combinations. See legend to Fig. 1.*

coli and *P. mirabilis* in concentrations of 6.2 μg or less/ml; enterococci and anaerobes were usually more resistant. Minocycline inhibited 60% of anaerobes, 50% of *E. coli,* and 40% of enterococci in concentrations of 1.6 μg or less/ml; *Klebsiella, Enterobacter, P. mirabilis,* and *P. aeruginosa* were usually resistant to those concentrations. Most isolates were either susceptible to only one drug or to neither drug; only 13 isolates, including 10 strains of *E. coli* and 1 strain each of *Klebsiella, Clostridium,* and *Peptostreptococcus,* were susceptible to both drugs.

The presence or absence of synergy could not be determined for 1 strain of enterococcus, 11 strains of *B. fragilis,* 8 strains of *Clostridium,* and 1 strain of *Peptostreptococcus,* which had MICs of minocycline that were 0.02 μg or less/ml because the lowest concentration tested was 0.01 μg/ml. Among the other strains tested, the combination was synergistic for 24 (69%) of the 35 *Enterobacteriaceae,* none of the 5 *P. aeruginosa,* 2 (22%) of the 9 enterococci, 3 (20%) of the 15 *B. fragilis,* 4 (67%) of the 6 *Clostridium,* and 2 (22%) of the 9 anaerobic cocci. Synergy was considered to be of potential clinical significance for 12 (60%) of the *E. coli,* 3 (30%) of the *Klebsiella* and *Enterobacter,* 1 (11%) of the enterococci, 2 (13%) of the *B. fragilis,* 4 (67%) of the *Clostridium,* and 2 (22%) of the anaerobic cocci. There was no evidence of antagonism within the range of concentrations tested.

DISCUSSION

In the present study 88% of the *Enterobacteriaceae* and *P. aeruginosa,* 40% of the enterococci, and 62% of the anaerobes tested were susceptible to gentamicin or minocycline or both. Among the 70 susceptible isolates, 21 (primarily *B. fragilis* and *Clostridium*) were inhibited by 0.02 μg or less of minocycline per ml, and the presence or absence of synergy could not be determined. Significant synergy was demonstrated for 20 (41%) of the remaining susceptible isolates and for 4 (13%) of the 30 resistant isolates. Significant synergy was most commonly observed among strains of *E. coli* and *Clostridium*; two isolates of each were resistant to both antibiotics alone but susceptible to the combination. There were no instances of antagonism.

On the basis of the in vitro data, the treatment of mixed intra-abdominal sepsis with gentamicin and minocycline would seem reasonable. Minocycline is active against a higher percentage of anaerobes, particularly *B. fragilis,* than is tetracycline (1, 4–6; Fass et al., in press) and, in the present study, acted synergistically with gentamicin against a number of strains tested, particularly *E. coli* and *Clostridium*. Since *E. coli* is the most common gram-negative facultative pathogen isolated from patients with intra-abdominal sepsis and is not consistently susceptible to the concentrations of gentamicin achieved after recommended dosage (Fass et al., in press), this synergy could be of considerable clinical significance. The combination of gentamicin and minocycline would not be expected to be ideal, however, since a significant number of organisms, particularly enterococci, *B. fragilis,* and anaerobic cocci, which were resistant to both drugs alone, were usually resistant to the combination as well.

ACKNOWLEDGMENTS

We thank Beth Ann Bailey for her excellent technical assistance.

This study was supported by a grant from Lederle Laboratories.

LITERATURE CITED

1. **Chow, A. W., V. Patten, and L. B. Guze.** 1975. Comparative susceptibility of anaerobic bacteria to minocycline, doxycycline, and tetracycline. Antimicrob. Agents Chemother. 7:46–49.
2. **Fass, R. J., C. A. Rotilie, and R. B. Prior.** 1974. Interaction of clindamycin and gentamicin in vitro. Antimicrob. Agents Chemother. 6:582–587 (Erratum 7:226).
3. **Gorbach, S. L., and J. G. Bartlett.** 1974. Anaerobic infections. N. Engl. J. Med. **290**:1177–1184, 1237–1245.
4. **Lerner, P. I.** 1974. Susceptibility of pathogenic actinomycetes to antimicrobial compounds. Antimicrob. Agents Chemother. 5:302–309.
5. **Rotilie, C. A., R. J. Fass, R. B. Prior, and R. L. Perkins.** 1975. Microdilution technique for antimicrobial susceptibility testing of anaerobic bacteria. Antimicrob. Agents Chemother. 7:311–315.
6. **Staneck, J. L., and J. A. Washington II.** 1974. Antimicrobial susceptibilities of anaerobic bacteria: recent clinical isolates. Antimicrob. Agents Chemother. 6:311–315.

Antimicrobial Agents and Chemotherapy, July 1976, p. 38–44 Vol. 10, No. 1

Printed in U.S.A.

Characterization and Quantitation of Experimental Surgical-Wound Infections Used to Evaluate Topical Antibacterial Agents

R. J. McRIPLEY* and R. R. WHITNEY

Department of Microbiology, The Squibb Institute for Medical Research, Princeton, New Jersey 08540

Received for publication 9 February 1976

Reproducible experimental surgical-wound infections in mice for use in the evaluation of topical antibacterial agents are described. The experimental wound was created on the backs of mice by means of a midline incision and was infected by means of cotton sutures monocontaminated with *Staphylococcus aureus* or *Pseudomonas aeruginosa*. The course of these wound infections was followed by quantitation of surface bacteria through use of a surface rinse technique. Surface wound counts of the infecting organisms thus obtained appeared to reflect the dynamics of the total wound count, as determined by homogenization of biopsied tissue. Treatment of infected wounds with a placebo cream had only a slight effect on surface wound counts and on mortality in the case of the *S. aureus* infection but enhanced markedly the lethality of the *P. aeruginosa* infection.

The search for new drugs effective as topical antibacterial agents requires the careful and systematic evaluation of drugs not only in vitro but also in vivo, *i.e.*, in the control and management of experimental infections. Several model infections for evaluating topical antibacterial agents have been developed in laboratory animals (5–7, 9, 18, 19, 21) and in humans (3, 14, 15, 20). Although many of the models have proved to be effective in assessing topical agents, most of them do not lend themselves easily to a mass screening of potential agents. This paper describes and characterizes a relatively simple surgical-wound model in mice in which potential topical antibacterial drugs can be evaluated easily and expeditiously against *Staphylococcus aureus* and *Pseudomonas aeruginosa* wound infections.

MATERIALS AND METHODS

Animals. Female CF-1 mice, 18 to 20 g, purchased from a commercial source (Carworth Farms, New City, N.Y.) were used in all experiments. Mice were maintained, 10 to a cage, on wire, in temperature- and humidity-controlled quarters and were allowed food and water ad libitum.

Test organisms. *S. aureus* SC 2406 (phage type 53/77/84/85) and *P. aeruginosa* SC 8822, clinical isolates from the departmental culture collection, were used as test organisms. The two organisms were maintained on brain heart infusion (BHI) agar (BBL) slants stored at 4 C, with transfers to fresh slants made monthly. For each experiment, a fresh slant was inoculated from the appropriate stock culture and incubated at 37 C for 18 h. After incubation, the growth was removed from the slant by washing with 0.1 M phosphate buffer, pH 7.2, and the resulting suspension was adjusted to a concentration of 2.0×10^9 cells/ml by use of a Klett-Summerson colorimeter with a 540-nm filter and a previously prepared standard curve. The suspension was then appropriately diluted and used for the contamination of sutures or the direct seeding of the experimental wounds.

Preparation of contaminated sutures. Commercial cotton thread (Coats and Clark's, mercerized, size 8) monocontaminated with *S. aureus* or *P. aeruginosa* was used as the suture material to initiate and potentiate the experimental infection. The thread was cut into 5-cm segments and placed in boiling water for 3 min. After removal from the water, the segments were allowed to cool and the excess water was removed by blotting with sterile paper towels. The segments were then dropped into a test tube containing 8 ml of the appropriate dilution of the *S. aureus* or *P. aeruginosa* suspension, mixed on a Vortex mixer for 10 s, and allowed to soak in the suspension for 30 min. During this time period, approximately 10^3 cells were adsorbed on each segment of thread. Since the adsorption of the cells was directly related to the concentration of organisms in the suspension, segments containing different numbers of cells could be prepared merely by varying the concentration of the test organism in the soak suspension. After the soak period, the segments were removed from the tube and blotted dry. The number of organisms adsorbed on each suture was ascertained by shaking a suture in a test tube containing 2 ml of sterile distilled water on a twist-action shaker (model N8, New Brunswick Scientific Co.) for 45 min at the lowest setting. Previous studies had shown that this procedure eluted more than

90% of the adsorbed organisms. After the bacteria had been eluted from the suture, the resulting suspension was diluted and plated on the appropriate agar medium.

Experimental wound and infection. The procedures used to produce the experimental wound and infections have been described previously (18). One day prior to infection, mice were anesthetized by an intraperitoneal injection of sodium pentobarbital (30 mg/kg). The backs of the mice were closely shaved with a fine-tooth electric clipper. On the day of infection superficial surgical wounds were produced on the backs of reanesthetized mice by making a longitudinal midline incision, 2.3 ± 0.2 cm in length and extending down to the panniculus carnosus. The skin on either side of the incision was retracted, and the wound was infected either by direct seeding or by the insertion of a contaminated segment of thread (suture) through the skin with a suturing needle in such a way that the suture lay diagonally across the panniculus, with the ends extending slightly from the skin. The ends of the suture were secured with rubber cement. The wound eventually covered approximately 6% of the total body surface of a mouse (Fig. 1).

Treatment of wounds. For some experiments, the open wounds were treated topically with an emulsion-type cream base placebo that contained promulgen, protopet, sorbitol solution, silicone antifoam, distilled water, and methyl and ethyl parabens as preservatives. Approximately 400 mg of this placebo cream was applied with a tongue depressor over the entire wound and suture twice daily on the day of infection, 0.25 and 5.5 h after infection, and twice daily thereafter for a predetermined number of days.

Quantitation of bacteria in wounds. Several methods were used to follow the course of an infection, as reflected in the dynamics of wound counts of the test organism.

Surface bacterial counts were made by a surface rinse technique. At predetermined times after infection, mice were sacrificed with CO_2; the suture, if present, was removed from the wounds. Each wound was cultured by placing a sterile test tube (22 mm in diameter) containing 5 ml of distilled water in an inverted position on the back of a mouse in such a manner that more than 90% of the wound was tightly enclosed by the mouth of the tube. The mouse and the test tube, held together with the tube upright, were shaken vigorously 25 times to remove the infecting organisms from the surface of the wound. Washings were appropriately diluted and then, because of the possibility of contamination, were plated on selective media, staphylococcus agar no. 110 (BBL) for *S. aureus* and MacConkey agar (BBL) for *P. aeruginosa*. In some cases washings were also plated on BHI agar (Difco). Plates were incubated for 24 to 48 h at 37 C, and then colony counts were performed.

Tissue bacterial counts were obtained by homogenizing weighed biopsy samples from infected wounds. Samples were homogenized for 3 min in a microblender (Eberbach); the homogenates were then diluted and plated on the appropriate selective agar medium, as described above.

The number of viable test organisms on sutures removed from infected wounds was determined as described earlier.

Evaluation of systemic involvement. Because the experimental wound infections often led to generalized infections, various organs were cultured over a period of time to characterize the magnitude and extent of the systemic involvement. At predetermined intervals after infection, mice were bled from the retro-orbital sinus or by cardiac puncture and sacrificed by CO_2; liver, spleen, and kidney were removed aseptically. The organs were rinsed with sterile saline, blotted dry, and then minced. Small samples of the macerated tissue were incubated in BHI broth or were used to make impression smears on BHI agar to ascertain the absence or presence of the challenge organism or of any other bacteria. Blood was cultured directly in BHI pour plates or was streaked on BHI agar. In the case of the *S. aureus* infection, isolated organisms resembling staphylococci microscopically and culturally were phage typed to insure that the strain of *S. aureus* used for the infection was the same as that recovered.

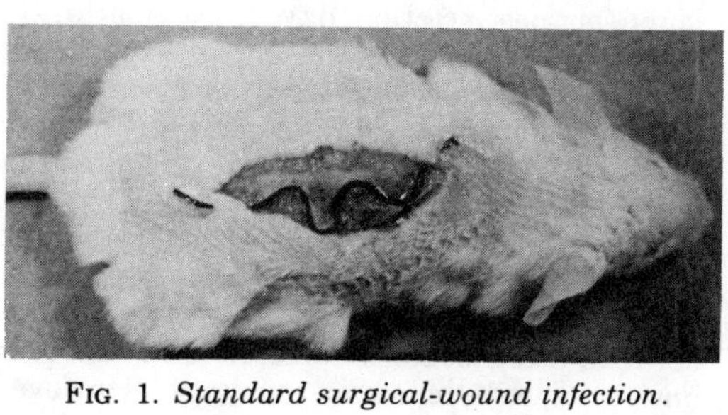

FIG. 1. *Standard surgical-wound infection.*

RESULTS

Grossly, the uninfected experimental surgical wound in the mouse presented the usual clinical picture associated with an uninfected open-type wound. Immediately after the incision had been made, there was only minimal bleeding, and it ceased spontaneously. Slight edema and erythema were evident during the early stages of wound healing, which progressed rapidly to almost complete repair in approximately 2 to 3 weeks. Microscopically, the uninfected wound initially demonstrated the classical signs of inflammation: edema, extravasated erythrocytes and leukocytes, dilated capillaries, etc. No deaths occurred as a result of the surgical procedure. When the wound had been infected with *S. aureus* or *P. aeruginosa*, clinical signs of infection were present but were not striking. Slight edema and erythema were observed around the margins of the wound, and suppuration was noted occasionally beneath the retracted skin. Wound healing generally required 3 weeks from the time of infection. No deaths occurred in mice infected with *S. aureus*; only a few deaths were recorded in mice infected with *P. aeruginosa*.

When *S. aureus* was used as the test organism, two methods were employed to infect the experimental wound, direct seeding and the insertion of contaminated sutures. As can be seen in Table 1, during a period of 4 days there was no significant difference in bacterial counts in mice infected in these two ways with the same size inoculum. The peak count of *S. aureus* in the wounds appeared to occur earlier in mice infected by direct seeding. More important, however, was the fact that slightly less variation between individual counts of mice in the same group occurred when contaminated sutures were used to initiate the infection. Because of this finding, contaminated sutures were used to produce wound infections in all subsequent experiments.

To determine the smallest inoculum of *S. aureus* that could initiate the experimental infection, sutures were soaked in predetermined concentrations of the test organism that would yield 10, 10^3, and 10^5 cells/suture after adsorption and were then evaluated in the experimental wound. The results (Table 2) indicate that 10 *S. aureus* cells/suture were insufficient to induce an infection, whereas an inoculum of 10^3 or 10^5 cells could elicit the infection. The use of an inoculum of 10^5 cells, as could be expected, initially produced slightly higher wound counts than did the use of 10^3 cells, but by 3 days after infection the counts were essentially equivalent. Since the inoculum of 10^3 cells/suture was sufficient to produce proliferation of the test organism in wounds, this inoculum was selected for use in the model infection.

As previously noted, mice infected with *P. aeruginosa* occasionally died, apparently as a result of the infection; this finding suggested systemic involvement leading to a generalized infection. The possibility of systemic involvement after the start of wound infections with

TABLE 1. *Comparison of seeding versus insertion of contaminated sutures for producing the S. aureus wound infection*

Days after infection	Mean surface count ($\times 10^6$)[a]	
	Infected with sutures[b]	Infected by seeding[b]
1	2.2 ± 0.5	5.2 ± 1.2
2	8.7 ± 1.2	15.9 ± 4.2
3	12.2 ± 2.1	11.7 ± 3.0
4	8.3 ± 0.9	7.2 ± 2.0

[a] Mean ± standard error of surface counts from five mice.

[b] Infection initiated with 1.0×10^3 *S. aureus* cells.

TABLE 2. *Effect of inoculum size on the production of an experimental staphylococcal wound infection as reflected by surface wound counts*

Days after infection	Mean surface count ($\times 10^6$)[a]		
	10 cells/ suture	10^3 cells/ suture	10^5 cells/ suture
1	NI[b]	3.4 ± 0.4	8.4 ± 1.4
2	NI	6.8 ± 1.2	22.5 ± 1.5
3	NI	15.9 ± 2.1	18.2 ± 2.1
6	NI	4.5 ± 0.8	3.2 ± 1.0
7	NI	1.1 ± 0.7	2.6 ± 1.4

[a] Mean ± standard error of surface counts from five mice.

[b] NI, No infection; surface counts $< 1.0 \times 10^3$ organisms.

either *P. aeruginosa* or *S. aureus* was investigated. At various intervals after infection, selected organs and blood were cultured to determine the absence or presence of the test organism. The results (Table 3) were somewhat surprising in that both infections exhibited some degree of systemic involvement very soon after suture insertion. In the *P. aeruginosa* infection, at 3 days after infection almost 75% of the mice demonstrated the presence of the organism in liver, kidney, and spleen although blood cultures were, for the most part, negative throughout the course of the experiment. *P. aeruginosa* persisted in the organs for up to 7 days but thereafter was rarely isolated. A few deaths were recorded during the first 2 weeks after infection, but none occurred after this period. *P. aeruginosa* was isolated from all internal organs cultured of mice that died, indicating generalized infection.

In the case of the *S. aureus* infection, the test organism was found in the liver, spleen, and kidney of most mice within 24 h after infection and persisted therein for 1 to 2 weeks. However, when the organs were cultured 2 weeks after infection, *S. aureus* was isolated only occasionally. No staphylococci were isolated when organs were cultured at the 3- and 4-week postinfection intervals. A few positive blood cultures were obtained only during the first week of infection, with the largest number found on postinfection day 1. No mortalities were recorded during the entire experiment. All *S. aureus* cells isolated from blood and organs were phage typed to insure that the organisms isolated were of the same strain as that used for the infection.

It should be noted that earlier studies, in which blood from the retro-orbital plexus was cultured, had indicated a much higher incidence of positive blood cultures than was demonstrated with cardiac puncture. However, these earlier data were not valid because, as was found later, the blood from the retro-orbital plexus was contaminated with pseudomonads from the hair surrounding the eye and from the conjunctivitis that is especially common in *P. aeruginosa*-infected animals. Thus, only the data obtained from the cardiac puncture blood cultures are presented in Table 3.

Because the signs of infection were not striking with either test organism, the course of the wound infections was followed through changes in the population dynamics of the infecting organisms. Three different quantitation techniques were used: (i) the classical biopsy homogenization method, (ii) a surface rinse technique, and (iii) a suture culture technique. A comparison of the wound counts obtained via the three techniques is shown in Fig. 2. As would be expected, the homogenization technique yielded the largest wound counts, since both surface and tissue-associated organisms were quantitated, in contrast to only the surface organisms that were assessed by the surface rinse and suture culture techniques. In the *P. aeruginosa* infection, changes in the total wound population of the pseudomonads, as

TABLE 3. *Localization of infecting organisms after the initiation of superficial wound infections*

Infecting organism	Days after infection	No. of positive cultures/total cultures made				Cumulative mortality[a]
		Liver	Spleen	Kidney	Blood	
P. aeruginosa	1	4/15	2/15	4/15	0/15	0/40
	2	6/15	2/15	7/15	0/15	0/40
	3	13/15	10/15	10/15	3/15	2/40
	4	10/15	7/15	7/15	1/15	3/40
	7	6/15	7/15	7/15	0/15	5/40
	14	1/15	2/15	1/15	0/15	7/40
	21	0/15	0/15	0/15	0/15	7/40
	28	0/15	0/15	0/15	0/15	7/40
S. aureus	1	15/15	15/15	14/15	6/15	0/36
	2	14/15	15/15	14/15	1/15	0/36
	3	13/15	12/15	14/15	3/15	0/36
	4	15/15	14/15	15/15	3/15	0/36
	7	10/15	10/15	11/15	0/15	0/36
	14	1/15	1/15	0/15	0/15	0/36
	21	0/15	0/15	0/15	0/15	0/36
	28	0/15	0/15	0/15	0/15	0/36

[a] Number of mice dead/total infected.

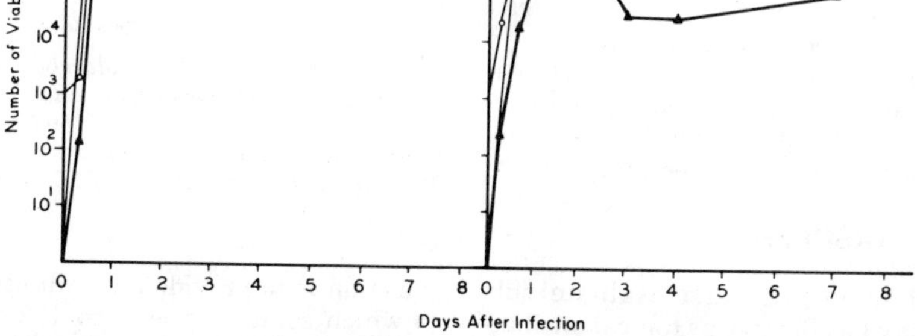

FIG. 2. *Quantitation of test organisms in experimental wound infections by three different methods. Symbols:* ●, *mean number of bacteria per gram of tissue (homogenization procedure);* ▲, *mean number of bacteria per wound surface (surface rinse technique);* ○, *mean number of bacteria per suture (suture culture method). Each point represents results from a minimum of 10 mice.*

demonstrated by the tissue (and surface) counts obtained by the homogenization technique, were quite accurately reflected by the results of the surface rinse technique. Wound counts obtained from the quantitation of pseudomonads eluted from wound-associated sutures to some extent also reflected the dynamics of the infection; however, sutures could not be retained in the wounds in adequate numbers for testing longer than 4 days. The same relationship between the different methods of quantitation was also observed in the *S. aureus* infection. Tissue and surface bacterial counts beyond the day 7 postinfection interval were generally too diverse to provide meaningful results and, therefore, are not presented.

The effect of a cream base vehicle on the two wound infections was investigated since test compounds must be formulated in some type of topical vehicle to be evaluated in the model. The cream base vehicle employed was selected because studies in vitro had indicated that it did not support the growth of either test organism when incubated at 37 C for several days in the presence of inocula equivalent to those used in the model infections. In addition, it was apparently compatible with various types of antibacterial agents, as indicated by the results of drug-release studies (unpublished data). The effect of treatment with the vehicle, utilized as a placebo cream, on the wound infections is shown in Fig. 3. The cream base treatment produced a marked effect on the *P. aeruginosa* infection, elevating the wound counts by more than 2 $\log_{10}$ during the first 3 days after infection. By day 4, most of the mice had died as a result of the enhanced infection. In the *S. aureus* infection, the application of the placebo cream produced only a moderate increase in wound counts. These results were also demonstrated with other topical creams and ointments (unpublished data).

As is shown in Fig. 4, treatment with the placebo cream produced only a slight increase in the mortality resulting from the *S. aureus* infection but enhanced mortality markedly in the case of the *P. aeruginosa* infection. All treated mice had died by 2 weeks after infection, with a majority of the deaths occurring during the first 5 days after infection.

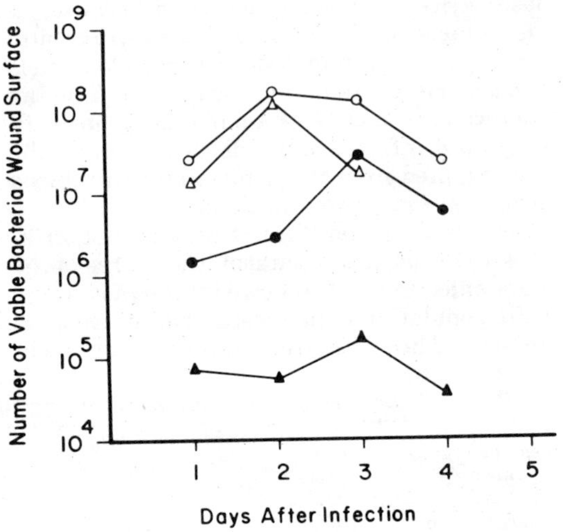

FIG. 3. *Effect of topical treatment with placebo cream on wound counts of P. aeruginosa and S. aureus in experimental wound infections. P. aeruginosa:* △, *placebo treated;* ▲, *untreated. S. aureus:* ○, *placebo treated;* ●, *untreated. Each point represents the mean count from 10 mice.*

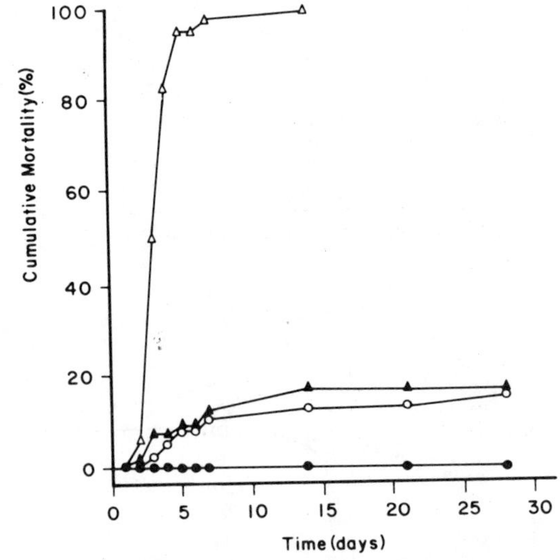

FIG. 4. *Effect of topical placebo cream treatment on mortality in P. aeruginosa and S. aureus wound infections. P. aeruginosa infection:* △, *placebo treated;* ▲, *untreated. S. aureus:* ○, *placebo treated;* ●, *untreated. A minimum of 36 mice was used for each test group.*

DISCUSSION

In an effort to identify and evaluate substances that may be effective as topical antibacterial agents in humans, many experimental infections in laboratory animals have been developed (5, 7, 9, 18, 21). However, if a model infection is to provide an evaluation of efficacy to which some degree of confidence can be attached, then it must satisfy several conditions: (i) because the model infection should simulate or approximate naturally occurring infections in humans, the pathogenesis of infection must be known; (ii) the infection should be reproducible, readily controlled, and provide some measurable end point; (iii) it should be sensitive enough to permit detection of bacteriostatic, as well as of bactericidal, substances; (iv) clinically active antibacterial agents should demonstrate efficacy in the model; and (v) results from the model infection should provide a high degree of predictability of efficacy in humans. Moreover, if the model is to be used for screening purposes, it must meet additional requirements: (i) the model infection should be relatively simple to produce; (ii) the infection must be easily observed and quantitated; and (iii) it should be easy to evaluate several compounds at one time in an adequate number of animals. Many experimental models fail to meet the requirements that are necessary for a model to be truly relevant. The results described in this study and those presented in the following paper (13) indicate that most of the criteria are met in the surgical-wound model. It should be noted, however, that the extensive systemic involvement resulting from the experimental wound infections is rarely observed in clinical cases.

Since both gram-positive and gram-negative organisms are encountered in various skin and wound infections, *S. aureus* and *P. aeruginosa* were selected as representative test organisms for the wound model. The selection of these test organisms is even more appropriate since they are often the causative agents of open wound infections in humans. The rationale for using contaminated sutures to initiate the experimental infections was based on reported observations that: (i) contaminated sutures produce infections in laboratory animals; (ii) a relatively small number of *S. aureus* cells (10^3) adsorbed on certain types of sutures can initiate an experimental infection in a closed wound; and (iii) various suture materials induce a foreign body response (1, 10). However, the results of our study indicated no difference between the course of the experimental infections elicited by placement of contaminated sutures and that initiated by direct seeding of wounds. This finding can probably be explained by the fact that most of the effects of suture-initiated infections were demonstrated in subcutaneous infections and not the open wound infection that is utilized in our model. Nonetheless, we decided to utilize the suture method of eliciting infection because a slight problem was encountered in the direct seeding of wounds. No matter how meticulously the 0.02-ml inoculum was applied, there was occasionally some runoff. The greater variation in wound counts in mice infected by direct seeding probably occurred as a consequence of runoff of inoculum.

In wound infections, either naturally occurring or experimental, some means must be employed to follow the course of the infection and evaluate the effectiveness of therapy. One procedure that has been utilized, both in animals and humans, is the quantitation of bacteria in infected tissues. Various methods and techniques have been devised for this quantitation, ranging from the classical tissue homogenization method (11) to various types of surface-sampling techniques using moist swabs (4), gauze pads (2), impression pads (8), suture counts (18), and other more elaborate procedures (17, 19). To utilize the experimental surgical-wound infections for screening purposes, it was necessary to have a method of quantitation that would be facile to perform and yet would yield accurate results. The surface rinse technique that was devised seemed to meet these requirements. Large numbers of wounds could be cultured in a relatively short period, and the resulting counts compared quite favorably with those obtained after homogenization of biopsied tissues.

The surface rinse technique collects only the superficially localized bacteria in the wound, whereas the homogenization method assesses both surface and tissue-localized organisms. Consequently, higher wound counts, indicative of the invasiveness of the infecting organism, are obtained via the homogenization method. However, wound counts obtained by the surface rinse technique, although lower, appear to reflect accurately the dynamics of the total wound count, surface- and tissue-localized bacteria, in the course of an infection. The homogenization method is not really suitable for use in screening for topical antibacterials because of the considerable amount of time required to evaluate a large number of tissue samples. Because the surface wound counts correlate well with the total wound counts, we decided to employ the surface rinse technique in evaluating potential topical agents. It should be mentioned that counts from wound-associated sutures to some extent also follow the dynamics of the wound bacterial population, but it was almost impossible to retain the sutures for more than 3 to 4 days in most mice.

One problem occasionally encountered in the model infection was contamination. As would be expected, the open wounds sometimes became contaminated with gram-positive and gram-negative organisms from skin, hair, and feces. However, these contaminating organisms, mainly gram-positive cocci, attained a population peak of only 5.0×10^4 in uninfected wounds, considerably less than counts obtained by either of the test organisms, and were rarely isolated from internal organs. To circumvent potential problems in colony counting that might be caused by contaminants, selective media were employed.

Since many topical antibacterial agents are generally formulated in cream or ointment vehicles for application to wounds or other skin infections, the effect of a commonly employed cream vehicle on the experimental infections was investigated. Although the placebo cream exhibited a moderate effect on the *S. aureus* infection, it affected the *P. aeruginosa* infection markedly, producing significant increases in wound counts and mortality. These results were not surprising, since it is known that many gram-negative organisms flourish in moist areas on the surface of a human body (16). The placebo cream, containing a high concentration of water, either increased the moisture content of the wound or prevented water loss from the wound per se, thereby creating a better environment for the growth of *P. aeruginosa*. The enhanced growth of the organism resulted in elevated wound counts, augmented invasiveness, and, consequently, increased mortality. This effect of the placebo cream can be duplicated with other cream and ointment bases or other procedures that keep the infected wound hydrated. The fact that the cream base vehicle used in this study does not support the growth of either test organism indicates that the higher bacterial counts found in placebo-treated mice represent microbial growth in the wound and not in the vehicle per se.

The application of the model infection to the evaluation of topical antibacterial agents is described in the following paper (13).

ACKNOWLEDGMENTS

We are grateful to D. Hsieh and R. Schwind for assistance in supplementary studies, to R. George and A. Hellwig for technical assistance, and to H. Gadebusch and D. Frost for critical review of the manuscript.

LITERATURE CITED

1. **Alexander, J. W., J. Z. Kaplan, and W. A. Altemeier.** 1967. Role of suture materials in the development of wound infection. Ann. Surg. 165:192–199.
2. **Brentano, L., and D. L. Gravens.** 1967. A method for the quantitation of bacteria in burn wounds. Appl. Microbiol. 15:670–671.
3. **Duncan, W. C., M. McBride, and J. M. Knox.** 1970. Experimental production of infections in humans. J. Invest. Dermatol. 54:319–323.
4. **Georgiade, N. G., M. C. Lucas, W. M. O'Fallon, and S. Osterhout.** 1970. A comparison of methods for the quantitation of bacteria in burn wounds. I. Experimental evaluation. Am. J. Clin. Pathol. 53:35–39.
5. **Glotzer, D. J., W. S. Goodman, and L. H. Geronimus.** 1970. Topical antibiotic prophylaxis in contaminated wounds. Arch. Surg. 100:589–593.
6. **Godschmidt, F.** 1972. Reproducible topical staphylococcal infection in rats. Appl. Microbiol. 23:130–134.
7. **Gray, F. J., and E. E. Kidd.** 1963. Topical chemotherapy in prevention of wound infection. Surgery 54:891–899.
8. **Holt, R. J.** 1966. Pad culture studies on skin surfaces. J. Appl. Bacteriol. 29:625–630.
9. **Hopson, W. B., L. G. Britt, R. J. Sherman, and C. P. Ledes.** 1967. Topical antibiotics in the prevention of experimental wound infection. J. Surg. Res. 8:261–277.
10. **James, R. C., and C. J. MacLeod.** 1961. Induction of staphylococcal infections in mice with small inocula introduced on sutures. Br. J. Exp. Pathol. 42:266–277.
11. **Lawrence, J. C., and H. A. Lilly.** 1972. A quantitative method for investigating the bacteriology of skin: its application to burns. Br. J. Exp. Pathol. 53:550–559.
12. **Mack, R. M., and J. R. Cantrell.** 1967. Quantitative studies of the bacterial flora of open skin wounds: the effect of topical antibiotics. Ann. Surg. 166:886–895.
13. **McRipley, R. J., and R. R. Whitney.** 1976. Responsiveness of experimental surgical-wound infections to topical chemotherapy. Antimicrob. Agents Chemother. 10:45–51.
14. **Marples, R. R., and A. M. Kligman.** 1974. Methods for evaluating topical antibacterial agents on human skin. Antimicrob. Agents Chemother. 5:323–329.
15. **Marples, R. R., A. Rebora, and A. M. Kligman.** 1973. Topical steroid antibiotic combinations. Arch. Dermatol. 108:237–240.
16. **Noble, W. C., and J. A. Savin.** 1971. Gram-negative infections of the skin. Br. J. Dermatol. 85:286–289.
17. **Robson, M. C., and J. P. Heggers.** 1969. Bacterial quantitation of open wounds. Mil. Med. 134:19–24.
18. **Russell, H. E., D. P. Gutekunst, and R. E. Chamberlain.** 1968. Evaluation of furazolium chloride in topical treatment of model infections in laboratory animals, p. 497–501. Antimicrob. Agents Chemother. 1967.
19. **Saymen, D. G., P. Nathan, I. A. Holder, E. O. Hill, and B. G. MacMillan.** 1972. Infected surface wound: an experimental model and a method for the quantitation of bacteria in infected tissues. Appl. Microbiol. 23:509–514.
20. **Singh, G., R. R. Marples, and A. M. Kligman.** 1971. Experimental *Staphylococcus aureus* infections in humans. J. Invest. Drmatol. 57:149–162.
21. **Tabernero, E., E. Gauithero, and N. Ercoli.** 1974. Therapeutic action of antimicrobial agents in localized infections of mice. Chemotherapy (Basel) 20:52–60.

ANTIMICROBIAL AGENTS AND CHEMOTHERAPY, July 1976, p. 45-51

Vol. 10, No. 1
Printed in U.S.A.

Responsiveness of Experimental Surgical-Wound Infections to Topical Chemotherapy

R. J. McRIPLEY* AND R. R. WHITNEY

Department of Microbiology, The Squibb Institute for Medical Research, Princeton, New Jersey 08540

Received for publication 9 February 1976

Topical agents freshly formulated in a cream base vehicle as well as commercial topical preparations were used to evaluate in mice the responsiveness of experimental surgical wounds infected with *Staphylococcus aureus* or *Pseudomonas aeruginosa* to chemotherapy. The responsiveness of the infections to therapy or the efficacy of a topical agent was assessed primarily by means of wound counts of the infecting organism before and after the employment of an immediate (prophylactic) or delayed (therapeutic) treatment regimen. From tests of several concentrations of an agent formulated in the vehicle, a median effective dose could be determined. In the case of the lethal *P. aeruginosa* infection, a median protective dose could be determined. Both infections were found to be quite susceptible to treatment with those topical agents that demonstrated good activity in vitro against the test organisms. The results of the investigation indicated that the model infections were suitable for the screening of potential topical agents in vivo.

In the preceding paper experimental surgical-wound infections in mice were described and characterized (6). In addition, a rapid method for quantitating bacteria in the wound infections was presented. In this paper the response of the surgical-wound infections to chemotherapy with various topical antimicrobial agents is explored. Freshly formulated antibacterial agents, commonly administered topically, as well as commercial topical antimicrobial products were employed in the study. These topical formulations were used not only for evaluating the responsiveness of the experimental infections to chemotherapy but also for demonstrating how, using standardized methodology, the model infections can be employed to assess various measures of topical efficacy.

MATERIALS AND METHODS

Antibacterial agents. The antibiotics and chemicals used in this study were gentamicin sulfate, 634 μg/mg (Schering Corp.); polymyxin B sulfate, 7,956 U/mg (Pfizer Laboratories); neomycin sulfate, 654 μg/mg (E. R. Squibb & Sons); zinc bacitracin, 47.7 U/mg (Commercial Solvents); gramicidin, 943 μg/mg (E. R. Squibb & Sons); nitrofurazone (Eaton Laboratories); and triclobisonium chloride (Roche Laboratories). The agents were supplied as powders or crystals and, for testing in vivo, were formulated at the desired concentration on a weight basis in an emulsion-type cream base vehicle containing promulgen, protopet, sorbitol solution, silicone antifoam, distilled water, and methyl and ethyl parabens.

Commercial products. These products, with the active ingredients listed, were purchased on the open market: Neosporin ointment (Burroughs Wellcome Co.), consisting of (per gram) 5,000 U of polymyxin B sulfate, 400 U of zinc bacitracin, and neomycin sulfate equivalent to 3.5 mg of neomycin base; Mycolog cream (E. R. Squibb & Sons), consisting of (per gram) 100,000 U of nystatin, 0.25 mg of gramicidin, and neomycin sulfate equivalent to 2.5 mg of neomycin base, including 0.1% triamcinolone acetonide; Polysporin ointment (Burroughs Wellcome Co.), consisting of (per gram) 10,000 U of polymyxin B sulfate and 500 U of zinc bacitracin; Furacin topical cream (Eaton Laboratories), consisting of 0.2% nitrofurazone; Garamycin cream (Schering Corp.), consisting of 0.1% gentamicin sulfate; and Triburon ointment (Roche Laboratories), consisting of 0.1% triclobisonium chloride.

Evaluation of antibacterial activity in vitro. Minimal inhibitory concentrations (MIC) were determined by the conventional twofold dilution method, using antibiotic assay broth (BBL) as previously described (3). Aliquots from all tubes showing no visible growth were plated on antibiotic assay seed agar (BBL) to determine the minimal bactericidal concentration (MBC). Antibacterial agents were dissolved in 0.05 M phosphate buffer, pH 7.0, prior to being evaluated in vitro.

Evaluation of efficacy in vivo. Details of the experimental *Staphylococcus aureus* and *Pseudomonas aeruginosa* surgical-wound infections were presented in the preceding paper (6). The efficacy of test formulations in the experimental infections was assessed by two methods: (i) inhibition or reduction of viable wound counts of both test organisms, and (ii) in the case of the *P. aeruginosa* infection, protection from the lethal effect of the infection. When quantitation of viable organisms was utilized, two treatment regimens were employed: (i) immediate (prophylactic) treatment and (ii) delayed (therapeutic) treatment. With the immediate-treatment regimen, which was initiated prior to the actual establishment of wound infections, each wound was treated topically with 0.4 g of formulation 15 min after the insertion of sutures and then 6 h later. The delayed-treatment regimen, which commenced after wound infections were established, consisted of two treatments administered 24 and 30 h after suture insertion. With both regimens, wounds were cultured 18 h after the final treatment using the surface rinse technique (6), and counts of viable infecting organisms were made by conventional methods. Ten mice were used for evaluating the efficacy of each formulation. When the immediate-treatment regimen was used, the efficacy of a formulation was based on its ability to inhibit the establishment of wound infections as reflected by the populations of test organisms in wounds after treatment relative to those obtained in placebo-treated wounds. The difference between the means of the two populations was assumed to represent the inhibition produced by an active agent in the formulation. When the delayed-treatment regimen was used, a formulation's efficacy was assessed by the reduction in the bacterial wound counts produced by treatment relative to pretreatment counts of the test organism.

In evaluating the protective efficacy of test formulations against the lethal *P. aeruginosa* infection, all mice, 10/group, were treated with cream base immediately after infection. After 6 h, treatment with test formulations commenced. Each mouse was treated topically with 0.4 g of formulation. Treatment continued twice daily for the next 2 days. Throughout the course of therapy, mice were closely observed to ascertain whether the topically applied formulations were being ingested. Mice were held for observation a total of 2 weeks, with deaths being recorded daily.

The median effective dose (ED_{50}) or the median protective dose (PD_{50}) of an antibacterial agent was determined by the method of Reed and Muench (8) and was based on a minimum of three dosage levels at fourfold increments.

Detection of drug activity in serum and wound washings. At 18 h after the termination of therapy, blood and wound washings were obtained from noninfected mice treated with each test drug at the highest concentration used in the study. The washings and the collected sera were passed through 0.45-μm membrane filters (Millipore Corp.) prior to being tested for drug activity. Aliquots of washings and sera were incubated at 37 C in the presence of known concentrations of *P. aeruginosa* or *S. aureus* (10^3 to 10^5 colony-forming units/ml). At various intervals during the incubation period, samples were removed from each mixture, diluted appropriately, and cultured quantitatively on brain heart infusion agar. The mean concentration of viable organisms determined for each group of test mixtures was compared with those concentrations found with control mixtures that contained sterile washings or sera from placebo-treated or untreated mice. In addition, aliquots of wound washings and bacterial inocula containing 50 to 300 viable organisms were placed on brain heart infusion agar plates and spread over the surface of the agar. The plates were incubated at 37 C for 48 h. The number of colonies formed after incubation was compared with control counts obtained when washings were omitted.

RESULTS

The activity in vitro of several antibacterial agents, commonly utilized topically, against the two test organisms used in the surgical-wound infections is shown in Table 1. The results indicate that the agents tested varied considerably in their activity against the test organisms. Against *S. aureus*, triclobisonium and gentamicin were the most active agents tested, exhibiting MIC values of <1.0 μg/ml. Nitrofurazone and neomycin also demonstrated good activity, whereas gramicidin and polymyxin B were less active. Against *P. aeruginosa*, gentamicin and polymyxin B were the most active agents. Neomycin and triclobisonium were also active, whereas the other agents were essentially inactive. With the exception of the activity of neomycin and gentamicin against *P. aeruginosa*, MBC values for the various agents were not markedly different from MIC values.

Several commercial topical preparations were evaluated in the experimental infections to determine the responsiveness of the infections to treatment with products specifically marketed for use against local infections. The results (Table 2) indicate that most of the products were efficacious against the *S. aureus* infection. All the products except the nitrofurazone formulation were extremely effective in inhibiting the growth of the test organism in the wound when the immediate-treatment schedule was followed; the nitrofurazone prod-

TABLE 1. *Activity in vitro of selected antibacterial agents used in commercial topical products*

Test organism	Antibacterial agent	MIC (μg/ml)	MBC (μg/ml)
S. aureus (SC 2406)	Gentamicin sulfate	0.78	1.6
	Gramicidin	18.7	25
	Neomycin sulfate	6.25	12.5
	Nitrofurazone	9.4	12.5
	Polymyxin B sulfate	37.5	75
	Triclobisonium chloride	0.6	1.6
	Zinc bacitracin	6.25	12.5
P. aeruginosa (SC 8822)	Gentamicin sulfate	0.6	3.1
	Gramicidin	>100	>100
	Neomycin sulfate	9.4	50
	Nitrofurazone	>100	>100
	Polymyxin B sulfate	1.6	3.1
	Triclobisonium chloride	25	75
	Zinc bacitracin	>100	>100

TABLE 2. *Activity of selected commercial topical products against experimental surgical-wound infections in mice*

Experimental infection	Formulation	Mean inhibition[a] (log_{10})	Mean reduction[b] (log_{10})
S. aureus	Gentamicin cream	5.02 ± 0.24[c]	3.40 ± 0.25
	Neomycin-gramicidin-nystatin-triamcinolone acetonide cream	5.82 ± 0.19	3.85 ± 0.43
	Nitrofurazone cream	2.85 ± 0.23	0
	Polymyxin B-bacitracin-neomycin ointment	5.54 ± 0.18	3.92 ± 0.40
	Triclobisonium chloride ointment	4.99 ± 0.59	3.77[d]
P. aeruginosa	Gentamicin cream	5.33 ± 0.14	2.29 ± 0.33
	Neomycin-gramicidin-nystatin-triamcinolone acetonide cream	4.42 ± 0.32	0.43 ± 0.25
	Nitrofurazone cream	0.36 ± 0.09	0
	Polymyxin B-bacitracin-neomycin ointment	4.02 ± 0.21	0.69 ± 0.03
	Triclobisonium chloride ointment	2.59 ± 0.28	0.49 ± 0.14

[a] Inhibition relative to the mean concentration of viable test organisms in placebo-treated wounds; immediate treatment.

[b] Reduction relative to the mean wound concentration of viable test organisms prior to treatment; delayed treatment.

[c] Mean ± standard error of a minimum of three experiments.

[d] Tested only once; product is no longer commercially available.

uct was less effective than the other products. In the more stringent evaluation that occurred when treatment was delayed, all the products except the nitrofurazone preparation produced a significant reduction in the *S. aureus* wound count. The products were more diversified in their activity against the experimental *P. aeruginosa* infection. In the evaluation of prophylactic activity, i.e., with the immediate-treatment schedule, gentamicin and the two combination products were quite effective, the triclobisonium ointment was moderately active, and the nitrofurazone cream was essentially inactive. However, under the rigorous assessment of bactericidal efficacy that occurred when treatment was delayed, only the gentamicin formulation was efficacious.

To evaluate further the effectiveness of the experimental infections in assessing the efficacy of topical antibacterial agents, several of the agents used in commercial products were formulated at various concentrations near the "use" level in a compatible cream base vehicle and were tested in the model infections. The results of this abbreviated dose response study are presented in Table 3. In general, the two infections were quite responsive to therapy with the various series of formulations and demonstrated approximately 2 log_{10} differences in bacterial wound counts when treated with two or three 10-fold decrements of the agent being evaluated. Neomycin formulations were the notable exception to this observation, exhibiting modest differences in wound counts in the *S. aureus* infection when applied prophylactically and in the *P. aeruginosa* infection when applied therapeutically. As was expected, with delayed treatment, larger concentrations of the various agents were required to produce significant responses in the infections than were required with the immediate-treatment regimen.

For a definitive comparison of the efficacy of different antibacterial agents in the experimental infections, a method of assessing activity based on the ED_{50} was employed. At least three concentrations of an agent, formulated at four- to fivefold increments in the cream base vehicle, were tested. The ED_{50} was defined as the concentration that produced a 3 log_{10} inhibition or reduction in the wound count of the infecting organism in 50% of mice. The results of a typical experiment are presented in Table 4. Against the *S. aureus* infection, gentamicin and neomycin demonstrated equivalent activity when the immediate-treatment schedule was followed; however, gentamicin was more efficacious than neomycin when delayed treatment was employed. Bacitracin was not as efficacious as either of the other two antibiotics. Against the *P. aeruginosa* infections, polymyxin B was the most efficacious agent, demonstrating the same ED_{50} with both the immediate- and delayed-treatment schedules. Gentamicin was more active than neomycin but less active than polymyxin B.

In using inhibition and reduction of bacterial wound counts as criteria of formulation effi-

TABLE 3. *Effect of concentration on the activity of selected antibacterial agents in surgical-wound model infections in mice*

Experimental infection	Test drug	Concn (%)	Mean inhibition[a] (log_{10})	Mean reduction[b] (log_{10})
S. aureus	Gentamicin sulfate	0.1	5.16 ± 0.36[c]	2.88 ± 0.22
		0.01	2.40 ± 0.70	0.36 ± 0.15
		0.001	0.96 ± 0.05	
	Neomycin sulfate	0.5	4.90 ± 0.05	3.30 ± 0.37
		0.05	3.84 ± 0.20	1.59 ± 0.25
		0.005	2.37 ± 0.71	
	Zinc bacitracin	1.0		0.43 ± 0.30
		0.5	4.49 ± 0.27	
		0.05	1.80 ± 0.32	
P. aeruginosa	Gentamicin sulfate	0.5		2.80 ± 0.45
		0.1	4.92 ± 0.16	
		0.05		0.49 ± 0.24
		0.01	2.23 ± 0.42	
		0.001	0.42 ± 0.15	
	Neomycin sulfate	2.0		2.87 ± 0.11
		1.0	4.50 ± 0.22	
		0.2		1.25 ± 0.28
		0.1	1.47 ± 0.21	
	Polymyxin B sulfate	0.05	5.20 ± 0.63	3.55 ± 0.17
		0.005	1.40 ± 0.20	0.43 ± 0.18

[a] Inhibition relative to the mean concentration of viable test organisms in placebo-treated wounds; immediate treatment.
[b] Reduction relative to the mean wound concentration of viable test organisms prior to treatment; delayed treatment.
[c] Mean ± standard error of two to four experiments.

TABLE 4. *ED_{50} of selected antibacterial agents against surgical-wound infections based on the inhibition or reduction in counts of viable infecting organisms*

Test drug	ED_{50} (%)			
	S. aureus infection		*P. aeruginosa* infection	
	Immediate treatment	Delayed treatment	Immediate treatment	Delayed treatment
Gentamicin sulfate	0.02	0.05	0.03	>0.50
Neomycin sulfate	0.02	0.22	0.33	≥2.00
Polymyxin B sulfate			0.02	0.02
Zinc bacitracin	0.30	>2.00		

cacy, it was possible that residual drug in wound washings or the systemic activity of a topically applied drug might account for the efficacy observed. To investigate these possibilities, the antibacterial activity of washings and sera from mice treated with high levels of the various drugs was compared with that of washings and sera from placebo-treated and untreated mice. No significant antibacterial activity was demonstrated with either washings or sera from any treated mice; quantitation of the two test organisms after various periods of exposure to the test or control washings and sera yielded identical results.

Since the *P. aeruginosa* infection is lethal when the infected wound is kept hydrated (7), it seemed possible to exploit this fact and use survival as a measure of efficacy in the evaluation of topical antibacterial agents that possess antipseudomonad activity in vitro. To test this possibility, several commercial topical agents were evaluated against the *P. aeruginosa* wound infection (Table 5). The two combination products and the gentamicin formulation were quite efficacious in the infection, producing >80% survival, as compared with 13% survival in placebo-treated controls. The triclobisonium ointment demonstrated slight activity and the nitrofurazone preparation was inactive in the model infection.

As a further means of comparing the efficacy of topical antibacterial agents in protecting mice against the lethal effect of a *P. aeruginosa* infection, the PD_{50} was determined for several of the agents. The results of a typical experiment are presented in Table 6. Polymyxin B and gentamicin were quite active, exhibiting PD_{50} values of <0.1%. Neomycin was also active but to a lesser extent than either polymyxin B or gentamicin. Nitrofurazone, as could

TABLE 5. *Effect of commercial topical products on survival in mice with surgical wounds infected with P. aeruginosa*

Formulation	% Survival[a]
Gentamicin cream	95.3 ± 3.1
Polymyxin B-bacitracin-neomycin ointment	92.6 ± 5.3
Polymyxin B-bacitracin ointment	84.0 ± 6.0
Triclobisonium chloride ointment	36.7 ± 8.3
Nitrofurazone cream	9.5 ± 0.5
Untreated control	13.0 ± 3.2

[a] Mean ± standard error of two to four experiments.

TABLE 6. *PD_{50} of selected antibacterial agents in mice infected with P. aeruginosa*

Antibacterial agent	PD_{50} (%)
Polymyxin B sulfate	0.03
Gentamicin sulfate	0.05
Neomycin sulfate	0.13
Nitrofurazone	>1.00

be expected from its lack of activity in vitro and in vivo against *P. aeruginosa* in earlier studies, was not active at the concentrations tested.

DISCUSSION

Although there is some controversy as to the effectiveness of topical chemotherapy in certain types of local infections, there are several clinical situations in which topical therapy is apparently beneficial (1, 2, 5, 7). Topical antimicrobial formulations are widely used in the field of dermatology (9). Because problems related to the development of resistance, sensitization, toxicity, and other undesirable effects have been encountered with several of the substances commonly used topically, the search has continued for new and more efficacious substances that can be utilized as topical chemotherapeutic agents.

The model infections described herein have been established for use as a screening tool for identifying and evaluating substances that may be employed as topical antibacterial agents. By utilizing standardized materials and methods, we have sought to eliminate some of the variables associated with the evaluation of topical antibacterial formulations, with the ultimate aim of bringing the most efficacious candidates to clinical trials in which the final assessment of efficacy must be made.

The primary purpose of this study was to evaluate the response of the model infections to treatment with various topical antimicrobial agents and preparations, most of which are employed in the clinic. Since topical agents may be either synthetic compounds or antibiotics, representatives of both types were included in this study. The results obtained indicate that the infections are quite responsive to treatment with efficacious topical agents of various potencies. In addition, various levels of efficacy could be detected, as determined by inhibition or reduction of bacterial wound counts and, in the case of the *P. aeruginosa* infection, by the survival of lethally infected mice. Furthermore, the responsiveness of the experimental infections to treatment with various concentrations of the commercial topical agents allowed the determination of ED_{50}. Although an ED_{50} was arbitrarily defined, its determination permits a more definitive and valid comparison of the activities of various agents than does the use of single concentrations of agents. In the case of the *P. aeruginosa* infection, the determination of PD_{50} also aids in the evaluation of the topical efficacy of test substances. Results obtained from the screening of newly synthesized compounds indicate that the model infections are indeed useful in assessing the topical efficacy of potential agents (unpublished data).

For most of the topical agents employed in this study, there appeared to be some correlation between activities in vitro and in vivo. Agents that exhibited low MICs against a particular test organism in vitro usually demonstrated good efficacy when the immediate (prophylactic)-treatment schedule was followed for the experimental infection with that same organism; conversely, agents inactive in vitro showed little or no efficacy in vivo. The correlation was also observed with MBCs. Agents that demonstrated low MBCs in vitro were found to be efficacious when the delayed (therapeutic)-treatment schedule was followed; agents with high MBCs usually showed no activity in vivo. Thus, to some extent, the efficacy of an agent could be predicted from its activity in vitro.

Our experience to date in evaluating new compounds has revealed several potential agents that exhibited marked activity in vitro but were relatively ineffective in the experimental infections (unpublished data). Other investigators have made similar observations (4). Although both evaluations, in vitro and in vivo, involve direct contact between the antibacterial agent and the microorganism, the conditions in the infected wound are more complex than those found in the test tube and may affect adversely the activity of an antibacterial agent. For example, an agent markedly active in vitro may be inactivated or neutralized in the wound by the presence of serum, tissue fluids, enzymes, or other substances not present in the test tube. Thus, potential topical agents must be evaluated in vivo under simulated clinical conditions before their true topical efficacy can be ascertained.

One criticism commonly leveled when topical chemotherapy is studied in animals is that the topically administered drug has probably been ingested by the animals. Obviously, this can be a serious problem, but in our experience it is only occasionally encountered. For example, in this study, only mice treated with the commercial gentamicin formulation were observed ingesting it from the backs of cagemates. Because the ingestion of agents that are active when administered orally can interfere drastically with the evaluation of the substance as a topical agent, measures must be taken to prevent such ingestion. In the case of the gentamicin formulation, the problem was resolved by isolating the treated mice in small individual cages in which movement was severely restricted. Other means of preventing ingestion are the use of restrainers, collars, or coverings for the treatment site or the addition to the formulation of some inert chemical that discourages ingestion. It should be emphasized that the problem of ingestion occurs only infrequently with most of the commonly used topical preparations and vehicles.

Other criticisms sometimes raised when the efficacy of a topical formulation is evaluated culturally are that the activity observed may be due to residual drug and drug carry-over or to systemic activity resulting from topical absorption. In some instances these criticisms may be valid. Therefore, in evaluating topical chemotherapy on a cultural basis, it is necessary to demonstrate that these factors are not involved in the efficacy produced. Simple measures such as those employed in this study can be used to eliminate the possibility that drug carry-over and systemic activity have participated in the cultural results. In the case of residual drug and drug carry-over, there are various preventive measures that can be taken to reduce or abolish their involvement in the cultural evaluation. For example, substantial amounts of residual formulation should be removed prior to culturing a lesion, there should be a definite interval between the termination of therapy and the beginning of cultural evaluations, and the cultural procedures should employ several dilutions before plating.

Admittedly, the quantity of formulation applied to each wound as part of the experimental procedure is somewhat large, being analogous to applying 1.5 kg of formulation on a 77-kg human. However, we have found that it is necessary to apply a formulation in the experimental wound rather heavily in order to obtain a therapeutic response. Since the mice are caged in groups of 10, there is, obviously, some loss of formulation from the treated site. But, as the data show, the variation in bacterial wound counts between mice in a group is less than might be expected considering the conditions employed.

It should be noted that antimicrobial agents formulated for topical usage, in contrast to parenterally and orally administered agents, are often used at the same concentration in both animals and humans. The amount of drug applied and the frequency of treatment are usually determined by the size, type, and nature of the superficial infection being treated and not by the species of the host. Thus, in this study commercial topical antimicrobial preparations, intended for human use, were applied "as is" on the infected surgical wounds. In addition, freshly prepared formulations were made with the antimicrobial agent incorporated within the range of the "use concentration."

The surgical-wound model, in addition to its use in the evaluation of the topical antibacterial activity of test substances, has several other applications. For example, a subjective evaluation of the effect of a particular substance on wound healing can be made by examining the gross appearance of the wound at various intervals after treatment. Moreover, the application of the test material to the denuded suface of the wound can reveal topical absorption and toxicity. Finally, the model infections can be used to evaluate the activity of a substance that has been administered parenterally (unpublished data).

Although the surgical-wound model can provide useful and valuable information about the effect of topical treatment in mice, as mentioned previously, the ultimate determination of topical efficacy and safety must be made in humans.

ACKNOWLEDGMENTS

We are indebted to H. Basch for MIC and MBC determinations, to D. Hsieh and R. Schwind for help in animal studies, to R. George and A. Hellwig for technical assistance, and to H. Gadebusch and D. Frost for critical review of the manuscript.

LITERATURE CITED

1. **Belzer, F. O., O. Salvatierra, Jr., R. T. Schweizer, and S. L. Kountz.** 1973. Prevention of wound infections by topical antibiotics in high risk patients. Am. J. Surg. **126:**180–185.
2. **Bingham, R., W. H. Fleenor, and S. Church.** 1974. The local use of antibiotics to prevent wound infection. Clin. Orthop. Relat. Res. **99:**194–200.

3. **Gadebusch, H. H., and H. I. Basch.** 1974. A new antimicrobial nitrofuran, *trans*-5-amino-3[2-(5-nitro-2-furyl)vinyl] Δ^2-1,2,4-oxadiazole: antibacterial, antifungal, and antiprotozoan activity in vitro. Antimicrob. Agents Chemother. **6**:263-267.
4. **Grunberg, E., and R. J. Schnitzer.** 1959. Experimental approach to topical antibacterial therapy. Ann. N.Y. Acad. Sci. **82**:114-118.
5. **Hummel, R. P., B. G. MacMillan, and W. A. Altemeier.** 1970. Topical and systemic antibacterial agents in the treatment of burns. Ann. Surg. **172**:370-384.
6. **McRipley, R. J., and R. R. Whitney.** 1976. Characterization and quantitation of experimental surgical-wound infections used to evaluate topical antibacterial agents. Antimicrob. Agents Chemother. **10**:38-44.
7. **Moncrief, J. A.** 1973. Burns. N. Engl. J. Med. **288**:444-454.
8. **Reed, L. J., and H. Muench.** 1938. A simple method of estimating fifty percent end points. Am. J. Hyg. **27**:493-499.
9. **Sauer, G. S.** 1973. Manual of skin diseases. J. B. Lippincott Co., Philadelphia.

ANTIMICROBIAL AGENTS AND CHEMOTHERAPY, July 1976, p. 52-56
Vol. 10, No. 1

Cefazolin in the Treatment of Acute Enteric Fever

MARWAN UWAYDAH[1]

Departments of Medicine and Bacteriology and Virology, American University Hospital, Beirut, Lebanon

Received for publication 11 November 1975

Cefazolin was used in the treatment of nine patients with acute enteric fever proven by positive blood cultures. In seven patients the causative organism was *Salmonella typhi* and in two it was *Salmonella paratyphi* B. Minimal inhibitory and minimal bactericidal concentrations of cefazolin against the nine isolates ranged between 1.95 and 3.90 μg/ml. Cefazolin was administered either intramuscularly or intravenously in a daily dose of 3 to 6 g for 11 to 16 days. The mean peak serum antibiotic concentration after a 0.5-g intravenous injection was 64.4 μg/ml, and the mean trough concentration, 3 h later, was 12.7 μg/ml. The highest serum inhibitory dilution at peak level was frequently 1/64, and at trough level it was 1/16 to 1/32. The acute infection was satisfactorily controlled in all patients. Phlebitis, complicating intravenous therapy, in five out of eight patients, was the only side effect observed. Relapse of typhoid fever, as documented by positive blood culture, occurred in one patient 11 days after treatment course was completed. More extensive clinical studies are required before drawing any conclusions regarding the efficacy of cefazolin in acute enteric fever.

Interest in the antimicrobial therapy of acute enteric fever has been revived after the occurrence of outbreaks caused by chloramphenicol-resistant *Salmonella typhi* in Mexico, the United States, and other parts of the world (1, 4, 11). Only two additional antimicrobial agents, ampicillin and cotrimoxazole, are generally considered useful in the treatment of this infection (8, 17). Recently, Pillay et al. claimed amoxycillin to be another alternative therapeutic agent (12). Some of the chloramphenicol-resistant *S. typhi* isolates were also found to be resistant to ampicillin and sulfonamides (1, 11), and it is uncertain whether cotrimoxazole will prove effective in infections caused by organisms highly resistant to sulfonamides.

It is a well-recognized, yet poorly understood, fact that not all antimicrobial agents active in vitro against *S. typhi* or *S. paratyphi* are necessarily effective in the treatment of the clinical disease (5, 8). This lack of correlation between the results of the in vitro and the in vivo studies may have been related to a number of factors, including the patterns of serum antibacterial activity achieved with the dosage regimens used. The possibility that inadequate serum antibiotic concentration was an important cause of the relatively high incidence of treatment failures reported with oral, but not parenteral, ampicillin therapy has not been altogether excluded (9, 11, 14). These issues and their practical implications have been discussed previously (16).

Cefazolin, when compared with other cephalosporin antibiotics, has been demonstrated to yield significantly higher and better sustained blood levels after either intramuscular (i.m.) or intravenous (i.v.) administration (10). Preliminary in vitro studies conducted in this laboratory have shown that the minimal inhibitory concentrations (MIC) of this antibiotic against eleven locally isolated strains of chloramphenicol and ampicillin-susceptible *S. typhi* and *S. paratyphi* B ranged between 0.80 and 3.12 μg/ml, suggesting that very high serum antibacterial activity against salmonellae may be expected in patients receiving the recommended antibiotic dosage. The purpose of this study was to evaluate the efficacy of cefazolin in the treatment of acute enteric fever, as monitored by serum antibiotic level and serum inhibitory activity determinations.

MATERIALS AND METHODS

Only patients with acute enteric fever, proven by positive blood cultures, were selected for this study. Blood for culture was collected in tryptose phosphate broth (BBL), and bottles were incubated at 37 C. Rectal swabs were streaked on salmonella-shigella (BBL) and MacConkey agar (Difco) plates and were inoculated in Selenite cystine broth (BBL). Final identification of *Salmonella* was based on carbohydrate fermentation patterns and slide agglutination tests, according to standard procedures (6). Suscep-

[1] Address reprint requests to: Dr. Marwan Uwaydah, c/o Dr. Morton Swartz, Chief, Infectious Disease Unit, Massachusetts General Hospital, Boston, MA 02114.

tibility of isolates to cefazolin, ampicillin, and chloramphenicol was determined by the Kirby-Bauer disk agar diffusion technique (3) and by the serial twofold dilution technique in Mueller-Hinton broth (BBL) (7), using as an inoculum a 10^{-4} dilution of overnight broth culture (final concentration, approximately 10^5 organisms/ml). After overnight incubation, the lowest antibiotic concentration inhibiting visible growth was recorded as the MIC value. All clear tubes were subcultured on MacConkey agar plates using a 0.01-ml calibrated loop. The lowest concentration from which no more than one colony grew was considered as the minimal bactericidal concentration.

Cefazolin (Kefzol, Eli Lilly & Co.) was administered either i.v. or i.m. in a daily dose of 3 to 6 g. Treatment was continued for 11 to 16 days, and patients were examined daily for evaluation of their clinical response. Blood cultures were obtained from all patients 6 and 24 h after initiating antibiotic therapy and whenever indicated thereafter. Blood samples were obtained from every patient on two or three different occasions during treatment for determining serum cefazolin concentrations and serum antibacterial activity against the infecting organism. On every occasion, two blood samples were collected to detect peak levels (10 to 15 min after the i.v. dose and 60 min after the i.m. dose) and trough levels (just before the next dose).

Assay of cefazolin concentrations was performed by the two-layer cylinder-plate method using antibiotic medium 5 (Difco) after adjusting its pH to 6.0. A *Bacillus subtilis* spore suspension (Difco) served as the test organism. Serum antibacterial activity was determined by the twofold dilution technique (2). For comparative purposes, both pooled normal human serum and Mueller-Hinton broth (BBL) were used as diluents. The inoculum was a 10^{-4} dilution of an overnight broth culture (final concentration, approximately 10^5 organisms/ml). After overnight incubation, the highest serum dilution inhibiting visible growth was recorded. Clear tubes were subcultured on MacConkey agar plates using a 0.01-ml calibrated loop. The highest dilution from which no more than one colony grew was regarded as the highest bactericidal dilution. Other laboratory tests done on every patient before, during, and after the treatment course included urinalysis, complete blood count, blood urea nitrogen, and serum creatinine. In addition, serum electrolyte and liver function tests were done whenever indicated.

RESULTS

Patients. Nine patients, five females and four males, ranging in age between 15 and 32 years, were selected for this trial. All presented with the classic clinical picture of acute enteric fever. The duration of the febrile illness prior to initiating antibiotic therapy varied between 4 and 12 days, and the peak temperatures ranged between 39.7 and 41.0 C. Pretreatment blood cultures from seven patients grew *S. typhi*, and from the other two *S. paratyphi* B grew. Serum creatinine values were normal in all subjects. Leukocyte counts were either normal or low, consistent with the diagnosis of acute enteric fever. None of the patients showed evidence of intestinal hemorrhage or perforation.

In vitro susceptibility tests. All *Salmonella* isolates recovered from the nine patients proved to be susceptible to cefazolin, ampicillin, and chloramphenicol. The results of inhibition zone sizes, together with MIC and minimal bactericidal concentration values of the three antibiotics against the nine isolates, are given in Table 1. It is clear that the inhibitory concentrations are readily achievable in sera of patients receiving the regularly recommended dosages of any of the three antibiotics. In contrast to the bacteriostatic effect of chloramphenicol, the bactericidal effects of cefazolin and ampicillin were demonstrated by MIC and minimal bactericidal concentration values that were essentially identical.

Treatment regimens. In eight patients, cefazolin was administered initially by the i.v. route. In four patients this was continued until treatment was completed, but in the rest the occurrence of severe pain necessitated a change to the i.m. route 8 to 14 days after starting therapy. One patient received the antibiotic i.m. throughout the entire treatment course. Probenicid was given to one patient (number 8) in a dose of 0.5 g every 6 h, starting on day 6 of cefazolin therapy. The details of the antibiotic regimens are summarized in Table 2.

Serum cefazolin concentrations and serum antibacterial activity. Serum peak and trough cefazolin concentrations and highest serum bacteriostatic and bactericidal dilutions are outlined in Table 2. The mean peak serum cefazolin concentration after a 0.5-g i.v. injection was 64.4 μg/ml and the mean trough concentration, 3 h later, was 12.7 μg/ml. Thus, serum antibiotic concentration was continuously maintained well above the MIC value against the infecting organism. This was also confirmed by the results of serum inhibitory activity determinations. The serum inhibitory dilution (static effect) at peak level was frequently 1/64, and at trough level it was either 1/16 or 1/32. Serum antibacterial activity was more pronounced when the samples were diluted in pooled normal serum rather than in broth. This may be attributed to the nonspecific inhibitory factors present in normal serum, which itself produced bacteriostatic and bactericidal effects in a dilution of 1/4 (in broth). The mean serum cefazolin concentration after a 1.0-g i.v. dose was about twice that obtained with a 0.5-g dose. The only exception was encountered in the first

TABLE 1. *Susceptibility of seven S. typhi and two S. paratyphi B isolates to cefazolin, ampicillin, and chloramphenicol as determined by disk agar and broth dilution techniques*

Patient	Organism	Cefazolin			Ampicillin			Chloramphenicol		
		Zone size (mm; 30-μg disk)	MIC (μg/ml)	MBC[a] (μg/ml)	Zone size (mm; 10-μg disk)	MIC (μg/ml)	MBC (μg/ml)	Zone size (mm; 30-μg disk)	MIC (μg/ml)	MBC[b] (μg/ml)
1	*S. typhi*	32.0	1.95	1.95	32.5	0.98	0.98	32.7	1.95	31.25
2	*S. typhi*	27.3	1.95	1.95	27.7	0.98	0.98	31.0	1.95	7.81
3	*S. typhi*	28.0	1.95	1.95	28.2	0.98	0.98	30.4	3.90	62.50
4	*S. paratyphi* B	25.5	1.95	1.95	23.2	0.98	3.90	26.7	3.90	31.25
5	*S. typhi*	28.5	1.95	1.95	30.0	0.98	0.98	32.3	1.95	31.25
6	*S. typhi*	27.1	1.95	1.95	28.0	0.98	0.98	31.0	0.98	15.62
7	*S. typhi*	31.8	3.90	3.90	33.0	0.98	0.98	32.0	1.95	62.50
8	*S. paratyphi* B	25.0	3.90	3.90	25.3	0.98	1.95	29.5	3.90	15.62
9	*S. typhi*	27.3	1.95	1.95	33.0	0.98	0.98	31.5	3.90	62.50

[a] MBC, Minimal bactericidal concentration.

[b] Values may represent concentrations required to carry over enough chloramphenicol in the inoculum to the plate to inhibit growth thereon, and thus they do not necessarily indicate true "bactericidal" activity.

TABLE 2. *Dosage regimen, peak and trough serum antibiotic concentrations, and serum antibacterial activity determinations in nine enteric fever patients treated with cefazolin*

Patient	Dosage regimen	Treatment day	Cefazolin serum concn (μg/ml)		Serum antibacterial activity (reciprocal)							
					Diluent-broth				Diluent-normal serum			
					Peak		Trough		Peak		Trough	
			Peak	Trough	Static	Cidal	Static	Cidal	Static	Cidal	Static	Cidal
1	0.5 g i.v. every 3 h for 14 days; then 0.5 g i.m. every 6 h for 2 days	1	60.0	12.6	64	32	32	32	≥64	≥64	≥64	≥64
		4	59.0	17.0	32	32	16	8	≥64	≥64	≥64	≥64
		11	59.0	13.2	≥64	64	16	4	≥64	32	≥64	4
2	0.5 g i.v. every 3 h for 10 days; then 0.5 g i.m. every 6 h for 1 day	2	55.0	12.9	64	32	32	16	≥64	≥64	≥64	≥64
		4	59.0	14.7	≥64	8	32	8	≥64	≥64	≥64	≥64
		11	78.0	9.3	≥64	32	32	2	≥64	32	≥64	16
3	0.5 g i.v. every 3 h for 8 days; then 0.5 g i.m. every 6 h for 4 days	1	66.0	13.8	≥64	≥64	32	8	≥64	≥64	≥64	≥64
		7	93.0	11.7	≥64	≥64	16	16	≥64	≥64	≥64	≥64
4	0.5 g i.v. every 3 h for 7 days; then 1.0 g i.v. every 4 h for 4 days	4	56.0	9.9	≥64	32	16	4	≥64	4	≥64	2
		7	64.0	12.0	64	16	16	4	≥64	≥64	≥64	8
5	0.5 g i.v. every 4 h for 13 days	2	62.0	5.5	32	32	8	8	≥64	≥64	≥64	≥64
		8	62.0	5.3	≥64	32	8	8	≥64	≥64	≥64	≥64
6	1.0 g i.v. every 4 h for 9 days; then 1.0 g i.m. every 6 h for 4 days	2	150.0	27.9	≥64	≥64	≥64	16	≥64	≥64	≥64	≥64
		9	94.0	29.1	≥64	≥64	≥64	16	≥64	≥64	≥64	≥64
7	1.0 g i.v. every 4 h for 11 days	2	49.0	6.8	≥64	32	16	16	≥64	≥64	≥64	≥64
		7	115.0	9.0	≥64	≥64	32	16	≥64	≥64	≥64	16
8	1.0 g i.v. every 4 h for 13 days	4	110.0	9.8	≥64	32	8	4	≥64	2	≥64	2
		7[a]	150.0	48.0	≥64	≥64	≥64	16	≥64	32	≥64	8
		11[a]	175.0	48.0	≥64	32	32	16	≥64	16	≥64	8
9	0.5 g i.m. every 4 h for 13 days	2	52.0	21.9	32	32	16	16	≥64	64	≥64	64
		8	51.0	9.9	32	32	16	16	≥64	≥64	≥64	≥64

[a] Patient was receiving 0.5 g of probenicid by mouth every 6 h.

sample from patient 7. Trough antibiotic concentrations 4 h after injection varied widely, but adequate inhibitory activity was maintained. Administration of probenicid resulted in substantially increased trough serum antibiotic concentration and inhibitory activity (patient 8, samples 2 and 3).

Response to therapy and post-treatment follow-up. The acute infection was satisfactorily controlled in all nine patients. Details per-taining to clinical illness and response to therapy are outlined in Table 3. Definite subjective improvement was consistently observed within 2 to 3 days of antibiotic treatment. All blood cultures taken 6 and 24 h after beginning therapy remained sterile. The first drop in rectal temperature to 37.9 C or less occurred within 2 to 8 days, with a mean interval of 4.3 days. Three patients who did not develop frank evidence of phlebitis at the i.v. injection site and one patient who received the antibiotic by the i.m. route alone remained completely afebrile after 3 to 11 days of treatment, with a mean interval of 6.5 days. The other patients continued to have irregular spikes of fever which persisted until phlebitis subsided, indicating that this was probably the cause, particularly since all systemic symptoms related to the typhoidal illness were absent and repeated blood cultures were negative. No other side effects of cefazolin were noted.

After discontinuation of treatment, all patients were followed-up for a period of 5 to 8 weeks. Relapse of typhoid fever, as documented by positive blood culture, occurred in one patient (number 1) 11 days after the treatment course was completed. The relapse was successfully controlled with cotrimoxazole. There was no change in the in vitro susceptibility pattern of the *S. typhi* isolated during the relapse as compared to that recovered previously. The other patients remained afebrile and asymptomatic. Rectal swabs for stool cultures were obtained on single occasions from seven patients 2 to 3 weeks after treatment was completed, and all were negative for salmonellae.

DISCUSSION

Of the several cephalosporin antibiotics available for clinical use, none had been shown to be of therapeutic value in enteric fever. The results of this preliminary study indicate that cefazolin is effective in controlling the infection, since all nine patients studied responded satisfactorily to this antibiotic. Only one patient showed a relapse within the follow-up period of 5 to 8 weeks. Phlebitis complicating i.v. therapy in five out of eight patients was the only untoward effect observed. This precluded the use of the temperature curve as a reliable index for evaluating treatment response.

The reasons for the superior efficacy of chloramphenicol over other antimicrobial agents in the treatment of enteric fever have not been elucidated. A noticeable characteristic of this antibiotic is its prolonged serum half-life, so that dosage administration every 6 to 8 h results in its accumulation (15). This might suggest that well-sustained serum antibacterial activity is advantageous for satisfactory control of the typhoidal infection. Studies conducted in this laboratory on typhoid patients receiving chloramphenicol in a dose of 750 mg by mouth every 6 h revealed that the peak inhibitory serum dilution was 1/16 to 1/32 and the trough inhibitory dilution was 1/8 to 1/16. These results are similar to the data obtained with cefazolin reported in this study, although the peak inhibitory activity produced by cefazolin was frequently higher.

The relative efficacy of cefazolin in acute enteric fever and specific recommendations regarding its optimal dosage regimen should await more extensive studies that would consider, among other parameters, the incidence of the chronic carrier state after acute infection. In this respect, cefazolin offers the advantage of reaching bile in very high concentrations (13). Possibly, the high frequency and severity of troublesome phlebitis complicating treatment

TABLE 3. *Clinical and bacteriological responses in nine enteric fever patients treated with cefazolin*

Patient	Age (yr)	Sex	Duration of illness prior to treatment (days)	Duration of treatment before subjective improvement noted (days)	Duration of treatment before first drop in rectal temp to 37.9 C or less (days)	Duration of treatment before complete defervescence (days)	Blood cultures obtained after starting treatment (all negative)	Phlebitis
1	32	M	8	2	5	9	6 h, days 2 + 3	Present
2	17	M	12	2	3	5	6 h, days 2 + 3	Absent
3	15	F	5	2	3	3	6 h, day 2	Absent
4	20	F	4	3	8	12	6 h, days 2 + 7	Present
5	15	F	12	2	2	12	6 h, day 2	Present
6	17	M	7	2	7	17	6 h, days 2 + 7	Present
7	20	M	10	2	5	7	6 h, day 2	Absent
8	29	F	6	2	3	13	6 h, days 2 + 9	Present
9	15	F	7	3	3	11	6 h, days 2 + 4	(Cefazolin administered i.m.)

may be reduced by using different methods of parenteral administration. The value of probenicid in maintaining high trough serum antibacterial activity should be weighed against the possible side effects of this drug. Determinations of serum antibiotic concentration and serum antibacterial activity should reveal useful information for monitoring therapy. The procedure for determining serum inhibitory activity requires better standardization in respect to technical details and interpretation of static and cidal end points (2). If this could be established, the test may serve to lay down general guidelines for predicting whether an antimicrobial agent is likely to be effective in enteric fever and in what dosage regimen it should be used, as indicated by the MIC value against the infecting organism and the pharmacokinetic characteristics of the drug in question.

ACKNOWLEDGMENTS

I thank Shaké Albarian for exellent technical assistance. Cefazolin (Kefzol) used in this study was supplied by Eli Lilly & Co., Beirut, Lebanon.

LITERATURE CITED

1. **Anderson, E. S., and H. R. Smith.** 1972. Chloramphenicol resistance in the typhoid bacillus. Br. Med. J. 3:329–331.
2. **Barry, A. L., and L. D. Sabath.** 1974. Special tests: bactericidal activity and activity of antimicrobics in combination, p. 431–435. *In* E. H. Lennette, E. H. Spaulding, and J. P. Truant (ed.), Manual of clinical microbiology, 2nd ed. American Society for Microbiology, Washington, D.C.
3. **Bauer, A. W., W. M. M. Kirby, J. L. Sherris, and M. Turck.** 1966. Antibiotic susceptibility testing by a standardized single disk method. Am. J. Clin. Pathol. 45:493–496.
4. **Butler, T., N. N. Linh, K. Arnold, and M. Pollack.** 1973. Chloramphenicol-resistant typhoid fever in Vietnam associated with R factor. Lancet 2:983–985.
5. **Dawkins, A. T., Jr., and R. B. Hornick.** 1967. Evaluation of antibiotics in a typhiod model, p. 6–10. Antimicrob. Agents Chemother. 1966.
6. **Edwards, P. R., and W. H. Ewing.** 1972. Identification of Enterobacteriaceae, 3rd ed. Burgess Publishing Co., Minneapolis.
7. **Ericsson, H. M., and J. C. Sherris.** 1971. Antibiotic sensitivity testing. Report of an international collaborative study. Acta Pathol. Microbiol. Scand. Suppl. 217:65–67.
8. **Garrod, L. P., H. P. Lambert, and F. O'Grady.** 1973. Antibiotic and chemotherapy, 4th ed. Churchill Livingstone, Edinburgh.
9. **Kaye, D., H. Rocha, L. Eyckmans, A. Prata, and E. W. Hook.** 1967. Comparison of parenteral ampicillin and parenteral chloramphenicol in the treatment of typhoid fever. Ann. N.Y. Acad. Sci. 145:423–428.
10. **Kirby, W. M. M., and C. Regamey.** Pharmacokinetics of cefazolin compared with four other cephalosporins. J. Infect. Dis. 128(Suppl.):S341–S346.
11. **Overturf, G., K. I. Marton, and A. W. Mathies, Jr.** 1973. Antibiotic resistance in typhoid fever: chloramphenicol resistance among clinical isolates of *Salmonella typhosa* in Los Angeles, 1972. Epidemiologic and bacteriologic characteristics. N. Engl. J. Med. 289:463–465.
12. **Pillay, N., E. B. Adams, and D. North-Coombes.** 1975. Comparative trial of amoxycillin and chloramphenicol in treatment of typhoid fever in adults. Lancet 2:333–334.
13. **Ram, M. D., and S. Watanatittan.** 1973. Levels of cefazolin in human bile. J. Infect. Dis. 123(Suppl.):S361–S363.
14. **Robertson, R. P., M. F. Abdel-Wahab, and F. O. Raasch.** 1968. Evaluation of chloramphenicol and ampicillin in salmonella enteric fever. N. Engl. J. Med. 278:171–176.
15. **Snyder, M. J., and T. E. Woodward.** 1970. The clinical use of chloramphenicol. Med. Clin. North Am. 54:1187–1197.
16. **Uwaydah, M.** 1975. Choice of antimicrobial agents in enteric fever. J. Antimicrob. Chemother. 1:135–137.
17. **Uwaydah, M., R. Matossian, and M. Balabanian.** 1975. Cotrimoxazole compared to chloramphenicol in the treatment of enteric fever. Scand. J. Infect. Dis. 7:123–126.

ANTIMICROBIAL AGENTS AND CHEMOTHERAPY, July 1976, p. 57-63
Vol. 10, No. 1

Specific Inactivation of Herpes Simplex Virus by Silver Nitrate at Low Concentrations and Biological Activities of the Inactivated Virus

FUMIO SHIMIZU,* YOSHINOBU SHIMIZU, AND KATSUO KUMAGAI

Department of Microbiology, Tohoku University School of Dentistry, Sendai, Japan

Received for publication 29 January 1976

The infectivities of herpes simplex virus types 1 and 2 were inactivated by silver nitrate at concentrations of 30 μM or less, which did not affect at all the infectivities of hemagglutinating virus of Japan, vesicular stomatitis virus, poliovirus, vaccinia virus, and adenovirus. The inactivated virus retained the capability of adsorbing to the cell, with an adsorption kinetics quite similar to that of intact virus, and of inducing the concanavalin A agglutinability in the infected cells, whereas it lost completely the capability of producing viral antigens and other cytopathic changes.

Salts of heavy metal ions such as silver, mercury, or copper are bactericidal at very low concentrations, under which conditions they act by combining with sulfhydryl groups. Such sulfhydryl reagents have also been shown to inactivate the infectivity of many viruses. This reaction has been used by many previous investigators to obtain information on the superficial structure of viruses and the early stages of virus multiplication (1, 2, 4, 7).

It has been reported that the infectivity of herpes simplex virus (HSV) is almost completely diminished when the virus is treated with the compounds at concentrations as low as 10^{-4} to 10^{-5} M (7, 10). Thus, in vitro and in vivo effects of compounds such as silver nitrate (5) or silver sulfadiazine (3) on HSV infection have recently been investigated to evaluate them as local chemotherapeutic agents.

The present communication is concerned with further studies on the in vitro effect of silver nitrate on the infectivity of HSV. The inactivation kinetics of HSV by the compound and the specific inactivation of HSV at low concentrations of the compound, which did not affect the infectivity of other viruses, are described. It is also shown that the inactivated virus retained the capability to interact with the cellular membranes, although they did not undergo a growth cycle.

MATERIALS AND METHODS

Viruses. Two types of HSV (type 1, Miyama strain; type 2, UW 268 strain), vaccinia virus (IHD strain), adenovirus (type 5), hemagglutinating virus of Japan (HVJ; Fushimi strain), vesicular stomatitis virus (Indiana strain), and poliovirus (type 1, Mahoney strain) were used. Both types of HSV were propagated in African green monkey kidney cells and centrifuged at 1,400 × *g* for 15 min. Titers of the stock HSV-1 and -2 were 2 × 10^7 and 10^7 plaque-forming units/ml, respectively. Partially purified HSV-1 was prepared by centrifugation of the crude virus onto a cushion of 60% (wt/wt) sucrose in tris(hydroxymethyl)aminomethane(Tris) - hydrochloride buffer through a layer of 5% sucrose in Tris-hydrochloride at 64,000 × *g* for 90 min at 4 C. The viral preparation at the interface between 5 and 60% sucrose layers was rinsed at once and resuspended in the buffer. Adenovirus was propagated in HEp-2 cells, and the titer was $10^{6.8}$ 50% tissue culture infectious doses ($TCID_{50}$)/ml. Vesicular stomatitis virus and vaccinia virus were propagated in rabbit kidney cells (RK13), and their titers were 10^7 and $10^{7.5}$ $TCID_{50}$/ml, respectively. Poliovirus was prepared in human embryonic lung cells, and the titer was $10^{7.2}$ $TCID_{50}$/ml. HVJ was prepared in the chorioallantoic cavity of 11-day-old embryonated chicken eggs, and the titer was $10^{9.6}$ 50% egg infectious doses/ml. All the viruses were stored at −80 C until used.

Tissue culture cells. Monolayer cultures of chicken embryo, RK13, African green monkey kidney, HEp-2, and human embryonic lung cells were grown in Eagle minimum essential medium (MEM) supplemented with 10% heat-inactivated bovine serum, penicillin (100 U/ml), and streptomycin (100 μg/ml). The growth medium for monolayer cultures of 3T3 mouse cells was MEM containing 10% calf serum, penicillin, and streptomycin.

Infectivity assay. All the viruses other than HVJ were assayed by counting plaque-forming units or $TCID_{50}$ per milliliter, using African green monkey kidney or human embryonic lung cells. HVJ was assayed by hemagglutinin titration.

Reagents and radioisotopes. The reagents used were obtained from the following sources. Silver nitrate ($AgNO_3$), silver iodide (AgI), and reduced glutathione (R-glutathione) were from Wako Chemical Industries, Tokyo. Potassium iodide (KI) was from Junsei Chemicals, Tokyo. $AgNO_3$ was dissolved in distilled water at 100 μg/ml, and lower concentrations were prepared by diluting the solution with MEM. KI and AgI were diluted with MEM to the desired concentrations. R-glutathione was dissolved in Tris buffer, and the pH was adjusted to 7.4. [^{3}H]thymidine (specific activity, 10 Ci/mmol) was obtained from New England Nuclear Corp.

Inactivation of viruses by silver nitrate. In most experiments, inactivation of viruses with $AgNO_3$ was performed by adding 1.0 ml of 2×10^5 plaque-forming units or 2×10^5 50% egg infectious doses (HVJ) of viruses per ml to 1.0 ml of a 60 μM $AgNO_3$ solution and agitating the mixture at 37 C for varying times. For controls, 1.0 ml of phosphate-buffered saline (PBS), pH 7.2, was added to the virus suspension before agitation at 37 C. At intervals, serial dilutions into MEM were made, and their virus titers were assayed by counting plaque-forming units or $TCID_{50}$.

Preparation of labeled HSV. Monolayer cultures of 2×10^7 African green monkey kidney cells were infected with HSV-1 at an input multiplicity of 6. After a 2.5-h adsorption period at 37 C, cell sheets were washed three times with PBS to remove the unadsorbed virus and flooded with 30 ml of fresh medium. After 4 h of incubation, [^{3}H]thymidine in MEM was then added to monolayer cultures to a concentration of 4 μCi/ml. The cultures were incubated at 37 C until the cytopathic effect became evident (about 24 h). After centrifugation of the culture medium at $4{,}000 \times g$ at 4 C for 15 min to remove cell debris, the supernatant fluid was harvested. The virus was purified by the cushion ultracentrifugation method in a sucrose gradient (20 to 70%), and 1.0-ml fractions of virus were collected from the top to the bottom. The fractions were assayed for infectivity and radioactivity.

ConA agglutination tests. The methods used were essentially those of Inbar and Sacks (6). For agglutination assays, chicken embryo cells were infected with HSV inactivated by 30 μM $AgNO_3$ or with noninactivated HSV. After an adsorption period of 90 min at 37 C, the cell sheets were washed three times with culture medium to remove the unadsorbed virus and flooded with 6 ml of fresh medium. Six hours after infection, the cell sheets were washed with Ca- and Mg-free PBS, prewarmed to 37 C, and then brought into single cell suspensions with 0.02% disodium versenate solution (ethylenediaminetetraacetate). The cells were then washed with saline and suspended with PBS at a concentration of 10^6 cells/ml, and 0.3-ml samples of cell suspension were transferred to 15-mm plastic trays to which was added either 0.3 ml of concanavalin A (ConA) or 0.3 ml of saline. The mixture was rocked gently several times by hand at room temperature and then examined for cell agglutination under an inverted microscope after 45 min.

Tests for hemadsorption of sensitized erythrocytes. Sensitization of sheep erythrocytes with rabbit anti-sheep erythrocyte serum and hemadsorption on cover slip cultures were carried out as described by Watkins (12). Briefly, a 1% suspension of erythrocytes was mixed with an equal volume of anti-erythrocyte serum (1 hemagglutination unit), and the mixture was incubated at 37 C for 30 min. The erythrocytes were washed three times with glucose veronal buffer and used as a 0.5% suspension for hemadsorption tests. After removing the culture medium, the cover slip cultures, in petri dishes, were gently rinsed three times with glucose veronal buffer. Two milliliters of a suspension of sensitized erythrocytes was then added. After incubation for 2 h at room temperature, the cover slip cultures were gently washed two times with glucose veronal buffer to remove nonadsorbed erythrocytes, and hemadsorption was then examined microscopically.

Fluorescent staining. The antibodies to HSV used were rabbit antisera from rabbits immunized with partially purified virus preparations of HSV-1, Miyama strain. The fluorescein isothiocyanate-conjugated sera used were sheep anti-rabbit gamma globulin (Behringwerke, Uppsala, Sweden).

Production of HSV antigens in the cells was detected by the indirect method. Smear preparations of infected cells fixed with acetone were first covered with an appropriate dilution of antiserum and incubated for 60 min in a moist chamber at 37 C. At this time the preparations were removed, washed with PBS, covered with fluorescein isothiocyanate-conjugated serum, and then reincubated at 37 C for 60 min.

To detect HSV-induced surface antigens, infected monolayer cultures were washed three times with glucose veronal buffer and incubated with the antiserum for 30 min at 4 C. The antiserum was removed by washing, and the cells were stained with a 1:8 dilution of fluorescein isothiocyanate-conjugated serum.

RESULTS

Kinetics of inactivation of HSV by $AgNO_3$. The first experiment was performed to investigate the rate of inactivation of HSV-1 during exposure to $AgNO_3$. A total of 10^5 $TCID_{50}$ of HSV per ml was treated with 30 μM $AgNO_3$ for up to 120 min at 37 C in a water bath and tested for the titers of residual virus. HSV was rapidly inactivated with time (Fig. 1). After 60 min, the virus was almost completely inactivated.

To investigate whether the inactivation of HSV by $AgNO_3$ was dependent upon the amounts of test virus, we exposed different infectivities of HSV to 30 μM $AgNO_3$ for 60 min at 37 C and tested for the titers of residual virus (Fig. 2). When the unpurified virus preparation was used as a test virus, less than 10^6 $TCID_{50}$ of HSV per ml was completely inactivated upon exposure to the compound, whereas 10^7 $TCID_{50}$ of the virus per ml lost no virus titers. Although the inactivation by $AgNO_3$ of unpurified HSV thus appeared to be dependent on the virus titers, partially purified virus at 10^7 $TCID_{50}$/ml was completely inactivated by the same concentration of the compound (Fig. 2). The protein concentrations of unpurified and purified prep-

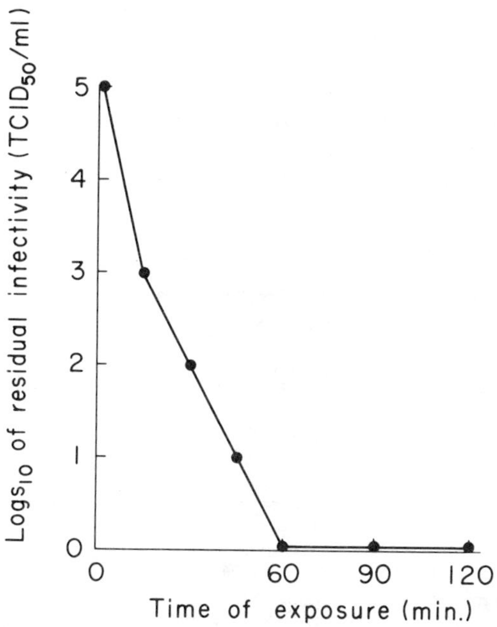

FIG. 1. *Effect of exposure time on inactivation of HSV-1 by silver nitrate.*

arations, both of which contained 10^7 $TCID_{50}$/ml, were 2.7 and 0.2 mg/ml, respectively, as determined by the method of Lowry et al. (8). These results, therefore, suggest that lack of inactivation by $AgNO_3$ of the unpurified virus at 10^7 $TCID_{50}$/ml may be due to the presence of the proteins at concentrations that would inhibit the effect of $AgNO_3$ on the virus. When the purified virus at 10^7 $TCID_{50}$/ml, after addition of bovine serum albumin at a final concentration of 0.8%, was tested for inactivation by $AgNO_3$, no inactivation was observed (Fig. 2). Thus, it was concluded that $AgNO_3$ at 30 μM can inactivate HSV independently of the virus titers, at least up to 10^7 $TCID_{50}$/ml.

Effect of $AgNO_3$ on different viruses. After studying the inactivation kinetics of HSV-1 by $AgNO_3$, the compound was tested for its effect on different viruses, including HSV-2. A total of 10^5 $TCID_{50}$ or 10^5 50% egg infectious doses (HVJ) of viruses per ml were treated with $AgNO_3$ at different concentrations (less than 30 μM) for 60 min at 37 C and then tested for the titers of residual virus. There was a marked contrast between the results for HSV (types 1 and 2) and those for the other viruses (Fig. 3). Both HSV-1 and -2 underwent at least a 10^4-fold loss of titer when treated with 15 or 30 μM $AgNO_3$. By contrast, the other viruses, irrespective of whether they were enveloped or non-enveloped and deoxyribonucleic acid or ribonucleic acid viruses, were not reduced in titer by treatment with the same concentrations of this reagent.

The protein concentrations contained in the test preparations were calculated for each virus by the estimation of the concentrations of undiluted samples and were found to be as low as 27, 28, 0.2, 70, 97, 83, and 140 μg/ml for HSV-1 and -2, HVJ, vesicular stomatitis virus, vaccinia virus, and polio- and adenoviruses, respectively. These results indicate that non-inactivation by $AgNO_3$ of the viruses other than HSV may be due to the insensitivity to the compound of the virus itself, in contrast to the case of an undiluted preparation of HSV-1 at 10^7 $TCID_{50}$/ml, in which non-inactivation of HSV is possibly due to the diminution of the $AgNO_3$ effect by the nonviral proteins. Thus, it is concluded that $AgNO_3$ at a concentration of 30 μM was specific to herpesviruses and could not inactivate other test viruses.

Inhibition of $AgNO_3$ effect by different reagents. An experiment was performed to test whether the inactivation effect of $AgNO_3$ is due to the binding of ionized Ag to the sulfhydryl groups in the virus (Table 1). The results clearly show that no inactivation of HSV was obtained with $AgNO_3$ after it was reacted with a sulfhydryl compound, R-glutathione, or with KI, the reaction of which with $AgNO_3$ results in formation of AgI. In addition, AgI per se, which is an extremely low-ionizing compound, could not inactivate HSV at all. These results indicate that this specific inactivation of HSV by

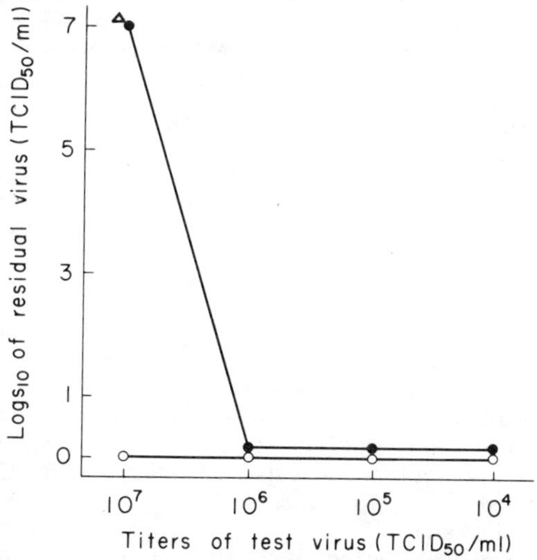

FIG. 2. *Loss of infectivity of HSV of various infectivities by silver nitrate. Symbols:* ●, *crude virus;* ○, *purified virus;* △, *purified virus after addition of bovine serum albumin.*

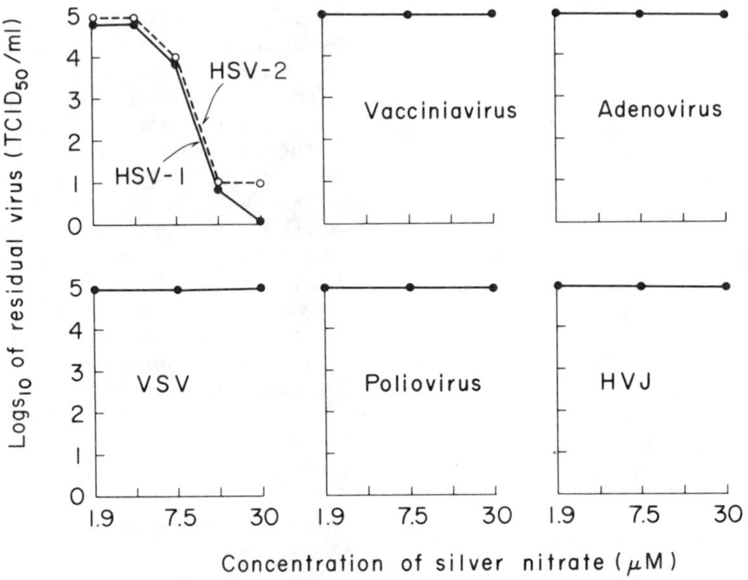

FIG. 3. *Effect of silver nitrate on various viruses.*

TABLE 1. *Inhibition by different reagents of the $AgNO_3$ effect on HSV-1*

Compounds added to HSV[a]	Residual virus[b]	
	PFU/ml	% of control
$AgNO_3$	<10	<0.02
$AgNO_3$ + R-glutathione[c]	4.8×10^4	88.9
$AgNO_3$ + KI[c]	4.3×10^4	79.5
AgI	3.9×10^4	72.2
MEM	5.4×10^4	

[a] Final concentrations of $AgNO_3$, R-glutathione, KI, and AgI in the virus preparations were 30, 10^3, 300, and 0.006 μM, respectively.

[b] Residual virus was assayed after exposure of the virus to the compound at 37 C for 60 min. PFU, Plaque-forming units.

[c] $AgNO_3$ and R-glutathione or $AgNO_3$ and KI were incubated at room temperature for 5 min after mixing and then were added to the virus preparation.

$AgNO_3$ may be due to the binding of ionizing Ag to the sulfhydryl groups in the virus.

Biological activities retained in $AgNO_3$-inactivated HSV. To investigate the steps by which replication of the $AgNO_3$-treated virus was prevented, we tested whether the inactivated virus retained some biological activities to the cells.

First, we tested the ability of the virus to adsorb to the cell surface. [^{3}H]thymidine-labeled HSV (12,000 counts/min per ml), which possessed an infectivity of 7×10^5, was divided into two equal portions. Infectivity of one portion of the virus was completely inactivated by exposure to 30 μM $AgNO_3$ at 37 C for 60 min. The other portion was incubated in PBS at 37 C for 60 min and served as an intact virus. Both virus preparations were diluted fourfold in MEM, and 1 ml of each was then inoculated into approximately 4×10^5 3T3 cells and incubated at 37 C. At intervals, radioactivities in the supernatant fluids and the cells were counted in a liquid scintillation spectrometer (Fig. 4). The results clearly show that the radioactivity of inactivated virus decreased in the supernatant fluids and increased in the cells, with time, at rates almost identical to those of intact virus. Simultaneously, the infectivity residues in the supernatant fluids were assayed in the cultures infected with intact virus (Fig. 4). The results show that the rates of decrease in radioactivities of both the intact and inactivated viruses were similar to that of the decrease in infectivity. This indicates that the HSV inactivated with $AgNO_3$ retained almost fully the activity of adsorbing to the cells.

A further attempt was made to test whether infection with the inactivated virus can induce the early surface changes and synthesis of viral antigens observed in the cells infected with intact HSV. The results clearly show that neither a hemadsorption phenomenon nor cell fusion and polykaryocytes occurred in the cells infected with the inactivated virus (Table 2). Neither surface nor intracellular viral antigens, as detected by immunofluorescence tests, were observed (Table 2).

Tevethia et al. have reported that, soon after

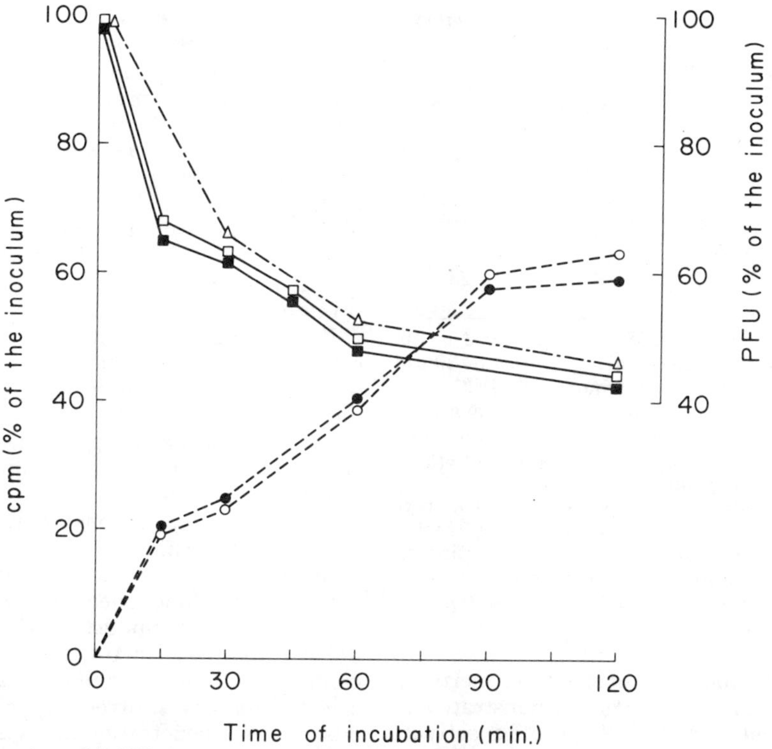

FIG. 4. *Adsorption of $AgNO_3$-inactivated HSV to the cells. Symbols: Circles represent the radioactivity in the cells—●, cells infected with $AgNO_3$-inactivated HSV; ○, cells infected with intact virus. Squares represent the radioactivity in the culture fluids—■, $AgNO_3$-inactivated HSV; □, intact virus. Triangles represent the infectivity in the supernatant fluids of the cultures infected with intact virus.*

infection, the cells infected with HSV showed agglutinability by ConA before production of infectious virus (11). We thus examined the agglutinability by ConA of cells infected with the $AgNO_3$-inactivated virus. The results clearly show that the chicken embryo cells infected with inactivated virus, as well as the cells infected with intact virus, were agglutinated in the presence of 250 μg of ConA per ml, by which the noninfected cells tested as a control were not agglutinated at all (Table 3). Hence, it would seem that infection of the inactivated virus underwent the early steps that produce certain cell surface changes responsible for ConA agglutinability, but not other surface changes and viral antigens.

DISCUSSION

It is well known that many agents exist that have potent antiviral properties against extracellular HSV (7) and that mercaptide-forming sulfhydryl reagents are a group of potent inactivators (9). The present report has shown that the inactivation of HSV by $AgNO_3$ is also probably attributable to the formation of mercaptides of Ag with the SH base of the virion components. Previous investigators have reported that the infectivities of many viruses other than HSV were also inactivated by 10^{-3} to 10^{-5} M mercuric compounds such as mercuric

TABLE 2. *Surface changes and antigen production in cells infected with intact and $AgNO_3$-inactivated HSV*[a]

Surface changes and antigen production	HSV[b]			
	Intact		$AgNO_3$-inactivated	
	6 h	20 h	6 h	20 h
Hemadsorption	1+	3+	0	0
Surface antigens	1+	4+	0	0
Intracellular antigens	1+	4+	0	0
Cell fusion and polykaryocytes	0	3+	0	0

[a] HSV-1 containing 5×10^5 $TCID_{50}$/ml, and its preparation inactivated by 30 μM $AgNO_3$ were diluted to one-fifth in MEM and inoculated into 10^5 3T3 cells. The infected cells were cultivated at 37 C and tested for their surface changes and production of viral antigens 6 and 20 h after infection.

[b] Positive reactions were graded form 1+ to 4+ depending upon the degree of reaction: 4+, almost all the cells were positive; 1+, less than one-fourth of the total cells were positive.

TABLE 3. *Agglutination by ConA of chicken embryo cells infected with $AgNO_3$-inactivated HSV-1*

Cells infected with:	Agglutination by ConA (μg/ml)		
	500	250	0
Intact HSV[a]	+++	++	−
$AgNO_3$-inactivated HSV[a]	++	++	−
Not infected (7.5 μM $AgNO_3$)[b]	−	−	−
Not infected	−	−	−

[a] A 1-ml amount of HSV-1 containing 2×10^6 $TCID_{50}$/ml and its preparation inactivated by 30 μM $AgNO_3$ were diluted to one-fourth in MEM. Two milliliters of each was inoculated into the monolayers of 10^6 chicken embryo cells in plastic petri dishes. The infected cells were then tested for agglutination by ConA as described in the text.

[b] To test whether $AgNO_3$ per se, of which trace amounts probably are residue in the $AgNO_3$-treated virus preparation, could induce ConA agglutinability, the cells were incubated in the presence of 7.5 μM $AgNO_3$ for 6 h at 37 C and then tested for their ConA agglutinability.

chloride, *p*-chloromercuribenzoate, or merthiolate (9). We have, however, demonstrated in this paper that 10^{-5} M $AgNO_3$ could inactivate specifically the infectivity of HSV at exposure times that did not affect the infectivity of other deoxyribonucleic acid or enveloped viruses or of ribonucleic acid or non-enveloped viruses tested so far. The biochemical basis for the differential inactivation of herpesviruses and other viruses is unknown. However, it was concluded that the sulfhydryl groups of the HSV virion may play an important role, more so than those in other viruses, in keeping the superficial structure required for the infectivity of the virus.

The present experiments have also demonstrated that $AgNO_3$ did not affect the rate of attachment of HSV to host cells. Philipson and Choppin (4, 9) have demonstrated that treatment with mercuric chloride and *p*-chloromercuribenzoate prevented the hemagglutination by many Echo- and Coxsackie viruses and the attachment of Echo-7 virus to host cells. In contrast, treatment with such sulfhydryl reagents have been shown not to have any effect on hemagglutination by fowl plague virus and other myxoviruses (9) and on attachment of fowl plague and vaccinia viruses to host cells (1). These results and our findings thus strongly suggest the possibility that the sulfhydryl groups in the enveloped viruses, in contrast to those in the non-enveloped viruses, are not involved in the adsorption of the virus to host cells.

It appears that $AgNO_3$ may prevent the multiplication of HSV at a certain step(s) of infection soon after attachment. The present paper does not indicate a precise step(s) after attachment responsible for the abortion of infection. Allison has presented some evidence indicating that after treatment with mercurials the uncoating of the vaccinia virus may not occur, although the virus has been taken up by the cells (1). Whether a similar mechanism exists for the inactivation of HSV by $AgNO_3$ is under investigation.

It is interesting to note that infection of the cells with $AgNO_3$-inactivated virus could induce ConA agglutinability, whereas it produced no virus-determined surface changes. Tevethia et al. have reported that the surface change leading to the agglutination of HSV-infected cells is caused by a virus-determined function but not by a nonspecific change due to virus-cell interaction (11). This may not be the case here, since it seems unlikely that the inactivated virus functioned as a genome determined only for the induction of ConA agglutinability and not for the other virus-specific changes. It seems more likely that certain nonspecific changes occurred in the steps of virus adsorption or penetration that were responsible for the induction of the ConA agglutinability obtained in our study.

ACKNOWLEDGMENT

We wish to thank Shoko Tanabe for her excellent assistance in preparation of the manuscript.

LITERATURE CITED

1. **Allison, A. C.** 1962. Observations on the inactivation of viruses by sulfhydryl reagents. Virology 17:176–183.
2. **Allison, A. C., F. E. Buckland, and C. H. Andrewes.** 1962. Effects of sulfhydryl reagents on infectivity of some viruses. Virology 17:171–175.
3. **Chang, Te-Wen, and L. Weinstein.** 1975. In vitro activity of silver sulfadiazine against *Herpesvirus hominis*. J. Infect. Dis. **132**:79–81.
4. **Choppin, P. W., and L. Philipson.** 1960. The inactivation of enterovirus infectivity by the sulfhydryl reagent p-chloromercuribenzoate. J. Exp. Med. **113**: 713–734.
5. **Coleman, V. R., J. Wilkie, W. E. Levinson, T. Stevens, and E. Jawetz.** 1973. Inactivation of *Herpesvirus hominis* types 1 and 2 by silver nitrate in vitro and in vivo. Antimicrob. Agents Chemother. 4:259–262.
6. **Inbar, M., and L. Sachs.** 1969. Interaction of the carbohydrate-binding protein concanavalin A with normal and transformed cells. Proc. Natl. Acad. Sci. U.S.A. 63:1418–1425.
7. **Levinson, W., V. Coleman, B. Woodson, A. Rabson, J. Lanier, J. Whitcher, and C. Dawson.** 1974. Inactivation of herpes simplex virus by thiosemicarbazones and certain cations. Antimicrob. Agents Chemother. 5:398–402.
8. **Lowry, O. H., N. J. Rosebrough, A. L. Farr, and R. J. Randall.** 1951. Protein measurement with the Folin phenol reagent. J. Biol. Chem. **193**:265–275.

9. **Philipson, L., and P. W. Choppin.** 1960. On the role of virus sulfhydryl groups in the attachment of enteroviruses to erythrocytes. J. Exp. Med. 112:455–478.
10. **Sery, T. W., and F. P. Furgiuels.** 1961. The inactivation of herpes-simplex virus by chemical agents. Am. J. Ophthalmol. 51:42–57.
11. **Tevethia, S. S., S. Lowry, W. E. Rawls, J. L. Melnick, and V. McMillan.** 1972. Detection of early cell surface changes in herpes simplex virus infected cells by agglutination with concanavalin A. J. Gen. Virol. 15:93–97.
12. **Watkins, J. F.** 1964. Adsorption of sensitized sheep erythrocytes to HeLa cells infected with herpes simplex virus. Nature (London) 202:1364–1365.

ANTIMICROBIAL AGENTS AND CHEMOTHERAPY, July 1976, p. 64-74
Vol. 10, No. 1

Antiviral Activity of Arabinosyladenine and Arabinosylhypoxanthine in Herpes Simplex Virus-Infected KB Cells: Selective Inhibition of Viral Deoxyribonucleic Acid Synthesis in the Presence of an Adenosine Deaminase Inhibitor

PAULINE M. SCHWARTZ,[1] CHARLES SHIPMAN, JR., and JOHN C. DRACH*

The Dental Research Institute, Department of Oral Biology, School of Dentistry; Department of Microbiology, School of Medicine; and Interdepartmental Graduate Program in Medicinal Chemistry, The University of Michigan, Ann Arbor, Michigan 48109*

Received for publication 29 December 1975

The antiviral activity of the fraudulent nucleoside arabinosyladenine (ara-A) against herpes simplex virus (HSV) type 1 was increased nearly 20-fold by the adenosine deaminase inhibitor, coformycin. The combination of ara-A plus coformycin was 90 times more potent in blocking HSV replication than was arabinosylhypoxanthine (ara-H). In suspension culture both drugs were more active than they were in monolayer culture. Deoxyribonucleic acid (DNA) synthesis also was inhibited by the nucleosides. Depending upon the species of DNA examined, ara-A was 8 to 15 times more active in the presence of coformycin, and the combination was 35 to 70 times more potent than ara-H. Both drugs inhibited total DNA synthesis to the same extent in uninfected and HSV-infected KB cells. In contrast, viral DNA synthesis was three to six times more susceptible to inhibition than was cellular DNA synthesis. Inhibition of viral DNA synthesis was more pronounced in suspension culture than in monolayer culture. However, the method of cell propagation did not alter the degree to which the drugs inhibited DNA synthesis in uninfected KB cells. An index has been derived to quantitate the extent of the selective inhibition of viral or cellular DNA synthesis. Fifty percent inhibitory concentrations of a drug were calculated for uninfected KB DNA synthesis and viral DNA synthesis and expressed as a ratio. The logarithm of this ratio was termed the selective index and was positive if viral DNA synthesis was inhibited preferentially or negative if uninfected KB DNA synthesis was more strongly inhibited. Data from experiments performed in monolayer culture gave positive selective index values of 0.3, 0.5, and 0.4 for ara-A plus coformycin, ara-A, and ara-H, respectively. Values of 0.7 and 0.6 were obtained from suspension culture data for ara-A plus coformycin and ara-H, respectively. Considered collectively, the data presented in this communication establish that coformycin increased the potency of ara-A but did not increase its selectivity.

The fraudulent nucleoside 9-β-D-arabinofuranosyladenine (ara-A) is active against a broad spectrum of deoxyribonucleic acid (DNA) viruses, including herpes simplex virus (HSV) type 1 (4, 21, 25, 28). In cell culture ara-A significantly reduced viral replication at drug concentrations that had no cytotoxic effect in uninfected cultures (13, 25, 27). In experimental animals, ara-A has been shown to be effective against several DNA virus infections without significant host toxicity (9, 21, 28). Early clinical studies in humans have indicated its usefulness against herpetic keratitis and cases of disseminated herpes zoster infection without significant toxicity (18).

Deamination of ara-A by adenosine deaminase from many sources yields 9-β-D-arabinofuranosylhypoxanthine (ara-H) (4, 10). Although ara-H also is active against DNA viruses, it is considerably less active than ara-A (21, 25, 28). Consequently, inhibitors of adenosine deaminase have been developed to potentiate the activity of ara-A. Investigators at Parke, Davis and Co. first noted in 1967 that such an inhibitor (covidarabine [31]) increased

[1] Present address: LAC/USC Cancer Center, 1720 Zonal Ave., Los Angeles, Calif. 90033.

the antiviral potency of ara-A (25). This observation recently was confirmed by us (P. M. Schwartz, C. Shipman, Jr., and J. C. Drach, Prog. Abstr. Intersci. Conf. Antimicrob. Agents Chemother., 14th, San Francisco, Abstr. 33, 1974) using coformycin (15) and by Bryson and Conner (2) and Conner et al. (5) using covidarabine. Plunkett and Cohen (19) have reported that the antiproliferative activity of ara-A also could be increased through the use of erythro-9-(2-hydroxy-3-nonyl)adenine, another potent inhibitor of adenosine deaminase (22).

Based upon experience in both cell culture and whole animals, the activity of ara-A and ara-H seems to be selective. In animal models the drugs exhibit antiviral activity at nontoxic doses, and in cell culture the nucleosides appear to affect virus-infected cells to a greater extent than uninfected cells. For example, Sidwell and Huffman (27) found that ara-A inhibited HSV-induced cytopathic effects at drug levels that did not produce cytotoxic effects in uninfected cultures. Shannon et al. (24) reported significant inhibition of Gross murine leukemia virus-induced plaque formation by ara-A at concentrations that produced no cytotoxicity in uninfected cells. In part I of this series, Shipman et al. (26) established that the selective activity of ara-A and ara-H could be observed at the level of DNA synthesis. Specifically, HSV DNA synthesis was inhibited to a greater extent by ara-A and ara-H than was cellular DNA synthesis in synchronous cultures of KB cells.

As a concurrent approach to a more detailed understanding of the biochemical action of ara-A, we addressed two points not considered in the first part of this series (26): namely, (i) was the selective inhibition of viral DNA synthesis dependent upon the use of synchronized cell cultures and (ii) did ara-A act selectively if it was used in concert with an adenosine deaminase inhibitor? We now have examined the activity of ara-A and ara-H in asynchronous cultures of KB cells using the same strain of HSV as studied previously (26). Here we present evidence that ara-A and ara-H are selective inhibitors of viral DNA synthesis regardless of the method used for cell propagtion and that coformycin did not alter the selectivity of ara-A.

(This investigation is based on portions of a dissertation submitted by P. M. Schwartz in partial fullfillment of the requirements for the Ph.D. degree in Medicinal Chemistry.)

MATERIALS AND METHODS

Materials. Coformycin was provided through the courtesy of H. Umezawa, Institute of Microbial Chemistry, Tokyo, Japan. All other chemicals, radioisotopes, and sera were obtained as noted in the preceding communication (26).

Cell culture techniques. The source of cells and HSV; the routine growth and passage of BHK-21/4 cells and KB cells; the propagation and titration of HSV; and techniques used for the enumeration of cells, the determination of cell viability, and the detection of mycoplasma contamination have been described previously (26).

Statistical analyses. Dose-response relationships were constructed by linearly regressing probit values of the percentage of inhibition of DNA synthesis or plaque formation against log drug concentrations. The 50% inhibitory (I_{50}) concentrations and the 95% confidence intervals were calculated from the regression lines using the methods described by Goldstein (8). Identity of any two dose-response curves was tested using one-way covariance analysis (7) by calculating P values for the equality of the regressions and slopes. The slopes of all the pairs of dose-response curves compared in this study were similar ($P > 0.350$), consequently P values given in the text refer only to the comparison of regressions.

Protocol for studies in monolayer cultures. KB cells were planted in plastic tissue culture flasks (75-cm^2 surface area) (Falcon Plastics, Oxnard, Calif.) 18 to 24 h before infection with HSV. At the onset of experiments, logarithmically growing, replicate, monolayer cultures were 60 to 70% confluent and contained 4×10^6 to 6×10^6 cells per flask. The medium was decanted, and the cultures were infected with 10 plaque-forming units (PFU) of HSV per cell. The HSV was contained in 1.0 ml of minimal essential medium (MEM) with Hanks salts supplemented with 10% unheated calf serum. Mock-infected monolayer cultures received 1.0 ml of medium alone. After a 1-h adsorption period at 37 C, the cell sheet was rinsed twice with 5 ml of MEM with Hanks salts to remove unabsorbed virus, and 10.0 ml of medium containing [^{3}H]thymidine (dThd) (5 μM, 2 or 3 μCi/ml), 2× arginine and 10% heated calf serum (23) was added. Medium also contained ara-A, with or without 3.5 μM coformycin, or ara-H, as illustrated in Fig. 1. Drugs were added to the medium at the selected concentrations immediately before use. After a 12-h incubation at 37 C, 0.5 ml of 0.25 mM ethylenediaminetetraacetate was added to uninfected monolayer cultures, and after several minutes at 37 C flasks were shaken to suspend the cells. Infected monolayers were shaken to suspend cells, and 1.0-ml samples were removed and stored at −76 C for subsequent virus assay. Ethylenediaminetetraacete (0.45 ml) then was added to the remaining medium. Samples of the cells were utilized to determine cell number and viability. One hundred-microliter portions of the suspensions also were spotted in triplicate on filter paper circles which were processed for the determination of incorporated label as described previously (26). Data were tabulated on the basis of tritium incorporated into acid-insoluble material per 10^3 cells. Inhibition of DNA synthesis was determined at the various drug levels as a percentage of a control without drugs. Five-milliliter portions of infected cell suspensions were centrifuged at 600 × g for 5 min, and the pellets were stored at −76 C for subsequent sepa-

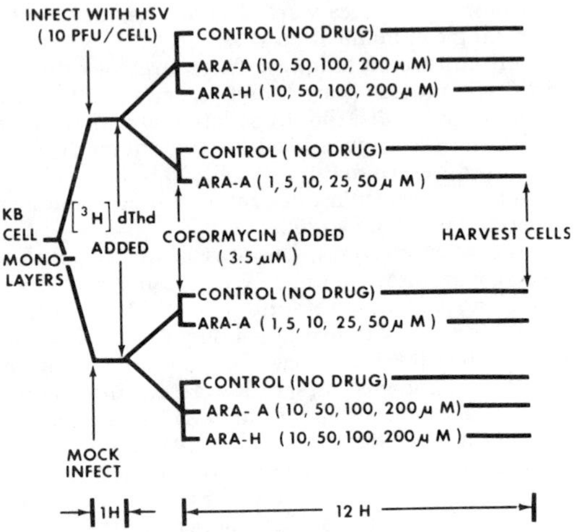

FIG. 1. *Experimental protocol for studies performed in monolayer cultures. In all experiments in volving ara-A plus coformycin, the inhibitor also was present in the corresponding control flasks.*

ration of viral and cellular DNA. After isopycnic centrifugation in CsCl gradients (see reference 26), the amount of label was proportioned between viral and cellular DNA on the basis of peak areas. Areas were determined by integration after the peaks were fully separated using a Dupont 310 curve resolver set to fit Lorentzian distribution curves.

Protocol for studies in suspension cultures. Suspension cultures of KB cells were grown and maintained as described previously (26). Logarithmically growing cultures were used in experiments 5 to 14 days after their initiation from a monolayer culture. The general protocol for experiments in suspension cultures was that depicted in Fig. 1 with the following differences: (i) no studies were performed with ara-A alone, and (ii) all experiments were modified to take advantage of multiple sampling times. Thus, 400 ml of cell suspension from a single spinner flask was centrifued at 300 × *g* for 10 min at 4 C. All but 5 ml of the supernatant was removed and the loose pellet was suspended by gentle swirling. Suspended cells were infected with HSV to give 2 or 3 PFU/cell in a total volume of approximately 5 ml. Infective center assays established that 82% of the cells were infected resulting in an actual multiplicity of infection (MOI) of 0.9 or 1.4. Both virus-infected and mock-infected suspensions were kept at room temperature for 1 h and swirled periodically. To remove unadsorbed virus, cells were resuspended in 30 to 50 ml of MEM with spinner salts, and centrifuged again. After removal of the supernatant medium, the virus- and mock-infected cells were resuspended at a final density of 2×10^5 to 3×10^5 cells/ml and split into four separate spinner flasks. Each flask contained 100 ml of MEM with spinner salts buffered with 10 mM HEPES [*N*-2-hydroxyethyl-piperazine-N'-2-ethanesulfonic acid] (pH 7.2 at 37 C), 2× arginine, 10% extensively heated calf serum (23), [^{3}H]dThd (5 μM, 3 μCi/ml), and selected concentrations of ara-A plus 3.5 μM coformycin or ara-H. The flasks were incubated at 37 C, and portions of the suspension were removed at selected times for the subsequent determination of cell number, cell viability, incorporated label, virus titer, and the separation of cellular and viral DNA species. Portion volumes and methods of determination were similar to those described in the preceding section.

RESULTS

The effects of ara-A and ara-H on virion replication and DNA synthesis were examined in asynchronous populations of KB cells so that a direct comparison could be made with the data obtained in synchronized cultures (26). Coformycin (3.5 μM) also was included in the experiments with ara-A to determine whether the selectivity observed previously might be a consequence of deamination of ara-A to ara-H.

Studies in suspension culture. Virion production was examined after HSV-infected KB cells were exposed to selected concentrations of the drugs for 12 h. During this time there was no decrease in viability of uninfected cells as measured by trypan blue dye exclusion. Ara-A in the presence of coformycin reduced HSV replication by 50% at a concentration of approximately 0.5 μM, whereas 68 μM ara-H was required to produce the same effect (Table 1, Fig. 2). Coformycin alone did not affect HSV replication at a concentration that completely blocked the deamination of ara-A (3.5 μM).

Incorporation of labeled dThd into acid-insoluble material was examined in these cultures and in corresponding mock-infected cultures. In the absence of drugs uninfected KB cells incorporated label at a constant rate during a 12-h period. HSV-infected cultures also incorporated label at this rate for 3 h, after which the rate increased owing to the synthesis of viral DNA (Fig. 3, inset). In the presence of drug, label incorporation was reduced at all times examined. On the basis of the percentage of label incorporated in the absence of drugs, maximal inhibition was observed from 6 to 12 h. Data obtained after a 12-h exposure to [^{3}H]dThd and drug is presented in Fig. 3. Comparisons of dose-response relationships as described in Materials and Methods revealed that total DNA synthesis was inhibited to the same extent in mock-infected and HSV-infected cultures by both drugs ($P = 0.383$ for ara-A plus coformycin and $P = 0.829$ for ara-H).

Lysates also were prepared from the HSV-infected cells and were subjected to isopycnic centrifugation in CsCl gradients to separate cellular and viral DNA. The amount of label incorporated into each DNA species increased for 12 h after virus adsorption both in the absence of drug and in the presence of 10 μM ara-

TABLE 1. *Inhibition of HSV replication and DNA synthesis by ara-A and ara-H*

Method of culture propagation	Parameter measured	50% inhibitory concentrations (μM) and corresponding 95% confidence interval[a]		
		Ara-A plus 3.5 μM coformycin	Ara-A	Ara-H
Monolayer	HSV replication	2.1 (1.0–4.6)	43 (29–65)	191 (137–265)
	Viral DNA synthesis	2.6 (2.0–3.3)	20 (13–30)	126 (88–182)
	Cellular DNA synthesis[b]	8.0 (6.1–10.5)	67 (34–129)	1790 (710–4,490)[c]
	Uninfected KB DNA synthesis	4.9 (4.4–5.4)	62 (45–85)	309 (165–578)
Suspension	HSV replication	0.5[d]		69[d]
	Viral DNA synthesis	0.9[d]		60[d]
	Cellular DNA synthesis[b]	5.1[d]		179[d]
	Uninfected KB DNA synthesis	5.0[d]		226[d]
Synchronized suspension[e]	HSV replication		15 (9.8–25)	33 (15–75)
	Viral DNA synthesis		7 (3.4–14)	18 (12–28)
	Cellular DNA synthesis[b]		37 (14–97)	45 (10–206)
	Uninfected KB DNA synthesis		86 (59–126)	253 (153–416)

[a] That range of values which, at the 95% confidence level, contains the true value.
[b] In HSV-infected KB cells.
[c] $r^2 < 0.2$ for fit of data points to dose-response curve.
[d] Not determined owing to insufficient data.
[e] Calculated from the data of Shipman et al. (26).

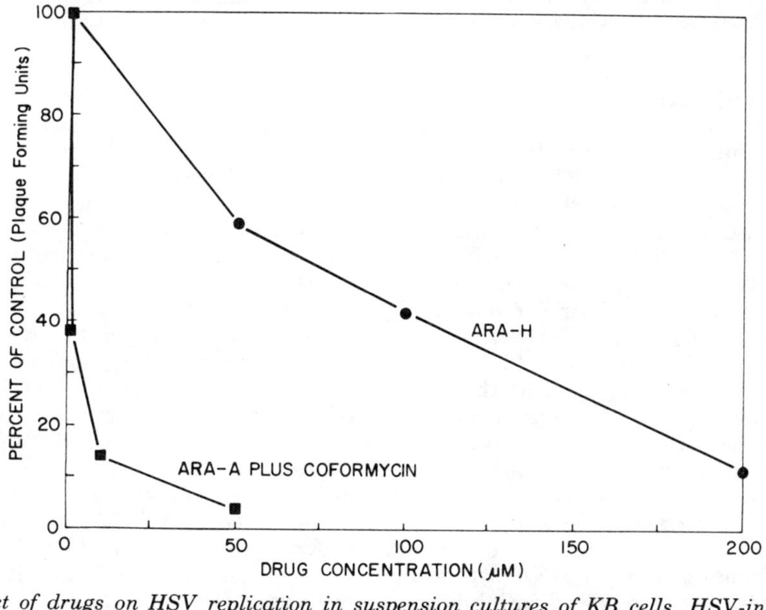

FIG. 2. *Effect of drugs on HSV replication in suspension cultures of KB cells. HSV-infected cultures contained no drug or selected concentrations of ara-A plus 3.5 μM coformycin or ara-H. Samples of virus-infected cells were disrupted by freeze-thawing and were assayed for plaque-forming ability on BHK-21/4 cells. Each assay was performed in triplicate, and the mean is expressed as a percentage of the number of plaques formed by samples from an infected culture without drug.*

A plus coformycin. No additional labeling occurred for up to 25 h. Figure 4 illustrates the separation of the two DNA species and shows the effects of ara-A plus 3.5 μM coformycin (Fig. 4A) and ara-H (Fig. 4B) on the amount of [^{3}H]dThd incorporated during 12 h of labeling. As is evident from the figure, viral DNA synthesis was inhibited to a significantly greater extent than was cellular DNA synthesis within the infected cell ($P = 0.022$ for both drugs). A

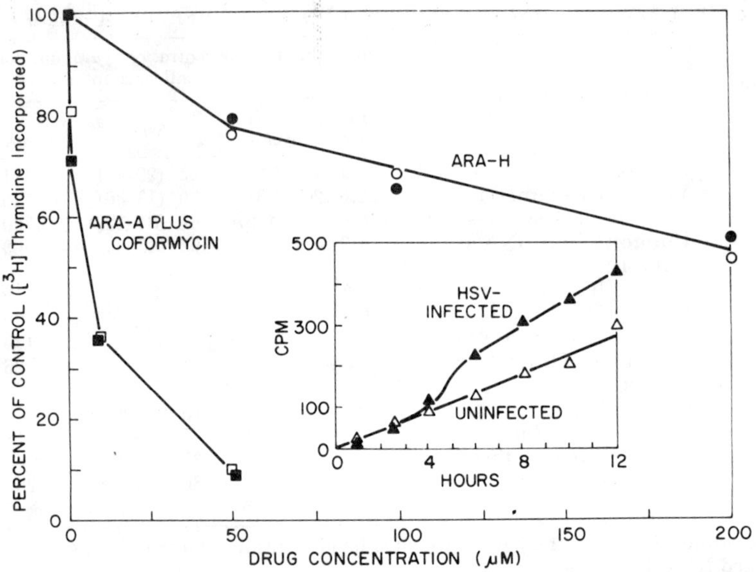

FIG. 3. *Effect of drugs on incorporation of [^{3}H]dThd into DNA of KB cells grown in suspension culture. HSV-infected cultures described in Fig. 2 (closed symbols) and corresponding mock-infected cultures (open symbols) were exposed to [^{3}H]dThd and drugs. Assays were performed in triplicate and expressed as a percentage of the amount of label incorporated by cultures that contained no drug. The amount of label incorporated per 10^3 cells in the absence of drug (the control cultures in the ara-A experiment) is shown in the inset.*

similar relationship existed between inhibition of viral DNA synthesis and inhibition of DNA synthesis in uninfected KB cells ($P = 0.025$ for ara-A plus coformycin, $P = 0.037$ for ara-H). I_{50} concentrations were calculated from dose-response relationships (see Materials and Methods) to quantitate the inhibition of DNA synthesis by the two drugs. These results, along with those for inhibition of HSV replication, are summarized in Table 1. Cellular DNA synthesis in HSV-infected cells required I_{50} concentrations approximately the same as those required in uninfected cells. In contrast, significantly lower concentrations of the two nucleosides were required for 50% inhibition of viral DNA synthesis.

There was close correspondence between the I_{50} concentration of ara-A plus coformycin required for inhibition of viral DNA synthesis and the I_{50} concentration required for inhibition of virion production. A similar relationship existed for ara-H (Table 1). Furthermore, virtually identical dose-response relationships existed for inhibition of viral DNA synthesis and inhibition of virion production by both drugs ($P = 0.776$ for ara-A plus coformycin, $P = 0.842$ for ara-H).

Studies in monolayer culture. Monolayer cultures of KB cells mock-infected or infected with HSV were used for more extensive comparisons of ara-A, with or without coformycin, and ara-H. The effect of a 12-h exposure to these drugs on HSV replication is presented in Fig. 5. Calculation of I_{50} concentrations from these data showed that in the presence of 3.5 μM coformycin, 2.1 μM ara-A was required to inhibit HSV production by 50%, whereas in the absence of the adenosine deaminase inhibitor 43 μM ara-A or 190 μM ara-H was required (Table 1).

Labeled dThd incorporation was measured in these and corresponding mock-infected cultures after the 12-h exposure to [^{3}H]dThd and drugs. Figure 6 illustrates the inhibition of label incorporation by each nucleoside. Comparison of dose-response curves shows that total DNA synthesis was inhibited to the same extent in mock-infected and HSV-infected cultures by ara-A plus coformycin ($P = 0.525$) or ara-H ($P = 0.692$). In contrast, ara-A inhibited total DNA synthesis in HSV-infected cultures to a greater extent than it inhibited DNA synthesis in uninfected cultures ($P = 0.015$). An I_{50} concentration of 31 μM was required in the former case, and a 62 μM concentration was required in the latter.

Viral and cellular DNA from the HSV-infected monolayer cultures was separated as detailed above, and drug effects were noted. In all cases examined, except in one experiment at 10 μM ara-H, viral DNA synthesis was inhibited more strongly than was cellular DNA synthesis (Fig. 7). All dose-response curves representing

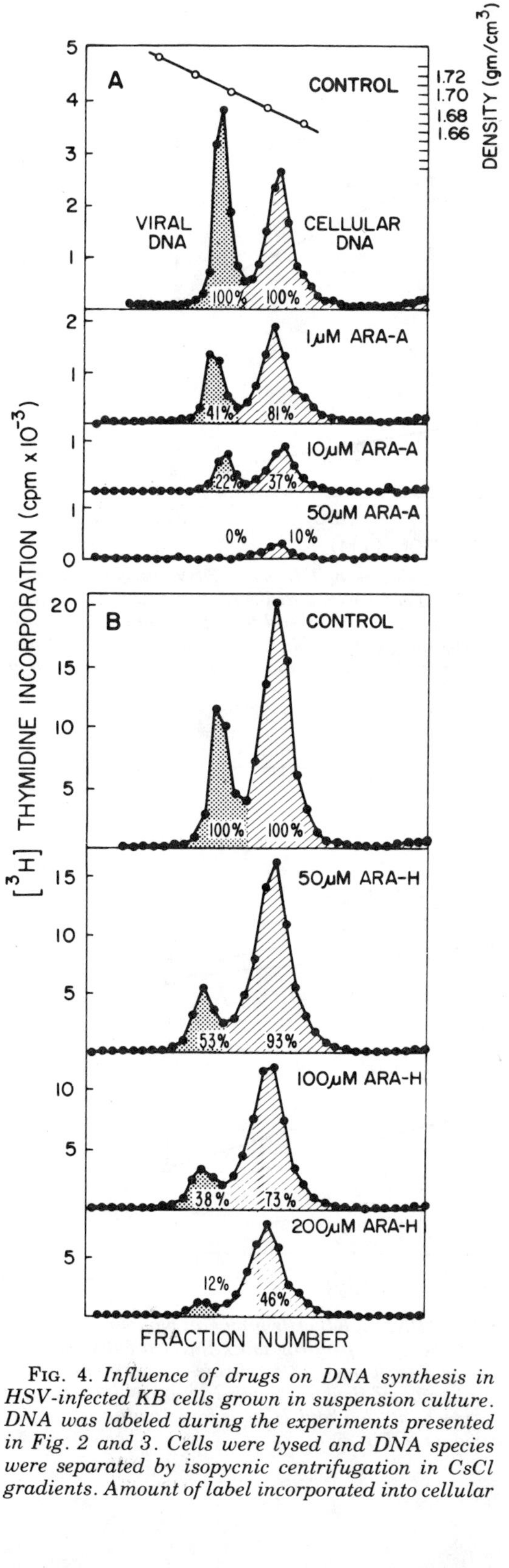

FIG. 4. *Influence of drugs on DNA synthesis in HSV-infected KB cells grown in suspension culture. DNA was labeled during the experiments presented in Fig. 2 and 3. Cells were lysed and DNA species were separated by isopycnic centrifugation in CsCl gradients. Amount of label incorporated into cellular and viral DNA in the presence of selected concentrations of ara-A plus 3.5 μM coformycin (A) or ara-H (B) is expressed as a percentage of the amount incorporated into the respective DNA species in cell cultures without drugs.*

inhibition of viral DNA synthesis differed significantly ($P \lesssim 0.014$) from the corresponding curves representing inhibition of cellular DNA synthesis (Fig. 7). Similar significant differences ($P \lesssim 0.023$) existed between inhibition of viral DNA synthesis and inhibition of DNA synthesis in uninfected KB cells (Fig. 6). As in suspension cultures, significantly lower concentrations of ara-A plus coformycin, ara-A, or ara-H were required for inhibition of viral DNA synthesis than were required for the same inhibition of cellular DNA synthesis in either uninfected or HSV-infected cells (Table 1).

Correspondence between inhibition of viral DNA synthesis and inhibition of HSV replication production was not as good as that observed in suspension cultures. I_{50} concentrations differed more widely (see Table 1), and dose-response curves were dissimilar ($P = 0.086$ and 0.010 for ara-A and ara-H, respectively). On the other hand there was agreement in I_{50} concentrations and dose-response curves ($P = 0.273$) for ara-A in the presence of coformycin.

DISCUSSION

Ara-A and ara-H inhibited the replication of HSV type 1 in KB cells. Experiments in monolayer culture demonstrated that the antiviral activity of ara-A was approximately four times greater than that of ara-H. The potency of ara-A, however, depends directly upon the rate of deamination to ara-H. This, in turn, depends upon the type of cells studied, the number of cells present, and the length of the incubation (29; C. Shipman, J. N. Sandberg, P. M. Schwartz, and J. C. Drach, Prog. Abstr. Intersci. Conf. Antimicrob. Agents Chemother., 15th, Washington, D.C., Abstr. 358, 1975). To eliminate these variables, the activity of ara-A was measured in the presence of coformycin, an adenosine deaminase inhibitor. Coformycin itself was devoid of antiviral activity at the concentration used in this study and in a study by Williams and Lerner (30). In the presence of coformycin, 2.1 μM ara-A inhibited viral replication by 50% compared with 43 μM ara-A required in its absence. Thus, ara-A plus coformycin was 90 times more effective as an antiviral agent than ara-H when assayed in monolayer cultures. In comparison, Bryson and Conner (2) reported that 1.8 μM ara-A plus covidarabine inhibited varicella zoster virus replication by 50% and the combination was 40- to 50-fold

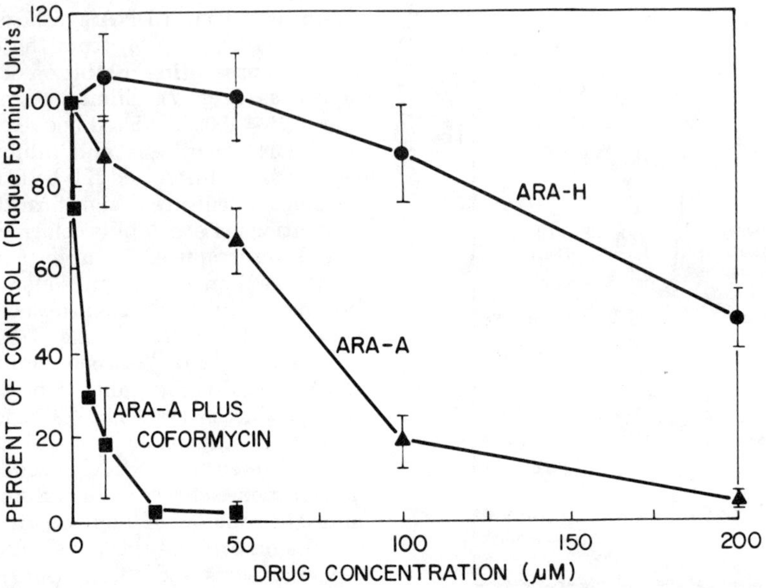

FIG. 5. *Effect of drugs on HSV replication in monolayer cultures of KB cells. HSV-infected cultures contained no drug or selected concentrations of ara-A plus 3.5 μM coformycin, ara-A alone, or ara-H. Portions from cultures were assayed for plaque-forming ability as described in the legend to Fig. 2. Data points with vertical bars represent the mean ± standard error of six (ara-A plus coformycin), three (ara-A), or four (ara-H) separate determinations. Points without bars are the means of two determinations. Each determination was performed in triplicate.*

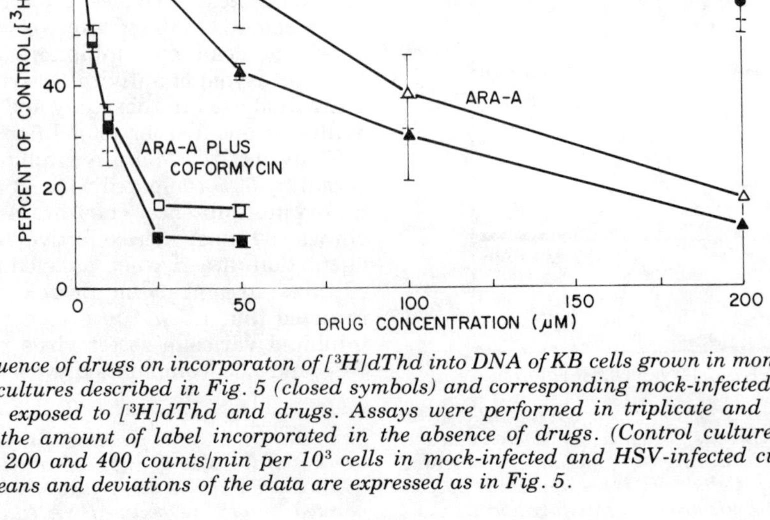

FIG. 6. *Influence of drugs on incorporaton of [^{3}H]dThd into DNA of KB cells grown in monolayer culture. HSV-infected cultures described in Fig. 5 (closed symbols) and corresponding mock-infected cultures (open symbols) were exposed to [^{3}H]dThd and drugs. Assays were performed in triplicate and expressed as a percentage of the amount of label incorporated in the absence of drugs. (Control cultures incorporated approximately 200 and 400 counts/min per 10^3 cells in mock-infected and HSV-infected cultures, respectively.) The means and deviations of the data are expressed as in Fig. 5.*

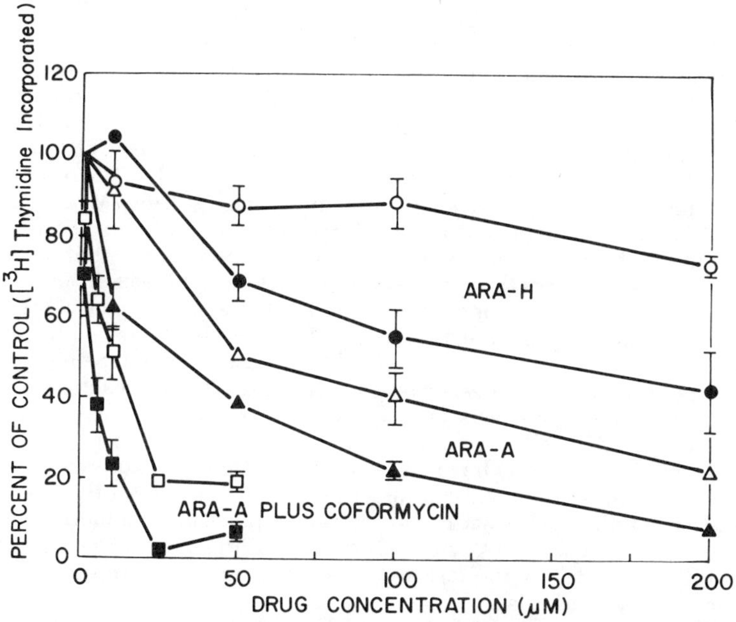

FIG. 7. *Effect of drugs on DNA synthesis in HSV-infected KB cells grown in monolayer culture. DNA was labeled in the experiments depicted in Fig. 5 and 6, and viral DNA was separated from cellular DNA by isopycnic centrifugation. The amount of label incorporated into viral DNA (closed symbols) and cellular DNA (open symbols) is expressed as a percentage of the amount incorporated into the respective DNA species in cell cultures without drugs. The means and deviations of the data are expressed as in Fig. 5.*

more potent than ara-H. Both ara-A and ara-H were more active in suspension cultures than they were in monolayer cultures (Table 1). Furthermore, comparisons with data obtained in the companion study (26) also showed that ara-A and ara-H had more antiviral activity in synchronized suspension cultures than in monolayer cultures. For example, the I_{50} concentration for ara-H in monolayer cultures was 191 μM compared with 33 μM in synchronized suspension cultures (without overlap of confidence intervals). The I_{50} concentration for ara-H in asynchronous suspension cultures (69 μM) also appeared to be lower than in monolayer cultures. No conclusions can be drawn, however, about similarities or differences in activity between synchronous and asynchronous suspension cultures without more data from the latter system. The reasons for the differences in drug potency between monolayer and suspension cultures are unknown but may reflect differences in the multiplicities of HSV infection. Monolayer cell sheets were infected at an MOI of 10 for 1 h at 37 C, whereas suspension cultures were infected at an MOI of 0.9 or 1.4 in a slurry for 1 h at room temperature. The former cultures produced 40 to 80 PFU/cell compared with a yield of 2 to 5 PFU/cell from the latter. Hence, the drugs were more active in cells infected at the lower multiplicity. Miller et al. (13) and Marks (12) also observed that ara-A was more effective in blocking replication of HSV or cytomegalovirus at lower MOIs.

Ara-A was a more potent inhibitor of DNA synthesis than was ara-H and was most potent in the presence of coformycin. Although there was some variation depending on the type of DNA synthesis examined or the culture conditions utilized, ara-A was two to six times more potent than ara-H and, in the presence of coformycin, was 35 to 70 times more potent. Differences in drug activities from monolayer to suspension cultures are most informative. As with inhibition of HSV replication, inhibition of viral DNA synthesis was more pronounced in suspension cultures than in monolayers. In contrast, the method of cell propagation did not alter the effectiveness of drugs on DNA synthesis in uninfected KB cells. For example, 126, 60, and 18 μM ara-H were required to inhibit viral DNA synthesis by 50% in monolayer, asynchronous, and synchronous suspension cultures, respectively (Table 1). The first and last values clearly are different, with no overlap of confidence intervals. However, 309, 226, and 253 μM ara-H were required to inhibit DNA synthesis in uninfected KB cells by 50%. Based upon the coincidence of confidence intervals, these values are virtually the same. Although our data are not as complete, a similar situation existed for the activity of ara-A, with or without coformycin. The relationship between the method of cell propagation and the effect of drugs on cellular DNA synthesis in HSV-infected cells is less clear. Cellular DNA synthesis appeared to be more susceptible to inhibition by ara-A and ara-H in synchronized cell cultures than it was in either asynchronous suspension or monolayer cultures. We are currently unable to explain this phenomenon.

In all experiments viral DNA synthesis was inhibited to a greater extent than was DNA synthesis in uninfected KB cells. To more clearly define this relationship, we have derived an index that quantitates the preferential inhibition of viral or cellular DNA synthesis. The I_{50} concentration of a drug for DNA synthesis in uninfected cells is divided by the I_{50} concentration for viral DNA synthesis. We have termed the logarithm of this ratio the selective index (SI) (additional details may be found in Drach and Shipman, Third Conf. on Antiviral Substances, New York Academy of Sciences, 1976). It is positive if viral DNA synthesis is inhibited preferentially and negative if uninfected cellular DNA synthesis is more strongly inhibited. Owing to the range of values defined by the 95% confidence intervals of the component I_{50} concentrations, differences of 0.1 to 0.2 units probably are not meaningful. Table 2 gives SI values for the cases presented in this and the prior communication (26). All values were positive and were similar for each nucleoside tested under the same culture conditions. Growth of cells in suspension cultures resulted in the greatest selectivity because of the increased drug sensitivity of viral DNA synthesis. On the other hand, inhibition of adenosine deaminase by coformycin did not affect the selectivity of ara-A even though it greatly increased the potency of the drug.

Bennett et al. (1) also have reported that ara-A acts selectively. Their observations were based, however, on a comparison between inhibition of DNA synthesis in uninfected HEp-2 cells and inhibition of total, not viral alone, DNA synthesis in HSV-infected cells. In this system ara-A inhibited dThd incorporation only in HSV-infected cells. The nearly complete lack of inhibition by 375 μM ara-A in uninfected HEp-2 cells is quite surprising and contrasts with our observation that 62 μM ara-A inhibited DNA synthesis in uninfected KB cells by 50%. The apparent lack of inhibition in HEp-2 cells may be explained on the basis of a threefold increase in the labeling of soluble dThd nucleotides (1). Our results also showed selectivity based on total DNA synthesis, but only with ara-A in the absence of coformycin. We speculate that the differential effect on total DNA synthesis was not the result of a selective action of the drug on a biochemical system, but rather was the result of a more extensive deamination of ara-A by the less perturbed uninfected cells.

The possibility that ara-A did not act selectively against viral DNA synthesis must be considered. In this and the prior (26) article the incorporation of [^{3}H]dThd into acid-precipitable material has been equated with DNA synthesis. We have not ruled out the possibility that the selective effect was the result of differential changes in the specific activity of [^{3}H]dThd that might accompany drug treatment or HSV infection. HSV infection does increase dThd nucleotide pools in mammalian cells (3, 16, 20), but for changes in pool sizes to explain the selective effect, it would be necessary for cellular and viral DNA to be synthesized from separate nuclear dThd nucleotide pools in HSV-infected cells which changed independently with changes in drug concentration. In a separate study we (Drach et al., unpublished observations) have found that 120 μM ara-A did not alter the labeling of dThd nucleotides in B-mix K-44/6 cells. The recent data of Müller et al. (W. E. G. Müller, R. K. Zahn, K. Bittlingmaier, and D. Falke, Ann. N.Y. Acad. Sci., in press) also support the conclusion that we measured a selective inhibition of DNA synthesis and not just of [^{3}H]dThd incorporation. The 5′-triphosphate of ara-A was found to be a more potent inhibitor of HSV DNA polymerase than of cellular DNA polymerases (K_i = 0.14, 7.4, and 5.6 μM, respectively, for HSV and α- and β-DNA polymerases). Such differences are adequate to account for the selectivity we have noted. Nonetheless, experimental determination of the specific activity of [^{3}H]dThd incorporated into DNA will be required to totally resolve the issue.

TABLE 2. *Selective indexes for ara-A and ara-H*

Method of culture propagation	SI value		
	Ara-A plus 3.5 μM coformycin	Ara-A	Ara-H
Monolayer	0.3	0.5	0.4
Suspension	0.7		0.6
Synchronized suspension[a]		1.1	1.1

[a] Calculated from the data of Shipman et al. (26).

If ara-A acted selectively against viral DNA synthesis, the additional question arises of whether or not this action was responsible for the differential effects on virion and cell viability. Several studies (see reference 25) have demonstrated antiviral activity for ara-A at dose levels that were not cytotoxic to uninfected cells. As discussed previously (26), this differential sensitivity could arise because HSV-induced enzymes involved in DNA metabolism were preferentially susceptible to ara-A or its nucleotides, thereby resulting in selective toxicity to HSV-infected cells. Nonetheless, other mechanisms also may be operative. The greatest antiviral effects occurred when ara-A was added from 2 h before to 3 h after virus adsorption (1, 26), indicating that if ara-A was present during viral DNA synthesis then antiviral activity was expressed. When ara-A is used without adenosine deaminase inhibitors, it is metabolized, and therefore is present only for a limited time. This restricted exposure of HSV-infected cells to ara-A apparently is adequate to decisively inhibit viral DNA synthesis and hence virion replication. Uninfected cells, on the other hand, recover from a limited exposure to ara-A. We (C. Shipman, J. Novack, and J. C. Drach, Fed. Proc. 32:699, 1973) have observed that B-mix K-44/6 cells inhibited by 600 μM ara-A resumed growth after the removal of the drug. Similarly Cohen et al. (6, 17) found that L cells resumed multiplication after a 9- or 10-h exposure to 200 μM ara-A. Müller et al. (14) also noted that the inhibitory effect of ara-A was completely reversible over a limited concentration range. Furthermore, LePage (11) found the Ehrlich carcinoma ascites cells recovered their ability to synthesize DNA as ara-A levels declined in host animals. An entirely different situation may exist if the metabolism of ara-A is blocked. Even though we observed no decrease in cell viability (as measured by trypan blue dye exclusion) during the 12-h exposure of KB cells to ara-A plus coformycin, Plunkett and Cohen (19) have reported that cytostatic concentrations of ara-A become lethal to 99.9% of L cells in the presence of an adenosine deaminase inhibitor. Viability did not decline, however, until 24 to 36 h after the addition of up to 20 μM ara-A. It is conceivable, therefore, that, although KB cells appeared to be viable after the 12-h exposure to ara-A plus coformycin, irreversible damage had been done but would not be expressed until later in the replication cycle. If this were the case, then the selective inhibition of viral DNA synthesis in the presence of coformycin would not translate into selective action at the cellular level. Consequently, the selectivity of ara-A at the cellular level may depend not only upon selective inhibition of viral DNA synthesis, but also upon its subsequent metabolism to ara-H.

Selectivity of drug action in vivo, defined as the ability of ara-A to inhibit viral replication at nontoxic doses, probably is more complex. In addition to the two factors mentioned above, the total cellular and physiological disposition of the drug also would be involved. Therefore, it is of considerable interest to learn what contribution the selective inhibition of viral DNA synthesis makes to the overall selectivity of drug action in vivo. Our in vitro studies predict that in vivo ara-A plus coformycin should be more potent than ara-A, but no more selective (see Tables 1 and 2). The antiviral and toxicological evaluation of ara-A plus an adenosine deaminase inhibitor in experimental animals should provide an interesting test of this prediction.

ACKNOWLEDGMENTS

This work was supported by Public Health Service grant DE 02731 from the National Institute of Dental Research. P. M. S. was supported in part by Public Health Service training grant GM 02010 from the National Institute of General Medical Sciences and was an AFPE Pharmaceutical Manufacturers Association Fellow.

We thank Jean Sandberg and Sandra H. Smith for their excellent technical assistance and Charles J. Kowalski for his help with the statistical methods.

LITERATURE CITED

1. **Bennett, L. L., Jr., W. M. Shannon, P. W. Allan, and G. Arnett.** 1975. Studies on the biochemical basis for the antiviral activities of some nucleoside analogs. Ann. N. Y. Acad. Sci. **255**:342–358.
2. **Bryson, Y. D., and J. D. Connor.** 1976. In vitro susceptibility of varicella-zoster virus to adenine arabinoside and hypoxanthine arabinoside. Antimicrob. Agents Chemother. **9**:540–543.
3. **Cheng, Y. C., B. Goz, and W. H. Prusoff.** 1975. Deoxyribonucleotide metabolism in herpes simplex virus infected HeLa cells. Biochim. Biophys. Acta **390**:253–263.
4. **Cohen, S. S.** 1966. Introduction to the biochemistry of D-arabinosyl nucleosides. Progr. Nucl. Acid Res. Mol. Biol. **5**:1–88.
5. **Connor, J. D., L. Sweetman, S. Carey, M. A. Stuckey, and R. Buchanan.** 1974. Effect of adenosine deaminase upon the antiviral activity in vitro of adenine arabinoside for vaccinia virus. Antimicrob. Agents Chemother. **6**:630–636.
6. **Doering, A., J. Keller, and S. S. Cohen.** 1966. Some effects of D-arabinosyl nucleosides on polymer syntheses in mouse fibroblasts. Cancer Res. **26**:2444–2450.
7. **Fox, D. J., and K. E. Guire.** 1973. MIDAS: Michigan interactive data analysis systems, p. 59–60. The Statistical Research Laboratory of The University of Michigan. University of Michigan, Ann Arbor.
8. **Goldstein, A.** 1964. Analysis of a single curve with graded responses, p. 156–161. *In* Biostatistics: an introductory text. MacMillan Co., New York.
9. **Kurtz, S. M.** 1975. Toxicology of adenine arabinoside, p. 145–157. *In* D. Pavan-Langston, R. A. Buchanan, and C. A. Alford, Jr. (ed.), Adenine arabinoside: an anti-

viral agent. Raven Press, New York.

10. **LePage, G. A.** 1970. Alterations in enzyme activity in tumors and the implications for chemotherapy. Adv. Enzyme Regul. 8:323–332.

11. **LePage, G. A.** 1974. Manipulation of DNA synthesis in normal and neoplastic tissues with drugs. Adv. Enzyme Regul. 12:373–381.

12. **Marks, M. I.** 1974. Variables influencing the in vitro susceptibilities of herpes simplex viruses to antiviral drugs. Antimicrob. Agents Chemother. 6:34–38.

13. **Miller, F. A., G. J. Dixon, J. Ehrlich, B. J. Sloan, and I. W. McLean, Jr.** 1969. Antiviral activity of 9-β-D-arabinofuranosyladenine. I. Cell culture studies, p. 136–147. Antimicrob. Agents. Chemother. 1968.

14. **Müller, W. E. G., H. J. Rohde, R. Beyer, A. Maidhof, M. Lachmann, R. K. Zahn, and H. Taschner.** 1975. Mode of action of 9-β-D-arabinofuranosyladenine on the synthesis of DNA, RNA, and protein in vivo and in vitro. Cancer Res. 35:2160–2168.

15. **Nakamura, H., G. Koyama, Y. Iitaka, M. Ohno, N. Yagisawa, S. Kondo, K. Meada, and H. Umezawa.** 1974. Structure of coformycin, an unusual nucleoside of microbial origin. J. Am. Chem. Soc. **96**:4327–4328.

16. **Newton, A., P. P. Dendy, C. L. Smith, and P. Wildy.** 1962. A pool size problem associated with the use of tritiated thymidine. Nature (London) **194**:886–887.

17. **Ortiz, P. J., M. J. Manduka, and S. S. Cohen.** 1972. The lethality of some D-arabinosyl nucleotides to mouse fibroblasts. Cancer Res. 32:1512–1517.

18. **Pavan-Livingston, D., R. A. Buchanan, and C. A. Alford, Jr. (ed.).** 1975. Parenteral and ophthalmic studies, p. 197–416. *In* Adenine arabinoside: an antiviral agent. Raven Press, New York.

19. **Plunkett, W., and S. S. Cohen.** 1975. Two approaches that increase the activity of analogs of adenine nucleosides in animal cells. Cancer Res. 35:1547–1554.

20. **Roller, B., and G. H. Cohen.** 1976. Deoxyribonucleoside triphosphate pools in synchronized human cells infected with herpes simplex virus types 1 and 2. J. Virol. 18:58–64.

21. **Schabel, F. M., Jr.** 1968. The antiviral activity of 9-β-D-arabinofuranosyladenine (ara-A). Chemotherapy **13**:321–338.

22. **Schaeffer, H. J., and C. F. Schwender.** 1974. Enzyme inhibitors. 26. Bridging hydrophobic and hydrophilic regions on adenosine deaminase with some 9-(2-hydroxy-3-alkyl)adenines. J. Med. Chem. **17**:6–8.

23. **Schwartz, P. M., C. Shipman, Jr., R. H. Carlson, and J. C. Drach.** 1974. Thermal inactivation as a means of inhibiting the serum-associated deamination of 9-β-D-arabinofuranosyladenine in tissue culture media. Antimicrob. Agents Chemother. 5:337–343.

24. **Shannon, W. M., L. Westbrook, and F. M. Schable, Jr.** 1974. Antiviral activity of 9-β-D-arabinofuranosyladenine (ara-A) against Gross murine leukemia virus in vitro. Proc. Soc. Exp. Biol. Med. **145**:542–545.

25. **Shannon, W. M.** 1975. Adenine arabinoside: antiviral activity in vitro, p. 1–43. *In* D. Pavan-Langston, R. A. Buchanan, and C. A. Alford, Jr. (ed.), Adenine arabinoside: an antiviral agent. Raven Press, New York.

26. **Shipman, C., Jr., S. H. Smith, R. H. Carlson, and J. C. Drach.** 1976. Antiviral activity of arabinosyladenine and arabinosylhypoxanthine in herpes simplex virus-infected KB cells. I. Selective inhibition of viral DNA synthesis in synchronized suspension cultures. Antimicrob. Agents Chemother. **9**:120–127.

27. **Sidwell, R. W., and J. H. Huffman.** 1971. Use of disposable micro tissue culture plates for antiviral and interferon induction studies. Appl. Microbiol. **22**:797–801.

28. **Sloan, B. J.** 1975. Adenine arabinoside: chemotherapy studies in animals, p. 45–94. *In* D. Pavan-Langston, R. A. Buchanan, and C. A. Alford, Jr. (ed.), Adenine arabinoside: an antiviral agent. Raven Press, New York.

29. **Sweetman, L., J. D. Connor, R. Seshamani, M. A. Stuckey, S. Carey, and R. Buchanan.** 1975. Deamination of adenine arabinoside in cell cultures used for in vitro viral inhibition studies, p. 135–144. *In* D. Pavan-Langston, R. A. Buchanan, and C. A. Alford, Jr. (ed.), Adenine arabinoside: an antiviral agent. Raven Press, New York.

30. **Williams, B. B., and A. M. Lerner.** 1975. Antiviral activity of an adenosine deaminase inhibitor: decreased replication of herpes simplex virus. J. Infect. Dis. **131**:673–677.

31. **Woo, P. W. K., H. W. Dion, S. M. Lang, L. F. Dahl., and L. J. Durham.** 1974. A novel adenosine and ara-A deaminase inhibitor, (R)-3-(2-deoxy-β-D-erythropentofuranosyl)-3,6,7,8-tetrahydroimidazo [4,5-d] [1,3] diazepin-8-ol. J. Heterocycl. Chem. **11**:641–643.

ANTIMICROBIAL AGENTS AND CHEMOTHERAPY, July 1976, p. 75-79

Vol. 10, No. 1
Printed in U.S.A.

Susceptibility of *Prototheca* Species to Antifungal Agents

ESTER SEGAL, ARVIND A. PADHYE,* AND LIBERO AJELLO

Mycology Division, Center for Disease Control, Public Health Service, U.S. Department of Health, Education, and Welfare, Atlanta, Georgia 30333

Received for publication 27 February 1976

Twenty isolates of *Prototheca filamenta, Prototheca moriformis, Prototheca stagnora, Prototheca wickerhamii,* and *Prototheca zopfii* were tested for in vitro susceptibility to five commonly used antifungal agents: amphotericin B, 5-fluorocytosine, griseofulvin, miconazole, and nystatin. The results revealed resistance to griseofulvin of all the *Prototheca* isolates tested and an inhibitory effect on *P. filamenta* by high 5-fluorocytosine concentrations (minimal inhibitory concentration [MIC] = 12.5 to 100 μg/ml; minimal fungicidal or algacidal concentration [MFC/MAC] = 50 to 100 μg/ml). *P. filamenta* isolates were also susceptible to miconazole (MIC = 0.1 to 0.5 μg/ml, MFC/MAC = 0.5 to 1 μg/ml); isolates of the other *Prototheca* species varied in regard to miconazole activity from susceptible to resistant (MIC = 1 – >100 μg/ml, MFC/MAC = 5 – >100 μg/ml). The *Prototheca* isolates revealed an in vitro susceptibility to the polyene antifungal agents, amphotericin B, and nystatin (MIC = 0.09 to 3.12 μg/ml and 0.19 to 12.5 μg/ml, respectively; MFC/MAC = 0.19 to 25 μg/ml and 0.75 to 25 μg/ml, respectively).

Prototheca species are microscopic, achloric, heterotrophic organisms, reproducing asexually by cleavage to form endospores (4). Some investigators think that these organisms are related to fungi (3); others believe that they are achloric algae (13); still others believe that these organisms hold an intermediate position (1).

Members of the genus *Prototheca* are known to cause systemic and cutaneous disease in dogs, deer, and cattle (2, 19, 21). Since 1964 cases of cutaneous or disseminated protothecosis in humans have also been reported (5, 6, 10, 12, 15, 22).

The chemotherapy of protothecosis, generally carried out on an empirical basis (19), is usually reported to be unsatisfactory (15). Extensive studies on the in vitro susceptibility of *Prototheca* species have not been reported. We therefore thought that it would be advisable to test the in vitro activity of antifungal agents against *Prototheca* isolates. The results of that study are presented in this report.

MATERIALS AND METHODS

Test cultures. Twenty test cultures from the culture collection of the Mycology Division of the Center for Disease Control (Table 1) were used. They were isolates of the species *Prototheca filamenta, Prototheca moriformis* (designated as such for this study but considered by Sudman and Kaplan [20] as a synonym of *Prototheca zopfii*), *Prototheca stagnora, Prototheca wickerhamii,* and *Prototheca zopfii.* The test cultures were subcultured and maintained on an antibiotic-free Sabouraud's dextrose agar.

Antifungal agents. Five antifungal agents were used: amphotericin B and nystatin, both products of E. R. Squibb & Sons, New York, N.Y.; 5-fluorocytosine (5-FC), supplied by Hoffmann-La Roche, Inc., Nutley, N.J.; griseofulvin, obtained from United States Pharmacopeia Co. Inc., Rockville, Md.; and miconazole (miconazole nitrate salt), supplied by Janssen R & D, Inc., New Brunswick, N.J.

Susceptibility testing with 5-FC. The minimal inhibitory concentration (MIC) and minimal fungicidal or algacidal concentration (MFC/MAC) were determined by using the methods described by Shadomy (17) and as used in a previous study (16).

A liquid synthetic medium, composed of yeast nitrogen base (Difco Laboratories, Detroit, Mich.) supplemented with asparagine and dextrose, was used as the test medium. The testing system consisted of twofold serial dilutions of 5-FC, ranging from 100 to 0.05 μg/ml, in 1 ml of yeast nitrogen base. The inoculum of the cultures to be tested consisted of 0.05 ml of 10^5 to 3.5×10^5 organisms per ml of suspension. The test cultures were incubated for 48 h at 25 C, and the lowest 5-FC concentration inhibiting visible growth was considered the MIC. The tubes showing no visible growth and the MIC tubes were then plated on Sabouraud's agar and incubated for 48 h; the lowest 5-FC concentration in yeast nitrogen base that inhibited growth on the Sabouraud plates was considered the MFC/MAC. A *Saccharomyces cerevisiae* isolate, obtained from S. Shadomy, Virginia Commonwealth University, Richmond, Va., was used as the control culture.

Susceptibility testing with amphotericin B and nystatin. The amphotericin B and nystatin suscepti-

TABLE I. *Source of Prototheca isolates tested*

Species	Accession no.	Source
P. filamenta	B-1273	Skin; Ohio
	B-1568	Foot; Missouri
	B-1569	Bone marrow; Missouri
	B-1570	Missouri
	B-1658	Dr. Pore; West Virginia
P. moriformis (synonym of *P. zopfii*)	B-1266	NRRL[a] strain Y-6864
	B-1692	Algae collection; Indiana
P. stagnora	B-1277	Waste stabilization pond; Ohio
P. wickerhamii	B-1269	Soil; Illinois
	B-1275	Skin; Africa
	B-1278	Lavatory drain pipe; Illinois
	B-1280	Human intestine; Illinois
	B-1651	Dog; Minnesota
	B-2224	Cat; Georgia
P. zopfii	MCC-378	Raw sewage; California
	MCC-379	Raw sewage; California
	MCC-380	Raw sewage; California
	B-1272	Bovine mastitis; Ohio
	B-1270	Bovine mastitis; Ohio
	B-1413	Venezuela

[a] NRRL, National Regional Research Laboratory.

bility tests were performed by a broth dilution method based on the procedure described by Shadomy and Espinel-Ingroff (18). Amphotericin B and nystatin stock solutions were made up in dimethylsulfoxide (Me_2SO) and kept protected from light. The test system consisted of twofold dilutions (from 100 to 0.05 μg/ml) of amphotericin B and nystatin in 1 ml of antibiotic medium (M-20, Difco), inoculated with 0.05 ml of 10^5 to 3.5×10^5 organisms per ml of suspension, and incubated at 25 C for 48 h. The MIC and MFC/MAC were determined as described for 5-FC testing. *S. cerevisiae* was used as the control culture.

Susceptibility testing with miconazole. Susceptibility testing with miconazole was also carried out by the tube dilution method. A miconazole stock solution was made up in ethanol at a concentration of 10 mg/ml. The tests were performed in Sabouraud broth (1 ml/tube) by using miconazole concentrations starting from 100 μg/ml down to 0.1 μg/ml. The inocula of the test cultures, incubation temperature, incubation period, control culture, and determination of MIC and MFC/MAC were the same as described for 5-FC, amphotericin B, and nystatin testing.

Susceptibility testing with griseofulvin. Griseofulvin was dissolved in acetone at a concentration of 2 mg/ml. Susceptibility was determined using agar plates containing agar incorporated with griseofulvin in concentrations starting from 50 μg of medium per ml down to 0.9 μg of medium per ml (twofold dilutions). The inocula of the test cultures, prepared as previously described, were inoculated on Sabouraud-griseofulvin agar plates; these were incubated at 25 C for 72 h. *Trichophyton mentagrophytes* ATCC 28068 was used as the control culture. By this method the activity of griseofulvin could be established only in regard to its minimal cidal concentration (MFC/MAC).

RESULTS

Griseofulvin susceptibility. The in vitro susceptibility of the 20 *Prototheca* isolates to the five tested antifungal agents is summarized in Table 2. Griseofulvin had no inhibitory effect on the *Prototheca* cultures, since all of them grew on Sabouraud agar plates containing 50 μg of griseofulvin per ml; the control culture of *T. mentagrophytes*, however, was affected at a 6.25 μg of griseofulvin per ml concentration.

5-FC susceptibility. The activity of 5-FC on *Prototheca* species had a selective pattern; it did not affect isolates of *P. zopfii*, *P. wickerhamii*, *P. stagnora*, or *P. moriformis* but was effective on four of five *P. filamenta* isolates tested (Table 2). Even the *P. filamenta* that were affected by 5-FC, however, were inhibited only at high concentrations, namely, MIC levels ranging from 12.5 to 25 μg/ml and MFC/MAC levels ranging from 50 to 100 μg/ml, respectively, as compared to the control culture of *S. cerevisiae* whose MIC and MFC/MAC were 0.38 and 1.56 μg/ml, respectively.

Amphotericin B and nystatin susceptibility. All the *Prototheca* isolates were affected by both of the polyene compounds tested, amphotericin B and nystatin (Table 2). In the case of four isolates (three *P. zopfii* cultures and one *P. wickerhamii*), however, high concentrations of amphotericin B (12.5 or 25 μg/ml) were required to produce a cidal effect. Furthermore, as revealed by the data in Table 3, which summarizes the minimal and maximal sensitivity values of *Prototheca* species, the *P. zopfii* isolates apparently were less sensitive to amphotericin B than to members of the other species tested.

TABLE 2. *In vitro susceptibility*[a] *of Prototheca sp. to amphotericin B, 5-FC, griseofulvin, miconazole, and nystatin*

Species	Amphotericin B		5-FC		Griseofulvin		Miconazole		Nystatin	
	MIC[a]	MFC/MAC[a]	MIC	MFC/MAC	MIC	MFC/MAC	MIC	MFC/MAC	MIC	MFC/MAC
P. filamenta										
B-1273	0.75	1.56	25.0	50.0		>50.0	0.1	0.5	1.56	3.12
B-1568	0.75	0.75	25.0	50.0		>50.0	0.1	0.5	3.12	3.12
B-1569	0.75	1.56	25.0	100.0		>50.0	0.5	1.0	0.75	0.75
B-1570	0.19	0.19	>100.0	>100.0		>50.0	0.5	0.5	0.38	0.75
B-1658	0.38	0.38	12.5	50.0		>50.0	0.5	0.5	0.75	1.56
P. moriformis										
B-1266	0.75	0.75	>100.0	>100.0		>50.0	0.5	1.0	1.56	3.12
B-1692	0.38	0.38	>100.0	>100.0		>50.0	1.0	1.0	1.56	3.12
P. stagnora										
B-1277	0.19	1.56	>100.0	>100.0		>50.0	100.0	100.0	3.12	12.5
P. wickerhamii										
B-1269	0.09	0.19	>100.0	>100.0		>50.0	>100.0	>100.0	3.12	3.12
B-1275	0.38	0.38	>100.0	>100.0		>50.0	10.0	50.0	0.75	1.56
B-1278	0.19	0.38	>100.0	>100.0		>50.0	100.0	100.0	0.75	1.56
B-1280	1.56	3.12	>100.0	>100.0		>50.0	10.0	50.0	0.75	0.75
B-1651	1.56	12.5	>100.0	>100.0		>50.0	50.0	50.0	3.12	3.12
B-2224	0.19	0.38	>100.0	>100.0		>50.0	>100.0	>100.0	3.12	3.12
P. zopfii										
MCC-378	0.75	1.56	>100.0	>100.0		>50.0	10.0	50.0	0.75	1.56
MCC-379	0.75	12.5	>100.0	>100.0		>50.0	10.0	25.0	1.56	3.12
MCC-380	0.75	3.12	>100.0	>100.0		>50.0	1.0	5.0	1.56	3.12
B-1270	3.12	25.0	>100.0	>100.0		>50.0	10.0	>100.0	1.56	3.12
B-1272	0.19	0.75	>100.0	>100.0		>50.0	10.0	>100.0	0.75	0.75
B-1413	3.12	25.0	>100.0	>100.0		>50.0	10.0	>100.0	12.5	25.0
Controls										
S. cerevisiae	0.38	1.56	0.38	1.56			7.5	10.0	0.75	1.56
T. mentagrophytes (ATCC 28068)						6.25				

[a] Expressed as micrograms per milliliter.

TABLE 3. *Minimal and maximal susceptibility of Prototheca sp. to amphotericin B, miconazole, and nystatin*

Species	No. of isolates tested	Amphotericin B		Miconazole		Nystatin	
		MIC (μg/ml)	MFC/MAC (μg/ml)	MIC (μg/ml)	MFC/MAC (μg/ml)	MIC (μg/ml)	MFC/MAC (μg/ml)
P. filamenta	5	0.19–0.75	0.19–1.56	0.1–0.5	0.5–1.0	0.38–3.12	0.75–3.12
P. moriformis (synonym of *P. zopfii*)	2	0.38–0.75	0.38–0.75	0.5–1.0	1.0–1.0	1.56–1.56	3.12–3.12
P. stagnora	1	0.19	1.56	100.0	100.0	3.12	12.5
P. wickerhamii	6	0.09–1.56	0.19–3.12	10.0–100	50.0–>100	0.75–3.12	0.75–3.12
P. zopfii	6	0.19–3.12	0.75–25.0	1.0–10.0	5.0–>100	0.75–12.5	0.75–25.0

Judging from both the MIC and the MFC/MAC values, the *Prototheca* isolates were generally less susceptible to nystatin than to amphotericin B (Tables 2 and 3). On the other hand, three of four *P. zopfii* isolates with high MFC/MAC values for amphotericin B showed significantly lower MFC/MAC values for nystatin (Table 2).

Miconazole susceptibility. The results obtained by the miconazole susceptibility testing of *Prototheca* isolates (Tables 2 and 3) showed that miconazole had an inhibitory effect. However, there was some variation in regard to its activity among members of the same species, some being susceptible and others resistant (*P. zopfii* and *P. wickerhamii* isolates, Table 2). In addition, there were also differences in the sensitivity among the different *Prototheca* species (Table 3). Furthermore, although miconazole was inhibitory (MIC) to all the *P. zopfii* isolates tested, three of the isolates showed resistance to its cidal action (MFC/MAC) (Table 2).

DISCUSSION

The species *Prototheca* were divided by Arnold and Ahearn (1) on the basis of physiological characteristics into five species: *P. filamenta, P. moriformis, P. stagnora, P. wickerhamii,* and *P. zopfii,* with a number of strains having various designations such as *Prototheca segbwema* (isolated by Davies and Wilkinson [6] from human cutaneous protothecosis), which these investigators considered synonymous with *P. zopfii*. Based on antigenic properties Sudman and Kaplan (20) recognized only four species in the genus *Prototheca,* with *P. moriformis* being synonymous with *P. zopfii*. As noted, in this study we used the term *P. moriformis* for the two strains B-1266 and B-1692 (see Results), since they were designated as such when referred to the Center for Disease Control Mycology Culture collection. They should, however, be considered synonymous with *P. zopfii*.

Arnold and Ahearn (1) described *P. filamenta* as a new species. However, it was found to be different from other *Prototheca* species, and its classification within the genus *Prototheca* has been questioned (9). The antifungal susceptibility pattern of *P. filamenta,* as found in this study, is indeed different from the other *Prototheca* species. The *P. filamenta* cultures were the only *Prototheca* isolates affected at all by 5-FC; they were also very susceptible to miconazole, as compared to the susceptibility of isolates of other *Prototheca* species.

Miconazole is an imidazole nitrate substance that is inhibitory to dermatophytes and yeasts and reported to be useful in the topical treatment of dermatological and gynecological infections (7, 8, 14, 15). It has also been reported to have an in vitro activity on the etiological agents of certain deep mycoses (11, 15). The data obtained in this study in regard to miconazole activity show that some isolates of *P. zopfii* and *P. wickerhamii,* the two *Prototheca* species known to cause disease (19), are affected by it and that other isolates are resistant to it. It seems important, therefore, to test more clinical *Prototheca* isolates in regard to their susceptibility to miconazole before considering its topical use in cases of cutaneous protothecosis.

As judged by the data from this study, the two polyene antimycotics amphotericin B and nystatin are apparently the antimicrobial agents most effective in vitro against the *Prototheca* species.

ACKNOWLEDGMENTS

This study was supported by fellowship FO5 TW 2132 from the Fogarty International Center of the National Institutes of Health, Bethesda, Md.

We are grateful to W. Kaplan of the Mycology Division, Center for Disease Control for his advice throughout this investigation and to Janssen R & D, Inc., New Brunswick, N.J., for supplying Miconazole.

Ester Segal is a visiting scientist from the Department of Human Microbiology, Tel-Aviv University Medical School, Tel-Aviv, Israel.

LITERATURE CITED

1. **Arnold, P., and D. G. Ahearn.** 1972. The systematics of the genus *Prototheca* with a description of a new species *P. filamenta*. Mycologia 64:265–275.
2. **Carlton, W. W., and L. Austin.** 1973. Ocular protothecosis in a dog. Vet. Pathol. 10:274–280.
3. **Ciferri, O.** 1956. Thiamine deficiency of *Prototheca,* a yeast-like achloric alga. Nature (London) 178:1475–1476.
4. **Cooke, W. B.** 1968. Studies in the genus *Prototheca*. II. Taxonomy. J. Elisha Mitchell Sci. Sco. 84:217–220.
5. **Cox, E. G., J. D. Wilson, and P. Brown.** 1974. Protothecosis: a case of disseminated algae infection. Lancet 2:379–382.
6. **Davis, R. R., and J. L. Wilkinson.** 1964. Human protothecosis: supplementary studies. Ann. Trop. Med. Parasitol. 61:112–115.
7. **Gentles, J. C., G. R. Jones, and D. T. Roberts.** 1975. Efficacy of miconazole in the topical treatment of tinea pedis in sportsmen. Br. J. Dermatol. 93:79–84.
8. **Holt, R. J.** 1974. Recent developments in antimycotic chemotherapy. Infection 2:95–107.
9. **King, D. S., and S. C. Jong.** 1975. *Sarcinosporon:* a new genus to accomodate *Trichosporon inkin* and *Prototheca filamenta*. Mycotaxon 3:84–94.
10. **Klintworth, G. K., B. F. Fetter, and M. S. Nielsen, Jr.** 1968. Protothecosis, an algal infection; report of a case in man. J. Med. Microbiol. 1:211–216.
11. **Levine, H. B., D. A. Stevens, J. M. Cobb, and A. E. Gebhardt.** 1975. Miconazole in coccidioidomycosis. I. Assays of activity in mice and in vitro. J. Infect. Dis. 132:407–414.
12. **Mars, P. W., A. R. Rabson, J. J. Rippey, and L. Ajello.** 1971. Cutaneous protothecosis. Br. J. Dermol. 85(Suppl. 7):76–84.

13. **Nadakavukaren, J. M., and D. A. McCraken.** 1973. *Prototheca:* an alga or a fungus? J. Phycol. **9:**113–116.
14. **Proost, J. M., F. M. Maes-Dockx, M. O. Nelis, and J. M. Van Cutsen.** 1972. Miconazole in the treatment of mycotic vulvovaginitis. Am. J. Obstet. Gynecol. **112:**668–692.
15. **Rippon, J. W.** 1974. Medical mycology. The pathogenic fungi and the pathogenic actinomycetes, p. 459–464, 531–541. W. B. Saunders Co., Philadelphia.
16. **Segal, E., A. Romano, E. Eylan, and R. Stein.** 1975. Experimental and clinical studies of 5-fluorocytosine activity in *Candida* ocular infections. I. In vitro activity of 5-fluorocytosine on *Candida* species isolated from ocular infections. Chemotherapy **21:**358–366.
17. **Shadomy, S.** 1969. In vitro studies with 5-fluorocytosine. Appl. Microbiol. **17:**871–877.
18. **Shadomy, S., and A. Espinel-Ingroff.** 1974. Susceptibility testing of antifungal agents, p. 569–574. *In* E. H. Lennette, E. H. Spaulding, and J. P. Truant (ed.), Manual of clinical microbiology, 2nd ed. American Society for Microbiology. Washington, D.C.
19. **Sudman, S. M.** 1974. Protothecosis: a critical review. Am. J. Clin. Pathol. **61:**10–19.
20. **Sudman, S. M., and W. Kaplan.** 1973. Identification of the *Prototheca* species by immunofluorescence. Appl. Microbiol. **25:**981–990.
21. **Van Kruiningen, M. J.** 1970. Protothecal enterocolitis in a dog. J. Am. Vet. Med. Assoc. **157:**56–63.
22. **Lee, W-Sh., M. D. Lagios, and R. Leonards.** 1975. Wound infection by *Prototheca wickerhamii,* a saprophytic algapathogenic for man. J. Clin. Microbiol. **2:**62–66.

Antimicrobial Agents and Chemotherapy, July 1976, p. 80–82 Vol. 10, No. 1

Printed in U.S.A.

Gentamicin- and Cephalothin-Associated Rises in Blood Urea Nitrogen

W. LEE FANNING, DIETER GUMP, AND HERSHEL JICK[1] *

Infectious Disease Unit, Medical College of Vermont, Burlington, Vermont 05401, and Boston University School of Medicine, Waltham, Massachusetts 02154

Received for publication 28 January 1976

Standardized rates of drug-attributed rises in blood urea nitrogen were 8.6%, 2.9%, and 9.3%, respectively, in patients receiving gentamicin alone, cephalothin alone, and both drugs together. These results provide evidence against a substantial synergism between the two drugs in the production of impaired renal function.

Recently, case reports have appeared describing the development of impaired renal function in patients receiving both gentamicin and cephalothin, and it has been suggested that they may be synergistic in producing this effect (1, 3, 8, 12). To evaluate this possibility, the data collected by the Boston Collaborative Drug Surveillance Program (BCDSP) were examined.

(This paper was presented at the 15th Interscience Conference on Antimicrobial Agents and Chemotherapy in Washington, D.C., 24–26 September 1975.)

PATIENTS AND METHODS

The BCDSP has to date collected data on over 22,000 consecutive admissions to selected wards in nine hospitals. All patients were admitted to medical services, none had undergone surgery, and none had received anesthetic agents. The data routinely collected include detailed information on demographic characteristics, all drugs administered, and a record of any adverse events deemed by the attending physician to be related to the administration of any drug or combination of drugs. Thus, the event, rising blood urea nitrogen (BUN) attributed to a drug, was based on the attending physician's discovery and notation of this event during the clinical course of his patient. Further details of the program and its methods have been presented elsewhere (10).

As a first step in the evaluation of the effect of the combination of gentamicin and cephalothin in producing impaired renal function, all patients receiving these drugs alone or in combination were identified. From this group, patients receiving other nephrotoxic agents (i.e., kanamycin, colistin sulfate, polymixin B, amphotericin B, cephaloridine, or tetracycline) were excluded from further study. For all of the remaining patients who had developed a drug-attributed rising BUN, the records were studied in detail. For the purposes of the present evaluation, rising BUN was ascribed to the relevant antibiotic under study in those instances where it occurred at least 24 h after treatment was begun and not more than 24 h after it was stopped.

The following were evaluated as possible confounding factors: age, sex, hospital, admission BUN level, first discharge diagnosis, survival, drug dosage, route of drug administration, duration of antibiotic therapy, and concomitant administration of diuretics.

A total of 1,073 patients met the criteria for inclusion. Among these, 18% were 40 years of age or less, 26% were between 41 and 60 years, and 56% were over 60 years of age. Fifty-six percent were male. The admission BUN was less than 25 mg/100 ml in 63% of the group, between 25 and 50 mg/100 ml in 22%, and over 50 mg/100 ml in 15%. The overall mortality rate was 25%. The first recorded discharge diagnosis was neoplasm in 246 patients (23%), respiratory disease in 237 patients (22%), cardiovascular disease in 188 patients (18%), genitourinary disease in 82 patients (7%) and other diseases in 320 patients (30%).

The number of patients receiving gentamicin alone (group G) was 334, the number receiving cephalothin alone (group C) was 492, and the number receiving both together (group GC) was 247. The distributions of these groups by age, sex, hospital, and admission BUN were similar and, therefore, these factors were not controlled in further analyses. In addition, the distributions of patients with rising BUN and those without were similar with respect to discharge diagnosis and the concomitant administration of diuretics. There were, however, differences between the comparison groups with regard to survival and this factor was taken into account in evaluating the relationship. The mortality rate for groups G and C was 20%, whereas for group GC it was 40%. The frequency of BUN rise was 3.9% in those who lived and 8.8% in those who died.

RESULTS

The crude rate of drug-attributed rising BUN was 6.6% for group G, 2.0% for group C, and 9.3% for group GC (Table 1). Standardized (9)

[1] Address reprint requests to: Boston Collaborative Drug Surveillance Program, 400 Totten Pond Road, Waltham, Mass. 02154.

TABLE 1. *Frequency of rises in BUN among the compared groups*

Group	Frequency of rise in BUN					
	Gentamicin		Cephalothin		Both antibiotics	
Survivors	13/268	(4.9%)	5/392	(1.3%)	13/141	(9.2%)
Nonsurvivors	9/66	(13.6%)	5/100	(5.0%)	10/106	(9.4%)
All						
Crude	22/334	(6.6%)	10/492	(2.0%)	23/247	(9.3%)
Standardized[a]		8.6%		2.9%		9.3%

[a] Using the "both antibiotics" group as the standard.

for the survival distribution of group GC, the rates of rising BUN were 8.6, 2.9, and 9.3% for groups G, C, and GC, respectively.

The maximum rise of BUN averaged 59 (range 10 to 330), 76 (range 20 to 100), and 46 (range 10 to 120) mg/100 ml for groups G, C, and GC, respectively. In 17 cases data on changes in the plasma creatinine were available, and in each instance the plasma creatinine rose in proportion to the rise in BUN.

The frequency of drug-attributed rising BUN was 10.5% among 229 patients who received a daily dose of more than 180 mg of gentamicin. By contrast, the frequency among 352 patients who received 180 mg or less was 6.0% ($P <$ 0.05). The dose-response relationship was apparent both in group G and in group GC. There was no appreciable correlation between the frequency of rising BUN and route of administration of gentamicin.

The mean durations of treatment before the identification of rising BUN were 7, 8, and 6 days for groups G, C, and GC, respectively.

DISCUSSION

Both gentamicin and cephalothin have been shown to be nephrotoxic in animal studies (7, 11; O. Flandre and M. Jannon, Gentamicin, First Int. Symp., Paris, 1967). In rats, gentamicin causes pathological changes in the proximal tubules at a dose of 200 mg/kg per day, whereas for cephalothin a dose of 1,000 mg/kg per day is required and must be combined with glycerol or furosemide. Recent animal studies have failed to show a synergistic effect of the combination of gentamicin and cephalothin in the production of renal damage (6; W. Harrison, F. Silverblatt, and M. Turck, Progr. Abstr. Intersci. Conf. Antimicrob. Agents Chemother., 14th, San Francisco, Calif., Abstr. 70, 1974). Impaired renal function was attributed to gentamicin in 4.9% of 349 patients carefully monitored for antimicrobial toxicity (4) and in 6.5% of 77 courses of gentamicin after other A similar estimate for cephalothin given alone has not been reported previously, but this drug has been implicated in case reports as causing nephrotoxicity (2, 5, 13).

In the current clinical study, each reported instance of rising BUN was attributed to either gentamicin, cephalothin, or both, if it occurred 24 h or more after the relevant treatment was begun and not more than 24 h after it was stopped. Despite the absence of patients undergoing surgery and the exclusion of patients receiving other nephrotoxic drugs, it is possible that some of these events were not caused by antibiotic treatment and would have occurred in its absence. Indeed, in four instances the rising BUN occurred after an episode of hypotension, which may have contributed to the development of impaired renal function. Nevertheless, in the absence of other apparent causes, it is quite likely that a substantial majority of these events were caused by one of the treatments being evaluated. It should be noted that the events reported here were of substantial clinical significance since the mean rise in BUN for the entire series was of the order of 60 mg%.

Whereas the standardized rates of rising BUN patients receiving gentamicin alone and cephalothin alone were 8.6% and 2.9%, respectively, the rate for the recipients of both drugs (9.3%) was lower than the sum of these. Considering the statistical stability of these estimates, the results provide evidence against a substantial synergism between gentamicin and cephalothin in the production of rising BUN.

In the current study, treatments were not randomized. Furthermore, the evaluation of individual patients for rising BUN was certainly not standard since many physicians in many hospitals were involved. It is, therefore, possible that a real synergism between gentamicin and cephalothin was missed. For this to have occurred, it would require either that patients receiving both drugs were a priori less susceptible to developing drug-induced rising BUN or that the event was less likely to have been discovered in patients receiving the combination or both. None of these seems likely. Patients receiving both drugs seemed to have more severe illness and this would tend to raise the susceptibility to developing rising BUN. Also, it seems unlikely that patients receiving both drugs would be less carefully watched with regard to renal function as compared with patients receiving gentamicin alone. Nevertheless, such possibilities cannot be excluded entirely.

Because of the method of ascertainment, the observed rates of rising BUN reported in this study are likely to be underestimates of the true rates, as only those rises detected by the attending physicians and thought to be drug-related were recorded. However, as mentioned above, it is most unlikely that such under-reporting would be more pronounced in patients receiving both antibiotics, and therefore the failure to find an increased frequency of rising BUN in such patients cannot be reasonably explained on this basis.

Ten of 492 patients who received cephalothin alone developed a rising BUN after the drug was started and before its discontinuation. For the purposes of this study, the event was assigned to cephalothin since in each instance there was no other evident cause for the rise and cephalothin was suspected clinically to be the cause. However, in no instance could the drug be implicated with certainty, and these data therefore provide only suspicion that cephalothin alone may occasionally cause a rise in BUN.

In summary, the data indicate that no appreciable synergy exists between cephalothin and gentamicin in the production of impaired renal function. The rate with gentamicin correlates with daily dose but does not appear to correlate with route of administration or concomitant administration of diuretics.

ACKNOWLEDGMENTS

Hospitals which have participated in the Boston Collaborative Drug Surveillance Program are: Boston, Mass.—Lemuel Shattuck Hospital, Peter Bent Brigham Hospital, Boston City Hospital, VA Hospital, Massachusetts General Hospital, and University Hospital; Providence, R.I.—Roger Williams General Hospital; Syracuse, N.Y.—State University Hospital of the Upstate Medical Center; Tucson, Ariz.—Arizona Medical Center; Richmond, Va.—Virginia Commonwealth University Hospital; Canada—St. Joseph's Hospital, London, Ontario; Israel—Hadassah-Hebrew University Hospital, Jerusalem, Beilinson Medical Center, Petah Tiqva, and Asaf-Harofe Hospital, Zerifin; New Zealand—Auckland Hospital, Auckland, and Hutt Hospital, Wellington; Scotland—Western Infirmary and Stobhill General Hospital, Glasgow; Italy—Desio Hospital, Milan.

The Boston Collaborative Drug Surveillance Program has been supported by Public Health Service contract no. NO1-GM-4-2148 from the National Institute of General Medical Sciences; and in part by grants from the Food and Drug Administration; the Canadian Health Protection Branch; the Israeli Ministry of Health; the Hadassah Medical Organization; the Kupat-Holim; Auckland Hospital, Auckland, New Zealand; the Roger Williams General Hospital (Brown University Public Health Service grant no. GM-165-38-02 from the National Institute of General Medical Sciences); and the Scottish Home and Health Department.

LITERATURE CITED

1. **Bobrow, S. N., E. Jaffe, and R. Young.** 1972. Anuria and acute tubular necrosis associated with gentamicin and cephalothin. J. Am. Med. Assoc. **222**:1546–1547.
2. **Burton, J., N. Lichtenstein, R. Colvin, and E. Newton.** 1974. Acute renal failure during cephalothin therapy. J. Am. Med. Assoc. **229**:679–682.
3. **Cabanillas, F., R. Burgos, R. Rodriguez, and C. Baldizon.** 1975. Nephrotoxicity of combined cephalothin-gentamicin regimen. Arch. Intern. Med. **135**:850–852.
4. **Caldwell, J., and L. Cluff.** 1974. Adverse reactions to antimicrobial agents. J. Am. Med. Assoc. **230**:77–80.
5. **Carling, P., B. Idelson, A. Casano, E. Alexander, and W. McCabe.** 1975. Nephrotoxicity associated with cephalothin administration. Arch. Intern. Med. **135**:797–801.
6. **Dellinger, E., T. Murphy, V. Pinn, M. Barza, and L. Weinstein.** 1974. Protection by cephalothin against gentamicin induced nephrotoxicity in rats. Clin. Res. **22**:706A.
7. **Falco, F. G., H. M. Smith, and G. M. Arcieri.** 1969. Nephrotoxicity of aminoglycosides and gentamicin. J. Infect. Dis. **119**:406–409.
8. **Fillastre, J. P., R. Larmovier, G. Humbert, D. Dubois, J. Metayer, A. Delpech, J. Leroy, and M. Robert.** 1973. Acute renal failure associated with combined gentamicin and cephalothin therapy. Br. Med. J. **2**:396–397.
9. **Hill, A. B.** 1971. Principles of medical statistics, p. 201–209. Oxford University Press, New York.
10. **Jick, H., O. Miettinen, S. Shapiro, G. P. Lewis, V. Siskind, and D. Slone.** 1970. Comprehensive drug surveillance. J. Am. Med. Assoc. **213**:1455–1460.
11. **Linton, A., R. Borley, and D. Turnbull.** 1972. Relative nephrotoxicity of cephalosporin antibiotics in an animal model. J. Can. Med. Assoc. **107**:414–417.
12. **Masbernard, A., A. L'Ainee, C. Portal, C. L. Guidicelli, C. R. Lombard, and D'Audibert Caille Du Bourquet.** 1974. Nephrotoxicite de l'association cephalotine-gentamicine; etude clinique a propos de quatre observations. Ann. Med. Interne **125**:749–754.
13. **Pickering, M., G. Spooner, A. DeQuesada, and J. Cade.** 1970. Declining renal function associated with administration of cephalothin. South. Med. J. **63**:426–428.
14. **Wilfert, J. N., J. P. Burke, H. A. Bloomer, and C. B. Smith.** 1971. Renal insufficiency associated with gentamicin therapy. J. Infect. Dis. **124**:148–153.

ANTIMICROBIAL AGENTS AND CHEMOTHERAPY, July 1976, p. 83-88
Vol. 10, No. 1

Short-Term Storage of Six Penicillins and Cephalothin in Microdilution Trays for Antimicrobial Susceptibility Tests

A. L. BARRY,* L. J. EFFINGER, AND R. E. BADAL

*Department of Internal Medicine, School of Medicine, University of California, Davis, Davis, California 95616, and Clinical Microbiology Laboratory, University of California, Davis-Sacramento, Medical Center, Sacramento, California 95817**

Received for publication 8 March 1976

To perform microdilution antimicrobial susceptibility tests efficiently, broth dilutions of the antimicrobial drugs should be prepared in large batches and stored frozen until needed. Studies were carried out to document the stability of ampicillin, benzylpenicillin, carbenicillin, methicillin, oxacillin, nafcillin, and cephalothin in microdilution trays during storage at −20 and −60 C. No significant deterioration was noted after 21 days of storage, as detected by bioassay and by replicate minimal inhibitory concentration determinations with control organisms. No significant differences were noted moreover between trays stored for three weeks at −20 C and those stored at −60 C. The microdilution technique was found to be a highly reproducible method for quantitative determination of antimicrobial susceptibility.

Quantitative susceptibility tests can be performed efficiently with a microdilution technique (3–10), especially since the development of semiautomated equipment for preparing serial dilutions of the antimicrobial agent. Such semiautomated equipment can be used effectively only when large numbers of trays containing antimicrobial dilutions can be prepared at one time and held frozen until needed, rather than preparing fresh sets of dilutions each day. The present report documents the stability of ampicillin, benzylpenicillin, carbenicillin, methicillin, oxacillin, nafcillin, and cephalothin during short-term storage of microdilution trays at −20 and −60 C. These drugs were selected for study because they are notoriously unstable and most likely to become inactive during storage. To document the stability of these drugs, it was first necessary to estimate the accuracy and precision by which antibiotic dilutions could be prepared with our semiautomated system, an Autotiter IV (Canalco Ltd.).

MATERIALS AND METHODS

Antibiotic dilutions. Antibiotic powders were obtained from Canalco Ltd., Rockville, Md., and diluted in sterile distilled water to give stock solutions of the appropriate concentration. Serial dilutions were then prepared with an Autotiter IV (Canalco Ltd.), each well containing 50 μl of drug diluted in Mueller-Hinton broth (Difco). Each tray contained 16 series of seven doubling dilutions of antibiotics under study. The trays were either tested immediately or returned to the plastic bags in which they were received; each bag held a maximum of four trays plus an empty cover tray. The bags were then sealed with masking tape and stored in a Revco freezer (−60 C) or in a household freezer without automatic defrost (−20 C). After 1, 2, 3, or 4 weeks of storage, the trays were removed from the freezer and allowed to thaw at room temperature before testing.

Inoculation of antibiotic dilutions. To evaluate the performance of different antibiotic trays replicate tests were performed with the "Seattle" *Escherichia coli* or *Staphylococcus aureus* (originally obtained from a subculture of ATCC 25922 or ATCC 25923) strains. The inoculum was standardized by diluting an actively growing broth culture to match the turbidity of a MacFarland 0.5 standard as for the disk diffusion test of Bauer et al. (1). The adjusted suspension was then diluted 1:200 in Mueller-Hinton broth, and 50-μl drops were added to each well of a tray using a disposable dropping pipette (Cooke Engineering, Alexandria, Va.). After inoculation, the trays were sealed with sealing tape and placed in a 35 C incubator, with no more than two trays in a stack. After overnight incubation, the minimal inhibitory concentration (MIC) was determined as the lowest concentration that inhibited visible growth, as viewed by examining the trays from the bottom.

Bioassay. To directly estimate the concentration of ampicillin, penicillin, or carbenicillin in the trays, the large-plate assay technique of Bennett et al. (2) was adapted by using 0.25-inch (6.4-mm) filter paper disks (Schleicher and Schuell no. 740E) rather than filling wells cut from the agar. Nutrient agar (Difco) was seeded with *Bacillus subtilis* spore suspension (Difco) just before pouring into a large (30 by 30 cm) assay plate. The filter paper disks were charged with 10-μl volumes of antibiotic standard solutions or of an aliquot from the wells being assayed, and the moist disks were then applied directly to the assay plates. Each assay plate received 15 disks containing standard solutions (three with each of five different concentrations) and 3 disks prepared from each well to be assayed. A maximum of 64 disks could be tested on one assay plate. For each test plate, a standard curve was constructed and found to represent a straight line within the range of concentrations selected for testing. The concentration in each test well was calculated from the mean zone diameter, using the regression equation for the standard curve. With this test system, repeated tests with the standard solutions demonstrated an overall coefficient of variation of 5 to 6% for the three penicillins studied at the concentration selected for assaying microdilution trays. Variation between triplicate tests was minimal.

RESULTS

Accuracy and precision of antibiotic dilutions. Stock solutions of ampicillin trihydrate were prepared at a concentration of 80 μg/ml and then diluted serially with an Autotiter IV, filling 16 series of wells in each tray with the same stock solution. Once a week for three consecutive weeks, 10 trays were prepared from freshly prepared stock solutions. Trays 2 and 10 in each set were tested on the day of preparation, and the remaining trays were stored for later testing. The dilution in well 6 in each series (1.25 μg/ml) was sampled for bioassay, and all 16 wells on each of the freshly prepared trays were assayed in triplicate. The results of this experiment are summarized in Table 1. For each tray the mean value came close to being within 10% of the expected concentration. Variability was also minimal, with the overall coefficient of variation being 12.5%. An analysis of variance was utilized to compare variances between trays, between rows (loops), and between days. No significant differences could be identified.

A second experiment was then undertaken to extend these observations by adding tests with benzylpenicillin and carbenicillin and to repeat the tests with ampicillin. This time trays were prepared once a week for 4 consecutive weeks, and 12 wells were selected from each tray for bioassay. The results of these initial tests before storage of the trays are included in Table 2. As before, the mean concentration was generally within 10% of the expected value, and the coefficient of variation demonstrated an acceptable degree of precision.

Activity of penicillins after short-term storage. Trays containing ampicillin prepared in experiment 1 were stored for 1, 2, or 3 weeks at both −20 and −60 C. On week 4 of this experiment, all trays were removed from storage and tested simultaneously. Eight wells in each of the stored trays were assayed (Table 1). Even after 3 weeks of storage, the concentration of antibiotic in the trays was well within acceptable limits. The Student *t* test failed to reveal any significant differences between trays stored at −20 C and those held at −60 C or between the initial test values and those obtained after 7, 14, or 21 days of storage. Experiment 2 (Table 2) also failed to reveal any significant loss of activity during the storage of diluted penicillins in microdilution trays. Even after 21 days of storage, assays of all three penicillins demonstrated an acceptable degree of accuracy and precision.

Performance of stored microdilution trays.

TABLE 1. *Accuracy and precision of ampicillin microdilutions before and after short-term storage of diluted trays: bioassay of well 6 in a series of doubling dilutions (expected value = 1.25 μg/ml)*

Tray no.	Bioassay[a]		Time stored (days)	Storage temp (C)	Bioassay[b]	
	Mean (± 2SD)	CV (%)			Mean (± 2SD)	CV (%)
Week 1						
2	1.21 (1.0–1.4)	9.9	21	−20	1.23 (0.9–1.5)	12.1
10	1.17 (1.0–1.4)	8.9		−60	1.38 (1.0–1.7)	13.4
Week 2						
2	1.09 (0.8–1.4)	15.9	14	−20	1.47 (1.1–1.8)	11.7
10	1.13 (0.8–1.4)	13.0		−60	1.59 (1.2–1.9)	11.3
Week 3						
2	1.21 (0.9–1.5)	12.8	7	−20	1.64 (1.4–1.9)	7.0
10	1.26 (1.0–1.5)	11.0		−60	1.69 (1.4–2.0)	9.0
Total (96 wells)	1.18 (0.9–1.5)	12.5				

[a] Bioassay (16 wells per tray) was based upon triplicate tests from each well and expressed as micrograms per milliliter; before storage. SD, Standard deviation; CV, coefficient of variation.

[b] Bioassay (8 wells per tray) was based upon triplicate tests from each well and expressed as micrograms per milliliter; after storage.

TABLE 2. *Stability of three penicillins in microdilution trays*

Determination	Mean bioassay value[a] (μg/ml) of:		
	Benzylpenicillin (4 μg/ml)[b]	Carbenicillin (128 μg/ml)[b]	Ampicillin (2 μg/ml)[b]
Week 4			
Control for stored trays[c]	3.9 (7.8)[d]	117 (4.8)	1.8 (8.2)
Week 3			
Initial tests before storage	5.1 (7.8)	122 (4.2)	2.1 (10.4)
After 7 days at −20 C	3.7 (7.9)	126 (5.1)	1.8 (6.7)
After 7 days at −60 C	3.9 (11.4)	129 (4.6)	2.0 (8.4)
Week 2			
Initial tests before storage	3.7 (10)	122 (6.1)	1.8 (12.9)
After 14 days at −20 C	3.4 (4.8)	123 (6.0)	1.6 (3.4)
After 14 days at −60 C	3.5 (20.3)	132 (6.1)	1.9 (6.4)
Week 1			
Initial tests before storage	4.0 (7.9)	114 (8.0)	1.8 (7.4)
After 21 days at −20 C	2.9 (12.8)	114 (6.2)	1.4 (14.8)
After 21 days at −60 C	4.4 (7.9)	133 (7.0)	1.8 (6.6)

[a] Each bioassay was based on triplicate tests on 12 wells from trays tested before storage and 8 wells tested after storage.
[b] Expected concentration in wells selected for bioassay.
[c] Values from freshly prepared trays, prepared and tested on the day that stored trays were tested.
[d] Numbers in parentheses represent the coefficient of variation expressed as a percentage.

To further support the conclusions drawn from the above bioassay tests, the trays were inoculated with a standardized suspension of the "Seattle" *E. coli*, and multiple MIC determinations were made. Experiment 1 provided 288 MIC values with ampicillin (Table 3). The median MIC was 5.0 μg/ml, with variation no more than one doubling dilution on either side of the mean. The geometric mean for each set of freshly prepared trays was between 4.0 and 5.0 μg/ml. After storage of the trays, the MIC did not differ significantly from the initial tests before storage (chi-square test).

The performance of trays prepared in experiment 2 is summarized in Table 4. A total of 128 MICs was recorded for each of the three antibiotics before storage. The MICs were all within one doubling dilution above or below the mode and, except for one set of trays, with benzylpenicillin, the MICs all fell into a single dilution step on either side of the geometric mean. After storage of the trays for 3 weeks, no significant change could be detected in the MICs obtained with the standard control *E. coli*.

Experiment 3 was undertaken to study the performance of microdilution trays containing three semisynthetic penicillins and cephalothin after storage for as long as 28 days. These trays were inoculated with the "Seattle" strain of *S. aureus* and, for each drug, eight MICs were recorded each week before the trays were stored and again after 7, 14, 21, and 28 days of storage

TABLE 3. *Performance of ampicillin microdilution trays after short-term storage*

Tray storage		Geometric mean MIC[a]	% of tests[b]/MIC[a]			
Days	Temp (C)		1.25	2.5	5.0	10.0
0		4.7		8	92	
7	−20	5.0			100	
7	−60	4.8		6	94	
0		4.6		10	90	
14	−20	5.0			100	
14	−60	4.9		6	91	3
0		4.1		29	71	
21	−20	5.2			94	6
21	−60	5.1			97	3

[a] MIC (micrograms per milliliter) of "Seattle" *E. coli*.
[b] Based on 32 tests for each storage condition or for each set of "fresh" plates.

at −20 and −60 C. On week 5, when all stored trays were tested, sixteen MICs were determined with freshly prepared antimicrobial agents. In this way five different sets of unstored trays yielded 48 MIC values for each drug, and the geometric mean MIC is recorded in Table 5. Two methicillin MIC values were two dilution steps above the median; all other MICs were within one doubling dilution on either side of the median. Methicillin MICs

TABLE 4. *Performance of microdilution trays with three penicillins before and after storage at −20 and −60 C*

Determination	Geometric mean MICs[a] of:		
	Benzylpenicillin	Carbenicillin	Ampicillin
Week 4			
Control for stored trays[b]	65.4 (64–128)	16.3 (16–32)	4.4 (4–8)
Week 3			
Initial tests before storage	44.3 (32–128)	17.4 (16–32)	4.0 (4)[c]
After 7 days at −20 C	61.3 (32–64)	16.7 (8–32)	4.1 (4–8)
After 7 days at −60 C	38.0 (32–64)	21.7 (16–32)	3.8 (2–4)
Week 2			
Initial tests before storage	64.0 (64)	ND[d]	5.2 (4–8)
After 14 days at −20 C	64.0 (64)	32.0 (32)	4.6 (4–8)
After 14 days at −60 C	39.0 (32–64)	ND[d]	3.9 (2–4)
Week 1			
Initial tests before storage	61.3 (32–64)	5.2 (4–8)	4.4 (4–8)
After 21 days at −20 C	64.0 (64)	4.6 (4–8)	4.9 (4–8)
After 21 days at −60 C	36.4 (32–64)	3.9 (2–4)	3.9 (2–4)

[a] Each value was based on 32 MIC determinations with the "Seattle" *E. coli*. Numbers in parentheses represent minimum and maximum values. MICs expressed in micrograms per milliliter.
[b] MIC values determined on freshly prepared trays, prepared and tested on the day that stored trays were tested.
[c] Only one figure is presented when all 32 MICs were the same, i.e., minimum = maximum.
[d] ND, Data excluded; trays were contaminated.

TABLE 5. *Performance of microdilution trays with three semisynthetic penicillins and cephalothin before and after storage at −20 and −60 C*

Determination	Geometric mean MICs[a] of:			
	Methicillin	Oxacillin	Nafcillin	Cephalothin
Week 5				
Control for stored trays[b]	3.4 (2–4)	0.28 (0.25–0.50)	0.27 (0.12–0.50)	0.16 (0.12–0.25)
Week 4				
Initial tests before storage	2.0 (2)[c]	0.25 (0.25)	0.25 (0.25)	0.12 (0.12)
After 7 days at −20 C	2.0 (2)	0.25 (0.25)	0.25 (0.25)	0.15 (0.12–0.25)
After 7 days at −60 C	2.0 (2)	0.25 (0.25)	0.25 (0.25)	0.15 (0.12–0.25)
Week 3				
Initial tests before storage	2.0 (2)	0.21 (0.12–0.25)	0.35 (0.25–0.50)	0.16 (0.12–0.25)
After 14 days at −20 C	2.7 (2–4)	0.38 (0.25–0.50)	0.35 (0.25–0.50)	0.19 (0.12–0.25)
After 14 days at −60 C	2.7 (2–4)	0.30 (0.25–0.50)	0.35 (0.25–0.50)	0.18 (0.12–0.25)
Week 2				
Initial tests before storage	3.4 (2–8)	0.25 (0.25)	0.25 (0.25)	0.18 (0.12–0.25)
After 21 days at −20 C	2.0 (2)	0.32 (0.25–0.50)	0.38 (0.25–0.50)	0.16 (0.12–0.25)
After 21 days at −60 C	2.0 (2)	0.25 (0.25)	0.25 (0.25)	0.16 (0.12–0.25)
Week 1				
Initial tests before storage	2.0 (2)	0.15 (0.12–0.25)	0.18 (0.12–0.25)	0.10 (0.06–0.12)
After 28 days at −20 C	4.4 (4–8)	0.35 (0.25–0.50)	0.30 (0.25–0.50)	0.15 (0.06–0.12)
After 28 days at −60 C	2.6 (2–4)	0.18 (0.12–0.25)	0.18 (0.12–0.25)	0.15 (0.06–0.25)

[a] Each value was based on eight MIC determinations with the "Seattle" *S. aureus*. Numbers in parentheses represent minimum and maximum values. MIC, expressed as micrograms per milliliter.
[b] Mean of 16 MIC values determined on freshly prepared trays, prepared and tested on the day that stored trays were tested.
[c] Only one figure is presented when all MIC values were the same, i.e., minimum = maximum.

obtained from trays stored 28 days at −20 C differed significantly ($P < 0.001$) from those obtained before storage (chi-square test), but no significant differences were seen after 21 days of storage at −20 C. No significant changes were seen with cephalothin, oxacillin, or nafcillin or with methicillin stored at −60 C. Since these experiments were terminated after 28 days, it is not possible to determine the shelf life for the semisynthetic penicillins. The apparent inactivation of methicillin after 28 days at −20 C, but not at −60 C, deserves further investigation before firm conclusions can be drawn. However, we can conclude that the antibiotics included in this study may be stored frozen for at least 21 days without significant loss of activity.

DISCUSSION

The data reported in the present study clearly demonstrate the high degree of accuracy and precision by which a series of seven doubling dilutions of antibiotic can be prepared with an Autotiter IV system. More recently, we have obtained indirect evidence suggesting that there may be a cummulative error that decreases the accuracy and precision of the antimicrobic dilutions if the machine is programmed to continue the dilutions to a full 14 dilution steps. Fortunately, such an extensive series of doubling dilutions is rarely required for most quantitative susceptibility tests. Even though we documented extremely good results, there are enough factors that can influence performance of this mechanical system to necessitate constant monitoring of samples from each batch of trays in order to properly control the test system (4–7). This can be done most efficiently by including one or more control organisms with each series of tests; the results should be no more than one dilution step above or below the mean for each drug.

The stability of diluted antimicrobics frozen in 50-μl volumes has been observed by others (2, 4). The more quantitative data included in the present studies were limited to tests with only three penicillins that are notoriously unstable. Additional tests with three semisynthetic penicillins and a cephalosporin were added to further support our conclusions. Additional tests with other antimicrobial agents and more prolonged storage periods will be needed to make specific recommendations concerning maximal shelf life of the trays. From our experience with the more labile antimicrobial drugs, we can conclude that the trays may be stored at least 3 weeks without loss of activity. In practice, many antimicrobics can be stored longer than 3 weeks without altering the concentration enough to affect the end points seen with the control organisms.

In addition to the inactivation of an antimicrobial agent during storage, the actual concentration of drugs in the microdilution trays may be increased by a loss of moisture due to evaporation that may occur during the freeze-thaw cycle. For that reason, the shelf life will depend upon the way in which the trays are wrapped for storage; every precaution should be taken to minimize the loss of moisture from the frozen trays. The temperature at which the trays are stored (−20 or −60 C) did not influence the stability of the drugs during the first 3 weeks of storage.

Although freshly prepared stock solutions were used for each batch of trays included in the present study, a more convenient system could be developed if the stock solutions could be prepared in bulk and frozen aliquots could be stored until a set of trays is needed. The trays could then be frozen for a maximum of 2 to 3 weeks, but that would necessitate two freeze-thaw cycles which might alter the activity of some antimicrobial agents. We have performed preliminary studies that failed to demonstrate any change in the activity of concentrated stock solutions of ampicillin, benzylpenicillin, and carbenicillin after several freeze-thaw cycles. This observation needs to be confirmed and expanded to other antimicrobial agents before such an approach can be recommended as a standard procedure.

In summary, an Autotiter IV is capable of preparing dilutions of antimicrobial agents with a satisfactory degree of accuracy and precision, and the trays containing diluted antimicrobial drugs can be stored at −20 C or less for as long as 3 weeks without a significant loss of activity, at least with the more labile agents included in the present study.

LITERATURE CITED

1. **Bauer, A. W., W. M. M. Kirby, J. C. Sherris, and M. Turck.** 1966. Antibiotic susceptibility testing by a standardized disk method. Am. J. Clin. Pathol. **45**:493–496.
2. **Bennett, J. V., J. L. Brodie, E. J. Benner and W. M. M. Kirby.** 1966. Simplified, accurate method for antibiotic assay of clinical specimens. Appl. Microbiol. **14**:170–177.
3. **Gavan, T. L., and D. Butler.** 1974. An automated microdilution method for antimicrobial susceptibility testing, p. 88–93. *In* A. Balows (ed.), Current techniques for antibiotic susceptibility testing. Charles C Thomas, Publisher, Springfield, Ill.
4. **Gavan, T. L., and M. A. Town.** 1970. A microdilution method for antibiotic susceptibility testing. Am. J. Clin. Pathol. **53**:880–885.
5. **Gerlach, E. H.** 1974. Microdilution: a comparative study, p. 63–76. *In* A. Balows (ed.), Current tech-

niques for antibiotic susceptibility testing. Charles C Thomas, Publisher, Springfield, Ill.

6. **MacLowry, J. D., M. J. Jaqua, and S. T. Selepak.** 1970. Detailed methodology and implementation of a semiautomated serial dilution microtechnique for antimicrobial susceptibility testing. Appl. Microbiol. **20**:46–53.
7. **MacLowry, J. D., and H. H. Marsh.** 1968. Semi-automated microtechnique for serial dilution–antibiotic sensitivity testing in the clinical laboratory. J. Clin. Med. **72**:685–687.
8. **Marymont, J. H., and R. M. Wentz.** 1966. Serial dilution antibiotic sensitivity testing with the microtiter system. Am. J. Clin. Pathol. **45**:548–551.
9. **Tilton, R. C., L. Lieberman, and E. H. Gerlach.** 1973. Microdilution antibiotic susceptibility test: examination of certain variables. Appl. Microbiol. **26**:658–665.
10. **Tilton, R. C., and L. Newberg.** 1974. Standardization of the microdilution susceptibility test, p. 77–87. *In* A. Balows (ed.), Current techniques for antibiotic susceptibility testing. Charles C Thomas, Publisher, Springfield, Ill.

Antimicrobial Agents and Chemotherapy, July 1976, p. 89-95
Vol. 10, No. 1

Influence of Subtherapeutic Levels of a Combination of Neomycin and Oxytetracycline on *Salmonella typhimurium* in Swine, Calves, and Chickens

A. E. GIRARD,* A. R. ENGLISH, D. G. EVANGELISTI, J. E. LYNCH, and I. A. SOLOMONS
Medical Research Laboratories, Pfizer Central Research, Groton, Connecticut 06340

Received for publication 14 January 1976

Subtherapeutic levels of oxytetracycline plus neomycin in animal feeds did not bring about increases in the quantity, prevalence, or shedding of *Salmonella typhimurium* in swine, calves, or chickens. In fact, the medication generally reduced the proportion of animals carrying *S. typhimurium*. The medicated groups were fed rations containing oxytetracycline plus neomycin commencing 5 days prior to oral inoculation with *S. typhimurium* and continuing through a 28-day postinoculation period. Colonization of *S. typhimurium* occurred in all three animal species, as evidenced by clinical signs of infection and/or colony counts in feces. Only from swine and on only one occasion was a single resistant colony isolated. It is concluded that no evidence has been obtained which would implicate the continuous low-level feeding of oxytetracycline and neomycin for a 4-week period to a potential increased incidence of disease in animals or as a hazard to humans.

There has been general concern over the feeding of subtherapeutic levels of antibiotics to animals primarily because of a possible hazard to human health (4, 5). Recently (2) we reported on the influence of oxytetracycline on *Salmonella typhimurium* in animals. Generally the subtherapeutic use of oxytetracycline brought about a decrease in the percentage of animals carrying *S. typhimurium* and did not bring about any increase in the quantity, prevalence, or shedding of *S. typhimurium* in swine, calves, and chickens.

The studies reported here were undertaken to ascertain whether the continuous feeding of a combination of neomycin and oxytetracycline at subtherapeutic levels increases the quantity, prevalence, and duration of shedding of *S. typhimurium* in swine, calves, and chickens over that observed in nonmedicated controls. In addition, the susceptibility of *S. typhimurium* to neomycin, oxytetracycline, and several other antimicrobial agents used in human clinical medicine was determined before and during the course of these studies.

MATERIALS AND METHODS

Organism(s). The strains of *S. typhimurium* used were the same as those previously reported (2). All strains produced an acid butt with H_2S and an alkaline slant in triple sugar iron agar (TSI; Difco Laboratories, Detroit, Mich.), were urease negative, agglutinated with *Salmonella* group B antiserum (BBL, Cockeysville, Md.), and were susceptible to oxytetracycline, neomycin, kanamycin, gentamicin, ampicillin, cephalothin, streptomycin, and chloramphenicol.

Salmonella challenge. Swine and calves were fed 0.5 lb (approximately 226 g) of basal feed to which was added a 40-ml suspension of *S. typhimurium* containing $\sim 1.1 \times 10^{11}$ to 1.4×10^{11} organisms. The chickens were given the inoculum by delivering a slurry of *S. typhimurium* suspension in feed into the gullet. A plate count of the inoculum revealed that each chicken received $\sim 2.92 \times 10^{11}$ organisms.

Animals. All animals were purchased from commercial sources. At the start of the experiments, the Hampshire-Yorkshire Cross swine weighed an average of 9.1 kg, whereas Holstein calves' average weight was 85.7 kg, and the chicks, at 8 days of age, averaged 0.0798 kg.

Experimental diets. Groups designated T-1 were fed a ration of nonmedicated feed throughout the experimental period, whereas the T-2 groups were fed the same feed containing neomycin and oxytetracycline, commencing 5 days prior to *S. typhimurium* inoculation and throughout the remainder of the experimental period. No other medication was administered over the experimental period. Finished feeds were bioassayed for neomycin and oxytetracycline at the start and termination of each study according to established procedures (3). The levels of neomycin and oxytetracycline in each animal feed are presented in Table 1.

General. The methods and materials used in the maintenance of the animals and clinical records, as well as performance of pretest *Salmonella* screening, quantitation of *S. typhimurium* from inoculated animals, quantitation of pretest oxytetracycline-resistant *Escherichia coli*, antibiotic susceptibility, and statistical analysis, were the same as those previously reported (2). The oxytetracycline resistance in *E. coli* was examined after random lotting of animals but before the start of treatment.

RESULTS

Swine. Just prior to the start of the experiment, oxytetracycline-resistant *E. coli* represented an average of 5.4% of the total *E. coli* population in the infected controls and 19.7% in the medicated animals.

TABLE 1. *Levels of oxytetracycline and neomycin in each animal feed*

Animal	Nonmedicated feed (basal)	Amount of each antimicrobial added to feed (g/ton)
Swine	Pig grower ration	150[a]
Calf	Rough cattle finisher ration	94.9[b]
Chicken	Chick starter ration	200

[a] A 150-g portion of oxytetracycline plus 150 g of neomycin sulfate.

[b] Calculated to provide a level equivalent to 350 mg of each compound/head per day at the start of the experiment.

The viable *Salmonella* counts from the fecal samples are presented in Table 2. It is apparent that *S. typhimurium* colonized the swine gut in both the medicated and nonmedicated groups. Logarithms of the colony counts obtained over the seven sampling periods were averaged for each animal, and comparison (two-sample t test) showed that the quantity of *Salmonella* in the medicated group was significantly less than that in the nonmedicated controls having a value of $P < 0.001$.

The medicated group exhibited more *Salmonella*-free fecal specimens, 56/70 (10 swine/group × 7 samplings = 70 samples) compared to 17/70 for the control group. A statistical analysis of prevalence was performed by examining the overall gross patterns of shedding. A score was assigned to each animal using the number of days (out of 7) on which shedding occurred. For instance, animal no. 18 had a score of four, animal no. 36 had a score of three and animal no. 37 (in whom an apparent reinfection may have occurred on day 14) had a score of four (Table 2). Two-sample t tests were then run on these scores, and the rate of decrease in shedding was significantly ($P < 0.001$) more rapid in the neomycin-oxytetracycline group than in the nonmedicated controls.

TABLE 2. *S. typhimurium counts per gram[a] of swine feces*

Swine no.	Days (postinoculation)						
	2	4	7	10	14	21	28
T-1 group[b]							
1	4.19×10^7	1.90×10^6	9.17×10^3	5.99×10^4	4.04×10^3	8.02×10^3	2.50×10^2
4	2.45×10^7	4.59×10^6	2.25×10^4	0	0	0	0
9	2.76×10^6	1.38×10^5	1.96×10^5	4.81×10^4	1.69×10^4	5.59×10^3	2.36×10^2
12	5.34×10^4	3.39×10^4	2.24×10^3	0	1.39×10^3	0	1.86×10^2
18	3.38×10^5	2.84×10^3	1.64×10^4	1.00×10^4	0	0	0
23	2.60×10^6	7.14×10^3	4.07×10^4	1.85×10^3	2.25×10^3	9.96×10^5	0
27	2.50×10^5	1.25×10^5	4.43×10^4	4.81×10^4	2.25×10^4	2.25×10^4	7.07×10^3
29	3.10×10^5	6.96×10^3	3.46×10^4	2.48×10^4	2.67×10^4	1.54×10^3	1.20×10^5
36	3.38×10^5	1.14×10^4	0	0	0	0	3.32×10^4
37	9.77×10^6	7.77×10^4	2.02×10^3	0	1.13×10^3	0	0
T-2 group[c]							
1	6.49×10^4	0	0	0	0	0	0
8	1.52×10^7	0	1.90×10^5	4.24×10^4	0	0	0
13	0	0	0	0	0	0	0
15	7.78×10^5	4.20×10^4	4.07×10^2	0	1.70×10^4[d]	0	0
21	0	0	0	0	0	0	0
26	0	2.17×10^3	0	0	0	0	0
32	1.35×10^3	2.63×10^4	0	0	0	0	0
34	5.46×10^5	5.13×10^3	0	0	0	0	0
39	2.92×10^7	0	0	0	0	0	0
43	0	0	0	0	0	0	0

[a] Dry weight.

[b] Control nonmedicated group. The results of all control groups were previously published (2) and are presented here for the benefit of the reader.

[c] Neomycin- and oxytetracycline-medicated group.

[d] Resistant colony (one colony of five examined from a 10^{-3} dilution; see text for discussion).

The percentage of swine shedding *Salmonella* as a function of time is plotted in Fig. 1A, which shows a decrease in both groups with time. The rate of decrease in shedding is faster in the oxytetracycline-neomycin group. Since all animals were inoculated initially, the statistical analysis dealt with the rate at which *S. typhimurium* disappeared. A rate of change in the probability of shedding per day was computed across all 28 days of the trial for each animal. These rates were then compared with a two-sample t test. The rate of decrease in shedding was significantly ($P < 0.01$) more rapid in the medicated group than in the nonmedicated controls.

Susceptibility tests were performed with 57 isolates from the treated group (T-2) over the sampling periods during the 28-day postinoculation period. The only instance of antibiotic resistance was with one isolate (pig no. 15) that was found to be resistant to kanamycin, neomycin, and streptomycin, as defined in the Federal Register (1). There were no changes in the susceptibility of *S. typhimurium* to the other antibacterial agents tested. This resistant colony (Table 2) was one of five isolated from a 10^{-3} dilution of sample spread on an antibiotic-free medium. The resistant count then was $\sim 3.4 \times 10^3$. These results demonstrate that the subtherapeutic level of neomycin and oxytetracycline did not cause a significant increase in resistant *S. typhimurium*. No resistance was detected in the 232 *S. typhimurium* isolates recovered from the nonmedicated group.

Clinical signs of disease, body temperature, and diarrhea scores are plotted in Fig. 2A. The observations demonstrate that clinical signs of infection were established in swine. In fact, the animals were on the border line of a severe illness that would normally be treated with therapeutic doses of the antibiotic. The medicated group demonstrated a decrease in the severity of diarrhea but no reduction in temperature elevation. The performance values for feed conversion (Table 5) indicate that the medicated feed was better than the control nonmedicated feed in its efficiency.

Calves. During the first postinoculation week, disease symptoms were so severe that there was concern for the survival of the animals. By the second week the animals had a generally healthy appearance. It seemed then that the challenge was near the lethal dose and the illness acute in nature, since recovery and disappearance of *S. typhimurium* was rapid and complete. The fecal counts observed during the course of this study were not as high as anticipated, but a higher challenge may have been fatal. In fact, one animal in the nonmedicated group died on day 6 postinoculation. The necropsy report indicated the presence of *Pasteurella hemolytica* and *S. typhimurium*. *S. typhimurium* was cultured from the liver, spleen, lung, a lymph node, and the ileocecal junction. *P. hemolytica* was isolated from the lungs. Gross lesions were present in the lung probably due to pasteurellosis with the additional stress of the *S. typhimurium* challenge.

The oxytetracycline-resistant *E. coli* examined before the start of the experiment represented an average of 65.6% of the total *E. coli* population in the infected controls and 54.8% in the medicated animals.

The viable *Salmonella* counts obtained from the fecal samples are shown in Table 3. It is clear that the *S. typhimurium* population in the nonmedicated group decreased with time. *S. typhimurium* was detected in only two ani-

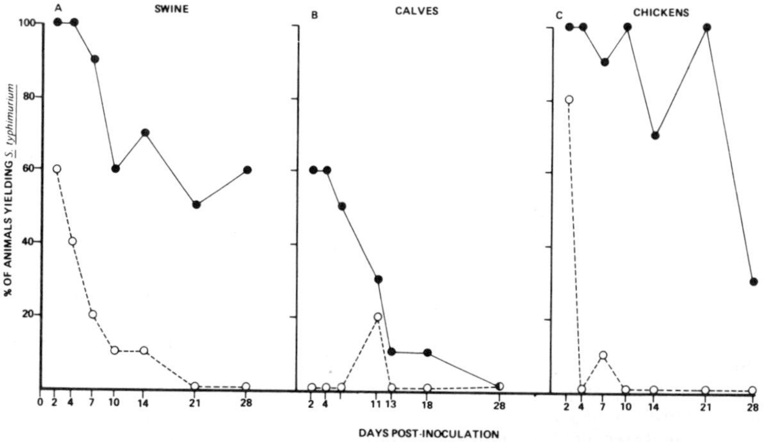

FIG. 1. *Percentage of animals shedding S. typhimurium. Symbols:* ●, *Nonmedicated controls;* ○, *oxytetracycline-neomycin treated.*

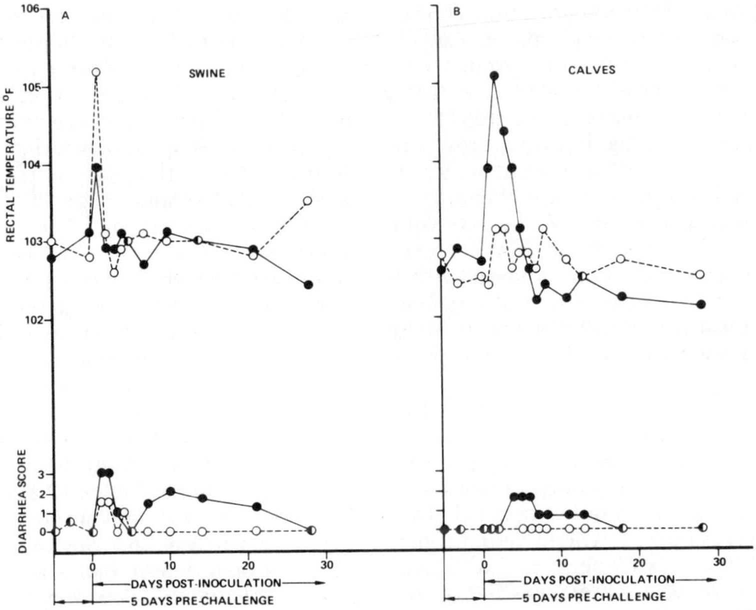

FIG. 2. *Temperature and diarrhea measurements (median values). Symbols:* ●, *Nonmedicated controls;* ○, *oxytetracycline-neomycin treated. Diarrhea was scored according to stool consistency with 0 as normal and 3 being a very loose consistency.*

TABLE 3. *S. typhimurium counts per gram[a] of calf feces*

Calf no.	Days (postinoculation)						
	2	4	6	11	13	18	28
T-1 group[b]							
12	8.89×10^6	2.60×10^7	6.96×10^7[c]				
26	0	0	0	0	0	0	0
27	0	0	0	0	0	0	0
31	2.16×10^2	0	0	0	0	0	0
34	2.43×10^2	4.96×10^7	5.67×10^4	0	0	0	0
36	5.46×10^5	6.90×10^6	8.32×10^5	8.60×10^3	6.93×10^3	4.79×10^3	0
39	1.69×10^4	3.37×10^4	7.39×10^3	3.94×10^2	0	0	0
41	0	0	0	0	0	0	0
42	2.93×10^4	8.16×10^7	5.00×10^5	2.29×10^2	0	0	0
44	0	1.31×10^4	0	0	0	0	0
T-2 group[d]							
14	0	0	0	0	0	0	0
17	0	0	0	0	0	0	0
19	0	0	0	4.78×10^4	0	0	0
24	0	0	0	0	0	0	0
33	0	0	0	0	0	0	0
37	0	0	0	5.86×10^3	0	0	0
43	0	0	0	0	0	0	0
48	0	0	0	0	0	0	0
49	0	0	0	0	0	0	0
51	0	0	0	0	0	0	0

[a] Dry weight.
[b] Control nonmedicated group.
[c] Died on postinoculation day 6.
[d] Neomycin- and oxytetracycline-medicated group.

mals of the medicated group and this detection was limited to one sampling period. A comparison of logarithms of the colony counts with a two-sample t test showed that the quantity of *Salmonella* in the medicated group was significantly ($P < 0.05$) less than that in the nonmedicated controls.

The medicated group exhibited many more *Salmonella*-free cultures (68/70) over the duration of the experiment than did the nonmedicated controls (44/66). A statistical analysis of the prevalence of *S. typhimurium* in the medicated versus the nonmedicated group revealed that there was a significant ($P < 0.05$) decrease in the medicated animals.

The percentage of calves shedding *S. typhimurium* as a function of time is plotted in Fig. 1B. Whereas the rate of decrease in shedding was faster in the neomycin-oxytetracycline group, statistical analysis of the rate of change in probability of shedding yielded no significant difference. A 95% confidence interval on the mean difference suggests that the difference in probability of shedding per day lies between 1.6% less to 0.10% more for the medicated group compared to the nonmedicated group.

There were no resistant organisms detected in the *S. typhimurium* population recovered from either the medicated or nonmedicated group.

Rectal temperature measurements and diarrhea scores are plotted in Fig. 2B. These observations demonstrate that clinical signs of infection were established in the nonmedicated calves and, as noted previously, the challenge was a near lethal one. The neomycin-oxytetracycline-medicated group showed a reduced temperature rise and better control of diarrhea compared with nonmedicated controls.

Chickens. The oxytetracycline-resistant *E. coli* examined before the start of the experiment represented an average of 30.0% of the total *E. coli* population in the infected controls and 14.9% in the medicated animals.

The viable *Salmonella* counts obtained from the fecal samples are shown in Table 4. A com-

TABLE 4. *S. typhimurium counts per gram[a] of chicken feces*

Calf no.	Days (postinoculation)						
	2	4	7	10	14	21	28
T-1 group[b]							
7	1.56×10^5	3.13×10^5	1.36×10^5	2.92×10^4	7.69×10^2	1.17×10^4	0
8	4.02×10^7	4.52×10^5	3.63×10^4	1.57×10^4	3.52×10^4	2.42×10^3	0
14	1.21×10^5	2.24×10^6	1.88×10^8	2.50×10^4	1.64×10^3	1.22×10^4	0
19	2.18×10^4	1.06×10^4	4.37×10^2	2.89×10^2	0	1.32×10^4	0
31	1.03×10^7	7.79×10^5	6.61×10^5	1.94×10^5	1.87×10^3	3.33×10^4	0
34	3.06×10^5	1.36×10^5	5.21×10^3	7.61×10^3	0	3.39×10^3	0
37	3.47×10^6	5.56×10^4	4.38×10^3	4.97×10^3	1.52×10^4	1.23×10^3	2.55×10^4
56	1.99×10^6	3.15×10^4	7.43×10^3	8.85×10^2	2.18×10^4	1.00×10^4	1.65×10^3
73	3.47×10^5	1.88×10^4	0	4.82×10^3	0	2.08×10^4	5.08×10^2
81	2.92×10^6	7.21×10^3	3.25×10^2	8.57×10^2	2.08×10^3	5.47×10^3	0
Environmental group							
18	0	0	0	0	0	0	0
58	0	0	0	0	0	0	0
85	0	0	0	0	0	0	0
T-2 group[c]							
3	3.13×10^2	0	0	0	0	0	0
21	0	0	0	0	0	0	0
25	2.15×10^4	0	0	0	0	0	0
49	1.43×10^4	0	0	0	0	0	0
57	0	0	0	0	0	0	0
71	4.95×10^3	0	0	0	0	0	0
83	1.35×10^5	0	0	0	0	0	0
87	3.74×10^3	0	0	0	0	0	0
90	5.71×10^3	0	1.86×10^2	0	0	0	0
92	1.47×10^6	0	0	0	0	0	0

[a] Dry weight.
[b] Control nonmedicated group.
[c] Neomycin- and oxytetracycline-medicated group.

parison between the two groups demonstrates the beneficial effects of this subtherapeutic dosage regimen of oxytetracycline and neomycin. The quantity of *S. typhimurium* was considerably less in the medicated group than in the control group. This observation was shown to be a statistically significant decrease, having a value of $P < 0.001$. The medicated group also yielded many more *Salmonella*-free cultures (61/70) over the duration of the experiment than did the nonmedicated controls (11/70) (Table 4). This was also shown to be statistically significant, having a value of $P < 0.001$.

The percentage of chickens shedding *S. typhimurium* as a function of time is plotted in Fig. 1C. All chickens in the nonmedicated group were shedding *S. typhimurium* on day 21; a dramatic decline was observed only on the final day of the experiment. In contrast, 8/10 animals of the medicated group were shedding *S. typhimurium* on day 2 postinoculation, and there was only one more occurrence of shedding in the medicated group during the remainder of the trial. The results demonstrate that the oxytetracycline-plus-neomycin treatment decreased the extent of colonization. The rate of decrease in shedding was significantly ($P < 0.001$) more rapid in the oxytetracycline-neomycin group than in the nonmedicated controls.

There was no increase in the development of resistance of *S. typhimurium* in the medicated animals (no resistant colonies among the 33 recovered from the medicated group).

The values calculated for feed conversion (Table 5) suggest that the medicated feed was approximately equal to the control nonmedicated feed in its efficiency.

DISCUSSION

Some of the difficulties involved in determining the proper inoculum size and route of challenge allowing colonization without death were presented in an earlier report (2). Clinical signs of disease were apparent in swine and calves when using *S. typhimurium* at a concentration of approximately 10^{11} cells/ml. Temperature elevation and/or diarrhea of varying degree were evident in both medicated and nonmedicated groups. The viable counts of *S. typhimurium* obtained from all the swine and calves provided evidence that the organism successfully colonized the intestines. No clinical signs of disease were observed in the two groups of chickens, even though colonization by *S. typhimurium* was also successful, utilizing an inoculum of $\sim 2.9 \times 10^{11}$/chicken.

The challenges used in these model studies were intentionally much more severe than would be found under practical field conditions. Animals with symptoms of disease, as observed in the swine and calf experiments, would normally be treated with larger doses of antibiotic (therapeutic rather than subtherapeutic drug levels).

The numbers of *S. typhimurium* in medicated swine, calves, and chickens did not increase over those observed in the nonmedicated controls. On the contrary, the quantity of *S. typhimurium* isolated from the medicated swine, calves, and chickens was significantly less than that of their nonmedicated counterparts. The degree of prevalence and shedding of *S. typhimurium* was not increased in the medicated swine and chickens. If one assumes that an increase in the animal *Salmonella* reservoir is a hazard to man, these data suggest that the use of subtherapeutic levels of oxytetracycline plus neomycin actually reduces the potential hazards of *S. typhimurium* to human and animal health.

Except for one isolate obtained from swine, there was no change in the susceptibility of the 97 *S. typhimurium* colonies isolated from all medicated animals. The results demonstrate that the subtherapeutic level of neomycin and oxytetracycline did not cause a significant increase in resistant *S. typhimurium*.

Accepting that food animals are usually fed antibiotic for more than 28 days, we feel that the results would not have been significantly

TABLE 5. *Weight, feed consumption, and feed conversion*

Animal	Treatment	Average daily gain (kg/animal)	Gain relative to control (%)	Feed efficiency (feed consumed/wt gain)	Feed efficiency relative to control (%)
Swine	Nonmedicated	0.328	100.0	2.342	100.0
Swine	Medicated	0.497	151.5	1.971	118.8
Calves	Nonmedicated	0.678	100.0	5.244	100.0
Calves	Medicated	1.193	176.0	3.604	145.5
Chickens	Nonmedicated	0.030	100	1.744	100.0
Chickens	Nonmedicated[a]	0.028	92.2	1.758	99.2
Chickens	Medicated	0.030	100	1.729	100.9

[a] This group (environmental controls) was not inoculated.

different had we extended the experimental period, since all treated and nontreated animals of all species demonstrated a general decline in shedding *Salmonella* as a function of time. The medicated animals included in these experiments were fed antibiotic throughout the studies, although there is usually a withdrawal period prior to marketing. The inclusion of a withdrawal period conceivably could have removed any differences observed between the treated and nonmedicated groups with regard to antibiotic resistance, because of the reduction of antibiotic selective pressure.

A significant increase in the reservoir of *Salmonella* in food animals is speculated to constitute an increased risk to human health. The results reported here indicate there was no significant increase in the quantity, prevalence, and shedding of *S. typhimurium* in the medicated group compared to nonmedicated inoculated controls. Although only one strain was employed, the data generally demonstrate that the subtherapeutic use of oxytetracycline and neomycin actually decreases the quantity, prevalence, and shedding of *S. typhimurium* in animals. No evidence that would associate the continuous low-level feeding of oxytetracycline plus neomycin with an increased incidence of salmonellosis in animals or humans has been obtained.

ACKNOWLEDGMENTS

We are grateful to William Babcock and the staff at the Pfizer Animal Health Center at Terre Haute, Ind., for performing the bioassays on the feed, collecting the fecal samples, and generally assisting in the logistical support of this study. We wish to thank David S. Salsburg, who did the statistical analysis of the data, and R. J. Borovoy and F. A. Meyer for their technical assistance.

LITERATURE CITED

1. **Edwards, C. C.** 1971. Antibiotic susceptibility discs. Drug efficacy study implementation. Fed. Regist. 36:6899–6902.
2. **Evangelisti, D. G., A. R. English, A. E. Girard, J. E. Lynch, and I. A. Solomons.** 1975. Influence of subtherapeutic levels of oxytetracycline on *Salmonella typhimurium* in swine, calves, and chickens. Antimicrob. Agents Chemother. 8:664–672.
3. **Grove, D. C., and W. A. Randall.** 1955. Assay methods of antibiotics. A laboratory manual, p. 50–52. Medical Encyclopedia, Inc., New York.
4. **Smith, H. W.** 1966. The incidence of infective drug resistance in strains of *Escherichia coli* isolated from diseased human beings and domestic animals. J. Hyg. 64:465–474.
5. **Smith, H. W.** 1970. The transfer of antibiotic resistance between strains of Enterobacteria in chicken, calves and pigs. J. Med. Microbiol. 3:165–180.

ANTIMICROBIAL AGENTS AND CHEMOTHERAPY, July 1976, p. 96-101 Vol. 10, No. 1

Inactivation of the Enveloped Bacteriophage $\phi 6$ by Butylated Hydroxytoluene and Butylated Hydroxyanisole

PAUL WANDA, JAMES CUPP, WALLACE SNIPES,* ALEC KEITH, TOM RUCINSKY,[1] LOUIS POLISH, AND JEFFREY SANDS

Biophysics Laboratory, Department of Biochemistry and Biophysics, The Pennsylvania State University, University Park, Pennsylvania 16802, and Physics Department and Molecular Biology Program, Lehigh University, Bethlehem, Pennsylvania 18015*

Received for publication 5 April 1976

Butylated hydroxytoluene (BHT) is a potent inactivator of the enveloped bacterial virus $\phi 6$ at concentrations as low as 3×10^{-5} M. The viral envelope is not removed by BHT treatment, in contrast to the effects of exposure to the detergent Triton X-100. BHT-treated viruses are morphologically indistinguishable from controls but are defective in their ability to attach to the host cell. Temperature at the time of exposure was found to be a crucial factor in the effectiveness of BHT against $\phi 6$. A precipitous drop in the degree of inactivation by 3×10^{-5} M BHT occurred when the temperature was lowered from 20 to 15 C. Calcium ions were found to potentiate the effect of BHT, particularly at lower temperatures where BHT alone was relatively ineffective. Barium and strontium, but not magnesium, were also effective in enhancing the activity of BHT. A structurally related molecule, butylated hydroxyanisole (BHA), was also found to inactivate $\phi 6$ virus, but higher concentrations were required than with BHT. Both BHT and BHA are commonly used as food additives, have apparent low toxicity to humans and other animals, and are potentially useful as antiviral agents.

It was recently reported from our laboratory that butylated hydroxytoluene (BHT) is a potent inactivator of lipid-containing viruses (11). This compound is generally recognized as safe by the Food and Drug Administration (5) and is widely used as an antioxidant in food and cosmetic preparations. The combination of effectiveness against viruses and apparent low toxicity to humans has generated considerable interest in the potential use of BHT as an antiviral agent, particularly for topical application to virus-infected areas of the skin. Consequently, we are characterizing the effects of BHT on lipid-containing viruses in vitro, hoping to improve our understanding of the mechanisms whereby BHT destroys viral infectivity.

In a detailed study of the effects of BHT on the bacterial virus PM2, it was found that virus particles are completely disrupted by BHT, with the viral deoxyribonucleic acid being released to the medium as a very slowly sedimentable material (1). Several factors which influence the inactivation of PM2 by BHT, including the initial virus titer, the time of exposure, and the presence of certain "protective" agents including surfactants, bovine serum albumin, and bacterial cells, were studied. Potentially important with regard to the use of BHT as an antiviral substance was the observation that its effectiveness is strongly dependent upon the solvent from which it is added to the culture medium.

Different viruses have different susceptibilities to BHT, and the most susceptible one studied thus far is the enveloped bacterial virus $\phi 6$. This virus is bounded by a rather loose membrane structure (3, 13) and has many similarities to several animal viruses. We have now studied in more detail the inactivation of $\phi 6$ by BHT, and the results of this research are described here. In addition, we report that the related food additive butylated hydroxyanisole (BHA) also inactivates $\phi 6$, although higher concentrations are required than for BHT. The chemical structures of BHT and BHA are given in Fig. 1. BHA, as shown, is a mixture of two isomers.

[1] Present address: Washington University Medical School, Cancer Center, St. Louis, Mo. 63130.

MATERIALS AND METHODS

Viruses and cells. Bacteriophage $\phi 6$ was discovered by Vidaver et al. (13). Our initial stocks of $\phi 6$ and its host, *Pseudomonas phaseolicola* strain HB10Y, were kindly provided by Anne Vidaver.

Media and culture methods. Two types of media were used for the culture of HB10Y and $\phi 6$. V me-

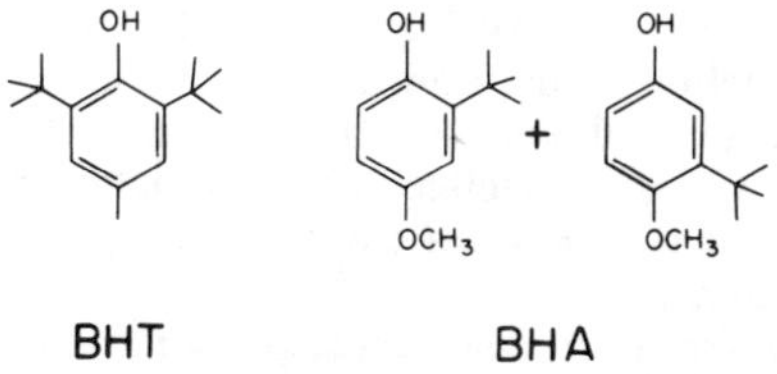

FIG. 1. *Structures of BHT and BHA.*

dium contained 10 g of tryptone, 5 g of yeast extract, 7 g of NaCl, 1.5 g of KCl, and 0.5 g of $MgSO_4 \cdot 7H_2O$ per liter of distilled water. V plates were composed of V medium hardened with 1.5% (wt/vol) agar (Difco Laboratories, Detroit, Mich.).

A defined but somewhat enriched medium, designated TBM21, contained 3 g of KCl, 6 g of NaCl, 2 g of NH_4Cl, 0.2 g of $MgSO_4 \cdot 7H_2O$, 0.05 g of KH_2PO_4, 5 g of glucose, and 12.1 g of tris(hydroxymethyl)-aminomethane (Tris) base per liter of distilled water. The pH was adjusted to 7.6 with concentrated HCl. Medium TBM21 also contains all the naturally occurring amino acids except tryptophan (20 mg of each per liter) and the purine nucleosides adenosine and guanosine (50 mg of each per liter).

A Tris-buffered dilution solution, designated TB, contained the same salts as TBM21 but lacked glucose and the additional amino acid and nucleoside supplements.

Sucrose gradient analysis. Sucrose gradients (15 to 35%) were prepared in 50% medium TBM21. Virus samples were layered on top of the gradients and centrifuged for 180 min at 25,000 rpm in a Beckman SW27 rotor. The tube was punctured, and fractions were collected for assay.

Electron microscopy. A parlodian-carbon-coated grid was floated on the virus sample for approximately 5 min and then transferred, with a drop of sample adhering, to a drop of 0.2 M sodium cacodylate buffer, pH 7.0, containing 1% glutaraldehyde. After 5 min the grid was washed twice with distilled water and stained by transferring to a drop of 1% phosphotungstic acid for 1 to 2 min. Excess fluid was removed with filter paper, and the sample was dried in air. Electron micrographs were obtained with a Philips EM300 operating at 60 kV.

Source of materials. Carrier free $H_3{}^{32}PO_4$ was obtained from New England Nuclear Corp., Boston, Mass. BHT was purchased from Aldrich Chemical Co., Milwaukee, Wis., under the name 2,6-di-tert-butyl-4-methylphenol. BHA was obtained from Sigma Chemical Co., St. Louis, Mo.

RESULTS

Sedimentation properties of BHT-treated virus. Samples of BHT-treated virus were analyzed on sucrose gradients to determine the degree to which the virus particles are disrupted by BHT treatment. In particular, we were interested to know whether or not the viral envelope is removed during BHT treatment. It is known that the detergent Triton X-100 removes the membrane envelope from $\phi6$, leaving only the inner icosahedral core (9). Therefore, Triton X-100-treated samples were also analyzed for comparative purposes.

A radioactively labeled virus stock was prepared in medium TBM21 supplemented with $^{32}PO_4$. After lysis cell debris was removed by low-speed centrifugation, and the virus was pelleted, resuspended in a small volume of medium TBM21, and purified on a sucrose gradient. The peak fractions of radioactivity (and plaque-forming units) were used in further experiments.

One sample of labeled virus was treated with 0.1 mM BHT for 30 min. This resulted in greater than 99% inactivation of the virus. Another sample was treated with 1% Triton X-100, again resulting in greater than 99% inactivation. The treated samples and an untreated control were layered onto sucrose gradients and analyzed as described in Materials and Methods. The results are shown in Fig. 2. For the control and the BHT-treated samples, the ^{32}P radioactivity forms a band centered about fraction 13 with very little radioactivity at the top of the gradient. In several experiments of this type, control and BHT-treated samples gave indistinguishable results, with never more than one fraction separating the peaks of radioactivity. Plating results showed that, for the control, the peaks of virus infectivity and ^{32}P radioactivity coincide, whereas the virus titer

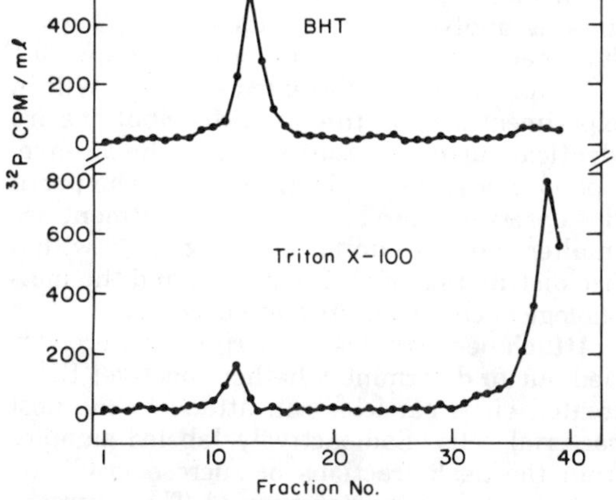

FIG. 2. *Sucrose gradient analysis of control, BHT-treated, and Triton X-100-treated samples of $\phi6$ virus. The direction of sedimentation in this figure is from right to left.*

in the peak fractions of the BHT-treated sample was less than 1% of that for the control. Thus, sucrose gradient analysis shows no observable difference in the sedimentation properties of inactive, BHT-treated virus and the untreated, infectious virus.

The sample treated with Triton X-100 gave a gradient profile with ^{32}P radioactivity in two positions. A band centered about fraction 12, much reduced in total radioactivity compared to bands of control and BHT-treated samples, contained the $\phi 6$ cores (see next section). The material near the top of the gradient was not characterized further but was most likely the phospholipid material released from the virion by Triton X-100 treatment.

These data indicate quite strongly that the envelope of the $\phi 6$ is not removed by BHT treatment under conditions where viral infectivity is reduced to less than 1%. This conclusion is further substantiated by data described in the following section.

Electron microscopy studies. Samples from the peak fractions of the gradients of Fig. 2 were prepared and examined by electron microscopy. These experiments were carried out to further establish that the $\phi 6$ envelope was intact in BHT-treated virus and to detect any noticeable morphological differences that might exist between treated and control samples. Electron micrographs showed that BHT-treated samples were indistinguishable from controls, whereas Triton X-100-treated samples were lacking the viral envelope. We have quantified these observations by measuring the diameter of a large number of particles from each sample and displaying the data as a size distribution (Fig. 3). The size of $\phi 6$ particles has been reported to vary from about 60 to 100 nm, with the average being about 80 nm (3). A least-squares analysis of the data of Fig. 3 gives diameters of 81.8 ± 6.3 nm for control and 80.1 ± 6.6 nm for the BHT-treated samples. Within experimental error, these size distributions are identical, further establishing that the $\phi 6$ envelope is intact after BHT treatment. The particles observed after Triton X-100 treatment are smaller and more uniform in geometry, with a size distribution of 65.5 ± 2.7 nm and the morphological characteristics of virus cores.

Attachment studies. Experiments were carried out to determine whether inactive, BHT-treated virus particles can attach to the host bacterial cells. Radioactively labeled samples from the peak fractions of sucrose gradients such as those of Fig. 2 were used. The control or BHT-inactivated virus were mixed with HB10Y cells and incubated at 25 C. At different times, samples were centrifuged to pellet host cells and attached virus, and the supernatants were assayed for radioactivity associated with unattached virus particles. These measurements were used to calculate the percentage of virus attachment.

Date from two separate experiments are shown in Table 1. Although there is some scatter in the data, it is clear that the process of attachment is defective in BHT-inactivated virus. These experiments, therefore, establish that the portion of the $\phi 6$ virus life cycle where BHT is effective is in the attachment of virus particles to the host cell. Little is known about the attachment process for $\phi 6$, and an under-

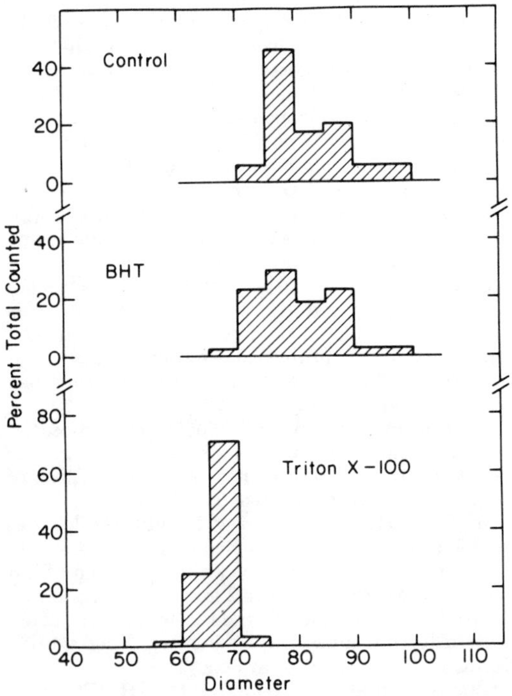

FIG. 3. *Size distribution of $\phi 6$ virus particles as determined from electron micrographs. The numbers of particles measured were 35, 44, and 65 for control, BHT-treated, and Triton X-100-treated samples, respectively. The horizontal axis is given in nanometers.*

TABLE 1. *Attachment of control and BHT-treated virus to host cells*

Time (min)	Expt	Attachment (%)	
		Control	BHT-treated
30	1	19	4
60	1	40	0
45	2	72	12
75	2	77	8

standing of the mechanism whereby BHT inhibits the specific virus-host cell interaction will require further investigations.

Temperature effects. The physical properties of membrane structures are strongly dependent on temperature. Hydrophobic molecules can partition more favorably into the hydrocarbon zones of membrane lipids at higher temperatures than at lower temperatures (12). We carried out experiments to determine the effects of temperature on the inactivation of $\phi 6$ by BHT. In one experiment virus survival was measured after different times of exposure to 0.05 mM BHT at 0 and 25 C. These results show a striking difference in survival at the two temperatures (Fig. 4). After a 5-min exposure at 25 C the survival is less than 0.1%, whereas a 2-h exposure at 0 C results in no more than 50% inactivation. We next determined the effects of a 30-min exposure to 0.03 mM BHT at various temperatures in the range 0 to 33 C; the results are shown in Fig. 5. Up to about 15 C there is very little inactivation under these conditions. A precipitous drop in survival occurs between 15 and 20 C, with greater than 99% inactivation at all temperatures above 20 C. These results make it clear that temperature is a crucial parameter in the inactivation of $\phi 6$ by BHT.

Effects of calcium ions. Several divalent ions, notably Ca^{2+}, interact strongly with membrane components and may therefore modify the response of membranes to other molecules. We investigated the effects of Ca^{2+} on the inactivation of $\phi 6$ by BHT and found a considerable modification of the antiviral activity of BHT in the presence of Ca^{2+}. At low temperatures, where 0.03 mM BHT is relatively inactive in the absence of added Ca^{2+}, the addition of Ca^{2+} in concentrations from about 5 to 50 mM greatly enhanced the inactivation by BHT. Ca^{2+} alone at these concentrations was without effect. The data of Fig. 5 illustrate the effect of 50 mM Ca^{2+} on BHT inactivation versus temperature. At 15 C, the percentage of survival is reduced from 88 to 2.5% by the addition of 50

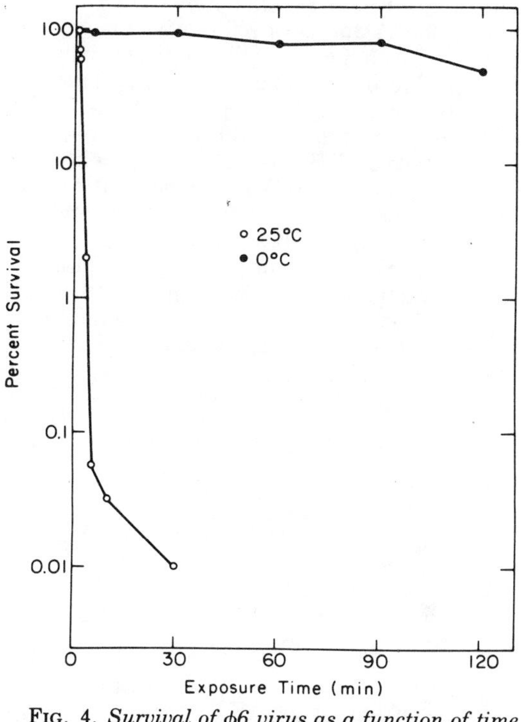

FIG. 4. *Survival of $\phi 6$ virus as a function of time of exposure to 0.03 mM BHT at 0 and 25 C. From a solution of 3 mM BHT in 95% ethanol, 0.1 ml was added to 5 ml of V medium and vortexed gently. Thirty seconds later (t = 0) 5 ml of a $\phi 6$ sample at about 2×10^{10} plaque-forming units per ml (in V medium) was added, and the mixture was again gently vortexed. At various times after mixing the virus and BHT suspensions, samples were diluted appropriately in TB buffer at the same temperature used for exposure and plated for plaque-forming units on V plates with HB10Y cells as an indicator host. Data are presented as percentage of survival compared to control samples in the absence of BHT.*

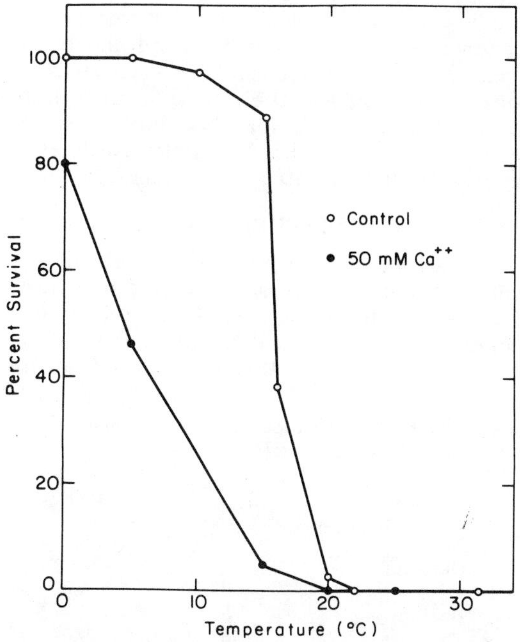

FIG. 5. *Survival of $\phi 6$ virus after exposure to 0.03 mM BHT for 30 min at different temperatures. Exposures were carried out in V medium as described in Fig. 4, with and without 50 mM added calcium chloride. The residual level of Ca^{2+} in V medium, as measured by flame photometry, is about 0.3 mM.*

mM Ca^{2+}. These observations may be of considerable importance in the design of antiviral preparations using BHT as the active agent.

In many systems barium and strontium, but not magnesium, can substitute for calcium in certain aspects of membrane structure and function (6, 7, 10). We have found similar results in the present work. Virus was exposed at 15 C to 0.03 mM BHT in the presence of ions at different concentrations. Data for ion concentrations of 5 and 50 mM, presented in Table 2, show similar enhancement of BHT activity by Ca^{2+}, Ba^{2+}, and Sr^{2+}, but much less enhancement by Mg^{2+}. At higher concentrations Mg^{2+} shows a mild potentiating effect, but this is smaller even at 50 mM than the effect of Ca^{2+} at 5 mM.

Inactivation of ϕ6 by BHA. BHA has some structural similarities to BHT and is about equally widespread as a food additive. Experiments were carried out to determine whether BHA is effective at inactivating ϕ6 virus. Figure 6, which presents data for a 30-min exposure to different concentrations of BHA and BHT, shows that BHA does inactivate ϕ6 but that somewhat higher concentrations are required as compared to BHT.

Samples of BHA-treated virus were analyzed on sucrose gradients as described in the BHT studies. No differences were observed in the sedimentation properties of control and BHA-treated samples under conditions where exposure to BHA reduced the plaque-forming units to less than 1%. This suggests similar mechanisms for BHT and BHA activity. No further analysis of BHA-treated virus was carried out.

DISCUSSION

The envelope of ϕ6 has been described as a "membranous, compressible, saclike structure" surrounding the virus core (13). Its fatty acid composition is nearly identical to that of the host cell, with 16- and 18-carbon, saturated and

TABLE 2. *Effect of divalent ions on the inactivation of ϕ6 by BHT at 15 C*

Ion	Concn added (mM)[a]	Survival (%)
None		88
Calcium	5	32
	50	4.5
Barium	5	47
	50	8.5
Strontium	5	30
	50	22.5
Magnesium	5	100
	50	42.5

[a] The residual levels of calcium and magnesium in V medium are about 0.3 and 3 mM, respectively.

monounsaturated fatty acids accounting for about 95% of the total fatty acids (13). Both the ϕ6 and the host cell have phosphatidylethanolamine and phosphatidylglycerol as their major phospholipids, but the proportions are quite different in the two cases. ϕ6 has an unusually high proportion of phosphatidylglycerol. This negatively charged phospholipid makes up about 57% of the total lipids (8).

Many organic solvents and surfactant substances will inactivate lipid-containing viruses, frequently by extracting or removing the membrane components. Our experiments show that BHT does not remove the ϕ6 envelope but inactivates the virus by a different mechanism. After BHT treatment, virus particles are unable to attach to host cells. Electron micrographs of crude lysates from untreated preparations reveal virus particles attached to pili of host bacterial cells (13). It is not known whether this association is due to specific attachment sites on the virus and cell or whether other polar or hydrophobic interactions of a less specific nature are involved. With regard to the effect of BHT on ϕ6 attachment the question remains as to whether BHT is interacting with the membrane lipids, proteins, or both. BHT has been shown to exert disordering effects on lipid alkyl chains in micellar structures (2) and in the hydrocarbon interior of membrane bilayers (4). Interactions of this type in the ϕ6 mem-

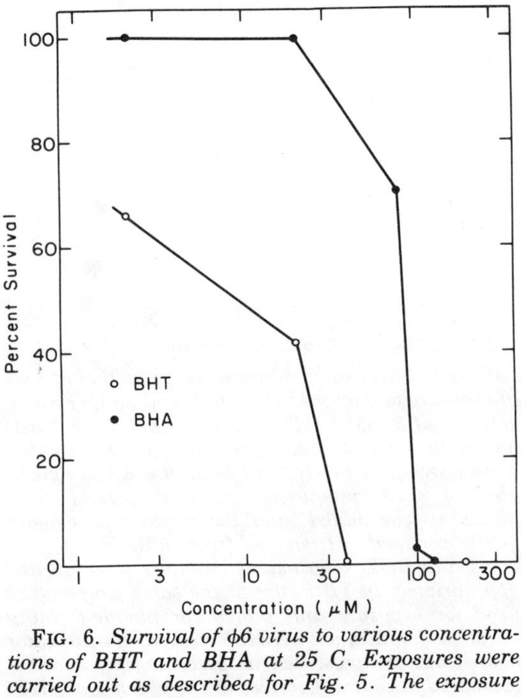

FIG. 6. *Survival of ϕ6 virus to various concentrations of BHT and BHA at 25 C. Exposures were carried out as described for Fig. 5. The exposure time was 30 min.*

brane could, in an indirect manner, alter the conformation or orientation of virus-attachment proteins through modifications of the lipid-protein interactions. Other possibilities are that the attachment sites are masked by BHT or that an attachment protein or glycoprotein is completely removed from the virion by BHT treatment. The proteins of $\phi 6$ have been characterized to some extent, including three proteins that are removed by Triton X-100 treatment and which, therefore, may be part of the envelope (9). Similar studies of BHT-treated virus would help elucidate the mechanism of BHT activity.

The reduced potency of BHT at lower temperatures may be due to a decrease in the ability of the BHT molecules to partition into the viral membrane. At low temperatures the alkyl chains of membrane phospholipids are more ordered, the interchain van der Waals forces are greater, and hydrophobic molecules with less favorable packing geometry are expected and have been found to have reduced partitioning into the hydrocarbon zones (12). BHT has very low solubility in aqueous media and was delivered to the virus in our experiments by adding the compound from a concentrated solution in ethanol. Under these conditions the kinetics of exchange of the BHT molecules into the viral membrane are no doubt quite complex.

The enhancement of BHT activity by calcium ions is not readily understandable. Calcium is generally thought to stabilize membrane structures, so it might be expected that the presence of calcium would dimiminish BHT activity. Although the nature of the potentiating effect of calcium remains open to question, some considerations in light of recent molecular studies of Ca^{2+}-phospholipid interactions seem appropriate. Ohnishi and Ito (6), using the spin label technique, have investigated the interaction of Ca^{2+} ions with negatively charged phospholipids in artificial membranes containing phosphatidylserine and phosphatidylcholine. These investigators found that Ca^{2+} induces a phase separation in the bilayer structure, such that regions of phosphatidylserine aggregates bridged by Ca^{2+} chelates coexist with a more fluid phase of phosphatidylcholine molecules. The strong binding of Ca^{2+} to the negative phospholipids provides very efficient charge neutralization, and the surface of the aggregated phase is described as being hydrophobic. Of particular interest is the fact that Ba^{2+} and Sr^{2+}, but not Mg^{2+}, ions induced similar phase separations. The $\phi 6$ membrane contains a large proportion of negatively charged phosphatidylglycerol, and similar phase separations could occur in the presence of Ca^{2+} ions. The resulting hydrophobic surface of the Ca^{2+}-phosphatidylglycerol aggregates might then promote the exchange of BHT into the viral membrane, thereby increasing virus inactivation. Modifications of BHT activity by Ca^{2+} and other ions is an area that requires further investigation.

The data presented here for the inactivation of $\phi 6$ by BHA is the first report that this substance has antiviral properties. For $\phi 6$, BHA is less active than BHT at comparable concentrations. It may be that other viruses, with different membrane structures, will be equally or more susceptible to BHA than BHT. In light of the apparent low toxicity of BHA, this substance may deserve further study as a potential antiviral agent.

ACKNOWLEDGMENTS

This research was supported by ERDA contract no. E(11-1)2311 and by grant BMS 74-05587 from the National Science Foundation.

LITERATURE CITED

1. **Cupp, J., P. Wanda, A. Keith, and W. Snipes.** 1975. Inactivation of the lipid-containing bacteriophage PM2 by butylated hydroxytoluene. Antimicrob. Agents Chemother. 8:698–706.
2. **Eletr, S., M. A. Williams, T. Watkins, and A. D. Keith.** 1974. Perturbation of the dynamics of lipid alkyl chains in membrane systems: effect on the activity of membrane-bound enzymes. Biochim. Biophys. Acta 339:190–201.
3. **Ellis, L. F., and R. A. Schlegel.** 1974. Electron microscopy of *Pseudomonas* $\phi 6$ bacteriophage. J. Virol. 14:1547–1551.
4. **Hammerstedt, R., R. Amman, T. Rucinsky, W. Snipes, P. Morse II, J. Lepock, and A. Keith.** 1976. Characterization of bovine sperm membranes using spin labels and electron spin resonance spectroscopy: effect of butylated hydroxytoluene and cold shock on membrane structure. Biol. Reprod. 14:381–397.
5. **Kermode, G. O.** 1972. Food additives. Sci. Am. 226:15–21.
6. **Ohnishi, S., and T. Ito.** 1974. Calcium induced phase separations in phosphatidylserine-phosphatidylcholine membranes. Biochemistry 13:881–887.
7. **Okada, Y., and F. Murayama.** 1966. Requirement of calcium ions for the cell fusion reaction of animal cells by HVJ. Exp. Cell Res. 44:527–551.
8. **Sands, J. A.** 1973. The phospholipid composition of bacteriophage $\phi 6$. Biochem. Biophys. Res. Commun. 55:111–116.
9. **Sinclair, J. F., A. Tzagoloff, D. Levine, and L. Mindich.** 1975. Proteins of bacteriophage $\phi 6$. J. Virol. 16:685–695.
10. **Snipes, W., J. Cupp, J. A. Sands, A. Keith, and A. Davis.** 1974. Calcium requirement for assembly of the lipid-containing bacteriophage PM2. Biochim. Biophys. Acta 339:311–322.
11. **Snipes, W., S. Person, A. Keith, and J. Cupp.** 1975. Butylated hydroxytoluene inactivates lipid-containing viruses. Science 187:64–66.
12. **Tinberg, H. M., L. Packer, and A. Keith.** 1972. Role of lipids in mitochondrial energy coupling: evidence from spin labeling and freeze-fracture electron microscopy. Biochim. Biophys. Acta 283:193–205.
13. **Vidaver, A. K., R. K. Koski, and J. L. Van Etten.** 1973. Bacteriophage $\phi 6$: a lipid-containing virus of *Pseudomonas phaseolicola*. J. Virol. 11:799–805.

ANTIMICROBIAL AGENTS AND CHEMOTHERAPY, July 1976, p. 102-105

Vol. 10, No. 1
Printed in U.S.A.

Susceptibility of *Acinetobacter calcoaceticus* var. *anitratus* (*Herellea vaginicola*) to Minocycline

J. Z. MONTGOMERIE,[1]* M. J. PICKETT, R. N. YOSHIMORI, A. W. CHOW, AND L. B. GUZE

Departments of Medicine and Pathology, Harbor General Hospital, Torrance, California 90509; Research and Medical Service, Veterans Administration Hospital (Wadsworth), Los Angeles, California 90073; and Departments of Medicine and Bacteriology, University of California at Los Angeles School of Medicine, Los Angeles, California 90024

Received for publication 30 December 1975

The in vitro activity of minocycline against *Acinetobacter calcoaceticus* var. *anitratus (Herellea vaginicola)* was examined. All strains of *A. anitratus* were inhibited by minocycline at concentrations of 0.4 μg/ml or less. The strains studied were considerably more susceptible to minocycline than tetracycline. No difference between the susceptibility to minocycline and tetracycline was seen with *Escherichia coli, Klebsiella pneumoniae, Enterobacter* and *Proteus* sp. A regression line of the log minimal inhibitory concentration (MIC) values and the diameter of the zone of inhibition, determined by the Kirby-Bauer technique, showed good linear correlation for minocycline. Comparison of the disk diffusion results and MICs indicated that an inhibitory zone size of 19 mm produced by a 30-μg minocycline disk was equivalent to a MIC of 3.1 μg/ml, a serum concentration achieved by oral administration of the drug. When the zone of inhibition was greater than 19 mm, however, there was poor correlation with the MIC for *Enterobacteriaceae*.

Nosocomial infections due to gram-negative bacilli have been increasing in recent years. Among the less common gram-negative bacilli has been a group identified by its failure to ferment carbohydrates. *Acinetobacter calcoaceticus* var. *anitratus* (syn. *Acinetobacter anitratus* or *Herellea vaginicola*) is a species within the genus *Acinetobacter*, a member of the nonfermentative bacilli (6). It has been noted to be susceptible to kanamycin and colistin, whereas the susceptibility patterns to other antibiotics have been variable (2, 3, 5, 7). Steigbigel et al. (10) observed that seven strains of *A. anitratus* were very susceptible to minocycline. To determine the significance of this finding, we have examined the susceptibility of 42 clinical isolates of *A. anitratus* to minocycline.

MATERIALS AND METHODS

Bacteria. Eighteen strains of *A. anitratus*, described in a previous study (5), were used. In addition, 25 strains were obtained from the clinical microbiology laboratory at the UCLA Medical Center. Strains of *Escherichia coli* (40), *Klebsiella pneumoniae* (43), *Enterobacter* (42), and *Proteus* sp. (41) isolated from blood cultures were obtained from the clinical microbiology laboratory at Harbor General Hospital, Torrance, Calif.

Antibiotic susceptibility. Antibiotic disk susceptibility tests were carried out on Mueller-Hinton agar (MHA) using the Kirby-Bauer technique (1). Each strain was tested in duplicate. *E. coli* ATCC 25922 and *Staphylococcus aureus* ATCC 25923 were examined as control organisms. Minimal inhibitory concentrations (MIC) were measured by the Steers replicating technique (8) in MHA. Twofold dilutions of antibiotic were added to MHA at 50 C to give appropriate final concentrations of the antibiotic. The agar was poured and dried for 15 min. Overnight microbial cultures in Trypticase soy broth were diluted and adjusted using a McFarland standard, so that approximately 10^5 cell units were delivered to the surface of the agar with the replicator. The regression line of the diameter of the zone of inhibition and the log MIC values of minocycline were plotted with the zone of inhibition as the independent variable.

RESULTS

The cumulative percentage of *A. anitratus*, *E. coli*, *K. pneumoniae*, *Enterobacter*, and *Proteus* sp. susceptible to minocycline and tetracycline is shown in Fig. 1. *A. anitratus* strains were very susceptible to minocycline, since all strains had a MIC of 0.4 μg/ml or less. The strains studied were considerably more susceptible to minocycline than tetracycline. This difference was not seen with the other bacteria studied, *E. coli*, *K. pneumoniae*, *Enterobacter*,

[1] Present address: Division of Infectious Disease, Rancho Los Amigos Hospital, Downey, Calif. 90242.

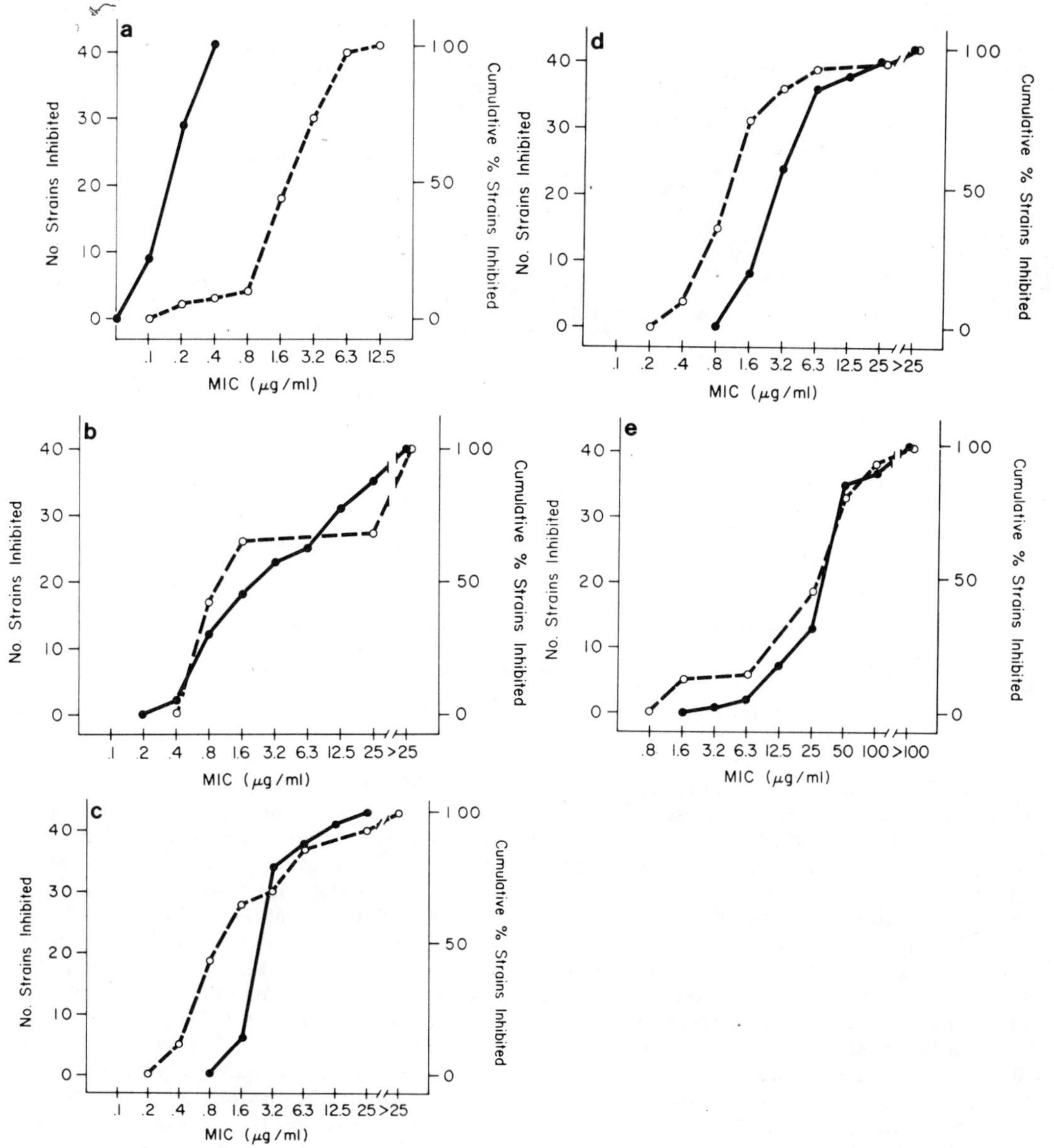

FIG. 1. *Cumulative percentage of (a) A. anitratus, (b) E. coli, (c) K. pneumoniae, (d) Enterobacter sp., and (e) Proteus sp. susceptible to minocycline (●) and tetracycline (○).*

and *Proteus* sp. The MIC for *E. coli* ATCC 25922 was 0.8 µg of minocycline or tetracycline per ml. The MIC for *S. aureus* ATCC 25923 was 0.2 µg of minocycline per ml. The regression line of the diameter of the zone of inhibition and the log MIC values of minocycline for strains of *A. anitratus*, *E. coli*, *K. pneumoniae*, *Enterobacter*, and *Proteus* sp. are shown in Fig. 2. Strains that had no inhibitory zone around the disks were excluded. The regression line has a correlation coefficient of 0.93.

DISCUSSION

The strains of *A. anitratus* we examined were very susceptible to minocycline and apparently more susceptible than the strains examined by Steigbigel et al. (10) and Washington et al. (11). More recently, Maderazo et al. (4) observed that all but one strain of *A. anitratus* was inhibited by 0.007 µg of minocycline per ml. Unfortunately, the technique for measuring MICs has not been adequately standard-

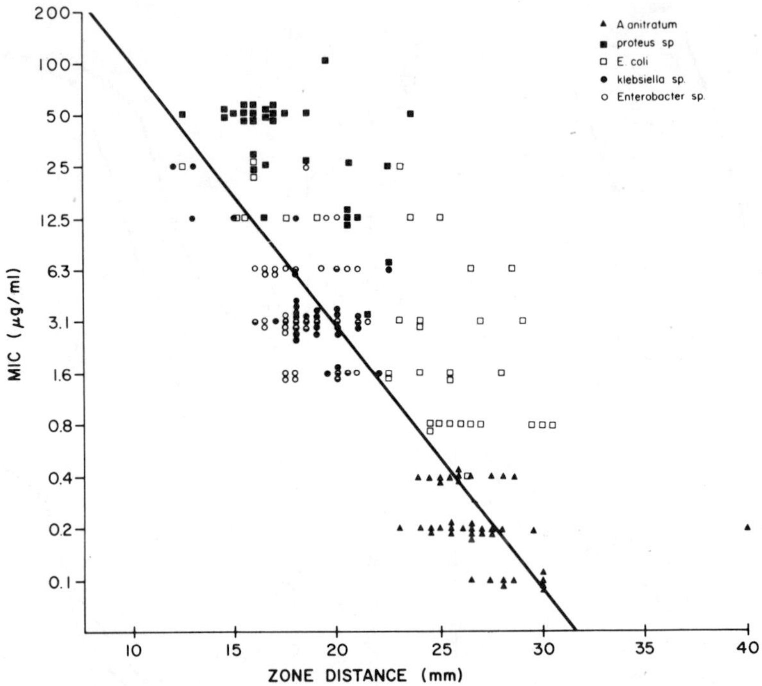

FIG. 2. *Regression line of the $\log_2$ of the MIC and diameter of the zone of inhibition of minocycline using a 30-μg disk (linear correlation coefficient of 0.93).*

ized, and this difference may only reflect differences in technique and media used. Washington et al. (11) found that the susceptibility of bacteria to minocycline was markedly affected by the media used. We have compared the brain heart infusion tube dilution technique with the agar dilution technique on MHA, using a Steers replicator. *A. anitratus* was less susceptible to minocycline on MHA, the MIC to minocycline being approximately one twofold dilution lower on brain heart infusion than on MHA (unpublished data).

The data from our regression line for minocycline indicated that an inhibitory zone size of 19 mm with a 30-μg minocycline disk was equivalent to a MIC of 3.1 μg/ml, a concentration obtainable in serum by oral administration of appropriate doses of minocycline (9). However, using this breakpoint (19 mm), there was considerable discrepancy in MICs, since one-third of the *Enterobacteriaceae* showing zone sizes of 19 mm or greater had MICs >3.1 μg/ml. On the basis of these data, we would recommend caution in the interpretation of minocycline disk tests for *Enterobacteriaceae*.

The antibiotic susceptibility of *A. anitratus* measured by the broth dilution method showed that this organism was considerably more susceptible to minocycline than to tetracycline. This is consistent with the finding of Steigbigel et al. (10), who observed that seven strains of *A. anitratus* were considerably more susceptible to minocycline than to any of the other analogues. Doxycycline ranked second. Maderazo et al. (4) also found tetracycline to be less active than minocycline against *A. anitratus*. The difference in susceptibility of *A. anitratus* to minocycline and tetracycline was not observed with the strains of *E. coli*, *K. pneumoniae*, *Enterobacter*, and *Proteus* sp. studied.

Other studies (2, 3, 5, 7) have indicated that the aminoglycosides or the polypeptide colistin may be the antibiotics of choice for infections due to *A. anitratus*. In general, this organism has been resistant to ampicillin and cephalothin. Our results suggest that minocycline might be useful in the treatment of infections with *A. anitratus*.

ACKNOWLEDGMENTS

We thank Michael Fox, Department of Biomathematics, UCLA, for statistical analysis. We acknowledge the excellent technical assistance of Judith Cook, Christine Edmonds, and Ricki Miller.

This work was supported by a grant from Lederle Laboratories.

LITERATURE CITED

1. **Bauer, A. W., W. M. Kirby, J. C. Sherris, and M. Turck.** 1966. Antibiotic susceptibility testing by a standardized single disk method. Am. J. Clin. Pathol. 45:493–496.

2. **Daly, A. K., B. Postic, and E. H. Kass.** 1962. Infections due to organisms of the genus Herellea. Arch. Int. Med. 110:580–591.
3. **Elston, H. R., and K. C. Hoffman.** 1966. Identification and clinical significance of Achromobacter (Herellea) anitratus in urinary tract infections. Am. J. Med. Sci. 251:75–80.
4. **Maderazo, E. G., R. Quintiliani, R. C. Tilton, R. Bartlett, N. C. Joyce, and V. T. Andriole.** 1975. Activity of minocycline against *Acinetobacter calcoaceticus* var. *anitratus* (syn. *Herellea vaginicola)* and *Serratia marcescens*. Antimicrob. Agents Chemother. 8:54–57.
5. **Pederson, M. M., E. Marso, and M. J. Pickett.** 1970. Nonfermentative bacilli associated with man. III. Pathogenicity and antibiotic susceptibility. Am. J. Clin. Pathol. 54:178–192.
6. **Pickett, M. J., and C. R. Manclark.** 1970. Nonfermentative bacilli associated with man. I. Nomenclature. Am. J. Clin. Pathol. 54:155–163.
7. **Reinranz, J. B., B. B. Ways, and J. P. Sanford.** 1965. In vitro sensitivity determination on *Herellea* and *Flavobacterium* species, p. 451–456. Antimicrob. Agents Chemother. 1964.
8. **Steers, E. E., B. S. Foltz, B. S. Graves and J. Riden.** 1959. An inocula replicating apparatus for routine testing of bacterial susceptibility to antibiotics. Antibiot. Chemother. (Basel) 9:307–311.
9. **Steigbigel, N. H., W. C. Reed, and M. Finland.** 1968. Absorption and excretion of five tetracycline analogues after single oral doses in normal young men. Am. J. Med. Sci. 255:296–312.
10. **Steigbigel, N. H., C. W. Reed, and M. Finland.** 1968. Susceptibility of common pathogenic bacteria to seven tetracycline antibiotics in vitro. Am. J. Med. Sci. 255:179–195.
11. **Washington, J. A., P. K. W. Yu, and W. F. Martin.** 1970. In vitro antibacterial activity of minocycline and effect of agar medium utilized in its susceptibility testing. Appl. Microbiol. 19:259–263.

ANTIMICROBIAL AGENTS AND CHEMOTHERAPY, July 1976, p. 106-111 Vol. 10, No. 1

Beta-Lactamase Activity in Anaerobic Bacteria

A. ELISE WEINRICH AND VICTOR E. DEL BENE*

Department of Medicine, Division of Infectious Diseases and Immunology, Medical University of South Carolina, Charleston, South Carolina 29401

Received for publication 5 February 1976

A diverse group of anaerobic bacteria representing a spectrum of resistance to β-lactam antibiotics was studied to characterize their β-lactamase activity and relate it to resistance. The *Bacteroides fragilis* organisms had moderate resistance and produced a cephalosporinase with low activity. The *Clostridium ramosum* was intermediate in resistance and had intermediate, inducible β-lactamase activity. The *B. clostridiiformis* organism was highly resistant, produced a potent inducible penicillinase, and had a barrier to the penicillin substrates. Only the β-lactamase of *C. ramosum* fit Richmond's classification (class IV). Although there was a rough correlation between β-lactamase activity and antibiotic resistance, other mechanisms are undoubtedly involved in determining resistance levels.

The ability of an organism to hydrolyze the β-lactam ring is thought to play a significant role in its resistance to various β-lactam antibiotics. β-Lactamases of aerobic bacteria have been extensively investigated. Those from gram-positive organisms are characterized as predominately inducible, extracellular penicillinases rather than cephalosporinases. β-Lactamases of gram-negative bacteria have more recently been found to have a wide spectrum of characteristics which are the basis for an extensive classification of these diversified enzymes (9). However, the role of β-lactamase in the antibiotic resistance of gram-negative facultative bacilli has still not been completely resolved (3).

Anaerobic bacteria have been shown to have β-lactamase activity, but the character of this activity and its contribution to the resistance of these organisms has not been completely determined. Holt and Stewart (4) found no activity in eight *Bacteroides* strains, but Pinkus et al. (7) found that half of the *Bacteroides fragilis* organisms in their study produced a penicillinase, and that a greater number of resistant strains showed this activity than did susceptible strains. Kanazawa et al. (5) demonstrated penicillinase activity by means of a biological method in nine strains of bacteroides, but none was found in 21 strains of clostridia. In a letter published in *Lancet*, Okubadejo et al. (6) stated that they found no β-lactamase activity in approximately 60 strains of *B. fragilis*. Anderson and Sykes (1) found no activity in nine *B. fragilis* organisms with moderate minimal inhibitory concentrations (MICs) but did find a noninducible β-lactamase that hydrolyzed cephaloridine more than penicillin in a highly resistant organism. Del Bene and Farrar (2) investigated 10 strains of *B. fragilis* and found cephalosporinase activity which was generally not inducible, showed no substrate barrier, and was inhibited by a sulfhydryl reagent and cloxacillin.

This study was undertaken to characterize the β-lactamase activity of a diverse group of anaerobic bacteria selected for their resistance to β-lactam antibiotics. An attempt was made to classify these β-lactamases and to assess the role that they may play in the antibiotic resistance of the organisms.

MATERIALS AND METHODS

Bacterial strains. Twelve strains of anaerobic bacteria were studied, 10 *Bacteroides fragilis*, 1 *Bacteroides clostridiiformis*, and 1 *Clostridium ramosum*. Two of the strains of *B. fragilis* which were previously reported (2) to possess cephalosporinase activity were restudied here. The remaining *B. fragilis* strains, the *B. clostridiiformis*, and the *C. ramosum* strains were isolated from clinical specimens and were supplied by T. Wilkins. All 12 organisms were characterized in our laboratory by the biochemical and gas chromatographic methods described in the Virginia Polytechnic Institute *Anaerobe Laboratory Manual* (13).

Antibiotic susceptibility tests. The minimal inhibitory concentration (MIC) of penicillin G, ampicillin, carbenicillin, cephaloridine, cefazolin, cefamandole, and cefoxitin was found for each organism by the agar plate dilution method. Inoculum was prepared from a turbid culture grown for 18 h in Schaedler broth (Baltimore Biological Laboratory, with 0.05 μg of menadione added) in an anaerobic incubator. Inoculum diluted 1:10-fold was delivered to the surface of prereduced Schaedler agar by means of the Steers-Foltz replicator (10). The agar plates contained serial twofold dilutions of the antibiotics tested. Agar plates without antibiotics were inoculated before and after inoculation of the antibiotic-containing plates and served as growth controls. Experiments were read after 24 h of incubation.

Preparation of crude enzyme fractions. Each organism was grown for 18 h at 37 C in Schaedler broth (modified by the addition of menadione, 0.05 μg/ml) under anaerobic conditions with shaking. A simultaneous culture containing penicillin G at a 0.5 MIC concentration was also prepared for induction studies. The cells were then harvested by centrifugation at 12,000 × *g* for 30 min at 4 C and resuspended in 0.75 mM phosphate buffer (pH 7) at 0.01 the volume of the original culture. A portion of the concentrated fraction of bacterial cells was treated by sonication (Branson Sonifier, Inc.) at 100 W for 3 min at 5 C to disrupt the cells. Studies of enzymatic activity were performed on intact and broken cells with and without induction by penicillin or cefoxitin.

Measurement of β-lactamase activity. The alkalimetric assay was performed with 1.2 mM substrate antibiotic and 0.25 ml of enzyme preparation in 0.75 mM phosphate buffer. The reaction mixture (initial total volume 25.25 ml) was maintained at pH 7 (37 C) with 0.01 M NaOH in an automated pH-stat (Metrohm Herisau, Brinkmann Instruments).

Calculations were made on the basis of 1 mol of titratable acid produced per mol of penicillin substrate hydrolyzed and 2 mol of acid per mol of cephalosporin substrate hydrolyzed. Rates of activity were expressed as micromoles of substrate hydrolyzed per hour per milligram of bacterial protein. The protein was determined by a modification of the biuret reaction (8). Each enzyme preparation was tested with the following substrates: penicillin G, ampicillin, carbenicillin, cephaloridine, cefazolin, cefamandole, and cefoxitin.

The iodometric paper chromatographic assay for penicillinase activity was also performed with each enzyme preparation (7).

Studies of enzyme inhibition. Crude enzyme preparations were partially clarified by centrifugation and the supernatant was used as the source of enzyme. The inhibitors cloxacillin (0.12 mM), cefoxitin (0.12 mM), and *para*-chloromercuribenzoate (pCMB, 0.1 mM) were preincubated with the enzyme for 10 min at 37 C before addition of the substrate (1.2 mM) which was the most susceptible to hydrolysis by that enzyme.

RESULTS

Antimicrobial susceptibility studies. All the *B. fragilis* strains were moderately resistant to the β-lactam antibiotics. The individual MICs and the median MIC for each substrate are shown in Table 1. In general, the *B. fragilis* organisms showed moderate resistance to the antibiotics tested (MICs of approximately 40 μg/ml), with slightly greater resistance to cephaloridine and slightly less resistance to cefoxitin.

C. ramosum was more susceptible than the *B. fragilis* strains to all cephalosporins except cefoxitin, but its susceptibility to penicillin, carbenicillin, and ampicillin was significantly less than that of the *B. fragilis* strains.

B. clostridiiformis was the most resistant of the organisms tested. Its MIC of penicillin, carbenicillin, and ampicillin was 2,500 μg/ml for each drug. Its susceptibility to the cephalosporins (with the exception of cefamandole) was similar to that seen for *B. fragilis*.

β-Lactamase activity. The 12 organisms studied had a wide variation in their rates of enzymatic hydrolysis of the substrates (Table 2). The absolute rates of hydrolysis shown by

TABLE 1. *Minimal inhibitory concentrations (MIC) of β-lactam antibiotics for anaerobic bacteria*

Organism	MIC (μg/ml)						
	Penicillin	Ampicillin	Carbenicillin	Cephaloridine	Cefazolin	Cefamandole	Cefoxitin
B. fragilis							
no. 10	20	10	20	20	10	40	20
no. 11	20	40	20	20	20	40	5
no. 25	80	80	80	80	80	80	40
no. 27	20	80	20	20	20	40	20
no. 30	80	80	80	80	80	80	40
no. 31	20	40	40	80	40	80	40
no. 32	20	40	40	20	40	80	20
no. 33	20	40	20	20	40	40	20
no. 41	40	40	80	80	40	40	40
no. 42	40	40	80	80	80	40	40
Median MIC	40	40	40	50	40	40	30
C. ramosum							
no. 79	300	160	300	10	20	20	>160
B. clostridiiformis							
no. 7	2,500	2,500	2,500	40	80	160	20

the *B. fragilis* organisms were measurable, but quite low. The β-lactamase from each of the eight *B. fragilis* organisms was predominately a cephalosporinase, with little or no penicillinase activity. Cephaloridine was the most rapidly hydrolyzed, and cefazolin was hydrolyzed slightly less rapidly than cephaloridine. The hydrolysis rates of cefamandole and cefoxitin were similar, both being hydrolyzed less readily than cefazolin. (The two strains not shown in the table had no detectable β-lactamase activity regardless of substrate.) In contrast, the *C. ramosum* enzyme hydrolyzed both penicillins and cephalosporins at approximately the same rates. Hydrolyses of penicillin and ampicillin were about 15 times that of the *B. fragilis* enzymes and the rates of hydrolysis of cephaloridine, cefazolin, and cefamandole were about twice those of *B. fragilis* enzymes. *B. clostridiiformis* produced an enzyme that was the most active of those studied. Its activity against penicillin was 60 times that of the *C. ramosum* enzyme and 600 times that of the *B. fragilis* enzymes. Ampicillin and carbenicillin were also more readily hydrolyzed by this enzyme than by the others studied. Despite its generally high activity, this enzyme did not hydrolyze cefoxitin at all.

Attempts to induce the *B. fragilis* organisms with penicillin were generally unsuccessful. Previous exposure of *C. ramosum* to penicillin (Table 3) resulted in a 25-fold increase in the hydrolysis of penicillin, 200-fold for ampicillin, 10-fold for cephaloridine, 40-fold for cefamandole, and 15-fold for cefazolin. The rate of cefoxitin hydrolysis was not affected. Since the absolute values for this organism's hydrolysis rates are at times relatively small, the magnitudes of the induction factors may not be accurate, but it is clear that the β-lactamase activity of this organism is stimulated upon induction. Previous exposure to penicillin of *B. clostridiiformis* resulted in a twofold increase in hydrolysis of penicillin, ampicillin, carbenicillin, and cephaloridine. The hydrolysis of cefamandole and cefazolin was not increased, and cefoxitin remained resistant to hydrolysis.

Since cefoxitin was the least hydrolyzed of all substrates studied, its effect as an inducing agent was compared with that of penicillin in

TABLE 2. *Rates of hydrolysis of β-lactam antibiotics by induced and disrupted enzyme preparations of anaerobic bacteria*

Organism	Hydrolysis[a]						
	Penicillin	Ampicillin	Carbenicillin	Cephaloridine	Cefazolin	Cefamandole	Cefoxitin
B. fragilis[b]							
no. 10	0.33	0.91	0.22	0.31	0.54	0.46	0.43
no. 25	0	0	0	0.50	0.22	0.02	0
no. 27	0.29	1.13	0	0.09	0	0.10	0.26
no. 30	0.03	0.14	0.14	3.27	1.06	0.15	0.36
no. 31	0.21	0.35	0.30	2.54	1.89	0.55	0.40
no. 32	0.41	0.29	0.24	0.76	0.48	0.67	0.30
no. 41	0.69	0.44	1.68	4.09	2.36	1.06	0.51
no. 42	0.35	0.29	0.23	2.29	1.08	0.43	0.39
C. ramosum							
no. 79	7.21	18.00	0.14	7.25	4.78	1.58	0.05
B. clostridiiformis							
no. 7	450.70	394.37	15.21	7.98	1.56	1.41	0

[a] Micromoles hydrolyzed per hour per milligram of protein.
[b] Two strains (not shown) had no activity.

TABLE 3. *Effect of previous exposure to penicillin[a] on hydrolysis of various substrates*

Strain no.	Induction factor[b]						
	Penicillin	Ampicillin	Carbenicillin	Cephaloridine	Cefazolin	Cefamandole	Cefoxitin
C. ramosum							
no. 79	25.0	200		10.4	14	40	0
B. clostridiiformis							
no. 7	2.5	1.9	2	1.8	1	1	0

[a] Inducing concentration = 0.5 MIC for each strain.
[b] Induction factor = rate of hydrolysis induced/rate of hydrolysis uninduced.

two strains (Table 4). *B. clostridiiformis*, when grown in the presence of penicillin, had a two- to threefold increase in its ability to hydrolyze penicillin and cephaloridine. When cefoxitin was used as the inducer, however, the hydrolysis of penicillin and cephaloridine increased 7- to 10-fold. Neither penicillin nor cefoxitin were effective inducers of the *B. fragilis* enzyme against either substrate.

In general, the β-lactamases produced by the *B. fragilis* organisms were not associated with a substrate barrier (crypticity factor) except with two substrates, carbenicillin and cefoxitin (Table 5). The enzyme preparation from *C. ramosum* exhibited no increase in activity when the cells were disrupted. The *B. clostridiiformis* enzyme had a consistent substrate barrier of 2.5-fold with all three penicillin substrates.

Confirmation that the activity detected against penicillin was indeed β-lactamase was achieved by means of a specific iodometric paper chromatographic analysis. This method showed that the *B. fragilis* enzyme preparations hydrolyzed the penicillin substrate at a slower rate than did *B. clostridiiformis* preparations, but all organisms showed complete conversion of penicillin to penicilloic acid by 48 h. In addition, the activity of four representative enzyme preparations was lost after incubation at 60 C for 1 h.

Substrate profile and inhibition studies. The majority of the *B. fragilis* enzyme preparations hydrolyzed cephaloridine>cefazolin> cefamandole>cefoxitin, with only minor variations in this order of substrate preference (Table 6) except for strain 32, which had this order virtually reversed. There was no general pattern of preference shown by these organisms for penicillin substrates. The enzyme from *C. ramosum* hydrolyzed penicillins and cephalosporins comparably. Ampicillin was hydrolyzed> penicillin>carbenicillin, and cephaloridine was hydrolyzed>cefazolin>cefamandole>cefoxitin. The *B. clostridiiformis* enzyme hydrolyzed both ampicillin and penicillin at approximately equal rates. Although carbenicillin was not hydrolyzed as rapidly as ampicillin and penicillin, the absolute rate of hydrolysis

TABLE 4. *Effect of previous exposure to penicillin or cefoxitin on hydrolysis of substrates*

Inducing drug	MIC inducing concentration	Hydrolysis (μmol/h per mg)			
		B. clostridiiformis (no. 7)		*B. fragilis* (no. 42)	
		Penicillin	Cephaloridine	Penicillin	Cephaloridine
None		78	2	0	2.2
Penicillin	1/4	118	3	0	2.1
Penicillin	1/2	200	4	0.3	1.0
Penicillin	3/4	217	4.5	0	0
Penicillin	1	194	4	0.2	0.5
Cefoxitin	1/4	612	14		
Cefoxitin	1/2	562	14	0.1	0.2
Cefoxitin	3/4	807	15		
Cefoxitin	1	733	15	0	0

TABLE 5. *Effect of disruption of uninduced cells on rate of hydrolysis of β-lactam antibiotics*

Organism	Crypticity factor[a] for substrates						
	Penicillin	Ampicillin	Carbenicillin	Cephaloridine	Cefazolin	Cefamandole	Cefoxitin
B. fragilis							
no. 30	∞	1	2.8	1	1	1	3.1
no. 41	1	1	1.2	1	1	1	1
no. 42	∞	1	1	1	1	1	6.2
no. 10		1.8	2.3	1	1	1	1.9
no. 27	2	1	1	1	1	1.4	1.6
no. 31	1	1	15	1	1	1	1
no. 32	1	1	1	1	1	1	1.8
C. ramosum							
no. 79	1	1.2	1	1	∞	1	1
B. clostridiiformis							
no. 7	2.5	2.5	2.5	1.2	1	1	1

[a] Crypticity factor = (rate of hydrolysis broken)/(rate of hydrolysis intact).

TABLE 6. *Relative rates of hydrolysis of β-lactam antibiotics by anaerobic bacteria*

Organism	Relative rates of hydrolysis[a]						
	Penicillin	Ampicillin	Carbenicil-lin	Cephalori-dine	Cefazolin	Cefaman-dole	Cefoxitin
B. fragilis[b]							
no. 10	100	335	50	380	285	165	170
no. 27	100	565	0	360	70	100	70
no. 30	100	0	0	3,575	2,525	200	1,250
no. 31	100	3,800	1,500	11,200	7,200	2,700	1,800
no. 32	100	265	135	120	100	220	400
no. 41	100	320	760	1,670	815	345	335
no. 42	100	0	100	3,755	1,710	355	280
C. ramosum[c]							
no. 79	100	255	2	100	65	3	0
B. clostridiiformis[c]							
no. 7	100	88	3	2	0.4	0.3	0

[a] Hydrolysis of penicillin = 100.
[b] Two *B. fragilis* strains had negligible activity, so the entire substrate profile was not done.
[c] Substrate profile based upon values for induced, disrupted preparations.

of carbenicillin by the enzyme preparation from *B. clostridiiformis* exceeded that of any of the other organisms. As with the majority of the *B. fragilis* organisms and *C. ramosum*, cephaloridine was hydrolyzed>cefazolin>cefamandole>cefoxitin.

The enzymes were further characterized by determining their response to inhibitors (Table 7). The *B. fragilis* enzymes' activity was inhibited by cloxacillin, pCMB, and cefoxitin. The activity of the *C. ramosum* enzyme was inhibited by pCMB and cefoxitin. (This enzyme was capable of hydrolyzing cloxacillin which precluded its use as an inhibitor.) The *B. clostridiiformis* enzyme was not inhibited by any of the three substances, even when the concentrations of the inhibitor and substrate were equal.

Relationship between MIC and rates of hydrolysis. The *B. fragilis* enzyme preparations had very low rates of hydrolysis, usually less than 1 μmol/h per mg of protein. Their MICs ranged from 5 to 80 μg/ml, with most median MICs at 40 μg/ml. The substrate most readily hydrolyzed by these organisms was cephaloridine, and there was a decline in activity (from 4.0 to 0 μmol) with a declining MIC (from 80 to 20 μg/ml) when cephaloridine was used as the substrate. Del Bene and Farrar (2) also found a correlation between hydrolysis rates and MIC for the substrate cephaloridine. With all other antibiotics, however, no such pattern was demonstrated.

C. ramosum had moderately high resistance to penicillin and ampicillin (MIC, 300 and 160 μg/ml, respectively), and its enzyme hydrolyzed 7 μmol of penicillin and 18 μmol of ampicillin/h per mg. Despite MICs of 300 μg of carbenicillin and >160 μg of cefoxitin per ml, its enzyme hydrolyzed these antibiotics minimally (0.14 and 0.05 μmol/h per mg, respectively). Although this organism showed substantial rates of hydrolysis of cephaloridine, cefazolin, and cefamandole (7.3 to 1.6 μmol/h per mg), it was inhibited by lower concentrations of these antibiotics (10 to 20 μg/ml) than the *B. fragilis* strains.

TABLE 7. *Inhibition of the hydrolysis of β-lactam antibiotics*

Organism	Inhibition (%)		
	Cloxacillin	*p*-Chloro-mercuri-benzoate	Cefoxitin
B. fragilis			
no. 27	45	81	50
no. 30	46	91	90
no. 31	60	83	83
no. 41	47	79	63
C. ramosum			
no. 79		74	94
B. clostridiiformis			
no. 7	0	0	0

B. clostridiiformis was the most resistant organism studied. Its MIC for penicillin, ampicillin, and carbenicillin was 2,500 μg/ml, and its enzyme was the most active of those studied (450 μmol, 394 μmol, and 15 μmol/h per mg, respectively). Although less active against the cephalosporins, substantial hydrolysis of cefamandole, cefazolin, and cephaloridine (range of 1 to 7 μmol/h per mg) and substantial resistance (MIC, 40 to 160 μg/ml) was demonstrated. Although it did not hydrolyze cefoxitin, its MIC for cefoxitin was 20 μg/ml.

DISCUSSION

Anaerobic bacteria selected for their resistance to β-lactam antibiotics were found to produce β-lactamases which contribute to this resistance.

The antimicrobial resistance of the organisms studied was significantly greater than that normally found in anaerobic bacilli. *B. clostridiiformis* had marked resistance characteristics, particularly with the penicillins. *C. ramosum* was resistant to the penicillins at intermediate concentrations. *B. fragilis* strains were less resistant than *B. clostridiiformis* and *C. ramosum* but were generally more resistant than strains commonly encountered. This is especially true for cefoxitin (11, 12).

The β-lactamase activity demonstrated in the study organisms paralleled their relative resistance to β-lactam antibiotics. *B. clostridiiformis* showed the greatest β-lactamase activity, *C. ramosum* was intermediate, and the *B. fragilis* strains were the least active.

Additional factors contributing to the very high levels of resistance of *B. clostridiiformis* to the penicillins were its substrate barrier and its inducibility. Similarly, with *C. ramosum* the resistance to penicillins was associated with the ability to induce increased β-lactamase activity for the penicillin substrates. In both strains, resistance to the cephalosporins was not as great as to the penicillins and the induction factors were not as prominent.

Only one of the anaerobic bacteria studied produced an enzyme that could be classified using the criteria of Richmond and Sykes (9). This enzyme was derived from *C. ramosum* and satisfies the criteria designated for class IV β-lactamases (9). Class IV β-lactamases hydrolyze both penicillins and cephalosporins relatively equally and are inhibited by pCMB. They are usually resistant to inhibition by cloxacillin, and some have been shown to hydrolyze cloxacillin as the enzyme from *C. ramosum* did. The characteristics of the β-lactamase activity of the *B. fragilis* strains (namely, predominantly cephalosporinase activity which was inhibited by pCMB and cloxacillin) are different from any in Richmond's groups. These same characteristics were previously found with other β-lactamases from *Bacteroides* (1, 2). The enzyme from *B. clostridiiformis* was highly unusual since it was not affected by any of the inhibitors. Iodometric analysis of end products, however, confirmed the specific β-lactamase activity of this enzyme.

In some instances, β-lactamase activity certainly seems to be playing an important role in the resistance of anaerobic bacteria to β-lactam antibiotics. In other instances, additional mechanisms contributing to resistance must be involved.

ACKNOWLEDGMENTS

We thank Mary Rogers for identifying the organisms, Diane Delamar for performing the iodometric paper chromatographic analyses, and Sandra Petit for typing the manuscript.

This research was supported by South Carolina Allocations for Biomedical Research and by Merck Institute, Rahway, N. J.

Antibiotics were generously supplied by the Eli Lilly and Merck Sharpe and Dohme pharmaceutical companies.

LITERATURE CITED

1. **Anderson, J. E., and R. B. Sykes.** 1973. Characterization of a β-lactamase obtained from a strain of *Bacteroides fragilis* resistant to β-lactam antibiotics. J. Med. Microbiol. **6**:201–206.
2. **Del Bene, V. E., and W. E. Farrar, Jr.** 1973. Cephalosporinase activity in *Bacteroides fragilis*. Antimicrob. Agents Chemother. **3**:369–372.
3. **Farrar, W. E., Jr., and J. M. Krause.** 1970. Relationship between β-lactamase activity and resistance of *Enterobacter* to cephalothin. Infect. Immun. **2**:610–616.
4. **Holt, R. J., and G. T. Stewart.** 1964. Production of amidase and β-lactamase by bacteria. J. Gen. Microbiol. **36**:203–213.
5. **Kanazawa, Y., T. Kuramata, and S. Miyanura.** 1970. Inactivation of chemotherapeutic agents by anaerobes, p. 388–393. *In* Progress in antimicrobial and anticancer chemotherapy. Proceedings of Sixth International Congress of Chemotherapy. University of Tokyo Press, Tokyo.
6. **Okubadejo, O. A., P. J. Green, and D. J. H. Payne.** 1973. Bacteroides in the blood. Lancet **i**:147.
7. **Pinkus, G., G. Veto, and A. I. Braude.** 1968. *Bacteroides* penicillinase. J. Bacteriol. **96**:1437–1438.
8. **Platt, T.** 1972. Protein purifications, p. 381–382. *In* J. H. Miller (ed.), Experiments in molecular genetics. Cold Spring Harbor Laboratory, Cold Spring Harbor, N.Y.
9. **Richmond, M. H., and R. B. Sykes.** 1973. The β-lactamases of gram-negative bacteria and their possible physiological role, p. 31–87. *In* A. S. Rose and D. W. Tempest (ed.), Advances in microbial physiology, vol. 9. Academic Press Inc., London.
10. **Steers, E., E. L. Foltz, and B. S. Graves.** 1959. An inocula replicating apparatus for routine testing of bacterial susceptibility to antibiotics. Antibiot. Chemother. **9**:307–311.
11. **Sutter, V. L., and S. M. Finegold.** 1975. Susceptibility of anaerobic bacteria to carbenicillin, cefoxitin, and related drugs. J. Infect. Dis. **131**:417–422.
12. **Tally, F. P., N. V. Jacobus, J. G. Bartlett, and S. R. Gorbach.** 1975. Susceptibility of anaerobes to cefoxitin and other cephalosporins. Antimicrob. Agents Chemother. **7**:128–132.
13. **Virginia Polytechnic Institute.** 1972. Outline of clinical methods in anaerobic bacteriology. *In* Anaerobe laboratory manual, 2nd ed. Virginia Polytechnic Institute and State University, Blacksburg.

ANTIMICROBIAL AGENTS AND CHEMOTHERAPY, July 1976, p. 112-118
Vol. 10, No. 1
Printed in U.S.A.

Susceptibility Testing of Anaerobic Bacteria with 100-μg Carbenicillin Disks

W. W. LASLIE[1]* AND D. W. LAMBE, JR.

Department of Pathology and Laboratory Medicine, Emory University, Atlanta, Georgia 30322

Received for publication 23 February 1976

A total of 245 strains of anaerobic bacteria were examined for their susceptibility to carbenicillin by the disk test method and by minimum inhibitory concentration (MIC) determinations. Standard-curve studies with a strain of *Bacteroides fragilis* subsp. *fragilis* that was minimally susceptible to carbenicillin and *Escherichia coli* (ATCC 25922) demonstrated that a disk containing 100 μg of carbenicillin was suitable for testing susceptibility of anaerobes to carbenicillin. Thus, the diameter of zones around the 100-μg carbenicillin disks and MIC values were determined under the following test conditions: Mueller-Hinton agar supplemented with sheep blood, vitamin K_1, and hemin; an incubation temperature of 35 C; and an atmosphere of 80% N_2, 10% H_2, and 10% CO_2. The strains were separated into two populations by correlating zone diameters and geometric mean MICs. The disk test more clearly separated the resistant and susceptible populations and was more reproducible than the MIC test. Thus, a statistical analysis based on the distribution of zone diameters of susceptible and resistant strains was used to derive an interpretive scheme for anaerobic bacteria tested with 100-μg carbenicillin disks. The following interpretive scheme is recommended for testing anaerobes with 100-μg disks of carbenicillin: resistant, 8 mm or less; indeterminate, 9 to 12 mm; and susceptible, 13 mm or greater.

Until the last few years, anaerobic organisms were rarely implicated as causative agents of human infection, although *Bacteroides* species had been accepted as a potential cause of infection since 1897 (39). Recent advances in culturing and identifying nonsporulating anaerobes have led to increased awareness of the role of these organisms in the disease process, and it is now well recognized that anaerobic bacteria are involved in a significant number of human infections (9, 10, 13, 19, 27, 28, 42).

This recognition of the role of anaerobes in the disease process has stimulated interest in the susceptibility of these organisms to antimicrobial agents. Recently, Nobles (25) reported a high mortality rate among patients with *Bacteroides fragilis* septicemia who received no effective antibiotic therapy, yet Lambe et al. (18) found a high survival rate among patients infected with *B. fragilis* subsp. *fragilis* if the patients received proper antibiotic therapy. *B. fragilis* has become increasingly resistant to certain antibiotics such as tetracycline (20, 38). Only chloramphenicol has been consistently effective in treating infections, including septicemias, caused by anaerobic bacteria (4). Clindamycin has also been recommended for treatment of *B. fragilis* infections (11), but both chloramphenicol and clindamycin produce adverse effects that limit their usefulness (6, 8, 12, 30, 31, 33, 40). Carbenicillin is relatively nontoxic, and in vitro data (3, 5, 16, 25, 34, 41) indicate that most anaerobes are susceptible to this agent. Furthermore, one in vivo study has demonstrated a high rate of success in treating anaerobic infections with carbenicillin (23).

The purpose of the present study was to derive an interpretive scheme by the disk test method for evaluating the susceptibility of rapidly growing anaerobic bacteria to carbenicillin. The standard method that we proposed previously for antibiotic susceptibility testing of anaerobes (26) was used in this study. We developed this method initially because it most closely duplicated the Bauer-Kirby (1) antibiotic susceptibility test for rapidly growing aerobes. Population characteristics were analyzed to determine the interpretive scheme for the 100-μg carbenicillin disk test.

MATERIALS AND METHODS

Bacterial strains. There were 245 strains of anaerobic bacteria used in this study. Of these, 141 strains were *B. fragilis*, and the subspecies of *B.*

[1] Present address: Laboratory of Pathology, New England Deaconess Hospital, Boston, Mass. 02215.

fragilis represented included 67 *B. fragilis fragilis*, 35 *B. fragilis thetaiotaomicron*, 27 *B. fragilis distasonis*, and 12 *B. fragilis vulgatus*. Of the 245 strains tested, 86 were anaerobic cocci, which included *Peptococcus magnus* (seven strains), *Peptostreptococcus anaerobius* (27 strains), *Peptococcus prevotii* (17 strains), *Peptococcus asaccharolyticus* (23 strains), *Streptococcus constellatus* (three strains), *Streptococcus intermedius* (eight strains), and *Streptococcus morbillorum* (one strain). Other anaerobes included *Bacteroides* group PS (proteolytic-saccharolytic) (one strain), *Bacteroides oralis* (one strain), *Bacteroides ruminicola* (one strain), *Fusobacterium necrophorum* (two strains), *Fusobacterium nucleatum* (one strain), *Fusobacterium russii* (one strain), *Fusobacterium varium* (two strains), *Actinomyces israelii* (one strain), *Actinomyces viscosus* (one strain), *Actinomyces naeslundii* (one strain), *Bifidobacterium adolescentis* (two strains), *Eubacterium lentum* (two strains), *Eubacterium limosum* (one strain), and *Lactobacillus acidophilus* (one strain). These strains were isolated from clinical specimens submitted to Emory University Hospital; these strains were identified by the method described by Holdeman and Moore (14).

Anaerobiosis. All work was performed in an anaerobe chamber (Coy Manufacturing Co., Ann Arbor, Mich.) with an atmosphere of 80% N_2, 10% H_2, and 10% CO_2 (Matheson Gas Products, Atlanta, Ga.).

Media. Stock cultures of the test organisms were maintained in brain heart infusion broth (Difco) supplemented with vitamin K_1 (0.00005%) (Sigma) and hemin (0.0005%) (K & K Laboratories, Plainview, N.Y.). The inoculum was diluted with Mueller-Hinton broth (MHB) (Difco) containing vitamin K_1 and hemin (VKH). Zone size determinations and minimum inhibitory concentration (MIC) determinations were made on Mueller-Hinton agar (MHA) (Difco) supplemented with VKH and 5% defibrinated sheep blood (Nolan Biological Laboratories, Inc., Tucker, Ga.). Purity plates consisted of brain heart infusion agar supplemented with VKH and 5% defibrinated sheep blood. All broth media were prepared outside the anaerobe chamber and placed in the anaerobe chamber while warm. The agar plates were prepared outside the anaerobe chamber, allowed to solidify, and then placed inside the anaerobe chamber; the plates were used within a few hours after preparation.

Antibiotics. Carbenicillin powder (Pfizer, Inc., New York, N.Y.) was dissolved in sterile distilled water. Antibiotic disks (Pfizer, Inc., New York, N.Y.) had a content of 100 μg of carbenicillin.

Antibiotic disk method. The disk method described by Overman et al. (26) was used in this study. MHA plates supplemented with blood and VKH were prepared on the day of use. The medium was adjusted to pH 7.4 before autoclaving; the pH was rechecked after autoclaving and adjusted to pH 7.4 if necessary. After autoclaving, 30 ml of the medium was poured into sterile petri dishes (100 by 15 mm). An inoculum was prepared by growing a culture for 24 h in brain heart infusion broth-VKH at 35 C. The culture was adjusted to one-half the turbidity of a no. 1 McFarland nephelometer standard using MHB-VKH as the diluent. Sterile cotton swabs were inserted into the diluted culture; the swabs were pressed against the tube wall to remove excess inoculum, and the MHA plates were then swabbed evenly in three directions. After the surface of the medium was allowed to dry for 3 to 5 min, disks were placed on the surface of the medium. The plates were inverted and incubated anaerobically at 35 C for 24 h. A vernier caliper was used to measure the zone diameter, which included the diameter of the disk. The zone diameter was recorded to the nearest millimeter. For some cultures, an inner zone of diminished growth was observed; the zone diameter was measured to the inner edge of this zone. Only those strains which gave clearly readable zones in 24 h were included in this study. The reproducibility of the test was determined by performing the test on three different days.

MIC determinations. One milliliter of each twofold antibiotic dilution ranging from 4,096 to 0.062 μg/ml was placed in each of two sterile petri dishes. MHA supplemented with VKH and blood (19 ml) was pipetted into each dish. After the medium had solidified, the plates were placed in an anaerobe chamber.

The inocula were prepared by growing the cultures in brain heart infusion broth supplemented with VKH for 22 h at 35 C. The cultures were adjusted to one-half the turbidity of a no. 1 McFarland nephelometer standard by using MHB-VKH as the diluent. A 1:10 dilution was prepared by using an Oxford automatic pipette to deliver 1 ml of the diluted culture to 9 ml of MHB-VKH. A Steers replicating device (32) was used to transfer the diluted cultures to the surface of the MHA plates.

After the inoculum had dried, the plates were inverted and incubated at 35 C for 22 h. The MIC was recorded as the lowest concentration of antibiotic that completely inhibited the growth of each organism as viewed macroscopically.

Standard curve. Antibiotic disks were prepared in our laboratory according to the following protocol. Gelman filter sheets (Scientific Products, Atlanta, Ga.) were punched with a two-hole punch (Punchodex) to yield disks with a diameter of 6 mm. The blank disks were placed in glass petri plates (15 by 150 mm) and autoclaved for 15 min. The disks were allowed to dry overnight at room temperature. Sterile disks were then placed on sterile nylon screens in petri dishes (15 by 90 mm). Various concentrations (in 20-μl amounts) of the antibiotic were applied to each disk, resulting in 11 different disk contents ranging from 1.5 to 800 μg. All disks were lyophilized (Virtis) overnight. All disks were used within 1 week of preparation.

Each disk content was tested seven times against a strain of *Escherichia coli* (ATCC 25922) and a carbenicillin-susceptible strain of *B. fragilis* subsp. *fragilis*; this *B. fragilis* strain produced a zone diameter close to the range ultimately defined as indeterminate. The antibiotic disk method described above was modified so that a large glass plate (38 by 26.7 cm) containing the medium was flooded with the appropriately diluted culture. The inoculum was evenly distributed over the surface of the medium by gently rocking the plate. Excess fluid was removed with a Pasteur pipette. After the surface of the medium had dried, seven disks of each content (77 total disks) were placed on the surface of the medium. One plate containing *E. coli* and one plate containing *B. fragilis* were incubated anaerobically at 35 C for 24 h. Zone diameters around each disk were measured with a vernier caliper, and the readings from the replicated studies were averaged for each organism to give a value that could be used in plotting a standard curve.

RESULTS

The standard curves of carbenicillin for *B. fragilis* subsp. *fragilis* and *E. coli* are shown in Fig. 1. The results were plotted with the zone diameters on the abscissa and disk content on a log scale on the ordinate. This standard curve was useful in determining the appropriate disk content to be used for antibiotic susceptibility testing (7, 21, 22). With the standard curve, it was possible to assess two criteria required for the selection of the proper disk content: (i) the effect of antibiotic deterioration on the size of the zone diameter and (ii) the disk content that produced a zone size that was not too large for use in a single petri plate in conjunction with other antibiotic disks. There was a linear relationship from 25 to 400 μg for both organisms tested. The portion of the line between 25 and 400 μg was examined for linearity, because a disk content of 50 μg or less was insufficient to separate resistant and susceptible populations; thus, 25 μg was chosen as the lower limit of the range. Since the carbenicillin disk will be used in conjunction with other antimicrobial disks, the disk content ultimately chosen should not produce zone diameters that are exceedingly large. Thus, disks with a content greater than 400 μg would not be practical. Thus, within that range, for *B. fragilis*, a twofold reduction in disk content resulted in about a 4-mm reduction in zone size. One hundred-microgram disks, which fell on this linear segment and were commercially available, were then selected for the disk test method.

The correlation between MIC values and zone diameters around 100-μg carbenicillin disks for 245 anaerobic bacteria is shown in Fig. 2. The results suggested the existence of two distinct populations of organisms with respect to the coordinates and zone diameters for MICs. The separation of the two populations for carbenicillin was not as great as for tetracycline against the five subspecies of *B. fragilis* (26) or for *B. fragilis* (35). When the zone diameters and MICs for 141 strains of four subspecies of *B. fragilis* were correlated separately, the phenomenon of bimodality was also observed. Excluding *B. fragilis*, all of the other anaerobic bacteria tested appeared to be members of the susceptible population, except for two strains of *P. anaerobius*. The two strains of *P. anaerobius* were susceptible by zone size determination but had MICs greater than the achievable serum level for carbenicillin. Because of the nonrandom occurrence of the bimodal distribution, the interpretation of the disk test was based on

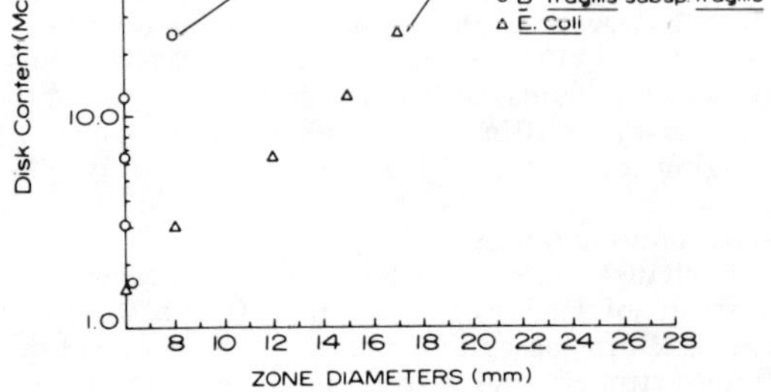

FIG. 1. *Standard curve of carbenicillin for E. coli (ATCC 25922) and B. fragilis subsp. fragilis (Emory University Hospital no. N-1216-72A) (the coefficient of correlation [r] for the B. fragilis strain was 0.9187; for the E. coli strain, r was 0.8786).*

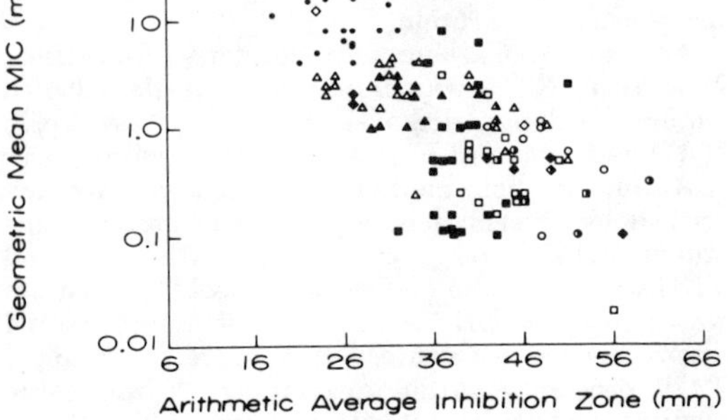

FIG. 2. *Correlation of MIC values and zone diameters of anaerobic bacteria around 100-μg carbenicillin disks.*

zone size characteristics of the two populations rather than by regression line analysis.

Both MIC and zone size data were used to classify the susceptibility of strains. The distribution of zone diameters for the 245 anaerobes tested is shown in Fig. 3. The bimodality of the population distribution was more apparent in the distribution of the zone diameters (Fig. 3) than in the distribution of the MICs (Fig. 4): 4 mm separated the two populations by the disk test, whereas there was no clear separation between the two populations by the MIC test alone.

An interpretive scheme was established by calculating the probability of outcomes in the area between the two zone sizes (Table 1). Calculations were then made to determine the probability that a given zone was produced by a strain of either the susceptible or resistant population. Thus, only 61 out of 10,000 susceptible strains would produce a zone of 8 mm, whereas 17 out of 100 resistant strains would produce a zone this size. Based on these data, there was a relative chance of 96% that a strain producing a zone diameter of 8 mm or less would be resistant. In contrast, there was a relative chance of 95% that a strain producing a zone diameter of 13 mm or greater would belong to the susceptible population and only a 5% chance that such a strain would belong to the resistant population. Since we wished to make correct decisions at least 95% of the time, those strains producing zones of 9 to 12 mm were termed "indeterminate." This type of statistical analysis was also calculated separately on the 141 strains of *B. fragilis* and the 86 strains of the anaerobic cocci. It was found that the susceptibility of none of the strains of *B. fragilis* and only one coccus would have been misclassified by using the interpretive scheme for all the anaerobes tested, rather than the interpretive scheme de-

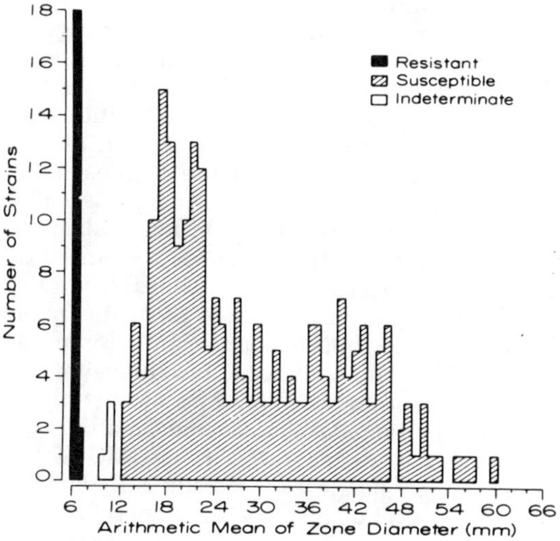

FIG. 3. *Distribution of the arithmetic mean of zone diameters with 245 strains of anaerobic bacteria tested with carbenicillin.*

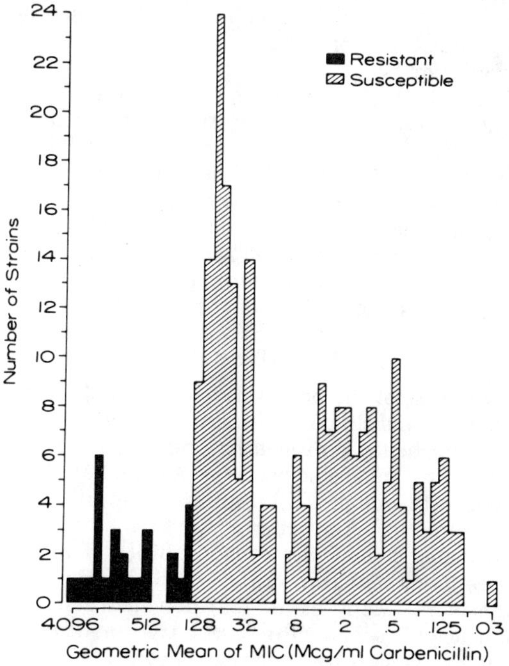

FIG. 4. *Distribution of MIC values of carbenicillin for 245 strains of anaerobic bacteria.*

TABLE 1. *Probabilities of obtaining zone diameters from strains in resistant and susceptible populations*

Recorded zone size (mm)	Actual range of measurements (mm)	Probability that zone was produced by a strain of either population		Relative chance (%)	
		Susceptible	Resistant	Susceptible	Resistant
8	7.5–8.4	0.00610	0.16828	3.62	96.38
9	8.5–9.4	0.00715	0.10243	6.98	93.02
10	9.5–10.4	0.00832	0.04669	17.82	82.18
11	10.5–11.4	0.00946	0.01462	64.71	35.29
12	11.5–12.4	0.01084	0.00343	68.36	31.64
13	12.5–13.4	0.01236	0.00060	95.13	4.87

veloped for each of the two groups. Thus, by using the test conditions outlined, the following interpretive scheme is recommended for carbenicillin against all anaerobes that grow sufficiently to produce a zone of inhibition in 24 h: resistant, 8 mm or less; indeterminate, 9 to 12 mm; and susceptible, 13 mm or greater.

For the MIC and zone size methods, a comparison of the reproducibility of tests performed at different times is shown in Table 2. Zone size and MIC determinations were made on 3 separate days. A table of random numbers was used to select 60 strains in the susceptible population for calculation of the coefficient of variation. The reproducibility of the two testing methods was studied by examining the difference in the arithmetic mean of the zone diameters and MICs of the strain and each of the three separate results contributing to these averages. It was not possible to determine the reproducibility of the strains in the resistant population because most strains in this population had a mean zone diameter of 6 mm.

For those strains in the susceptible population, the MIC test was approximately 10-fold more variable than the disk test. Thus, as noted by others (2, 26), the disk test separates populations more clearly and is more reproducible than determination of MICs. Therefore, use of the disk test reduces the chance of misclassifying the susceptibility of the strains.

DISCUSSION

Because of the potential toxicity of chloramphenicol and clindamycin, an effective, alternative antibiotic is needed for treating infections caused by anaerobic bacteria. A member of the relatively safe penicillin group of antibiotics is carbenicillin. A number of workers have demonstrated the in vitro susceptibility of anaerobes to carbenicillin (3, 5, 16, 25, 34, 41). Furthermore, Meny et al. (23) demonstrated the efficacy of carbenicillin in the treatment of infections caused by anaerobic bacteria.

Although some workers do not recommend routine susceptibility testing of anaerobic bacteria, the changing susceptibility pattern of these organisms now dictates that clinical laboratories should routinely perform antibiotic susceptibility testing of anaerobes (26, 35). To accomplish this objective, guidelines for a standard method for susceptibility testing of anaerobes were proposed by Overman et al. (26). Differences in interpretive schemes exist among various workers (17, 26, 29, 36, 41), but these differences result from the use of different inoculum sizes, media, atmospheric conditions and statistical methods for analyzing data.

Many workers have derived their interpretive schemes through regression line analysis. In reports of antimicrobial susceptibility testing of anaerobes by Kwok et al. (17), Sapico et al. (29), Sutter et al. (34, 35, 36) and Wilkins et al. (41), considerable variation about the regression line was shown. As noted previously (26), regression line analysis is valid only if the variables are normally distributed along the regression line. Furthermore, in linear regression, emphasis is placed on the MIC test; as we and others (2, 26) have shown, the MIC test is not only less reproducible than the disk test but has been successful in separating resistant and susceptible populations even when geometric mean values have been used. Statistical difficulties inherent in the use of linear regression for relating MICs to zone diameters have been noted by others (24). We believe that the use of the regression line to develop interpretive schemes in certain studies (17, 29, 34, 35, 36, 41) can be questioned for the reasons cited.

Previously, Bennett et al. (2) and others (26) recommended the use of population analysis to determine interpretive schemes for an antibiotic if two criteria are met: bimodality must occur, and the two populations of strains must be separated by an MIC value that is comparable to a clinically obtainable blood level of the antibiotic in question. Our strains met these two criteria: bimodality occurred, and the two populations were separated by an MIC of 128 μg/ml, which is accepted as a clinically obtainable blood level of carbenicillin. Therefore, we used the population analysis to derive the interpretive scheme for the anaerobic strains and carbenicillin.

In clinical laboratories, 50-μg disks were originally employed in performing the Bauer-Kirby susceptibility testing of aerobes with carbenicillin. However, it was noted by some workers (22) that strains which were susceptible by MIC criteria were resistant by zone diameter measurements around the 50-μg disks. This discrepancy was probably due to the use of disks with too low a content of antibiotic. Matsen et al. (22) performed standard-curve studies with aerobic bacteria and demonstrated that there was no theoretical reason for limiting the

TABLE 2. *Reproducibility of antibiotic susceptibility tests*

Population susceptible by:	Standard deviation	Arithmetic avg	Coefficient of variation (%)
Disk test	2.0	27.3	7.3
MIC	33.3	43.5	76.6

content of carbenicillin disks to 50 μg. One hundred-microgram disks were then made available by the manufacturer.

Earlier work with 50-μg carbenicillin disks and anaerobes in our laboratory (unpublished data) and the work of others (41) demonstrated the inability of disks of this content to adequately separate resistant and susceptible populations. As was demonstrated by Matsen et al. (22) with aerobes and carbenicillin, a linear relationship between zone diameters and disk content was noted in the range of 10 to 150 μg; our work with anaerobes and carbenicillin in standard-curve studies showed a linear relationship in the range of 25 to 400 μg. A disk content that falls on or above the linear portion of the standard curve must be used in an attempt to minimize the effect of deterioration of the antibiotic in the disks on zone size reduction and interpretive errors.

There are several criteria that a disk content must satisfy before it is selected as the optimal disk mass for use in antibiotic susceptibility testing. First, standard-curve studies should be performed to determine the effect of antibiotic deterioration on zone diameters as well as to determine the absolute zone size produced by minimally susceptible strains. Once a disk content is considered it should be studied for its ability to separate resistant and susceptible populations. This is followed by the development of interpretive schemes. Since manufacturers are permitted tolerances of 60 to 140% of stated contents, it is thus important to again review the standard curve to ensure that a 40% decrease in content (100 to 60%) would not cause minimally susceptible strains to be erroneously labeled resistant. One hundred-microgram disks satisfied this requirement. Furthermore, the selected disk mass must give reproducible results. Only a variation of 7.3% in zones was observed with the 100-μg carbenicillin disks in our studies. For these and other reasons, we recommend the use of 100-μg carbenicillin disks for antibiotic susceptibility testing of anaerobes.

Under test conditions different from ours and with the use of 50-μg carbenicillin disks and regression line analyses, Wilkins et al. (41) recommended that anaerobic organisms with zone sizes greater than 18 mm be considered susceptible. With our test conditions and 100-μg carbenicillin disks, those strains producing zone diameters of 13 mm or greater were considered susceptible.

Between 1 January 1975 and 31 December 1975, the clinical laboratory of Emory University Hospital isolated and tested 411 anaerobic strains with 100-μg carbenicillin disks. Of these 411 strains, 91% (375 of 411 strains) were susceptible to carbenicillin using the test method that we proposed. A total of 257 of the 411 strains isolated were susceptible to carbenicillin; these strains included anaerobic cocci, *Bifidobacterium* species, *Eubacterium* species, *Fusobacterium* species, *Lactobacillus* species, and *Bacteroides* species, excluding *B. fragilis*. A total of 154 strains of four subspecies of *B. fragilis* were isolated during this time period. Of these strains, 77% (118 strains) were susceptible, 10% (15 strains) were indeterminate, and 13% (21 strains) were resistant. By MIC criteria, Tally et al. (37) reported that 60% of 33 strains of *B. fragilis* were susceptible to carbenicillin at achievable blood levels. A total of 129 anaerobes other than *B. fragilis* were tested by Tally et al. (37); 99% were susceptible to carbenicillin at 128 μg/ml.

The CO_2 content in the atmosphere used for antibiotic disk susceptibility testing is important since CO_2 content can alter zone diameters around antimicrobial disks (15). Earlier work in our laboratory (26) demonstrated less variation in zone size with use of 10% CO_2 in the atmosphere than with higher concentrations of CO_2.

Therefore, with changing antimicrobial susceptibility patterns of anaerobes and with the availability of interpretive schemes that have been derived for various antimicrobial agents, we propose that clinical laboratories should routinely perform anaerobic antimicrobial susceptibility testing for clinically significant anaerobic isolates with appropriate, clinically useful antibiotics.

ACKNOWLEDGMENTS

We very much appreciate the critical review of this manuscript by John V. Bennett. Appreciation is also expressed to Carolyn R. Ramsey and Kay A. Bishop for expert technical assistance.

This work was supported by a grant from Pfizer Diagnostics.

LITERATURE CITED

1. **Bauer, A. W., W. M. M. Kirby, J. C. Sherris, and M. Turck.** 1966. Antibiotic susceptibility testing by a standardized single disk method. Am. J. Clin. Pathol. 45:493–496.
2. **Bennett, J. V., H. M. Camp, and I. C. Eickhoff.** 1968. Rapid sulfonamide disc sensitivity test for meningococci. Appl. Microbiol. 16:1056–1060.
3. **Blazevic, D. J., and J. M. Matsen.** 1974. Susceptibility of anaerobic bacteria to carbenicillin. Antimicrob. Agents Chemother. 5:462–465.
4. **Bodner, S. J., M. G. Koenig, and J. S. Goodman.** 1970. Bacteremic *Bacteroides* infections. Ann. Intern. Med. 73:537–544.
5. **Bodner, S. J., M. G. Koenig, L. L. Treanor, and J. S. Goodman.** 1972. Antibiotic susceptibility testing of

Bacteroides. Antimicrob. Agents Chemother. 2:57–60.

6. **Carey, W. D., and M. Brotman.** 1974. Clindamycin colitis: an emerging problem. West. J. Med. 121:504–507.
7. **Chabbert, Y. 1949.** Titrage de la sensibilite des germes aerobies aux antibiotiques par la methode de la cupule en gilose. Ann. Inst. Pasteur Paris 76:68–71.
8. **Cohen, L. E., C. J. McNeil, and R. F. Wells.** 1973. Clindamycin-associated colitis. J. Am. Med. Assoc. 223:1379–1381.
9. **Danielsson, D., D. W. Lambe, Jr., and S. Persson.** 1972. The immune response in a patient to an infection with *Bacteroides fragilis* ss. *fragilis* and *Clostridium difficile*. Acta. Pathol. Microbiol. Scand. Sect. B 80:709–712.
10. **Danielsson, D., D. W. Lambe, Jr., and S. Persson.** 1974. Immune response to anaerobic infections, p. 173–191. *In* A. Balows, R. M. DeHaan, V. R. Dowell, and L. B. Guze (ed.), Anaerobic bacteria: role in disease. International Conference on Anaerobic Bacteria, Center for Disease Control, 1972. Charles C Thomas Publisher, Springfield, Ill.
11. **Douglas, R. L., and J. W. Kislak.** 1973. Treatment of *Bacteroides fragilis* bacteremia with clindamycin. J. Infect. Dis. 128:569–571.
12. **Ersler, A. J., and M. M. Wintrobe.** 1962. Detection and prevention of drug-induced blood dyscrasias. J. Am. Med. Assoc. 181:114–119.
13. **Gorbach, S. L., and J. G. Bartlett.** 1974. Anaerobic infections (first of three parts). N. Engl. J. Med. 290:1177–1184.
14. **Holdeman, L. V., and W. E. C. Moore (ed.).** 1972. Anaerobe laboratory manual. Virginia Polytechnic Institute Anaerobe Laboratory, Blacksburg.
15. **Ingham, H. R., J. B. Selkan, A. A. Codd, and J. H. Hale.** 1970. The effect of carbon dioxide on the sensitivity of *Bacteroides fragilis* to certain antibiotics in vitro. J. Clin. Pathol. 23:254–258.
16. **Kislak, J. W.** 1972. The susceptibility of *Bacteroides fragilis* to 24 antibiotics. J. Infect. Dis. 125:295–299.
17. **Kwok, Y. Y., F. P. Tally, V. L. Sutter, and S. M. Finegold.** 1975. Disk susceptibility testing of slow-growing anaerobic bacteria. Antimicrob. Agents Chemother. 7:1–7.
18. **Lambe, D. W., Jr., D. Danielsson, D. H. Vroon, and R. K. Carver.** 1975. Immune response in eight patients infected with *Bacteroides fragilis*. J. Infect. Dis. 131:499–508.
19. **Marcoux, J. A., R. J. Zabransky, J. A. Washington III, W. E. Wellmann, and W. T. Martin.** 1970. Bacteroides bacteremia. Minn. Med. 53:1169–1176.
20. **Martin, W. J., M. Gardner, and J. A. Washington III.** 1972. In vitro antimicrobial susceptibility of anaerobic bacteria isolated from clinical specimens. Antimicrob. Agents Chemother 1:148–158.
21. **Matsen, J. M.** 1971. In vitro evaluation of nifuratrone, p. 260–266. Antimicrob. Agents Chemother. 1970.
22. **Matsen, J. M., M. E. Lund, and D. C. Brooker.** 1974. Comparison and evaluation of carbenicillin disks in diffusion susceptibility testing. Antimicrob. Agents Chemother. 5:599–606.
23. **Meny, R., C. D. Webb, and W. Fiedelman.** 1975. Carbenicillin therapy of anaerobic infections. Curr. Ther. Res. Clin. Exp. 17:478–487.
24. **Metzler, C. M., and R. M. DeHaan.** 1974. Susceptibility tests of anaerobic bacteria: statistical and clinical considerations. J. Infect. Dis. 130:588–594.
25. **Nobles, E. R., Jr.** 1973. *Bacteroides* infections. Ann. Surg. 177:601–606.
26. **Overman, S. B., D. W. Lambe, Jr., and J. V. Bennett.** 1974. Proposed standardized method for testing and interpreting susceptibility of *Bacteroides fragilis* to tetracycline. Antimicrob. Agents Chemother. 5:357–361.
27. **Rotheram, E. B., Jr., and S. F. Schick.** 1969. Nonclostridial anaerobic bacteria in septic abortion. Am. J. Med. 46:80–89.
28. **Saksena, D. S., M. A. Block, M. C. McHenry, and J. P. Truant.** 1968. Bacteroidaceae: anaerobic organisms encountered in surgical infections. Surgery 63:261–267.
29. **Sapico, F., Y. Y. Kwok, V. L. Sutter, and S. M. Finegold.** 1972. Standardized antimicrobial disc susceptibility testing of anaerobic bacteria: in vitro susceptibility of *Clostridium perfringens* to nine antibiotics. Antimicrob. Agents Chemother. 2:320–325.
30. **Sissons, J. G., J. M. Boulton-Jones, and D. K. Peters.** 1974. Clindamycin and pseudomembranous enterocolitis. Lancet 1:172.
31. **Smiley, R. K., G. E. Cartwright, and M. M. Wintrobe.** 1952. Fatal aplastic anemia following chloramphenicol (chloromycetin) administration. J. Am. Med. Assoc. 149:914–918.
32. **Steers, E., E. L. Foltz, B. S. Graves, and J. Riders.** 1959. An inocula replicating apparatus for routine testing of bacterial susceptibility to antibiotics. Antibiot. Chemother. 9:307–311.
33. **Stroehlein, T. H., R. E. Sedlock, H. N. Hoffman, and A. D. Newcomer.** 1974. Clindamycin-associated colitis. Mayo Clin. Proc. 49:240–243.
34. **Sutter, V. L., and S. M. Finegold.** 1975. Susceptibility of anaerobic bacteria to carbenicillin, cefoxitin, and related drugs. J. Infect. Dis. 131:417–422.
35. **Sutter, V. L., Y. Y. Kwok, and S. M. Finegold.** 1972. Standardized antimicrobial disc susceptibility testing of anaerobic bacteria. I. Susceptibility of *Bacteroides fragilis* to tetracycline. Appl. Microbiol. 23:268–275.
36. **Sutter, V. L., Y. Y. Kwok, and S. M. Finegold.** 1973. Susceptibility of *Bacteroides fragilis* to six antibiotics determined by standardized anti-microbial disc susceptibility testing. Antimicrob. Agents Chemother. 3:188–193.
37. **Tally, F. P., N. V. Jacobus, J. G. Bartlett, and S. L. Gorbach.** 1975. In vitro activity of penicillins against anaerobes. Antimicrob. Agents Chemother. 7:413–414.
38. **Thornton, G. F., and J. A. Cramer.** 1971. Antibiotic susceptibility of *Bacteroides* species, p. 509–513. Antimicrob. Agents Chemother. 1970.
39. **Tynes, B. S., and W. B. Frommeyer, Jr.** 1962. Bacteroides septicemia. Ann. Intern. Med. 56:12–26.
40. **Wells, R. F., L. E. Cohen, and C. J. McNeil.** 1974. Clindamycin and pseudomembranous colitis. Lancet 1:66.
41. **Wilkins, T. D., L. V. Holdeman, I. J. Abramson, and W. E. C. Moore.** 1972. Standardized single-disc method for antibiotic susceptibility testing of anaerobic bacteria. Antimicrob. Agents Chemother. 1:451–459.
42. **Zabransky, R. J., J. A. Johnston, and K. J. Hauser.** 1973. Bacteriostatic and bactericidal activities of various antibiotics against *Bacteroides fragilis*. Antimicrob. Agents Chemother. 1:148–158.

Antimicrobial Agents and Chemotherapy, July 1976, p. 119-122
Vol. 10, No. 1

Printed in U.S.A.

Antiviral Action and Cellular Toxicity of Four Thymidine Analogues: 5-Ethyl-, 5-Vinyl-, 5-Propyl-, and 5-Allyl-2′-Deoxyuridine

YUNG-CHI CHENG,* BARBARA A. DOMIN, RAM A. SHARMA, AND MIROSLAV BOBEK

Department of Experimental Therapeutics and Grace Cancer Drug Center, Roswell Park Memorial Institute, New York State Department of Health, Buffalo, New York 14263

Received for publication 3 February 1976

5-Ethyl-, 5-vinyl-, 5-propyl-, and 5-allyl-2′-deoxyuridine (dUrd) had antiviral activity against herpes simplex type 1 and type 2 grown in HeLa TK$^-$ cells, in the order 5-vinyl-dUrd, 5-ethyl-dUrd, 5-propyl-dUrd, 5-allyl-dUrd, but they were inactive against a TK$^-$ mutant of herpes simplex type 1. The antiviral activity of these compounds could be partially reversed by thymidine. Except for 5-vinyl-dUrd, they were not toxic to WI-38 and HeLa TK$^-$ cells at a concentration of 25 μM. All four analogues inhibited the growth of herpes simplex type 1-transformed HeLa TK$^-$ cells at a concentration of 1 μM.

Herpesviruses are responsible for many diseases in man, and recent evidence also suggests a strong correlation between herpes infections and the incidence of certain human malignancies (4). One characteristic of herpes simplex type I (HSV-1) and type II (HSV-2) is that they can induce virus-specific thymidine kinases (TK) in some human cells after infection. These viral TK's are different from the cytoplasmic and mitochondrial TK's of human cells not only with respect to their physical and chemical properties, such as electrophoretic mobility, activation energy, and salt sensitivity, but also in substrate specificity (Y. C. Cheng, submitted for publication; L. S. Lee and Y. C. Cheng, submitted for publication). This fact suggested to us that specific anti-HSV-1 and HSV-2 agents that specifically utilize viral TK might be developed.

The approach taken in this laboratory is to seek analogues of thymidine that could act as alternative substrates for viral TK but would not be substrates for normal mammalian cell TK's. Such analogues could be trapped inside the cells either as monophosphates or triphosphates to exert adverse effects on viral replication. Analogues of this nature would have no inhibitory effects on the growth of the uninfected cells.

Recently our laboratory purified TK's from HSV-1- and HSV-2-infected HeLa TK$^-$ cells (Y. C. Cheng and M. Ostrander, J. Biol. Chem., in press) as well as from the cytoplasmic and mitochondrial fractions of acute myelocytic leukemic blast cells (L. S. Lee and Y. C. Cheng, J. Biol. Chem., in press). A previous study on the binding specificity of some pyrimidine 2′-deoxyribonucleosides showed that 5-ethyl-, 5-propyl-, and 5-allyl-deoxyuridine (dUrd) had good binding affinity to HSV-1- and HSV-2-specific TK's (K_m of thymidine to K_i of analogue less than 0.2) but much poorer affinity for either human cytosol or mitochondrial TK's (K_m of thymidine to K_i of analogue larger than 0.005) and that 5-vinyl-dUrd had a high binding affinity to both viral and human mitochondrial TK's. For instance, the K_i of 5-ethyl-dUrd for human cytosol, human mitochondrial, HSV-1 (strain KOS), and HSV-2 (strain 333) TK's was 82, 305, 0.7, and 0.3 μM, respectively. The K_i of 5-vinyl-dUrd for human cytosol, human mitochondrial, HSV-1 (strain KOS), and HSV-2 (strain 333) TK's was 35, 1.7, 0.5, and 0.5 μM, respectively (Cheng and Lee, submitted for publication). This communication reports the results of a comparative study on the antiviral and cytotoxic effects of all four analogues and suggests that selective affinity to various TK's is responsible for their differential activity. Some studies on the biological activity of 5-ethyl-, 5-vinyl-, and 5-allyl-dUrd have been reported previously by other investigators (2, 7, 9–11).

MATERIALS AND METHODS

Cells and viruses. The stock viruses, HSV-1 (strains KOS and B2006) and HSV-2 (strain 333), were kindly given to us by W. Munyon of this institute (1, 3). Both the KOS and 333 strains of herpes simplex viruses but not the B2006 strain could induce TK in injected HeLa TK$^-$ cells. TK activities in those infected cells peak 12 h postinfection for strain KOS and 16 h postinfection for strain 333.

A viral suspension of low multiplicity (0.1 plaque-forming unit [PFU]/cell) was added to a 150-cm² confluent CV-I monolayer culture, and adsorption was allowed to proceed for 1 h. Forty milliliters of Eagle minimum essential medium containing 5% calf serum was then added, and the cells were incubated at 37 C for 24 h, followed by incubation at 34 C for 48 h (HSV-1) or 24 h (HSV-2). At the end of the incubation period, cells and medium were kept frozen at −70 C until titration. The yield of virus under these conditions was at least 5×10^9 PFU/ml for HSV-2.

HeLa TK^- (BU25), HSV-1 (strain KOS)-transformed HeLa TK^- cells, and CV-I cells were kindly given to us by W. Munyon and were grown as previously reported (1). WI-38 cells were obtained from Flow Laboratories (Rockville, Md.) and were free of mycoplasm.

Confluent HeLa TK^- cells (25 cm²) were used as host cells for virus infection. After a 1-h adsorption of virus with 10 PFU/cell, cell layers were rinsed twice with phosphate-buffered saline and 4 ml of Eagle minimum essential medium supplemented with 10% calf serum; various concentrations of drugs were then added, and the cells were incubated for 28 h at 37 C. At the end of the incubation they were stored frozen at −70 C until titration.

The various cell lines were grown at 37 C in different media (1) containing the analogues, and the cells were grown for three generations. The cytotoxic effect of the drugs is expressed as percentage of growth inhibition at the end of the third generation.

Materials. 5-Vinyl-2′-dUrd was synthesized as described by Sharma and Bobek (8). Briefly, catalytic hydrogenation of 1-(2-deoxy-3,5-di-*O*-*p*-toluoyl-*β*-D-erythropentofuranosyl)-5-vinyl uracil over 10% Pd-C in ethyl acetate, followed by removal of the protecting groups with sodium methoxide, yielded 5-ethyl-2′-dUrd. This material was identical in its melting point and ultraviolet spectrum to 5-ethyl-2′-dUrd prepared by Swierkowski and Shugar (11). 5-Allyl-2′-dUrd was kindly supplied by James F. Holland from Mount Sinai School of Medicine New York, N.Y. This material was purified by silica gel chromatography in ethyl acetate and finally recrystallized from ethyl acetate. 5-Propyl-2-dUrd was prepared by catalytic hydrogenation of 5-allyl-2′-dUrd on 5% Pd-C in methanol.

RESULTS

Antiviral activities. The effects of 5-ethyl-, 5-vinyl-, 5-propyl-, and 5-allyl-dUrd on the replication of HSV-1 (strain KOS) and HSV-2 (strain 333) in HeLa TK^- cells were compared with those of 5-iododeoxyuridine (Fig. 1). All analogues significantly inhibited the production of both types of virus. For HSV-1, 5-vinyl-dUrd was the most inhibitory, followed by 5-ethyl-, 5-propyl-, and 5-allyl-dUrd (Fig. 1A). For HSV-2, 5-ethyl- and 5-vinyl-dUrd were equally potent, followed by 5-propyl- and 5-allyl-dUrd (Fig. 1B). Preincubation of the two viral strains with 100 μM concentrations of any

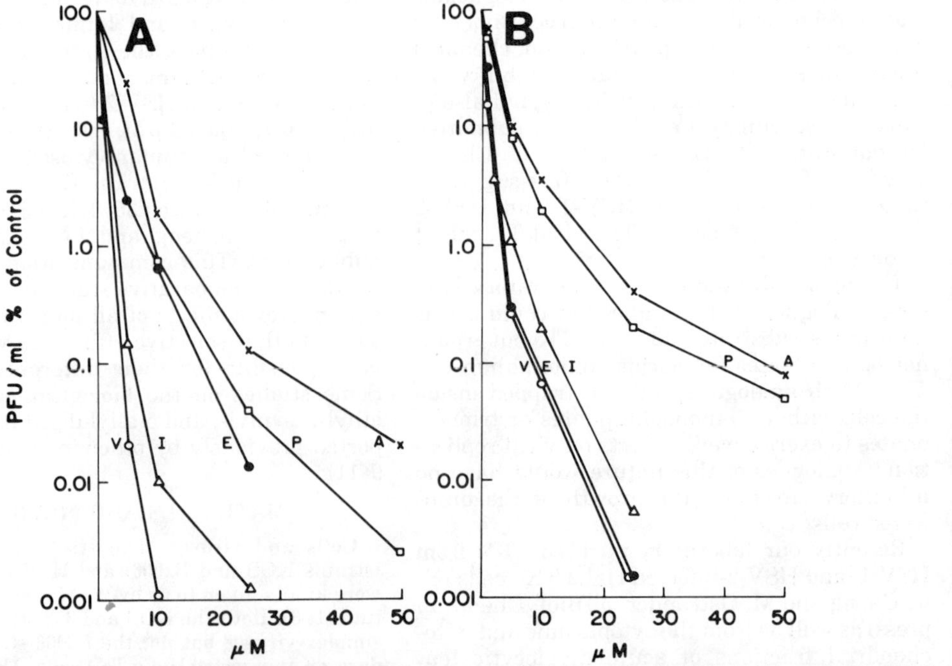

FIG. 1. *Effect of 5-ethyl-dUrd (E), 5-vinyl-dUrd (V), 5-propyl-dUrd (P), 5-allyl-dUrd (A), and 5-I-dUrd (I) on the replication of HSV-1 (A) and HSV-2 (B) in HeLa TK⁻ cells as a function of drug concentration. The experimental details are described in the text.*

of the four analogues for 1 h did not result in viral inactivation (data not shown).

Both HSV-1 (strain KOS) and HSV-2 (strain 333) induced TK in HeLa TK⁻ cells after infection. A mutant of HSV-1, strain B2006, that could not induce TK activity in HeLa TK⁻ cells was used for comparative tests of the antiviral activity of all four analogues. At 30 μM 5-ethyl- or 5-vinyl-dUrd and 100 μM 5-propyl- and 5-allyl-dUrd, no inhibition of B2006 growth in HeLa TK⁻ was observed.

The anti-HSV-1 (strain KOS) and HSV-2 (strain 333) activities of these four analogues in HeLa TK⁻ cells could be partially reversed by thymidine. The concentration of thymidine used, 25 μM, by itself had no activity against the growth of HSV-1 or HSV-2 in HeLa TK⁻ cells (Table 1).

Cytotoxicity. Three human cell lines were chosen for examining the cytotoxicity of the analogues: (i) HeLa TK⁻ cells, which are deficient in cytoplasmic TK but have mitochondrial TK (5); (ii) HSV-I (strain KOS)-transformed HeLa TK⁻ cells, which possess HSV-1-specific TK (5); (ii) HSV-1 (strain KOS)-transformed (1); and (iii) WI-38 cells, which have both types of human TK. The results (Table 2) are expressed in three ways: no inhibition, less than 50% growth inhibition, or larger than 50% inhibition after three generations of cell growth. The cytotoxic effect of 25 μM 5-vinyl-dUrd against either WI-38 cells or HeLa TK⁻ cells did not become apparent until the cells were incubated with this analogue for at least one generation. Under these conditions and for the same length of inhibition, 5-ethyl-, 5-propyl-, and 5-allyl-dUrd did not effect the growth of WI-38 and HeLa TK⁻ cells. In contrast, all four analogues at a concentration of 1 μM inhibited the growth of HSV-1-transformed HeLa TK⁻ cells even during the first generation of cell growth.

DISCUSSION

In summary, each of these four thymidine analogues, all of which had relatively good affinity for either HSV-1 (strain KOS)- or HSV-2 (strain 333)-induced TK (Cheng, submitted for publication), also showed significant antiviral activity against both types of viruses. An HSV-1 mutant (B2006) that lacked the ability to induce TK in infected cells was not inhibited by any of the analogues. The antiviral effects of these analogues could be partially reversed by thymidine. 5-Vinyl-dUrd, which has good affinity for human mitochondrial TK (Lee and Cheng, submitted for publication), inhibited

TABLE 1. *Reversal of antiviral activities of 5-ethyl-, 5-vinyl-, 5-propyl-, and 5-allyl-dUrd by thymidine*[a]

Compound	PFU/ml (% of control)	
	HSV-1 (KOS)	HSV-2 (333)
None	100	100
5-Ethyl-dUrd (10 μM)	0.7	0.08
5-Ethyl-dUrd (10 μM) Thymidine (25 μM)	5.5	9.7
5-Vinyl-dUrd (10 μM)	0.001	0.07
5-Vinyl-dUrd (10 μM) Thymidine (25 μM)	0.09	1.27
5-Propyl-dUrd (25 μM)	0.05	0.1
5-Propyl-dUrd (25 μM) Thymidine (25 μM)	1	1
5-Allyl-dUrd (25 μM)	0.1	0.5
5-Allyl-dUrd (25 μM) Thymidine)25 μM)	3	5
Thymidine (25 μM)	106	150

[a] Conditions of the experiments are described in the text.

TABLE 2. *Effects of 5-ethyl-, 5-vinyl-, 5-propyl-, and 5-allyl-dUrd on cell growth after three generations*[a]

Compound	Concn (μM)	Cell line	Growth inhibition		
			None	<50%	>50%
5-Ethyl-dUrd	25	HeLa TK⁻	+		
5-Vinyl-dUrd	25	HeLa TK⁻		+	
5-Propyl-Urd	25	HeLa TK⁻	+		
5-Allyl-dUrd	25	HeLa TK⁻	+		
5-Ethyl-dUrd	25	WI-38	+		
5-Vinyl-dUrd	25	WI-38		+	
5-Propyl-dUrd	25	WI-38	+		
5-Allyl-dUrd	25	WI-38	+		
5-Ethyl-dUrd	1	HSV-1-transformed HeLa TK⁻		+	
5-Vinyl-dUrd	1	HSV-1-transformed HeLa TK⁻			+
5-Propyl-dUrd	1	HSV-1-transformed HeLa TK⁻		+	
5-Allyl-dUrd	1	HSV-1-transformed HeLa TK⁻		+	

[a] Conditions of growth of the various cell lines are described in the text. Growth inhibition was calculated by the fold increase in number in the control cells minus that in the drug-treated cells divided by the fold increase in number in the control cells.

both HeLa TK⁻ and WI-38 cell growth, but only after the first generation. There was no inhibition of cell growth in the first generation. The delay in 5-vinyl-dUrd toxicity could be due to a number of factors. For instance, this compound might specifically disturb mitochondrial deoxyribonucleic acid replication, and cells could therefore sustain their growth for one generation. While this manuscript was in preparation, the delayed type of toxicity exerted by 5-vinyl-dUrd against Ehrlich ascites carcinoma cells was reported (6). The selective biological effects of 5-ethyl-, 5-propyl-, and 5-allyl-dUrd on cells having viral TK seem to suggest that the action of the three analogues depends on the presence of the viral TK. Whether they act at the monophosphate or triphosphate level to exert their activities is still under investigation.

ACKNOWLEDGMENT

This investigation was supported by American Cancer Society grant 77031-01.

LITERATURE CITED

1. **Davis, D. B., W. Munyon, R. Buchsbaum, and R. Chawda.** 1974. Virus type-specific thymidine kinase in cells biochemically transformed by herpes simplex virus types 1 and 2. J. Virol. 13:140–145.
2. **Holland, J. F., R. Korn, J. O'Malley, H. J. Minnemeyer, and H. Tiechalmann.** 1967. 5-Allyl-2'-deoxyuridine inhibition of nucleoside phosphorylase in HeLa cells containins Mycoplasma. Cancer Res. 27:1867–1873.
3. **Hughes, R. G., Jr., and W. H. Munyon.** 1975. Temperature-sensitive mutants of herpes simplex virus type 1 defective in lysis but not in transformation. J. Virol. 16:275–283.
4. **International symposium on human tumors associated with herpes viruses.** 1974. Cancer Res. 34:1083–1244.
5. **Kit, S., D. R. Dubbs, and P. M. Frearson.** 1966. HeLa cells resistant to bromodeoxyuridine and deficient in thymidine kinase activity. Int. J. Cancer 1:19–30.
6. **Langen, P., and D. Barwolff.** 1975. In the mode of action of 5-vinyl-2'-deoxyuridine. Biochem. Pharmacol. 24:1907–1910.
7. **Martenet, A.-C.** 1975. The treatment of experimental deep herpes simplex keratitis with 5-ethyl-deoxyuridine and iodo-deoxycytidine. Ophthalmic Res. 7:170–180.
8. **Sharma, R. A., and M. Bobek.** 1975. Synthesis of 5-vinyluridine and 5-vinyl-2'-deoxyuridine as new pyrimidine nucleoside analogs. J. Org. Chem. 40:2377–2379.
9. **Singh, S., I. Willers, H. W. Goedde, and K. K. Gauri.** 1974. 5-Ethyl-2'-deoxyuridine: absence of effects on the chromosomes of human lymphocytes and fibroblasts in culture. Humangenetik 24:135–139.
10. **Swierkowski, K. M., T. K. Jasinska, and J. A. Steffan.** 1973. 5-Ethyl-2'-deoxyuridine: evidence for incorporation into DNA and evaluation of biological properties in lymphocyte cultures grown under conditions of amethopterine-exposed thymidine deficiency. Biochem. Pharmacol. 22:85–93.
11. **Swierkowski, K. M., and D. Shugar.** 1969. A nonmutagenic thymidine analog with antiviral activity. 5-Ethyldeoxyuridine. J. Med. Chem. 12:533–534.

ANTIMICROBIAL AGENTS AND CHEMOTHERAPY, July 1976, p. 123-127
Vol. 10, No. 1

R Factor-Mediated Antibiotic Resistance in *Serratia marcescens*

ROBERT C. COOKSEY, GRACE M. THORNE, AND W. EDMUND FARRAR, JR.*

Department of Basic and Clinical Immunology and Microbiology, and Department of Medicine, Medical University of South Carolina, Charleston, South Carolina 29401*

Received for publication 9 February 1976

Nineteen of 39 multiresistant strains of *Serratia marcescens* isolated from clinical sources transferred antibiotic resistance to *Escherichia coli* or *Klebsiella pneumoniae* recipients. Marcesins and/or phage prevented effective resistance transfer to *E. coli* and attempts to select marcescin-resistant mutants of the *E. coli* recipient strain were unsuccessful. Transfer of resistance was demonstrated for all drugs tested except nalidixic acid. Approximately 90% of donors resistant to tobramycin, ampicillin, or carbenicillin transferred resistance to these drugs. High levels of transferred resistance (minimal inhibitory concentration, >2,500 μg/ml) were demonstrated particularly for ampicillin, carbenicillin, and kanamycin. Transmissibility of *Serratia* R factors was greatest betwween isogeneic strains of *E. coli* K-12. Comparative rates of spontaneous loss of R factor-mediated resistance indicated that *Serratia* R factors are less stable in *E. coli* and *K. pneumoniae* transcipients than in the indigenous hosts.

The incidence of hospital-associated infections caused by *Serratia marcescens* has increased significantly in recent years (3, 4, 13). Investigations of drug resistance in this species have shown *Serratia* to have resistance to a broader range of therapeutic agents than other *Enterobacteriaceae* (5, 7, 9, 13). The contribution of R factors to the multiple resistance of *Serratia* was studied in 1969 by Medeiros and O'Brien (8) who found that 21 of 22 multiple-resistant isolates transferred at least part of their resistance. They also concluded that multiple drug resistance is more prevalent in *Serratia* than in any other commonly isolated member of the *Enterobacteriaceae*, and that R factors not only mediated resistance to drugs to which the strain was previously susceptible but also conferred additional degrees of resistance to drugs to which the organism was already resistant.

Recently, 236 strains of *Serratia marcescens* obtained from Europe, Canada, and the United States were tested for R factor compatibility groups and transferability to *Escherichia coli* (7). Only 27 strains transferred resistance; the R factors found belonged either to compatibility groups notable for their wide generic host range or to groups found only in *Serratia*.

In this study 39 multiresistant strains of *S. marcescens* isolated from clinical sources were studied to evaluate the prevalence, antibiotic resistance patterns, transmissibility, and stability of R factors in *S. marcescens* and in *E. coli* and *Klebsiella pneumoniae* transcipients.

MATERIALS AND METHODS

Donors. From a collection of 102 strains of *S. marcescens* isolated from clinical sources at three medical centers (1), 39 multiresistant strains were selected for study. These strains were either resistant to antibiotics to which most strains in the collection were susceptible (streptomycin and kanamycin minimal inhibitory concentrations [MICs] ≥ 80 μg/ml; chloramphenicol MIC ≥ 30 μg/ml; gentamicin and tobramycin MICs ≥ 16 μg/ml) or were resistant to unusually high levels of ampicillin or tetracycline (MIC ≥ 500 μg/ml).

Recipients. Antibiotic-susceptible laboratory strains of *E. coli* K-12 and clinical strains of *K. pneumoniae* were selected as mating recipients. The recipient organisms and their selection markers are listed in Table 1.

Conjugation. R factor transfer experiments were performed by the method described by Datta and Hedges (2). Approximately 10^7 donor cells and 10^8 recipient cells were mixed and incubated at 37 C in a total volume of 2 ml of Penassay broth (Difco Laboratories, Detroit, Mich.), usually for 24 to 72 h with 1 ml of fresh broth added every 24 h. (Preliminary experiments had indicated that in some instances the frequency of resistance transfer was so low that a long period of mixed cultivation was necessary.) Mating mixtures were plated on antibiotic-containing or nutritionally selective media. Resistant progeny were tested by agar dilution methods for transferred patterns and levels of resistance.

Experiments to determine frequency of resistance transfer were performed as described above except that mating pairs were disrupted after 1 h by vigorous agitation. Transfer frequency was expressed as the number of resistant transcipients per donor cell.

Bacteriocin production. When results of mating

TABLE 1. *Recipient organisms*

Species	Strains	Markers	Source
E. coli K-12	CSH27	Nal^R, *trp, thi,* F^-	Cold Spring Harbor Laboratory
E. coli K-12	W1485-29	Nal^R, *lac*	Spontaneous mutant (Cold Spring Harbor Laboratory)
E. coli K-12	W1485-25	Rif^R	Spontaneous mutant
E. coli K-12	W1485-88	Nal^R, Rif^R, *lac*	Spontaneous mutant
K. pneumoniae	KB5	Amp^R, $Carb^R$	Diagnostic Bacteriology Laboratory, Medical University of South Carolina
K. pneumoniae	KB5-B1	Amp^S (MIC, 4 μg/ml), $Carb^S$ (MIC, 40 μg/ml), Rif^R	Spontaneous Rif^R mutant of the Amp^S $Carb^S$ derivative of KB5

experiments indicated that the *Serratia* donor was producing substances which were lethal to the intended *E. coli* recipient, selection of *E. coli* resistant to the presumptive bacteriocin was attempted. Bacteriocin lysates were made according to the method of Traub et al. (12) and spotted onto lawns of *E. coli* CSH 27 (Nal^R). Colonies found growing inside the zones of inhibition were retested against the same lysates before reincubation with the *Serratia* donor.

Spontaneous loss of resistance. Multiresistant strains of *S. marcescens* and *E. coli* and *K. pneumoniae* transcipients bearing *Serratia* R factors were grown for 24 h at 37 C in Penassay broth on a roller drum. The cultures were then diluted and plated for isolated colonies on Trypticase soy agar medium (BBL, Cockeysville, Md.). After subsequent incubation, 350 to 500 colonies of each strain were replica plated onto Trypticase soy agar medium containing single antimicrobial agents. Colonies failing to grow on drug-containing plates were picked, and the organisms were examined for loss of resistance markers.

RESULTS

Each of the 39 strains was incubated in mixed cultivation with *E. coli* CSH-27 (Nal^R). Only three strains (S3, S4, and S46) transferred resistance to this recipient. Death of the recipient due to production of marcescin and/or lytic phage by the *Serratia* donor was suspected as a cause for the failure of transfer in the majority of these matings (see later section).

Thirty-seven of the 39 multiresistant *Serratia* were incubated with *K. pneumoniae* strains KB5 or the derivative KB5-B1. Transfer of resistance was observed with 17 strains (Table 2). No decline in viability of recipients was observed in any of these experiments, indicating the resistance of *K. pneumoniae* to marcescins and/or phage. Two donors (MDA20 and MDA761) transferred complete as well as partial resistance patterns to KB5-B1. The resistance pattern of *Serratia* N-12 segregated into two distinct patterns upon transfer, suggesting the possible existence of two R factors in this strain.

The proportion of *Serratia* strains that transferred antibiotic resistance to *K. pneumoniae* or *E. coli* is shown in Table 3. At least 88% of strains resistant to tobramycin, ampicillin, or carbenicillin transferred resistance to these drugs. The lowest frequency of transfer was for chloramphenicol; only 29% of donors transferred resistance.

Levels of resistance in *E. coli* and *K. pneumoniae* transcipients for nine antibiotics were compared with those of the *Serratia* donors. The highest levels of resistance in *E. coli* CSH-27 transcipients were to ampicillin, carbenicillin, and kanamycin. With the exception of these drugs and tetracycline, resistance levels in *E. coli* CSH-27 transcipients were lower than in the *Serratia* donors. When resistance levels in *Klebsiella* transcipients were compared with those of the *Serratia* donors, it was found that low (MIC = 10 to 80 μg/ml) and high (MIC = 2,500 to 5,000 μg/ml) levels of resistance to ampicillin were found in both organisms. Levels of resistance to the other drugs were generally less in *K. pneumoniae* than in *S. marcescens*. However, high-level kanamycin resistance (MIC > 5,000 μg/ml) was observed in *K. pneumoniae* transcipients of R factors from three of four *Serratia* with high-level kanamycin resistance. High levels of resistance to the β-lactam drugs and kanamycin were maintained in two of three *E. coli* W1485 transcipients receiving *Serratia* R factors from *K. pneumoniae*. In one case (N-12) the levels of resistance to chloramphenicol and to tetracycline were greater in *E. coli* K-12 than in the *K. pneumoniae* donor.

Frequency of transfer of *Serratia* R factors from various donor organisms to *E. coli* W1485 was determined by 1-h matings. The results of 1-h matings between five *E. coli* and one *K. pneumoniae* donors and *E. coli* W1485 recipients are shown in Table 4. The highest transfer frequency was demonstrated between isogenic strains of *E. coli*. Lower frequencies of transfer were observed in 1-h matings between *E. coli*

TABLE 2. *Transfer of resistance from S. marcescens to K. pneumoniae KB5 or KB5-B1*

Serratia donors	Donor patterns[a]	*K. pneumoniae* recipient	Patterns transferred
SC13[b]	AmCbCr*Tc*Kn*Sm*Tb*GmCm*Su*Nx*	KB5	AmCbCrKnTbSu
MDA359[b]	AmCbCrTcKnSmTbGm*Cm*Su*Nx*	KB5	AmCbCrTcKnSmTbGmSu
MDA1296[b]	AmCbCr*TcKnSmTbGmSu*	KB5	AmCbCr
MDA575[b]	AmCbCrTcKnSmTbGm*Cm*Su*Nx*	KB5	AmCbCrTcKnSmTbGmSu
MDA829[b]	AmCbCrTcKnSmTbGm*Cm*Su*Nx*	KB5	AmCbCrTcKnSmTbGmSu
SC33[b]	Am*Cr*Tc*Sm*	KB5-B1	AmTc
SC39[b]	Am*Cr*Tc*Sm*	KB5-B1	AmTc
MDA22	Am*CbCrTc*Kn	KB5-B1	AmKn
MDA20[b]	AmCbCrKnSmTbGmSu	KB5-B1	AmCbCrKnSmTbGmSu
S10[b]	*AmCbCrKn*Sm*GmSu*	KB5-B1	Sm
S3	AmCb*CrTc*KnSmTb	KB5-B1	AmCbKnSmTb
N18[b]	AmCb*Cr*Tc*Sm*	KB5-B1	AmCbTc
S7	AmCbCr*Tc*Sm*Su*	KB5-B1	AmCbCrSm
N22	AmCb*Cr*TcKnSmGmCm*Su*	KB5-B1	AmCbTcKnSmCm
			AmCbTcKnSmGm
N-12[b]	AmCbCrTcKnSmTbGmCmSu*Nx*	KB5-B1	AmCbCrTcSmTbGmCm
			AmCbTcCm
			AmCbCm
			TcKnTbGmCmSu
			KnTbGmSu
			KnTbGm
			AmCbCrTcSm
MDA761[b]	AmCbCrTcKnSmTbGmSu	KB5-B1	AmCbCrTcKnSmTbGmSu
			AmCbCrKnTbGmSu
			AmCbKnSmTbGmSu
			AmCbCrKnTbGm
			AmCbSmSu
			SmSu
MDA576[b]	AmCbCrTcKnSmTbGm*Cm*Su*Nx*	KB5-B1	AmCbCrTcKnSmTbGmSu
			AmCbCrTcKnTbGmSu
			AmCbTcKnSmTbGmSu
			AmCbCrKnTbGmSu

[a] Abbreviations: Cm, chloramphenicol; Tc, tetracycline; Am, ampicillin; Cb, carbenicillin; Cr, cephalothin; Sm, streptomycin; Kn, kanamycin; Tb, tobramycin; Gm, gentamicin; Su, sulfisoxazole; and Nx, nalidixic acid. No transfer was demonstrated for resistance markers italicized.

[b] Produced marcescin-like activity against *E. coli* K-12.

TABLE 3. *Number of S. marcescens transferring resistance*

Antibiotic	No. transferred/ no. resistant	%
Tobramycin	9/10	90
Ampicillin	17/19	89
Carbenicillin	15/17	88
Kanamycin	12/15	80
Gentamicin	8/12	67
Streptomycin	12/18	67
Tetracycline	11/17	65
Sulfisoxazole	9/14	64
Cephalothin	10/19	53
Chloramphenicol	2/7	29

CSH-27 and *E. coli* W1485 and between *K. pneumoniae* and *E. coli*, suggesting the possibility of interstrain and interspecies mating barriers.

In 19 of 28 mating mixtures of *S. marcescens* and *E. coli* the recipient *E. coli* was killed by bacteriocins produced by the donor. Among the nine strains of *Serratia* not causing lethality were the three strains successfully transferring resistance to *E. coli* CSH-27. The remaining six *Serratia* did not transfer resistance to *E. coli* or *K. pneumoniae*. Twelve of 19 marcescin-producing *Serratia* strains transferred resistance to *K. pneumoniae*, and no decline in viability of either parental strain was observed with any of 37 mating mixtures of *Serratia* and *K. pneumoniae*. No death of recipients was observed with any mating mixtures between *K. pneumoniae* and *E. coli* or between strains of *E. coli*, indicating that marcescin production was not transferred in association with *Serratia* R factors. Bacteriocin lysate induced by mitomycin C at 33 C were prepared for eight *Serratia* known to kill *E. coli*, but none of the *E. coli* CSH-27 mutants resistant to the lysates showed increased survival when mixed with marcescin-producing *Serratia* strains.

The stability of resistance markers in *Serratia* donors and in their transcipients was also studied. None of the four *Serratia* tested exhibited any loss of resistance after 24-h broth passage, indicating relative R factor stability in the original host strain (Table 5). In the transcipients there were notable losses of resistance, especially to cephalothin, carbenicillin, ampicillin, and tetracycline.

DISCUSSION

In this study 19 of 39 multiresistant strains of *S. marcescens* transferred resistance to recipient strains of *K. pneumoniae* or *E. coli*. *K. pneumoniae* proved to be a better recipient than *E. coli* for *Serratia* R factors; only 3 of 39 strains transferred resistance to *E. coli*. Nineteen of 28 *S. marcescens* strains examined were found to produce bacteriocins lethal for the intended *E. coli* K-12 recipient (6).

Most strains of *S. marcescens* did not transfer the complete resistance pattern. Transcipients were usually found to exhibit various combinations of resistance markers. Mating experiments with one strain (N-12) yielded two types of transcipients, each possessing a separate portion of the original resistance pattern, suggesting that in this donor strain two distinct R factors were present.

Other factors may have interfered with our ability to demonstrate transfer of resistance. The transfer systems of some *Serratia* R factors have recently been shown to be temperature sensitive, since transfer occurs at 22 C but not at 37 C (10). Transfer of R factors is more efficient between organisms that are closely related phylogenetically. The frequency of intergeneric transfer using *Serratia* donors was always low. Higher frequencies were found in mating experiments between *Klebsiella* donors and *E. coli* recipients and between *E. coli* donors and *E. coli* recipients. The highest fre-

TABLE 4. *Frequency of transfer of Serratia R factors from K. pneumoniae and E. coli transcipients to E. coli W1485*

Donor	Donor pattern[a]	*E. coli* recipient	Pattern transferred[a]	Transfer frequency[b]
W1485 (MDA576)-2	AmCbCrTcKnSmTbSu	W1485-25	AmCbCrTcKnSmTbSu	1.4×10^{-2}
W1485 (MDA761)-1	AmCbCrTcKnSmTbSu	W1485-25	AmCbCrTcKnSmTbSu	3.7×10^{-2}
W1485 (N12)-2	TcCm	W1485-25	TcCm	2.8×10^{-2}
CSH 27 (S3)-1	AmCbTcKnSm	W1485-88	AmCbTcKnSm	1.5×10^{-3}
			Sm	2.9×10^{-3}
CSH 27 (S43)-2	TcKnSm	W1485-88	TcKnSm	6.3×10^{-6}
			Sm	1.4×10^{-5}
KB5B1 (MDA20)	*AmCbCrKn*Sm*TbGmSu*	W1485-29	Sm	1.3×10^{-5}

[a] Abbreviations: Am, ampicillin; Cb, carbenicillin; Cr, cephalothin; Tc, tetracycline; Kn, kanamycin; Sm, streptomycin; Tb, tobramycin; Gm, gentamicin; Cm, chloramphenicol; and Su, sulfisoxazole. No resistance transfer was demonstrated for resistance markers italicized.

[b] Number of recipient cells with pattern per donor cell.

TABLE 5. *Spontaneous loss of resistance from four R⁺ strains of S. marcescens and from E. coli and K. pneumoniae transcipients*

Host strain	Resistance pattern[a]	Resistance markers lost[b]
MDA576	AmCbCrTcKnSmTbGmCmSuNx	None (0/500)
KB5B1 (MDA576)-1	AmCbCrTcKnSmTbGmSu	Cr (72/421)
W1485 (MDA576)-1	AmCbCrTcKnSmTbGmSu	Cb (19/350), Cr (11/350), Sm (9/350), Tb (7/350)
MDA761	AmCbCrTcKnSmTbGmSu	None (0/460)
KB5B1 (MDA761)-1	AmCbCrTcKnSmTbGmSu	Am (182/450), Cb(182/450), Tc (197/450)
W1485 (MDA761)-1	AmCbCrTcKnSmTbSu	Am (145/425), Cb (267/425), Cr (9/425), Tc (238/425)
MDA829	AmCbCrTcKnSmTbGmCmSuNx	None (0/440)
KB5 (MDA829)	AmCbCrTcKnSmTbGmSu	Cr (436/480), Kn (2/480), Tb (6/480), Gm (10/480)
MDA20	AmCbCrKnSmTbGmSu	None (0/425)
KB5B1 (MDA20)	AmCbCrKnSmTbGmSu	Cr (171/412), Tb (13/412), Gm (56/412)

[a] Abbreviations: Am, ampicillin; Cb, carbenicillin; Cr, cephalothin; Tc, tetracycline; Kn, kanamycin; Sm, streptomycin; Tb, tobramycin; Gm, gentamicin; Cm, chloramphenicol; and Nx, nalidixic acid.

[b] Number of susceptible colonies per number of colonies tested.

quencies of transfer were found in experiments in which the *E. coli* donors and recipients were isogenic.

With a few exceptions, levels of resistance to most drugs were higher in *Serratia* organisms than in *K. pneumoniae* or *E. coli*. This may indicate a higher degree of intrinsic resistance in *S. marcescens* or may possibly be related to the presence of multiple copies of R factors in the *Serratia* host.

Medeiros and O'Brien (8) reported that R factors were less stable in *S. marcescens* than in other species of *Enterobacteriaceae*. Our findings are different, in that the R factors we studied were quite stable in *S. marcescens* but less so in either *K. pneumoniae* or *E. coli* hosts. Schaefler et al. have reported a similar experience (11). This was not surprising to us as R factors have been shown to have definite host preferences (2, 14) and selection in favor of stable R factor-host combinations presumably takes place in antibiotic-containing environments such as hospitals, where nearly all serious *Serratia* infections occur.

ACKNOWLEDGMENTS

We appreciate the kindness of E. R. Bannister, J. A. Shulman, and Dieter Gröschel in providing us with bacterial strains.

LITERATURE CITED

1. **Cooksey, R. C., E. R. Bannister, and W. E. Farrar, Jr.** 1975. Antibiotic resistance patterns of clinical isolates of *Serratia marcescens*. Antimicrob. Agents Chemother. 7:396–399.
2. **Datta, N., and R. W. Hedges.** 1972. Host ranges of R factors. J. Gen. Microbiol. 70:453–460.
3. **Dodson, W. H.** 1968. *Serratia marcescens* septicemia. Arch. Intern. Med. 121:145–150.
4. **Ewing, W. H., J. G. Johnson, and B. R. Davis.** 1962. The occurrence of *Serratia marcescens* in nosocomial infections. Center for Disease Control, Atlanta, Ga.
5. **Greenup, P., and D. J. Blazevic.** 1971. Antibiotic susceptibilities of *Serratia marcescens* and *Enterobacter liquefaciens*. Appl. Microbiol. 22:309–314.
6. **Hannon, Y., and Y. Perón.** 1961. Etude de la propriete dans le genre *Serratia*. Ann. Inst. Pasteur. 100:818–821.
7. **Hedges, R. W., V. Rodriguez-Lemoine, and N. Datta.** 1975. R factors from *Serratia marcescens*. J. Gen. Microbiol. 86:88–92.
8. **Medeiros, A. A., and T. O'Brien.** 1969. Contribution of R factors to the antibiotic resistance of hospital isolates of *Serratia*, p. 30–35. Antimicrob. Agents Chemother. 1968.
9. **Oberhofer, T. R., and R. Hajkowski.** 1970. Evaluation of nonlactose-fermenting members of the *Klebsiella-Enterobacter-Serratia* division. Am. J. Clin. Pathol. 54:726–732.
10. **Rodriguez-Lemoine, V., A. E. Jacob, R. W. Hedges, and N. Datta.** 1975. Thermosensitive production of their transfer systems by group S plasmids. J. Gen. Microbiol. 86:111–114.
11. **Schaefler, S., J. Winter, A. Catelli, J. Greene, and B. Toharski.** 1971. Specific distribution of R factors in *Serratia marcescens* strains isolated from hospital infections. Appl. Microbiol. 22:339–343.
12. **Traub, W. H., E. A. Raymond, and T. S. Startsman.** 1971. Bacteriocin (marcescin) typing of clinical isolates of *Serratia marcescens*. Appl. Microbiol. 21:837–840.
13. **Wilfert, J. N., F. F. Barrett, W. H. Ewing, M. Finland, and E. H. Kass.** 1970. *Serratia marcescens:* biochemical, serological, and epidemiological characteristics and antibiotic susceptibility of strains isolated at Boston City Hospital. Appl. Microbiol. 19:345–352.
14. **Yoshikawa, M., S. Nagashima, and S. Matsushima.** 1971. Genetical distinction of R factors derived from Shigellae and Salmonella. Jpn. J. Microbiol. 15:425–436.

ANTIMICROBIAL AGENTS AND CHEMOTHERAPY, July 1976, p. 128-131 Vol. 10, No. 1

Printed in U.S.A.

Antimicrobial Susceptibility of Group B Streptococci Isolated from a Variety of Clinical Sources

CAROL J. BAKER,* BETTE J. WEBB, AND FRED F. BARRETT

Departments of Pediatrics and Microbiology and Immunology, Baylor College of Medicine, Houston, Texas 77030*

Received for publication 1 March 1976

The minimal inhibitory concentration of 10 antibiotics for 244 isolates of group B streptococci was determined. Susceptibility to penicillin G, ampicillin, cephalothin, chloramphenicol, and carbenicillin was uniform. Tetracycline and bacitracin resistance among these isolates was frequent (87.5 and 97.9%, respectively). Three strains (1.2%) failed to be inhibited by 100 μg of lincomycin or clindamycin per ml. Susceptibility of these 244 strains to the agents tested was unrelated to source of the isolate, year of isolation, or strain serotype. No apparent change in the suceptibility of group B streptococci to penicillin G has occurred during the past 2 decades.

Strains of group B *Streptococcus* have become increasingly frequent isolates from neonates and infants with serious bacterial infection during the past decade (1, 2, 4, 8). Because this microbial species has previously been noted to be uniformly susceptible to the penicillins (7, 9), penicillin G has been the recommended drug of choice for the treatment of group B streptococcal infections (3, 7). However, two recent reports suggest that certain strains are relatively resistant to penicillin G (M. J. Severin and J. L. Wiley, Prog. Abstr. Intersci. Conf. Antimicrob. Agents Chemother., 14th, San Francisco, Calif., Abstr. 251, 1974) or ampicillin (15), an observation that is believed to be related to time and that has important therapeutic implications if confirmed. In addition, serious puerperal infections and skin infection among diabetics have been associated with group B streptococci (2, 7), and certain patients with these infections require antimicrobial therapy with drugs alternative to penicillin G because of a history of allergy to the penicillins. Lincomycin and clindamycin may be useful for these patients on the basis of their uniformly good in vitro activity against Lancefield group B strains of streptococci (11). However, relatively few strains have been tested in vitro to clindamycin, and no data are available to date regarding its efficacy in the treatment of group B streptococcal infections.

In the present study we determined the antimicrobial susceptibility of 244 strains of group B streptococci isolated from a variety of clinical sources between 1970 and 1975 as a means of defining resistance to penicillin G, useful alternative antibiotics for the treatment of penicillin-allergic patients, and differences in the susceptibility of isolates on the basis of strain serotype, or source and year of isolation.

MATERIALS AND METHODS

Two hundred and forty-four strains of group B streptococci were studied. These strains were isolated from the following patient groups: (i) blood or cerebrospinal fluid isolates from 45 infants and 5 adults (50 strains); (ii) vaginal isolates from 80 nonpregnant college women and 32 parturients at delivery (112 strains); (iii) throat, umbilical, or external auditory canal isolates from 34 asymptomatically, colonized neonates (34 strains); and (iv) vaginal or urethral isolates from 28 women and 20 men enrolled in a venereal disease clinic (48 strains). These strains were isolated in several geographical areas. Most of the "significant" isolates were from Houston, as were all the strains from asymptomatic pregnant women and neonates. All isolates from venereal disease clinic patients were from Boston, and all isolates from college women were from Rhode Island. Grouping and serotyping of these isolates were performed by the capillary precipitin method (12) with hyperimmune rabbit antisera prepared against formalinized vaccines of standard strains.

Agar plate dilution tests of quantitative antibiotic susceptibility were performed on Mueller-Hinton agar (Difco Laboratories, Detroit, Mich.) containing 5% defibrinated sheep blood. Agar plates containing serial twofold dilutions of antibiotic at final concentrations from 0.00625 to 100 μg/ml were inoculated by using the replicator technique of Steers et al. (14). The inoculum consisted of an undiluted overnight culture in Todd-Hewitt broth (Difco Laboratories) delivered in an aliquot of 0.002 ml; the inoculum was estimated to contain 10^7 viable organisms. The minimal inhibitory concentration (MIC) was defined as the lowest concentration of antibiotic in which no growth was visible after incubation of the agar plates for 18 h at 37 C. Control plates without antibiotic were inoculated in a similar fashion in each series of tests to assess strain viability, and a reference strain of group B *Streptococcus* was included to assure reproducibility. Thirty-one of the isolates for which the MIC of penicillin G was ≥0.1 μg/ml were simultaneously tested, using identical methods and an inoculum of approximately 10^4 as well as 10^7 viable organisms on the same test day. The antibiotics tested were penicillin G, ampicillin, carbenicillin, cephalothin, chloramphenicol, gentamicin, bacitracin, lincomycin, clindamycin, and tetracycline.

Standard epidemiological data, including the source and serotype of the isolate, the year of isolation, and the diagnosis of the patient, were recorded for each strain tested. These data were then correlated with in vitro susceptibility by appropriate statistical methods.

RESULTS

The results for the susceptibility of these 244 group B streptococci to 10 antibiotics are depicted graphically in Fig. 1 and are summarized in Table 1. Penicillin G was the most active antimicrobial agent tested; the median MIC was 0.05 μg/ml (0.083 units/ml). When inoculum size was decreased to 10^4 viable organisms, the median MIC of strains to penicillin decreased to 0.025 μg/ml. All the strains tested were susceptible to penicillin G, ampicillin, cephalothin, chloramphenicol, and carbenicillin, in descending order of activity. Resistance to gentamicin at a concentration of 12.5 μg/ml was uniform, and 97.1% of strains were not inhibited by bacitracin at a concentration of 3.1 μg or less per ml.

Lincomycin and clindamycin were quite active against these 244 strains of group B *Streptococcus*. All but three isolates (1.2% of strains) were inhibited by a concentration of 0.2 μg or less of lincomycin and 0.1 μg or less of clindamycin per ml. The three resistant strains failed to have their growth inhibited by 100 μg of either agent per ml, and cross-resistance to erythromycin (disk diffusion method [5], zone of 6 mm) was uniform. These clindamycin-resistant strains were isolated from a neonate with septicemia (1972), a woman with puerperal sepsis (1973), and a vaginally colonized, asymptomatic parturient (1974).

Of the antimicrobial agents tested, tetracycline was the only one for which there were significant numbers of both resistant and susceptible strains (87.5 and 12.5%, respectively). No relationship between susceptibility to tetracycline and the source, or the serotype of an isolate or its year of isolation was apparent.

To detect increasing resistance to penicillin G among the isolates tested on the basis of strain, serotype, or year of isolation, strains with an MIC of ≥0.1 μg/ml were analyzed (Tables 2 and 3). It was apparent that serotype of infecting strain was unrelated to penicillin susceptibility, since the distribution of serotypes for strains inhibited at a concentration of ≥0.1 μg/ml was not significantly different from that among strains inhibited at a concentration of <0.1 μg of penicillin G per ml. The relatively large number of type III strains tested (40.9%) was accounted for by the fact that 36 (72%) of the 50 strains isolated from blood or cerebrospinal fluid cultures of patients with significant infection contained the type III polysaccharide.

Although the number of strains isolated between 1970 and 1973 was small (29), the median

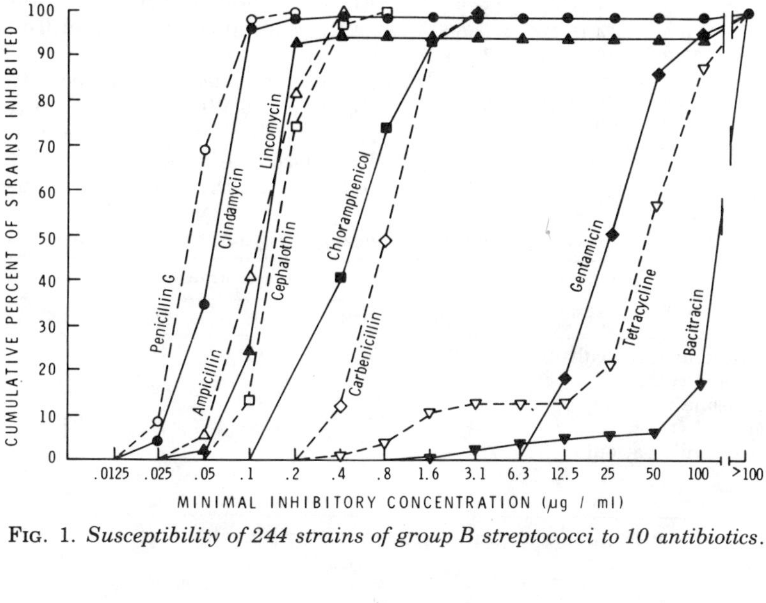

FIG. 1. *Susceptibility of 244 strains of group B streptococci to 10 antibiotics.*

and range of MICs to penicillin G were not significantly different from those among strains isolated in 1974 and 1975 ($\chi^2 = 2.36$, $P = 0.2$). However, no definite conclusions can be made from these data regarding shift in penicillin G susceptibility for the 6-year period during which these strains were isolated because of small numbers (Table 3). Since all but eight strains isolated before 1974 were from patients with significant infection, usually neonates, no correlation between penicillin susceptibility and source of isolate could be ascertained.

TABLE 1. *Susceptibility of 244 strains of group B streptococci to 10 antibiotics*

Antibiotic	MIC (μg/ml)	
	Range	Median
Penicillin G	0.025–0.2	0.05[a]
Ampicillin	0.05–0.4	0.2
Carbenicillin	0.4–3.1	0.8
Cephalothin	0.1–0.8	0.2
Lincomycin[b]	0.05–>100	0.1
Clindamycin	0.025–>100	0.1
Tetracycline	0.4–>100	50
Chloramphenicol	0.4–3.1	0.8
Bacitracin	1.6–>100	>100
Gentamicin	12.5–>100	25

[a] Equivalent to 0.083 units/ml.
[b] Forty-five of 50 "significant" patient isolates were tested.

TABLE 2. *Relationship of serotype of group B Streptococcus to MIC of penicillin G*

Serotype	No. of total strains tested[a]	% of strains	No. (%) of strains with MIC ≤0.1 μg/ml	No. (%) of strains with MIC <0.1 μg/ml
Ia	16	6.8	1 (1.4)	15 (9.0)
Ib	15	6.3	4 (5.7)	11 (6.6)
Ic	41	17.3	9 (12.9)	32 (19.1)
II	67	28.3	27 (38.6)	40 (23.9)
III	97	40.9	29 (41.4)	68 (40.7)
NT[b]	1	0.4	0	1 (0.7)

[a] Seven strains were not serotyped.
[b] NT, Nontypable.

DISCUSSION

Lancefield group B strains of streptococci have been previously shown to have uniform susceptibility to penicillin (7, 8, 10, 13), although the concentrations required for their inhibition are 4 to 10 times those necessary for the inhibition of group A streptococci (2, 7, 13). The report by Severin and Wiley (Prog. Abstr. Intersci. Conf. Antimicrob. Agents Chemother., 14th, San Francisco, Calif., Abstr. 251, 1974) of increasing resistance of strains to penicillin G over the past few years was not observed in the present study. The median MIC of penicillin G for these 244 strains of group B streptococci was 0.05 μg/ml (0.083 units/ml), the same as that reported by Jones et al. (10) in 1957 for 56 strains of group B streptococci. It is apparent that the size of the inoculum will affect the MIC of group B streptococci to penicillin G in agar dilution tests. A twofold lower concentration of penicillin G was required to inhibit growth of strains when the inoculum was decreased to approximately 10^4 viable organisms. The effect of inoculum size may account, in part, for the susceptibility of strains to penicillin G at lower concentrations reported by Matsen and Coghlan (13) (range, 0.001 to 0.026 μg/ml), compared to that noted in the present study (range, 0.025 to 0.2 μg/ml), since an inoculum of 10^1 less was used in the earlier work. The observation that 100% of the 244 strains were inhibited by penicillin G at a concentration of 0.2 μg or less per ml was also reported by Anthony and Concepcion in their study of 511 group B streptococci isolated from a variety of clinical sources (2). This degree of susceptibility does not seem to support the hypothesis (Severin and Wiley, Prog. Abstr. Intersci. Conf. Antimicrob. Agents Chemother., 14th, San Francisco, Calif., Abstr. 251, 1974) that a gradual shift in the penicillin G susceptibility of

TABLE 3. *Relationship between year of isolation and susceptibility of group B streptococci to penicillin G*

Source of isolate	No. of strains isolated by:					
	1970	1971	1972	1973	1974	1975
Cerebrospinal fluid or blood cultures	4 (2)[a]	5 (1)	8 (1)	4 (1)	25 (0)	4 (0)
Asymptomatic parturients					12 (4)	20 (9)
Asymptomatic neonates			8 (8)		22 (16)	4 (0)
College women					23 (4)	57 (2)
Venereal disease clinic patients						
Men						28 (10)
Women					8 (6)	12 (10)

[a] Number in parentheses is number of strains with an MIC to penicillin G of ≤0.1 μg/ml (0.17 units/ml).

group B streptococci has occurred during the past 2 decades. However, it should be emphasized that it is possible for geographical variation in the antimicrobial susceptibilities of group B streptococci to occur and that relative or true penicillin G resistance could emerge in the future. Therefore, continued laboratory surveillance of the susceptibility of these organisms to penicillin G is recommended.

Bacitracin susceptibility was similar to that noted by other investigators (1.2%) (7, 13). Of interest was the observation that 1 to 2% of these serologically confirmed isolates of group B streptococci were nonhemolytic on sheep blood agar medium, a previously reported (2, 13) but not often recognized occurrence. Tetracycline resistance was common among the isolates tested (87.5%) and appears to have increased significantly during the past 2 decades (15 to 44%) (7, 10).

An unexpected finding on the basis of previous reports (7, 8, 11, 13) was the observation that 1.2% of the 244 strains were resistant to lincomycin and clindamycin, although these two antimicrobial agents were quite active against the majority of strains tested. Cross-resistance with erythromycin was complete. The rate of resistance to these two drugs is similar to that noted in two recent reports (2, 6) but was not detected in studies of erythromycin (7, 10) and lincomycin (7) prior to 1970. The occurrence of strains resistant to lincomycin and clindamycin may limit their theoretical usefulness for the treatment of patients with significant group B streptococcal infection and documented penicillin allergy. Chloramphenicol susceptibility was uniform in this and previous studies (7, 13), and this agent may be useful in the treatment of penicillin-allergic patients with life-threatening infections or meningitis due to group B *Streptococcus*.

ACKNOWLEDGMENT

We are indebted to N. Byrd for helpful criticism and to Gaynelle Straley for her assistance in the preparation of the manuscript.

This research was supported by a grant from the Upjohn Co.

LITERATURE CITED

1. **Ablow, R. C., S. G. Driscoll, E. L. Effmann, I. Gross, C. J. Jolles, R. Vany, and J. B. Warshaw.** 1976. A comparison of early onset group B streptococcal neonatal infection and the respiratory-distress syndrome of the newborn. N. Engl. J. Med. 294:65–70.
2. **Anthony, B. F., and N. F. Concepcion.** 1975. Group B *Streptococcus* in a general hospital. J. Infect. Dis. 132:561–567.
3. **Baker, C. J.** 1976. Neonatal sepsis, meningitis and pneumonia, p. 526–529. *In* S. S. Gellis and B. M. Kagan (ed.), Current pediatric therapy. W. B. Saunders Co., Philadelphia.
4. **Baker, C. J., F. F. Barrett, R. C. Gordon, and M. D. Yow.** 1973. Suppurative meningitis due to streptococci of Lancefield group B: a study of 33 infants. J. Pediatr. 82:724–729.
5. **Bauer, A. W., W. M. Kirby, J. C. Sherris, and M. Turck.** 1966. Antibiotic susceptibility testing by a standardized single disc method. Am. J. Clin. Pathol. 36:493–496.
6. **Dixon, J. M. S., and A. E. Lipinski.** 1972. Resistance of group A beta hemolytic streptococci to lincomycin and erythromycin. Antimicrob. Agents Chemother. 1:333–339.
7. **Eickhoff, T. C., J. O. Klein, A. K. Daly, D. Ingall, and M. Finland.** 1964. Neonatal sepsis and other infections due to group B beta-hemolytic streptococci. N. Engl. J. Med. 271:1221–1228.
8. **Finn, P. D., and F. A. Holden.** 1970. Observations and comments concerning the isolation of group B β-hemolytic streptococci from human sources. Can. Med. Assoc. J. 103:249–252.
9. **Howard, J. B., and G. H. McCracken, Jr.** 1974. The spectrum of group B streptococcal infections in infancy. Am. J. Dis. Child. 128:815–818.
10. **Jones, W. F., Jr., H. A. Feldman, and M. Finland.** 1957. Susceptibility of hemolytic streptococci other than those of group D, to eleven antibiotics *in vitro*. Am. J. Clin. Pathol. 27:159–169.
11. **Karchmer, A. W., R. C. Moellering, Jr., and B. K. Watson.** 1975. Susceptibility of various serogroups of streptococci to clindamycin and lincomycin. Antimicrob. Agents Chemother. 7:164–167.
12. **Lancefield, R. C.** 1934. Serologic differentiation of specific types of bovine hemolytic streptococci (group B). J. Exp. Med. 59:441–458.
13. **Matsen, J. M., and C. R. Coghlan.** 1972. Antibiotic testing and susceptibility patterns of streptococci, p. 189–204. *In* L. W. Wannamaker and J. M. Matsen (ed.), Streptococci and streptococcal diseases, recognition, understanding, and management. Academic Press Inc., New York.
14. **Steers, E., E. L. Foetz, and B. S. Graves.** 1959. Inocula replicating apparatus for routine testing of bacterial susceptibility to antibiotics. Antibiot. Chemother. 9:307–311.
15. **Whitworth, T. C., and S. H. Sell.** 1973. Beta-hemolytic *Streptococcus* group B in neonates. Clin. Res. 20:106.

Antimicrobial Agents and Chemotherapy, July 1976, p. 132-138
Vol. 10, No. 1

Laboratory Evaluation of 3-(5-Tetrazolyl)Penam, a New Semisynthetic Beta-Lactam Antibacterial Agent with Extended Broad-Spectrum Activity

ARTHUR R. ENGLISH,* JAMES A. RETSEMA, AND JOHN E. LYNCH
Medical Research Laboratores, Pfizer Inc., Groton, Connecticut 06340

Received for publication 3 March 1976

In the new agent 3-(5-tetrazolyl)penam, hereafter referred to as CP-35,587, the carboxyl function at C3 in the penicillin nucleus has been replaced with the 5-tetrazolyl moiety. Marked changes in spectrum and resistance to gram-negative β-lactamases, particularly with regard to *Klebsiella pneumoniae* isolates, were conferred by this modification. The anti-*Klebsiella* activity clearly distinguishes the antibacterial spectrum of CP-35,587 from any known broad-spectrum penicillin. Compared to orally active cephalosporins, the spectrum advantage of CP-35,587 encompasses *Enterobacter, Serratia marcescens, Citrobacter, Providencia, Haemophilus influenzae*, and *Streptococcus faecalis*, both in vitro and in murine infections produced by many of the above-named microorganisms. Thus, CP-35,587 combines and extends the antibacterial activity of broad-spectrum penicillins and orally active cephalosporins.

At one time it was believed that the antibacterial activity of penicillin required the presence of a carboxyl group at C3. However, it was later found that the carboxamido group at the C3 locus possesses interesting antibacterial activity per se (4), and α-methoxy-*n*-propyl penicillinamide was effective against experimental infections in mice produced by penicillin G-resistant and penicillin-susceptible staphylococci (5).

This paper describes the microbiological properties of 3-(5-tetrazolyl)penam, hereafter referred to as CP-35,587, in which the C3 carboxyl of penicillin has been replaced with a 5-tetrazolyl group (W. C. Barth, West German patent 2449863, 1975) and which exhibited broad-spectrum activity with particularly good activity against *Klebsiella* species.

MATERIALS AND METHODS

Microorganisms. The microorganisms used to assess the spectrum and initial activity of CP-35,587 were primarily pathogenic strains well adapted to growth under laboratory conditions. To supplement these microorganisms, fresh clinical isolates were obtained from hospitals in several geographical areas in the eastern United States.

Antibiotics. CP-35,587, a white, water-soluble crystalline solid, was used either as the sodium salt or in the zwitterion form (Fig. 1). Ampicillin trihydrate, amoxicillin, cephaloridine, and cephalexin used in various phases of these studies were commercial products of, respectively, Bristol Laboratories, Beecham-Massengill, and Eli Lilly & Co. Appropriate antibiotic dilutions were made in sterile bacteriological medium.

Experimental animals. Male and female mice used in these experiments were purchased from Blue Spruce Farms in Altamont, N.Y. The average weight of the mice used in the chemotherapeutic studies was 13 g; the average weight of those used in pharmacokinetic studies was 25 g. Dogs used in pharmacokinetic studies were purebred beagles.

MICs. Minimum inhibitory concentrations (MIC) of the antibiotics were determined by a standard dilution method in brain heart infusion agar in which the multiple inoculator described by Steers et al. was used (3, 10). The standard inoculum contained approximately 20,000 organisms. Incubation was for 18 h at 37 C. Single colonies were disregarded in MIC determinations. The procedure for MIC determinations in broth, which utilized an inoculum of about 10^6 cells/ml, has been described previously (2).

Bactericidal studies. Bactericidal properties of CP-35,587 and the other antibiotics were evaluated in killing-curve experiments. These were initiated by diluting cultures, which had been grown overnight on a rotary shaker, 100-fold in brain heart infusion broth containing the appropriate concentration of antibiotic. During incubation at 37 C on a rotary shaker, samples were removed at various times and diluted at 2-log intervals, and 0.1 ml was plated out in triplicate on brain heart infusion agar plates. After overnight incubation, colonies were counted and recorded as viable colony-forming units.

β-Lactamase studies. The hydrolysis of CP-35,587, penicillins, and cephalosporins was determined, respectively, by the microiodometric method of Novick and by decreases in ultraviolet absorbance

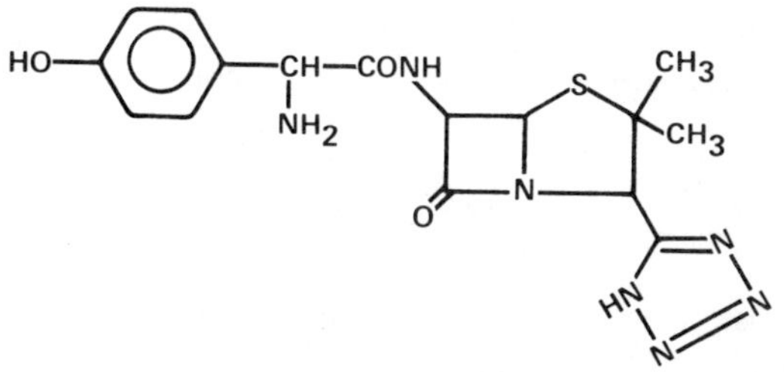

FIG. 1. *Structure of CP-35,587, 3-(5-tetrazolyl)-penam.*

(7, 8). Conditions were identical for both assays, i.e., 0.5 M potassium phosphate, pH 6.5, at 37 C. The penicilloic acid of CP-35,587 was prepared by incubation with a purified *Bacillus cereus* penicillinase. The resulting product was found to obey the Novick equation (7) for determination of penicillin hydrolysis. Cell-free extracts containing β-lactamases were prepared by sonication of harvested and washed cultures, which had been grown in brain heart infusion broth on a rotary shaker incubator. When indicated, the de novo synthesis of β-lactamases was induced by growing a log-phase culture in the presence of a sublethal concentration of ampicillin for 1.5 h before harvesting. Induced cell-free extracts were dialyzed overnight at 4 C against a 1,000-fold greater volume of buffer (0.005 M sodium cacodylate, pH 6.5, and 0.001 M 2-mercaptoethanol). Protein was determined by the biuret method (6).

Experimental infections in mice. Acute systemic infections in mice were produced by intraperitoneal inoculation of standardized bacterial cultures suspended in 5% hog gastric mucin. The challenge dose was generally 1 to 10 lethal doses, i.e., 1 to 10 times the number of organisms needed to kill 100% of the mice within a 4-day period. The dosage regimen for all experimental infections was initiated 0.5 h postchallenge, with subsequent dosing at 4 and 24 h. After 4 days, a 50% protective dose value, expressed in milligrams per kilogram, was calculated by a probit method (1). The 50% protective dose is defined as the dose of antibiotic, in milligrams per kilogram, that will protect 50% of the treated mice from the otherwise lethal infection.

Pharmacokinetic studies in mice and dogs. CP-35,587 and the other antibiotics were administered in a water–carboxymethyl-cellulose–Tween diluent. Mouse whole blood samples were collected via the intra-orbital sinus bleeding technique (9). Serum from dogs was removed from clotted blood samples obtained via jugular vein puncture. Biological assays were performed using a conventional large-plate disk assay, with *Micrococcus lutea* (ATCC 9341) as the assay organism. Standard curves for the assay of mouse whole blood and dog sera were prepared in the respective fluid from normal animals.

Serum-binding studies. The binding of CP-35,587 and other antibiotics to human and dog serum proteins was determined in an ultrafiltration procedure. The various antibiotics were added to serum samples to approximate 50 μg/ml. After zero-time portions were removed, the samples were incubated at 37 C for 1 h and then ultrafiltrated with conical ultrafiltration cones (Centriflo, CF 50A, Amicon Corp., Lexington, Mass.; cutoff level molecular weight, 50,000) for 30 min at 4 C. Initial antibiotic concentration in serum (zero-time sample) and the residual concentration in ultrafiltrate were determined by bioassay procedures using standard curves prepared in, respectively, serum or ultrafiltrate.

RESULTS

MIC values of CP-35,587 against large numbers of clinically isolated microorganisms of diverse genera are summarized in Table 1. Amoxicillin and cephalexin are included for comparison. CP-35,587 was active against nearly all of the microorganisms studied, the most striking feature being the degree of activity against *Klebsiella pneumoniae* isolates. MIC values for CP-35,587 compared favorably (50 and 75% end points) with those of cephalexin and clearly distinguish the novel spectrum and degree of activity of CP-35,587 from that of any known penicillin. The further extension of the CP-35,587 spectrum over that of amoxicillin is indicated by activity against *Enterobacter, Proteus morgani,* and *Serratia* species. The spectrum advantage of CP-35,587 over cephalexin included the three genera mentioned above for amoxicillin and, in addition, *Streptococcus faecalis, Citrobacter, Providencia,* and *Haemophilus influenzae*.

Based on MIC values, which included those for 50 and 75% of the gram-negative isolates studied, CP-35,587 generally was more active than amoxicillin and cephalexin. CP-35,587 was more active against gram-positive organisms than was cephalexin but was not as active against gram-positive bacteria as ampicillin. MIC values of all antibiotics against 90% of the gram-negative isolates were routinely higher than those at the 50 and 75% end points. This increase in MICs probably resulted from a few multiply resistant isolates carrying R-factor present in each genus.

A 100-fold increase in inoculum size (from 200 to 20,000 cells) in a series of gram-negative microorganisms was without significant effect on agar dilution MIC values of CP-35,587. A further increase of 10 times (200,000 cells) generally produced a rise in MIC from the original, which represented a single twofold dilution in concentration. In general, similar data were obtained with ampicillin and cephalexin.

The bactericidal activity of CP-35,587 with high inocula ($>3 \times 10^7$ cells/ml) is clearly evident in the killing-curve experiments described by Fig. 2. CP-35,587 was bactericidal against *K. pneumoniae, Escherichia coli,* and *Serratia marcescens*. At equal concentrations amoxicil-

TABLE 1. *Activity of CP-35,587 against fresh clinical cultures*

Organism	No. of isolates tested	MIC value (μg/ml) to inhibit 50, 75, or 90% of strains tested								
		CP-35,587			Amoxicillin			Cephalexin		
		50%	75%	90%	50%	75%	90%	50%	75%	90%
Klebsiella pneumoniae	57	6.25	12.5	100	200	200	>200	6.25	6.25	6.25
Escherichia coli	32	6.25	12.5	>200	6.25	100	>200	6.25	12.5	12.5
Enterobacter	31	25	50	>200	200	>200		100	>200	
Serratia marcescens	23	25	25	100	100	>200	>200	>200		
Citrobacter	16	12.5	25	>200	100	>200	>200	25	25	100
Providencia	10	50	200	200	100	>200		50	>200	
Salmonella typhimurium	16	6.25	12.5	12.5	1.56	3.12	200[a]	3.12	12.5	25
Proteus mirabilis[b]	15	12.5	12.5	12.5	0.78	1.56	3.12	25	25	100
Proteus vulgaris[b]	16	100	>200	>200	>200			>200		
Pseudomonas aeruginosa	29	200	>200		>200			>200		
Hemophilus influenzae[b]	10	1.56	3.12	3.12	0.39	3.12	3.12[a]	6.25	12.5	25[c]
Staphylococcus aureus	31	12.5	25	50	12.5	50	50[a, d]	6.25	12.5	25
Staphylococcus epidermidis	9	1.56	3.12	3.12	0.1	0.39	1.56[a]	1.56	1.56	3.12
Streptococcus faecalis	29	1.56	1.56	1.56	0.78	1.56	1.56[a]	100	100	200
Streptococcus pyogenes[b]	4[e]			0.05			0.0078[a]			0.39
Streptococcus pneumoniae[b]	3[e]			0.05			0.00039[a]			0.78

[a] Ampicillin tested instead of amoxicillin.
[b] Mean value of three determinations. Medium for swarming *Proteus* strain was brain heart infusion (BHI) broth, instead of BHI agar. Medium for *H. influenzae* was BHI broth and agar enriched with 5% (vol/vol) Fildes and 2% (vol/vol) IsoVitaleX. Medium for *S. pyogenes* and *S. pneumoniae* was BHI agar plus 5% blood. *H. influenzae*, *S. pyogenes*, and *S. pneumoniae* cultures grown overnight were diluted 10-fold for use as inoculum. Incubations were for 18 h at 37 C except for *H. influenzae,* which was incubated for 40 h at 37 C.
[c] Cefazolin tested instead of cephalexin.
[d] Note that approximately 80% of the strains were resistant to ampicillin.
[e] In the case of eight or less strains, the MIC value given is the amount required to inhibit 90% of the strains.

lin was bactericidal against only *E. coli* and cephalexin was bactericidal against only *K. pneumoniae*. The lack of bactericidal activity of cephalexin (5 μg/ml) against *E. coli* was confirmed with a second strain.

The resistance of CP-35,587 to hydrolysis by crude β-lactamase preparations from diverse gram-negative bacteria and *S. aureus* is presented in Table 2. Ampicillin and cephalexin data are included for comparison. CP-35,587 was highly refractory to the β-lactamase preparations from most strains of *K. pneumoniae* tested, one of two strains of *E. coli,* and representative strains of *S. marcescens* and *Enterobacter* sp. Hydrolysis of CP-35,587 did occur with single strains of *K. pneumoniae* (53A077) and *E. coli* (51A129). Both of these cultures are multiply antibiotic-resistant clinical isolates and probably contain β-lactamases mediated by transferable R-factors. Both cultures had MIC values of 200 μg/ml (Table 2). The *E. coli* strain, 51A002, which does not hydrolyze CP-35,587, is not a multiply antibiotic-resistant isolate. It is apparent, therefore, that the β-lactamase present in this monoresistant (ampicillin) isolate and the typical *K. pneumonia* strains is quite different than the β-lactamase(s) present in the multiply resistant strains 51A129 and 53A077. Although some hydrolysis of CP-35,587 occurred with *Proteus, Pseudomonas,* and *S. aureus,* the hydrolysis rates were significantly less than that of one or both of the other antibiotics.

CP-35,587 proved to be a very effective therapeutic agent against experimental infections produced by a variety of gram-negative pathogens and *S. aureus* in mice. These data, accompanied by comparative values for amoxicillin and cephalexin, are presented in Table 3. In agreement with in vitro data, CP-35,587 showed good activity against experimental infections produced by five *K. pneumoniae* isolates. Neither amoxicillin nor ampicillin protected against these infections. Its efficacy against ampicillin-resistant *Klebsiella* clearly distinguishes CP-35,587 from any known penicillin.

The activity of CP-35,587 was also noteworthy against infections produced by *Proteus, S. marcescens,* and *Enterobacter* sp. Dependent upon the infections under study, either amoxicillin or cephalexin, or both, were inactive. Therefore, the spectrum of CP-35,587 is an extension of the combined spectra of amoxicillin plus cephalexin. Oral and subcutaneous activities were quite similar, although the parenteral

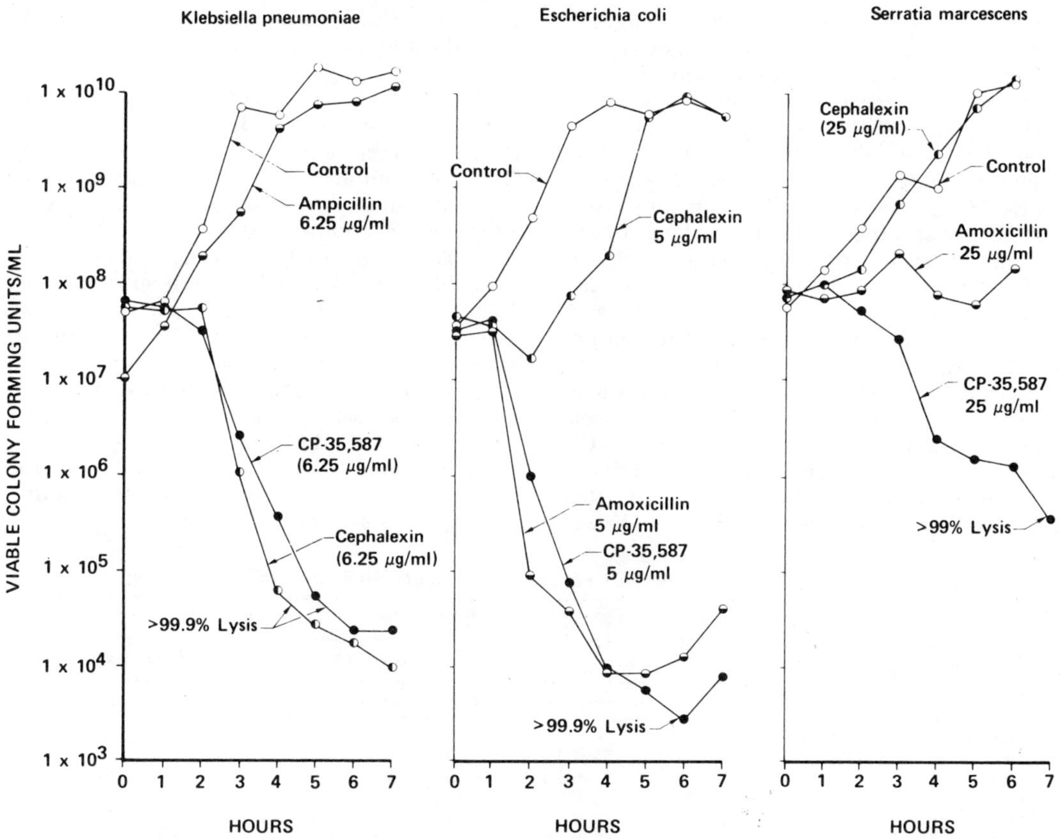

FIG. 2. *Bactericidal activity of CP 35,587 compared with ampicillin or amoxicillin and cephalexin.*

TABLE 2. *Comparative β-lactamase resistance of CP-35,587 and other semisynthetic β-lactam antibiotics*[a]

Source of β-lactamase (cell-free extracts)	Hydrolysis rate (µmol/h/mg of protein)		
	Ampicillin	CP-35,587	Cephalexin
Klebsiella pneumoniae			
53A015[b]	326	<1	<1
53A009[b]	156	<1	<1
53A079[b]	578	2	NT[c]
53A077[b, d]	6,147	7,118	<1
Escherichia coli, ampicillin resistant			
51A002[b]	712	<1	NT
51A129[b, d]	25,200	27,250	<1
Serratia marcescens 63A017[e]	<1	<1	222
Enterobacter aerogenes 67A026[e]	<1	<1	340
Enterobacter cloacae 67B003[e]	<1	<1	14
Proteus morgani 57G001[e]	7.0	8.0	290
Proteus vulgaris 57A060[e]	709	159	990[f]
Pseudomonas aeruginosa 52A104[e]	119	148	610
Staphylococcus aureus ampicillin-resistant 01A400[e]	1,160	290	<1

[a] Assays were carried out as described in Materials and Methods. All strains have MIC values of ≥50 µg of ampicillin per ml. Substrate concentration was 62 µM or 25 µg of CP-35,587 per ml.

[b] These cultures contained constitutive β-lactamases.

[c] NT, Not tested.

[d] Organisms resistant to CP-35,587 (MIC >200 µg/ml).

[e] To obtain appreciable β-lactamase activity, these cultures had to be induced.

[f] Substrate was cephaloridine, not cephalexin.

50% protective dose was generally somewhat lower. The activity of CP-35,587 against the various experimental infections studied (Table 3) is generally greater or equivalent to that shown by amoxicillin or cephalexin. Cephalexin, however, did have greater activity against the infections produced by *Klebsiella*.

CP-35,587, like amoxicillin and ampicillin, was rapidly absorbed after oral and subcutaneous administration to mice (Table 4). Peak concentrations were detected in the first time sample studied, i.e., 15 min. Oral administration of CP-35,587 and ampicillin led to approximately equivalent blood concentrations, and blood concentrations of the three antibiotics appeared to be very similar after subcutaneous administration. The elimination rate of CP-35,587 was more rapid than those of amoxicillin and ampicillin after intravenous administration. However, blood levels of CP-35,587, as well as those of the other antibiotics, were still detectable 120 min post-drug administration (Table 4).

CP-35,587 and amoxicillin gave similar serum concentrations and urinary recoveries after oral administration of 20 mg/kg to dogs (Table 5). Similarly, CP-35,587 compared favorably with ampicillin in these parameters after intravenous administration of 10 mg/kg to dogs. Table 6 presents serum and urine excretion values for CP-35,587 after subcutaneous dosage of 5 and 20 mg/kg to dogs. Peak serum concentrations were detected 1 h postdosing. Percentage of urinary recovery after subcutaneous dosing was quite similar to that after intravenous dosing, which suggests excellent absorption by the former route.

Serum-binding values for CP-35,587 in dog and human sera were higher than those of ampicillin but were quite similar to those of car-

TABLE 3. *CP-35,587 activity against experimental infections in mice*[a]

Experimental infection	PD_{50} (mg/kg) and 95% confidence limits					
	CP-35,587		Amoxicillin		Cephalexin	
	Oral	s.c.	Oral	s.c.	Oral	s.c.
Klebsiella pneumoniae						
53A009	89 ± 30	65 ± 34	>200[b]	>200[b]	28 ± 14	30 ± 15
53A028	88 ± 16	71 ± 8.5	>200	>200	12 ± 1.5	8.6 ± 4.8
53A099	79 ± 20	70 ± 29	>200	>200	17 ± 4	21 ± 5
53A082	70 ± 23	35 ± 9.6	>200	>200	11 ± 2.8	7.7 ± 2.3
53A079	89 ± 39	61 ± 18	>200	>200	11 ± 2.3	7.7 ± 2.3
Proteus vulgaris						
57A060	110 ± 38	91 ± 34	>200	>200	>200	>200
57A061	74 ± 26	90 ± 27	220	165	140	140
Serratia marcescens						
63A017	84 ± 26	68 ± 33	96 ± 29	110 ± 47	>200	>200
63A026	150 ± 50	125 ± 31	117 ± 27	91 ± 24	>200	>200
Enterobacter aerogenes 67A040	93 ± 40	80 ± 32	>200	>200	74 ± 2.6	120 ± 38.4
Enterobacter cloacae 67B046	67 ± 35	50 ± 29	32 ± 6	25 ± 6	73 ± 34	72 ± 23
Escherichia coli 51A266	28.8 ± 6.5	23.8 ± 4.8	16.1 ± 2.9	5.7 ± 1.9	6.4 ± 1.1	5.2 ± 0.9
Staphylococcus aureus 01A005	7.0 ± 1.8	9.0 ± 2.0	4.5 ± 1.1	4.3 ± 1.5		

[a] PD_{50}, 50% protective dose; s.c., subcutaneous.

[b] Ampicillin was also inactive in dosages up to 200 mg/kg against these five isolates. In most instances, no mice were alive at the dosage indicated.

TABLE 4. *Cp-35,587: oral, subcutaneous, and intravenous administration to mice*[a]

Sample time (min)	Mean whole blood concn (μg/ml) and SEM[b]								
	Oral			Subcutaneous			Intravenous		
	CP-35,587	Amoxicillin	Ampicillin	CP-35,587	Amoxicillin	Ampicillin	CP-35,587	Amoxicillin	Ampicillin
0	0	0	0	0	0	0	0	0	0
1							23.0 ± 1.75	24.7 ± 2.75	21.5 ± 2.19
15	1.77 ± 0.15	2.99 ± 0.25	1.34 ± 0.18	5.49 ± 0.33	5.40 ± 0.30	8.41 ± 0.50	3.75 ± 1.38	12.5 ± 0.80	7.18 ± 0.51
30	1.56 ± 0.21	2.98 ± 0.31	1.52 ± 0.20	3.54 ± 0.34	3.98 ± 0.43	5.48 ± 0.50	1.37 ± 0.46	7.50 ± 0.10	4.36 ± 0.37
60	0.84 ± 0.18	1.70 ± 0.17	0.71 ± 0.14	1.59 ± 0.29	1.59 ± 0.21	1.80 ± 0.41	0.52 ± 0.03	3.60 ± 0.15	1.81 ± 0.24
90	0.34 ± 0.11	0.70 ± 0.14	0.17 ± 0.10	0.52 ± 0.18	0.58 ± 0.08	0.53 ± 0.20	0.24 ± 0.03	2.0 ± 0.05	1.01 ± 0.19
120	0.13 ± 0.06	0.31 ± 0.09	0.19 ± 0.09	0.32 ± 0.13	0.23 ± 0.04	0.20 ± 0.10	0.12 ± 0.05	1.2 ± 0.15	0.64 ± 0.13

[a] Antibiotic dosage was 20 mg/kg.

[b] Mean value of 15 to 20 mice; SEM, standard error of the mean.

TABLE 5. *CP-35,587: antibiotic concentrations in serum and urinary excretion in dogs*[a]

Sample time (h)	Oral (20 mg/kg)				Intravenous (10 mg/kg)			
	Serum (μg/ml)		Urine (mg)		Serum (μg/ml)		Urine (mg)	
	CP-35,587	Amoxicillin	CP-35,587	Amoxicillin	CP-35,587	Ampicillin	CP-35,587	Ampicillin
0	0	0	0	0	0	0	0	0
0.5	11.50 ± 1.87	11.00 ± 1.52	7.60	2.25	8.61 ± 0.99	11.3 ± 1.0	25.6	27.6
1	8.80 ± 2.59	8.08 ± 0.66	12.90	12.45	7.54 ± 0.25	6.48 ± 0.79	10.9	12.1
2	4.80 ± 2.09	5.52 ± 0.88	10.90	13.35	1.72 ± 0.14	1.18 ± 0.19	4.6	14.1
3	2.40 ± 1.03	3.14 ± 0.44	5.90	3.30	0.88 ± 0.23	0.40 ± 0.00	2.9	0.8
4	1.84 ± 0.98	1.80 ± 0.34	3.05	3.20	0.68 ± 0.04	0.16 ± 0.03	1.9	0.6
6	0.68 ± 0.38	0.56 ± 0.10	4.75	3.45	0.11 ± 0.03	0.06 ± 0.05	1.3	0.5
6–24			3.95	0.75			1.0	0.2
% Urinary recovery			19.60	16.8			42.3	49.0

[a] Mean values with standard error of the mean for 1 to 2 dogs.

TABLE 6. *CP-35,587: antibiotic concentrations in serum and urinary excretion after subcutaneous administration to dogs*[a]

Sample time (h)	Serum concn (avg values, μg/ml)		Urine excretion (avg values, mg)	
	5 mg/kg	20 mg/kg	5 mg/kg	20 mg/kg
0	0	0	0	0
0.5	6.55 ± 0.76	19.25 ± 3.68	1.9	1.5
1	6.74 ± 0.50	21.20 ± 2.93	3.9	9.6
2	4.06 ± 0.29	12.80 ± 0.80	8.0	14.5
3	2.40 ± 0.20	9.59 ± 0.58	5.0	17.2
4	1.69 ± 0.23	7.54 ± 0.86	3.2	16.6
6	0.84 ± 0.18	2.44 ± 0.38	2.4	13.2
6–24			1.6	9.2
% Urinary recovery			44.6 ± 6.67	42.1 ± 3.70

[a] Mean values with standard error of the mean for 2 to 4 dogs.

benicillin (Table 7). CP-35,587, as well as the other two antibiotics, was bound to a higher extent in human serum than in dog serum.

DISCUSSION

The spectrum of CP-35,587 is more extensive than that of any known broad-spectrum penicillin for it encompasses the majority of clinically isolated *K. pneumoniae*. In contrast to orally active cephalosporins, the spectrum of CP-35,587 includes *Enterobacter, Serratia, H. influenzae,* and *S. faecalis*. This spectrum conferred excellent oral and parenteral activity against experimental infections in mice produced by many of the above-named microorganisms.

Factors other than the presence of a β-lactamase may account for resistance to a β-lactam antibiotic; however, in many instances there is a strong correlation between resistance to β-lactam antibiotics and the ability of an organism to elaborate a β-lactamase. CP-35,587 is very refractory to β-lactamases produced by a variety of gram-negative microorganisms, and this probably serves as the explanation for its expanded spectrum (Table 2). In addition, mice experimentally infected with four of these same strains were successfully protected with CP-35,587 (Table 3).

TABLE 7. *CP-35,587 serum-binding studies*

Antibiotic	% Binding[a]	
	Dog	Human
CP-35,587	27.9 ± 0.81	54.2 ± 1.21
Carbenicillin	23.0 ± 1.01	43.0 ± 0.76
Ampicillin	18.0 ± 0.99	22.4 ± 1.21

[a] Mean value with standard error of the mean.

CP-35,587 is well absorbed after oral or parenteral administration to mice and beagles. Dependent upon the route of administration, CP-35,587, in general, compared favorably with ampicillin or amoxicillin.

The serum-binding value of CP-35,587 for human serum compared favorably with that of other clinically useful β-lactam antibiotics.

LITERATURE CITED

1. **Batson, H. E.** 1957. An introduction to statistics in the medical sciences, p. 64–67. Burgess Publishing Co., Minneapolis.
2. **English, A. R., J. A. Retsema, V. A. Ray, and J. E.**

Lynch. 1972. Carbenicillin indanyl sodium, an orally active derivative of carbenicillin. Antimicrob. Agents Chemother. 1:185–191.

3. **Ericsson, H. M., and J. C. Sherris.** 1971. Antibiotic sensitivity testing—report of international collaborative study. Acta. Pathol. Microbiol. Scand. Sect. B 217(Suppl.):64–68.
4. **Hoogmartens, J., P. J. Claes, and H. Vanderhaeghe.** 1974. Total synthesis of Bisnorpenicillin V. J. Med. Chem. 17:389–392.
5. **Huang, H. T., T. A. Seto, J. M. Weaver, A. R. English, T. J. McBride, and G. M. Shull.** 1964. Antibiotic properties of α-substituted penicillin amides against penicillin-resistant staphylococci, p. 493–499. Antimicrob. Agents Chemother. 1963.
6. **Layne, E.** 1957. Spectrophotometric and turbidimetric methods for measuring proteins, p. 447–454. *In* S. P. Colowick and N. O. Kaplan (ed.), Methods in enzymology, vol. 3. Academic Press Inc., New York.
7. **Novick, R. P.** 1962. Micro-iodometric assay for penicillinase. Biochem. J. 83:236–240.
8. **O'Callaghan, C. H., P. W. Muggleton, and C. W. Ross.** 1969. Effects of β-lactamase from gram-negative organisms on cephalosporins and penicillins, p. 57–63. Antimicrob. Agents Chemother. 1968.
9. **Salem, H., M. H. Grossman, and D. L. J. Bilbey.** 1963. Micro-method for intravenous injection and blood sampling. J. Pharm. Sci. 52:794–795.
10. **Steers, E., E. L. Foltz, and B. S. Graves.** 1959. An inocula replicating apparatus for routine testing of antibiotic susceptibility to antibiotics. Antibiot. Chemother. 9:307–311.

ANTIMICROBIAL AGENTS AND CHEMOTHERAPY, July 1976, p. 139-145
Vol. 10, No. 1

In Vitro Comparison of Netilmicin, a Semisynthetic Derivative of Sisomicin, and Four Other Aminoglycoside Antibiotics

S. A. KABINS,* C. NATHAN, AND S. COHEN

Departments of Microbiology and Medicine, Michael Reese Hospital and Medical Center, and the Pritzker School of Medicine, University of Chicago, Chicago, Illinois 60616*

Received for publication 13 February 1976

One hundred isolates of *Pseudomonas* and *Enterobacteriaceae*, of which 85 were chosen because of their resistance to gentamicin or amikacin, were tested for susceptibility to netilmicin (SCH 20569), a new semisynthetic derivative of sisomicin, and to four other aminoglycosides. Tests were performed in Mueller-Hinton agar and, with 43 of these isolates, also in Mueller-Hinton broth. Most isolates of *Escherichia coli*, *Klebsiella*, *Enterobacter*, *Citrobacter*, and *Serratia* that were gentamicin resistant proved to be susceptible to netilmicin and amikacin. Tests of representative isolates of this group showed that they owed their resistance to the production of aminoglycoside-adenylylating enzymes. Four isolates of *Serratia*, detected by their resistance to amikacin, were also highly resistant to netilmicin but were susceptible to gentamicin. These isolates produced aminoglycoside-acetylating enzymes. Gentamicin-resistant *Proteus* and *Providencia* were, in general, highly resistant to netilmicin but were susceptible to amikacin. These isolates also produced aminoglycoside-acetylating enzymes. Most gentamicin-resistant strains of *Pseudomonas* were resistant to netilmicin, either by enzymatic aminoglycoside modification or by other undefined mechanisms. Thus, like amikacin, netilmicin extends the aminoglycoside susceptibility pattern of *Enterobacteriaceae* to include gentamicin-resistant isolates that produce aminoglycoside-adenylylating enzymes. It is ineffective against strains, some of them susceptible to amikacin, gentamicin, or tobramycin, that produce aminoglycoside-acetylating enzymes.

The purpose of this study was to compare the susceptibility of clinical isolates of *Pseudomonas* and *Enterobacteriaceae* to netilmicin (SCH 20569), a new semisynthetic derivative of sisomicin developed by the Schering Corp. Netilmicin is *O*-2,6-diamino-2,3,4,6-tetradeoxy-α-D-glycerohex-4-enopyranosyl-(1 → 4)-*O*-[3-deoxy-4-*C*-methyl-3-(methylamino)-β-L-arabinopyranosyl-(1 → 6)]-2-deoxy-1-*N*-ethyl-D-streptamine. It is being prepared for clinical testing in humans (J. A. Waitz, personal communication, Schering Corp., Bloomfield, N.J.). For comparison, we also determined the susceptibility of our bacteria to gentamicin, tobramycin, sisomicin, and amikacin.

MATERIALS AND METHODS

Organisms. Ninety-three of the one hundred strains selected for study were isolated in our diagnostic microbiology laboratory between January 1971 and September 1974. Eighty-five were resistant either to gentamicin or amikacin by repeated standard Kirby-Bauer disk tests. The 100 strains included 36 isolates of *Pseudomonas aeruginosa*, 10 other *Pseudomonas* species (5 *P. maltophilia*, 2 *P. cepacia*, 1 *P. acidovorans*, 1 *P. putida*, and 1 unidentified species), 18 *Escherichia coli*, 9 *Klebsiella pneumoniae*, 9 *Enterobacter* (7 *E. cloacae*, 2 *E. liquefaciens*), 8 *Serratia marcescens*, 4 *Providencia* (not speciated), 2 *Proteus mirabilis*, 1 *P. vulgaris*, 1 *P. rettgeri*, and 2 *Citrobacter freundii*. Included among these strains were *P. aeruginosa* GN315 and A20897, and *Pseudomonas* species strain A20621, obtained from K. E. Price, Bristol Laboratories. These strains produced the aminoglycoside acetyltransferase AAC(6')-4 (for nomenclature see section on enzymatic assays) (4, 11). Also included were *E. coli* K-12 carrying the R factor R5, which produces a similar enzyme, and *E. coli* K-12 carrying the R factor JR66, which produces aminoglycoside adenylyltransferase AAD(2"). Both strains were obtained from J. Davies, University of Wisconsin (2, 3). Our isolates, *P. aeruginosa* strain POW and *C. freundii* strain WIL (previously erroneously identified as *E. coli*), were earlier shown to produce gentamicin adenylyltransferases determined by R factors (5, 8, 9). Two *P. aeruginosa*, strains Pre and Kru, were clinical isolates obtained from S. Lerner, University of Chicago.

Antibiotics. The aminoglycosides used in this study were laboratory standard preparations. Gentamicin (a mixture of approximately equal parts gentamicin C_1, C_{1a}, and C_2), sisomicin, and netilmicin were supplied by J. A. Waitz of the Schering Corp.; tobramycin was supplied by R. S. Griffith, Eli Lilly & Co.; amikacin (BB-K8), a semisynthetic kanamycin derivative, was obtained from G. E. Wright, Bristol Laboratories.

Quantitative determination of aminoglycoside susceptibility. The standard assay for microbial inhibition was performed with each of the five aminoglycosides by an agar dilution technique. For this purpose serial twofold dilutions of the aminoglycosides in duplicate Mueller-Hinton agar (BBL) plates were inoculated with 10^{-2} and 10^{-5} dilutions of an overnight growth at 37 C in Mueller-Hinton broth (Difco) (approximately 10^4 and 10^1 organisms) by means of a Steers-Foltz apparatus. The minimal inhibitory concentration (MIC) was defined as the lowest concentration of antibiotic that prevented any visible growth of the organisms after overnight incubation at 37 C. The MIC values would have been unchanged in 97% of the tests performed if the MIC end point had been defined as a 90% reduction in number of colonies formed. Tests performed with inocula of 10^4 and 10^1 organisms showed the same MIC of netilmicin, or one differing by only one dilution, with 85 of the 100 strains examined.

Twenty-five isolates of *P. aeruginosa*, one *P. putida*, and seventeen isolates of *Enterobacteriaceae* representative of the different susceptibility patterns shown in the agar dilution tests were assayed with gentamicin and netilmicin for MIC and for minimal bactericidal concentration (MBC) by a broth dilution procedure. For this purpose, serial twofold dilutions of aminoglycosides in duplicate tubes containing 1 ml of Mueller-Hinton broth were inoculated with 0.1 ml of a 10^{-3} dilution of an overnight growth (approximately 10^5 organisms). The MIC was defined as the lowest concentration of antibiotic in those tubes showing no turbidity after 18 h of incubation at 37 C. MIC was also determined after 42 h. After 18 h of incubation, the contents of nonturbid tubes were subcultured with a 0.01-ml loop to antibiotic-free Mueller-Hinton agar. The MBC was defined as the lowest concentration of antibiotic that permitted the growth of 10 or fewer colonies.

Single lots of Mueller-Hinton broth and agar were used for these studies. Samples of each were analyzed for total Mg^{2+} and Ca^{2+} concentrations with an atomic absorption spectrophotometer by S. Natelson, Department of Biochemistry, Michael Reese Hospital. The agar contained (per liter) 63 mg of Ca^{2+} and 18 mg of Mg^{2+}, whereas the broth contained 7 and 3 mg/liter, respectively.

To compare the effects of the different antibiotics in tests of each type (i.e., agar MIC, broth MIC or MBC), the results of each test were recorded separately as susceptible if the organisms were inhibited in an MIC test or killed in an MBC test by 5 μg or less of gentamicin, tobramycin, sisomicin, or netilmicin per ml and by 10 μg or less of amikacin per ml. Strains that required 20 μg or more of the former antibiotics per ml or 40 μg of amikacin per ml for inhibition or killing were considered resistant. Organisms requiring 10 μg of one of the former agents per ml or 20 μg of amikacin per ml for inhibition or killing were considered intermediate. These values were selected on the basis of the therapeutic drug concentrations attained in serum by treatment with gentamicin, tobramycin, sisomicin, and amikacin. The resistant, susceptible, and intermediate values selected for netilmicin were the same as those for gentamicin and sisomicin, in view of the close chemical relation between these agents.

Enzymatic assays. From prior unpublished studies on 32 of the gentamicin- or amikacin-resistant strains used in this study, information was available on results of adenylylation and acetylation assays by sonic extracts of the bacteria against aminoglycosides selected from the following: gentamicin C_1, C_{1a}, and C_2, gentamicin A, sisomicin, tobramycin, amikacin, kanamycin A, kanamycin B, neomycin B, and paromomycin. The assays were performed according to published methods (1, 2, 6, 9). Bacteria whose extracts gave at least five times the counts per minute of a similarly processed extract of a comparable antibiotic-susceptible strain were considered to acetylate or adenylylate the substrate significantly.

The enzymatic nomenclature was taken from the Commission on Chemoresistance, International Society of Chemotherapy (S. Mitsuhashi, personal communication, Gunma Univ., Maebashi City, Japan). The enzymes carried by our isolates had substrate specificities similar to or the same as the following: AAD(2″), aminoglycoside 2″-nucleotidyltransferase (gentamicin adenylyltransferase); AAC(6′)-4, aminoglycoside 6′-acetyltransferase-4 (6′*N*-gentamicin acetyltransferase or kanamycin acetyltransferase); AAC(3), aminoglycoside 3-acetyltransferase (3*N*-gentamicin acetyltransferase I); AAC(2′)-2, aminoglycoside 2′-acetyltransferase-2 (2′*N*-gentamicin acetyltransferase II).

RESULTS

***Enterobacteriaceae*: MICs and MBCs.** Aminoglycoside susceptibility patterns were similar among the 36 isolates of *E. coli*, *K. pneumoniae*, and *Enterobacter* studied by the agar dilution method (Fig. 1). In general, the majority of the gentamicin-resistant isolates were susceptible to netilmicin and amikacin. They were resistant to tobramycin and were resistant or intermediate to sisomicin. Only 8% of the isolates were resistant to netilmicin, and 14% were resistant to amikacin. Fig. 2 shows that 24 of the 36 isolates of *Enterobacteriaceae* were resistant to gentamicin but susceptible to netilmicin, whereas only one isolate was resistant to netilmicin but susceptible to gentamicin. Five isolates that were either intermediate or resistant to gentamicin had similar MICs with netilmicin. The susceptibility of two gentamicin-resistant *C. freundii* isolates, not shown in Fig. 1, resembled the pattern predominant in this group of bacteria: these isolates were susceptible to netilmicin and amikacin.

Two patterns of susceptibility to aminoglyco-

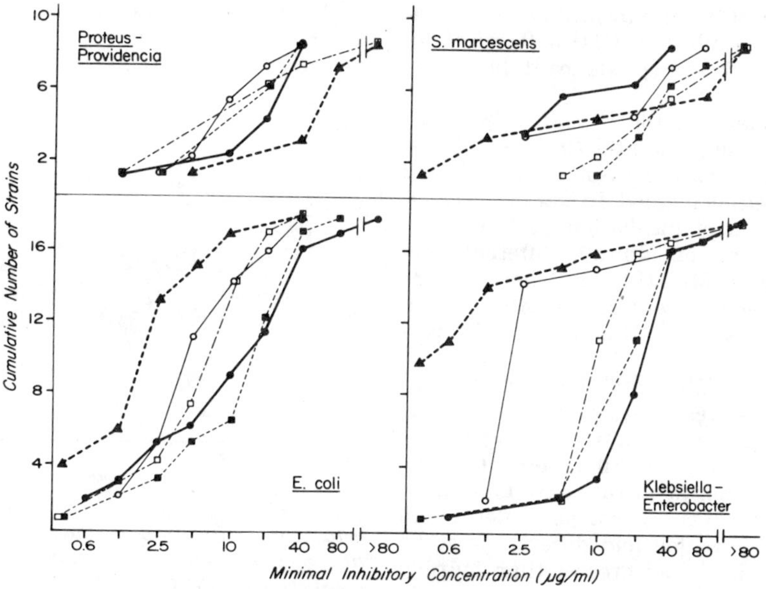

FIG. 1. *MICs of aminoglycosides tested with Enterobacteriaceae by the agar dilution method using as an inoculum a 10^{-2} dilution of an overnight growth. Antibiotics tested were gentamicin (●), amikacin (○), sisomicin (□), tobramycin (■), and netilmicin (▲).*

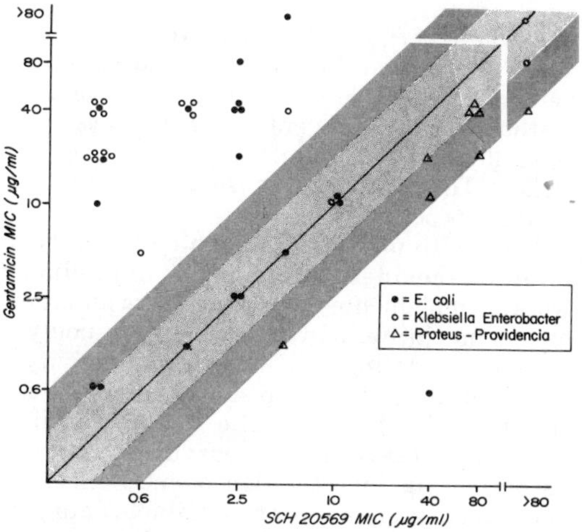

FIG. 2. *Comparative MICs of gentamicin and netilmicin for E. Coli, Klebsiella-Enterobacter, and Proteus-Providencia organisms. Note that the scale is logarithmic. The boundary between the two shaded lines indicates results that differ by twofold. The boundary between the shaded and the unshaded zones indicates results that differ by fourfold.*

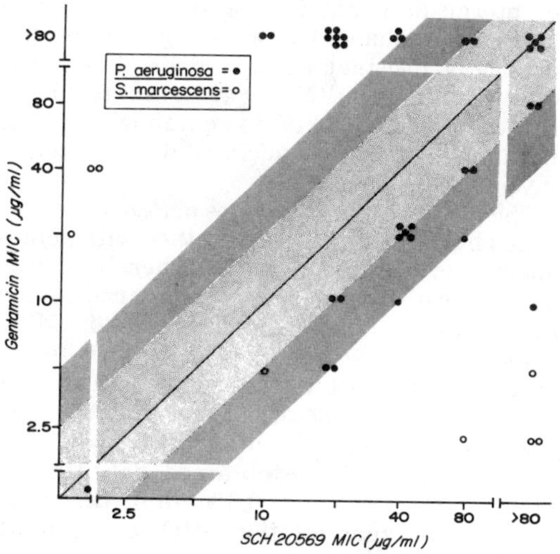

FIG. 3. *Comparative MICs of gentamicin and netilmicin for isolates of P. aeruginosa and S. marcescens tested by the agar dilution method. Note the logarithmic scales. For significance of shaded zones, see Fig. 2.*

sides were found by agar dilution tests among isolates of *Serratia marcescens* (Fig. 3). Three isolates that were resistant to gentamicin were susceptible to netilmicin. Four isolates that were susceptible to gentamicin were resistant to netilmicin. One isolate was nearly equally susceptible to both agents. Seven of the eight isolates were resistant or intermediate to tobramycin and sisomicin (Fig. 1). The gentamicin-resistant isolates were susceptible to amikacin, whereas the four gentamicin-susceptible isolates that were resistant to netilmicin were also resistant to amikacin.

Most of the *Proteus* and *Providencia* isolates scored by the agar dilution method were resistant to gentamicin, netilmicin, tobramycin, and sisomicin (MIC <10 μg/ml), but for the most part were susceptible or intermediate to amikacin (MIC ≤20 μg/ml) (Fig. 1). One *P. mirabilis* isolate was equally susceptible to all the agents tested.

Thirteen isolates of the *E. coli, Klebisella, Enterobacter* group, two of the *Proteus* isolates, and two of the *Providencia* isolates were tested by the tube dilution method. In 88% of the tests, MICs after 18 h of incubation at 37 C were identical to or only one dilution different from the agar dilution MIC (Fig. 4). There was 88 and 86% agreement (within one dilution) between 18-h and 42-h MICs and MBCs, respectively.

***P. aeruginosa*: MICs and MBCs.** Nearly all of the gentamicin-resistant isolates were resistant or intermediate to netilmicin in agar dilution MIC tests (Fig. 3). Fifty percent of the isolates gave either identical or twofold different MICs with gentamicin and netilmicin whereas 22% gave fourfold different results. Nine (25%) isolates had greater than fourfold higher MICs with gentamicin, whereas only one (3%) had a greater than fourfold higher MIC with netilmicin. Amikacin was the most effective agent tested: only 55% were resistant or intermediate (Fig. 5). The superiority of amikacin was enhanced if we compared the frequency of resistant isolates alone. Eight percent were resistant (MIC ≥40 μg/ml) to amikacin, compared with 81% to gentamicin, 92% to netilmicin, 72% to sisomicin, and 50% to tobramycin (MIC ≥20 μg/ml).

The MICs for the 25 isolates of *P. aeruginosa* tested by the broth dilution method with gentamicin and netilmicin were generally lower than those obtained by the agar dilution method and enhanced the differences in MICs between those two agents (Fig. 4). Forty-eight percent of the isolates tested were scored as resistant to gentamicin, whereas only 8% were scored as resistant to netilmicin (Fig. 5). For isolates in which we obtained definite end points (i.e., ≤80 and ≥0.6 μg/ml), the mean ratio of the agar dilution MIC to the broth dilution MIC was 6.

Judged by the MBC test, most of these 25 isolates of *P. aeruginosa* would be classified as resistant both to gentamicin and netilmicin (Table 1). The MBCs were four- to eightfold higher than the tube dilution MICs. They were, however, comparable to the MIC values obtained by agar dilution. Table 1 also shows that MIC values obtained by the tube dilution test were similar after 18 or 42 h of incubation.

***Pseudomonas* species: MICs and MBCs.** With 9 of the 10 isolates selected for study, the agar dilution MICs of all five aminoglycosides were equal to or greater than 80 μg/ml. With

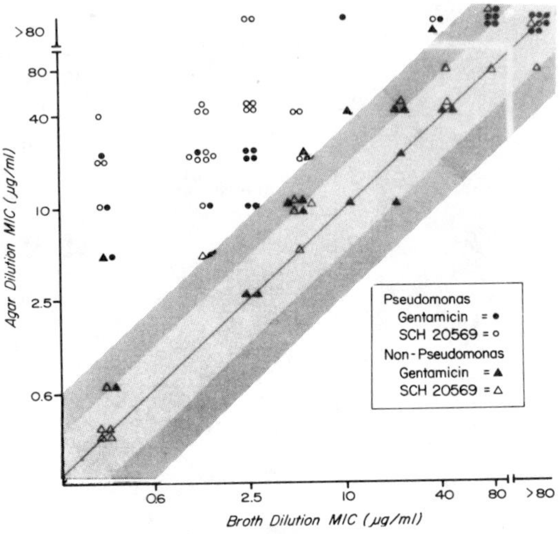

FIG. 4. *Comparative MICs of gentamicin and netilmicin, determined by the agar and tube dilution methods with Pseudomonas aeruginosa and non-Pseudomonas organisms. Note the logarithmic scales. For significance of shaded zones see Fig. 2. Non-Pseudomonas isolates include: E. coli, Klebsiella, Enterobacter, Proteus, and Providencia tested with gentamicin (▲) and with netilmicin (△).*

one isolate of *P. putida*, MICs were 10, 20, and 40 μg of amikacin, tobramycin, and netilmicin per ml, respectively. By the broth dilution method, the MICs of gentamicin and netilmicin were 40 and <0.6 μg/ml, respectively, for this isolate. The MBC for this isolate was 10 μg of netilmicin per ml.

Tests with organisms capable of modifying aminoglycosides. From prior unpublished work, supplemented by some determinations on netilmicin, we had data on the aminoglycoside-adenylylating and -acetylating activity of 32 strains from the group submitted for susceptibility determinations. The strains had been selected for assay of these enzymatic activities as part of an investigation of mechanisms of gentamicin resistance. The available data gave evidence of a correlation between the enzymatic activities of the isolates examined and the results of the susceptibility tests.

The 10 *Enterobacteriaceae* isolates that were resistant or intermediate to gentamicin and produced the enzyme AAD(2″) were susceptible to netilmicin and amikacin (Table 2). The four gentamicin-resistant isolates of *P. aeruginosa* that also produce this enzyme had netilmicin MICs that were only 10 to 20 μg/ml (resistant or intermediate) (Table 2) and, in addition, by the broth dilution tests had MICs of <0.6 to 1.2 μg/ml (susceptible). All but one of the 14 adenylylating isolates were resistant or intermediate to tobramycin and sisomicin. The adenylylating isolates included 7 of the 24 *Enterobacteriaceae* that were resistant to gentamicin and susceptible to netilmicin in Fig. 2 and 4 of the 9 *Pseudomonas* isolates in Fig. 3 that had greater than fourfold higher MICs with gentamicin than with netilmicin. The remaining 17 *Enterobacteriaceae* and 5 *Pseudomonas* isolates in these two groups were not assayed, but we think it likely that they also produced AAD(2″). Other adenylylating isolates include *C. freundii* strain WIL and two of the three *Serratia* shown in Fig. 3 that were resistant to gentamicin and susceptible to netilmicin.

Fifteen of the 32 assayed isolates produced enzymes with substrate specificities resembling those of three classes of aminoglycoside acetyltransferases (4), namely AAC(6′)-4, AAC(3), and AAC(2′) (6, 14) (Table 2). All of these 15 isolates, which included *P. aeruginosa, S. marcescens, Proteus, Providencia,* and *E. coli* K-12, were highly resistant to netilmicin, having MICs of 40 or more μg/ml (Table 2). Eight isolates that produce acetylating enzymes representative of each of the three classes of aminoglycoside acetyltransferases acetylated netilmicin. With two exceptions, the 15 acetylating isolates were also resistant to sisomicin and tobramycin.

In contrast to the nearly uniform resistance of the acetylating strains to the aminoglycosides cited above, three *Providencia* strains and one *Proteus* strain were susceptible to amikacin, and one *Proteus* and two *Pseudomonas* isolates were intermediate. The remaining acetylating isolates were resistant to amikacin, and most of them produced enzymes either known to be AAC(6′)-4 or closely resembling it. AAC(6′)-4 is the only enzyme known to acetylate amikacin. Five isolates that produced this enzyme were susceptible to gentamicin. They included four isolates of *Serratia* that were resistant to netilmicin (Fig. 3) and one strain of *E. coli* K-12 carrying R5 (Fig. 2). In addition, *P. aeruginosa* GN315, which had a higher MIC to

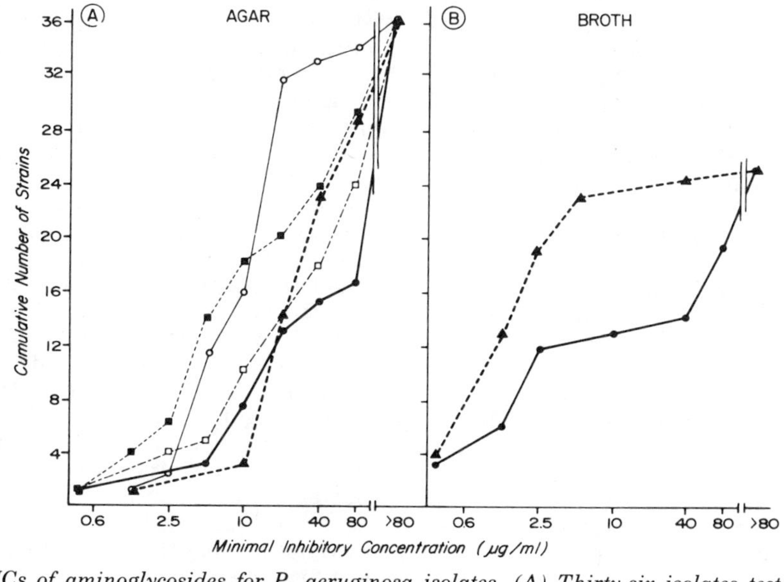

FIG. 5. *MICs of aminoglycosides for P. aeruginosa isolates. (A) Thirty-six isolates tested by the agar dilution method; (B) 25 isolates tested by the broth dilution method. For antibiotics tested see Fig. 1.*

TABLE 1. *MICs and MBCs of netilmicin and gentamicin against Pseudomonas aeruginosa*[a]

Antibiotic	Determination	Cumulative no. of isolates with MIC or MBC (μg/ml) of:									
		<0.6	0.6	1.2	2.5	5	10	20	40	80	>80
Gentamicin	MIC (18 h)	3	3	6	12	12	13	13	14	19	25
	MIC (42 h)	2	2	4	8	12	12	13	13	14	25
	MBC	0	0	0	0	4	9	12	12	12	25
Netilmicin	MIC (18 h)	4	4	13	19	23	23	23	24	24	25
	MIC (42 h)	0	0	3	10	19	21	23	23	24	25
	MBC	0	0	0	0	0	8	17	21	22	25

[a] MIC and MBC were determined by the broth dilution method (see Materials and Methods).

TABLE 2. *Relation of aminoglycoside-modifying enzymes to MIC*

Enzyme[a]	Organism	No. of isolates	MIC by agar dilution (μg/ml)				
			Gentamicin	Netilmicin	Sisomicin	Tobramycin	Amikacin
AAD(2″)	Coliforms[b]	8	10–40	<0.6–2.5	5–20	10–40	1.2–10
	P. aeruginosa	4	>80	10–20	40–>80	10–80	5
	S. marcescens	2	20–40	<0.6–1.2	10–20	10–20	2.5–5
AAC(6′)-4	*E. coli* K-12-R5	1	0.6	40[c]	5	40	40
	P. aeruginosa strain GN315	1	10	>80[c]	80	80	40
	P. aeruginosa[d]	2	>80	>80	>80	>80	20–>80
	S. marcescens	4	2.5–5	>80[e]	40–>80	40–80	40–80
AAC(3)	*P. aeruginosa* strain Pre	1	>80	>80[c]	80	5	20
AAC(2′)-2	*Proteus*[b]	3	10–40	40–>80[c]	20–>80	20–40	10–40
	Providencia	3	20–40	40–80[c]	20	20	2.5–10

[a] Enzymatic nomenclature is given in Materials and Methods.
[b] Coliforms include: *E. coli*, *Klebsiella*, *Enterobacter*, and *Citrobacter* species. *Proteus* include: *P. mirabilis*, *P. vulgaris*, and *P. rettgeri*. All were clinical isolates except for one strain, *E. coli* K-12 (JR66).
[c] Extracts from these isolates acetylated netilmicin.
[d] *P. aeruginosa* A20897 and *Pseudomonas* species strain A20521.
[e] Extracts from one of these isolates acetylated netilmicin; the other isolates were not tested.

netilmicin than to gentamicin, carried this enzyme (Fig. 3). AAC(6′)-4 does not acetylate gentamicin C_1, a component of the gentamicin complex. The unimpaired activity of gentamicin C_1, together with possible residual antibiotic activity of the acetylated components, may account for the effectiveness of gentamicin against these organisms (4).

Three isolates resistant to netilmicin (one *P. aeruginosa* strain Kru, one *E. coli*, and one *K. pneumoniae*) had previously been found not to acetylate or adenylylate gentamicin. In contrast to the organisms that were resistant by virtue of their enzymatic modification of aminoglycosides, these isolates were uniformly resistant to all five of the aminoglycosides tested, with MICs of nearly identical magnitude. Resistance in these isolates may be caused by restricted access of these agents to their site of action, as has been demonstrated for streptomycin resistance in some strains of *P. aeruginosa* (13).

DISCUSSION

Our data suggest that many gentamicin-resistant *E. coli*, *Klebsiella*, *Enterobacter*, *Citrobacter*, and *Serratia* were susceptible to netilmicin and to amikacin. Gentamicin-resistant *Proteus* and *Providencia* were, in general, resistant to netilmicin but were susceptible to amikacin. Amikacin-resistant *Serratia* were also resistant to netilmicin but were susceptible to gentamicin.

P. aeruginosa and the other *Pseudomonas* isolates occupy a special position, because their MICs varied with experimental conditions. A systematic difference between broth and agar dilution MIC has been observed with *P. aeruginosa* and other aminoglycosides, attributed to the higher concentration of the divalent cations Mg^{2+} and Ca^{2+} in Mueller-Hinton agar than in Mueller-Hinton broth (7, 12). Since the concentration of these cations in agar more closely approximates that of serum, it has been suggested that the data obtained in agar may be of more clinical significance (7, 12).

The foregoing results of susceptibility determinations are in general accord with those of others (J. A. Waitz and G. H. Miller, Prog. Abstr. Intersci. Conf. Antimicrob. Agents Chemother., 15th, Washington, D.C., Abstr. 92, 1975; and J. J. Rahal, Jr., M. S. Simberkoff, and K. Kagan, Prog. Abstr. Intersci. Conf. Antimicrob. Agents Chemother., 15th, Washington, D.C., Abstr. 93, 1975).

In general, strains harboring a gentamicin-adenylylating enzyme were resistant to gentamicin but susceptible to netilmicin. In our experience, these enzymes have been found most frequently in *E. coli*, *Klebsiella*, *Enterobacter*, and *Citrobacter*. Thus, it seems likely that netilmicin may prove to be a therapeutically useful agent against many isolates of these genera. The *P. aeruginosa* isolates that harbored adenylylating enzymes conceivably might respond to therapy with netilmicin, especially if found in the urine, since in 80% of the isolates, MICs did not exceed 20 μg/ml, even by agar dilution.

Preliminary experiments in our laboratory indicate that netilmicin is not refractory to attack by AAD-(2″), when tested at saturating concentrations of substrate. A possible remaining mechanism for the susceptibility of adenylylating bacteria to this antibiotic is a low affinity of netilmicin for AAD-2(2″) at concentrations comparable to the MIC for susceptible bacteria. Confirming preliminary observations of J. A. Waitz (personal communication), we have found that at least one adenylylating enzyme, AAD-(2″) from *E. coli* K-12 carrying JR66, adenylylated netilmicin at concentrations of 1 to 5 μg/ml to an appreciably lesser extent than gentamicin C_1 or the gentamicin complex. An additional mechanism, as yet untested, is that the adenylylated netilmicin retains antibiotic activity.

A number of varieties of aminoglycoside acetyltransferases with somewhat different substrate specificities are known to exist in bacteria (4). From our observations and those of others, it seems likely that our collection included at least three different varieties of acetyltransferase. The bacteria that harbored any of these enzymes were, in general, highly resistant to netilmicin. In contrast to the results with the adenylyltransferase enzyme, our preliminary experiments indicate that netilmicin at concentrations of 1 to 5 μg/ml is acetylated, as well as gentamicin C_1 or C_{1a}, by each of the three varieties of acetyltransferases encountered in our collection. Judging by the isolates we have examined, resistance to netilmicin owing to acetyltransferase activity is relatively infrequent in *Escherichia, Klebsiella,* and *Enterobacter,* but is common in *Proteus, Providencia,* and *Pseudomonas.*

Thus, it appears that netilmicin, like amikacin, may prove effective against *Enterobacteriaceae* and possibly some *Pseudomonas* strains that are resistant to gentamicin owing to aminoglycoside-adenylylating enzymes. The therapeutic ineffectiveness of netilmicin against bacteria possessing aminoglycoside-acetylating enzymes may be mitigated by the susceptibility of some of these bacteria to amikacin and, in a few instances, to gentamicin and tobramycin.

ACKNOWLEDGMENTS

This study was supported by a grant from the Schering Corp., Bloomfield, N.J., and by the Medical Research Institute Council, Michael Reese Hospital and Medical Center.

LITERATURE CITED

1. **Benveniste, R., T. Yamada, and J. Davies.** 1970. Enzymatic adenylylation of streptomycin and spectinomycin by R factor-resistant *Escherichia coli*. Infect. Immun. 1:109–119.
2. **Benveniste, R., and J. Davies.** 1971. R-factor-mediated gentamicin-resistance: a new enzyme which modifies aminoglycoside antibiotics. FEBS Lett. 14:293–296.
3. **Benveniste, R., and J. Davies.** 1971. Enzymatic acetylation of aminoglycoside antibiotics by *Escherichia coli* carrying an R-factor. Biochemistry 10:1787–1796.
4. **Benveniste, R., and J. Davies.** 1973. Mechanisms of antibiotic resistance in bacteria. Annu. Rev. Biochem. 42:471–506.
5. **Bryan, L. E., M. S. Shahrabadi, and H. M. Van Den Elzen.** 1974. Gentamicin-resistance in *Pseudomonas aeruginosa*: R-factor-mediated resistance. Antimicrob. Agents Chemother. 6:191–199.
6. **Brzezinska, M., R. Benveniste, J. Davies, P. J. L. Daniels, and J. Weinstein.** 1972. Gentamicin-resistance in strains of *Pseudomonas aeruginosa* mediated by enzymatic N-acetylation of the deoxystreptamine moiety. Biochemistry 11:761–765.
7. **Gilbert, D. N., E. Kutscher, P. Ireland, J. A. Barnett, and J. P. Sanford.** 1971. Effect of the concentrations of magnesium and calcium on the *in vitro* susceptibility of *Pseudomonas aeruginosa* to gentamicin. J. Infect. Dis. 124(Suppl.):S37–S45.
8. **Kabins, S. A., C. R. Nathan, and S. Cohen.** 1971. R-factor-mediated resistance to gentamicin in a clinical isolate of *Escherichia coli*. J. Infect. Dis. 124(Suppl.):565–567.
9. **Kabins, S., C. Nathan, and S. Cohen.** 1974. Gentamicin-adenylyltransferase activity as a cause of gentamicin-resistance in clinical isolates of *Pseudomonas aeruginosa*. Antimicrob. Agents Chemother. 5:565–570.
10. **Kawabe, H., T. Naito, and S. Mitsuhashi.** 1975. Acetylation of amikacin, a new semisynthetic antibiotic by *Pseudomonas aeruginosa* carrying R-factor. Antimicrob. Agents Chemother. 7:50–54.
11. **Kawabe, H., S. Kondo, H. Umezawa, and S. Mitsuhashi.** 1975. R-factor-mediated aminoglycoside antibiotic resistance in *Pseudomonas aeruginosa*: a new aminoglycoside 6′-*N*-acetyltransferase. Antimicrob. Agents Chemother. 7:494–499.
12. **Reller, L. B., F. D. Schoenknecht, M. A. Kenny, and J. C. Sherris.** 1974. Antibiotic susceptibility testing of *Pseudomonas aeruginosa*: selection of a control strain and criteria for magnesium and calcium content in media. J. Infect. Dis. 130:454–463.
13. **Tseng, Jui Teng, L. E. Bryan, and H. M. Van Den Elzen.** 1972. Mechanisms and spectrum of streptomycin-resistance in a natural population of *Pseudomonas aeruginosa*. Antimicrob. Agents Chemother. 2:136–141.
14. **Yamaguchi, M., S. Mitsuhashi, F. Kobayashi, and H. Zenda.** 1974. A 2′-N-acetylating enzyme of aminoglycosides. J. Antibiot. 27:507–515.

Antimicrobial Agents and Chemotherapy, July 1976, p. 146–149 Vol. 10, No. 1

Printed in U.S.A.

In Vitro Antimicrobial Activity of Cinoxacin Against 2,968 Clinical Bacterial Isolates

R. N. JONES* and P. C. FUCHS

Department of Pathology, Kaiser Foundation Hospital Laboratories, Portland, Oregon 97217, and Department of Pathology, St. Vincent Hospital and Medical Center, Portland, Oregon 97225*

Received for publication 9 February 1976

Cinoxacin demonstrated effective in vitro antimicrobial activity against the *Enterobacteriaceae*, but negligible activity against *Pseudomonas aeruginosa* and gram-positive cocci. The activity of cinoxacin was slightly greater than that of nalidixic acid.

A number of synthetic organic acids containing cinnoline ring structures have been investigated for antimicrobial activity (3, 8). Of these compounds, cinoxacin (1-ethyl-1,4-dihydro-4,oxo-[1,3]dioxolo[4,5-g]cinnogine-3-carboxylic acid) was chosen for clinical and expanded in vitro investigation. Cinoxacin (Lilly compound 64715) possesses many characteristics similar to nalidixic acid and oxolinic acid. Preliminary in vitro bacterial susceptibility studies indicate a similar gram-negative antibacterial activity to that of nalidixic acid (2, 5, 7).

This study presents in vitro broth dilution susceptibility data for cinoxacin against 2,968 clinical bacterial isolates plus a direct comparison of cinoxacin and nalidixic acid minimal inhibitory concentration (MIC) and minimal bactericidal concentration (MBC) results against the most prevalent urinary tract isolates.

MATERIALS AND METHODS

Bacterial cultures. Organisms used in the study were obtained from the Clinical Microbiology Division of the Kaiser Foundation Hospital Laboratories, Oregon Region. A total of 2,968 bacterial isolates including 1,621 urinary tract isolates conforming to the quantitative criteria of Kass (4) were tested. Each isolate was identified by the replicator plate method described by Fuchs (1), utilizing 17 to 24 biochemical tests.

Susceptibility testing. MICs of all antimicrobial agents were determined by the broth microdilution technique. Mueller-Hinton broth (Difco) was used in previously prepared well plastic trays (8 by 10; Micro-Media Systems, Inc., Campbell, Calif.). The antimicrobial agents were injected into the wells in 100-μl volumes. Organisms were grown to stationary phase (10^9 organisms/ml) in brain heart infusion broth and then diluted 1:100 in sterile water. An automatic tray inoculator delivered 5 μl of this dilution to each 100-μl well; final inoculum concentration was 5×10^5 organisms/ml.

In the inoculum size studies, organisms were inoculated as above, using similar equipment and three inoculum concentrations, 10^7, 10^5, and 10^3 organisms/ml.

MIC end points were defined as the lowest broth concentration totally inhibiting organism growth (clear well) after 15 to 18 h of incubation at 35 C. Determination of the MBC was performed by subculturing 1 μl of both turbid and clear wells into Mueller-Hinton broth. The MBC was defined as the lowest subcultured broth concentration revealing no growth (clear well) after overnight incubation at 35 C. This represents a three-log minimum-kill (99.9%) end point.

RESULTS AND DISCUSSION

The cumulative percentage of gram-negative bacilli inhibited by increasing cinoxacin concentrations is shown in Table 1. Among the 2,139 strains tested, *Escherichia coli*, *Citrobacter diversus*, *Proteus morganii*, and *Proteus vulgaris* exhibited the greatest susceptibility. Ten of the thirteen tabulated *Enterobacteriaceae* species showed greater than 90% inhibition of strains at 16 μg/ml. Only *Proteus mirabilis*, *Proteus rettgeri*, and *Providencia* species demonstrated a relative resistance to cinoxacin. All *P. morganii* and *P. vulgaris* strains were inhibited by 4 μg/ml in contrast to 67 and 0% for *Proteus rettgeri* and *Providencia* species, respectively. Only 12 of 210 pseudomonas isolates had MIC values of 64 μg/ml or less. However, 43 of the 57 non-*Enterobacteriaceae*, non-pseudomonas gram-negative isolates had MIC values of 64 μg/ml or less.

The data in Table 2 confirm the poor cinoxacin antimicrobial activity against gram-positive organisms. Of note, however, was the 26 to 28% inhibitory response of staphylococcus isolates. Only 2 of 191 streptococcus strains had MIC values of 64 μg/ml or less.

The comparison of cinoxacin and nalidixic acid MICs and MBCs is shown in Table 3. The six organism species tested represent six of the

TABLE 1. *Susceptibility (MICs) of clinical isolates of gram-negative bacilli to cinoxacin*

Organism	No. of isolates	Cumulative % susceptible at MIC of:						
		1.0	2	4	8	16	32	64
Escherichia coli	1,383	25	78	96	99	99	99	99
Citrobacter freundii	28		25	61	97	100		
C. diversus	11	27	73	91	100			
Klebsiella pneumoniae	166	1	25	81	99	100		
Enterobacter cloacae	50	6	24	72	88	96		98
E. aerogenes	17		6	65	88	94	100	
E. agglomerans	15	27	47	73	100			
Serratia marcescens	11	18		73	100			
Proteus mirabilis	123	1	9	30	76	87	89	90
P. morganii	13	77	100					
P. rettgeri	12	17	34	67	73	75	92	100
P. vulgaris	5	20	80	100				
Providencia species	6					50	83	100
Pseudomonas aeruginosa	197		1	1	2			3
Pseudomonas species[a]	13	8					16	44
Acinetobacter anitratus (Herellea)	25				4	8	20	64
Acinetobacter lwoffi	9				11	33	55	100
Moraxella species	9	22		44			88	
Others[b]	46	30	74	87			89	91

[a] Includes *Pseudomonas maltophilia* (6), *P. stutzeri* (3), *P. cepacia* (2), and *Pseudomonas* species (2).
[b] Includes *Pasteurella multocida* (4), *Aeromonas hydrophilia* (3), enteropathogenic *E. coli* (3), *Shigella* species (22), *Salmonella enteritidis* (7), and one strain each of EF4, Ve type 2, Vd, 11K type 1, *Achromobacter xylosoxidans*, *Flavobacterium* species, and gram-negative bacillus NOS.

TABLE 2. *Susceptibility (MICs) of clinical isolates of gram-positive cocci to cinoxacin*

Organism	No. of isolates	Cumulative % susceptible at MIC of:						
		1	2	4	8	16	32	64
Staphylococcus aureus	415					1	3	26
S. epidermidis	223					1	3	28
Streptococcus faecalis	172							1
Streptococcus[a] group D (not *S. faecalis*)	7							
Streptococcus, beta-hemolytic[b]	4							
Streptococcus, viridans group	8							13

[a] Includes *S. faecium* (5), *S. durans* (1), and *S. bovis* (1).
[b] Includes *S. agalacteae* (1) and beta streptococcus not group A, B, or D (3).

eight more frequently encountered urinary tract pathogens (*Staphylococcus epidermidis* and *Enterobacter* species not included). In direct comparison, cinoxacin was slightly more active than nalidixic acid against the group.

The effect of the inoculum size on the cinoxacin MIC results is shown in Table 4. Slight increases in the mean MIC values were demonstrated for all tested species with increasing inoculum concentrations. However, four- to eightfold increase in MBCs was found for both cinoxacin and nalidixic acid with an inoculum size of 10^7 organisms/ml (not shown). At the highest concentration tested (64 μg/ml), 87% of the 1,621 urinary tract isolates were inhibited by cinoxacin. This concentration was considerably below the 250- to 500-μg/ml concentration of drug easily reached in the urine on usual dosages (6). With a higher testing range, the percentage of organisms inhibited may approach those of nitrofurantoin (94% inhibited at 128 μg/ml) and trimethoprim/sulfamethoxazole (98% inhibited at 4/76 μg/ml). If the gram-positive urinary microbes were eliminated, the cinoxacin efficacy of 96% at 64 μg/ml was comparable to that of the other two antimicrobial agents tested in parallel.

Cinoxacin appears to have definite advantages over nalidixic acid, including higher serum and urine concentrations, expanded *Enterobacteriaceae* antimicrobial activity, and a greater homogeneity of susceptible bacterial populations (8). More studies are needed to clarify the significance of antagonizing factors

TABLE 3. *Comparison of MICs and MBCs of cinoxacin and nalidixic acid for six prevalent urinary tract pathogens*

Organism	No. of isolates	Antibiotic[a]	MIC or MBC	Cumulative % susceptible at concn (μg/ml) of: 1	2	4	8	16	32	64
Escherichia coli	25	CX	MIC	8	72	92	100			
			MBC	4	44	88	100			
		NA	MIC	16	76	88	100			
			MBC	12	68	88	100			
Klebsiella pneumoniae	25	CX	MIC			76	96	100		
			MBC			68	92	100		
		NA	MIC			42	88	100		
			MBC			32	84	100		
Proteus mirabilis	25	CX	MIC		12	84	92		96	100
			MBC		4	84	92			100
		NA	MIC			56	100			
			MBC			48	96	100		
Indole-positive *Proteus* species[b]	10	CX	MIC	20	90	100				
			MBC		80	100				
		NA	MIC	10	60	70	90	100		
			MBC	10	40	70	90	100		
Pseudomonas aeruginosa	10	CX	MIC							20
			MBC							10
		NA	MIC						30	
			MBC							20
Streptococcus faecalis	25	CX	MIC							
			MBC							
		NA	MIC							
			MBC							

[a] CX, Cinoxacin, NA, nalidixic acid.
[b] Includes *P. morganii* (4), *P. rettgeri* (4), and *P. vulgaris* (2).

TABLE 4. *Effect of inoculum size on cinoxacin in MICs for prevalent urinary tract pathogens*

Organism (no.)	Inoculum size	No. of isolates with MIC at: ≤1	2	4	8	16	32	64	>64
Escherichia coli (10)	10^3	1	6	3					
	10^5	1	5	2	2				
	10^7		6	2	2				
Klebsiella pneumoniae (10)	10^3			9		1			
	10^5			8	1	1			
	10^7			7	2	1			
Proteus mirabilis (10)	10^3		6	2			2		
	10^5		2	5	1		1	1	
	10^7		1	5	2		1	1	
Indole-positive *Proteus* species[a] (10)	10^3	5	5						
	10^5	2	7	1					
	10^7	2	6	2					
Pseudomonas aeruginosa (10)	10^3							2	8
	10^5							2	8
	10^7								10
Streptococcus faecalis (10)	10^3							1	9
	10^5								10
	10^7								10

[a] Indole-positive strains: *P. morganii* (4), *P. rettgeri* (4), and *P. vulgaris* (2).

(8), effects of high cinoxacin concentration on heretofore resistant strains, and in vivo utility in urinary and non-urinary infection.

ACKNOWLEDGMENTS

We thank Eli Lilly & Co. for the financial grant to investigate cinoxacin.

Additional appreciation is given to Rollie Packer, MT(ASCP), for technical help.

LITERATURE CITED

1. **Fuchs, P. C.** 1975. The replicator method for identification and biotyping of common bacterial isolates. Lab. Med. 6:6–11.

2. **Giamarellou, H., and G. G. Jackson.** 1975. Antibacterial activity of cinoxacin in vitro. Antimicrob. Agents Chemother. 7:688–692.
3. **Holmes, D. H., P. W. Ensminger, and R. S. Gordee.** 1974. Cinoxacin: effectiveness against experimental pyelonephritis in rats. Antimicrob. Agents Chemother. 6:432–436.
4. **Kass, E. H.** 1960. The role of asymptomatic bacteria in the pathogenesis of pyelonephritis, p. 390–411. *In* E. L. Quinn and E. H. Kass (ed.), Biology of pyelonephritis. Little Brown and Co., Boston.
5. **Kurtz, S., and M. Turck.** 1975. In vitro activity of cinoxacin, an organic acid antibacterial. Antimicrob. Agents Chemother. 7:370–373.
6. **Lilly Research Laboratories.** 1974. Clinical pharmacology of cinoxacin. Lilly Research Laboratory, Indianapolis, Ind.
7. **Lumish, R. M., and C. W. Norden.** 1975. Cinoxacin: in vitro antibacterial studies of a new synthetic organic acid. Antimicrob. Agents Chemother. 7:159–163.
8. **Wick, W. E., D. A. Preston, W. A. White, and R. S. Gordee.** 1973. Compound 64716, a new synthetic antibacterial agent. Antimicrob. Agents Chemother. 4:415–420.

Antimicrobial Agents and Chemotherapy, July 1976, p. 150–156 Vol. 10, No. 1
 Printed in U.S.A.

Phleomycin-Induced Solubilization of Deoxyribonucleic Acid in Uninfected and T Bacteriophage-Infected *Escherichia coli* B

KAREN SHIVE AND C. F. EARHART*

Department of Microbiology, The University of Texas at Austin, Austin, Texas 78712

Received for publication 3 February 1976

Phleomycin (PM) induces rapid solubilization of deoxyribonucleic acid (DNA), inhibition of cellular mass increase, and loss of viability when added either to growing cultures of *Escherichia coli* B or an endonuclease I-defective derivative of B. Nonetheless, bacteriophage of the T-even series are produced, albeit to a reduced extent, when PM is added with phage or after infection to *E. coli* cells. Bacteriophage T4 infection inhibits the ability of PM to bring about the solubilization of DNA; this effect appears to account for most of the resistance of T-even phage replication to PM. The patterns of inhibition of phage yields obtained when PM is added at infection suggest that glucosylation of T-even phage DNA may also have a protective effect. However, PM induces the solubilization of glucosylated and nonglucosylated DNA at approximately the same rate and thermal denaturation studies indicate that the antibiotic binds both types of DNA equally well. The latter experiments also provided evidence that PM dissociates from DNA at temperatures greater than 80 C.

Phleomycin (PM) is an inhibitor of deoxyribonucleic acid (DNA) synthesis that consists of a mixture of at least 11 related glycopeptidic antibiotics (13). Degradation of DNA is observed when PM is added to cultures of prokaryotic cells, such as *Escherichia coli* (8, 21) and *Bacillus subtilis* (26); after exposure of eukaryotic cells to the drug, inhibition of DNA synthesis (32) and chromosome breakage (18) have been noted. The effect of PM on bacteriophage replication has been studied in only two systems. Addition of PM soon after infection with PBS2, a *B. subtilis* phage whose DNA contains uracil instead of thymine, or ϕX174 inhibits phage DNA synthesis and no progeny phage are produced (24, 25). (One report in which PM was shown to inhibit the multiplication of the ribonucleic acid phage R23 and phage T2 [34] was performed with a PM lot [no. 616] which has since been shown to contain a nitrile contaminant in sufficient concentration to inhibit cellular respiration [22].)

There is substantial evidence that PM binds to DNA (13, 22), but the subsequent mechanism by which PM brings about breaks in DNA strands has not been determined precisely. Two hypotheses, presented here in their most general forms, have been put forth: (i) PM is capable of acting alone to produce strand breaks (21, 30) and (ii) PM-stimulated nuclease activity causes the damage (8, 10, 22, 26). In both *B. subtilis* (26) and *E. coli* (8, 21) the ability of PM to act is energy dependent. Studies on the mechanism of PM-induced damage are complicated by the possibility that even within the same species the type of damage generated may not be identical. Thus, excisionless mutants of *E. coli* B (10), but not *E. coli* K-12 (21), are unsusceptible to low concentrations (≤ 2 μg/ml) of PM and *rec* mutants of K-12 are more susceptible to low PM concentrations than is the parental strain (21).

Our interest in PM was stimulated by the report of Farrell and Reiter (8) in which it was suggested that the activity involved in PM-induced DNA degradation is similar to, if not the same as, that activated by colicin E2. Of particular interest was the observation that T4 infection blocks both E2-induced and PM-stimulated solubilization of bacterial DNA. These studies were thus begun to study the effect of PM on T4 replication and, as endonuclease I has been implicated in colicin E2 action (1), to determine if endonuclease I has a role in PM action. We show here (i) that T-even phage are able to replicate in the presence of PM and (ii) that endonuclease I-deficient *E. coli* B cells are as susceptible to PM inhibition as are *end*$^+$ cells.

MATERIALS AND METHODS

Phage and bacterial strains. Bacteriophage T4D_0, T4*am*N82 (gene 44, defective in DNA synthesis), T4*am*N94 (gene 46, defective in the ability to degrade host DNA), and T7 were from the collection of this laboratory. T2 was obtained from E. B. Goldberg and T6 was provided by T. Matney.

E. coli strains B, B40suI, CR63, and ER22, a derivative of *E. coli* B that lacks endonuclease I *(end)* (6), were from the culture collection of this laboratory. L. Snyder sent us the strains W4597, which is defective in uridinediphosphate glucose pyrophosphorylase (9), and K803 Met$^-$, *rgl*$^-$ (35).

Media and other solutions, enzymes, and reagents. Tryptone-sodium chloride broth, plates, top agar, dilution fluid, and wash fluid have been described previously (5). SSC (0.015 M NaCl plus 0.015 M sodium citrate) buffer (pH 7.0) has also been described (17). S medium was identical to that previously described (27) except that the concentration of Na_2SO_4 was reduced to 10^{-4} M.

Egg white lysozyme (grade I, crystallized three times) was obtained from Sigma Chemical Co., and deoxyribonuclease I (bovine pancreas) and ribonuclease A (bovine pancreas) were purchased from Worthington Biochemicals Corp. Phleomycin, lot no. 64L1238, was a gift from W. T. Bradner of Bristol Laboratories. It was prepared in advance to 1.0 mg/ml in water or SSC and frozen until used. Each batch was tested for activity by noting the extent of inhibition of optical density increase of *E. coli* B growing in broth. The radiochemicals [*methyl*-^{3}H]thymidine (79 mCi/mg) and [2-^{14}C]thymine (476 μCi/mg) were purchased from Amersham/Searle, Arlington Heights, Ill.

Construction and preparation of phage stocks. The double mutant T4*am*N82*am*N94 was prepared using our modifications (A. D. Beckey, M.S. thesis, University of Texas at Austin, 1974) of previously described procedures (3, 31).

T4 particles with nonglucosylated DNA (T4* phage) were prepared on W4597 by the method of Shedlovsky and Brenner (28) and assayed on K803. All other phage stocks were clonally derived by infecting the appropriate host with a single plaque and, when required, the lysates were purified as reported (5).

Infection of cells. Assays for unadsorbed phage were carried out 2 min after infection; in all cases, the corrected multiplicity of infection was between five and ten phage/cell. Tryptophan (50 μg/ml) was added immediately before infection when experiments were conducted in S medium.

Radioisotopic labeling of DNA. The methods used for labeling bacterial and phage DNA have been described (5).

Assay of DNA solubilization. Our adaptation (16) of the procedure of Barbour and Clark (2) was utilized to assay for DNA solubilization.

Extraction of phage DNA. DNA was obtained from purified phage particles (8 × 10^{11} in 5 ml of SSC) by three extractions with 2.5 ml of SSC-saturated phenol (11). Subsequent dialysis against SSC was carried out in treated dialysis tubing (33) as described by Mandel and Marmur (17). When required, the concentration of SSC in DNA solutions was reduced by exhaustive dialysis against 0.2× SSC. Specific absorbances of 0.0181 $cm^2/\mu g$ and 0.020 $cm^2/\mu g$ at 260 nm were used for quantitative determinations of glucosylated and nonglucosylated DNA, respectively (33).

Thermal denaturation of DNA. The procedures described by Mandel and Marmur (17) were used. Corrections for solvent expansion at high temperatures were not made, however. PM showed no change in absorbance over the temperature range used.

RESULTS

Effect of PM on cellular mass increase, viability, and DNA stability. These experiments with uninfected cells were conducted to provide reference data for comparisons with events in infected cells, to make possible comparisons of our lot of PM with those used by other investigators, and to examine the effects of PM on *end*$^+$ and *end*$^-$ cells. The ability of various concentrations of PM to inhibit *E. coli* B and *E. coli* ER22 (*end*) growth is shown in Fig. 1. A low concentration of PM (2 μg/ml) permits a subsequent mass increase of approximately 150%; higher concentrations of PM result in growth inhibition in less than one generation and, at concentrations of 50 μg/ml and higher, a decrease in the turbidity of the cultures occurs. Despite the fact that there is a substantial mass increase after a growing culture is treated with 2 μg of PM per ml, cells exposed to this concentration of antibiotic are killed rapidly (Fig. 2). Results of these viability studies are in good agreement with the work of Grigg (10), who showed that only 0.6% of *E. coli* B cells survived 40 min of exposure to 2 μg of PM per ml, and are also consistent with results obtained in *E. coli* K-12 strains (21).

The ability of PM to induce DNA degradation

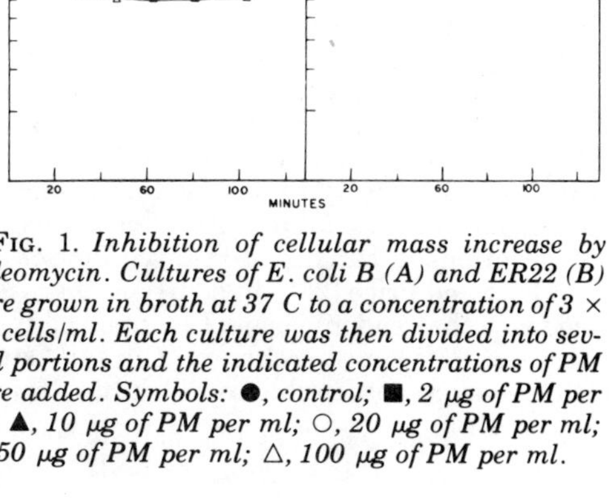

FIG. 1. *Inhibition of cellular mass increase by phleomycin. Cultures of E. coli B (A) and ER22 (B) were grown in broth at 37 C to a concentration of 3 × 10^8 cells/ml. Each culture was then divided into several portions and the indicated concentrations of PM were added. Symbols:* ●, *control;* ■, *2 μg of PM per ml;* ▲, *10 μg of PM per ml;* ○, *20 μg of PM per ml;* □, *50 μg of PM per ml;* △, *100 μg of PM per ml.*

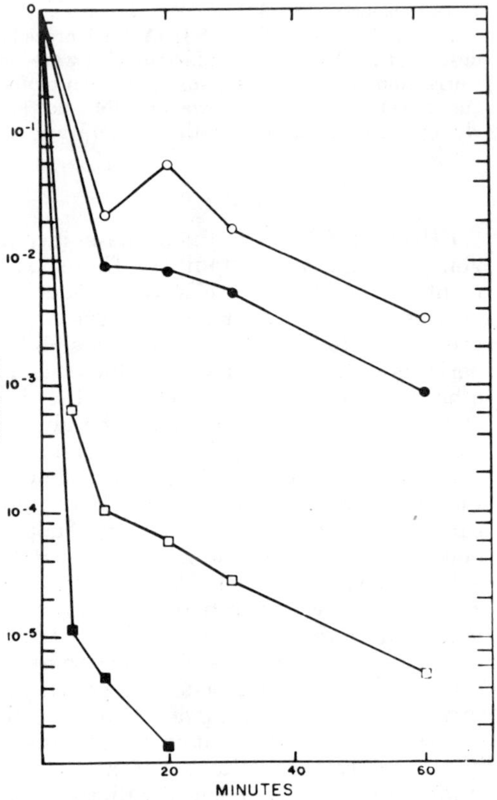

FIG. 2. *Effect of phleomycin on the viability of E. coli B and E. coli ER22 cells. Cultures of E. coli were grown in broth at 37 C to a concentration of 2 × 10^8 cells/ml. PM was added and samples were taken periodically thereafter. Appropriate dilutions were performed and pour plates were made to determine the viable cell count in each sample. Symbols: ○, E. coli B, 2 μg of PM per ml; ●, ER22, 2 μg of PM per ml; □, B, 20 μg of PM per ml; ■, ER22, 20 μg of PM per ml.*

These initial tests demonstrate that 20 μg of PM per ml is sufficient to cause both an immediate, drastic loss of cell viability and the rapid solubilization of DNA. The remainder of our experiments were carried out with this concentration of PM.

Replication of T-even phage in the presence of PM. Preliminary experiments demonstrated that T4, unlike bacteriophages φX174 (24) and PBS2 (25), is able to replicate to some extent when it and PM are simultaneously added to cells. The effect of adding PM at different times before or during the infective cycle on the burst sizes of four phage of the T series was investigated in subsequent experiments (Table 1). The results demonstrate that T2, T4, and T6 are able to replicate in the presence of PM, with T4 infections being most resistant to the inhibitory effect of PM. They also suggest that 3 min of infection with T-even phage confers additional protection against PM. (Phage DNA replication begins approximately 5 min after infection, under the conditions used in these experiments.) T7, on the other hand, is similar to the previously studied phages PBS2 and φX174 in that it is very susceptible to PM inhibition.

These results suggested that some property common only to T-even phage is able to provide partial protection against PM. As is well has been amply documented (8, 10, 21). The kinetics of DNA solubilization brought about by 20 μg of PM per ml in three *E. coli* strains are shown in Fig. 3. By 60 min, greater than 80% of the bacterial DNA is rendered acid soluble in all three strains.

It appears, on the basis of the results described above, that the PM lot in our possession is similar in biological activity to those used by Grigg (no. 648) (10) and by Farrell and Reiter (no. 909) (8). The PM used by Nakayama (21) was from the same lot as ours. (For discussions of variations in batches of PM, see Pietsch [22] and Post and Price [25].) In addition, there is no evidence that endonuclease I is involved in the action of PM. On the contrary, the *end*⁻ strain ER22 is more susceptible to PM killing than is *E. coli* B.

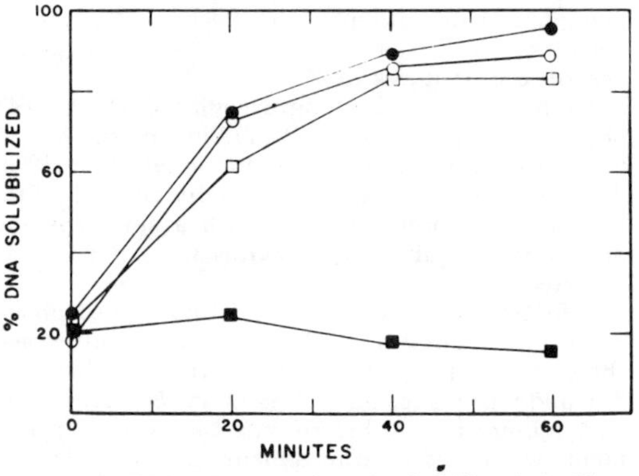

FIG. 3. *Phleomycin-induced solubilization of bacterial DNA. Cultures of E. coli were grown at 37 C in broth supplemented with 250 μg of deoxyadenosine per ml and 0.3 μCi of [³H] thymidine per ml to a concentration of 3 × 10^8 cells/ml. The cells were then harvested by centrifugation, washed once, and resuspended to the same concentration in prewarmed broth. The cultures were divided into two equal portions, one of which received 20 μg of PM per ml. Samples (1.0 ml) were taken into 0.2 ml of 30% trichloroacetic acid at 20-min intervals. Further processing of samples was as described (16). The control curve was obtained by averaging the results obtained from the untreated samples of the three bacterial strains. Symbols: ○, E. coli B; □, E. coli B40suI; ●, E. coli ER22; ■, no PM added.*

TABLE 1. *Inhibition of T-phage production[a] by addition of phleomycin before or during the multiplication cycle*

Phage	Host	Control burst size[b]	Phage yield[c] when PM was added		
			At infection	5 min preinfection	3 min postinfection
T4	B	147	6.3	1.3	16
T2	B	66	1	1.5	6
T6	B	149	1.4	0.2	4
T7	B	116	1	1	0.9
T4	K803	181	5.5	0.3	11.6
T4*	K803	159	1.2	0.2	9.1

[a] Cells were grown at 37 C in broth to a concentration of 3×10^8 cells/ml and then infected with phage at a multiplicity of 7.5.

[b] All samples were lysed with chloroform after 60 min of infection and the phage titer was then determined.

[c] Phage yields are presented as percentages of control burst size.

known, the DNA of T-even phage contains hydroxymethylcytosine (HMC) in place of cytosine (4) and the HMC bases are partially or totally glucosylated (15). The percentages of HMC glucosylation are 100%, 75%, and 75% for T4, T2, and T6, respectively (14); these values are in general agreement with the degree of PM resistance exhibited by these phage. Accordingly, the possibility that the glucosylation of T-even phage DNA was affording some protection from PM inhibition was tested. *E. coli* K803, which does not restrict nonglucosylated phage (T*), was infected with T4* in the presence of PM. As is evident from Table 1, only when PM was added simultaneously with the phage was the ability of T4* to replicate significantly less than that of T4.

The kinetics of development of T-even phage resistance to PM was studied in more detail. It was observed that the longer time cells are infected before the addition of PM, the closer to normal the final burst size is. For example, T2, T4, and T6 all yielded bursts of 30% or more of the normal value when PM was added 9 min postinfection (data not shown).

Solubilization of host and phage DNA in PM-treated cells. The possibility that glucosylated DNA is better protected than normal DNA from the degradative effects brought about by PM was tested as follows. The effect of PM on the solubilization of bacterial and phage DNA was monitored after infection of cells with T4*am*N82*am*N94, a phage which in Su^- hosts is unable either to synthesize significant amounts of phage DNA or to render host DNA acid soluble. Infections were carried out in both permissive and nonpermissive hosts and PM was added at several different times. The results are shown in Fig. 4. (In experiments carried out in the absence of PM, there was essentially no solubilization of host or phage DNA above the background level during either permissive or nonpermissive infections. Solubilization of host DNA in a permissive infection is not observed because nucleotides arising from degradation of host DNA are rapidly incorporated into phage DNA.) Two points can be made from the data. The earlier the PM was added, the greater was the extent of solubilization of both types of DNA. In fact, when the nonpermissive host was pretreated for 5 min before infection, degradation of both host and phage DNA approached the level of solubilization of bacterial DNA seen

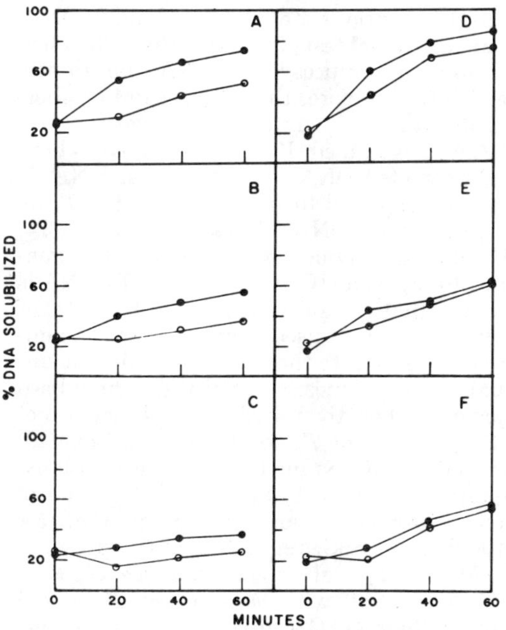

FIG. 4. *Phleomycin-induced solubilization of bacterial and parental T4 DNA after infection. Cultures of E. coli B (Su^-) and B40suI (Su^+) were grown at 37 C in broth supplemented with 250 μg of deoxyadenosine/ml and 0.3 μCi of [^{14}C]thymine/ml to a cell concentration of 3×10^8/ml. The cultures were harvested, washed once, and resuspended in prewarmed broth. After an additional 5 min of growth, PM (20 μg/ml) and [^{3}H]thymidine-labeled T4amN82amN94 were added as indicated. Samples were taken and processed as described in the legend for Fig. 3. Symbols: ●, bacterial DNA; ○, phage DNA. (A, B, C) Solubilization of DNA after infection of B40suI; PM was added 5 min before infection, at infection, and 3 min after infection, respectively. (D, E, F) Solubilization of DNA after infection of B; PM was added 5 min before infection, at infection, and 3 min after infection, respectively.*

in uninfected control cells (compare Fig. 3 with Fig. 4D). Also, in all cases host DNA was solubilized to a greater extent than parental phage DNA. The differences in percentages of solubilization were not great, however, and the experiments provide little evidence that glucosylated DNA is better able to withstand PM-stimulated solubilization than is nonglucosylated DNA. The data do indicate that T4 infection has a strong protective effect against PM-induced solubilization of both bacterial and phage DNA.

Effect of PM on the thermal denaturation curves of glucosylated and nonglucosylated DNA. It has been demonstrated (7, 20) that the melting temperature (T_m) for normal DNA is increased in the presence of PM; indeed, results of this type of experiment provided one of the earliest indications that PM does bind to DNA. As an additional test of the idea that PM is less able to bind to glucosylated DNA than to normal DNA, therefore, the effect of PM on thermal denaturation curves of the two types of DNA was examined. If PM is less able to bind to glucosylated DNA than to normal DNA, it would be expected to influence less the T_m of the glucosylated DNA. Three types of DNA, T4, T4*, and calf thymus, were studied; the guanine plus cytosine (G+C) content of T4 DNA is 34% and that of calf thymus is 39% (29). Calf thymus DNA was used because it has a similar G+C content to that of T4, contains no unusual sugar residues, and has the normal base cytosine rather than hydroxymethylcytosine. In SSC buffer, the T_m for T4 DNA is 84 C (29) and that of calf thymus DNA can be calculated (equation 1 of [17]) to be 85.3. The results of these experiments are shown in Fig. 5A through C; in SSC, regardless of the presence of PM, the T_m values for all three types of DNA agree well with those expected on the basis of their G+C content alone. However, when the ionic strength of the SSC buffer was reduced fivefold, such that the T_m values for T4 and calf thymus DNA could be calculated to be 72 and 74 C, respectively (equation 2 of [17]), the ability of PM to increase the T_m of DNAs became apparent (Fig. 5D–F). Nonetheless, PM had the same effect on all three DNA species. That is, at the concentration of 40 μg/ml, PM appears to affect glucosylated and nonglucosylated DNA molecules equally well.

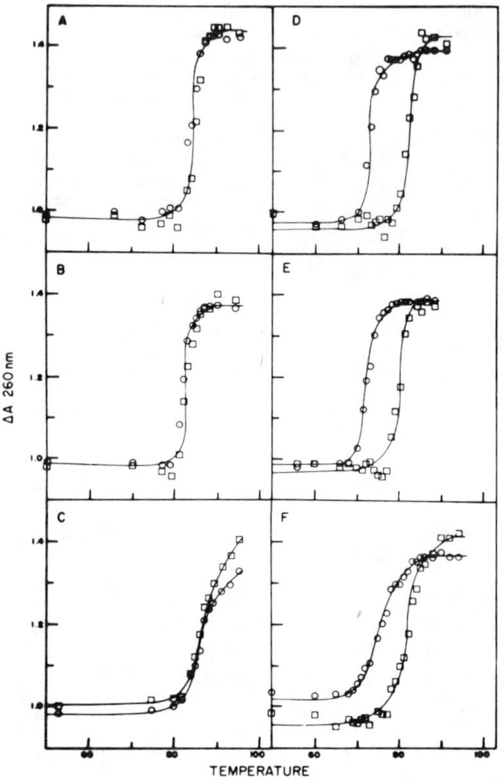

FIG. 5. *Influence of phleomycin on the thermal denaturation of DNA. (A–C) DNA was dissolved in SSC; (D–F) DNA was dissolved in 0.2× SSC. Denaturation profiles of T4, T4*, and calf thymus DNA are shown in A and D, B and E, and C and F, respectively. Symbols; ○, control; □, 40 μg of PM per ml.*

DISCUSSION

The principal finding arising from this work is the observation that T-even phage can replicate in the presence of PM. A previous study indicated that PM completely prevents the replication of T2 phage (34); this work has been seriously challenged, however, on the basis that the PM lot used was contaminated. The reasons for the unusual resistance of T-even phage growth to PM are not clear. More precise information is needed regarding the molecular mode of action of PM before a definitive explanation for this resistance can be determined but several factors are probably involved.

Data shown in Table 1 suggest that T4* phage are more susceptible to PM inhibition than are T4, particularly when PM is added before infection or simultaneously with the phage. The protective effect of glucosylation is conceptually easy to explain on the basis that glucose residues in T-even DNA sterically hinder and weaken the association between PM and DNA. However, we did not observe that glucosylated DNA was significantly more resistant to PM-stimulated solubilization than nonglucosylated (bacterial) DNA (Fig. 4) and we were unable to detect any differential effect of PM on melting curves of DNA from T4 and

T4* phage (Fig. 5). Speculations regarding the role of glucosylation in PM protection are further complicated by (i) the fact that, even during normal T-even phage infections, newly synthesized DNA is momentarily unglucosylated and (ii) recent data which suggests that glucosylation or HMC-glucosyl transferases have a role in T4 transcription (19) and in the production of T6 phage with normal structural properties (12).

The data presented in Fig. 4 show clearly that T4 infection prevents PM-induced solubilization of both host and phage DNA. This effect seems to be the most likely explanation for the resistance of T-even phage replication to PM. The basis for this protection could result from alterations in cellular permeability which occur after infection with T-even phage or the shut off upon infection of the nuclease(s) responsible for PM-induced degradation (8). We are unable to distinguish between these two possibilities. However, if envelope alterations which are brought about after infection are involved, the alteration is apparently not identical to that which accounts for superinfection exclusion, tolerance to ghosts, or resistance to lysis from without. The modification involved in these latter phenomena is complete by 5 min after infection, whereas PM resistance develops throughout the infective cycle.

Farrell and Reiter (8) have reported an experiment similar to that shown in Fig. 4E, except that only bacterial DNA was examined. They observed essentially no solubilization of host DNA after T4 infection in the presence of PM. The slight discrepancy between their observation and ours is probably accounted for by the fact that their results were obtained with cells growing in minimal medium; Grigg (10) has reported that cells growing in minimal medium are more resistant to PM than those growing in a rich medium, and we have observed that the inhibitory effects of PM on T4 growth are reduced from two- to fivefold when infections occur in S medium.

A second finding of this project concerns the effect of PM on thermal denaturation curves of DNA. In SSC, the usual solvent for T_m determinations, PM was found to have no effect on the T_m's of any of the three DNAs tested. However, when the ionic strength of the buffer was decreased and the T_m values thereby correspondingly reduced, the elevating effect of PM on T_m's (7, 20) was observed. Falaschi and Kornberg (7) noted that PM has no significant effect on DNA samples with T_m values of 80 C or higher. They suggested that this was either because there is poor binding of PM to DNA with low AT contents or that PM dissociated from DNA at higher temperatures. Our results, obtained from experiments in which the same DNA species were examined under two ionic conditions (Fig. 5), appear to exclude the former explanation.

Lastly, the possibility that endonuclease I is involved in the DNA degradation stimulated by PM was eliminated. Even at the low concentrations (2 μg/ml) of PM used in experiments that implicated *rec* mutants (21) and excision-defective strains (10) as having roles in PM-induced lethality, *end*$^+$ and *end* strains of *E. coli* B were approximately equally affected by PM. This observation is in agreement with recent evidence (21) that endonuclease I is not involved in PM action in *E. coli* K-12 strains.

ACKNOWLEDGMENTS

We gratefully acknowledge Judy Ing for her technical assistance and Linda Gaddy for her typing of this manuscript.

This investigation was supported by grant BMS75-07693 from the National Science Foundation, by Biomedical Science Support grant RR-07091 to The University of Texas, and by funds from The University of Texas Genetics Institute.

LITERATURE CITED

1. **Almendinger, R., and L. P. Hager.** 1972. Role for endonuclease I in the transmission process of colicin E_2. Nature (London) New Biol. 235:199–203.
2. **Barbour, S. D., and A. J. Clark.** 1970. Biochemical and genetic studies of recombination proficiency in *Escherichia coli*. I. Enzymatic activity associated with recB$^+$ and recC$^+$ genes. Proc. Natl. Acad. Sci. U.S.A. 65:955–961.
3. **Chase, M. C., and A. H. Doerman.** 1958. High negative interference over short segments of the genetic structure of bacteriophage T4. Genetics 43:332–353.
4. **Cohen, S. S.** 1968. Virus-induced enzymes. Columbia University Press, New York.
5. **Earhart, C. F.** 1970. The association of host and phage DNA with the membrane of *Escherichia coli*. Virology 42:429–436.
6. **Eigner, J., and S. Block.** 1968. Host-controlled restriction of T-even bacteriophages: relation of four bacterial deoxyribonucleases to restriction. J. Virol. 2:320–326.
7. **Falaschi, A., and A. Kornberg.** 1964. Phleomycin, an inhibitor of DNA polymerase. Fed. Proc. 23:940–945.
8. **Farrell, L., and H. Reiter.** 1973. Phleomycin-stimulated degradation of deoxyribonucleic acid in *Escherichia coli*. Antimicrob. Agents Chemother. 4:320–326.
9. **Fukasawa, T., K. Jokura, and K. Kurahashi.** 1962. A new enzymic defect of galactose metabolism in *Escherichia coli* K-12 mutants Biochem. Biophys. Res. Commun. 7:121–125.
10. **Grigg, G. W.** 1969. Induction of DNA breakdown and death in *Escherichia coli* by phleomycin. Mol. Gen. Genet. 104:1–11.
11. **Goldberg, E. B.** 1966. The amount of DNA between genetic markers in phage T4. Proc. Natl. Acad. Sci. U.S.A. 56:1457–1463.
12. **Hewlett, M. J., and C. K. Mathews.** 1975. Bacteriophage-host interaction and restriction of nonglucosylated T6. J. Virol. 15:776–784.
13. **Kersten, H., and W. Kersten.** 1974. Inhibitors of nucleic acid synthesis; biophysical and biochemical aspects. Springer-Verlag, New York.

14. **Kornberg, A.** 1974. DNA synthesis. W. H. Freeman and Co., San Francisco.
15. **Lehman, I. R., and E. A. Pratt.** 1960. On the structure of the glucosylated hydroxymethylcytosine nucleotides of coliphages T2, T4, and T6. J. Biol. Chem. 235:3254–3259.
16. **McIntosh, M. A., and C. F. Earhart.** 1975. Effect of Ribonuclease on the association of deoxyribonucleic acid with the membrane in *Escherichia coli*. J. Bacteriol. 122:592–598.
17. **Mandel, M., and J. Marmur.** 1968. Use of ultraviolet absorbance-temperature profile for determining the guanine plus cytosine content of DNA, p. 195–206. *In* L. D. Grossman and K. Moldave (ed.), Methods in enzymology, vol. 12b. Academic Press Inc., New York.
18. **Mattingly, E.** 1967. Induction of chromosome- and chromatid-type aberrations by phleomycin. Mutat. Res. 4:51–57.
19. **Montgomery, D. L., and L. R. Snyder.** 1973. A negative effect of β-glucosylation on T4 growth in certain RNA polymerase mutants of *Escherichia coli*: genetic evidence implicating pyrimidine-rich sequences of DNA in transcription. Virology 53:349–358.
20. **Nagai, K., H. Yamaki, H. Suzuki, N. Tanaka, and H. Umezawa.** 1969. The combined effects of bleomycin and sulfhydryl compounds on the thermal denaturation of DNA. Biochim. Biophys. Acta 179:165–171.
21. **Nakayama, H.** 1975. Phleomycin-induced lethality and DNA degradation in *Escherichia coli* K12. Mutat. Res. 29:21–33.
22. **Pietsch, P.** 1969. Phleomycin: biological and chemical variations in different batches. Microbios 4:387–392.
23. **Pietsch, P.** 1973. Biopolymers in drug technology: the use of DNA in purifying phleomycin. Biotechnol. Bioeng. 15:1039–1044.
24. **Pitts, J. D., and R. L. Sinsheimer.** 1965. Effects of phleomycin upon replication of bacteriophage ϕX174. J. Mol. Biol. 15:676–680.
25. **Post, L., and A. R. Price.** 1975. Inhibition of bacteriophage PBS2 replication in *Bacillus subtilis* by phleomycin. J. Virol. 15:363–371.
26. **Reiter, H., M. Milewskiy, and P. Kelley.** 1972. Mode of action of phleomycin on *Bacillus subtilis*. J. Bacteriol. 111:586–592.
27. **Roberts, R. B., P. H. Abelson, D. B. Cowie, E. T. Bolton, and R. J. Britten.** 1955. Studies of biosynthesis in *Escherichia coli*. Carnegie Institution of Washington publication 607. The Kirby Lithographic Co., Inc., Washington, D.C.
28. **Shedlovsky, A., and S. Brenner.** 1963. A chemical basis for the host induced modification of T-even bacteriophages. Proc. Natl. Acad. Sci. U.S.A. 50:300–305.
29. **Sober, H. A.** 1968. Handbook of biochemistry: selected data for molecular biology. The Chemical Rubber Co., Cleveland.
30. **Stern, R., J. A. Rose, and R. M. Friedman.** 1974. Phleomycin-induced cleavage of deoxyribonucleic acid. Biochemistry 13:307–312.
31. **Streisinger, G., J. Emrich, Y. Okada, A. Tsugita, and M. Inouye.** 1968. Direction of translation of the lysozyme gene of bacteriophage T4 relative to the linkage map. J. Mol. Biol. 31:607–612.
32. **Tanaka, N., H. Yamaguchi, and H. Umezawa.** 1963. Mechanism of action of phleomycin. I. Selective inhibition of the DNA synthesis in *E. coli* and HeLa cells. J. Antibiot. 16:86–91.
33. **Thomas, C. A., Jr., and J. Abelson.** 1966. The isolation and characterization of DNA from bacteriophage, p. 553–561. *In* G. L. Cantoni and D. R. Davies (ed.), Procedures in nucleic acid research. Harper and Row, New York.
34. **Watanabe, M., and J. T. August.** 1968. Replication of RNA bacteriophage R23. II. Inhibition of phage-specific RNA synthesis by phleomycin. J. Mol. Biol. 33:21–33.
35. **Wood, W. B.** 1966. Host specificity of DNA produced by *Escherichia coli*: bacterial mutations affecting the restriction and modification of DNA. J. Mol. Biol. 16:118–133.

ANTIMICROBIAL AGENTS AND CHEMOTHERAPY, July 1976, p. 157-163
Vol. 10, No. 1

Synergism of Cefazolin-Gentamicin Against Enterococci

MICHAEL BOURQUE, RICHARD QUINTILIANI,* AND RICHARD C. TILTON

*University of Connecticut, School of Medicine and Department of Laboratory Medicine, Farmington, Connecticut 06032, and Infectious Disease Division, Hartford Hospital, Department of Medicine, Hartford, Connecticut 06115**

Received for publication 23 February 1976

A miniaturized technique for detecting antibiotic synergy by using microliter volumes was perfected. With this microtiter serial dilution method, the effect of the previously untried combination of cefazolin and gentamicin on 10 strains of enterococci was evaluated. At clinically achievable concentrations, the combination of cefazolin and gentamicin was found to be synergistic against all 10 strains when the data were plotted in the form of an isobologram. These results were compared with the conventional method of detecting synergy in vitro, namely, the determination of the rate of killing of the microorganisms with the antibiotics, singly and in combination. Similar results were also observed. These findings indicate that the microtiter serial dilution technique is a useful method for the routine determination of drug synergy. Moreover, in a patient with penicillin hypersensitivity and enterococcal infection, the combination of cefazolin and gentamicin should be considered for possible therapy.

As microorganisms are encountered that are resistant to certain antibiotics, the use of drug combinations in certain clinical situations has proved valuable. Of particular interest in recent years has been the phenomenon of drug synergism.

Drug synergism, as defined, implies the ability of two antimicrobial drugs acting together to produce a bactericidal activity greater than the sum of the effects produced by each of the drugs independently (6, 11).

Unfortunately, most of the quantitative techniques for detecting drug synergy are laborious and impractical for routine use in clinical laboratories. One purpose of this study was to compare a microtiter method with the conventional method of detecting synergy. The greater efficiency and economy of the microtiter method might implement synergy assays as a routine procedure.

The combination of penicillin and streptomycin has been widely used in the treatment of enterococcal infections since the discovery that these drugs were at times synergistic against such organisms. In recent years, however, this combination of drugs has been found to be ineffective against increasing numbers of enterococci (10, 20, 21), and, hence, an alternative drug regimen would be very valuable.

The combination of penicillin and gentamicin has been shown to be synergistic in its killing action against virtually all strains in vitro (4, 15, 20). Because recent clinical studies have confirmed the in vivo efficacy of gentamicin and penicillin against enterococcal infections, it has been suggested by some investigators that this combination be the initial treatment of choice (17, 19).

However, occasional patients will present such unique circumstances as penicillin allergy. More toxic antibiotics, such as vancomycin, have been successfully used as alternatives in some of these patients (2), but new forms of safe and effective therapy are needed. Cephalosporin derivatives are similar to the penicillins in molecular structure and antibacterial activity, but cross-sensitivity between these compounds and penicillin only rarely occurs (1, 16). For these reasons it was decided to investigate the in vitro activity of a cephalosporin derivative, cefazolin, combined with gentamicin.

In this study, two major goals were attained: a test of the performance of the microtiter serial dilution synergy technique, as well as an evaluation of this previously untried drug combination against enterococci.

MATERIALS AND METHODS

Bacteria. Seven strains of enterococci were obtained from routine cultures of urine, wounds, and blood performed in the clinical microbiology laboratory at John Dempsey Hospital of the University of Connecticut. An additional three strains of enterococci were obtained from the Connecticut Department of Health Laboratory and from the clinical laboratory at Hartford. All 10 enterococci were *Streptococcus faecalis*. All strains of enterococci were confirmed in the clinical laboratory by routine techniques. The nonenterococcal group D streptococcus *(S. bovis)* was not included in this study due to its uniform susceptibility to penicillin.

Media and antibiotics. Culture media used were Mueller-Hinton broth (MHB) (BBL) and Mueller-Hinton agar. Antibiotics used in this study were obtained from the hospital pharmacy as injectable solutions without preservative. These antibiotics consisted of gentamicin sulfate (Schering Laboratories) and cefazolin sodium (Eli Lilly & Co.). Stock solutions of the antibiotics were prepared in concentrations of 1,280 μg/ml. These solutions were frozen and stored in 2-ml aliquots at −20 C. The potency of these antibiotics was checked weekly by comparing the minimal inhibitory concentration (MIC) of each drug alone, by using a standard enterococcus, with the MIC of that strain each week thereafter. No variation in the MIC was noted throughout the length of this study.

Microdilution assay for antibiotic synergy. The checkerboard tube dilution technique described by Sabath (11) was adapted to the microtiter system (8) using Autotiter plates containing 120 wells (Ames Co.). After the addition of 50 μl of growth media (MHB) to each of 64 wells (8 × 8 square), antibiotics were serially diluted with a 50-μl spiral loop, horizontally and vertically. Eight rows in one direction contained twofold dilutions of cefazolin in decreasing concentrations ranging from 32 to 0.25 μg/ml, whereas the eight rows in the other direction contained serial twofold dilutions of gentamicin ranging in concentrations from 32 to 0.25 μg/ml. The final result was 64 wells, each containing a different concentration of the cefazolin-gentamicin combination (see Fig. 1). Two additional rows contained twofold serial dilutions of cefazolin and gentamicin alone in final concentrations of from 32 to 0.25 μg/ml. An overnight broth culture of the particular strain was standardized with a nephelometer to 1 × 10^8 organisms per ml and then diluted to a final inoculum size of 5 × 10^4 colony-forming units per ml. One row in each Autotiter plate contained only MHB and bacteria as a growth control, while a second row contained only MHB as a contamination control. Bacteria and antibiotic solutions were added to the wells of the Autotiter tray with a calibrated 50-μl pipette. The final volume in each well was 100 μl.

Each Autotiter tray was sealed with plastic transparent tape and incubated at 37 C for 18 to 24 h. After incubation, the trays were examined for evidence of growth by using the Autotray Viewer (Astec, Inc.). The turbidity of the wells containing only enterococci and broth was used for comparison in determining the end points of growth. The lowest concentration of antibiotics showing complete inhibition of growth was read as the MIC (micrograms per milliliter).

For determination of bactericidal end points, samples were removed from each row with a 0.01-ml platinum-calibrated loop, from the end point well and from the other five wells on either side. These samples were plated out on Mueller-Hinton agar and observed for evidence of growth after incubation at 37 C for 18 to 24 h. The lowest dilution in which there was no growth was read as the minimum bactericidal concentration (MBC) in micrograms per milliliter.

The MIC and MBC of each antibiotic, alone and in combination, were recorded and plotted as an isobologram on an arithmetic scale. Concave curves represent synergistic action of the two drugs, a straight line joining the ordinate and abscissa axes represents an additive effect, and a convex outward curve represents antagonism of the two drugs (11).

Growth curve and assay for synergy. The rate of killing of the enterococci by cefazolin and gentamicin, alone and in combination, was determined for all 10 strains by performing serial colony counts. Overnight broth cultures for each strain were standardized with a nephelometer to 1 × 10^8 organisms

		1	2	3	4	5	6	7	8	9	10	11
A	C	32	16	8	4	2	1	.5	.25		32	0
	G	32	32	32	32	32	32	32	32		0	32
B	C	32	16	8	4	2	1	.5	.25		16	0
	G	16	16	16	16	16	16	16	16		0	16
C	C	32	16	8	4	2	1	.5	.25		8	0
	G	8	8	8	8	8	8	8	8		0	8
D	C	32	16	8	4	2	1	.5	.25		4	0
	G	4	4	4	4	4	4	4	4		0	4
E	C	32	16	8	4	2	1	.5	.25		2	0
	G	2	2	2	2	2	2	2	2		0	2
F	C	32	16	8	4	2	1	.5	.25		1	0
	G	1	1	1	1	1	1	1	1		0	1
G	C	32	16	8	4	2	1	.5	.25		.5	0
	G	.5	.5	.5	.5	.5	.5	.5	.5		0	.5
H	C	32	16	8	4	2	1	.5	.25		.25	0
	G	.25	.25	.25	.25	.25	.25	.25	.25		0	.25

FIG. 1. *Diagram of an Autotiter tray with the different concentrations of antibiotics in each well. C, Cefazolin; G, gentamicin in micrograms per milliliter.*

per ml and diluted, and 2-ml aliquots of these organisms were added to a series of tubes to reach a final inoculum size of approximately 5 × 10^5 organisms per ml. Antibiotics were added, singly and in combination, to these tubes so that the final concentration would be as follows: cefazolin, either 32 μg/ml (five strains) or 16 μg/ml (five strains); gentamicin, either 4, 2, or 1 μg/ml. The concentrations of gentamicin were chosen to be less than the MIC (previously determined for each particular strain by the microtiter serial dilution technique) for, in order to demonstrate a synergistic effect, unimpaired growth in the presence of gentamicin alone was required. Each strain was therefore tested against the two antimicrobials singly and against two to three distinct concentrations of gentamicin in combination with a single concentration of cefazolin. An additional test tube contained only MHB and bacteria and served as a growth control. The final total volume in each tube was 4 ml.

The tubes were incubated at 37 C for 4, 8, and 24 h. One-milliliter samples were removed at each time period, 10-fold serial dilutions were made, and colony counts were performed on Mueller-Hinton agar. The plates were then incubated at 37 C and the colonies were counted after 24 h of incubation. According to the criterion used by Watanakunakorn (15), the combination of antibiotics was considered synergistic when the number of colonies surviving the combined killing action was at least 1 $\log_{10}$ less than the number of colonies surviving with the most effective of the antibiotics alone.

RESULTS

The MIC and MBC of cefazolin and gentamicin, alone and in combination, against 10 strains of enterococci are illustrated in Fig. 2 and 3. The lines joining the MICs and MBCs of the various combinations (isobols) for all 10 strains are distinctly concave and, according to the criteria of Sabath (11), represent synergy of the two antibiotics. Due to the overlap of many of the isobols in Fig. 2 and 3, Fig. 4 has been included to present a clearer visualization of a single isobol from a single strain (15). The concave nature of the curve signifies synergy. These results are summarized in Table 1.

The activity of cefazolin and gentamicin alone and in combination against the 10 strains

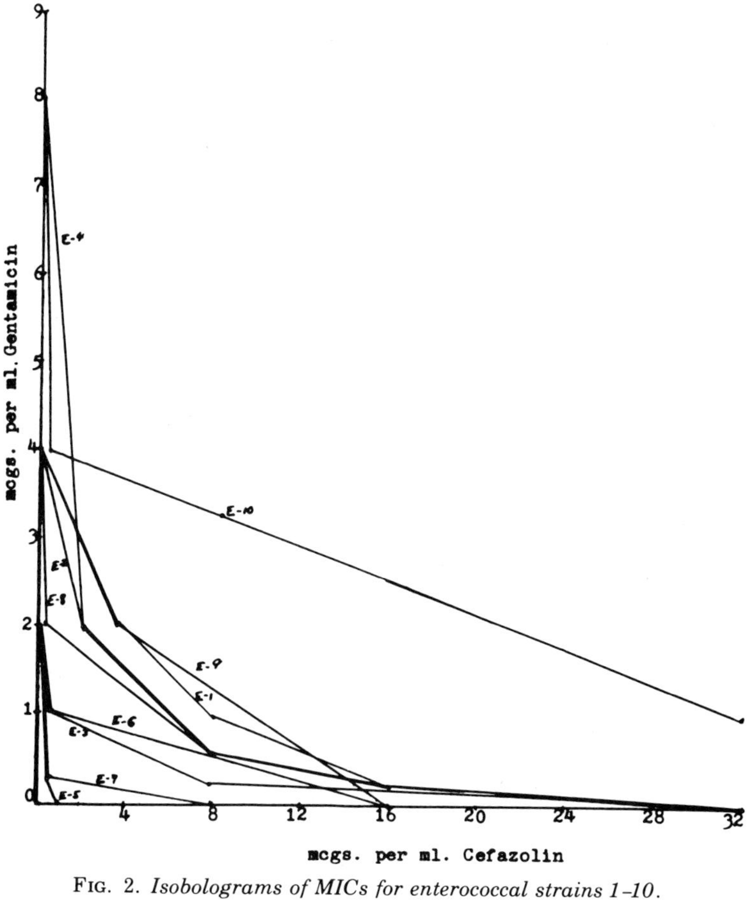

FIG. 2. *Isobolograms of MICs for enterococcal strains 1–10.*

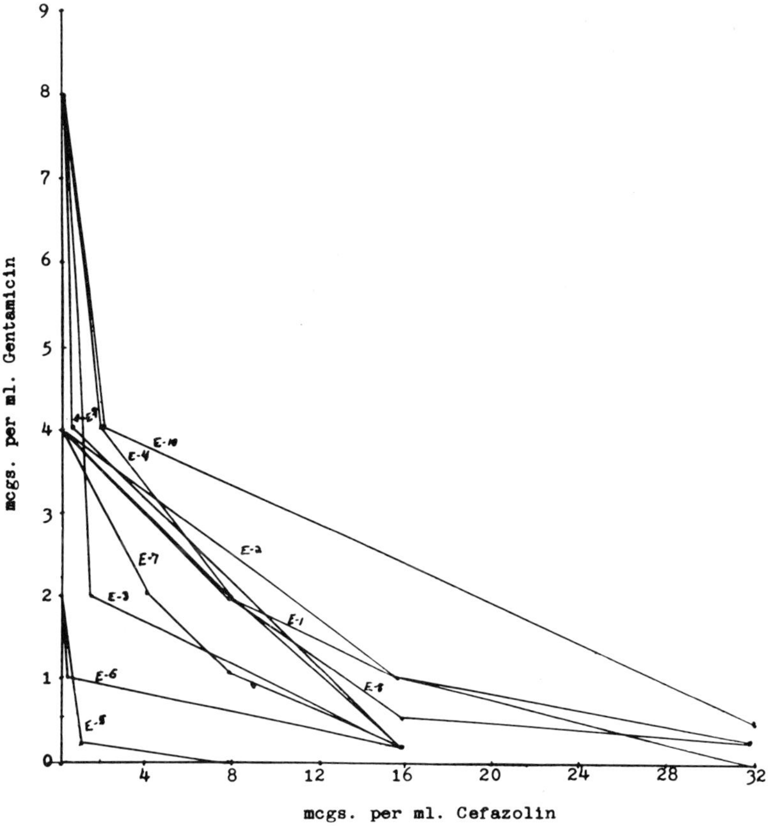

FIG. 3. *Isobolograms of MCBs for enterococcal strains 1–10.*

of enterococci was evaluated in broth culture. The results are presented in Table 2. Using the criteria of synergy as a decrease in viable cell numbers after 24 h of incubation by at least a factor of 10, when the combination of drugs is compared to the most effective of the antibiotics alone, all 10 strains (100%) demonstrated synergy. An example of a growth curve showing synergy (enterococcus no. 4) is presented in Fig. 5. The concentrations of gentamicin (4 and 2 μg/ml) were chosen because the MIC of gentamicin for this particular strain was found to be 8 μg/ml by a previous determination, and, in order to demonstrate the synergistic effect, unimpaired growth in the presence of gentamicin alone was required.

DISCUSSION

Two methods for evaluating synergy between cefazolin and gentamicin were evaluated in this study. The microtiter serial dilution method yields results that indicate whether there is synergy, antagonism, or an additive effect of antibiotic combinations. This technique also provides quantitative data in the form of the MIC and MBC of each antibiotic for the microorganisms being considered. This method proved to be a rapid, efficient, and economical method of assay for synergy. With the availability of equipment that will automate this miniaturized checkerboard technique, routine determinations of antibiotic synergy may soon be feasible in many clinical laboratories.

The conventional large-volume, broth dilution technique with the plotting of growth curves used in the second part of this study is a cumbersome, time-consuming, and expensive technique. The results of this study show a good agreement between these two techniques. Because many other studies have also attested to the accuracy and reproducibility of the microdilution technique when compared to the broth dilution method (3, 7, 13), serious consideration should be given to its implementation.

The exact mechanism of the penicillin-streptomycin synergy against the enterococci is not known. However, it has been shown that penicillin increases the uptake of radioactive streptomycin by enterococci, presumably as a result of injury to the cell wall (9). However, despite

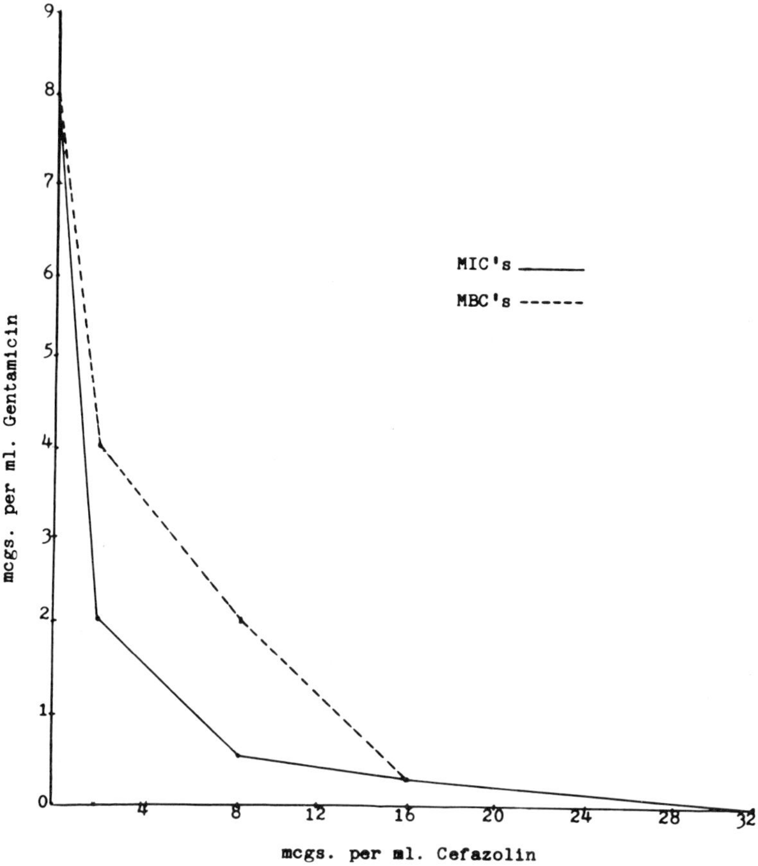

FIG. 4. *Isobologram of MICs and MBCs for enterococcal strain no. 4.*

TABLE 1. *Summary of isobolograms for detecting synergism between cefazolin and gentamicin against 10 enterococcal strains*

Antibiotic activity	No. of enterococcal strains		
	Shape of isobologram		
	Concave	Linear	Convex
MIC	10	0	0
MBC	10	0	0

TABLE 2. *Effectiveness of combination of cefazolin and gentamicin against 10 strains of enterococci as determined by growth curves*

No. of enterococcal strains				
0–1[a]	1–2	2–3	3–4	4–5
0	6	2	0	2

[a] Numbers show fold $\log_{10}$ decrease in the number of surviving colonies. Decrease in viable cell count after 24 h by the combination was compared with the most effective of the antibiotics used alone. In all cases, the most effective antibiotic alone was cefazolin since the aminoglycoside concentration was chosen to be less than the MIC.

penetration into the cell by streptomycin, increasing numbers of enterococcal strains remain unaffected by even high levels of this antibiotic when combined with penicillin (3, 10). This high level of resistance has been found to be ribosomally mediated (21).

To date, because ribosomally mediated resistance has not been observed with gentamicin and because virtually all strains of enterococci are susceptible to the synergistic bactericidal effects of the combination of gentamicin and penicillin (15, 20), this combination emerges as an attractive choice in the therapy of enterococcal endocarditis (17). However, it must be stressed that in vitro evidence of synergism is not always predictive of therapeutic success and, hence, 20 to 40 million U of penicillin G intravenously plus 1 g of streptomycin intramuscularly probably remains the preferred selection in the initial treatment of enterococcal endocarditis; however, if the clinical response is poor, then prompt consideration

15

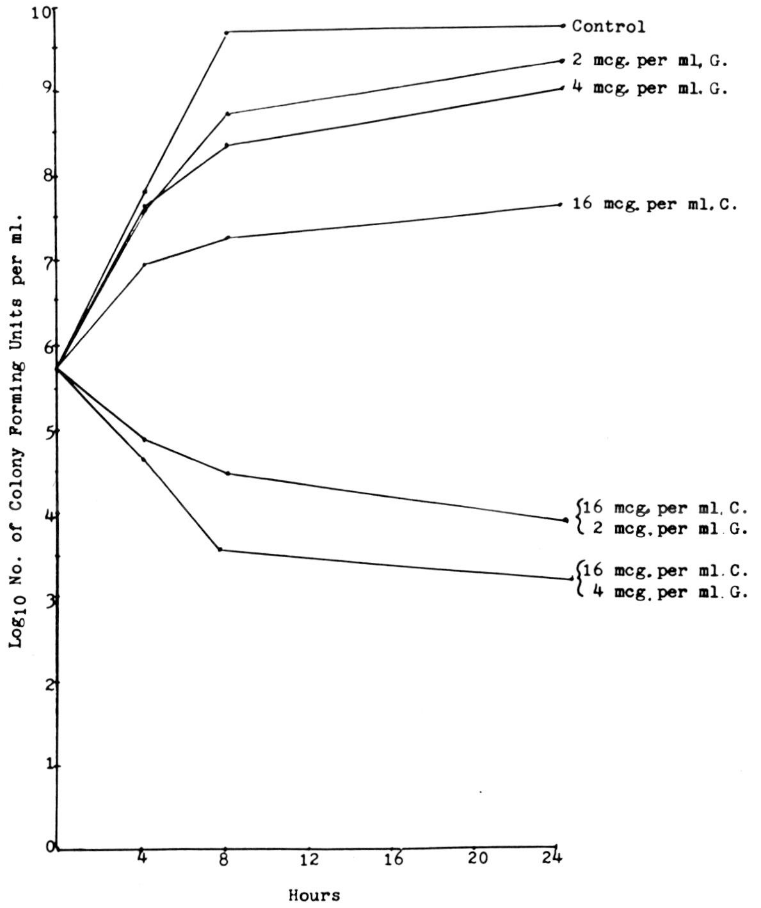

FIG. 5. *Effect of two different concentrations of gentamicin alone and in combination with cefazolin against enterococcal strain no. 4. C, Cefazolin; G, gentamicin.*

should be given to the replacement of the streptomycin with gentamicin in appropriate dosage (19).

In patients allergic to the penicillins, treatment of systemic enterococcal infections becomes more complex. In the past, various therapeutic approaches have been tried, such as substituting a more toxic agent for penicillin, attempting to desensitize the patient, or using corticosteroids and antihistamines to depress the allergic response (5).

Since cephalosporin derivatives have become available, they represent a potentially useful alternative to penicillin treatment of enterococcal infections. These antibiotics are relatively nontoxic and have an antibacterial spectrum similar to penicillin G, and cross-hypersensitivity reactions between the penicillins and the cephalosporins only rarely occur (1, 16). Previous studies have shown the combination of cephalothin, another cephalosporin derivative, and streptomycin to be a relatively ineffective combination against enterococci (12). However, the results of more recent studies clearly demonstrate the superiority of gentamicin against enterococci when coupled with other antibiotics (15, 20). The results of this present study using two different techniques show a marked synergistic effect when gentamicin was combined with the cephalosporin derivative cefazolin. At clinically achievable concentrations of these antibiotics, synergy was demonstrated with all 10 strains, with a 100% correlation of the results between the two techniques. Our results were not surprising since it has been shown in a previous study that the combination of cephalothin and gentamicin was also synergistic against strains of enterococci (18).

These in vitro results suggest that cefazolin offers promise as a penicillin substitute for the treatment of enterococcal endocarditis.

LITERATURE CITED

1. **Apicella, M., R. L. Perkins, and S. Saslow.** 1966. Treatment of bacterial endocarditis with cephalosporin derivatives. N. Engl. J. Med. **51**:266–276.
2. **Friedberg, C. K., K. M. Rosen, and P. A. Bienstock.** 1968. Vancomycin therapy for enterococcal and *Streptococcal viridans* endocarditis. Arch. Intern. Med. **122**:134–140.
3. **Gavan, T. L., and M. A. Town,** 1970. A microdilution method for antibiotic susceptibility testing. Am. J. Clin. Pathol. **53**:880–885.
4. **Glew, R. H., R. C. Moellering, Jr., and C. Wennerstein.** 1975. Comparative synergistic activity of nafcillin, oxacillin, and methicillin in combination with gentamicin against enterococci. Antimicrob. Agents Chemother. **7**:828–832.
5. **Grieco, M. H., M. R. Dubin, J. L. Robinson, and M. J. Schwartz.** 1964. Treatment of bacterial endocarditis with cephalosporin derivatives in penicillin allergic patients. Ann. Intern Med. **60**:204.
6. **Jawetz, E.** 1968. Combined antibiotic actions: some definitions and correlations between laboratory and clinical results, p. 203–209. Antimicrob. Agents Chemother. 1967.
7. **MacLowry, J. D., and H. A. Marsh.** 1968. Semiautomatic microtechnique for serial dilution antibiotic sensitivity testing in the clinical laboratory. J. Lab. Clin. Med. **72**:685–687.
8. **Marymont, J. H., and R. M. Wertz.** 1966. Serial dilution antibiotic sensitivity testing with the microtiter system. Am. J. Clin. Pathol. **45**:548–551.
9. **Moellering, R. C., Jr., A. Weinberg, R. Zimmerman, and C. Wennerstein.** 1970. Antibiotic synergism against group D streptococci. Clin. Res. **18**:445.
10. **Moellering, R. C., Jr., C. Wennerstein, T. Medrek, and A. N. Weinberg.** 1971. Prevalence of high-level resistance to aminoglycosides in clinical isolates of enterococci, p. 335–340. Antimicrob. Agents Chemother. 1970.
11. **Sabath, L. D.** 1968. Synergy of antibacterial substances by apparently known mechanisms, p. 210–217. Antimicrob. Agents Chemother. 1967.
12. **Simon, N.** 1917. Antimicrobial susceptibility of group D hemolytic streptococci. Am. J. Med. Sci. **253**:14–18.
13. **Tilton, R. C., L. Lieberman, and E. H. Gerlach.** 1973. Microdilution antibiotic susceptibility test: examination of certain variables. Appl. Microbiol. **26**:658–665.
14. **Toala, P., A. McDonald, C. Wilcox, et al.** 1969. Susceptibility of group D streptococcus (enterococcus) to 21 antibiotics in vitro, with special references to species differences. Am. J. Med. Sci. **258**:416.
15. **Watanakunakorn, C. P.** 1971. Penicillin combined with gentamicin or streptomycin synergism against enterococci. J. Infect. Dis. **124**:581–596.
16. **Weinstein, L.** 1970. Antibiotics. *In* L. S. Goodman, and A. Gilman (ed.), The pharmacological basis of therapeutics, 4th ed. Macmillan, New York.
17. **Weinstein, A. J., and R. C. Moellering, Jr.** 1973. Penicillin and gentamicin therapy for enterococcal infections. J. Am. Med. Assoc. **223**:1030–1032.
18. **Weinstein, A. J., and R. C. Moellering, Jr.** 1975. Studies of cephalothin: aminoglycoside synergism against enterococci. Antimicrob. Agents. Chemother. **7**:522–529.
19. **Weinstein, L., and J. Schlesinger.** 1973. Treatment of infective endocarditis. Prog. Cardiovasc. Dis. **16**:275–302.
20. **Wilkowske, C. J., R. Facklam, J. A. Washington, and J. E. Geraci.** 1971. Antibiotic synergism: enhanced susceptibility of group D streptococci to certain antibiotic combinations, p. 195–200. Antimicrob. Agents Chemother. 1970.
21. **Zimmerman, R., R. C. Moellering, Jr., and A. N. Weinberg.** 1971. Enterococcal resistance to antibiotic synergism, p. 517–521. Antimicrob. Agents Chemother. 1970.

ANTIMICROBIAL AGENTS AND CHEMOTHERAPY, July 1976, p. 164-172
Vol. 10, No. 1

Acute Diffuse Interstitial Nephritis Related to Chemotherapy of Tuberculosis

WILLIAM J. STONE,* JAMES A. WALDRON, JOHN H. DIXON, JR., R. KIRBY PRIMM, AND ROBERT G. HORN

Departments of Medicine and Pathology, Veterans Administration Hospital, and Vanderbilt University School of Medicine, Nashville, Tennessee 37203*

Received for publication 30 December 1975

Acute renal insufficiency developed in three patients receiving chemotherapy for tuberculosis. It is proposed that acute diffuse interstitial nephritis related to the drugs was responsible for the renal injury. Recovery of renal function was slow and incomplete. Physicians administering chemotherapy to patients with tuberculosis must be aware of the potential nephrotoxicity of the common treatment regimens.

Acute diffuse interstitial nephritis (ADIN) is a distinct clinicopathological entity comprising fever, decreasing renal function, hematuria, proteinuria, peripheral blood eosinophilia, and on histological examination mononuclear and eosinophilic infiltration of the renal interstitium without vasculitis or glomerulonephritis. ADIN usually occurs as a complication of an acute bacterial infection or hypersensitivity reaction to a drug (1, 2, 14). Bacterial infections that have been implicated in the development of ADIN include streptococcal sepsis, syphilis, leptospirosis, diphtheria, and brucellosis (2, 14). A number of drugs have been reported to cause this form of renal injury, most commonly penicillins, sulfonamide antibiotics, and sulfonamide diuretics (1, 10, 14).

ADIN has been reported as a toxic complication of rifampin therapy (4, 8, 12) but has not been commonly attributed to isoniazid, ethambutol, or streptomycin (1, 2, 5, 6, 10, 14). In two of the three cases reported herein, the clinical and, in one, the histopathological picture of ADIN occurred during the course of antituberculous therapy not including rifampin. The third patient was receiving isoniazid and rifampin when ADIN developed. These cases are reported to suggest that this form of renal injury may complicate antituberculous chemotherapy and to alert physicians to the necessity of monitoring renal function in patients being treated for tuberculosis.

CASE REPORTS

First case. A 52-year-old man was admitted to the Nashville Veterans Administration Hospital because of weakness, chills, productive cough, a chest X ray suggestive of cavitary tuberculosis, and a sputum smear positive for acid-fast bacilli. Multiple initial sputum and urine cultures were positive for *Mycobacterium tuberculosis*. A urine analysis was normal, except for three to four leukocytes per high-power field. The serum creatinine was 1.4 mg/100 ml, and an intravenous pyelogram (IVP) was normal soon after admission.

The patient was treated with isoniazid (Kasar Laboratories), ethambutol (Myambutol; Lederle), and streptomycin (Tubex; Wyeth) beginning 8 May 1973. He regained his sense of well-being within 2 weeks of admission. Streptomycin was discontinued after 4 weeks because of vestibular toxicity. Urine cultures obtained on and after day 3 of treatment were negative for *M. tuberculosis*. Sputum cultures remained positive until week 16. The drug therapy is summarized in Table 1.

Renal insufficiency (serum creatinine of 4.8 mg/100 ml) was first noted during week 9 of hospitalization. Examination of the urine revealed 10 to 25 erythrocytes per high-power field, many coarse granular casts, and occasional tubular epithelial cells. Drug therapy at this time consisted of isoniazid, ethambutol, pyridoxine (50 mg daily), and one multiple vitamin capsule daily. No other drugs were being given. Despite the absence of symptoms and physical findings, renal function continued to deteriorate. The creatinine clearance fell from 65 ml/min on day 14 of hospitalization to 11 ml/min on day 97. Hypercalcemia (10.6 to 11.7 mg/100 ml) and peripheral blood eosinophilia were also noted (Fig. 1). The fluctuating eosinophil count may have been related to its computation from the total leukocyte count and the percentage of peripheral eosinophils. Proteinuria of 1 g/24 h was measured on one occasion. An IVP demonstrated no abnormalities except delayed excretion of contrast material. There was no evidence of obstruction and the kidneys were normal in size and contour.

Renal biopsy was performed during week 11. Examination by light microscopy revealed a homogenous pattern of interstitial infiltration by lymphoid cells and eosinophils, increase in intertubular connective tissue, and mild tubular atrophy (Fig. 2). The process was diffuse although more marked in some areas than in others. No areas of calcification were seen. All glomeruli were well preserved and free from lesions. Examination by electron microscopy revealed a predominantly lymphocytic interstitial infiltrate (Fig. 3). Dense deposits were observed within the tubular basement membrane, finely granular in character and consistent with morphological descriptions of immune complex deposits, including those seen in renal tubular disease in humans (3, 7). In some instances, interstitial foci of lymphocytes were found adjacent to tubular basement membrane deposits (Fig. 4). No glomerular abnormalities were seen. Immunofluorescent microscopy demonstrated small granular deposits of complement (C'_3) along the tubular basement membrane. There was no glomerular staining and no evidence of deposition of antitubular basement membrane antibody.

The renal function of the patient slowly returned toward normal, but eosinophilia persisted (Fig. 1). Ethambutol and then isoniazid were discontinued. At the time of discharge, the antituberculous regimen consisted of rifampin and pyrazinamide, the patient felt well, and all cultures were negative for *M. tuberculosis*. However, significant renal insufficiency was still present (serum creatinine of 2.4 mg/100 ml

TABLE 1. *Antituberculous drug therapy*

Drug	Hospital days received	Dosage (g/day)
Case 1		
Ethambutol	1–64	1.6
	65–134	1.2
Isoniazid	1–191	0.3
Streptomycin	1–26	1.0
Rifampin	65–260	0.6
para-Aminosalicylic acid	142–157	6.0–15.0
Pyrazinamide	192–260	1.25–1.5
Case 2		
Ethambutol	1–73	1.2
Isoniazid	1–125	0.3
Streptomycin	1–15	1.0
Rifampin	73–125	0.6
Case 3		
Isoniazid	2–56	0.3
Streptomycin	70–200	0.3
Rifampin	2–58	0.6
Pyrazinamide	129–200	2.0

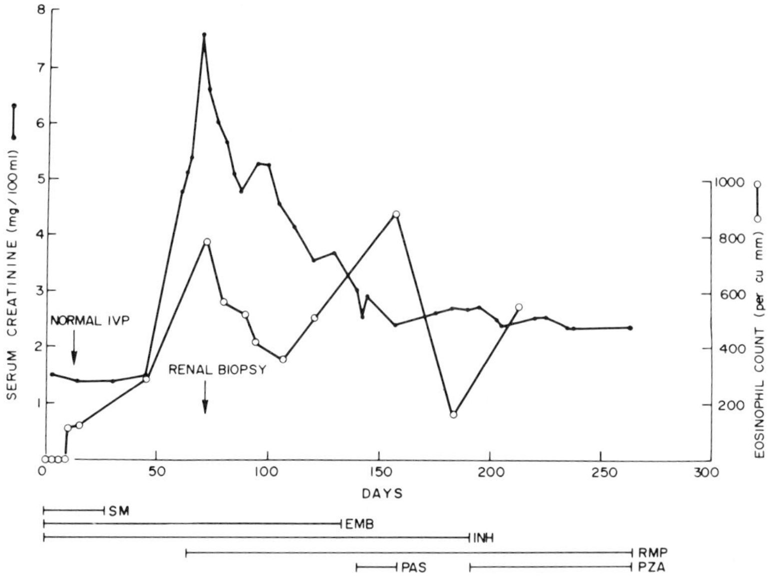

FIG. 1. *Clinical course of the first patient in relation to drugs received. Note the sudden appearance of eosinophilia and renal insufficiency while the patient was being given only isoniazid and ethambutol. SM, Streptomycin; EMB, ethambutol; INH, isoniazid; RMP, rifampin; PAS, para-aminosalicylic acid; PZA, pyrazinamide.*

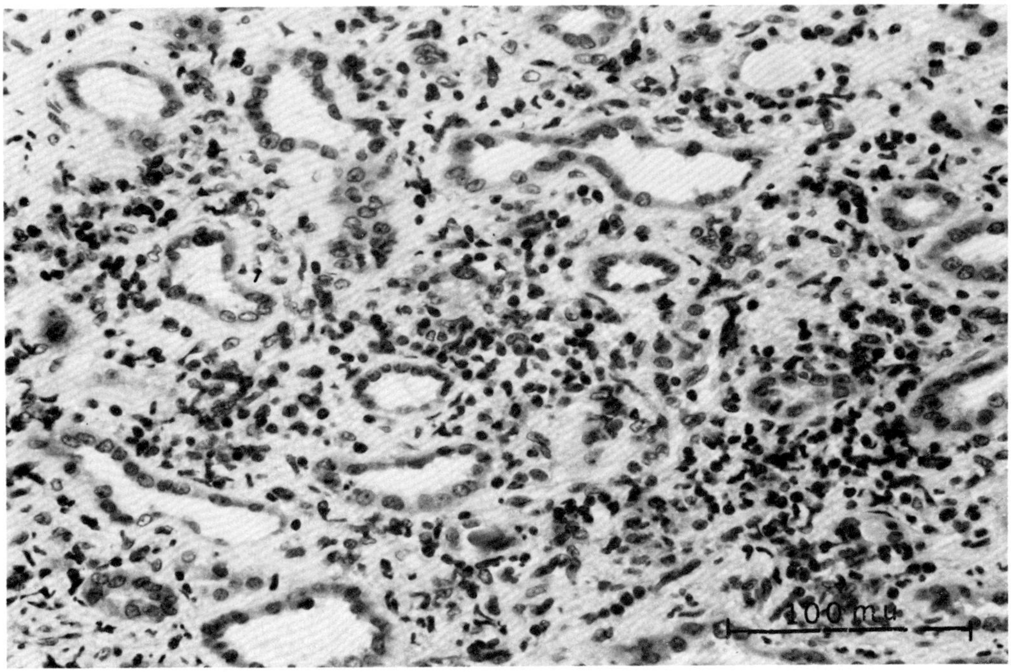

FIG. 2. *Interstitium of the kidney shows moderate fibrosis, a diffuse lymphoid infiltrate, and moderate tubular atrophy. Hematoxylin and eosin stain. ×320.*

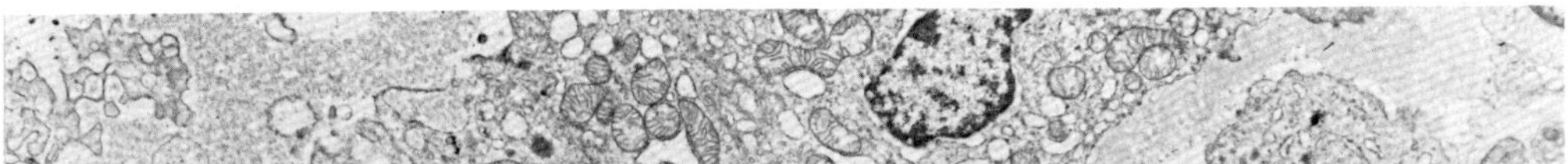

FIG. 3. *Three lymphocytes are present in the interstitium (I), adjacent to the basement membrane (arrows). Uranyl acetate and lead citrate. ×4,600. Ep, Tubular epithelium; L, lymphocytes.*

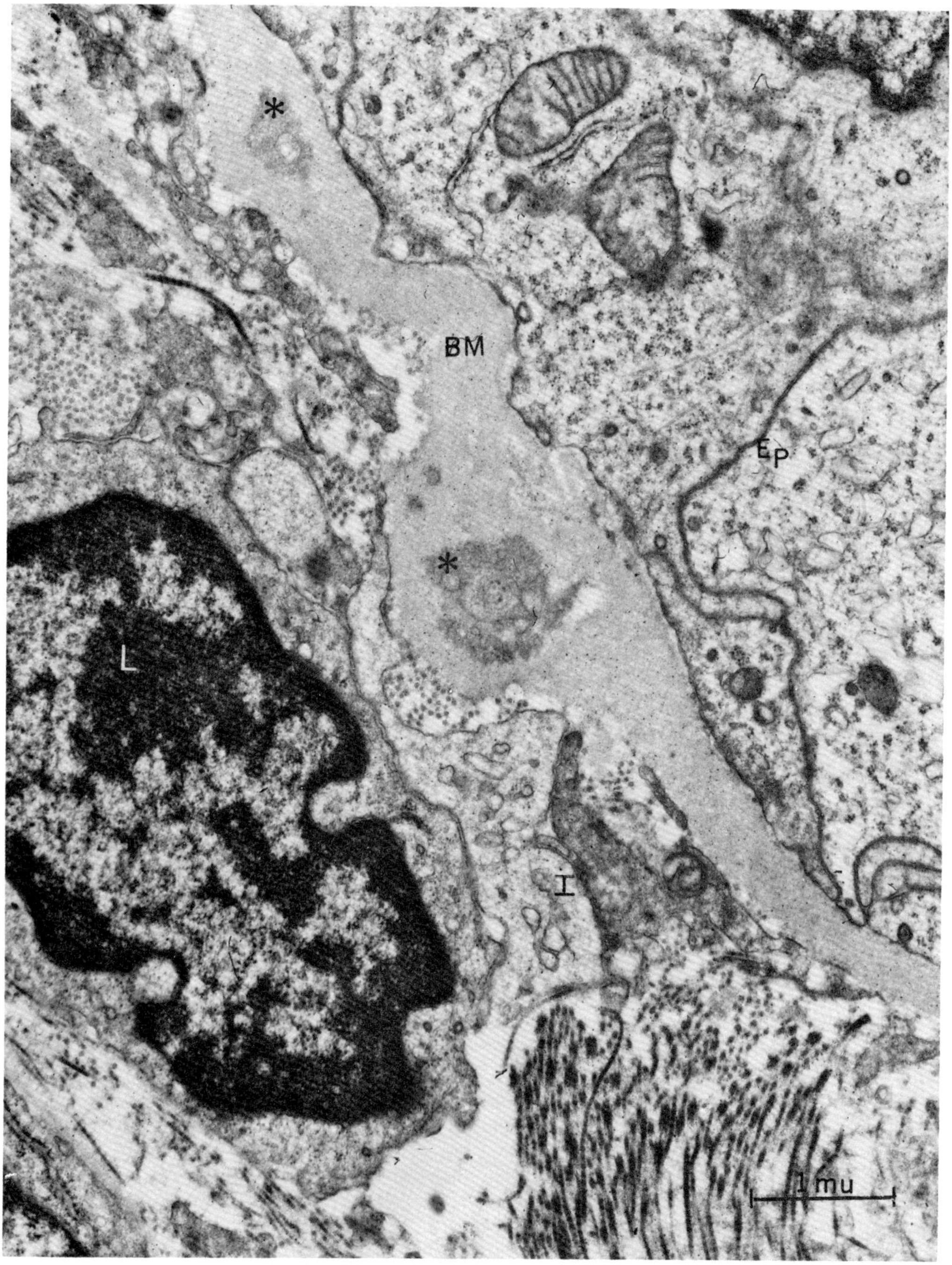

FIG. 4. *Two deposit-like densities (asterisks) are present within the basement membrane (BM) of the tubular epithelium (Ep). A lymphocyte (L) is present in the adjacent interstitium (I). Uranyl acetate and lead citrate. ×19,000.*

and creatinine clearance of 32 ml/min). After 26 months his serum creatinine was 1.9 mg/100 ml.

Comment. This patient developed an acute loss of renal function at a time when he was clinically well and apparently recovering from his tuberculous infection. He had not received streptomycin for 5 weeks when this occurred.

There was no evidence of urinary tract obstruction. Discounting the two vitamin preparations, only ethambutol and/or isoniazid would seem to have been responsible for the renal dysfunction and histological picture of ADIN. Since this relationship had not been hitherto appreciated, the drug regimen was not altered for a significant period of time. This may have resulted in the incomplete recovery of renal function.

Second case. A 56-year-old man was admitted to the Nashville Veterans Administration Hospital because of night sweats, weight loss, dyspnea on exertion, productive cough, and a chest X ray compatible with cavitary tuberculosis. Initial sputum examinations revealed numerous acid-fast bacilli, and sputum cultures were subsequently positive for *M. tuberculosis*. Cultures of urine and bone marrow were negative. Routine analysis of the urine was unremarkable, the serum creatinine was 1.0 mg/100 ml, and the creatinine clearance was 79 ml/min.

Treatment was initiated with streptomycin, isoniazid, and ethambutol on 28 May 1974. The trade names of the drugs used were the same as those in Case 1. Streptomycin was discontinued after 2 weeks, when a skin rash developed. The rash was treated with hydroxyzine hydrochloride (Atarax, Roerig), 25 mg four times daily for 8 days. Sputum cultures remained positive until month 4 of therapy. The drug dosage and duration are listed in Table 1.

The patient was first noted to have developed renal insufficiency (serum creatinine of 6.5 mg/100 ml and creatinine clearance of 16 ml/min) during week 9 of hospitalization. Renal function had not been tested for the 4 preceding weeks. He had not received hydroxyzine hydrochloride for 5 weeks. His drug therapy at this time included ethambutol, isoniazid, pyridoxine hydrochloride (50 mg daily), ferrous sulfate (300 mg thrice daily), and one multiple vitamin capsule daily. No other drugs were being given. Urine analysis showed eight to ten leukocytes and three to four coarse granular casts per high-power field. An IVP showed no significant abnormalities. A mild hypercalcemia (10.9 to 11.3 mg/100 ml) was also noted at this time. A 24-h urine protein excretion was 2.2 g. Peripheral blood eosinophilia and the course of his renal insufficiency are shown in Fig. 5. Since the eosinophil count was computed by multiplying the total leukocyte count by the percentage of eosinophils, the drop in eosinophilia on about day 60 was thought to be insignificant. Permission for renal biopsy was not obtained. Rifampin was substituted for ethambutol during week 11. The hypercalcemia and urinary sedi-

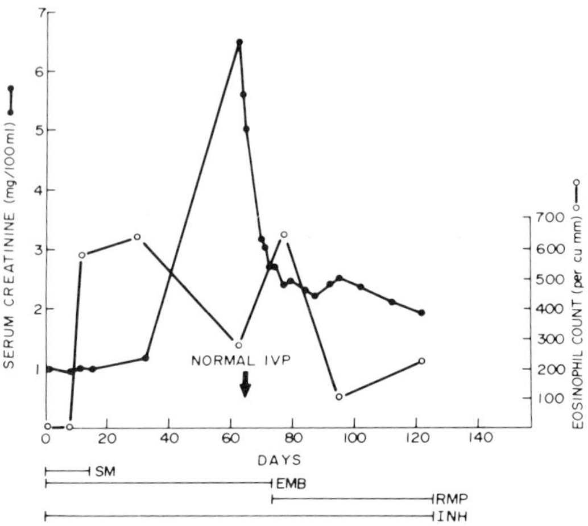

FIG. 5. *Clinical course of the second patient in relation to drugs received. Abbreviations are the same as those in the legend to Fig. 1.*

ment abnormalities gradually disappeared. The patient was discharged to outpatient follow-up of his pulmonary tuberculosis after 18 weeks of hospitalization. The serum creatinine was 1.9 mg/100 ml, and the creatinine clearance was 38 ml/min at discharge. After 17 months his serum creatinine was 1.7 mg/100 ml.

Comment. This patient was almost identical to the one described in the first case report. Unfortunately, he refused to have a renal biopsy. A skin rash antedated the development of acute renal insufficiency as has been seen with methicillin-induced ADIN (1), which further strengthens our contention. Other than vitamins and iron, he was receiving only isoniazid and ethambutol when renal dysfunction appeared, and there was no evidence of urinary tract obstruction at any time. Withdrawal of the drugs probably causing ADIN was delayed, another agent known to cause ADIN (rifampin) was added, and total recovery of renal function did not occur.

Third case. A 56-year-old man was admitted to the Nashville Veterans Administration Hospital because of fever, weight loss, a chest X ray suggestive of miliary tuberculosis, and a positive PPD skin test. Liver biopsy and bone marrow aspirate revealed granulomas and acid-fast bacilli. A sputum smear was also positive for acid-fast bacilli. On day 2 of hospitalization (26 March 1975), treatment was initiated with isoniazid (Kasar Laboratories) and rifampin (Rifadin; Dow) (Table 1 and Fig. 6). Acetaminophen (Tylenol, McNeil) was used as an antipyretic from days 3 through 6 in a dose of 650 mg every 4 h. Sputum cultures remained positive until week 11 of hospitalization. An initial IVP

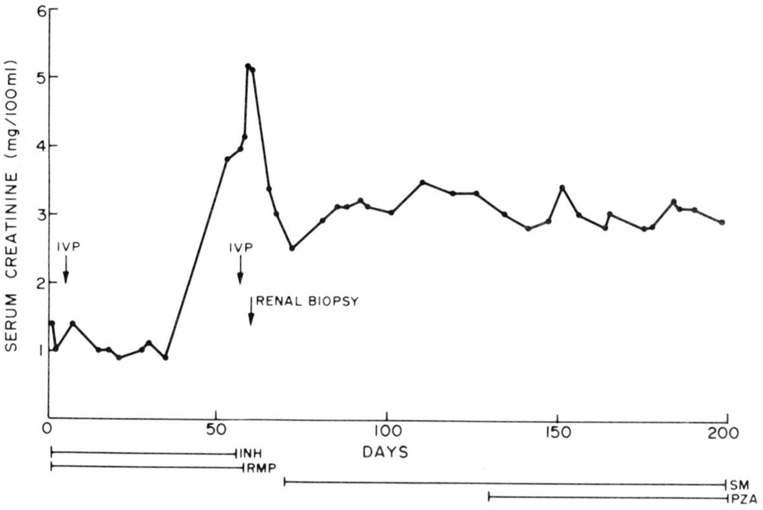

FIG. 6. *Clinical course of the third patient in relation to drugs received. Abbreviations are the same as those in the legend to Fig. 1.*

was normal, except for a minor irregularity of the right upper pole calyx. One urine culture on day 2 was positive for *M. tuberculosis,* but three subsequent urine cultures between days 3 and 50 were negative. On day 8 he was placed on 10 mg of prednisone every 8 h because of constitutional symptoms and high fever, but this had to be discontinued 10 days later because of signs of acute pancreatitis. On day 53 of hospitalization, the creatinine clearance was noted to have decreased from an admission value of 85 to 23 ml/min. Serial serum creatinine determinations are shown in Fig. 6. There was no increased peripheral blood eosinophilia at any time during his course. Glycosuria and hyperchloremic acidosis were transiently present during week 8. Another IVP was unremarkable except for delayed excretion of contrast material. A renal biopsy on day 60 demonstrated a diffuse, heavy infiltrate of inflammatory cells around tubules in both the cortex and medulla (Fig. 7 and 8). Lymphocytes predominated, but many eosinophils and plasma cells were also seen. There was marked interstitial edema with little fibrosis. Glomeruli and blood vessels appeared normal. No granular deposits or linear staining were demonstrated by immunofluorescent studies with antisera to immunoglobulin A (IgA), IgG, IgM, C'_3, and C'_4. No deposits were seen on electron microscopy. All antituberculous therapy was stopped. Other drugs administered prior to this included pyridoxine, aluminum-magnesium hydroxide (Riopan, Maalox, Amphojel), a multiple vitamin capsule, folic acid, and vitamin B_{12}. No other drugs were given. By day 70 his creatinine clearance had improved to 35 ml/min. Streptomycin was begun because of continued fever. Pyrazinamide was added to the regimen on day 129. At about this time an asymptomatic elevation of the serum calcium (11.4 to 13.2 mg/100 ml) was noted but was never well explained. On a low calcium diet and off multiple vitamins (400 U of vitamin D per tablet), this had stabilized at 12 mg/100 ml at the time of discharge on day 205. He was afebrile and was continued on streptomycin, 1 g intramuscularly twice weekly, and pyrazinamide, 1 g twice daily. Recovery of renal function was incomplete (Fig. 6), with creatinine clearances of 30 ml/min at discharge and 37 ml/min 5 months later.

Comment. The chemotherapy this patient received for tuberculosis consisted of only isoniazid and rifampin. He was on no other medications, except vitamins and antacids, when acute loss of renal function occurred. Although rifampin has been reported to cause ADIN (4, 8, 12), this case is included to emphasize the fact that this type of nephrotoxicity can accompany more than one drug regimen for tuberculosis.

DISCUSSION

Renal insufficiency complicating tuberculous infection may be due to (i) advanced parenchymal disease, in which case the intravenous pyelogram is almost always abnormal (15); (ii) obstructive uropathy as a result of urethral cicatrization (implicating drug-induced healing of superficial mucosal lesions); (iii) rarely, streptomycin-induced acute tubular necrosis; and (iv) as mentioned, ADIN complicating drug ther-

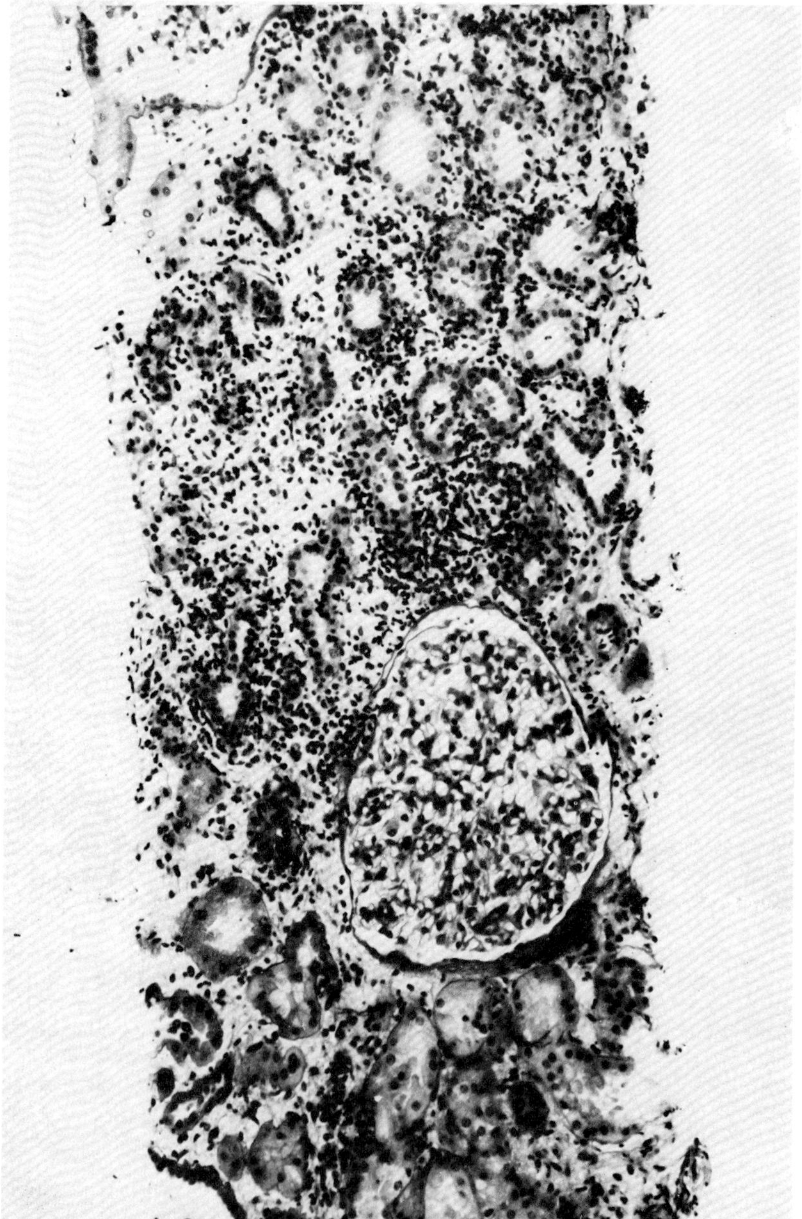

FIG. 7. *Renal interstitium is edematous and heavily infiltrated with lymphoid cells. The glomerulus shows no abnormalities. Periodic acid-Schiff stain. ×160.*

apy. The evidence is substantial against the first three situations in all of the three cases reported herein. The combination of clinical and histological data provides strong support for the presumptive diagnosis of ADIN in all.

As mentioned above, rifampin has been reported to cause ADIN (4, 8, 12), and Rich (13) has attributed one case to streptomycin and isoniazid therapy. In the first two patients reported, it seems unlikely that rifampin could have initiated the process. In these two cases it is possible that streptomycin may have been

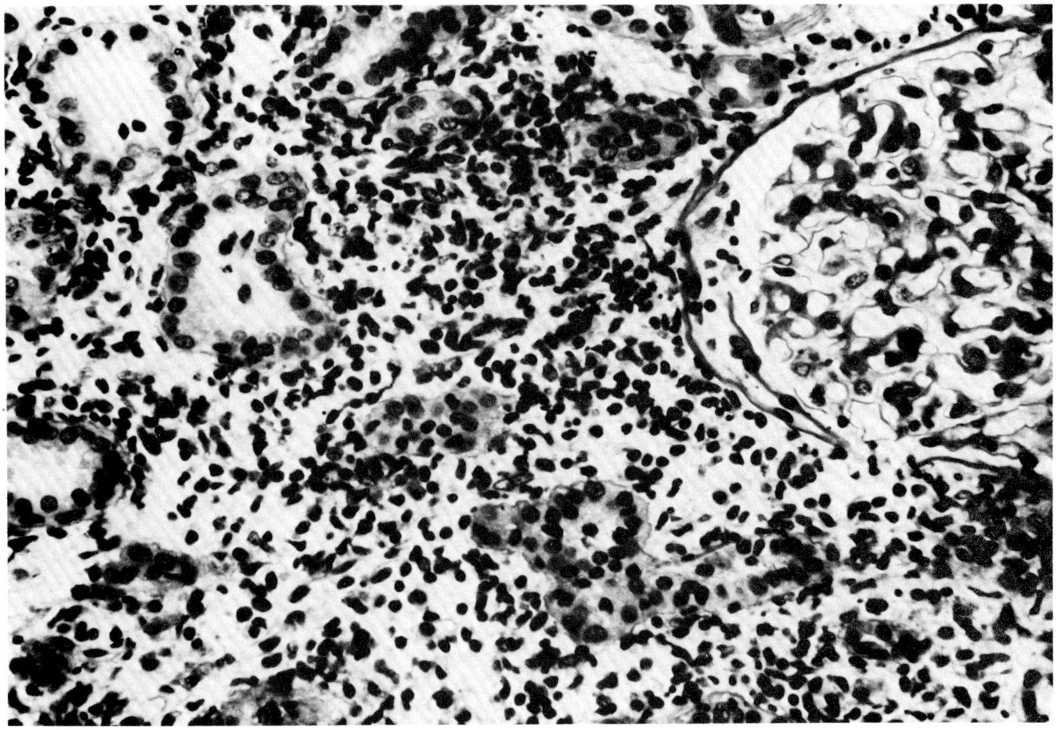

FIG. 8. *A normal glomerulus and marked inflammatory cell infiltration of the interstitium are pictured. Periodic acid-Schiff stain. ×330.*

the responsible agent, although neither patient had received streptomycin for several weeks at the onset of renal insufficiency. However, it is worth emphasis that streptomycin given as a single agent has never been reported to cause ADIN, and, further, neither have any of the related aminoglycoside antibiotics, which, when they are responsible for renal insufficiency, produce the clinical and histological picture of acute tubular necrosis (9, 11).

By elimination it seems reasonable to suggest that isoniazid and/or ethambutol may have produced the observed abnormalities in the first two patients. It is recognized that the evidence presented is only suggestive and by no means conclusive, especially since recovery in these two cases appeared to commence while the agents were still being administered. However, the concept that drug-induced ADIN progresses as long as the offending agent is being administered is itself largely based on circumstantial evidence and is by no means rigorously established, since in almost all instances drugs are discontinued when the diagnosis is made. However, at least one patient with methicillin-induced ADIN demonstrated improvement in renal function while still receiving the drug (1).

ADIN is a more frequent form of renal injury than is commonly recognized by most physicians, is being described as a complication of an increasing number of drugs, and is poorly understood in terms of pathogenesis and natural history. This, together with the frequency with which isoniazid and ethambutol are administered, would seem to justify raising the possibility that these drugs may also cause this serious and potentially irreversible type of renal failure.

LITERATURE CITED

1. **Baldwin, D. S., B. B. Levin, R. T. McCluskey, and G. R. Gallo.** 1968. Renal failure and interstitial nephritis due to penicillin and methicillin. N. Engl. J. Med. **279**:1245–1252.
2. **Chazan, J. S., S. Garella, and A. Esparza.** 1972. Acute interstitial nephritis. A distinct clinicopathologic entity? Nephron **9**:10–26.
3. **Churg, J., and E. Grishman.** 1972. Ultrastructure of immune deposits in renal glomeruli. Ann. Intern. Med. **76**:479–486.
4. **Cordonnier, D., and J. M. Muller.** 1972. Acute renal failure after rifampicin. Lancet **2**:1364–1365.
5. **Goldman, A. L., and S. S. Braman.** 1972. Isoniazid: a review with emphasis on adverse effects. Chest **62**:71–77.
6. **Hoeprich, P. D.** 1972. Antimicrobics and anthelminthics for systemic therapy, p. 177–205. *In* P. D. Hoeprich (ed.), Infectious diseases, 1st ed. Harper & Row, Publishers, Inc., Hagerstown, Md.
7. **Klassen, J., G. A. Andres, J. C. Brennan, and R. T. McCluskey.** 1972. An immunologic renal tubular le-

sion in man. Clin. Immunol. Immunopathol. 1:69–83.

8. **Kleinknecht, D., J. C. Homberg, and G. Decroix.** 1972. Acute renal failure after rifampicin. Lancet 1:1238–1239.
9. **Kovnat, P., E. Labovitz, and S. P. Levison.** 1973. Antibiotics and the kidney. Med. Clin. North Am. 57:1045–1063.
10. **Lyons, H., V. W. Pinn, S. Cortell, J. J. Cohen, and J. J. Harrington.** 1973. Allergic interstitial nephritis causing reversible renal failure in four patients with idiopathic nephrotic syndrome. N. Engl. J. Med. 288:124–128.
11. **McDermott, W.** 1947. Toxicity of streptomycin. Am. J. Med. 2:491–500.
12. **Minetti, L., G. Barbiano di Belgiojoso, G. Civati, A. Durante, F. Ratti, and C. Rovati.** 1974. Drug induced hypersensitivity nephritis. Proc. Eur. Dial. Transplant Assoc. 11:526–532.
13. **Rich, A. R.** 1958. Tissue reactions produced by sensitivity to drugs, p. 196–208. *In* M. L. Rosenheim and R. Moulton (ed.), Sensitivity reactions to drugs. Blackwell Scientific Publications, Oxford.
14. **Simenhoff, M. L., W. R. Guild, and G. J. Dammin.** 1968. Acute diffuse interstitial nephritis. Am. J. Med. 44:618–625.
15. **Wechsler, H.** 1971. Renal tuberculosis, p. 1309-1317. *In* Maurice B. Strauss and Louis G. Welt (ed.), Diseases of the kidney, 2nd ed. Little, Brown and Co., Boston.

ANTIMICROBIAL AGENTS AND CHEMOTHERAPY, July 1976, p. 173-175 Vol. 10, No. 1

Printed in U.S.A.

NOTES

Triple Crossover Study on Absorption and Excretion of Ampicillin, Talampicillin, and Amoxycillin

L. VERBIST

Department of Microbiology, Academisch Ziekenhuis St. Rafaël, University of Leuven, B-3000, Belgium

Received for publication 8 March 1976

Talampicillin and amoxycillin were shown to be absorbed twice as well as ampicillin in a triple crossover experiment.

In recent years a number of ampicillin derivatives have been synthesized that result in higher drug concentrations in serum after oral administration (1-9). A previous triple crossover study showed that equivalent doses of amoxycillin and pivampicillin gave rise to a twofold and threefold increase of drug serum concentrations in serum, respectively, as compared with ampicillin (8).

The present study compares the absorption and excretion of equivalent doses of talampicillin, the phthalidyl ester of ampicillin, and of amoxycillin with a double dose of ampicillin in 10 healthy volunteers in a randomized crossover fashion. Ampicillin (1,000 mg), talampicillin (742 mg), or amoxycillin (500 mg) was administered after an overnight fast, and breakfast was allowed 2 h later. Blood samples were obtained before and at 1, 1.5, 2, 4, and 6 h after drug administration. Urine samples were collected between 0 to 3, 3 to 6, and 6 to 9 h after drug administration. The antibiotic concentrations were determined with an agar well method using *Bacillus subtilis* ATCC 6633 as the test organism. Further details of this method have been described in a previous paper (8).

All samples were stored at −20 C until the series was complete and were assayed in duplicate on the same day. The calculated regression lines of the standards in serum and saline had a correlation coefficient for ampicillin of $r = 0.977$ and $r = 0.999$, respectively, and for amoxycillin of $r = 0.997$ and $r = 0.995$.

The mean drug concentrations in serum are graphically presented in Fig. 1, which indicates that the curves for the three drugs are superimposed, although there is an earlier peak with talampicillin and slightly more persistent levels with ampicillin and amoxycillin.

The average of the individual peak drug concentrations in serum (Table 1) of talampicillin (7.41 μg/ml) and amoxycillin (6.78 μg/ml) were somewhat higher than those obtained after an equivalent double dose of ampicillin (6.20 μg/ml).

The surface of the "area under the curve" was geometrically calculated for each volunteer as previously described (8). Dividing this surface value by the total time in hours resulted in an average drug concentration in serum per hour over a 6-h period. This provided an excellent therapeutic index for comparison since it took into account early as well as late drug concentrations in the serum. These values were found similar for all three drugs, namely, 3.05 μg/ml for ampicillin, 2.62 μg/ml for talampicillin, and 3.06 μg/ml for amoxycillin (Table 1). The mean cumulative quantities of active compounds recovered from urine and expressed as a percentage of the administered dose are shown in Fig. 2. On the average, 41.5% of the ampicillin dose, 65.6% of the talampicillin dose, and 65.7% of the amoxycillin dose were excreted in 9 h. With each antibiotic, at least two-thirds of the excreted dose was recovered during the first 3 h, and more than 98% was recovered within 6 h.

Similar results have been obtained with amoxycillin in a previous study, namely, a mean peak drug concentration in serum of 8.3 μg/ml, an average serum level per hour of 3.1 μg/ml, and a urinary recovery of 64.2% (8). However, the urinary recovery of ampicillin (41.5% of a 1,000-mg dose) in this study was nearly twice as high as in the previous study (21.8% of a 500-mg dose). Since the major difference between both studies was the delay between drug administration and breakfast (30 min in the first study, 2 h in the present study), it may be concluded that food intake had a major adverse influence on the absorption of ampicillin but not on amoxycillin.

The differences in absorption between the three antibiotics can be evaluated on the basis

TABLE 1. *Drug concentrations in serum and recovery in urine*

Drug	Peak concn in serum (μg/ml)			Avg concn in serum/h (μg/ml)			Recovery (%) in urine (0 to 9 h)		
	Mean	SD[a]	V	Mean	SD	V	Mean	SD	V
Ampicillin (1,000 mg)	6.20 (3.3–10.7)[b]	2.57	0.41	3.05 (2.0–5.1)	1.07	0.35	41.5 (23.2–68.1)	15.1	0.36
Talampicillin (742 mg)[c]	7.41 (5.2–10.1)	1.59	0.21	2.62 (1.9–3.6)	0.55	0.21	65.5 (56.5–76.3)	6.4	0.10
Amoxycillin (500 mg)	6.78 (4.2–10.1)	1.94	0.29	3.06 (2.2–4.4)	0.67	0.22	65.7 (40.9–93.9)	14.5	0.22

[a] SD, Standard deviation; V = standard deviation/mean, dispersion coefficient.
[b] Extreme values are given in parentheses.
[c] Equivalent to 500 mg of ampicillin.

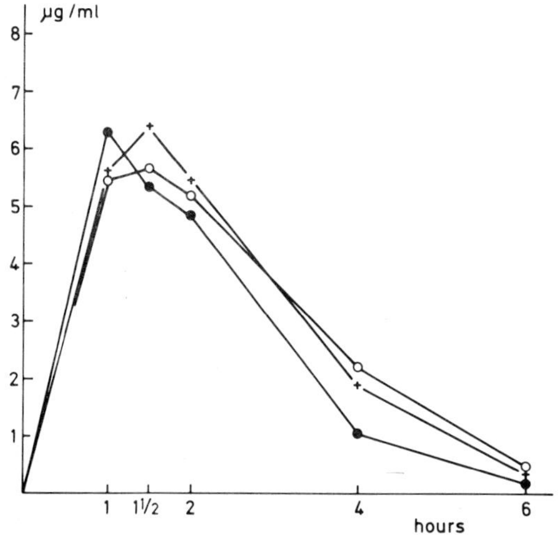

FIG. 1. *Mean drug concentrations in serum after oral administration of: (○) ampicillin, 1,000 mg; (+) amoxycillin, 500 mg; (●) talampicillin, 742 mg (equivalent to 500 mg of ampicillin).*

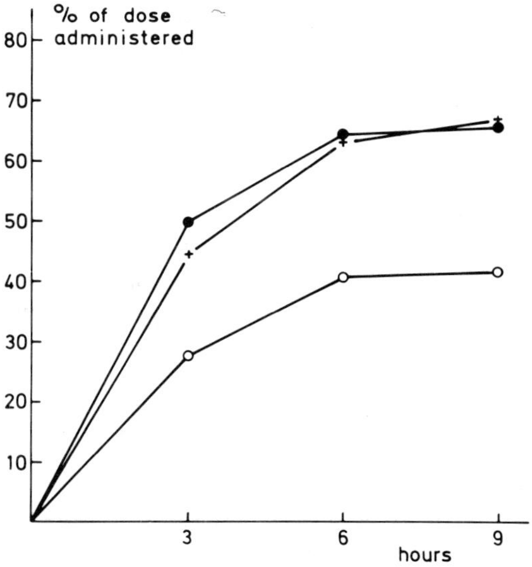

FIG. 2. *Cumulative renal excretion of active compounds after oral administration of: (○) ampicillin, 1,000 mg; (+) amoxycillin, 500 mg; (●) talampicillin, 742 mg (equivalent to 500 mg of ampicillin).*

of three main criteria: the average of the individual peak serum levels, the average serum level per hour over a 6-h period, and the percentage of recovery of active compounds in urine within 9 h (Table 1). From these data it is obvious that talampicillin and amoxycillin are absorbed twice as well as ampicillin since half the equivalent dose provides approximately the same antimicrobial activity in serum.

The degree of uniformity of individual data within the same group of subjects is best expressed by the dispersion coefficient, calculated by the formula V = standard deviation/mean: the smaller this dispersion coefficient, the less variability within the values of the individuals. As measured on the dispersion coefficient of all three criteria, the uniformity was highest with talampicillin and lowest with ampicillin. This greater uniformity in absorption of amoxycillin, and especially of talampicillin, over ampicillin is a further advantage of these antibiotics with regard to the reliability of an oral chemotherapy.

This investigation has been supported by a grant from Continental Pharma.

The technical assistance of Claire Van Ourti is gratefully acknowledged.

LITERATURE CITED

1. **Bodey, G. P., and J. Nance.** 1972. Amoxycillin: in vitro and pharmacological studies. Antimicrob. Agents Chemother. 1:358–362.
2. **Clayton, J. P., M. Cole, S. W. Elson, and H. Ferres.** 1974. BRL.8988 (talampicillin), a well-absorbed oral form of ampicillin. Antimicrob. Agents Chemother. 5:670–671.
3. **Croydon, E. A. P., and R. Sutherland.** 1971. α-Amino-*p*-hydroxybenzylpenicillin (BRL 2333), a new semisynthetic penicillin: absorption and excretion in man, p. 427–430. Antimicrob. Agents Chemother. 1970.
4. **Foltz, E. L., J. W. West, I. H. Breslow, and H. Wallick.** 1971. Clinical pharmacology of pivampicillin, p.

442–454. Antimicrob. Agents Chemother. 1970.
5. **Jordan, M. C., J. B. de Maine, and W. M. M. Kirby.** 1971. Clinical pharmacology of pivampicillin as compared with ampicillin, p. 438–444. Antimicrob. Agents Chemother. 1970.
6. **Neu, H. C., and E. B. Winshell.** 1971. Pharmacological studies of 6[D(−)α-amino-*p*-hydroxyphenylacetamido]penicillanic acid in humans, p. 423–426. Antimicrob. Agents Chemother. 1970.
7. **Sutherland, R., and G. N. Robinson.** 1971. α-Amino-*p*-hydroxybenzylpenicillin (BRL 2333), a new semisynthetic penicillin: in vitro evaluation, p. 411–415. Antimicrob. Agents Chemother. 1970.
8. **Verbist, L.** 1974. Triple crossover study on absorption and excretion of ampicillin, pivampicillin, and amoxycillin. Antimicrob. Agents Chemother. 6:588–593.
9. **von Daehne, W., W. O. Godtfredsen, K. Roholt, and L. Tybring.** 1971. Pivampicillin, a new orally active ampicillin ester, p. 431–437. Antimicrob. Agents Chemother. 1970.

ANTIMICROBIAL AGENTS AND CHEMOTHERAPY, July 1976, p. 176-178 Vol. 10, No. 1
 Printed in U.S.A.

Photoinactivation of Venezuelan Equine Encephalitis Virus Mediated by Tetracyclines

JOSE ESPARZA,* CARMEN I. PIÑA, AND ERNESTO NOVO

Instituto Venezolano de Investigaciones Científicas, Centro de Microbiología y Biología Celular, Apartado 1827, Caracas, Venezuela

Received for publication 1 March 1976

Demethylchlortetracycline and, to a lesser extent, chlortetracycline were found to mediate the in vitro photoinactivation of Venezuelan equine encephalitis virus.

Viruses can be rendered sensitive to visible light when treated with dyes such as acridine orange, proflavine, neutral red, and others (11). Dyes bind to the virus nucleic acid, acting as light absorbers for photochemical reactions in which molecular oxygen takes part, resulting in the inactivation of nucleic acid infectivity (6, 9). Phenomena of photosensitization have been described in a variety of biological systems, including drug-induced photosensitivity in humans (7). Treatment with the antibiotic demethylchlortetracycline (DMCT) results in a high frequency of sun-induced reactions, manifested as exaggerated sunburn-type lesions, which disappear soon after discontinuation of the drug (3, 8). Phototoxicity of DMCT has also been demonstrated using tissue culture techniques (5). The ability of DMCT and other tetracyclines to induce photosensitization in Venezuelan equine encephalitis virus is described in this report.

Vero cells, maintained in disposable tissue culture flasks (Falcon Plastics, Oxnard, Calif.), were inoculated with Venezuelan equine encephalitis virus, using a multiplicity of infection of 0.1 plaque-forming unit/cell. The virus used was the TC-83 strain, subjected in our laboratory to several passages in different cell lines. After a 1-h absorption at 37 C, infected cultures were washed once with phosphate-buffered saline. Cells were maintained in Eagle medium with a double concentration of vitamins and amino acids, 2% lactalbumin hydrolysate, 0.66% yeast extract, 0.16% sodium bicarbonate, 1.4% ovalbumin (fraction V), 100 U of penicillin per ml, 100 μg of streptomycin per ml, and 2.5 μg of amphotericin B per ml (2). In some experiments, DMCT (no. 48151, lot 338; a gift of Cyanamid de Venezuela, Caracas) was added to the maintainance medium to a final concentration of 1, 10, 50, or 100 μg/ml. After the addition of the drug, all handling of the cultures was done in the dark.

Infected cultures were incubated at 37 C through 72 h postinfection and harvested by one cycle of freezing and thawing. Suspensions were centrifuged at 2,000 rpm for 15 min, and 1-ml aliquots of supernatant fluid were dispensed into glass test tubes. Samples were exposed 10 cm from three "daylight-type" fluorescent lighting tubes (15 W each), giving a total of 5,000 lx of illumination. After light exposure for 30, 60, or 90 min, samples were immediately assayed in Vero cells by a plaque formation method using an agarose-containing, serum-free overlay (2).

Concentrations of DMCT up to 50 μg/ml present in the maintainance medium were nontoxic for the cells and resulted in normal virus yields. A concentration of 100 μg/ml induced a cytopathic effect in uninfected cultures and resulted in a 10-fold decrease in the yield of infectious virus. When virus grown in the presence of 1 to 10 μg of DMCT per ml was exposed to light, no significant inactivation of infectivity was observed. However, virus grown in the presence of 50 or 100 μg of DMCT per ml was readily inactivated by visible light (Fig. 1A). After 90 min of light exposure, a drop in the infectivity titer of 4 to 6 logs was observed when using 50 and 100 μg of DMCT per ml, respectively. Virus grown in the absence of DMCT expressed a slight decrease in titer, probably due to an intrinsic photosensitivity of the virus or to photosensitizing agents present in tissue culture medium (1). Control suspensions, containing virus grown in the presence of DMCT but not exposed to light, were not inactivated.

Virus grown in the absence of DMCT and mixed with the drug immediately prior to light exposure was also found to become photosensitive (Fig. 1B), being inactivated at a rate comparable to that observed with virus grown in the presence of the drug.

The ability of other tetracyclines to induce photosensitization was studied by mixing the

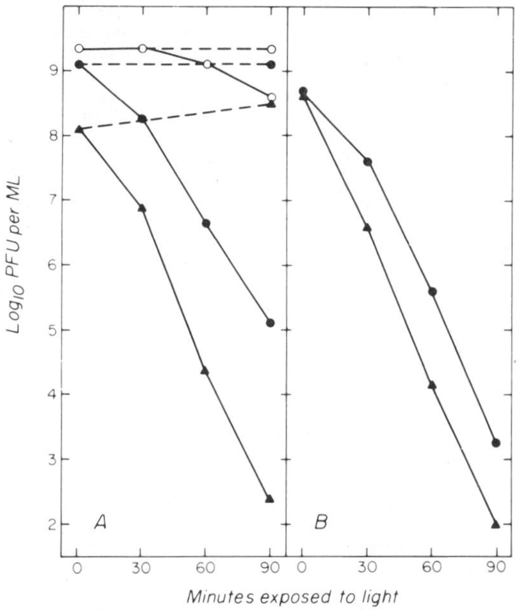

FIG. 1. *Photosensitization of Venezuelan equine encephalitis (VEE) virus by DMCT. (A) Photoinactivation of VEE virus grown in the presence of DMCT. (B) Photoinactivation of VEE virus grown in the absence of DMCT and mixed with the drug immediately prior to light exposure. Symbols: ○, no DMCT; ●, 50 μg of DMCT per ml; ▲, 100 μg of DMCT per ml. Solid lines represent samples exposed to light; broken lines represent samples kept in the dark.*

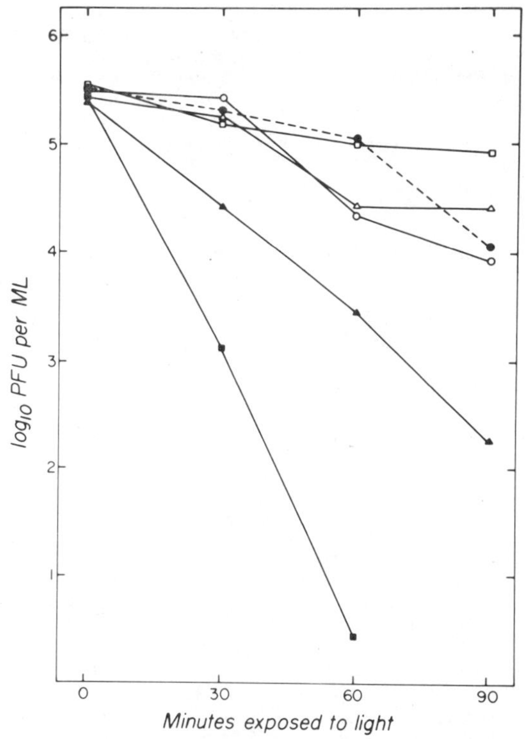

FIG. 2. *Photosensitization of Venezuelan equine encephalitis virus by different tetracyclines. Symbols: ●, control; □, oxytetracycline; △, tetracycline hydrochloride; ○, tetracycline crystalline; ▲, chlortetracycline; ■, DMCT.*

virus with the drugs at a final concentration of 100 μg/ml and exposing to light as described. Besides DMCT, only chlortetracycline was found to mediate virus photoinactivation, but at a slower rate than DMCT (Fig. 2).

The experiments described indicated that DMCT and, to a lesser extent, chlortetracycline act as sensitizer agents in the in vitro photoinactivation of Venezuelan equine encephalitis virus. The mechanism(s) of photoinactivation of Venezuelan equine encephalitis virus by tetracyclines is not known at present. The site of action of the drug remains to be established: the ability of DMCT and chlortetracycline to induce photosensitization when virus and drug are mixed in vitro seems to indicate that the possible site(s) of action could be exposed in the viral envelope or, alternatively, that the drug could penetrate through the envelope and capsid to bind an active site in the virus ribonucleic acid.

In this regard, it is interesting to note that it has recently been reported that chlortetracycline sensitizes tobacco mosaic virus ribonucleic acid to near- and middle-ultraviolet light (10).

The demonstration of tetracycline-induced virus photosensitization suggests that this biologically simple system could be used in the study of the mechanisms of drug-induced phototoxicity. It should be pointed out that photoreactive dyes are now being used in clinical medicine for the treatment of surface viral infections (4).

LITERATURE CITED

1. **Appleyard, G.** 1967. The photosensitivity of Semliki Forest and other viruses. J. Gen. Virol. 1:143–152.
2. **Bergold, G. H., and R. Mazzali.** 1968. Plaque formation by arboviruses. J. Gen. Virol. 2:273–284.
3. **Blank, H., S. I. Cullen, and P. M. Catalano.** 1968. Photosensitivity studies with Demethylchlortetracycline and Doxycycline. Arch. Dermatol. 97:1–2.
4. **Felber, T. D., E. B. Smith, J. M. Knox, C. Wallis, and J. L. Melnick.** 1973. Photodynamic inactivation of Herpes simplex. Report of a clinical trial. J. Am. Med. Assoc. **223**:289–292.
5. **Freeman, R. G., W. Murtishaw, and J. M. Knox.** 1970. Tissue culture techniques in the study of cell photobiology and phototoxicity. J. Invest. Dermatol. **54**:164–169.
6. **Fukunaga, T., N. Ishikawa, A. Igarashi, and K. Fukai.** 1967. Photodynamic inactivation of Japanese Encephalitis virus. Biken J. **10**:1–9.
7. **Harber, L. C., and R. L. Baer.** 1972. Pathogenic mechanisms of drug-induced photosensitivity. J. Invest. Dermatol. **58**:327–342.

8. **Harber, L. C., T. A. Tromovitch, and R. L. Baer.** 1961. Studies on photosensitivity due to Demethylchlortetracycline. J. Invest. Dermatol. 37:189–193.
9. **Hiatt, C. W., E. Kaufman, J. J. Helprin, and S. Baron.** 1960. Inactivation of viruses by photodynamic action of Toluidine blue. J. Immunol. 84:480–484.
10. **Murphy, T. M.** 1975. Inactivation of Tobacco Mosaic virus ribonucleic acid by near- and middle-ultraviolet light: sensitization by sulfanilamide and chlortetracycline. Biochem. Biophys. Res. Commun. 65:1108–1114.
11. **Wallis, C., and J. L. Melnick.** 1965. Photodynamic inactivation of animal viruses: a review. Photochem. Photobiol. 4:159–170.

ANTIMICROBIAL AGENTS AND CHEMOTHERAPY, July 1976, p. 179–181 Vol. 10, No. 1

Absence of Penicillin-Degrading Enzymes in Penicillin-Resistant Strains of *Neisseria gonorrhoeae*

J. L. BEEBE,[1]* P. LIGETI, AND T. J. WLODKOWSKI

Department of Microbiology, Cornell University Medical College, New York, New York 10021

Received for publication 16 March 1976

Penicillin-resistant and -susceptible strains of *Neisseria gonorrhoeae* were evaluated for the presence of enzymes capable of degrading penicillin by incubation of [^{14}C]benzylpenicillin with resting-cell suspensions of *N. gonorrhoeae* followed by extraction and chromatography of the labeled antibiotic. No degradative activity was observed.

The current investigations of penicillin resistance in *Neisseria gonorrhoeae* have not resulted in any reports of a penicillinase or beta-lactamase. Engelkirk and Schoenhard (2) presented physical evidence for a plasmid, a common site of resistance determinants in other bacteria. In addition, a number of reports have appeared that present data suggesting that resistance to penicillin, streptomycin, tetracycline, and spectinomycin, which is frequently observed in clinical isolates of *N. gonorrhoeae*, is multigenic in origin and primarily associated with chromosomal genetic determinants (4–7, 10).

Rodriguez and Saz (9) examined whole cells and osmotically shocked cells for presence of a beta-lactamase. They used a microiodometric enzyme assay for the beta-lactamase and attempted to detect the product of a possible amidase by infrared spectroscopy. They failed to detect either enzyme in resistant strains of *N. gonorrhoeae*.

In this report we describe an examination of penicillin-resistant and -susceptible strains of *N. gonorrhoeae* by a technique that allows the detection of a beta-lactamase, an amidase, or virtually any other enzyme capable of catalytically degrading the penicillin molecule. The method uses whole cells and minimizes some of the negative aspects of the largely arbitrary selection of the parameters of pH, ionic strength, substrate concentration, and method of enzyme preparation, which accompany in vitro enzyme determinations, and may enhance the likelihood of detection of some of the aforementioned enzymes.

Table 1 shows the minimal inhibitory concentrations for a number of antibiotics of the strains of *N. gonorrhoeae* chosen for this study. Minimal inhibitory concentrations were determined by the plate dilution technique according to the procedure described by Gavin et al. (3) and using a Steers replicator (12).

Inocula for experiments were prepared by growth of *N. gonorrhoeae* on GC medium-base agar with hemoglobin and 1% supplement B (Difco) for 18 to 24 h at 35 C in a candle jar, followed by inoculation into a medium of the following composition: proteose peptone no. 3 (Difco), 15 g; K_2HPO_4, 0.4 g; KH_2PO_4, 0.1 g; soluble starch, 0.1 g; NaCl, 5 g; and distilled water, 1,000 ml. To this medium was added 10 ml of supplement B or IsoVitaleX enrichment (BBL) per liter after autoclaving. Inoculated medium, 100 ml in 250-ml flasks, was incubated at 35 C in a water bath shaker at 90 oscillations/min for 12 to 18 h. Experiments were initiated by harvest of liquid culture-grown cells by centrifugation, resuspension in fresh liquid medium to an optical density at 600 nm of 0.15, and inoculation of a flask of fresh medium at a rate of 5 ml/100 ml of medium. After 2 h of shaking at 35 C, penicillin G, potassium salt (Pfizer), was added to a final concentration of 0.05 μg/ml for susceptible strains (005 and 009) and 0.5 μg/ml for the resistant strains (F19 and 62168M). No untoward effect on cell growth was observed with the addition of inducer penicillin at these concentrations. Incubation was continued for an additional 2 h, after which the cells were harvested by centrifugation at 1,300 $\times g$ for 10 min. The cell pellets were washed twice in normal saline, or were not washed, and resuspended in (i) 0.1 M potassium phosphate buffer, pH 7.0, (ii) 0.1 M tris(hydroxymethyl)-aminomethane buffer, pH 7.0, or (iii) liquid medium without added supplement to an optical density of 0.3 to 0.35. [^{14}C]benzylpenicillin, potassium salt (specific activity, 54 μCi/μmol; Amersham/Searle), dissolved in distilled water at 50 μCi/ml, was added to a 50-ml cell suspension after an additional 2 to 4 h of incubation. The mixtures were incubated at room temperature and 30 C for periods up to 3 h. The label

[1] Present address: Clinical Microbiology Service, Columbia-Presbyterian Medical Center, New York, N.Y. 10032.

TABLE 1. *Minimal inhibitory concentrations (MIC) of N. gonorrhoeae strains*

Antibiotic	MIC (μg/ml)			
	005	009	F19	62168M
Penicillin G	0.02	0.02	1.66	1.8
Ampicillin	0.02	0.02	0.40	0.63
Nafcillin	0.31	0.63	5.0	5.0
Penicillin V	0.02	0.16	5.0	5.0
Cloxacillin	0.12	0.08	10.0	10.0
Oxacillin	0.02	0.04	10.0	
Methicillin	0.05	0.04	10.0	10.0
Cephalothin	0.12	0.24	5.0	5.0
Cephaloridine	1.25	0.8	10.0	10.0
Erythromycin	0.08	0.31	0.8	0.24
Tetracycline	0.16	0.31	0.8	1.8
Streptomycin	7.5	10.0	10.0	10.0
Chloramphenicol	0.63	0.24	0.8	3.75

was then extracted with methylisobutyl ketone according to the procedure of Preuss and Johnson (8). Most of the cells were removed by a brief centrifugation. Ammonium sulfate was added to 80% saturation to the supernatant. The pH of the solution was lowered to 5.5 by dropwise addition of dilute HCl and then extracted three times in a counter-current fashion with methylisobutyl ketone. The solvent phases were pooled and reduced under high vacuum at 40 C to a small volume. The efficiency of recovery of label was approximately 85%, the balance of the label remaining unrecovered in cells and separation interphases.

Controls included (i) uninoculated medium containing penicillinase (BBL) at 4,000 U/ml and (ii) uninoculated medium, both of which contained labeled penicillin at 1 μCi/ml and were incubated and extracted in a manner identical to that of the cell suspensions.

Extracts were chromatographed on Silica Gel G thin-layer plates (250 μm; 20 by 20 cm, Analtech) in a single dimension in an ascending fashion. Solvent systems used were (i) acetone-glacial acetic acid, 19:1 (vol/vol), (ii) *n*-butanol-glacial acetic acid-water, 60:20:20 (vol/vol/vol), and (iii) methanol-isopropanol, 7:3 (vol/vol) (11). Developed chromatograms were dried and exposed to Kodak RP14 X-ray film for 24 h to 3 weeks. Table 2 shows the chromatographic mobilities of benzylpenicillin and its derivatives and those of the labeled penicillin after incubation with resting-cell suspensions of the various strains of *N. gonorrhoeae* and the controls. The integrity of the labeled penicillin was verified by co-chromatography with unlabeled penicillin, which was visualized on chromatographs by sulfuric acid charring (1). Use of either phosphate or tris(hydroxymethyl)aminomethane buffers for cell suspensions resulted in progressive autolysis of cells during subsequent incubation periods, and these buffers were not used further. Washing had no effect manifest in the results of these experiments. Resting-cell suspensions in unsupplemented liquid medium exhibited no striking change in appearance or optical density for up to 6 h of incubation. The activity of 1 U of penicillinase can be detected by a 48-h radioautographic exposure. Less activity can be detected by longer exposures or liquid scintillation counting of chromatograph fractions.

TABLE 2. *Chromatographic mobility of benzylpenicillin G and degradation products*

Antibiotic	R_f[a]		
	AA	BAW	MIP
Benzylpenicillin G (Pen G)	0.96	0.74	0.83
Benzylpenicilloic acid	0.95	0.57	0.76
6-Aminopenicillanic acid	–[b]	0.20[c]	–
Phenylacetic acid	–	0.95[c]	–
PenG + penicillinase	0.96	0.74, 0.57	0.83, 0.76
PenG + medium	0.96	0.74	0.83
PenG + strain 005	0.96	0.74	0.83
PenG + strain 009	0.96	0.74	0.83
PenG + strain F19	0.96	0.74	0.83
PenG + strain 62168M	0.96	0.74	0.83

[a] Solvent systems: AA, acetone-glacial acetic acid, 19:1 (vol/vol); BAW, *n*-butanol-glacial acetic acid-water, 60:20:20 (vol/vol/vol); MIP, methanol-isopropanol, 7:3 (vol/vol).

[b] –, Not useful for this separation.

[c] Values are from Stahl (11).

The results show that [^{14}C]benzylpenicillin may be incubated with resting-cell suspensions of penicillin-resistant and -susceptible strains of *N. gonorrhoeae* and then reextracted without chromatographically detectable alteration. The activity of an amidase would enzymatically cleave the aromatic phenylacetate moiety of the labeled penicillin, resulting in the appearance of a highly mobile entity on chromatograms. The activity of a beta-lactamase would result in the appearance of benzylpenicilloic acid, a compound with an R_f significantly different from benzylpenicillin in two of the three chromatographic systems used. Evidence for these degradation products was not observed even after prolonged exposures of the chromatographs to X-ray film.

This data and that of Rodriguez and Saz (9) indicate that penicillin resistance does not involve production of an enzyme capable of degrading this antibiotic.

This investigation was supported by New York City Health Research Council Grant U-2462.

We are grateful to Bristol Laboratories, Abbot Laboratories, Sterling Drug, Inc., Wyeth Laboratories, American Cyanamid, Eli Lilly & Co., Inc., and Pfizer, Inc. for the samples of the antibiotics used in this study, and to R. Weaver of the Center for Disease Control for the penicillin-resistant strains of *N. gonorrhoeae*. The technical assistance of Margret Yamamoto is gratefully acknowledged.

LITERATURE CITED

1. **Ansell, G. B., and J. N. Hawthorne.** 1964. Phospholipids – chemistry, metabolism and function, p. 411–419. Elsevier Publishing Co., Amsterdam.
2. **Engelkirk, P. G., and D. E. Schoenhard.** 1973. Physical evidence of a plasmid in *Neisseria gonorrhoeae*. J. Infect. Dis. **127**:197–200.
3. **Gavan, T. L., E. L. Cheatle and H. W. McFadden, Jr.** 1971. Antimicrobial susceptibility testing. American Society for Clinical Pathology, Chicago.
4. **Maier, T. W., H. R. Beilstein, and L. Zubrzycki.** 1974. Multiple antibiotic resistance in *Neisseria gonorrhoeae*. Antimicrob. Agents Chemother. **6**:22–28.
5. **Maier, T. W., L. Zubrzycki, M. B. Coyle, M. Chila, and P. Warner.** 1975. Genetic analysis of drug resistance in *Neisseria gonorrhoeae:* production of increased resistance by the combination of two antibiotic resistance loci. J. Bacteriol. **124**:834–842.
6. **Maness, M. J., G. C. Foster, and P. F. Sparling.** 1974. Ribosomal resistance to streptomycin and spectinomycin in *Neisseria gonorrhoeae*. J. Bacteriol. **120**:1293–1299.
7. **Maness, M. J., and P. F. Sparling.** 1973. Multiple antibiotic resistance due to a single mutation in *Neisseria gonorrhoeae*. J. Infect. Dis. **128**:321–330.
8. **Pruess, D. L., and M. J. Johnson.** 1965. Enzymatic deacylation of ^{35}S-benzylpenicillin. J. Bacteriol. **90**:380–383.
9. **Rodriguez, W., and A. K. Saz.** 1975. Possible mechanisms of decreased susceptibility of *Neisseria gonorrhoeae* to penicillin. Antimicrob. Agents Chemother. **7**:788–792.
10. **Sparling, P. F., F. A. Sarubbi, Jr., and E. Blackman.** 1975. Inheritance of low-level resistance to penicillin, tetracycline, and chloramphenicol in *Neisseria gonorrhoeae*. J. Bacteriol. **124**:740–749.
11. **Stahl, E. (ed.).** 1965. Thin layer chromatography. Academic Press Inc., New York.
12. **Steers, E., F. Foltz, B. S. Graves, and J. Riden.** 1959. An inocula replicating apparatus for routine testing of bacterial susceptibility to antibiotics. Antiobiot. Chemother. **9**:307–311.

ANTIMICROBIAL AGENTS AND CHEMOTHERAPY, July 1976, p. 182-184 Vol. 10, No. 1

Nalidixic Acid Inhibition of Post-Ultraviolet Recovery in *Escherichia coli* K-12: Requirement for *recBC* Function

MICHAEL A. PURDY* AND K. LEMONE YIELDING

Laboratory of Molecular Biology, University of Alabama, Birmingham, Alabama 35294

Received for publication 10 February 1976

Various repair-deficient mutants of *Escherichia coli* K-12 were tested for the impairment of post-ultraviolet survival by nalidixic acid. These studies have shown that the target of this nalidixic acid effect is dictated by the *recB* and *recC* genes and may be due to the binding of nalidixic acid to exonuclease V. Furthermore, this effect cannot be correlated with either recombination proficiency or excision repair alone.

Although nalidixic acid inhibits deoxyribonucleic acid (DNA) synthesis, it has no effect on purified DNA enzymes (2, 5, 10) and differs from many other inhibitors in that it apparently does not bind to DNA (1). Early studies suggested that the drug interfered with assembly of large DNA from smaller DNA fragments (4), but recent experiments have emphasized that synthesis is blocked only at the growing fork (11).

We reported that non-bactericidal levels of nalidixic acid decreased post-ultraviolet (post-UV) survival in *Escherichia coli* B, TAU-bar, and ts-7 and increased the temperature sensitivity of ts-7 (8). The finding that photoreactivation abolished the post-UV effect of nalidixic acid (9) clearly implicated pyrimidine dimers in the impairment of survival, but the liquid-holding recovery was not inhibited by nalidixic acid in the holding medium. In fact, a period of liquid holding prior to plating on nalidixic acid increased the actual numbers of colonies that did not survive because of the drug. These findings suggested that liquid-holding recovery produced a "repaired" state that still required function of some nalidixic acid-sensitive target for full survival of the organism after UV irradiation.

The bacterial mutations used in these studies are listed in Table 1 with a summary of their characteristics. The *uvrA6* mutant is unable to excise pyrimidine dimers (7) but is fully competent for recombination repair. Recombination repair has been postulated to be composed of two pathways (3). One pathway uses the *recBC* gene products and the other is comprised of the *recFKL* gene products, with the *recA* gene product being a necessary component of both pathways. The *recA13* mutant is unable to carry out recombination repair (12). The *recB* and *recC* genes code for the subunits of an adenosine 5'-triphosphate-requiring deoxyribonuclease used in recombination repair (6). These strains display a wide range in UV sensitivity associated with changes in recombination proficiency or the ability to perform excision repair.

The cells were grown to late-log phase in peptone broth (10 g of peptone [Difco]), diluted to appropriate density with 0.9% NaCl, irradiated with a model 6281-K10 UV lamp (Arthur H. Thomas Co.) at 253 nm at a dose rate of 4 ergs/mm^2 per s (J-225 UV meter; Ultraviolet Products, Inc.), and plated on peptone agar with and without added nalidixic acid. The cells were incubated under dark conditions at 37 C for 48 h. At the end of this time period the surviving colonies on each plate were counted to obtain a dose response curve.

All K-12 strains were tested for post-UV survival, with and without added nalidixic acid, and the critical strains were tested for the bactericidal drug effects in the absence of irradiation. Since the various mutants used differ in their sensitivity to UV irradiation, each was examined both at comparable UV dose rates and at comparable post-UV survival levels for the effects of the drug. The *recA* mutant was significantly impaired in post-UV survival at a nalidixic concentration of 10^{-6} M, which is comparable to previous experiments with *E. coli* B (Fig. 1). *uvrA*, which exhibits about the same UV sensitivity as the *recA* mutant, was affected at 0.1 this drug concentration to an even greater extent. Each strain having either a *recB*$^-$, *recC*$^-$, or *recBC*$^-$ genotype was not impaired in post-UV survival by the drug, despite wide ranges in basic UV sensitivity. Thus, neither recombination nor excision proficiency alone can be correlated with nalidixic acid sensitivity.

The inhibition of post-UV survival did not

TABLE 1. *Bacterial mutations used*

Strain	Repair mutation	Source[a]	UV sensitivity[b]	Recombination proficiency	Excision repair	Post-UV nalidixic acid effect
X1648	*recC22*	R.C.	−0.504	Limited	+	−
X1646	*recB21 recC22*	R.C.	−0.610	Limited	+	−
AB2470	*recB21*	B.B.	−1.167	Limited	+	−
AB2500	*uvrA6*	B.B.	−3.074	Complete	−	++
AB2487	*recA13*	B.B.	−3.323	None	+	+
JC5544	*recA13 recC22*	B.B.	−6.276	None	+	−
JC5495	*recA13 recB21*	B.B.	−8.021	None	+	−

[a] The strains used were generously supplied to us by Roy Curtiss (R.C.) of this institute and by Barbara Bachmann (B.B.), Department of Microbiology, Yale School of Medicine, New Haven, Conn.
[b] Expressed as the natural logarithm of the survival at a dose of 40 ergs/mm².

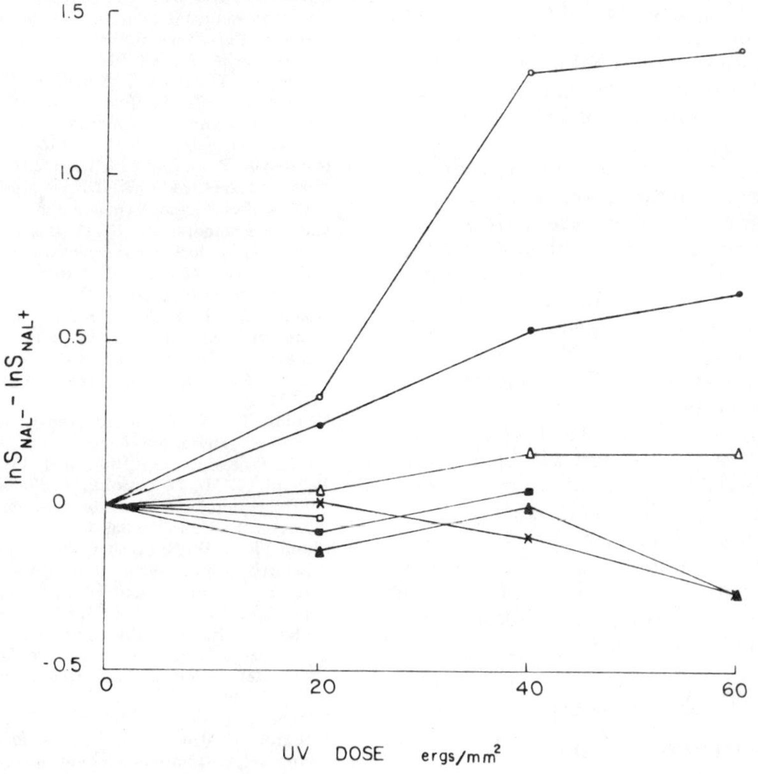

FIG. 1. *ln S without nalidixic acid minus ln S with nalidixic acid versus dose of UV light. Symbols: ○, AB2500 (uvrA6) with 10^{-7} M nalidixic acid (Nal); ●, AB2487 (recA13) with 10^{-6} M Nal; △, X1648 (recC22) with 10^{-6} M Nal; ▲, AB2470 (recB21) with 10^{-6} M Nal; ×, X1646 (recB21 recC22) with 10^{-6} M Nal; ■, JC5544 (recA13 recC22) with 10^{-6} M Nal; □, JC5495 (recA13 recB21) with 10^{-6} M Nal. Survival levels of less than 0.09% (ln S ~ −7) were not included in the computation of the values used.*

appear to result simply from interaction with the bactericidal target, since our studies were carried out at non-bactericidal levels (Table 2). Furthermore, the bactericidal effect was essentially the same in all the tested strains (Table 2). That the bactericidal potency was not increased toward *uvrA* nor decreased in the *recB* and *recC* mutants suggests that the drug targets dictating post-UV sensitivity may be different from the bactericidal effect.

From these data it can be inferred that the site of action for the impairment of post-UV survival by nalidixic acid depends on the *recB* and *recC* gene products. It has been reported that the gene product of the *recB* and *recC* genes is an adenosine 5′-triphosphate-requiring

TABLE 2. *Bactericidial effect of nalidixic acid*

Strain	% Survival of mutants at nalidixic acid concn (M) of:				
	10^{-7}	10^{-6}	10^{-5}	10^{-4}	10^{-3}
AB2500 (*uvrA6*)	100	100	15	0.22	0
X1648 (*recC22*)	100	100	4.3	~0.03	0
AB2470 (*recB21*)	100	100	<0.01	0	0

deoxyribonuclease (exonuclease V) composed of two nonidentical subunits, each subunit being the product of one of these two *rec* genes (6, 13). Our data indicate that nalidixic acid interacts with or requires the complete enzyme and not merely the individual subunits for its effect on UV survival. Only the mutants *(uvrA* and *recA)* containing the complete *recBC* deoxyribonuclease showed impairment of post-UV survival by nalidixic acid, whereas both single mutants *(recB*$^-$ or *recC*$^-$*)* and the double mutant *(recB*$^-$ *recC*$^-$*)* were insensitive.

These experiments indicate that neither UV sensitivity, recombination proficiency, nor excision repair proficiency alone are critical to the drug effect described. Experiments now in progress with suppressor strains of *recBC* mutants having fully restored recombination ability and/or restored UV resistance should provide a further test of this conclusion. Similarly, a test of the drug effect with *recFKL* mutants will evaluate the importance of the *recFKL* branch of the recombination pathway, and *uvrA6 recB*$^-$ or *uvrA6 recC*$^-$ mutants will be of interest to test the possible dominant effect of *uvrA6* in dictating nalidixic acid sensitivity. Finally, a direct test of the conclusions that the *recBC* gene products are nalidixic acid targets will require examination of the isolated ATP-requiring DNase in vitro for drug binding and changes in kinetic properties.

This work was supported by Public Health Service grant no. CA-17629 from the National Cancer Institute.

LITERATURE CITED

1. **Bourguignon, G. J., M. Levitt, and R. Sternglanz.** 1973. Studies on the mechanism of action of nalidixic acid. Antimicrob. Agents Chemother. **4**:479–486.
2. **Boyle, J. V., T. M. Cook, and W. A. Goss.** 1969. Mechanisms of action of nalidixic acid on *Escherichia coli*. J. Bacteriol. **97**:230–236.
3. **Clark, A. J.** 1973. Pathways of genetic recombination of bacteria and their viruses. Biochem. Soc. Trans. **1**:234–236.
4. **Eberle, H., and W. J. Masker.** 1971. Effect of nalidixic acid on semiconservative replication and repair synthesis after ultraviolet irradiation in *Escherichia coli*. J. Bacteriol. **105**:908–912.
5. **Gefter, M., Y. Hirota, T. Kornberg, J. Wechsler, and C. Barnoux.** 1971. Analysis of DNA polymerases II and III in mutants of *Escherichia coli* K-12. Proc. Natl. Acad. Sci. U.S.A. **68**:3150–3152.
6. **Goldmark, P. J., and S. J. Linn.** 1972. Purification and properties of the *recBC* DNase of *Escherichia coli* K-12. J. Biol. Chem. **247**:1849–1860.
7. **Howard-Flanders, P., R. P. Boyce, and L. Theriot.** 1966. Three loci in *Escherichia coli* K-12 that control the excision of pyrimidine dimers and certain other mutagen products from DNA. Genetics **53**:1119–1136.
8. **Nishida, M., Y. Mishima, J. Kawada, and K. L. Yielding.** 1975. Enhancement by nalidixic acid of the thermal susceptibility of the Ts-7 mutant of *Escherichia coli* TAU-Bar. Antimicrob. Agents Chemother. **8**:384–386.
9. **Nishida, M., N. Nakanura, and K. L. Yielding.** 1976. Inhibition by nalidixic acid of post-UV survival of *E. coli*. Proc. Soc. Exp. Biol. Med. **151**:271–274.
10. **Pedrini, A. M., D. Geroldi, A. Siccardi, A. Falaschi.** 1972. Studies on the mode of action of nalidixic acid. Eur. J. Biochem. **25**:359–365.
11. **Simon, T. J., W. E. Masker, and P. C. Hanawalt.** 1974. Selective inhibition of semiconservative DNA synthesis by nalidixic acid in permeabilized bacteria. Biochim. Biophys. Acta **349**:271–274.
12. **Willetts, N. S., A. J. Clark, and B. Low.** 1969. Genetic location of certain mutations conferring recombination deficiency in *Escherichia coli*. J. Bacteriol. **97**:244–249.
13. **Wright, M., and G. Buttin.** 1971. The isolation and characterization from *Escherichia coli* of an adenosine triphosphate-dependent deoxyribonuclease directed by *recB*, *C* genes. J. Biol. Chem. **246**:6543–6555.

ANTIMICROBIAL AGENTS AND CHEMOTHERAPY, July 1976, p. 185-187 Vol. 10, No. 1

Printed in U.S.A.

Inhibition of L5178Y Cells in Culture by Methotrexate and Antibiotics

P. L. CHELLO[1]* AND H. W. BRUCKNER[2]

Departments of Pharmacology and Medicine, Yale University School of Medicine, New Haven, Connecticut 06510

Received for publication 4 February 1976

Methotrexate, tetracycline, gentamicin, streptomycin, and penicillin inhibited the growth of L5178Y murine leukemia cells in culture with I_{50} (concentration of drug that caused a 50% inhibition of growth at 72 h) values of 0.0028 μg/ml (6.2×10^{-9} M), 7.9 μg/ml, 200 μg/ml, 1,700 μg/ml, and 3,000 μg/ml (5,000 U/ml), respectively. At concentrations achieved clinically or utilized in the laboratory, the antibiotics did not alter the I_{50} of methotrexate.

The folate antagonist methotrexate is utilized for the chemotherapy of leukemia and other malignancies. Due to the low resistance of the leukemic patient to bacterial and viral infections, sustained use of antibiotics is required. In mice, antibiotics alter the metabolism of methotrexate by intestinal flora (12), increase its intestinal excretion (12), and increase methotrexate toxicity (H. Bruckner, Fed. Proc. **28**:263, 1969). Little is known concerning the effect antibiotics have on the susceptibility of the leukemic cell to methotrexate. Zager et al. (11) showed that antibiotics did not significantly alter the uptake of the antifolate by L1210 murine leukemia cells in vitro. However, these studies were of short duration and did not permit evaluation of the effect of prolonged exposure to antibiotics on the ability of methotrexate to inhibit cell growth or metabolism.

The L5178Y murine leukemia cell in culture was used as a model to investigate this question. The parameter examined was the I_{50} (concentration of drug that caused a 50% inhibition of growth at 72 h) for methotrexate in the presence and the absence of antibiotics. Penicillin, streptomycin, tetracycline, and gentamicin were chosen as representative of antibiotics used clinically and in the laboratory. The ability of these compounds to inhibit growth was also determined.

L5178Y cells were grown in Fischer medium (4), 10% with respect to horse serum, as described previously (1). Methotrexate (Lederle Laboratories, Pearl River, N.Y.), potassium penicillin G (E. R. Squibb and Sons, Inc., New York), streptomycin sulfate (General Biochemicals, Chagrin Falls, Ohio), tetracycline (Tetrachel; Rachelle Laboratories, Inc., Long Beach, Calif.), and gentamicin (Garamycin; Schering Corp., Bloomfield, N.J.) were prepared in medium plus serum. All solutions were resterilized by passage through 0.22-μm Swinnex filters (Millipore). Cultures in the logarithmic stage of growth were harvested, resuspended, and exposed to drug(s) for 72 h. Growth of controls minus methotrexate and antibiotics was monitored every 24 h to verify that the growth pattern was normal. At 72 h, cell counts were taken and averaged, and the means were plotted against drug concentration. Counts from triplicate tubes within the same experimental group agreed within 10%. Each experiment was repeated at least twice.

The inhibition of L5178Y cells by methotrexate and/or antibiotics is shown in Table 1. Methotrexate had an I_{50} of 0.0028 μg/ml (6.2×10^{-9} M), which is in agreement with reported values (3). Each of the antibiotics also inhibited L5178Y growth. On a basis of micrograms per milliliter, tetracycline was the most potent (I_{50} = 7.9 μg/ml), followed in order of decreasing efficacy by gentamicin (I_{50} = 200 μg/ml), streptomycin (I_{50} = 1,700 μg/ml), and penicillin (I_{50} = 3,000 μg/ml). Inhibition by tetracycline, gentamicin, and streptomycin was not surprising since these antibiotics produce metabolic alterations at various parts of the protein synthetic apparatus of bacteria (10) and each has known clinical cytotoxicity (6, 8, 9). However, the concentrations necessary to produce inhibition, with the exception of tetracycline, limit the practicality of these observations. The I_{50} for tetracycline is similar to serum levels of 3 to 5

[1] Present address: Sloan-Kettering Institute for Cancer Research, Donald S. Walker Laboratory, 145 Boston Post Road, Rye, N.Y. 10580.

[2] Present address: Department of Medicine, Mount Sinai School of Medicine, Fifth Avenue and 100th Street, New York, N.Y. 10021.

TABLE 1. *Inhibition of L5178Y cells by methotrexate and antibiotics*

Drug tested	Concn tested (μg/ml)	Additions to medium[a]	I_{50} (μg/ml)[b]
Methotrexate	4.5×10^{-6}–4.5	None	0.0028
Penicillin	0.006–6,000	None	3,000
Streptomycin	0.010–10,000	None	1,700
Tetracycline	0.044–440	None	7.9
Gentamicin	0.010–1,000	None	200
Methotrexate	4.5×10^{-6}–4.5	Penicillin (60)	0.0028
Methotrexate	4.5×10^{-6}–4.5	Streptomycin (100)	0.0027
Methotrexate	4.5×10^{-6}–4.5	Tetracycline (4.4)	0.0031
Methotrexate	4.5×10^{-6}–4.5	Gentamicin (5.0)	0.0028
Penicillin	0.006–6,000	Streptomycin (100)	3,000
Streptomycin	0.010–10,000	Penicillin (60)	1,600
Tetracycline	0.044–440	Penicillin (60), streptomycin (100)	7.5
Gentamicin	0.010–1,000	Penicillin (60), streptomycin (100)	190
Tetracycline	0.044–440	Penicillin (60), streptomycin (100), gentamicin (5.0)	7.4
Gentamicin	0.010–1,000	Penicillin (60), streptomycin (100), tetracycline (4.4)	195
Methotrexate	4.5×10^{-6}–4.5	Penicillin (60), streptomycin (100)	0.0027
Methotrexate	4.5×10^{-6}–4.5	Penicillin (60), streptomycin (100), tetracycline (4.4)	0.0030
Methotrexate	4.5×10^{-6}–4.5	Penicillin (60), streptomycin (100), gentamicin (5.0)	0.0026
Methotrexate	4.5×10^{-6}–4.5	Penicillin (60), streptomycin (100), tetracycline (4.4), gentamicin (5.0)	0.0025

[a] Numbers in parentheses indicate concentration in micrograms per milliliter added to the medium.

[b] Geometric mean calculated from at least two experiments.

μg/ml maintained after oral administration of 500 mg every 6 h or to the peak of 5 to 10 μg/ml obtained after 250 mg intravenously (6, 9). The findings may prove relevant to the clinical cytotoxicity of tetracycline (6, 9). The values for gentamicin and streptomycin, however, were 50 to 70 times greater than peak clinical levels of 3 to 4 and 25 to 30 μg/ml achieved with intramuscular administration of 40 mg of gentamicin/m^2 (5, 8) or 1 g of streptomycin, respectively (8). Assuming 1 U to be equivalent to 0.6 μg (7), the I_{50} for penicillin (5,000 U/ml) was 600 times the serum level of 8 U/ml achieved after 5×10^5 U intramuscularly (7).

For drug interaction studies, noninhibitory levels of each antibiotic were used. Penicillin and streptomycin were utilized at 60 μg/ml (100 U/ml) and 100 μg/ml, respectively. Although these concentrations were higher than observed clinically (7, 8), they conformed to levels in the original formulation of Fischer medium (4) and widely used in biochemical studies with L5178Y cells (1–3). The levels of gentamicin and tetracycline were similar to those observed clinically (5, 6, 8, 9). The inclusion of streptomycin with penicillin or penicillin with streptomycin did not alter the respective I_{50} values. Penicillin and streptomycin did not alter the efficacy of either tetracycline or gentamicin. Gentamicin plus penicillin-streptomycin did not alter the I_{50} for tetracycline, nor did tetracycline in combination with penicillin-streptomycin change the gentamicin findings. Variation in I_{50} values due to additional antibiotics was not significant when analyzed by analysis of variance.

Growth with these noninhibitory levels of antibiotics, singly or in combination, did not alter the I_{50} for methotrexate. Differences were not significant when analyzed by analysis of variance. Thus, although antibiotics may cause one or more subtle metabolic alterations, e.g., a decreased uptake of methotrexate by penicillin (11), they do not appear to grossly affect the long-term susceptibility of the dividing cell to the antifolate, as measured by the I_{50}.

We wish to thank Charlene A. McQueen and Lisa M. DeAngelis for excellent technical assistance.

This work was supported by Public Health Service grant CA-08010 from the National Cancer Institute.

LITERATURE CITED

1. **Chello, P. L., and J. R. Bertino.** 1973. Dependence of 5-methyl-tetrahydrofolate utilization by L5178Y murine leukemia cells *in vitro* on the presence of hydroxycobalamin and transcobalamin II. Cancer Res. 33:1898–1904.
2. **Chello, P. L., and J. R. Bertino.** 1976. Effect of methionine deprivation on L5178Y murine leukemia cells in culture. Interference with the antineoplastic effect of methotrexate. Biochem. Pharmacol. 25:889–892.
3. **Fischer, G. A.** 1961. Increased levels of folic acid reductase as a mechanism of resistance to amethopterin in leukemia cells. Biochem. Pharmacol. 7:75–80.
4. **Fischer, G. A., and A. C. Sartorelli.** 1963. Development, maintenance, and assay of drug resistance. Methods Med. Res. 10:247–262.
5. **Rodriguez, V., G. P. Bodey, M. Valdivieso, and R.**

Feld. 1975. Clinical pharmacology of sisomicin. Antimicrob. Agents Chemother. **7**:38–41.

6. **Weinstein, L.** 1965. Antibiotics. IV. The tetracyclines: chlortetracycline, oxytetracycline, tetracycline, and demethylchloretetracycline, p. 1242–1259. *In* L. S. Goodman and A. Gilman (ed.), The pharmacological basis of therapeutics. The Macmillan Co., New York.
7. **Weinstein, L.** 1975. Antimicrobial agents: penicillins and cephalosporins, p. 1130–1166. *In* L. S. Goodman and A. Gilman (ed.), The pharmacological basis of therapeutics. The Macmillan Co., New York.
8. **Weinstein, L.** 1975. Antimicrobial agents: streptomycin, gentamicin, and other aminoglycosides, p. 1167–1182. *In* L. S. Goodman and A. Gilman (ed.), The pharmacogogical basis of therapeutics. The Macmillan Co., New York.
9. **Weinstein, L.** 1975. Antimicrobial agents: tetracyclines and chloramphenicol, p. 1183–1200. *In* L. S. Goodman and A. Gilman (ed.), The pharmacological basis of therapeutics. The Macmillan Co., New York.
10. **Weisblum, B., and J. Davies.** 1968. Antibiotic inhibitors of the bacterial ribosome. Bacteriol. Rev. **32**:493–528.
11. **Zager, R. F., S. A. Frisby, and V. T. Oliverio.** 1973. The effects of antibiotics and cancer chemotherapeutic agents on the cellular transport and antitumor activity of methotrexate in L1210 murine leukemia. Cancer Res. **33**:1670–1676.
12. **Zaharko, D. S., H. Bruckner, and V. T. Oliverio.** 1969. Antibiotics alter methotrexate metabolism and excretion. Science **166**:887–888.

Antimicrobial Agents and Chemotherapy, July 1976, p. 188-190
Vol. 10, No. 1

In Vitro Activity of Josamycin and Rosamicin Against *Bacteroides fragilis* Compared with Clindamycin, Erythromycin, and Metronidazole

JEROME SANTORO, DONALD KAYE, AND MATTHEW E. LEVISON*

Department of Medicine, The Medical College of Pennsylvania, Philadelphia, Pennsylvania 19129

Received for publication 19 February 1976

The inhibitory and bactericidal activities of josamycin and rosamicin against 29 clinical isolates of *Bacteroides fragilis* were compared with those of clindamycin, erythromycin, and metronidazole by a broth dilution technique. Josamycin and rosamicin had similar inhibitory activity to metronidazole and clindamycin. Rosamicin had similar bactericidal activity to clindamycin but was less bactericidal than metronidazole (the most bactericidal agent tested). Josamycin was slightly more bactericidal than erythromycin (the least bactericidal agent tested), but less so than rosamicin and clindamycin.

Josamycin and rosamicin, two new macrolide antibiotics, have been reported to be active against strains of *Bacteroides fragilis* (9, 10). The following study was undertaken to compare the in vitro activity of these antibiotics with erythromycin, a commonly used macrolide, and with clindamycin and metronidazole, compounds with known in vitro activity and clinical usefulness against *B. fragilis* (6, 11, 12).

Twenty-nine clinical isolates of *B. fragilis* (12 strains of *B. fragilis* subsp. *fragilis*, 11 of *B. fragilis* subsp. *thetaiotaomicron*, and 6 of *B. fragilis* subsp. *vulgatus*) were identified and subspeciated by the methods of the Virginia Polytechnic Institute (4). The susceptibility of the organisms to the antimicrobial agents was determined by a broth dilution method in freshly prepared heart infusion broth. Approximately 10 mg each of rosamicin (kindly supplied by Schering Corp., Bloomfield, N.J.), josamycin (kindly supplied by Endo Laboratories, Inc., Garden City, N.Y.), and erythromycin (kindly supplied by Eli Lilly & Co., Indianapolis, Ind.) was initially dissolved in about 0.01 ml of 70% ethanol; then sterile distilled water was added to make a solution of 1,000 μg/ml. Clindamycin (kindly supplied by The Upjohn Co., Kalamazoo, Mich.) and metronidazole (kindly supplied by Searle, Chicago, Ill.) were dissolved directly in distilled water to make solutions of 1,000 μg/ml. The antimicrobial agents were diluted in twofold steps in tubes containing 0.5 ml of prereduced heart infusion broth. The tubes were then stored overnight in GasPak jars (BBL). This anaerobic system provides an atmosphere of 0.5 to 2.7% CO_2 (3). The pH of the broth was 7.2 both before and after the attainment of anaerobiosis. The pH was measured by placing a pH electrode through the lid of a GasPak system, which was sealed with stopcock grease. Readings were made only when the redox indicator assured a reduced atmosphere.

The bacterial inoculum for each tube was 0.5 ml of a 10^{-4} dilution of an 18-h culture of each strain in prereduced heart infusion broth. The minimal inhibitory concentration was considered to be the lowest concentration of antimicrobial that prevented turbidity after 48 h of incubation at 37 C in GasPak jars. At 48 h, 0.01 ml was removed from each tube without visible growth by use of a sterile platinum loop and streaked on prereduced plates of Trypticase soy agar containing 5% sheep erythrocytes. After incubation at 37 C for 48 h in GasPak jars, the plates were examined, and the lowest concentration of antimicrobial agent that resulted in $\leq$1 colony was taken as the minimal bactericidal concentration.

Inhibitory activity of the antimicrobial agents. As shown in Fig. 1 and 2, josamycin, rosamicin, clindamycin, and metronidazole had similar inhibitory activity, and all were more active than erythromycin. At 0.8 μg of antimicrobial per ml, 100% of strains were inhibited by josamycin and metronidazole, 93% were inhibited by rosamicin, 97% were inhibited by clindamycin, and 76% were inhibited by erythromycin. One hundred percent of the strains were inhibited by 1.6 μg of rosamicin or clindamycin per ml. Erythromycin at 3.1 μg/ml inhibited 97% of the strains (Fig. 1). These results indicating the degree of inhibitory activity of clindamycin, erythromycin, and metronidazole against *B. fragilis* are similar to those reported in previous studies (5, 11, 12). In studies by others (9, 10), josamycin and rosamicin showed inhibitory activity against strains of *B. fragilis* similar to that observed in the present study.

Bactericidal activity of the antimicrobial agents. Metronidazole has been reported to be consistently bactericidal against 19 strains of *B. fragilis* tested in concentrations of ≤6.25 μg/ml, and clindamycin has been shown to be bactericidal against 6 of 19 strains in a concentration of 1.56 μg/ml (7). The bactericidal activity of the macrolides against *B. fragilis* has not been previously studied. In the present study, metronidazole was the most bactericidal of the compounds tested: 97% (28 of 29 strains) were killed by 1.6 μg/ml of metronidazole, and 100% were killed by 3.1 μg/ml. Rosamicin and clindamycin showed similar bactericidal activity: 83% (24 of 29 strains) were killed by 1.6 μg of rosamicin per ml, and 76% (22 of 29 strains) were killed by 1.6 μg of clindamycin per ml. Erythromycin and josamycin were the least bactericidal, with only 28% (8 of 29 strains) killed by 1.6 μg of erythromycin per ml, and 59% (17 of 29 strains) killed by 1.6 μg of josamycin per ml (Fig. 1 and 2).

Relative activity against subspecies of *B. fragilis*. *B. fragilis* subsp. *thetaiotaomicron* has been reported to be relatively resistant to josamycin, erythromycin, clindamycin, and metronidazole when compared to other subspecies (S. S. Long, S. Miller, and R. M. Swenson, Prog. Abstr. Intersci. Conf. Antimicrob. Agents Chemother., 15th, Washington, D.C., Abstr. 381, 1975). In the present study, no appreciable differences in either minimal inhibitory or

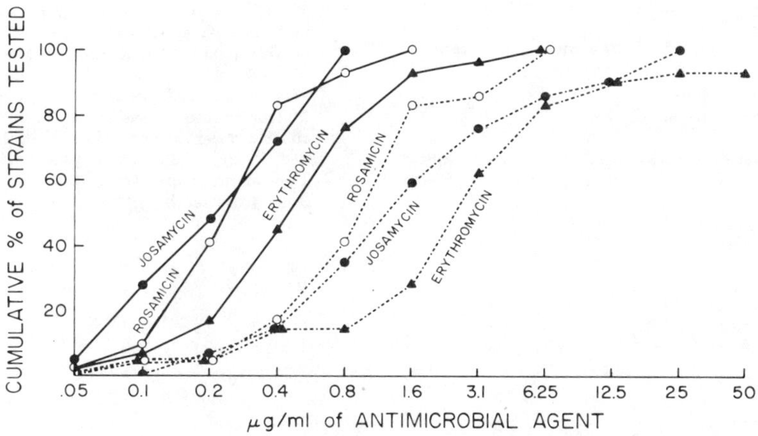

FIG. 1. *Cumulative percentage of 29 isolates of B. fragilis inhibited (solid lines) and killed (dashed lines) by increasing concentrations of the macrolide antibiotics, josamycin (●), rosamicin (○), and erythromycin (▲).*

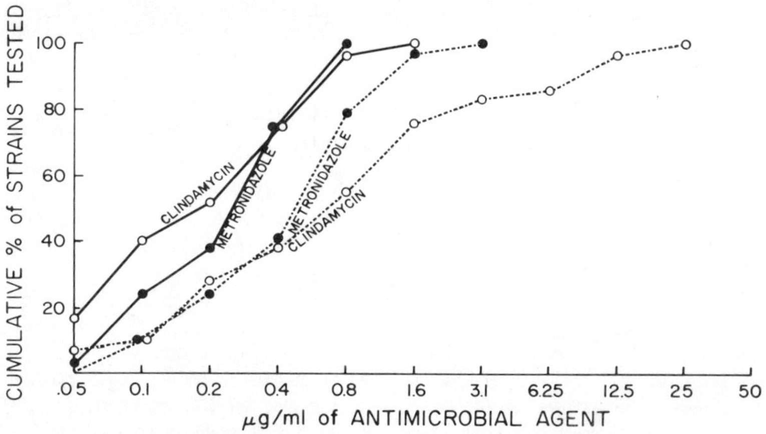

FIG. 2. *Cumulative percentage of 29 isolates of B. fragilis inhibited (solid lines) and killed (dashed lines) by increasing concentrations of clindamycin (○) and metronidazole (●).*

minimal bactericidal activity were noted for any of the antimicrobial agents against subspecies of *B. fragilis* identified ($P > 0.05$, chi-square test), as has been similarly reported for clindamycin and other antibiotics (2).

Peak concentrations of josamycin in serum obtained after oral administration of 0.5 g every 6 to 8 h (M. A. Sande, L. J. Strausbaugh, J. M. Gwaltney, and J. A. Dilworth, Prog. Abstr. Intersci. Conf. Antimicrob. Agents Chemother., 15th, Washington, D.C., Abstr. 16, 1975) or a single dose of 1.25 g (1) consistently exceed 1.5 μg/ml. Rosamicin has not been administered to humans (8). However, if rosamicin proves to be nontoxic and if the concentrations of rosamicin in serum are similar to those produced by the other macrolides, both josamycin and rosamicin may prove to be useful in infections caused by *B. fragilis*.

This study was supported in part by Endo Laboratories, Inc., Garden City, N.Y., and Schering Corp., Bloomfield, N.J.

We gratefully acknowledge the technical assistance of Virginia Simpson and Evan Zimmer.

LITERATURE CITED

1. **Bergan, T., and B. Øydvin.** 1972. Pharmacokinetics of josamycin—a new macrolide antibiotic. Pharmacology 7:36–50.
2. **Blafevic, D.** 1976. Antibiotic susceptibility of subspecies of *Bacteroides fragilis*. Antimicrob. Agents Chemother. **9**:481–484.
3. **Ferguson, I. R., K. D. Phillips, and P. V. Tearle.** 1975. An evaluation of the carbon dioxide component in the Gas Pak anaerobic system. J. Appl. Bacteriol. **39**:167–173.
4. **Holdeman, L. S., and W. E. C. Moore.** 1973. Anaerobic laboratory manual. Virginia Polytechnic Institute and State University, Blacksburg, Va.
5. **Kislak, J. W.** 1972. The susceptibility of *Bacteroides fragilis* to 24 antibiotics. J. Infect. Dis. **125**:295–299.
6. **Levison, M. E., J. L. Bran, and K. Ries.** 1974. Treatment of anaerobic bacterial infections with clindamycin-2-phosphate. Antimicrob. Agents Chemother. **5**:276–280.
7. **Nastro, L. J., and S. M. Finegold.** 1972. Bactericidal activity of five antimicrobial agents against *Bacteroides fragilis*. J. Infect. Dis. **126**:104–107.
8. **Schering Corp.** 1972. Informational booklet for the investigational drug, Sch 14947 (Rosamicin). Schering Corp., Bloomfield, N.J.
9. **Strausbaugh, L. J., J. A. Dilworth, J. M. Gwaltney, and M. A. Sande.** 1976. In vitro susceptibility studies with josamycin and erythromycin. Antimicrob. Agents Chemother. **9**:546–548.
10. **Sutter, V. L., and S. M. Finegold.** 1976. Rosamicin: in vitro activity against anaerobes and comparison with erythromycin. Antimicrob. Agents Chemother. **9**:350–351.
11. **Talley, F. P., V. L. Sutter, and S. M. Finegold.** 1972. Metronidazole vs. anaerobes. In vitro data and initial clinical observations. Calif. Med. **117**:22–26.
12. **Tally, F. P., V. L. Sutter, and S. M. Finegold.** 1975. Treatment of anaerobic infections with metronidazole. Antimicrob. Agents Chemother. **7**:672–675.

ANTIMICROBIAL AGENTS AND CHEMOTHERAPY, Aug. 1976, p. 191-195
Vol. 10, No. 2

Printed in U.S.A.

Inducible Oxacillin-Hydrolyzing Penicillinase in *Aeromonas hydrophila* Isolated from Fish

TETSUO SAWAI,* KAYOKO MORIOKA, MAYUMI OGAWA, AND SABURO YAMAGISHI
Faculty of Pharmaceutical Sciences, Chiba University, Chiba, Japan

Received for publication 9 March 1976

An inducible penicillinase was shown to be present in a strain of *Aeromonas hydrophila* subsp. *hydrophila* isolated from freshwater fish. Enzyme induction was observed with benzylpenicillin or 6-aminopenicillanic acid, and the enzyme was cell bound. The penicillinase was purified 50-fold from a crude cell extract. The molecular weight was estimated to be 23,000 by gel filtration. The pH and temperature optima for the enzyme activity were 8.0 and 35°C, respectively. The penicillinase showed a unique substrate profile by hydrolyzing oxacillin about twice as rapidly as benzylpenicillin. The enzyme activity was weakly inhibited by sodium chloride but was not affected by *p*-chloromercuribenzoate. The property of penicillinase production by the *A. hydrophila* strain could not be transferred to *Escherichia coli* and also could not be eliminated from the bacteria by ethidium bromide treatment.

Beta-lactamase (EC 3.5.2.6, penicillin β-lactam amidohydrolase) is a hydrolytic enzyme produced by species representing many bacterial genera. Although a physiological role for the enzyme in bacterial metabolism has not been determined, the enzyme plays its most important role in the drug resistance of many pathogenic bacteria to beta-lactam antibiotics. Many beta-lactamases are thought to be species specific. In addition to these enzymes, beta-lactamases mediated by a gene(s) borne on R plasmids are widely distributed among gram-negative bacteria.

Since the discovery of R plasmids specifying ampicillin resistance (1), we have studied the penicillinases mediated by R plasmids as well as the species-specific beta-lactamases of various gram-negative bacteria (10, 14, 18–20, 22, 23). One of the purposes of these studies has been to elucidate the phylogenetic relationship between the plasmid- and the chromosome-mediated beta-lactamases. The penicillinases mediated by R plasmids have been classified for convenience into two groups, i.e., type I and II, according to their enzymological and immunological properties (10, 18, 23). Our previous studies demonstrated a striking similarity in enzymological and immunological properties between the species-specific penicillinases of the *Klebsiella* group and type I R plasmid penicillinases (18, 20). However, we could not find a species-specific penicillinase similar to type II penicillinase, which has a unique substrate specificity able to hydrolyze methicillin and oxacillin and its derivatives.

Recently, we have extended our survey to gram-negative bacteria that are not of human origin. One of them is *Aeromonas hydrophila*, isolated from freshwater fishes by Aoki and Egusa (4). This paper presents data concerning an inducible penicillinase of *A. hydrophila* that shows an unusual substrate specificity able to hydrolyze the semisynthetic penicillins, which are resistant to many beta-lactamases.

MATERIALS AND METHODS

Bacterial strains, media, and growth conditions. *A. hydrophila* subsp. *hydrophila* 67-P-24 and Y-62 were isolated by T. Aoki and S. Egusa from freshwater fishes in Japan (4) and kindly made available to us. The two strains had previously been reported by the original collectors to be *Aeromonas liquefaciens*. The strains were again characterized in this laboratory by means of their biological and biochemical properties, as interpreted by Schubert (21). The strains grew in nutrient broth at 37°C but could not grow in nutrient broth containing 7.5% (wt/vol) sodium chloride at 37°C. They could grow with ammonium sulfate and glucose as the sole source of nitrogen and carbon and also could utilize L-arginine, L-asparagine, or L-histidine as the sole source of carbon. The strains fermented glucose and glycerol with the production of gas and were positive to the Voges-Proskauer test; they were tested for production of 2,3-butanediol dehydrogenase and were found to be positive. Both strains are resistant to ampicillin but susceptible to chloramphenicol, tetracycline, streptomycin, and kanamycin.

Nutrient broth and heart infusion broth were used for bacterial cultivation in liquid medium, and heart infusion agar was used for the determination of bacterial resistance to antibiotics. The media used were all products of Eiken Chemical Co., Tokyo, Japan. Bacterial cultivation was performed at 30°C.

Beta-lactam antibiotics. Penicillins and cephalosporins were kindly provided by the following pharmaceutical companies: benzylpenicillin, ampicillin, phenethicillin, methicillin, and 6-amino-penicillanic acid, Meiji Seika Co., Tokyo, Japan; cloxacillin and oxacillin, Bristol Laboratories, Inc., Syracuse, N.Y.; cephalothin, Shionogi Pharmaceutical Co., Osaka, Japan; cephaloridine, Torii Pharmaceutical Co., Tokyo, Japan; carbenicillin, Fujisawa Pharmaceutical Co., Osaka, Japan.

Determination of penicillinase activity. Penicillinase activity was determined iodometrically at 30°C in 0.1 M phosphate buffer (pH 7.5) by a modification of Perret's method (16). The microiodometric assay method devised by Novick (15) was used with slight modification for kinetic measurements of the enzyme reaction. Penicillinase activity was expressed in units; one unit of the enzyme activity was defined as the activity that hydrolyzes 1 μmol of benzylpenicillin per min under the conditions described above.

Since ampicillin is more readily hydrolyzed than benzylpenicillin, it was used in the experiments for determination of optimum pH, optimum temperature, molecular weight, and effect of inhibitors.

Determinations of protein. The concentration of protein in column eluates was followed by measuring the absorbancy at 280 nm. Bovine serum albumin was used as the protein standard. For more accurate estimations, the method of Lowry et al. (13) was used.

Estimation of molecular weight. The molecular weight of penicillinase was estimated by gel filtration through a Sephadex G-75 column (1.2 by 75 cm) according to the method of Andrews (2). Ovalbumin, α-chymotrypsinogen, and cytochrome *c* were used as the internal standard proteins. All the standard proteins were the products of C. F. Boehringer & Soehne GmbH, Mannheim, Germany.

Polyacrylamide gel electrophoresis. Analytical disc polyacrylamide gel electrophoresis was performed with 7.5% gel (0.5 by 7 cm) and tris(hydroxymethyl)aminomethane-glycine buffer at pH 8.7. Electrophoresis was carried out at a constant current of 3 mA/tube at 5°C for 2 h, and the gel was stained with 0.25% Coomassie brilliant blue. The stained protein band, which corresponded to penicillinase, was identified by the position of penicillinase activity in a non-stained gel. For detection of penicillinase activity in the gel, the non-stained gel was cut into 2-mm slices, and the enzyme was extracted from the slices with 0.1 M phosphate buffer (pH 7.5).

Assay of bacterial resistance to penicillins and cephaloridine. The determination of levels of bacterial resistance to antibiotics was performed according to procedures described previously (10), except that the temperature of bacterial growth was 30°C.

Transfer test. Transfer of ampicillin resistance by cell-to-cell contact from *A. hydrophila* 67-P-24 to *Escherichia coli* was examined by the method described previously (10). Briefly, *E. coli* 58-161 F$^-$ Nal^r (resistant to nalidixic acid) was used as a recipient strain. After overnight incubation of the donor strain with the recipient cells in heart infusion broth at 30°C, portions of the mixed culture were plated on heart infusion agar containing 50 μg of nalidixic acid and 800 or 1,600 μg of ampicillin per ml. The plates were incubated at 30°C for 48 h. Because penicillinase from the donor cell inactivates ampicillin in the selective medium, 800 μg of ampicillin per ml was found to be the minimal concentration for inhibiting the growth of the *E. coli* strain when mixedly plated with the donor strain.

RESULTS

A. hydrophila strains 67-P-24 and Y-62 were selected from the stock cultures of T. Aoki and S. Egusa as representatives of highly ampicillin-resistant and less resistant strains, respectively. Levels of resistance to ampicillin and other beta-lactam antibiotics in the two strains are shown in Table 1. Strain 67-P-24 is resistant to both the penicillins and cephaloridine. Strain Y-62 shows higher susceptibility to the antibiotics, especially to cephaloridine, than strain 67-P-24, although from a clinical point of view it may be considered as a strain resistant to the clinically used penicillins.

Transfer of the ampicillin resistance gene from strain 67-P-24 to *E. coli* could not be detected, although about 10^8 recipient cells were examined. Ampicillin resistance was stable during long storage of the organism in cooked meat medium and could not be eliminated by treatment with ethidium bromide, according to the procedures described by Bouanchaud et al. (7).

Penicillinase activity in organisms growing exponentially in nutrient broth was assayed after sonically disrupting the cells. The enzyme activity of strain 67-P-24 was 0.11 units/mg (dry weight) of bacteria, and we could not detect measurable penicillinase activity in the culture of strain Y-62. When benzylpenicillin at a subinhibitory concentration (50 μg/ml) was added

TABLE 1. *Levels of resistance to beta-lactam antibiotics in A. hydrophila strains 67-P-24 and Y-62*

Drug	Drug resistance (μg/ml)[a]	
	67-P-24	Y-62
Benzylpenicillin	400	200
Ampicillin	400	50
Carbenicillin	400	25
Oxacillin	1,600	200
6-Aminopenicillanic acid	100	12.5
Cephaloridine	50	6.3

[a] The level of drug resistance is expressed as the maximum concentration of drug that allows visible growth of bacteria after 18 h of incubation at 30°C.

to the logarithmic-phase culture of 67-P-24, the specific enzyme activity at 1 h after addition of the inducer was 1.7 units. Although we did not perform a quantitative assay, penicillinase activity was also found in the culture of strain Y-62 after induction with benzylpenicillin. 6-Aminopenicillanic acid, known as the most effective inducer for a cephalosporinase of *Pseudomonas aeruginosa* (17), was also an effective inducer, comparable to benzylpenicillin.

Figure 1 shows the kinetics of induced penicillinase synthesis in strain 67-P-24 growing exponentially. By addition of benzylpenicillin as inducer, a marked increase in enzyme activity occurred after a lag period of less than 15 min. The produced enzyme was rarely released into the growth medium and appeared to be cell bound, similar to other beta-lactamases of gram-negative bacteria.

From cells of strain 67-P-24 induced for 2 h with benzylpenicillin (100 μg/ml) the enzyme was extracted and purified by the procedures summarized in Table 2. Although the enzyme was purified 50-fold from the crude cell extract, the purified enzyme preparation gave three minor protein bands other than the major band corresponding to penicillinase activity in an acrylamide gel.

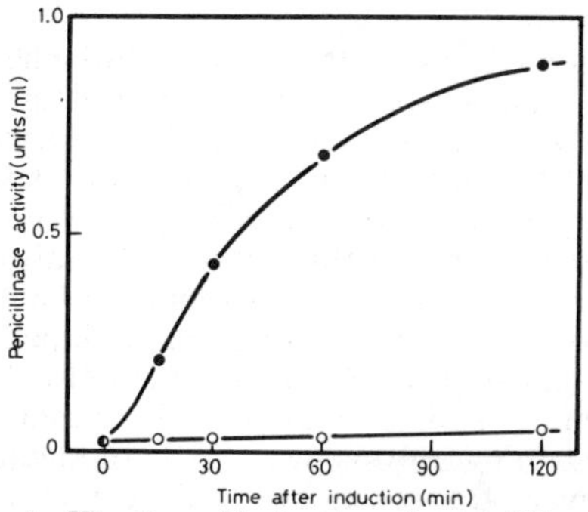

FIG. 1. *Kinetics of induction of penicillinase synthesis by benzylpenicillin in A. hydrophila 67-P-24. A bacterial culture grown overnight in nutrient broth at 30°C was diluted fivefold with fresh broth and incubated with shaking at the same temperature. When the optical density of the culture at 610 nm reached about 0.4 (in mid-exponential growth phase), benzylpenicillin was added to the culture to a final concentration of 50 μg/ml and incubation was continued. Portions of the culture were removed at the indicated times, and penicillinase activity was assayed after sonically disrupting the cells. Symbols:* ●, *induced culture;* ○, *uninduced culture.*

The pH activity plot for the partially purified penicillinase, using ampicillin as a substrate, is shown in Fig. 2A. The enzyme has an optimum pH of 8.0. The temperature activity curve of the enzyme at pH 7.5 is shown in Fig. 2B, and the optimum temperature for the enzyme activity is 35°C.

The relative activities (relative V_{max}) of the enzyme from strain 67-P-24 at substrate saturation for seven penicillins and two cephalosporins are given in Table 3, together with the Michaelis constants (K_m) for some of these substrates. The K_m values were obtained from Lineweaver-Burk plots (12). The penicillinase has a unique substrate profile that shows a highly hydrolytic activity and a high affinity against oxacillin. Oxacillin is known as a semisynthetic penicillin resistant to hydrolysis by many beta-lactamases. Two other semisynthetic penicillins, cloxacillin and methicillin, which are resistant to many known beta-lactamases, are also effectively hydrolyzed by the enzyme. Another striking characteristic of the penicillinase is that the enzyme is able to hydrolyze ampicillin at a high rate, about five times that of benzylpenicillin. The crude enzyme preparation from *A. hydrophila* Y-62 also showed a substrate profile similar to that of the enzyme of strain 67-P-24.

The molecular weight of the enzyme was estimated by gel filtration experiments on Sephadex G-75. The average of two measurements gave a molecular weight of 23,000 ± 1,000 for the penicillinase of strain 67-P-24.

p-Chloromercuribenzoate and sodium chloride were examined for their inhibitory effect on the activity of the enzymes from the strains

TABLE 2. *Summary of purification of penicillinase from A. hydrophila 67-P-24*

Step	Penicillinase activity recovered (units)	Penicillinase sp act (units of protein)	Purification	Recovery (%)
Ultrasonic disintegration followed streptomycin treatment and dialysis	1,500[a]	3.67	1	100
Chromatography on carboxymethyl-Sephadex C-50 (0.2 M NaCl, stepwise)	1,033	25.0	6.8	69
Gel filtration on Sephadex G-75	1,000	90.0	24.5	67
Chromatography on carboxymethyl-Sephadex C-50 (0 to 0.4 M NaCl, gradient)	450	183	50	30

[a] Extracted from cells cultured in 2 liters of medium.

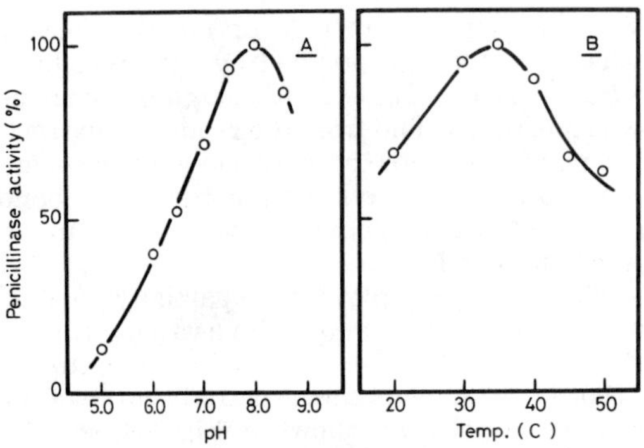

FIG. 2. *Effects of pH and temperature on penicillinase activity. Effects of pH (A) and temperature (B) on the activity of the penicillinase of A. hydrophila 67-P-24 were measured with ampicillin as a substrate. (A) Acetate buffer (0.1 M) was used at pH 5.0, and 0.1 M phosphate buffer was used for the range pH 6.0 to 8.5. (B) The penicillinase in 0.1 M phosphate buffer, pH 7.5, containing 8 mM of the substrate was incubated for 10 min at the indicated temperature, and reaction rates were determined iodometrically.*

67-P-24 and Y-62 (crude enzyme preparation) according to the procedures described previously (23). *p*-Chloromercuribenzoate did not show an inhibitory effect on either of the enzyme activities at a concentration of 1 mM. In the presence of 100 mM sodium chloride, both enzymes were 25 to 30% inhibited in their activities against ampicillin. Chloride ion is known to be a specific inhibitor for the type II penicillinase mediated by R plasmid (23).

DISCUSSION

Aoki and Egusa demonstrated that most of the *Aeromonas* strains isolated from freshwater fishes and soft-shelled turtles cultured in farm ponds in Japan were highly resistant to ampicillin (4). They reported that the ampicillin resistance in *Aeromonas* failed to transfer to *E. coli* by conjugation, although sulfanilamide, tetracycline, and chloramphenicol resistances on R plasmids were transferable from various species to *E. coli* (3, 5, 6). Therefore, they suggested that ampicillin resistance may be an innate resistance in this species.

We have also failed to demonstrate transferability of ampicillin resistance in strain 67-P-24. Furthermore, it was observed that the ampicillin resistance was not lost from the organism after long storage of the strain in cooked-meat medium or by treatment of the organism with ethidium bromide. The penicillinase characterized in this paper may be a species-specific beta-lactamase of *A. hydrophila*. Although the ampicillin resistance cannot be attributed only to

TABLE 3. *Substrate profiles and kinetic properties of penicillinases from A. hydrophila*

Substrate	Penicillinase of 67-P-24: Relative rate of hydrolysis (%)[b]	Penicillinase of 67-P-24: K_m (μM)	Penicillinase of Y-62[a] (Relative rate of hydrolysis [%])[b]
Benzylpenicillin	100	14	100
Ampicillin	534	143	441
Phenethicillin	243		208
Oxacillin	212	33	
Cloxacillin	90	77	75
Methicillin	32	154	
6-Aminopenicillanic acid	48		91
Cephaloridine	95		183
Cephalothin	49		50

[a] Crude extract from cells of strain Y-62.

[b] The rate of hydrolysis was determined at 30°C in 0.1 M phosphate buffer (pH 7.5) with a substrate concentration of 8 mM. The rates given are expressed as the percentage of hydrolysis of benzylpenicillin.

the penicillinase, the close relationship between the levels of ampicillin resistance and the enzyme activity to ampicillin observed in strains 67-P-24 and Y-62 suggests that the enzyme plays a significant role in the high ampicillin resistance of this species. It is also interesting to note that beta-lactam antibiotics have not been used in fish culturing in Japan.

Oxacillin, its derivatives, and methicillin are known as semisynthetic penicillins that are resistant to hydrolysis by many beta-lactamases. However, these semisynthetic penicillins are subject to hydrolysis by two specific beta-lactamases, i.e., beta-lactamase II produced by *Bacillus cereus* 569/H (11) and penicillinases mediated by R plasmids RGN238 and R1818 (9, 10, 23). Recently, Dale and Smith (8) classified the oxacillin-hydrolyzing penicillinases of R plasmids into two main groups. Enzymes of the first group, including the enzyme of R plasmid RGN238, hydrolyze methicillin about three times as rapidly as benzylpenicillin and have a relatively lower molecular weight (about 24,000). Enzymes of the second group, which include the enzyme of R plasmid R1818, have relatively lower activity against methicillin and a very high molecular weight, 41,000 to 46,000. These two group-specific enzymes are produced constitutively in the host organisms. When the penicillinase of *A. hydrophila* was compared with the enzymes of R plasmids, it was found to have a substrate profile intermediate between those of the two enzymes of R plasmids and a molecular weight close to the enzymes of the first group. The most significant difference between the enzymes of *A. hydrophila* and R plasmids is in inducibility. The penicillinase presented in this paper is, to our knowledge, the only inducible penicillinase that has been found in gram-negative bacteria.

As demonstrated by Dale and Smith (8), the oxacillin-hydrolyzing penicillinases mediated by R plasmids are not homogeneous, and it is possible to classify them into seven subgroups. Our investigation revealed the existence of an oxacillin-hydrolyzing penicillinase that may be chromosomally mediated. More detailed comparison of the penicillinase with the oxacillin-hydrolyzing penicillinases of R plasmids is a subject of deep interest in connection with the origin of the genetic determinants for the enzymes on R plasmids. A comparison of physicochemical and immunological properties of the two enzymes is in progress.

ACKNOWLEDGMENTS

We are grateful to T. Aoki and S. Egusa for providing bacterial strains.

LITERATURE CITED

1. **Anderson, E. S., and N. Datta.** 1965. Resistance to penicillins and its transfer in Enterobacteriaceae. lancet I:407–409.
2. **Andrews, P.** 1964. Estimation of the molecular weights of proteins by Sephadex gel-filtration. Biochem. J. 91:222–233.
3. **Aoki, T.** 1974. Studies of drug-resistant bacteria isolated from water of carp-ponds and intestinal tracts of carp. Bull. Jpn. Soc. Sci. Fish (In Japanese) 40:247–254.
4. **Aoki, T., and S. Egusa.** 1971. Drug sensitivity of *Aeromonas liquefaciens* isolated from freshwater fishes. Bull. Jpn. Soc. Sci. Fish. 37:176–185.
5. **Aoki, T., S. Egusa, Y. Ogata, and T. Watanabe.** 1971. Detection of resistance factors in fish pathogen *Aeromonas liquefaciens*. J. Gen. Microbiol. 65:343–349.
6. **Aoki, T., S. Egusa, O. Yada, and T. Watanabe.** 1972. Studies of drug resistance and R factors in bacteria from pond-cultured Salmonids. I. Amago (*Oncorhynchus rhodurus macrostomus*) and Yamane (*Oncorhynchus masou ishikawae*). Jpn. J. Microbiol. 16:233–238.
7. **Bouanchaud, D. H., M. R. Scavizzi, and Y. A. Chabbert.** 1969. Elimination by ethidium bromide of antibiotic resistance in Enterobacteria and Staphylococci. J. Gen. Microbiol. 54:417–425.
8. **Dale, J. W., and J. T. Smith.** 1974. R-factor-mediated β-lactamases that hydrolyze oxacillin: evidence for two distinct groups. J. Bacteriol. 119:351–356.
9. **Datta, N., and P. Kontomichalou.** 1965. Penicillinase synthesis controlled by infectious R factors in *Enterobacteriaceae*. Nature (London) 208:239–241.
10. **Egawa, R., T. Sawai, and S. Mitsuhashi.** 1967. Drug resistance of enteric bacteria. XII. Unique substrate specificity of penicillinase produced by R factors. Jpn. J. Microbiol. 11:173–178.
11. **Kuwabara, S., and E. P. Abraham.** 1967. Some properties of two extracellular β-lactamases from *Bacillus cereus* 569/H. Biochem. J. 103:27c–30c.
12. **Lineweaver, H., and D. Burk.** 1934. The determination of enzyme dissociation constants. J. Am. Chem. Soc. 56:658–666.
13. **Lowry, O. H., N. J. Rosebrough, A. L. Farr, and R. J. Randall.** 1951. Protein measurement with the Folin phenol reagent. J. Biol. Chem. 193:265–275.
14. **Matsumoto, H., T. Sawai, T. Tazaki, S. Yamagishi, and S. Mitsuhashi.** 1972. Characterization of the chromosomally mediated penicillinase in *Klebsiella pneumoniae*. Jpn. J. Microbiol. 16:169–176.
15. **Novick, R. P.** 1962. Micro-iodometric assay for penicillinase. Biochem. J. 83:236–240.
16. **Perret, C. J.** 1954. Iodometric assay of penicillinase. Nature (London) 174:1012–1013.
17. **Rosselet, A., and W. Zimmermann.** 1973. Mutants of *Pseudomonas aeruginosa* with impaired β-lactamase inducibility and increased sensitivity to β-lactam antibiotics. J. Gen. Microbiol. 76:455–457.
18. **Sawai, T., S. Mitsuhashi, and S. Yamagishi.** 1968. Drug resistance of enteric bacteria. XIV. Comparison of β-lactamases in gram-negative rod bacteria resistant to α-aminobenzylpenicillin. Jpn. J. Microbiol. 12:423–434.
19. **Sawai, T., T. Takahashi, S. Yamagishi, and S. Mitsuhashi.** 1970. Variant of penicillinase mediated by an R factor in *Escherichia coli*. J. Bacteriol. 104:620–629.
20. **Sawai, T., S. Yamagishi, and S. Mitsuhashi.** 1973. Penicillinases of *Klebsiella pneumoniae* and their phylogenetic relationship to penicillinases mediated by R factors. J. Bacteriol. 115:1045–1054.
21. **Schubert, R. H. W.** 1974. Genus II. *Aeromonas* Kluyver and van Niel 1936, 398, p. 345–348. *In* R. E. Buchanan and N. E. Gibbons (ed.), Bergey's manual of determinative bacteriology, 8th ed. The Williams & Wilkins Co., Baltimore.
22. **Yaginuma, S., T. Sawai, S. Yamagishi, and S. Mitsuhashi.** 1973. Biochemical properties of a cephalosporin β-lactamase from *Pseudomonas aeruginosa*. Jpn. J. Microbiol. 17:141–149.
23. **Yamagishi, S., K. O'Hara, T. Sawai, and S. Mitsuhashi.** 1969. The purification and properties of penicillin β-lactamases mediated by transmissible R factors in *Escherichia coli*. J. Biochem. 66:11–20.

Antimicrobial Agents and Chemotherapy, Aug. 1976, p. 196-199
Vol. 10, No. 2

Printed in U.S.A.

In Vitro Effects of Low Concentrations of Penicillin and Sulfadiazine on *Streptococcus mutans*

H. G. WELD[1] AND H. J. SANDHAM*

Department of Preventive Dentistry, Faculty of Dentistry, University of Toronto, Toronto, Ontario M5G 1G6, Canada

Received for publication 28 August 1975

Investigations were conducted to determine the in vitro effects of low levels of penicillin and sulfadiazine on the growth, plaque formation, and agglutination of *Streptococcus mutans* and on the synthesis and activity of enzymes synthesizing extracellular polymers. The concentrations tested were equivalent to those expected in the saliva of subjects receiving oral therapy with the agents. Penicillin at 0.5 ng/ml and sulfadiazine at 1 μg/ml substantially inhibited in vitro plaque formation. At these concentrations, sulfadiazine but not penicillin also inhibited growth of the organism. Neither antimicrobial agent affected the agglutination of *S. mutans* with dextran or the synthesis or activity of enzymes synthesizing extracellular polymers. The effect of sulfadiazine on plaque formation was attributed, at least in part, to the inhibitory action of that agent on *S. mutans* growth.

Streptococcus mutans has been strongly implicated as a causative agent in dental caries both because of its ability to cause caries in animals and because of its association with caries in humans (5). A property of *S. mutans* that is believed to contribute to its cariogenicity is its ability to form sticky extracellular polyglucans from sucrose, thereby enabling the organisms to adhere to the teeth (7). Thus, in theory, agents which could interfere with the ability of *S. mutans* to form adherent deposits on teeth might reduce caries experience in humans.

In earlier studies, children receiving 200,000 U of penicillin G orally per day for the prophylaxis of rheumatic fever showed up to 56% fewer new carious lesions than their untreated siblings (8, 9). The present in vitro study sought to determine whether penicillin G, at the concentrations that would be expected in the salivas of such individuals, affects activities of *S. mutans* that might be related to the cariogenicity of that organism. The activities examined were growth, formation of adherent plaques on steel wires, agglutination, and the formation and activity of enzymes capable of producing extracellular polymers from sucrose.

Because sulfadiazine (1 g/day) is also currently used in the prophylaxis of rheumatic fever, parallel in vitro studies were carried out to determine whether that agent might also affect the activities of *S. mutans*. At the present time there is no information on whether sulfadiazine therapy has any effect on caries in humans. As with penicillin, the concentrations examined were those expected to occur in the salivas of treated subjects.

[1] Present address: Faculty of Dentistry, McGill University, P. O. box 6070, Montreal, Quebec H3C 3G1, Canada.

MATERIALS AND METHODS

Microorganisms. Type strains of *S. mutans* tested included OMZ-61 (serotype *a*), BHT (serotype *b*), JC-2, Ingbritt (serotype *c*), SL-1, 6715 (serotype *d*), and LM-7 (serotype *e*) (2, 13, 14). Fresh isolates were obtained from children who were untreated siblings of outpatients at the Toronto Hospital for Sick Children.

Selection of concentrations of antimicrobial agents. The antimicrobial agents were tested at a range of concentrations chosen to include those expected to occur in saliva. Since previous workers studying the effect of long-term penicillin therapy on caries (8, 9) did not report the salivary penicillin levels in their subjects, it was necessary to estimate the levels from other information in the literature. The oral administration of 200,000 U of penicillin G has been shown to result in a serum level of approximately 0.12 μg/ml (11). Inasmuch as salivary penicillin levels are approximately 1% of serum levels (1), we estimated the maximum salivary concentration from 200,000 U of penicillin G to be between 1 and 2 ng/ml. The concentrations tested ranged from 0.5 to 48 ng/ml.

The sulfadiazine concentrations tested, 1 and 10 μg/ml, were both within the range of reported salivary excretion levels (3, 17).

Effects of penicillin and sulfadiazine on the growth of *S. mutans*. Inocula were prepared by growing *S. mutans* strains for 24 h in Mueller-Hinton broth (Difco Laboratories, Detroit, Mich.) supplemented with 0.1% glucose and 0.25% K_2HPO_4 (6). This, as well as all subsequent incubations, was carried out in airtight containers at 37°C in an atmosphere of 95% nitrogen and 5% carbon dioxide.

A 0.20-ml portion of the culture was inoculated into duplicate test tubes containing 5.7 ml of Mueller-Hinton broth supplemented with 1% glucose, 0.25% K_2HPO_4, and 0.1 ml of the antibiotic solution to be tested. Optical densities of the cultures were read at 550 nm with a spectrophotometer (Turner model 350; G. K. Turner Associates, Palo Alto, Calif.) at regular intervals during incubation.

Effects on plaque formation. Plaque formation in vitro was tested quantitatively using the methods of McCabe et al. (10) and Miller and Kleinman (12). In preparation for each experiment, bacterial strains were grown for 24 h in Mueller-Hinton broth supplemented with 1% glucose and 0.25% K_2HPO_4. The culture (0.20 ml) was then inoculated into cotton-stoppered test tubes containing 4.9 ml of Mueller-Hinton broth supplemented with 0.25% K_2HPO_4, 1 ml of a filter-sterilized 30% sucrose solution, and 0.1 ml of the antimicrobial agent. Antimicrobial solutions were prepared daily from sterile frozen stock solutions and freshly autoclaved distilled water.

Each test tube contained a length of stainless steel wire (20 gauge) which projected 32 to 33 mm into the broth. After 24 h of incubation, the wires were aseptically transferred into tubes containing fresh broth and agent. Nine consecutive daily transfers were performed to allow adequate plaque accumulation. The coated portions of the wires were then cut off, oven dried at 80°C for 24 h, and weighed. After weighing, the wires were cleaned and reweighed to determine the net dry weight of the deposit.

Effects on the agglutination of washed cells. The effect of low levels of penicillin and sulfadiazine on the agglutination of washed cells of *S. mutans* by high-molecular-weight dextran was assessed by the method of Gibbons and Fitzgerald (6). Strains were grown overnight in a Trypticase salts medium (6) containing separately autoclaved 0.2% glucose. Organisms were harvested by centrifugation at 10,800 $\times g$ and washed twice with 0.9% sodium chloride. They were then resuspended in 0.067 M phosphate buffer (pH 7.0) to make a suspension containing approximately 2×10^9 cells/ml.

To carry out the agglutination testing, 0.3 ml of the cell suspension was combined with 0.1 ml of either distilled water or a dilution of penicillin or sulfadiazine. Then 0.2 ml of a solution containing 100 μg of dextran per ml (molecular weight, 2×10^6; from *Leuconostoc mesenteroides*; Sigma Chemical Co., St. Louis, Mo.) was added. The mixtures were incubated in a water bath at 35°C for 2 h, and agglutination was recorded visually on a scale from no agglutination (−) to marked agglutination (4+). Controls containing cells alone and cells plus penicillin or sulfadiazine were also included.

Effects on the activity of cell-bound enzymes synthesizing polymers from sucrose. Cell-bound enzymes capable of synthesizing polymers from sucrose were isolated from *S. mutans* strains JC-2 and 10-1 grown for 18 h in a Trypticase salts medium containing 0.2% glucose (7) supplemented with 0.01% sucrose to enhance cell-bound dextransucrase activity (16). The cells were harvested by centrifugation at 10,800 $\times g$, washed twice with 0.9% sodium chloride, and resuspended at a 50-fold concentration in 0.067 M phosphate buffer (pH 7.0). To release the enzymes from the surfaces of the cells, the cell suspension was treated with a sonic probe (Biosonik IV, Bronwill Scientific Co., Rochester, N.Y.) for 90 s at maximum power and centrifuged, and the supernatant containing the enzyme was collected.

Duplicate reaction mixtures, each containing 0.2 ml of the enzyme preparation, 1.75 ml of phosphate buffer, 0.05 ml of sulfadiazine, and 1.0 ml of a 0.5% sucrose solution, were incubated in a water bath for 2 h at 35°C. Enzyme activity was measured turbidimetrically according to the method of Gibbons and Nygaard (7).

Effects on the synthesis of cell-bound enzymes synthesizing extracellular polymers. Cultures were grown for 18 h in Mueller-Hinton broth supplemented with 0.25% K_2HPO_4, 0.2% glucose, 0.01% sucrose, and appropriate concentrations of penicillin or sulfadiazine, and growth was assessed spectrophotometrically. Control cultures were also grown without the antibiotics.

Harvesting of the cells, preparation of enzyme suspensions, and determination of enzyme activity were performed as previously described, except that the 0.05-ml additions of the antimicrobial agents were replaced by an equal volume of phosphate buffer.

Statistical analysis. In each experiment, data were obtained from several *S. mutans* strains in the absence of the antimicrobial agent and at several concentrations of the agent. For each strain, the data obtained in the presence and absence of a given concentration of the agent were considered to be paired data. The findings for several strains of *S. mutans* at a given concentration of agent in each experiment provided a paired set of data. The difference between treatment and control data was tested for significance using the paired *t* test (15).

RESULTS

Effects of penicillin and sulfadiazine on growth. Growth of two type strains (JC-2 and Ingbritt) and two fresh isolates (12-1 and 14-1) was studied in the presence of low concentrations of penicillin G. Bacterial growth after 24 h in the presence of the highest penicillin concentration tested (24 ng/ml) did not differ significantly from that in the absence of penicillin ($P > 0.5$).

Growth of 12 strains, including 6 type strains and 6 fresh isolates, was studied in the presence of low levels of sulfadiazine (Table 1). A concentration of 1 μg/ml, which is well within the reported range of salivary excretion levels, resulted in a mean inhibition of growth of 19.1%, which was significant at $P < 0.005$. The degree of inhibition differed markedly between strains, with the greatest inhibition demonstrated by strain SL-1 and no inhibition by strain Ingbritt. At a sulfadiazine concentration of 10 μg/ml the mean inhibition was 22.7%, significant at $P < 0.001$.

Effects on plaque formation. Both penicillin and sulfadiazine substantially inhibited in vitro plaque formation (Table 2). At the lowest concentrations tested, 0.5 ng of penicillin per ml and 1 μg of sulfadiazine per ml, which were well within the limits of expected salivary excretions levels, mean inhibitions of 45.0 and 45.3% were observed, significant at $P < 0.005$ and $P < 0.01$, respectively. In the case of sulfadiazine, the inhibition of plaque formation (45.3%) was more than twice the inhibition of growth (19.1%) observed in the experiments described in the previous section. Increasing the concentration of penicillin 90-fold (to 18 ng/ml) and that of sulfadiazine 10-fold (to 10 μg/ml) produced greater inhibitions of plaque formation than did the lowest concentrations, but the increases in inhibition were not proportional to the increases in concentration of the antimicrobial agents.

Differences were observed in the absolute amount of plaque formed in different experiments. The mean dry weight for plaques in the controls was 19 mg, with a range of 8 to 38 mg in different tests. Despite this variability in the overall amount of plaque formed, the effects of the agents were comparable in each experiment.

Other effects. All *S. mutans* strains tested (type strains 6715 and JC-2 and fresh isolates 10-1 and 12-1) agglutinated strongly (4+) in the presence of dextran but failed to agglutinate in its absence. The dextrain-induced agglutination was unaffected by the presence of 0.5 to 48 ng of penicillin G per ml or 1 and 10 μg of sulfadiazine per ml.

Furthermore, the activity of polymer-forming enzymes after their liberation from cells of the two strains of *S. mutans* tested, JC-2 and 10-1, was unaffected by penicillin at 1 or 18 ng/ml or by sulfadiazine at 1 or 10 μg/ml. Findings ranged from 6% inhibition to 4% stimulation of activity.

The synthesis of cell-bound, polymer-forming enzymes per wet weight of cells was similarly unaffected by low levels of the agents.

DISCUSSION

The most notable observation in the present study was the marked inhibition of in vitro plaque formation by *S. mutans* in the presence of the very low concentrations of both penicillin

TABLE 1. *Effect of sulfadiazine on the growth of S. mutans*

Strains	Relative growth with sulfadiazine (μg/ml)[a]: 1	10
Type strains		
JC-2	92	80
Ingbritt	104	100
OMZ-61	83	68
BHT	87	75
LM-7	89	80
SL-1	53	47
Fresh isolates		
12-1	90	81
14-1	57	34
7-1	81	78
8-1	93	92
10-1	79	74
13-1	63	58

[a] Growth at 24 h, expressed as a percentage of growth in the absence of sulfadiazine.

TABLE 2. *Effect of penicillin and sulfadiazine on in vitro plaque formation*

Strain	No. of plaques	Relative amounts of plaque formation[a] in the presence of: Penicillin G (ng/ml)							Sulfadiazine (μg/ml)	
		0.5	1	3	6	9	18	36	1	10
Type strain JC-2										
Expt 1	2			55	55	46	36		61	54
Expt 2	4			35	35	43	18		52	47
Expt 3	4	43	52	30		29	24	14		
Expt 4	4	58	58	52		40	34	17		
Fresh isolate 10-1										
Expt 1	2			59	67	52	31		71	58
Expt 2	4			42	48	35	24		35	33
Expt 3	4	69	68	70		82	53	41		
Expt 4	4	50	39	39		26	14	9		

[a] Dry weight of plaque expressed as a percentage of that formed in the absence of antimicrobial agents.

and sulfadiazine that might be expected in the saliva of patients on long-term antimicrobial therapy. In the case of penicillin, the diminution of plaque formation was not associated with evidence of a decreased rate of *S. mutans* growth, interference with dextran-mediated agglutination, interference with the synthesis, or activity of cell-bound, polymer-synthesizing enzymes. Therefore, for the present, the effect of penicillin on in vitro plaque formation by *S. mutans* remains unexplained.

The inhibitory effect of sulfadiazine on *S. mutans* growth appeared to be responsible, at least in part, for its inhibitory effect on in vitro plaque formation. However, the finding that plaque formation was inhibited to a greater degree than was growth suggests that other, presently unidentified, factors may have also been involved.

The inhibitory effect of 1 μg of sulfadiazine per ml on *S. mutans* growth was also unexpected, since in susceptibility tests reported elsewhere (18) we found that *S. mutans* was resistant to a concentration of sulfadiazine 3,000 times higher. Apparently sulfadiazine, even at higher concentrations, causes only a partial inhibition of growth which is undetectable by susceptibility testing procedures that are only able to detect complete abolition of growth. These observations point to the possibility that an antimicrobial agent might reduce dental caries, even though susceptibility tests indicate that *S. mutans* is resistant to the agent.

The findings have additional implications for clinical studies. The observed inhibition of *S. mutans* plaque formation by penicillin could explain the inhibitory effect on caries of long-term daily administration of penicillin observed in clinical studies (8, 9). Additionally, the observed effect of sulfadiazine on plaque formation suggests that the possible effect of that agent on dental caries should be clinically evaluated.

ACKNOWLEDGMENTS

The suggestions and criticisms of R. C. Burgess, R. Ellen, and H. Onose are gratefully acknowledged. This study was assisted under the Province of Ontario Health Research grant no. P. R. 446.

LITERATURE CITED

1. **Bender, I. B., R. S. Pressman, and S. G. Tashman.** 1953. Studies on excretion of antibiotics in human saliva. I. Penicillin and streptomycin. J. Am. Dent. Assoc. **46**:164–170.
2. **Bratthall, D.** 1970. Demonstration of five serological groups of streptococcal strains resembling *Streptococcus mutans*. Odontol. Revy **21**:143–152.
3. **Devine, L. F., R. C. Knowles, W. E. Pierce, R. O. Peckinpaugh, C. R. Hagerman, and R. I. Lytle.** 1969. Proposed model for screening antimicrobial agents for potential use in eliminating meningococci from the nasopharynx of healthy carriers, p. 307–314. Antimicrob. Agents Chemother. 1968.
4. **Ericsson, H. M., and J. C. Sherris.** 1971. Antibiotic sensitivity testing: report of an international collaborative study. Acta Pathol. Microbiol. Scand. Suppl. 217.
5. **Gibbons, R. J., P. F. DePaola, D. M. Spinell, and Z. Skobe.** 1974. Interdental localization of *Streptococcus mutans* as related to dental caries experience. Infect. Immun. **9**:481–488.
6. **Gibbons, R. J., and R. J. Fitzgerald.** 1969. Dextran-induced agglutination of *Streptococcus mutans*, and its potential role in the formation of microbial dental plaques. J. Bacteriol. **98**:341–346.
7. **Gibbons, R. J., and M. Nygaard.** 1968. Synthesis of insoluble dextran and its significance in the formation of gelatinous deposits by plaque-forming streptococci. Arch. Oral Biol. **13**:1249–1262.
8. **Handelman, S. L., J. R. Mills, and R. R. Hawes.** 1966. Caries incidence in subjects receiving long-term antibiotic therapy. J. Oral Ther. Pharmacol. **2**:338–345.
9. **Littleton, N. W., and C. L. White.** 1964. Dental findings from a preliminary study of children receiving extended antibiotic therapy. J. Am. Dent. Assoc. **68**:520–525.
10. **McCabe, R. M., P. H. Keyes, and A. Howell, Jr.** 1967. An *in vitro* method for assessing the plaque forming ability of oral bacteria. Arch. Oral Biol. **17**:1653–1656.
11. **McCarthy, C. G., G. Wallmark, and M. Finland.** 1961. *In vitro* activity of various penicillins. Am. J. Med. Sci. **241**:143–159.
12. **Miller, C. H., and J. L. Kleinman.** 1974. Effect of microbial interactions on *in vitro* plaque formation by *Streptococcus mutans*. J. Dent. Res. **53**:427–434.
13. **Mukasa, H., and H. D. Slade.** 1974. Mechanism of adherence of *Streptococcus mutans* to smooth surfaces. II. Nature of the binding site and the adsorption of dextran-levan synthetase enzymes on the cell-wall surface of the streptococcus. Infect. Immun. **9**:419–429.
14. **Perch, B., E. Kjems, and T. Ravn. T.** 1974. Biochemical and serological properties of *Streptococcus mutans* from various human and animal sources. Acta Pathol. Microbiol. Scand. **82**:357–370.
15. **Snedecor, G. W., and W. G. Cochran.** 1967. Statistical methods, 6th ed., p. 91–97. Iowa State University Press, Ames.
16. **Spinell, D. M., and R. J. Gibbons.** 1974. Influence of culture medium on the glucosyl transferase- and dextran-binding capacity of *Streptococcus mutans* 6715 cells. Infect. Immun. **10**:1448–1451.
17. **Stephen, K. W., and C. F. Speirs.** 1972. Oral environmental source of antibacterial drugs. The importance of gingival fluid, p. 76–83. *In* T. MacPhee (ed.), Host resistance to commensal bacteria: the response to dental plaque. Churchill-Livingstone, Edinburgh.
18. **Weld, H. G., and H. J. Sandham.** 1976. Effect of long-term therapies with penicillin and sulfadiazine on *Streptococcus mutans* and lactobacilli in dental plaque. Antimicrob. Agents Chemother. **10**:200–204.

Antimicrobial Agents and Chemotherapy, Aug. 1976, p. 200-204
Vol. 10, No. 2

Effect of Long-Term Therapies with Penicillin and Sulfadiazine on *Streptococcus mutans* and Lactobacilli in Dental Plaque

H. G. WELD[1] AND H. J. SANDHAM*

Department of Preventive Dentistry, Faculty of Dentistry, University of Toronto, Toronto, Ontario M5G 1G6, Canada

Received for publication 28 August 1975

Plaque samples were obtained from 13 children receiving long-term therapy with benzathine penicillin for the prevention of rheumatic fever recurrences, 31 children receiving oral sulfadiazine for the same purpose, and 29 untreated siblings. The therapies were found to have no effect upon the proportions of *Streptococcus mutans* or lactobacilli in dental plaque, upon the percentage of children harboring the organisms, nor upon the susceptibility of the organisms to penicillin and sulfadiazine. Of the *S. mutans* strains tested, 97% had a minimal inhibitory concentration of penicillin G of less than 48 ng/ml and, of the lactobacillus strains tested, 96.8% had a minimal inhibitory concentration of less than 1,600 ng/ml. All strains of both organisms were profoundly resistant to sulfadiazine.

Children receiving 200,000 U of oral penicillin daily for rheumatic fever prophylaxis have been reported to experience reductions in the incidence of dental caries of up to 56% as compared with their untreated siblings (13, 18). Handelman and Hawes have reported that the oral penicillin therapy had no effect on the number of salivary lactobacilli (12) and that the penicillin resistances of the total flora, the streptococci, and the staphylococci in the salivas of the antibiotic users were higher than those in the untreated siblings (11). They did not study the effect of oral penicillin on *Streptococcus mutans*; consequently, it is not known whether the caries-inhibiting effect of that agent (13) resulted from its action on that organism. Furthermore, they did not examine the dental plaque flora, which is more intimately associated with the development of the carious lesion than is the salivary flora.

Treatment currently used at the Toronto Hospital for Sick Children for the prevention of rheumatic fever recurrences consists of either a monthly injection of 1.2×10^6 U of benzathine penicillin or a daily oral administration of 1 g of sulfadiazine. This report describes a study of the effects of these therapies on the proportions and antimicrobial susceptibility of *S. mutans* and lactobacilli isolated from dental plaque. *S. mutans* was selected because it is a plaque organism that has been strongly implicated as an etiological factor in dental caries (8). Lactobacilli have been implicated in dental caries etiology for many years (15).

[1] Present address: Faculty of Dentistry, McGill University, P. O. box 6070, Montreal, Quebec H3C 3G1, Canada.

MATERIALS AND METHODS

Study groups. The subjects examined were outpatients of the Division of Cardiology, Hospital for Sick Children, Toronto, and their siblings. All children attending the clinic in the 8-month period from June 1974 to February 1975 and whose parents consented were included in the study. The experimental groups consisted of a group of 13 children receiving one injection of benzathine penicillin per month and a second group of 31 receiving daily oral sulfadiazine. A group of 29 siblings served as controls. All subjects were between 7 and 21 years of age. An attempt was made to equalize the ages of children in the treatment and control groups by asking the parent to bring in the sibling nearest in age to the treated child.

Plaque sampling. Because many children in the penicillin group received their injections from private practitioners, it was not possible to standardize the time interval between the penicillin injection and plaque sampling. In the majority of cases the interval was between 2 weeks and 1 month. The plaques of sulfadiazine children were sampled approximately 6 h after they had received the drug.

Three plaque samples were obtained from each of the subjects: one from occlusal pits and fissures, one from vestibular smooth surfaces, and one from approximal surfaces. Each sample consisted of plaque pooled from all of the posterior teeth in the mandibular left quadrant. If two or more teeth were missing, the mandibular right quadrant was used. To minimize salivary contamination, all surfaces were briefly air dried with a rubber bulb syringe before sampling.

Samples, collected with sterile sharp explorers (Stardent no. 5, Star Dental Manufacturing Co., Philadelphia, Pa.), were immediately placed into reduced transport fluid (25).

Microbiological methods. Plaque samples, returned to the laboratory within 2 h of collection, were dispersed under a 95% nitrogen-5% carbon dioxide mixture with a sonic probe (Biosonik IV, Bronwill Scientific Inc., Rochester, N.Y.) for 10 s at maximum power. Sample tubes were cooled in an ice water bath during the dispersion.

Tenfold serial dilutions in reduced transport fluid were plated in duplicate on brain heart infusion agar (Difco) supplemented with 5% defibrinated sheep blood (BHI-blood agar), on mitis salivarius (MS) agar (Difco), and on Rogosa SL agar (Difco). These media were used for the enumeration of total cultivable flora, of total streptococci and *S. mutans* proportions, and of lactobacilli, respectively. A plate of mitis salivarius-bacitracin (MSB) agar (9) was also inoculated to obtain adequate numbers of *S. mutans* for susceptibility testing.

All bacteria in the study were grown in airtight containers in an atmosphere of 95% nitrogen and 5% carbon dioxide at 37°C. MS and MSB agar plates were incubated for 18 h; BHI-blood agar and Rogosa SL plates were incubated for 72 h. MS and MSB agar plates were subsequently incubated aerobically at room temperature for 24 h before counting (16).

Enumeration. Counting was carried out on plates containing between 75 and 150 colonies, whenever possible. On MS agar, both rough and mucoid colonies of *S. mutans* were counted (4, 14). On Rogosa SL agar, *Lactobacillus* colonies were counted as described previously (15).

Susceptibility testing. To assess susceptibility of the organisms to penicillin and sulfadiazine, colonies were chosen at random from the MSB and Rogosa SL plates. Nine colonies of *S. mutans* and six to nine colonies of lactobacilli were picked per subject, placed into 1 ml of Mueller-Hinton broth (Difco) supplemented with 0.1% glucose and 0.25% K_2HPO_4, and incubated for 18 h as described above. A suspension containing approximately 10^7 colony-forming units/ml was distributed with a replicator (model R-2, Bio-Tech Co., Lynden, Ontario) onto plates of Mueller-Hinton medium (Difco), supplemented with 5% defibrinated sheep blood and dilutions of potassium penicillin G (Connaught Laboratories Ltd., Toronto), or sulfadiazine (Solu-Diazine, Poulenc, Montreal). Control plates free of the antimicrobial agents were also inoculated. The plates were incubated for 18 h and qualitatively assessed for growth (+) or no growth (−) (5). The lowest concentration of antimicrobial agent preventing growth was considered to be the minimal inhibitory concentration (MIC).

Analysis of data. Quantitative data, such as the age and sex of the subjects and duration of therapy and the frequency of isolation and prevalence of streptococci and *S. mutans*, were compared by means of *t* tests. Qualitative data, such as the proportions of subjects and surfaces harboring either lactobacilli or *S. mutans*, were compared by means of chi-square tests of confidence (22). Effects of age, sex, and duration of therapy on *S. mutans* proportions in plaque were analyzed by regression analysis (22).

RESULTS

Study groups. Despite our efforts to equalize the ages in the treatment and control groups, the mean ages of children in the treatment groups were approximately 2 years greater than that of the control group. The mean age in years, standard errors, and ranges of ages in the various groups were as follows: penicillin group, 14.3 ± 0.73 (7.4 to 18.5); sulfadiazine group, 14.5 ± 0.50 (9.8 to 20.4); and control group, 12.5 ± 0.52 (7.5 to 20.0).

The mean duration of therapy was greater in the sulfadiazine group (6.1 ± 0.47 years; range, 1 to 13 years) than in the penicilllin group (4.1 ± 0.80 years; range, 1 to 8 years). In the sulfadiazine group, the numbers of males and females were nearly equal (51.8% males), but in the penicillin group males predominated (69.2%) and in the control group females predominated (58.6%).

Effect of therapy on the frequency of isolation of streptococci. Comparing the mean percentages of streptococci in the plaques of subjects from the treatment and control groups (Table 1), the only statistically significant difference observed was that plaques from the penicillin-treated children contained a higher proportion of streptococci than did plaques from the control group ($t = 2.49$; $P < 0.05$). The differences on specific surfaces between either treatment group and the control group were not statistically significant.

Effect on the incidence and prevalence of *S. mutans*. *S. mutans* numbers, expressed as a percentage of the total streptococci (Table 2), in the groups receiving therapy did not differ significantly from those in the control group when either all plaques or plaques from specific tooth surfaces were compared. A lack of effect of therapy was also observed when *S. mutans* numbers were expressed as the percentage of the total cultivable flora.

The proportions of *S. mutans* present on the occlusal surfaces in all groups (approximately 30% of the total streptococci) were greater than those for the vestibular and approximal surfaces (between 2.1 and 7.4%).

Statistical analyses showed no significant correlation between (i) proportions of *S. mutans* in plaques of control children and age of the children, (ii) proportions of *S. mutans* in the plaques and sex of the subjects, (iii) proportions of *S. mutans* in plaques of subjects in each of the treatment groups and length of therapy, and (iv) the percentage of subjects harboring *S. mutans* in one or more of their plaque samples and drug therapy. The percentage of children with *S. mutans*-infected plaque did not differ significantly among the control group (93.1%), the penicillin group (84.6%), and the sulfadiazine group (87.1%).

Effect on the incidence and prevalence of lactobacilli. The percentage of the children harboring lactobacilli in one or more of their plaque samples (approximately 30%) did not differ significantly between treatment and control groups ($P > 0.05$). The percentage of specific tooth surfaces harboring lactobacilli also did not differ between groups. Neither age of subjects nor duration of therapy had any demonstrable effect on the proportions of subjects harboring lactobacilli.

Drug administration also had no effect on the proportions of lactobacilli, either in all plaques or in plaques from specific surfaces. The proportions of lactobacilli in plaques were low; in 61.3% of the samples from which lactobacilli were identified, they comprised less than 0.01% of the total cultivable flora. In no instance did they comprise more than 4.0% of the flora.

Effect on the susceptibility of *S. mutans* and lactobacilli. A total of 80 strains of *S. mutans* from subjects receiving penicillin and 168 strains from control subjects were compared for their susceptibility to penicillin; no significant differences in susceptibility were observed. An MIC of 24 or 48 ng of penicillin per ml was observed for 100 and 96.4% of isolates from the respective groups. The growth of the remaining strains was prevented by 100 ng/ml.

All 18 strains of lactobacilli isolated from the penicillin group had an MIC of 1,600 ng of penicillin per ml, more than 30-fold higher than that of *S. mutans*. Most of the 34 *Lactobacillus* strains isolated from the control group also had an MIC of 1,600 ng/ml, but 8.8% had an MIC of 100 ng/ml and 29.4% had an MIC of 400 ng/ml. None of the lactobacilli had an MIC greater than 1,600 ng/ml.

A total of 76 isolates of *S. mutans* and 59 isolates of lactobacilli were obtained from all study groups and tested for their susceptibility to sulfadiazine; all demonstrated a high level of resistance by growing in the presence of concentrations greater than 3.0 mg/ml.

DISCUSSION

The results of this study do not support the possibility that long-term therapy with benzathine penicillin or with sulfadiazine might decrease the cariogenicity of the plaque microflora. Neither drug caused a significant alteration in the proportions of *S. mutans* or lactobacilli, the organisms most commonly implicated as etiological agents in dental caries (8, 15).

The lack of effect of the benzathine penicillin therapy on the proportions of these bacteria in plaque, despite the high susceptibility to penicillin demonstrated by the organisms in vitro (see also 1, 6, 7), suggests that the therapy results in negligible levels of penicillin in saliva. The lack of development of resistance by the organisms to penicillin supports this contention. A similar conclusion was reached by previous workers (23) on the basis of findings that benzathine penicillin has an effect on the

TABLE 1. *Percentages of streptococci in the total cultivable flora of plaque samples from children receiving various therapies*

Group	Streptococci (%) on tooth surfaces:			
	All	Occlusal	Vestibular	Approximal
Penicillin	34.7 ± 4.3[a]	47.1 ± 8.4	31.9 ± 6.6	25.2 ± 6.3
Sulfadiazine	26.7 ± 2.0	28.7 ± 3.3	27.4 ± 3.6	24.1 ± 3.7
Control	22.7 ± 2.2	27.7 ± 5.1	20.8 ± 3.0	21.2 ± 3.8

[a] Mean ± standard error.

TABLE 2. *Percentages of S. mutans in the total streptococci of plaque samples from children receiving various therapies*

Group	*S. mutans*[a] (%) on various tooth surfaces:			
	All	Occlusal	Vestibular	Approximal
Penicillin	14.6 ± 4.0[b]	30.8 ± 9.7	5.5 ± 3.3	7.4 ± 3.7
Sulfadiazine	12.1 ± 2.5	29.9 ± 6.1	2.1 ± 1.1	4.4 ± 1.9
Control	15.4 ± 2.7	32.7 ± 6.2	6.3 ± 2.7	7.1 ± 2.7

[a] Expressed as a percentage of the total cultivable streptococci.
[b] Mean ± standard error.

penicillin resistance of the flora in the throat, saliva, and gingival margin (2, 19, 23).

In contrast, Handelman and Hawes (11) have observed that, in children receiving daily oral penicillin, the penicillin resistance of the salivary flora, including the streptococci, is higher than that in untreated siblings. This suggests that the caries inhibitory effect of the therapy (13) was associated with appreciable salivary levels of the agent. They did not determine the penicillin resistance of lactobacilli in their subjects, but their observation that the numbers of lactobacilli were unaltered by the therapy suggests that organism was resistant to the concentration of penicillin present in the saliva. Since they did not examine the antibiotic resistance or numbers of *S. mutans*, the possibility that the caries inhibitory effect of the therapy (13) was due to its effect on that organism is unknown. Nevertheless, our observations that *S. mutans* is approximately 30-fold more susceptible to penicillin than are lactobacilli and that *S. mutans* is more intimately involved with the initiation of the carious lesion (15) lend weight to that premise.

The mean length of time that the patients receiving benzathine penicillin had been under therapy in our study, 4.1 years, was considerably longer than that of the subjects receiving oral penicillin in the study of Handelman and Hawes (11) and should have been adequate to demonstrate any long-term effect. On the other hand, the small number of patients available in our study would have prevented the detection of small differences between the experimental groups. Imbalances were also present in ages and sex between the control and experimental groups but did not appear to significantly affect the results.

An unexpected finding in the present study, that the penicillin group demonstrated a higher proportion of streptococci than did the controls, suggests that, if penicillin had an effect on the plaque flora, it was on components of the flora other than the streptococci. The reason for this observation is not apparent at the present time.

Long-term sulfadiazine therapy did not have a significant effect on the proportions of *S. mutans* or lactobacilli in plaque. The result with *S. mutans* was particularly surprising since an earlier study (26), using an in vitro quantitative assessment of *S. mutans* growth, had shown that low levels of sulfadiazine (1 to 10 μg/ml) inhibited growth, even though the organisms were resistant to the agent as judged by usual qualitative susceptibility testing procedures (3, 20, 21). It would seem that, if such an inhibition occurs in vivo, it was not of sufficient magnitude to significantly alter the proportions of that organism in plaque.

Whether the lack of effect of sulfadiazine therapy in our study may have been due in part to a lack of patient compliance was not determined. Lack of patient compliance to long-term therapeutic regimes is a well-known problem (24, 27, 28).

The apparent lack of effect of prolonged benzathine penicillin and sulfadiazine therapies on the proportions of *S. mutans* and lactobacilli in plaque suggests, but does not prove, that the therapies are ineffective in reducing dental caries activity. More substantial proof must be provided by clinical caries studies.

The present study also confirmed previous reports that occlusal pits and fissures are a major reservoir of *S. mutans* in permanent teeth (15), that the majority of young people are infected with that organism (15), and that lactobacilli are a numerically minor component of dental plaque over noncarious sites, although they are present in the plaques of a substantial number of children (10, 15, 17).

ACKNOWLEDGMENTS

We thank R. D. Rowe, Langford Kidd, R. B. Ross, and the staff of the Division of Cardiology, Toronto Hospital for Sick Children, for their cooperation in the study. The assistance of J. Bennett in administering the clinical aspects of the study, R. P. Ellen and R. C. Burgess in reviewing the manuscript, G. W. Thompson in the statistical analyses, and M. Villari in typing is gratefully acknowledged.

This study was assisted under the Province of Ontario Health Research grant no. P.R. 446. Interim support at the beginning of the study was provided by the R. Samuel McLaughlin Foundation. H.G.W. was the recipient of a fellowship from the Canadian Fund for Dental Education.

LITERATURE CITED

1. **Baker, C. N., and C. Thornsberry.** 1974. Antimicrobial susceptibility of *Streptococcus mutans* isolated from patients with endocarditis. Antimicrob. Agents Chemother. 5:268–271.
2. **Bentley, D. W., T. Frank, and J. J. Hahn.** 1971. Penicillin-resistant oral streptococci, p. 277–279. Antimicrob. Agents Chemother. 1970.
3. **Carlsson, J.** 1968. A numerical taxonomic study of human oral streptococci. Odontol. Revy **19**:137–160.
4. **Edwardsson, S.** 1970. The caries-inducing property of variants of *Streptococcus mutans*. Odontol. Revy **21**:153–157.
5. **Ericsson, H. M., and J. C. Sherris.** 1971. Antibiotic sensitivity testing: report of an international collaborative study. Acta Pathol. Microbiol. Scand. Sect. B; Suppl. 217.
6. **Fitzgerald, R. J.** 1972. Inhibition of experimental dental caries by antibiotics. Antimicrob. Agents Chemother. **1**:296–302.
7. **Fitzgerald, R. J., H. A. Zander, and H. V. Jordan.** 1950. The effects of a penicillin dentifrice on oral lactobacilli. J. Am. Dent. Assoc. **41**:62–65.
8. **Gibbons, R. J., and J. van Houte.** 1973. On the formation of dental plaques. J. Periodontol. **44**:347–360.
9. **Gold, O. G., H. V. Jordan, and J. van Houte.** 1973. A selective medium for *Streptococcus mutans*. Arch. Oral Biol. **18**:1357–1364.

10. **Green, G. E., M. C. Dodd, and H. S. Inverso.** 1957. Comparative microflora of developing dental plaques in caries-immune and susceptible individuals. J. Dent. Res. **36**:331–337.
11. **Handelman, S. L., and R. R. Hawes.** 1964. The effect of long-term antibiotic therapy on the antibiotic resistance of the salivary flora. J. Oral Ther. Pharmacol. **1**:23–44.
12. **Handelman, S. L., and R. R. Hawes.** 1965. The effect of long-term systemic antibiotic administration on the numbers of salivary organisms. Arch. Oral Biol. **10**:353–360.
13. **Handelman, S. L., J. R. Mills, and R. R. Hawes.** 1966. Caries incidence in subjects receiving long-term antibiotic therapy. J. Oral Ther. Pharmacol. **2**:338–345.
14. **Ikeda, T., T. Mukasa, S. Yagi, K. Ochiai, Y. Doi, T. Shiota, and H. J. Sandham.** 1975. The characteristics of *Streptococcus mutans* PS-14. Nihon Univ. J. Oral Sci. **1**:202–208.
15. **Ikeda, T., H. J. Sandham, and E. L. Bradley, Jr.** 1973. Changes in *Streptococcus mutans* and lactobacilli in plaque in relation to the initiation of dental caries in Negro children. Arch. Oral Biol. **18**:555–566.
16. **Jordan, H. V., B. Krasse, and A. Moller.** 1968. A method of sampling human dental plaque for certain "caries-inducing" streptococci. Arch. Oral Biol. **13**:919–927.
17. **Krasse, B.** 1954. The relationship between lactobacilli, Candida and streptococci and dental caries. Odontol. Revy **5**:241–261.
18. **Littleton, N. W., and C. L. White.** 1964. Dental findings from a preliminary study of children receiving extended antibiotic therapy. J. Am. Dent. Assoc. **68**:520–525.
19. **Patterson, P. Y., and G. M. Madden.** 1969. Occurrence and erythromycin susceptibility of penicillin-resistant viridans streptococci in rheumatic fever patients on oral penicillin prophylaxis, p. 323–325. Antimicrob. Agents Chemother. 1968.
20. **Perch, B., E. Kjems, and T. Raun.** 1974. Biochemical and serological properties of *Streptococcus mutans* from various human and animal sources. Acta Pathol. Microbiol. Scand. **82**:357–370.
21. **Rogers, A. H.** 1969. The proportional distribution and characteristics of streptococci in human dental plaque. Caries Res. **3**:238–248.
22. **Snedecor, G. W., and W. G. Cochran.** 1967. Statistical methods, 6th ed. Iowa State University Press, Ames.
23. **Spencer, W. H., III, C. Thornsberry, M. D. Moody, and N. K. Wenger.** 1970. Rheumatic fever chemoprophylaxis and penicillin-resistant gingival organisms. Ann. Intern. Med. **73**:683–687.
24. **Stollerman, G. H., J. H. Rusoff, and I. Hirschfeld.** 1953. Prophylaxis against group A streptococci in rheumatic fever patients by the use of single monthly injections of N,N[1] dibenzylethylenediamine dipenicillin G (bicillin). Antibiot. Annu. **1**:114–118.
25. **Syed, S. A., and W. J. Loesche.** 1972. Survival of human dental plaque flora in various transport media. Appl. Microbiol. **24**:638–644.
26. **Weld, H. G., and H. J. Sandham.** 1976. In vitro effects of low concentrations of penicillin and sulfadiazine on *Streptococcus mutans*. Antimicrob. Agents Chemother. **10**:196–199.
27. **Wood, H. F., A. R. Feinstein, A. Taranta, J. A. Epstein, and K. Simpson.** 1964. Rheumatic fever in children and adolescents. II. Comparative effectiveness of three prophylaxis regimes in preventing streptococcal infections and rheumatic recurrences. Ann. Intern. Med. **60** (Suppl. 5):31–46.
28. **Wood, H. F., G. H. Stollerman, A. R. Feinstein, I. Hirschfeld, J. H. Rusoff, A. Taranta, R. C. Hoas, and J. A. Epstein.** 1957. A controlled study of three methods of prophylaxis against streptococcal infection in a population of rheumatic children. I. Streptococcal infections and recurrences of acute rheumatic fever in the first two years of the study. N. Engl. J. Med. **257**:394–398.

ANTIMICROBIAL AGENTS AND CHEMOTHERAPY, Aug. 1976, p. 205-210
Vol. 10, No. 2

Amikacin in Newborn Infants: Comparative Pharmacology with Kanamycin and Clinical Efficacy in 45 Neonates with Bacterial Diseases

JORGE B. HOWARD, GEORGE H. McCRACKEN, JR.,* HUGO TRUJILLO, AND EDGAR MOHS

Department of Pediatrics, The University of Texas Health Science Center at Dallas, Southwestern Medical School, Dallas, Texas 75235; Universidad de Antioqua, Departmento de Pediatria, Medellin, Colombia; and Hospital Nacional de Ninos, San Jose, Costa Rica*

Received for publication 8 March 1976

The pharmacokinetic properties of amikacin (BBK8) were similar to those of kanamycin in newborn infants. Peak serum concentrations of both drugs were in the range of 15 to 25 μg/ml with the exception of kanamycin in babies weighing greater than 2,000 g at birth where peak levels were 12.5 to 15 μg/ml. Volumes of distribution, plasma clearances, and serum half-life values were comparable for the two drugs. The clinical and bacteriological responses to amikacin therapy were assessed in 45 neonates with bacterial diseases. A case fatality rate of 26% was observed in infants with septicemia and/or meningitis, whereas no deaths occurred among 22 infants with urinary tract and mucocutaneous infections. Cultures from infected sites were sterile within 72 h of initiating amikacin therapy in 47% of the infants, continued positive for greater than 72 h in 31%, and were not reevaluated during therapy in 22%. The clinical response was judged to be satisfactory in 92% of the surviving infants. The efficacy of amikacin was comparable to that of kanamycin or gentamicin in neonatal bacterial diseases.

Aminoglycosides are frequently administered to neonates to prevent or treat gram-negative bacterial infections. As a result, emergence of coliforms resistant to these drugs has developed in some nurseries. For example, streptomycin resistance was noted in the early 1960s, and kanamycin-resistant *Escherichia coli* and *Klebsiella* strains were observed within the past 5 years (5–8). Gentamicin has been used in many neonatal units. Significant resistance to this agent has been demonstrated recently in an infant intensive care unit (5) and can be anticipated in other centers where the antibiotic is used extensively. Therefore, it is imperative that the pharmacology, efficacy, and safety of new aminoglycosidic drugs which offer promise for treatment of neonatal bacterial diseases be evaluated.

The purpose of the present communication is to review our experience in newborn infants with a new aminoglycoside, amikacin (BBK8). Previously published data from our laboratory showed that amikacin susceptibilities of gram-negative bacilli and *Staphylococcus aureus* were comparable to those for kanamycin, with the exception that over 90% of *Pseudomonas aeruginosa* were susceptible to 15 μg or less of amikacin per ml (6). Five kanamycin-resistant *E. coli* strains isolated from cerebrospinal fluid (CSF) of neonates with meningitis were inhibited and killed by 5 μg or less of amikacin per ml.

Pharmacological studies in 48 babies demonstrated mean serum levels of 17 to 20 μg/ml at 30 min and of 3.3 to 5.3 μg/ml at 12 h after a 7.5-mg/kg amikacin dose (6). Accumulation of drug in serum and acute renal or hematological toxicity were not observed after repeated doses for 5 to 7 days. Urinary amikacin concentrations were 50 to 650 μg/ml, and the average 12-h urinary excretion of drug was 30 to 50% of the administered dose. Serum half-life values were inversely correlated with postnatal age and ranged from 3 to 9 h.

In this paper we present the comparative pharmacokinetic properties of amikacin and kanamycin in neonates and the clinical efficacy of amikacin in 45 infants with bacterial infections. The pharmacological data are based in part on our previously published studies of amikacin (6) and kanamycin (7).

MATERIALS AND METHODS

Antimicrobial assay. Concentrations of amikacin and kanamycin in serum and CSF were assayed by a modification of the micromethod of Simon and Yin

(13) using *Bacillus subtilis* as the test organism. Standard antibiotic curves were prepared in an identical fashion to test samples.

Serum half-life determinations. The equation for the regression line of the log of serum antibiotic concentrations was calculated by the method of the least mean squares. The half-life was determined by dividing the $\log_{10}2$ by the slope of the line.

Drug distribution and plasma clearance. The volumes of distribution (V_D) of amikacin and kanamycin expressed in milliliters per kilogram were calculated using the formula:

$$V_D = \frac{\text{Dosage (mg/kg)}}{AUC \times K} \times 1{,}000$$

where (K) is the elimination rate constant and AUC represents the area under the serum concentration-time curve which is formulated by successive trapezoidal approximation (4). Plasma clearance (C_p) in ml/min per 1.73 m^2 was determined using the formula:

$$C_p = \frac{\text{Total dosage}}{AUC} \times \frac{1{,}000\ \mu g}{60\ \text{min}} \times \frac{1.73\ \text{m}^2}{\text{SA}}$$

where (SA) is surface area in m^2.

Study patients. Pharmacological studies were performed in patients selected from the nurseries of Parkland Memorial Hospital, Dallas. Written informed parental consent was obtained for all infants. Serum samples for bioassay were collected by heel-stick technique. Eleven infants who were receiving amikacin intramuscularly were given one dose intravenously over a 20-min period and multiple serum samples after both routes of administration were obtained on successive days.

The clinical efficacy of amikacin was studied in 19 infants cared for at the Hospital Infantil San Vincente de Paul in Medellin, Columbia, in 17 infants at the Hospital Nacional de Ninos in San Jose, Costa Rica, and in 9 infants at Parkland Memorial Hospital in Dallas. The parents of all patients were fully informed about the study and written consent was obtained before therapy. Penicillin G or ampicillin was given in combination with amikacin to 22 patients. It is customary to administer a penicillin and an aminoglycoside as initial therapy for neonatal infections until the pathogen has been identified. The clinical and bacteriological responses of these infants were evaluated and a complete blood count, urinalysis, blood urea nitrogen and/or serum creatinine were obtained at the beginning and completion of therapy.

RESULTS

Serum and CSF concentrations. Complete serum concentration-time curves for amikacin and kanamycin have been presented elsewhere (6, 7). Mean serum amikacin levels 30 min after a 7.5-mg/kg dose were 17 to 20 μg/ml for all infant groups irrespective of birth weight and age (Fig. 1). By contrast, average serum kanamycin concentrations 30 min after a 7.5-mg/kg dose were 17 to 22 μg/ml in low-birth-weight (less than 2,000 g) infants and 12.5 to 15 μg/ml in infants who weighed 2,000 g or greater at birth. Concentrations of both drugs were comparable 12 h after a dose with the exception of a higher mean kanamycin concentration in low-birth-weight infants who were 1 to 4 days of age.

Serum amikacin levels were measured in 11 infants after intravenous and intramuscular 7.5-mg/kg doses were administered on successive days (Fig. 2). Peak serum concentrations were 13.6 to 40 μg/ml (mean, 21.1 μg/ml) after the intramuscular dose. By contrast, the peak

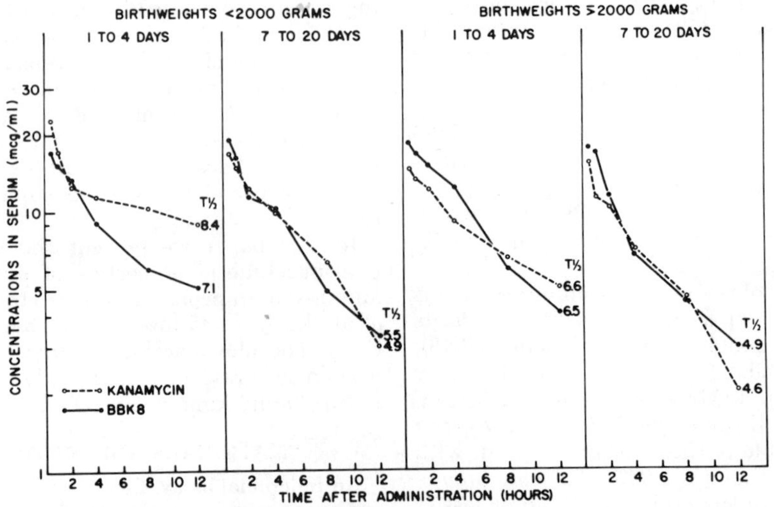

FIG. 1. *Serum concentration-time curves for amikacin (BBK8) and kanamycin after 7.5-mg/kg doses administered intramuscularly to neonates according to birth weight and postnatal age.*

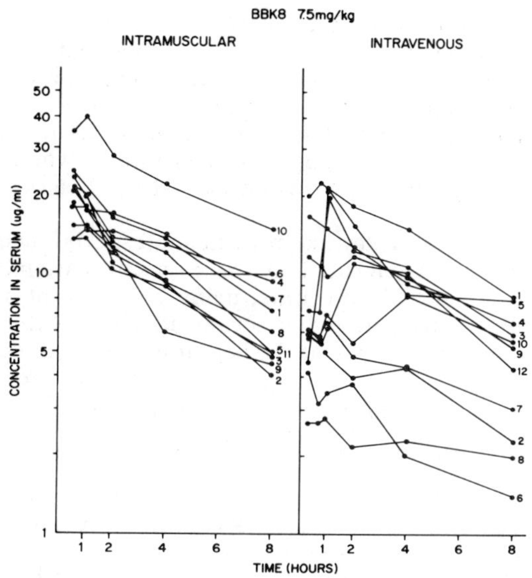

FIG. 2. *Serum amikacin (BBK8) concentration-time curves after 7.5-mg/kg doses administered intramuscularly and intravenously to 11 neonates. Numbers in parentheses refer to individual patients and are shown so that the curves after both routes of administration in the same patient can be compared.*

serum values in five infants who received amikacin intravenously over a 20-min period ranged from 2.8 to 7.0 μg/ml (mean, 5.4 μg/ml), and the slopes of the serum concentration-time curves were less acute compared with those for the same infants after the intramuscular dose (Fig. 2). The curves after intravenous amikacin in the other six infants were comparable to those after intramuscular administration. Four of the five infants with low serum concentrations after the intravenous dose had birth weights of 1,920 g or less (1,080 to 1,920 g), whereas only two of the six infants with peak serum levels in the expected range had similar birth weights. The intravenous dose was administered in a peripheral vein by the same physician (J. Howard), and the time during which the drug was given and the actual mechanics of administering the drug were identical for all infants.

Fifteen ventricular fluid specimens were obtained from five infants with meningitis and ventriculitis who received amikacin intraventricularly as well as intramuscularly. Ventricular fluid amikacin concentrations 12 h after 1- or 2-mg intraventricular doses and 2 to 8 h after the intramuscular doses were 4.5 to 11.6 μg/ml (mean, 7.3 μg/ml). Five CSF specimens were obtained from the lumbar intrathecal space of three infants who received parenteral therapy only. Amikacin concentrations 1 to 12 h after a 7.5-mg/kg intramuscular dose ranged from 0.8 to 9.2 μg/ml (mean, 4.4 μg/ml).

Serum half-life. The serum half-life values for amikacin and kanamycin were inversely correlated with gestational and chronological ages and ranged from 7 to 8 h in low-birth-weight babies who were under 4 days of age to 4 to 5 h in the larger babies who were greater than 7 days of age (Fig. 1 and Table 1).

Volume of distribution and plasma clearance. The calculated distribution volumes of the two aminoglycosides were similar with exception of the larger kanamycin values in newborn infants 1 to 4 days of age (Table 1). The plasma clearance values were similar for amikacin and kanamycin throughout the neonatal period and correlated inversely with the serum half-life values.

Clinical efficacy. Clinical and bacteriological responses were evaluated in 45 neonates with documented bacterial diseases. The bacterial pathogens associated with these illnesses are shown in Table 2. Miscellaneous pathogens included one each of the following: *Proteus mirabilis, Haemophilus influenzae* type b, *Straphylococcus epidermidis,* and a gram-negative rod that was not identified. Two patients had mixed cultures with two organisms: *E. coli* and *Klebsiella* species from the urine of one infant and *S. aureus* and *E. coli* from an abscess cavity of a second baby.

Fifteen infants had septicemia documented by positive blood cultures on at least one occasion before antimicrobial therapy (Table 3). Four infants (27%) died; death occurred within 48 h of initiating amikacin therapy in two patients. The clinical response of the 11 surviving infants was assessed as satisfactory in 10 infants and unsatisfactory in the 11th patient. The bacteriological response was prompt (blood cultures sterile within 72 h of initiating amikacin) in seven (47%) of the 15 septic infants, delayed (cultures positive with the same pathogen for greater than 72 h) in one infant, and unknown in the remaining seven patients.

Meningitis was diagnosed in eight infants. Two infants died. The first infant's course was complicated by *E. coli* Kl ventriculitis, and despite intraventricular amikacin therapy the patient died on the 18th hospital day. The second patient had a meningomyelocele which became infected with *P. aeruginosa*. Parenteral carbenicillin and amikacin therapy combined with daily intraventricular administration of 1 mg of amikacin for 10 days were ineffective, and the infant died on the 26th hospital day. The bacteriological response to therapy was delayed in seven infants, and the clinical response was satisfactory in five of six surviving patients.

Four infants had acute urinary tract infections that were diagnosed from culture of urine obtained from suprapubic bladder aspiration. The urine was sterile within 72 h of initiating amikacin in three infants; repeat culture from the fourth infant was not obtained during therapy. All four infants had satisfactory clinical courses.

Eighteen infants had mucocutaneous infections (Table 3). Sixteen of the neonates were from Medellin where purulent rhinitis and omphalitis are frequently encountered. *E. coli* was the pathogen in 12 (71%) of these patients. Eleven of 18 (61%) infants showed prompt bacteriological responses, and the lesions responded satisfactorily to amikacin therapy in 17 babies. The single clinical failure was an infant with otitis media caused by *P. aeruginosa*.

Safety of amikacin in neonates. Amikacin was well tolerated in the 45 study patients. Complete blood counts, urinalyses, and blood urea nitrogen, and/or serum creatinine values were determined at the beginning and comple-

TABLE 1. *Pharmacokinetic properties of kanamycin and amikacin in newborn infants*

Infant groups		Vol of distribution (ml/kg)		Plasma clearance (ml/min/1.73 m²)		Serum half-life (h)	
Birth weight	Age (days)	Kanamycin	Amikacin	Kanamycin	Amikacin	Kanamycin	Amikacin
<2,000 g	1 to 4	715	563	23.0	21.3	8.6	7.1
	4 to 7	519	568	24.2	22.8	6.7	6.1
	>7	547	502	25.4	24.6	5.2	5.5
≥2,000 g	1 to 4	623	509	29.3	27.0	5.7	6.5
	4 to 7	460	567	36.3	29.8	5.0	5.1
	>7	497	594	45.5	36.4	3.8	4.9

TABLE 2. *Bacteria isolated from 45 study patients*

Organisms	No. of isolates	Septicemia	Meningitis	Urinary tract infection	Mucocutaneous infection
Escherichia coli	26	6	4	4	12
Klebsiella-Enterobacter	8	5	0	1	2
Pseudomonas aeruginosa	6	0	2	0	4
Staphylococcus aureus	2	1	0	0	1
Miscellaneous[a]	5	3	2	0	0
Total	47[b]	15	8	5	19

[a] Includes *Salmonella* sp. (1), *Proteus mirabilis* (1), *H. influenzae* type b (1), *S. epidermidis* (1), and one gram-negative rod that was not identified.

[b] Two organisms were isolated from cultures of two patients.

TABLE 3. *Clinical and bacteriological responses of 45 infants treated with amikacin*

Condition	No. of patients	Died[a]		Bacteriological response			Clinical response of survivors	
		<48 h	>48 h	Prompt <72 h	Delayed >72 h	Unknown	Satisfactory	Unsatisfactory
Septicemia	15	2	2	7	1	7	10	1
Meningitis	8		2		7	1	5	1
Urinary tract infection	4			3		1	4	
Mucocutaneous infection[b]	18			11	6	1	17	1
Total	45	2	4	21	14	10	36	3

[a] Deaths recorded according to time after initiation of therapy.

[b] Includes purulent rhinitis (five patients), omphalitis (nine patients), wound infection (two patients), otitis media (one patient), and chest wall abscess (one patient).

tion of amikacin therapy in 39 infants. There was no evidence of acute hematological or renal toxicity after 5 to 24 days (mean, 10.6 days) of therapy; ototoxicity was not evaluated.

DISCUSSION

As anticipated from studies in normal adult volunteers (3), the pharmacokinetic properties of amikacin were similar to those of kanamycin in newborn infants. Serum concentration-time curves after 7.5-mg/kg doses were comparable for the two aminoglycosides with the exception of lower peak serum kanamycin levels in the larger birth-weight babies. The distribution volumes of these two aminoglycosides were similar to the bromide spaces (2) and the ticarcillin volumes (11) measured in babies, suggesting that these antibiotics distribute within the calculated extracellular fluid space of neonates (1). Plasma clearances and serum half-life values were almost identical for the two drugs and most likely reflect the low but increasing glomerular filtration rates characteristic of the newborn period (14).

We are unable to explain why 5 of 11 infants achieved peak serum levels of only 3 to 7 μg/ml after an intravenous amikacin dose and considerably higher concentrations (15 to 40 μg/ml) after intramuscular administration. It is unlikely that the peak serum values were missed because samples were obtained at zero time and at 10, 20, 45, 60, 120, and 480 min after initiation of the 20-min intravenous injection. It is possible that the distribution of amikacin after intravenous administration in these babies was different than that after an intramuscular dose.

The clinical and bacteriological efficacy of amikacin was comparable to that of kanamycin or gentamicin in neonatal bacterial diseases caused by susceptible pathogens. Two of the six deaths occurred within 48 h of admission to the hospital and both infants had evidence of disseminated intravascular coagulation before initiation of therapy. The case fatality rate of 26% (6 of 23 infants) in neonatal septicemia and meningitis caused principally by gram-negative organisms was less than the rates (40 to 60%) recorded in the literature (10, 12). The bacteriological response to amikacin therapy was prompt in 21 (47%) infants, delayed in 14 (31%), and indeterminate in 10 (22%) infants. Delayed sterilization of CSF cultures observed in seven of eight infants with meningitis was not unexpected in view of our previous experience with neonatal gram-negative enteric meningitis (9).

The clinical responses of the 39 survivors was judged to be satisfactory in 36 (92%) infants and unsatisfactory in three infants. Although the terms satisfactory and unsatisfactory are inexact, subjective descriptions, it is difficult to be more objective because most neonates with bacterial diseases have few distinctive signs that can be evaluated on a daily basis. Thus, pediatricians use poor feeding, diminished suck, lethargy, irritability, and other nonspecific findings to assess the clinical responses of neonates to antimicrobial therapy. In this context, we conclude that amikacin was as effective as kanamycin or gentamicin for therapy of neonatal bacterial diseases.

A dosage schedule of 10 mg of amikacin per kg given initially followed by 7.5-mg/kg doses administered intramuscularly every 12 h results in peak serum concentrations of 15 to 25 μg/ml without accumulation of drug in serum. Intravenous amikacin should be used only when the intramuscular route is contraindicated such as in babies with bleeding disorders or sclerema. Serum concentrations must be monitored in such infants to be certain that peak values are within the therapeutic and safe range. Amikacin should not be used routinely in newborn and young infants until there are long-term follow-up studies establishing its safety with regard to cochlear and vestibular function.

ACKNOWLEDGMENTS

This investigation was supported in part by grants from The John A. Hartford Foundation, Inc. and Bristol Laboratories.

LITERATURE CITED

1. **Cassady, G.** 1966. Plasma volume studies in low birthweight infants. Pediatrics **38**:1020–1027.
2. **Cassady, G.** 1970. Bromide space studies in infants of low birthweight. Pediatr. Res. **4**:14–24.
3. **Clarke, J. T., R. D. Libke, C. Regamy, and W. M. Kirby.** 1974. Comparative pharmacokinetics of amikacin and kanamycin. Clin. Pharmacol. Ther. **15**:610–616.
4. **Dost, F. H.** 1968. Grundlagen der Pharmacokinetic, p. 155–190. Georg Thieme Verlog, Stuttgart.
5. **Franco, J. A., D. V. Eitzman, and H. Baer.** 1973. Antibiotic usage and microbial resistance in an intensive care nursery. Am. J. Dis. Child. **126**:318–321.
6. **Howard, J. B., and G. H. McCracken.** 1975. Pharmacological evaluation of amikacin in neonates. Antimicrob. Agents Chemother. **8**:86–90.
7. **Howard, J. B., and G. H. McCracken.** 1975. Reappraisal of kanamycin usage in neonates. J. Pediatr. **86**:949–956.
8. **McCracken, G. H.** 1971. Changing pattern of the antimicrobial susceptibilities of *Escherichia coli* in neonatal infections. J. Pediatr. **78**:942–947.
9. **McCracken, G. H.** 1972. The rate of bacteriologic response to antimicrobial therapy in neonatal meningitis. Am. J. Dis. Child. **123**:547–553.

10. **McCracken, G. H., and H. R. Shinefield.** 1966. Changes in the pattern of neonatal septicemia and meningitis. Am. J. Dis. Child. **112**:33–39.
11. **Nelson, J. D., S. Shelton, and H. Kusmiesz.** 1975. Clinical pharmacology of ticarcillin in the newborn: relation to age, gestational age and weight. J. Pediatr. **87**:474–479.
12. **Overall, J. C.** 1970. Neonatal bacterial meningitis. J. Pediatr. **76**:499–511.
13. **Simon, H., and E. J. Yin.** 1970. Microbioassay of antimicrobial agents. Appl. Microbiol. **19**:573–579.
14. **Winberg, J.** 1959. The 24-hour true endogenous creatinine clearance in infants and children without renal disease. Acta Pediatr. Scand. **48**:443–452.

Antimicrobial Agents and Chemotherapy, Aug. 1976, p. 211-214 Vol. 10, No. 2

Printed in U.S.A.

Comparison of Direct and Standardized Antimicrobial Susceptibility Testing of Positive Blood Cultures

JAMES E. JOHNSON and JOHN A. WASHINGTON II*

Mayo Clinic and Mayo Foundation, Rochester, Minnesota 55901

Received for publication 11 March 1976

In an effort to determine the feasibility and accuracy of performing direct susceptibility tests from positive blood cultures, minimal inhibitory concentrations (MICs), determined by the agar dilution method, of direct and standardized tests with seven antibiotics were compared. Results were analyzed as to the number of very major (change in MIC from susceptible in preliminary direct testing to resistant in final standardized testing), major (change in MIC from resistant to susceptible), and minor (change in MIC without change in interpretation) discrepancies. The results for gram-positive cocci and for gram-negative bacilli were 5, 6, and 82 of 162 strains tested and 3, 12, and 79 of 90 strains tested, respectively. Of the total number of susceptibility tests compared, major and very major discrepancies occurred in only 1 and 2.4% of instances with gram-positive and -negative isolates, respectively. The majority of discrepancies were noted with *Staphylococcus epidermidis* (four very major, five major), *Klebsiella* (two very major, four major), and *Alcaligenes* (five major). The antibiotics most often exhibiting discrepancies were penicillin, ampicillin, and cephalothin. The results indicate that preliminary susceptibility testing directly from positive blood culture bottles is generally both feasible and accurate.

It has been stated that preliminary antimicrobial susceptibility testing may be done directly from a positive blood culture bottle (3; R. C. Bartlett, P. D. Ellner, and J. A. Washington II, *Cumitech I*, American Society for Microbiology, Washington, D.C.). Although many laboratories follow this practice with positive blood cultures, they almost always confirm their results by using a standardized procedure on the isolated microorganism (2).

This study was undertaken to determine the feasibility and accuracy of performing direct susceptibility tests from positive blood cultures by comparing results of direct and standardized susceptibility tests obtained by the agar dilution method.

MATERIALS AND METHODS

Standardized susceptibility tests were performed by the agar dilution test with expanded dilution steps (Table 1), according to procedures described elsewhere (8). In the direct tests, an attempt was made to adjust the turbidity of the broth removed from positive blood culture bottles (tryptic soy, Difco Laboratories) to match that of one-half of a McFarland no. 1 barium sulfate standard by adding a sample of the broth to 2 ml of Mueller-Hinton broth (Difco Laboratories) and incubating the mixture at 35°C for 2 to 4 h. Gram-positive organisms were tested with cephalothin, chloramphenicol, clindamycin, erythromycin, oxacillin, and penicillin. Gram-negative organisms were tested with ampicillin, cephalothin, chloramphenicol, gentamicin, kanamycin, and tetracycline. Ampicillin was also tested against enterococci, and carbenicillin was tested against the pseudomonads. All antibiotics were mixed in Mueller-Hinton agar (BioQuest).

Interpretation. Discrepancies between the direct and standardized methods were classified as minor, major, and very major. A minor discrepancy was one in which a change in minimal inhibitory concentration (MIC) was noted without a corresponding change in interpretation of susceptibility or resistance, or, rarely, in which a change occurred from a susceptible or a resistant MIC to an intermediate MIC. A discrepancy was considered to be major if the organism was resistant by direct testing and susceptible by the standard method. Discrepancies were considered to be very major when organisms were found to be susceptible by direct testing and resistant by the standardized method. Clinically oriented MIC guidelines were used for defining levels of resistance and susceptibility (Table 2).

RESULTS

A summary of the results comparing direct and standardized susceptibility tests according to antibiotics is shown in Table 3. The overall correlation was 87.9%. Most of the discrepancies were in the minor category, and only 8 (0.5%) very major and 18 (1.2%) major discrepancies were observed. Agreement between the two methods was 98.3% if minor discrepancies

TABLE 1. *Concentrations of antimicrobials tested against bacterial isolates by agar dilution method*

Antimicrobial	Concn (μg/ml)									
	0.1	0.5	1.0	3.0	5.0	10.0	20.0	50.0	100	200
Ampicillin			X		X	X	X			
Carbenicillin								X	X	X
Cephalothin			X		X	X	X			
Chloramphenicol					X	X	X			
Clindamycin			X		X	X				
Erythromycin	X		X		X					
Gentamicin			X	X	X	X				
Kanamycin			X		X	X				
Oxacillin			X		X	X				
Penicillin	X	X	X		X					
Tetracycline			X		X	X				

TABLE 2. *Clinically oriented interpretative criteria of MICs*

Antimicrobial	MIC (μg/ml)	
	Resistant	Susceptible
Ampicillin		
Gram-negative and enterococci	>20	<10
Carbenicillin		
Pseudomonas aeruginosa	>200	<100
Cephalothin	>20	≦10
Chloramphenicol	>20	≦10
Clindamycin	>5	≦1
Erythromycin	>5	≦1
Gentamicin	>5	≦3
Kanamycin	>10	≦5
Oxacillin	>10	≦5
Penicillin G		
Staphylococci	>0.1	≦0.1
Tetracycline	>5	≦5

were regarded as insignificant. Changes in MIC and in interpretation of results were most frequently noted with penicillin and ampicillin.

When the results comparing the two test methods were analyzed according to the microorganism tested, some differences were noted (Tables 4 and 5). In tests of the gram-positive organisms, most discrepancies were noted with penicillin. The overall agreement of results for penicillin was 69.1%, with 4.3% of the discrepancies being due to major or very major changes. *Staphylococcus epidermidis* was the organism most commonly associated with discrepant results, 4 very major, 5 major, and 57 minor discrepancies being observed among the 93 strains tested. Of 30 strains of *Staphylococcus aureus* tested, 1 very major, 1 major, and 8 minor discrepancies were noted. No major or very major discrepancies were noted with group D streptococci or other gram-positive organisms. One hundred and sixty-two strains of gram-positive cocci were tested against six antibiotics, and only 11 major or very major discrepancies were observed. Eleven group D streptococci were also tested against ampicillin. No discrepancies of any type were observed.

The results obtained with 90 strains of gram-negative organisms were also compared against six antibiotics. A total of 15 major or very major discrepancies occurred in this group. The organisms most commonly involved were *Klebsiella*, which had two very major and four major discrepancies of 14 strains tested, and *Alcaligenes* spp., in which five major discrepancies were observed with four strains tested. The antibiotics most often involved in the discrepancies with gram-negative organisms were ampicillin and cephalothin. Twelve isolates of the *Pseudomonas* group of organisms were also tested with carbenicillin, with only one minor discrepancy noted.

DISCUSSION

In this study of 1,536 antibiotic comparisons, there was an overall agreement of 87.9% in results. The vast majority of the discrepancies observed, however, were minor and might have been attributed to test variability, as they generally reflected a one-dilution difference and did not significantly alter the interpretation of susceptibility or resistance applied to the MIC. There were only 26 major or very major discrepancies of 1,536 antibiotic test comparisons, resulting in 98.3% agreement in results when only these two significant groups of discrepancies are considered.

On the other hand, if one examines the data according to the strains tested, a slight difference in percent agreement is seen. Of a total of 252 strains compared, 128 (50.8%) strains provided results that were in complete agreement in both test systems. If minor discrepancies are disregarded, the results obtained with 233 (92.5%) of the strains agreed. Nineteen (7.5%) strains demonstrated the 26 major and very

TABLE 3. *Summary of results comparing direct and standardized susceptibility testing according to antimicrobial agent*[a]

Antimicrobial	No. of tests	No. (%) in agreement	No. (%) with discrepancies		
			VM	MA	MI
Ampicillin	102	80 (78.5)	3 (2.9)	4 (3.9)	15 (14.7)
Carbenicillin	12	11 (91.7)	0 (0)	0 (0)	1 (8.3)
Cephalothin	252	230 (91.3)	0 (0)	3 (1.2)	19 (7.5)
Chloramphenicol	252	219 (86.9)	0 (0)	0 (0)	33 (13.1)
Clindamycin	162	159 (98.1)	0 (0)	0 (0)	3 (1.9)
Erythromycin	162	145 (89.5)	1 (0.6)	1 (0.6)	15 (9.3)
Gentamicin	90	83 (92.2)	0 (0)	1 (1.1)	6 (6.7)
Kanamycin	90	80 (88.9)	0 (0)	0 (0)	10 (11.1)
Oxacillin	162	156 (96.3)	0 (0)	2 (1.2)	4 (2.5)
Penicillin	162	112 (69.1)	4 (2.5)	3 (1.9)	43 (26.5)
Tetracycline	90	74 (82.2)	0 (0)	4 (4.5)	12 (13.3)

[a] VM, Very major = susceptible by direct, resistant by standardized method; MA, major = resistant by direct, susceptible by standardized method; MI, minor = change in MIC without change in interpretation.

TABLE 4. *Discrepancies between direct and standardized susceptibility tests for gram-positive organisms*[a]

Antibiotic	*S. aureus*	*S. epidermidis*	Streptococci, group D	Other	% Agreement[b]	
					Overall	VM, MA
Ampicillin			0,0,0/11		100	100
Cephalothin	0,0,0/30[c]	0,0,0/93	0,0,1/11	0,0,0/28	99.4	100
Chloramphenicol	0,0,5/30	0,0,6/93	0,0,3/11	0,0,2/28	90.1	100
Clindamycin	0,0,0/30	0,0,0/93	0,0,3/11	0,0,0/28	98.1	100
Erythromycin	1,0,1/30	0,1,12/93	0,0,1/11	0,0,1/28	89.5	98.8
Oxacillin	0,0,0/30	0,2,2/93	0,0,2/11	0,0,0/28	96.3	98.8
Penicillin	0,1,2/30	4,2,37/93	0,0,1/11	0,0,3/28	69.1	95.7

[a] VM, Very major = susceptible by direct, resistant by standardized method; MA, major = resistant by direct, susceptible by standardized method. Minor change, Change in MIC without change in interpretation.

[b] Average: Overall = 91.8%; VM, MA = 99.0%.

[c] Each entry represents the number of very major, major, and minor discrepancies/total number of strains tested.

TABLE 5. *Discrepancies between direct and standardized susceptibility tests for gram-negative organisms*[a]

Antibiotic	*E. coli*	*Klebsiella*	*Enterobacter*	*Serratia*	*Proteus*	*Pseudomonas*	*P. aeruginosa*	*Alcaligenes*	% Agreement[b]	
									Overall	VM, MA
Ampicillin	0,0,2/44[c]	2,1,7/14	1,0,1/6	0,0,1/5	0,0,2/5	0,0,2/7	0,0,0/5	0,3,0/4	75.6	92.2
Carbenicillin						0,0,1/7	0,0,0/5		91.7	100
Cephalothin	0,1,9/44	0,1,7/14	0,0,1/6	0,0,0/5	0,0,0/5	0,0,0/7	0,0,0/5	0,1,1/4	76.7	96.7
Chloramphenicol	0,0,3/44	0,0,6/14	0,0,1/6	0,0,0/5	0,0,2/5	0,0,3/7	0,0,0/5	0,0,2/4	81.1	100
Gentamicin	0,0,2/44	0,0,0/14	0,0,0/6	0,0,0/5	0,0,0/5	0,1,1/7	0,0,1/5	0,0,2/4	92.2	98.9
Kanamycin	0,0,3/44	0,0,5/14	0,0,1/6	0,0,0/5	0,0,1/5	0,0,0/7	0,0,0/5	0,0,0/4	88.9	100
Tetracycline	0,0,6/44	0,2,5/14	0,0,0/6	0,0,0/5	0,0,0/5	0,1,1/7	0,0,0/5	0,1,0/4	82.3	95.6

[a] VM, Very major = susceptible by direct, resistant by standardized method; MA, major = resistant by direct, susceptible by standardized method. Minor change, Change in MIC without change in interpretation.

[b] Average: Overall = 84.1%; VM, MA = 97.6%.

[c] Each entry represents the number of very major, major, and minor discrepancies/total number of strains tested.

major discrepancies noted. Of these, six strains of *S. epidermidis* and three strains of *Alcaligenes* were involved. Both of these organisms are generally considered to be contaminants of blood cultures, indicating that only 10 strains (4%) representing "significant" isolates demonstrated major or very major shifts in susceptibility. In like manner, if one were to remove the 15 major discrepancies observed with these nine organisms, an overall agreement of 99.3% is noted for antibiotic test comparisons.

A number of positive blood cultures were not included in this study, either because the organisms were initially detected on subculture or because of polymicrobial bacteremia. Recently, our laboratory has instituted a procedure for the early subculture of blood cultures on the day they are collected (4). This has resulted in there being fewer gram-negative isolates that could be subjected to direct testing in this study, as these organisms tended to be detected initially on the chocolate blood agar plate used for subcultures. Polymicrobial bacteremia was infrequent during the course of this study and occurred in fewer than 2% of all positive blood cultures. Nevertheless, it is important to reiterate that susceptibility testing data are valid only when they are derived from pure cultures, as has been emphasized by Shahidi and Ellner (6) and by Barry et al. (1).

Fourteen of the 26 major and very major discrepancies were contained in the penicillin-related group of antimicrobial agents. Penicillin G and ampicillin were involved in seven instances each. Therefore, if direct susceptibility testing is done, one must exercise caution in interpreting the results with this group of antibiotics. Even so, there was approximately 95% agreement between direct and standardized susceptibility tests for each of these antibiotics.

In analyzing our data, it was quite evident that multiple discrepancies tended to occur that may well have been related to differences in inoculum density (1; A. W. Bauer, *in* H. P. Kuemmerle and P. Preziosi (ed.), *Third International Congress of Chemotherapy*, vol. 1, p. 466–479). Although we attempted to standardize the inoculum in the direct tests, it was not infrequently difficult to do so because of the presence of erythrocytes in the blood culture broth. Centrifugation of the broth at 700 rpm to eliminate the erythrocytes failed to improve the degree of agreement between the direct and standard tests, and this practice was discontinued after a brief trial. The organisms most commonly causing difficulty with adjustment of the inoculum density were the gram-positive cocci, because they tended to grow as colonies on the surface of the blood-broth interface in the bottle. This problem may well have been responsible for most of the discrepancies observed with *S. aureus* and *S. epidermidis*.

It is possible that some of the discrepancies noted between direct and standard testing could be related to the reproducibility of the agar dilution test itself. Because of experimental error and biological variation in antimicrobial susceptibility tests, their reproducibility might, even under ideal circumstances, not be expected to exceed 98% (7). Duplicate standardized susceptibility tests were not included in this study; however, internal quality control specimens submitted to our susceptibility testing laboratory as unknowns have never demonstrated a major or very major discrepancy in more than 5 years of testing. In like manner, the daily control organisms used in our laboratory have shown only one minor discrepancy in the past 2 months, indicating the high degree of reproducibility of the agar dilution test.

The degree of reproducibility and comparability observed with agar dilution tests may differ from that noted for disk diffusion methods. However, a study in our laboratory comparing direct and standardized disk diffusion susceptibility tests on urine specimens produced results similar to those obtained in this study (5).

In conclusion, the results of this study indicate that preliminary antimicrobial susceptibility testing directly from positive blood culture bottles is generally both feasible and accurate.

LITERATURE CITED

1. **Barry, A. L., L. J. Joyce, A. P. Adams, and E. J. Benner.** 1973. Rapid determination of antimicrobial susceptibility for urgent clinical situations. Am. J. Clin. Pathol. **59**:693–699.
2. **Bartlett, R. C.** 1973. Contemporary blood culture practices, p. 15–35. *In* A. C. Sonnenwirth (ed.), Bacteremia: laboratory and clinical aspects. Charles C Thomas, Publisher, Springfield, Ill.
3. **Bartlett, R. C., C. Fitzgerald, R. Maggio, D. Miller, R. Quintiliani, J. Redys, G. Thornton, A. von Graevenitz, and W. Vincent.** 1975. Report of the ad hoc committee on medical microbiology laboratory utilization. Conn. Med. **39**:499–505.
4. **Harkness, J. L., M. Hall, D. M. Ilstrup, and J. A. Washington II.** 1975. Effects of atmosphere of incubation and of routine subcultures on detection of bacteremia in vacuum blood culture bottles. J. Clin. Microbiol. **2**:296–299.
5. **Hollick, G. E., and J. A. Washington, II.** 1976. Comparison of direct and standardized disk diffusion susceptibility testing of urine cultures. Antimicrob. Agents Chemother. **9**:804–809.
6. **Shahidi, A., and P. D. Ellner.** 1969. Effect of mixed cultures on antibiotic susceptibility testing. Appl. Microbiol. **18**:766–770.
7. **Thornsberry, C., T. L. Gavan, J. C. Sherris, A. Balows, J. M. Matsen, L. D. Sabath, F. Schoenknecht, L. D. Thrupp, and J. A. Washington II.** 1975. Laboratory evaluation of a rapid, automated susceptibility testing system: report of a collaborative study. Antimicrob. Agents Chemother. **7**:466–480.
8. **Washington, J. A., II.** 1974. Laboratory procedures in clinical microbiology. Little, Brown & Co., Boston.

ANTIMICROBIAL AGENTS AND CHEMOTHERAPY, Aug. 1976, p. 215-218 Vol. 10, No. 2

Printed in U.S.A.

Indirect Method for Assessing the Penetration of Beta-Lactamase-Nonsusceptible Penicillins and Cephalosporins in *Escherichia coli* Strains

M. H. RICHMOND,* D. C. CLARK, AND SANDRA WOTTON

Department of Bacteriology, University of Bristol, Bristol BS8 1TD, England

Received for publication 9 February 1976

Escherichia coli UB1005 and two mutants of this strain (DC2 and DC3) have been used to assess indirectly the relative ability of various β-lactam antibiotics to penetrate the outer layers of *E. coli*. Benzylpenicillin, ampicillin, methicillin, cloxacillin, cephaloridine, cephalothin, and cephalexin have been examined. The results confirm those obtained with other methods and show that, among the compounds studied here, cephalosporins seem to penetrate more readily than penicillins.

One important feature that affects the activity of β-lactam antibiotics against gram-negative bacteria is their ability to pass through the outer layers of the organisms to their targets in the inner membrane (4, 14). Unfortunately, direct measurements on penetration, for example, by following the uptake of radiolabeled antibiotics, are unreliable because of the high levels of nonspecific adsorption (3, 5, 18). As a result, indirect methods must be used.

One such method depends on a determination of "crypticity." For β-lactam antibiotics, this property is measured as the extent to which the β-lactamase activity of a bacterial culture increases when the permeability barriers in the cell envelope are disrupted (14, 15). The validity of this method for assessing penetration is based on the assumption that the passage of the compound to the β-lactamase in the periplasmic space reflects the properties of the barrier(s) that the antibiotic also encounters on its way to its target in the bacterial inner membrane (15).

Although useful under certain circumstances, crypticity determinations do have a number of important disadvantages (14, 17). Perhaps the most serious in the context of this work is that the method can only be used to evaluate substances against which enzyme used in the test is active. Since many of the latest generation of β-lactam compounds (notably, some cephalosporins [C. H. O'Callaghan, R. B. Sykes, D. M. Ryan, R. D. Foord, and P. W. Muggleton, J. Antibiot., in press] and most cephamycins [11]) are resistant to the enzymes available for use, the crypticity method is unlikely to have much long-term practical value.

This paper describes the evaluation of a series of mutant *Escherichia coli* strains that can be used to provide an alternative method of assessing the penetration of the outer layers of *E. coli* by β-lactam antibiotics, including those resistant to β-lactamases.

MATERIALS AND METHODS

Mutant strains and their isolation. Both mutants used in these studies (DC2 and DC3) were obtained from *E. coli* strain UB1005 (alias EC1005), a nalidixic acid-resistant mutant of *E. coli* W1655 (7), as isolates abnormally susceptible to chloramphenicol. On examination they proved to be abnormally susceptible to penicillins as well (see Results). Mutagenesis was performed with *N*-methyl-*N'*-nitro-*N*-nitrosoguanidine under standard conditions (1), and the treated bacteria were selected by penicillin selection in liquid medium containing 1 μg of chloramphenicol and 200 μg of ampicillin per ml. After overnight growth at 37°C, the surviving bacteria in this culture were plated on unsupplemented nutrient agar to give single colonies, and these colonies were then replica plated onto nutrient agar containing 1 μg of chloramphenicol per ml. Colonies growing on the master plates, but not on the replicas, were then picked, and their properties were checked in detail.

Crypticity measurements. The theoretical basis of this measurement has been discussed in detail elsewhere (14, 17). In practice, the value is obtained by measuring the activity of a bacterial suspension against a given penicillin or cephalosporin both before and after disruption and dividing the activity of the broken preparation by the unbroken activity (14). Thus, crypticity = activity in milligrams (dry weight) of broken bacteria/activity in milligrams (dry weight) of intact bacteria.

Strain UB1005, and the mutants DC2 and DC3 derived from it, expressed less than 0.1 unit of β-lactamase activity/mg (dry weight) of bacteria when enzyme activity was assayed with either benzylpenicillin or cephaloridine. To measure the crypticity of such strains towards β-lactam antibiotics, it was therefore necessary to transfer the gene(s) needed to specify the synthesis of an appropriate periplasmic β-lactamase into them. The enzyme chosen in this case was the type IIIa β-lactamase (6, 15), an enzyme known to have a periplasmic location in *E. coli* (8–10). The necessary genetic information to produce this enzyme was transferred to strain UB1005, and to the mutants DC2 and DC3, by mating with *E. coli* W3110(RP1) as donor under standard conditions for an overnight mating experiment at 37°C (7). After this period, the mating mixture was plated on agar containing 40 μg of nalidixic acid and 50 μg of carbenicillin per ml to select recipient clones that had received the R plasmid.

Crypticity measurements were carried out as follows. A culture of the strain under test was grown exponentially in nutrient broth at 37°C with shaking until a bacterial density of about 10^8 organisms/ml had been reached. The culture was then centrifuged at 5,000 × *g* for 15 min to collect bacteria, and these were resuspended to a density of about 10 mg (dry weight)/ml in 0.1 M KH_2PO_4/K_2HPO_4 buffer, pH 7.0. A sample was removed from this suspension for assay of β-lactamase activity of the intact bacteria, and the remainder of the suspension was disrupted for 5 min in an ultrasonic disintegrator (25Kc/s, Mullard Instruments, Crawley, England). After disruption, the suspension was stored on ice until required for assay. The assay of the intact bacteria was carried out as soon as possible to minimize leakage of enzyme from the bacteria.

β-Lactamase assays. All β-lactamase assays were carried out by the iodometric method (12) using substrate concentrations of 2.5 mg/ml dissolved in 0.1 M KH_2PO_4/K_2HPO_4 buffer, pH 7.0. The results of these assays were calculated on the assumption that, after hydrolysis, 1 mol of a penicillin reacts with eight equivalents of iodine solution, whereas the equivalent value for a hydrolyzed cephalosporin is four (2).

RESULTS

Comparative properties of UB1005 and the mutants DC2 and DC3. Although DC2 and DC3 were isolated as abnormally susceptible mutants on agar containing chloramphenicol, they also showed reduced minimum inhibitory concentration (MIC) values for a range of other antibiotics when compared with strain UB1005. Among these were several penicillins, notably, ampicillin and cloxacillin. The only β-lactam compounds tested that were not more active against the mutants than against the parental strain were cephaloridine, cephalothin, and cephalexin. These results are summarized in Table 1 (see also Fig. 1).

Crypticity determinations on UB1005 and on DC2 and DC3. Since the mutants DC2 and DC3 were more susceptible than UB1005 to a range of antibiotic substances, it seemed possible that the mutants were altered in a broadly nonspecific way to allow freer access of these substances to their targets in the bacterial cell. One method of confirming that this was so for β-lactam compounds was to determine the crypticity values of the mutants towards an appropriate penicillin and to compare it with the equivalent value for strain UB1005.

Crypticity determinations suffer a number of shortcomings, but their accuracy is greatest when used for comparative purposes with an enzyme that has an affinity for the antibiotic being used in the test of greater than 5×10^{-4} M and when the enzyme activity of the unbroken bacteria is high enough to be measured accurately (17). In *E. coli* K-12 these conditions are best met when the plasmid RP1 is used with benzylpenicillin as substrate. Accordingly, the crypticity values for strain UB1005 (RP1-1) and for the mutants DC2 (RP1-1) and DC3 (RP1-1) were determined with benzylpenicillin as substrate. Table 2 shows the results of these measurements. Strain UB1005 (RP1-1) gave a crypticity value of 55 with benzylpenicillin in this test, whereas DC2 (RP1-1) and DC3 (RP1-1) gave values of 2.5 and 20, respectively. These results suggest, therefore, that the abnormal susceptibility of DC2 and DC3 to benzylpenicillin arises from a reduced ability to prevent this antibiotic from passing through the outer layers of the cell envelope to its target in the bacterial inner membrane.

TABLE 1. *MIC values obtained with E. coli UB1005 and with the mutants DC2 and DC3 against a range of antibacterial substances*

Antibiotic	MIC (μg/ml)[a]		
	UB1005	DC3	DC2
Chloramphenicol	8	1	0.5
Benzylpenicillin	25	10	1.2
Ampicillin	8	4	0.5
Cloxacillin	500	32	2.0
Cephaloridine	2	2	2
Cephalothin	2	2	1
Novobiocin	200	25	5
Rifampin	16	8	4
Tetracycline	4	2	1

[a] MIC values were obtained by plating bacteria as single colony-forming units on the surface of agar containing the antibiotic in question.

TABLE 2. *Crypticity values for E. coli UB1005 (RP1) and the mutant strains DC2 (RP1) and DC3 (RP1)*

Substrate	Crypticity value		
	UB1005 (RP1)	DC2 (RP1)	DC3 (RP1)
Benzylpenicillin	55	20	2.5
Cephaloridine	1.7	1.2	1.2

Table 1 also shows that, unlike the results with penicillins, DC2 and DC3 were no more susceptible to cephaloridine than was strain UB1005, and it was therefore important to see whether the crypticity of the mutants to this antibiotic was altered or not. The crypticity values for strains DC2 (RP1-1) and DC3 (RP1-1) were therefore measured with cephaloridine as substrate, and the results were compared with that obtained with strain UB1005 (RP1-1). With this substrate no difference in crypticity between the parental and either of the mutant strains could be detected (Table 2), and this observation was consistent with the similar MIC values obtained with the three strains in the presence of cephaloridine.

Use of DC2 and DC3 to compare the penetration of various penicillins and cephalosporins. The implication of these results is that certain β-lactam antibiotics (notably, cephaloridine) can pass freely through the envelope of unmutated *E. coli* strains, whereas penicillins are impeded, in some cases severely. Moreover, substrates that show a range of different MIC values with UB1005, DC2, and DC3 must also be impeded by this barrier, whereas, in contrast, those that show a similar MIC against these three strains are indifferent to the barrier. Mutants DC2 and DC3 may therefore be used, in conjunction with strain UB1005, in a standard test to determine whether penicillins and cephalosporins are impeded in their entry into *E. coli*.

Figure 1 shows the results obtained with the three test strains and a range of penicillins and cephalosporins. The crypticity values of the test strains towards benzylpenicillin has been used as an index of the extent to which the cells' penetration barrier has been impaired by mutation. In practice, two broad types of response have been obtained (see Fig. 1a and b). Figure 1a shows the results obtained with penicillins. With methicillin and cloxacillin the difference in MIC between UB1005 and the mutant DC2 is about 250-fold, and this argues that these compounds are powerfully excluded from unmutated *E. coli*. Furthermore, the high level of activity of the penicillins against DC2 argues that both these penicillins would be very active against naturally occurring *E. coli* strains if the antibiotics were able to reach their target in the bacterial inner membrane. Figure 1a also contains results for benzylpenicillin and ampicillin. These compounds are also substantially more active against DC2 than against UB1005, although the difference is not as marked as with methicillin and cloxacillin.

Figure 1b shows the results obtained with cephaloridine, cephalexin, and cephalothin. In this case, the mutant strains were no more than twice as susceptible as strain UB1005, and even this minimal difference was not observed with cephaloridine. In contrast to the penicillins, therefore, these three cephalosporins seem to exercise a similar effect on *E. coli* whether or not the barrier to penicillin entry is damaged. Furthermore, this behavior argues that cephaloridine, cephalexin, and cephalothin express their full potential in inhibiting cell wall synthesis in *E. coli* when tested against naturally occurring strains.

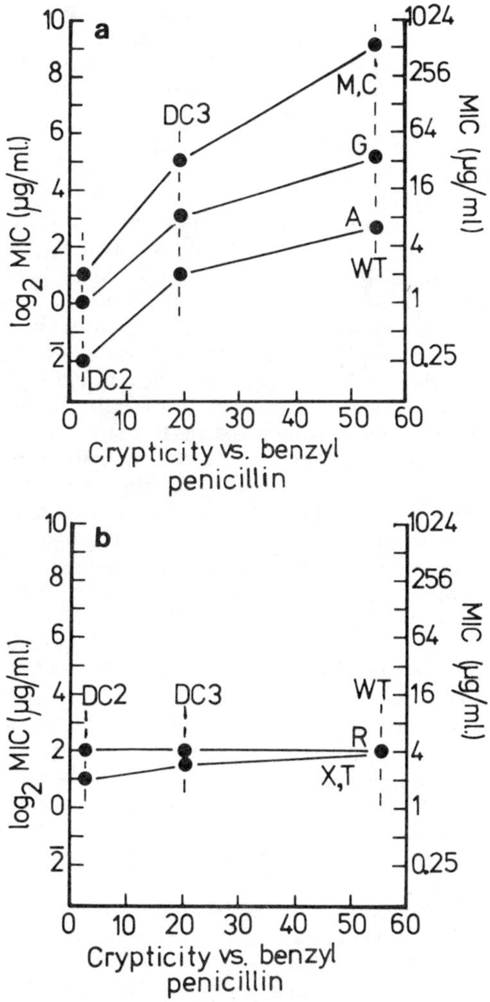

FIG. 1. *Relative MIC values obtained with β-lactam antibiotics acting on UB1005 and the mutants DC2 and DC3. WT, strain UB1005. (a) Penicillins: A, ampicillin; G, benzylpenicillin; C, cloxacillin; M, methicillin. (b) Cephalosporins: R, cephaloridine; T, cephalothin; X, cephalexin. The crypticity values used in these figures were determined using UB1005 (RP1), DC2 (RP1), and DC3 (RP1).*

DISCUSSION

The activity of β-lactam antibiotics on a gram-negative bacterial strain depends on three main properties: first, its inherent activity against the enzymes in the bacterial inner membrane that are related to peptidoglycan biosynthesis (D,D-transpeptidase and carboxypeptidase); second, its ability to pass through the outer layers of the bacterial cell envelope to reach its target; and third, its ability to resist hydrolysis by β-lactamases that the antibiotic may encounter on the way to its target. Any full evaluation of a new β-lactam antibiotic, therefore, requires measurements to be made on each of these three crucial processes.

Methods for assessing the effect of β-lactamases on new β-lactam antibiotics have already been well worked out (16), and effective in vitro test systems are also available to evaluate the action of these compounds directly on transpeptidase and carboxypeptidase enzyme systems from the inner membrane (13). Only with the measurements of penetration are methods still less than adequate, largely because the β-lactam group of antibiotics are so reactive chemically that attempts to measure their uptake by conventional radiolabeling methods give levels of nonspecific adsorption so high that interpretation of the results is very difficult on a routine basis (3, 5, 18).

The method for assessing penetration described here is an advance on the "crypticity method" used hitherto (4, 14, 15, 17). Not only is it less sensitive to the growth conditions of the culture, but it can also be used for β-lactam antibiotics completely nonsusceptible to β-lactamase hydrolysis, and this ability is likely to be of increasing importance as more β-lactamase-nonsusceptible penicillins and cephalosporins are developed. Another advantage of the method described here is that the determination only involves the measurement of MIC values on agar plates, a technique widely available in microbiology laboratories. The main disadvantage of the method is that the measurement is indirect, and compounds are evaluated in comparison with antibiotics whose properties must be known in detail in advance. With β-lactam actibiotics this limitation is not too severe, since a number of penicillins and cephalosporins (such as ampicillin, cephaloridine, and cephalothin) are widely available and have already been studied extensively.

ACKNOWLEDGMENTS

This work was supported by a grant from the Medical Research Council to M.H.R. D.C. was supported by a grant from the Science Research Council.

We are extremely grateful to G. Rolinson, of Beecham Research Ltd., for a generous gift of ampicillin, to P. W. Muggleton, of Glaxo Research Ltd., for cephaloridine and cephalexin, and to G. Shedden, of Ely Lilly, for cephalothin.

LITERATURE CITED

1. **Adelberg, E. A., and C. C. Chen.** 1965. Optimal conditions for mutagenesis by N-methyl-N'-nitro-N-nitrosoguanidine in *Escherichia coli* K12. Biochem. Biophys. Res. Commun. **18**:788–790.
2. **Alicino, J. F.** 1961. Iodometric assay of natural and synthetic penicillins, 6-aminopenicillanic acid and cephalosporin C. Anal. Chem. **33**:648–649.
3. **Blumberg, P. M., and J. L. Strominger.** 1974. Interaction of penicillin with the bacterial cell: penicillin-binding proteins and penicillin-sensitive enzymes. Bacteriol. Rev. **38**:291–335.
4. **Boman, H. G., K. Nordström, and S. Normark.** 1974. Penicillin resistance in *Escherichia coli* K12: synergism between penicillinases and a barrier in the outer part of the envelope. Ann. N.Y. Acad. Sci. **235**:569–585.
5. **Cooper, P. D.** 1956. Site of binding of radiopenicillin. Bacteriol. Rev. **20**:28–48.
6. **Datta, N., and M. H. Richmond.** 1966. The purification and properties of a penicillinase whose synthesis is mediated by an R-factor in *Escherichia coli*. Biochem. J. **98**:204–209.
7. **Grinsted, J., J. R. Saunders, L. C. Ingram, R. B. Sykes, and M. H. Richmond.** 1972. Properties of an R factor which originated in *Pseudomonas aeruginosa* 1822. J. Bacteriol. **110**:529–537.
8. **Heppel, L. A.** 1971. The concept of periplasmic enzymes, p. 224–247. *In* L. Rothfield (ed.), The structure and function of biological membranes. Academic Press Inc., New York.
9. **Neu, H. C.** 1968. The surface location of penicillinases in *Escherichia coli* and *Salmonella typhimurium*. Biochem. Biophys. Res. Commun. **32**:258–263.
10. **Neu, H. C., and J. Chou.** 1967. Release of surface enzymes in *Enterobacteriaceae* by osmotic shock. J. Bacteriol. **94**:1934–1935.
11. **Onishi, H. R., D. R. Daoust, Z. B. Zimmerman, D. Handlin, and E. O. Stapley.** 1974. Cefoxitin, a semisynthetic cephamycin antibiotic: resistance to β-lactamase inactivation. Antimicrob. Agents Chemother. **5**:38–48.
12. **Perret, C. J.** 1954. The iodometric assay for penicillinase. Biochem. J. **83**:236–240.
13. **Pollock, J. J., M. Nguyen-Disteche, J-M. Ghuysen, and M. R. J. Salton.** 1974. Discussion paper: the DD-carboxypeptidase-transpeptidase system in *Escherichia coli* strain 44. Ann. N.Y. Acad. Sci. **235**:225–235.
14. **Richmond, M. H., and N. A. C. Curtis.** 1974. The interplay of β-lactamases and intrinsic factors in the resistance of Gram-negative bacteria to penicillins and cephalosporins. Ann. N.Y. Acad. Sci. **235**:553–568.
15. **Richmond, M. H., and R. B. Sykes.** 1973. The Gram-negative bacteria and their possible physiological role, p. 31–88. *In* A. H. Rose and D. W. Tempest (ed.), Advances in microbial physiology, vol. 9. Academic Press Inc., London.
16. **Ross, G. W., and C. H. O'Callaghan.** 1975. β-Lactamase assays, p. 69–85. *In* J. H. Hash (ed.), Methods in enzymology, vol. 43. Academic Press Inc., New York.
17. **Rosselet, A., F. Knüsel, and W. Zimmermann.** 1972. Phenotypic expression of β-lactamase activity in different strains carrying the TEM R-factor, p. 231–243. *In* V. Krcmery, L. Rosival, and T. Watanabe (ed.), Bacterial plasmids and antibiotic resistance. Springer-Verlag, Berlin.
18. **Schmidt, R., and R. Plapp.** 1972. Binding of ^{14}C-penicillin G to *Proteus mirabilis*. Arch. Mikrobiol. **83**:246–260.

ANTIMICROBIAL AGENTS AND CHEMOTHERAPY, Aug. 1976, p. 219-222 Vol. 10, No. 2

Printed in U.S.A.

Comparative Study of Seven Cephalosporins: Susceptibility to Beta-Lactamases and Ability to Penetrate the Surface Layers of *Escherichia coli*

M. H. RICHMOND AND SANDRA WOTTON

Department of Bacteriology, University of Bristol, Bristol BS8 1TD, England

Received for publication 1 March 1976

The properties of cefazolin, cefoxitin, cefamandole, and cefuroxime have been compared with those of cephaloridine, cephalothin, and cephalexin. The properties included for examination are the susceptibility to a range of β-lactamases commonly encountered in gram-negative species and the ability of a β-lactam antibiotic to penetrate the outer layers of *Escherichia coli*. Of the antibiotics tested, cefamandole was the most active in its antibiotic activity but had the disadvantage that it was sensitive to hydrolysis by type IVc β-lactamase. Cefoxitin and cefuroxime were slightly less active than cefamandole but were effectively resistant to all the β-lactamases used in the test.

The activity of a penicillin or cephalosporin against gram-negative bacteria seems to depend on three main properties: first, the ability of the antibiotic to inhibit peptidoglycan synthesis in the bacterial inner membrane (12, 20); second, its ability to penetrate through the outer layers of the bacterial envelope to reach its target (1, 7, 15); and third, its ability to survive in the presence of any β-lactamase it may meet on the way to its target (1, 7, 15).

A previous paper has already described the use of some mutant strains of *Escherichia coli* K-12 both to assess the ability of a given penicillin or cephalosporin to penetrate to the inner membrane of gram-negative bacteria and to give some idea of the ability of the antibiotic to inhibit peptidoglycan synthesis (14). These mutant strains (DC2 and DC3) have now been used, in conjunction with the parental *E. coli* strain (UB1005), to assess the properties of cefazolin (10), cefoxitin (9, 11, 22), cefamandole (23), and cefuroxime (C. H. O'Callaghan, R. B. Sykes, D. M. Ryan, R. D. Foord, and P. W. Muggleton, J. Antibiot., in press) and to compare them with three well-established therapeutic cephalosporins: cephaloridine, cephalothin, and cephalexin.

Although more than 14 distinct types of β-lactamase have been detected among ampicillin-resistant strains of gram-negative species (16, 17), an adequate idea of the resistance to β-lactamase hydrolysis can be obtained by studying the response of a penicillin or cephalosporin antibiotic against semipurified preparations of four enzymes: type Ia β-lactamase, an enzyme predominantly active against cephalosporins (6, 16); type Id enzyme, a cephalosporinase encountered in the very great majority of clinical isolates of *Pseudomonas aeruginosa* (16, 19, 21); type IIIa enzyme, a broad-spectrum β-lactamase commonly specified by R plasmids in a wide range of gram-negative species (2); and type IVc enzyme, a β-lactamase with a broad spectrum of activity including cloxacillin, a penicillin that inhibits type IIIa enzyme (8, 16). This paper compares the properties of the seven cephalosporins examined here against these four types of β-lactamase.

An overall assessment of the compounds from these three points of view shows that cefoxitin and cefuroxime are certainly the most resistant to β-lactamase hydrolysis, whereas cefuroxime and cefamandole show the highest activity against peptidoglycan biosynthesis in the mutant DC2.

MATERIALS AND METHODS

Strains. The studies on penetration have been carried out with *E. coli* UB1005 (a nalidixic acid-resistant mutant of *E. coli* W1655) and with two susceptible mutants of this strain, DC2 and DC3 (14). The origin and characteristics of this parental strain and its mutant derivatives have been described previously (5).

Preparation of β-lactamases. Type Ia, Id, IIIa, and IVc β-lactamases were prepared from *Enterobacter cloacae* P99 (3), *P. aeruginosa* 18S/H (F. Flett, N. A. C. Curtis, and M. H. Richmond, submitted for publication), *E. coli* (R_{TEM}) (2), and *Klebsiella aerogenes* 1082E (8), respectively. The enzymes were partially purified from *E. cloacae* P99 and *E. coli* (R_{TEM}) by the methods described previously (13, 17). *P. aeruginosa* 18S/H is a constitutive mutant of *P. aeruginosa* 18S isolated by treatment of the parental strain with *N*-methyl-*N'*-nitro-*N*-nitrosoguanidine under conventional conditions, followed by repeated subculture of the strain on a series of agar plates containing increasing concentrations of carbenicillin. The lowest concentration used was 50 μg/ml and the highest was 2,500 μg/ml (M. H. Richmond and F. Flett, unpublished data). Type Id enzyme was isolated in partially purified form from this strain as follows. A culture of *P. aeruginosa* 18S/H growing exponentially in nutrient broth was centrifuged when the culture had reached a density of approximately 2 mg (dry weight) of organisms per ml. After sedimentation the bacteria were resuspended to a density of about 50 mg (dry weight) of bacteria per ml in 0.1 M Na_2HPO_4/KH_2PO_4 buffer, pH 7.0. This bacterial suspension was then disrupted in an ultrasonic disintegrator for 5 min, the bacteria being cooled in an ice bath while treatment proceeded. After disruption, the cell debris was removed by centrifugation, first at 5,000 × *g* for 10 min and then at 33,000 × *g* for 20 min, and the supernatant was collected. Such enzyme preparations contained about 200 units of enzyme activity per ml when assayed against cephaloridine as substrate.

Type IVc enzyme, prepared from *K. aerogenes* 1082E (8), was a gift from G. W. Ross (Glaxo Research Ltd., Greenford, Middlesex, England).

β-Lactamase assays. Estimations of β-lactamase activity were carried out by the spectrophotometric method described by Ross and O'Callaghan (18) using substrate concentrations of 10^{-4} M.

MIC determinations. The susceptibility of *E. coli* UB1005, and of the mutants DC2 and DC3, to the cephalosporins tested in this study, was measured by inoculating single colony-forming units onto a range of nutrient agar plates containing increasing concentrations of the cephalosporin in question. The recorded minimum inhibitory concentration (MIC) value is the lowest concentration at which no growth occurred after overnight incubation at 35°C.

Cephalosporins. Cephaloridine, cephalexin, cefazolin, and cefuroxime were gifts from P. W. Muggleton (Glaxo Research Ltd., Greenford, Middlesex, England), and cephalothin and cefamandole were given by W. I. H. Shedden (Lilly Research Centre, Ltd., Windlesham, England). The cefoxitin was provided partly by E. O. Stapley (Merck, Sharp and Dohme, Rahway, N.J.) and partly by Warren Wick (Eli Lilly & Co., Indianapolis, Ind.).

RESULTS

Susceptibility to β-lactamase hydrolysis. The susceptibility of the seven cephalosporins to the four β-lactamases used in these studies was examined in Na_2HPO_4/KH_2PO_4 buffer, pH 7.0, at 37°C, and the results are summarized in Table 1. The relative rate of hydrolysis of each cephalosporin has been related to an arbitrary value of 100 for each enzyme. It must be stressed, however, that the choice of this value for the rate of cephaloridine hydrolysis does not imply that the absolute rate of cephaloridine hydrolysis by the four enzymes is the same.

Type Ia enzyme is known to be relatively active against cephaloridine, cephalothin, and cephalexin (16), and activity against cefazolin was also detected in this study. On the other hand, cefoxitin, cefuroxime, and cefamandole were all substantially resistant to hydrolysis by this enzyme. Of these three compounds, cefamandole showed slight susceptibility, but even in this case a given amount of the antibiotic remained unhydrolyzed for more than 1,000 times as long as an equivalent amount of cephaloridine.

The enzyme from *P. aeruginosa* (type Id) is also known to be active against cephalosporins (16), and, as with the type Ia enzyme, cephaloridine, cephalothin, cephalexin, and cefazolin were hydrolyzed at appreciable rates (Table 1). Cefoxitin, cefuroxime, and cefamandole, on the other hand, were very resistant to hydrolysis. Overall, therefore, the two type I enzymes (Ia and Id) have very similar properties towards the seven cephalosporins tested here.

Type IIIa enzyme has a broad spectrum of activity, including both penicillins and cephalosporins (16). Among the cephalosporins the enzyme shows its greatest activity against cephaloridine, but cephalothin and cefazolin are also hydrolyzed to a significant extent. Unlike type Ia and Id enzymes, however, cefamandole is also hydrolyzed, and with this enzyme it is only cefoxitin, cefuroxime, and, to a lesser extent, cephalexin that are resistant to hydrolysis (Table 1).

Type IVc enzyme is already known to have a broad spectrum of activity against both penicillins and cephalosporins, including cloxacillin

TABLE 1. *Relative rates of hydrolysis by β-lactamases*

Antibiotic	Rate of hydrolysis[a]			
	Ia	Id	IIIa	IVc
Cephaloridine	100	100	100	100
Cephalothin	100	60	25	68
Cephalexin	12.5	70	0.5	0.5
Cefazolin	45	110	15	75
Cefoxitin	0	0.1	0	0
Cefamandole	0.1	0	20	60
Cefuroxime	0	0	0.1	1.3

[a] An arbitrary value of 100 was assumed for the rate of hydrolysis of cephaloridine by each enzyme. The sources of the enzymes are as follows: type Ia, *E. cloacae* (17); type Id, *P. aeruginosa* (Flett et al., submitted for publication); type IIIa, *E. coli* (R_{TEM}) (13); type IVc, *K. aerogenes* 1082E (8). The absolute activities of these four enzymes against cephaloridine are as follows (all values quoted as enzyme units per microgram of enzyme protein, using cephaloridine as substrate): type Ia, 8.7 (17); type Id, 13.8 (unpublished data); type IIIa, 170 (13); type IVc, 8.1 (unpublished data).

(8, 11). Its spectrum of activity against the seven compounds tested here is broadly very similar to that of type IIIa enzyme, save that some hydrolysis of cefuroxime is detectable with this enzyme even though the rate is still only about 1% of that found with cephaloridine (Table 1). In summary, therefore, only cefoxitin and cefuroxime show substantial resistance to all the β-lactamases examined here, and even cefuroxime is hydrolyzed, albeit very slowly, by type IVc enzyme.

Studies with *E. coli* UB1005 and the mutants DC2 and DC3. A previous paper (14) has described the use of these three *E. coli* strains indirectly to assess the ability of β-lactam antibiotics to penetrate to their target in the inner membrane of gram-negative bacteria. Antibiotics that show the same MIC value against *E. coli* UB1005 and its two mutant derivatives appear not to be hindered in their penetration through the outer layers of the *E. coli* envelope, whereas compounds that show different MIC values against the three strains seem to be so hindered. Moreover, the activity of the antibiotics against the most susceptible of the mutants (DC2) gives an indirect measure of the potential effectiveness of that antibiotic as an inhibitor of peptidoglycan biosynthesis in *E. coli*.

Figure 1 summarizes the effect of the seven cephalosporin derivatives studied here. In this figure the activity of the antibiotic (measured as MIC) is plotted against the "crypticity" values of the three strains when determined with benzylpenicillin, an indirect measure of the extent to which β-lactam penetration is altered in these strains (14, 15). Cephaloridine, cephalothin, and cephalexin are known to be equally effective against these three *E. coli* isolates (14) and therefore seem to pass unhindered to their target in the inner membrane (14). Cefazolin also falls into this category, since its activity against the mutant DC2 is the same as that against the parental strain (Fig. 1). Cefoxitin, cefuroxime, and cefamandole, on the other hand, are all affected to a greater or lesser extent by the mutational changes in DC2 and DC3. Cefoxitin shows the smallest difference, whereas cefuroxime and cefamandole are both affected substantially and to the same extent. Indeed, both these compounds are about 50 times more active against DC2 than against UB1005.

Since the mutant DC2 has a very low crypticity to all penicillins and cephalosporins whose activity in this respect can be tested (14), it can be argued that the susceptibility of this mutant to β-lactam antibiotics may reflect the inherent activity of these compounds against the peptidoglycan-synthesizing system in *E. coli*. If this

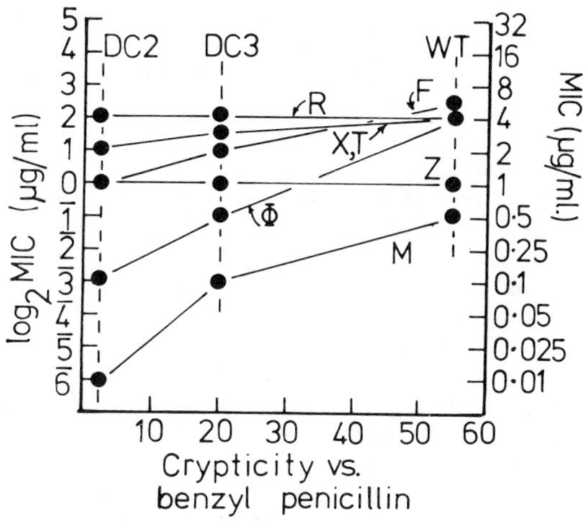

FIG. 1. *MIC values obtained with cephaloridine (R), cephalothin (T), cephalexin (X), cefazolin (Z), cefoxitin (F), cefuroxime (ϕ, and cefamandole (M) acting on E. coli UB1005 and the mutants DC2 and DC3. The "crypticity values" used in this figure were determined using benzylpenicillin and strains UB1005(RP1), DC2(RP1), and DC3(RP1) as described previously (14).*

is the case, then cefuroxime and cefamandole would seem inherently to be by far the most active among these seven cephalosporins tested here, with cefamandole showing an MIC against DC2 of about 0.01 μg/ml (Fig. 1).

DISCUSSION

Penicillinases and cephalosporinases play an important part in the resistance to β-lactam antibiotics of the increasing number of resistant isolates of gram-negative bacteria now being made in hospital clinics (4). Although cephaloridine, cephalothin, cephalexin, and cefazolin all seem to penetrate the outer layers of *E. coli* well, and therefore express their inherent activity against peptidoglycan synthesis to the full, these compounds are all hydrolyzed rapidly by all types of enzymes. Cefamandole is hydrolyzed at a substantial rate by both type IIIa and type IVc enzyme, but cefoxitin and cefuroxime show almost total resistance to all the enzymes (11; O'Callaghan et al., in press). Indeed, cefoxitin is so stable that it is difficult to detect any hydrolysis that is unequivocally due to β-lactamase action. These observations certainly confirm those published elsewhere (11).

The development of molecules as resistant to β-lactamase hydrolysis as cefoxitin and cefuroxime raises the question as to whether these compounds yet represent the ideal solution to the problem of β-lactamase-specified resistance among members of the *Enterobacteriaceae*. It seems from the studies published here that they do. Even the very slow hydrolysis of cefuroxime by type IVc enzyme is unlikely to have great clinical significance, since a given amount of this antibiotic has about 1,000 times more stability than cephaloridine even under the most disadvantageous conditions. Of course, new types of β-lactamase may emerge after the use of such compounds in clinics, but they do not seem prevalent at the moment. Although the problem of β-lactamase hydrolysis may well have been solved with cefoxitin and cefuroxime, neither molecule is yet perfect either as an inhibitor of peptidoglycan synthesis in gram-negative bacteria or in its ability to penetrate the surface layers of these bacteria. Among all the compounds studied here, β-lactamase resistance only seems to have been achieved at the expense of the free penetration characteristic of cephaloridine, cephalexin, cephalothin, and cefazolin. Thus, both cefoxitin and cefuroxime are a good deal more active against the mutant DC2 than against the wild type from which it was derived.

If one has to decide which of the seven compounds examined here has the optimal properties with respect to all the parameters of activity that have been measured in this study, then cefoxitin and cefuroxime seem to have first place, with the slight edge perhaps going to cefuroxime because of its greater in vitro activity is an antibiotic against *E. coli* K-12. Cefamandole is the most active of the compounds, and this is even more clearly the case with DC2, but has the defect of susceptibility to one of the β-lactamases (type IVc). However, it must be stressed that the parameters studied here are only a few of the many that are involved in determining the clinical effectiveness of a β-lactam antibiotic.

ACKNOWLEDGMENTS

This work was supported by a grant from the Medical Research Council to M.H.R. We are grateful to Glaxo Research Ltd., to Lilly Research Centre Ltd., and to Merck, Sharp and Dohme for gifts of the cephalosporins used in this study.

LITERATURE CITED

1. **Boman, H. G., K. Nordström, and S. Normark.** 1974. Penicillin resistance in *Escherichia coli* K12: synergism between a barrier in the outer part of the envelope. Ann. N.Y. Acad. Sci. 235:569–587.
2. **Datta, N., and M. H. Richmond.** 1966. The purification and some properties of a penicillinase whose synthesis is mediated by an R-factor in *Escherichia coli*. Biochem. J. 98:204–209.
3. **Goldner, M., D. G. Glass, and P. C. Fleming.** 1968. Characteristics of *Aerobacter* β-lactamase. Can. J. Microbiol. 14:139–145.
4. **Greenwood, D., and F. O'Grady.** 1975. Resistance categories of enterobacteria to β-lactam antibiotics. J. Infect. Dis. 132:233–240.
5. **Grinsted, J., J. R. Saunders, L. C. Ingram, R. B. Sykes, and M. H. Richmond.** 1972. Properties of an R-factor which originated in *Pseudomonas aeruginosa* 1822. J. Bacteriol. **110**:529–537.
6. **Hennessey, T. D., and M. H. Richmond.** 1968. The purification and some properties of a β-lactamase (cephalosporinase) synthesized by *Enterobacter cloacae*. Biochem. J. **109**:469–473.
7. **Leive, L.** 1974. The barrier function of the Gram-negative envelope. Ann. N.Y. Acad. Sci. **235**:109–129.
8. **Marshall, M. J., G. W. Ross, K. V. Chandler, and A. M. Harris.** 1972. Comparison of the substrate specificities of the β-lactamases from *Klebsiella aerogenes* 1082E and *Enterobacter cloacae* P99. Appl. Microbiol. **23**:765–769.
9. **Miller, A. K., E. Celozzi, Y. Yong, B. A. Pelak, D. Hendlin, and E. O. Stapley.** 1974. Cefoxitin, a semisynthetic cephamycin antibiotic: in vivo evaluation. Antimicrob. Agents Chemother. **5**:33–37.
10. **Nishida, M., T. Matsubara, T. Murakawa, Y. Mine, and Y. Yokota.** 1970. Cephazolin, a new semisynthetic cephalosporin antibiotic. II. *In vitro* and *in vivo* antibacterial activity. J. Antibiot. **23**:137–148.
11. **Onishi, H. R., D. R. Daoust, S. B. Zimmerman, D. Hendlin, and E. O. Stapley.** 1974. Cefoxitin, a semisynthetic cephamycin antibiotic: resistance to beta-lactamase inactivation. Antimicrob. Agents Chemother. **5**:38–48.
12. **Pollock, J. J., M. Nguyen-Distèche, J-M. Ghuysen, R. Linder, and M. R. J. Salton.** 1974. The DD-carboxypeptidase-transpeptidase system in *Escherichia coli* mutant strain 44. Ann. N.Y. Acad. Sci. **235**:225–235.
13. **Richmond, M. H.** 1975. β-Lactamase (*E. coli* R^{+}_{TEM}), p. 672–677. *In* J. H. Hash (ed.), Methods in enzymology, vol. 43, Antibiotics. Academic Press Inc., New York.
14. **Richmond, M. H., D. C. Clark, and S. Wotton.** 1976. Indirect method for assessing the penetration of beta-lactamase-nonsusceptible penicillins and cephalosporins in *Escherichia coli* strains. Antimicrob. Agents Chemother. **10**:215–218.
15. **Richmond, M. H., and N. A. C. Curtis.** 1974. The interplay of β-lactamases and intrinsic factors in the resistance of Gram-negative bacteria to penicillins and cephalosporins. Ann. N.Y. Acad. Sci. **235**:553–568.
16. **Richmond, M. H., and R. B. Sykes.** 1973. The β-lactamases of Gram-negative bacteria and their possible physiological role, p. 31–88. *In* A. H. Rose and D. Tempest (ed.), Advances in microbial physiology, vol. 9. Academic Press Inc., London.
17. **Ross, G. W.** 1975. β-Lactamase (*Enterobacter species*), p. 678–686. *In* J. H. Hash (ed.), Methods in enzymology, vol. 43, Antibiotics. Academic Press Inc., New York.
18. **Ross, G. W., and C. H. O'Callaghan.** 1975. β-Lactamase assays, p. 69–86. *In* J. H. Hash (ed.), Methods in enzymology, vol. 43, Antibiotics. Academic Press Inc., New York.
19. **Sabath, L., M. Jago, and E. P. Abraham.** 1965. Cephalosporinase and penicillinase activities of a β-lactamase from *Pseudomonas pyocyanea*. Biochem. J. **96**:739–752.
20. **Strominger, J. L., E. Willoughby, T. Kamiryo, P. M. Blumberg, and R. R. Yocum.** 1974. Penicillin sensitive enzymes and penicillin-binding components in bacterial cells. Ann. N.Y. Acad. Sci. **235**:210–224.
21. **Sykes, R. B., and M. H. Richmond.** 1971. R-factors, beta-lactamase and carbenicillin-resistant *Pseudomonas aeruginosa*. Lancet **ii**:342–344.
22. **Wallick, H., and D. Hendlin.** 1974. Cefoxitin, a semisynthetic cephamycin antibiotic: susceptibility studies. Antimicrob. Agents Chemother. **5**:25–32.
23. **Wick, W., and D. A. Preston.** 1972. Biological properties of three 3-heterocyclic-thiomethyl cephalosporin antibiotics. Antimicrob. Agents Chemother. **1**:221–234.

ANTIMICROBIAL AGENTS AND CHEMOTHERAPY, Aug. 1976, p. 223-228 Vol. 10, No. 2

Printed in U.S.A.

Comparison of Tetracycline Action on *Staphylococcus aureus* and *Escherichia coli* by Microbial Kinetics

SAMUEL M. HEMAN-ACKAH

Department of Pharmacy, College of Pharmacy and Pharmacal Sciences, Howard University, Washington, D.C. 20001

Received for publication 7 August 1975

Cultures of tetracycline-treated *Staphylococcus aureus* exhibited monophasic steady-state growth curves similar to that observed for tetracycline-treated *Escherichia coli*. Apparent growth rate constants of the respective drug-treated cultures showed the same formal dependence on drug concentration, which was linear at a low concentration but asymptotically approached zero at higher concentration levels and implied the saturation of a limited number of receptor sites engaged in microbial protein synthesis. The relative potency of tetracycline action of *S. aureus*/*E. coli* was 6.50:1 at 37.5°C and pH 7.05. This is attributed to relative differences in drug permeation and/or binding affinity for biophase receptors in the respective organisms. It is concluded from kinetic dependencies of growth inhibition of the cultures that tetracycline has the same mode of action on *S. aureus* and *E. coli*. It is bacteriostatic at concentrations below the minimal inhibitory concentration level but bactericidal at the higher concentration levels.

Tetracycline is a broad-spectrum antibiotic, which is active against gram-positive cocci and some gram-negative organisms, in addition to rickettsias and clamydia (15). It has been shown to bind to the 30S ribosomal subunit (5, 18, 22, 23, 29) and to inhibit the formation of peptide linkages in microbial protein synthesis (4, 21, 27, 29). Tetracycline is reported to produce bacteriostatic effects on microorganisms, even though high concentrations of the drug have shown bactericidal effects (15).

The relative potency of the tetracyclines against susceptible and resistant strains of organisms (15) has been attributed to differences in the drug permeation through cell membranes, which result in increased ability of susceptible strains to accumulate the drug in the biophase (6–8, 19, 25, 28). Since tetracycline is more active against *Staphylococcus aureus* than against *Escherichia coli* (15), it would be expected that the drug would have a higher partitioning and/or binding affinity for biophase receptors in the former than in the latter organism.

Studies on the action of tetracycline against *E. coli* by the kinetics of microbial growth (2, 10–14, 24) permitted not only the characterization of drug-receptor interactions in the biophase but also an elucidation of the possible mode of tetracycline action on the cells. Recently, comparative studies on the action of some drugs on *S. aureus* and *E. coli* by microbial growth kinetics (16) have revealed relative differences in the kinetics and dependencies related to modes of drug action on gram-positive and gram-negative organisms. This paper presents the results of similar studies on tetracycline action. It considers the functional dependency of kinetic parameters, derived from growth inhibition of the cultures, on tetracycline concentrations, the inoculum size, broth constituents, and other varying conditions. In addition, the modes of tetracycline action in the subinhibitory concentration range and at high concentrations above the minimal inhibitory concentration (MIC) values are considered.

MATERIALS AND METHODS

Antibiotics. Assayed samples of tetracycline hydrochloride (U.S.P.), supplied by courtesy of the Upjohn Co., were used for the experiments. The concentrations employed in all experiments refer to the hydrochloride salt of the antibiotic. Stock solutions were aseptically prepared by membrane filtration and stored at 4°C.

Culture media. Broth was antibiotic medium 3 (Difco Laboratories) rehydrated to peptone broth (U.S.P.). The broth was clarified by initial filtration through 22-μm membrane filters (HA type; Millipore Corp.) and finally through 0.45-μm membrane filters (HA type; Millipore Corp.). It was sterilized by autoclaving at 15 lb/in^2 for 15 min. The pH of the broth was 7.05 ± 0.05. Nutrient agar was broth containing 1.5% agar (Difco Laboratories) and was sterilized by autoclaving at 15 lb/in^2 for 15 min.

Bacterial cultures. Replicate cultures of *S. au-*

reus (ATCC 6538) and *E. coli* (ATCC 12407) on nutrient agar slants were stored at 4°C and used for daily experiments. When required, a 15- to 18-h growth of the respective culture in broth was diluted 50-fold (*S. aureus*) or 100-fold (*E. coli*) in 50 ml of fresh broth contained in a 125-ml, loosely capped Erlenmeyer flask. They were grown aerobically at 37.5°C in a thermostatically controlled shaker water bath (model R. W. 65, New Brunswick Scientific Co.) to a cell count of 2×10^7/ml. A portion of this culture (1.0 ml of *S. aureus* cultures per 50 ml of broth or 1.0 ml of *E. coli* culture per 100 ml of broth) was added to a bulk amount of broth contained in a 500-ml Pyrex flask fitted with a 50-ml dispenser to form the "seeded" broth. This was incubated at 37.5°C for 30 min with intermittent shaking. Quantities (50 ml) of the "seeded" broth were then aseptically transferred with the aid of the dispenser into replicate sterile Erlenmeyer flasks and maintained at 37.5°C in the shaker water bath. A portion (0.5 ml) of the suitably diluted tetracycline solution was added to each culture to yield a desired concentration of the antibiotic. The solution was added when the culture in the flask reached the logarithmic phase of growth at a cell concentration of 2.0×10^6/ml. The culture without antibiotic served as the control.

Viable count methods. Samples (1.0 ml) of drug-free and drug-treated cultures were withdrawn at 30-min intervals and diluted serially in sterile 0.9% NaCl and finally in broth to a cell concentration of 50 to 150/ml. Portions (1.0 ml) from the final broth dilution were plated in each of three replicate sandwich agar plates and incubated at 37.5°C for 48 h. The bacterial colonies were counted on the colony counter (Lab-line Instruments, Inc.).

Total count methods. Samples (0.25 to 1.0 ml) of drug-free and drug-treated cultures were withdrawn at 30-min intervals and diluted in Formol-saline to obtain counts within a range of 2,000 to 70,000 counts/50 μl on a particle-size counter (Coulter counter, model ZB1, Coulter Electronics Co.) that was equipped with a 30-μm orifice. The settings of the instrument were: 1/aperture current, 1.0; 1/amplification, 1/2; gain, 8.0; matching switch, 40 K; lower threshold, 5; and upper threshold, at maximum. The Formol-saline diluent was 0.85% sodium chloride in 1.0% formaldehyde, filtered twice through a 0.2-μm membrane filter (GA-8 type, Metricel), which promptly arrested growth of the culture sample without lytic or clumping effects on the cells.

RESULTS

Shape of growth curves. The steady-state generation of *S. aureus* and *E. coli* cultures affected with graded concentrations of tetracycline demonstrated linear semilogarithmic plots in accordance with the expression:

$$\log N = \log N_0 + k_{app}\, t/2.303 \qquad (1)$$

where N is the number of organisms per milliliter at anytime (t), N_0 is the number of organisms per milliliter at some initial time (0), and k_{app} is the apparent generation rate constant. In all cases, the tetracycline-treated cultures showed an initial lag phase of approximately 30 min before emerging into a steady-state phase of growth. Figure 1 shows typical monophasic generation curves of tetracycline-affected *S. aureus*, determined by the total count method. The curves are similar to those obtained for *E. coli* and confirm previous observations (2, 10–14, 16, 24).

Functional dependency of apparent growth rate constants on drug concentrations. The relationship between the k_{app} and the tetracycline concentration is plotted in Fig. 2. There was a linear dependency in the low concentration range from 0 to 0.075 μg/ml for tetracycline action on *E. coli* (curve A) and from 0 to 0.02 μg/ml for its action on *S. aureus* (curve B) in accordance with the expression (2, 10–13, 24):

$$k_{app} = k_0 - k_t\, T \qquad (2)$$

where k_t is the specific inhibitory rate constant and T is tetracycline concentration. In the absence of drug, $k_{app} = k_0$, which is the growth rate constant of drug-free culture. At the

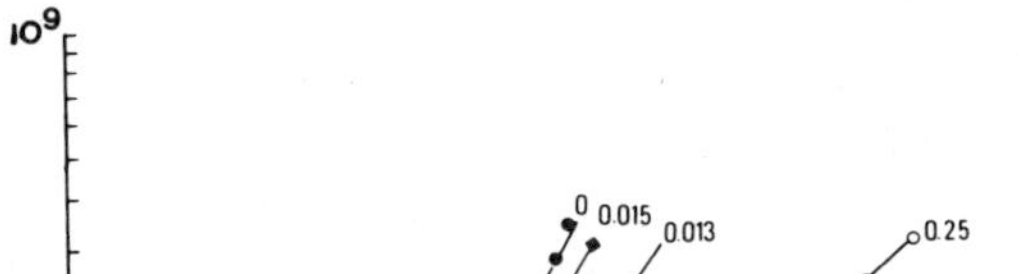

FIG. 1. *Typical growth curves of S. aureus in antibiotic medium 3 at pH 7.05 and 37.5°C in the absence and presence of graded concentrations of tetracycline, obtained by the total count method. The curves are labeled according to drug concentrations (micrograms per milliliter).*

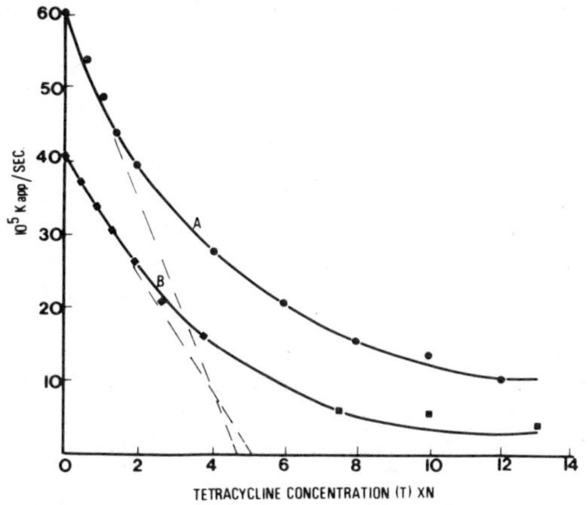

FIG. 2. *Dependence of apparent growth rate constant, k_{app}, for S. aureus and E. coli on concentrations of tetracycline at pH 7.05 and 37.5°C. The actual concentrations are multiplied by a factor, n, where n = 20 in curve A for E. coli (●) and n = 100 in curve B for S. aureus (■).*

higher concentration levels, the k_{app} was not a linear function of increasing tetracycline concentration but asymptotically approached zero. The plots of $T/(k_0 - k_{app})$ versus T (Fig. 3) were reasonably linear for the action of tetracycline concentrations >0.075 μg/ml on *E. coli* (curve A) and >0.02 μg/ml on *S. aureus* (curve B), but showed deviations at the lower concentration levels. This implied quantitative adherence of the action of tetracycline on *E. coli* and *S. aureus* to an expression previously derived from a saturation kinetic model (13):

$$T/(k_0 - k_{app}) = T(k_a/k_b) + 1/k_a \qquad (3)$$

where k_a and k_b are constants of proportionality related to the tetracycline partition through cell membranes and its binding affinity for biophase receptors. At the MIC, when $k_{app} = 0$, equation 3 simplifies to:

$$T_m = 1/(k_a/k_0 - k_b) \qquad (4)$$

where T_m is the MIC for tetracycline.

The values of k_a and k_b, derived from the slopes and intercepts of the plots in Fig. 3, and the T_m, calculated in accordance with equation 4, are given in Table 1.

Effect of the counting method on growth curves. Semilogarithmic plots of total and viable counts versus time for the action of selected concentrations of tetracycline, 0, 0.014, 0.06, 0.30, 0.60, and 1.20 μg/ml, respectively, on *S. aureus* are shown in Fig. 4. Parallel growth curves were obtained from the plots of the total and viable counts on cultures treated with low concentrations (0 to 0.06 μg/ml) of tetracycline (curves A_1, A; B_1, B; and C_1, C). The total count was 70 to 80% of the viable count at each concentration level. Cultures treated with high concentrations, 0.30 μg/ml or greater, showed coincidence of plots for the total counts that remained constant for the entire period of the drug-bacteria contact time (curves D, E, and F). The corresponding plots for the viable count showed an exponential decrease with time as a function of the tetracycline concentration (curves D_1, E_1, and F_1).

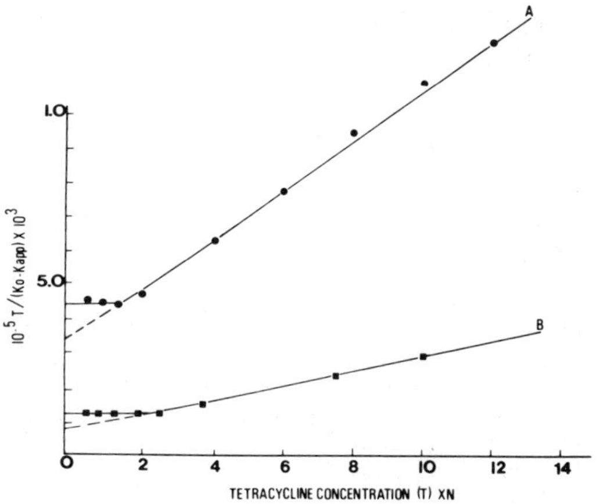

FIG. 3. *Applicability of saturation kinetic model to the dependency of apparent growth rate constants, k_{app}, for drug-treated cultures at high concentrations of tetracycline. The actual concentrations are multiplied by a factor of n, where n = 20 in curve A for E. coli (●) and n = 100 in curve B for S. aureus (■).*

TABLE 1. *Kinetic parameters derived[a] from tetracycline inhibition of S. aureus and E. coli cultures*

Kinetic parameter	*S. aureus*	*E. coli*
$10^5\ k_t$ (ml/μg per s)[b]	807.69	255.32
$10^5\ k_a$ (ml/μg per s)[c]	1,250.00	294.10
k_b (ml/μg)[c]	26.67	4.20
$10^5\ k_a/k_b$ (s^{-1})[c]	47.62	70.00
$(k_a/k_b)/k_0$[c]	1.19	1.17
MIC[d]	0.22	1.43
θ_m[e]	0.85	0.86

[a] Derived from the data of Fig. 2.

[b] Calculated from the plot of k_{app} versus T for the action of 0–0.02 μg of tetracycline per ml on *S. aureus* or 0–0.75 μg of tetracycline per ml on *E. coli* in accordance with the expression in equation 2.

[c] Estimated from the slopes and intercepts of the plots of $T/(k_0 - k_{app})$ versus T for the action of tetracycline on *S. aureus* at concentrations > 0.02 μg/ml or for its action on *E. coli* at concentrations >0.075 μg/ml according to the expression in equation 3.

[d] Calculated from the expression in equation 4.

[e] Calculated from the expression in equation 10.

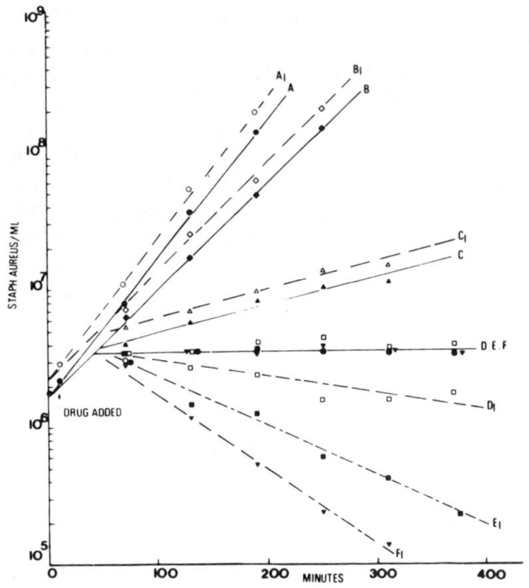

FIG. 4. *Growth curves of S. aureus at pH 7.05 and 37.5°C in the presence and absence of tetracycline, obtained by total count (——) and viable count (- - -) methods. The curves and respective drug concentrations (micrograms per milliliter) are A, A_1, 0.0; B, B_1, 0.014; C, C_1, 0.06; D, D_1, 0.30; E, E_1, 0.60; and F, F_1, 1.20.*

These observations clearly indicated that the action of tetracycline was bactericidal at concentrations above the MIC. Similar results were obtained for the action of tetracycline on *E. coli* (12).

Effect of changes in inoculum size and broth composition on apparent growth rates of tetracycline-treated cultures. The apparent growth rate constants for *S. aureus* cultures that were treated with 0, 0.01, 0.02, 0.04, 0.06, and 0.08 μg of tetracycline per ml, respectively, did not show significant variations from those obtained at corresponding concentration levels in Fig. 2, when either (i) the inoculum size was changed 0.1- to 10.0-fold at the time of drug addition in a single-strength broth, or (ii) the broth composition was changed 0.5- to 2.0-fold with the organism population fixed at 2.0×10^6/ml at the time of drug addition.

DISCUSSION

There was no dependence of the apparent growth rate constants of drug-treated *S. aureus* on variations in the broth composition or the inoculum size at the time of drug addition, suggesting drug interaction with broth constituents or drug depletion/inactivation by microbial metabolic activities as was similarly observed (12) for the action of tetracycline on *E. coli*.

The parallelism of growth curves, obtained by the total and viable counts, indicates suitability of either method for determining growth rates of drug-free and drug-treated *S. aureus* cultures. It also provides evidence that there was no killing or lytic phenomenon superimposed on normal growth inhibition by the action of subinhibitory concentrations of tetracycline on *S. aureus*. Therefore, tetracycline exerts a "true bacteriostatic" action (3) on *S. aureus*, causing a decrease in the rate of cell multiplication, presumably by competitive binding on ribosomes to lower cell protein synthesis.

At concentrations above the inhibitory level, the total count remains invariant with time, but the viable count decreased logarithmically with time as a function of tetracycline concentration. If the death of the organism was due to effects of prolonged bacteriostasis, then the death rate should show deviation from the monomolecular law (17, 20, 26, 30). The fact that there is an exponential relationship between the viable count and drug-bacteria contact time suggests a bactericidal phenomenon.

The formal dependence of k_{app} on drug concentration for tetracycline-treated *S. aureus* is the same as the tetracycline-treated *E. coli* (Fig. 2) and suggests the same mechanism of action.

The relationship is described by a kinetic expression that is derived from model compartmental analysis (13) on the premise that: (i) the rate of increase in microbial numbers (dN/dt) is proportional to the net rate of protein synthesis (dp^1/dt) above a certain minimum rate (Δp) required for survival and the numbers of organisms (N) present, and (ii) the overall rate of protein synthesis (dp/dt) is proportional to the free or unbound fraction ($1 - \theta$) of total ribosomal sites, R_T, where θ is the fraction of total ribosomal sites bound by tetracycline. Therefore, the following equations are applicable:

$$dN/dt = k_m(dp^1/dt)N = k_m(dp/dt - \Delta p)N = k_{app}\,N \tag{5}$$

and

$$dp/dt = q\,(1 - \theta)R_T \tag{6}$$

where k_m and q are constants of proportionality, and k_{app} is the growth rate constant of tetracycline-treated cultures. θ is implicitly defined (9, 13) as follows:

$$\theta = K_1K_2T/(1 + K_1K_2T) \qquad (7)$$

where K_1 is tetracycline partition constant through cell membranes, and K_2 is the ribosomal affinity constant for tetracycline (T). A combination of equations 5, 6, and 7 yields:

$$k_{\text{app}} = k_0 - k_aT/(1 + k_bT) \qquad (8)$$

where $k_0 = q\ k_mR_T - k_m\ \Delta_p$ is the growth rate constant of the drug-free culture, $k_b = K_1K_2$, and $k_a = q\ k_mR_TK_1K_2$.
Therefore

$$(k_a/k_b)/k_0 > 1 \qquad (9)$$

Equation 8 may describe the functional dependency of the k_{app} on drug concentration for tetracycline-treated *S. aureus* and *E. coli*, respectively (Fig. 2). The action of low concentrations (0 to 0.02 μg/ml) of tetracycline on *S. aureus* or (0 to 0.75 μg/ml) of tetracycline on *E. coli* shows linear dependency of the k_{app} on drug concentration, possibly because few receptors interact with the drug and $k_b\ T \ll 1$, which therefore simplifies equation 8 to equation 2. At high concentrations (>0.02 μg of tetracycline per ml on *S. aureus* or >0.075 μg of tetracycline per ml on *E. coli*), a nonlinear dependency is applicable in accordance with equation 8. Arithmetical transformation of equation 8 is equation 3, for which linear plots of $T/(k_0 - k_{\text{app}})$ versus T are obtained in Fig. 3 from the data of Fig. 2 at the high concentration levels. This indicates quantitative adherence to a saturation kinetic model (13). Deviations occur in the low concentration range when the receptor sites are not saturated and the extent of growth inhibition ($k_0 - k_{\text{app}}$) is directly proportional to drug concentration. In earlier studies of tetracycline action on *E. coli*, a linear dependence of the k_{app} on drug concentration that could be quantified by equation 2 was reported (2, 10, 12, 13). The apparent discrepancy could be attributed to the fact that earlier studies did not employ a wider concentration than was presently investigated. Alternatively, the laboratory strain B/r of *E. coli* employed for earlier studies could be a substrain of *E. coli* (ATCC 12407), which is more susceptible to tetracycline action. Other workers (G. H. Miller, H. L. Smith, W. L. Rock, and S. Hedbert, J. Pharm. Sci., in press), using resistant strains of *E. coli*, have also reported a nonlinear dependency of the k_{app} on concentration that can be quantified by equation 8 at high concentration levels for various tetracyclines.

The values of k_a and k_b, calculated from the data of Fig. 3 in accordance with equation 3, are given in Table 1. The experimentally determined values of $(k_a/k_b)/k_0 > 1$ agree very well with theoretical predictions in equation 9. The calculated ratio of the k_b of *S. aureus/E. coli* is 6.35:1. The MIC values of tetracycline against the organisms calculated from k_a, k_b, and k_0, in accordance with equation 4, are also given in Table 1. The relative potency of tetracycline action, as determined by the MIC values, is of the order *S. aureus/E. coli* as 6.50:1. Although k_b is a parameter derived from K_1 and K_2, as defined in equation 7, K_1 and K_2 cannot be kinetically differentiated. However, the close agreement between the comparative values of k_b and the relative potency of tetracycline action on *S. aureus* and *E. coli* indicate that the drug partitioning through cell membranes and/or drug binding affinity for receptor sites are the determining factors for the differences shown in tetracycline activity against susceptible strains of organisms.

At the MIC level, the following is applicable:

$$\theta_m = K_1K_2T_m/(1 + K_1K_2T_m) = k_bT_m/(1 + k_bT_m) \qquad (10)$$

where θ_m is a fraction of total ribosomal sites bound by tetracycline. Therefore, $1 - \theta_m$ is the fraction engaged in the minimum rate of protein synthesis for survival. T_m is the MIC, as defined in equation 4. Table 1 shows that θ_m, calculated from kinetic parameters for the action of tetracycline, competitively binds 85% of transfer ribonucleic acid-binding sites to produce true bacteriostasis (12) on the organisms. At concentrations greater than the MIC, there must be a change in the overt mechanism of tetracycline action that results in a change from truly bacteriostatic to a highly bactericidal agent, as observed experimentally (Fig. 4).

ACKNOWLEDGMENTS

I thank Patricia Ann Wright for excellent technical assistance.

LITERATURE CITED

1. **Brock, T. D.** 1970. Biology of microorganisms, p. 17–61, 173–199. Prentice-Hall, Englewood Cliffs, N.J.
2. **Brown, M. R. W., and C. R. Garrett.** 1964. Kinetics and mechanisms of action of antibiotics. T. Reproducibility of *Escherichia coli* growth curves and dependence upon tetracycline concentrations. J. Pharm. Sci. 53:170–183.
3. **Cook, A. M.** 1964. Comparative studies of methods of

evaluating antibacterial substance. I. Evaluation of bacteriostatic action. J. Pharm. Pharmacol. 6:629-637.

4. **Cudliffe, E., and K. McQuillen.** 1967. Bacterial protein synthesis: the effects of antibiotics. J. Mol. Biol. 30:137-146.
5. **Franklin, T. J.** 1966. Mode of action of tetracycline. Symp. Soc. Gen. Microbiol. 16:192-212.
6. **Franklin, T. J.** 1967. Resistance of *Escherichia coli* to tetracyclines—changes in permeability to tetracyclines in *Escherichia coli* bearing transferable resistance factors. Biochem. J. 105:371-378.
7. **Franklin, T. J., and A. Godfrey.** 1965. Resistance of *Escherichia coli* to tetracyclines. Biochem. J. 94:54-60.
8. **Franklin, T. J., and B. Higginson.** 1970. Active accumulation of tetracycline by *Escherichia coli*. Biochem. J. 116:287-297.
9. **Garrett, E. R.** 1971. Drug action and assay by microbial kinetics, p. 271-352. *In* E. Jucker (ed.), Progress in drug research, vol. 15. Birkhauser Verlag, Basel, Switzerland.
10. **Garrett, E. R., and M. R. W. Brown.** 1963. The action of tetracycline and chloramphenicol alone and in admixture on the growth of *Escherichia coli*. J. Pharm. Pharmacol. 15:185T-191T.
11. **Garrett, E. R., and S. M. Heman-Ackah.** 1973. Microbial kinetics and dependence of individual and combined antibiotic inhibitors of protein biosynthesis. Antmicrob. Agents Chemother. 4:574-584.
12. **Garrett, E. R., and G. H. Miller.** 1965. Kinetics and mechanisms of action of antibiotics on micro-organisms III. Inhibitory action of tetracycline and chloramphenicol on *Escherichia coli* established by total and viable counts. J. Pharm. Sci. 54:427-431.
13. **Garrett, E. R., G. H. Miller, and M. R. Brown.** 1965. Kinetics and mechanisms of antibiotics on microorganisms. V. Chloramphenicol and tetracycline affected *Escherichia coli* generation rates. J. Pharm. Sci. 55:593-600.
14. **Garrett, E. R., and C. M. Won.** 1973. Effect of novobiocin and its combination with tetracycline, chloramphenicol, erythromycin, and lincomycin on the microbial generation of *Escherichia coli*. Antimicrob. Agents Chemother. 4:626-633.
15. **Garrod, L. P., and F. O'Grady.** 1971. Antibiotic and chemotherapy, 3rd ed., p. 147-165. E. & S. Livingstone, London.
16. **Heman-Ackah, S. M.** 1974. Microbial kinetics of drug action against Gram-positive and Gram-negative organisms. I. Effect of lincomycin on *Staphylococcus aureus and Escherichia coli*. J. Pharm. Sci. 63:1077-1084.
17. **Hinshelwood, C.** 1951. Decline and death of bacterial populations. Nature (London) 167:666-669.
18. **Igarashi, K., and A. Kaji.** 1970. Relationship between sites 1, 2 and acceptor, donor sites for the binding of aminoacyl RNA to ribosomes. Eur. J. Biochem. 14:41-46.
19. **Izaki, K., K. Kiuchi, and K. Arima.** 1966. Specificity and mechanism of tetracycline resistance in a multiple drug resistant strain of *Escherichia coli*. J. Bacteriol. 91:628-633.
20. **Jordan, R. C., and S. E. Jacobs.** 1944. Studies in the dynamics of disinfection. J. Hyg. 43:275-289.
21. **Laskin, I.** 1970. Molecular aspects of tetracycline activity, p. 441-444. *In* Hamao Umezawa (ed.), Progress in antimicrobial and antineoplastic chemotherapy. Proceedings of the 6th International Congress on Chemotherapy, vol. II. University Park Press, Baltimore, Md.
22. **Last, J. A.** 1969. Studies on the binding of tetracyclines to ribosomes. Biochim. Biophys. Acta 195:506-514.
23. **Maxwell, I. H.** 1968. Studies of the binding of tetracyclines to ribosomes *in vitro*. Mol. Pharmacol. 4:25-37.
24. **Miller, G. H., S. A. Khalil, and A. N. Martin.** 1971. Structure-activity relationships of tetracyclines. I. Inhibition of cell division and protein and nucleic acid syntheses in *Escherichia coli* W. J. Pharm. Sci. 60:33-40.
25. **Reynard, A. M., L. F. Nellis, and M. E. Beck.** 1971. Uptake of ^{3}H-tetracycline by resistant and sensitive *Escherichia coli*. Appl. Microbiol. 21:71-75.
26. **Rhan, O.** 1921. The size of bacteria as the cause of the logarithmic order of death. J. Gen. Physiol. 13:179-205.
27. **Sarker, S., and R. E. Thach.** 1968. Inhibition of formylmethionyl-transfer RNA binding to ribosomes by tetracyclines. Proc. Natl. Acad. Sci. 60:1474-1486.
28. **Sompolinsky, D., Y. Zaidenzaig, R. Zieglar-Schlomowitz, and N. J. Abramova.** 1970. Mechanism of tetracycline resistance in *Staphylococcus aureus*. J. Gen. Microbiol. 62:351-362.
29. **Weisblum, B.** 1969. Antibiotic inhibitors of the bacterial ribosome. Bacteriol. Rev. 32:493-528.
30. **Wilson, G. S., and A. A. Miles.** 1964. Principles of bacteriology and immunity, vol. 1, 5th ed., p. 152-172. Williams & Wilkins Co., Baltimore.

Antimicrobial Agents and Chemotherapy, Aug. 1976, p. 229-233 Vol. 10, No. 2

Printed in U.S.A.

Photoinactivation of Latent Herpes Simplex Virus in Rabbit Kidney Cells

J. J. KELLEHER* AND J. VARANI

Microbiology Department, University of North Dakota School of Medicine, Grand Forks, North Dakota 58201

Received for publication 16 March 1976

The photoinactivation of actively and nonactively growing herpes simplex virus by neutral red and proflavine was studied in rabbit kidney cells. Active virus growth was inhibited by both dyes under conditions which did not destroy the cells. Neutral red caused a much greater inhibition than proflavine. Neutral red also caused a reduction in the reactivation rate of latent virus when the infected cells were treated during the latent period. In the treated cultures that did reactivate virus, the average length of the latent period was increased over the control value. Proflavine treatment did not reduce the rate of reactivation of latent virus and did not increase the average latent period of the treated cultures.

Herpes simplex virus (HSV) is inactivated by photosensitizing dyes such as neutral red and proflavine after exposure to visible light (1, 11, 17). Experiments with other viruses have indicated that these dyes bind to the viral nucleic acid, resulting in the breakdown of guanine residues (3, 12–14, 18). A number of clinical studies and studies using laboratory animals concerning the therapeutic effects of neutral red and proflavine have been reported (2, 4, 5, 7–10, 16). These studies include cases of herpetic eye infections (7, 9, 16) and genital herpes lesions (4, 5) as well as primary and recurrent oral and skin lesions. The overall effectiveness of photosensitization therapy has yet to be proven, and potential hazards of the treatment have been brought up (11). In experimental studies virus has been inactivated by exposure to light both after extracellular virus was treated with dye (1, 17) and after virus was grown in cells treated with dye and then separated from the cellular material (11). In the present study we have treated cultures with neutral red and proflavine in an attempt to inactivate virus within the infected cells. We have treated cultures in which virus was actively growing and cultures in which virus was not actively growing and was considered to be latent (6). We have found that production of infectious virus could be reduced by neutral red treatment employing conditions that were tolerated by the cells and that reactivation of latent virus could also be inhibited under these conditions. Proflavine treatment was much less effective in reducing active virus growth and did not prevent the reactivation of latent virus.

MATERIALS AND METHODS

Cell cultures and virus. Primary rabbit kidney (RK) cells were used throughout this study. The preparation of cell cultures and the maintenance of the cells for long-term studies have been described in a previous report (6). The virus used in this study was the MS strain of HSV, a type 2 strain obtained from the American Type Culture Collection, Rockville, Md. The routine handling of virus including preparation of virus stocks, infection of RK cells, isolation, identification, and quantitation of the virus recovered from RK cells have all been previously described (6).

Latent infection. To establish latent infection RK cells were infected with a low multiplicity of virus (5,000 plaque-forming units [PFU] of virus per culture containing 10^6 cells) and incubated at 41°C for 2 to 6 days. Virus growth did not occur at 41°C, and the infectious virus disappeared at a logarithmic rate. After incubation at 41°C, the cultures were transferred to 37°C. Virus growth resumed in some of the infected cultures immediately after transfer to 37°C. However, there were extensive delays in many of the cultures at 37°C, before active virus growth resumed. The period of time during which virus growth was not observed at 37°C was defined as the lag period. Lag periods of 4 or more days indicated some delay in virus replication after transfer to 37°C, because virus growth could always be seen within 3 days when infectious virus was inoculated directly onto cells at 37°C. Of the 200 cultures initially infected and incubated at 41°C, 82 had lag periods of 4 or more days and 48 had lag periods of 7 or more days after transfer to 37°C. The longest lag period was 45 days, and the average lag period of the last 48 cultures was 15.3 days. When active virus growth resumed, a cytopathic effect (CPE) could always be seen. Infectious virus was recovered from the cultures at this time.

The virus was passed once in RK cells and neutralized by commercial anti-HSV serum. The details of this model latent infection have been previously reported (6).

Photosensitizing dyes. A sterile solution of neutral red dye (1:300) was purchased from Grand Island Biological Co. (Grand Island, N.Y.). This stock solution was diluted 1:1,000 with Earle balanced salt solution. Cultures containing 1 ml of maintenance medium were treated with 0.2 ml of the diluted dye. The cultures were then incubated in the dark for 2 h. After 2 h the dye was removed, and the cultures were washed once with Earle balanced salt solution. They were then exposed to light from three 6-watt, cool-white fluorescent bulbs at a distance of approximately 10 cm for a period of 2 h. Proflavine dye was obtained from Pfaltz & Bauer, Inc. (Corona, N.Y.). A 0.1% solution of dye was prepared in Earle balanced salt solution and filter sterilized. This stock solution was diluted 1:1,000 with Earle balanced salt solution, and cultures containing 1 ml of the maintenance medium were treated with 0.2 ml of the diluted dye. The proflavine-treated cultures were then handled in the same manner as the neutral red-treated cultures. The concentrations of dyes used were chosen because they were the highest concentrations that were tolerated by the cells under the conditions of the experiments. At the concentrations used, a few of the cells detached from the monolayers after exposure to light. However, most of the cells appeared normal, and the monolayers remained intact.

RESULTS

Effect of neutral red treatment on virus growth at 37°C. Cultures of RK cells were infected with approximately 500 PFU of virus (multiplicity of infection, 0.0005) and incubated at 37°C for 4 h to allow virus to adsorb. The cultures were then treated with neutral red and photosensitized as described in the Material and Methods section. After photosensitization, the cultures were incubated in the dark at 37°C along with untreated control cultures. By 48 to 72 h after infection the control cultures showed widespread CPE. CPE could also be seen in all treated cultures, although it was only seen in a few focal areas in each culture. The cultures were freeze-thawed three times and assayed for virus in RK cells. The cultures were wrapped in aluminum foil during handling to minimize their exposure to visible light. The neutral red treatment greatly reduced the amount of virus produced. In the control cultures 5×10^5 to 1.5×10^6 PFU of virus per ml were recovered, whereas in the neutral red-treated cultures only 17 to 20 PFU of virus per ml were recovered. Some of the neutral red-treated cultures were allowed to continue incubating in the dark for an additional 3 days. Virus spread throughout these cultures and eventually did infect all of the cells. Some cultures were treated with neutral red but were not exposed to visible light. No reduction in CPE was observed in these cultures and as much infectious virus was produced in these cultures as in the control cultures.

Effect of neutral red treatment on latent virus. Cultures of RK cells were infected with 5,000 PFU of virus and incubated at 41°C for 2 to 3 days. After incubation at 41°C the cultures were transferred to 37°C and separated into two groups. One group was kept as a control, and the other group was treated with neutral red and photosensitized as described in the Materials and Methods section. All cultures were then incubated in the dark at 37°C and examined daily for the appearance of CPE. From previous work (6) we knew that once CPE appeared, active virus growth was occurring and infectious HSV could be recovered from the cultures at this time. The date on which CPE first appeared was noted. The cultures that did not show CPE were routinely incubated up to 45 days before being discarded. At the conclusion of the experiment the overall reactivation rates and the average lag periods of the control and treated groups were determined (Table 1). In the control group virus was recovered from 124 of 164 cultures for a reactivation rate of 76%. The average lag period of the cultures in this group was 5.0 days. In the neutral red-treated group virus was recovered from 82 of 153 cultures for a 54% recovery rate. The average lag period of the cultures in this group was 10.7 days. The differences in the overall reactivation rates and average lag periods between the control group and treated group were both highly significant statistically ($P < 0.001$).

In one experiment the neutral red-treated cultures were not exposed to visible light. Virus was recovered from these cultures and from

TABLE 1. *Effects of neutral red treatment on the recovery of HSV from cells infected with latent virus*

Treatment[a]	No. of cultures treated	No. of cultures in which virus was recovered after incubation at 37°C (%)	Avg lag period (days)
None	164	124 (76%)	5.0
Neutral red	153	82 (54%)	10.7

[a] Cultures were infected with 5×10^3 PFU of virus and incubated at 41°C for 2 to 3 days. After incubation at 41°C, the cultures were transferred to 37°C. Half were kept as controls, and half were treated with neutral red and photosensitized as described in the Materials and Methods section. All cultures were incubated in the dark and examined daily for CPE. At the conclusion of the experiment, the recovery rates and average lag periods were determined.

matched control cultures at the same rate, and there was no significant difference in the average lag periods of these two groups. In another experiment cultures of RK cells were infected with virus and incubated at 41°C for 1 day. After 1 day the cultures were separated into two groups. One group was kept as a control, whereas the other was treated with neutral red and photosensitized. After photosensitization the cultures were immediately returned to 41°C incubation for an additional 2 days. The cultures were then transferred to 37°C, incubated in the dark, and examined daily for CPE. The photosensitization treatment followed by 41°C incubation affected the virus in the same manner as photosensitization followed by 37°C incubation. Virus was recovered from 17 out of 27 control cultures for a reactivation rate of 63% and from 5 out of 24 treated cultures for a reactivation rate of 21%. The average lag period of the treated cultures was increased from 3.8 to 5.6 days.

Effect of proflavine treatment on virus growth at 37°C. Cultures of RK cells were infected with approximately 500 PFU of virus (multiplicity of infection, 0.0005) and incubated at 37°C for 4 h.The cultures were then treated with proflavine and photosensitized. The treated cultures and untreated control cultures were then incubated in the dark at 37°C. By 48 h the control cultures showed widespread CPE. The amount of CPE observed in the proflavine-treated cultures was reduced, although the reduction was not as great as that seen with the neutral red treatment. The control and proflavine-treated cultures were freeze-thawed three times and assayed for infectious virus in RK cells. Again care was taken to keep the treated cultures from being exposed to visible light. The amount of virus produced in the treated cultures was reduced from the control value. In the control cultures 5.5×10^5 PFU of virus per ml were recovered, whereas in the proflavine-treated cultures only 5×10^4 PFU of virus per ml were recovered.

Effect of proflavine treatment on latent virus. Cultures of RK cells were infected with 5,000 PFU virus, incubated at 41°C for 2 to 3 days, and then transferred to 37°C. The cultures were separated into two groups; one group was kept as a control group and the other cultures were treated with proflavine and photosensitized as described in the Materials and Methods section. After photosensitization the cultures were incubated in the dark and observed daily for CPE. The date on which CPE was first observed was recorded and at the completion of the experiment the overall reactivation rates and the average lag periods of the control and treated groups were determined (Table 2). Unlike neutral red treatment, proflavine treatment did not reduce the overall reactivation rate. Virus was actually recovered from a higher percentage of the proflavine-treated cultures (70%) than from the control cultures (63%), although this difference was not statistically significant. In addition, the average lag period of the treated cultures was slightly reduced from the control value. This difference was statistically significant ($P < 0.001$).

DISCUSSION

The inactivation of viruses by the various photosensitizing dyes in the presence of visible light is thought to be the result of the dye binding to the viral nucleic acid and causing the breakdown of guanine residues in a photooxidation reaction (3, 12–14, 18). Extracellular HSV particles have been shown to be photosensitive either when extracellular virus is exposed to neutral red or proflavine (1,17) or when the virus is grown in cells in medium containing the dye (11). It was the aim of this study to look at the photosensitizing ability of these agents on virus within viable cells. In this type of study, the concentrations of dyes that can be used is limited by the inherent toxicity of these agents for the cells. In this study experiments were run to test the agents against actively growing virus and against virus in a nonproductive infection. Against actively growing virus both neutral red and proflavine were effective in reducing virus yields at dye concentrations tolerated by the cells. Proflavine treatment reduced production by about 90%. Neutral red was even more effective and caused a reduction of 4 to 5 logs.

TABLE. 2. *Effects of proflavine treatment on the recovery of HSV from cells infected with latent virus*

Treatment[a]	No. of cultures treated	No. of cultures in which virus was recovered after incubation at 37°C (%)	Avg lag period (days)
None	214	135 (63%)	6.9
Proflavine	214	150 (70%)	4.7

[a] Cultures were infected with 5×10^3 PFU of virus and incubated at 41°C for 2 to 3 days. After incubation at 41°C, the cultures were transferred to 37°C. Half were kept as controls and half were treated with proflavine and photosensitized as described in the Materials and Methods section. All cultures were incubated in the dark and examined daily for CPE. At the conclusion of the experiment, the recovery rates and average lag periods were determined.

A very important aspect of this study was to look at the effects of these agents on virus that was not actively multiplying. In the model latent infection that we used all attempts to demonstrate the presence of infectious virus have been negative. We have never been able to isolate infectious virus; the infected cells do not appear to be altered morphologically by the virus, and agents such as bromodeoxyuridine and iododeoxyuridine do not eliminate the virus from the cells (6, 15). In this study treatment of latent virus-infected cells with neutral red significantly reduced the number of cultures from which virus was recovered and also increased the average lag period of the cultures that eventually did begin producing virus. If the increase in the average lag period were the only finding, this could be due simply to the elimination of actively growing virus. When the cultures are transferred to 37°C some of the cultures begin producing infectious virus immediately and CPE is seen within 3 days. If this virus that is actively growing were eliminated, it would reduce the number of cultures with short lag periods. However, this should not reduce the overall reactivation rate, since these cultures would still contain nonactively growing virus in addition to the virus that is actively multiplying. The fact that we did see a reduction in the reactivation rate leads us to suspect that the neutral red treatment affects the latent virus in addition to the actively growing virus.

Furthermore, in one experiment cultures were photosensitized and then returned to a 41°C incubation for 2 days. This treatment also resulted in a reduction of the overall reactivation rate. Although we do not refer to nongrowing virus at 41°C as being latent, it definitely is not actively growing. Finally, it has been shown that free viral nucleic acid can be inactivated by photosensitization (12) so there is no theoretical reason why the nongrowing virus in our infection should be resistant to the treatment.

The apparent elimination of latent virus by the neutral red photosensitization treatment indicates that latent HSV in our model system is not necessarily completely resistant to chemical attack. These results are in contrast to our previous results with bromodeoxyuridine on the same model infection (15). In the previous study we found that the latent infection could be modified by prior treatment of the cells with bromodeoxyuridine, but that once the latent infection was established the reactivation rate could not be reduced by treatment. Even though neutral red treatment did reduce the reactivation rate, there was still a large amount of latent virus that was not affected by the neutral red treatment. A total of 82 of the 153 neutral red-treated cultures did eventually reactivate virus and, of these, 45 had lag periods of 7 or more days. Perhaps we might have been able to eliminate all of the virus if we were able to use a higher concentration of dye and a longer exposure to visible light.

When proflavine was used in place of neutral red, the overall reactivation rate was not reduced. In fact, virus was recovered from a few more of the proflavine-treated cultures than control cultures. We also observed a slight shortening of the average lag period of the proflavine-treated cultures. This reduction was actually statistically significant ($P < 0.001$), although we hesitate at this point to say that virus reactivations were induced by the proflavine treatment.

It is not possible to explain the different results observed with the two dyes. The mechanisms of action of the two dyes may, in fact, be different, or it may be that neutral red is able to penetrate the cell more easily than proflavine. The concentration of dyes used was limited by their toxicity for the cell cultures. We were able to use a slightly higher concentration of neutral red in these experiments. Perhaps if a higher concentration of proflavine could have been used, we would have obtained results similar to those obtained with neutral red.

With regard to the therapeutic usefulness of photosensitization treatment for herpetic infections, the questions regarding effectiveness and safety remain to be answered. It appears from this study, however, that substantially different results may be obtained when different agents are used. In this study neutral red was more effective than proflavine in inhibiting active virus growth in RK cells. Furthermore, neutral red reduced the number of latent virus reactivations and prolonged the average lag period before reactivations occurred. Proflavine did not have these affects.

ACKNOWLEDGMENTS

This study was supported in part by Public Health Service research training grant 5T 01 GM 0 1097 from the National Institute of General Medical Sciences and by grant 5 S01 RR05407 from the Division of Research Resources.

LITERATURE CITED

1. **Chang, T. W., and L. Weinstein.** 1975. Photodynamic inactivation of Herpesvirus hominis by methylene blue. Proc. Soc. Exp. Biol. Med. 148:291–293.
2. **Felber, T. D., E. B. Smith, J. M. Knox, C. Wallis, and J. L. Melnick.** 1973. Photodynamic inactivation of herpes simplex. Report of a clinical trial. J. Am. Med. Assoc. 223:289–292.

3. **Freifelder, D., and R. B. Uretz.** 1966. Mechanism of photoinactivation of coliphage T7 sensitized by acridine orange. Virology **30**:97–103.
4. **Friedrich, E. G.** 1973. Relief for herpes vulvitis. Obstet. Gynecol. **41**:74–77.
5. **Kaufman, R. H., H. L. Gardner, D. Brown, C. Wallis, W. E. Rawls, and J. L. Melnick.** 1973. Herpes genitalis treated by photodynamic inactivation of virus. Am. J. Obstet. Gynecol. **117**:1144–1146.
6. **Kelleher, J. J., J. Varani, and W. W. Nelson.** 1975. Establishment of a nonproductive herpes simplex virus infection in rabbit kidney cells. Infect. Immun. **12**:128–133.
7. **Lanier, J. D., J. P. Whitcher, C. R. Dawson, and J. O. Oh.** Proflavine and light in the treatment of experimental herpetic ocular infections. Antimicrob. Agents Chemother. **6**:613–619.
8. **Lefebvre, E. B., and E. E. McNellis.** 1973. Photoinactivation of herpes simplex. J. Am. Med. Assoc. **224**:1039.
9. **Moore, C., C. Wallis, J. L. Melnick, and M. D. Kuns.** 1972. Photodynamic treatment of herpes keratitis. Infect. Immun. **5**:169–171.
10. **Myers, M. G., M. N. Oxman, J. E. Clark, and K. A. Arndt.** 1975. Failure of neutral-red photodynamic inactivation in recurrent herpes simplex virus infections. N. Engl. J. Med. **293**:945–949.
11. **Rapp, F., J. H. Li, and M. Jerkofsky.** 1973. Transformation of mammalian cells by DNA-containing viruses following photodynamic inactivation. Virology **55**:339–346.
12. **Sastry, K. S., and M. P. Gordon.** 1966. The photodynamic inactivation of tobacco mosaic virus and its ribonucleic acid by acridine orange. Biochim. Biophys. Acta **129**:32–41.
13. **Sastry, K. S., and M. P. Gordon.** 1966. The photosensitized degradation of guanosine by acridine orange. Biochim. Biophys. Acta **129**:42–48.
14. **Simon, M. I., and H. V. Vunakis.** 1964. The dye-sensitized photooxidation of purine and pyrimidine derivatives. Arch. Biochem. Biophys. **105**:197–206.
15. **Varani, J., and J. J. Kelleher.** 1975. Effects of 5-bromodeoxyuridine and 5-iododeoxyuridine on a latent herpes simplex virus infection. Antimicrob. Agents Chemother. **8**:18–21.
16. **Varnell, E. D., and H. E. Kaufman.** 1973. Photodynamic inactivation with proflavine: quantitative comparison with iodo-deoxyuridine. Infect. Immun. **7**:518–519.
17. **Wallis, C., and J. L. Melnick.** 1965. Photodynamic inactivation of animal viruses: a review. Photochem. Photobiol. **4**:159–170.
18. **Waskell, L. A., K. S. Sastry, and M. P. Gordon.** 1966. Studies on the photosensitized breakdown of guanosine by methylene blue. Biochim. Biophys. Acta **129**:49–53.

ANTIMICROBIAL AGENTS AND CHEMOTHERAPY, Aug. 1976, p. 234-240
Vol. 10, No. 2

Printed in U.S.A.

Hydroxyquinolines Inhibit Ribonucleic Acid-Dependent Deoxyribonucleic Acid Polymerase and Inactivate Rous Sarcoma Virus and Herpes Simplex Virus

WOLFGANG ROHDE,[1] PETER MIKELENS, JEAN JACKSON, JANE BLACKMAN, JACK WHITCHER, AND WARREN LEVINSON*

Department of Microbiology and Proctor Foundation for Research in Ophthalmology, University of California, San Francisco, California 94143

Received for publication 12 March 1976

8-Hydroxyquinoline and several of its derivatives inactivate the transforming ability of Rous sarcoma virus and inhibit its ribonucleic acid-dependent deoxyribonucleic acid polymerase activity. The copper complex of these metal-binding ligands is as active as the free ligand. The activity of the 8-hydroxyquinolines is approximately 50-fold more effective than another group of metal-binding compounds that we have tested, the thiosemicarbazones. In contrast to the potency of the 8-hydroxyquinolines to inactivate Rous sarcoma virus, no intracellular inhibition of transformation could be demonstrated at a concentration that did not affect the growth and appearance of the cells. Cellular deoxyribonucleic acid synthesis was inhibited to a greater extent than was ribonucleic acid or protein synthesis. The phenomenon of "concentration quenching" was observed with high concentrations of drug, causing less inhibition of deoxyribonucleic acid synthesis than was observed with lower concentrations. Herpes simplex virus type 1 was inactivated also by the 8-hydroxyquinolines and their copper complexes. No intracellular inhibition of plaque formation was observed. Treatment with 8-hydroxyquinoline sulfate had no effect on the resolution of herpetic keratitis in rabbits. Some 8-hydroxyquinolines bind to deoxyribonucleic acid in the presence of copper, a phenomenon that may be important in their antiviral activity.

N-methyl isatin β-thiosemicarbazone (M-IBT) (Methisazone) inhibits the ribonucleic acid (RNA)-dependent deoxyribonucleic acid (DNA) polymerase of Rous sarcoma virus (RSV) and inactivates its malignant transforming ability (15). Copper is involved in the action of this drug since ethylenediaminetetraacetic acid prevents the antiviral effect (15), copper synergizes it (15), and a preformed, purified M-IBT-copper chelate complex is equally effective as is the free ligand (W. Kaska and W. Levinson, unpublished data). In addition, M-IBT-copper complexes, but not M-IBT alone, inhibit transfection by purified lambda phage DNA in *Escherichia coli* (16). Also, we have shown that the copper chelating agent orthophenanthroline inhibits the RNA-dependent DNA polymerase of RSV (21).

In view of this activity, we wished to determine whether other copper-binding ligands act in a similar manner. For this purpose we chose to investigate 8-hydroxyquinoline (8-HQ) and some of its derivates. 8-HQ is the only one of seven isomeric monohydroxyquinolines that has antibacterial activity and the only one that forms chelate complexes with divalent metal ions (4). The inhibitory activity of 5×10^{-6} M 8-HQ against *Staphylococcus aureus* was markedly enhanced by the presence of 4×10^{-5} M copper sulfate (20). Other cations were much less effective. 8-HQ possesses inhibitory activity in eukaryotic cells also since it inhibits RNA synthesis in yeast (9) and the copper (II) bischelate of the halogenated 5,7-derivative has antifungal activity (10). Recently, it was shown that 8-HQ inhibits the RNA-dependent DNA polymerase of avian myeloblastosis virus (6).

In this report, we show that 8-HQ and several of its derivatives inactivate the transforming ability of RSV and inhibit its RNA-dependent DNA polymerase. The nucleic acid of the virion may be the site of action since, in the presence of copper, these drugs bind to DNA. 8-HQ, its 5-chloro-7-iodo-derivative (Entervioform), and their copper complexes inactivate the infectivity of herpes simplex virus (HSV) type 1. Chicken embryo cell DNA synthesis is in-

[1] Present address: Institut fur Virologie, Justus Liebig Universitaet, D-6300 Giessen, German Federal Republic.

hibited to a greater extent by 5-chloro-8-iodo-8-HQ than is RNA and protein synthesis.

MATERIALS AND METHODS

Virus and cells. The B-77 strain (group C) of RSV was propagated in chicken embryo cells as described in reference 7, and its transforming ability was assayed by focus formation as described in reference 17. The HSV type I was propagated and assayed in Vero cells (14).

RNA-dependent DNA polymerase assay. The enzyme assay used to evaluate these drugs has been described (15). Some experiments used the non-metal-chelating HEPES (*N*-2-hydroxyethylpiperazine-*N*′-2-ethanesulfonic acid) buffer rather than tris(hydroxymethyl)aminomethane (Tris) buffer, which chelates copper (11). No significant difference between the results using the two buffers was seen.

Nucleic acid-binding assay. The nucleic acid-binding assay has been described (18a).

Chemicals. The sources of the chemicals used in this study were: 5-chloro-7-iodo-8-HQ, 5,7-diiodo-8-HQ, 5,7-dichloro-8-HQ, 5-chloro-8-HQ, quinolines, and M-IBT from K and K Laboratories; 8-HQ-copper, 5-nitro-8-HQ, 7-iodo-5-sulfonic acid-8-HQ, 5-sulfonic acid-8-HQ, 8-mercaptoquinoline, 8-aminoquinoline, and 8-HQ sulfate salt from Sigma Chemical Co.; 8-HQ from Matheson, Coleman and Bell; 8-hydroxyquinaldine from Aldrich; 8-nitroquinoline from Eastman Kodak; and 5-chloro-7-iodo-8-HQ-copper and M-IBT-copper from W. Kaska, Univ. of California-Santa Barbara.

RESULTS

Inhibition of RNA-dependent DNA polymerase of RSV. The inhibitory activity of 8-HQ and its copper complex is depicted in Fig. 1. It can be seen that the inhibitory dose$_{50}$ (ID$_{50}$) for both compounds is 2×10^{-7} M, that little if any inhibition occurs at 5×10^{-8} M, and that greater than 90% inhibition occurs with the copper salt at 5×10^{-7} M. The inhibitory activity of M-IBT, our standard reference compound, and its copper complex is shown in Fig. 2. The ID$_{50}$ for M-IBT is 1.5×10^{-5} M and that for the copper complex is 7×10^{-6} M. The inhibition by the hydroxyquinoline compounds is approximately 50-fold more effective than that by the thiosemicarbazones.

The kinetics of inactivation of enzyme activity by 10^{-5} M 8-HQ is illustrated in Fig. 3. Fifty percent inhibition occurs at approximately 9 min, and 90% occurs at 40 min.

The data in Table 1 describe the inhibitory activity of 8-HQ and several of its derivatives in the presence and absence of equimolar copper sulfate. The 5-nitro- and 5-chloro-substituted compounds are the most active. They are approximately four times better than is the parent compound. The 5-chloro-7-iodo, 5,7-dichloro, and 5,7-diiodo are approximately as active as the parent 8-HQ. The 5-sulfonic acid and the 2-methyl-derivatives are much less active. 8-

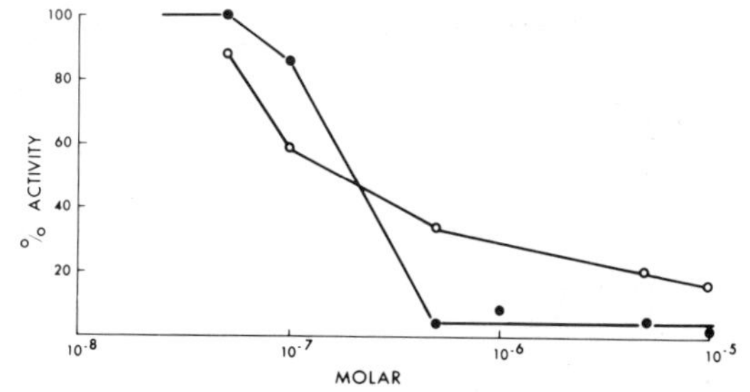

FIG. 1. *Inhibition of RNA-dependent DNA polymerase by 8-HQ and its copper complex. A total of 5 μl of purified B-77 strain of RSV, suspended in 200 μl of solution A (see below), was exposed to the drug by the addition of 2 μl of solution and incubated at 37°C for 15 min. A total of 20 μl of solution B (see below) was added, and the reaction mixture was incubated at 37°C for 60 min. Acid-precipitable counts were obtained by the addition of 0.5 ml of 0.01 M sodium pyrophosphate and 2 ml of 3.5% perchloric acid in 0.01 M sodium pyrophosphate. The precipitate was filtered onto glass fiber filters, dried, and counted in a liquid scintillation spectrometer. Solution A contained 10 mM phosphate buffer, pH 7.4, 150 mM NaCl, 10 mM $MgCl_2$, and 25 μM deoxyadenosine 5′-triphosphate, deoxyguanosine 5′-triphosphate, and deoxycytidine 5′-triphosphate. Solution B contained 90 μl of [^{3}H]thymidine 5′-triphosphate (17 Ci/mmol), 45 μl of 1% Nonidet P-40 and 5 μl of 2-mercaptoethanol. The final concentrations of these reagents in the reaction mixture were 7.5 μCi/ml, 0.03%, and 0.3%, respectively. Stock solutions of drugs in 100% Me_2SO were used. No inhibition of enzyme activity was observed with 1% Me_2SO. Symbols: ○, 8-HQ; ●, 8-HQ-copper complex.*

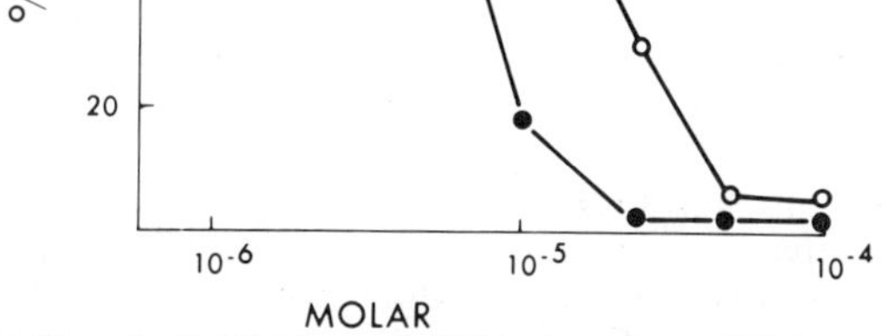

FIG. 2. *Inhibition of RNA-dependent DNA polymerase by M-IBT and its copper complex. The enzyme assay was performed in the same manner as described in the legend to Fig. 1. Symbols: ○, M-IBT; ●, M-IBT-copper complex.*

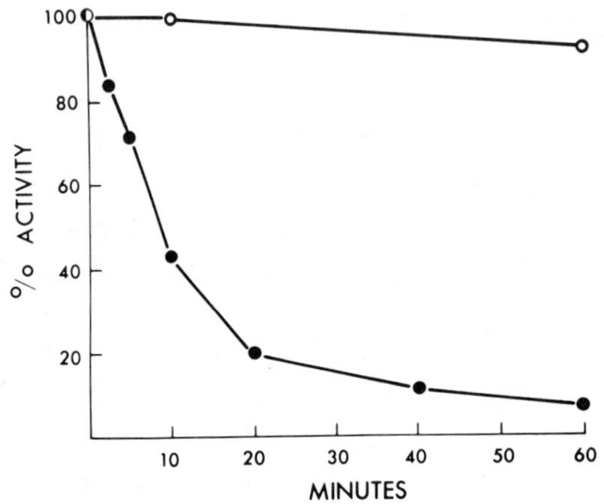

FIG. 3. *Kinetics of inhibition of enzyme activity by 8-HQ. The enzyme assay was performed in the same manner as described in the legend to Fig. 1, except that the samples were taken at 10-min intervals after the addition of the drug. Symbols: ○, 1% Me_2SO; ●, 10^{-5} M 8-HQ.*

TABLE 1. *Effect of quinoline derivatives on RNA-dependent DNA polymerase of RSV*[a]

Compound	ID_{50} (M)	
	No addition	+ $CuSO_4$ (1:1)
8-HQ	2×10^{-7}	2×10^{-7}
5-NO_2-8-HQ	5×10^{-8}	3×10^{-8}
5-Chloro-8-HQ	5×10^{-8}	6×10^{-8}
5-Chloro-7-iodo-8-HQ	2×10^{-7}	1×10^{-7}
5,7-Dichloro-8-HQ	9×10^{-8}	2×10^{-7}
5,7-Diiodo-8-HQ	9×10^{-8}	1×10^{-7}
2-CH_3-8-HQ	9×10^{-7}	4×10^{-7}
5-SO_3H-8-HQ	6×10^{-6}	5×10^{-6}
5-SO_3H-7-iodo-8-HQ	9×10^{-6}	2×10^{-6}
8-SH-quinoline	1×10^{-6}	2×10^{-7}
8-NH_2-quinoline	3×10^{-6}	9×10^{-7}
8-NO_2-quinoline	No[b]	No
Quinoline	No	No
M-IBT	1.5×10^{-5}	7×10^{-6}
$CuSO_4$	7×10^{-6}	

[a] The enzyme assay was performed in the same manner as described in the legend to Fig. 1.
[b] No, No ID_{50} below 100 μM.

HQ is significantly more active than the 8-sulfhydryl- and 8-amino-derivatives. The 8-nitro-derivative and quinoline itself have no activity at the highest concentration tested. The addition of copper sulfate to the reaction did not have an appreciable effect on the inhibition of enzyme activity, except in the case of the 8-mercapto-derivative, which was enhanced five-fold. Preformed, purified copper complexes of 8-HQ and its 5-chloro-7-iodo-derivative are as active as the free ligands alone (data not shown).

An experiment was performed to determine the rapidity with which 8-HQ inhibited an enzyme reaction that had already started. The data in Fig. 4 indicate that, when the 8-HQ-copper complex is added 10 min after synthesis has begun, incorporation of [^{3}H]thymidine 5′-triphosphate is inhibited gradually. In contrast, the addition of the M-IBT-copper complex causes a prompt inhibition of [^{3}H]thymidine 5′-triphosphate incorporation. The addition of 10% Me_2SO as a solvent control inhibited incorporation in a gradual but significant manner. It appears that the M-IBT-copper complex acts rapidly to inhibit elongation of the DNA, whereas the 8-HQ-copper complex does not.

Inactivation of RSV-transforming ability. Several of the active compounds were evaluated for their ability to inactivate the transforming ability of RSV. The data in Table 2 demonstrate that these compounds are also effective inactivators of transformation by RSV. Both the free ligands and the copper complexes inactivated transforming ability by 99% at 4×10^{-8} M, and the copper complexes possessed 50% activity at 4×10^{-9} M. The hydroxyquinolines are vastly more active than is M-IBT. A comparison of this data with that in Table 1

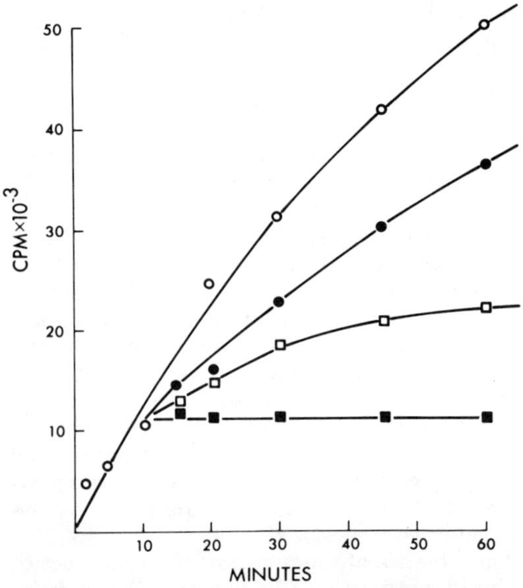

FIG. 4. *Kinetics of inhibition of enzyme activity after synthesis for 10 min. The enzyme assay was performed in the same manner as described in the legend to Fig. 1, except that HEPES buffer was used instead of Tris buffer, the drug was not added until 10 min after solution B was added, and samples were taken at 10-min intervals. Symbols: ○, none; ●, 10% Me_2SO; □, 8-HQ-copper complex; ■, M-IBT-copper complex.*

TABLE 2. *Inactivation of RSV transformation by hydroxyquinolines*[a]

Compound	M	Inhibition (%)
8-OH-quinoline	4×10^{-8}	99
8-OH-quinoline-copper	4×10^{-8}	99
8-OH-quinoline-copper	4×10^{-9}	50
5-Chloro-7-iodo-8-OH-quinoline	4×10^{-8}	99
5-Chloro-7-iodo-8-OH-quinoline-copper	4×10^{-8}	99
5-Chloro-7-iodo-8-OH-quinoline-copper	4×10^{-9}	50
M-IBT	4×10^{-5}	99
M-IBT	4×10^{-6}	50
$CuSO_4$	2×10^{-6}	50

[a] The virus was exposed to the drug in the same manner as described in the legend to Fig. 1 and incubated at 37°C for 15 min, at which time a 5-μl portion was taken and a 1:100 dilution was assayed for focus formation as described previously (17).

indicates that focus formation is significantly more sensitive to these drugs than is polymerase activity.

Inhibition of transformation by RSV. In view of the ability of the 5-chloro-7-iodo-derivative to inactivate transformation, we determined whether it could inhibit focus formation when the cells were exposed to the drugs after the 30-min adsorption and penetration period of viral infection. The drugs were included in the agar-growth medium overlay for the entire 6-day assay period. Variable results were obtained. A 50 and 75% inhibition were observed at 2 and 4 μM, respectively, in some experiments but not in others. Cell growth was visibly decreased at 8 μM.

Inhibition of cellular DNA, RNA, and protein synthesis by 5-chloro-7-iodo-HQ. In view of the finding that cell growth was visibly affected by 5-chloro-7-iodo-HQ at 8 μM, experiments were performed to determine whether DNA, RNA, or protein synthesis was inhibited in chicken embryo cells. The data expressed in Fig. 5 indicate that, after 1 h of exposure to the drug at 20 μM, DNA synthesis is inhibited 97%, RNA synthesis is inhibited 91%, and protein synthesis is inhibited 83%. At all drug concentrations tested, DNA synthesis was inhibited to the greatest extent. The effect of the drug at higher concentrations (40 and 80 μM) is aberrant since these amounts inhibit less well than does 20 μM. This relative loss of activity at higher concentrations is similar to the effect of this compound on the RNA-dependent DNA polymerase; viz., at 4×10^{-7} and 1×10^{-6} M the enzyme is 95% inhibited, but at 4×10^{-6} M virtually no inhibition was obtained. This unusual effect has been observed in other systems, and a possible explanation is described below.

Inactivation of HSV. The inactivation of RSV, an RNA tumor virus, prompted us to attempt to extend the antiviral spectrum to other classes of viruses. Table 3 shows that HSV type I is significantly inactivated by 8-HQ, the 5-chloro-7-iodo-derivative, and their preformed copper complexes. Using the compounds listed in Table 3, no inhibition of plaque formation was seen at any drug concentration (between 4 and 8 μM) that did not visibly alter cell growth (data not shown).

In view of the marked inactivation of herpes simplex infectivity by 8-HQs, we tested the ability of the water-soluble salt 8-HQ sulfate to ameliorate the course of herpes keratitis in rab-

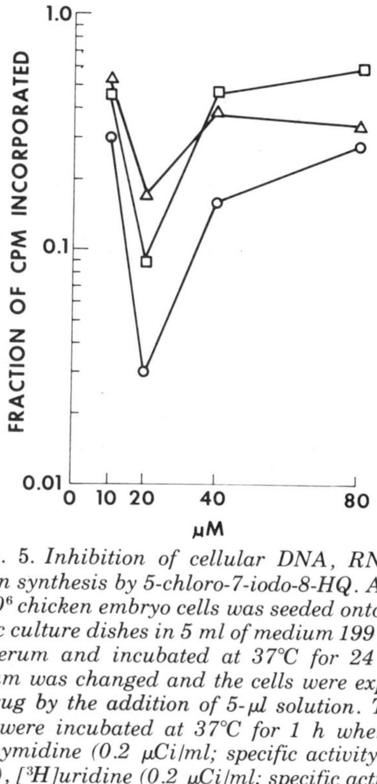

FIG. 5. *Inhibition of cellular DNA, RNA, and protein synthesis by 5-chloro-7-iodo-8-HQ. A total of 1×10^6 chicken embryo cells was seeded onto 50-mm plastic culture dishes in 5 ml of medium 199 plus 4% calf serum and incubated at 37°C for 24 h. The medium was changed and the cells were exposed to the drug by the addition of 5-µl solution. The cultures were incubated at 37°C for 1 h when either [³H]thymidine (0.2 µCi/ml; specific activity, 13 Ci/mmol), [³H]uridine (0.2 µCi/ml; specific activity, 23 Ci/mmol), or [³H]reconstituted protein hydrolysate (4 µCi/ml) was added. The cultures were incubated for a further 30 min at 37°C when the medium was discarded, and the cells were washed with Tris-buffered saline and solubilized with 1 ml of 1% sodium dodecyl sulfate in Tris-buffered saline with 10^{-3} M ethylenediaminetetraacetic acid. The acid-precipitable radioactivity was determined by adding 5 ml of 10% trichloroacetic acid at 4°C, filtering onto glass fiber filters, and counting in a liquid scintillation spectrometer. Symbols: ○, DNA; □, RNA; △, protein.*

TABLE 3. *Inactivation of HSV*[a]

Compound	M	Inhibition (%)
8-HQ	4×10^{-7}	75
8-HQ-copper	4×10^{-7}	80
5-Chloro-7-iodo-8-HQ	4×10^{-8}	90
5-Chloro-7-iodo-8-HQ-copper	4×10^{-8}	95

[a] A 1-μl amount of a solution of the compounds was added to 1 ml of a 1:200 dilution of HSV type 1 in phosphate-buffered saline. After incubation at 37°C for 15 min, a 1:100 dilution of the virus in medium 199 + 15% calf serum was made, and a 0.2-ml portion was assayed for plaque-forming ability.

bits (14). The infection was initiated by instilling 2 drops of a HSV type I (PH strain) suspension (titer, 2×10^7 plaque-forming units/ml) in both eyes of New Zealand white rabbits. After 72 h, when corneal lesions were visible by slit-lamp examination, the treatment of one eye of each rabbit with 0.1% (wt/vol) 8-HQ sulfate in 50% polyethylene glycol 4000 (2 drops every 2 h for 14 h) was begun and continued for 5 days. The control eye of each animal was treated with the suspending vehicle alone. The course of the disease was followed by daily slit-lamp examinations and by HSV infectivity assays three times a week. No effect of the drug on the course of the disease or on the amount of herpesvirus produced was observed.

Binding of hydroxyquinolines to DNA. We have demonstrated that M-IBT-copper complexes bind to DNA and RNA and have postulated that their antiviral effect may be due to their ability to bind to nucleic acid (18a). We have, therefore, determined whether the 8-HQs bind to DNA. The data in Table 4 indicate that 5-chloro-7-iodo-8-HQ (40 μM) in the presence of $CuSO_4$ (10 μM) is approximately as good as an M-IBT-copper complex in its ability to bind DNA. The 5-chloro-7-iodo-HQ (40 μM) without added copper complex is significantly less active. The preformed complex of 5-chloro-7-iodo-8-HQ and copper is markedly more active than both the free ligand and the ligand to which exogenous $CuSO_4$ is added. This may be a function of the complex being in the correct ratio of ligand to metal (either 1:1 or 2:1) for DNA binding. 8-HQ, with or without added copper, possesses much less DNA-binding ability than its 5-chloro-7-iodo-derivative. The 8-HQ-copper complex is as active as 8-HQ to which exogenous copper is added.

DISCUSSION

The results presented in this paper extend the spectrum of metal-binding ligands that inhibit RNA-dependent DNA polymerase and inactivate the transforming ability of RSV to include 8-HQ, several of its derivatives, 8-mercaptoquinoline, and 8-aminoquinoline. Other metal-binding ligands, which have the same activities, are M-IBT and other isatin β-thiosemicarbazones (15), ortho-phenanthroline (21), and isonicotinic acid hydrazide, which is the drug of choice for tuberculosis (W. Levinson, manuscript submitted for publication).

8-HQ is known to chelate copper (4), and the ability of the drug to inhibit *S. aureus* is enhanced by copper (20). However, no enhancement of the activity of 8-HQ to inhibit the RNA-dependent DNA polymerase was seen when equimolar copper was added. This could be due to the presence of sufficient copper or other first transition series metal either in the solutions or in the virion itself to form an active chelate complex. The finding of copper in the vaccinia virion lends support to the conjecture that the metal may be in the virus particle (13).

A study has been made of 8-HQ derivatives that chelate metals using a precipitation assay (5). Of the derivatives tested in Table 1 of this report, it was found that 8-HQ, its 5-NO_2, 5-chloro-5,7-dichloro-, 5-chloro-7-iodo-, and 2-CH_3-derivatives, and 8-mercaptoquinoline formed precipitates with copper and other metals. All of these strongly inhibit the RNA-dependent DNA polymerase. The two 5-sulfonic

TABLE 4. *Binding of hydroxyquinolines to DNA*[a]

Compound	μM	$CuSO_4$ (μM)	cpm bound (%)
None		0	3
M-IBT	50	10	100
5-Chloro-7-iodo-HQ	10	10	11
5-Chloro-7-iodo-HQ	20	10	63
5-Chloro-7-iodo-HQ	40	10	92
5-Chloro-7-iodo-HQ	40	0	29
5-Chloro-7-iodo-HQ-copper	0.6	0	8
5-Chloro-7-iodo-HQ-copper	1.2	0	52
5-Chloro-7-iodo-HQ-copper	2.4	0	79
8-HQ	200	0	1
8-HQ	100	50	10
8-HQ	200	500	30
8-HQ-copper	200	0	30

[a] Reactions contained ^{3}H-labeled HeLa cell DNA (275 ng) in 0.5 ml of 0.05 M phosphate buffer, pH 8.0. Appropriate volumes of drug solutions in 100% Me_2SO were then added. After incubation at 4°C for 5 min, the solutions were filtered through 0.45-μM membrane filters (Millipore), dried, and counted in a Beckman liquid scintillation spectrometer. No filter retention was seen with 10 μl of Me_2SO, the largest volume added.

acid derivatives were found to cause a color change (but no precipitate) only with ferrous and ferric ions; these compounds inhibit enzyme activity but are not as active as those that form definite precipitates. The 8-NH_2-quinoline does not cause a color change or precipitate with any metal, yet it is an enzyme inhibitor. The reason for this discrepancy is not clear. Quinoline itself does not change color or precipitate and does not inhibit the enzyme. The 5,7-diiodo-derivative was not tested in the precipitation assay.

Our initial interpretation of the correlation between the inactivation of RSV-transforming ability and the inhibition of its RNA-dependent DNA polymerase was one of cause and effect. However, since transforming ability is significantly more sensitive than is enzyme activity, we speculate that there may be an additional inactivating event of an unknown nature occurring.

The failure of these compounds to inhibit transformation of chicken cells after infection by RSV can be attributed to their lack of selective toxicity; e.g., the drugs significantly inhibit cellular processes as well. Another possibility is that virus-specific DNA synthesis is completed since the drug is added to the culture after the adsorption period. This explanation is unlikely since we have found recently that several thiosemicarbazone derivatives do inhibit transformation by RSV when added after the adsorption period.

The data in Table 4 demonstrate that the copper complexes of 8-HQ and its 5-chloro-7-iodo-derivative bind to DNA, significantly more so than do the free ligands. The binding of the drug to nucleic acid could be important in the inhibition of the RNA-dependent DNA polymerase, but the lack of correlation of the extent of binding to the activity of the compounds calls this supposition into question. For example, the ID_{50} of 8-HQ and 5-chloro-7-iodo-HQ are the same (Table 2), yet their ability to retain DNA on the filter is markedly different (Table 4).

A second puzzling aspect of the DNA-binding data is the markedly enhanced ability of the preformed copper complex of 5-chloro-7-iodo-8-HQ compared with the free ligand to which equimolar copper was added. This raises the question of the relationship between the stoichiometry of the copper complex and its antiviral activity. It has been shown previously (3, 8) that the 2:1 and 1:1 ligand-metal complexes have different biological and chemical effects. It is possible, therefore, that the preformed complex has a different ratio from that formed in the binding assay by mixing equimolar ligand and copper. In addition, these reports indicate that only the 1:1 complex possesses antibacterial and antifungal activity. These findings may explain the results shown in Fig. 5; e.g., as the concentration of ligand is increased, the inactive 2:1 complex is formed in greater amounts, which results in the observed loss of activity. This phenomenon has been given the term "concentration quenching" (2).

In addition to the possibility that these drugs act by binding to the viral nucleic acid, an alternative explanation for the ability of these drugs to inhibit the RNA-dependent DNA polymerase is that the drug binds to the enzyme. Since zinc is known to be present in the enzyme, it has been proposed that metal-binding ligands inhibit by binding to this atom (6, 21). The results presented in this report cause us to question this interpretation. Since we have shown that the preformed copper complex is equally as effective as the free ligand and it has been reported previously that the stability constant for the copper complex is 10^3- to 10^4-fold greater than for the zinc complex (1), it seems unlikely that the ligand in the copper complex form can bind to the zinc in the enzyme.

Lastly, it is interesting to note two recent findings regarding compounds similar to those described here. First, 4-nitroquinoline-1-oxide is a chemical carcinogen that is known to cause covalent bond breakage in DNA, increased integration of simian virus 40 DNA into cellular DNA, and increased transformation of CHO cells by simian virus 40 (12). Second, 5,8-dioxo-6-amino-7-chloroquinoline inhibits protein synthesis in *E. coli* apparently by preventing the charging of transfer RNA (19). In both cases an interaction of the drugs with nucleic acids either is or may be important in the mode of action.

LITERATURE CITED

1. **Albert, A.** 1953. Quantitative studies of the avidity of naturally occurring substances for trace metals. Biochem. J. **54**:646–654.
2. **Albert, A.** 1973. Selectivity toxicity, p. 371. Chapman and Hall, London.
3. **Albert, A., M. Gibson, and S. Rubbo.** 1953. The influence of chemical constitution on anti-bacterial activity. 6. The bactericidal action of 8-hydroxyquinoline (oxine). Br. J. Exp. Pathol. 34:119–130.
4. **Albert, A., and W. Gledhill.** 1947. The choice of a chelating agent for inactivating trace metals. Biochem. J. **41**:529–533.
5. **Albert, A., and D. Magrath.** 1947. The choice of a chelating agent for inactivating trace metals. Biochem. J. **41**:534–545.
6. **Auld, D., H. Kawaguchi, D. Livingston, and B. Vallee.** 1974. RNA dependent DNA polymerase from avian myeloblastosis virus: a zinc metalloenzyme. Proc. Natl. Acad. Sci. U.S.A. **71**:2091–2095.

7. **Bishop, J. M., W. Levinson, N. Quintrell, D. Sullivan, L. Fanshier, and J. Jackson.** 1970. The low molecular weight RNA's of Rous sarcoma virus. Virology **42**:182–195.
8. **Block, S.** 1956. Reversal of fungitoxicity of copper-8-quinolinate. J. Agric. Food Chem. **4**:1042–1046.
9. **Fraser, R., and J. Creanor.** 1974. Rapid and selective inhibition of RNA synthesis in yeast by 8-hydroxyquinoline. Eur. J. Biochem. **46**:67–73.
10. **Gershon, H.** 1974. Anti-fungal activity of bischelates of 5,7-, and 5,7, halogenated 8-quinolinols with copper (II). J. Med. Chem. **17**:824–827.
11. **Hanlon, D., D. Watt, and E. Westhead.** 1966. The interaction of divalent metal ions with Tris buffer in dilute solution. Anal. Biochem. **16**:225–233.
12. **Hirai, K., V. Defendi, and L. Diamond.** 1974. Enhancement of SV40 transformation and integration by 4-nitroquinoline 1-oxide. Cancer Res. **34**:3497.
13. **Joklik, W.** 1962. The purification of four strains of pox virus. Virology **18**:9–18.
14. **Levinson, W., V. Coleman, B. Woodson, A. Rabson, J. Lanier, J. Witcher, and C. Dawson.** 1974. Inactivation of herpes simplex virus by thiosemicarbazones and certain cations. Antimicrob. Agents Chemother. **5**:398–402.
15. **Levinson, W., A. Faras, B. Woodson, J. Jackson, and J. M. Bishop.** 1973. Inhibition of RNA dependent DNA polymerase of Rous sarcoma virus by thiosemicarbazones and several cations. Proc. Natl. Acad. Sci. U.S.A. **70**:164–168.
16. **Levinson, W., and R. Helling.** 1976. Inactivation of lambda phage infectivity and lambda deoxyribonucleic acid transfection by *N*-methyl-isatin β-thiosemicarbazone-copper complexes. Antimicrob. Agents. Chemother. **9**:160–163.
17. **Levinson, W., and H. Rubin.** 1966. Radiation studies of avian tumor viruses and Newcastle disease virus. Virology **28**:533–542.
18. **McNew, G., and H. Gershon.** 1971. The fungitoxic mechanisms of quinoline compounds and their chelates in inhibition and destruction of microbial cell, p. 107–120. *In* W. Hugo (ed.), Inhibition and destruction of antimicrobial cells. Academic Press Inc., New York.
18a. **Mikelens, P., B. Woodson, and W. Levinson.** 1976. Association of nucleic acids with complexes of N-methyl isatin beta thiosemicarbazone and copper. Biochem. Pharmacol. **25**:821–827.
19. **Ogilvie, A., K. Wiebauer, P. Spitlbarth, and W. Kersten.** 1975. Inhibition of leucyl t-RNA synthetase in *E. coli* by the cytostatic drug 5, 8 dioxo 6-amino 7-chloroquinoline. Biochim. Biophys. Acta **407**:357–364.
20. **Rubbo, S., A. Albert, and M. Gibson.** 1950. The influence of chemical constitution on anti-bacterial activity. 5. The anti-bacterial action of 8-hydroxyquinoline. Br. J. Exp. Pathol. **31**:425–441.
21. **Valenzuela, P., R. Morris, A. Faras, W. Levinson, and W. Rutter.** 1973. Are all nucleotidyl transferases metalloenzymes? Biochem. Biophys. Res. Commun. **53**:1036–1041.

ANTIMICROBIAL AGENTS AND CHEMOTHERAPY, Aug. 1976, p. 241-244 Vol. 10, No. 2

Comparative Activity In Vitro of Ticarcillin, BL-P1654, and Carbenicillin

THEODORE C. EICKHOFF* AND JOSEPHINE M. EHRET

Division of Infectious Disease, Department of Medicine, University of Colorado Medical Center, Denver, Colorado 80220

Received for publication 16 March 1976

The activity of ticarcillin, BL-P1654, and carbenicillin was compared in vitro using a microtiter tube dilution test in Mueller-Hinton broth against 50 recent clinical isolates each of *Staphylococcus aureus*, *Staphylococcus epidermidis*, *Escherichia coli*, *Klebsiella* species, *Enterobacter* species, *Proteus* species, and *Pseudomonas aeruginosa*. Bactericidal end points were determined using a modified Steers replicator. Ticarcillin was generally two to four times more active against all organisms tested except *S. epidermidis* against which BL-P1654 was most active. Median minimum inhibitory concentrations in micrograms per milliliter were for *S. aureus*: ticarcillin (6.2), carbenicillin (12.5), BL-P1654 (25); for *S. epidermidis*: BL-P1654 (1.6), ticarcillin (3.2), carbenicillin (3.2); for *E. coli*: ticarcillin (3.2), BL-P1654 (6.2), carbenicillin (6.2); for *Klebsiella* sp.: >100 for all three drugs; for *Enterobacter* sp.: ticarcillin (3.2), carbenicillin (6.2), BL-P1654 (12.5); for *Proteus* sp.: ticarcillin (1.6), carbenicillin (1.6), BL-P1654 (3.2); for *P. aeruginosa*: ticarcillin (31), BL-P1654 (62), carbenicillin (125). Bactericidal end points were dependent on both the drug and the species but were in general no more than twofold more than the minimum inhibitory concentration with the exception of BL-P1654 against *P. aeruginosa*. BL-P1654 was bactericidal for only 60% of the strains tested at a concentration of 500 μg/ml.

Carbenicillin has been found, in the years since its introduction, to be a remarkably useful drug in certain patients with infections caused by *Pseudomonas aeruginosa*, *Serratia marcescens*, and other selected susceptible pathogens. However, the emergence of carbenicillin-resistant strains and the risk of electrolyte and coagulation problems associated with high-dose therapy of sytemic infections have limited its clinical use.

BL-P1654 is the sodium salt of 3-guanylureido-phenyl-acetamino-penicillanic acid, with a spectrum similar to that of carbenicillin. BRL-2288, ticarcillin, is the disodium salt of α-carboxy-3-thienylmethyl penicillin, also with a spectrum similar to that of carbenicillin. We compared the in vitro activity of these three drugs against a number of recent clinical isolates.

MATERIALS AND METHODS

Fifty isolates each of *Staphylococcus aureus*, *Staphylococcus epidermidis*, *Escherichia coli*, *Klebsiella* species, *Enterobacter* species, *Proteus* species, *Pseudomonas aeruginosa*, and 10 isolates of enterococci were studied. The organisms were isolated in the Clinical Microbiology Laboratory of Colorado General Hospital, University of Colorado Medical Center, having been recovered from specimens of blood, urine, sputum, and other infected sites submitted from patients and were identified by standard methods under the direction of L. Barth Reller. Minimum inhibitory concentrations were carried out using microtiter tube dilution tests in Mueller-Hinton broth, adding 0.05 ml of a 10^{-4} dilution of an overnight Mueller-Hinton broth culture of each organism to be tested to 0.05 ml of diluted antibiotic in a microtiter plate (Cooke Engineering Co.). The minimum inhibitory concentrations were read after 18 h of incubation at 37°C. Bactericidal end points were determined using a Steers replicator (13) with the head modified to possess 96 specifically spaced inoculating rods corresponding in position to the location of the reservoirs in a microtiter plate (Cooke Engineering Co.). This was used to deliver approximately 0.003 ml from each well onto Mueller-Hinton agar plates. Bactericidal end points (no growth) were read after 24 h of incubation at 35°C in ambient air. Tests of *P. aeruginosa* were carried out in Difco Mueller-Hinton broth corrected to contain 3.8 meq of calcium per liter and 2.6 meq of magnesium per liter. Tests of enterococci were carried out in Trypticase soy broth.

The effect of inoculum size on bacteriostatic and bactericidal end points was studied in 5 strains of *S. aureus*, 10 strains of enterococci, and 10 strains of *P. aeruginosa*, using 10^{-2} and 10^{-5} dilutions of overnight broth cultures.

Sodium BL-P1654, disodium carbenicillin, and disodium ticarcillin were supplied by Bristol Laboratories, J. B. Roerig Division of Chas. Pfizer & Co., Inc., and Beecham-Massengill Pharmaceuticals, respectively.

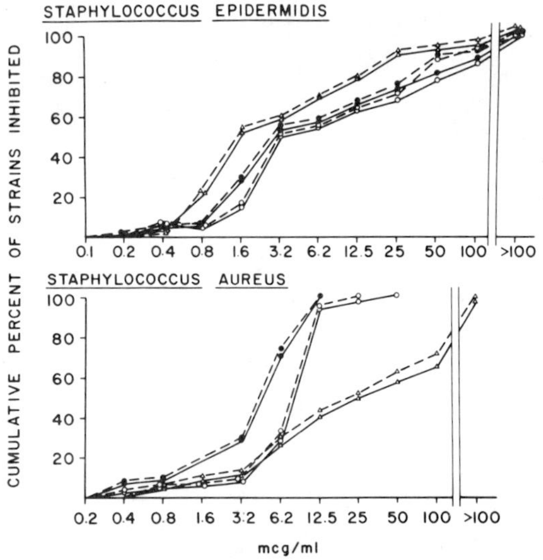

FIG. 1. *Susceptibility of S. epidermidis and S. aureus to carbenicillin, ticarcillin, and BL-P1654. Symbols: ---, minimum inhibitory concentration; –, minimal bactericidal concentration; ○, carbenicillin; ●, tricarcillin; △, BL-P1654.*

RESULTS

The activity of the three penicillins against staphylococci is shown in Fig. 1. Against 50 strains of *S. epidermidis*, BL-P1654 was the most active, being a little more than twice as active as the other two drugs. Bactericidal end points were virtually the same as bacteriostatic end points.

Against 50 strains of *S. aureus*, ticarcillin was most active, being about twice as active as carbenicillin. BL-P1654 was remarkably ineffective against staphylococci that were inhibited and killed by 6 to 12 μg of either ticarcillin or carbenicillin per ml. Again, the bactericidal and bacteriostatic end points were identical.

Figure 2 demonstrates that against the 50 strains of *E. coli* ticarcillin was the most active drug tested, by a factor of two- to fourfold. BL-P1654 and carbenicillin were essentially identical in their activity against *E. coli*.

Against 50 *Enterobacter* sp., ticarcillin was again the most active drug tested, but against the strains that required a concentration greater than 25 μg/ml for inhibition, there was little difference among the three drugs.

Against 50 strains of *Klebsiella* sp., none of the three drugs had any appreciable activity at concentrations as great as 100 μg/ml.

Of the 50 strains of *Proteus* sp., eight strains

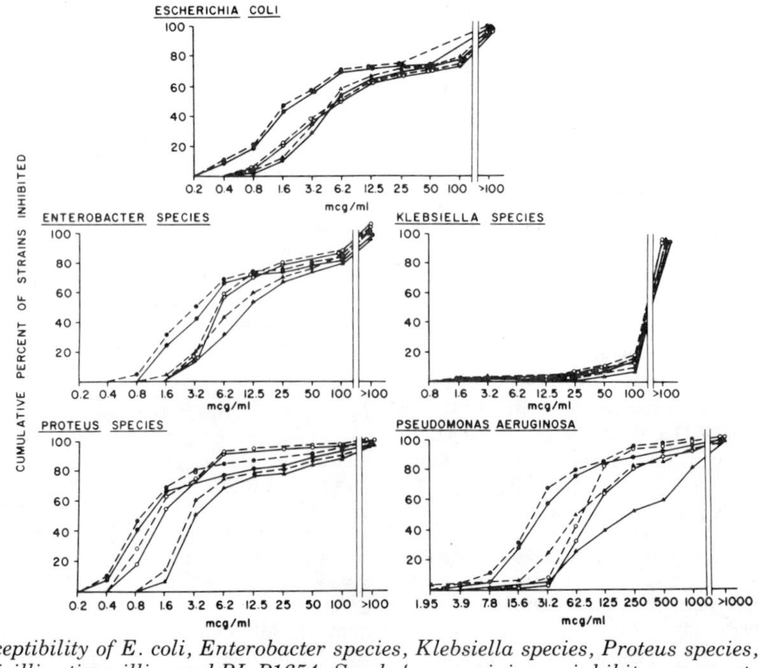

FIG. 2. *Susceptibility of E. coli, Enterobacter species, Klebsiella species, Proteus species, and P. aeruginosa to carbenicillin, ticarcillin, and BL-P1654. Symbols: ---, minimum inhibitory concentration; —, minimal bactericidal concentration; ○, carbenicillin; ●, ticarcillin; △, BL-P1654.*

were indole positive, the remainder were indole negative. No significant difference was found between the two groups. Ticarcillin was again the most active of the drugs tested, but never differed by more than one twofold dilution from carbenicillin (Fig. 2).

Against 50 strains of *P. aeruginosa* ticarcillin was almost fourfold as active as carbenicillin. It is of particular interest that there was little difference in the bacteriostatic and bactericidal end points for ticarcillin in contrast to the observations for BL-P1654. In fact, at a concentration of 500 μg/ml, BL-P1654 was bactericidal for only 60% of strains of *P. aeruginosa*.

The effect of inoculum size on bacteriostatic and bactericidal end points was variable. Against *S. aureus*, the effect was marked (Table 1). Against the 10 strains of enterococci the effect was variable (Fig. 3). In the case of carbenicillin, for example, a bacteriostatic effect was achieved even against a heavy inoculum at low concentrations, but concentrations of 16 to 125 μg/ml were required to kill enterococci with a light inoculum, and a heavy inoculum could not be killed by a concentration of 1,000 μg/ml. In the case of BL-P1654, a light inoculum was both inhibited and killed by low concentrations, but concentrations of 16 to 125 μg/ml were required to inhibit a heavy inoculum and much higher concentrations were needed to achieve a bactericidal effect. Similarly, with ticarcillin, concentrations of 8 to 62 μg/ml were required to inhibit and kill a light inoculum. The same concentrations were also inhibitory against a heavy inoculum. The heavy inoculum could not be killed, however, by a concentration of 1,000 μg/ml. With *P. aeruginosa* the effect of the inoculum size was quite marked, particularly with BL-P1654 (Fig. 4). Most of the strains showed at least a fourfold increase in the BL-P1654 minimum inhibitory concentrations with heavier inocula. A greater discrepancy between the minimum inhibitory concentration and minimum bactericidal concentration was also noted at the 10^{-2} dilution. None of the drugs tested effectively killed a heavy inoculum of *P. aeruginosa*, though all of them were effective in killing a light inoculum.

DISCUSSION

On the basis of these in vitro studies, we concluded, as have other investigators (1, 7, 14) that ticarcillin compares favorably with carbenicillin. We found ticarcillin to be two to four times more active than carbenicillin against all organisms tested except *S. epidermidis* and enterococci, suggesting that perhaps lower doses of ticarcillin, as compared with the usual doses of carbenicillin might be clinically effective.

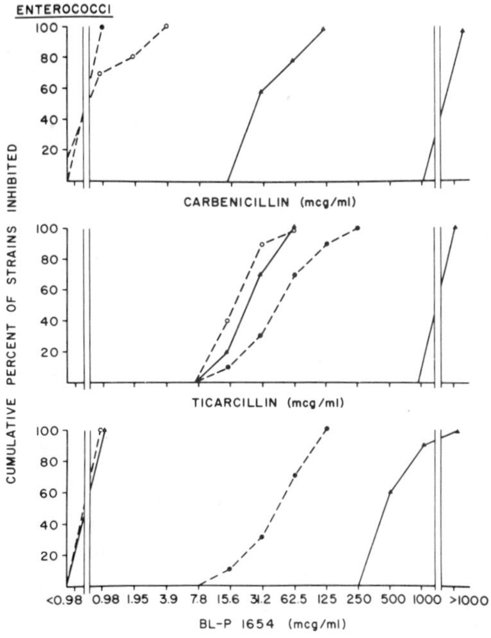

FIG. 3. *Effect of inoculum size on the susceptibility of enterococci when tested against carbenicillin, ticarcillin, and BL-P1654. Symbols: minimum inhibitory concentration at 10^{-2} (●) and 10^{-5} (○) dilutons; minimal bactericidal concentrations at 10^{-2} (▲) and 10^{-5} (△) dilutions.*

TABLE 1. *Inoculum effect on the susceptibility of penicillinase-producing staphylococci (S. aureus)[a]*

Strain	Ticarcillin (concn)				BL-P 1654 (concn)				Carbenicillin (concn)			
	10^{-2}		10^{-5}		10^{-2}		10^{-5}		10^{-2}		10^{-5}	
	MIC	MBC	MIC	MBC	MIC	MBC	MIC	MBC	MIC	MBC	MIC	MBC
1	0.9	7.8	0.9	0.9	0.9	0.9	0.9	0.9	0.9	0.9	0.9	0.9
2	3.9	62.5	0.9	0.9	0.9	15.6	0.9	0.9	0.9	250	0.9	0.9
3	62.5	62.5	3.9	3.9	250	500	1.8	3.9	62.5	62.5	31.2	31.2
4	31.2	31.2	15.6	15.6	1,000	1,000	7.8	7.8	31.2	31.2	7.8	7.8
5	15.6	500	0.9	1.8	1,000	>1,000	3.9	7.8	15.6	500	3.9	3.9

[a] Abbreviations: MIC, minimum inhibitory concentration (micrograms per milliliter); MBC, minimal bactericidal concentration (micrograms per milliliter).

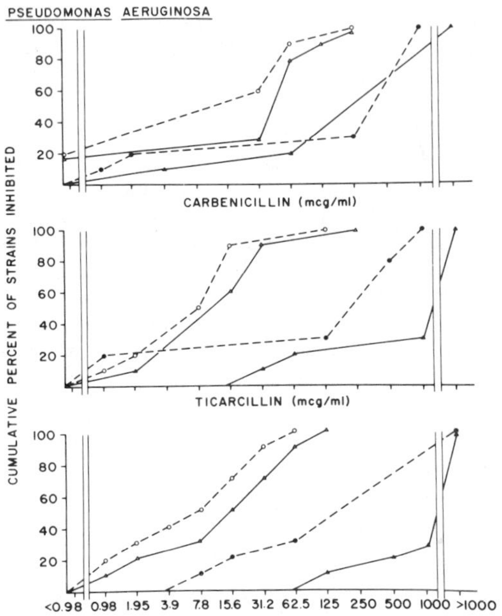

FIG. 4. *Effect of inoculum size on the susceptibility of P. aeruginosa when tested against carbenicillin, ticarcillin, and BL-P1654. Symbols: minimum inhibitory concentration at 10^{-2} (●) and 10^{-5} (○) dilutions; minimal bactericidal concentration at 10^{-2} (▲) and 10^{-5} (△) dilutions.*

Pharmacologically, carbenicillin and ticarcillin seem to be comparable (3, 4, 6, 11), and early clinical studies have shown promise (9, 10, 15). Therefore, ticarcillin would seem to merit further laboratory and clinical investigation to ascertain whether it offers a real advantage over carbenicillin in terms of cost, clinical effectiveness, and side effects.

Our second conclusion was that BL-P1654 was generally slightly less active than either ticarcillin or carbenicillin except against enterococci and *S. epidermidis*. We found, as have others (2, 5, 8, 12) that there was a marked discrepancy between the bacteriostatic and the bactericidal concentrations of BL-P1654 when tested against *P. aeruginosa*.

ACKNOWLEDGMENT

This work was supported by a grant from Beecham Pharmaceutical Co., Bristol, Tenn.

LITERATURE CITED

1. **Bodey, G. P., and B. Deerhake.** 1971. In vitro studies of α-carboxyl-3-thienylmethyl penicillin, a new semisynthetic penicillin. Appl. Microbiol. **21**:61–65.
2. **Bodey, G. P., and D. Stewart.** 1969. In vitro studies of a new semisynthetic penicillin 6-(D-α-sulfoaminophenylacetamido)-penicillanic acid. Appl. Microbiol. **18**: 76–79.
3. **Brown, C. H., III, E. A. Natelson, M. W. Bradshaw, C. P. Alfrey, Jr., and T. W. Williams, Jr.** 1975. Study of the effects of ticarcillin on blood coagulation and platelet function. Antimicrob. Agents Chemother. **7**:652–657.
4. **Klastersky, J., A. Henri, and D. Daneau.** 1974. Ticarcillin, a new semisynthetic penicillin active on *Pseudomonas aeruginosa in vitro* activity and blood levels in man. J. Clin. Pharm. **14**:172–175.
5. **Kurtz, S., K. Holmes, and M. Turck.** 1975. Disparity between inhibitory and killing effects of BL-P1654. Antimicrob. Agents Chemother. **7**:215–218.
6. **Libke, R. D., J. T. Clarke, E. D. Ralph, R. P. Luthy, and W. M. Kirby.** 1975. Ticarcillin vs. carbenicillin: clinical pharmacokinetics. Clin. Pharm. Ther. **17**:441–446.
7. **Neu, H. C., and E. B. Winshell.** 1971. Semisynthetic penicillin 6-[D(−)-α-carboxy-3-thienylacetamido] penicillanic acid active against *Pseudomonas* in vitro. Appl. Microbiol. **21**:66–70.
8. **Overturf, G. D., R. Ressler, and J. Wilkins.** 1974. Comparative in vitro evaluation of BL-P1654 and carbenicillin against *Pseudomonas*. Antimicrob. Agents Chemother. **6**:643–646.
9. **Pines, A., G. Khaja, H. Raafat, and K. S. Sreedharan.** 1974. Preliminary clinical experience with ticarcillin (BRL 2288) in 101 patients treated for severe respiratory infections. Chemotherapy **20**:39–44.
10. **Rodriguez, V., G. P. Bodey, N. Horikoshi, J. Inagaki, and K. B. McCredie.** 1973. Ticarcillin therapy of infections. Antimicrob. Agents Chemother. **4**:427–431.
11. **Rodriguez, V., J. Inagaki, and G. P. Bodey.** 1973. Clinical pharmacology of ticarcillin (α-carboxyl-3-thienylmethyl penicillin, BRL-2228). Antimicrob. Agents Chemother. **4**:31–36.
12. **Sanders, C. C., and W. E. Sanders, Jr.** 1975. BL-P1654: a bacteriostatic penicillin? Antimicrob. Agents Chemother. **7**:435–440.
13. **Steers, E. E., L. Foltz, B. S. Graves, and J. Riden.** 1959. An inocula replicating apparatus for routine testing of bacterial susceptibility to antibiotics. Antibiot. Chemother. **9**:307–311.
14. **Wald, E. R., H. C. Standiford, B. A. Tatem, F. M. Calia, and R. B. Hornick.** 1975. BL-P1654, ticarcillin, and carbenicillin: in vitro comparison alone and in combination with gentamicin against *Pseudomonas aeruginosa*. Antimicrob. Agents Chemother. **7**:336–340.
15. **Wise, R., and D. S. Reeves.** 1974. Clinical and laboratory investigations on ticarcillin, an anti-pseudomonal antibiotic. Chemotherapy **20**:45–51.

ANTIMICROBIAL AGENTS AND CHEMOTHERAPY, Aug. 1976, p. 245-248 Vol. 10, No. 2
 Printed in U.S.A.

A New Cephalosporin with a Dual Mode of Action

CYNTHIA H. O'CALLAGHAN,* R. B. SYKES, AND SUSAN E. STANIFORTH

Glaxo Research Ltd., Greenford, Middlesex, England

Received for publication 26 April 1976

A cephalosporin, (6R,7R)-7-[(2R)-2-hydroxy-2-phenylacetamido]-3-(pyrid-2-yl-*N*-oxide)thiomethylceph-3-em-4-carboxylic acid (MCO), that could lead to a novel approach to the problem of β-lactamase destruction is described. The compound is slightly more resistant to some β-lactamases than is cephalothin, but it is still hydrolyzed by many to a varying degree. Hydrolysis of the β-lactam bond of a cephalosporin releases the 3-substituent, which in MCO is itself an antibacterial agent, 2-mercaptopyridine-*N*-oxide. Thus, MCO has a dual mode of action, and bacteria that do not produce an effective amount of a β-lactamase are inhibited by the intact cephalosporin, whereas those that do hydrolyze it are inhibited by the released antibacterial compound.

β-Lactamases from a wide range of bacteria can attack most currently available cephalosporins and inactivate them by hydrolyzing the β-lactam ring. For this reason, these cephalosporins cannot be used to treat infections due to gram-negative organisms that produce large amounts of β-lactamases. One way of overcoming this problem is to alter the substituents on the cephalosporin nucleus so that the compounds are more resistant to attack by β-lactamases. Although cephalosporins with resistance to some types of β-lactamase from gram-negative organisms have been known for many years (8), the early compounds were of no therapeutic value because they had very little antibacterial activity. Recently, cephalosporins with both resistance to β-lactamases and activity against a wider range of bacteria have been described (10, 12).

An alternative solution to the problem has been considered whereby antibacterial activity might be retained, even though the β-lactam ring of the cephalosporin were to be broken. When the β-lactam ring is hydrolyzed, the substituent at position 3 is expelled from the cephalosporin molecule (6); if that group possessed antibacterial activity of its own, this would still be available after the destruction of the cephalosporin moiety.

A cephalosporin meeting these requirements has been synthesized in our laboratories. The 7-acyl group of the compound is D-mandeloyl, a group that also appears in cefamandole (12), and the 3-substituent is 2-mercaptopyridine-*N*-oxide (Fig. 1), which is also known as omadine; as the zinc salt, zinc pyrithione, it is used as an antiseptic in toiletries such as shampoos. The properties of the cephalosporin analogue are described in this paper.

MATERIALS AND METHODS

(6R,7R)-7-[(2R)-2-hydroxy-2-phenylacetamido]-3-(pyrid-2-yl-*N*-oxide)thiomethylceph-3-em-4-carboxylic acid (MCO) (Fig. 1) was prepared in our laboratories as a creamy white crystalline solid with a molecular weight of 473; as the sodium salt, it is approximately 20% soluble in water.

Organisms. Most of the organisms tested were recent clinical isolates. The bacteria were maintained on nutrient agar slopes, and the fungi were maintained on Sabouraud maltose agar.

MIC determinations. (i) Bacteria. Minimum inhibitory concentrations (MICs) were determined by an agar dilution technique. Serial twofold dilutions of freshly prepared antibiotic solution were made into Oxoid no. 1 nutrient agar and poured into petri dishes. The plates were inoculated with a replicate inoculating device (Denley Instruments Ltd., Bolney, Sussex, England), with inocula containing approximately 10^5 colony-forming units of bacteria. The MIC, in micrograms per milliliter, was read after 18 h of incubation at 37°C as the lowest concentration that inhibited growth. All bacterial cultures were tested for β-lactamase production, using the chromogenic cephalosporin 87/312 described by O'Callaghan et al. (7).

(ii) Fungi and yeasts. The MICs of fungi and yeasts were determined in Sabouraud maltose broth, as described by Holt (4).

Stability studies with β-lactamases. β-Lactamases from *Klebsiella aerogenes* K1, *Enterobacter cloacae* P99, *Escherichia coli* TEM$^+$, *E. coli* RGN_{238}, and *Pseudomonas aeruginosa* 67/70 were prepared in a partially purified form as described by O'Callaghan et al. The activity of each enzyme preparation against MCO was estimated photometrically, using the decrease in optical density at 263 nm to determine the rate of hydrolysis of the compound (9).

Determination of 2-mercaptopyridine-*N*-oxide. MCO was incubated at 2 mg/ml in M/20 phosphate buffer at pH 7 with equal volumes of *K. aerogenes* K1 β-lactamase containing between 10 and 0.15 en-

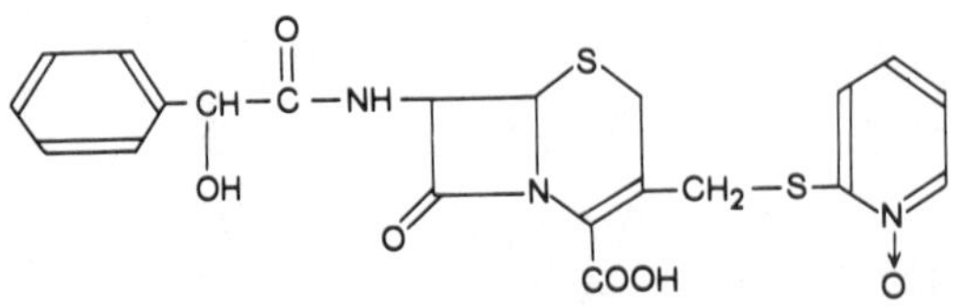

FIG. 1. *Structure of MCO.*

zyme units for 1 h at 37°C. One unit of β-lactamase activity is defined as that amount of enzyme capable of hydrolyzing 1 μmol of MCO in 1 h at 37°C; 2.5 units will hydrolyze 1,000 μg of MCO in 1 h. The samples were filtered after incubation in an Amicon microultrafiltration system 8MC, using a UM10 membrane, to remove enzyme protein. 2-Mercaptopyridine-*N*-oxide was then estimated either polarographically or by a colorimetric method.

(i) Polarographic method. 2-Mercaptopyridine-*N*-oxide contains a free sulfhydryl group that can be easily oxidized to give an anodic wave on the polarograph at −0.16 V at pH 2 and at −0.28 V at pH 4, 6, and 8 with reference to a standard calomel electrode. The anode was a dropping mercury electrode with characteristics t = 2.8 s, m = 1.6 mg/s, and h = 65 cm.

A calibration curve of the concentration of 2-mercaptopyridine-*N*-oxide in pH 7 M/20 phosphate buffer against the height of the anodic step gave a straight line, the minimum amount detectable being 2×10^{-4} M (25 μg/ml).

(ii) Chemical method. Dalziel and Thompson (1) used the reaction of 2-mercaptopyridine-*N*-oxide with iron salts to form colored complexes that could be used for the estimation of iron in solution. The black iron complex $(C_5H_4NOS)_3Fe$ is precipitated from weakly acidic solutions. To a known volume of 2-mercaptopyridine-*N*-oxide solution was added an equal volume of 0.01 M solution of ferric nitrate in 0.1 N sulfuric acid. The violet color or precipitate was extracted with a volume of chloroform equal to twice the volume of the original solution. The optical density of this solution was measured at 550 nm in a 1-cm cell. The calibration curve was a straight line, the least amount of 2-mercaptopyridine-*N*-oxide detectable being 2.5×10^{-4} M (31.8 μg/ml). No reaction was obtained with untreated MCO. Values from solutions incubated with β-lactamase were read from the calibration curve.

RESULTS

Antibacterial activity. The in vitro activity of MCO against a selection of organisms is summarized in Table 1, in comparison with cephalothin. The results are expressed as geometric mean MICs, and it is evident that the compound has both greater intrinsic activity and a wider antimicrobial spectrum than does cephalothin. Apart from the strains of *E. coli*, most of the organisms are β-lactamase producers.

Stability to β-lactamase. A comparison of the rates of destruction of cephalothin and MCO by five partially purified enzymes of classes I, III, and IV from gram-negative organisms (11) was made using the spectrophotometric method. The results are given in Table 2; for each enzyme, the resistance of cephalothin is given the arbitrary value of 1. The increase in resistance to class I enzymes, from *E. cloacae* and *P. aeruginosa,* was greater than for the class III and IV enzymes, where the improvement was only marginal. However, MCO was not wholly stable to any of the enzymes tested.

Expulsion of the 3-substituent after attack by β-lactamases. It has previously been shown that attack on the β-lactam ring of a cephalosporin by a β-lactamase is accompanied by expulsion of the substituent at position 3 if this is a leaving group, such as acetoxy (3) pyridyl, or azido (6), obviously able to accept an electron. Solutions of MCO, before and after incubation with *K. aerogenes* K1 β-lactamase, were examined by two methods for the presence of free 2-mercaptopyridine-*N*-oxide. *K. aerogenes* enzyme was chosen because it was the one to which MCO was most susceptible. The various strengths of enzyme were chosen to give a spread from complete hydrolysis in the 1-h period of incubation at 37°C to little or no decomposition in that time. The liberated 3-substituent was estimated by two methods, and the results are given in Table 3.

Treatment with 5 or 2.5 enzyme units/ml

TABLE 1. *Geometric mean MICs in comparison with cephalothin*

Organism	No. of strains tested	Geometric mean MIC (μg/ml) of: MCO	Cephalothin
Staphylococcus aureus	25	2.7	1.2
Escherichia coli	24	1.8	9.2
Citrobacter freundii	8	11	50
Enterobacter cloacae	4	3.4	250
Enterobacter hafniae	10	3.7	74
Klebsiella aerogenes	13	16	>250
Proteus rettgeri	2	2	>250
Proteus morganii	1	4	>250

TABLE 2. *Stability to β-lactamases*

Source of β-lactamase	Class	Increase in resistance over cephalothin
K. aerogenes K1	IV	1.7
E. cloacae P99	I	18.6
E. coli TEM	III	2.7
E. coli RGN 238	III	4.3
P. aeruginosa 67/70	I	8.8

produced complete hydrolysis of MCO; smaller amounts of enzyme produced only partial hydrolysis of the compound, as shown by the decreasing amounts of 2-mercaptopyridine-*N*-oxide liberated. The two methods of estimating the amount of 2-mercaptopyridine-*N*-oxide produced during incubation with the β-lactamase agreed quite well and corresponded to the change in ultraviolet absorption at the λ_{max} for the β-lactam ring. The polarographic method depends on the presence of the free -SH group only, whereas the chemical method depends on both the -SH group and the *N*-oxide group. The agreement between the two methods indicates that 2-mercaptopyridine-*N*-oxide was expelled intact from the cephalosporin after β-lactamase hydrolysis of the β-lactam ring of MCO. Incubation of cefazolin and cefamandole with 5 enzyme units of β-lactamase resulted in their total decomposition, and the polarographic method showed that their respective 3-substituents were expelled intact in stoichiometric proportions. The chemical method could not be applied to 2-mercapto-5-methyl-1,2,4-thiadiazole nor to 1-methyl-5-mercaptotetrazole, the 3-substituents of cefazolin and cefamandole, respectively, since these substances do not chelate iron.

Antibacterial activity of 2-mercaptopyridine-*N*-oxide. Unlike most groups substituted in position 3 of the cephalosporins, 2-mercaptopyridine-*N*-oxide had antibacterial activity in its own right. Its activity, compared with that of the intact cephalosporin MCO, is shown in Table 4. MCO had activity against all the strains tested, including those that produce a β-lactamase, although it was significantly less active against enzyme-producing organisms than against those with no β-lactamase. However, it had more activity against these organisms than would be explained by its marginally increased β-lactamase resistance. In contrast, 2-mercaptopyridine-*N*-oxide was active at the same high level against all strains, regardless of their β-lactamase activity. The possibility must, therefore, be considered that the intrinsic activity of the 2-mercaptopyridine-*N*-oxide substituent made some contribution to the total antibacterial activity of MCO.

Effect of β-lactamase treatment on the antimicrobial activity of MCO. The inhibitory action of MCO was tested against four β-lactamase-producing bacteria before and after it was destroyed by K1 β-lactamase, and the results are given in Table 5. Unlike other cephalosporins, MCO did not lose its antibacterial activity when it was hydrolyzed by β-lactamase; on the contrary, in some cases the activity was enhanced.

TABLE 3. *Amount of free 2-mercaptopyridine-N-oxide released from 1 mg of MCO by incubation with β-lactamase (K1)*

Enzyme units/ml (1 h at 37°C)	Amount of free 2-mercaptopyridine-*N*-oxide (μg/ml) measured by:	
	Polarographic method	Ferric nitrate method
5	268[a]	270
2.5	268	260
1.25	240	255
0.6	170	150
0.3	30	<25
0.15	<25	<25

[a] A 1,000-μg amount of MCO would theoretically produce 268 μg of 2-mercaptopyridine-*N*-oxide on total destruction.

TABLE 4. *Comparison of the in vitro antibacterial activities of MCO and 2-mercaptopyridine-N-oxide*

Organism	MIC (μg/ml) of:	
	MCO	2-Mercaptopyridine-*N*-oxide
E. coli TEM⁺	8	2
E. coli TEM⁻	2	2
E. cloacae P99	62	2
E. cloacae P99⁻	1	2
K. aerogenes K1	16	2
K. aerogenes K1⁻	1	2
P. morganii NCTC 235	0.5	8
P. mirabilis 431	2	8

TABLE 5. *Effect of β-lactamase treatment on the antimicrobial activity of MCO*

Organism	MIC (μg/ml) of:		
	MCO	MCO + enzyme	2-mercaptopyridine-*N*-oxide
E. cloacae P99	62	4	4
P. aeruginosa 150	500	8	4
P. aeruginosa 30/70	500	31	16
C. albicans	3	0.06	0.06
M. canis	16	3	0.8
T. mentagrophytes	62	1.5	0.8

Also, unlike other cephalosporins, MCO was active against yeasts and fungi such as *Candida albicans*, *Microsporum canis*, and *Trichophyton mentagrophytes*. When a solution of the compound was treated with the β-lactamase, these activities increased markedly.

DISCUSSION

The single property most limiting on the clinically useful antibacterial spectrum of most cephalosporins is their susceptibility to destruction by β-lactamases, which results in total loss of antibacterial activity. MCO represents a new approach to the problem of hydrolysis of cephalosporins by β-lactamases, whereby the intact compound not only has typical cephalosporin activity against non-β-lactamase-producing bacteria but also disruption of the β-lactam ring by a β-lactamase expels a 3-substituent, which then has antibacterial activity in its own right.

Like cefamandole (12), MCO has increased resistance to hydrolysis by some β-lactamases. Both compounds have a mandeloyl group at position 7, and their increased enzyme resistance is attributed to the small substituent (OH) on the α-carbon atom of the phenylacetamido-7-acyl group; this type of substitution has previously been shown to improve the resistance of such cephalosporin analogues (8) to β-lactamases, particularly to class 1 enzymes.

MCO has a mercaptoheterocyclic substituent at position 3, and this group is expelled intact from the molecule when the cephalosporin is hydrolyzed by β-lactamase. A similar result was obtained upon hydrolysis of two other cephalosporins, cefamandole and cefazolin, which also have mercaptoheterocyclic substituents at position 3. However, the groups in cefamandole (1-methyl-5-mercaptotetrazole) and cefazolin (2-mercapto-5-methyl-1,3,4-thiadizole) have no antibacterial activity of their own, whereas the group in MCO, 2-mercaptopyridine-*N*-oxide, is antibacterially active. MCO can, therefore, be regarded either as a cephalosporin antibiotic or, alternatively, as a substituted 2-mercaptopyridine-*N*-oxide derivative.

The antibacterial activity of MCO is, by and large, more characteristic of a cephalosporin than of an omadine derivative, but a more detailed study of its mode of action might reveal other effects on the bacterial cell. In addition, it is unique among the cephalosporins so far reported, in having activity against yeasts and fungi; against these organisms, it seems likely that it is acting as a substituted omadine. When the cephalosporin moiety was removed by β-lactamase hydrolysis, the residual activity against both bacteria and fungi could only be attributed to free omadine. The MCO molecule contains approximately 27% omadine by weight and, in general, there is good correlation between the antimicrobial activity of the equivalent amount of omadine and that of MCO after β-lactamase hydrolysis although, in some cases, there was a greater variation from the theoretical than expected. MCO gave good results in the treatment of experimental infections with β-lactamase-producing gram-negative organisms and non-enzyme-producing strains in laboratory animals (Ryan, unpublished data).

Although the novel principle of action of MCO is obviously effective, this particular cephalosporin is unlikely to have any useful therapeutic future as an antibiotic for systemic use because its 3-substituent, omadine, has undesirable toxic properties when given systemically (2, 5). These might not be manifested when omadine is attached to the cephalosporin structure, but there is the risk that they would become apparent if it was released by an attack of any kind on the β-lactam ring.

LITERATURE CITED

1. **Dalziel, J. A. W., and M. Thompson.** 1966. The solvent extraction and absorptiometric determination of iron with 2-mercaptopyridine-N-oxide. Analyst (London) **91**:98–101.
2. **Gucklhorn, I. R.** 1970. Antimicrobials in cosmetics. Manuf. Chem. **41**:30–33.
3. **Hamilton-Miller, J. M. T., G. G. F. Newton, and E. P. Abraham.** 1970. Products of aminolysis and enzymic hydrolysis of the cephalosporins. Biochem. J. **116**:371–384.
4. **Holt, R. J.** 1975. Laboratory tests of antifungal drugs. J. Clin. Pathol. **28**:767–774.
5. **Moe, R. A., J. Kinpan, and C. R. Linegan.** 1960. Toxicology of hydroxypyridinethione. Toxicol. Appl. Pharmacol. **2**:156–170.
6. **O'Callaghan, C. H., S. M. Kirby, A. Morris, R. E. Waller, and R. E. Duncombe.** 1972. Correlation between hydrolysis of the β-lactam bond of the cephalosporin nucleus and expulsion of the 3-substituent. J. Bacteriol. **110**:988–991.
7. **O'Callaghan, C. H., A. Morris, S. M. Kirby, and A. H. Shingler.** 1972. Novel method for detection of β-lactamases using a chromogenic cephalosporin substrate. Antimicrob. Agents Chemother. **1**:282–288.
8. **O'Callaghan, C. H., P. W. Muggleton, S. M. Kirby, and D. M. Ryan.** 1967. Inhibition of β-lactamase decomposition of cephaloridine and cephalothin by other cephalosporins, p. 337–343. Antimicrob. Agents Chemother. 1966.
9. **O'Callaghan, C. H., P. W. Muggleton, and G. W. Ross.** 1969. Effects of β-lactamase from gram-negative organisms on cephalosporins and penicillins, p. 57–63. Antimicrob. Agents Chemother. 1968.
10. **O'Callaghan, C. H., R. B. Sykes, D. M. Ryan, R. D. Foord, and P. W. Muggleton.** 1976. Cefuroxime, a new cephalosporin antibiotic. J. Antibiot. **29**:29–37.
11. **Richmond, M. H., and R. B. Sykes.** 1973. The β-lactamases of gram-negative bacteria and their possible physiological role. Adv. Microb. Physiol. **9**:31–88.
12. **Wick, W. E., and D. A. Preston.** 1972. Biological properties of three 3-heterocyclic-thiomethyl cephalosporin antibiotics. Antimicrob. Agents Chemother. **1**:221–234.

ANTIMICROBIAL AGENTS AND CHEMOTHERAPY, Aug. 1976, p. 249-252 Vol. 10, No. 2

Printed in U.S.A.

Dual-Action Cephalosporin Utilizing a Novel Therapeutic Principle

D. GREENWOOD* AND F. O'GRADY

Department of Microbiology, University of Nottingham, City Hospital, Nottingham NG5 1PH, England

Received for publication 26 April 1976

A new cephalosporin is described that overcomes, in a novel way, the general susceptibility of this group of agents to enterobacterial β-lactamases. The new compound carries a substituent that is released on cleavage of the β-lactam ring and then exhibits antibacterial activity in its own right. The possible therapeutic benefits of such an antibiotic are discussed.

Many cephalosporins have marked activity against a wide spectrum of gram-negative bacilli when tested by conventional minimum inhibitory concentration (MIC) methods using low inocula. When tested against dense populations of enterobacteria, however, their activity is much less impressive (1, 2, 11). This inoculum effect is particularly marked in those strains of enterobacteria that are resistant to ampicillin, and, when tested against dense populations of such strains, cephalosporins often cause only a transient antibacterial effect due to their relative susceptibility to enterobacterial β-lactamases (2, 4).

One approach to the enhancement of the antibacterial effect of this group of agents is to combine them with a β-lactamase inhibitor, and this can be very effective in vitro, providing a potent, broad-spectrum β-lactamase inhibitor is used (5).

A new cephalosporin synthesized by Glaxo Research Ltd. (9) offers a totally different solution to the problem. This compound, when attacked by β-lactamases, loses a substituent, omadine, normally carried at the 3-position of the cephalosporin molecule, which itself possesses antibacterial activity in the free, but not in the bound, state. The present paper discusses this novel principle and presents some results of in vitro tests that explore the potential of this type of agent.

MATERIALS AND METHODS

(6R,7R)-7-[(2R)-2-hydroxy-2-phenylacetamido]-3-(pyrid-2-yl-*N*-oxide) thiomethylceph-3-em-4-carboxylic acid (MCO) (Fig. 1) was synthesized and provided by Glaxo Research Ltd. Suitable concentrations were freshly prepared in sterile distilled water as required.

Sodium omadine was provided by Kingsley and Keith (Chemicals) Ltd. as a 40% solution.

Turbidimetric studies were made using the multichannel opacity monitoring device described by Mackintosh et al. (8). Strains of *Escherichia coli*, of which the response to β-lactam antibiotics has been extensively studied in previous investigations (2, 3, 6, 7), were grown in complete broth (2) in the opacity monitoring device. Antibacterial agent was added at a standard point (30% maximum opacity) in the mid-to-late logarithmic growth phase. Drug-induced morphological changes in the exposed bacteria were observed by interference contrast microscopy.

Cephalosporin MCO was also used to treat "bacterial cystitis" in a mechanical model that simulates the hydrokinetic features of a urinary bladder (3, 6, 10). In the model, 20 ml of a fully grown broth culture is diluted at 1 ml/min with fresh broth, simulating the diurnal flow of urine into the bladder. At preset intervals (1 h in the present experiments), a "micturition" episode empties the "bladder," leaving a residual 20-ml volume. In the present series of experiments, a single pulse of antibiotic, to achieve an initial concentration of 500 μg/ml, was added to the system after the fourth hourly micturition.

RESULTS

The MICs of cephalosporin MCO, a number of other β-lactam antibiotics, and sodium omadine, tested against several strains of *E. coli*, are shown in Table 1.

Figure 2 shows a typical continuous opacity trace of an ampicillin-susceptible strain of *E. coli* (ECSA 1) exposed to various concentrations of cephalosporin MCO. The morphological changes exhibited by the bacteria after 1 h of exposure are depicted in Fig. 3. Rapid lysis of the culture occurred at an antibiotic concentration of 128 μg/ml, a biphasic response (associated with part of the population lysing, part transforming to the spheroplast form, and part undergoing filamentation) was induced at 64 μg/ml, and a delayed lysis (associated with spheroplast formation and filamentation) occurred at 32 μg/ml. Little or no lysis occurred at lower concentrations although filamentation of the bacteria was demonstrated microscopically at antibiotic concentrations of less than 1 μg/ml. In striking contrast to the finding with other cephalosporins (2, 4, 7), no regrowth of cultures that had succumbed to antibiotic lysis occurred during the 20-h period of observation.

A typical continuous opacity trace obtained with an ampicillin-resistant *E. coli* strain (*Gen*) is shown in Fig. 4. With this strain, partial lysis occurred at an antibiotic concentration of 128 μg/ml, but again no regrowth was seen on prolonged incubation.

Data obtained from these experiments together with similar data obtained in experiments with other β-lactam agents are plotted for strains ECSA 1 and *Gen* in Fig. 5 and 6, which show the time elapsing after the addition of various concentrations of each antibiotic before lysis of the cultures occurred.

The effect of sodium omadine on an exponentially growing culture of *E. coli* ECSA 1 is shown in Fig. 7. A concentration of 4 μg/ml, equivalent to the conventionally determined MIC, caused an abrupt cessation of growth, with little subsequent increase in opacity over the period of observation.

Bladder model. The general form of the growth/dilution response of *E. coli* strains in the bladder model and the influence of β-lactam antibiotics upon the normal response have been described elsewhere (3, 6, 10). In the model, bacterial culture and antibiotic are subjected to dilution and periodic discharge. The hydrokinetic washout effect thus produced depends on the "urine" flow rate, the interval between micturition episodes, the residual volume of culture left after micturition, and the bacterial growth rate. An overnight bacterial culture, initially in the lag phase, enters a "fluctuating equilibrium" state (in which the same cycle of opacity changes occur between each micturition) after about 6 h of dilution and hourly micturition (3). In the equilibrium state the bacterial population is maintained at a near-climax level, in which the viable count is in excess of 10^8 organisms/ml. Antibiotic added as a single pulse after a micturition episode is subsequently diluted 1:4 during each hourly cycle, but in the case of β-lactam agents enzymatic destruction may also serve to reduce the concentration of active antibiotic (6).

Table 2 compares the ability of a single pulse (sufficient to achieve an initial concentration of 500 μg/ml) of MCO or of several other β-lactam agents to suppress growth of two strains of *E. coli* in the bladder model. One of these strains was *E. coli* ECSA 1, also used in the "static"

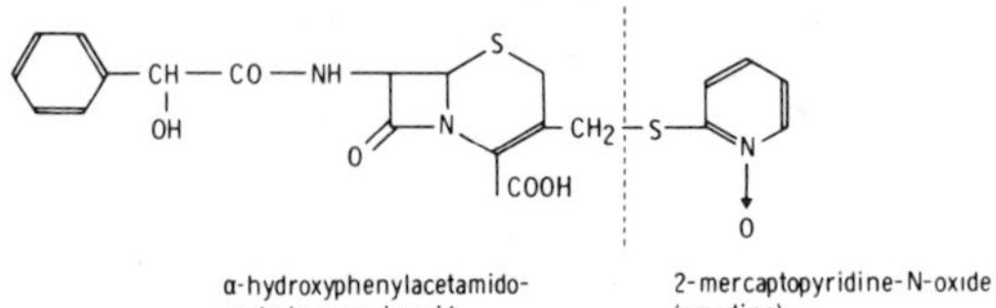

FIG. 1. *Structure of cephalosporin MCO.*

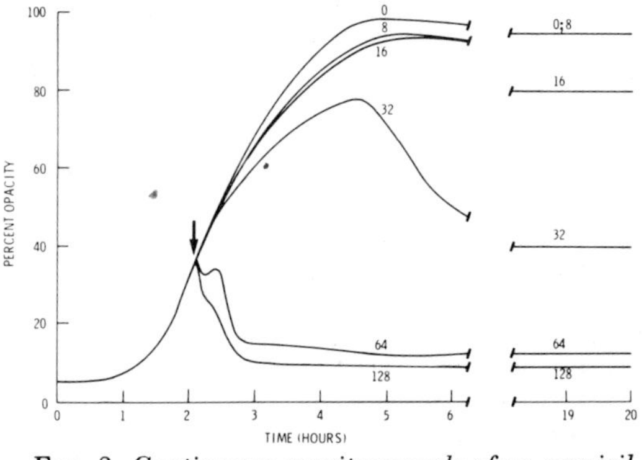

FIG. 2. *Continuous opacity records of an ampicillin-susceptible E. coli strain (ECSA 1). Numbers indicate the concentration (micrograms per milliliter) of cephalosporin MCO added at arrow.*

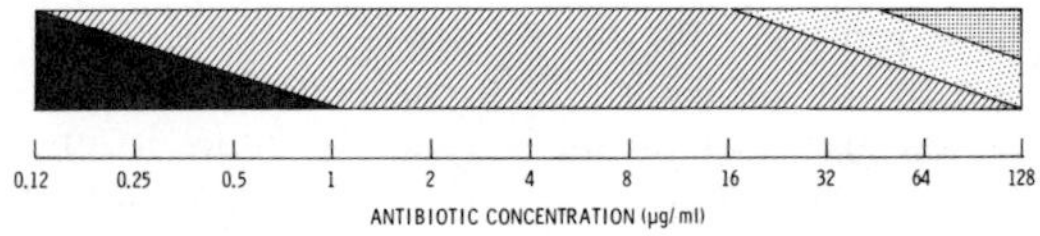

FIG. 3. *Morphological response profile of an ampicillin-susceptible E. coli strain (ECSA 1) after 1 h of exposure to cephalosporin MCO. Black = normal; hatching = filaments; light stippling = emergent spheroplasts; dense stippling = lysed cell debris.*

TABLE 1. *Comparison of the MICs of cephalosporin MCO, other β-lactam agents, and sodium omadine for several strains of E. coli*

Strain	MIC (μg/ml) of:						
	Ampicillin	Cephaloridine	Cephalothin	Cefazolin	Cephalexin	Cephalosporin MCO	Sodium omadine
ECSA 1	4	8	16	2	32	8	4
ECSA 2	4	4	8	1	16	2	4
Far	>500	8	8	8	8	32	4
Bur	>500	4	4	2	4	16	4
Gen	>500	16	8	4	8	32	2
Hos	>500	16	16	64	16	64	4

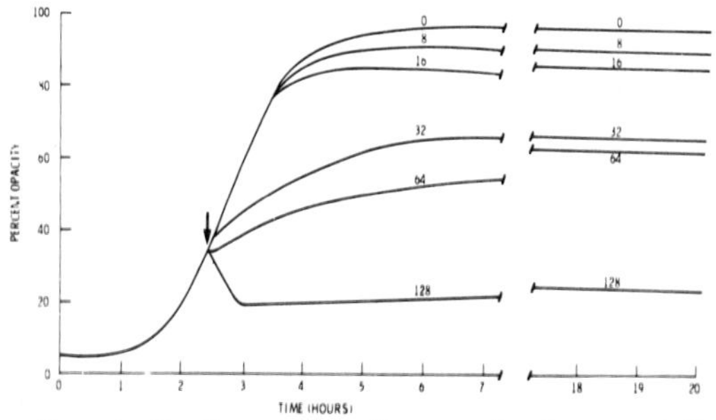

FIG. 4. *Continuous opacity records of an ampicillin-resistant E. coli strain (Gen). Numbers indicate the concentration (micrograms per milliliter) of cephalosporin MCO added at arrow.*

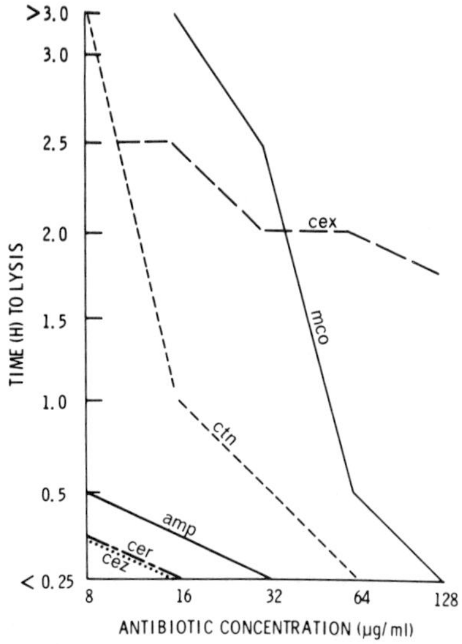

FIG. 5. *Comparison of the lytic activity of cephalosporin MCO and of several other β-lactam antibiotics, showing the time taken for lysis to occur when dense cultures of E. coli strain ECSA 1 were exposed to various concentrations of the antibiotics. amp, Ampicillin; cer, cephaloridine; ctn, cephalothin; cez, cefazolin; cex, cephalexin; mco, cephalosporin MCO.*

experiments; the second strain was an ampicillin-resistant *E. coli* strain (*Hos*) previously shown to be highly resistant to a number of other β-lactam agents in the conditions of the bladder model (6). The results are expressed as the time taken for the opacity to reattain the level at which antibiotic was added. Cephalosporin MCO suppressed the growth of the ampicillin-susceptible strain ECSA 1 for 10 h and that of the ampicillin-resistant strain *Hos* for 5.5 h—longer than any of the other β-lactam agents tested.

DISCUSSION

The in vitro activity of cephalosporins against gram-negative bacilli is generally mitigated by their susceptibility to enterobacterial β-lactamases, including the slow β-lactamase characteristic of ampicillin-susceptible *E. coli* strains (2, 4–7). The new cephalosporin, MCO, overcomes this disability by releasing, on cleavage of the β-lactam ring, a substituent, omadine, which on liberation exhibits antibacterial activity. Thus, although the compound is susceptible to enterobacterial β-lactamases, the initial antibacterial effect of the entire molecule is continued after its destruction by the omadine substituent.

We have previously argued (10) that the benefits of high-dose therapy with β-lactam agents may be confined to the first dose of a treatment schedule, in which a large part of the bacterial population is destroyed. Subsequent doses sup-

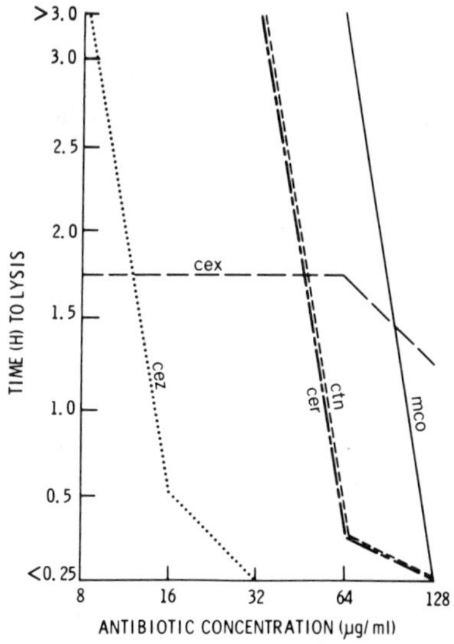

FIG. 6. *Comparison of the lytic activity of cephalosporin MCO and of several other β-lactam antibiotics, showing the time taken for lysis to occur when dense cultures of an ampicillin-resistant E. coli strain (Gen) were exposed to various concentrations of the antibiotics. Abbreviations are the same as those given in the legends to Fig. 5.*

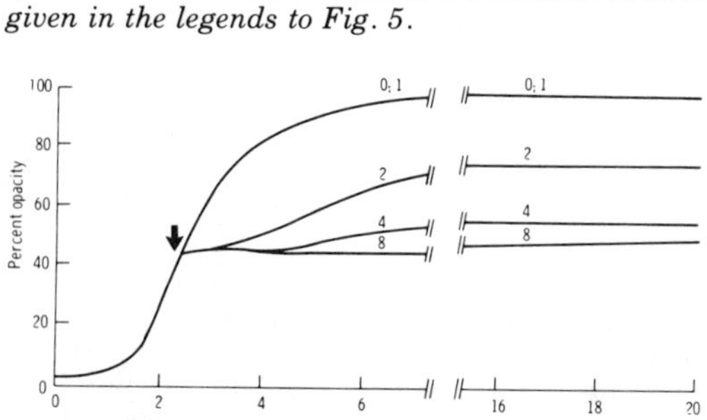

FIG. 7. *Continuous opacity records of an ampicillin-susceptible E. coli strain (ECSA 1). Numbers indicate the concentration (micrograms per milliliter) of sodium omadine added at arrow.*

TABLE 2. *Comparison of the times taken in the bladder model for bacterial cultures to reattain the opacity level at which antibiotic was added after exposure to cephalosporin MCO or to other β-lactam antibiotics*

Strain	Time (h) after antibiotic addition for opacity to reattain original level after a single pulse (500 μg/ml) of:					
	Ampicillin	Cephaloridine	Cephalothin	Cefazolin	Cephalexin	Cephalosporin MCO
ECSA 1	10	8	6.5	11	6	10
Hos	NL[a]	2	4	3	3.5	5.5

[a] NL, No lysis.

port intrinsic clearance mechanisms by maintaining a bacteriostatic effect on the persisting bacteria and need to be present in concentrations only just above the MIC. Cephalosporin MCO provides in a single antibiotic just such prompt bacterial lysis followed by a prolonged bacteriostatic effect, which is maintained even when the cephalosporin moiety is inactivated.

An important feature of a successful cephalosporin of this type must be the ability to destroy by lysis a greater part of the bacterial population before it is itself destroyed by β-lactamases. The minimum concentration level at which cephalosporin MCO caused rapid bacterial lysis was intermediate between that of highly lytic cephalosporins, such as cephaloridine, cephalothin, and cefazolin, and that of α-aminocephalosporins, cephalexin, cephradine, and cephaloglycin, which have little or no lytic activity at therapeutically useful concentrations (2, 7). Furthermore, the lytic activity of cephalosporin MCO, when tested against an ampicillin-resistant *E. coli* strain (Fig. 4 and 6), was very poor, probably indicating that its susceptibility to the more potent β-lactamases is such that it breaks down before extensive bacterial lysis develops.

On the other hand, limited lytic activity at low concentrations may not be an obstacle to use in situations, such as the urine, where high antibiotic concentrations may be achieved. In experiments in a mechanical model simulating the conditions of dilution and periodic discharge that obtain in the urinary bladder, the new cephalosporin was able to suppress growth of an ampicillin-susceptible strain of *E. coli* for as long as the highly active ampicillin and was more active than any other β-lactam agent tested against a very resistant *E. coli* strain (Table 2).

The pharmacokinetics and toxicity of this compound and its cleavage products have not been extensively studied, but toxicity of the omadine substituent is likely to militate against its therapeutic use. Nevertheless, the principle that underlies the antibacterial effect of this novel cephalosporin is one of considerable therapeutic interest.

ACKNOWLEDGMENTS

We thank Glaxo Research Ltd. for information about cephalosporin MCO, for donation of the compound, and for financial support. We also thank Kingsley and Keith (Chemicals) Ltd. for a gift of sodium omadine.

LITERATURE CITED

1. **Eykyn, S.** 1971. Use and control of cephalosporins. J. Clin. Pathol. 24:419–429.
2. **Greenwood, D., and F. O'Grady.** 1973. Comparison of the responses of *Escherichia coli* and *Proteus mirabilis* to seven β-lactam antibiotics. J. Infect. Dis. 128:211–222.
3. **Greenwood, D., and F. O'Grady.** 1974. The comparative performance of β-lactam antibiotics against ampicillin-sensitive *Escherichia coli* in conditions simulating those of the infected urinary bladder. Br. J. Exp. Pathol. 55:245–250.
4. **Greenwood, D., and F. O'Grady.** 1975. Resistance categories of enterobacteria to β-lactam antibiotics. J. Infect. Dis. 132:233–240.
5. **Greenwood, D., and F. O'Grady.** 1975. Potent combinations of β-lactam antibiotics using the β-lactamase inhibition principle. Chemotherapy (Basel) 21: 330–341.
6. **Greenwood, D., and F. O'Grady.** 1975. Response of ampicillin-resistant *Escherichia coli* to cephalosporins in an *in vitro* model simulating conditions of bacterial growth in the urinary bladder. Br. J. Exp. Pathol. 56:167–171.
7. **Greenwood, D., C. H. C. Teoh, and F. O'Grady.** 1975. Activity of cefazolin against dense populations of enterobacteria. Antimicrob. Agents. Chemother. 7:191–195.
8. **Mackintosh, I. P., F. O'Grady, D. Greenwood, B. W. Watson, T. C. Crichton, R. Piper, and A. Ferrer.** 1973. A twelve-channel bacterial growth monitoring system. Biomed. Eng. 8:514–515, 526.
9. **O'Callaghan, C. H., R. B. Sykes, and S. E. Staniforth.** 1976. A new cephalosporin with a dual mode of action. Antimicrob. Agents. Chemother. 10:245–248.
10. **O'Grady, F., I. P. Mackintosh, D. Greenwood, and B. W. Watson.** 1973. Treatment of "bacterial cystitis" in fully automatic mechanical models simulating conditions of bacterial growth in the urinary bladder. Br. J. Exp. Pathol. 54:283–290.
11. **Steigbigel, N. H., C. E. McCall, C. W. Reed, and M. Finland.** 1967. Antibacterial action of "broad"-spectrum penicillins, cephalosporins and other antibiotics against Gram-negative bacilli isolated from bacteremic patients. Ann. N.Y. Acad. Sci. 145:224–236.

ANTIMICROBIAL AGENTS AND CHEMOTHERAPY, Aug. 1976, p. 253-257
Vol. 10, No. 2

In Vitro Susceptibility of Common Clinical Anaerobic and Aerobic Isolates Against Josamycin

RICHARD E. REESE, ROBERT F. BETTS,* LOLA W. GOEDDE, AND R. GORDON DOUGLAS, JR.

Department of Medicine, University of Rochester School of Medicine, Rochester, New York 14642

Received for publication 3 February 1976

The in vitro susceptibility of 145 anaerobic clinical isolates and 96 gram-positive aerobic clinical isolates to josamycin, a new macrolide antibiotic, was studied using the agar dilution technique. Ninety-five of the aerobes were susceptible to 1.56 μg or less of josamycin per ml. The median minimal inhibitory concentration of these organisms was $\leq$0.39 μg/ml. The in vitro activity of josamycin against the anaerobes was compared with that of erythromycin, clindamycin, penicillin, and chloramphenicol. At concentrations $\leq$3.12 μg/ml, 100% of strains of *Bacteroides* species and *Bacteroides fragilis* were susceptible to josamycin. At low concentrations ($\leq$0.39 μg/ml), clindamycin was more active than josamycin against the anaerobes. However, at concentrations $\leq$3.12 μg/ml, the activities of josamycin and clindamycin were similar except against the *Fusobacterium* species, which was quite resistant to josamycin.

In recent years the clinical significance, diagnostic methods, and therapy of anaerobic infections have been emphasized (1, 5, 7). Because of the rare occurrence of aplastic anemia and the more common dose-related bone marrow suppression associated with the use of chloramphenicol (16) and the variable risk reported for clindamycin-associated colitis (6, 9, 15), other antimicrobial agents for treatment of anaerobic infections are being sought (5).

The macrolide antibiotics are active in vitro against anaerobic organisms. However, the activity of the most commonly used macrolide, erythromycin, is variable against most groups of anaerobes at concentrations achievable in the blood with oral therapy. Therefore, it is not recommended for use in anaerobic infections (7). With parenteral erythromycin, higher concentrations can be achieved in blood, but the difficulties in using erythromycin parenterally have limited the role of erythromycin in anaerobic infections. An unanswered question is whether other macrolides would absorb better and be more efficacious, as was observed when lincomycin was modified to yield clindamycin (4).

Josamycin is a macrolide antibiotic produced by *Streptomyces narbonensis* var. *josamyceticus*, which was isolated in Japan in 1964. In 1970, josamycin was marketed in Japan and later in Europe, where it has been used primarily for treatment of aerobic gram-positive infections (11). Information regarding its activity against anaerobes is limited (11, 12).

We, therefore, undertook an in vitro evaluation of josamycin to determine its activity against a variety of gram-positive and gram-negative anaerobic organisms and compared its activity with that of erythromycin, clindamycin, penicillin, and chloramphenicol. In addition, a number of aerobic gram-positive organisms were also tested.

(This paper was presented in part at the 15th Interscience Conference on Antimicrobial Agents and Chemotherapy, Washington, D.C., 25 September 1975.)

MATERIALS AND METHODS

Bacteria. All organisms tested (see Table 1) were recent clinical isolates. Aerobes were identified by routine methods in the clinical microbiology laboratory at Strong Memorial Hospital. The anaerobic isolates were identified by Gram stain, colony morphology, oxygen tolerance, high-potency antibiotic disk sensitivity testing (14), gas chromatography (8), and biochemical tests, using previously described Center for Disease Control patterns of identification (3). Identified anaerobic strains were maintained at -70°C until testing.

Antibiotics. Standard powders of chloramphenicol, erythromycin, clindamycin, and penicillin were used. Josamycin powder was supplied by Endo Laboratories, Inc., a subsidiary of E. I. DuPont de Nemours and Co., Garden City, N.Y.

Procedures. (i) Aerobic. Single-colony isolates were inoculated into Trypticase soy broth, which was then incubated overnight at 37°C. A 0.1-ml sample of the resultant suspension was diluted 1:1,000, and this dilution was inoculated onto plates containing 5% sheep erythrocytes in Mueller-Hinton agar containing serial twofold dilutions of the test antibiotics, using the replicating apparatus described by

Steers et al. (13). No sheep erythrocytes were added to the Mueller-Hinton agar plates for the staphylococci. The minimal inhibitory concentration was defined as the lowest concentration of antibiotic at which there was no growth or the occurrence of not more than a discrete colony of growth.

(ii) Anaerobic. A plastic glove box, which had an atmosphere of approximately 5% CO_2, 10% H_2, and 85% N_2, was used for the anaerobic studies. Organisms were inoculated separately into chopped meat-glucose broth. After 3 h of incubation, the undiluted suspension of organisms was applied to prereduced brain heart infusion agar containing 5% sheep erythrocytes and serial twofold dilutions of the test antibiotics, using a Steers replicator. One of four isolates (*Bacteroides fragilis, Peptococcus asaccharolyticus, Peptostreptococcus anaerobius,* and *Clostridium perfringens*) for which minimal inhibitory concentrations had previously been determined was run with each agar dilution experiment to serve as a control. Plates were incubated at 37°C and read at 24 and 48 h.

TABLE 1. *Aerobic and anaerobic clinical isolates studied*

Isolate	No. of strains
Aerobes	
Staphylococcus aureus	30
S. epidermidis	18
Streptococcus pneumoniae	10
S. pyrogenes	15
S. agalactiae	23
Anaerobes	
Peptococcus sp.	28
Peptostreptococcus sp.	15
Clostridium perfringens	18
Clostridium sp.	23
Bacteroides sp.	17
B. fragilis	30
Fusobacterium sp.	14

RESULTS

Anaerobic gram-positive organisms. A comparison of the activity of josamycin with the activities of the other test antibiotics against the gram-positive cocci and bacilli is shown in Table 2. Although the differences were not marked, at potentially achievable concentrations josamycin was as active or more active than erythromycin against these organisms. Clindamycin was consistently more active at low concentrations, but the total number of organisms that were susceptible to higher concentrations of either clindamycin or josamycin (≤3.12 μg/ml) was quite similar. Josamycin was either as active or more active than chloramphenicol but less active than penicillin against these gram-positive anaerobes (Table 2).

Anaerobic gram-negative organisms. The

TABLE 2. *Number of gram-positive anaerobes susceptible to indicated concentrations (micrograms per milliliter)*

Organism	Antibiotics	No. of anaerobes									
		≤0.024	0.048	0.097	0.195	0.39	0.78	1.56	3.12	6.25	≥12.5
Peptococcus sp. (28 strains)	Erythromycin	7			2	2	4	8	2	1	2
	Josamycin	1		4		1	19	1			2
	Clindamycin	5	3	2	7	7	2			1	1
	Chloramphenicol						2	6	10	8	2
	Penicillin	14	3	6		3		1		1	
Peptostreptococcus sp. (15 strains)	Erythromycin	3					3	3	2	1	3
	Josamycin	1		1	2	1	5	1	1	1	2
	Clindamycin	3		1	4	2	3	1	1		
	Chloramphenicol				1		2	2	1	7	2
	Penicillin	3	2	3	2	2	1			1	1
Clostridium perfringens (18 strains)	Erythromycin	3				1		7	7		
	Josamycin	3			1		1	6	7		
	Clindamycin	3	5	2		2	2	1	3		
	Chloramphenicol	1							8	9	
	Penicillin		1	3	4	2	5	3			
Clostridium sp. (23 strains)	Erythromycin		1	1	3	3	3	2	3	2	5
	Josamycin	2		1	1	3	5	5	3	1	2
	Clindamycin	5	1	1	1	1	3	4	2	1	4
	Chloramphenicol						1		7	8	7
	Penicillin		1	2	1	3	9	1	2	1	3

activity of the five antibiotics against the *Bacteroides* species and *B. fragilis* is compared in Fig. 1 and 2. Erythromycin paralleled josamycin but was slightly less active against the *Bacteroides* species as well as against *B. fragilis*. The macrolides at low concentrations were less active than clindamycin, especially against *B. fragilis*. Josamycin is also more active in vitro than chloramphenicol against *Bacteroides* species and *B. fragilis* strains (Fig. 1 and 2). Furthermore, josamycin is strikingly more active than penicillin against *B. fragilis*.

Josamycin was inactive against *Fusobacterium* species (Fig. 3). However, this group of organisms may have been unusually resistant. Less than one-half of the strains were susceptible to ≤0.39 μg of penicillin per ml, although over 70% were susceptible to ≤0.097 μg of clindamycin per ml.

Aerobic gram-positive organisms. The activity of josamycin against gram-positive organisms is shown in Table 3. Erythromycin is active against a higher percentage of gram-positive aerobic organisms at a lower concentration than is josamycin (not shown). Nevertheless, 95 of the 96 aerobic gram-positive organisms tested were susceptible to 1.56 μg or less of josamycin per ml. The only gram-positive aerobic organism that was not susceptible to josamycin was a strain of *Staphylococcus epidermidis* isolated from a patient with artificial valve endocarditis. This organism was also markedly resistant to clindamycin, erythromycin, and methicillin. However, methicillin-resistant strains of *S. epidermidis* isolated from five other patients with prosthetic valve endocarditis were susceptible to 0.39 μg or less of josamycin and clindamycin per ml, although they were markedly resistant to erythromycin.

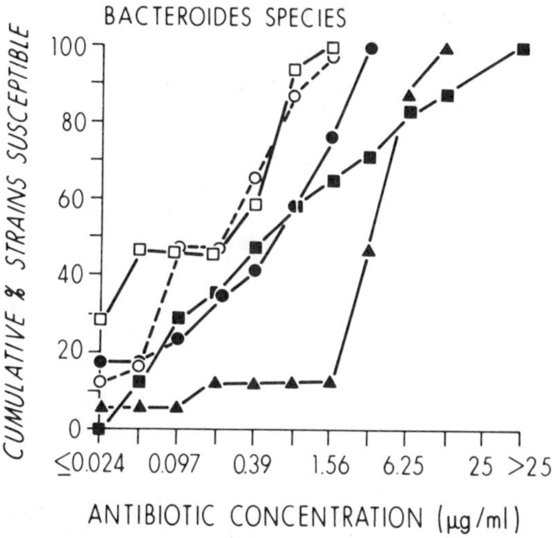

FIG. 1. *Cumulative percentage of Bacteroides sp. strains susceptible to varying concentrations of clindamycin (□), josamycin (○), erythromycin (●), penicillin (■), and chloramphenicol (▲).*

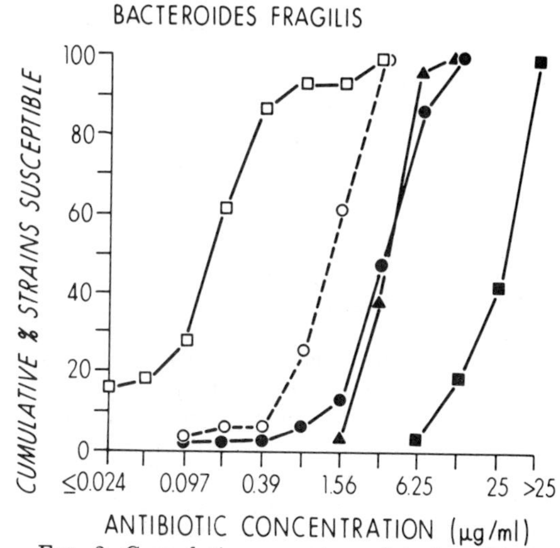

FIG. 2. *Cumulative percentage of strains of B. fragilis susceptible to varying concentrations of clindamycin (□), josamycin (○), erythromycin (●), penicillin (■), and chloramphenicol (▲).*

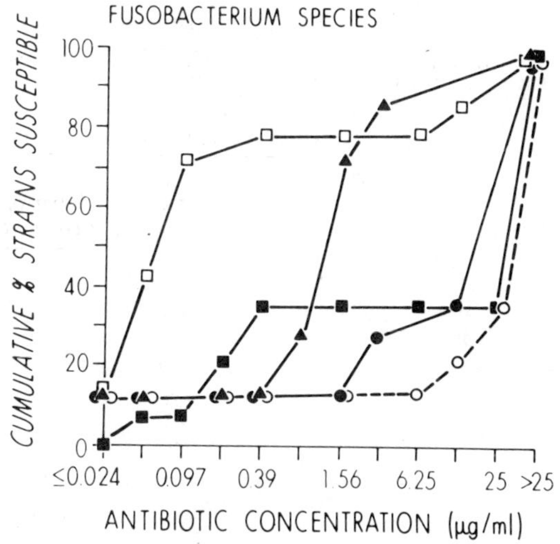

FIG. 3. *Cumulative percentage of strains of Fusobacterium sp. susceptible to varying concentrations of clindamycin (□), josamycin (○), erythromycin (●), penicillin (■), and chloramphenicol (▲).*

DISCUSSION

Our studies show that josamycin was active against a variety of gram-positive aerobes. Strausbaugh and colleagues (12) recently reported similar median minimal inhibitory concentrations of josamycin against *Streptococcus pneumoniae*, *Streptococcus pyrogenes*, and *Staphylococcus aureus*. Although josamycin was active against many gram-positive aerobes, it appeared to have no unique spectrum of activity.

Josamycin was quite active against the anaerobes, with the exception of *Fusobacterium* species. A mean of 75% of the gram-positive and other gram-negative anaerobes was inhibited by 1.56 μg or less of josamycin per ml. At 3.12 μg or less of josamycin per ml, 100% of *B. fragilis* were susceptible. These results confirm, and expand, previous data that revealed that josamycin was active against anaerobes, although only a small number of strains were tested in these studies (11, 12).

Presently, josamycin is available only as an oral preparation. After 750 mg of oral josamycin, mean peak serum concentrations range from 0.4 to 2.6 μg of josamycin per ml (2). At concentrations of ≤3.12 μg of antibiotic per ml, the activities of josamycin and clindamycin are similar (Table 4). At low concentrations (≤0.39 μg/ml) routinely achievable with oral therapy, many organisms would not be susceptible to josamycin. Our data suggest that, if there were an alternate form of josamycin, which assured at least moderately high concentrations in serum (≥3.12 μg/ml), then josamycin might be a useful antibiotic for treatment of anaerobic infections.

The anaerobes that were quite resistant to josamycin were the *Fusobacterium* species. Since these organisms are often involved in mixed anaerobic infections (5), it is not clear whether resistance of *Fusobacterium* species to josamycin would limit its potential role in suspected clinical anaerobic infections. However, somewhat unexpectedly, a majority of the 14 strains of *Fusobacterium* species tested was also resistant to penicillin. Members of the genus *Fusobacterium* isolated in this study were not identified as to species. Therefore, from our data it cannot be determined if one or several particular *Fusobacterium* species were more resistant than others to josamycin.

TABLE 3. *Gram-positive aerobes—susceptibilities to josamycin*[a]

Organism	MIC range (μg of josamycin/ml)	Median MIC
30 *Staphylococcus aureus*		
10 Penicillin susceptible	0.39–1.56	0.390
20 Pencillin resistant		
18 *S. epidermidis*		
9 Methicillin susceptible	≤0.024–0.78	0.195
9 Methicillin resistant	≤0.024–≥25	0.390
10 *Streptococcus pneumoniae*	≤0.024–0.195	0.097
15 *S. pyrogenes*	0.097–0.39	0.195
23 *S. agalactiae*	0.390–0.78	0.390

[a] Agar dilution minimal inhibitory concentrations (MIC).

TABLE 4. *Comparison of activity of josamycin and clindamycin at low and moderate antibiotic concentrations*

Organisms	No. of strains	Clindamycin		Josamycin	
		0.39 μg/ml	3.12 μg/ml	0.39 μg/ml	3.12 μg/ml
Peptococcus sp.	28	24	26	6	26
Peptostreptococcus sp.	15	10	15	5	12
Clostridium perfringens	18	12	18	4	18
Clostridium sp.	23	9	18	7	20
Bacteroides sp.	17	10	17	11	17
B. fragilis	30	26	30	2	30
Fusobacterium sp.	14	11	11	2	2

ACKNOWLEDGMENTS

We wish to thank Richard Robertson, David Bentley, Paula Migneault, and Judy Fitzgerald for their help in obtaining the clinical isolates, and Judy Closson and Margaret Christy for their help in preparing this manuscript.

This work was supported by a research grant from E. I. DuPont De Nemours and Co., Newark, Del.

LITERATURE CITED

1. **Balows, A., R. M. DeHaan, V. R. Dowell, and L. B. Guze (ed.).** 1972. Anaerobic bacteria—role in disease. Charles C Thomas Co., Springfield, Ill.
2. **Bergan, T., and B. Oydvin.** 1972. Pharmacokinetics of Josamycin—a new macrolide antibiotic. Pharmacology **7**:36–50.
3. **Dowell, V. R., Jr., and T. M. Hawkins.** 1974. Laboratory methods in anaerobic bacteriology. Center for Disease Control manual, DHEW publication no. (CDC) 74-8272, Atlanta.
4. **Fass, R. J.** 1974. Lincomycin and clindamycin, p. 83–94. *In* B. M. Kagan (ed.), Antimicrobial therapy. W. B. Saunders Co., Philadelphia.
5. **Finegold, S. M., J. Bartlett, A. W. Chow, D. J. Flora, S. L. Gorbach, E. J. Harder, and F. P. Tally.** 1975. Management of anaerobic infections. Ann. Intern. Med. **83**:375–389.
6. **Frankel, R. I.** 1975. Clindamycin-efficacy and toxicity. West. J. Med. **122**:526–530.
7. **Gorbach, S. L., and J. C. Bartlett.** 1974. Anaerobic infection. N. Engl. J. Med. **290**:1177–1184, 1237–1245, 1289–1294.
8. **Holdeman, L. V., and W. E. C. Moore (ed.).** 1972. Anaerobic laboratory manual. Virginia Polytechnic Institute and State University, Blacksburg.
9. **Keefee, E. B., R. M. Katon, T. T. Chan, C. S. Melnyle,**

and J. A. Benson, Jr. 1974. Pseudomembranous enterocolitis: resurgence related to newer antibiotic therapy. West. J. Med. **121**:462–472.
10. **Marr, J. J., M. D. Sans, and F. J. Tedesco.** 1975. Bacterial studies of clindamycin-associated colitis. Gastroenterology **69**:352–358.
11. **Osono, T., and H. Umezawa.** 1971. Josamycin, a new macrolide antibiotic of resistance non-inducing type, p. 41–120. *In*. S. Mitsuhasi (ed.), Drug action and drug resistance in bacteria. University of Tokyo Press, Tokyo.
12. **Strausbaugh, L. J., J. A. Dilworth, J. M. Gwaltney, Jr., and M. A. Sande.** 1976. In vitro susceptibility studies with josamycin and erythromycin. Antimicrob. Agents Chemother. **9**:546–548.
13. **Steers, E., E. L. Foltz, and B. J. Graves.** 1959. An inocula replicating apparatus for routine testing of bacterial susceptibility to antibiotics. Antibiot. Chemother. **9**:307–311.
14. **Sutter, V. L., H. R. Attebery, J. E. Rosenblatt, K. S. Bricknell, and S. M. Finegold.** 1972. Manual of anaerobic bacteriology. Department of Continuing Education in Health Sciences University Extension and the School of Medicine, University of California, Los Angeles.
15. **Tedesco, F. J., R. W. Barton, and D. J. Alpers.** 1974. Clindamycin-associated colitis: a prospective study. Ann. Intern. Med. **81**:429–433.
16. **Yunis, A. A.** 1973. Chloramphenicol-induced bone marrow suppression. Semin. Hematol. **10**:225–234.

ANTIMICROBIAL AGENTS AND CHEMOTHERAPY, Aug. 1976, p. 258-264

Vol. 10, No. 2
Printed in U.S.A.

New Plasmid-Mediated Nucleotidylation of Aminoglycoside Antibiotics in *Staphylococcus aureus*

F. LE GOFFIC,* A. MARTEL, M. L. CAPMAU, B. BACA, P. GOEBEL, H. CHARDON, C. J. SOUSSY, J. DUVAL, AND D. H. BOUANCHAUD

Centre d'Etude et de Recherche de Chimie Organique Appliquée, Centre National de la Recherche Scientifique, 94320 Thiais, Service de Bactériologie, Centre Hospitalier Universitaire Henri-Mondor, 94010 Créteil, and Institut Pasteur (Service de Bactériologie Médicale), 75015 Paris, France*

Received for publication 12 April 1976

A wild-type strain of *Staphylococcus aureus*, which inactivates a wide variety of aminoglycosides (except the gentamicin components), has been found to harbor a plasmid (RAp01) that mediates the biosynthesis of a nucleotidyltransferase. This enzyme modifies the 4'-hydroxy function of these antibiotics. The plasmid has been studied, the enzyme responsible for this resistance pattern has been isolated by affinity chromatography, and its kinetics and physicochemistry have been characterized. The target of this enzyme has also been located by demonstrating the structure of one inactivated compound, 4'-(*O*)-adenylyltobramycin.

A wide variety of plasmid-mediated enzymes that inactivate aminoglycosides by three types of reactions has been found in gram-negative bacteria (1, 11). Until recently, resistance of gram-positive bacteria to aminoglycosides has scarcely been examined; however, inactivation of kanamycin by a resistant strain of *Staphylococcus aureus* has been reported (5). This phenomenon was later demonstrated to be plasmid mediated (16). A lividomycin phosphotransferase has also been isolated from *S. aureus* strains (7). The phosphorylated product of this drug was found to be identical to that of *Escherichia coli* carrying an R plasmid that confers lividomycin resistance (8). Recently (15), a new plasmid has been found in another strain of *S. aureus*. It directs the inactivation of a wide variety of aminoglycosides by acetylation and adenylation (F. Le Goffic and A. Martel, unpublished data). We have also described recently a strain of *S. aureus* harboring a new nucleotidyltransferase that has been partially characterized; however, the origin of this enzyme was not clearly demonstrated (F. Le Goffic, B. Baca, C. J. Soussy, and J. Duval, Ann. Microbiol. Inst. Pasteur, in press).

We now report the characterization of a plasmid-mediated nucleotidyltransferase obtained from another clinical isolate of *S. aureus*. This strain is strongly resistant to paromomycin, neomycin, butyrosin, kanamycin, and tobramycin and slightly resistant to lividomycin and amikacin, but susceptible to gentamicin components. A plasmid mediating this resistance, referred to as RAp01, has been identified by ultracentrifugation and "curing" experiments (2). The aminoglycoside-modifying enzyme has been isolated, purified by affinity chromatography, and characterized.

MATERIALS AND METHODS

Bacterial strains. The resistant strain, an *S. aureus* referred to as Ap01, was a Chapman-positive and coagulase-positive strain; it had been isolated from an abscess and blood culture in the Hospital of Aix (France). Another strain of *S. aureus* (RN1304) was used in this study; it carries a tetracycline resistance plasmid referred to as T169 (13). "Curing" experiments were performed as previously described (2).

Chemicals and antibiotics. [^{14}C]adenosine 5'-triphosphate (ATP), [^{14}C]guanosine 5'-triphosphate (GTP), and [^{3}H]uridine 5'-triphosphate (UTP) were obtained from the Radiochemical Center, Amersham, England; [^{3}H]thymidine and [^{14}C]thymidine were from Commissariat à l'Energie Atomique (France); ATP, GTP, UTP, and ethidium bromide were purchased from Calbiochem. The antibiotics were provided by the following laboratories: gentamicin, sisomicin, gentamicin A: Unilabo; tobramycin and apramycin: Eli Lilly; kanamycin and amikacin: Allard-Bristol; neomycin: Upjohn; paromomycin and butyrosin: Parke, Davis & Co.; lividomycin: Roger Bellon; ribostamycin: Delalande; streptomycin and dihydrostreptomycin: Rhône-Poulenc.

Susceptibility to aminoglycoside antibiotics. The minimal inhibitory concentration (MIC) of various aminoglycoside antibiotics on *S. aureus* Ap01 and other strains was determined by the agar dilution method by using a Steer apparatus (10^4 to 10^5 bacteria per spot).

Enzymatic assays. The phosphocellulose (1, 11)

paper binding assay, which uses [^{14}C]nucleotidyltriphosphate, was employed in all assays during the enzyme extraction, purification, substrate studies, and electrofocusing experiments.

Enzyme preparation. *S. aureus* Ap01 (wild-type strain and a "cured" susceptible variant) was grown in Trypticase soy broth (Difco). The cells were collected by centrifugation and washed in buffer "A" [10 mM $MgCl_2$, 10 mM tris(hydroxymethyl)aminomethane [Tris], 60 mM NH_4Cl, 6 mM β-mercaptoethanol, pH 7.5] at 4°C. The cells were collected by centrifugation and disrupted by grinding in a mortar with 2.5 parts (wt/wt) of alumina powder. Broken cells were suspended in buffer A (2 ml/1 g), and cell debris were removed by centrifugation at 20,000 × *g* for 30 min. The enzyme was purified by ultracentrifugation of the supernatant for 2 h at 200,000 × *g*, followed by affinity chromatography on a column of immobilized kanamycin (10, 12), or directly by affinity chromatography as shown in Fig. 1.

Isolation of RAp01 plasmid DNA. For isolation of deoxyribonucleic acid (DNA) the resistant strain and a susceptible clone "cured" of RAp01 were grown in Trypticase soy broth and labeled for two generations in midlog phase with [^{3}H]thymidine and [^{14}C]thymidine, respectively. A culture of strain RN1304, carrying the T169 plasmid for tetracycline resistance, was also labeled with [^{14}C]thymidine. The cells were washed and treated by lysostaphin in 2.5 M NaCl (pH 7.0), as described by Novick and Bouanchaud (13), and then lysed with Sarkosine (Sigma) (6). The lysates were sheared with a 5-ml syringe equipped with a B-D Yale microlance (21G1/2) and then mixed with cesium chloride plus ethidium bromide (4). These mixtures were centrifuged for 48 h at 42,000 rpm in a Beckman 50Ti fixed-angle rotor (L2-65B Spinco ultracentrifuge). The resistant gradients were collected, and 10-μl portions were counted in 8 ml of a butyl-PBD-toluene-Triton X-100 scintillation liquid. In other cases, drops from the gradients were collected on 2.4-cm glass-fiber filters

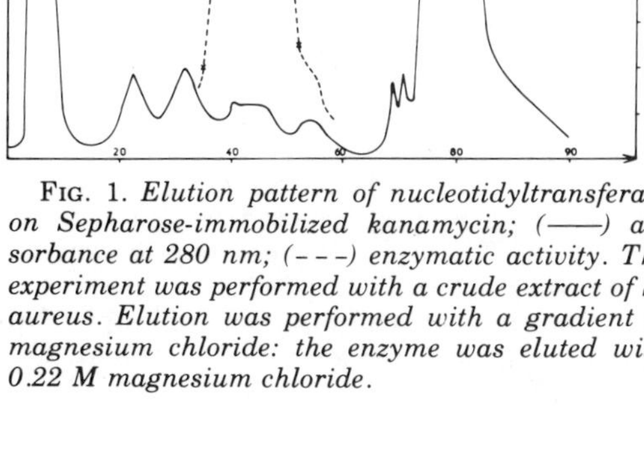

FIG. 1. *Elution pattern of nucleotidyltransferase on Sepharose-immobilized kanamycin; (——) absorbance at 280 nm; (- - -) enzymatic activity. The experiment was performed with a crude extract of S. aureus. Elution was performed with a gradient of magnesium chloride: the enzyme was eluted with 0.22 M magnesium chloride.*

(Whatman GF/C), which were dried and then washed twice in 5% trichloroacetic acid and twice in 95% ethanol and dried again. They were then counted in an Intertechnique scintillation counter.

Sucrose density gradients. Those fractions containing RAp01 or T169 DNA were pooled, and ethidium bromide was removed by five isopropanol extractions. DNA samples were dialyzed twice against 10^{-2} M Tris-10^{-3} M ethylenediaminetetraacetic acid (pH 7.5). Convenient volumes of RAp01 (^{3}H) and T169 (^{14}C) were mixed and layered onto 10 to 30% neutral sucrose gradients in 10^{-2} M tris, 10^{-3} M ethylenediaminetetraacetic acid, and 1 M NaCl (pH 7.4) and then sedimented at 20°C in a Beckman SW41 rotor at 45,000 rpm for 2 h. In other experiments, 5 to 20% sucrose gradients were used and sedimented for 1.5 h. The gradients were collected by dripping onto filters and counted as previously described.

Electrofocusing determination. The isoelectric point of the enzyme was determined using an LKB apparatus. The ampholines had a pH range from 3 to 10. The maximum energy applied to the column was 1.5 W. The enzymatic activity was located by using tobramycin and butyrosine B as substrates and [^{14}C]ATP as coenzyme.

Structural determination. The proton magnetic resonance and ^{13}C spectra were determined in D_2O at 90 mH_Z using a Brucker Instrument. The mass spectra were determined on a MS30 spectrometer at 28 eV and 200°. Per *N*-acetylated and per *O*-silylated derivatives were prepared (4) and used in this study.

RESULTS

The resistance pattern of *S. aureus* Ap01 to deoxystreptamin antibiotics is shown in Table 1 and compared with patterns of resistance conferred by reference plasmids that mediate inactivation of aminoglycoside antibiotics. This pattern is unusual and different from that associated with any of the previously described mechanisms of aminoglycoside inactivation (9).

Extracts of *S. aureus* Ap01 were prepared and assayed for their ability to catalyze modification of tobramycin, kanamycin, and other aminoglycosides. With [^{14}C]ATP as cofactor, it was found that an adenylphosphotransferase activity was present in the enzymatic preparations, whereas neither phosphorylation nor acetylation activity was detected.

The enzyme preparation was found to be stable on repeated freezing and thawing and could be purified by affinity chromatography on a column of Sepharose 4B-kanamycin using a gradient of MgCl as eluent (10, 12). The elution pattern of this enzyme is illustrated in Fig. 1. This enzyme is plasmid mediated as described below. We propose ANT(4′)I as a designation.

Isolation of plasmid DNA and size of RAp01 DNA molecules. A typical result obtained from dye-buoyant equilibrium centrifugation can be seen in Fig. 2a. The wild-type strain DNA gives

TABLE 1. *MICs of deoxystreptamine antibiotics for S. aureus Ap01 and reference plasmids*[a]

Strain[b]	R plasmid	MIC (μg/ml)[c]								
		BUT	LIV	NEO	PAR	KAN	TOB	GEN	SIS	AMI
S. aureus Ap01	RAp01	64	8	32	128	64	64	0.25	0.25	8
S. aureus Ap01	"Cured"	1	2	0.5	0.5	2	0.25	0.25	0.25	1
E. coli K-12		2	4	4	4	1	1	0.5	0.25	1
	R176	0.5	2	1	4	8	16	128	64	0.25
	R55	2	4	2	4	64	32	64	32	1
	R135	2	4	4	4	2	1	64	32	1
	R5	2	8	2	4	16	8	0.5	4	2
	R112	2	1,000	500	1,000	500	0.5	0.4	0.5	2
	JR66	250	4	500	1,000	1,000	128	64	16	4

[a] *S. aureus* Ap01 is susceptible to all other antibiotics, such as β lactamin and pristinamycin.
[b] The original strains CS2R5, JR66/W677, and LA290 R112 were obtained from H. Umezawa, J. Davies, and Y. A. Chabbert.
[c] BUT, Butyrosine; LIV, lividomycin; NEO, neomycin; GEN, gentamicin; SIS, sisomicin; AMI, amikacin.

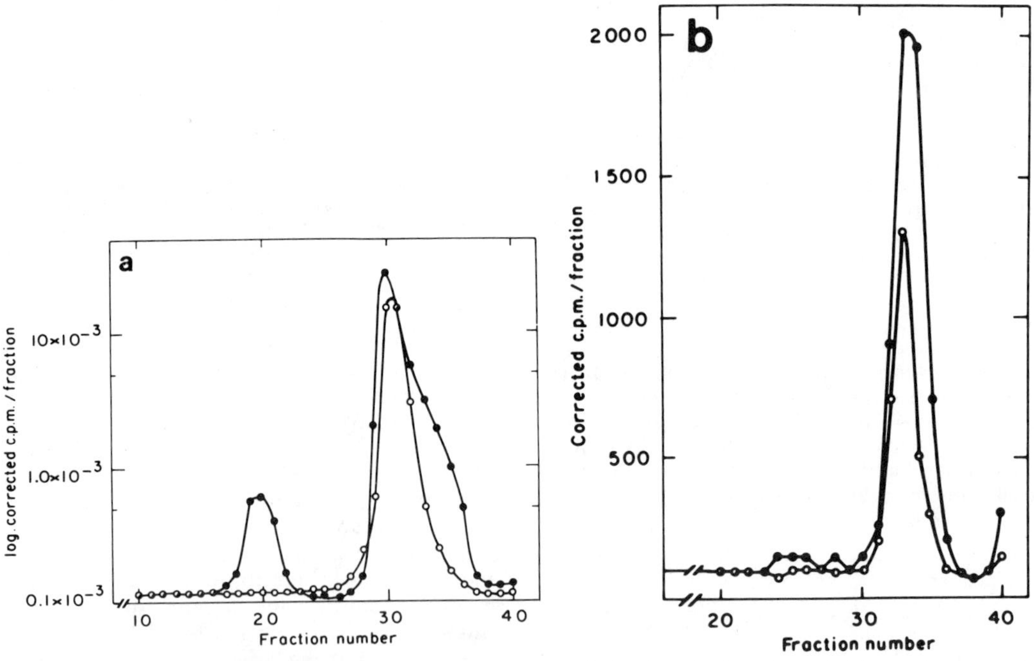

FIG. 2. *(a) Dye-buoyant density gradient analysis of the DNA of strain S. aureus Ap01 carrying plasmid RAp01 ([³H]thymidine; ●) and of a "cured" susceptible variant ([¹⁴C]thymidine; ○). Counts were corrected for double label. (b) Sedimentation analysis of RAp01 plasmid in neutral sucrose gradient (5 to 20%). Symbols: (●) RAp01 ([³H]thymidine labeled); (○) T169 ([¹⁴C]thymidine labeled).*

rise to a satellite peak, which represents 5% (±2%) of total DNA. This peak is not observed in a spontaneous susceptible variant of the wild type strain.

Analysis of plasmid DNA in neutral sucrose gradients demonstrated that RAp01 molecules were homogenous in size. After a 12-h dialysis, no form II (open circles) was observed (Fig. 2b). The sedimentation constant (and size) of form I (covalently closed circular) molecules were determined by using plasmid T169 (19.4*S*, 1.4 μm) as a reference. The sedimentation behavior of both plasmids can be seen in Fig. 2b. No detectable difference in velocity and size of RAp01 and T169 was observed in 10 to 30% sucrose gradients sedimented for 1.5 h (data not shown). The size of RAp01 can be estimated at 1.4 μm (molecular weight, 2.7 × 10⁶).

Estimation of the number of copies of RAp01 molecules per genome equivalent. Using the size of 1.4 μm for RAp01 molecules and previous estimations of the amount of chromosomal DNA per *S. aureus* cell (11, 15), we estimated at 50 to 70 the number of copies per cell, which is a minimum estimate, because a variable proportion of plasmid DNA is not detected in the assay procedure.

Preparation and purification of adenylylated tobramycin. The substrate activities (Table 2) of ANT(4')I suggest that the enzyme modifies the 4'-hydroxyl group, since the only compounds that are not substrates are the gentamicin components (gentamicin C_1, C_2, C_{1a}, sisomicin), whereas gentamicin A remains a substrate of the enzyme. The fact that neamine, kanamycin A or B, and tobramycin are also excellent substrates for this nucleotidylating enzyme further suggests that the modification might occur on the 4'-hydroxyl group of aminoglycoside antibiotics.

To confirm this hypothesis, tobramycin was inactivated by the *S. aureus* Ap01 enzyme by incubation with [^{14}C]ATP. The resulting mixture was purified by ion-exchange chromatography, as previously described, and the adenylylated tobramycin was eluted from a Biorex 70 column with 1.5 M NaCl (9). After application on a second Biorex column (ammonium form) and elution with 0.14 M ammonium bicarbonate, the product was collected and shown to be homogenous by thin-layer chromatography on silica gel.

Properties and structure determination of adenylyl tobramycin. Thin-layer chromatography on silica gel (methanol-ammoniac, 3:1) showed that *O*-[^{14}C]adenylyltobramycin produced by ANT(4')I was a single component (R_f −0.6) clearly distinct from tobramycin (R_f 0.35).

Elemental analysis of the inactivated product was as follows: calculated for $C_{28}H_{49}N_{15}O_{10}P \cdot 5\ H_2O$: C 37,92; H 6,70; N 15,79; P 3,49; found: C 37,37; H 5,91; N 15,55; P 3,11. This first result suggests that an adenosine 5'-monophosphate (AMP) residue is introduced on tobramycin. This is clearly proved by the ultraviolet spectrum, which has a maximum absorption at 260 nm.

The proton magnetic resonance spectrum is quite complex; however, two singlet hydrogen resonances are observed at 8.6 and 8.4 ppm. These signals are, respectively, those ($H—C_2$; $H—C_8$) of the adenine residue. An additional doublet is present at 6.3 ppm ($J_{H,H}$: 5 H_Z) due to the anomeric hydrogen of adenosine moiety.

The ^{13}C spectrum has been compared with those of tobramycin and AMP. The results are shown in Table 3 and demonstrate clearly that both residues, tobramycin and adenosine, are present in the inactivated product. The precise position of the AMP residue cannot be determined by this method.

The inactivated product was confirmed as 4'-

TABLE 2. *Efficiency of different aminoglycosides as substrates for ANT(4')I*[a]

Antibiotic	% Antibiotic adenylylated in assay
Kanamycin B	100
Kanamycin A	45
Amikacin	50
Tobramycin	90
Gentamicin B	70
Gentamicin A	35
Neamine	90
Neomycin B	30
Neomycin C	20
Paromomycin	15
Lividomycin	65
Butyrosin A	80
Butyrosin B	110
Ribostamycin	80
Gentamicin C_1	0
Gentamicin C_2	0
Gentamicin C_{1A}	0
Sisomicin	0
Apramycin	0

[a] All experiments were performed at pH 7.5 for 15 min at 37°C.

TABLE 3. *^{13}C nuclear magnetic resonance signals with tobramycin, ATP, and inactivated tobramycin*[a]

Tobramycin	Inactivated tobramycin	AMP
	159.4	
	154.8	155.9
	152.2	153.3
	138.9	149.3
	128.2	140.8
	99.8	118.9
99.2	99.2	
87.5	86.8	87.9
85.9	83.7	85.1
74.03	83.04	
73.3	74.4	75.4
71.8	73.8	71.4
71.3	72.4	
68.9	68.5	
66	66.5	64.4
60.1	64.5	
53.9	59.6	
50.2	54.3	
49.2	52.3	
49.0	48.1	
41.5	40.8	
35.1	30.7	
35.9		

[a] Spectra were determined in D_2O solution on a Brucker instrument.

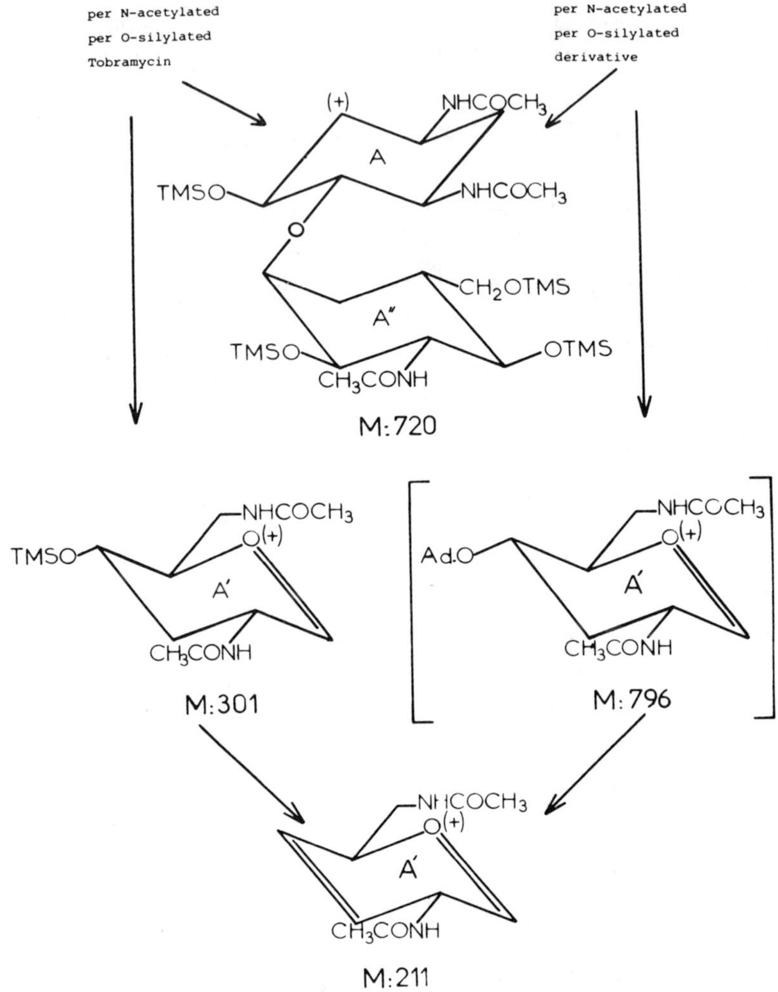

FIG. 3. *Structure of the two main fragments found in the mass spectrum of inactivated tobramycin after per O-silylation and per N-acetylation.*

(*O*)-adenyltobramycin by the analysis of mass spectra of both per *N*-acetylated-per *O*-silylated tobramycin and the inactivated compound.

The mass spectrum of per *N*-acetylated-per *O*-silylated tobramycin harbors three characteristic peaks at *m/e* 720, *m/e* 301, and *m/e* 211, which locate, respectively, ion (A-A″), ion (A′), and an ion coming from the elimination of trimethylsylanol (TMSOH) in ion (A′) (Fig. 3). The mass spectrum of per *N*-acetylated-per *O*-silylated-inactivated tobramycin reveals two characteristic peaks at *m/e* 720 and *m/e* 211. The peak characteristic of the adenylylated (A′) residue is missing in this spectrum (ion between brackets of *m/e* 796). However, this labile moiety gives, by elimination of AMP residue, a sharp peak at *m/e* 211. This proves clearly that the AMP group is located on the 4′-HO function of the molecule.

Characteristics of the enzymatic nucleotidylation of aminoglycoside antibiotics. A number of aminoglycosides with 4′-hydroxyl group were tested as substrates and were found to vary in their susceptibility to the enzyme (Table 2). Compounds without the 4′-hydroxyl function were not substrates. Three cofactors, [^{14}C]ATP, [^{14}C]GTP, and [^{3}H]UTP, were also used as potential nucleotidyl donors. The results are summarized in Table 4.

The influence of pH on the activity of this new nucleotidyltransferase was studied. The activity was optimum at pH 6 for amikacin and pH 4.5 for tobramycin (Fig. 4). Such effects have also been found for AAC(6′) and AAC(2′)

TABLE 4. *Efficiency of three cofactors as nucleotidyl donors for ANT(4')I*[a]

Cofactors	% Antibiotic adenylylated in assay
ATP	100
GTP	144
UTP	76

[a] All experiments were performed at 37°C for 10 min in veronal buffer (pH 5) containing 10 mM $MgCl_2$ and 10 mM dithiothreitol. Tobramycin, 5 nmol, was incubated with 50 nmol of cofactor and 20 μl of the enzyme.

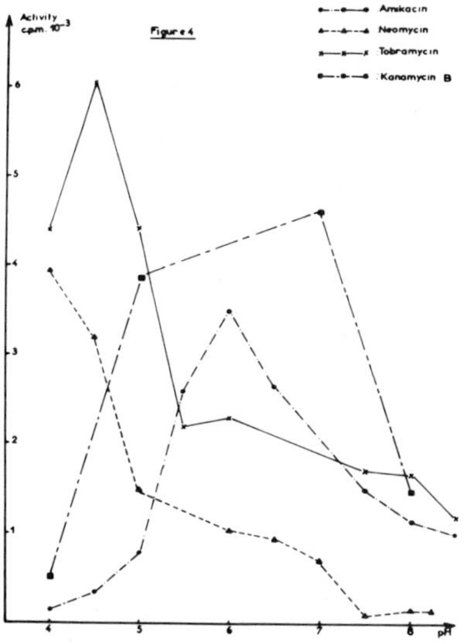

FIG. 4. *pH dependence of adenylation reactions with ANT(4')I. Reaction mixtures were prepared at the indicated pH using the appropriate veronal buffer. Symbols: (○) amikacin; (△) neomycin; (×) tobramycin; (■) kanamycin B.*

and are not clearly explained.

The isoelectric point of the enzyme was also determined. The enzymatic activity was located by using two antibiotics. Its value was pI 5.1 (Fig. 5).

DISCUSSION

S. aureus Ap01 is a naturally occurring strain highly resistant to five classical aminoglycosidic drugs (kanamycin, neomycin, paromomycin, tobramycin, and butyrosine) and slightly resistant to lividomycin and amikacin. The gene(s) which mediates resistance to these antibiotics has been shown to be located on a plasmid, referred to as RAp01. The resistance characters are lost spontaneously and simultaneously at a rather high frequency (10^{-2} to 10^{-3} per cell). No extrachromosomal DNA is found in susceptible clones. RAp01 is a small plasmid (1.4 μm, or 2.7×10^6 daltons), which encodes a nucleotidyltransferase, responsible for the inactivation of aminoglycosidic antibiotics. Like other small plasmids in *S. aureus,* as well as in coliform bacteria, RAp01 appears to replicate under relaxed control, with a minimal estimate of 50 copies of plasmid per cell.

The nucleotidyltransferase has been partially purified and examined. The determination of the isoelectric point of this enzyme by using two different substrates in the detection of the activity suggests that the enzymatic preparation is homogenous. At that stage of purification, it was possible to compare the efficiency of different substrates to bind covalently an AMP or a nucleotidyl residue. The results, which are summarized in Table 2, show that there are requirements for the fitting of the substrates to the active site of the enzyme.

The deoxystreptamine moiety is the first requirement for the compound to be a substrate: streptomycin, dihydrostreptomycin, or apramycin are not adenylylated. A number of functions appear also to be important. The 2'-amino group, found, for instance, in kanamycin B or tobramycin, apparently promotes esterification; kanamycin A, which lacks this function at the 2' site, is not a very good substrate for this enzyme. The enzyme has another striking feature. An hydroxyaminobutyric acid arm lo-

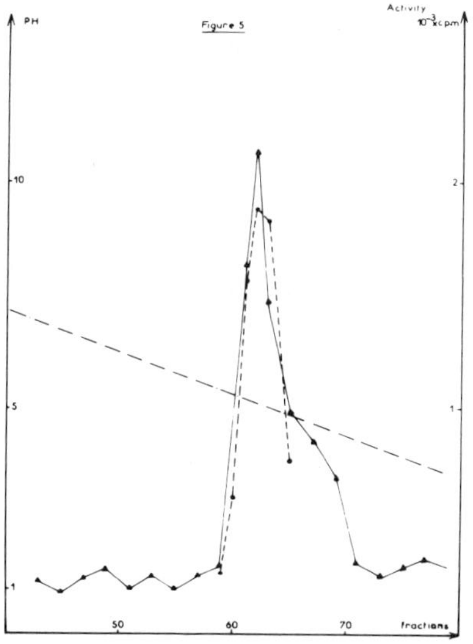

FIG. 5. *Isoelectric point determination of ANT(4')I. Enzymatic activity was detected by the chemical phosphocellulose paper binding assay. Enzymatic activity found with tobramycin (- - -); enzymatic activity found with butyrosine (——).*

cated on the 1-NH_2 function, which until now made amikacin resistant to almost every enzyme known, is inefficient in the enzymatic assay: amikacin is as good a substrate as kanamycin A, and ribostamycin is a worse substrate than butyrosine A or B. The structure of the nucleotidyl donor is not very critical; ATP, GTP, or UTP is well recognized by the enzyme, as shown in Table 4. A comparison of Tables 1 and 2 shows an apparent paradox for lividomycin and amikacin resistance. *S. aureus* Ap01 is slightly resistant to these antibiotics, but these drugs are adenylylated to the same extent as butyrosine. This can perhaps be explained by the fact that the MIC values are dependent not only on substrate susceptibility and rate of enzymatic inactivation, but also on the rate of accumulation by the whole cell.

It can be concluded that the plasmid-mediated enzyme described here represents a new class of nucleotidyltransferases, which are able to inactivate aminoglycosides possessing a 4′-hydroxyl group, even if they harbor an hydroxyaminobutyric acid arm residue at the 1-amino site.

ACKNOWLEDGMENTS

This work was supported in part by grants from le Centre National de la Recherche Scientifique, l'Institut National de la Santé et de la Recherche Médicale (CRAT–75.4.442.50), la Fondation pour la Recherche Médicale Française, et la Fondation de l'Industrie Pharmaceutique pour la Recherche (contract 75-04).

We wish to thank Gilda Bieth for excellent technical assistance.

LITERATURE CITED

1. **Benveniste, R., and J. Davies.** 1973. Mechanisms of antibiotics resistance in bacteria. Annu. Rev. Biochem. 42:471–506.
2. **Bouanchaud, D. H., M. R. Scavizzi, and Y. A. Chabbert.** 1969. Elimination by ethidium bromide of antibiotic resistance in enterobacteria and staphylococcus. J. Gen. Microbiol. 54:417–425.
3. **Davies, J. E., and R. Rownd.** 1972. Transmissible multiple drug resistance in Enterobacteriaceae. Science 76:758–768.
4. **Dejongh, D. C., E. B. Hills, J. D. Hribar, S. Hanessian, and T. Chang.** 1973. A mass spectral investigation of derivatives of kanamycin A. Tetrahedron 29:2707–2713.
5. **Doi, O., M. Miyamoto, N. Tanuka, and H. Umezawa.** 1968. Inactivation and phosphorylation of kanamycin by drug-resistant *Staphylococcus aureus*. Appl. Microbiol. 16:1282–1284.
6. **Ingram, L. C., M. R. Richmond, and R. B. Sykes.** 1973. Molecular characterization of R factors implicated in the carbenicillin resistance of a sequence of *Pseudomonas aeruginosa* strains isolated from burns. Antimicrob. Agents Chemother. 3:279–288.
7. **Kobayashi, F., K. Tomoynki, E. Junji, Y. Yoko, and S. Mitsuhashi.** 1973. Lividomycin resistance in *Staphylococcus* by enzymatic phosphorylation. Antimicrob. Agents Chemother. 4:1–5.
8. **Kondo, S., H. Yamamoto, H. Nuganawa, H. Umezawa, and S. Mitsuhashi.** 1972. Isolation and characterisation of lividomycin A inactivated by *Pseudomonas aeruginosa* and *Escherichia coli* carrying R factor. J. Antibiot. 25:483–485.
9. **Le Goffic, F., A. Martel, and J. Witchitz.** 1974. 3-N enzymatic acetylation of gentamicin, tobramycin, and kanamycin by *Escherichia coli* carrying an R factor. Antimicrob. Agents Chemother. 6:680–684.
10. **Le Goffic, F., and N. Moreau.** 1973. Purification by affinity chromatography of an enzyme involved in gentamicin inactivation. FEBS Lett. 29:289–291.
11. **Le Goffic, F., and N. Moreau.** 1975. Enzymes actives sur les antibiotiques aminosidiques, p. 147–175. *In* Actualités de chimie thérapeutique, 3ème série. Edifor, France.
12. **Le Goffic, F., N. Moreau, and M. Chevreau.** 1973. Purification par chromatographie d'affinité d'une acétyltransférase et d'une phosphotransférase inactivant les antibiotiques aminosidiques. Biochimie 55:1183–1185.
13. **Novick, R. P., and D. H. Bouanchaud.** 1971. Extrachromosomal nature of drug resistance in *Staphylococcus aureus*. Ann. N.Y. Acad. Sci. 181:279–294.
14. **Novick, R. P., L. Wyman, D. H. Bouanchaud, and E. Murphy.** 1975. Plasmid life circles in *Staphylococcus aureus*, p. 115–129. *In* D. Schlessinger (ed.), Microbiology–1974. American Society for Microbiology, Washington, D.C.
15. **Soussy, C. J., D. H. Bouanchaud, J. Fouace, A. Dublanchet, and J. Duval.** 1975. A gentamicin resistant plasmid in *Staphylococcus aureus*. Ann. Microbiol. Inst. Pasteur 126B:91–94.
16. **Stiffler, P. M., H. M. Sweeney, M. Schneider, and S. Cohen.** 1974. Isolation and characterization of a kanamycin resistance plasmid from *Staphylococcus aureus*. Antimicrob. Agents Chemother. 6:516–520.

ANTIMICROBIAL AGENTS AND CHEMOTHERAPY, Aug. 1976, p. 265-273
Vol. 10, No. 2
Printed in U.S.A.

Nutrition of *Bacillus brevis* ATCC 9999, the Producer of Gramicidin S[1]

E. J. VANDAMME[2] AND A. L. DEMAIN*

Department of Nutrition and Food Science, Massachusetts Institute of Technology, Cambridge, Massachusetts 02139

Received for publication 5 April 1976

The nutrition of the gramicidin S (GS) producer *Bacillus brevis* ATCC 9999 was studied with respect to growth and antibiotic production. In a complex medium containing yeast extract and peptone, only glycerol, D-fructose, and *meso*-inositol contributed to growth, whereas other hexoses, pentoses, polyols, polysaccharides, and organic acids were inactive. Glycerol and fructose were inhibitory to GS formation; inositol had no effect. In chemically defined media containing a mixture of five amino acids (glutamine, methionine, proline, arginine, and histidine) necessary for good growth, again only glycerol, D-fructose, and *meso*-inositol served as effective carbon sources for growth. With respect to antibiotic formation, inositol was much poorer than glycerol or fructose. In the presence of glycerol and the five amino acids, addition of 0.1% L-phenylalanine specifically stimulated GS production. Growth kinetics in this defined medium showed two phases: early and rapid growth at the expense of the amino acid mixture, followed by glycerol utilization after a diauxic lag of 2 to 3 h; inositol utilization suffered a much longer lag period. GS formation was initiated after the diauxic lag. Ammonium sulfate was the best individual nitrogen source, but the combination of the five growth-stimulatory amino acids was more potent for GS production. The level of potassium phosphate influenced GS production. High levels stimulated the growth rate but progressively inhibited GS production. Methionine was the best sulfur source. A defined medium (F3/6) that supported rapid exponential growth ($\mu = 0.53\ h^{-1}$) followed by progressively slower growth over a 30- to 40-h period was devised containing fructose, six amino acids, and mineral salts. GS formation was initiated as the cells left the exponential growth phase and reached high levels (1,500 mg of GS per liter; 0.19 mg of GS/mg of dry cell weight) after 40 to 50 h of incubation.

The biosynthesis of the cyclic decapeptide antibiotic gramicidin S (GS) by certain strains of *Bacillus brevis* has been the subject of extensive research in the last decade (15, 16, 18). These studies have led to the discovery of a nonribosomal process for peptide biosynthesis. GS, which consists of two identical pentapeptides (DPhe-LPro-LVal-LOrn-LLeu), is synthesized by two enzymes in the presence of adenosine 5′-triphosphate and Mg^{2+}. Synthetase II (molecular weight, 100,000) activates and racemizes L-phenylalanine, whereas synthetase I (molecular weight, 280,000) activates L-proline, L-valine, L-ornithine, and L-leucine. In sequence, each amino acid is translocated from its activation site to its specific thiol site prior to peptide formation. Elongation to a pentapeptide occurs with the aid of the cofactor 4′-phosphopantetheine, which is tightly bound to synthetase I. Subsequently, two pentapeptides cyclize to form GS. The two synthetases are produced during the transition period between log phase and stationary phase and then rapidly disappear (19).

A comparative survey of the nutrition of mesophilic *Bacillus* species (13, 20) established the following as characteristic nutritional patterns for *B. brevis*: growth in the absence of vitamins but a requirement for mixtures of amino acids. Since then, only a few reports on the nutritional requirements of *Bacillus* species have been published (1, 27).

Three strains of *B. brevis* have been used for studies on GS biosynthesis: the Nagano strain in Japan, strain GB (7) in the Soviet Union,

[1] Contribution no. 2957 of the Department of Nutrition and Food Science, Massachusetts Institute of Technology, Cambridge, MA 02139.

[2] Present address: Laboratory of General and Industrial Microbiology, University of Gent, 9000-Gent, Belgium.

and ATCC 9999 in the rest of the world. Most studies have been done with complex media. Chemically defined media for the ATCC 9999 strain were used by Eikhom et al. (5), Gevers et al. (8), and recently by Matteo et al. (19), but GS production was low under such conditions. The GB strain has been the subject of intensive nutritional research, and chemically defined media have been developed which support high GS production (14, 25, 28, 29). However, these media are not suitable for the ATCC 9999 strain. We felt that a chemically defined medium supporting a reasonably high level of GS production by strain ATCC 9999 was important for an understanding of the dynamics of growth and GS formation and of the regulatory mechanisms involved in the biosynthesis of this secondary metabolite. In the present report, we discuss our work on the nutrition of *B. brevis* ATCC 9999 which has resulted in the development of such a defined medium.

MATERIALS AND METHODS

Details concerning the maintenance of *B. brevis* ATCC 9999 and the preparation of spores were given previously (19). The spore suspension contained 6 × 10^8 spores per ml by viable cell counts. Fermentations in complex medium utilized spores germinated in the germination medium of Matteo et al. (19). In the case of defined media, the germination medium was the same as the respective fermentation medium. Conditions employed for germination, fermentation, and GS assays were as described previously (19).

The basal complex fermentation medium was the YP medium (5% yeast extract, 5% peptone [Difco]) of Matteo et al. (19). The starting chemically defined medium was their G2T5 medium (Table 1). Compositions of the key media developed in these studies are given in Table 1. In all cases, the pH was adjusted to 7.4 with 1 N HCl before autoclaving at 121°C for 20 min. Phosphate buffers and carbon sources were autoclaved separately. Growth and GS production took place at 37°C in 500-ml baffled Erlenmeyer flasks at 250 rpm on a rotary shaker (2-inch [ca. 5 cm] diameter orbit). After inoculation with cells from the germination media, the flasks were examined at various times up to 120 h. In the best media, however, the fermentation was complete by 48 h. For growth, pH, and GS determinations, a small amount of whole broth was removed from the flasks. Growth was measured with a Klett-Summerson colorimeter using a red filter, after appropriate dilutions. It was found that 250 Klett units correspond to 1 g of dry cell weight (DCW) per liter.

RESULTS

Effect of carbon sources in complex medium. At the start of our investigation, the complex medium that was best for GS production was YP medium (19). It yielded rapid and extensive growth and high levels of GS. In view of the finding (19) that addition of glucose did not increase growth or antibiotic formation, we decided to examine a wide range of carbon sources.

Before testing carbon sources, we studied the effect of lowering the concentration of yeast extract and peptone in YP medium. However, this resulted in decreased growth and antibiotic formation followed by extensive lysis of the culture. In full-strength YP medium, we observed a short lag phase followed by exponential growth over a period of 3 to 4 h at a specific growth rate of 1.2 h^{-1}. Growth then slowed down and cell density reached a maximum at 24 h. During this time, pH rose from neutrality to 8.2 to 9.0. GS formation began at the end of

TABLE 1. *Composition of chemically defined media used in this study*

Component	Amt/liter					
	G2T5	G2T6	1%G2T6	G3T6	G3/6	F3/6
D-Fructose						10 g
Glycerol	25 g	25 g	10 g	10 g	10 g	
$(NH_4)_2SO_4$	12 g	12 g	12 g			
K_2HPO_4	6.5 g	6.5 g	6.5 g	6.5 g	6.5 g	6.5 g
KH_2PO_4	1.7 g	1.7 g	1.7 g	1.7 g	1.7 g	1.7 g
$MgCl_2 \cdot 6H_2O$	203 mg	203 mg	203 mg	203 mg	203 mg	203 mg
$CaCl_2 \cdot 2H_2O$	103 mg	103 mg	103 mg	103 mg	103 mg	103 mg
$MnCl_2 \cdot 4H_2O$	10 mg	10 mg	10 mg	10 mg	10 mg	10 mg
$FeCl_3 \cdot 6H_2O$	0.27 mg	0.27 mg	0.27 mg	0.27 mg	0.27 mg	0.27 mg
Tris	12 g	12 g	12 g	12 g		
L-Proline	1.5 g	1.5 g	1.5 g	1.5 g	1.5 g	1.5 g
L-Histidine	1.3 g	1.3 g	1.3 g	1.3 g	1.3 g	1.3 g
L-Glutamine	1.3 g	1.3 g	1.3 g	1.3 g	1.3 g	1.3 g
L-Methionine	0.5 g	0.5 g	0.5 g	0.5 g	0.5 g	0.5 g
L-Arginine	3.0 g	3.0 g	3.0 g	3.0 g	3.0 g	0.3 g
L-Phenylalanine		1.0 g	1.0 g	1.0 g	1.0 g	1.0 g

exponential phase, and the antibiotic was produced rapidly throughout the transition between the logarithmic and stationary phases (Fig. 1).

The effects of polysaccharides, disaccharides, hexoses, pentoses, polyols, and acids are shown in Table 2. All sugars tested failed to stimulate growth with the exception of fructose. The only other effective carbon sources were glycerol and *meso*-inositol. Of these three carbon sources, only inositol increased growth without inhibiting GS formation. None of the growth-stimulatory carbon sources increased the rate of growth, only its extent.

Effect of carbon sources in chemically defined medium. Prior to the studies in this laboratory, there had been only a limited amount of work done on development of chemically defined media for GS production by *B. brevis* ATCC 9999. Eikhom et al. (5) used a defined medium containing glutamate as the major carbon source, the five constituent amino acids of GS, eight vitamins, and mineral salts. Although GS production only amounted to ca. 200 mg/liter in this medium, it has been widely used for enzyme studies (6, 17, 18). Previous work in our laboratory led to the development of a simple, defined medium containing glycerol, ammonium sulfate, and mineral salts

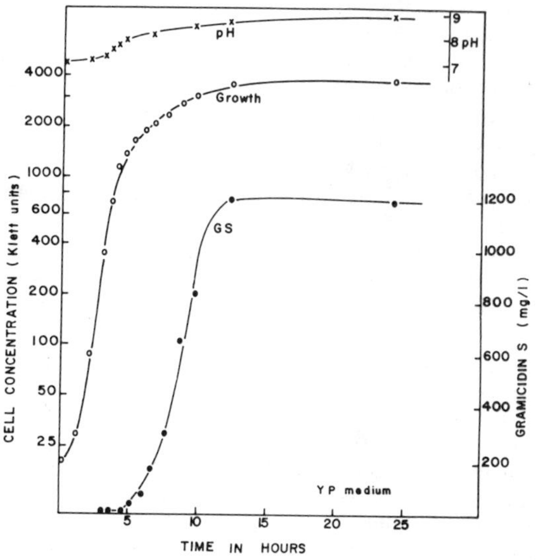

FIG. 1. *Pattern of the GS fermentation in complex medium YP.*

TABLE 2. *Effect of carbon sources[a] on growth in complex (YP) medium*

Type	Growth stimulatory effect	Ineffective effect	Growth inhibitiory effect
Polysaccharides		Soluble starch	
		Dextrin	
Disaccharides		D-Lactose	
		D-Maltose	
		Sucrose	
		D-Cellobiose	
		D-Trehalose	
Hexoses	D-Fructose	D-Glucose	L-Sorbose
		D-Galactose	
		D-Mannose	
Pentoses		L-Rhamnose	L-Arabinose
			D-Ribose
			D-Xylose
Polyols	Glycerol		
	meso-Inositol	D-Mannitol	
		Sorbitol	
		meso-Erythritol	
Organic acids		Sodium lactate	
		Sodium tartrate	Sodium acetate
			Sodium citrate
			Sodium succinate
			Sodium oxalate
			Sodium pyruvate
			Sodium α-ketoglutarate

[a] All carbon sources were tested at 2.5% (wt/vol).

suitable for chemostat studies and of an enriched defined medium (G2T5) supporting rapid and extensive growth (19). This latter medium contained glycerol, ammonium sulfate, five growth-stimulatory amino acids (L-glutamine, L-methionine, L-proline, L-arginine, and L-histidine), tris(hydroxymethyl)aminomethane (Tris) buffer, and mineral salts; only the proline is a component of the GS molecule. Despite extensive growth, medium G2T5 supported only poor GS production (230 mg/liter; 0.046 mg/mg of DCW).

As a basal defined medium, medium G2T5 less glycerol was used for further examination of the carbon nutrition of *B. brevis* ATCC 9999. This basal medium was found to be capable of supporting a small amount of growth (1.4 g of DCW/liter) but no detectable GS production (<20 mg/liter; <0.02 mg/mg of DCW). Carbon sources were added at the 2.5% level, and their effects on growth and GS production were determined. As observed in the complex medium, a large number of carbohydrates, polyalcohols, and organic acids failed to support growth. Again, glycerol, D-fructose, and inositol were the best carbon sources; a small amount of growth with little to no GS formation was supported by some organic acids (Table 3).

TABLE 3. *Effect of carbon sources added to chemically defined medium G2T5 less glycerol*

Additive at 2.5% (wt/vol)[a]	DCW (g/liter)	GS (mg/liter)	GS (mg/mg of DCW)
None	1.4	<20	<0.020
Glycerol[b]	8.8	230	0.046
meso-Inositol	7.0	140	0.030
Sodium pyruvate	3.0	20	0.007
Sodium lactate	2.2	<20	<0.010
Sodium succinate	2.1	<20	<0.010

[a] Growth was not increased by starch, dextrin, sucrose, D-lactose, D-maltose, D-trehalose, D-cellobiose, D-glucose, D-galactose, D-mannose, L-arabinose, L-rhamnose, sorbitol, D-mannitol, sodium acetate, sodium citrate, sodium α-ketoglutarate, or sodium tartrate. Growth was inhibited by L-sorbose and D-xylose.

[b] Medium G2T5.

Impressed by the excellent growth and GS production in the complex medium, we also tested amino acids as major carbon sources. Some were fairly good for growth. The best was L-valine, which yielded 5.8 g of DCW/liter, with GS amounting to 80 mg/liter and 0.014 mg/mg of DCW. Unfortunately, it is difficult to compare them with carbohydrates since amino acids also supply nitrogen and *B. brevis* has a complicated pattern of nitrogen nutrition (see below), with amino nitrogen being favored over inorganic nitrogen. L-Glutamine, L-alanine, and L-arginine were the best single amino acids serving as carbon sources for specific production of GS (0.046, 0.039, and 0.029 mg of GS/mg of DCW, respectively). However, they supported only little growth, and thus their volumetric GS titers (120, 130, and 60 mg/liter, respectively) were not as impressive as that obtained with glycerol.

Effect of utilizable carbon soruces in the presence of L-phenylalanine. L-Phenylalanine, the substrate of GS synthetase II, stimulates GS production, acting as a limiting precursor rather than a regulatory effector (4). In the absence of carbohydrate, phenylalanine did not increase GS production either at a low (0.1%) or a high (2.5%) concentration in the present studies. In the presence of glycerol at 2.5%, L-phenylalanine markedly stimulated GS production (580 mg/liter; 0.108 mg/mg of DCW) without affecting growth, its optimum concentration being 0.1%. The medium containing phenylalanine was called G2T6.

The effect of varying the concentration of glycerol from 0.5 to 5% in medium G2T6 showed 1% to be optimal. In the same experiments, similar concentrations of *meso*-inositol were examined. Although 1% was also the best concentration of inositol, performance in inositol was much poorer than that observed with glycerol. With medium modifications that featured elimination of all amino acids or all except phenylalanine, again glycerol was superior to inositol. Similarly, when ammonium salts were eliminated from the medium and the nitrogen source was the amino acid mixture, glycerol was the better carbon source. Performance on inositol was not improved relative to glycerol even when the carbon source for inoculum development was changed to inositol. Experiments comparing glycerol and fructose will be described below.

At this stage in our studies, we adopted medium 1%G2T6, containing 1% glycerol, for further work. This medium supported production of 670 mg of GS/liter and 0.116 mg of GS/mg of DCW.

Nitrogen nutrition. Medium 1%G2T6 contained the following nitrogenous constituents: $(NH_4)_2SO_4$, five growth-stimulatory amino acids (histidine, proline, glutamine, arginine, and methionine), and one amino acid stimulating GS formation (phenylalanine). To determine the effect of nitrogen sources on growth and GS formation, the $(NH_4)_2SO_4$ and the five growth-stimulatory amino acids were removed, and nitrogen sources were tested in this basal medium. Elimination of only the $(NH_4)_2SO_4$

TABLE 4. *Effect of nitrogen sources on growth and GS formation in medium 1%G2T6 less $(NH_4)_2SO_4$ and 5AA* [a]

Variation	Additive[a]	DCW (g/liter)	GS (mg/liter)	GS (mg/mg of DCW)
1	None[b]	0.6	<20	<0.030
2	$(NH_4)_2SO_4$	3.4	100	0.039
3	NH_4Cl	1.3	<20	<0.020
4	$(NH_4)_2HPO_4$	1.4	<20	<0.020
5	NH_4NO_3	1.4	<20	<0.020
6	5AA[c]	6.2	670	0.114
7	$(NH_4)_2SO_4$ + 5AA[d]	6.7	670	0.116
8	Sheffield acid-hydrolyzed casein	8.3	740	0.098
9	L-Glutamine	1.0	<20	<0.020
10	L-Valine	1.5	<20	<0.020
11	L-Arginine	1.8	<20	<0.020
12	Ammonium oxalate	2.4	<20	<0.010
13	Ammonium succinate	2.0	20	0.014
14	Ammonium lactate	1.4	<20	<0.020
15	Urea	1.3	<20	<0.020

[a] Not utilized were ammonium sulfamate, potassium nitrate, L-histidine, L-proline, L-methionine, and ammonium acetate. Ammonium citrate inhibited growth.

[b] The basal medium contained 1% glycerol, Tris, mineral salts, 0.1% L-phenylalanine [medium 1%G2T6 less $(NH_4)_2SO_4$ and five amino acids]. Nitrogen sources other than the five growth-stimulatory amino acids were added at a nitrogen level equivalent to that of 12 g of $(NH_4)_2SO_4$/liter.

[c] 5AA refers to the five growth-stimulatory amino acids: L-histidine, 1.3 g/liter; L-proline, 1.5 g/liter; L-glutamine, 1.3 g/liter; L-arginine, 3.0 g/liters; L-methionine, 0.5 g/liter.

[d] 1%G2T6 medium.

from medium 1%G2T6 had no effect as long as the five amino acids were still present (Table 4, variation 6 versus 7). On the other hand, elimination of the five amino acids drastically limited growth (variation 7 versus 2). The small amount of growth (0.6 g of DCW/liter) in the basal medium (variation 1) was evidently due to the presence of 0.1% L-phenylalanine. In the presence of $(NH_4)_2SO_4$ (variation 2), there was moderate growth (3.4 g of DCW/liter) and GS formation (100 mg/liter; 0.039 mg/mg of DCW). All other ammonium salts tested, inorganic or organic, were poorer than $(NH_4)_2SO_4$ (variations 3, 4, 5, 12, 13, and 14 versus 2). Six amino acids were tested individually: L-valine and the five amino acids previously found to stimulate growth. None was impressive alone as a major nitrogen source; three are listed in Table 4 (variations 9 through 11). Together, the five amino acids were extremely potent (variation 6) and were even better than casein hydrolysate (variation 8) with respect to specific GS production.

For further studies, ammonium sulfate was eliminated from the medium, and the five growth-stimulatory amino acids were included at their original concentration, which was found to be optimal. The new medium was called G3T6. Fermentation dynamics in this medium are shown in Fig. 2 along with those of modified media in which glycerol was omitted or replaced with inositol. These results indicate that *B. brevis* ATCC 9999 grew initially at the expense of the amino acid mixture followed by a lag period. The lag was rather short in the case of glycerol but was considerably longer in the case of inositol. These experiments also show that GS formation was initiated only after the diauxic lag.

Phosphorus nutrition. Phosphorus sources were compared at 50 mM with the mixture of K_2HPO_4 and KH_2PO_4 present in medium G3T6. $(NH_4)_2HPO_4$ and $NH_4H_2PO_4$ were comparable to potassium phosphate with respect to extent of growth and GS formation, but growth was slower. The ammonium salt of acetyl phosphate was similar to ammonium phosphate in supporting growth, but GS formation was somewhat depressed. Adenylic acid (2′,3′) was not utilized by *B. brevis*. Inorganic pyrophosphate (PP_i) was interesting in that it supported more rapid growth than did any other phosphorus compound, but GS formation was inhibited by about 65%. This inhibition could be due to the fact that pyrophosphate is an end product of GS biosynthesis:

$$\text{10 amino acids} + \text{10 ATP} \xrightarrow[\text{Mg}^{2+}]{\text{GS synthetases I and II}} \text{1 GS} + \text{10 AMP} + \text{10 PP}_i$$

An examination of the effect of potassium phosphate concentrations on fermentation dynamics (Fig. 3) suggested that GS formation is under phosphate control. The rate of growth was higher at 100 to 300 mM potassium phosphate than at the control concentration of 50 mM, yet GS formation was progressively inhibited by these higher levels of phosphate. Whether this is due to a genuine regulatory effect of phosphate, to a potassium effect, or to the slight pH differences shown in Fig. 3 remains to be established. At levels lower than 50 mM (not shown), pH values dropped to 5.0 to 5.5 and growth was inhibited markedly.

It is interesting that, although the growth rate was lower at 50 mM phosphate than at higher levels, the ultimate cell level was highest at 50 mM and progressively lower as phosphate concentration was raised. At 500 mM, there was a 20-h lag in growth followed by a high growth rate. The final extents of growth, originally determined by absorbance measurements, were confirmed by actual DCW determi-

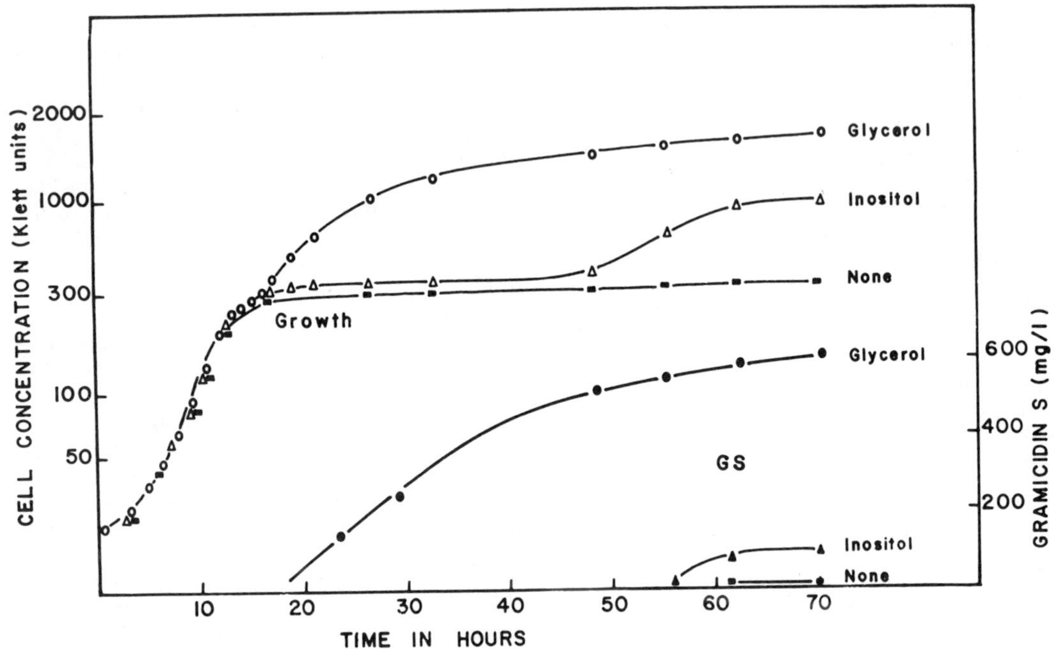

FIG. 2. *Pattern of GS fermentation in defined medium containing glycerol (G3T6), in the same medium lacking glycerol, and in the same medium with inositol replacing glycerol.*

nations. At 500 mM phosphate, where no GS was produced, the cells grew as long filaments.

Sulfur nutrition. In G3T6 medium, the only source of sulfur was the amino acid L-methionine. Addition of K_2SO_4 at concentrations of 100 mM and above progressively inhibited both growth and GS formation. At a lower level of K_2SO_4 (25 mM), where the additive was not toxic, it showed no beneficial effect on GS formation. When we attempted to replace the amino acid with K_2SO_4, production of GS was depressed. For this reason, we continued to use methionine as the sole sulfur source.

Effect of Tris. At an early stage in this laboratory's nutritional investigation of *B. brevis* ATCC 9999, Matteo et al. (19) found Tris to be a beneficial additive to the glycerol-ammonium sulfate-mineral salts medium with respect to both growth and GS production. Since G3T6 medium contained amino acids that have chelating and buffering properties, we decided to determine whether Tris was still needed. We found that elimination of Tris (medium G3/6) markedly improved both growth and GS formation.

Fructose versus glycerol. The effectiveness of fructose as a carbon source was compared with that of glycerol in the medium lacking Tris. Fructose was found to be a better source of carbon for GS formation. The final medium developed in this study (F3/6) supported production of approximately 1,500 mg of GS/liter and 0.19 mg of GS/mg of DCW (Fig. 4).

DISCUSSION

At present, we lack the data to attribute the inhibitory effect of glycerol and fructose on GS production in complex medium to catabolite repression of GS synthetases. Polypeptide antibiotics are usually produced in association with sporulation in bacilli (22, 23), and sporulation appears to be controlled by catabolite repression (24). Although evidence is accumulating that the relationship between antibiotic formation and sporulation is not an obligatory one (3, 10–12, 21), both processes could be regulated by the same metabolic controls. As we found in all of our defined media experiments, inositol was a poorer carbon source than glycerol and fructose and thus we would expect it to be less repressive or not repressive at all. However, before concluding that metabolic regulation is responsible, enzyme studies must be done. It is possible, for example, that inhibition of GS formation could be due to a trivial factor such as pH. Growth in YP medium plus 2.5% glycerol or fructose decreased the pH one to two units below that observed in YP medium, whereas the decrease observed with 2.5% inositol was usually less than one pH unit. On the other hand, 1% glycerol was also inhibitory to GS production; yet pH was only decreased by about 0.5 pH unit.

It is of interest to compare our results on the utilization of glycerol, fructose, and *meso*-inositol with those of Soviet investigators who used *B. brevis* var. GB. Korshunov and Egorov (14) found glucose to be the best sugar and glycerol the best polyol for growth and GS production; they did not test fructose. We have seen a complete inability of glucose to serve as a carbon source for *B. brevis* ATCC 9999. Even when inocula were developed by germinating spores in chemically defined medium containing glucose, we did not observe subsequent glucose utilization. Udalova and Fedorova (25) found growth and GS formation to be best with glycerol or inositol; glucose and starch supported less growth and no GS formation; fructose was not examined. Among the organic acids, lactic (25), succinic (14), fumaric, and malic acids (29) have been reported to increase GS production. We found lactate and succinate to increase growth somewhat but did not test fumarate and malate. The marked stimulation of GS formation by addition of lactic acid to a glycerol-based defined medium (25) was not observed by us.

We found the best nitrogen source to be a mixture of five amino acids (L-histidine, L-proline, L-glutamine, L-arginine, and L-methionine); $(NH_4)_2SO_4$ had no effect in their presence. Individual amino acids or ammonium salts of organic acids were rather poor for growth and GS formation. On the other hand, beneficial effects of amino acids and ammonium salts of organic acids on growth and GS

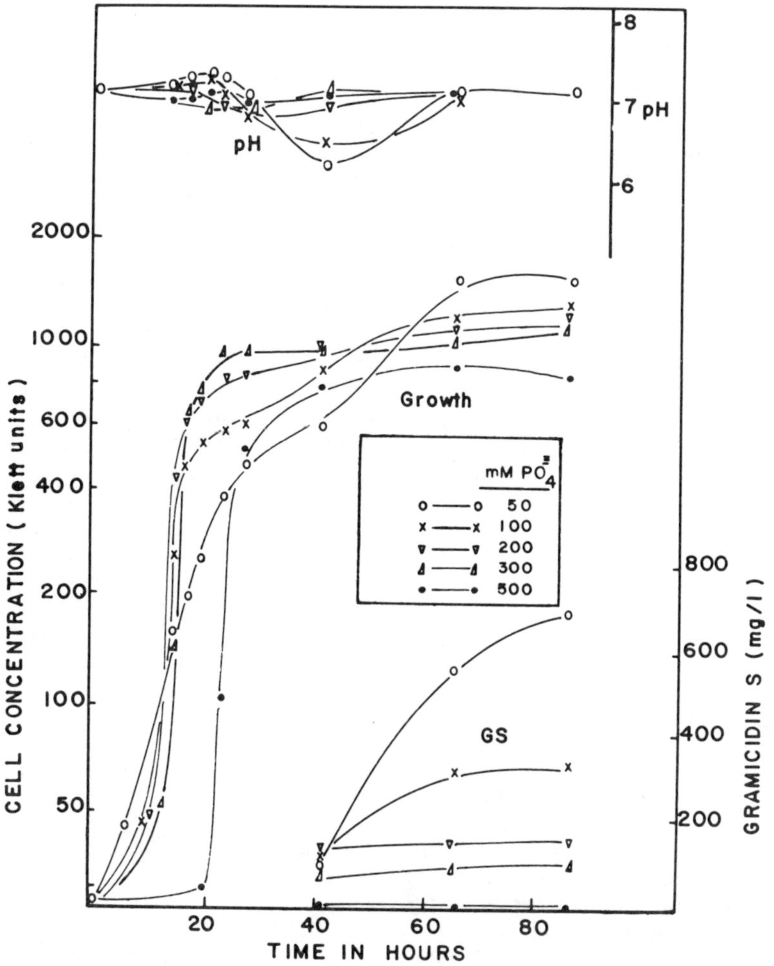

FIG. 3. *Effect of concentration of potassium phosphate on growth and GS production in medium G3T6.*

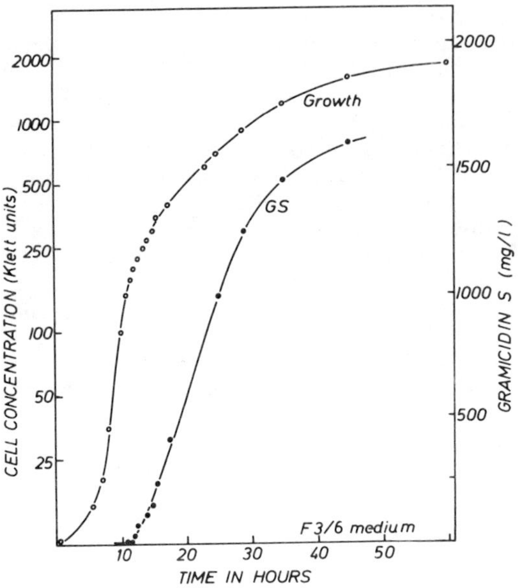

FIG. 4. *Pattern of GS fermentation in defined medium F3/6.*

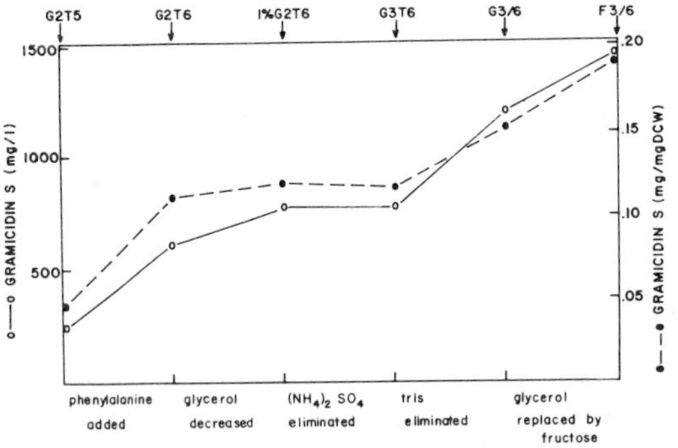

FIG. 5. *GS production in the media developed in this study.*

formation have been reported for *B. brevis* GB (14, 25, 28, 29).

The effect of inorganic phosphate in our studies indicated that GS formation was controlled by phosphate. Concentrations (100 to 300 mM) supporting the highest growth rates showed poor GS formation. Soviet investigators reported optimum phosphate levels for GS formation by *B. brevis* GB to be 10 to 60 mM (14) and 30 mM (25) but did not report a specific inhibition effect of higher concentrations on GS biosynthesis. Many antibiotic fermentations are subject to phosphate inhibition at growth-optimal concentrations of inorganic phosphate (2, 26). In the case of bacitracin formation, Haavik (9) contends that the effect is due to pH changes, but definitive experiments with pH control are needed to support his claim.

The final medium developed in this study contains fructose, five growth-stimulatory amino acids, phenylalanine to increase GS formation, and mineral salts. Figure 5 shows the improvements obtained at various stages of this study. Certain steps did not markedly improve GS production but did simplify the medium. The ability of medium F3/6 to support production of 1,500 mg of GS/liter and 0.19 mg of GS/mg of DCW (Fig. 4) may be compared with that of the complex YP medium (Fig. 1). Although higher figures were reported earlier (19), our recent experiments show the production of 1,300 mg of GS/liter and 0.10 mg/mg of DCW in the complex medium. This discrepancy is probably due to the use of different batches of the complex ingredients. The growth rate in F3/6 is 0.53 h^{-1} compared with 1.2 h^{-1} in YP. It is interesting that F3/6 does not show the diauxic growth characteristic of our earlier defined media (cf. Fig. 2 and 4). Our conclusion is that the F3/6 chemically defined medium is superior to any defined or complex medium developed previously for GS production by *B. brevis* ATCC 9999 and is much more suitable for studies on the regulation of GS synthetase formation.

We are somewhat puzzled about the differences between the performance of strain ATCC 9999 here and the reported behavior of Soviet strain GB in some of the media developed in the U.S.S.R., since strain GB is thought to be the original source of ATCC 9999. One possibility could be the occurrence of genetic changes during the many transfers that these cultures have undergone since 1944.

ACKNOWLEDGMENTS

We gratefully acknowledge the support of the National Science Foundation (grant GI-34284). E.J.V. was a recipient of a NATO fellowship and was also supported through the Belgian Ministry of National Education.

We are indebted to T. Wakazawa of Meiji Seika Kaisha, Ltd. for gifts of gramicidin S. Technical assistance was provided by Jordan Kreidberg.

LITERATURE CITED

1. **Demain, A. L.** 1958. Minimal media for quantitative studies with *Bacillus subtilis*. J. Bacteriol. 75:517–522.
2. **Demain, A. L.** 1972. Cellular and environmental factors affecting the synthesis and excretion of metabolites. J. Appl. Chem. Biotechnol. 22:345–362.
3. **Demain, A. L.** 1974. How do antibiotic-producing microorganisms avoid suicide? Ann. N.Y. Acad. Sci. 234:601–612.
4. **Demain, A. L., and C. C. Matteo.** 1976. Phenylalanine stimulation of gramicidin S formation. Antimicrob. Agents Chemother. 9:1000–1003.
5. **Eikhom, T. S., J. Jonsen, S. Laland, and T. Refsvik.**

1963. On the biosynthesis of gramicidin S. Biochim. Biophys. Acta 76:465–468.
6. **Eikhom, T. S., and S. Laland.** 1965. The effect of actinomycin D on the production of gramicidin S in whole cells of *Bacillus brevis*. Biochim. Biophys. Acta 100:451–458.
7. **Gause, G. F., and M. G. Brazhnikova.** 1944. Gramicidin S. Origin and mode of action. Lancet 247:715–716.
8. **Gevers, W., H. Kleinkauf, and F. Lipmann.** 1968. The activation of amino acids for biosynthesis of gramicidin S. Proc. Natl. Acad. Sci. U.S.A. 60:269–276.
9. **Haavik, H. I.** 1974. Studies on the formation of bacitracin by *Bacillus licheniformis*: effect of inorganic phosphate. J. Gen. Microbiol. 84:226–230.
10. **Haavik, H. I., and O. Froyshov.** 1975. Function of peptide antibiotics in producer organisms. Nature (London) 254:79–82.
11. **Haavik, H. I., and S. Thomassen.** 1973. A bacitracin-negative mutant of *Bacillus licheniformis* which is able to sporulate. J. Gen. Microbiol. 76:451–454.
12. **Kambe, M., Y. Imae, and K. Kurahashi.** 1974. Biochemical studies on gramicidin S non-producing mutants of *Bacillus brevis* ATCC 9999. J. Biochem. 75:481–493.
13. **Knight, B. C. J. G., and H. Proom.** 1950. A comparative survey of the nutrition and physiology of mesophilic species in the genus *Bacillus*. J. Gen. Microbiol. 4:508–538.
14. **Korshunov, V. V., and N. S. Egorov.** 1962. A synthetic medium for cultivation of *Bacillus brevis* var. G.B. and gramicidin S production. Mikrobiologiya 31:515–519.
15. **Kurahashi, K.** 1974. Biosynthesis of small peptides. Annu. Rev. Biochem. 43:445–459.
16. **Laland, S. G., and T. L. Zimmer.** 1973. The protein thiotemplate mechanism of synthesis for the peptide antibiotics produced by *Bacillus brevis*. Essays Biochem. 9:31–57.
17. **Leung, D. C., and R. M. Baxter.** 1972. Substrate-derived reversible and irreversible inhibitors of the multienzyme I of gramicidin S biosynthesis. Biochim. Biophys. Acta 279:34–47.
18. **Lipmann, F.** 1973. Nonribosomal polypeptide synthesis of polyenzyme templates. Acc. Chem. Res. 6:361–367.
19. **Matteo, C. C., M. Glade, A. Tanaka, J. Piret, and A. L. Demain.** 1975. Microbiological studies on the formation of gramicidin S synthetases. Biotechnol. Bioeng. 17:129–142.
20. **Proom, H., and B. C. J. G. Knight.** 1955. The minimal nutritional requirements of some species in the genus *Bacillus*. J. Gen. Microbiol. 13:474–480.
21. **Ray, B., and S. K. Bose.** 1971. Polypeptide antibiotic-negative sporeformer mutants of *Bacillus subtilis*. J. Gen. Appl. Microbiol. 17:491–498.
22. **Sadoff, H. L.** 1972. The antibiotics of *Bacillus* species: their possible roles in sporulation. Prog. Ind. Microbiol. 11:3–27.
23. **Sarkar, N., and H. Paulus.** 1972. Function of peptide antibiotics in sporulation. Nature (London) New Biol. 239:228–230.
24. **Schaeffer, P.** 1969. Sporulation and the production of antibiotics, exoenzymes, and exotoxins. Bacteriol. Rev. 33:48–71.
25. **Udalova, T. P., and R. I. Fedorova.** 1965. The effect of different nutrient compounds on the formation of gramicidin by *Bacillus brevis* var. G.B. Mikrobiologiya 34:631–635.
26. **Weinberg, E. D.** 1974. Secondary metabolism: control by temperature and inorganic phosphate. Dev. Ind. Microbiol. 15:70–81.
27. **White, P. J.** 1972. The nutrition of *Bacillus megaterium* and *Bacillus cereus*. J. Gen. Microbiol. 71:505–515.
28. **Zharikova, G. G.** 1965. Effect of amino acids on the development of *Bacillus brevis* var. G. B. and on the biosynthesis of gramicidin S. Prikl. Biokhim. Mikrobiol. 1:83–89.
29. **Zharikova, G. G., A. B. Silaev, and I. V. Sushkova.** 1963. Effect of certain organic acids and amino acids on the biosynthesis of gramicidin S. Antibiotiki (Kiev) 8:425–430.

ANTIMICROBIAL AGENTS AND CHEMOTHERAPY, Aug. 1976, p. 274-276 Vol. 10, No. 2

Susceptibility of *Streptococcus mutans* to Antimicrobial Agents

JOSEPH J. FERRETTI* AND MARGIE WARD

Department of Microbiology and Immunology, The University of Oklahoma Health Sciences Center, Oklahoma City, Oklahoma 73190

Received for publication 23 February 1976

Fifty strains of *Streptococcus mutans*, including defined strains and clinical isolates, were tested for susceptibility to 20 different antimicrobial agents. Minimal inhibitory concentrations were determined by a liquid microtiter procedure. Antibiotics that were most effective in concentrations below 0.1 μg/ml included penicillin, ampicillin, erythromycin, cephalothin, and methicillin. Antibiotics effective in concentrations between 0.1 μg and 10 μg/ml included rifampin, lincomycin, thiostrepton, spiromycin, vancomycin, streptolydigan, novobiocin, tetracycline, chloramphenicol, spectinomycin, and gentamicin. Antibiotics effective at higher concentrations ranging from 10 μg/ml to 400 μg/ml included the aminoglycosides kanamycin, neomycin, streptomycin, and kasugamycin. Although most antibiotics exhibited inhibitory effects in a narrow range of concentrations, antibiotics such as tetracycline, thiostrepton, and spiromycin had a 1,000-fold range from the lowest to highest concentrations required for growth inhibition.

Interest in the organism *Streptococcus mutans* is closely associated with its involvement in dental caries. This organism is also involved as a causative agent of endocarditis (1, 3). Knowledge of the antibiotic susceptibility patterns of *S. mutans* is of importance for proper therapy in the cases of endocarditis because *S. mutans* endocarditis has been in some instances confused with group D enterococcal endocarditis (3). In one recent report, approximately 5% of streptococcal endocarditis isolates studied were *S. mutans*. (2).

Baker and Thornsberry (2) have reported the patterns of susceptibility of *S. mutans*, isolated from patients with endocarditis, to 11 antibiotics. In this study we have determined the susceptibility of 50 strains of *S. mutans*, isolated from dental plaque, to 20 different antimicrobial agents.

MATERIALS AND METHODS

Bacterial strains. The bacterial strains used in this study were obtained from the dental clinics of the University of Oklahoma College of Dentistry and from C. Schaechtele, the University of Minnesota. Of the 50 strains of *S. mutans*, 6 were defined strains representing each known serotype and included the following: LM7, SL-1, 6715, Ingbritt, BHT, and OMZ-61. The remaining strains were isolated from samples of dental plaque and were identified according to (i) colony morphology on Mitis Salivarius agar, (ii) fermentation of mannitol and sorbitol, and (iii) extracellular polysaccharide production in 5% sucrose broth.

Antibiotics. The antibiotics used and the sources from which they were obtained were: erythromycin, kanamycin, neomycin, novobiocin, and tetracycline (Sigma Chemical Co., St. Louis, Mo.); ampicillin, kasugamycin, and methicillin (Bristol Laboratories, Syracuse, N.Y.); lincomycin, spectinomycin, and streptolydigan (Upjohn Co., Kalamazoo, Mich.); cephalothin and vancomycin (Eli Lilly & Co., Indianapolis, Ind.); penicillin and streptomycin (Nutritional Biochemical Corp., Cleveland, Ohio); rifampin (Becton-Dickinson & Co., Rutherford, N.J.); chloramphenicol (Parke, Davis & Co., Detroit, Mich.); spiromycin (Rhodia Inc., New York); gentamicin (Schering Laboratories, Bloomfield, N.J.); and thiostrepton (E. R. Squibb & Sons, New York).

Media. The standard liquid medium used in this study was proteose peptone broth. It contained 6% proteose peptone no. 3 (Difco), 0.3% NaCl, and 0.38% Na_2HPO_4. After sterilization the broth was completed by the addition of three more components at the following final concentrations: 0.02% $CaCl_2$, 0.05% glucose, and 5% normal horse serum (GIBCO). Trypticase soy broth (BBL) was also used in the initial portions of the study.

Susceptibility tests. Each strain of *S. mutans* was streaked onto Mitis Salivarius agar plates, incubated at 37°C in an anaerobic jar for 24 h, and then allowed to incubate at 37°C aerobically for an additional 24 h. Several colonies with similar morphology were picked and inoculated into proteose peptone broth. After overnight incubation at 37°C, 0.1 ml of each culture was inoculated into a tube containing 10 ml of proteose peptone broth. To sterile microdilution plates containing appropriate serial dilutions of antibiotic in proteose peptone broth, 0.05 ml of the overnight diluted culture was added. Each plate was covered with clear plastic and incubated at 37°C for 48 h. Unless otherwise specified, all incubations were performed aerobically. In instances when anaerobic conditions were maintained, anaerobic Gas-Pak (BBL) jars were utilized. The minimal inhibitory concentration (MIC) was the lowest concentration of antibiotic that caused complete inhibition of growth.

RESULTS

Growth of the various strains of *S. mutans* was supported best in proteose peptone broth containing 5% horse serum. In comparison with other media, including Trypticase soy broth, growth of all bacterial strains was sufficient in 24 h to determine the MIC of a particular antibiotic within one dilution. To insure that maximal growth occurred, however, final MICs were routinely determined after 48 h of incubation.

There was some question whether there were any differences in growth or inhibition by antibiotics when the organism was incubated under aerobic or anaerobic conditions. To answer this question the MICs of several antibiotics (cephalothin, methicillin, and vancomycin) were determined with 50 different strains of *S. mutans* incubated under both aerobic and anaerobic conditions. The results from these experiments are given in Table 1. The average MICs obtained for each antibiotic were essentially identical with either aerobic or anaerobic incubation and indicated that the atmosphere had little effect on the growth of the organism or its susceptibility to antibiotics.

The MICs for inhibition of the 50 strains, plotted as a function of the percentage of susceptible strains, are shown in Fig. 1 through 3. In Fig. 1 the concentration of antibiotics ranged from 0.0005 to 2 μg/ml and included penicillin, ampicillin, erythromycin, cephalothin, methicillin, rifampin, and lincomycin. The inhibitory concentrations of most of the antibiotics covered a 10-fold range from the lowest to highest concentration required for growth inhibition. With two of the antibiotics, rifampin and lincomycin, there was a 250-fold range from the lowest to highest concentration required for growth inhibition.

In Fig. 2 the concentration of antibiotics ranged from 0.01 to 10 μg/ml and included streptolydigan, thiostrepton, spiromycin, kanamycin, and novobiocin. A 1,000-fold range in the concentration for inhibition of growth was observed with thiostrepton and spiromycin.

In Fig. 3 the concentration of antibiotics ranged from 0.05 to 400 μg/ml and included tetracycline, chloramphenicol, spectinomycin, gentamicin, kanamycin, neomycin, streptomycin, and kasugamycin. A 1,000-fold range in the concentrations of tetracycline required for inhibition of growth was observed, whereas there was a more narrow range of inhibition for all other antibiotics.

DISCUSSION

The purpose of this investigation was to test the susceptibility of strains of *S. mutans* iso-

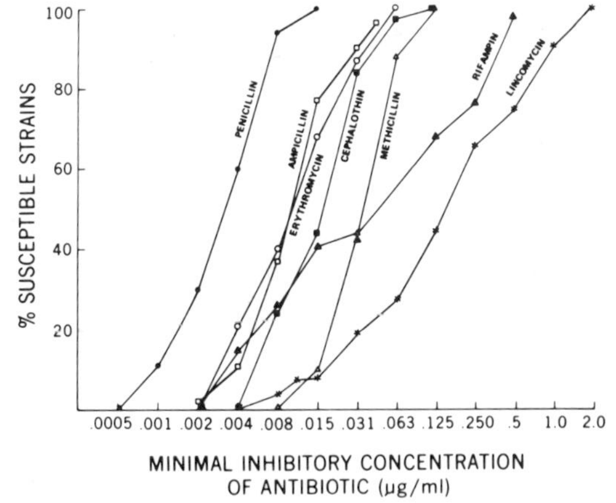

FIG. 1. *Susceptibility of S. mutans strains to penicillin (●), erythromycin (○), ampicillin (□), cephalothin (■), rifampin (▲), methicillin (△), and lincomycin (*).*

TABLE 1. *Minimal inhibitory concentrations (MICs) of three antibiotics for 50 strains of S. mutans incubated under aerobic and anaerobic conditions*

Antibiotic	Percentage of strains with MIC (μg/ml) of:									
Cephalothin	(0.25)	(0.125)	(0.063)	(0.031)	(0.015)	(0.008)	(0.004)	(0.002)	(0.001)	(0.0005)
Aerobic	0	0	4	13	40	19	24	0	0	0
Anaerobic	0	0	2	15	36	30	15	2	0	0
Methicillin	(0.25)	(0.125)	(0.063)	(0.031)	(0.015)	(0.008)	(0.004)	(0.002)	(0.001)	(0.0005)
Aerobic	0	0	13	43	34	10	0	0	0	0
Anaerobic	0	0	11	45	42	2	0	0	0	0
Vancomycin	(10)	(5)	(2.5)	(1.25)	(0.625)	(0.313)	(0.157)	(0.08)	(0.04)	(0.02)
Aerobic	0	0	0	2	4	28	36	28	2	0
Anaerobic	0	0	0	2	8	26	21	32	11	0

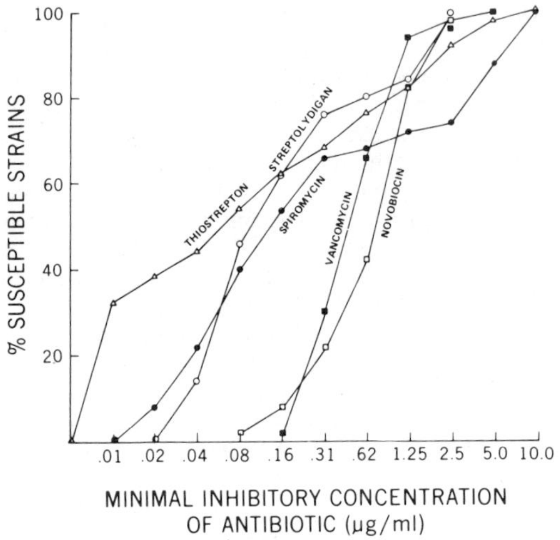

FIG. 2. *Susceptibility of S. mutans strains to spiromycin (●), streptolydigan (○), novobiocin (□), vancomycin (■), and thiostrepton (△).*

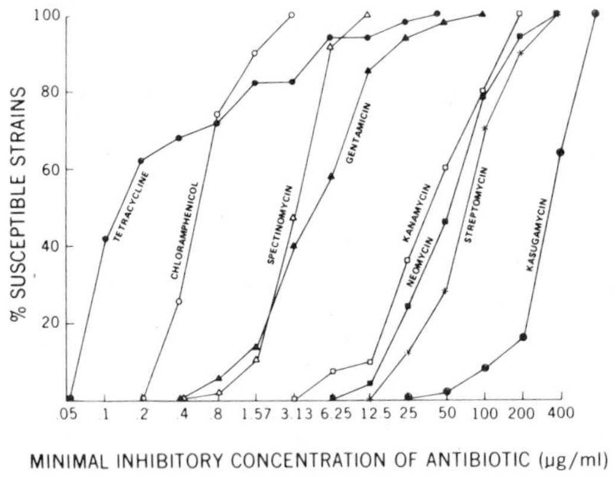

FIG. 3. *Susceptibility of S. mutans strains to tetracycline (●), chloramphenicol (○), gentamicin (▲), spectinomycin (△), kanamycin (□), neomycin (■), streptomycin (*), and kasugamycin (⊙).*

lated from dental plaque to 20 different antimicrobial agents. In a previous study of 11 antibiotics, Baker and Thornsberry (2) determined the antimicrobial susceptibility patterns of strains of *S. mutans* known to cause endocarditis. The MICs observed in our study are in essential agreement with those observed by Baker and Thornsberry and indicate that there is no difference in the susceptibility patterns of *S. mutans* isolated from endocarditis patients and from dental plaque. This observation is significant as it excludes the possibility that antimicrobial resistance has been induced in the endocarditis strains due to prior chemotherapy. Further, it excludes antimicrobial susceptibility patterns as contributory to the ability of plaque-forming organisms to establish infection in the heart. The results of this study also increase the number of antimicrobial agents with known efficacy against these organisms.

Antimicrobial agents that were particularly effective at low concentrations (below 0.1 µg/ml) included penicillin, ampicillin, erythromycin, cephalothin, and methicillin. Each of these antibiotics inhibited all of the strains tested in a narrow concentration range. Two antibiotics that inhibited *S. mutans* at low concentrations, rifampin and lincomycin, had a 250-fold concentration range of effectiveness. Even more striking were the wide ranges of effectiveness of tetracycline, thiostrepton, and spiromycin. Each of these antibiotics had a 1,000-fold range from the lowest to highest concentrations required for growth inhibition.

Among group A streptococci there has been a world-wide increase in the number of tetracycline-resistant strains observed (4, 6). Since tetracycline is a frequently used antibiotic, the incidence of tetracycline resistance among *S. mutans* may also be increasing. However, the other two antibiotics with wide ranges of MICs, thiostrepton and spiromycin, are not frequently used and one would not expect much increase in the incidence of resistant organisms. There was no evidence of multiple drug resistance among any of the strains of *S. mutans* used in this study.

ACKNOWLEDGMENT

This work was supported by Public Health Service grant DE03697 from the National Institute of Dental Research.

LITERATURE CITED

1. **Abercombie, G. F., and W. M. Scott,** 1928. A case of infective endocarditis due to Streptococcus mutans. Lancet *2:*697–699.
2. **Baker, C. N., and C. Thornsberry.** 1974. Antimicrobial susceptibility of *Streptococcus mutans* isolated from patients with endocarditis. Antimicrob. Agents Chemother. 5:268–271.
3. **DeMoor, C. E., J. D. DeStoppelaar, and J. van Houte.** 1972. The occurrence of *S. mutans* and *S. sanguis* in the blood of endocarditis patients. Caries Res. 6:73.
4. **Fallon, R. J.** 1974. Tetracycline-resistant group A streptococci. Br. Med. J. 3:741.
5. **Neefe, L. I., J. H. Chretien, E. C. Delaha, and V. F. Garagusi.** 1974. *Streptococcus mutans* endocarditis. J. Am. Med. Assoc. **230:**1298–1299.
6. **Ubakata, K., M. Konno, and R. Fujii.** 1973. Group A beta-hemolytic streptococci resistant to tetracycline, chloramphenicol, macrolides, lincomycin, and clindamycin. Jpn. J. Pediatr. **26:**1451–1458.

Antimicrobial Agents and Chemotherapy, Aug. 1976, p. 277-282 Vol. 10, No. 2

Printed in U.S.A.

Renal Extraction of Gentamicin in Anesthetized Dogs

PETER J. S. CHIU,* ARTHUR BROWN, GEORGE MILLER, AND JAMES F. LONG

Schering Corporation, Research Laboratories Division, Bloomfield, New Jersey 07003

Received for publication 25 February 1976

The tubular handling of gentamicin (G) and its intrarenal distribution were determined to elucidate the mechanism of G accumulation in the kidney. At a serum level of 11.1 ± 0.5 μg/ml (10 animals), as maintained by constant infusion for 5 h, serum Na^+ and K^+, arterial pressure, effective renal plasma flow and glomerular filtration rate remained undisturbed. The clearance values in milliliters per minute for G, inulin, and *p*-aminohippuric acid were 40.3 ± 1.8, 49.9 ± 2.8, and 132 ± 14, respectively. The ratio of clearance of G to clearance of inulin was 0.82 ± 0.04 ($P < 0.005$), suggesting net reabsorption of G by the renal tubules. The renal cortex/serum ratio for G was 11.9 ± 2.1, and the medulla/serum ratio was 2.7 ± 0.4, indicating greater uptake of G by the cortex. The extraction ratio of *p*-aminohippuric acid was 0.74 ± 0.03. In contrast, the extraction ratio of G was 0.20 ± 0.03, which was significantly lower than that of inulin (0.30 ± 0.04). It is concluded that the accumulation of G in the cortex was due to tubular reabsorption. Probably some of the reabsorbed G became trapped in the epithelial cells after crossing the luminal membrane, whereas some returned to the circulation.

Gentamicin, an aminoglycoside antibiotic, is potentially nephrotoxic, particularly with excessive blood levels or in subjects with preexistent renal insufficiency (16). Gentamicin-induced nephrotoxicity has been documented in man (10, 25, 37), as expressed by elevations in blood urea nitrogen and serum creatinine levels. In rats (11, 19) and dogs (3), histopathological studies have shown that gentamicin caused tubular necrosis in the proximal convoluted tubule. Renal biopsy in patients also revealed tubular damage (25). As the kidney is the major route of elimination of gentamicin, its functional status is important in the development of nephrotoxicity in human subjects (8, 12, 29).

The clearance value for gentamicin has been found similar to glomerular filtration rate in dogs (3, 32) and man (14). It has also been established that there is significant correlation between the serum half-life of gentamicin and the glomerular filtration rate (12). Prolonged serum half-life is usually seen in patients with severe renal insufficiency (14, 21) or in animals with partial nephrectomy (15). In animals and human subjects with normal kidney function, the bulk of gentamicin administered appeared in the urine within 24 h (3, 7, 14, 26, 30).

Gentamicin uptake by the renal tissue was found in animals (H. Whalig, Proc. Int. Congr. Chemother., 8th, Athens, Greece, Abstr. A-14, 1973) as well as in man (1). In addition, prolonged half-life of gentamicin has been observed in rat kidney (22). The presence of tubular transport of gentamicin coupled with its concentration in the renal tissue may be related to its nephrotoxicity and/or delayed excretion (24; H. Whalig, Proc. Int. Congr. Chemother., 8th, Athens, Greece, Abstr. A-74, 1973).

We studied the tubular handling of gentamicin and intrarenal distribution by clearance techniques and tissue analysis, respectively, in an attempt to elucidate the mechanism of gentamicin accumulation in the kidney. Further, the effects of gentamicin on rrenal hemodynamics and electrolyte excretion were determined.

(This work has been published in abstract form [Annu. Meet. Am. Soc. Nephrol., 8th, Washington, D.C., 1975, p. 75].)

MATERIALS AND METHODS

Mongrel dogs of either sex were fasted overnight and were anesthetized with Nembutal (30 mg/kg, intravenously [i.v.]) on the day of each experiment. The animals were breathing spontaneously during each experiment. A suprapubic incision was made, and both ureters were cannulated with polyethylene tubing for urine collection. The left femoral artery was cannulated for measurement of blood pressure. The spermatic or ovarian vein was cannulated for sampling renal venous blood. The animals were given 400 to 500 ml of physiological saline to replace fluid loss and to ensure adequate urinary flow. The animals were given a priming injection of inulin, *p*-aminohippuric acid (PAH) and, except in the control animals, gentamicin (2.0 mg/kg, i.v.). An i.v. infusion immediately followed which contained sustaining doses of PAH and inulin in physiological saline at a rate of 4.0 ml/min. Except in the control experiments, gentamicin (30 mg/ml) was given in this infusion at a dose of 3.0 mg/kg per h. At least 1 h was allowed for equilibration before sample collections so that a steady-state blood level of the compounds could be attained. Urine samples were then taken every 25 min. Blood samples were drawn at the beginning and the end of each urine collection period; plasma from heparinized portions was used to determine PAH and inulin levels, and serum from nonheparinized portions was used to determine electrolytes and gentamicin. At the end of each experiment, both kidneys were excised. Portions of cortex and inner medulla were analyzed for gentamicin. Urine and blood samples were analyzed for PAH (5) and inulin (9). Sodium and potassium concentrations were determined with flame photometry.

Gentamicin in serum and urine was assayed by the cylinder-plate method with *Bacillus subtilis* (ATCC 6633) as the test organism (28). Tissue samples were weighed, diluted 1:5 with 0.1 M phosphate buffer (pH 8), and homogenized in a Tissumax homogenizer. The homogenates were assayed microbiologically in a manner similar to the serum level determination, except that the standard curve was prepared from control tissue homogenates.

Calculations. (i) Clearances. The clearance values of each compound was obtained by the equation $U_X V/P_X$, where U_X and P_X are the urinary and total plasma concentrations of compound X, respectively. V represents the urinary flow rate in milliliters per minute. Clearance rates of PAH and inulin were used to measure effective renal plasma flow and glomerular filtration, respectively.

(ii) Extraction ratio. The renal extraction ratio was calculated by dividing the arteriovenous concentration difference by the arterial concentration, or $(Pa - Pv)/Pa$, where Pa and Pv are the concentrations in arterial and renal venous plasma, respectively.

(iii) Fractional excretion of Na^+ or K^+. The fractional excretion of Na^+ or K^+ was calculated by the equation $(U_X \cdot V/GFR \cdot P_X) \times 100$, where U_X and P_X are urinary and serum concentrations of the electrolytes, and GFR is glomerular filtration.

All data were subjected to statistical analyses. The Student t test for independent and dependent variables was used to make appropriate comparisons.

RESULTS

Effect of gentamicin on serum electrolytes and blood pressure. At a serum level of 11.1 ± 0.5 μg/ml (N=10), as maintained by constant infusion for 5 h (Fig. 1), all animals demonstrated stable arterial blood pressure. The concentrations of serum sodium and potassium remained undisturbed and were similar to untreated animals (data not shown).

Urine and electrolyte excretion. No differences were discerned between the gentamicin and saline groups with respect to urinary flow (Table 1) and excretion of sodium and potassium. Mild natriuresis and kaliuresis in these animals were indications of physiological responses to moderate extracellular fluid volume expansion associated with the saline infusion.

Inulin and PAH clearances. The inulin and PAH clearances were quite stable throughout the experiments in animals treated with gentamicin, as shown in Fig. 2. The mean values of the two parameters did not differ from those of the animals receiving only saline (Table 2). Thus, gentamicin did not seem to show any adverse effects on the renal hemodynamics under the conditions of the present study.

Renal clearance of gentamicin. The clearance values of gentamicin were consistently less than inulin clearance values in all animals (Fig. 3); the difference between the mean values of the two parameters was statistically sig-

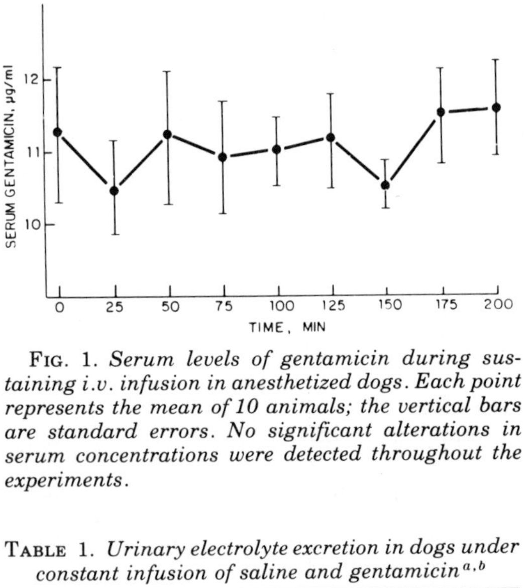

FIG. 1. *Serum levels of gentamicin during sustaining i.v. infusion in anesthetized dogs. Each point represents the mean of 10 animals; the vertical bars are standard errors. No significant alterations in serum concentrations were detected throughout the experiments.*

TABLE 1. *Urinary electrolyte excretion in dogs under constant infusion of saline and gentamicin*[a,b]

Electrolyte determination	Saline group (N = 7)	Gentamicin group (N = 10)
V (ml/min)[c]	1.6 ± 0.2	1.7 ± 0.2
$U_{Na}V$ (μeq/min)[c]	108 ± 18	127 ± 29
$U_K V$ (μeq/min)[c]	37.1 ± 5.0	40.4 ± 5.4
FE_{Na} (%)[d]	1.8 ± 0.4	1.8 ± 0.4
FE_K (%)[d]	22.7 ± 2.8	23.1 ± 3.3

[a] All values represent means ± standard error.

[b] None of the differences between values was significant.

[c] $U_{Na}V$ and $U_K V$ are absolute rate of urinary excretion of Na^+ and K^+, respectively. V is the urine flow rate.

[d] FE_{Na} and FE_K represent the percentage of filtered Na^+ and K^+ being excreted in the urine, respectively.

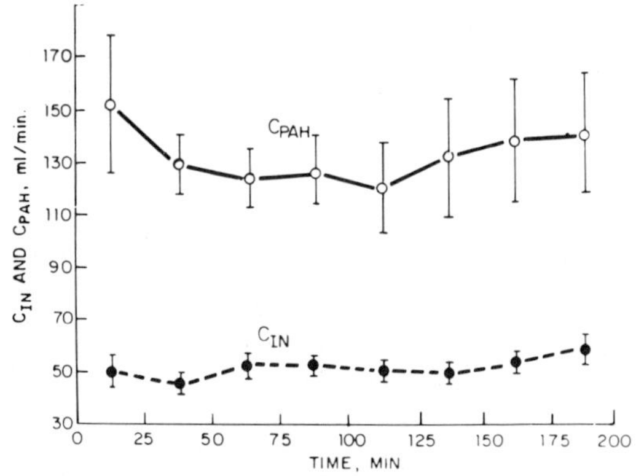

FIG. 2. *Effect of gentamicin on clearances of PAH (C_{PAH}) and inulin (C_{In}) in anesthetized dogs. C_{PAH} and C_{In} measure effective renal plasma flow and glomerular filtration rate, respectively. Each point represents the mean value of 10 animals; the vertical bars represent standard errors.*

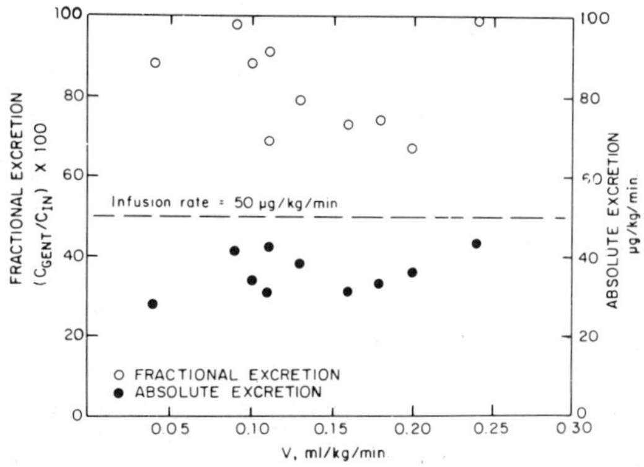

FIG. 3. *Urine flow rate versus urinary excretion of gentamicin in anesthetized dogs. Symbols: (○) fractional excretion of gentamicin; (●) absolute rate of excretion, of which all are less than the sustaining infusion rate (- - -). Each circle represents mean of eight consecutive clearance values per animal.*

nificant (Table 2). The ratio of clearance of gentamicin to clearance of inulin was 0.82 ± 0.04 ($P < 0.005$), significantly less than unity, suggesting that some gentamicin was reabsorbed by the renal tubule after being filtered (Table 2). The percentage of administered gentamicin that appeared in the urine was 71.2 ± 3.4; the fractional excretion and absolute excretion rate were independent of urine flow rate (Fig. 3).

Renal extraction ratios. The extraction ratios of PAH appeared unaffected by gentamicin (Table 3), since they were similar to control values obtained in this study and to values in the literature for dogs (27, 33). The normal extraction ratios and clearance values in drug-treated animals (Table 2), therefore, indicated that the presence of the drug did not interfere with the tubular secretion of PAH. On the other hand, the extraction ratio for gentamicin was significantly lower than the extraction ratio for inulin, presenting further evidence that the compound underwent tubular reabsorption.

Renal tissue and urine antibiotic levels. The concentration of gentamicin in the renal cortex was 12 times as much as the serum level (Table 4). In contrast, the medullary concentration of gentamicin was less than 3 times the serum level. The mean urinary concentration of gentamicin was 310 ± 74 µg/ml and was over 10 times as much as the medullary concentration.

DISCUSSION

The present finding that gentamicin clearance was 82.5% of inulin clearance suggested the existence of tubular reabsorption. Since at concentrations of up to 5 mg/ml about 30% gen-

TABLE 2. *Renal handling of gentamicin in anesthetized dogs*[a]

Determination	Saline group (N = 7)	Gentamicin group (N = 10)
C_G (ml/min)[b]		40.3 ± 1.8
C_{In} (ml/min)[b]	46.7 ± 4.4	49.9 ± 2.8
C_{PAH} (ml/min)[b]	108 ± 6	132 ± 14
FE_G (%)[c]		82.5 ± 3.7[d]
U_GV (µg/kg per min)[e]		35.6 ± 1.7
V (ml/kg per min)[e]	0.14 ± 0.03	0.14 ± 0.02

[a] All values represent means ± standard error.

[b] C_G, C_{In}, and C_{PAH}, Clearance values for gentamicin, inulin, and PAH, respectively.

[c] FE_G, Percentage of filtered gentamicin being excreted in the urine.

[d] Mean value is significantly ($P < 0.005$) less than 100%.

[e] U_GV, Absolute rate of urinary excretion of gentamicin. V is the urine flow rate.

TABLE 3. *Extraction ratios of gentamicin, inulin, and PAH in anesthetized dogs*[a,b]

Determination	Saline group (N = 7)	Gentamicin group (N = 7)
Inulin	0.29 ± 0.05[c]	0.30 ± 0.04
PAH	0.69 ± 0.03	0.74 ± 0.03
Gentamicin		0.20 ± 0.03[d]

[a] Extraction ratio = $(Pa - Pv)/Pa$, where Pa and Pv are the femoral arterial and renal venous concentrations of the individual compounds, respectively.

[b] All values represent means ± standard error.

[c] Mean value of four animals; measurements of venous inulin in the other three animals were not done.

[d] Significantly different from the mean exctraction ratio for inulin ($P < 0.05$).

TABLE 4. *Gentamicin in serum, kidney, and urine of anesthetized dogs*[a]

Tissue examined	Gentamicin concn[b]	Ratio[c]
Serum (μg/ml)	10.4 ± 0.3	(C/S) 11.9 ± 2.1
Cortex (μg/g)[d]	122.8 ± 22.1	(M/S) 2.7 ± 0.4
Medulla (μg/g)[d]	28.2 ± 4.0	(C/M) 4.8 ± 0.8
Urine (μg/ml)	310 ± 74	

[a] All values represent means ± standard error of seven dogs.

[b] Gentamicin (2 mg/kg, i.v.) was given and followed by sustaining infusion at a rate of 3.0 mg/kg per h, the total dose administered being approximately 200 mg per animal over a period of 5 h.

[c] C/S and M/S, Cortex to serum and medulla to serum concentration ratios, respectively. C/M is cortex to medulla ratio. Serum concentrations of gentamicin are shown on Fig. 1.

[d] Tissue concentration is based on the wet weight of tissues.

tamicin was reported to be protein bound in human sera (6, 31), some authors suggested tubular secretion of gentamicin (8, 14), because in their experiments gentamicin clearance exceeded inulin clearance, after corrections were made for presumed serum protein binding. Since only the free form is available for filtration, the clearance value of gentamicin may be underestimated by using the total serum concentration in our calculations. However, a recent report (13) showed that at a concentration close to therapeutic level (5 μg/ml) and measured under physiological conditions of temperature and pH, serum protein binding of gentamicin was absent. Naumann and Auwärter (26) also found no evidence of serum protein binding of gentamicin with concentrations of 2.5 and 5.0 μg/ml. It is probable that protein binding was negligible at serum levels around 10 μg/ml, as existed in the present experiments.

In contrast with PAH, which is profusely secreted by the proximal tubule and has a high extraction ratio (33), gentamicin has a very low extraction ratio. This value is even less than that for inulin, which is neither reabsorbed nor secreted (Table 2). It appeared that some of the filtered gentamicin was reabsorbed by the renal tubule and returned to the peritubular capillary network; the low extraction ratio was due to a smaller arteriovenous concentration difference relative to the arterial concentration. The finding provides additional evidence that gentamicin reabsorption occurs in the proximal tubule. The possibility of net tubular secretion can be ruled out at this point.

Although there are active transport systems in the proximal tubule of the nephron for exogenous organic compounds, passive reabsorption of many of these compounds occurs in the distal nephron and is influenced by the lipid solubility and pKa of the specific organic acid or base under consideration, in addition to urine flow and urine pH. Alterations in urine pH (23) and urine flow (17) did not influence urinary excretion of gentamicin in human subjects. In the present study the excretion of gentamicin was found to be independent of urine flow rate as well. The findings are suggestive of minimal nonionic back-diffusion of gentamicin in the distall nephron in spite of the great differences between the urinary and medullary concentrations (Table 4).

Gentamicin demonstrated preferential accumulation in the renal cortex (Table 4). Based on the whole-kidney weight of the dog (approximately 60 g), it is estimated that the cortex contained about 4 mg of the compound, less than 2% of the administered dose. It seems evident that there is a reabsorptive mechanism for gentamicin in the proximal tubule, the major portions of which are situated in the cortex. High affinity of gentamicin for kidney cell particulates has been reported (20), and the filtered compound was probably bound to the intracellular substances after crossing the luminal membrane, and concentration buildup ensued. Accumulation of gentamicin in the renal tissue occurs in animals (H. Whalig, Proc. Int. Congr. Chemother., 8th, Athens, Greece, Abstr. A-74, 1973) and man (1). Furthermore, Luft and Kleit (22) observed a half-life of 109 h in the kidney of rats after a single subcutaneous injection of gentamicin, 10 mg/kg (cf. serum half-life: 0.5 h). In addition, the drug was found in serum and in urine for more than a week after the last dose in uremic patients (24). Delayed excretion of gentamicin also occurred in mice and dogs (H. Whalig, Proc. Int. Congr. Chemother., 8th, Athens, Greece, Abstr. A-74, 1973). Bergan et al. (2) found that the clearance of gentamicin, even after correction was made for 30% protein binding, was markedly below the creatinine clearance in eight patients with chronic pyelonephritis. The authors suggested that the apparent enhancement of gentamicin reabsorption might provide a physiological correlate to the possibly increased incidence of nephrotoxicity in these patients with reduced kidney function. Although the relationship between the intracellular existence of this aminoglycoside antibiotic and its nephrotoxicity remains unclear, it is of interest to note that cephaloridine, a cephalosporin antibiotic, resembles gentamicin in that it accumulates in the renal cortex and also causes acute necrosis of the proximal tubule (35). In contrast to gentamicin, cephaloridine is transported into the proximal tubular cell at the peritubular membrane, but does not move readily across the luminal membrane into the tubular fluid. Further studies did suggest that the nephrotoxicity of cephaloridine was related to its renal cortical transport, with high intracellular concentrations of drug (34).

Under the conditions of the present study, gentamicin did not appear to interfere with kidney function, as the animals had normal glomerular filtration and effective renal plasma flow (Table 2) in addition to slight natriuresis in response to the moderate extracellular fluid volume expansion with saline (Table 1). Serum levels as high as 30 to 40 μg/ml have been tested previously (32). It appears that the nephrotoxicity of gentamicin cannot be demonstrated in short-term experiments on anesthetized dogs with apparent normal kidney function, although dogs are known to be markedly sensitive to the nephrotoxic effects of aminoglycoside antibiotics (3).

In conclusion, the present data have provided evidence that gentamicin undergoes filtration and reabsorption in the kidney. That the bulk of filtered drug is excreted in the urine indicates that the renal clearance of gentamicin mainly depends on filtration rate (Fig. 3). Only a small fraction of filtered drug is reabsorbed by the proximal tubule. A portion of reabsorbate might have returned to the circulation, as shown by the low extraction ratio of the compound, whereas some was trapped in the epithelial cells, leading to cortical accumulation.

LITERATURE CITED

1. **Alfthan, O., O. Renkonen, and A. Sivonen.** 1973. Concentration of gentamicin in serum, urine and urogenital tissue in man. Acta Pathol. Microbiol. Scand. (B) 81(Suppl. 241):92–94.
2. **Bergan, T., E. K. Brodwall, and A. Oyri.** 1971. Renal excretion of gentamicin in chronic pyelonephritis. Acta Med. 189:1–5.
3. **Black, J., B. Calesnick, D. Williams, and M. J. Weinstein.** 1964. Pharmacology of gentamicin, a new broad-spectrum antibiotic. p. 138–152. Antimicrob. Agents Chemother. 1963.
4. **Brayton, R. G., and D. B. Louria.** 1964. Gentamicin in gram-negative urinary and pulmonary infections. Arch. Intern. Med. 114:205–212.
5. **Brun, C.** 1951. A rapid method for the determination of para-aminohippuric acid in kidney function tests. J. Lab. Clin. Med. 37:955–958.
6. **Bulger, R. J., S. Sidell, and W. M. M. Kirby.** 1963. Laboratory and clinical studies of gentamicin, a new broad-spectrum antibiotic. Ann. Intern. Med. 59:593–604.
7. **Chisholm, G. D., J. S. Calnan, P. M. Waterworth, and N. D. Reis.** 1968. Distribution of gentamicin in body fluids. Br. Med. J. 2:22–24.
8. **Cutler, R. E., A. M. Gyselynck, W. P. Fleet, and A. W. Forrey.** 1972. Correlation of serum creatinine concentration and gentamicin half-life. J. Am. Med. Asoc. 219:1037–1041.
9. **Davidson, W. D., and M. A. Sackner.** 1963. Simplification of the anthrone method for the determination of inulin in clearance studies. J. Lab. Clin. Med. 62:351–356.
10. **Falco, F. G., H. M. Smith, and G. M. Arcieri.** 1969. Nephrotoxicity of aminoglycosides and gentamicin. J. Infect. Dis. 119:406–409.
11. **Flandre, O., and M. Damon.** 1967. Experimental study of the nephrotoxicity of gentamicin in rats. *In* Gentamicin: 1st international symposium. Paris.
12. **Gingell, J. C., and P. M. Waterworth.** 1968. Dose of gentamicin in patients with normal renal function and renal impairment. Br. Med. J. 2:19–22.
13. **Gordon, R. C., C. Regamey, and W. M. M. Kirby.** 1972. Serum protein binding of the aminoglycoside antibiotics. Antimicrob. Agents Chemother. 2:214–216.
14. **Gyselynck, A. M., A. Forrey, and R. Cutler.** 1971. Pharmacokinetics of gentamicin: distribution and plasma and renal clearance. J. Infect. Dis. 124(Suppl.):70–76.
15. **Hatala, M., J. Moravek, and O. Shuck.** 1975. Gentamicin pharmacokinetics in rats with reduced renal parenchyma. Int. J. Clin. Pharmacol. 11:1–6.
16. **Hewitt, W. L.** 1974. Gentamicin: toxicity in perspective. Postgrad. Med. J. 50(Suppl.):55–61.
17. **Jao, R. L., and G. G. Jackson.** 1964. Gentamicin sulfate, new antibiotic against gram-negative bacilli—laboratory, pharmacological, and clinical evaluation. J. Am. Med. Assoc. 189:817–822.
18. **Katz, Y. J.** 1958. Some factors affecting renal lymphatic pressure. Circ. Res. 6:452–455.
19. **Kosek, J. C., R. I. Mazze, and M. J. Cousins.** 1974. Nephrotoxicity of gentamicin. Lab. Invest. 30:48–57.
20. **Kunin, C. M., W. A. Craig, M. Kornguth, and R. Monson.** 1973. Influence of binding on the pharmacologic activity of antibiotics. Ann. N.Y. Acad. Sci. 226:214–224.
21. **Lockwood, W. R., and J. D. Bower.** 1973. Tobramycin and gentamicin concentrations in the serum of normal and anephric patients. Antimicrob. Agents Chemother. 3:125–129.
22. **Luft, F. C., and S. A. Kleit.** 1974. Renal parenchymal accumulation of aminoglycoside antibiotics in rats. J. Infect. Dis. 130:656–659.
23. **Mariel, C., P. Veyssier, J. C. Pechere, and E. De Cerner.** 1972. Urinary pH and excretion of gentamicin. Br. Med. J. 2:406.
24. **Milman, N.** 1973. Gentamycinnefropati. Ugeskr. Laeg. 135:1861–1865.
25. **Milman, F.** 1974. Renal failure associated with gentamicin therapy. Acta Med. Scand. 196:87–91.
26. **Naumann, V. P., and W. Auwärter.** 1968. Pharmakologische and therapeutische Eigenschaften von Gentamycin. Arzneim. Forsch. 18:1119–1123.
27. **Norby, L. H., and G. F. DiBona.** 1975. The renal vascular effects of meglumine diatrizoate. J. Pharmacol. Exp. Ther. 193:932–940.
28. **Oden, E. M., H. Stander, and M. J. Weinstein.** 1964. Microbiological assay of gentamicin, p. 8–13. Antimicrob. Agents Chemother. 1963.
29. **O'Grady, F.** 1971. Antibiotics in renal failure. Br. Med. Bull. 27:142–147.
30. **Regamey, C., R. C. Gordon, and W. M. M. Kirby.** 1973. Comparative pharmacokinetics of tobramycin and gentamicin. Clin. Pharmacol. Ther. 14:396–403.
31. **Riff, L. J., and G. G. Jackson.** 1971. Pharmacology of

gentamicin in man. J. Infect. Dis. 124(Suppl.):98–105.
32. **Schultze, R. G., R. E. Winters, and J. Kauffman.** 1971. Possible nephrotoxicity of gentamicin. J. Infect. Dis. 124(Suppl.):145–147.
33. **Smith, J.** 1951. The kidney. Oxford University Press, New York.
34. **Tune, B. M.** 1975. Relationship between the transport and toxicity of cephalosporins in the kidney. J. Infect. Dis. **132:**189–194.
35. **Tune, B. M., and M. Fernholt.** 1973. Relationship between cephaloridine and p-aminohippurate transport in the kidney. Am. J. Physiol. **225:**1114–1117.
36. **Whelton, A., and W. G. Walker.** 1974. Intrarenal antibiotic distribution in health and disease. Kidney Int. **6:**131–137.
37. **Wilfert, J. N., J. P. Burke, H. A. Bloomer, and C. B. Smith.** 1971. Renal insufficiency associated with gentamicin therapy. J. Infect. Dis. **124**(Suppl.):148–155.

ANTIMICROBIAL AGENTS AND CHEMOTHERAPY, Aug. 1976, p. 283-287
Vol. 10, No. 2

Pharmacokinetic Interpretation of Cephradine Levels in Serum After Intravenous and Extravascular Administration in Humans

ELISABETH S. RATTIE, PETER D. BERNARDO, AND LOUIS J. RAVIN*

Research and Development Division, Smith Kline and French Laboratories, Philadelphia, Pennsylvania 19101

Received for publication 17 February 1976

Pharmacokinetic parameters were calculated from intravenous data based upon a two-compartment open model. These parameters were subsequently used to determine the absorption rates and bioavailability of cephradine administered intramuscularly and orally. The results indicate that cephradine obeys dose-independent kinetics and that biological availability is complete from all dosage forms.

Cephradine, a semisynthetic cephalosporin derivative chemically designated as 7-[D-2-amino(1,4 - cyclohexadien - 1 - yl)acetamido] - 3-methyl-8-oxo-5-thia-1-azabicyclo[4.2.0]oct-2-ene-2-carboxylic acid, is structurally similar to cephalexin (Fig. 1). The compound is well absorbed from the gastrointestinal tract irrespective of the presence of food (3) and is effective in the treatment of both animal (1, 6) and human bacterial infections (4, 5). Cephradine is acid stable (1) and, after oral administration in mice, is rapidly absorbed and excreted virtually unchanged in the urine (10). Binding of cephradine to human plasma proteins is reversible and is less than 20% in vitro (7). The purpose of this paper is to elucidate the pharmacokinetics in humans and to determine the bioavailability of the drug administered intramuscularly and orally at various dosage levels in capsule and suspension forms.

MATERIALS AND METHODS

Intravenous administration. Each of eight fasting, normal, adult male subjects, ranging in age from 22 to 39 years and weighing between 145 and 188 pounds (ca. 65.8 and 85.3 kg), was given a single 1,000-mg dose of cephradine intravenously. Blood samples were taken prior to drug administration and at 5, 15, 30, 60, 120, 240, and 360 min after administration.

Urine samples were collected prior to drug administration and for the time periods 0 to 2, 2 to 4, and 4 to 6 h after injection of the drug.

Blood and urine samples were collected, frozen, and then analyzed for drug concentration by a *Bacillus subtilis* agar disk plate method (2).

Intramuscular administration. Each of 20 fasting, normal, adult male subjects, ranging in age from 20 to 60 years and weighing between 145 and 195 pounds (ca 65.8 and 86.5 kg), received a single 1,000-mg dose of cephradine intramuscularly. Blood samples were obtained prior to drug administration and at 15, 30, 45, 60, 90, 120, 150, 180, 240, and 360 min after injection.

Urine samples were collected prior to drug administration and for the time periods 0 to 2, 2 to 4, and 4 to 6 h after injection of the drug.

Blood and urine samples were collected, frozen, and then analyzed as described in the intravenous study.

Oral administration. A crossover study was carried out in 20 normal, adult male subjects ranging in age from 21 to 54 years and weighing between 140 and 208 pounds (ca. 63.5 and 94.3 kg). On test day 1, each subject was given either a single 250-mg or a 500-mg capsule according to a randomized dosing schedule. The subjects fasted 8 h before and 3 h after administration of the drug. Blood samples were taken prior to drug ingestion and at 30, 60, 90, 120, 180, and 360 min after administration. Urine samples were collected prior to drug administration and for the time periods 0 to 3, 3 to 6, 6 to 12, and 12 to 24 h after ingestion of the drug. After 1 week, the subjects were crossed over so that those who received a 250-mg capsule were given a 500-mg capsule and vice-versa.

In an additional study, 22 normal, adult male subjects, ranging in age from 21 to 50 years and weighing between 145 and 190 pounds (ca. 65.8 and 86.2 kg), received a single 1,000-mg (two 500-mg capsules) dose. Each subject fasted 8 h before and 3 h after drug administration. Blood samples were taken prior to drug ingestion and at 30, 60, 120, 180, 360, 480, and 600 min after administration.

Urine samples were collected prior to drug administration and for the time periods 0 to 3, 3 to 6, 6 to 12, and 12 to 24 h after ingestion of the drug.

Blood and urine samples were collected, frozen, and then analyzed as described in the intravenous study.

Each of 24 normal female subjects, ranging in age

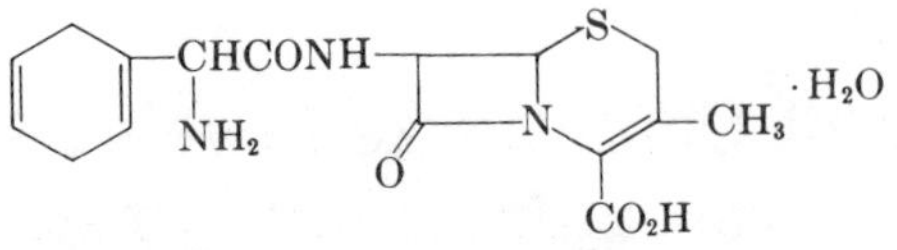

FIG. 1. *Structure of cephradine.*

from 20 to 52 years and weighing between 108 and 170 pounds (ca. 49.0 and 77.1 kg), was given 10 ml of cephradine oral suspension equivalent to 500 mg of cephradine. Each subject fasted 8 h before and 3 h after drug administration.

In another study 18 normal female subjects, ranging in age from 21 to 52 years and weighing between 139 to 199 pounds (ca. 63.1 and 90.3 kg), were given a single 5-ml dose of cephradine oral suspension equivalent to 250 mg of cephradine. Each subject fasted 8 h before and 3 h after drug administration. Blood samples were taken prior to drug ingestion and at 30, 60, 90, 120, 180, and 360 min after drug administration in both studies.

Urine samples were also collected prior to drug administration and for the 6-h period after ingestion of the drug.

Blood and urine samples were collected, frozen, and then analyzed as described in the intravenous study.

RESULTS

Intravenous administration. The average serum levels of cephradine obtained from the data of eight subjects dosed intravenously with 1,000 mg are shown in Fig. 2. It can be seen that the serum level declines in a biexponential manner. Therefore, the data can be fitted mathematically with a two-compartment model according to equation 1.

$$C_p = Ae^{-\alpha t} + Be^{-\beta t} \qquad (1)$$

The serum concentrations were used as input data for a digital computer (model PD12) program to provide a biexponential least-square regression fit to the data from which the coefficients A and B and the hybrid rate constants α and β were determined. The area under the serum level curve was calculated by using the expression $(A/\alpha) + (B/\beta)$ and determined by the trapezoidal rule. The parameters of equation 1 are as follows: A, 89; B, 27.8; α, 4.948; β, 0.809; $C_p{}^o$, 116.8; calculation of area, 52.32; area determined by trapezoidal rule, 52.65. The values are in close agreement. Utilizing these values, the rate constants k_{12}, k_{21}, and k_{el} and the serum $t_{1/2}$ were calculated: k_{12}, 1.731/h; k_{21}, 1.796/h; k_{el}, 2.23/h; $t_{1/2}$, 0.85 h.

The serum-tissue distribution of cephradine was estimated by calculating the fraction of the administered intravenous dose in the peripheral and central compartments at various times from known equations (8). Figure 3, a plot of the fractional serum-tissue distribution for the intravenous dose of cephradine, illustrates that the compound is well distributed throughout the tissue compartment.

Intramuscular administration. All data obtained from the intramuscular and oral routes of administration were fitted based upon a two-compartment open model. Assuming a first-order absorption process, the model is described by equation 2 (9).

$$C_p = \frac{k_a D}{V_p}\left[\left\{\frac{k_{21}-\alpha}{(k-\alpha)(\beta-\alpha)}\right\}e^{-\alpha t} + \left\{\frac{k_{21}-\beta}{(k-\beta)(\alpha-\beta)}\right\}e^{-\beta t} + \left\{\frac{k_{21}-k}{(\alpha-k)(\beta-k)}\right\}e^{-kt}\right] \qquad (2)$$

In each case the absorption rate constants were determined utilizng the pharmacokinetic parameters obtained from the intravenous data.

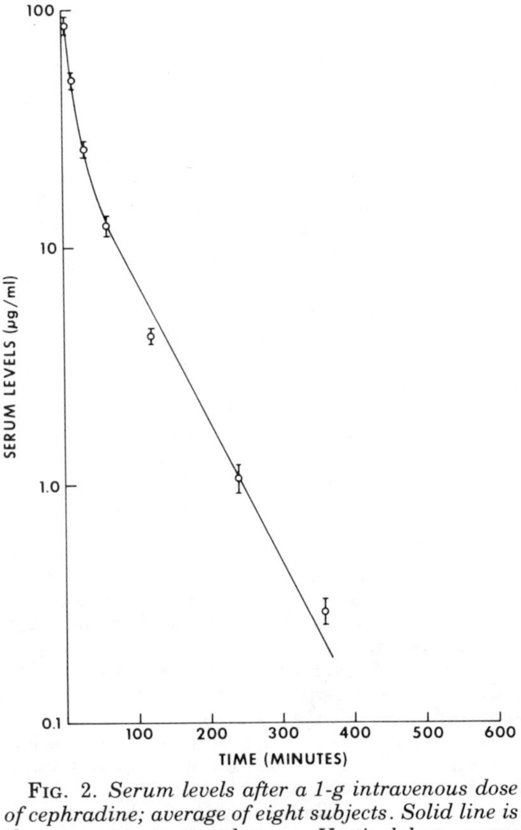

FIG. 2. *Serum levels after a 1-g intravenous dose of cephradine; average of eight subjects. Solid line is the computer-generated curve. Vertical bars represent the standard deviation of the mean.*

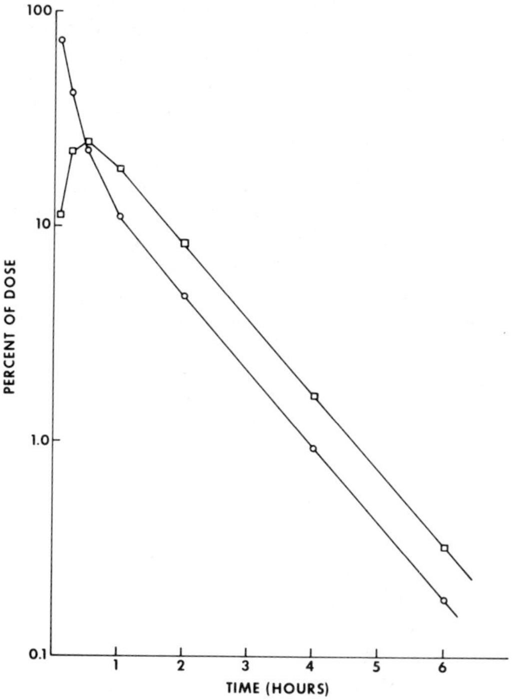

FIG. 3. *Percentage of cephradine dose estimated in the peripheral compartment (□) and in the central compartment (○) after a 1-g intravenous dose (average of eight subjects).*

Semilog plots of the average serum levels of cephradine (20 subjects) after a 1,000-mg intramuscular dose versus time are shown in Fig. 4. The averages are a good representation of the data of all the individual subjects. Cephradine was rapidly absorbed by this route, as noted by the attainment of peak serum levels of 19.66 ± 5.70 μg/ml after 30 min. Good agreement was also obtained between the computer-generated curve and the experimental data after administration by the intramuscular route. Table 1 contains the values for the absorption rate constant and the area under the serum level curve. Ninety-seven percent of the administered dose was accounted for by this route of administration.

Oral administration. Semilog plots of average serum levels versus time after oral administration of 250, 500, and 1,000 mg of cephradine as capsules are shown in Fig. 5. Again, good agreement was obtained between the computer-generated curve and the experimental data. Rapid absorption is obvious, with peak serum concentrations being obtained in approximately 30 min. The absorption rate constants and the area under the serum level curves are also shown in Table 1. The absorption rate constants were in good agreement, and 92, 92, and 104% of the administered dose for the 250-, 500-, and 1,000-mg capsules, respectively, were accounted for by this route of administration.

Semilog plots of the average serum levels

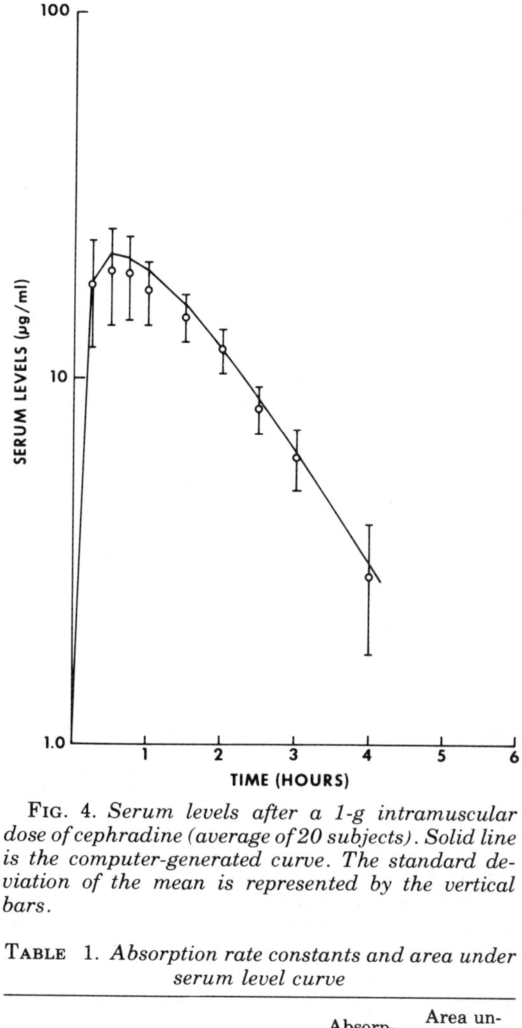

FIG. 4. *Serum levels after a 1-g intramuscular dose of cephradine (average of 20 subjects). Solid line is the computer-generated curve. The standard deviation of the mean is represented by the vertical bars.*

TABLE 1. *Absorption rate constants and area under serum level curve*

Route of administration	Dose (mg)	Absorption rate constant k_a (per h)	Area under serum level curve (μg/h/ml)
Intravenous	1,000		52.65
Intramuscular	1,000	1.1	50.97
Oral (capsule)	250	1.5	12.10
Oral (capsule)	500	1.1	24.29
Oral (capsule)	1,000	1.0	54.78
Oral (suspension)	250	3.0	13.70
Oral (suspension)	500	2.8	30.05

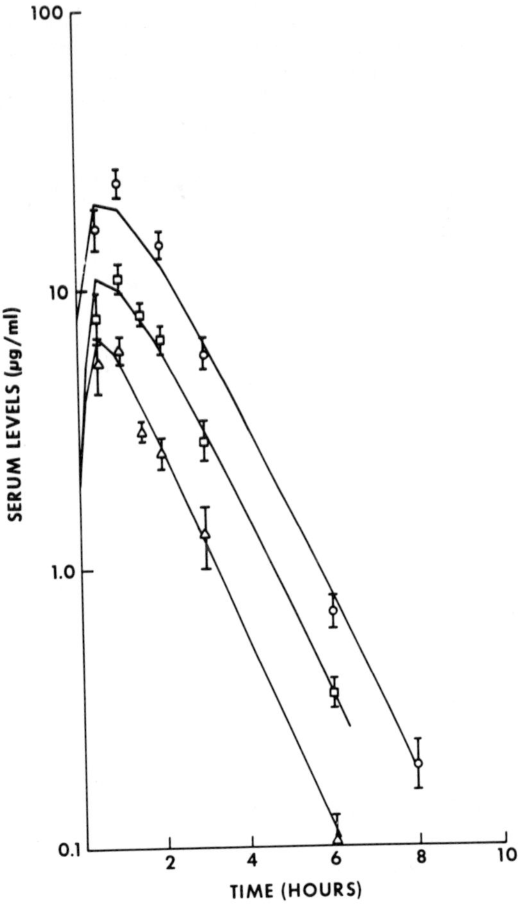

FIG. 5. *Average serum levels after oral administration of 250-, 500-, and 1,000-mg cephradine capsules, respectively. Symbols: ○, 1,000 mg; □, 500 mg; △, 250 mg. Solid lines are the computer-generated curves. Vertical bars represent the standard deviation of the mean.*

versus time after administration of 250 and 500 mg of cephradine as a suspension are shown in Fig. 6. A good fit is seen between the computer-generated curve and the experimental data. The oral suspension is rapidly absorbed, with peak serum concentrations being attained in less than 30 min. Since the oral suspension is essentially a saturated solution of cephradine, it is not surprising that peak levels are achieved earlier with this dosage form. The absorption rate constants and the area under the serum level curves are shown in Table 1. The data indicate that cephradine is completely available from this dosage form.

The relationships among the areas under serum level-time curves, the urine output of drug activity, and the bioavailability of various dosage forms of cephradine are only meaningful if the drug obeys dose-independent kinetics. Cephradine was found to obey dose-independent kinetics. This is illustrated in Fig. 7, which is a plot of the area under the serum level curves versus the total amount of drug eliminated for cephradine administered intravenously, 800 mg; intramuscularly, 770 mg; orally in capsules, 905, 495, and 245 mg for the 1,000-, 500-, and 250-mg strengths; orally in suspension, 363 and 225 mg for the 500- and 250-mg doses. Consequently, the bioavailability of extravascular dosage forms of cephra-

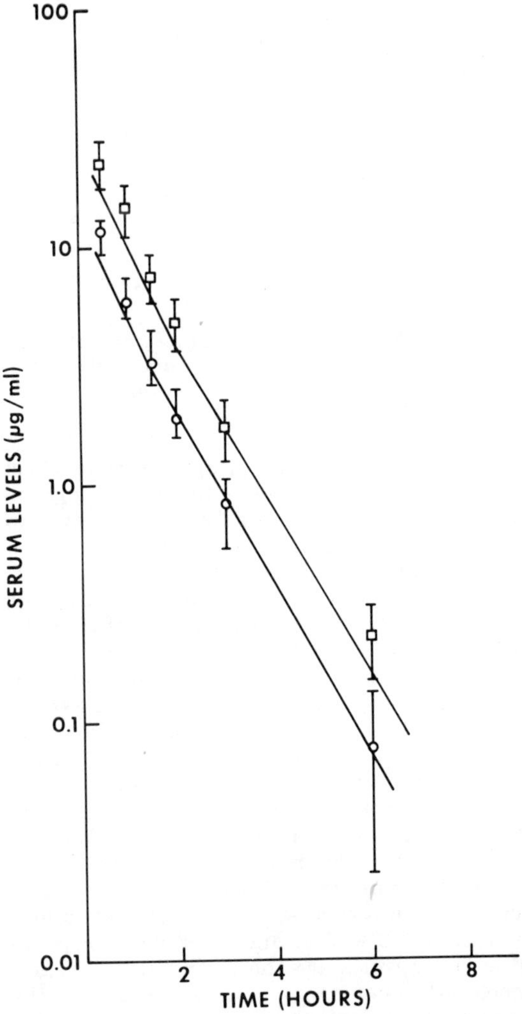

FIG. 6. *Average serum levels after oral administration of 250 and 500 mg of cephradine suspension. Symbols: □, 500 mg; ○, 250 mg. Solid lines are the computer-generated curves. The standard deviation of the mean is represented by the vertical bars.*

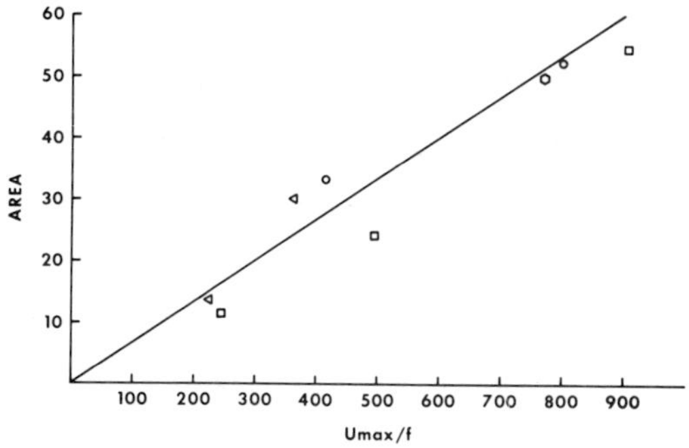

FIG. 7. *Plot illustrating dose-independent kinetics for cephradine over the dose range studied. The slope of the line is the reciprocal of the total clearance rate of cephradine. Symbols:* ○, *intravenous;* ⬡, *intramuscular;* □, *capsules;* △, *suspension.*

dine may be evaluated by comparing the area under the serum level-time per milligram of extravascular dose with the area per milligram of intravenous dose if the doses are within the range of 250 to 1,000 mg. Since dose-independent kinetics is obeyed, the slope of the plot in Fig. 7 is equal to the reciprocal of the total clearance rate of the drug from the body. A total clearance rate of 14.8 liters/h calculated from the slope of Fig. 7 compares favorably with the total clearance rate of 14.9 liters/h calculated from the pharmacokinetic parameters for cephradine determined in the intravenous study. The mean apparent volume of distribution, v_0, also calculated from these parameters was found to be 22.53 liters/1.73 m^2.

DISCUSSION

The pharmacokinetic parameters for cephradine were determined after intravenous administration. This was achieved by using a two-compartment open model. These parameters were subsequently used to determine the rate of absorption and the extent of cephradine bioavailability after extravascular administration. Cephradine is rapidly absorbed from all dosage forms. The oral suspension shows earlier peak levels, which is consistent, in part, with the characteristics of this dosage form. Cephradine is essentially completely absorbed from all the dosage forms and has a serum half-life of approximately 50 min.

The pharmacokinetic parameters determined from these studies can serve as guidelines in establishing proper dosage regimens during the clinical use of cephradine.

ACKNOWLEDGMENTS

The intravenous and oral data included in this paper were obtained through the courtesy of E. R. Squibb & Co.

We would like to thank Harry B. Kostenbauder, University of Kentucky College of Pharmacy, for his comments during the preparation of this manuscript.

LITERATURE CITED

1. **Gadebusch, H. W., G. J. Miraglia, H. I. Basch, et al.** 1972. Cephradine: a new orally absorbed cephalosporin antibiotic. Adv. Antimicrob. Antineoplast. Chemother. 1:1059–1062.
2. **Grove, D. C., and W. A. Randall.** 1955. Assay methods of antibiotics: a laboratory manual. Medical Encyclopedia, Inc., New York.
3. **Harvengt, C., P. DeSchepper, F. Lamy, et al.** 1973. Cephradine absorption and excretion in fasting and non-fasting volunteers. J. Clin. Pharmacol. 13:36–40.
4. **Klastersky, J., D. Daneua, and D. Weerts.** 1973. Cephradine: antibacterial activity and clinical effectiveness. Chemotherapy 18:191–204.
5. **Landa, L.** 1972. Cephradine in the treatment of intestinal infections caused by Shigella or Salmonella organisms. Curr. Ther. Res. Clin. Exp. 14:496–502.
6. **Miraglia, G. J., K. J. Renz, and H. H. Gadebusch.** 1973. Comparison of chemotherapeutic and pharmacodynamic activities of cephradine, cephalothin, and cephaloridine in mice. Antimicrob. Agents Chemother. 3:270–273.
7. **Neiss, E.** 1973. Cephradine – a summary of preclinical studies and clinical pharmacology. J. Irish Med. Assoc. 66(Suppl.):1–12.
8. **Riegelman, S., J. C. K. Loo, and M. Rowland.** 1968. Shortcomings in pharmacokinetic analysis by conceiving the body to exhibit properties of a single compartment. J. Pharm. Sci. 57:117–123.
9. **Wagner, J. G.** 1971. Biopharmaceutics and relevant pharmacokinetics. Drug Intelligence Publications, Hamilton, Ill.
10. **Weliky, I., H. H. Gadebusch, K. Kripalani, P. Arnow, and E. C. Schreiber.** 1974. Cephradine: absorption, excretion, and tissue distribution in animals of a new cephalosporin antibiotic. Antimicrob. Agents Chemother. 5:49–54.

ANTIMICROBIAL AGENTS AND CHEMOTHERAPY, Aug. 1976, p. 288-292
Vol. 10, No. 2

Printed in U.S.A.

In Vitro Evaluation of the New Oral Cephalosporin Cefatrizine: Comparison with Other Cephalosporins

C. CAROLINE BLACKWELL,* EARL H. FREIMER, AND GREGORY C. TUKE

Department of Medicine and Department of Microbiology, Medical College of Ohio at Toledo, Toledo, Ohio 43614*

Received for publication 23 February 1976

Cefatrizine (BL-S640), a semisynthetic, orally administered cephalosporin, was found to have an in vitro spectrum of activity comparable to those of four other cephalosporins tested. It is as effective as cephalexin, the other orally administered cephalosporin evaluated, against most species, and it appears to be more effective than cephalexin against many *Enterobacter*, *Haemophilus*, and *Proteus* strains isolated in our hospital. It is not inactivated by the plasmid-determined β-lactamases of 14 strains of ampicillin-resistant *Salmonella typhimurium* or the ampicillin resistance determinant of an *H. influenza* strain from the Center for Disease Control. No synergy was observed between cefatrizine and gentamicin, kanamycin, carbenicillin, or polymyxin when tested against selected strains.

The need for an effective orally administered cephalosporin has been apparent for sometime. Cefatrizine (CF), BL-S640, is a new semisynthetic cephalosporin that is absorbed well from the gastrointestinal tract (2). The other orally administered cephalosporin in present use, cephalexin (CX), has less antibacterial activity than other members of this group of compounds: cephalothin (KF), cephaloridine (CL), cefazolin (CZ), and cephaloglycin (3, 7). In conjunction with clinical trials of this new cephalosporin, sensitivities of 272 local bacterial isolates were determined and compared for CF, KF, CL, CX, and CZ. In addition, *Enterobacter*, *Pseudomonas*, and *Serratia* strains were tested for synergistic effects of CF with other antibiotics.

MATERIALS AND METHODS

Antibiotic agents. CF propylene glycolate (Bristol Laboratories, Syracuse, N.Y.) was supplied as the crystalline dipolar ion for use in antibiotic susceptibility testing (2). KF, CL, CX, CZ, all from Lilly Research Laboratories, Eli Lilly & Co., Indianapolis, Ind., were used for comparative studies. Gentamicin sulfate (Garamycin, Schering Corp., Bloomfield, Mass.), disodium carbenicillin (Pyopen, Beecham-Massengil, Bristol, Tenn.), polymyxin sulfate (Aerosporin, Burroughs-Wellcome), and kanamycin sulfate (Kantrex, Bristol Laboratories) were used in synergy studies. All stock solutions of antibiotics were prepared daily.

Bacterial isolates. Standard strains of *Escherichia coli* ATCC 25922 and *Staphylococcus aureus* ATCC 25923 were used in each trial as controls. Representative strains of gram-negative (190 isolates) and gram-positive (82 isolates) organisms were obtained from the clinical laboratory of the Hospital of the Medical College of Ohio at Toledo. All were stored in sterilized skimmed milk at −60°C. The strains to be tested were thawed and subcultured on solid medium to insure adequate growth. In addition, seven strains of *Neisseria meningitidis* and an ampicillin-resistant *Haemophilus influenzae* strain sent to us from the Center for Disease Control, Atlanta, Ga., were included.

Susceptibility studies. Minimal inhibitory concentrations (MICs) were determined by standard methods (6). Todd-Hewitt broth (BBL) was used to test *Streptococcus* species. Tryptic soy broth (Difco) was tried, but more reproducible results were obtained with the Todd-Hewitt medium. Clear GC medium used for *Neisseria gonorrhoeae* was composed of: soluble starch, 1 g; KH_2PO_4, 1 g; KCl, 5 g; K_2HPO_4, 4 g; proteose peptone, 15 g; water, 1 liter; glucose (20%, wt/vol), 25 ml; $NaHCO_3$ (4.2%, wt/vol), 10 ml; and supplement B (Difco), 10 ml. Mueller-Hinton medium (Difco) with 1% supplement B was used for *H. influenzae* and *N. meningitidis*. Mueller-Hinton medium without any supplement was used for all other strains tested. Twofold serial dilutions of the antibiotics were prepared (128 to 0.125 μg/ml). Tubes were inoculated with 10^5 organisms per ml and were incubated at 37°C for 18 to 24 h. *Neisseria*, *Streptococcus*, and *Haemophilus* strains were incubated in 10% CO_2. The MIC was recorded as the lowest concentration of antibiotic at which there was no visible growth.

Broth from tubes in which there was no visible growth was inoculated to an agar plate by using a calibrated platinum loop (3-mm diameter), and the lowest concentration at which there was 99.9% killing of the inoculum was recorded as the minimal bactericidal concentration (MBC). Duplicate plates were inoculated with 0.1 ml of an appropriate dilution to determine the number of colony-forming units in the inoculum. Disk susceptibilities to each of the cephalosporins were determined by the Kirby-Bauer method (1). Zone sizes, indicating susceptibility or resistance, were recorded for KF, CL, CX and CZ. The size of the zone surrounding the CF disk was recorded in millimeters.

Synergy studies. Synergy studies were performed on *Serratia*, *Pseudomonas*, and *Enterobacter* species by the agar dilution method. Plates containing antibiotic (0.125 to 128 μg/ml) or antibiotic plus one of three concentrations of CF (0.25, 2, or 16 μg/ml) were inoculated with a Steers replicator (9). Approximately 100 to 300 colony-forming units per spot were inoculated by each prong of the replicator. Plates were prepared each day from fresh stock solutions of antibiotics and dried for 2 h in an incubator before inoculation. The inoculated plates were incubated for 18 to 24 h at 37°C. Growth of fewer than five colonies per inoculum indicated susceptibility.

RESULTS

Activity of cephalosporins against gram-negative isolates. Table 1 records the MICs for some of the more common gram-negative organisms. Each strain was tested at least twice under the conditions described above. Most strains of *E. coli* and *Klebsiella* were inhibited by low concentrations (≤8 μg/ml) of BL-S640: 81% of *E. coli* and 70% of *K. pneumoniae* tested. As predicted, based on previous studies by other workers (5, 8, 10, 11), *Serratia* and *Pseudomonas* species were uniformly resistant to >128 μg of each of the cephalosporins per ml. Each of 15 strains of *S. typhimurium*, 14 of which contained plasmids mediating resistance to ampicillin, was inhibited by 8 μg of BL-S640 per ml. Forty-two percent of the *Proteus* species tested were inhibited at this concentration of CF; similar values were found for KF (42%) and CZ (47%). CL and CX appeared less effective in their abilities to inhibit these strains. CF was not as effective against *Enterobacter* at 8 μg/ml (31% of strains inhibited) as CZ (50%) but definitely more so than the other three cephalosporins. Both *N. meningitidis* and *gonorrhoeae* were inhibited by low concentrations of CF. All isolates of *H. influenzae* were inhibited by 8 μg of CF and KF per ml. CL and CZ inhibited 89% of the strains, but only 22% of the strains had MICs of 8 μg/ml or less with CX. An ampicillin-resistant strain (25 to 50 μg of ampicillin per ml) from the Center for Disease Control was sensitive at 8 μg of BL-S640 per ml, 2 μg of KF per ml, 8 μg of CL per ml, 16 μg of CX per ml, and 8 μg of CZ per ml. MBCs were usually within one or two dilutions of the MIC. With disks containing 30 μg of CF per ml, the zone of inhibition ranged from 0 to 30 mm. The strains that were susceptible to 8 μg/ml or less usually had zones ranging from 18 to 30 mm. The majority of strains that were resistant to 8 μg/ml or greater had zones ranging from 0 to 16 mm.

Activity of cephalosporins against gram-positive isolates. Emphasis, reflected in the numbers of each species tested, was on the organisms that are frequently resistant to antibiotics in common use. Each strain of *Streptococcus pyogenes* and *Streptococcus pneumoniae* was sensitive to concentrations of CF readily obtainable in serum (Table 2). For both *S. pyogenes* and *S. pneumoniae*, the diameter of the zone of inhibition surrounding the disk containing 30 μg of CF per ml ranged from 20 to 30 mm. The MBC was usually the same as the MIC or within one- or two-tube dilutions of the MIC.

One strain of methicillin-resistant *S. aureus*, DU 4916, was resistant to >128 μg of each of the cephalosporins tested per ml, except for CL (MIC = 16 μg/ml). Zone diameters for those staphylococcal strains susceptible to ≤8 μg of CF per ml ranged from 18 to 40 mm. Those that required >8 μg of BL-S640 per ml had a diameter of 16 mm or less. MBC values varied; not all MBCs were within the one- or two-tube dilution range of the MIC. The only consistent observation for *S. aureus* was that size of the original inoculum influenced the MBC value; larger inocula usually resulted in higher values for both the MIC and MBC.

The enterococci were resistant to these compounds, 16 μg/ml being the lowest MIC. The MBC was not reached at the concentrations used. Zone diameters determined by the Kirby-Bauer method ranged from 10 to 16 mm, the majority being 14 or 15 mm.

Synergy studies. *Enterobacter*, *Pseudomonas*, and *Serratia* strains were tested for synergistic effects of CF with other antibiotics. *Pseudomonas* and *Serratia* were examined for susceptibilities to gentamicin and carbenicillin and for the effect of the addition of CF at three concentrations (0.25, 2, and 16 μg/ml). As in the tube dilution experiments, each of the strains was resistant to CF. All but two strains, both *Pseudomonas*, were inhibited by 1 μg of gentamicin per ml; these two strains required 2 μg/ml. No synergistic effect was noted for the majority of the strains; in fact, in several instances, a slightly antagonistic effect was seen in the presence of CF. There was a slight amount of growth, a thin film or a few tiny colonies, on plates containing both gentamicin and CF, but no growth on gentamicin alone. The results obtained with carbenicillin were

TABLE 1. *MICs of cephalosporins of gram-negative organisms*

Organism and no. of isolates	Antibiotic	No. of isolates susceptible at a cephalosporin concn (μg/ml) of:											
		0.125	0.25	0.5	1	2	4	8	16	32	64	128	>128
Enterobacter sp. (16)	CF							5	3	1	2	1	4
	KF								4	3	1		8
	CL							1	1		3	3	8
	CX								4	2	4	1	5
	CZ					1	3	4	1		1	1	5
Escherichia coli (47)	CF				3	9	17	9	5	2			2
	KF					1	4	16	17	5	2		2
	CL					1	22	17	5	1	1		
	CX						2	27	15	1			2
	CZ				9	24	7	5	2				
Haemophilus influenzae (9)	CF					3		6					
	KF				6	3							
	CL					4	1	3	1				
	CX							2	6	1			
	CZ					4	1	3	1				
Klebsiella pneumoniae (18)	CF				4	5	2	3	1			1	2
	KF				2	3	5	3	1		1	1	1
	CL						7	5	2	2			2
	CX						2	10	3	1			2
	CZ					8	3		4	1			2
Neisseria gonorrhoeae (10)	CF	4	6										
	KF	1	8	1									
	CL	9	1										
	CX	7	3										
	CZ	10											
N. meningitidis (7)	CF	4	1	2									
	KF	1	1	4	1								
	CL			1			1	5					
	CX			1	3	3							
	CZ	1		3	3								
Pseudomonas aeruginosa (31)	CF												31
	KF												31
	CL												31
	CX												31
	CZ												31
Proteus sp. (19)	CF							8	8	1			2
	KF						1	7	7		1		3
	CL							4	10	1	1		3
	CX							1	13	3			2
	CZ							9	6	1	1		2
Salmonella typhimurium (15)	CF				1	6	3	5					
	KF					3	2	2	3	4	1		
	CL						5	4	4	2			
	CX						1	11	3				
	CZ					3	4						
Serratia marcescens (7)	CF												7
	KF												7
	CL												7
	CX												7
	CZ												7

TABLE 2. *MICs of cephalosporins of gram-positive organisms*

Organism and no. of isolates	Antibiotics	No. of isolates susceptible at a cephalosporin concn (μg/ml) of:											
		0.125	0.25	0.5	1	2	4	8	16	32	64	128	>128
Staphylococcus aureus (52)	CF		1	2	13	12	17	6					1
	KF	4	6	19	19	2	1						1
	CL	22	12	11	6			1					
	CX	1	1	11	12	10	14	2					1
	CZ	1	5	19	14	8	4						1
Enterococci (13)	CF								1	5	7		
	KF									10	3		
	CL								12	1			
	CX											11	2
	CZ									10	3		
Streptococcus pneumoniae (6)	CF		2	3	1								
	KF	2	4										
	CL	6											
	CX						3	3					
	CZ												
S. pyogenes (10)	CF	8	2										
	KF	7	3										
	CL	10											
	CX			1	9								
	CZ	1	9										

similar to those obtained with gentamicin. No synergy between the two antibiotics was observed, but there was very slight, if any, antagonism.

Enterobacter strains were tested for synergistic effects of gentamicin, kanamycin, and polymyxin B with CF. Again, no significant synergistic effect was observed with any of the antibiotics tested.

DISCUSSION

Our findings with isolates from the clinical laboratory of the Medical College of Ohio Hospital are in agreement with reports of other groups (5, 8, 10, 11) that CF is a broad-spectrum antimicrobial agent effective against pyogenic, gram-positive cocci and many members of the *Enterobacteriaceae*. It is not inactivated by the β-lactamases from 14 strains of *S. typhimurium* or the ampicillin resistance determinants of *H. influenzae*. Its in vitro activity compared well with the activities of the four other cephalosporins tested (5, 8). Against the gram-negative organisms, it was as active as CZ and usually more active than CX or KF (Table 1). These findings generally parallel those obtained by Watanakunakorn et al. (11), who used the agar dilution method. Our MIC values for *N. meningitidis* and *N. gonorrhoeae* appear to be somewhat lower than those reported by Leitner et al. (5). This may be due to differences in the methods used; Stilwell et al. (10) observed that CF appeared less active in broth than in agar. The MICs of CF against our strains are similar to those obtained by Overturf using the broth dilution method. Overturf reported lower MICs for *H. influenzae*, ranging from 1.60 to 3.13 μg/ml (8). The present study found MICs that ranged from 2 to 8 μg/ml. Since the medium used by both groups was the same, Mueller-Hinton broth containing 1% supplement B, differences may reflect variations in the local strains.

The MICs in these studies were somewhat higher for the streptococci, but this may reflect the differences in the media. Our data agree with the findings of Kayser (4), who reported that CL was the most effective cephalosporin tested against *S. aureus*.

CZ is certainly as effective as CX, the orally administered cephalosporin, in most species evaluated, and it appears to be more effective than CX against many strains of *Enterobacter*, *Haemophilus*, and *Proteus* isolated in our hospital.

ACKNOWLEDGMENTS

This study was supported by a grant-in-aid from Bristol Laboratories, Syracuse, N.Y.

We thank Cheryl Zimmerman for her assistance in preparation of this manuscript.

LITERATURE CITED

1. **Bauer, A. W., W. M. M. Kirby, J. C. Sherris, and M. Turck.** 1966. Antibiotic susceptibility testing by a standardized single disc method. Am. J. Clin. Pathol. 45:493–496.
2. **Bristol Laboratories.** 1974. Basic data brochure, oral BL-S640 PG. Bristol Laboratories, Syracuse, N.Y.
3. **Finland, M.** 1972. Oral and parenteral cephalosporins: the place of cephalexin in antibacterial therapy. Drugs 3:1–8.
4. **Kayser, F. H.** 1971. *In vitro* activity of cephalosporin antibiotics against gram positive bacteria. Postgrad. Med. J. 47(Suppl.):14–18.
5. **Leitner, F., R. E. Buck, M. Misiek, T. A. Pursiano, and K. B. Price.** 1975. BL-S640, a cephalosporin with a broad spectrum of antibacterial activity: properties in vitro. Antimicrob. Agents Chemother. 7:298–305.
6. **Lennette, E. H., E. H. Spaulding, and J. P. Truant (ed.).** 1974. Manual of clinical microbiology, p. 407–442. American Society for Microbiology, Washington, D.C.
7. **Levison, M. E., W. D. Johnson, T. S. Thornhill, and D. Kaye.** 1969. Clinical and *in vitro* evaluation of cephalexin. J. Am. Med. Assoc. 209:1331–1336.
8. **Overturf, G. D., R. L. Ressler, P. B. Marengo, and J. Wilkins.** 1975. In vitro evaluation of BL-S640, a new oral cephalosporin antibiotic. Antimicrob. Agents Chemother. 8:305–310.
9. **Steers, E. E., E. L. Foltz, and B. S. Graves.** 1959. Inocula replicating apparatus for routine testing of bacterial susceptibility to antibiotics. Antibiot. Chemother. 9:307–311.
10. **Stilwell, G. A., H. G. Adams, and M. Turck.** 1975. In vitro evaluation of a new oral cephalosporin, cefatrizine (BL-S640). Antimicrob. Agents Chemother. 8:751–753.
11. **Watanakunakorn, C., T. Bannister, and C. Glozbecker.** 1975. Susceptibility of clinical isolates of *Enterobacteriaceae* to BL-S640, a new oral cephalosporin. Antimicrob. Agents Chemother. 7:381–385.

ANTIMICROBIAL AGENTS AND CHEMOTHERAPY, Aug. 1976, p. 293-298
Copyright © 1976 American Society for Microbiology

Vol. 10, No. 2
Printed in U.S.A.

Mode of Action of a Purified Antitumor Protein from the Proteinaceous Crystal of *Bacillus thuringiensis* subsp. *thuringiensis* on Yoshida Ascites Sarcoma Cells

S. S. S. V. PRASAD[1]* AND Y. I. SHETHNA

Microbiology and Cell Biology Laboratory, Indian Institute of Science, Bangalore 560012, India

Received for publication 23 March 1976

A purified antitumor protein from the proteinaceous crystal of *Bacillus thuringiensis* subsp. *thuringiensis* inhibits the growth of Yoshida ascites sarcoma both in vivo and in vitro. Exogenous respiration of the tumor cells was unaffected by the protein at a concentration as high as 500 μg/ml. The antitumor protein inhibits the uptake and incorporation of labeled precursors into macromolecules. However, the ratio of incorporation over uptake is not affected by the protein. Further, the protein brings about the leakage of 260-nm-absorbing material, proteins, and ^{32}P-labeled cellular constituents from the Yoshida ascites sarcoma cells. The results show that the action of the antitumor protein appears to alter the cellular permeability of the tumor cells.

During sporulation *Bacillus thuringiensis* produces a crystalline material which is liberated into the medium when the sporangium is lysed (6). This unique crystal was composed of an alkali-soluble protein with a molecular weight of 200,000, which is highly toxic for lepidopterous insect larvae (1) and is the least toxic for mammals (8, 18). Recently, we have reported antitumor activity against Yoshida ascites sarcoma (YAS) with a high therapeutic index for this crystal preparation (18). We have also observed that this crystal brings about long-lasting antitumor immunity (21) and enhances the nonspecific immune response (20). Further, the purification, crystallization, and characterization of the biologically active protein subunit of the crystals have been achieved (19).

The only biological activity of the crystal known until recently was its insecticidal activity. The exact insecticidal mode of action of the crystal is poorly understood because of the unresolved identity of the toxic protein subunit of the crystal. The available evidence suggests that the crystal toxin alters the membrane permeability of the insect gut wall, resulting in the impairment of ion transport and the leakage of alkaline gut contents into acidic hemocoel. The resulting pH change brings about paralysis and death of the insect larvae (3, 4, 16). However, the antitumor mode of action of this toxic protein has not yet been elucidated. The purification of the active protein subunit made it possible to study its mode of action on tumor cells, which is being reported here.

MATERIALS AND METHODS

Chemicals. The following radioactive chemicals were obtained from Bhabha Atomic Research Centre, Bombay, India: [^{3}H]thymidine (specific activity, 10,500 mCi/mmol); [^{14}C]phenylalanine (specific activity, 312 mCi/mmol); [^{14}C]glucose (specific activity, 229 mCi/mmol); and [^{32}P]orthophosphoric acid (specific activity, 5 mCi/mmol). [^{14}C]uridine (specific activity, 55.3 mCi/mmol) was purchased from New England Nuclear Corp., Boston, Mass.; medium 199 with Hanks basal salts solution (HBSS) was purchased from V.P. Chest Institute, New Delhi, India. All the other chemicals were of analytical grade.

Animals. Inbred Wistar A/Iisc rats weighing around 100 to 120 g were used in all the studies. The animals were given a diet of "pellet" food (Hindustan Lever Ltd., Bombay) and water ad libitum.

Tumor. YAS, a rapidly developing, chemically induced tumor (25) was maintained in isogenic Wistar rats (A/Iisc) by serial intraperitoneal (i.p.) transfer of 2×10^7 tumor cells, once in 4 days. The details about the morphology and chromosomal characteristics of the tumor have been described earlier (2, 22).

Purification of antitumor protein. Pure antitumor protein from crystals was obtained as previously described (19). The lyophilized sample was dissolved in cold Krebs phosphate buffer at pH 7.4, so that the required concentrations were contained in 0.2 ml of suspension.

Antitumor activity in vivo. Experimental animals were injected i.p. with 3×10^7 actively dividing

[1] Present address: Department of Developmental Therapeutics, M.D. Anderson Hospital and Tumor Institute, The University of Texas System Cancer Center, Houston, Tex. 77030.

YAS cells. Treatment consisted of a single or multiple i.p. dose of protein preparation given 24 h after tumor transplantation. Regular observations were made on the weights and the general behavior of the animals.

Collection of YAS cells. YAS cells were collected asceptically from the peritoneal cavity of 3-day-old, tumor-bearing rats in 10 volumes of cold saline. The cells were then washed with cold Krebs phosphate buffer by repeated centrifugations (1,000 × *g*) at 0°C until the tumor cells were free from contaminating erythrocytes. The tumor cells were then suspended in the original volume, and a count was made by the trypan blue dye exclusion method (17). The concentration of YAS cells was adjusted to 3 × 10^6 viable cells/ml in cold Krebs phosphate buffer.

Cell multiplication. The YAS cell multiplication was studied by short-term cell culture as described earlier (9), using medium 199 with HBSS and 40% heat-inactivated calf serum. Viable YAS cells (10^5/ml) were inoculated into the medium along with different concentrations of the antitumor protein. In another set [^{3}H]thymidine (2 μCi/ml) was added along with the protein. The culture tubes were then incubated at 37°C, and the viable count and the incorporation of [^{3}H]thymidine into deoxyribonucleic acid (DNA) were determined at regular intervals. Viable counts were made by the trypan blue dye exclusion method. The incorporation of [^{3}H]thymidine into DNA was estimated by taking a 0.2-ml sample and precipitating it with an equal volume of 10% trichloroacetic acid. The mixture was then filtered under suction on Whatman no. 1 filter paper disks, the precipitate was washed with 5% trichloroacetic acid, ethanol-ether (1:1), and ether successively, and radioactivity was determined in a Beckman LS-100 liquid scintillation counter.

Respiration studies. Studies on respiration were carried out using standard manometric techniques (24). YAS cells were washed as described before and suspended in Krebs phosphate buffer. Warburg flasks contained the following in final volume of 3.2 ml: 1 ml of 0.2 M glucose and 3 × 10^7 YAS cells/ml in the main compartment. The center well contained 0.2 ml of 20% KOH. The antitumor protein was used in appropriate amounts to give the desired concentrations. The flasks were equilibrated for 10 min at 37°C, and the oxygen uptake was measured.

Uptake of [^{14}C]glucose by YAS cells. The uptake of glucose from the medium (medium 199 without serum) by YAS cells was determined by adding [^{14}C]glucose (1 μCi/ml) to the YAS cell suspension (3 × 10^6 cells/ml) in a final volume of 2 ml. The antitumor protein was added at desired concentrations and incubated at 37°C in a water bath for 2 h. The period of incubation was standardized by several preliminary experiments. Samples were taken out at the end of the incubation, and YAS cells were filtered under suction on Whatman no. 1 filter paper disks and then washed with excess of Krebs phosphate buffer. The filter paper disks were then dried under an infrared lamp, and the radioactivity was determined.

Uptake and incorporation of labeled precursors into DNA, RNA, and proteins of YAS cells. The YAS cells (3 × 10^6 viable cells/ml) were incubated at 37°C for 2 h with various concentrations of the antitumor protein along with either [^{3}H]thymidine (1 μCi/ml), [^{14}C]uridine (1 μCi/ml), or [^{14}C]phenylalanine (1 μCi/ml) in a total volume of 2 ml. At the end of the incubation period the uptake of the labeled precursors by YAS cells was determined as described earlier for [^{14}C]glucose. The incorporation of [^{3}H]thymidine, [^{14}C]uridine, and [^{14}C]-phenylalanine into DNA, ribonucleic acid (RNA), and protein, respectively, was estimated according to Mans and Novelli (13). The reaction was stopped by the addition of an equal volume of 10% cold trichloroacetic acid. The mixture was then filtered under suction on Whatman no. 1 filter paper disks, and the precipitate was washed with 5% trichloroacetic acid, ethanol-ether (1:1), and ether successively, and the radioactivity was determined.

Cell permeability studies. The tumor cells (3 × 10^7 cells/ml) were exposed to the antitumor protein at various concentrations in a water bath at 37°C. At different time intervals samples were removed, and the cell exudates were examined for 260-nm-absorbing materials by measuring the absorbance. Proteins were determined by the method of Lowry et al. (12).

In vivo ^{32}P labeling of tumor cells. Actively growing, 3-day-old tumor cells were labeled in vivo by the administration of ^{32}P label as *ortho*-phosphoric acid (0.5 mCi/animal) i.p. After 2 h of ^{32}P administration, rats were sacrificed by cervical dislocation, and the tumor cells were collected in cold saline and processed as described earlier. The labeled tumor cells were then incubated at 37°C for 2 h in the presence of different concentrations of the antitumor protein. At the end of the incubation period, the cell exudates were obtained by centrifugation, and the radioactivity was determined.

RESULTS

Effect of purified antitumor protein on YAS in vivo. The results on the antitumor activity of the pure protein are presented in Table 1. A single dose of 1 mg/kg brought about an increased survival period of the treated animals, whereas a split dose administration of 0.1 mg/kg given for 5 days resulted in the complete regression of the tumor. At a lower dose of 0.05 mg/kg, 60% of the treated animals died with a prolonged survival period of 28 days, in contrast to 10 days in case of controls.

Effect of antitumor protein on in vitro YAS cell multiplication. The results of this experiment are depicted in Fig. 1. The viability of the cells and the incorporation of the [^{3}H]-thymidine into DNA were adversely affected in the presence of the protein. Maximum effect was seen at 20 h with a protein concentration of 1 mg/ml. There was 60% reduction in the viable count and 54% decrease in the incorporation of [^{3}H]thymidine into DNA at this concentration. After 24 h there was a slight increase in both the viable count and DNA synthesis.

Effect of antitumor protein on respiration of YAS cells. The antitumor protein did not show a significant effect on the exogenous respiration of the tumor cells. Even at a concentration of 1 mg of protein/ml, there was only a 20% reduction in the total microliters of oxygen consumed after 210 min.

TABLE 1. *Effect of purified antitumor protein from the proteinaceous crystal of B. thuringiensis on YAS cells in rats*

Dose[a]	No. of injections	Survival period (days) ± standard error	Survivors[b]	No. of survivors after 90 days
2.5	1	30 ± 2.0	6/6	0
1	1	32 ± 1.3	6/6	0
0.5	5[c]	90[d]	6/6	6
0.2	5	90	6/6	6
0.1	5	90	6/6	6
0.05	5	28 ± 3.0	6/6	2
Control	1	9 ± 1.2	0/6	0
	5	10 ± 1.5	0.6	0

[a] Milligrams of protein per kilogram given i.p. 24 h after tumor transplantation; controls injected with saline.

[b] Survivors at the time of the death of the controls.

[c] Split dose treatment administered at the rate of one dose per day for 5 days.

[d] Surviving until the end of the experiment.

Effect of antitumor protein on the uptake of [^{14}C]glucose by YAS cells. The results indicate that there was a dose-dependent inhibition of the [^{14}C]glucose uptake by YAS cells (Table 2). Maximum inhibition of 82% was observed at a protein concentration of 1 mg/ml.

Effect of antitumor protein on the uptake and incorporation of labeled presursors into macromolecules of YAS cells. (i) [^{3}H]thymidine. The data revealed that there was an inhibition of both uptake and incorporation of [^{3}H]thymidine into DNA of YAS cells in the presence of the antitumor protein (Table 3). At a protein concentration of 0.5 mg/ml, the percentages of uptake and incorporation were 31.5 and 38.7%, respectively. However, the protein did not affect the ratio of incorporation over uptake.

(ii) [^{14}C]uridine. The protein brought about a decrease in the uptake and incorporation of

TABLE 2. *Effect of antitumor protein on the uptake of [^{14}C]glucose by YAS cells*[a]

Concn (mg/ml)	cpm[b]/3 × 10^6 viable cells	Uptake (%)	Inhibition (%)
0	18,200	100	0
0.25	15,341	84.3	15.7
0.5	7,234	39.8	60.2
1.0	3,262	18	82

[a] In all the experiments the measurements were made at the end of 2 h of incubation period at 37°C.

[b] cpm, Counts per minute.

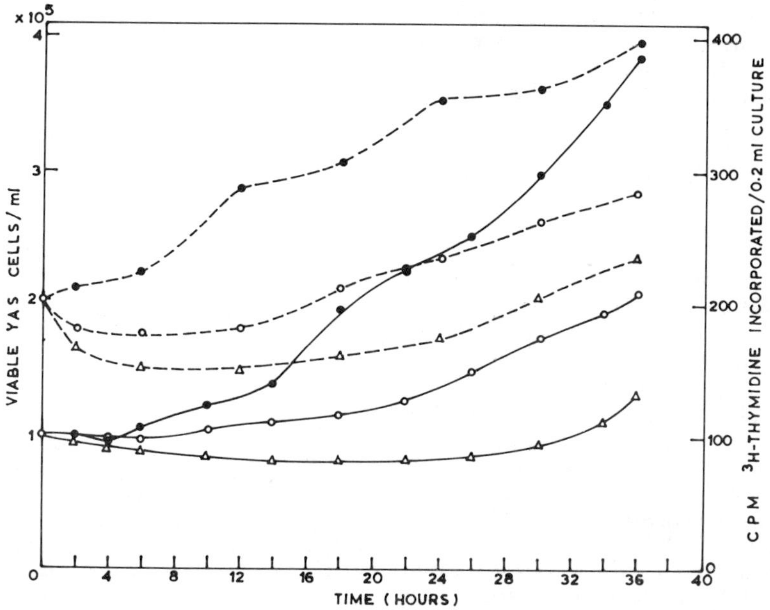

FIG. 1. *Effect of antitumor protein on cell multiplication and DNA synthesis of YAS cells in vitro. Solid lines, [^{3}H]thymidine incorporation; dotted lines, cell viability;* ●, *control,* ○, *0.5 mg,* △, *1.0 mg.*

TABLE 3. *Effect of antitumor protein on [³H]-thymidine uptake and incorporation into DNA of YAS cells*

Concn (mg/ml)	Uptake (3 × 10⁶ viable cells)		Incorporation (3 × 10⁶ viable cells)		Ratio of incorporation over uptake
	cpm[a]	%	cpm	%	
0	3,442	100	435	100	12.7
0.01	2,513	73.0	393	90.2	15.6
0.05	2,344	68.1	374	86.0	15.9
0.1	1,859	54	357	82	19.2
0.25	1,650	47	311	77.5	18.0
0.50	1,091	31.5	169	38.7	15.4

[a] cpm, Counts per minute.

TABLE 4. *Effect of antitumor protein on the uptake and incorporation of [¹⁴C]uridine into RNA of YAS cells*

Concn (mg/ml)	Uptake (3 × 10⁶ viable cells)		Incorporation (3 × 10⁶ viable cells)		Ratio of incorporation over uptake
	cpm[a]	%	cpm	%	
0	4,560	100	2,210	100	48.4
0.01	3,420	75	2,055	93	60.0
0.05	3,101	68.0	1,858	84.1	55.7
0.10	2,873	63.0	1,600	72.4	55.6
0.25	2,374	52.1	1,348	61.0	56.7
0.50	1,961	43.0	1,090	49.32	55.5

[a] cpm, Counts per minute.

[¹⁴C]uridine into RNA of tumor cells (Table 4). Maximum effect was seen at a concentration of 1 mg/ml, wherein the percentages of uptake and incorporation were 33.5 and 35.7%, respectively, of the control. The ratio of incorporation over uptake was not inhibited.

(iii) [¹⁴C]phenylalanine. The uptake and incorporation of [¹⁴C]phenylalanine were also inhibited by the antitumor protein without inhibiting the ratio of incorporation over uptake (Table 5). At a protein concentration of 1 mg/ml, 54.1 and 53.8% of uptake and incorporation were observed, respectively.

Effect of antitumor protein on cell permeability. The leakage of various cellular constituents like 260-nm-absorbing materials and proteins as affected by the antitumor protein are shown in Fig. 2 and 3, respectively. The leakage of 260-nm-absorbing materials was directly proportional to the concentration and time of exposure of the antitumor protein. The viability of the tumor cells was not affected by the protein within the incubation period of 2 h at all the doses tested.

The leakage of proteins also showed the same pattern as the 260-nm-absorbing materials. The leakage of ³²P-labeled cellular constituents is shown in Table 6. There was a leakage of 23.5% of the labeled constituents over the control at a concentration of 1 mg/ml.

DISCUSSION

The in vitro and in vivo data presented in this study clearly reveal the potent tumor inhibitory activity of the toxic protein from the proteinaceous crystal of *B. thuringiensis*. The effectiveness of the split dose administration may be due to the rapid removal of the protein from the system. The detoxification of the protein after 24 h of incubation may also be the reason for the increase in the viable count and

TABLE 5. *Effect of antitumor protein on the uptake and incorporation of [¹⁴C]phenylalanine into protein of YAS cells*

Concn (mg/ml)	Uptake (3 × 10⁶ viable cells)		Incorporation (3 × 10⁶ viable cells)		Ratio of incorporation over uptake
	cpm[a]	%	cpm	%	
0	5,500	100	4,200	100	76.3
0.01	4,730	86.0	3,868	92.1	81.7
0.05	4,472	81.3	3,705	88.2	82.8
0.10	4,070	74	3,465	82.5	85.1
0.25	3,823	69.5	3,285	78.2	85.9
0.50	3,480	63.3	3,053	71.6	87.0

[a] cpm, Counts per minute.

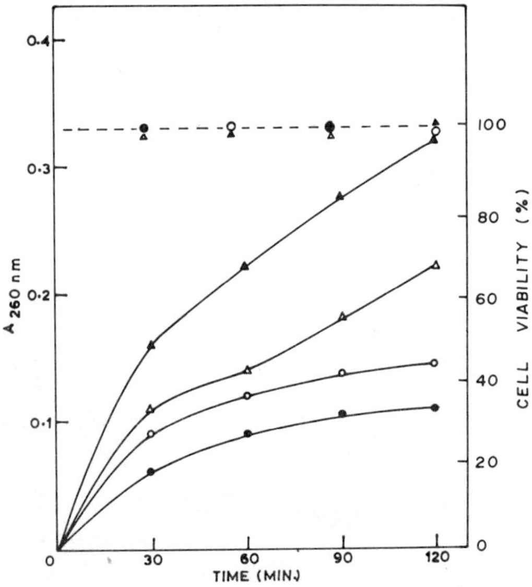

FIG. 2. *Effect of antitumor protein on the leakage of 260-nm-absorbing materials from YAS cells. Solid lines, Absorbancy at 260 nm; dotted lines, percentage of cell viability; ●, control, ○, 0.25 mg, △, 0.5 mg, ▲, 1.0 mg.*

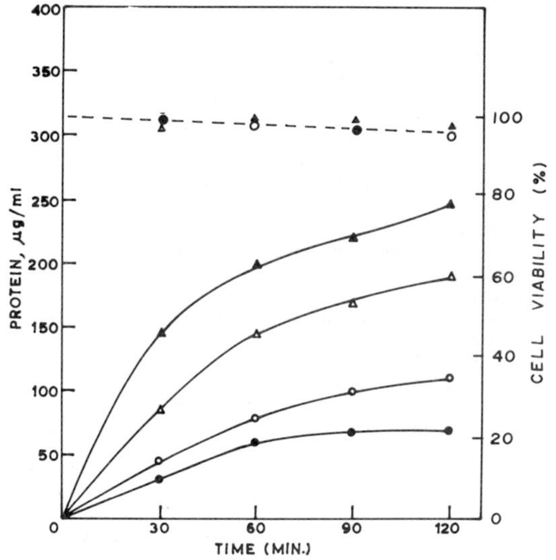

FIG. 3. *Effect of antitumor protein on the leakage of proteins from YAS cells. Solid lines, Protein (micrograms per milliliter); dotted lines, percentage of cell viability;* ●, *control;* ○, *0.25;* △, *0.5 mg;* ▲, *1.0 mg.*

TABLE 6. *Effect of antitumor protein on the leakage of* ^{32}P *from in vivo labeled YAS cells*

Concn (mg/ml)	Cell viability[a]	Leakage of ^{32}P (cpm)[b]	Leakage (%)
0	98	40,000	0
0.25	95	44,100	10.2
0.5	96.5	46,002	15
1.0	94.2	49,411	23.5

[a] Cell viability was determined at the end of the incubation period (2 h) by the trypan blue dye exclusion method (17).

[b] cpm, Counts per minute.

DNA synthesis in vitro. These results suggest that continuous exposure of the tumor cells to the toxic protein is necessary for its action.

The antitumor protein failed to inhibit exogenous respiration, but there is considerable inhibition of the [^{14}C]glucose uptake by the tumor cells. Further, the uptake and incorporation of [^{3}H]thymidine, [^{14}C]uridine, and [^{14}C]phenylalanine into DNA, RNA, and protein fractions of the tumor cells are also inhibited by the antitumor protein. However, the ratio of incorporation over uptake is not affected in all the cases. Further, there is a selective inhibition of uptake over the incorporation at all the doses tested. These observations suggest that the toxic protein may be damaging the integrity of the cell membrane. This is further confirmed by the rapid leakage of essential cellular constituents, like proteins and nucleotides from the tumor cells exposed to this toxic protein, without affecting the cell viability.

A vast amount of literature is available in the area of membrane-active antibacterial (5, 7, 15) and antifungal agents (11, 23). However, very few antitumor agents elicit their action by affecting the membrane function of the cells (10, 14). Membrane-active agents affect the membrane integrity and functions, thereby producing an initial rapid loss of high- and low-molecular-weight metabolites from the metabolic pool of the cell. Antifungal antibiotics like polyenes specifically combine with sterol components in the membrane of susceptible organisms, resulting in the structural disruption of membrane and the loss of essential metabolites from the cell.

The data presented here on the purified antitumor protein from the proteinaceous crystal of *B. thuringiensis* suggest that its mode of action is mainly on the cell membrane of the tumor cells, which is similar to the action of the whole crystal in the insect system. However, the elucidation of the exact site of action of this purified protein on the cell membrane of the tumor cells needs further investigation.

ACKNOWLEDGMENTS

We thank University Grants Commission, New Delhi, for the award of a special grant and the council of Scientific and Industrial Research, New Delhi, for awarding a Senior Research Fellowship to one of us (S.S.S.V.P.).

LITERATURE CITED

1. **Angus, T. A.** 1956. Extraction, purification and properties of Bacillus sotto toxin. Can. J. Microbiol. **2**:416–426.
2. **Belur, P. S., and M. Sirsi.** 1969. Chromosomal analysis of Yoshida ascites sarcoma in rats. Curr. Sci. **7**:156–158.
3. **Fast, P. G., and T. A. Angus.** 1965. Effect of parasporal inclusions of *Bacillus thuringiensis* var *sotto* Ishiwata on the permeability of the gut wall of *Bombyx mori* (Linnaeus) larvae. J. Invertebr. Pathol. **7**:29–32.
4. **Fast, P. G., and I. K. Morrison.** 1972. The δ-endotoxin of *Bacillus thuringiensis*. IV. The effect of δ-endotoxin on ion regulation by mid-gut tissue of *Bombyx mori* larvae. J. Invertebr. Pathol. **20**:208–211.
5. **Few, A. V., and I. H. Schulman.** 1953. The absorption of polymyxin E by bacteria and baterial cell walls and its bactericidal action. J. Gen Microbiol. **9**:454–466.
6. **Hannay, C. L., and P. C. Fitz-James.** 1955. Protein crystals of *Bacillus thuringiensis* Berliner. Can. J. Microbiol. **1**:694–710.
7. **Hugo, W. B., and S. F. Bloomfield.** 1971. Studies on the mode of action of the phenolic antibacterial agent fentichlor against *Staphylococcus aureus* and *Escherichia coli*. II. The effects of fentichlor on the bacterial membrane and the cytoplasmic constituents of the cell. J. Appl. Bacteriol. **34**:569–578.
8. **International Mineral and Chemical Corp.** 1969. Technical bulletin. Crop Aid Products Dept., International Mineral and Chemical Corp., Ill.

9. **Ishidate, M., Y. Sakurai, H. Imamura, and A. Moriwaki.** 1959. Studies on carcinostatic substances. XX. Studies on the culture of Yoshida sarcoma cells *in vitro*. Chem. Pharm. Bull. 7:690–694.

10. **Kameda, Y., K. Matsui, H. Kato, T. Yamada, and H. Sagai.** 1972. Antitumor activity of *Bacillus natto*. III. Isolation and characterization of a cytolytic substance on Ehrlich ascites carcinoma cells in the culture medium of *Bacillus natto* KMD1126. Chem. Pharm. Bull. 20:1551–1557.

11. **Kinsky, S. C.** 1967. Polyene antibiotics, p. 122–141. *In* D. Gottlieb and P.D. Shaw (ed.), Antibiotics, vol. I. Springer-Verlag, New York.

12. **Lowry, O. H., N. J. Rosebrough, A. L. Farr, and R. J. Randall.** 1951. Protein measurement with the Folin phenol reagent. J. Biol. Chem. 193:265–275.

13. **Mans, R. J., and G. D. Novelli.** 1961. Measurement of the incorporation of radioactive amino acids into protein by a filter-paper disk method. Arch. Biochem. Biophys. 94:48–53.

14. **Mondovi, B., R. Strom, A. F. Agro, P. Caiafa, P. De Sole, A. Bozzi, G. Rotillo, and A. R. Fanelli.** 1971. Effect of polyenic antibiotics on Ehrlich ascites and Novikoff hepatoma cells. Cancer Res. 31:505–509.

15. **Newton, B. A.** 1953. The release of soluble constituents from washed cells of *Pseudomonas aeruginosa* by the action of polymyxin. J. Gen. Microbiol. 9:654–664.

16. **Pendelton, I. R.** 1970. Sodium and potassium fluxes in *Philosamia ricini* during *Bacillus thuringiensis* protein crystal intoxication. J. Invertebr. Pathol. 16:313–314.

17. **Phillips, H. J., and J. E. Terryberry.** 1957. Counting actively metabolizing tissue cultured cells. Exp. Cell Res. 13:341.

18. **Prasad, S. S. S. V., H. Lalitha Kumari, and Y. I. Shethna.** 1973. Inhibitory activity of the parasporal crystal of *Bacillus thuringiensis* var *thuringiensis* on Yoshida ascites sarcoma. Curr. Sci. 42:568–570.

19. **Prasad, S. S. S. V., and Y. I. Shethna.** 1974. Purification, crystallization and partial characterization of the antitumor and insecticidal protein subunit from the δ-endotoxin of *Bacillus thuringiensis* var *thuringiensis*. Biochim. Biophys. Acta 363:558–566.

20. **Prasad, S. S. S. V., and Y. I. Shethna.** 1975. Enhancement of immune response by the proteinaceous crystal of *Bacillus thuringiensis* var *thuringiensis*. Biochem. Biophys. Res. Commun. 62:517–523.

21. **Prasad, S. S. S. V., and Y. I. Shethna.** 1976. Induction of antitumor immunity by the proteinaceous crystal of *Bacillus thuringiensis* var *thuringiensis*. Ind. J. Exp. Biol., in press.

22. **Reddy, V. V. S., and M. Sirsi.** 1969. Effect of *Abrus precatorius* L. on experimental tumors. Cancer Res. 29:1447–1451.

23. **Sreedhara Swamy, K. H., M. Sirsi, and G. Ramananda Rao.** 1974. Studies on the mechanism of action of miconazole: effect of miconazole on respiration and cell permeability of *Candida albicans*. Antimicrob. Agents Chemother. 5:420–425.

24. **Umbreit, W. W., R. H. Burris, and J. F. Sbauffer.** 1957. Manometric techniques. Burgess Publishing Co., Minneapolis.

25. **Yoshida, T.** 1952. Studies on an ascites (reticuloendothelial cell?) sarcoma of the rat. J. Natl. Cancer Inst. 12:947–969.

ANTIMICROBIAL AGENTS AND CHEMOTHERAPY, Aug. 1976, p. 299-306
Vol. 10, No. 2
Printed in U.S.A.

Genetic Basis of Streptococcin A-FF22 Production

J. R. TAGG[1] AND L. W. WANNAMAKER*

Departments of Pediatrics and Microbiology, Medical School, University of Minnesota, Minneapolis, Minnesota 55455

Received for publication 16 March 1976

Spontaneous, low-frequency loss of ability to produce streptococcin A-FF22 (SA) by group A streptococcus strain FF22 was observed. The proportion of non-SA-producing (SA^-) derivatives occurring in strain FF22 cultures grown in Todd Hewitt broth supplemented with 1% of yeast extract (THBY) was increased on treatment with ethidium bromide, acriflavin, or rifampin. The highest incidence of SA^- organisms, however, was found in untreated THBY cultures that had been aging by incubation at 37°C for several months. The possibility of selective effects in these experiments, operating to enhance the apparent frequency of SA^- bacteria, was discounted. The survival of SA^- derivatives in association with populations of SA^+ bacteria was dependent upon the use of culture conditions inimical to SA activity, since a consistent finding was that the loss of ability to produce SA was associated with loss of immunity to the killing action of this bacteriocin. Whereas selective killing of SA^- derivatives was evident in mixed cultures of SA^+ and SA^- strains in tryptic soy broth, no such effect was demonstrable in THBY. In these experiments, elimination of SA^- cells seemed directly related to the presence of active SA. Purified clones of SA^- substrains did not seem revertible to SA production, either spontaneously or on treatment with nitrosoguanidine. It is suggested that the property of production of SA by group A streptococcus strain FF22, together with that of host cell immunity to the homologous bacteriocin, may be mediated by plasmid-borne genetic determinants.

Streptococcin A-FF22 (SA; formerly called streptocin A) is a bacteriocin produced by group A streptococcus strain FF22 (20-22). In the course of studies of this bacteriocin, it was observed that non-SA-producing (SA^-) variants occasionally appeared during the routine transfer of stock cultures of the parent strain. An investigation of the genetic basis of this phenomenon is the subject of the present study. The findings suggest that the genes determining both the production of, and immunity to, SA may possibly be located on a single plasmid.

(This paper was presented in part at the 75th Annual Meeting of the American Society for Microbiology, New York, N.Y., 1975 [abstract no. H-94, p. 111].)

MATERIALS AND METHODS

Bacterial strains. The prototype SA-producing (SA^+) organism, group A streptococcus strain FF22, has been described before (21) and has been identified serologically as T type 3/13 and M type 52. Incorporation of the host strain designation (FF22) allows complete specification of the bacteriocin as streptococcin A-FF22.

SA^- derivatives of strain FF22 were numbered consecutively upon isolation, together with a prefix designating the specific chemical "curing" agent utilized; rifampin (RIF), ethidium bromide (EB), and acriflavine (AF). Spontaneous SA^- substrains were identified by the prefix SPON.

Indicator strains used for the detection of SA were *Micrococcus luteus* and *Staphylococcus aureus* CIT. These indicator organisms are extremely susceptible to SA and have also been utilized in an investigation of bacteriocin production by group B streptococci (23). SA-resistant strains used in adsorption experiments were *Escherichia coli* and *S. aureus* 502A. Group A streptococcus strains M28, M57, and M58 were specific prototype-M strains from our departmental culture collection. Group A streptococcus strain FF38, an M-type 13 strain susceptible to SA, has been described previously (21). Spontaneous streptomycin-resistant mutants were selected on blood agar containing 1 mg of streptomycin per ml. All strains were stored at −70°C or in the lyophilized state.

Media and chemicals. Bacteriological media was obtained from Difco. Sodium dodecyl sulfate (SDS) and AF were from Fisher Scientific Co., Fairlawn, N.J. RIF was from Sigma Chemical Co., St. Louis, Mo., and EB, B grade, was from Calbiochem, San Diego, Calif. Mitomycin C was from Sigma Chemical Co., and *N*-methyl-*N'*-nitro-*N*-nitrosoguanidine

[1] Present address: Department of Microbiology, University of Otago, Dunedin, New Zealand.

(NTG) from Aldrich Chemical Co. Inc., Milwaukee, Wis.

Demonstration of SA production. It was determined that the most sensitive and convenient method for the testing of bacteriocin production was replicative stab inoculation. By use of tooth picks, individual colonies were inoculated in a regular grid pattern, first onto blood agar medium and then also on blood agar freshly seeded with a susceptible indicator lawn. These indicator lawns were prepared by spreading with a swab charged with logarithmic growth-phase cultures grown in Todd Hewitt broth (THB). From 36 to 64 colonies were tested for bacteriocin production on each lawn (Fig. 1). Bacteriocin production was evidenced by the development of inhibition zones within the lawn surrounding stabs of SA^+ organisms. Recovery of the test strains for additional studies was from the primary stab cultures on unseeded medium. Apparent SA^- clones were inoculated into 3-ml volumes of THB, incubated at 37°C for 6 h, and then streaked on blood agar to obtain single colonies. Repicking and further cycles of purification were repeated until pure, stable SA^- clones were obtained.

Loss of SA production. Preliminary experiments were conducted to establish optimal test conditions for the demonstration of the elimination of bacteriocin production by strain FF22.

An important consideration was the possible counter-selective effect of bacteriocin produced by SA^+ cells against any SA^- segregants that had concomitantly lost their host cell immunity to the killing action of SA. Our earlier studies (22) had shown that the composition of the growth medium and conditions of incubation of the SA producer strain have a great influence on the yield of SA. For the present purposes, it was desirable to select culture conditions that were not conducive to the production or persistence of biologically active SA. Preliminary experiments confirmed our previous finding that THB is relatively poor for SA production (22) and showed that when THB is supplemented with 1% yeast extract (THBY), no extracellular SA activity can be detected at any stage of the growth of SA^+ cultures under the conditions used in the present study. By comparison, it was found that when tryptic soy broth (TSB) was used as the growth medium, active SA accumulates in the supernatant, and no SA^- segregants can be detected in experiments involving either the aging of SA^+ cultures or their

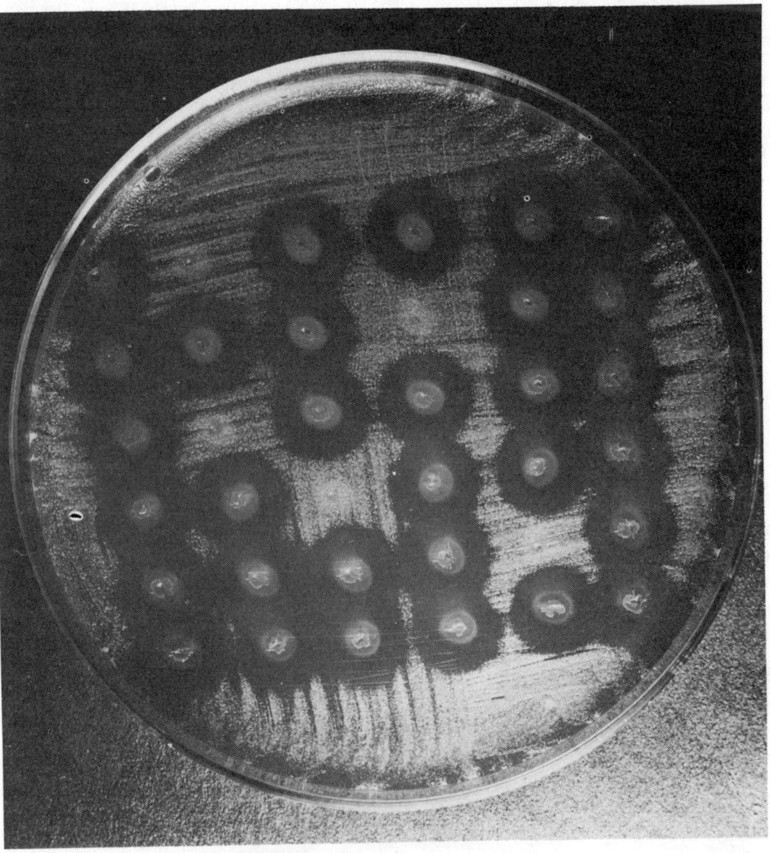

FIG. 1. *Detection of SA production after stab inoculation of individual clones into a lawn culture of M. luteus on blood agar medium. Failure to inhibit the growth of the indicator lawn by five of the test inocula indicates SA^- phenotype.*

treatment with curing agents. THBY was chosen as appropriate for use in the latter experiments. The general procedures adopted were as follows.

A single SA$^+$ colony was inoculated into 5 ml of THBY and incubated at 37°C for 18 h. Then: (i) to demonstrate spontaneous loss of SA, 0.1-ml portions were seeded into 25-ml volumes of fresh prewarmed THBY and incubated at the appropriate temperatures. Samples, at 24 h and various intervals thereafter, were plated on blood agar to obtain single colonies, and these were tested individually for the production of SA. (ii) To determine the effect of exposure to chemical curing agents, 0.1-ml portions were inoculated into 25-ml volumes of THBY containing concentrations (per milliliter) in the range of 0.01 to 0.05 μg of RIF, 0.02 to 0.4 μg of EB, 0.1 to 1.0 μg of AF, and 1.0 to 4.0 μg of SDS. The appropriate ranges of test doses of these chemicals were predetermined to be those inhibitory to the growth of strain FF22, such that viable cell counts (after incubation at 37°C for 24 h) were less by a factor of 10^2 to 10^3 colony-forming units (CFU) per ml compared with control cultures grown in the absence of the curing agents. Samples of the treated and control cultures were plated on blood agar, and individual colonies were treated as above. Variations of this procedure that were evaluated but later abandoned because of failure to increase the apparent rate of curing included: pretreatment of the 18-h seed culture with mitomycin C (1 μg/ml) or ultraviolet irradiation (99% kill dose); incubation of the test cultures at elevated (40°C) temperature; variation in sampling time within the range 4 to 48 h; treatment of the cultures with sonic oscillation before plating to shorten chains containing mixtures of SA$^+$ and SA$^-$ units; and incorporation of the test chemical within solid medium.

Characterization of SA$^-$ strains. Representative SA$^-$ strains were serotyped to identify M and T antigens, and the content of M protein was determined by the classical method (13) of assessing the ability of the organisms to resist phagocytosis when rotated in fresh human blood.

Possible "back mutation" of SA$^-$ strains to SA$^+$ phenotype was tested by exposing selected strains to 100 μg of NTG per ml, using previously described procedures (1).

A crude preparation of SA having a titer of 32 when assayed using *M. luteus* as indicator was obtained by established techniques (18), and this was used to test the susceptibility and also the adsorptive capacity of the parent FF22 strain and its SA$^-$ derivatives. Susceptibility of the organisms to SA was determined by titration of the bacteriocin on blood agar lawn cultures of the test strains prepared from 1:20 dilutions of overnight THB cultures.

For demonstration of adsorption, the organisms from 25-ml THB cultures grown 18 h at 37°C were washed twice in phosphate buffer (pH 7.2) and then resuspended in 1.5 ml of the buffer. Then, to 0.4 ml of cell suspension was added 0.1 ml of a SA preparation of titer 20 (assayed on *M. luteus*). Incubation was at 37°C for 60 min, after which the organisms were pelleted by centrifugation. The supernatant fluid was titrated for bacteriocin activity after heating at 80°C for 10 min. Crude SA is stable to heating under these conditions (18). Organisms used in some adsorption experiments were first killed by heating at 80°C for 30 min. Controls consisted of the bacteriocin and the cell suspension, appropriately diluted in THB.

The relative susceptibility of parent and SA$^-$ derivatives to growth inhibition by the curing agents was tested in two ways: (i) by drop testing with serial (THBY) dilutions of the different chemicals onto lawn cultures and estimating susceptibility as the end point of interference with growth of the lawn; (ii) by comparing the growth characteristics of the organisms in THBY supplemented with the curing agents in concentrations originally used to produce those SA$^-$ organisms.

Growth of mixed cultures of SA$^+$ and SA$^-$ strains. To aid differentiation between the two cell populations in mixed cultures, streptomycin-resistant mutants of the SA$^-$ cultures were utilized. Separate cultures of the SA$^+$ and SA$^-$ strains were established in either TSB or THBY at 37°C for 18 h. Portions, 0.5 ml, containing approximately 5×10^7 CFU of each strain were seeded into 25 ml of the appropriate prewarmed broths both independently (controls) and together (test). Incubation was at 37°C for 24 h, and 0.1-ml duplicate samples were withdrawn at intervals for viable counts on blood agar and on streptomycin blood agar. Counts for SA$^-$ organisms were estimated on streptomycin medium, and the SA$^+$ counts were determined by difference.

RESULTS

Spontaneous elimination of SA. Occasional, irreversible loss of ability to produce SA was observed on repeated subculture of group A streptococcus strain FF22. The extent of spontaneous elimination of SA upon long-term incubation of the producer strain in THBY cultures was tested at 30, 35, and 40°C. Table 1 summarizes the results of one such experiment. Repeat experiments of this type have given essentially similar results, although the maximum percentages of SA$^-$ cells sometimes showed considerable variation in different cultures incubated under similar conditions. For example, the greatest proportion of SA$^-$ cells in cultures incubated at 35°C has varied from a low of 20% to a high of 90%. Nevertheless, a consistent finding was the observation of very little increase in the proportion of SA$^-$ segregants until after about 3 weeks of incubation, followed by a sharp increase between 4 and 5 weeks. The reason for the relatively low rate of loss of SA at 30°C is not apparent. Incubation at the elevated temperature of 40°C did not seem to enhance either the time course or the frequency of appearance of SA$^-$ derivatives when compared with cultures incubated at 35°C. In the experiment documented in Table 1, a subculture was

TABLE 1. *Loss of SA synthesis by cells in aging broth cultures of group A streptococcus strain FF22*

Sample time (week)	% SA⁻ organisms[a] at temp					
	30°C		35°C		40°C	
	Original	Subculture[b]	Original	Subculture	Original	Subculture
0	0		0		0	
1	0		0		0	
2	0	0	1	0	0	0
3	0	0	3	3	0	0
4	1	0	4	1	0	0
5	ND[c]	ND	29	3	28	2
6	ND	1	54	33	ND	ND
7	1	1	60	80	33	3
8	2	0	68	62	44	20
9	1	2	82	88	69	28

[a] A total of 100 to 140 colonies was tested in each sample.
[b] Made from original culture at 2 weeks.
[c] ND, Not determined.

taken at 2 weeks from each of the established broths into fresh THBY medium at each of the temperatures. It was found that the pattern of appearance of SA^- derivatives was similar in each subculture to that observed with the corresponding primary culture (Table 1). There was little loss of ability to produce SA in the subcultures incubated at 30°C; however, after subculture at 35°C, the incidence of SA^- strains increased appreciably from 4 to 5 weeks.

Induced elimination of SA. Several of the chemical curing agents tested were found to give increased yields of SA^- derivatives by comparison with untreated control (THBY) cultures of strain FF22. Table 2 lists the aggregated results from numerous experiments. The curing rates obtained were low. RIF appeared to give the greatest yield of cured derivatives. SDS did not give rise to any SA^- organisms. It was significant that none of these chemicals appeared to eliminate bacteriocin production at a level comparable with that obtained by long-term incubation of the producer strain.

Origin of SA^- derivatives. A number of tests were conducted to establish whether the SA^- strains may have had some selective survival advantage under the test conditions.

Portions from cell-free membrane (Millipore Corp.) filtrates of 48-h- and 2-month-aged THBY cultures of strain FF22 were tested for capacity to support the growth of SA^+ strains and spontaneous SA^- derivatives (SPON1 and SPON6). Daily viable counts indicated that the growth and survival characteristics of the SA^- strains were similar to those of the SA^+ bacteria in each of the filtrates.

Possible selective effects of the chemical curing agents were tested by titrating preparations of each of the chemicals on lawn cultures of the parent and the corresponding SA^- substrains. By this procedure, it was found that the parent and the derivatives invariably had similar susceptibility to killing by the particular test chemicals. In other tests, growth curves of the parent and of SA^- substrains in the presence of test doses of the various curing agents were compared. These tests, e.g., the one illustrated in Fig. 2, indicated that the cured derivatives did not appear to have any selective growth advantage under the conditions of the test.

Stability of SA^- strains. All of the SA^- strains that had been obtained by exposure of actively multiplying SA^+ cultures to chemical

TABLE 2. *Elimination of SA in group A streptococcus strain FF22 by use of curing agents*

Treatment	Total colonies tested	No. of SA⁻ clones	Elimination (%)
Untreated	3,100	3	0.09
EB	620	3	0.48
AF	980	8	0.82
RIF	1,450	16	1.10
SDS	408	0	0

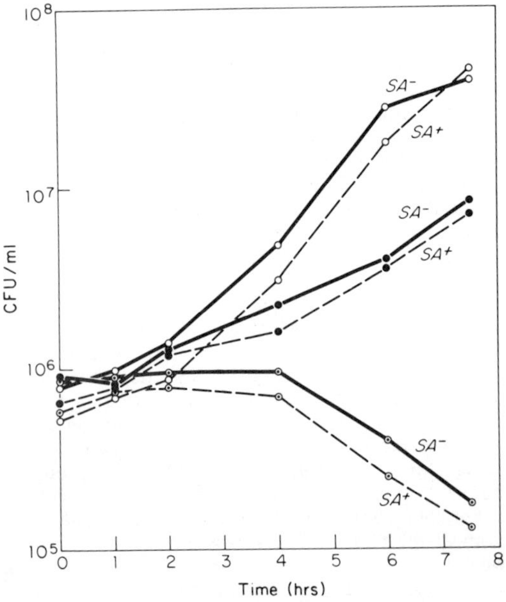

FIG. 2. *Growth curves of group A streptococcus strain FF22 (SA^+) and its cured derivative, strain EB1 (SA^-), in THBY containing 0.4 μg of EB per ml (⊙), 0.1 μg of EB per ml (●), and with no supplement (○).*

curing agents appeared to be stable on primary isolation, with no evidence of reversion of bacteriocin production upon repeated subculture. By comparison, almost 50% of the colonies appearing to be SA⁻ on preliminary isolation from prolonged incubation experiments were found to give rise to mixtures of SA⁺ and SA⁻ colonies on continued testing. Occasionally, it was necessary to repeat three or four cycles of purification from the original SA⁻ clones to obtain pure cultures of SA⁻ derivatives that failed to revert on continued subculture.

Four SA⁻ derivatives (EB1, AF1, SPON1, SPON6) were subcultured weekly for 4 months on blood agar and showed no evidence of reversion to bacteriocin production. In addition, strains EB1, SPON1, and SPON6 were treated with (per ml) 100 μg of the potent mutagen NTG, in an attempt to demonstrate reversion by back mutation. None of 2,000 tested colonies of EB1, or 1,000 each of SPON1 and SPON6, showed evidence of reversion to SA⁺ phenotype.

Characteristics of SA⁻ derivatives. No relationship between the loss of SA and colony appearance or production of hemolysis on blood agar was apparent. All 20 SA⁻ derivatives that were examined by serotyping had the characteristic 3/13 T pattern of the parental culture. Determination of M protein production indicated that all of 15 tested SA⁻ strains that had been obtained by exposure to curing agents were still M positive. Two of 20 examined SA⁻ cultures that had been obtained from aged cultures were M negative.

Little specificity was found in the adsorption of SA (Table 3). The extent of adsorption was similar by use of the parent SA⁺ strain, two M-positive SA⁻ derivatives (EB1, SPON1), one M-negative SA⁻ substrain (SPON6), and two unrelated organisms that are not susceptible to SA (*E. coli* and *S. aureus* 502A). Similar results were obtained with use of either viable or heat-killed organisms.

In spite of the similar adsorptive capacity of the parent and SA⁻ substrains, considerable difference was found in the susceptibility of these strains to the inhibitory action of SA. All of 20 spontaneous and 15 induced SA⁻ cultures tested were found to be 16 to 32 times more susceptible to SA than the parent strain when examined by the drop dilution method of titration.

Thus, both after exposure to curing agents and in aged cultures, it appeared that producer cell immunity to the homologous bacteriocin had consistently been lost together with ability to produce the bacteriocin. Concomitant loss of both functions gave support to the contention that both determinants may be located on a single plasmid and did not seem consistent with a point mutation origin of SA⁻ strains in these experiments.

TABLE 3. *Adsorption of SA to susceptible and resistant bacteria*[a]

Test organism	Susceptibility to SA killing action	SA titer in supernatant
Group A streptococcus		
Strain M57	Susceptible	2
Strain EB1	Susceptible	2
Strain SPON1	Susceptible	2
Strain SPON6	Susceptible	1
Strain FF22	Resistant	2
Escherichia coli	Resistant	1
Staphylococcus aureus		
Strain 502A	Resistant	2
Strain CIT	Susceptible	1
None (control)		4

[a] Viable, washed cells incubated with SA for 30 min at 37°C.

Treatment of the producer strain with NTG was found to give rise to SA⁻ derivatives, the majority of which differed significantly from those described above. Of 20 such SA⁻ substrains, 18 were found to retain parental-strain levels of resistance to the bacteriocin, whereas the other two were 16 times more susceptible and appeared to correspond phenotypically to the SA⁻ strains obtained by aging or use of curing agents. Reexposure of representative SA⁻ SA-resistant mutants to NTG induced reversion to the SA⁺ SA-resistant phenotype, indicating the occurrence of back mutation. Aging of cultures of the SA⁻ SA-resistant mutants gave rise to SA⁻ SA-susceptible derivatives, and these were not revertible to SA⁺ phenotype on reexposure to NTG. Although it was not the subject of a special study, the frequency of appearance of SA⁻ SA-susceptible derivatives in aging SA⁻ SA-resistant cultures seemed similar to the observed frequency of appearance of SA⁻ SA-susceptible derivatives arising on aging of SA⁺ SA-resistant cultures.

Growth of SA⁺ and SA⁻ organisms in mixed cultures. Figure 3 shows growth curves representing the pure and the mixed growth of strain FF22 (SA⁺) and its SA⁻ derivative EB1 in TSB medium at 37°C. The parent strain exhibited similar growth in both pure and mixed cultures, achieving a maximum population of 2×10^8 CFU per ml at 10 to 12 h after inoculation. By comparison, the SA⁻ strain was markedly inhibited by growth in association, with a strong decrease in viability after 6 h of incubation. A complete kill was effected within 10 h of

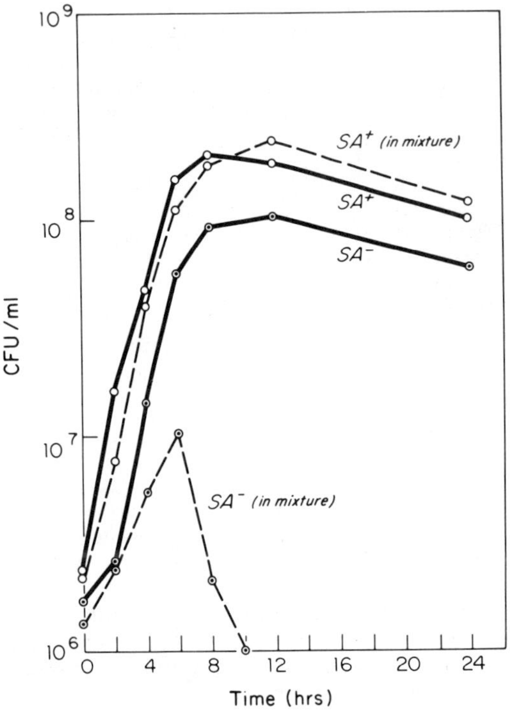

FIG. 3. *Growth characteristics of group A streptococcus strain FF22 (SA+) and its cured derivative, strain EB1 (SA−), in pure cultures (——) and in mixed culture (- - -).*

seeding the cultures. TSB was suitable for use in this experiment, since it is excellent for the production of SA (22). No inhibition of SA^- strains occurred in mixed cultures in either THB or THBY medium.

DISCUSSION

The reported data seem consistent with the interpretation that the genetic determinants of SA production and immunity are located on a plasmid in group A streptococcus strain FF22. Many, but not all (15), studies of the genetic basis of bacteriocin production have indicated the involvement of plasmids (18). Although most studies have been of bacteriocins of gram-negative species, exceptions include those of some of the staphylococcal bacteriocins (5, 10). Information of this kind about the streptococcal bacteriocins is lacking, although production of the bacteriocin-like antibiotic "nisin" by *Streptococcus lactis* was recently shown possibly to be plasmid determined (11).

In general, the replication and inheritance of plasmids is precisely controlled and the occurrence of plasmid-negative progeny is a rare event. However, under particular growth conditions or upon exposure to chemical curing agents, the rate of elimination of some plasmids may be substantially increased. In the present study, it was found that aging of a SA^+ culture in THBY at 35°C for a minimum of 4 to 5 weeks promoted the widespread loss of SA. Other reports have also documented the spontaneous loss of ability to produce bacteriocin on prolonged storage of staphylococci (10, 12, 17), *Lactobacillus helveticus* (25) and group B streptococci (24). In other studies, the elimination of plasmid deoxyribonucleic acid having determinants of multiple antibiotic resistance was demonstrated in group D streptococci (3, 8) and in a strain of *Staphylococcus epidermidis* (19) in the course of lengthy incubation of cultures. In these studies, as we have found for the loss of SA, the rate of elimination by aging of cultures was far greater than that obtained by exposure to curing agents. Malke has noted that in some strains of group A streptococci, chemical curing agents have little effect on the stability of resistance to erythromycin and lincomycin (14). It was presumed, from other indirect evidence, that the genetic determinants of these properties were plasmid borne.

The reason why SA elimination is promoted in aged cultures has not been determined. The importance of using culture conditions unfavorable to the production of active SA is clear. No SA^- segregants could be detected in media such as TSB which are suitable for SA production. Our previous studies (22) of the requirements for SA formation indicated an inverse correlation between the production of active SA and that of streptococcal proteinase. In the present investigation, the yield of active SA was shown to be particularly poor in THBY medium. The enhancing effect of yeast extract on proteinase elaboration has been documented in earlier investigations (4).

Although we were unable to detect the presence of levels of SA that are inhibitory to SA^- strains in filtrates of young THBY cultures of SA^+ bacteria, it is possible that under the test conditions sufficient SA may be present to select against the SA^- segregants. The role of some producer cell-bound form of SA in this effect cannot yet be dismissed. Alternatively, it may be speculated that a metabolite formed during aging of the culture facilitates plasmid elimination.

The failure of incubation at elevated temperature (40°C) to promote greater loss of SA is in marked contrast to studies of the staphylococcins, in which growth at elevated temperatures has been shown to promote elimination of bacteriocinogenic factors (5, 10). The observation of occasional concomitant loss of M protein in SA^-

derivatives obtained from aged broths is of interest in view of the recent report (1) that M protein and serum opacity factor of group A streptococci may also be plasmid determined. Apparently, however, in group A streptococcus strain FF22, the determinants for M and for SA are not co-eliminated, and it is unlikely that they are located on the same plasmid.

Control tests indicated that the appearance of SA^- clones is not due to selection of SA^- organisms. Extensive tests failed to demonstrate the spontaneous or NTG-induced reversion of SA^- clones obtained from cultures either aged or exposed to curing agents. Since it is a characteristic of plasmids that cured cells are unable to regain functions linked to that plasmid by means of mutation, this can be taken as good indirect evidence against the occurrence of point mutation or phase variations in the present investigations. It seems that loss of a plasmid is the most likely interpretation of the observed facts. Strong supportive evidence is accrued from the concomitant loss of immunity to SA in SA^- substrains. In this regard, a difference between the antibiotic "nisin" and SA is apparent, since the loss of nisin production was not associated with loss of immunity to nisin (11). On the other hand, investigations of several colicins (18) and of a staphylococcin (5) have indicated that the genes determining immunity to a particular bacteriocin are located on the same plasmid that determines production of the bacteriocin. This immunity, presumably operating via the synthesis of specific immunity substances, is a necessary property to ensure the survival of bacteriocinogenic organisms and is different from bacteriocin resistance, which is due to loss of the specific bacteriocin receptor.

The lack of adsorption specificity of SA is of interest. Although most of the bacteriocins produced by strains of gram-negative species appear to have considerable specificity of attachment to susceptible bacteria (18), studies of some bacteriocins produced by staphylococci (7, 9) and lactobacilli (25) have clearly shown that adsorption may be quite nonspecific, being unrelated to the susceptibility of different bacteria to the killing action of bacteriocins.

The demonstration in the present study that the adsorption of bacteriocin activity from solution is comparable with use of either viable or heat-killed bacteria may be taken as indirect evidence that the removal of SA is attributable to adsorption of the bacteriocin and not to its enzymic inactivation. Streptococcal proteinase (6) and other known streptococcal enzymes are inactivated under the conditions of heating at 80°C for 30 min.

To the best of our knowledge, there have only been four other studies reported that relate to the presence of plasmids in group A streptococci, three of which show association with antibiotic resistance markers (2, 14, 16) and the other relating to M protein and serum opacity factor production (1).

Our recent studies (unpublished data) have demonstrated that the determinants of SA production and immunity are co-transducible. Presently we are attempting to isolate and characterize the bacteriocinogenic factor.

ACKNOWLEDGMENTS

We thank Christine Windler for excellent technical assistance and Paul Cleary for advice on curing techniques and for critical review of the manuscript.

This work was supported by Public Health Service grant AI 08724 from the National Institute of Allergy and Infectious Diseases. J.R.T. was supported by a Career Investigator Fellowship from the American Heart Association. L.W.W. is a Career Investigator of the American Heart Association.

LITERATURE CITED

1. **Cleary, P. P., Z. Johnson, and L. W. Wannamaker.** 1975. Genetic instability of M protein and serum opacity factor of group A streptococci: evidence suggesting extrachromosomal control. Infect. Immun. **12**:109–118.
2. **Clewell, D. B., and A. E. Franke.** 1974. Characterization of a plasmid determining resistance to erythromycin, lincomycin, and vernamycin B_α in a strain of *Streptococcus pyogenes*. Antimicrob. Agents Chemother. **5**:534–537.
3. **Clewell, D. B., Y. Yagi, and B. Bauer.** 1975. Plasmid-determined tetracycline resistance in *Streptococcus faecalis*: evidence for gene amplification during growth in presence of tetracycline. Proc. Natl. Acad. Sci. U.S.A. **72**:1720–1724.
4. **Cohen, J. O.** 1969. Effect of culture medium composition and pH on the production of M protein and proteinase by group A streptococci. J. Bacteriol. **99**:737–744.
5. **Dajani, A. S., and Z. Taube.** 1974. Plasmid-mediated production of staphylococcin in bacteriophage type 71 *Staphylococcus aureus*. Antimicrob. Agents Chemother. **5**:594–598.
6. **Elliott, S. D.** 1945. A proteolytic enzyme produced by group A streptococci with special reference to its effect on the type-specific M antigen. J. Exp. Med. **81**:573–592.
7. **Gagliano, V. J., and R. D. Hinsdill.** 1970. Characterization of a *Staphylococcus aureus* bacteriocin. J. Bacteriol. **104**:117–125.
8. **Jacob, A. E., and S. J. Hobbs.** 1974. Conjugal transfer of plasmid-borne multiple antibiotic resistance in *Streptococcus faecalis* var. *zymogenes*. J. Bacteriol. **117**:360–372.
9. **Jetten, A. M., and G. D. Vogels.** 1972. Nature and properties of a *Staphylococcus epidermidis* bacteriocin. J. Bacteriol. **112**:243–250.
10. **Jetten, A. M., and G. D. Vogels.** 1973. Characterization and extrachromosomal control of bacteriocin production in *Staphylococcus aureus*. Antimicrob. Agents Chemother. **4**:49–57.
11. **Kozak, W., M. Rajchert-Trzpil, and W. T. Dobrzański.** 1974. The effect of proflavin, ethidium bromide and an elevated temperature on the appearance of nisin-negative clones in nisin-producing strains of *Streptococcus lactis*. J. Gen. Microbiol. **83**:295–302.

12. **Lachowicz, T.** 1965. Investigations on staphylococcins. Zentralbl. Bakteriol. Parasitenkd. Infektionskr. Hyg. Abt. 1 Orig. **196**:340–351.

13. **Lancefield, R. C.** 1957. Differentiation of group A streptococci with a common R antigen into three serological types, with special reference to the bactericidal test. J. Exp. Med. **106**:525–544.

14. **Malke, H.** 1974. Genetics of resistance to macrolide antibiotics and lincomycin in natural isolates of *Streptococcus pyogenes*. Mol. Gen. Genet. **135**:349–367.

15. **Mindich, L.** 1966. Bacteriocins of *Diplococcus pneumoniae*. 1. Antagonistic relationships and genetic transformations. J. Bacteriol. **92**:1090–1098.

16. **Nakae, M., M. Inoue, and S. Mitsuhashi.** 1975. Artificial elimination of drug resistance from group A beta-hemolytic streptococci. Antimicrob. Agents Chemother. **7**:719–720.

17. **Parker, M. T., and L. E. Simmons.** 1959. The inhibition of *Corynebacterium diphtheriae* and other gram-positive organisms by *Staphylococcus aureus*. J. Gen. Microbiol. **21**:457–476.

18. **Reeves, P.** 1972. The bacteriocins. Molecular biology, biochemistry and biophysics, vol. 11. Springer-Verlag, New York.

19. **Rosendorf, L. L., and F. H. Kayser.** 1974. Transduction and plasmid deoxyribonucleic acid analysis in a multiple antibiotic-resistant strain of *Staphylococcus epidermidis*. J. Bacteriol. **120**:679–686.

20. **Tagg, J. R., R. S. D. Read, and A. R. McGiven.** 1971. Bacteriocine production by group A streptococci. Pathology **3**:277–278.

21. **Tagg, J. R., R. S. D. Read, and A. R. McGiven.** 1973. Bacteriocin of a group A streptococcus: partial purification and properties. Antimicrob. Agents Chemother. **4**:214–221.

22. **Tagg, J. R., A. S. Dajani, L. W. Wannamaker, and E. D. Gray.** 1973. Group A streptococcal bacteriocin. Production, purification, and mode of action. J. Exp. Med. **138**:1168–1183.

23. **Tagg, J. R., A. S. Dajani, and L. W. Wannamaker.** 1975. Bacteriocin of a group B streptococcus: partial purification and characterization. Antimicrob. Agents Chemother. **7**:764–772.

24. **Tzannetis, S., A. Poulaki-Tsontou, and J. Papavassiliou.** 1974. Bacteriocine production in group B streptococci. Pathol. Microbiol. **41**:51–57.

25. **Upreti, G. C., and R. D. Hinsdill.** 1975. Production and mode of action of lactocin 27: bacteriocin from a homofermentative *Lactobacillus*. Antimicrob. Agents. Chemother. **7**:139–145.

ANTIMICROBIAL AGENTS AND CHEMOTHERAPY, Aug. 1976, p. 307-317
Vol. 10, No. 2

Printed in U.S.A.

Comparative Pharmacokinetics and Metabolism of Cephapirin in Laboratory Animals and Humans

B. E. CABANA,[1] D. R. VAN HARKEN,* AND G. H. HOTTENDORF
Research Division, Bristol Laboratories, Syracuse, New York 13201

Received for publication 17 December 1975

Comparative drug disposition studies in mice, rats, dogs, and humans indicate that cephapirin, a new semisynthetic cephalosporin antibiotic that exhibits broad-spectrum antimicrobial activity, is metabolized to desacetylcephapirin in these species. Pharmacokinetic analyses of the concentrations of cephapirin and desacetylcephapirin in plasma and urine reveal that the rate and extent of deacetylation decreases from rodents to dogs to humans. The kinetic analyses also suggest that the kidney performs a role not only in the excretion but also in the metabolism of cephapirin to desacetylcephapirin.

Cephapirin, sodium 7-(pyrid-4-yl-thioacetamido)cephalosporante (Fig. 1), is a new semisynthetic 7-aminocephalosporanic acid derivative that exhibits a broad spectrum of antimicrobial activity (2, 3, 5) and in humans exhibits a similar pharmacokinetic profile to that of cephalothin (1). These results (1) were based on total bioactivity in serum, as determined by the cup-plate assay (6), and failed to take into account any possible differences in drug metabolism. In mice, rats, dogs, and humans, cephapirin has been shown to be metabolized to a bioactive desacetyl metabolite, and it has been suggested that the kidney performs a role not only in the excretion of the parent compound and desacetyl metabolite but also in the metabolism of cephapirin to desacetylcephapirin (B. E. Cabana and D. R. Van Harken, 5th Int. Congr., Pharmacol., San Francisco, Calif., Abstr. 209, p. 35, 1972; B. E. Cabana, D. R. Van Harken, L. W. Dittert, and J. T. Doluisio, Prog. Abstr. Intersci. Conf. Antimicrob. Agents Chemother., 12th, Atlantic City, N.J., Abstr. 147, p. 77, 1972). This report consists of a detailed analysis of the comparative metabolic and pharmacokinetic profile of cephapirin in laboratory animals and humans.

MATERIALS AND METHODS

Swiss Webster mice and Miller rats weighing approximately 30 and 200 g, respectively, and four beagle dogs (mean weight, 8.2 kg) were employed in the metabolic studies. Pooled blood samples were taken in fasted mice by exsanguination after decapitation and from the dorsal aorta in fasted rats under ether anesthesia. Urine collection was achieved after water hydration diuresis by use of small rodent metabolism cages. In dogs, blood samples were taken from the saphenous vein by means of an intravenous (i.v.) catheter (Bardic, Intercath). The dogs were fasted overnight and hydrated (30 ml/kg) 15 to 30 min prior to drug administration. Continuous urine collection was achieved by means of Lucite-coated, stainless-steel cannulae surgically implanted within the bladder of the female dogs. The bladder cannulae were permanently implanted in dogs within 1 to 2 months of running the studies. The dogs had normal creatinine clearance (4 ml/min per kg) at the time of the study.

Ten fasted, healthy male volunteers (mean weight, 66 kg) were employed for the human metabolic studies. The drug was administered by the i.v. route into the median cubital vein over a 5-min period. Blood specimens (20 ml) were drawn immediately before and at 5 min, 0.5, 1.0, 1.5, 2, 3, and 4 h after drug administration, and urine was collected at 1, 2, 4, and 6 h after drug administration. A water diuresis was maintained throughout the urine collection period by oral administration of 600 ml of tap water 20 min prior to drug administration and subsequent administration of 300 ml of water at 1 and 3 h after dosing.

Blood specimens taken from the laboratory animals and men were placed in heparinized tubes (Vacutainers) and kept in an ice bath until centrifuged. Shortly thereafter, the blood specimens were spun down at approximately 1,000 × *g* in a refrigerated centrifuge (5°C), and the plasma samples were quickly frozen in a dry ice-acetone bath and kept frozen until bioassayed. The urine specimens were collected in flasks placed in an ice bath (5°C). All urine specimens were immediately frozen (−20°C) until bioassayed.

Plasma and urine samples were assayed for microbiological activity in terms of the free acid of the parent drug by means of the cup-plate assay (14), employing *Sarcina lutea* as the test organism (6). The identification of the microbiologically active metabolic products of cephapirin present in plasma and urine specimens was obtained by bioautography on *Bacillus subtilis* and *S. lutea* seeded agar plates

[1] Present address: Division of Biopharmaceutics, Bureau of Drugs, Food and Drug Administration, Rockville, MD 20852.

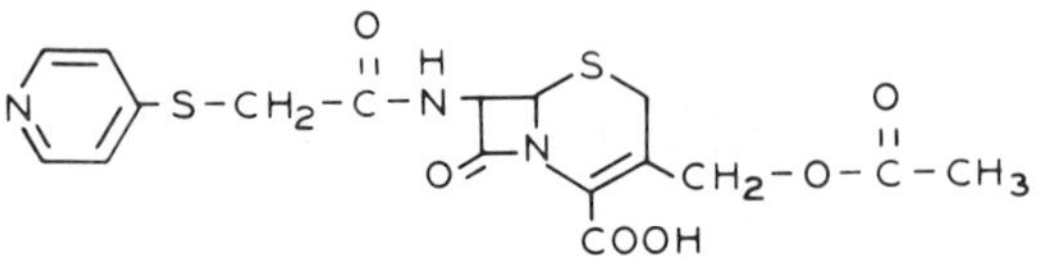

BL-P1322 (CEPHAPIRIN)

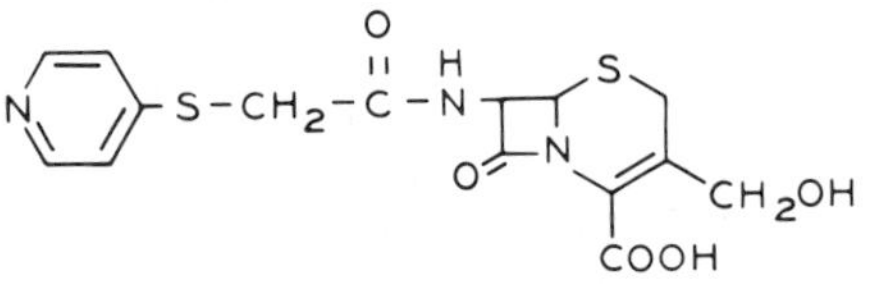

DESACETYL - BL-1322
(DESACETYL-CEPHAPIRIN)

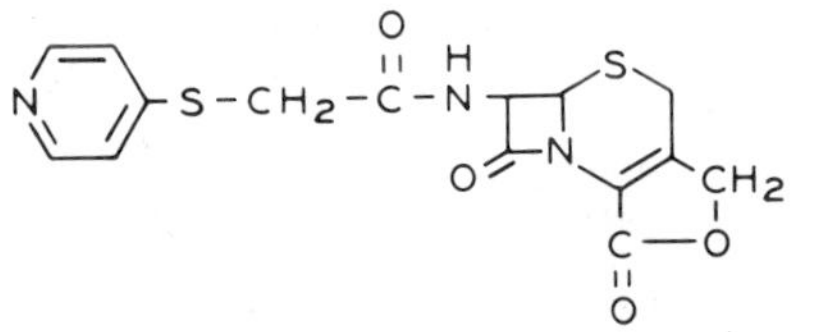

BL-P1322 (LACTONE)

FIG. 1. *Structures of cephapirin and corresponding metabolites isolated from rat urine after parenteral administration of cephapirin.*

at pH 6.0 (Fig. 2) after chromatography on Whatman no. 1 paper strips (100 mm in width) employing *n*-butanol-acetic acid-water (60:15:25) or butanol-ethanol-water (8:2:10, top phase) as the solvent system. The metabolites found in the urine and plasma samples were compared with chemically synthesized products employing the same solvent system. Quantitation of cephapirin and desacetylcephapirin was achieved by differential bioautography as described below.

Quantitative differential assays for cephapirin and desacetylcephapirin were achieved by means of descending paper strip chromatography employing butanol-ethanol-water (8:2:10, top phase) as the solvent system, followed by bioautography on *B. subtilis* agar seeded plates at pH 6.0. The size of inoculum and plates employed were similar to the official assay technique (8, 14). The chromatographic system used was Whatman no. 1 paper developed in *n*-butanol-ethanol-water (8:2:10, top phase). When this solvent system was employed, cephapirin and desacetylcephapirin had R_f values of 0.43 and 0.34, respectively (Fig. 2). The plasma samples were diluted with an equal volume of acetone to break protein binding and to reduce plasma esterase activity. The amount spotted on the Whatman paper strips varied from 10 to 100 μl, depending on the total microbiological activity. The Whatman paper strips were allowed to dry for about 30 to 60 min prior to incubation on the agar plates. Preliminary studies indicated that desacetylcephapirin was very stable, even at room temperature in acetone-precipitated plasma. This was not the case with cephapirin and, therefore, all plasma and urine samples were kept in an ice bath prior to bioassays. The urine samples were diluted with pH 6.0 phosphate buffer (1%) and spotted in 5 to 20-μl volumes. Quantitation was achieved by plotting the area of zone of inhibition (square millimeters) as a function of log concentration of drug (Fig. 3). The lower limit of detectability by bioautography on *B. subtilis* agar plates was approximately 0.03 μg for cephapirin and 0.05 μg for desacetylcephapirin, which generally was spotted in 10-μl portions. Linear relationships were obtained with both drugs at concentrations of up to 0.1 μg/μl (or 1.0 μg/10 μl; Fig. 3). In all instances, an attempt was made to dilute the plasma and urine

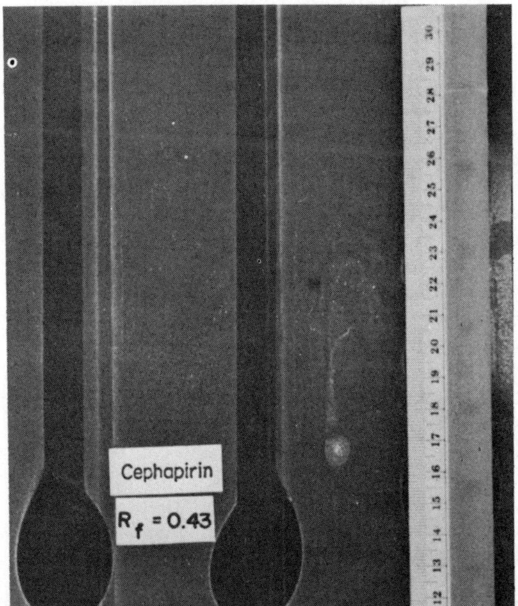

FIG. 2. *Bioautograph of cephapirin and desacetylcephapirin on B. subtilis seeded agar plates employing n-butanol-ethanol-water (8:2:10, top phase) as the chromatographic solvent system.*

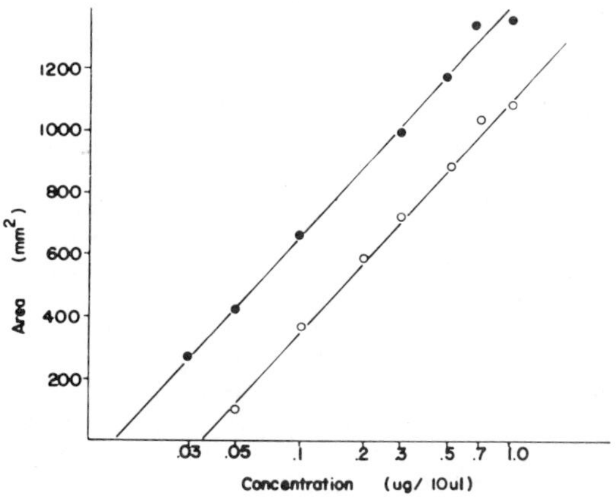

FIG. 3. *Area of zone inhibition on B. subtilis seeded agar plates versus log concentration of cephapirin (●) and desacetylcephapirin (○).*

samples and spot the appropriate portions such that they would approximate a reference standard (0.1 μg/10 μl) for cephapirin and (0.3 μg/10 μl) for desacetylcephapirin. The lower limit of detectability, when expressed in terms of plasma concentrations, was 0.3 μg/ml of plasma for cephapirin and 0.5 μg/ml for desacetylcephapirin. Cephapirin (lot 10611-9-15; bipotency, 942 μg/mg) and desacetylcephapirin (lot 10589-5-II) were employed as standards.

During the course of these studies, it was discovered that the concentration of cephapirin could be determined by the difference between the cup-plate assay (total bioactivity against *S. lutea*) and the desacetylcephapirin (S-335) bioautography assay as illustrated in equation 1. This procedure was facilitated by the fact that desacetylcephapirin had a biopotency of 0.54 ± 0.03 relative to cephapirin when assayed against *S. lutea*.

$$C_{\text{cephapirin}} = \text{cup-plate bioactivity versus } S.\ lutea - 0.54 \times C_{\text{S-335}} \quad (1)$$

where $C_{\text{S-335}}$ is the plasma concentration of desacetylcephapirin determined from the bioautography assay. The use of equation 1 was shown to give cephapirin plasma concentrations similar to those obtained with direct bioautography. This procedure was used to avoid the necessity of repeating the bioautography assay for higher concentrations of cephapirin and to avoid a saturation in the diffusion process on agar plates with relatively high concentrations of the parent drug. Whenever possible (sufficient sample permitting), the two assay methods were run simultaneously to assure the reliability of the assay procedures.

Kinetic analyses of the plasma concentration and cumulative urinary excretion data were performed with a Fortran 4 computer program (12) run on an IBM 360/30 digital computer and kinetic programs run on a G.E. Mark II Time Sharing computer. Nonlinear regression analyses of the plasma concentration-time curves and the least-squares estimations of the nonlinear parameters were determined by the method of Marquardt (11). The kinetic equations and the model describing the drug concentrations in plasma after i.v. and intramuscular administration were recently published (4, 16, 17, 20). The intrinsic absorption rate was determined by the method of Loo and Riegelman (10).

RESULTS

Identification of urinary excretion products. The pharmacokinetic evaluation of the metabolic characteristics of cephapirin in laboratory animals and humans required identification of the urinary excretion products. Paper strip chromatography followed by bioautography as described above indicated the presence of cephapirin (R_f = 0.43) and desacetylcephapirin (R_f = 0.30) in the urine of mice, dogs, and humans (Fig. 2). The urine of rats contained a trace amount of a third microbiologically active component (cephapirin lactone), having a greater mobility (R_f = 0.65) than cephapirin. The structures of cephapirin, desacetylcephapirin, and cephapirin lactone are presented in Fig. 1.

Metabolism and urinary excretion of cephapirin in mice. Summarized in Table 1 are the mean concentrations of cephapirin, desacetylcephapirin, and cup-plate bioactivity obtained in plasma of 30 mice 30 min after subcutaneous administration of 200-mg/kg doses of cephapirin. Also included in Table 1 are the mean cumulative urinary excretions of the same agents obtained in two groups of 15 mice over a 20-h period after subcutaneous administration of 200 mg of cephapirin per kg. It should be particularly noted that the rate of deacetylation of cephapirin in mice was very rapid, resulting in plasma levels of desacetylcephapirin approximately threefold that of the parent compound within 30 min of drug administration. It should

TABLE 1. *Plasma concentrations and urinary excretion of cephapirin and desacetylcephapirin in mice after subcutaneous administration of a 200-mg/kg dose of cephapirin*

Determination	Plasma concn[a,b]	Urinary excretion (% of dose)[c]
Cephapirin	33.1 ± 1.1	20.0
Desacetylcephapirin	106.7 ± 9.3	39.8
Cup-plate bioactivity[d]	105	31.3

[a] Time = 30 min.

[b] Micrograms per milliliter ± standard error; N = 30.

[c] Percentage of dose excreted in 24 h.

[d] Bioactivity is expressed in terms of cephapirin.

also be noted that the use of cephapirin as a standard to determine cup-plate bioactivity (6) in plasma and urine specimens underestimated the actual amounts of antibiotic present in plasma and urine specimens. Thus, for instance, the cumulative urinary excretion determined by the cup-plate assay (6) accounted for only 31% of the dose (Table 1), but the differential bioautography assay indicated that about 60% of the dose was actually excreted in the urine as microbiologically active products. Of the total amount of drug excreted in mice, cephapirin and desacetylcephapirin accounted for about 20 and 40% of the dose, respectively.

Metabolism and urinary excretion of cephapirin in rats. The intraperitoneal administration of cephapirin to rats at doses of 200 and 1,000 mg/kg resulted in mean plasma concentrations of 58 and 753 μg/ml, respectively, 30 min after dosing, which declined exponentially over a 4- to 6-h period (Table 2). The plasma concentrations of desacetylcephapirin during the same period were approximately 40% those of cephapirin. The plasma half-lives of cephapirin and its desacetyl metabolite in rats were approximately 0.6 to 0.9 h. Significantly higher plasma concentrations of cephapirin were achieved with the 1,000-mg/kg dose than expected from comparison of the peak plasma levels obtained after the 200-mg/kg dose. The higher plasma concentrations observed were not due to a greater bioavailability but rather presumed to be due to a decrease in metabolic clearances. This hypothesis is supported by the fact that the cumulative percent excretion of total drug was the same for both doses (Table 3). Approximately 30 to 34% of the administered dose of cephapirin was excreted in the urine of rats over an 8-h period at both doses. Assuming equal bioavailabilities, the plasma clearances (Cl_p) over a 6-h period after intraperitoneal administration of 200- and 1,000-mg/kg doses were 41.5 and 22.3 ml/min per kg, respectively. During that same period, the renal clearances of cephapirin were 2.2 and 1.8 ml/min per kg, respectively. The excretion of desacetylcephapirin accounted for approximately 80% of the total excretion. When expressed in terms of cephapirin employing the cup-plate assay, only approximately 18 to 22% of the administered dose can be accounted for in the urine of rats rather than 30 to 34% actually present. The difference is due to the fact that desacetylcephapirin has about 54% of the bioactivity of cephapirin when assayed against *S. lutea*. Despite the much greater concentrations of cephapirin (twofold relative to desacetylcephapirin) in plasma (Table 2), significantly more desacetylcephapirin was excreted (Table 3) in the rats.

Pharmacokinetics and metabolism of cephapirin in beagle dogs. After i.v. administration of cephapirin to beagle dogs at doses of 30 mg/kg, the concentrations of cephapirin in plasma decreased biexponentially very rapidly over the next 2 to 3 h (Table 4 and Fig. 4). Simultane-

TABLE 2. *Plasma concentrations of cephapirin and desacetylcephapirin in rats after intraperitoneal administration of cephapirin at doses of 200 and 1,000 mg/kg*

Dose (mg/kg)	Time (h)	Plasma concn[a]		
		Cephapirin	Desacetylcephapirin	Cup-plate bioactivity[b]
200	0.5	58.4 ± 10.8	24.6 ± 9.2	71.6 ± 12.8
	1.0	30.8 ± 2.3	16.8 ± 2.0	39.9 ± 2.8
	2.0	13.9 ± 3.6	8.9 ± 4.1	18.8 ± 5.5
	4.0	3.3 ± 2.3	1.9 ± 0.7	3.9 ± 1.8
1,000	0.5	753.2 ± 29.0	353.8 ± 17.5	945.0 ± 22.5
	1.0	304.6 ± 45.1	167.5 ± 23.2	395.0 ± 50.6
	2.0	85.6 ± 33.5	44.0 ± 18.7	108.8 ± 42.4
	4.0	6.7 ± 2.3	5.3 ± 1.0	7.8 ± 2.2
	6.0	1.5 ± 0.8	0.8 ± 0.3	1.8 ± 0.6

[a] Micrograms per milliliter ± standard error; $N = 8$.
[b] Bioactivity is expressed in terms of cephapirin.

TABLE 3. *Cumulative urinary excretion of cephapirin and desacetylcephapirin in rats after intraperitoneal administration of cephapirin at doses of 200 and 1,000 mg/kg*

Dose (mg/kg)	Time (h)	Urinary excretion[a]		
		Cephapirin	Desacetylcephapirin	Cup-plate bioactivity[b]
200	24	5.2 ± 0.7	28.1 ± 4.4	17.8 ± 3.1
1,000	24	8.1 ± 0.8	26.3 ± 4.4	22.4 ± 1.8

[a] Percentage of dose ± standard error; $N = 16$.
[b] Bioactivity is expressed in terms of cephapirin.

TABLE 4. *Mean concentration of cephapirin and desacetylcephapirin in plasma after i.v. administration of cephapirin to beagle dogs at a dose of 30 mg/kg*

Time	Concn[a]		
	Cephapirin	Desacetylcephapirin	Cup-plate bioactivity[b]
5 min	92.3 ± 14.6	9.9 ± 4.6	104.0 ± 11.4
15 min	52.0 ± 6.8	14.5 ± 3.6	56.8 ± 5.8
30 min	26.9 ± 2.9	13.9 ± 2.5	33.5 ± 3.7
45 min	15.1 ± 0.8	14.2 ± 1.8	20.6 ± 2.3
1.0 h	10.5 ± 2.2	11.9 ± 2.3	12.6 ± 2.6
1.5 h	3.8 ± 0.8	7.5 ± 0.9	5.6 ± 0.6
2.0 h	2.1 ± 0.5	4.0 ± 1.2	3.2 ± 0.5
3.0 h	0.6 ± 0.2	<1.0	0.6 ± 0.1
4.0 h	0.2 ± 0.1	<1.0	0.2 ± 0.1

[a] Micrograms per milliliter ± standard error.
[b] Bioactivity is expressed in terms of cephapirin.

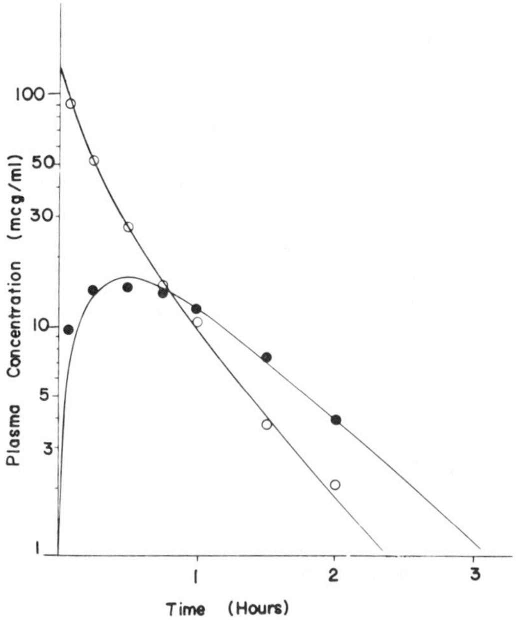

FIG. 4. *Mean concentrations of cephapirin (○) and desacetylcephapirin (●) in plasma of beagle dogs after i.v. administration of cephapirin at doses of 30 mg/kg.*

ously, the concentrations of desacetylcephapirin in plasma rapidly increased, achieving peak levels of 14 to 15 μg/ml within 30 min of dosing. Beyond 1 h, the concentrations of desacetylcephapirin in plasma were about twice those of cephapirin. Despite the lower plasma levels of desacetylcephapirin during h 1, the urinary excretion rate of the desacetyl metabolite significantly exceeded that of cephapirin (Table 5). Approximately 32 and 66% of the administered dose was excreted as cephapirin and desacetylcephapirin, respectively, in 8 h after i.v. administration of cephapirin, thus accounting for about 98% of the dose. It should be noted that the total microbiological activity grossly underestimated the actual amount of antibiotics excreted (Table 5).

Kinetic analyses of the plasma concentration data revealed that the mean plasma concentrations of cephapirin were best described by the following biexponential equation:

$$C_{\text{cephapirin}} = A_1 e^{-\alpha t} + B_1 e^{-\beta t} \quad (2)$$

where $A_1 = 76.69$ μg/ml, $\alpha = 5.77\ \text{h}^{-1}$, $B_1 = 51.55$ μg/ml, and $\beta = 1.67\ \text{h}^{-1}$.

The biexponential equation 2 can best be interpreted in terms of the two-compartmental, open-system model (Fig. 5). The model consists of a central plasma compartment (V_p) and a peripheral tissue compartment (V_T) between which cephapirin is in a state of complete equilibrium only under steady-state conditions (18).

The kinetic model invokes not only the drug distribution profile of cephapirin but also its metabolism. Summarized in Table 6 are the rate constants governing distribution (K_1 and K_{-1}) to and from tissue fluids, the rate constant governing drug elimination (K_2), and the respective volumes of drug distribution, V_p and V_t (illustrated). Also included in Table 6 are the total area under the plasma concentration-time curve, the plasma half-life of cephapirin, and the apparent volume of drug distribution (V_D). Thus, after i.v. administration to beagle dogs, cephapirin appears to be rapidly distributed (half-life for drug distribution = 0.12 h) within the extracellular fluids (V_p = 23% of body volume) and to some extent within the peripheral tissue compartment (V_T = 9% of body volume). The apparent volume of drug distribution was approximately 32% of the body volume and the plasma half-life in the dogs was approximately 0.4 h. The plasma half-life of desacetylcephapirin during the β-elimination phase was about 0.6 h, and the area under the plasma concentration-time curve was about 25 μg·h per ml or about 60% that of cephapirin (Table 6).

Given the following kinetic model (Fig. 5), the rate constants governing the urinary excretion (*ke*) and metabolism (*km*) of cephapirin (Table 6) are given by the following equations:

$$ke = fe \cdot K_2 = \frac{Xe}{\text{dose}} \cdot K_2 \quad (3)$$

and

$$km = fm \cdot K_2 = \frac{Xme}{\text{dose}} \cdot K_2 \quad (4)$$

where *Xe* and *fe* are the total amounts and

TABLE 5. *Cumulative urinary excretion of cephapirin and desacetylcephapirin after i.v. administration of cephapirin to beagle dogs at a dose of 30 mg/kg*

Time (h)	%[a] of dose excreted ± SE		
	Cephapirin	Desacetyl-cephapirin	Cup-plate bioactivity[b]
0.5	20.9 ± 3.1	27.9 ± 4.6	35.2 ± 4.0
1.0	27.0 ± 4.1	44.3 ± 4.3	48.4 ± 5.5
1.5	28.8 ± 3.9	53.5 ± 5.8	54.6 ± 6.5
2.0	30.3 ± 3.9	60.4 ± 4.7	58.8 ± 6.2
4.0	31.0 ± 3.9	64.8 ± 4.8	61.5 ± 6.5
6.0	31.1 ± 3.9	65.8 ± 4.8	61.9 ± 6.5
8.0	32.0 ± 4.0	65.9 ± 4.9	62.0 ± 6.5

[a] Percent molar excretion is expressed in terms of the administered dose. SE, Standard error.
[b] Bioactivity is expressed in terms of cephapirin.

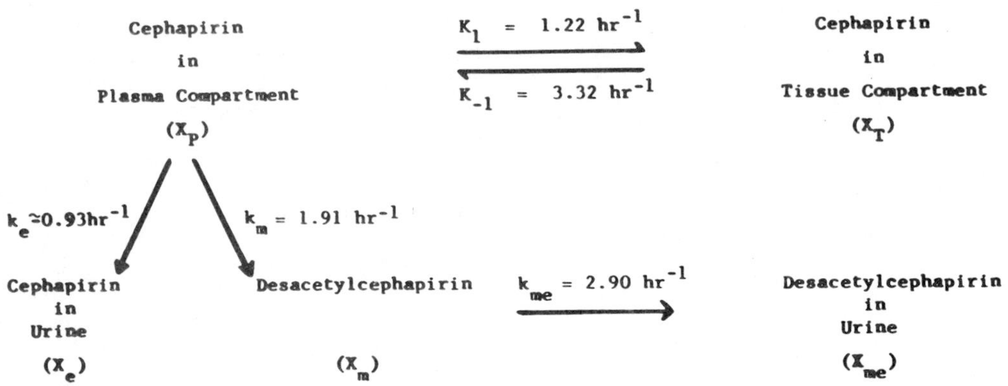

FIG. 5. *Two-compartment, open-system model describing the distribution and elimination of cephapirin in beagle dogs.*

TABLE 6. *Parameters for the two-compartment, open-system model estimated from concentration of cephapirin in plasma after i.v. administration of 30 mg/kg to dogs*[a]

Parameter	Value
K_1 (h^{-1})	1.22
K_{-1} (h^{-1})	3.32
K_2 (h^{-1})	2.90
Km (h^{-1})	0.91
Ke (h^{-1})	0.93
Kme (h^{-1})	2.90
V_P (liters/kg)	0.23
V_T (liters/kg)	0.09
V_D (liters/kg)	0.32
Half-life (h)	0.41
Area (μg·h per ml)	44.16

[a] Equation: $C_{\text{cephapirin}} = 76.69e^{-5.77t} + 51.55e^{-1.67t}$

molar fraction of cephapirin excreted at time infinity, respectively, and Xme and fm are the total amounts and molar fraction of cephapirin metabolized to descetylcephapirin. The use of equation 4 assumes that the desacetylcephapirin formed in the dogs is totally recovered in the urine. This assumption was considered valid since about 98% of the dose was recovered in the urine (Table 5). Therefore, in the beagle dogs, the rate constants governing excretion (ke) and metabolism (km) of cephapirin were 0.93 h^{-1} and 1.91 h^{-1}, respectively. It would appear that the deacetylation of cephapirin to desacetylcephapirin plays a major role in the elimination of cephapirin in the dogs.

The urinary excretion rate of cephapirin in the dogs is given by:

$$\frac{dXe}{dt} = ke \cdot Xp \qquad (5)$$

where Xp is the total amount of cephapirin in the central plasma compartment at any given time t.

Since Xp at any time t is given by:

$$Xp = \text{dose}\,(C_1\, e^{-\alpha t} + C_2\, e^{-\beta t}) \qquad (6)$$

where $C_1 = A_1/Cp^0$ and $C_2 = B_1/Cp^0$ (from equation 2) and Cp^0 (zero time plasma concentration $= A_1 + B_1$) = 128.24 μg/ml, equation 4 may be written as:

$$\frac{dXe}{dt} = ke\ \text{dose}\,(C_1\, e^{-\alpha t} + C_2\, e^{-\beta t}) \qquad (7)$$

Integration of equation 7, solving for the constant of integration and rearranging, yields:

$$Xe = ke\ \text{dose}\ \frac{C_1}{\alpha}(1 - e^{-\alpha t}) + \frac{C_2}{\beta}(1 - e^{-\beta t}) \qquad (8)$$

where Xe is the cumulative amount of cephapirin excreted at any time t. Although the plasma half-life of desacetylcephapirin was similar to that previously reported for cephapirin ($t_{1/2}$ = 0.5 h), an attempt was made to compute the excretion rate (kme) of desacetylcephapirin in dogs by plotting the rate of excretion ($dXme/dt$) in milligrams per hour against the mean interpolated amount of metabolite (Xme) present in the plasma during the excretion period (Fig. 6) as described by Martin (13). With the exception of the value obtained during the initial 30 min, the excretion rate of desacetylcephapirin was directly proportional to the plasma concentration. The regression coefficient describes the renal clearance of desacetylcephapirin (Cl_R) in the dogs, which was approximately 6 liters/h of 100 ml/min. The renal clearance of desacetylcephapirin (Cl_R) in the dogs was also computed from its area under the plasma concentration-time curve (area = 25.1 μg·h per ml) employing the following equation:

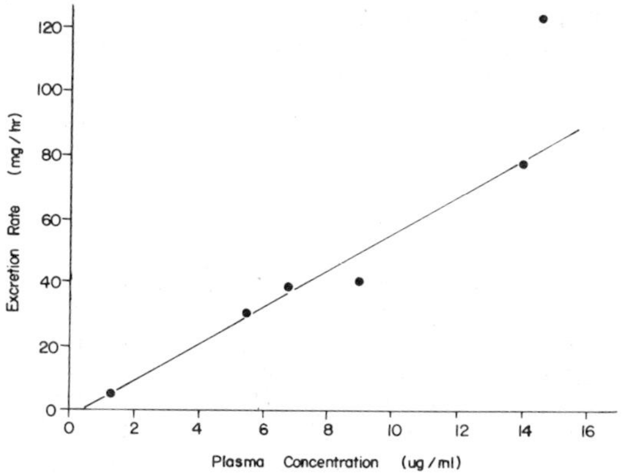

FIG. 6. *Plot of the urinary excretion rate of desacetylcephapirin in beagle dogs as a function of the corresponding plasma concentration. The regression line is equal to the renal clearance value in liters per hour.*

$$Cl_R = \frac{Xme}{\text{area}} \qquad (9)$$

A value of 5.8 liters/h or 96.7 ml/min was obtained by this method.

Assuming that the plasma compartment volume for desacetylcephapirin is about the same as that previously determined for cephapirin (V_p = 23% of body volume in the dogs), an estimate of the rate constant (*kme*) for excretion of desacetylcephapirin is given by:

$$kme = \frac{Cl_R}{V_p} \qquad (10)$$

where Cl_R is the renal clearance of desacetylcephapirin in milliliters per hour. Under the assumption, the rate constant *kme* would be 2.90 h^{-1}. Thus, it would appear that desacetylcephapirin is cleared by the kidneys at approximately the same rate as cephapirin and, therefore, would not be a rate-limiting step in the kinetic model.

Having thus defined the rate constants that govern the distribution of cephapirin to and from tissue fluids (K_1, K_{-1}) and its excretion (*ke*) as well as the rate constants that govern the rate of formation (*km*) and excretion (*kme*) of desacetylcephapirin in dogs, it is possible to test the appropriateness of the kinetic model (Fig. 5) by the combined use of digital and analogue computers employing previously described equations. Figure 7 illustrates the use of the kinetic model in describing the pharmacokinetic profile of cephapirin in dogs. It should be particularly noted that the observed plasma levels of cephapirin and the urinary excretion of cephapirin and desacetylcephapirin were in excellent agreement with the predicted computer plots, indicating that the kinetic model adequately described the kinetic profile of cephapirin in dogs. However, it should also be noted that there is a significant disagreement between the observed plasma levels of desacetylcephapirin and the computer-predicted plots. The latter findings suggest that the present kinetic model (Fig. 5) is inadequate in describing the kinetic profile of desacetylcephapirin. The present kinetic model predicted significantly higher plasma levels of desacetylcephapirin than were observed during the initial h 1. The tendency would be to assume that the observed discrepancy is due to faulty computation of the rate constants that govern the rate of formation (*km*) and elimination (*kme*) of desacetylcephapirin. It should be noted, however, that the magnitude of *km* is governed strictly by the molar fraction (*fm*) of desacetylcephapirin recovered in the urine (equation 3), and the rate constant (*kme*) was computed from renal clearance values for desacetylcephapirin determined by two separate methods. An alternate explanation might be a source of desace-

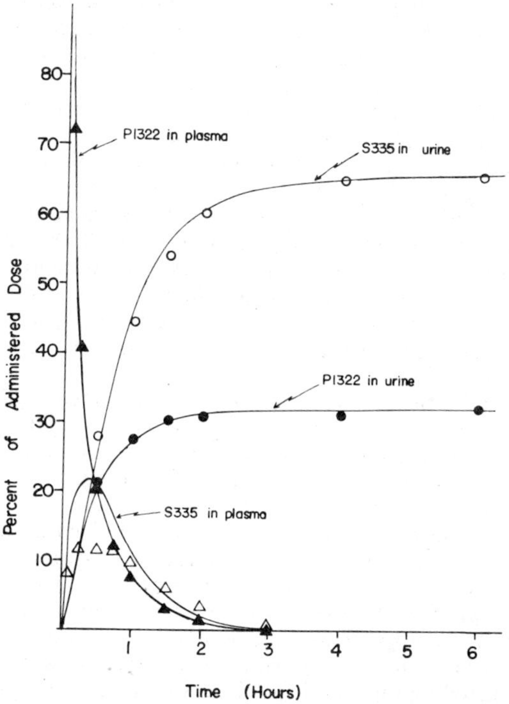

FIG. 7. *Observed and computer-predicted plots of the concentrations of cephapirin (P1322) (▲) and desacetylcephapirin (S335) (△) in plasma and cumulative urinary excretion of cephapirin (●) and desacetylcephapirin (○) in beagle dogs after rapid i.v. bolus.*

tylcephapirin that does not originate within the plasma compartment (V_p). The lack of proportionality between the excretion rate and the plasma concentrations during the initial 30 min suggests the possibility of a first pass effect occurring within the kidney, which results in the metabolism of cephapirin to desacetylcephapirin within the canine kidney. This hypothesis is further supported by the fact that, despite the lower plasma levels of metabolite during h 1, significantly more metabolite than parent drug was excreted during this initial period. This hypothesis will be further supported and discussed at length in dealing with human excretion data.

Pharmacokinetics and metabolism of cephapirin in humans. Summarized in Table 7 and illustrated in Fig. 8 are the mean concentrations of cephapirin and desacetylcephapirin in plasma of 10 human volunteers administered a 1.0-g i.v. bolus of cephapirin. It can be readily seen that the levels of desacetylcephapirin in plasma were extremely low and in some instances undetectable and that the concentrations of cephapirin in the plasma closely approximated the cup-plate activity (Table 7). Despite the extremely low levels of desacetylcephapirin in plasma, approximately 45.3% of the dose was excreted as the desacetyl metabolite (Table 8). The urinary excretion of cephapirin accounted for about 48.5% of the dose. The cup-plate assay (expressed in terms of parent drug) grossly underestimated the total amounts of antibiotics excreted, accounting for only 69.2% of the dose, whereas bioautographic assays, in fact, accounted for 93.8% of the dose. The large discrepancy was due to the presence of desacetylcephapirin in the urine, which has about 54% of the bioactivity of cephapirin, employing *S. lutea* as the test organism.

Kinetic analyses of the plasma concentrations of cephapirin beyond the early drug distribution phase revealed that the plasma half-life of cephapirin in humans was about 0.5 h. Similarly, the half-life of desacetylcephapirin was about 0.43 h, and the "apparent" volume of distribution (V_D) of cephapirin in humans was about 0.23 liter/kg. The renal clearance (Cl_R) of cephapirin (computed from an equation analogous to equation 9) was about 342 ml/min, indicating that cephapirin was secreted by the renal tubules. A similar attempt with the desacetylcephapirin excretion data revealed a total lack of proportionality in the excretion rate and observed plasma concentrations of desacetylcephapirin. Kinetic analysis of the cumulative excretion of desacetylcephapirin during h 1 after drug administration indicated that the effective renal clearance value for that period was about 2,700 ml/min. The mean renal clearance over the 6-h period was about 1,800 ml/min. This renal clearance

TABLE 7. *Mean concentration of cephapirin and desacetylcephapirin in plasma after i.v. administration of a 1.0-g dose of cephapirin to humans*

Time	Concn[a]		
	Cephapirin	Desacetyl-cephapirin[b]	Cup-plate bioactivity[c]
5 min	63.6 ± 5.2	2.5	65.0 ± 5.3
0.5 h	10.2 ± 0.8	1.9	11.1 ± 0.8
1.0 h	3.0 ± 0.3	1.0	3.5 ± 0.4
1.5 h	1.7 ± 0.2	0.3	1.9 ± 0.2
2.0 h	0.9 ± 0.1	ND[d]	0.9 ± 0.1
3.0 h	0.4 ± 0.05		0.4 ± 0.05
4.0 h	0.2 ± 0.02		0.2 ± 0.02

[a] Micrograms per milliliter ± standard error; N = 8.

[b] Desacetylcephapirin was detectable in three patients at 5 min, five patients at 0.5 h, and two patients at 1.5 h.

[c] Bioactivity is expressed in terms of cephapirin.

[d] ND, Not determined.

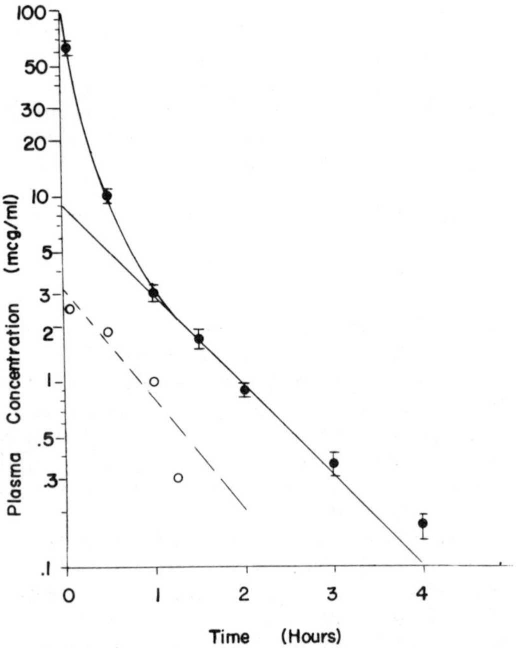

FIG. 8. *Semilogarithmic plots of the concentration of cephapirin (●) and desacetylcephapirin (○) in plasma of human volunteers after a rapid i.v. bolus of a 1.0-g dose of cephapirin.*

TABLE 8. *Cumulative urinary excretion of cephapirin and desacetylcephapirin after i.v. administration of cephapirin to humans*

Time (h)	Excretion (%)[a] ± SE		
	Cephapirin	Desacetyl-cephapirin	Cup-plate bioactivity[b]
1.0	40.5	32.4	55.8
2.0	46.4	40.7	64.9
4.0	48.3	44.6	68.6
6.0	48.5	45.3	69.2

[a] Percent excretion is expressed in terms of administered dose (1 g). SE, Standard error. $N = 8$.

[b] Bioactivity is based on a cephapirin reference standard.

value is totally unphysiological, even assuming renal tubular secretion, since renal plasma flow in humans is about 600 to 800 ml/min. In view of the total lack of proportionality between urinary excretion of desacetylcephapirin and the corresponding plasma concentration, no attempt was made to fit the data to the previously described model (Fig. 5).

DISCUSSION

Comparative metabolic studies performed in mice, rats, dogs, and humans suggest that the biotransformation of cephapirin was qualitatively similar in these species. The fate of cephapirin was similar to that reported for cephalothin (17, 18) and involved metabolism to its desacetyl metabolite and renal excretion of the parent drug and metabolite. Circulating desacetylcephapirin was found in plasma of all species in varying amounts after parenteral administration of cephapirin.

A method was devised, employing paper chromatography followed by bioautography on *B. subtilis* seeded agar plates, that permitted quantitation of both cephapirin and desacetylcephapirin in plasma and urine. The pharmacokinetic data presented herein conclusively showed that, with the exception of human plasma which contained very little desacetyl metabolite, the use of the cup-plate assay on *S. lutea* seeded agar plates grossly underestimated the actual amounts of antibiotics present in the plasma and urine specimens. This was particularly evident in dealing with urinary recovery of antibiotics when in some instances the cup-plate assay accounted for only about 50 to 60% of the actual amount of drug present, as determined by the bioautography assay (Tables 1 and 5). The large discrepancy observed was due to the fact that the desacetylcephapirin present in the urine specimens had a 54% activity relative to cephapirin when assayed on *S. lutea* plates. The use of the bioautography assay permitted the pharmacokinetic characterization of cephapirin in the laboratory animals and humans.

Although no qualitative differences in the biotransformation of cephapirin were noted among species, pharmacokinetic analyses of the plasma concentration and urinary excretion data revealed that the rate and extent of metabolism of cephapirin to its desacetyl metabolite decreased from rodents to dogs to humans. The kinetic analyses also suggested that, in rats, dogs, and humans, the kidney performed a role not only in excretion but also in the metabolism of cephapirin to desacetylcephapirin. These conclusions concerning rats and dogs are largely based on the disproportionate amount of desacetylcephapirin excretion in these species relative to plasma concentrations (see Tables 2 to 5). Although the circulating desacetylcephapirin was cleared at approximately the same rate as cephapirin ($t_{1/2}$ = 0.5 h) in dogs, significantly more desacetyl metabolite was excreted (Table 5) in the urine. The renal metabolism hypothesis is further supported by recent published data obtained in rats by Shimizu (19) on cephapirin and cephalothin. Significantly higher concentrations (threefold) of desacetyl metabolites of these two cephalosporin antibiotics were found in the kidney when compared with the serum levels (19).

A kinetic model was used to describe the distribution and elimination of cephapirin in beagle dogs (Fig. 6). Although the model was adequate in describing the concentrations of cephapirin in plasma and the urinary excretion of cephapirin and desacetylcephapirin in the dogs (Fig. 7), it failed to adequately predict the concentrations of desacetylcephapirin in plasma, which were disproportionately low relative to its corresponding urinary excretion. After an i.v. bolus of cephapirin to beagle dogs at a dose of 30 mg/kg, cephapirin was rapidly distributed to the central plasma compartment and tissue fluids, achieving an "apparent" volume of distribution (V_d) of approximately 320 ml/kg or 32% of the body volume. Cephapirin is thereafter eliminated by excretion and metabolism (the latter occurring in the plasma compartment and presumably in the kidneys) at a rapid rate (half-life = 0.44 h). The renal clearances (Cl_r = 100 ml/min) of cephapirin and desacetylcephapirin were similar in dogs and exceeded the glomerular filtration rate (4 ml/min per kg), indicating active renal tubular secretion.

The kinetic data obtained in human volunteers suggest that cephapirin is handled in a similar manner as in dogs. As in the beagle dogs, the plasma half-life of cephapirin was about 0.5 h and the renal clearance of cephapirin (Cl_r) = 342 ml/min) exceeded glomerular filtration, indicating that active tubular secretion was occurring. The "apparent" volume of drug distribution of cephapirin (V_d = 230 ml/kg) comprised about 23% of the body volume, suggesting that cephapirin is distributed primarily in the extracellular fluids and to some small extent within tissue fluids.

Although qualitative similarity exists in the kinetic profile of cephapirin in humans and in common laboratory animals, there are subtle unique differences in humans. A major difference is the rate of deacetylation of cephapirin within the central plasma compartment. Extremely low levels (<2 μg/ml) of desacetylcephapirin were obtained in plasma after i.v. administration of a 1.0-g bolus. The cephapirin plasma concentrations approximate the cup-plate bioactivity only in humans (Table 7) and not in dogs and rodents. Despite the low levels of circulating desacetylcephapirin, approximately 45% of the dose was excreted as the desacetyl metabolite in the urine. In contrast to cephapirin, which was cleared at a rate of 342 ml/min, the renal clearance of desacetylcephapirin ($Cl_r \simeq$ 1,800 ml/min) significantly exceeded renal plasma flow (600 to 800 ml/min). Kinetic analyses of the human data showed that the previously described kinetic model (Fig. 6) was totally inadequate in describing the metabolic profile of cephapirin in humans. A suitable kinetic model (6) was devised that takes into account not only tissue distribution and urinary excretion of cephapirin but also its deacetylation within the kidneys.

Kidney metabolism of drugs has recently been shown by Wan and Riegelman (21, 22) and Wan et al. (23) for a number of drugs, and Rennick (15) has recently postulated that renal metabolism may be an integral part of the renal tubular transport system for these drugs. The results reported herein indicate that renal metabolism of cephapirin does occur in humans, and comparative metabolic studies in rats and dogs suggest that a similar drug elimination mechanism may occur in these species. Kirby et al. (7) have recently reported that, in contrast to normal volunteers, high levels of circulating desacetylcephalothin were obtained in uremic patients. Those findings suggest that deacetylation of cephalothin must occur to a great extent within the plasma compartment (i.e., via plasma or liver esterases) and manifests itself particularly in uremic patients. The present findings suggest that renal metabolism of cephapirin must play a major role in the elimination of this drug in normal subjects. The effects of uremia on cephapirin elimination remain as yet undefined.

LITERATURE CITED

1. **Axelrod, J., R. R. Meyers, and S. Z. Hirschman.** 1972. Cephapirin: pharmacology in normal human volunteers. J. Clin. Pharmacol. **12**:84–88.
2. **Bodner, S. J., and M. G. Koenig.** 1972. Clinical and *in vitro* evaluation of cephapirin: a new parenteral cephalosporin. Am. J. Med. Sci. **263**:43–51.
3. **Bran, J. L., M. E. Levison, and D. Kaye.** 1972. Clinical and in vitro evaluation of cephapirin, a new cephalosporin antibiotic. Antimicrob. Agents Chemother. **1**:35–40.
4. **Cabana, B. E., D. R. Van Harken, G. H. Hottendorf, J. T. Doluisio, W. O. Griffen, Jr., D. W. A. Bourne, and L. W. Dittert.** 1975. The role of the kidney in the elimination of cephapirin in man. J. Pharmacokinet. Biopharm. **3**:419–438.
5. **Chisholm, D. R., F. Leitner, M. Misiek, G. E. Wright, and K. E. Price.** 1970. Laboratory studies with a new cephalosporanic acid derivative, p. 244–246. Antimicrob. Agents Chemother. 1969.
6. **Grove, D. C., and W. A. Randall.** 1955. Assay methods of antibiotics – a laboratory manual. Medical Encyclopedia, Inc., New York.
7. **Kirby, W. M. M., J. D. DeMaine, and W. S. Serill.** 1971. Pharmacokinetics of the cephalosporins in healthy volunteers and uremic patients. Postgrad. Med. J. **47** (Suppl):41–46.
8. **Kirshbaum, A., and B. Arret.** 1967. Outline of details for official microbiological assays of antibiotics. J. Pharm. Sci. **56**:511–515.
9. **Lee, C. C., E. B. Herr, Jr., and R. C. Anderson.** 1963. Pharmacological and toxicological studies on cephalothin. Clin. Med. **70**:1123–1138.
10. **Loo, J. C. K., and S. Riegelman.** 1968. New method for calculating the intrinsic absorption rate of drugs. J. Pharm. Sci. **57**:918–927.
11. **Marquardt, D. W.** 1963. An algorithm for least squares estimation of non-linear parameters. J. Soc. Ind. Appl. Math. **11**:431.
12. **Marquardt, D. W.** 1966. Least squares estimation of non-linear-parameters. IBM Share Program Library, no. 3094.
13. **Martin, B. K.** 1967. Treatment of data from urinary excretion. Nature (London) **214**:247–249.
14. **Office of Federal Register.** 1972. Code of federal regulations, Title 21, p. 234–240. U.S. Government Printing Office, Washington, D.C.
15. **Rennick, B. R.** 1972. Renal excretion of drugs: tubular transport and metabolism. Annu. Rev. Pharmacol. **12**:141–156.
16. **Riegelman, S., J. Loo, and M. Rowland.** 1968. Shortcomings in pharmacokinetic analysis by conceiving the body to exhibit properties of a single compartment. J. Pharm. Sci. **57**:117–127.
17. **Riegelman, S., J. Loo, and M. Rowland.** 1968. Concept of a volume of distribution and possible errors in evaluation of the parameter. J. Pharm. Sci. **57**:128–133.
18. **Riggs, D. S.** 1963. Mathematical approach to physiolog-

ical problems, p. 203–209. The Williams & Wilkins Co., Baltimore.

19. **Shimizu, T.** 1975. Serum level and urinary excretion of parent antibiotics and desacetyl forms after parenteral administration of cephalothin and cephapirin. Jpn. J. Antibiot. 28:628–633.
20. **Wagner, J. G., and J. I. Northam.** 1967. Estimation of volume of distribution and half-life of a compound after rapid intravenous injection. J. Pharm. Sci. **56**:529–531.
21. **Wan, S. H., and S. Riegelman.** 1972. Renal contribution to overall metabolism of drugs. I. Conversion of benzoic acid to hippuric acid. J. Pharm. Sci. **61**:1278–1284.
22. **Wan, S. H., and S. Riegelman.** 1972. Renal contribution to overall metabolism of drugs. II. Biotransformation of salicylic acid to salicyluric acid. J. Pharm. Sci. **61**:1284–1287.
23. **Wan, S. H., B. Von Lehmann, and S. Riegelman.** 1972. Renal contribution to overall metabolism of drugs. III. Metabolism of p-aminobenzoic acid. J. Pharm. Sci. **61**:1288–1292.

ANTIMICROBIAL AGENTS AND CHEMOTHERAPY, Aug. 1976, p. 318-321 Vol. 10, No. 2

Printed in U.S.A.

Treatment of Murine Coccidioidomycosis with Polymyxin B

M. S. COLLINS* AND D. PAPPAGIANIS

Department of Medical Microbiology, School of Medicine, University of California, Davis, California 95616

Received for publication 12 April 1976

An agar dilution method was employed to test the susceptibility of 12 strains of *Coccidioides immitis* to polymyxin B (PB). After 3 days of incubation, eight strains were markedly inhibited by 5.0 μg of PB per ml and four strains did not grow. PB at 10 μg/ml inhibited the growth of all strains through 20 days of incubation. To determine whether PB has anticoccidioidal activity in vivo, mice in groups of 30 were infected intraperitoneally with a mean lethal dose (LD_{50}) or 20 LD_{50} of arthrospores of *C. immitis* ATCC 28868 (Silveira). Treatment by intraperitoneal injection of PB (2.5 mg/kg) was begun 2 or 5 days after challenge. By 40 days after infection, 47 and 7% of the untreated mice challenged with an LD_{50}, respectively, were alive. Of mice infected with an LD_{50} or 20 LD_{50} and treated with PB beginning 2 days after the challenge, 90% of each group were alive by day 40. Initiation of PB therapy 5 days after infection permitted survival of 84% of the mice infected with an LD_{50}; however, only 27% of the mice infected with 20 LD_{50} survived by day 40. In this latter group there was evidence that PB prolonged life since 56% of the treated mice were alive by day 15 as compared with 30% of the controls. PB in vivo was fungistatic since the majority of treated mice had *C. immitis* in the liver, lungs, and spleen.

Polymyxin B (PB) has been shown to inhibit the growth of the spherule and mycelial phases of *Coccidioides immitis* in vitro (2, 3). Anticoccidioidal activity was associated with the strongly basic charge of the decapeptide moiety of PB. The rapid loss of cytoplasmic materials from spherules suspended in water when PB was added suggested that PB inhibited growth of *C. immitis* in vitro by damaging the cytoplasmic membrane. Because the low concentrations of PB that inhibited the growth of *C. immitis* also potentiated the anticoccidioidal activity of amphotericin B in vitro, we suggested that PB might be a useful adjunct to amphotericin B therapy in selected cases of coccidioidomycosis (3).

In the present study our observations on the anticoccidiodal activity of PB were extended to two in vivo situations. In addition we have determined the susceptibility to PB in vitro of 12 strains of *C. immitis*, 11 of which were isolated from humans with serious coccidioidal disease.

MATERIALS AND METHODS

Fungi. The 12 strains of *C. immitis* employed in this study were maintained in the mycelial phase by periodic transfer on glucose-yeast extract agar slants. Arthrospores were harvested by washing the slants with sterile distilled water. Spore concentration was determined by direct count in a hemocytometer. A 0.2-ml portion of spore suspension was added to 0.2 ml of Gram iodine plus 0.1 ml of 37% formaldehyde. The portions were held overnight to insure killing of spores and counted the next day. The spore suspensions were then adjusted to 2.5×10^4 spores/ml of distilled water.

Experimental animals. In experiment 1, male mice (NAMRU strain) were used. At the time of challenge they were 23 weeks old and their average weight was 38.9 g, with a standard deviation of 1.7 g. Female mice employed in experiment 2 were 6 weeks old at the time of challenge. Their average weight was 27.4 g, with a standard deviation of 0.9 g. Mice were caged in groups of 9 or 10. Food and water were available ad libitum.

Drug. A 50-mg amount of sterile PB (lot 142-K, Burroughs Wellcome) was solubilized in 10 ml of distilled water. Further dilutions were made in sterile distilled water and promptly used. The stock solution of PB (5 mg/ml) was stored at −16°C for no longer than 2 weeks.

Anticoccidioidal activity of PB in vitro. The susceptibility of 12 strains of *C. immitis* to PB was determined by an agar dilution method. Sabouraud dextrose agar (SDA) was prepared in 100-ml volumes by solidification of the broth with 0.85% Ionagar no. 2 (Colab). Purified agar was used because bacteriological grade agar abolishes the anticoccidioidal activity of PB (2). After the medium was autoclaved and cooled to 50°C, sterile PB solution was added, and 50-ml volumes were poured into two petri dishes (15 by 200 mm). After solidification, the plates were inoculated in a pattern with 0.03 ml of each of the 12 spore suspensions. The plates were incubated at 34°C. The minimum inhibitory concentration of PB was considered to be the concentration that completely suppressed growth, as determined by viewing the plates with the unaided eye.

Anticoccidioidal activity of PB in mice. Potential therapeutic efficacy of PB in experimental murine coccidioidomycosis was investigated in two separate experiments. In the initial experiment, 29 male mice were infected intraperitoneally with 4,600 arthrospores of *C. immitis* ATCC 28688 (Silveira strain). Ten controls remained uninfected. On days 3 to 8, 10, and 11 after infection, 19 of the infected mice were treated by intraperitoneal injection of 100 μg of PB (approximately 2.5 mg of PB per kg of body weight) in a 0.2-ml volume. The remaining 10 infected mice received 0.2 ml of water only. In experiment 2, 6-week-old female mice were divided into three groups: a group of 90 mice received 120 arthrospores intraperitoneally, 90 mice received 2,300 spores, and 30 mice remained uninfected. Treatment by intraperitoneal injection of 0.2 ml of PB solution (2.5 mg/kg) or of water was begun 2 or 5 days after infection and continued daily until day 17 after infection. The presence of *C. immitis* in mice alive 40 days after challenge with arthrospores was determined by culture of the liver, lungs, and spleen on Mycosel (BBL) agar.

The significance of protection afforded mice by PB therapy was assessed by the uncorrected chi-square test.

RESULTS

Anticoccidioidal activity of PB in vitro. The SDA plates were first examined after 3 days of incubation. The 12 strains of *C. immitis* grew without inhibition on plates containing 1.25 μg of PB per ml. At 2.5 μg/ml, all strains were partially inhibited. At 5.0 μg of PB per ml of SDA, eight strains, including ATCC 28688 (Silveira), were markedly inhibited and four strains did not grow. No strain grew at 10 μg of PB per ml of SDA. After 5 days of incubation, all strains grew at 5.0 μg of PB per ml; none grew at 10 or 20 μg of PB per ml. This inhibition persisted through 20 days of incubation.

Anticoccidiodal activity of PB in mice. In the initial experiment, the older mice challenged with 4,600 arthrospores were significantly protected ($P < 0.05$) by PB therapy (Fig. 1). By day 11, 50% of the control mice that received injection of water only were dead and, by day 40, 90% (9 of 10) were dead. Mice treated with PB had a cumulative mortality of 53% (10 of 19) by day 26. There were no additional deaths by day 40.

In experiment 2, by day 40 after challenge, 53% (16 of 30) and 93% (28 of 30) of the 6-week-old mice challenged with 120 and 2,300 spores, respectively, and treated with water were dead (Fig. 2). PB therapy beginning 2 days after challenge significantly reduced mortality since only 10% ($P < 0.05$) and 13% ($P < 0.05$) of mice challenged with 120 or 2,300 spores, respectively, died by day 40. PB therapy beginning 5 days after challenge permitted survival of 90% (27 of 30) of the mice infected with 120 spores ($P < 0.05$); however, only 27% (8 of 30) of the mice infected with 2,300 spores survived. Although mortality by day 40 of this latter group of mice was not significantly lower than that of the controls ($0.05 < P < 0.1$), there was evidence

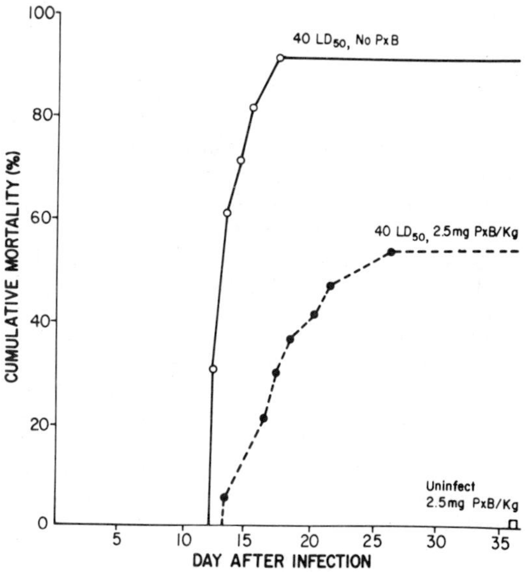

FIG. 1. *Mice were treated with polymyxin B 3 to 8, 10, and 11 days after infection with 40 LD_{50} of arthrospores of C. immitis.*

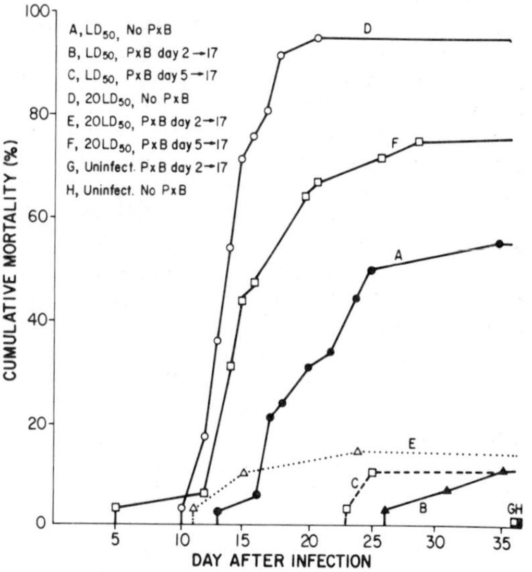

FIG. 2. *Mice were treated with polymyxin B 2 to 17 or 5 to 17 days after infection with an LD_{50} or 20 LD_{50} of arthrospores of C. immitis.*

that PB therapy prolonged life, since 56% of the treated mice were alive at day 15 as compared with 30% of the controls ($P < 0.05$).

A comparison of the weights of mice at the time of challenge and at 10 days after challenge revealed that infection was probably less severe in mice receiving PB. At each challenging dose, the weight loss of untreated mice exceeded that of PB-treated mice. Mice receiving treatment 2 days after challenge showed less weight loss than did mice treated 5 days after challenge (Table 1).

PB was fungistatic rather than fungicial since, despite apparent good health as was evident by level of activity, sleekness of coat, and weight gain by day 40, the majority of mice harbored *C. immitis* in their livers, lungs, and spleens. In both experiments the uninfected controls that received PB remained in apparent good health.

DISCUSSION

The results presented in this study indicate that PB has anticoccidioidal activity in vivo. In the preliminary study, mice challenged with approximately 40 mean lethal doses (LD_{50}) of arthrospores received eight injections of PB beginning 3 days after challenge. This regimen permitted survival by day 40 of nearly 50% (9 of 19) of the mice, whereas only 10% (1 of 10) of the untreated infected controls survived. Although a small number of mice were employed in this initial experiment, the differences in survival between the untreated and the PB-treated mice were significant.

Mice in experiment 2 were challenged with an LD_{50} or 20 LD_{50}. PB treatment began 2 or 5 days after challenge. Interestingly, in terms of survival by day 40, it mattered little whether the mice received an LD_{50} or 20 LD_{50}, provided that treatment with PB commenced 2 days after challenge. Treatment that was begun 5 days after challenge permitted survival of 90% of the mice challenged with an LD_{50}; however, mice challenged with 20 LD_{50} were only equivocally protected. A measure of protection was nonethless evident in this latter group because, when compared with the untreated infected controls, the PB-treated mice showed less weight loss at day 10 and lived significantly longer.

Tarbet et al. (11) studied the development of coccidioidal disease after injection of mycelial fragments into the peritoneal cavity of mice. Small aggregates of immature spherules, mycelial fragments, and polymorphonuclear cells were seen by day 2. These aggregates were covered with mucoid material and not yet firmly adherent to tissue surfaces. By day 5, the fungus was found within masses of amorphous material, which resulted from the death and disintegration of phagocytic cells. These purulent lesions were firmly adherent to tissue surfaces. Endosporulating spherules were not seen by Tarbet et al. until 6 to 7 days after challenge. Other investigators (7, 9, 10) have shown that only 2 to 4 days are required for endosporulating spherules to develop when arthrospores (not mycelial fragments) are deposited in the lungs.

The significant protection afforded mice by initiation of PB therapy 2 days after challenge likely depended upon at least two factors. First, fungal numbers by day 2 probably had not yet increased beyond the challenging dose. Second, diffusion of PB into the vicinity of the fungus was likely not yet prevented by the cellular response of the host. PB diffuses very poorly in tissues (8) and is strongly bound by pus (1); hence, the extensive cellular response of the host that develops in the peritoneal cavity by day 5 (11) would limit diffusion of the antibiotic into coccidioidal lesions.

Because the majority of PB-treated mice that survived to day 40 harbored *C. immitis* in their tissues, it can be assumed that the anticoccidioidal activity of PB was limited to inhibiting the growth of the fungus. This assumption was

TABLE 1. *Weight changes in mice infected with C. immitis and treated with polymyxin B*

Treatment group	No. of mice on day 1/day 10	Inoculum arthrospores (i.p.)[a]	Mean wt on day 1 (g)	Mean wt on day 10 (g)	Wt change (%)
Polymyxin B, day 2 → 17	30/30	120	27.7	28.0	+1.1
Polymyxin B, day 5 → 17	30/30	120	27.9	26.6	−4.7
Water only	30/30	120	27.4	25.9	−5.5
Polymyxin B, day 2 → 17	30/30	2,300	27.3	26.3	−3.7
Polymyxin B, day 5 → 17	30/29	2,300	26.8	24.9	−7.1
Water only	30/29	2,300	26.9	23.0	−14.5
Polymyxin B, day 2 → 17	20/20	0	28.1	28.5	+1.4
Water only	10/10	0	26.7	26.4	−1.1

[a] i.p., Intraperitoneal.

supported by the observation that in the two groups of PB-treated mice challenged with an LD_{50} the first death did not occur until 6 days after the drug was discontinued; however, by this time, 33% of the untreated infected controls were dead.

In an earlier study we demonstrated that PB potentiated the anticoccidioidal activity of amphotericin B in vitro (3). At that time, it was suggested that in special cases of coccidioidomycosis PB might be a useful adjunct to amphotericin B therapy. In most serious cases of coccidioidomycosis, the fungus is located deep within the tissues. Because of the limited diffusion of PB through tissues (8), it is doubtful that high concentrations of the antibiotic could be obtained in the vicinity of the fungus. In meningitis, however, *C. immitis* is located in the basilar meninges and the brain substance is infrequently involved (6). Intrathecal administration of 5 mg of PB could bathe the meninges with cerebrospinal fluid containing approximately 30 to 50 μg of PB per ml. Concentrations of this magnitude exceed by severalfold the concentration (10 μg/ml) required to inhibit in vitro the 12 strains of *C. immitis* employed in this study. Furthermore, these concentrations are approximately 12 to 20 times greater than concentrations, e.g., 2.5 μg/ml, that enhanced the anticoccidioidal activity of amphotericin B against the spherule phase of *C. immitis* in vitro (3). It should be noted that administration of 5 mg of PB per day by the intrathecal route has been successfully employed in the therapy of meningitis caused by *Pseudomonas aeruginosa* (4, 5), thus indicating that PB is not without antimicrobial activity in cerebrospinal fluid.

Coccidioidal meningitis remains a life-threatening complication of infection with *C. immitis*. Because amphotericin B must be administered for extended periods of time, serious problems of dose-related toxicity frequently arise. The demonstration that PB is active against *C. immitis* in vivo and our prior demonstration that PB potentiates the anticoccidioidal activity of amphotericin B against the spherule phase of *C. immitis* in vitro (3) warrant additional studies to determine whether PB might be a useful adjunct to amphotericin B in the treatment of coccidioidal meningitis.

ACKNOWLEDGMENTS

This investigation was supported by the U.S. Army Medical Research and Development Command under research contract no. DADA 17-69-C-9061. Michael S. Collins, a Bank of America-Giannini Foundation Fellow, is grateful for their support.

We wish to thank Lorraine Hobbs and Barbara Birdsall for their technical assistance.

LITERATURE CITED

1. **Bryant, R. E., and D. Hammond.** 1974. Interaction of purulent material with antibiotics used to treat *Pseudomonas* infection. Antimicrob. Agents Chemother. 6:702–707.
2. **Collins, M. S.** 1975. Inhibition of growth of *Coccidioides immitis* on Sabouraud medium containing polymyxin B. J. Clin. Microbiol. 1:335–336.
3. **Collins, M. S., and D. Pappagianis.** 1975. Inhibition of *Coccidioides immitis* in vitro and enhancement of anticoccidioidal effects of amphotericin B by polymyxin B. Antimicrob. Agents Chemother. 7:781–787.
4. **Furey, W., I. Ciric, and R. H. Parker.** 1971. Monitoring of intrathecal polymyxin B dosage during treatment of *Pseudomonas* meningitis. Ill. Med. J. 139:506–510.
5. **Geelhoed, G. W., and A. S. Ketcham.** 1973. *Pseudomonas* meningitis complicating radical resection for radiorecurrent cancer of the paranasal sinuses: report of two patients successfully treated with intrathecal polymyxin. J. Surg. Oncol. 5:365–374.
6. **Huntington, R. W., W. J. Waldmann, J. A. Sargent, H. O'Connel, R. Wybel, and D. Croll.** 1967. Pathologic and clinical observations on 142 cases of fatal coccidioidomycosis with necropsy, p. 143–167. *In* L. Ajello (ed.), Coccidioidomycosis. University of Arizona Press, Tucson.
7. **Kong, Y. M., D. C. Savage, and H. B. Levine.** 1966. Enhancement of immune responses in mice by a booster injection of *Coccidioides* spherules. J. Immunol. 95:1048–1056.
8. **Kunin, C. M., and A. Bugg.** 1971. Binding of polymyxin to tissues: the major determinant of distribution and persistence in the body. J. Infect. Dis. 124:394–400.
9. **Savage, D. C., and S. H. Madin.** 1968. Cellular responses in lungs of immunized mice to intranasal infection with *Coccidioides immitis*. Sabouraudia 6:94–102.
10. **Sinski, J. T., and P. J. Sato.** 1966. Onset of coccidioidomycosis in mouse lung after intravenous injection. Mycopathologia 30:41–46.
11. **Tarbet, J. E., E. T. Wright, and V. D. Newcomer.** 1952. Experimental coccidioidal granuloma. Developmental stages of sporangia in mice. Am. J. Pathol. 28:901–917.

ANTIMICROBIAL AGENTS AND CHEMOTHERAPY, Aug. 1976, p. 322-324 Vol. 10, No. 2

Printed in U.S.A.

Susceptibility of *Haemophilus influenzae* Type b to Cefatrizine, Ampicillin, and Chloramphenicol

THOMAS BROTHERTON, TRACY LEES, AND RALPH D. FEIGIN*

Edward Mallinckrodt Department of Pediatrics, Washington University School of Medicine, and Division of Infectious Diseases, St. Louis Children's Hospital, St. Louis, Missouri 63110*

Received for publication 6 April 1976

The susceptibility of 269 isolates of *Haemophilus influenzae* type b to cefatrizine (BL-S640), ampicillin, and chloramphenicol was evaluated by disk diffusion susceptibility tests, using a modified Bauer-Kirby method. Broth dilution susceptibility tests were performed on 88 of these isolates, including all isolates resistant by disk to cefatrizine or ampicillin. Six of the isolates were resistant by disk to cefatrizine (zone size, <16 mm), four were resistant to ampicillin (zone size, <19 mm), and none were resistant to chloramphenicol (zone size, <17 mm). Only two of the six isolates of *H. influenzae* that were resistant to cefatrizine by disk were resistant to more than 4 μg of drug per ml. The four organisms resistant to ampicillin on disk were resistant, when tested by the broth method, to >128 μg/ml. These four ampicillin-resistant *H. influenzae* were susceptible to <4 μg of cefatrizine per ml. The two isolates resistant to >4 μg of cefatrizine per ml were susceptible to 0.5 and 2 μg of ampicillin, respectively, per ml. The activity of cefatrizine appears to be comparable in vitro to ampicillin against *H. influenzae*.

Cefatrizine (BL-S640) is a new semisynthetic cephalosporin compound which is water soluble and well absorbed by animals after oral administration (4). In vitro, cefatrizine appears to be four- to eightfold more active than cephalexin against most gram-positive bacteria, as well as against *Escherichia coli* and *Klebsiella*, *Salmonella*, and *Shigella* sp., and approximately 16-fold more active against *Proteus mirabilis* and *Proteus vulgaris* strains (1, 3, 5, 7). It is also inhibitory in concentrations theoretically achievable in humans against many strains of cephalexin-resistant *Enterobacter* sp. and *P. vulgaris* (6) but is inactive against *Pseudomonas aeruginosa*, *Serratia marcescens*, and methicillin-resistant staphylococci (1, 3, 5–7).

Efficacy trials of oral cefatrizine have been initiated in adults and, most recently, in children with cervical lymphadenitis and otitis media. Thus, specific information regarding the susceptibility of *Haemophilus influenzae* to cefatrizine is required. In previous studies in which the susceptiblity of *H. influenzae* to cefatrizine has been evaluated, results have been somewhat contradictory (1, 3, 5, 7). A relatively small number of isolates have been tested, however.

MATERIALS AND METHODS

Between July 1974 and January 1976 *H. influenzae* type b were recovered on 269 occasions from the blood (55), cerebrospinal fluid (21), fluid obtained by needle tympanocentesis (17), or the throat (176) of children at St. Louis Children's Hospital. These isolates came from 263 patients (in six cases, positive blood and cerebrospinal fluid isolates were obtained from the same individual). These isolates were identified on the basis of their requirements for both hemin (x factor) and nicotinamide adenine dinucleotide (v factor), indole production, and lack of hemolysis on tryptic soy agar with 5% rabbit blood. The identity was confirmed by agglutination with type-specific antisera (Hyland Laboratories).

Disk diffusion susceptibility tests were performed on all isolates, using a modified Bauer-Kirby technique (2) against cefatrizine (30 μg), ampicillin (10 μg), and chloramphenicol (30 μg). Mueller-Hinton agar supplemented with 1% IsoVitaleX and 1% hemoglobin was streaked with a broth culture (Mueller-Hinton broth with 10% Fildes extract) that had been adjusted to equal 0.5 McFarland standard. The appropriate antimicrobial disks were then dropped onto the inoculated plates. The plates were incubated in 5% CO_2 at 35°C for 18 h. Zone sizes were measured to determine the susceptibility of the organism to the antimicrobial agent.

Broth dilution susceptibility tests were performed on 88 of these isolates, using Mueller-Hinton broth with 10% Fildes extract. The inoculum was adjusted to approximately 10^5 organisms/ml. Results were determined after a period of 18 h in an aerobic incubator. Cefatrizine-resistant organisms were defined as those for which the minimal inhibitory concentration (MIC) of cefatrizine was greater than 4 μg/ml, ampicillin-resistant organisms were defined as those for which the MIC of ampicillin was greater than 2 μg/ml, and chloramphenicol-resistant organisms were defined as those for which the MIC of chloramphenicol was greater than 8 μg/ml.

Cefatrizine is presently being evaluated by us at St. Louis Children's Hospital in children with cervical lymphadenitis. A daily dose of 40 mg/kg per day is administered in four divided oral doses. Concentrations of cefatrizine in serum are measured at 30 min and at 1, 2, 4, and 6 h after the initial dose of 10 mg/kg.

RESULTS

Six of 269 isolates of *H. influenzae* were resistant by disk to cefatrizine (zone size, <16 mm). Four of these isolates were resistant to ampicillin (zone size, <19 mm). None of these isolates was resistant to chloramphenicol (zone size, <17 mm).

Results of broth dilution susceptibility tests (88 isolates) against cefatrizine, ampicillin, and chloramphenicol, including all isolates that proved to be resistant by disk to cefatrizine or ampicillin, are shown in Table 1. Eighty-five of the 88 *H. influenzae* tested were inhibited and killed by 4.0 μg of cefatrizine per ml. The MIC and minimal bactericidal concentration of cefatrizine was 16 μg/ml for one isolate; the MICs and minimal bactericidal concentrations of cefatrizine were 32 and 64 μg/ml and 4 and 8 μg/ml, respectively, for two other resistant isolates. Eighty-four of the isolates were inhibited and killed by 2.0 μg or less of ampicillin per ml. The MIC and minimal bactericidal concentration of ampicillin was >128 μg/ml for the four resistant *H. influenzae* isolates. None of the strains of *H. influenzae* tested was resistant to concentrations of chloramphenicol that generally can be achieved in vivo. The susceptitiliby of *H. influenzae* to cefatrizine, as measured by the Bauer-Kirby technique (2) and by the broth dilution procedure, is shown in Table 2.

Six *H. influenzae* were resistant to cefatrizine by disk diffusion susceptibility tests; only two of these isolates were resistant to more than 4.0 μg of cefatrizine per ml. The four organisms that appeared to be resistant to ampicillin by disk proved to be resistant by broth dilution tests at >128 μg of ampicillin per ml. These findings were confirmed by the Center for Disease Control, Atlanta, Ga. The four isolates of *H. influenzae* resistant to ampicillin were susceptible to cefatrizine at <4 μg/ml. The two isolates resistant to cefatrizine at 16 and 32 μg/ml, respectively, were susceptible to ampicillin in concentrations of 0.5 and 2 μg/ml.

TABLE 2. *Frequency of isolates: disk susceptibility zone sizes compared with MICs of cefatrizine*

Zone size (mm)	No. of isolates	MIC (88 isolates)	
		MIC (μg/ml)	Isolates
15	1	32	1
16	5	2–16	5
17	8	2–4	2
18	26	2	18
19	19	2	5
20	22	1–2	6
21	26	1–2	8
22	27	1–2	10
23	31	1–2	4
24	32	1–2	4
25	21	1–2	6
26	16	1–2	7
27	22	0.13–1	4
28	7	0.063–0.25	2
29	0		
30	2	0.063–0.13	2
31	0		
32	1	0.063	1
33	1	0.063	1
34	0		
35	0		
36	0		
37	0		
38	2	0.032	2

TABLE 1. *Susceptibility of H. influenzae isolates to cefatrizine, ampicillin, and chloramphenicol*

Drug[a]	Parameter	No. of strains													
		0.032[b]	0.063	0.13	0.25	0.5	1	2	4	8	16	32	64	128	>128
CEF	MIC	2	4	2	1	6	26	43	2	0	1	1	0	0	0
	MBC[c]	1	5	2	0	7	23	44	3	1	1	0	1	0	0
AMP	MIC	7	5	3	17	38	12	2	0	0	0	0	0	0	4
	MBC	6	6	2	16	40	11	3	0	0	0	0	0	0	4
CHL	MIC	3	6	19	18	21	12	0	3	6	0	0	0	0	0
	MBC	3	5	20	18	20	13	0	2	7	0	0	0	0	0

[a] CEF, Cefatrizine; AMP, ampicillin; CHL, chloramphenicol.
[b] Antibiotic concentration (micrograms per milliliter).
[c] MBC, Minimal bactericidal concentration.

The activity of cefatrizine against *H. influenzae* appears to be comparable in vitro to that of ampicillin.

Concentrations of cefatrizine in serum have been measured in 11 children with cervical lymphadenitis. Concentrations of this antibiotic peaked at 1 h after the initial dose (mean, 4.72 μg/ml; range, 3.5 to 7.6 μg/ml). Concentrations at 2 h were virtually identical to those obtained 1 h after a dose. At 6 h (immediately prior to a second dose) the concentration in serum was 1.19 μg/ml (mean), and a range of 0.3 to 3.0 μg/ml was noted.

DISCUSSION

Only six isolates of *H. influenzae* were resistant to cefatrizine by the disk susceptibility test method. Thus, the activity of cefatrizine did not appear to differ significantly from that of ampicillin. All four ampicillin-resistant *H. influenzae* strains were susceptible to cefatrizine. These data are in agreement with information reported by most other investigators who have tested the susceptibility of smaller numbers of *H. influenzae* isolates (3, 5, 7). In one report, however, Actor and associates (1) reported that 6.3 to 12.5 μg of cefatrizine per ml was required to inhibit 90% of the *H. influenzae* isolates tested by them. The number of isolates of *H. influenzae* utilized in their study was not stated. The activity of cefatrizine against *H. influenzae* was not compared with that of ampicillin or chloramphenicol, drugs frequently used in the treatment of *H. influenzae* infections in clinical practice.

Concentrations of cefatrizine in serum after administration of a 10-mg/kg dose orally peaked at values that were twofold in excess of the MIC of 84 of the 88 *H. influenzae* isolates tested in this study. These data, coupled with the in vitro studies described above, document that it is possible to achieve concentrations of cefatrizine in serum that may prove efficacious in the treatment of *H. influenzae* infections.

ACKNOWLEDGMENTS

We express our appreciation to Bristol Laboratories, Syracuse, N.Y., for their support of these investigations. We thank Philip R. Dodge for his critical review and Judy Rodgers for help in the preparation of this manuscript.

LITERATURE CITED

1. **Actor, P., J. V. Uri, L. Phillips, C. S. Sachs, J. R. Guarino, I. Zajoe, D. A. Berges, G. L. Dunn, J. R. E. Hoover, and J. A. Weisbach.** 1975. Laboratory studies with cefatrizine (SK & F 60771) A new broad-spectrum orally-active cephalosporin. J. Antibiot. 25:594–601.
2. **Bauer, A. W., W. M. M. Kirby, J. C. Sherris, and M. Turck.** 1966. Antibiotic susceptibility testing by a standardized simple disc method. Am. J. Clin. Pathol. 45:493–496.
3. **Leitner, F., R. E. Buck, M. Misiek, T. A. Pursiano, and K. E. Price.** 1975. BL-S640, a cephalosporin with a broad spectrum of antibacterial activity: properties in vitro. Antimicrob. Agents Chemother. 3:298–305.
4. **Leitner, F., D. R. Chisholm, Y. H. Tsai, G. E. Wright, R. G. Deregis, and K. E. Price.** 1975. BL-S640, a cephalosporin with a broad spectrum of antibacterial activity: bioavailability and therapeutic properties in rodents. Antimicrob. Agents Chemother. 7:306–310.
5. **Overturf, G. D., R. L. Ressler, P. B. Marengo, and J. Wilkins.** 1975. In vitro evaluation of GL-S640, a new oral cephalosporin antibiotic. Antimicrob. Agents Chemother. 8:305–310.
6. **Watanakunakorn, C., T. Bannister, and C. Glotzbecker.** 1975. Susceptibility of clinical isolates of *Enterobacteriaceae* to BL-S640, a new oral cephalosporin. Antimicrob. Agents Chemother. 7:381–385.
7. **Yourassowsky, E., E. Schoutens, and M. P. Vanderlinden.** 1975. Comparative inhibitory activity of BL-S640 and two other cephalosporins. J. Antibiot. 28:590–593.

ANTIMICROBIAL AGENTS AND CHEMOTHERAPY, Aug. 1976, p. 325-332 Vol. 10, No. 2

Printed in U.S.A.

Specific Action of 4-Nitropyridine 1-Oxide on *Escherichia coli* K-12 Pro+ Strains Leading to the Isolation of Proline-Requiring Mutants: Isolation and Characterization of Pro− Mutants

MANABU INUZUKA,[1*] HIROSHI MIYANO, AND MUNEMITSU TOMOEDA[2]

Department of Chemistry, Faculty of Pharmaceutical Sciences, Kanazawa University, Takara-machi, Kanazawa 920, Japan

Received for publication 26 March 1976

A specific action of 4-nitropyridine 1-oxide on *Escherichia coli* K-12 Pro+ strains leading to highly efficient, selective isolation of Pro− mutants is described. Incubation of Pro+ cells with a sublethal concentration of 4-nitropyridine 1-oxide in Penassay broth gave Pro− mutants, which lacked either the biosynthetic pathway of proline from glutamic acid to glutamyl γ-phosphate (*proB*−) or the pathway from glutamyl γ-phosphate to glutamic γ-semialdehyde (*proA*−) or both. Pro− mutants, which have the metabolic block between Δ^1 pyrroline-5-carboxylate (the cyclized dehydration product of glutamic γ-semialdehyde) and proline (*proC*−) were not found among survivors. Treatment of Pro+ cells with *N*-methyl-*N'*-nitro-*N*-nitrosoguanidine led to isolation of all three types of Pro− mutants, suggesting that the action of 4-nitropyridine 1-oxide on Pro+ cells is apparently distinct from the action of *N*-methyl-*N'*-nitro-*N*-nitrosoguanidine. F-duction and interrupted mating experiments led to determination of the correlation between proline loci and the biosynthetic pathway of proline from glutamic acid.

4-Nitroquinoline 1-oxide has been known to show characteristic biological activities (14), similar to those revealed by acridine dyes (23), such as bactericidal action (2), prophage induction from lysogenic bacteria (13), mutagenic actions toward bacteria (28), and carcinogenicity (26). On the other hand, 4-nitropyridine 1-oxide (4NPO), a pyridine analogue of 4-nitroquinoline 1-oxide, has been known to exhibit little biological activity (14); for instance, the compound is inactive for induction of prophage (13) and shows only very weak carcinogenicity (3).

During the course of a series of investigations on the structure and biological activities of compounds with pyridine, quinoline and acridine skeletons, we found that 4NPO can effectively act on *Escherichia coli* K-12 Pro+ strains, leading to the isolation of proline-requiring (Pro−) mutants in large numbers. We found that Pro− mutants isolated by this method have a metabolic block between glutamic acid (Glu) and glutamic γ-semialdehyde (GSA) in the biosynthetic pathway from Glu to proline and may be characterized as *proA*− and/or *proB*−. The major mechanism of the action of 4NPO was shown to be selection; i.e., 4NPO is more toxic for *pro*+ cells than for *proA*− and *proB*− (but not for *proC*−) cells. This paper describes the standard method of isolation of Pro− mutants by treatment of *Escherichia coli* K-12 Pro+ cells with 4NPO and the genetic and biochemical characterizations of Pro− mutants isolated. Further evidence on the metabolism of 4NPO by Pro+ or Pro− cells and mechanism of selective specificity of the agent toward Pro+ and Pro− cells reported in the accompanying paper (19). A preliminary report has appeared (17).

[1] Present address: Department of Biology, University of California, San Diego, La Jolla, CA 92093.

[2] Present address: Research and Development Division, Eisai Co., 4 Koishikawa, Bunkyo 112, Tokyo, Japan.

MATERIALS AND METHODS

Bacterial strains. The bacterial strains used in this work were *E. coli* K-12 and *Salmonella typhimurium* LT-2 derivatives (Table 1). Pro− mutants other than those isolated by treatment with 4NPO were obtained by treatment with *N*-methyl-*N'*-nitro-*N*-nitrosoguanidine (NTG) or by ultraviolet irradiation. W strains of *E. coli* and JM strains of *S. typhimurium* were supplied by Y. Hirota, Osaka University, and T. Miyake, Keio University, respectively.

Materials and media. 4NPO (27), NTG (24), and Δ^1-pyrroline 5-carboxylic acid (PC) (34) were synthe-

TABLE 1. *Bacterial strains used*

Strain	Relevant genotype[a]	Origin or source
E. coli K-12		
W3110	F^-	
W3630	F^- *mal-5*$^-$	
W3747	F^+13 (F-*lac*$^+$ *proC*$^+$ *ade*$^+$) *met*$^-$	
W4573	F^- *ara-2*$^-$ *lac-85*$^-$ *gal-2*$^-$ *mal-1*$^-$ *mtl*$^-$ *xyl-2*$^-$ *str*^{r}	
JE177	F^- R^+_{100-1} (*str*^{r} *cml*^{r} *tet*^{r} *sul*^{r}) *mal-5*$^-$	W3630
JE1031	HfrH *met*$^-$ *thi*$^-$	
JE2133[b]	F^- *ara-2*$^-$ *proA1*$^-$ *lac85*$^-$ *gal-2*$^-$ *mal-1*$^-$ *mtl*$^-$ *xyl-2*$^-$ *str*^{r}	W4573
JE2265[c]	F^- *ara-2*$^-$ *tonB proA1*$^-$ *tsx lac-85*$^-$ *gal-2*$^-$ *mal-1*$^-$ *mtl*$^-$ *xyl-2*$^-$ *str*^{r}	JE2133
KE113[b]	F^- *ara-2*$^-$ *proB3*$^-$ *lac-85*$^-$ *gal-2*$^-$ *mal-1*$^-$ *mtl*$^-$ *xyl-2*$^-$ *str*^{r}	W4573
KE114[d]	F^- *ara-2*$^-$ *lac-85*$^-$ *proC36*$^-$ *gal-2*$^-$ *mal-1*$^-$ *mtl*$^-$ *xyl-2*$^-$ *str*^{r}	W4573
KE125[d]	F^- *ara-2*$^-$ *proB17*$^-$ *lac-85*$^-$ *gal-2*$^-$ *mal-1*$^-$ *mtl*$^-$ *xyl-2*$^-$ *str*^{r}	W4573
KE126[d]	F^- *ara-2*$^-$ *proA18*$^-$ *lac-85*$^-$ *gal-2*$^-$ *mal-1*$^-$ *mtl*$^-$ *xyl-2*$^-$ *str*^{r}	W4573
χ646	F′ORF-206 (F-*lac*$^+$ *proB*$^+$ *proA*$^+$) *lacy*$^-$	(11)
S. typhimurium LT-2		
JM108[e]	*proA*$^-$	pro-27
JM109[e]	*proC*$^-$	pro-150

[a] Genetic symbols are those used by Taylor and Trotter (31).

[b] Isolated after 4NPO treatment of W4573 and characterized as *pro*$^-$.

[c] Derived from JE2133 by spontaneous mutation to resistance to phage T_1 and T_6.

[d] Isolated after treatment with NTG followed by penicillin screening and characterized as *pro*$^-$.

[e] Kindly supplied by T. Miyake (25).

sized in our laboratory according to the literature. Dihydrostreptomycin sulfate (SM) was purchased from Takeda Chemical Ind., Osaka.

Penassay broth (Difco) was used for cultivation of microorganisms, 4NPO treatment, and conjugation experiments. Synthetic Davis glucose medium (12) was used for penicillin screening techniques. A complete EMB-glucose-agar medium was used for scoring survivors after 4NPO treatment. Synthetic Davis glucose-agar medium and EM-glucose-agar medium (20) were used for characterization of auxotrophic mutants. Synthetic Davis sugar-agar media (Davis-arabinose, Davis-lactose, and Davis-galactose) with necessary supplements were used for characterizing sugar fermentation and for selection of prototrophic recombinant colonies. Glucose salt mineral medium (34) was used for the accumulation of biosynthetic intermediates from glutamic acid to proline. Antibiotics were added as indicated. Tris(hydroxymethyl)aminomethane - malate (TM) buffer (1) was used for NTG treatment. The pH of media was 7.0 unless otherwise noted.

Method for selective isolation of Pro$^-$ mutants by treatment of Pro$^+$ strain with 4NPO. A clone of Pro$^+$ strain was inoculated into 5 ml of Penassay broth and incubated at 37°C overnight, at which time the titer of the culture had reached about 5×10^8 cells per ml. The culture was diluted 10^{-3}, and 0.2 ml of the diluted culture was added to 100 ml of Penassay broth together with 0.1 to 0.5 ml of 0.1% aqueous 4NPO. After the mixed culture was incubated on a reciprocal shaker at 37°C for 20 to 26 h, 0.1 ml of the culture was plated after appropriate dilutions on EMB-glucose-agar medium. Colonies appearing on this medium were replica-plated onto Davis glucose-agar with or without 40 μg of L-proline per ml.

Isolation of Pro$^-$ mutants by NTG treatment of Pro$^+$ strain. NTG treatment and penicillin screening methods were carried out by the procedures of Adelberg et al. (1) and Lederberg and Zinder (21). Pro$^+$ cells harvested from exponential-growth-phase culture (ca. 10^8 cells per ml) were suspended in TM buffer (pH 7.0) containing 300 μg of NTG per ml, and the mixture was incubated at 37°C for 30 min. Cells were harvested and suspended in Penassay broth (ca. 10^7 cells per ml), and the culture was incubated at 37°C overnight. Cells were collected by centrifugation and treated with 300 units of penicillin G potassium (Takeda Chemical Ind., Osaka, Japan) per ml in Davis-glucose at 37°C for 6 h. Pro$^-$ mutants formed were characterized by replica plating on Davis glucose-agar supplemented with or without 40 μg of L-proline per ml. Auxotrophic mutants other than *pro*$^-$ were characterized similarly.

Cross-feeding test. Cross-feeding testing was performed for syntrophism between *pro*$^-$ mutants of *E. coli* and *proA* and *proC* mutants of *S. typhimurium* LT2, which possess metabolic blocks in the pathway of proline biosynthesis, i.e., JM108 *proA*$^-$, which is unable to synthesize GSA (or its cyclized form, PC), and JM109 *proC*$^-$, which lacks the reducing enzyme for PC.

A streak across a Davis glucose-agar plate was made with a loopful of Pro$^-$ culture to be tested. Perpendicular to this streak, a loopful culture of JM108 or JM109 was spread so that the streaks were separated at one end by about 3 mm. After incubation at 37°C for 48 h, areas of growth of cells around the cross of the two streaks were checked. By this test, *proA*$^-$ and *proB*$^-$ could be distinguished from *proC*$^-$.

Assay for accumulation of biosynthetic intermediates of proline in Pro$^-$ mutants. Accumulation of PC in *proC*$^-$ cells was assayed by the method of Strecker (29) and Tristram and Thurston (33). To distinguish *proA*$^-$ from *proB*$^-$, accumulation of glutamohydroxamic acid was assayed by the method of Grossowicz et al. (15).

Infection with and elimination of F factors. The F13 (F *lac*$^+$ *proC*$^+$ *ade*$^+$) and F′ORF-206 (F *lac*$^+$ *proB*$^+$

proA$^+$) factors were transferred from appropriate F′ (donor) strains into F$^-$ (recipient) strains by mixing equal volumes of exponential-phase cultures of F′ (ca. 4 × 10^8 cells/ml) and F$^-$ (ca. 2 × 10^7 cells/ml) cultures, respectively, and the mixed culture was incubated at 37°C for 1 h. Elimination of F factors from male cells was carried out with acridine orange (16) or sodium dodecyl sulfate (32).

P1 transduction. The method of transduction described by Lenox (22) was generally followed. Recipient bacteria were grown in L broth to a concentration of 2 × 10^8 to 3 × 10^8 cells per ml. The culture was chilled and centrifuged, and the cells were harvested and suspended in 1/50 volume of L broth. The cell suspension was mixed with a few milliliters of P1 *vir* lysate containing 2.5 × 10^{-3} M $CaCl_2$ to give a multiplicity of infection of 0.1 to 0.3. This adsorption mixture was kept at 37°C for 20 min and then centrifuged. The pellet was washed with synthetic Davis medium without glucose and resuspended in the same medium, and portions were spread on suitable plates for selection of transductants.

Mating procedures. A 1-ml portion of JE1031 (Hfr-H) culture and 10 ml of Pro$^-$ F$^-$ recipient culture derived from W4573 (*str*^{r}) strain (cell titer of each exponential-phase culture, 2 × 10^8 to 3 × 10^8 cells per ml) were mixed and incubated without shaking at 37°C for 5 min. A 0.5-ml portion of the mixed culture was diluted without shearing into 50 ml of fresh Penassay broth prewarmed at 37°C, and the diluent was further incubated at the same temperature. Samples of 2 ml were removed from the mating mixture at certain intervals and transferred to sterilized tubes. The samples were violently agitated on an S-5 Mixer (Taiyo Corp.) for 30 s to separate mating partners. Samples were then immediately withdrawn for plating on selective media using soft agar plus SM at 100 μg/ml. Selection of *pro*$^+$*str*^{r}, *lac*$^+$*str*^{r}, and *gal*$^+$*str*^{r} recombinants were made on Davis glucose-agar plus SM, Davis lactose plus SM and L-proline, and Davis galactose plus SM and L-proline, respectively.

RESULTS

Selective isolation of proline-requiring mutants of *E. coli* K-12 by treatment with 4NPO. W4573 Pro$^+$ strain (inoculum size, 10^3 cells per ml) was incubated with 4NPO at various concentrations in Penassay broth at 37°C for 24 h. Survivors were analyzed for the proline growth requirement. Representative results are shown in Table 2. It was found that proline-requiring (Pro$^-$) mutants were isolated among survivors in very large numbers after treatment with 4NPO at sublethal concentrations, i.e., 2 or 3 μg/ml. Pro$^-$ cells thus obtained were stable after many generations, and spontaneous reverse mutation rates of those Pro$^-$ mutants to Pro$^+$ were 10^{-8} to 10^{-10}. Formation of auxotrophic mutants other than Pro$^-$ was not observed.

4NPO was found to act on *E. coli* K-12 and three derivatives, W3630, W3110 and JE177

TABLE 2. *Elective isolation of pro$^-$ mutants of E. coli K-12 W4573*

Expt no.	Inoculum size (cells/ml)	4NPO concn (μg/ml)	Viable counts (cells/ml)	No. of *pro*$^-$/no. of colonies tested	% *pro*$^-$
1	1.1 × 10^3	0	6.6 × 10^9	0/186	0
		1.0	6.7 × 10^9	0/256	0
		2.0	1.8 × 10^6	41/149	27.5
		3.0	1.4 × 10^4	102/130	78.5
2	1.8 × 10^3	0	4.6 × 10^9	0/193	0
		1.0	5.4 × 10^9	0/242	0
		2.0	2.5 × 10^4	201/231	87.0
		3.0	1.1 × 10^2	0/10	0
3	2.9 × 10^3	0	6.7 × 10^9	0/269	0
		1.0	6.0 × 10^9	0/234	0
		2.0	6.2 × 10^3	395/469	84.2
		3.0	1.3 × 10^3	34/113	30.1

(R100-1$^+$), although the frequency of Pro$^-$ mutants formed varied from strain to strain (Table 3). In every case, however, the isolation frequency of Pro$^-$ cells was maximum when Pro$^+$ cells were treated with sublethal concentrations of 4NPO. In further experiments, strain W4573 was mainly used.

Effects of inoculum size of Pro$^+$ cells, nutrient conditions of the medium, and incubation temperature were checked. Experiments with W4573 (Pro$^+$) cells showed that when 4NPO at 2.0 μg/ml in Penassay broth was used, apposite inoculum size of Pro$^+$ cells was 10^3 to 10^4 cells per ml. It was not possible to obtain Pro$^-$ mutants when the nutrient medium was substituted with a synthetic Davis glucose medium supplemented with 40 μg of L-proline per ml. With respect to incubation temperature, an optimum temperature for the 4NPO treatment was 37°C; at 4°C, formation of Pro$^-$ mutants was not observed. The results suggested that growth of the cells is essential for the action of 4NPO. It was further found that treatment of W3110 Pro$^+$ cells with ultraviolet irradiation or NTG prior to the addition of 4NPO increased the frequency of Pro$^-$ formation 3.8- or 6.9-fold, respectively.

Kinetics of the 4NPO treatment. An overnight culture (ca. 5 × 10^8 cells/ml) of W4573 Pro$^+$ was appropriately diluted in Penassay broth with or without 2.0 μg of 4NPO per ml to give cell concentrations of 10^4 cells/ml. The cultures were incubated with shaking at 37°C, and the survivors were analyzed at intervals. Representative results are shown in Fig. 1. In 4NPO broth, the titer of Pro$^+$ cells, after a lag of 2 h, rapidly decreased to 10^{-2} in 6 h. Then, the cell titer of the culture began to increase exponentially, when a substantial fraction of survivors

TABLE 3. *Effect of strains on the isolation of pro⁻ mutants by 4NPO treatment*

E. coli strain	4NPO concn (μg/ml)	% pro^{-a}							
W4573	2.0	59.9	0	0	27.5	69.4	87.0	84.2	0
	3.0	0	0	0	78.5	—	0	30.1	—
K-12	3.0	73.4	17.7	0	2.3	0	0		
	4.0	50.0	47.9	30.5	—	14.0	0		
	5.0	71.6	0	0	0	—	0		
	6.0	7.5							
W3630	1.0	18.5	8.9	38.5	0.9	17.9			
	2.0	59.3	53.2	—	100	—			
	3.0	—	0	0	93.9	1.7			
W3110	3.0	0	0	0	0	0	0		
	4.0	0	0	32.8	0	0	0		
JE177	1.0	42.9	0						
	1.5	34.5	—						
	2.0	57.8	100						
	2.5	99.5	100						
	3.0	—	11.6						

[a] Two to eight experiments were carried out using each strain. Each culture contained about 10^4 to 10^8 cells per ml; the number of colonies tested in each experiment was about 200. Results are expressed as (number of *pro* mutants)/(number of colonies tested) × 100.

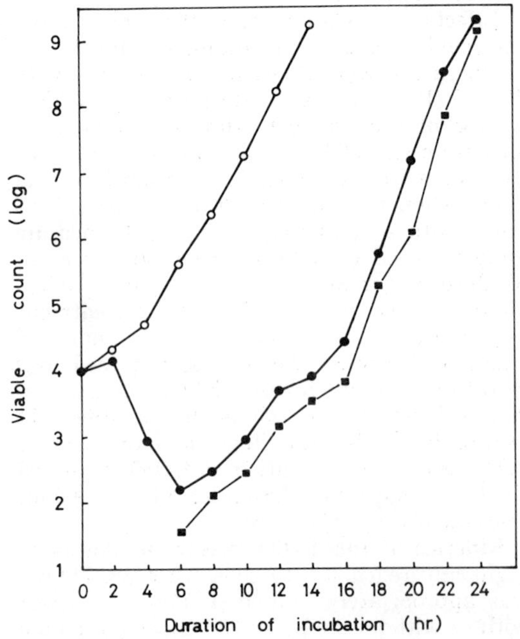

FIG. 1. *Kinetics of 4NPO treatment of W4573 pro⁺. An overnight culture (ca. 5 × 10^8 cells/ml) of W4573 pro⁺ was appropriately diluted in Penassay broth with or without 2.0 μg of 4NPO per ml to give cell concentrations of 10^4 cells/ml. The cultures were incubated with shaking at 37°C, and plating with suitable dilutions at intervals was on EMB-glucose-agar. Colonies were replica plated onto Davis glucose-agar with or without L-proline (40 μg/ml) to examine the frequency of pro⁻ cells. Symbols: ○, viable count without 4NPO; ●, viable count with 4NPO; ■, viable count of pro⁻ cells formed in the culture with 4NPO.*

was found to be Pro⁻ cells. Frequencies of Pro⁻ cells after 2, 6, 12, and 18 h of incubation were 0, 29, 31.3, and 31.7%, respectively. In broth without 4NPO, Pro⁺ cells began to grow exponentially immediately after incubation started; Pro⁻ cells were not isolated among survivors.

Biochemical characterization of Pro⁻ mutants. It has been reported that in enteric bacteria, proline is synthesized from glutamic acid via the following pathways, governed by three *pro* genes, *proA*, *proB*, and *proC* (4, 5, 6, 29, 30, 35): Glu → GP → GSA → PC → proline.

To determine which step of proline biosynthesis is blocked in proline-requiring mutants isolated after the 4NPO treatment, the growth response of 58 Pro⁻ clones obtained independently by 4NPO treatment of W4573 Pro⁺ to Glu, PC, proline, hydroxyproline, ornithine, arginine, and α-ketoglutaric acid in Davis glucose medium was first tested. All Pro⁻ mutants tested could grow in the presence of either PC or proline but not by other supplements. The result indicated that those Pro⁻ mutants have a metabolic block(s) between Glu and GSA.

Second, further characterization of Pro⁻ mutants as either those having metabolic block between Glu and Gp or GP and GSA was carried out by examining possible accumulation of GP identified as γ-glutamohydroxamic acid.

The Pro⁻ mutants were classified into two types, i.e., those that are capable of synthesizing GP and those that are not (Fig. 2a).

Examination of possible accumulation of PC in Pro⁻ mutants was also carried out (Fig. 2b). As expected, accumulation of PC was not observed in ten Pro⁻ clones tested as in W4573 Pro⁺.

Thirdly, the syntrophism test of 58 Pro⁻ mutants and authentic *proA* and *proC* strains of *S. typhimurium*, JM108 and JM109, was carried out. All the mutants were cross-fed not by JM109 *proA*⁻ but by JM109 *proC*⁻. The result further supported the previous observation that the Pro⁻ mutants tested cannot synthesize GSA or PC and may be genetically *proA* or *proB*.

The results, together with those obtained with Pro⁻ mutants isolated after treatment of W4573 *Pro*⁺ cells with NTG, are summarized in Table 4. A remarkable difference existed between the results obtained by treatment with 4NPO and NTG; whereas the NTG treatment led to isolation of all three types of *pro*⁻ mutants, *A*, *B*, and *C*, the treatment with 4NPO specifically afforded either *proA* and/or *proB* but never *proC*.

Genetic characterization of Pro⁻ mutants. As discussed above, three *pro* genes, *A*, *B*, and *C*, have been genetically identified with respect to proline biosynthesis in *E. coli* (7–10, 31). Moreover, it has been suggested that *proA* and *proB* genes correspond to biosynthetic pathways prior to GSA, and that *proC* is the structural gene for PC reductase. Chromosomal

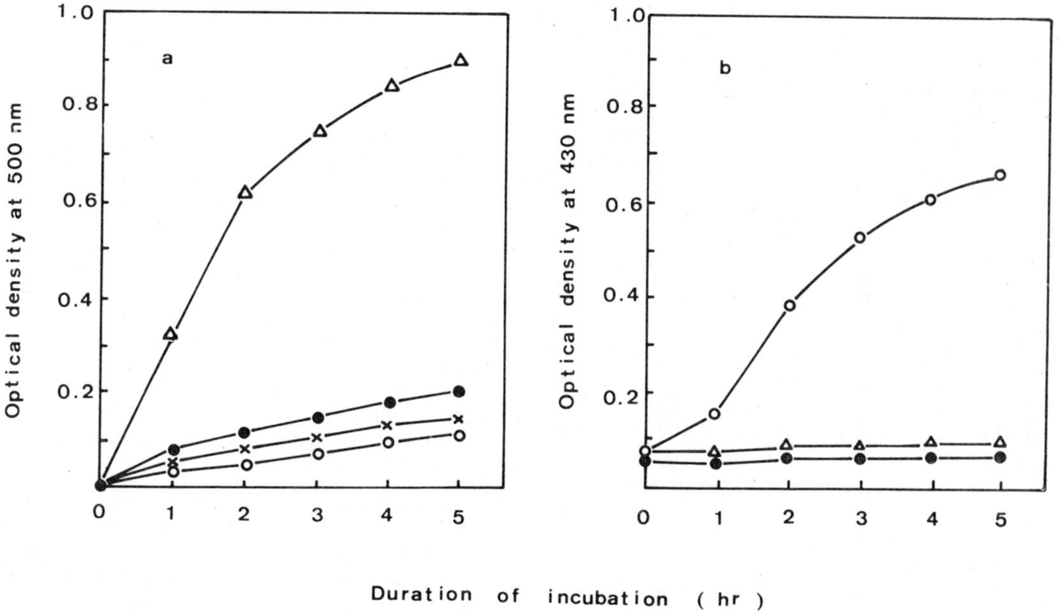

FIG. 2. *Accumulation of (a) GP and (b) PC. For procedure, see Materials and Methods. (a) Incubation was initiated by the addition of* L*-Glu and hydroxylamine into Pro⁻ or Pro⁺ cell suspensions. Symbols:* ●, *W4573 pro⁺;* △, *JE2133 pro⁻ (4NPO);* ×, *KE113 pro⁻ (4NPO);* ○, *KE114 pro⁻ (NTG). (b) Incubation was initiated by the addition of* L*-Glu into Pro⁻ and Pro⁺ cells suspensions. Symnbols as in (a).*

TABLE 4. *Classification of pro⁻ mutants by biochemical analysis*

Lacking steps in proline biosynthesis	No. of *pro*⁻ (4NPO treatment)		No. of *pro*⁻ (NTG treatment)	
	By syntrophism	By accumulation of intermediates	By syntrophism	By accumulation of intermediates
Glu → GP	58 (100%)	2 (20%)	27 (84%)	2 (25%)
GP → GSA		8 (80%)		5 (63%)
PC → proline	0 (0%)	0 (0%)	5 (16%)	1 (12%)
Total no. of clones examined	58	10	32	8

mapping of *pro* genes of proline-requiring mutants obtained by 4NPO treatment was then carried out to correlate without ambiguity proline loci and biosynthetic processes for proline in *E. coli*.

(i) F-duction of *pro* gene. For F-duction experiments, strains W3747 harboring F13 (F lac^+ $proC^+$ ade^+) (18) and χ646 harboring F′ORF-206 (F lac^+ $proB^+$ $proA^+$) (11) were used as F′ strains. Cultures (ca. 2×10^8 cells per ml) of W3747 ($F13^+$) and Pro^- Lac^- mutants in the exponential phase were mixed in a ratio of 10:1. After incubation at 37°C for 1 h, the mixture was plated on EMB-lactose-agar plus 100 μg of SM per ml, where only recipient bacteria could grow. Lac^+Str^r colonies grown on the plate were picked at random from EMB-lactose-agar and replica plated on Davis glucose-agar. When the Pro^- mutant KE114 obtained by the NTG treatment and characterized as having the metabolic block between PC and proline was used as recipient, all Lac^+Str^r F-ductants formed were Pro^+. When the Pro^- mutant JE2133 or KE113 obtained by the 4NPO treatment and characterized as having the block between GP and GSA or Glu and GP, respectively, was used as recipient, all Lac^+Str^r F-ductants were Pro^-. F-duction experiments with χ646 (F lac^+ $proB^+$ $proA^+$) as F′ strain further indicated that Pro^+ F-ductants were formed by the cross of χ646 with Pro^- mutants JE2133, KE113, and KE125 (which possess the same metabolic block as JE2133), as recipient but not with KE114. The result indicated that mutation sites of Pro^- mutants isolated after 4NPO treatment are not located on F13 but are on F′ORF-206.

(ii) Interrupted-mating experiments. Preliminary experiments of the cross of JE1031 (HfrH) as donor and JE2265 (pro^- $ara\text{-}2^-$ *tonB* *tsx* $lac\text{-}85^-$ $gal\text{-}2^-$ str^r), which was obtained by 4NPO treatment and has the metabolic block between GP and GSA, suggested that the location of the *pro* gene is between *tonB* and *lac*. Interrupted-mating experiments were carried out to determine the chromosomal location of *pro* (Glu → GP) and *pro* (Gp → PCA) genes. Figure 3 shows the kinetics of recombinant formation of interrupted mating of JE1031 (HfrH *pro* (Glu → GP) and *pro* (GP → PC) genes. GP] $lac\text{-}85^-$ $gal\text{-}2^-$ str^r). Average interlocus distance between *pro* (Glu → GP) and *lac-85* was 3.4 min, and the distance between *pro* and *gal-2* was 6.3 min. In the same manner, interrupted mating of JE1031 HfrH and JE2133 pro^- (GP → GSA) was carried out. The result indicated that the average distance between *pro* (GP → GSA) and *lac-85* was 5.3 min. This evidence indicates that the interlocus distance between *pro* (GP → GSA) and *pro* (Glu → GP)

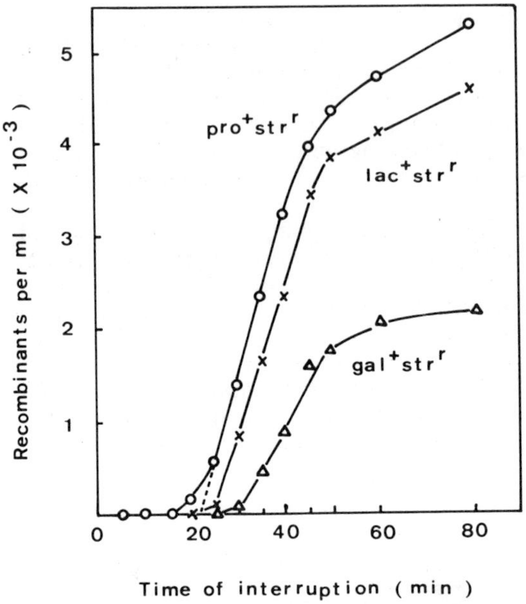

FIG. 3. *Kinetics of recombinant formation in an interrupted-mating cross of JE1031 HfrH and KE113 pro^- (Glu → GP). Cultures in the exponential growth phase of JE1031 and KE113 were mixed at a ratio of 1:10 and incubated without shaking at 37°C for 5 min. Mixed cultures were diluted 10^{-2} without shearing into fresh Penassay broth prewarmed at 37°C, and the diluent was further incubated. Samples removed from the mating mixture at certain intervals were violently agitated on a mixer for 30 s. After suitable dilutions, pro^+ str^r, lac^+str^r, and gal^+str^r recombinants were selected on Davis glucose-agar plus SM at 100 μg/ml, Davis lactose-agar plus SM and L-proline, and Davis galactose-agar plus SM and L-proline, respectively.*

is about 1.9 min, and the gene order of loci involving three *pro* is *ara*, *tonB*, *pro* (GP → GSA), *pro* (Glu → GP), *lac*, *pro* (PC → proline), *tsx*, and *gal*. It is concluded that *pro* (GP → GSA) and *pro* (Glu → GP) correspond to *proA* and *proB*, respectively, in the genetic map of *E. coli* by Taylor and Trotter (31). Transduction experiments with phage P1 *vir* further revealed a close linkage between *proA* and *proB* loci the number of transductants between $proA^-$ and $proB^-$ were consistently smaller (one-fifth to one-tenth) than those of transductants between *proA* or *proB* and *proC* or with wild type (data not shown). Frequencies of cotransduction between *proA1* or *proB3* or *lac-85* mutations in JE2133 or KE113 were shown to be less than 0.21 and 0.40%, respectively.

DISCUSSION

The results showed that 4NPO, which is known to exhibit little biological activity, can act on *E. coli* K-12 Pro^+ strains, leading to

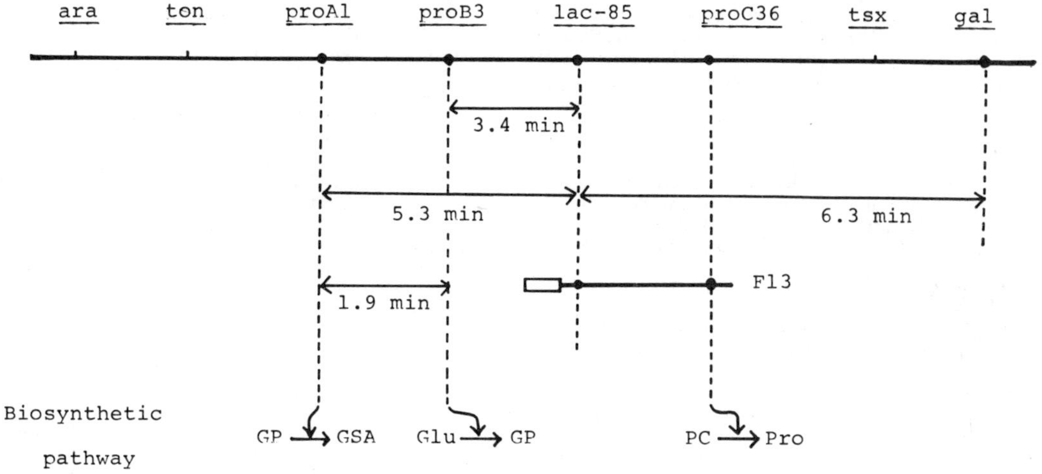

FIG. 4. *Correlation between loci and processes of the biosynthetic pathway of proline. Results are from the interrupted-matings crosses of JE1031 HfrH × KE113 F⁻ proB⁻ (Glu → GP) and JE1031 × JE2133 F⁻ proA⁻ (GP → GSA) and from F-duction of proC gene from W3747 F13⁺ to KE114 proC⁻ (PC → proline).*

highly efficient, selective isolation of Pro^- mutants. It was also shown that isolation of Pro^- mutants was highest when a sublethal concentration of 4NPO in Penassay broth was used (Tables 2 and 3). Kinetic studies of the 4NPO treatment of W4573 Pro^+ (Fig. 1) showed that after a short lag time, the titer of Pro^+ cells quickly decreased 10^{-2} to 10^{-3}. Then the cell titer began to again increase exponentially; Pro^- mutants appeared among survivors, and their cell titer increased thereafter. The results suggest that the agent might have a selective affinity toward Pro^+ and Pro^- cells; i.e., the agent is more toxic for Pro^+ than for Pro^-.

Biochemical characterization of Pro^- mutants thus formed indicated that all the Pro^- mutants lack the biosynthetic pathway of proline from Glu to GP and/or from GP to GSA. Pro^- mutants that have the metabolic block between PC and Pro were not found among the survivors. On the other hand, Pro^- mutants obtained by treatment with NTG could be classified into all three types of mutants (Fig. 2 and Table 4). This observation indicates that the specific action of 4NPO on Pro^+ cells is apparently distinct from the action of NTG.

Three genes, *proA*, *proB*, and *proC*, have been mapped close to *lac* on the chromosome of *E. coli* (7–10, 31). However, the correlation of *proA* and *proB* with the biosynthetic pathway of proline has not been completely settled. Results of F-duction and interrupted-mating experiments (Fig. 3 and 4) led us to the following conclusions. Pro^- mutants obtained after 4NPO treatment are *proA* (or *pro-1*) and/or *proB* (or *pro-2*) (but not *proC*) by the system of Taylor and Trotter (31) or of Curtiss (10). *proA*⁻ and *proB*⁻ genes have the metabolic block between GP and GSA and between Glu and GP, respectively. The correlation of three *pro* genes and their functions in the biosynthesis of proline from glutamic acid can therefore be summarized as Glu $\xrightarrow{proB}$ GP $\xrightarrow{proA}$ GSA $\xrightarrow[\text{dehydration}]{\text{nonenzymatic}}$ PC $\xrightarrow{proC}$ proline.

The data in Table 3 suggested that there was some strain effect on the efficiency of the action of 4NPO. It was further observed that the frequency of Pro^- cells isolated after 4NPO treatment fluctuated with every strain used. Pretreatment of bacteria with UV light or NTG prior to treatment with 4NPO apparently increased the frequency of formation of Pro^- mutants. These results, together with those of kinetic experiments, lead us to suggest that the mechanism of the specific action of 4NPO may be the selection of *proA*⁻ and *proB*⁻ cells that arose spontaneously in the Pro^+ culture. Further results on the metabolism of 4NPO and possible mechanisms of the specific action of 4NPO are dealt with in the accompanying paper (19).

ACKNOWLEDGMENTS

We are deeply indebted to Y. Hirota of the National Institute of Genetics, Mishima, Japan, for his encouragement and valuable advice in beginning the present investigation and Y. Sugino of the Faculty of Science, Osaka University, Osaka, Japan, for his valuable discussions. Our thanks are due to Y. Hirota, Y. Sugino, R. Curtiss III, University of Alabama, Birmingham, Ala., and T. Miyake, Keio University, Tokyo, Japan, for supplying bacterial strains.

This investigation was supported by a Grant-in-Aid for Scientific Research from the Ministry of Education, Science and Culture, Japanese government, and a grant from Kaisei-Kai Scientific Foundation, Tokyo.

LITERATURE CITED

1. **Adelberg, E. A., M. Mandel, and G. Chein Ching Chen.** 1965. Optimal conditions for mutagenesis by N-methyl-N'-nitro-N-nitrosoguanidine in *Escherichia coli* K12. Biochem. Biophys. Res. Commun. **18**:788–795.
2. **Albert, A.** 1951. The acridines, p. 251–280. Edward Arnold & Co., London.
3. **Araki, M., C. Koga, and Y. Kawazoe.** 1971. Carcinogenicity of 4-nitroquinoline 1-oxide analogs: pyridine series. Gann **62**:325–327.
4. **Baich, A.** 1969. Proline synthesis in *Escherichia coli*: a proline-inhibitable glutamic acid kinase. Biochim. Biophys. Acta **192**:462–467.
5. **Baich, A.** 1971. The biosynthesis of proline in *Escherichia coli*: phosphate-dependent glutamate γ-semialdehyde dehydrogenase (NADP), the second enzyme in the pathway. Biochim. Biophys. Acta **44**:129–134.
6. **Baich, A., and D. J. Pierson.** 1965. Control of proline biosynthesis in *Escherichia coli*. Biochim. Biophys. Acta **104**:397–404.
7. **Berg, C. M., and J. J. Rossi.** 1974. Proline excretion and indirect suppression in *Escherichia coli* and *Salmonella typhimurium*. J. Bacteriol. **118**:928–939.
8. **Broda, P.** 1974. Modified map positions for *lac* and the *pro* markers in *Escherichia coli* K-12. J. Bacteriol. **117**:747–752.
9. **Condamine, H.** 1971. Mutants des voies de biosynthese et de degradation de la proline chez *E. coli* K12. Ann. Inst. Pasteur Paris **120**:9–22.
10. **Curtiss, R., III.** 1965. Chromosomal aberations associated with mutations to bacteriophage resistance in *Escherichia coli*. J. Bacteriol. **89**:28–40.
11. **Curtiss, R., III, L. J. Charamella, D. R. Stallions, and J. A. Mays.** 1968. Parental functions during conjugation in *Escherichia coli* K-12. Bacteriol. Rev. **32**:320–348.
12. **Davis, B. D., and E. S. Mingloli.** 1950. Mutants of *Escherichia coli* requiring methionine or vitamin B12. J. Bacteriol. **60**:17–28.
13. **Endo, H., M. Ishizawa, and T. Kamiya.** 1963. Induction of bacteriophage formation in lysogenic bacteria by a potent carcinogen, 4-nitroquinoline 1-oxide, and its derivatives. Nature (London) **198**:195–196.
14. **Endo, H., T. Ono, and T. Sugimura.** 1971. Chemistry and biological actions of 4-nitroquinoline 1-oxide. Recent Results Cancer Res. **34**:1–98.
15. **Grossowicz, N., E. Wainfan, E. Borek, and H. Waelsch.** 1950. The enzymatic formation of hydroxamic acids from glutamine and asparagine. J. Biol. Chem. 187:111–125.
16. **Hirota, Y.** 1960. The effect of acridine dyes on mating type factors in *Escherichia coli*. Proc. Natl. Acad. Sci. U.S.A. **46**:57–64.
17. **Hirota, Y., M. Inuzuka, and M. Tomoeda.** 1966. Elective selection of proline-requiring mutants. J. Bacteriol. **91**:2392.
18. **Hirota, Y., and P. H. A. Sneath.** 1961. F' and F-mediated transduction in *Escherichia coli* K-12. Jpn. J. Genet. **36**:307–318.
19. **Inuzuka, M., H. Toyama, H. Miyano, and M. Tomoeda.** 1976. Specific action of 4-nitropyridine 1-oxide on *Escherichia coli* K-12 Pro^+ strains leading to the isolation of proline-requiring mutants: mechanism of action of 4-nitropyridine 1-oxide. Antimicrobial Agents Chemother. **10**:333–343.
20. **Lederberg, J.** 1950. Isolation and characterization of biochemical mutants of bacteria. Methods Med. Res. **3**:5–22.
21. **Lederberg, J., and N. Zinder.** 1948. Concentration of biochemical mutants of bacteria with penicillin. J. Am. Chem. Soc. **70**:4267–4268.
22. **Lenox, E. S.** 1955. Transduction of linked genetic characters of the host by bacteriophage P1. Virology **1**:190–206.
23. **Lerman, L. S.** 1964. Acridine mutagens and DNA structure. J. Cell. Comp. Physiol. **64**(Suppl. 1):1–18.
24. **Mckay, A. F., and G. G. Wright.** 1947. Preparation and properties of N-methyl-N-nitroguanidine. J. Am. Chem. Soc. **69**:3028–3030.
25. **Miyake, T., and M. Demerec.** 1960. Proline mutants of *Salmonella typhimurium*. Genetics **45**:754–762.
26. **Nakahara, W., F. Fukuoka, and T. Sugimura.** 1957. Carcinogenic action of 4-nitroquinoline-N-oxide. Gann **48**:129–137.
27. **Ochiai, E., M. Ishikawa, and K. Arima.** 1943. Nitration of pyridine N-oxide and its analogues. J. Pharm. Soc. Japan **63**:79.
28. **Okabayashi, T., M. Ide, A. Yoshimoto, and M. Otsubo.** 1965. Mutagenic activity of 4-nitroquinoline 1-oxide and 4-hydroxyaminoquinoline 1-oxide on bacteria. Chem. Pharm. Bull. **13**:610–611.
29. **Strecker, H. J.** 1957. The interconversion of glutamic acid and proline. L. The formation of Δ^1-pyrroline-5-carboxylic acid from glutamic acid in *Escherichia coli*. J. Biol. Chem. **225**:825–834.
30. **Strecker, H. J.** 1962. The interconversion of glutamic acid proline. V. The reduction of Δ^1-pyrroline-5-carboxylic acid to proline. J. Biol. Chem. **237**:2255–2260.
31. **Taylor, A. L., and C. D. Trotter.** 1972. Linkage map of *Escherichia coli* strain K-12. Bacteriol. Rev. **34**:155–175.
32. **Tomoeda, M., M. Inuzuka, N. Kubo, and S. Nakamura.** 1968. Effective elimination of drug resistance and sex factors in *Escherichia coli* by sodium dodecyl sulfate. J. Bacteriol. **95**:1078–1089.
33. **Tristram, H., and C. F. Thurston.** 1966. Control of proline biosynthesis by proline and proline analogues. Nature (London) **212**:74–75.
34. **Vogel, H. J., and B. D. Davis.** 1952. Glutamic γ-semialdehyde and Δ^1-pyrroline-5-carboxylic acid, intermediates in the biosynthesis of proline. J. Am. Chem. Soc. **74**:109–112.
35. **Yoshinaga, H., Y. Takeda, and S. Okumura.** 1967. Glutamate kinase activity in *Brevibacterium flavum*: relationship between L-proline and L-glutamine. Biochem. Biophys. Res. Commun. **27**:143–149.

Antimicrobial Agents and Chemotherapy, Aug. 1976, p. 333-343 Vol. 10, No. 2

Printed in U.S.A.

Specific Action of 4-Nitropyridine 1-Oxide on *Escherichia coli* K-12 Pro$^+$ Strains Leading to the Isolation of Proline-Requiring Mutants: Mechanism of Action of 4-Nitropyridine 1-Oxide

MANABU INUZUKA,[1]* HIROMI TOYAMA, HIROSHI MIYANO, AND MUNEMITSU TOMOEDA[2]

Department of Chemistry, Faculty of Pharmaceutical Sciences, Kanazawa University, Takara-machi, Kanazawa 920, Japan

Received for publication 26 March 1976

Possible mechanisms involved in the action of 4-nitropyridine 1-oxide (4NPO) on *Escherichia coli* K-12 *pro*$^+$ cells in Penassay broth leading to the selective isolation of *proA*$^-$ and/or *proB*$^-$ mutants but not *proC*$^-$ mutant were studied. Reconstruction experiments between *pro*$^+$ and *pro*$^-$ cells, together with experiments on the bactericidal action of 4NPO on *pro*$^+$ and *pro*$^-$ cells, indicated that 4NPO is more toxic for *pro*$^+$ and *proC*$^-$ cells than for *proA*$^-$ and *proB*$^-$ cells. These results, coupled with data indicating little mutagenicity of 4NPO on *E. coli* cells, led us to conclude that the selection of *proA*$^-$ and/or *proB*$^-$ cells that arose spontaneously in the *pro*$^+$ culture is a possible mechanism for the action of 4NPO. Examination of 4NPO sensitivity of *pro*$^+$ transductants derived from *proA*$^-$ and *proB*$^-$ cells with P1 *vir* phage and *pro*$^+$ cells as donor and of *pro*$^+$ spontaneous revertants derived from those *pro*$^-$ cells suggested that 4NPO-sensitive gene(s) should be on, or very close to, the *proA* and *proB* loci and that both products of *proA* and *proB* genes may be involved in the sensitivity of bacteria to 4NPO. The fact that the 4NPO-sensitive allele is dominant over the 4NPO-resistant allele further indicated the possible correlation between gene products of *proA* and *proB* and the 4NPO sensitivity of bacteria. Experiments on metabolic conversion of 4NPO with bacterial cells proved that the major metabolic pathway of the agent is reduction to (possibly via 4-nitroso-) 4-hydroxylamino- and 4-amino-pyridine 1-oxides, and then to 4-aminopyridine. Investigation of the effect of structural modification of 4NPO on the elective selection of Pro$^-$ mutants in Pro$^+$ culture further suggested that the structural feature indispensable for the action of the agent is the hydroxyl-amino or its more oxidized state at the 4 position and the *N*-oxide moiety at the 1 position on the pyridine skeleton. Action of 4NPO in minimal medium was found to be bacteriostatic on *pro*$^+$ cells but not on *pro*$^-$ cells, leading to the formation of long nonseptate multinucleate filament cells on *pro*$^+$ cells. Possible biochemical mechanisms of the selective toxicity of 4NPO for *pro*$^+$ and *pro*$^-$ cells are discussed.

We have found that 4-nitropyridine 1-oxide (4NPO) can act on *Escherichia coli* K-12 Pro$^+$ strains, leading to highly efficient isolation of proline-requiring (Pro$^-$) mutants (7, 8). All Pro$^-$ mutants thus isolated have been characterized as those defective in the pathway of proline biosynthesis from glutamic acid (Glu) to glutamic γ-semialdehyde (GSA), determined genetically by *pro* genes *A* and *B*; Pro$^-$ mutants that possess the metabolic block between Δ^1-pyrroline 5-carboxylic acid (PC), the cyclized product of GSA, and proline, determined genetically by *pro* gene *C*, were never isolated by this method. Further genetic study of *pro* mutants *A* and *B* obtained by 4NPO treatment together with *proC* mutants isolated by treatment with *N*-methyl-*N'*-nitro-*N*-nitrosoguanidine (NTG) have provided evidence that *proA*, *proB*, and *proC* genes code for the steps between glutamyl γ-phosphate (GP) and GSA, Glu and GP, and PC and proline, respectively.

We describe in this paper possible mechanisms involved in the phenomenon. Much of the effect of the agent was proved to be selective; 4NPO is more toxic for *pro*$^+$ or *proC*$^-$ cells than for *proA*$^-$ or *proB*$^-$ cells in 4NPO broth

[1] Present address: Department of Biology, University of California, San Diego, La Jolla, CA 92093.

[2] Present address: Research and Development Division, Eisai Co., 4 Koishikawa, Bunkyo 112, Tokyo, Japan.

and selects *proA*⁻ or *proB*⁻ mutants in the culture. As 4NPO showed little mutagenicity on Pro^+ cells, spontaneous mutation of Pro^+ cells to Pro^- (possibly all the *pro* mutants *A*, *B*, and *C*) cells and selection of *pro*⁻ *A* and/or *B* mutants thus formed might be the major driving force in the action of 4NPO. Evidence indicating dominance of 4NPO susceptibility over 4NPO resistance of bacteria was also obtained. Besides 4NPO, 4-nitrosopyridine 1-oxide (4NSPO) and 4-hydroxylaminopyridine 1-oxide (4HAPO) but not 4-aminopyridine 1-oxide (4APO) were found to be effective for the selection of Pro^- mutants in the Pro^+ culture. Structural elucidation of metabolic intermediates of 4NPO in the bacterial culture indicated that 4NPO is metabolized, possibly via 4NSPO, to 4HAPO and 4APO. This evidence suggests 4HAPO as a possible proximate compound in the action of 4NPO.

MATERIALS AND METHODS

Bacterial strains. The bacterial strains used were *E. coli* K-12 derivatives (Table 1). Pro^- mutants were isolated after treatment of appropriate Pro^+ strains with 4NPO or NTG. Strain W4573 (Pro^+) was kindly supplied by Y. Hirota, Osaka University, Osaka, Japan. The phage strain used for transduction experiments was P1 *vir*.

Materials and media. All the pyridine and quinoline derivatives used in this investigation, i.e., 4NPO (13), 4NSPO (16), 4HAPO (16), 4APO (15), 2NPO (2), 4,4′-azoxypyridine 1,1′-dioxide (15), 4,4′-azopyridine 1,1′ dioxide (AZO) (15), pyridine 1-oxide (PO) (13), 4-nitropyridine (4NP) (5), 4-nitrolutidine 1-oxide (4NLO), (4) 4-nitroquinoline 1-oxide (4NQO) (14) and 4-hydroxylaminoquinoline 1-oxide (4HAQO) (17) (Fig. 1), were synthesized in our laboratory according to the literature.

For 4NPO treatment, Penassay broth (Difco) was used as medium. Media for other experiments have been described previously (8).

Treatment of Pro^+ strains with 4NPO and its derivatives. An overnight culture of Pro^+ strain in Penassay broth was diluted to 10^3 cells/ml in 100 ml of the same broth containing 2 μg of 4NPO per ml or appropriate sublethal concentrations of 4NPO derivatives. After the culture was incubated at 37°C for 20 to 26 h, survivors were plated on EMB/glucose-agar medium, and the colonies grown on the plate were analyzed for proline requirement.

Metabolism of 4NPO by Pro^+ or Pro^- cells. Pro^+ or Pro^- cells were harvested from a 100-ml overnight culture of Davis minimal glucose broth supplemented with 40 μg of L-proline per ml. These cells

TABLE 1. *Bacterial strains of E. coli K-12 used*

Strain	Genetic characteristic[a]	Origin or source
W4573	F⁻ *ara-2*⁻ *lac-85*⁻ *gal-2*⁻ *mal-1*⁻ *mtl*⁻ *xyl-2*⁻	
JE2133[b]	As W4573, also *proA1*⁻	W4573
JE2147	As W4573, also *lac*⁺	W4573
JE2149	As JE2133, also *proA1*⁺ *lac*⁺	JE2133
JE2157	As JE2133, also *proA1*⁺	JE2133
KE113[b]	As W4573, also *proB3*⁻	W4573
KE114[c]	As W4573, also *proC36*⁻	W4573
KE115[c]	As W4573, also *proAB*⁻ *proC22*⁻	W4573
KE125[c]	As W4573, also *proB17*⁻	W4573
KE126[c]	As W4573, also *proA18*⁻	W4573
KE134[c]	As W4573, also *proC205*⁻	W4573
KE135[c]	As W4573, also *proC106*⁻	W4573
χ646[d]	F′ *proA*⁺ *proB*⁺ *lacY*⁺/*lacY*⁻	(1)
KE343[e]	As JE2133, also F′ *proA*⁺ *proB*⁺ *lacY*⁺/*proA1*⁻	JE2133 × χ646
KE344[f]	As JE2133	KE343
KE345[g]	As JE2133, also F′ *proA*⁻ *proB*⁺ *lacY*⁺/*proA1*⁻	KE343
JE2214	F⁻ *proAB*⁻	
JE1673	F⁻ *proC*⁻ *ara-2*⁻ *leu*⁻ *lac-2*⁻ *pur*⁻ *thi*⁻ *gal-2*⁻ *mtl*⁻ *mal*⁻ *str*ʳ	
AB1899NM	F⁻ *lon*⁻ *thr-1*⁻ *leu-6*⁻ *proA2*⁻ *his-4*⁻ *thi-1*⁻ *argE3*⁻ *ara-14*⁻ *lacY1*⁻ *galK2*⁻ *xyl-5*⁻ *mtl-1 tsx-33 strA31 sup-37*, nonmucoid	
W3110thy⁻	F⁻ *lp*ˢ *thy*⁻	

[a] Genetic symbols are those used by Taylor and Trotter (21). *proA*⁻ or *proB*⁻ that can grow in minimal medium containing PC but that has not been characterized as either *proA*⁻ or *proB*⁻ is herein tentatively designated *proAB*⁻.

[b] Isolated by 4NPO treatment of W4573 and characterized as *pro*⁻ (8).

[c] Isolated after treatment with NTG followed by penicillin screening and characterized as *pro*⁻ (8).

[d] Kindly supplied by R. Curtiss III (1).

[e] Derived from JE2133 by infection of F *proA*⁺ *proB*⁺ *lacY*⁺ factor with χ646 as the donor.

[f] Derived from KE343 by elimination of F′ factor by the treatment with acridine orange.

[g] Isolated by 4NPO treatment of KE343.

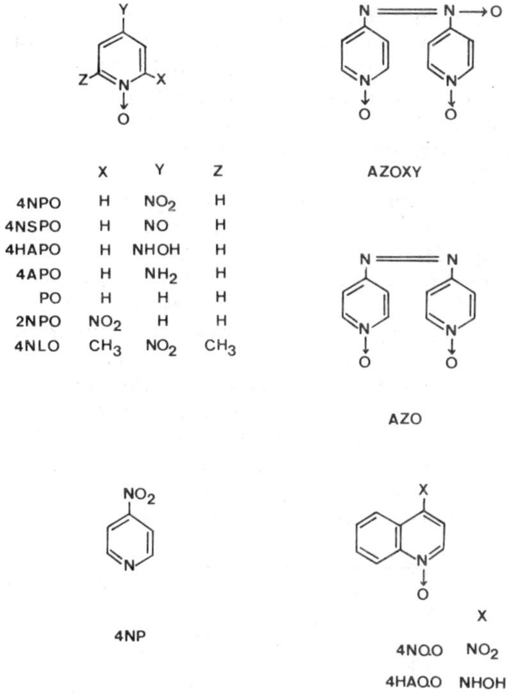

FIG. 1. *Structural features of 4-nitropyridine 1-oxide derivatives used.*

were suspended in 100 ml of Davis minimal glucose broth containing 40 μg of L-proline per ml and 8 μg of 4NPO per ml to give a cell concentration of 2×10^8 cells per ml. The suspension was incubated at 37°C; 2-ml samples were removed at intervals and quickly cooled to 0°C. Then an equivalent volume of ice-cold 10% trichloroacetic acid solution was added to these samples. The mixture was maintained at 0°C for 10 min, and then the ultraviolet spectra of supernatants obtained by centrifugation (3,000 rpm, 10 min) were measured with an Hitachi EPS-2U spectrophotometer using the uninoculated media as a reference solution.

Separation, purification, and identification of metabolites of 4NPO by Pro+ or Pro− cells. Pro+ or Pro− cells (ca. 15 g, wet weight) obtained from overnight culture in 1,000 ml of Davis minimal glucose broth containing 40 μg of L-proline per ml were suspended in 1,000 ml of the same broth. A 100-mg portion of 4NPO was added to the suspension, and the mixture was incubated at 37°C on a reciprocal shaker until the absorption maxima shifted to those of expected metabolites of 4NPO, i.e., 280 nm for 4HAPO, 273 nm for 4APO, and 261 nm for 4AP. The suspension was then cooled to 0°C, acidified with 12 N HCl, and centrifuged to separate cells and cellular debris. The supernatant fraction was concentrated to a small volume below 40°C under reduced pressure and was extracted with 99% ethanol. The extract was evaporated below 40°C under reduced pressure to give solid metabolites as the hydrochloric acid salt. If necessary, the crude product was chromatographed on silica gel with ether-methanol (1:1) as eluent. Metabolites thus obtained were converted to their corresponding picrates and recrystallized from water. The structures of metabolites were characterized by mixed melting point determination, elemental microanalysis, and comparison of ultraviolet and infrared spectra and R_f values of thin-layer chromatography with those of authentic specimens.

RESULTS

Reconstruction experiments between Pro+ and Pro− strains. To investigate the presence or absence of selective toxicity of 4NPO between Pro+ and Pro− cells, reconstruction experiments were carried out between JE2149 (*pro+ lac+*) and JE2133 (*proA− lac−*). Overnight cultures (ca. 5×10^8 cells/ml) of *pro+* and *pro−* strains were diluted in Penassay broth with and without 2 μg/ml of 4NPO to give cell concentration of about 10^3 cells/ml. Equal volumes of *pro+* and *pro−* cultures were mixed, the mixture was incubated at 37°C with shaking, and survivors were analyzed at intervals with *lac* as the distinguishing marker. The frequency of production of *pro− lac+* cells from *pro+ lac+* cells was also determined. Representative results are shown in Fig. 2. In the 4NPO medium, *pro−* cells began to grow after a lag of as long as 3 h, at a slower rate (generation time, ca. 42 min) than cells in broth without 4NPO (ca. 21 min). The viable count of *lac+* (originally *pro+*) cells, on the other hand, began to decrease after the same lag time and reached a minimum cell titer (10^{-2} of the inoculum) after 6 h. Then, the cell titer of survivors began to increase at a similar rate as that of *pro−* cells. The frequencies of *lac+ pro−* cells in the whole *lac+* cells after 5, 6, 8, 10, and 12 h of incubation were found to be 3.7, 37.5, 83.3, 75.9, and 66.5%, respectively. The results indicated that 4NPO exhibits higher toxicity toward *pro+* than *proA−* in the culture. This did not occur in the medium without 4NPO. Similar results were obtained with JE2157 *pro+ lac−* and JE2147 *proA− lac+*.

Sensitivity of *proA−*, *proB−*, *proC−* and *pro+* cells to 4NPO. Overnight cultures (ca. 5×10^8 cells/ml) of strains W4573 *pro+*, JE2133 *proA−*, KE113 *proB−* obtained by 4NPO treatment, and KE114 *proC−* isolated after NTG treatment were appropriately diluted in Penassay broth containing various concentrations of 4NPO to give cell titer of about 10^3 cells per ml. During incubation at 37°C for as long as 24 h, survivors were counted at certain intervals on EMB-glucose agar. Results are shown in Fig. 3. Sublethal concentrations of 4NPO toward *pro+* and *pro−* were 2.0 μg/ml for *pro+* and *proC−* and 4.0 to 5.0 μg/ml for *proA−* and *proB−*. Figure 4

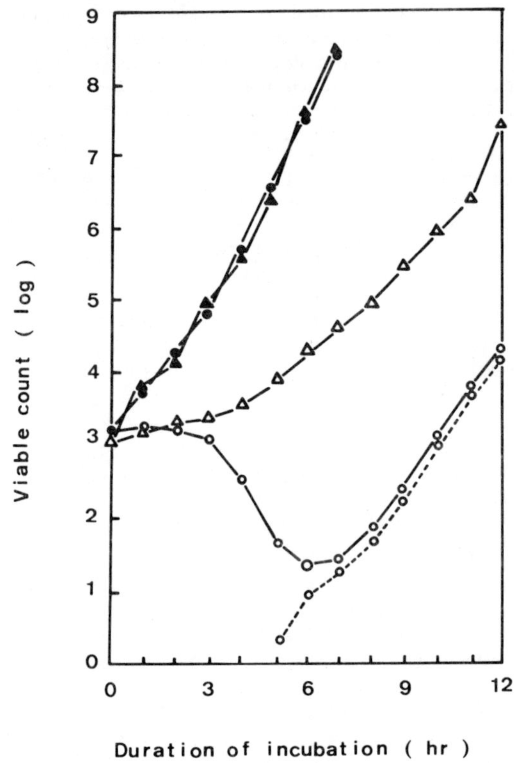

FIG. 2. *Reconstruction experiments between E. coli K12 JE2149 (pro⁺ lac⁺) and JE2133 (proA1⁻ lac-85⁻). Overnight cultures (ca. 5 × 10⁸ cells/ml) of pro⁺ and pro⁻ strains were diluted 2 × 10⁻⁶ in Penassay broth with or without 2.0 μg of 4NPO per ml. Equal volumes of pro⁺ (1.5 × 10³ cells/ml) and pro⁻ (1.6 × 10³ cells/ml) cultures were mixed and incubated at 37°C with shaking. Plating with appropriate dilutions at certain intervals was on EMB-lactose-agar. From 20 to 270 lac⁺ colonies were arbitrarily chosen and characterized as pro⁺ or pro⁻ by the replica-plating method. Symbols: ●, viable count of lac⁺ pro⁺ without 4NPO; ▲, viable count of lac⁻ pro⁻ without 4NPO; ○, viable count of lac⁺ pro⁺ plus lac⁺ pro⁻ with 4NPO; △, viable count of lac⁻ pro⁻ with 4NPO; ---○---, viable count of lac⁺ pro⁻ formed in 4NPO medium.*

shows the resulting kinetics for 4NPO treatment (2 μg/ml in Penassay broth) of *pro*⁺ and *pro*⁻ cells. 4NPO was found to be more toxic for *pro*⁺ and *proC*⁻ than for *proA*⁻ and *proB*⁻ cells. Namely, after 6 h of incubation, *proA*⁻ and *proB*⁻ cells showed about a 1,000-fold greater resistancy to 4NPO than *pro*⁺ and *proC*⁻ cells. 4NPO sensitivity of *proA*⁻, *proB*⁻, or *proAB*⁻ *proC*⁻ cells obtained by NTG treatment of W4573, KE125, or KE115 was further checked; these *pro*⁻ mutants were as resistant to 4NPO as *proA*⁻ and *proB*⁻ mutants isolated by 4NPO treatment. JE2214 *proAB*⁻ and JE1673 *proC*⁻, whose derivation was different than W4573, were resistant and sensitive to 4NPO, respectively. This evidence indicates that whatever the isolation method, *proA*⁻ and *proB*⁻ mutants are most resistant to 4NPO than *pro*⁺ mutants.

To examine 4NPO sensitivity patterns of auxotrophic mutants other than Pro⁻, Met⁻ Pro⁺, His⁻ Pro⁺, and Tyr⁻ Pro⁺ mutants obtained by NTG treatment of W4573 were inoculated into Penassay broth (100 ml) with and without 2.0 μg of 4NPO per ml and incubated at 37°C with shaking. Results indicated that these auxotrophs are as sensitive as W4573 *pro*⁺ and *proC*⁻ derived from W4573. This observation further supported selection of *proA*⁻ and/or *proB*⁻ in the *Pro*⁺ culture as a possible mechanism for the specific action of 4NPO.

Sensitivity to 4NPO of Pro⁺ revertants and

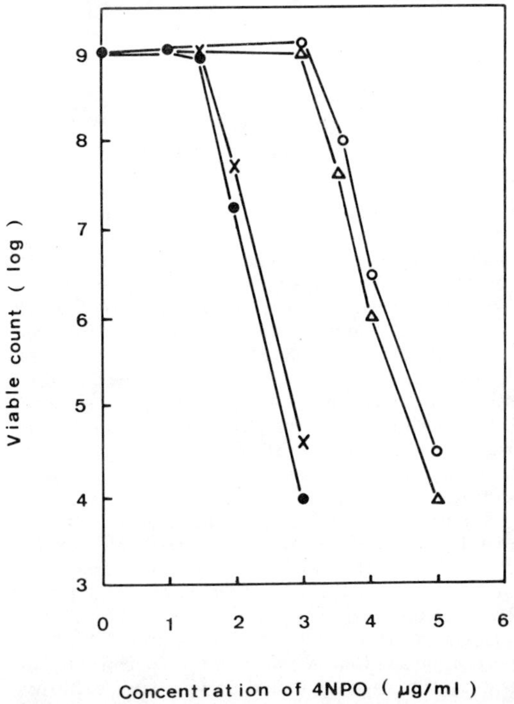

FIG. 3. *Lethal concentration of 4NPO on the viability pro⁺ and pro⁻ cells. Overnight cultures (ca. 5 × 10⁸ cells/ml) of pro⁺ and pro⁻ cells were appropriately diluted in Penassay broth (10 ml) containing 1.0 to 6.0 μg of 4NPO per ml to give a cell concentration of about 10³ cells/ml. After incubation at 37°C for 24 h with shaking, plating with suitable dilution was on EMB-glucose-agar. Symbols: ●, viable count of W4573 pro⁺; ○, viable count of JE2133 proA1⁻; △, viable count of KE113 proB3⁻; ×, viable count of KE114 proC36⁻.*

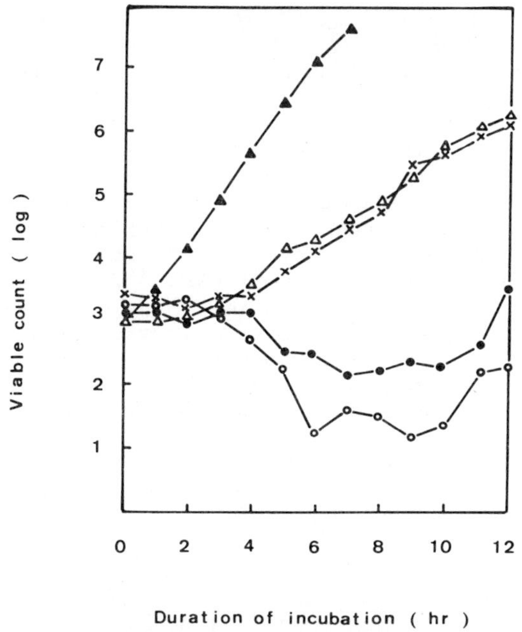

FIG. 4. *Sensitivity of pro+ and pro− cells to 4NPO. W4573 pro+, JE2133 proA1−, KE113 proB3−, and KE135 proC− cells (ca. 10^3 cells/ml) in Penassay broth (100 ml) with or without 2.0 μg of 4NPO per ml were incubated at 37°C with shaking. Symbols: ○, viable count of W4573 with 4NPO; △, JE2133 with 4NPO; ×, KE113 with 4NPO; ●, KE135 with 4NPO; ▲, pro+ and pro− cells tested without 4NPO.*

Pro+ transductants derived from various Pro− strains. To examine whether the observed higher sensitivity to 4NPO of Pro+ cells might be coded by *proA* and/or *proB* genes or some gene(s) linked very closely to these *pro* genes, Pro+ spontaneous revertants and Pro+ transductants were isolated from various Pro− strains, and their 4NPO sensitivity was checked. Spontaneous reverse mutation rates from Pro− to Pro+ were found to be 2×10^{-8} to 5×10^{-10}. Pro+ transductants were obtained with P1 *vir* as transducing phage and W4573 *pro+* as donor strain.

4NPO sensitivity of the Pro+ strains was examined as follows. An overnight culture of Pro+ or Pro− cells to be tested was inoculated with a cell titer of 10^3 cells per ml into Penassay broth containing 2.0 μg of 4NPO per ml. The culture was incubated at 37°C with shaking, and survivors were counted at certain intervals. Strains showing the same kinetics of growth as W4573 *pro+* were classified as 4NPO sensitive (4NPO^s^), and strains showing the same kinetics of growth of JE2133 *proA−* were classified as 4NPO resistant (4NPO^r^). Growth response of Pro+ and Pro− strains in Davis glucose minimal medium was also tested.

Results are summarized in Table 2. As expected, KE126 *proA−* and KE125 *proB−* derived from W4573 by NTG treatment were just as resistant to 4NPO as *proA−* and *proB−* strains obtained by 4NPO treatment. Pro+ spontaneous revertants derived from *pro−* strains obtained by NTG treatment, and which could grow in Davis-glucose minimal medium at a rate similar to that of W4573 *pro+*, were found to have recovered 4NPO sensitivity. All Pro+ transductants derived from these *pro−* strains were also found to be 4NPO sensitive. Many of the spontaneous Pro+ revertants derived from *proA−* and *proB−* strains obtained by 4NPO

TABLE 2. *4NPO sensitivity of spontaneous Pro+ revertants and Pro+ transductants derived from Pro− cells*

Strain	Isolation method[a]	Growth responses in D-glucose minimum medium[b]	4NPO sensitivity[c]
W4573 (*pro+*)		++	s
JE2133 (*proA−*)	4NPO	−	r
JE2133 *proA+*	Spont	++	s
		+	r
JE2133 *proA+*	P1 *vir*	++	s
KE113 (*proB−*)	4NPO	−	r
KE113 *proB+*	Spont	+	r
KE113 *proB+*	P1 *vir*	++	s
KE126 (*proA−*)	NTG	−	r
KE126 *proA+*	Spont	++	s
KE126 *proA+*	P1 *vir*	++	s
KE125 (*proB−*)	NTG	−	r
KE125 *proB+*	Spont	++	s
KE125 *proB+*	P1 *vir*	++	s
KE135 (*proC−*)	NTG	−	s
KE135 *proC+*	Spont	++	s
KE135 *proC+*	P1 *vir*	++	s

[a] 4NPO, NTG: isolated from W4573 by 4NPO and NTG treatments, respectivey, and characterized as *proA−*, *proB−*, and *proC−*, Spont: obtained as *pro+* by spontaneous reversion from each *pro−* strains. P1 *vir:* derived from each *pro−* strains by transuction with P1 *vir* and with W4573 as donor strain.

[b] Growth responses in D-glucose minimum medium was classified as follows: ++, same amount of growth as W4573 (*pro+*); +, less growth than original *pro+*; −, no growth.

[c] s, 4NPO-sensitive strain that shows the same kinetics of growth in 4NPO medium as the original W4573 (*pro+*); r, 4NPO-resistant strain that shows the same growth curve in 4NPO medium as JE2133 (*proA−*).

treatment had also recovered equal 4NPO sensitivity as Pro$^+$ and *proC*$^-$. These results indicated that the gene(s) determining the sensitivity to 4NPO (4NPO^s gene) of bacteria would be in the *proA* or *proB* loci or would be located so close to these *pro* genes that *pro* and 4NPO^s genes could be co-transduced by P1 *vir*.

Dominance of 4NPO sensitivity over 4NPO resistance of *pro* genes. To investigate the dominant or recessive character of *pro* genes for 4NPO sensitivity, the F′*proA*$^+$ *proB*$^+$ plasmid was transferred from χ646 to JE2133 *proA*$^-$, and 4NPO sensitivity of the resulting heterozygote *proA*$^-$/F′*proA*$^+$ *proB*$^+$ was checked. The heterozygote was found to show a similar sensitivity to 4NPO as W4573 *pro*$^+$ (Fig. 5). This F′ strain was then treated with acridine orange (6) or sodium dodecyl sulfate (22) to give F$^-$ *proA*$^-$; This F$^-$ had recovered resistance to 4NPO. Similar results were obtained with the heterozygotes of KE113 *proB*$^-$, KE125 *proB*$^-$, or KE126 *proA*$^-$ and F′ *proA*$^+$ *proB*$^+$. Furthermore, *proA*$^-$/F′ *proA*$^-$ *proB*$^+$ and *proB*$^-$/F′ *proA*$^+$ *proB*$^-$ cells derived from the above-mentioned heterozygotes by treatment with 4NPO also recovered the character of 4NPO resistance. The results revealed that the *4NPO*^{s} allele is dominant over the *4NPO*^{r} allele.

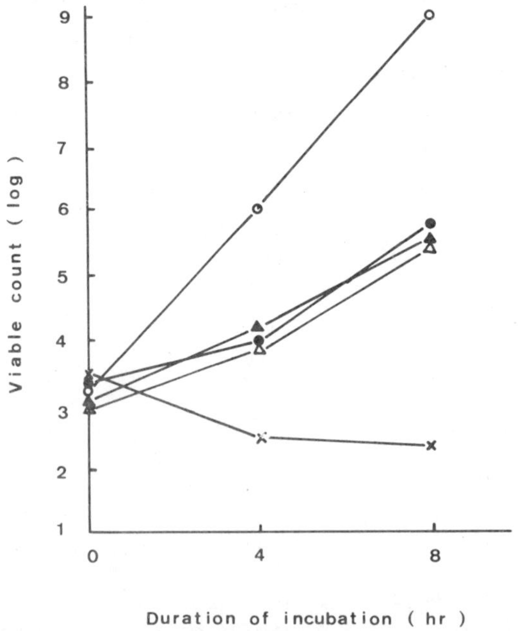

FIG. 5. *Dominance of sensitivity over resistance to 4NPO of pro*$^+$ *and pro*$^-$ *strains. JE2133 proA1*$^-$*, its heterozygote KE343 proA1*$^-$*/F′proA*$^+$ *proB*$^+$*, KE344 proA1*$^-$ *obtained from KE343 by elimination of F plasmid with acridine orange, and KE345 proA1*$^-$*/F′proA*$^-$ *proB*$^+$ *derived from KE343 by the 4NPO treatment were used. They were incubated in Penassay broth (10 ml) with or without 2.0 μg of 4NPO per ml at 37°C with shaking. Symbols:* ●*, viable count of JE2133 with 4NPO;* ×*, viable count of KE343 with 4NPO;* ▲*, viable count of KE344 with 4NPO;* △*, viable count of KE345 with 4NPO;* ○*, viable count of cells being tested without 4NPO.*

Mutagenicity of 4NPO. With respect to possible mechanisms for the action of 4NPO, the mutagenic action of 4NPO on strain W4573 from recessive valine sensitivity (Val^s) to dominant valine resistance (Val^r) (20) was checked. Treatments with 4NQO and ultraviolet irradiation, which are known to exhibit potent mutagenicities on bacteria, were used as control experiments. A refreshed exponential-phase culture (ca. 6×10^8 to 8×10^8 cells/ml) of W4573 Val^s in Penassay broth was centrifuged, and precipitates were washed twice with saline. The cells were suspended in the original volume of Penassay broth, Davis glucose broth, or 0.06 M phosphate buffer (pH 7.2), and 4NPO or 4NQO was added to the suspension to give the desired concentration. After incubation at 37°C for 2 h, 4 ml of sample was centrifuged, washed with 2 ml of saline, and suspended in 1 ml of saline. The suspension was serially diluted and plated on EMB-glucose agar for counting survivors and on DM-glucose agar with 20 μg of L-proline per ml and 40 μg of L-valine per ml for determination of the number of Val^r mutants formed. In preparation for UV irradiation, Val^s cells to be irradiated were suspended in saline instead of Penassay broth.

Representative results are shown in Table 3. 4NPO did not induce any remarkable mutation from Val^s to Val^r, as 4NQO and ultraviolet irradiation had done. It was further shown in other experiments that 4NPO does not induce any remarkable mutation of strain W3110 from *str*^{s} to *str*^{r} nor reverse mutation from JE2133 *proA*$^-$ to *proA*$^+$. Moreover, 4HAPO, a reduced metabolite of 4NPO, did not show potent mutagenicity under those conditions. The results are in accord with previous observations (3).

Rates of spontaneous mutation from Pro$^+$ to Pro$^-$ cells, which might be correlated to the eventual efficiency of isolation of Pro$^-$ mutants from Pro$^+$ culture by treatment with 4NPO, were determined by the penicillin-screening method. W4573 *pro*$^+$ cells (2.8×10^8 cells per ml) were incubated in Davis glucose broth containing 300 U of penicillin G per ml at 37°C for 8 h. Whereas the viable count of Pro$^+$ cells decreased 9.2×10^{-4}, that the Pro$^-$ cells did not under this condition. Survivors grown on EMB-glucose agar were replica plated on Davis glucose agar plates with and without L-proline. Only 2 out of 5,655 colonies tested were Pro⁻ mutants that had the metabolic block between Glu and GSA. Six auxotrophs other than Pro⁻ were also formed. The rate of spontaneous mutation from W4573 *pro*+ to *proA*⁻ and/or *proB*⁻ was calculated to be 3×10^{-7}.

Metabolic conversion of 4NPO by Pro+ and Pro⁻ cells. Possible metabolic conversions of 4NPO by Pro+ and Pro⁻ cells were examined. First, changes of ultraviolet absorption spectra of supernatant fluid of the 4NPO broth inoculated with W4573 *pro*+ cells were examined. Results with *pro*+ cells (Fig. 6) indicated that the ultraviolet absorption maximum of 4NPO at 315 nm shifts to shorter wave length according to the duration of incubation time. Namely, incubation of 4NPO with *pro*+ cells for 12 min caused a decrease of optical density at 315 nm and the appearance of a new peak at 290 nm. After incubation for 18 min, 3 h, and 24 h, the absorption maximum of the supernatant shifted to 280 nm, 275 nm, and 260 nm, respectively. Similar spectral changes were observed when 4NPO was incubated with JE2133 *proA*⁻, KE113 *proB*⁻, or KE135 *proC*⁻, and, furthermore, *pro*+ *chl*⁻ or *proA*⁻ *chl*⁻ cells that were derived from W4573 or JE2133, respectively, and which were nitrate reductase activity-defective mutants. The results suggested that 4NPO might be metabolically reduced to 4HAPO showing $\lambda_{max}^{H_2O}$ 280 nm, 4APO showing $\lambda_{max}^{H_2O}$ 277 nm, and 4AP showing $\lambda_{max}^{H_2O}$ 261 nm.

Next, isolation of metabolites of 4NPO was attempted. A 100-mg portion of 4NPO was added to Davis glucose minimal medium supplemented with L-proline containing about 15 g (wet weight) of Pro+ cells, and the mixture was shaken at 37°C. The ultraviolet absorption maximum of the supernatant fluid was shifted to 280 nm, 277 nm, and 261 nm, respectively, the mixture was cooled to 0°C, and metabolites

TABLE 3. *Mutagenicity of 4NPO toward strain W4573 from valine sensitivity to valine resistance*

Agent	Conc of agents (µg/ml)	Survival (%)	Val^r mutants (per 10^8 survivors)	Relative mutation rate
4NPO	0	100	1.89	1.00
	100	77.4	1.22	0.65
	250	98.1	0.72	0.38
	500	44.0	1.25	0.66
	750	55.3	2.82	1.49
	1,000	42.7	1.85	0.98
4NQO	2.5	72.9	6.46	3.42
	5.0	99.4	6.50	3.44
	7.5	46.8	20.2	10.7
	10	41.2	25.0	13.2
UV irradiation[b]	0[c]	100	2.88	1.00
	10	23.9	9.74	3.4
	20	17.1	27.0	9.4
	30	4.74	77.3	26.8

[a] The inoculum was 6.4×10^8 cells/ml in Penassay broth. Incubation was carried out at 37°C for 2 h.
[b] The inoculum was 1.7×10^8 cells/ml.
[c] Time of irradiation (seconds).

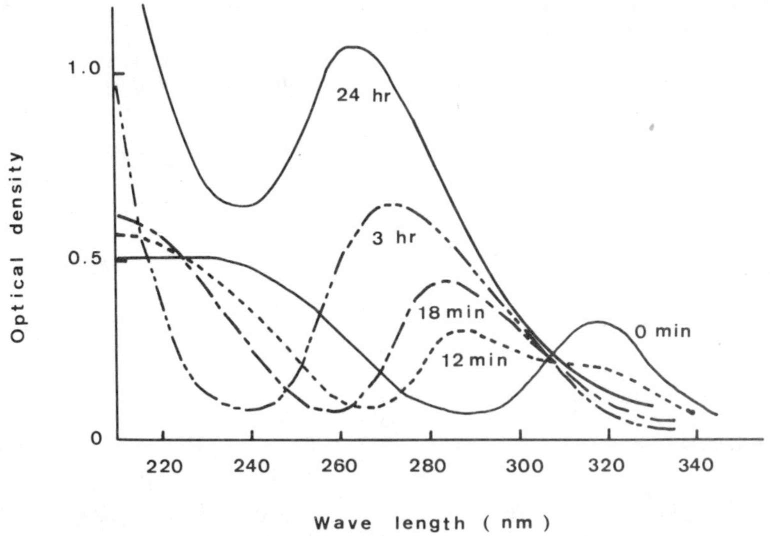

FIG. 6. *Changes of ultraviolet absorption spectrum of 4NPO in Pro+ culture. For procedure, see Materials and Methods. Absorption maxima of authentic specimens were as follows: 4NPO, 315 nm; 4HAPO, 280 nm; 4APO, 277 nm; 4AP, 261 nm.*

were extracted and purified as described above. The structures of metabolites thus isolated were characterized as 4HAPO, 4APO, and 4AP, respectively (Table 4). A discrepancy between melting points of a metabolite characterized as 4APO and its authentic specimen was observed; the metabolite may not have been fully purified from some unknown contaminants that had little effect on the other properties of 4APO. The results indicated that the reduction of the nitro group of 4NPO proceeds equally in Pro^+ and Pro^- cultures, and that the further reduction of the *N*-oxide bond also occurs (Fig. 7).

Metabolic reduction of 4NPO in Pro^+ culture under anaerobic condition was further carried out. Results indicated that 4NPO can be reduced at a 2.2 times faster rate than that observed under aerobic conditions.

The metabolic conversion process of 4NPO by JE2133 *proB*⁻ cells in synthetic minimal medium was also investigated. 4NPO was found to be reduced to 4HAPO and 4APO as in Penassay broth.

Structural modification of 4NPO and elective isolation of Pro^- mutants. It has been shown that 4NPO is reduced by Pro^+ and Pro^- cells to 4HAPO, 4APO, and 4AP. To investigate which metabolite might be a proximate compound or a compound most close to it for the phenomenon, W4573 *pro*⁺ was incubated in Penassay broth with each 4NPO derivative of the series shown in Fig. 1. Representative results are shown in Table 5. Isolation of Pro^- mutants was observed with 4NSPO (12 μg/ml) and 4HAPO (40 μg/ml) but not with AZOXY, AZO, 4APO, PO, and 2NPO. The results suggest that the nitro, nitroso, or hydroxylamino group at the 4 position and the *N*-oxide moiety

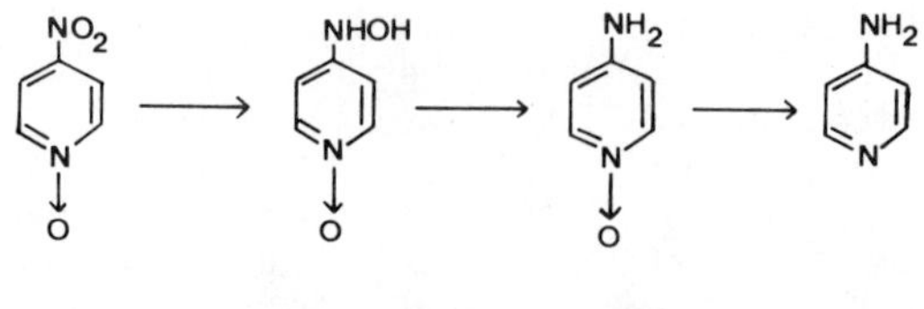

4NPO 4HAPO 4APO 4AP

FIG. 7. *Metabolic conversion process of 4NPO in bacterial culture.*

TABLE 5. *Action of 4NPO derivatives on W4573 (Pro^+) strain leading to the isolation of Pro^- mutants*[a]

Compound	Concn of agent (μg/ml)	Viable count (cells/ml)	Frequency (%) of Pro^- colonies
4-Nitropyridine 1-oxide (4NPO)	0		0
	2		100
4-Nitrosopyridine 1-oxide (4NSPO)	12	6.4×10^4	10.6
4-Hydroxylamino-pyridine 1-oxide (4HAPO)	90	1.3×10^5	30.8
	100	8.6×10^3	11.0
4,4′-Azoxypyridine 1,1′-dioxde (AZOXY)	50	1.4×10^3	0
4,4′-Azopyridine 1,1′-dioxide (AZO)	40	5.2×10^2	0
4-Aminopyridine 1-oxide (4APO)	500	2.2×10^9	0
4-Nitropyridine (4NP)	25		0
Pyridine 1-oxide (PO)	1,000	4.0×10^9	0
2-Nitropyridine 1-oxide (2NPO)	12.5	1.4×10^2	0
4-Nitrolutidine 1-oxide (4NLO)	20	4.0×10^6	0.3
	25	1.6×10^3	95.7
4-Nitroquinoline 1-oxide (4NQO)	0.8	1.7×10^8	29.6
4-Hydroxylamino-quinoline 1-oxide (4HAOO)	40	4.2×10^9	2.0

[a] Incubation of strain W4573 (Pro^+) with each compound was carried out in Penassay broth (100 ml) at a cell concentration of 10^3 cells/ml at 37°C for 24 h.

TABLE 4. *Characterization of metabolites of 4NPO by pro*⁺ *and pro*⁻ *cells*

Compounds	Source	Melting point (°C)[a] (decomp.)	Ultraviolet spectra		Elemental analysis			Yield (%)
			$\lambda_{max}^{H_2O}$ (nm)	ε[b]	C	H	N	
4HAPO Picrate	Metabolic product	172–174	280	21,700	37.59	2.63	20.21	21
			358	14,600				
	Authentic specimen	172–174	280	23,200	37.19	2.55	19.72	
			358	14,800				
4APO Picrate	Metabolic product	189–194	275	21,800	38.85	2.67	20.44	10
			358	15,200				
	Authentic specimen	204–206	277	21,400	38.95	2.67	20.65	
			358	13,800				
4AP Picrate	Metabolic product	218–220	260	22,200	40.53	2.75	21.03	25
			358	12,800				
	Authentic specimen	217–218	261	22,200	40.87	2.81	21.67	
			358	13,200				

[a] Melting points were taken on a kofler-type hot stage, and are uncorrected.

[b] Molecular intensity.

at the 1 position on the pyridine (and possibly quinoline) skeleton are indispensable for the action of the agent.

It is noted that 4NPO is more efficient than 4NQO in such action, and that every agent acts on Pro$^+$ cells most efficiently at a sublethal concentration of the agent.

Reconstruction experiments with these active 4NPO derivatives, i.e., 4HAPO, 4NSPO, 4NLO and 4NQO, were carried out between JE2149 *pro*$^+$ *lac*$^-$ and JE2133 *proA*$^-$ *lac*$^+$ and showed higher toxicity of the compounds toward *pro*$^+$ cells than *pro*$^-$ cells, as was the case with 4NPO.

Bacteriostatic action of 4NPO toward pro$^+$ cells in minimal medium. As mentioned above, the bacteriocidal action and selective toxicity of 4NPO toward *pro*$^+$ cells were observed in a complete medium, Penassay broth. To check further the mechanisms of the specific action of the agent, reconstruction experiments of the 4NPO treatment between JE2149 (*pro*$^+$ *lac*$^+$) and KE113 (*proA*$^-$ *lac*$^-$) JE2133 (*proB*$^-$ *lac*$^-$), or KE134 (*proC*$^-$ *lac*$^-$) were carried out in a synthetic minimal medium, Davis glucose minimal medium, supplemented with 20 μg of L-proline per ml. Results (Fig. 8) indicated that whereas 4NPO at a concentration of 2.5 μg/ml acted on *pro*$^+$ cells bacteriostatically for as long as 35 h, the agent allowed the growth of *proA*$^-$, *proB*$^-$, and *proC*$^-$ cells, although with longer generation times compared with those without the agent. Similar results were obtained when each strain was treated independently with 4NPO. When the minimum medium further supplemented with 0.1% Casamino Acids was used, however, *proC* cells showed 4NPO sensitivity, similar to *pro*$^+$ cells.

The observation of bacteriostatic action of 4NPO on *pro*$^+$ cells in synthetic minimal medium led to an examination of morphological features of *pro*$^+$ cells in the medium. An overnight culture of W4573 (*pro*$^+$) with a cell concentration of 10^3 cells per ml was incubated in 1 liter of Davis glucose minimal medium containing 40 μg of L-proline per ml and 2.5 μg of 4NPO per ml. After incubation with shaking for 24 h, the culture was filtered with suction through a Sartorius membrane filter (pore size, 0.45 μm). The cells collected on the filter were suspended in 1 ml of Davis glucose minimal medium. The nuclear apparatus of the cells was stained with Giemsa solution (Merck) after the cells were treated with 1 N hydrochloric acid at 60°C for 5 min to remove ribonucleic acid. Observation with a phase-contrast microscope (Nikon) revealed that *pro*$^+$ cells exposured to 4NPO had formed long nonseptate multinucleate filaments, the longest ones being 312 μm in length. Nuclear materials were distributed throughout the length of these filaments. Filament formation of *pro*$^+$ cells was not observed in the medium without 4NPO. The average cell length per nucleus of 30 long filamentous *pro*$^+$ cells was 3.9 μm, and that of the normal cells growing in the medium without 4NPO was 1.4 μm. Formation of filamentous cells, however, was not observed when JE2133 (*proA*$^-$) cells were incubated with and without 2.5 μg of 4NPO per ml.

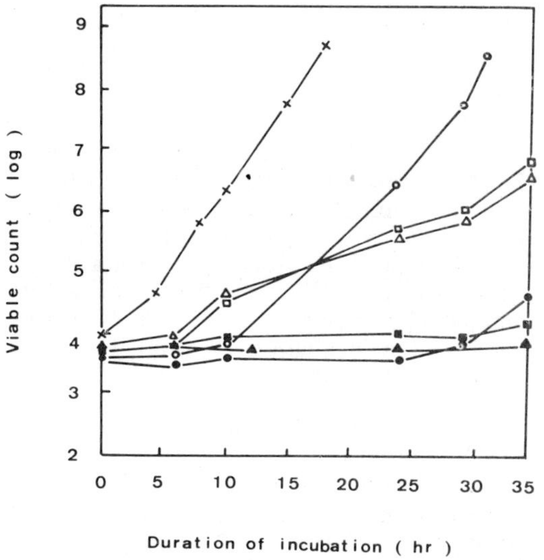

FIG. 8. *Reconstruction experiments between JE2149 (pro$^+$ lac$^+$) and JE2133 (proA1$^-$ lac-85$^-$), KE113 (proB3$^-$ lac-85$^-$), or KE134 (proC$^-$ lac-85$^-$) in Davis-glucose minimal medium containing 40 μg of L-proline per ml. Overnight cultures of pro$^+$ and pro$^-$ strains were diluted to give cell concentration of ca. 10^4 cells/ml in Davis glucose minimal medium containing L-proline with or without 2.5 μg of 4NPO per ml. Equal volumes of pro$^+$ and pro$^-$ cultures were mixed and incubated at 37°C with shaking. Plating with suitable dilutions was EMB-lactose-agar. Symbols: □, viable count of JE2133 with 4NPO; △, viable count of KE113 with 4NPO; ○, viable count of KE134 with 4NPO; ■, ▲, ●, viable count of JE2149 with 4NPO; ×, viable count of pro$^+$ and pro$^-$ cells without 4NPO.*

As control experiments, UV irradiation of AB 1899NM (*lon*$^-$) strain and thymine starvation of W3110 *thy*$^-$ strain were carried out, and the filamentous cells formed were analyzed by the nuclear staining method. The average cell length per nucleus was 1.2 μm in the filaments formed by the UV irradiation method and 2.7 μm in those isolated after thymine starvation. These results suggested that the action of 4NPO on *pro*$^+$ cells in minimal medium might be similar to the effect of thymine starvation on *thy*⁻ cells (inhibition of deoxyribonucleic acid biosynthesis) rather than the effect of UV irradiation on *lon*⁻ cells (inhibition of septum formation).

When filamentous cells derived from *pro*$^+$ cells by treatment with 4NPO were transferred into fresh minimal medium without the agent, they immediately began to regrow with the same kinetics of growth as *pro*$^+$ cells in the medium without 4NPO; the frequency of filamentous cells among total cells decreased by one-half after incubation for one generation time (data not shown).

DISCUSSION

We have found that 4NPO can act on *E. coli* K-12 Pro$^+$ strains in Penassay broth, leading to highly efficient isolation of Pro$^-$ mutants (7, 8). The Pro$^-$ cells thus isolated were *proA*$^-$ and/or *proB*$^-$ deficient in the biosynthetic pathway of proline, i.e., the process from Glu to GSA. With respect to possible mechanisms involved in the action of 4NPO, reconstruction experiments between *pro*$^+$ and *proA*$^-$ cells indicated that 4NPO is more toxic for *pro*$^+$ cells than for *proA*$^-$ cells (Fig. 2). Additional reconstruction experiments between *pro*$^+$ and *proB*$^-$, together with experiments on the bacteriocidal action of 4NPO on *pro*$^+$, *proA*$^-$, *proB*$^-$, and *proC*$^-$ cells in Penassay broth, further confirmed the higher sensitivity of *pro*$^+$ and *proC*$^-$ than *proA*$^-$ and *proB*$^-$ toward 4NPO (Fig. 3 and 4). Auxotrophic mutants other than *pro*$^-$ were found to have similar 4NPO sensitivity as *pro*$^+$ cells. These data indicate that the possible mechanism for the specific action of 4NPO may be the selective toxicity of the agent between *pro*$^+$ and *proA*$^-$ or *proB*$^-$ but no *proC*$^-$ cells. The fact that only *proA*$^-$ and *proB*$^-$ cells could be isolated by treatment of Pro$^+$ cells with 4NPO is in accord with the mechanism suggested.

Possible correlations between "4NPO-sensitive gene(s)" and *proA* or *proB* genes were then studied (Table 2). All *pro*$^+$ transductants derived from *proA*$^-$ and *proB*$^-$ cells with P1 *vir* phage and W4573 *pro*$^+$ as donor recovered sensitivity to 4NPO. Spontaneous Pro$^+$ revertants derived from *proA*$^-$ and *proB*$^-$ cells, on the other hand, were classified into two types, i.e., those fully growing in Davis glucose minimal medium and showing sensitivity to 4NPO and those growing rather slowly in the medium and showing resistance to 4NPO (data not shown). The latter type of *pro*$^-$ mutants may be those under the suppression of proline requirement by mutation of arginine requirement (11). These results suggest that *4NPO*^{s} gene(s) should be on or very close to the *proA* and *proB* loci and that both products of the *proA* and *proB* genes may be involved in the observed sensitivity of bacteria to 4NPO. The results of the dominance test using *pro*$^-$/F′ *proA*$^+$ *proB*$^+$ heterozygotes revealed that the 4NPO-sensitive allele is dominant over the 4NPO-resistant allele (Fig. 5). This suggests that gene product(s) of *proA* and/or *proB* may be associated in some way with the 4NPO sensitivity of Pro$^+$ cells, for example, by interference with 4NPO or more likely with its metabolite(s) to form a toxic substance(s) for the bacterial cell.

4NPO was found not to induce any remarkable mutation on strain W4573 (Table 3). This indicates that *proA*$^-$ and *proB*$^-$ cells formed from *pro*$^+$ cells by spontaneous mutation might be selected by 4NPO. The fact that the rate of spontaneous mutation from *pro*$^+$ to *proA*$^-$ and/or *proB*$^-$ was 3×10^{-7} may be in agreement with an already observed large fluctuation of frequency of *pro*$^-$ production by 4NPO treatment (8).

Considering 4NPO as an analogue of proline (10), the following answers to the question of why *proA*$^-$ and *proB*$^-$ cells show resistance to 4NPO are possible. First, *pro*$^+$ and *proC*$^-$ cells may incorporate much more 4NPO as a toxic substance than *proA*$^-$ and *proB*$^-$ cells do. This explanation was disproved by experiments incorporating [^{3}H]4NPO into the *pro*$^+$ and *pro*$^-$ cells; no significant difference between the incorporation rates of ^{3}H was observed between *pro*$^+$ and *pro*$^-$ (Inuzuka and Tomoeda, unpublished data). A second possible explanation is that whereas *pro*$^+$ and *proC*$^-$ cells are less efficient in metabolizing 4NPO as a detoxication process, *proA*$^-$ and *proB*$^-$ cells can metabolize 4NPO at a higher rate. Again, experiments on metabolic conversion of 4NPO with bacterial cells showed no significant differences in reduction rates of the agent to 4HAPO and 4APO by *pro*$^+$, *proA*$^-$, *proB*$^-$, or *proC*$^-$ cells. Moreover, the reducing enzyme responsible for the metabolism of 4NPO may be DT diaphorase, as reported in the case of metabolic reduction of 4NQO (18). This further suggests that the second explanation is unlikely. And third, intermediate(s) of proline biosynthetic pathway between Glu and Pro, which can be synthesized in *pro*$^+$ and *proC*$^-$ but not in *proA*$^-$ and *proB*$^-$, may be in some respect associated with the toxicity of 4NPO toward bacterial cells. With respect to this question, additional effect of PC on the toxicity of 4NPO toward bacterial cells was examined. However, no effect of PC at concentrations as high as 500 μg/ml in Penassay broth or Davis glucose minimal medium containing L-proline was observed.

It is interesting to note that 4NPO acted bacteriostatically on *pro*+ cells but not on *pro*− cells in minimal medium, leading to the formation of long nonseptate multinucleate filamentous cells. Comparison of the results with those of filament formation of *lon*− cells with UV irradiation and of *thy*− cells by thymine starvation suggested that 4NPO-induced formation of filamentous cells might result from possible inhibition of DNA synthesis of bacterial cells by the agent. However, further experiments should be conducted before any decisive explanation can be given.

ACKNOWLEDGMENTS

We thank Y. Hirota of the National Institute of Genetics, Mishima, Japan, Y. Sugino of Osaka University, Osaka, Japan, and N. Otsuji of Kyushu University, Fukuoka, Japan, for supplying bacterial strains.

This investigation was supported by a Grant-in-Aid of Scientific Research from the Ministry of Education, Science and Culture, Japan, and a grant from Kaisei-Kai Scientific Foundation, Tokyo, Japan.

LITERATURE CITED

1. **Berg, C. M., and P. Curtiss III.** 1967. Transposition derivatives of an Hfr strain of *Escherichia coli* K-12. Genetics **56**:503–525.
2. **Brown, E. V.** 1957. Preparation and reactions of 2-nitropyridine 1-oxides. J. Am. Chem. Soc. **79**:3565–3566.
3. **Endo, H., T. Ono, and T. Sugimura.** 1971. Chemistry and biological actions of 4-nitroquinoline 1-oxide. Recent Results Cancer Res. **34**:1–98.
4. **Evans, R. F., and H. C. Brown.** 1962. 4-Nitro-2,6-lutidine 1-oxide. J. Org. Chem. **27**:1665–1667.
5. **Hamana, M.** 1951. Ueber die Reduktion der aromatischen tetriaeren Aminoxyden mittels Phosphortrichlorid. J. Pharm. Soc. Jpn. **71**:263–266.
6. **Hirota, Y.** 1960. The effect of acridine dyes on mating type factors in *Escherichia coli*. Proc. Natl. Acad. Sci. U.S.A. **46**:57–64.
7. **Hirota, Y., M. Inuzuka, and M. Tomoeda.** 1966. Elective selection of proline-requiring mutants. J. Bacteriol. **91**:2392.
8. **Inuzuka, M., H. Miyano, and M. Tomoeda.** 1976. Specific action of 4-nitropyridine 1-oxide on *Escherichia coli* K-12 Pro+ strains leading to the isolation of proline-requiring mutants: isolation and characterization of Pro− mutants. Antimicrob. Agents Chemother. **10**:325–332.
9. **Kato, R., A. Takahashi, and T. Oshima.** 1970. Characteristics of nitro reduction of the carcinogenic agent, 4-nitroquinoline N-oxide. Biochem. Pharmacol. **19**:45–55.
10. **Kay, W. W., and A. F. Gronlund.** 1969. Isolation of amino acid transport-negative mutants of *Pseudomonas aeruginosa* and cells with repressed transport activity. J. Bacteriol. **98**:116–123.
11. **Kuo, T., and B. A. D. Stocker.** 1969. Suppression of proline requirement of *proA* and *proAB* deletion mutants in *Salmonella typhimurium* by mutation to arginine requirement. J. Bacteriol. **98**:593–598.
12. **Lennox, E. S.** 1955. Transduction of linked genetic characters of the host by bacteriophage P1. Virology **1**:190–206.
13. **Ochiai, E., M. Ishikawa, and K. Arima.** 1943. Nitration of pyridine N-oxide and its analogues. J. Pharm. Soc. Jpn. **63**:79.
14. **Ochiai, E., M. Ishikawa, and Z. Sai.** 1943. Nitration of quinoline N-oxide. J. Pharm. Soc. Jpn. **63**:280–282.
15. **Ochiai, E., and M. Katada.** 1943. Reduction of 4-nitropyridine N-oxide. J. Pharm. Soc. Jpn. **63**:186–191.
16. **Ochiai, E., and H. Mitarashi.** 1963. Darstellung von 4-Hydroxylaminopyridin-1-oxyd aus 4-Nitropyridin-1-oxyd. Annu. Rep. Itsuu Lab. **13**:19–23.
17. **Ochiai, E., A. Ohta, and H. Nomura.** 1957. Polarisation der heteroxyklischen Ringe mit aromatischem Charakter. Chem. Pharm. Bull. **5**:310–313.
18. **Okabayashi, T., and A. Yoshimoto.** 1962. Reduction of 4-nitroquinoline 1-oxide by microörganisms. Chem. Pharm. Bull. **12**:1221–1226.
19. **Piéchaud, M., J. Puig, F. Pichinoty, E. Azoulay, and L. Le Minor.** 1967. Mutations affectant la nitrate-réductase a et dáutres enzymes bactériennes dóxydoréduction. Ann. Inst. Pasteur Paris **112**:24–37.
20. **Ramakrishnan, T., and E. A. Adelberg.** 1964. Regulatory mechanisms in the biosynthesis of isoleucine and valine. I. Genetic derepression of enzyme formation. J. Bacteriol. **87**:566–573.
21. **Taylor, A. L., and C. D. Trotter.** 1972. Linkage map of *Escherichia coli* strain K-12. Bacteriol. Rev. **34**:115–175.
22. **Tomoeda, M., M. Inuzuka, N. Kubo, and S. Nakamura.** 1968. Effective elimination of drug resistance and sex factors in *Escherichia coli* by sodium dodecyl sulfate. J. Bacteriol. **95**:1078–1089.

ANTIMICROBIAL AGENTS AND CHEMOTHERAPY, Aug. 1976, p. 344-346 Vol. 10, No. 2

Printed in U.S.A.

Effect of Gentamicin on Growth of Viral, Chlamydial, and Rickettsial Agents in Mice and Embryonated Eggs

LENDELL A. WHITE,* HENRIETTA E. HALL, T. TZIANABOS, AND W. ADRIAN CHAPPELL

Viral and Rickettsial Products Branch, Biological Products Division, Bureau of Laboratories, Center for Disease Control, Atlanta, Georgia 30333

Received for publication 17 March 1976

Gentamicin, at concentrations up to 500 μg/ml, showed no effect on the replication, yield, or infectivity of seven viruses or on the agents of psittacosis and meningopneumonitis when grown in mice or embryonated eggs. At the 500 μg/ml level, lymphogranuloma venereum cultures had a slight reduction in infectivity. *Rickettsia akari* demonstrated susceptibility at the 5 μg/ml level, whereas *R. rickettsii*, *R. mooseri*, and *R. canada* grown in embryonated eggs were susceptible in varying degrees to gentamicin at or above the 50 μg/ml concentration.

Gentamicin sulfate, an aminoglycoside antibiotic, is readily soluble in water, autoclavable, and highly stable at wide pH and temperature ranges. It has been reported (4, 6, 11) to inhibit the in vitro growth of a wide range of gram-positive and gram-negative bacteria. Other investigators (5, 7) have described the effectiveness of gentamicin in eliminating mycoplasmas from cell cultures. Its use in virological studies with cell cultures as reported by Schafer et al. (10) showed neither cytotoxic effects nor virucidal activity at concentrations as high as 2,000 μg/ml. The routine recommended dose of 50 μg/ml in cell cultures was found to be bactericidal for a wide range of organisms. Wentworth (12) described the use of 10 μg of gentamicin per ml for the isolation in McCoy cell cultures of subgroup A *Chlamydia* from clinical specimens. Acute and subacute toxicity studies conducted in mice by Black et al. (1) revealed that the lethal dose of gentamicin sulfate administered by parenteral routes exceeded 400 mg/kg of body weight.

These reports led us to consider applying gentamicin in the large-scale production of viral, chlamydial, and rickettsial diagnostic reagents from fluids and tissues of mice and embryonated chicken eggs. Penicillin and streptomycin are routinely used to control contamination in the production of viral reagents; however, these antibiotics cannot be used in the production of chlamydial and rickettsial reagents. The purpose of this report is to describe the effect of gentamicin on the replication of several viral, rickettsial, and chlamydial agents in mice and embryonated eggs.

MATERIALS AND METHODS

Organisms. The viruses included in these investigations consisted of influenza A/England/42/72 (H3N2); influenza B/Hong Kong/5/72; Newcastle disease virus, strain Roakin; mumps, strain Enders; parainfluenza type 1, strain Sendai; eastern equine encephalomyelitis, strain NJ/60; and rabies, strain CVS.

The chlamydial agents included were those of psittacosis, strain DD-34; meningopneumonitis, strain Francis; and lymphogranuloma venereum, strain JH.

The four rickettsiae included were *Rickettsia akari*, strain Hartford; *R. rickettsii*, strain Shelia Smith; *R. mooseri*, strain Wilmington; and *R. canada*.

Host systems. Embryonated eggs were obtained from chicken flocks maintained on antibiotic-free feed. The viral agents and psittacosis were grown in the allantoic cavity of either 8- or 10-day-old eggs incubated at 33 to 35°C. The other chlamydiae were grown in the yolk sacs of 8-day-old eggs incubated at 36°C. The rickettsial agents were cultivated in the yolk sacs of 5- to 6-day-old eggs at 35°C.

Random-bred, ICR, weanling mice weighing approximately 15 to 18 g were inoculated intracranially with 0.03 ml of rabies, psittacosis, or meningopneumonitis agents. Eastern equine encephalomyelitis was titrated in 2-day-old suckling mice inoculated intracranially with 0.02 ml.

Effect of gentamicin. Gentamicin reagent solution, equivalent to 10 mg of antibiotic per ml, was purchased from Schering Corporation (Port Reading, N.J.). The viability of stock seed cultures was determined after exposure to gentamicin at final concentrations of either 5, 50, or 500 μg/ml. No additional antibiotics were included in the diluents. Phosphate-buffered saline, pH 7.2, was the diluent for the viral and chlamydial titrations; a sucrose phosphate buffer (2) was used with the rickettsiae.

Cultures were treated with gentamicin by making serial 10-fold dilutions in the diluent containing the desired gentamicin concentration. These dilutions were incubated at 4°C for 2 h and then inoculated into the appropriate host into either 10 embryonated eggs or 8 mice per dilution. Control cultures without gentamicin exposure were titrated in the same manner.

The median infective dose and the median lethal dose (LD_{50}) were calculated by the method of Reed and Muench (8). The egg median infective dose of the orthomyxoviruses and paramyxoviruses was determined by hemagglutination titrations (3) of the allantoic fluids from individual eggs. Tolerance tests were performed with various concentrations of gentamicin up to 5,000 μg/ml in eggs and mice of the corresponding age and under the same incubation conditions as with the infective materials.

RESULTS

No deaths or toxic reactions were observed in embryonated eggs inoculated with gentamicin in concentrations as high as 5,000 μg/ml by either the allantoic, amniotic, or yolk sac routes. Suckling and weanling mice receiving either intraperitoneal or intracranial injections also exhibited no adverse effects.

A comparison of the infectivity titers of seven viruses with and without treatment with three concentrations of gentamicin is presented in Table 1. Two different cultures of each viral agent were titrated in eggs. For each virus, no substantial differences were observed among viral titrations. The results of these titrations confirmed previous reports that viral growth was not inhibited by gentamicin.

Psittacosis and meningopneumonitis infectivity titers were determined in both eggs and weanling mice; LGV, however, was titered only in embryonated eggs. The results of replicate titrations of the chlamydial agents are presented in Table 2. Variations in the LD_{50} titers between the untreated and gentamicin-treated psittacosis and meningopneumonitis cultures were slight in both host systems and were not attributed to the effect of the antibiotic. Titer reductions of $10^{0.9}$ and $10^{1.1}$ occurred in the LGV titrations treated with 500 μg of gentamicin per ml. No effect was observed with the lower gentamicin concentrations.

The results of the gentamicin treatment of the rickettsia cultures are summarized in Table 3. After treatment with 500 μg of gentamicin per ml the four rickettsiae tested showed a reduction in infectivity ranging from $10^{1.4}$ to $10^{2.8}$. The *R. akari* cultures were susceptible to

TABLE 2. *Effect of gentamicin on chlamydial agents*

Agent (strain)	Host	Titer (LD_{50}/ml)			
		Concn of gentamicin (μg/ml)			
		0	5	50	500
Psittacosis (DD34)	Eggs	5.4[a,b]	5.4	5.4	5.4
		5.3[b]	5.4	5.5	5.1
	Mice	2.8	3.0	3.0	2.3
		5.0	4.6	4.3	4.8
Meningopneumonitis (Francis)	Eggs	5.8	6.1	5.8	5.7
		6.5	6.7	6.0	6.5
	Mice	7.1	6.8	6.7	6.9
		5.9	5.7	5.5	5.3
Lymphogranuloma venereum (JH)	Eggs	5.9	5.8	5.8	5.0
		5.6	6.0	5.7	4.5

[a] Expressed as $\log_{10}$ LD_{50}/ml.
[b] Results from duplicate experiments.

TABLE 1. *Effect of gentamicin on infectivity of viruses*

Virus (strain)	Host	Expt no.	Infectivity titer			
			Concn of gentamicin (μg/ml)			
			0	5	50	500
Influenza A/England/42/72	Egg	A	7.7[a]	7.7	7.9	7.9
		B	7.5	7.5	7.9	7.8
Influenza B/Hong Kong/5/72	Egg	A	7.5	7.3	7.9	8.0
		B	7.3	7.4	7.4	7.4
Newcastle disease (Roakin)	Egg	A	8.5	8.2	8.4	8.4
		B	8.8	8.5	8.3	8.3
Parainfluenza Type 1 (Sendai)	Egg	A	8.0	8.1	8.1	8.3
		B	8.3	7.9	8.1	8.2
Mumps virus (Enders)	Egg	A	3.6	3.1	3.7	3.4
		B	6.1	5.6	6.1	5.9
Rabies virus (CVS)	Weanling mice	A	6.7[b]	6.4	7.0	6.4
Eastern equine encephalomyelitis (NJ/60)	Suckling mice	A	10.6	10.2	10.1	10.4

[a] Expressed as $\log_{10}$ median infective dose per ml.
[b] Expressed as $\log_{10}$ LD_{50}/g.

TABLE 3. *Reduction in LD_{50} titers of rickettsiae grown in embryonated eggs after gentamicin treatment*

Agent	LD_{50}/ml without gentamicin	Decrease in LD_{50} after treatment: Gentamicin concn (μg/ml) 5	50	500
Rickettsia akari	7.9[a,b]	1.7	1.8	2.7
	6.7[b]	1.6	3.0	1.5
R. rickettsii	4.8	0.2	0.7	1.4
	6.3	0.0	0.8	1.9
R. mooseri	7.9	0.4	1.6	2.8
	3.5	0.0	0.7	1.4
R. canada	5.2	0.2	0.3	1.6
	5.8	0.6	0.7	1.6

[a] Expressed as $\log_{10}$ LD_{50}/ml.
[b] Results from duplicate experiments.

all gentamicin concentrations and showed titer decreases ranging from $10^{1.5}$ to $10^{3.0}$. The 5 μg/ml level caused insignificant effects on the other three rickettsiae. Although a slightly greater titer reduction was observed at the 50 μg/ml level, it was still less than that obtained with the 500 μg/ml concentration.

DISCUSSION

The results of these studies indicate that, in general, up to 500 μg of gentamicin per ml may be used in the cultivation of viral and chlamydial agents. With the exception of the effect on LGV, this antibiotic concentration showed no effect upon the replication, yield, or infectivity of these agents. The LGV titrations treated with 500 μg/ml indicated that infectivity was reduced by approximately a factor of 10. This may be the maximum tolerance level for LGV, since lower concentrations were used without adverse effects. Wentworth (12) described the successful use of gentamicin for the isolation of subgroup A *Chlamydia* from clinical materials. A chlamydial strain assayed with increasing concentrations of streptomycin, vancomycin, or gentamicin ranging from 5 to 100 μg/ml did not demonstrate inhibition of infectivity at any concentration.

To some degree, all of the rickettsial agents were susceptible to gentamicin at or above the 50 μg/ml level. However, no reduction in infectivity other than that shown with *R. akari* was observed at the 5 μg/ml concentration. In addition to a reduction in the amount of infectivity at or above the 50 μg/ml level, a delay in the time of embryo death was observed consistently with all four rickettsiae. When compared to the time of death of the untreated rickettsiae, the embryo death was delayed approximately 24 h at the 50-μg level and by at least 48 h at the 500-μg level. Except with *R. akari*, a negligible delay in time of death was observed with cultures treated with 5 μg/ml. With the *R. akari* cultures, the time of death was delayed approximately 24 h in the end point dilutions. These results indicate that gentamicin even in low concentrations must be used with caution in the growth of rickettsiae in embryonated eggs.

Studies have indicated that gentamicin offers several advantages over the penicillin-streptomycin combination routinely used in the growth of viral agents. The satisfactory use of gentamicin in the treatment of diagnostic specimens submitted for virus isolation has been reported by several investigators (9, 10, 12). However, our results indicate that gentamicin should not be used in diagnostic specimens collected for the isolation of rickettsiae. The use of gentamicin to control contamination in the large-scale production of viral diagnostic reagents has shown no effects on either the complement-fixing or hemagluttinating titers of the antigens.

LITERATURE CITED

1. **Black, J., B. Calesnick, D. Williams, and M. J. Weinstein.** 1964. Pharmacology of gentamicin, a new broad-spectrum antibiotic, p. 138–147. Antimicrob. Agents Chemother. 1963.
2. **Bovarnick, M. R., J. C. Miller, and J. C. Snyder.** 1950. The influence of certain salts, amino acids, sugars, and proteins on the stability of rickettsiae. J. Bacteriol. 59:509–522.
3. **Hierholzer, J. C., M. T. Suggs, and E. C. Hall.** 1969. Standardized viral hemagglutination-inhibition test. II. Description and statistical evaluation. Appl. Microbiol. 18:824–833.
4. **Kirby, W. M. M., and H. C. Standiford.** 1969. Gentamicin: in vitro studies. J. Infect. Dis. 119:361–363.
5. **Perlman, D., S. B. Rahman, and J. B. Semar.** 1967. Antibiotic control of *Mycoplasma* in tissue culture. Appl. Microbiol. 15:82–85.
6. **Rabinovich, S., I. S. Synder, and I. M. Smith.** 1964. Preliminary report on in vitro and clinical studies with gentamicin, p. 164–168. Antimicrob. Agents Chemother. 1963.
7. **Rahman, S. B., J. B. Semar, and D. Perlman.** 1967. Antibiotic resistance in *Mycoplasma* isolates from tissue culture. Appl. Microbiol. 15:970.
8. **Reed, L. J., and H. Muench.** 1938. A simple method for estimating fifty percent endpoints. Am. J. Hyg. 27:493–497.
9. **Rudin, A., A. Healey, C. A. Phillips, D. W. Gump, and B. R. Forsyth.** 1970. Antibacterial activity of gentamicin sulfate in tissue culture. Appl. Microbiol. 20:989–990.
10. **Schafer, T. W., A. Pascale, G. Shimonaski, and P. E. Came.** 1972. Evaluation of gentamicin for use in virology and tissue culture. Appl. Microbiol. 23:565–570.
11. **Waitz, J. A., and M. J. Weinstein.** 1969. Recent microbiological studies with gentamicin. J. Infect. Dis. 119:355–360.
12. **Wentworth, B. B.** 1973. Use of gentamicin in the isolation of subgroup A *Chlamydia*. Antimicrob. Agents Chemother. 3:698–702.

ANTIMICROBIAL AGENTS AND CHEMOTHERAPY, Aug. 1976, p. 347-353
Vol. 10, No. 2
Printed in U.S.A.

Chloramphenicol: an Enzymological Microassay

PAUL S. LIETMAN,* THOMAS J. WHITE,[1] AND WILLIAM V. SHAW[2]

Division of Clinical Pharmacology, Johns Hopkins University School of Medicine, Baltimore, Maryland 21205, and Department of Medicine and Department of Biochemistry, University of Miami School of Medicine, Miami, Florida 33152*

Received for publication 1 April 1976

A new assay for chloramphenicol in biological fluids has been developed that offers sensitivity, specificity, precision, accuracy, economy, and ease of performance. The assay is based on the enzymological acetylation of chloramphenicol catalyzed by an R factor-mediated enzyme. [^{14}C]acetyl coenzyme A serves as the donor of the labeled acetyl group, and the product, [^{14}C]acetoxychloramphenicol, is separated from the labeled precursor by utilizing its preferential extraction into benzene. The product is then quantified by liquid scintillation counting. This assay measures chloramphenicol concentrations in both plasma and other biological specimens and in the presence of other antibiotics, hemolysis, or jaundice. Its rapidity and ease of performance are useful for clinical laboratories, and its sensitivity allows determinations on 10 μl of plasma.

Plasma chloramphenicol levels are clinically useful in helping to skirt between ineffectiveness and toxicity in patients who respond in a heterogeneous manner to the drug.

Several methods for the quantification of chloramphenicol in biological fluids have been devised (1-7, 10, 11, 15), but to date none has been entirely satisfactory. We have developed an enzymological assay for chloramphenicol in biological fluids that offers sensitivity, specificity, precision, accuracy, economy, and ease of performance. This method is based on the specific acetylation of chloramphenicol with a radioactively labeled acetyl group derived from [^{14}C]acetyl coenzyme A and catalyzed by an R factor-mediated acetyltransferase. Both the reaction and the enzyme have been previously characterized (12-14). This report describes the adaptation of this reaction to a clinically useful assay.

(This paper was presented in part at the 73rd Annual Meeting of the American Society for Microbiology, 6-11 May 1973, Miami Beach, Fla.).

MATERIALS AND METHODS

Enzyme preparations. Chloramphenicol acetyltransferase was used as both a highly purified preparation (253 U/mg of protein) and a crude "osmotic shock fluid" (about 10 U/mg of protein). The former was purified as described previously (13) or can be prepared in high yield by a single-step procedure employing affinity chromatography (Y. Zaidenzaig and W. V. Shaw, FEBS Lett., in press). The crude osmotic shock fluid was prepared as follows. A strain of *Escherichia coli* (JR66/W677), harboring an R factor for chloramphenicol resistance, was subjected to osmotic shock by the method of Nossal and Heppel (8). This method was originally used because we had previously prepared an adenylylating enzyme for the measurement of gentamicin levels from the same strain of *E. coli*. The use of the shocking procedure is not meant to localize the intracellular distribution of the enzyme since we have no evidence that many intracellular enzymes as well as periplasmic enzymes were not released as we shocked the cells. the osmotic shock fluid was brought to a final concentration of 10 mM tris(hydroxymethyl)aminomethane (Tris)-hydrochloride (pH 7.8 at 5°C), 10 mM mercaptoethanol, and 5.0 mM magnesium chloride and was purified one step further by ammonium sulfate fractionation. The precipitate obtained between 30 and 60% saturation with ammonium sulfate contained all of the activity. This precipitate was suspended in 10 mM Tris-hydrochloride (pH 7.8 at 5°C) containing 0.2 M sodium chloride and 0.5 mM mercaptoethanol in a volume equal to 1/10 the volume of the original extract and dialzyed overnight (with one change of dialysate) against the same buffer at 4°C. This dialysis appears to remove substrates that serve as acceptors for the labeled acetate in reactions catalyzed by other enzymes present in the crude chloramphenicol acetyltransferase preparation. As prepared above, the shock fluid does not appear to catalyze the acetylation of substrates other than chloramphenicol in plasma or other biological fluids, nor does it catalyze the non-chloramphenicol-related degradation of acetyl coenzyme A when preincubated in the absence of chloramphenicol.

The activity of the enzyme preparations was measured in the assay system described below but with

[1] Present address: Department of Biochemistry, University of California, Berkeley, CA 94720.

[2] Present address: Department of Biochemistry, University of Leicester, University Road, Leicester, LE1 7RH, England.

an excess of chloramphenicol (0.12 mM) and with the enzyme diluted so that the incorporation of labeled acetate was linear with respect to both time and enzyme concentration. One unit of enzyme activity was taken to be the amount sufficient to monoacetylate 1 μmol of chloramphenicol per min under the conditions specified.

Quantification of chloramphenicol by gas-liquid chromatography. The method of Resnick et al. (10) was used for the measurement of chloramphenicol by gas-liquid chromatography with a Varian model 2100 equipped with a ^{63}Ni electron capture detector.

Antibiotics and miscellaneous materials. Chloramphenicol (DG-threo-1-*p*-nitrophenyl-2-dichloroacetamido-1,3-propandiol [lot 65211]) was purchased from Calbiochem, La Jolla, Calif. A stereoisomer of chloramphenicol, LG-threo-1-*p*-nitrophenyl-2-dichloroacetamido-1,3-propanediol (lot 4875-x535A), was the gift of Mildred Rebstock of Parke, Davis & Co., Ann Arbor, Mich. Chloramphenicol sodium succinate (lot P14163B) and thiamphenicol, the analogue of chloramphenicol with a methylsulfonyl group replacing the nitro group, were also gifts from Parke, Davis & Co. Sodium methicillin, ampicillin, tetracycline, and kanamycin sulfate were gifts from Bristol Laboratories, Syracuse, N.Y. Sulfisoxazole, erythromycin, oxytetracycline, neomycin, and streptomycin were purchased from Sigma Chemical Co., St. Louis, Mo. Sodium cephalothin, tobramycin, and phenoxymethyl penicillin were gifts from Eli Lilly & Co., Indianapolis, Ind. Rifampin was a gift from the Pitman-Moore Division of Dow Chemical Co., Indianapolis, Ind., the gentamicin complex was a gift from Schering Corp., Bloomfield, N.J., and clindamycin was from Upjohn, Kalamazoo, Mich.

Acetyl-1-[^{14}C]coenzyme A (lot 632-235), with a specific activity of 49.8 mCi/mmol, was purchased from New England Nuclear Corp., Boston, Mass. Acetyl coenzyme A trilithium trihydrate (lot 101229) was from Calbiochem. RP X-omat medical X-ray film was obtained from Eastman Kodak Co., Rochester, N.Y. β-glucuronidase (bacterial, type III, lot 80C-6880) was purchased from Sigma Chemical Co. The original strain of *E. coli* was a gift from Julian Davies of the University of Wisconsin.

RESULTS

Assay. The acetylation reaction is carried out in a final volume of 260 μl in 15-ml conical centrifuge tubes. The reaction contains, as final concentrations, 0.1 M Tris-hydrochloride (pH 7.8 at 37°C) and 0.2 mM [^{14}C]acetylcoenzyme A (1.5 mCi/mmol). Enzyme (0.5×10^{-3} to 1.25×10^{-3} U of activity corresponding to about 50 ng of protein) is added by adding 25 μl of a 1:100 dilution of a crude, dialyzed shock fluid prepared as above. Water is added to bring the volume of the mix to 250 ml. In practice, an assay mix of the above components is prepared for the appropriate number of samples to be analyzed, and 250 μl of this mix is added to each tube.

The reaction is initiated by the addition of 10 μl of plasma or water containing the chloramphenicol and is continued at 37°C for 30 min.

At the conclusion of the incubation period, the reaction mixture is extracted with three 1.0-ml portions of benzene by agitation on a Vortex mixer. Chloramphenicol, chloramphenicol monoacetate, and chloramphenicol diacetate are extracted quantitatively into benzene at an alkaline pH (pH > 7.5), while the acetate anion and acetyl coenzyme A remain in the aqueous phase. The tubes are centrifuged briefly after each addition of benzene (1 min at $1{,}000 \times g$), and the supernatant fluids are decanted with Pasteur pipettes into scintillation vials. Alternatively, the aqueous layer may be quickly frozen by dipping the lower portion of the tubes into an acetone-dry ice bath and the benzene layer, which remains unfrozen, may be poured directly into the scintillation vials. A 5-ml amount of a toluene-based scintillation fluid (toluene, 700 ml: ethanol, 300 ml; 2,5-diphenyloxazole, 3 g; *p*-bis-2-(5-phenyloxazolyl)benzene, 100 mg) is added to the pooled benzene phases, and the samples are counted at an efficiency of about 75% (as measured by the channels ratio method) in a Nuclear-Chicago model 6225 liquid scintillation counter.

The sensitivity of the assay can be improved by drying the benzene solution with mild heating under a stream of nitrogen of air. We have found this useful when measuring concentrations of less than 5 μg/ml.

Acetate incorporated into acetylated chloramphenicol was measured as counts per minute over control counts realized with reaction mixtures containing no antibiotic. These control counts, seen with control reaction mixtures containing 10 μl of plasma but lacking chloramphenicol, ranged from 30 to 50 cpm as compared with about 900 cpm above background for 10 μg of chloramphanicol per ml. This is no higher than the background on our instrument and indicates that there is no interference from benzene-extractable substrates present in plasma that might be nonspecifically acetylated.

The assay, as described above, utilizes only one part of the overall reaction, which proceeds through monoacetylation to diacetylation of the chloramphenicol. We can, by adjusting the amount of the enzyme in the reaction mixture, effect either a diacetylation or a monoacetylation of chloramphenicol. An example of a time course that was realized when 0.6 U of enzyme activity (600 times the usual amount) was provided to the system is shown in Fig. 1. An initial rapid reaction (monoacetylation) is followed by a slower second phase (diacetylation). By increasing the amount of enzyme still fur-

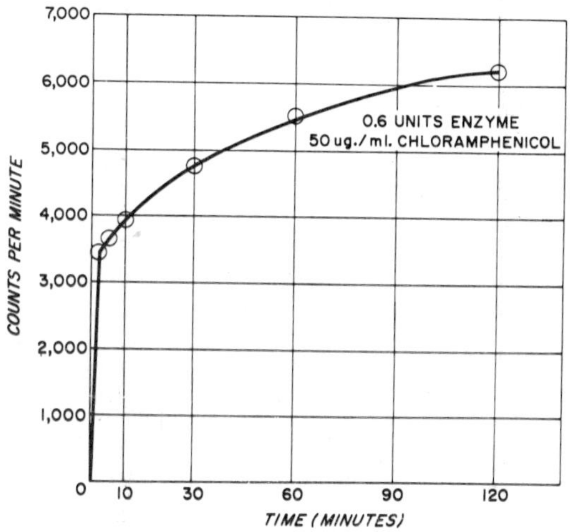

FIG. 1. *Time course of chloramphenicol diacetylation.*

ther, we have been able to construct a system that reaches complete diacetylation (>90%) in 3 h. Although this system offers the advantage of additional sensitivity because two labeled acetyl groups are added to each molecule of chloramphenicol, it suffers the disadvantages of requiring more incubation time (3 h) and considerably more enzyme. Furthermore, preliminary experiments suggested that chloramphenicol glucuronide served as a substrate, albeit a poor one, for this reaction.

We have, therefore, taken advantage of the finding that the rate of addition of the second acetyl group, under our conditions, is much slower than the rate of addition of the initial acetyl group (13). The time course of a typical monoacetylation reaction, utilizing 0.001 U of enzyme, is illustrated in Fig. 2. The slowness of the subsequent addition of a second acetyl group at this concentration of enzyme provides ample leeway for stopping the reaction. Thus, we have selected 30 min as our usual time for cessation of the reaction. Continuing the assay an additional 30 min would add only 4% to the result.

Stability of the enzyme. The activity of the dialyzed crude enzyme preparation was monitored in the frozen, frozen-thawed, and dilute frozen-thawed states. Preliminary results suggest that roughly half of the acetylating activity is lost in the first month of storage at −20°C, but the enzyme remains reasonably stable thereafter. Greater than 90% of the original activity of purified enzyme can be realized after 1 year if the enzyme is kept at −40°C in 50 mM Tris (pH 7.8), 0.1 mM mercaptoethanol, 0.2 M NaCl, and 0.1 mM chloramphenicol. Since such small amounts of enzyme are required in the assay and a typical preparation yields enough enzyme for about 8,000 assays, the 1 day required to prepare the dialyzed shock fluid should present no great inconvenience, even if it is necessary to repeat this preparation every 3 to 4 months.

Products. The products of the acetylation reaction that are extractable into benzene were verified by thin-layer chromatography using silica gel plates (Analtech) and a chloroform-methanol (90:10) solvent system (12). Labeled products were visualized by autoradiography and quantified by strip counting. Chloramphenicol-3-acetate (R_f = 0.60) is the main product of the monoacetylation assay along with very small amounts of chloramphenicol-1-acetate (R_f = 0.46) and chloramphenicol-1,3-diacetate (R_f = 0.83). Under conditions described above for diacetylation, there was a disappearance of the peaks at R_f = 0.60 and R_f = 0.46 and an accumulation of label at R_f = 0.83.

The benzene-extractable products of the monoacetylation and diacetylation systems were also subjected to analysis by gas-liquid chromatography. The benzene solution was evaporated as described, 100 μl of Tri-Sil (Applied Science) was added to form silylated derivates, and 0.5-μl samples were injected into the gas chromatograph. In the monoacetylation reaction, the peak corresponding to chloramphenicol disappeared with the subsequent appearance of a new peak of similar area at a longer retention time.

Standard curve. The dependence of the formation of product on chloramphenicol concentration was shown by standard curves made by assaying known amounts of chloramphenicol in water or acid-citrate-dextrose plasma. Conditions were selected such that the response was linear with chloramphenicol concentration from 1 to 50 μg/ml, using 10 μl of sample as shown in Fig. 3. The curve was similar whether

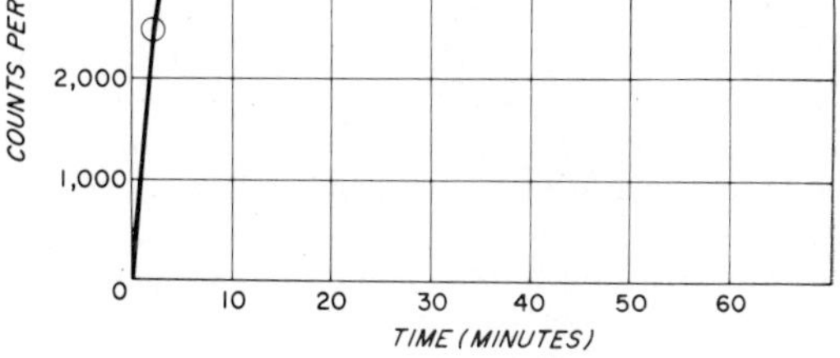

FIG. 2. *Time course of chloramphenicol monoacetylation.*

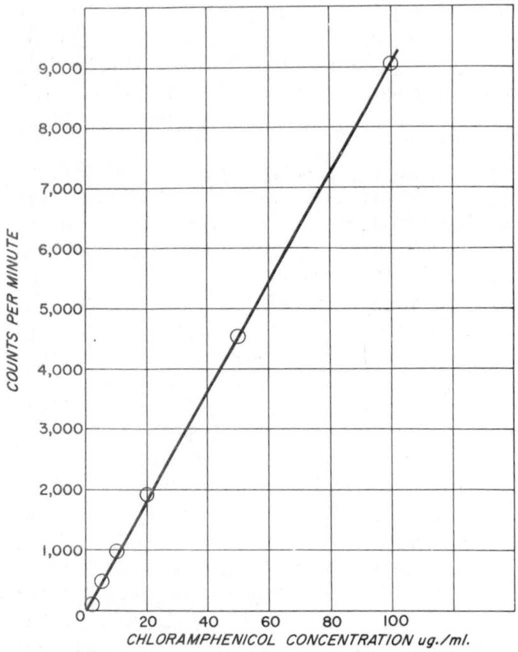

FIG. 3. *Standard curve of chloramphenicol.*

made in water or plasma.

Comparison of the enzymatic and gas-liquid chromatographic methods. The accuracy of the monoacetylation assay was substantiated by comparing the results with those obtained by the gas-liquid chromatographic method. The results on a series of 23 plasma samples from inpatients at The Johns Hopkins Hospital receiving chloramphenicol as part of their normal course of treatment are shown in Fig. 4. The correlation coefficient for these 23 samples is 0.98.

Specificity. A number of antibiotics, which might be used in conjunction with chloramphenicol at a clinical level, were tested for their ability to accept an acetyl group in the standard monoacetylation assay and for their ability to inhibit the acetylation of chloramphenicol that was present at a concentration of 50 μg/ml. The choice of drugs and the concentration at which each was tested are shown in Table 1. None of the drugs tested gave any radioactive counts extractable into benzene nor did they produce a decrease in the counts per minute found when incubated in the presence of chloramphenicol as compared with chloramphenicol alone. In addition, the formation of acetylated derivatives of the aminoglycoside antibiotics gentamicin, kanamycin, and tobramycin was examined by binding the reaction products to cation exchange resin loaded paper. No radioactivity was incorporated onto the paper disks under

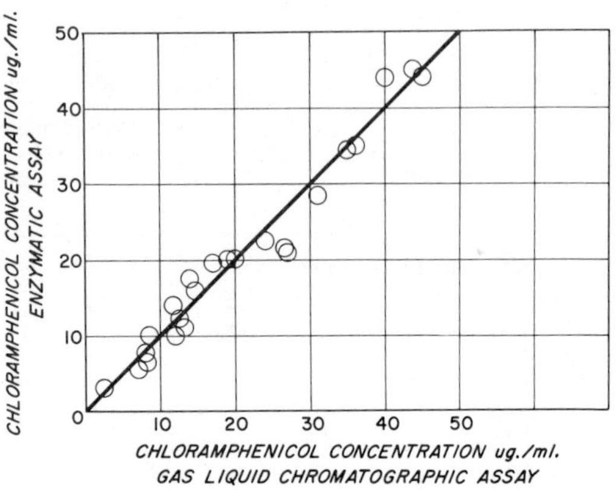

FIG. 4. *Chloramphenicol levels as measured by enzymatic and gas-liquid chromotographic methods.*

TABLE 1. *Antibiotics that are free from interference with the chloramphenicol assay*

Drug	Concn (μg/ml)
Methicillin	25
Ampicillin	25
Penicillin	5
Cephalothin	25
Tetracycline	5
Gentamicin	10
Kanamycin sulfate D	20
Tobramycin	20
Carbenicillin	125
Rifampin	10
Clindamycin	2
Sulfisoxazole	20
Erythromycin	2
Neomycin	10
Streptomycin	40
Oxytetracycline	5

conditions in which these drugs are known to be bound.

The results of the assay as applied to chloramphenicol sodium succinate, chloramphenicol glucuronide, and L-threo chlorampehnicol are shown in Table 2. Neither 1-threo chloramphenicol nor the sodium succinate ester of chloramphenicol was measured in the assay. Chloramphenicol glucuronide was also not detected. This conclusion is based on the fact that the enzymatic and gas-liquid chromatographic analyses of urine from a patient receiving chloramphenicol contained equal amounts of chloramphenicol; chloramphenicol glucuronide is known not to be measured by the chromatographic method. The addition of a known amount of chloramphenicol to the urine is accurately measured. The hydrolysis of chloramphenicol glucuronide by beta-glucuronidase yielded similar quantities when measured by

TABLE 2. *Inactivity of chloramphenicol assay for chloramphenicol succinate, chloramphenicol glucuronide, and L-threo chloramphenicol*

Sample	Chloramphenicol concn (μg/ml)	
	Enzymatic	GLC[a]
Chloramphenicol sodium succinate	0	0
L-threo chloramphenicol (50 μg/ml)	0	50
Control urine (without chloramphenicol)	0	ND[b]
Patient urine (2-g/day dose)	44	45
Patient urine + 10 μg of chloramphenicol "spike" per ml	54	ND
Patient urine treated with β-glucuronidase	240	250

[a] GLC, Gas-liquid chromatographic.
[b] ND, Not determined.

the enzymological or the chromatographic methods.

Thiamphenicol, an experimental drug similar in structure to chloramphenicol, was acetylated in the usual time period to an extent of about 40% of the amount expected for complete monoacetylation. Since this drug is not presently in clinical use in the United States and is unlikely to be used in conjunction with chloramphenicol in any case, its measurement should not interfere with the clinical usefulness of our assay.

Accuracy. The accuracy of the assay was assessed by adding a known amount of chloramphenicol to plasma already containing a measured level of chloramphenicol and repeating the assay. In a series of such "spiking" experiments on 10 different patient samples, the addition of 10 μg/ml was measured as an average of 11.5 μg/ml. We have not yet found the cause of the slightly higher values usually measured.

Reproducibility. The reproducibility of the assay was assessed by repeating the assay in duplicate 10 times on a single sample. The mean and standard deviation were 19.0 ± 0.8 μg/ml for one set of 10 samples. The same sample was also reassayed 10 times over a period of several weeks. The mean and standard deviation were 18.5 ± 0.8 μg/ml. All values presented in this paper are the averages of duplicate determinations.

Variation in standard curves. For a clinical assay, in which a large number of samples may need to be measured, it is of value to ascertain the necessity for generating a standard curve for each batch of samples. Eleven standard curves obtained over a 1-month period were compared and a mean standard curve was computed. The average deviation of points from the mean was ±7%. Therefore, once a standard curve has been established for a particular lot of radioactive acetyl coenzyme A, it should be sufficient to determine a background value and one standard concentration for comparison with the average standard curve.

Effects of hemolysis and jaundice. The accuracy of the assay was tested in the presence of plasma from hemolyzed blood and in jaundiced plasma obtained at an exchange transfusion. A 100-μg/ml standard of chloramphenicol in normal plasma was diluted to 20 μg/ml with normal, hemolyzed, or jaundiced plasma and the drug concentration was measured. Neither hemolyzed nor jaundiced plasma affected the determination of the chloramphenicol concentration since the chloramphenicol concentrations (in micrograms per milliliter) were as follows: normal plasma sample, 20; hemolyzed plasma, 20; and jaundiced plasma, 20.5.

Binding of chloramphenicol to serum proteins and erythrocytes. An assessment was made to determine whether the assay measures the free or total (free plus protein bound) chloramphenicol in plasma. Preliminary evidence, from the similarity of the extent of [^{14}C]acetate incorporation into chloramphenicol when standards were prepared in water and in plasma and from the similarity of values obtained by the enzymatic and gas-liquid chromatographic methods, indicated that the acetylation assay measures both free and bound drug. An equilibrium dialysis experiment was performed by suspending a dialysis bag containing 2 ml of plasma in 50 ml of a 0.1 M Tris buffer solution (pH 7.8) containing 20 μg of chloramphenicol per ml. The final concentrations of chloramphenicol inside and outside the dialysis bag were measured at equilibrium. If the assay measures only the free chloramphenicol, the concentration determined inside and outside the dialysis bag should have been equal. Since a higher level was measured inside the bag than in the dialysis solution (Table 3), the assay appears to measure both free and bound drug.

The effect of chloramphenicol binding to erythrocytes and its possible release upon hemolysis were also studied. Portions of a 100-μg standard of chloramphenicol per ml in plasma were diluted 1:5 with normal plasma and with whole blood. One of the blood samples was then incubated at 4°C for several hours to allow the chloramphenicol present to bind to the erythrocytes. Another blood sample containing chloramphenicol was hemolyzed by freezing and thawing, and then both samples were centri-

TABLE 3. *Chloramphenicol assay measuring plasma protein and bound and unbound chloramphenicol without interference from erythrocytes*

Determination	Chloramphenicol concn (μg/ml)	
	Enzymatic	GLC[a]
Equilibrium dialysis		
Final inside	35	36
Final outside	19.5	17
Binding to erythrocytes		
Normal plasma	20.5	
Blood + chloramphenicol, centrifuged	21.5	
Blood + chloramphenicol --→ hemolysis --→ centrifugation	20.5	

[a] GLC, Gas-liquid chromatographic.

fuged to remove intact erythrocytes or cell debris. The chloramphenicol concentrations of the supernatant fluids of each sample are shown in Table 3. Binding of chloramphenicol to erythrocytes with subsequent centrifugation or hemolysis does not affect the concentration of chloramphenicol measured in the supernatant.

Assay of chloramphenicol in biological fluids other than plasma. Chloramphenicol has been assayed by our method in plasma, serum, blood, cerebrospinal fluid, urine, peritoneal fluid after peritoneal dialysis, ascitic fluid, and synovial fluid. "Spiking" experiments on each of the fluids have failed to detect the presence of any inhibitory substances in these fluids that might interfere with the assay, and control experiments on plasma and urine in the absence of chloramphenicol suggest there are no natural substrates present that are acetylated and then extracted into benzene. Thus, the assay can be carried out on biological specimens from many sources.

DISCUSSION

Several methods have been described previously for the assay of chloramphenicol in biological fluids. Each of these has some advantages and each has limitations.

Perhaps, the most commonly used method continues to be the bioassay (3). Although the bioassay has the advantage of ease of performance, its sensitivity is limited, its precision appears to be variable, it requires at least several hours to complete, the specificity is poor in samples containing other antimicrobial agents, and specimens must be handled aspetically.

In an effort to improve on the bioassay, several colorimetric assays have been developed (1, 2, 4, 5, 9). Each of these measures the amine formed after reduction of the aromatic nitro group of chloramphenicol. Since chloramphenicol sodium succinate and chloramphenicol glucuronide both contain the nitro group, both are also measured and solvent extractions must be included to separate these from the chloramphenicol prior to the assay. Furthermore, none is designed to be done on a microscale, and all require at least 0.5 ml of blood for duplicate determinations.

Much greater sensitivity and specificity are provided by several gas-liquid chromatographic procedures utilizing either flame ionization (6, 7, 11) or electron capture (10, 15) detectors. These methods are time consuming, however, since a standard curve must be generated each day and a column must be dedicated to this assay.

The assay that we have developed overcomes each of the disadvantages of previous assays. Specificity is provided by the specificity of the enzyme that acetylates chloramphenicol but fails to acetylate any other known antibiotic (with the exception of the related thiamphenicol) or endogenous compound. Thus, chloramphenicol can be measured in the presence of other chemotherapeutic agents and other drugs without interference. We also have yet to find, in many hundreds of clinical assays, a plasma containing an inhibitor of the enzymatic reaction. Although this remains a theoretical possibility, it has not been realized to date. An appropriate degree of sensitivity is provided by the chosen specific activity of the [^{14}C]acetyl coenzyme A. Although greater sensitivity than we have used is possible with the use of acetyl coenzyme A of even high specific activity, our method allows the accurate determination of therapeutic concentrations of chloramphenicol with only 10 μl of plasma. Thus, our assay can be easily performed on the plasma recovered from two microhematocrit tubes. Counts that are double background are seen at levels of chloramphenicol of about 0.25 μg/ml, using 10 μl of plasma. The accuracy of our method, when compared with a gas chromatographic method or when considered in absolute terms, is excellent and the precision achieved is certainly comparable to or better than any other existing method. The time involved in the performance of the assay is small (about 2 h, including a standard curve) and the cost of the assay is low. The cost of our assay, excluding technician time, is estimated to be about 27¢ per tube. The disadvantages of our assay are minor. An enzyme must be prepared since, at the present time, the enzyme is not commercially available. This preparation takes little time, however, and the small amount used per assay coupled with the stability of the frozen enzyme allows one to perform about 1,000 assays from a single preparation that began with 900 ml of culture. Another potential disadvantage is the necessity for a liquid scintillation counter. Such instruments are, however, widely available and present in clinical laboratories in increasing numbers. The advantages of this new assay clearly outweigh the disadvantages, and we believe that it can be of great value in therapeutic monitoring.

ACKNOWLEDGMENTS

This work was supported by Public Health Service research grant AI 10741 from the National Institute of Allergy and Infectious Disease and was carried out in the Alan Bernstein Laboratories of Clinical Pharmacology, Johns Hopkins Hospital.

LITERATURE CITED

1. **Bessman, S. P., and S. Stevens.** 1950. A colorimetric method for the determination of chloromycetin in serum or plasma. J. Lab. Clin. Med. 35:129–135.
2. **Glazko, A. J., L. M. Wolf, and W. A. Dill.** 1949. Biochemical studies on chloramphenicol (chloromycetin). 1. Colorimetric methods for the determination of chloramphenicol and related nitro compounds. Arch. Biochem. 23:411–418.
3. **Hans, R., M. Galbraith, and W. C. Alegnani.** 1963. Chloramphenicol, p. 271–281. *In* F. Kavanagh (ed.), Analytical microbiology. Academic Press Inc., New York.
4. **Kakemi, K., T. Arita, and S. Ohashi.** 1962. Absorption and excretion of drugs. IV. Determination of chloramphenicol in blood. Yakugaku Zasshi 82:342–345.
5. **Levine, J., and H. Fischbach.** 1951. The chemical determination of chloramphenicol in biological materials. Antibiot. Chemother. 1:59–62.
6. **Margolis, M.** 1970. Analysis of antibiotics by gas chromatography. II. Chloramphenicol. J. Chromatogr. 47:341–347.
7. **Margolis, M.** 1974. GLC analysis of chloramphenicol: a collaborative study. J. Pharm. Sci. 63:435–437.
8. **Nossal, N. G., and L. A. Heppel.** 1966. The release of enzymes by osmotic shock from *Escherichia coli* in exponential phase. J. Biol. Chem. 241:3055–3062.
9. **O'Gorman Hughes, D. W., and L. K. Diamond.** 1964. Chloramphenicol in blood: simple chemical estimations in patients receiving multiple antibiotics. Science 144:296–297.
10. **Resnick, G. L., D. Corbin, and D. H. Sandberg.** 1966. Determination of serum chloramphenicol utilizing gas-liquid chromatography and electron capture spectrometry. Anal. Chem. 38:582–585.
11. **Shaw, P. D.** 1963. Gas chromatography of trimethylsilyl derivatives of compounds related to chloramphenicol. Anal. Chem. 35:1580–1582.
12. **Shaw, W. V.** 1967. The enzymatic acetylation of chloramphenicol by extracts of R factor-resistant *Escherichia coli*. J. Biol. Chem. 242:687–693.
13. **Shaw, W. V.** 1975. Chloramphenicol acetyltransferase from chloramphenicol-resistant bacteria, p. 737–755. *In* John H. Hash (ed.), Methods in enzymology, vol. XLIII, Antibiotics. Academic Press Inc., New York.
14. **Suzuki, Y., and S. Okamoto.** 1967. The enzymatic acetylation of chloramphenicol by the multiple drug-resistant *Escherichia coli* carrying R factor. J. Biol. Chem. 242:4722–4730.
15. **Yamamoto, M., S. Iguchi, and T. Aoyama.** 1967. Determination of chloramphenicol by gas-liquid chromatography. Chem. Pharm. Bull. 15:123–127.

ANTIMICROBIAL AGENTS AND CHEMOTHERAPY, Aug. 1976, p. 354-362
Vol. 10, No. 2
Printed in U.S.A.

Inhibition of *Neisseria gonorrhoeae* by a Bacteriocin from *Pseudomonas aeruginosa*

STEPHEN A. MORSE,* PATRICK VAUGHAN, DEANNE JOHNSON, AND BARBARA H. IGLEWSKI

Department of Microbiology and Immunology, University of Oregon Health Sciences Center, Portland, Oregon 97201

Received for publication 26 March 1976

Supernatants from broth-grown cultures of *Pseudomonas aeruginosa* PA 103 exhibited bactericidal activity against *Neisseria gonorrhoeae*. The concentration of the bactericidal substance increased significantly after induction by mitomycin C. Purification was effected by salt fractionation, chromatography on diethylaminoethyl-cellulose, and sedimentation by centrifugation at 100,000 × *g* for 90 min. Electron microscopy of this purified preparation revealed structures resembling R-type pyocins in both the contracted and uncontracted state. Pyocins in the contracted state were observed in association with the gonococcal cell surface. No loss of bactericidal activity was observed after treatment with proteolytic enzymes. Standard pyocin typing procedures identified the pyocin pattern as 611 131. The bactericidal activity of this pyocin was examined on various species of *Neisseria*. Out of 56 strains of *N. gonorrhoeae* from disseminated and nondisseminated infections, all were susceptible to pyocin 611 131. However, only 3 of 20 strains of *N. meningitidis* and 5 of 16 strains of *N. lactamica* were susceptible. The bactericidal activity that pyocin 611 131 has for *N. gonorrhoeae* and other species of *Neisseria* is significant because it departs from the expected specificity that heretofore has distinguished bacteriocins from most "classical" antibiotics.

Flynn and McEnteggart (11) reported the presence of bacteriocin-like activity in isolates of *Neisseria gonorrhoeae*. However, Knapp et al. (32) and Walstad et al. (47) were unable to demonstrate bacteriocinogeny in *N. gonorrhoeae*. The bacteriocin-like activity exhibited by many strains of *N. gonorrhoeae* was attributed to the production of inhibitory levels of free fatty acids and lysophosphatidylethanolamine (47). Substances from other organisms have also been reported to exhibit bacteriocin-like activity against *N. gonorrhoeae*. Volk and Kraus (46) reported the in vitro inhibition of *N. gonorrhoeae* by a meningococcal bacteriocin, and Geizer (12) reported the inhibition of gonococcal growth by unidentified substances produced by strains of *Vibrio cholerae, Escherichia coli, Aeromonas hydrophilia, Micrococcus* spp., and *Pseudomonas aeruginosa*. We have also observed a marked inhibition of gonococcal growth by culture supernatants of *P. aeruginosa*. The isolation, characterization, and identification of this inhibitory factor(s) are the subjects of this investigation.

MATERIALS AND METHODS

Organisms. Clinical isolates of *N. gonorrhoeae* were used in these studies. The specific properties of strains CS-7, JW-31, and 72H870 were previously reported (38, 40). Strains from disseminated gonococcal infections (DGI strains) were obtained from K. Holmes (U.S. Public Health Service Hospital, Seattle, Wash.). Additional clinical isolates from nondisseminated gonococcal infections were obtained from the Multnomah County Health Department, Portland, Ore. Known serological types of *N. meningitidis* were obtained from H. Schneider (Walter Reed Army Institute of Research, Washington, D.C.). Strains of *N. lactamica* and other species of *Neisseria* were obtained from D. Hollis and D. Kellogg, Jr. (Center for Disease Control, Atlanta, Ga.). The identity of all organisms was confirmed by cell morphology in Gram-stained smears, oxidase reaction, and the production of acid from specific carbohydrates (39). T-1 and T-4 colony types (31) from single clinical isolates were subcultured and maintained by selective passage.

A nonproteolytic strain of *P. aeruginosa* (PA-103) (34) was obtained from P. V. Liu (University of Kentucky, Lexington). This strain was used throughout this investigation as a source of R-type pyocin. The titer of the crude and purified pyocin preparations was determined using *P. aeruginosa* strain PS-7 (10) (obtained from E. Fisher, Portland State University, Portland, Ore.).

Medium. The basal medium contained the following per liter: proteose peptone no. 3 (Difco), 15 g; K_2HPO_4, 4 g; KH_2PO_4, 1 g; NaCl, 5 g; and soluble starch, 1 g. The final pH of the medium was 7.2.

When used for the production of R-type pyocins by *P. aeruginosa*, glycerol (1%, vol/vol) and monosodium glutamate (8.46 g/liter) were added after autoclaving. When used for the growth of *Neisseria* spp., a growth factor supplement (1%, vol/vol), identical in composition to IsoVitaleX enrichment (BBL) but lacking glucose, $NaHCO_3$ (42 mg/liter), and glucose (5 g/liter) were added after autoclaving. GC agar (Difco) plates containing glucose (5 g/liter) and growth factor supplement (1%, vol/vol) were used where indicated.

Induction and purification of R-type pyocins. An overnight culture of *P. aeruginosa* was centrifuged (2,100 × *g* for 10 min) and resuspended to 1/10 the original volume in a solution containing 0.85% NaCl and 0.1% cysteine hydrochloride at pH 6.5. A 1% (vol/vol) inoculum was used, and the cultures were incubated on a gyratory shaker at 37°C. When the turbidity of the culture reached approximately 150 Klett units, mitomycin C was added at a final concentration of 1 μg/ml. Incubation was continued until extensive lysis of the culture occurred (see Fig. 1). This lysis normally occurred within 3 h after the addition of mitomycin C. The mitomycin C-induced culture was centrifuged at 2,400 × *g* for 30 min to remove cellular debris, and the resulting supernatant was treated with chloroform (5%, vol/vol). This supernatant fraction was designated crude pyocin.

Crude pyocin preparations were further purified by a modification (14) of the method of Kageyama and Egami (29). Briefly, this procedure consisted of the slow addition of 1 M $MnCl_2$ (60 ml/liter of lysate), while stirring, to the crude pyocin preparation. After adjusting the pH to 7.5 with 1 M NaOH, the resulting precipitate was removed by centrifugation (2,400 × *g* for 15 min). The supernatant was designated partially purified pyocin.

Further purification was accomplished by the addition of $(NH_4)_2SO_4$ to 70% saturation and incubation overnight at 4°C. After centrifugation (2,400 × *g* for 30 min) at 4°C, the pellet containing the pyocin activity was dissolved in 50 ml of 0.01 M tris(hydroxymethyl)aminomethane (Tris)-hydrochloride (pH 7.5) containing 0.01 M $MgCl_2$ and 0.01 M $MgSO_4$ and dialyzed overnight at 4°C against 2 liters of the same buffer. If necessary, the preparation was clarified by centrifugation (2,400 × *g* for 15 min at 4°C). The pyocin preparation was then centrifuged at 100,000 × *g* for 90 min (type 40 rotor, Spinco model L2-65B ultracentrifuge). The gelatinous pellet was gently dissolved in 20 ml of buffer and chromatographed on diethylaminoethyl (DEAE)-cellulose (DE-52, Whatman Biochemicals Ltd., Kent, England) previously washed and equilibrated with the same buffer. An 8-ml sample of pyocin was applied to a column (1.5 by 28 cm) and allowed to adsorb for 1 h. The column was washed with 200 ml of buffer to remove material not adsorbing to the DEAE-cellulose. The pyocins were then eluted with 800 ml of an NaCl gradient (0 to 1.0 M) in 0.01 M Tris buffer containing 0.01 M $MgCl_2$ and $MgSO_4$. Five-milliliter fractions were collected and analyzed for absorbance at 280 nm and pyocin activity. The fractions exhibiting pyocin activity were pooled, dialyzed against 0.01 M Tris buffer containing 0.01 M $MgCl_2$ and 0.01 M $MgSO_4$ to remove NaCl, and then concentrated by ultracentrifugation (100,000 × *g* for 90 min). All chromatographic procedures were carried out at 4°C.

Pyocin typing. Pyocin typing was performed using the broth method as described by Jones et al. (27). The ALA set of 18 strains of *P. aeruginosa* (obtained from B. H. Minshew, University of Washington School of Medicine) was used for indicator strains (27). The pyocin type and pattern are reported by the notation described by Farmer and Herman (9).

Assay of pyocin activity. Organisms being tested for susceptibility to R-type pyocins were grown overnight on GC agar plates. A suspension of these organisms was prepared in a diluent consisting of 0.85% NaCl and 0.1% HCl (pH 6.4) and adjusted to a Klett reading of 50 to 60. GC agar plates were inoculated by means of a swab dipped into the cell suspension. Undiluted or serially diluted pyocin preparations (5 μl) were applied to the surface of the agar plate. All plates were incubated overnight at 37°C with increased CO_2 (5% CO_2) prior to being read. Pyocin titers are expressed as 200 times the highest dilution that shows complete inhibition.

ADP-ribosyl transferase activity. An enzyme mixture containing aminoacyl transferase activity was prepared from crude extracts of rabbit reticulocytes by a modification (6) of the method of Allen and Schweet (1). Adenosine diphosphate (ADP)-ribosyl transferase was measured by the procedure of Collier and Kandel (6). Briefly, the assay mixture in a total volume of 65 μl contained 50 mM Tris-hydrochloride (pH 8.2), 0.1 mM disodium ethylenediaminetetraacetic acid, 40 mM dithiothreitol, 25 μl of the reticulocyte enzyme mixture, 0.367 μM [^{14}C-adenine] nicotinamide adenine dinucleotide (Schwarz/Mann; specific activity, 136 mCi/mmol), and various amounts of purified pyocin preparation, *P. aeruginosa* exotoxin A, or diphtheria toxin fragment A as indicated. The reaction mixture was incubated at 25°C for 5 min and then stopped by the addition of 65 μl of 10% trichloroacetic acid. The acid-insoluble precipitates were collected, washed, and counted on a Nuclear-Chicago low background counter as previously described (20).

P. aeruginosa exotoxin A was produced and purified by the method of Liu (35) as previously described (19). Diphtheria toxin fragment A was kindly provided by R. J. Collier (Department of Bacteriology, University of California at Los Angeles). Protein was determined by the method of Lowry et al. (36) using bovine serum albumin as a standard.

Protease treatment of R-type pyocins. Purified pyocins were diluted to a final concentration of 1 × 10^4 U/ml in 0.01 M Tris-hydrochloride buffer (pH 7.5) containing 0.01 M $MgCl_2$ and 0.01 M $MgSO_4$. Protease from *Streptomyces griseus* (type VI, Sigma Chemical Co., St. Louis) or from *Bacillus subtilis* (type VIII, Sigma Chemical Co.) was added at a final concentration of 1.0 mg/ml. The susceptibility of the pyocin to trypsin was tested by preparing a similar dilution in 0.05 M Tris-hydrochloride buffer (pH 8.1) containing 0.01 M $CaCl_2$; trypsin (type III,

Sigma Chemical Co.) was added at a final concentration of 0.5 mg/ml. Controls diluted in the appropriate buffer were also included. All samples were incubated at 37°C for 3 h and then titered against *P. aeruginosa* strain PS-7 and *N. gonorrhoeae* JW-31.

Electron microscopy. Pyocins were prepared for examination in an electron microscope by the negative-staining technique of Brenner and Horne (4). Pyocin preparations were centrifuged at 100,000 × *g* for 1 h, and the pellet was resuspended in a small volume of 1 M $NH_4C_2H_3O_2$ (pH 7.0). Formvar-covered copper grids were placed onto a drop of the sample for 1 to 2 min and then blotted dry with filter paper. These grids were then placed onto a drop of 1.5% sodium phosphotungstate (pH 7.0) for 30 s. Excess fluid was removed with filter paper. Samples were examined in a Phillips EM-200 electron microscope at 60 kV.

The interaction of pyocins with cells of *N. gonorrhoeae* was observed by a similar procedure. At 30 min after the addition of pyocin to a liquid culture of *N. gonorrhoeae* 72H870, a sample was removed and treated as above. The negative-stained preparation was examined in an RCA electron microscope at 50 kV.

RESULTS

Purification and characterization of the inhibitory factor. Geizer (12) observed that the growth of *N. gonorrhoeae* was inhibited by a substance(s) produced during the growth of a strain of *P. aeruginosa*. We have confirmed this phenomenon and, further, have sought to isolate and identify the inhibitory substance(s). The inhibitory factor was produced in low concentration during the growth of *P. aeruginosa* strain PA-103 in a complex medium (Table 1). Addition of mitomycin C (1 μg/ml) caused extensive lysis of the culture within 3 h (Fig. 1) and resulted in a 16-fold increase in the concentration of the inhibitory factor (Table 1) as determined by titration on *P. aeruginosa* PS7 and *N. gonorrhoeae* strains JW-31 and DGI 1947. The titer of the inhibitory factor varied with different strains of *N. gonorrhoeae* (Table 1); no difference was observed with colonial variants of a single strain. The inducible nature of this factor suggested the involvement of a bacteriophage or bacteriophage product. However, no plaques were observed when dilution of supernatants from both induced and noninduced cultures were spotted on *N. gonorrhoeae* strain JW-31. Instead, the area of growth inhibition increased in turbidity with increasing dilution, suggesting the presence of a nonreplicating bacteriocin.

The inhibitory factor was partially purified from supernatants of mitomycin C-induced cultures of *P. aeruginosa* strain PA-103 by a procedure used for pyocin purification. Further purification was obtained by DEAE-cellulose chromatography (Fig. 1). The inhibitory factor was

TABLE 1. *Effect of mitomycin C on the production of gonococcal inhibitory factor by P. aeruginosa PA-103*[a]

Organism	Inhibitory titer (U/ml)	
	Non-induced	Induced
P. aeruginosa PS-7	2560	40,960
N. gonorrhoeae JW-31	2560	40,960
N. gonorrhoeae DGI 1947	640	10,240
N. gonorrhoeae 1138 (T-1)	ND[b]	5,120
N. gonorrhoeae 1138 (T-4)	ND	5,120

[a] Mitomycin C (1 μg/ml of medium), when serially diluted, ceased to inhibit the growth of these organisms at a >1:2 dilution (0.5 μg/ml).
[b] ND, Not determined.

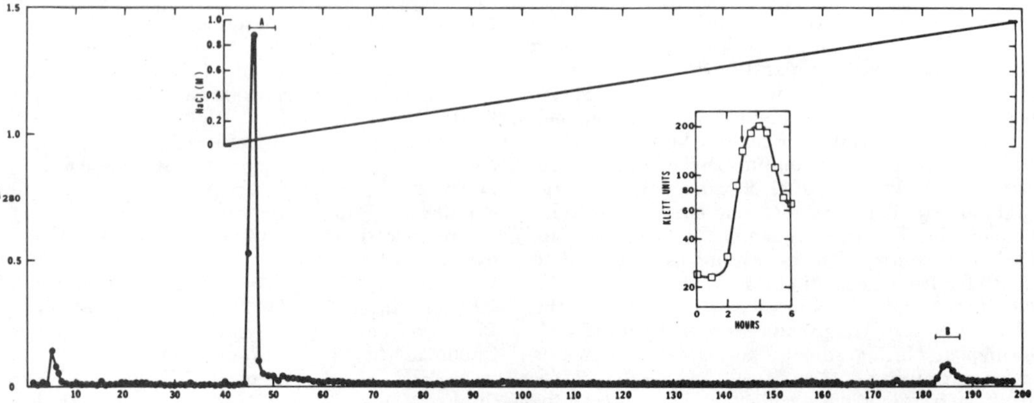

FIG. 1. *Purification of R-type pyocin (611 131) by DEAE-cellulose chromatography. Fractions containing inhibitory activity are indicated by A and B. Insert: induction of pyocin production in P. aeruginosa PA-103 by mitomycin C (1 μg/ml). The arrow indicates time of mitomycin C addition.*

eluted with an NaCl gradient of 0 to 1.0 M. Two peaks containing the inhibitory factor were observed. The major peak (A) eluted at an NaCl concentration of 0.06 M and contained more than 90% of the inhibitory activity. A minor peak (B) eluted at an NaCl concentration of 0.91 M and contained less than 10% of the activity. The fractions comprising peak A were pooled, dialyzed against 0.01 M Tris-hydrochloride buffer (pH 7.5) to remove the NaCl, and concentrated by ultracentrifugation (100,000 × *g* for 90 min). This preparation was used for the remainder of these studies.

Negative-stained preparations of the purified inhibitory factor were examined in the electron microscope. Particles resembling R-type pyocins were observed in both the uncontracted and contracted states (Fig. 2). In the uncontracted state, these particles measured 111.5 nm in length by 15.3 nm in width. In the contracted state, the particles consisted of an inner core (105 nm in length by 6.5 nm in width) surrounded by a contracted sheath (44.4 nm in length by 18.6 nm in width). Between 20 and 30% of the particles observed in these preparations were in the contracted state. Neither intact bacteriophage nor bacteriophage ghosts were seen in any of the negative-stained preparations.

The type of the pyocin in both partially purified and purified preparations was determined as described above. The results (data not shown) indicate that the pattern did not change during purification and suggest that one or more pyocin types were not removed during chromatography on DEAE-cellulose. The pyocin pattern is 611 131.

R-type pyocins may be differentiated from S-type pyocins by their resistance to proteolytic enzymes (24). Therefore, the effect of various proteolytic enzymes was examined on the inhibition of *P. aeruginosa* PS-7 and *N. gonorrhoeae* JW-31 by purified pyocin preparation. The results (not shown) indicate that the concentration did not decrease when compared with an untreated concentration of 1 × 10^4 U/ml. These data suggest that the inhibition of *N. gonorrhoeae* was not due to an S-type pyocin.

Many strains of *P. aeruginosa* produce a protein toxin (exotoxin A) that inhibits mammalian protein synthesis (20). The toxin catalyzes the transfer of the ADP-ribose moiety of nicotinamide adenine dinucleotide to elongation factor-2, resulting in an ADP-ribosyl-elonga-

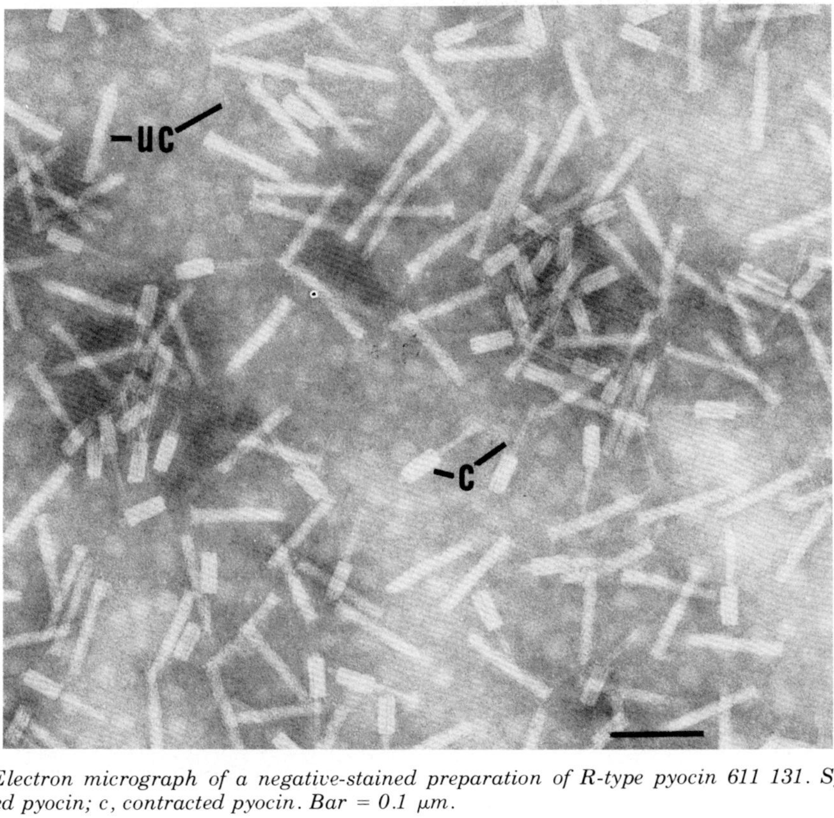

FIG. 2. *Electron micrograph of a negative-stained preparation of R-type pyocin 611 131. Symbols: uc, uncontracted pyocin; c, contracted pyocin. Bar = 0.1 μm.*

tion factor-2 complex which is inactive in peptide chain elongation (19, 20). The possibility that the inhibition of *N. gonorrhoeae* was due to the presence of this toxin in the pyocin preparation was investigated. The results (Table 2) show that neither the crude nor the purified preparation from *P. aeruginosa* strain PA-103 contains ADP-ribosyl transferase activity. Thus, it seems unlikely that the inhibitory effect of the pyocin preparation is due to exotoxin A.

Effect of R-type pyocin on the growth of *N. gonorrhoeae*. The effect of R-type pyocin on growing cells of *N. gonorrhoeae* strain 72H870 was examined by the addition of various concentrations of the purified preparation to exponentially growing cultures. Figure 3 shows a concentration-dependent inhibition of gonococcal growth by the addition of type 611 131 pyocin. At high pyocin concentrations, a complete inhibition of growth occurred within 1 h and was accompanied by extensive lysis of the culture. To ascertain whether a direct interaction occurred between the pyocin and susceptible cells of *N. gonorrhoeae*, samples were removed from the culture after 30 min and examined by electron microscopy. The results (Fig. 4) demonstrate the binding of pyocins to the surface of the cell. The pyocin-cell interaction appears to result in contraction of the pyocin. No significant association of type 611 131 pyocin occurred with the cell surface of a resistant organism (*N. ovis*). These data suggest that receptors are present on the cell surface of *N. gonorrhoeae*.

Inhibitory spectrum of pyocin type 611 131. Portions of the purified pyocin preparation were spotted on lawns prepared from clinical isolates of *N. gonorrhoeae*. Typical patterns of inhibition are shown in Fig. 5. The zone of inhibition was clearly evident in all strains examined. No difference was observed between colony types T-1 and T-4 from the same strain. A negative control of the producer strain, *P. aeruginosa* PA-103, was also included.

TABLE 2. *ADP-ribosyl transferase activity in preparations of R-type pyocin (611 131) from P. aeruginosa strain PA-103*

Additions	Protein (μg)	Acid-insoluble radioactivity (cpm)
Control[a]	0	121
Crude R-type pyocin	7.0	73
Purified R-type pyocin	5.0	96
Exotoxin A	0.01	2,788
Diphtheria toxin fragment A	0.01	2,839

[a] The control contained water in place of toxin or pyocin preparation.

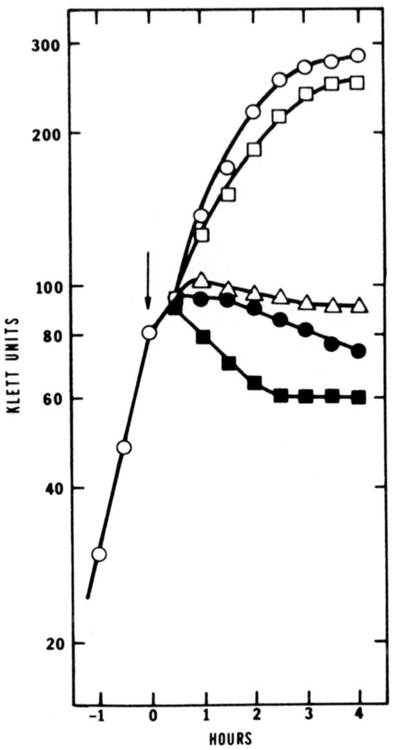

FIG. 3. *Effect of R-type pyocin (611 131) on the growth of N. gonorrhoeae strain 72H870. Purified pyocin was added to exponentially growing cultures (1.4 × 10^8 colony-forming units/ml) of strain 72H870. Symbols:* ○, *no additions;* □, *400 U of pyocin per ml;* △, *1,000 U of pyocin per ml;* ●, *4,000 U of pyocin per ml;* ■, *20,000 U of pyocin per ml.*

The inhibition of various *Neisseria* species by this pyocin is shown in Table 3. All isolates of *N. gonorrhoeae*, from both disseminated and nondisseminated infections, were inhibited. However, only 3 of 20 strains of *N. meningitidis* and 5 of 16 strains of *N. lactamica* were inhibited. No correlation was observed between the serological group and inhibition of *N. meningitidis*. None of the other five species tested was inhibited by this pyocin.

DISCUSSION

Bacteriocins are antibiotic substances produced by many species of bacteria which are thought to be inhibitory for strains of the same or closely related species (42). Bacteriocins are protein in nature and range from simple proteins (7, 33) to particles resembling bacteriophage components (3, 5, 14, 16, 22, 26). Bacteriocinogenic strains of *P. aeruginosa* produce several types of bacteriocins (17). The synthesis of these bacteriocins can be increased by mitomycin C treatment (17, 24, 28). These bacterio-

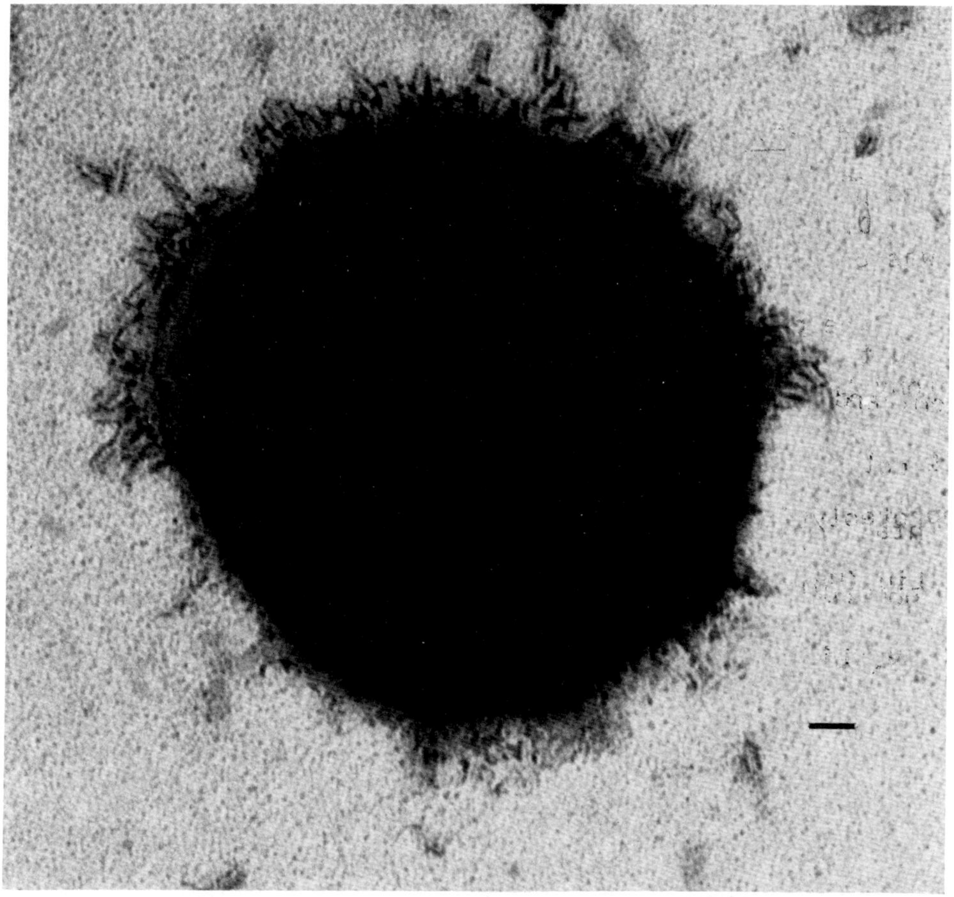

FIG. 4. *Interaction of R-type pyocin 611 131 with cells of N. gonorrhoeae strain 72H870. Bar = 0.1 μm.*

cins may be grouped into one of two types (3): the S-type bacteriocins, which are characterized by susceptibility to proteolytic enzymes and a lack of structure in electron microscopy, and the R-type bacteriocins, which are not susceptible to proteolytic enzymes and exhibit the appearance of bacteriophage components. The bacteriocins produced by *P. aeruginosa* are called pyocins (25).

In addition to resistance to proteolytic enzymes, R-type pyocins may be differentiated from S-type pyocins by their adsorption to DEAE-cellulose, molecular weight, rate of diffusion in agar, and neutralization by specific antiserum (24). R-type pyocins bear a close resemblance to the tails of T-even bacteriophage (14, 16, 18, 22, 28). Govan (14) reported that, regardless of the pyocinogenic strain used, the majority of the R-type particles measured approximately 100 by 15 nm in the uncontracted state; contracted particles consisted of a hollow inner core, approximately 100 by 7 nm, partially enclosed in a sheath measuring about 45 by 17 nm. Our findings indicate that the gonococcal inhibitory factor produced by *P. aeruginosa* PA-103 was an R-type pyocin. Several lines of evidence support this conclusion. The inhibitory factor was resistant to proteolytic enzymes and adsorbed to DEAE-cellulose. Sedimentation of the inhibitory factor by ultracentrifugation (100,000 × *g* for 90 min) suggests that this substance has a high molecular weight. The same susceptibility pattern (611 131) was always observed when the inhibitory factor was typed on the ALA strains of *P. aeruginosa*. Furthermore, electron microscopy revealed particles with the same morphology and size as those reported by Govan (14). No tail fibers were observed in negative-stained preparation of 611 131 as previously reported in other R-type pyocins (16, 18).

R-type pyocins may be found in both the contracted and uncontracted state (14, 16). Only uncontracted pyocins will adsorb to and kill

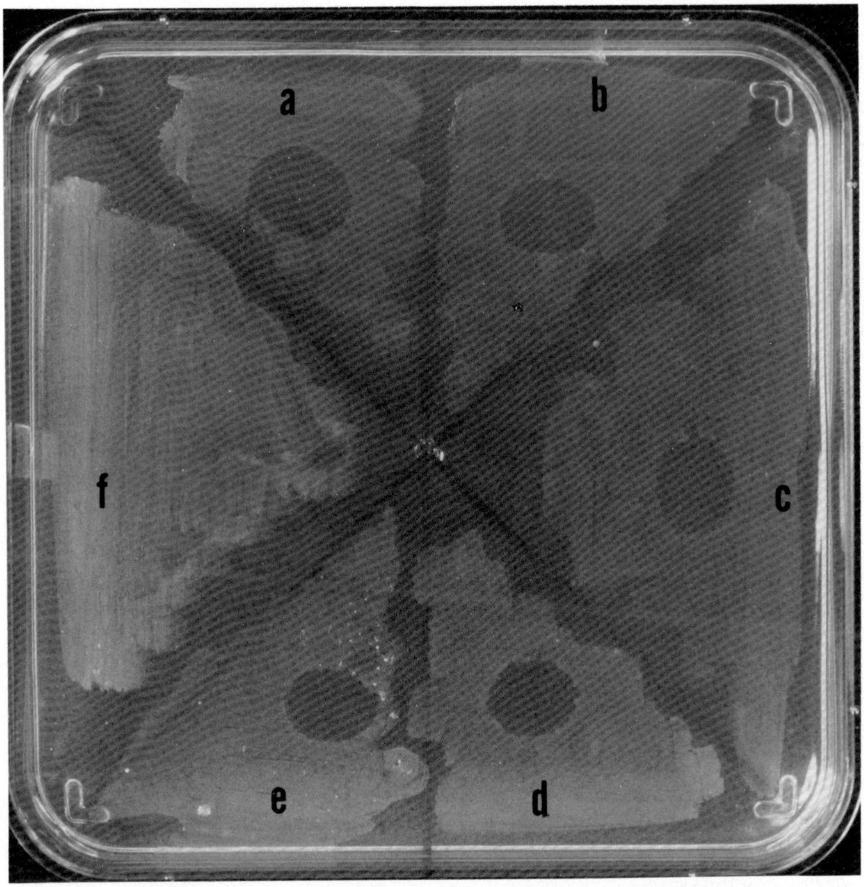

FIG. 5. *Inhibition of N. gonorrhoeae by an R-type pyocin (611 131). (a) N. gonorrhoeae strain JW-31; (b) N. gonorrhoeae strain 72H870; (c) N. gonorrhoeae strain 1138 (colony type T-1); (d) N. gonorrhoeae strain 1138 (colony type T-4); (e) N. gonorrhoeae strain CS-7; (f) P. aeruginosa strain PA-103.*

TABLE 3. *Susceptibility of various Neisseria species to purified R-type pyocin (611 131) from P. aeruginosa strain PA-103*

Species	Serogroup	No. of strains tested	No. of strains susceptible
N. gonorrhoeae		56	56
N. meningitidis	A	4	0
	B	5	1
	C	3	0
	X	3	0
	Y	1	1
	Z	2	1
	135	2	0
N. lactamica		16	5
N. mucosa		1	0
N. flava		1	0
N. subflava		1	0
N. ovis		1	0
N. flavescens		1	0

susceptible cells (14, 16); no adsorption to pyocin-resistant bacteria occurs (14). Lethal effects occur after the contraction of bound pyocins (14). We have demonstrated that R-type pyocin 611 131 adsorbs to the surface of *N. gonorrhoeae*. The presence of contracted pyocins on the gonococcus suggests that receptor sites on *N. gonorrhoeae* may be similar to those that exist on the cell surface of certain strains of *P. aeruginosa*. Of special interest are studies involving shared antigens between heterologous bacterial species. Minden et al. (37) demonstrated that *Pseudomonas* shared an indeterminate number of antigens with other gram-negative bacteria. The presence of naturally occurring antibodies to *N. gonorrhoeae* (13) suggests that this organism may also share antigenic determinants with heterologous bacterial species. This possibility is supported by the study of Robbins et al. (43), which showed that *N. meningitidis* groups A and C share capsular and noncapsular antigenic determinants with strains of *E. coli*.

The lipopolysaccharide (LPS) has been implicated as the receptor for R-type bacteriocins in *P. aeruginosa* (8, 14, 15, 21, 23) and in some strains of *Serratia marcescens* (45). The bacteriocin receptor in other strains of *S. marcescens* is reported to be proteinaceous (45). The receptor for pyocin 611 131 on *N. gonorrhoeae* has not as yet been identified. However, a receptor located on the O polysaccharide portion of the gonococcal LPS appears unlikely. We observed identical titers of 611 131 on T-1 and T-4 colonial variants from the same clinical isolate. Perry et al. (41) determined that LPS from T-1 cells contained a high-molecular-weight O polysaccharide that showed considerable variation between strains. This O polysaccharide was absent in T-4 cells. To the contrary, Stead et al. (44) were unable to detect O polysaccharide side chains in LPS isolated from either T-1 or T-4 cells. In addition, pyocin 611 131 inhibited strains of *N. gonorrhoeae* isolated during a 5-year period from Boston, Mass., Portland, Ore., and Seattle, Wash. Strains from these diverse locales would be expected to show variability in the composition of the O polysaccharide side chain as previously reported by Perry et al. (41). Alternatively, the receptor may reside in a common core region of the LPS. This core oligosaccharide may be sufficiently similar in *N. gonorrhoeae*, *N. meningitidis*, and *N. lactamica* to account for the inhibition observed in the latter two species. However, the possibility of a protein receptor cannot be excluded at this time.

A capsule may afford some measure of protection against the bactericidal activity of pyocin 611 131. The presence of a capsule in the resistant strains of *N. meningitidis* and *N. lactamica* has not been determined. This capsule could conceivably hinder the binding of the pyocin to its receptor. A similar phenomenon has been observed with respect to the inhibition of bacteriophage binding to encapsulated bacteria (48).

Allen and Kelly (2) observed that the titer of a given pyocin frequently varied with different strains of *P. aeruginosa*. These investigators proposed that the closeness of fit between the reactive portion of the pyocin and its receptor determined the potency of its bactericidal activity. An alternate hypothesis is that the variation in titer reflects the number of receptor sites per cell. Strains containing a large number of pyocin receptors per cell would exhibit a lower titer than would strains having fewer receptors per cell. Either hypothesis may explain the variation in titer observed with different strains of *N. gonorrhoeae*.

The mechanism of pyocin-induced killing of *N. gonorrhoeae* is not known. Kageyama et al. (30) identified a muramidase-like enzyme as a component of R-type pyocins. This enzyme could account for the rapid lysis of gonococcal cultures that were exposed to high concentrations of pyocin. However, other effects, such as an inhibition of macromolecular synthesis or other cell functions that may ultimately lead to cell lysis, cannot be eliminated at this time.

In summary, the results of this study indicate that the gonococcal inhibitory factor observed in culture supernatants of *P. aeruginosa* PA-103 is the R-type pyocin 611 131. The ability of pyocin 611 131 to inhibit *N. gonorrhoeae* suggests that either the definition of a bacteriocin with regards to species specificity needs to be reevaluated or that there is a much closer taxonomic relationship between *Neisseria* and *Pseudomonas* than heretofore suspected.

ACKNOWLEDGMENTS

This research was supported by grants from the Medical Research Foundation of Oregon and Phi Beta Psi Sorority.

LITERATURE CITED

1. **Allen, E. S., and R. S. Schweet.** 1962. Synthesis of hemoglobin in a cell-free system. J. Biol. Chem. 237:760–767.
2. **Allen, J. C., and P. C. Kelly.** 1975. Antigenic heterogeneity among pyocins of *Pseudomonas aeruginosa*. Infect. Immun. 12:318–323.
3. **Bradley, D. E.** 1967. Ultrastructure of bacteriophages and bacteriocins. Bacteriol. Rev. 31:230–314.
4. **Brenner, S., and R. W. Horne.** 1959. A negative staining method for high resolution electron microscopy of viruses. Biochim. Biophys. Acta 34:103–110.
5. **Coetzee, H. L., H. C. de Klerk, J. N. Koetzee, and J. A. Smit.** 1968. Bacteriophage tail-like particles associated with intraspecies killings of *Proteus vulgaris*. J. Gen. Virol. 2:29–36.
6. **Collier, R. J., and J. Kandel.** 1971. Structure and activity of diphtheria toxin. I. Thiol-dependent dissociation of a fraction of toxin into enzymatically active and inactive fragments. J. Biol. Chem. 246:1496–1503.
7. **Dandeau, J. P.** 1971. Chemical and immunological study of colicins E_1, K, A, and Q. Infect. Immun. 3:1–9.
8. **Dyke, J., and R. S. Berk.** 1974. Growth inhibition and pyocin receptor properties of endotoxin from *Pseudomonas aeruginosa*. Proc. Soc. Exp. Biol. Med. 145:1405–1408.
9. **Farmer, J. J., III, and L. G. Herman.** 1974. Pyocin typing of *Pseudomonas aeruginosa*. J. Infect. Dis. 130:543–546.
10. **Feary, T. W., E. Fisher, and T. N. Fisher.** 1963. Lysogeny and phage resistance in *Pseudomonas aeruginosa*. Proc. Soc. Exp. Biol. Med. 113:426–430.
11. **Flynn, J., and M. C. McEnteggart.** 1971. Bacteriocins from *Neisseria gonorrhoeae* and their possible role in epidemiological studies. J. Clin. Pathol. 25:60–61.

12. **Geizer, E.** 1968. Antibacterial substances produced by different bacteria inhibiting the growth of *Neisseria gonorrhoeae*. J. Hyg. Epidemiol. Microbiol. Immunol. 12:241–243.
13. **Glynn, A. A., and M. E. Ward.** 1970. Nature and heterogeneity of the antigens of *Neisseria gonorrhoeae* involved in the serum bactericidal reaction. Infect. Immun. 2:162–168.
14. **Govan, J. R. W.** 1974. Studies on the pyocins of *Pseudomonas aeruginosa:* morphology and mode of action of contractile particles. J. Gen. Microbiol. **80:**1–15.
15. **Govan, J. R. W.** 1974. Studies on the pyocins of *Pseudomonas aeruginosa:* production of contractile and flexous pyocins in *Pseudomonas aeruginosa*. J. Gen. Microbiol. **80:**17–30.
16. **Higerd, T. B., C. A. Baechler, and R. S. Berk.** 1969. Morphological studies on relaxed and contracted forms of purified pyocin particles. J. Bacteriol. **98:**1378–1389.
17. **Holloway, B. W., and V. Krishnapillai.** 1975. Bacteriophages and bacteriocins, p. 99–132. *In* P. H. Clarke and M. H. Richmond (ed.), Genetics and biochemistry of *Pseudomonas*. John Wiley and Sons, New York.
18. **Homma, J. Y., S. Goto, and H. Shionoya.** 1967. Relationship between pyocin and temperate phage of *Pseudomonas aeruginosa*. II. Isolation of pyocins from strain P 1-III and their characteristics. Jpn. J. Exp. Med. 37:373–393.
19. **Iglewski, B. H., L. P. Elwell, P. V. Liu, and D. Kabat.** 1976. ADP-ribosylation of elongation factor 2 by *Pseudomonas aeruginosa* exotoxin A and by diphtheria toxin, p. 62–69. *In* S. Shaltiel (ed.), Proceedings of the 4th International Symposium on the Metabolic Interconversion of Enzymes. Springer-Verlag, New York.
20. **Iglewski, B. H., and D. Kabat.** 1975. NAD-dependent inhibition of protein synthesis by *Pseudomonas aeruginosa* toxin. Proc. Natl. Acad. Sci. U.S.A. **72:**2284–2288.
21. **Ikeda, K., and F. Egami.** 1969. Receptor substance for pyocin R. I. Partial purification and chemical properties. J. Biochem. **65:**603–609.
22. **Ishii, S., Y. Nishi, and F. Egami.** 1965. The fine structure of a pyocin. J. Mol. Biol. **13:**428–431.
23. **Ito, S., and M. Kageyama.** 1970. Relationship between pyocins and a bacteriophage in *Pseudomonas aeruginosa*. J. Gen. Appl. Microbiol. **16:**231–240.
24. **Ito, S., M. Kageyama, and F. Egami.** 1970. Isolation and characterization of pyocins from several strains of *Pseudomonas aeruginosa*. J. Gen. Appl. Microbiol. **16:**205–214.
25. **Jacob, F.** 1954. Biosynthese induite et mode d'action d'une pyocine, antibiotique de *Pseudomonas pyocyanea*. Ann. Inst. Pasteur Paris **86:**149–160.
26. **Jayawardene, A., and H. Farkas-Himsley.** 1969. Vibriocin; a bacteriocin from *Vibrio comma*. I. Production, purification, morphology, and immunological studies. Microbios **1:**87–98.
27. **Jones, L. F., J. P. Zakanycez, E. T. Thomas, and J. J. Farmer III.** 1974. Pyocin typing of *Pseudomonas aeruginosa:* a simplified method. Appl. Microbiol. **27:**400–406.
28. **Kageyama, M.** 1964. Studies of a pyocin. I. Physical and chemical properties. J. Biochem. **55:**49–53.
29. **Kageyama, M., and F. Egami.** 1962. On the purification and some properties of a pyocin, a bacteriocin produced by *Pseudomonas aeruginosa*. Life Sci. **9:**471–476.
30. **Kageyama, M., K. Ikeda, and F. Egami.** 1964. Studies of a pyocin. III. Biological properties of the pyocin. J. Biochem. 55:59–64.
31. **Kellogg, D. S., Jr., W. L. Peacock, Jr., W. E. Deacon, L. Brown, and C. I. Pirkle.** 1963. *Neisseria gonorrhoeae*. I. Virulence genetically linked to clonal variation. J. Bacteriol. **85:**1274–1279.
32. **Knapp, J. S., S. Falkow, and K. K. Holmes.** 1975. Reevaluation of bacteriocinogeny in *Neisseria gonorrhoeae*. J. Clin. Pathol. **28:**274–278.
33. **Kramer, J., and H. Brandis.** 1975. Purification and characterization of two bacteriocins from *Streptococcus faecium*. J. Gen. Microbiol. **88:**93–100.
34. **Liu, P. V.** 1966. The roles of various fractions of *Pseudomonas aeruginosa* in its pathogenesis. II. Effects of lecithinase and protease. J. Infect. Dis. **116:**112–116.
35. **Liu, P. V.** 1973. Exotoxins of *Pseudomonas aeruginosa*. I. Factors that influence the production of exotoxin A. J. Infect. Dis. **128:**506–513.
36. **Lowry, O. H., N. J. Rosebrough, A. L. Farr, and R. J. Randall.** 1951. Protein measurement with the Folin phenol reagent. J. Biol. Chem. **193:**265–275.
37. **Minden, P., J. K. McClatchy, and R. S. Farr.** 1972. Shared antigens between heterologous bacterial species. Infect. Immun. **6:**574–582.
38. **Morse, S. A., and L. Bartenstein.** 1974. Factors affecting autolysis of *Neisseria gonorrhoeae*. Proc. Soc. Exp. Biol. Med. **145:**1418–1421.
39. **Morse, S. A., and L. Bartenstein.** 1976. Adaptation of the minitek system for the rapid identification of *Neisseria gonorrhoeae*. J. Clin. Microbiol. **3:**8–13.
40. **Morse, S. A., S. Stein, and J. Hines.** 1974. Glucose metabolism in *Neisseria gonorrhoeae*. J. Bacteriol. **120:**702–714.
41. **Perry, M. B., V. Daoust, B. B. Diena, F. E. Ashton, and R. Wallace.** 1975. The lipopolysaccharides of *Neisseria gonorrhoeae* colony types 1 and 4. J. Microbiol. **53:**623–629.
42. **Reeves, P.** 1965. The bacteriocins. Bacteriol. Rev. **29:**24–45.
43. **Robbins, J. B., R. L. Myerowitz, J. K. Whisnant, M. Argaman, R. Schneerson, Z. T. Handzel, and E. C. Gotschlich.** 1972. Enteric bacteria cross-reactive with *Neisseria meningitidis* groups A and C and *Diplococcus pneumoniae* types I and III. Infect. Immun. **6:**651–656.
44. **Stead, A., J. S. Main, M. E. Ward, and P. J. Watt.** 1975. Studies on lipopolysaccharides from strains of *Neisseria gonorrhoeae*. J. Gen. Microbiol. **88:**123–131.
45. **Traub, W. H., and I. Kleber.** 1974. Studies on group A (phage tail) bacteriocins of *Serratia marcescens*. IV. Preliminary characterization of receptors of subgroup II bacteriocins. Zentralbl. Bakteriol. Parasitenkd. Infektionskr. Hyg. Abt. I Orig. A **229:**490–502.
46. **Volk, J., and S. J. Kraus.** 1973. Asymptomatic meningococcal urethritis: possible protective value against gonococcal infection by bacteriocin production. Br. J. Vener. Dis. **49:**511–512.
47. **Walstad, D. L., R. C. Reitz, and P. F. Sparling.** 1974. Growth inhibition among strains of *Neisseria gonorrhoeae* due to production of inhibitory free fatty acids and lysophosphatidylethanolamine: absence of bacteriocins. Infect. Immun. **10:**481–488.
48. **Wilkinson, J. F.** 1958. The extracellular polysaccharides of bacteria. Bacteriol. Rev. **22:**46–73.

Antimicrobial Agents and Chemotherapy, Aug. 1976, p. 363-369
Vol. 10, No. 2

Formation of Methylated and Phosphorylated Metabolites During the Fermentation Process of Verdamicin

B. K. LEE,* R. G. CONDON, G. H. WAGMAN, and M. J. WEINSTEIN
Microbiological Sciences, Schering Corporation, Bloomfield, New Jersey 07003

Received for publication 19 April 1976

In an attempt to understand the biosynthetic processes leading to the formation of verdamicin (end product), we have examined the patterns of the formation of methylated and phosphorylated metabolites, which resulted from either the addition of L-[*methyl*-^{14}C]methionine or [^{32}P]KH_2PO_4 to the fermentation. Incorporation of label from L-[*methyl*-^{14}C]methionine into the bioactive sisomicin, verdamicin, and the chromatographically polar components increased with the progression of time. Two methylated bioinactive metabolites were found in the culture broth after removal of the methylated bioactive metabolites. In contrast to the bioactive metabolites, incorporation of the *methyl*-^{14}C label into the two methylated bioinactive metabolites decreased with the progression of time. A phosphorylated bioinactive metabolite (nonmethylated) was also found in the culture broth, fermented in the presence of [^{32}P]KH_2PO_4. The role of the phosphorylated metabolite in the biosynthesis of the bioactive metabolites cannot yet be explained.

The origins of the methyl groups of gentamicins and sisomicin have been studied and reported (2–4; B. K. Lee, R. G. Condon, G. H. Wagman, M. J. Weinstein, and E. Katz, manuscript in preparation). After recent findings in our laboratories that L-[*methyl*-^{14}C]methionine is an excellent methyl donor to verdamicin, as it is for the gentamicins and sisomicin, the patterns of the formation of both bioactive and nonbioactive methylated metabolites during the verdamicin fermentation processes were examined.

The accumulation of a phosphorylated streptomycin in the culture broth of *Streptomyces griseus* is known (5–7), and the subsequent hydrolysis of the phosphorylated antibiotic to streptomycin by an enzyme, produced in the cells of the same organism, has been reported (11). Uridine-5′-pyrophosphate derivatives were isolated from a penicillin-treated culture broth of *Staphylococcus aureus* (8–10). The verdamicin-producing *Micromonospora grisea* strain has been fermented in the presence of [^{32}P]KH_2PO_4, and a crude ^{32}P-labeled metabolite has been isolated from the spent portion of the fermentation broth.

MATERIALS AND METHODS

Strain. *M. grisea,* NRRL 3800, was used throughout the investigation.

Fermentation. Procedures similar to those described in reference 12 were used, except that 30 μCi of L-[*methyl*-^{14}C]methionine, 24 μCi of [^{32}P]KH_2PO_4, or 1.9 μCi of ^{14}C-labeled "B" fraction (as described in the following section) was added at 24 h after inoculation.

Fractionation of metabolites. After harvest of the fermentation broth (50 ml each in 300-ml flasks) at various time intervals (days 3, 5, and 7), 0.5 g of oxalic acid was added, and the pH of the broth was brought to 2.0 with 12 N H_2SO_4. The acidified fermentation broth was shaken for 1 h at 28°C and neutralized with concentrated NH_4OH. The neutralized broth was centrifuged, and 1.5 g of IRC-50 resin (Rohm and Haas) in NH_4^+ form was added to the supernatant. The mixture (resin and supernatant) was shaken for 1 h at 28°C, the solution was decanted into another flask, and the resin was washed three times with distilled water. The washed resin was eluted twice with 15-ml portions of 2 N NH_4OH, and the combined eluates were concentrated to dryness to obtain fraction designated "A." To the spent portion, which was decanted into another flask after the adsorption of the A fraction on the IRC-50 resin, 1.5 g of IR-120 resin (Rohm and Haas) in Na^+ form was added, and the mixture (resin and the spent portion) was shaken for 1 h at 28°C. The solution was decanted, and the resin was washed three times with distilled water. The washed resin was eluted twice with 15-ml portions of 2 N NH_4OH, and the combined eluates were concentrated to dryness to obtain the designated "B" fraction.

Bioassay and radioactivity assay. Previously described procedures (4, 12) were used.

Paper chromatography. Chromatograms of the A and the B fractions were developed in a descending system of the lower phase of chloroform-methanol-17% ammonia (2:1:1 by volume) and in an ascending system of *n*-propanol-pyridine-acetic acid-water

(15:10:3:12), respectively, on Whatman no. 1 filter paper.

RESULTS

Methylated metabolites in A fraction. After addition of L-[*methyl*-^{14}C]methionine at 24 h, a time course study of incorporation of label into the methylated metabolites showed a progressive increase of the incorporation into the A fraction, in contrast to that into the B fraction (see the section, Fractionation of metabolites, in Materials and Methods; Table 1). Five radioactivity peaks representing (i) the polar components, (ii) a bioinactive component (IA2), which migrated between the polar components and sisomicin, (iii) sisomicin, (iv) verdamicin, and (v) a least polar bioinactive component (IA1) were observed (Table 2, Fig. 1 and 2). Radioactivity incorporated into all of the five peaks increased in parallel with the progression of time. The early (3-day) sample showed only three radioactivity peaks, representing the polar components, the IA2 component, and sisomicin. The other two peaks, representing verdamicin and the IA1 component, showed up in the late samples (Fig. 2).

Methylated metabolites in B fraction. There were at least five ninhydrin-positive bioinactive metabolites present in the B fraction, and two (components 2 and 5) of the five were methylated metabolites (Fig. 3). The weight of the B fraction was approximately seven to eight times greater than that of the A fraction in all cases. Of 30 μCi of radioactive methionine added at 24 h, 3.83 μCi was incorporated into the B fraction of the 3-day sample. This represents a 32-fold ratio of the radioactivity as compared with that found in the A fraction. The ratio of the radioactivity incorporated, respectively, into the B and A fractions decreased from 32:1 in day 3, to 6:1 in day 5, and to 4:1 in day 7 (Table 2, Fig. 2 and 3). In other words, both methylated components 2 and 5 in the B fraction showed the highest radioactivity in the early stage of the fermentation, but lost radioactivity gradually as the fermentation progressed further. The loss of the radioactivity was much greater in the case of component 2, as compared with component 5 (Table 1, Fig. 3).

Phosphorylated metabolite in B fraction. Of 24 μCi of [^{32}P]KH_2PO_4 added at 24 h, 0.08 μCi was found to be incorporated into the B fraction of a 7-day sample. Out of the five ninhydrin-positive metabolites present in the B fraction, only one radioactive component (B. K. Lee et al., manuscript in preparation) was detectable (Fig. 4). Thus, component 4 was phosphorylated and ninhydrin positive, but a nonmethylated metabolite.

Bioconversion of B fraction to A fraction. When a verdamicin fermentation was conducted in the presence of *methyl*-^{14}C-labeled B fraction (28.9 mg, containing 1.9 μCi of radioactivity) added at 24 h, radioactivity incorporated

TABLE 1. *Fractionation of metabolites*

Duration of fermentation[a] (days)	Fraction A				Fraction B			
	Wt (mg)	Bioactivity (mg)	Radioactivity		Wt (mg)	Bioactivity (μg)	Radioactivity	
			nCi	%[b]			nCi	%
3	8.1	0.18	120	0.4	58.3	0	3,830	12.8
5	7.9	1.82	390	1.3	66.9	0	2,200	7.4
7	8.0	2.04	510	1.7	61.2	0	2,020	6.7

[a] Fermentation was conducted in 50 ml of medium in a 300-ml flask containing 30 μCi of L-[*methyl*-^{14}C]methionine added at 24 h.
[b] Percentage of radioactivity incorporated.

TABLE 2. *Radioactivity incorporated into the components of the A and the B fractions*

Duration of fermentation (days)	Fraction A										Fraction B			
	IA1 component		Verdamicin		Sisomicin		IA2 component		Polar components		Component 2		Component 5	
	nCi	%[a]	nCi	%	nCi	%	nCi	%	nCi	%	nCi	%	nCi	%
3	0	0	0	0	10	9.2	3	2.8	95	88.0	2,220	58.0	1,610	42.0
5	19	5.0	0	0	50	13.2	11	2.9	300	79.0	740	33.6	1,460	66.4
7	45	8.5	46	8.7	120	22.7	17	3.2	300	56.8	670	33.2	1,350	66.8

[a] Percentage of radioactivity distribution.

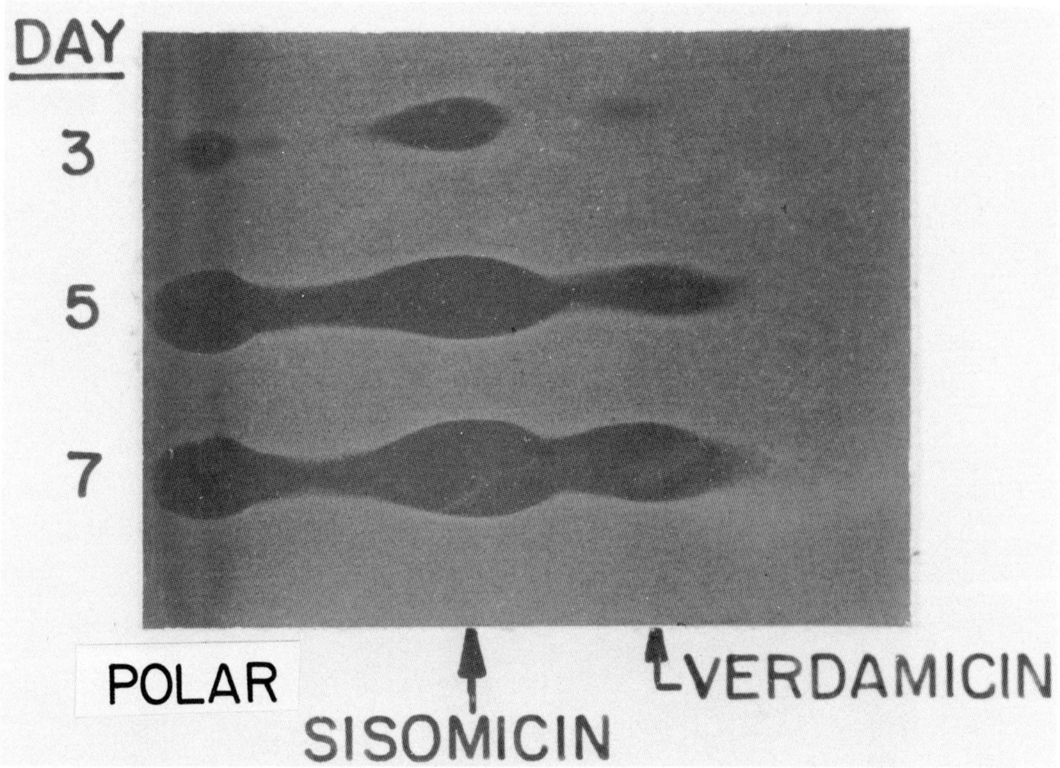

FIG. 1. *Bioautogram of A fractions, developed in a descending system of the lower phase of chloroform-methanol-17% ammonia (2:1:1, by volume) on Whatman no. 1 paper. Top to bottom, Verdamicin, sisomicin, polar components. Left to right, 3-, 5-, and 7-day samples.*

into the A fraction and the residual radioactivity in the B fraction were 0.024 μCi and 0.9 μCi, respectively. Sixty-seven and thirty-three percent of the radioactivity in the A fraction were distributed into the polar components and the IA2 component, respectively (Fig. 5).

DISCUSSION

At least five methylated ninhydrin-positive components were seen in the A fraction. Two methylated ninhydrin-positive components, and a phosphorylated but nonmethylated ninhydrin-positive component, were found in the B fraction. Among these components, only the mixture of the polar components, sisomicin, and verdamicin of the A fraction were bioactive. In contrast with the sisomicin fermentation, no bioactive components, corresponding to the two isomers of 4″-C-desmethyl-sisomicin (1), were detectable.

In the early stage of fermentation, high incorporation of label from L-[*methyl*-^{14}C]methionine into components 2 and 5 of the B fraction was observed. The radioactivity incorporated into these two components decreased with the progression of time, and the decreasing rate in component 2 was much greater than in component 5. When the isolated *methyl*-^{14}C-labeled fraction B was added to a verdamicin fermentation broth, 1% of the label in the B fraction was incorporated into the polar components and the IA2 component of the A fraction. Presumably, these results suggest that the methylated components 2 and 5 of the B fraction may be utilized as precursors for the polar components and the IA2 component of the A fraction.

In the early stage of the fermentation, the radioactive polar components and traces of the radioactive IA2 component and sisomicin appeared in the A fraction. During fermentation, a trace amount of the radioactive IA1 component was detectable in addition to those three (previously noted) radioactive components. At the end of the fermentation, a substantial amount of radioactive verdamicin appeared, and radioactivity, incorporated into the five methylated components of the A fraction, was detected in the increasing order: the polar com-

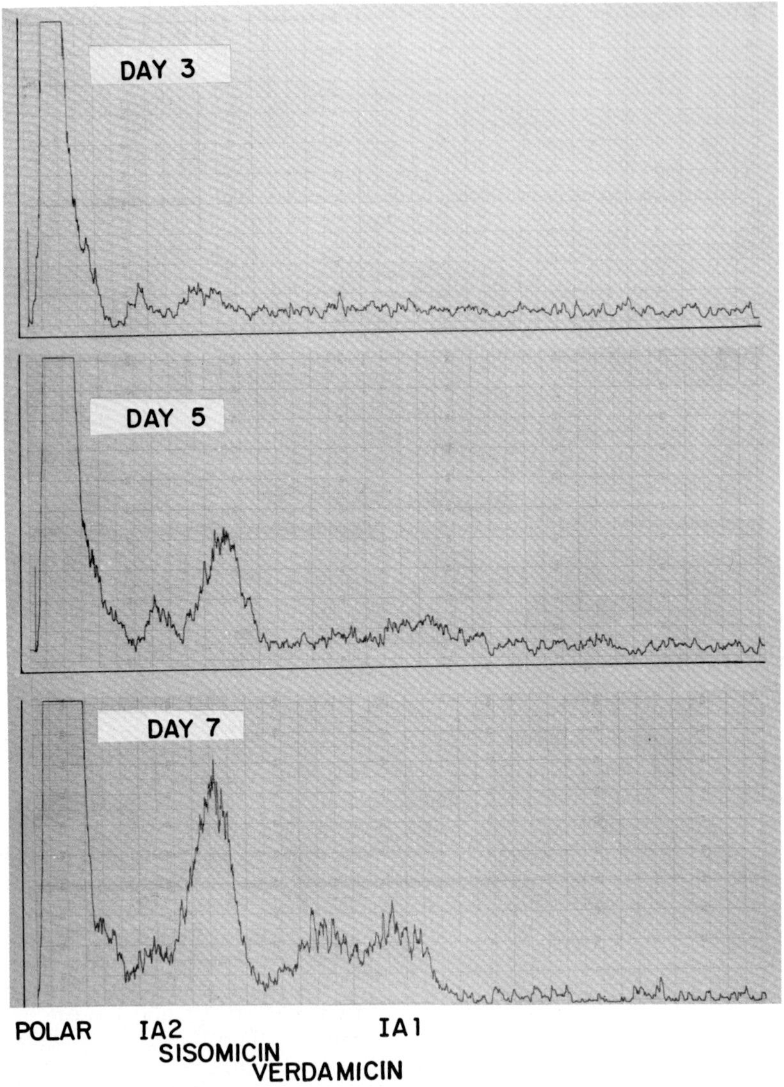

FIG. 2. *Radioactivity scans of A fractions developed in chloroform-methanol-ammonia. Top to bottom, 3-, 5-, and 7-day samples. Left to right, Polar components, IA2 component, sisomicin, verdamicin, and the IA1 component.*

FIG. 3. *Radioactivity scans of ninhydrin-treated B fractions developed in an ascending system of n-propanol-pyridine-acetic acid-water (15:10:3:12, by volume) on Whatman no. 1 paper. Top to bottom, Respective radioactivity scans and the ninhydrin-treated metabolites of the B fractions of 3-, 5-, and 7-day samples. Left to right, Components 5 (radioactive), 4, 3, 2 (radioactive), and 1.*

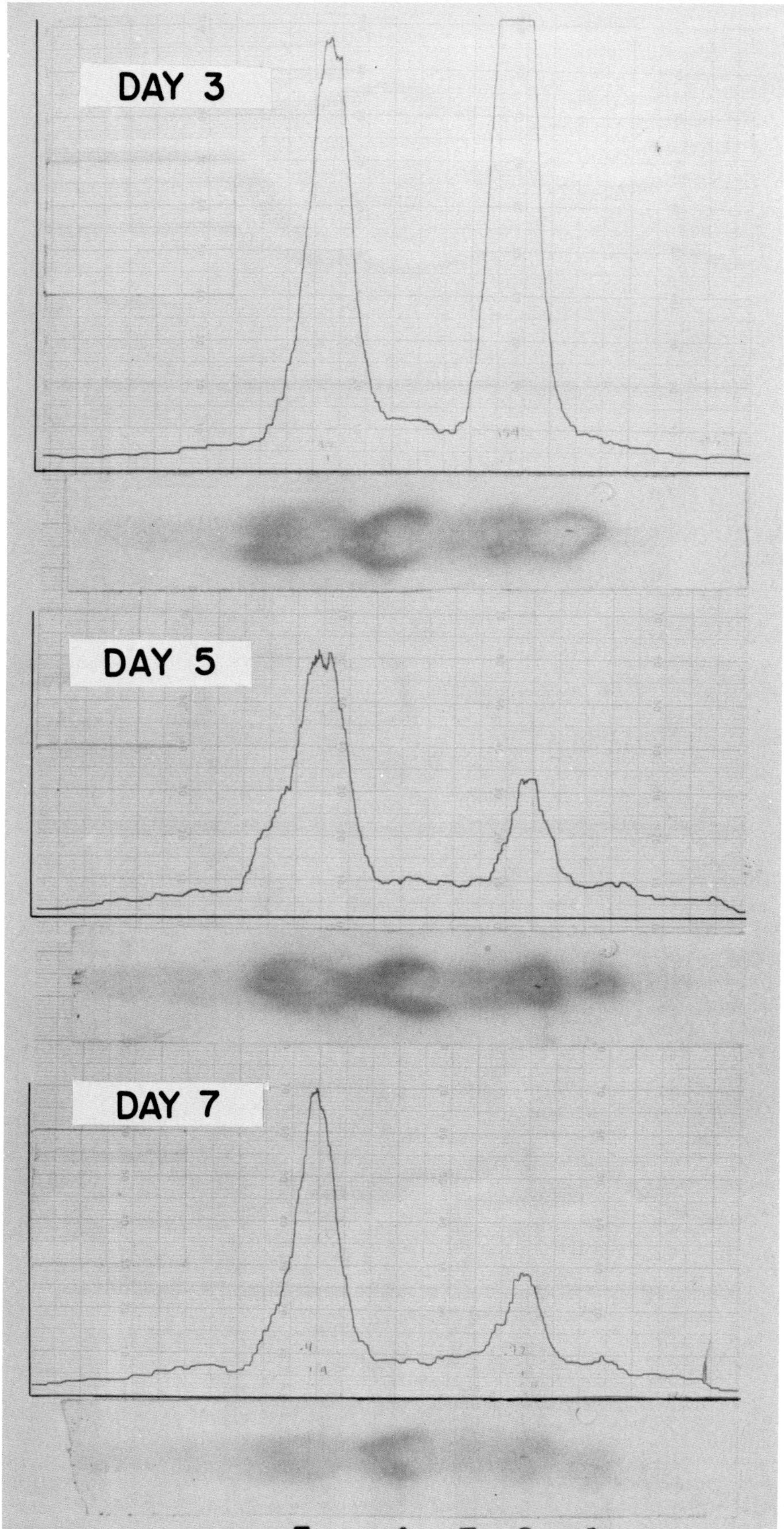

DAY 3
DAY 5
DAY 7
5 4 3 2 1

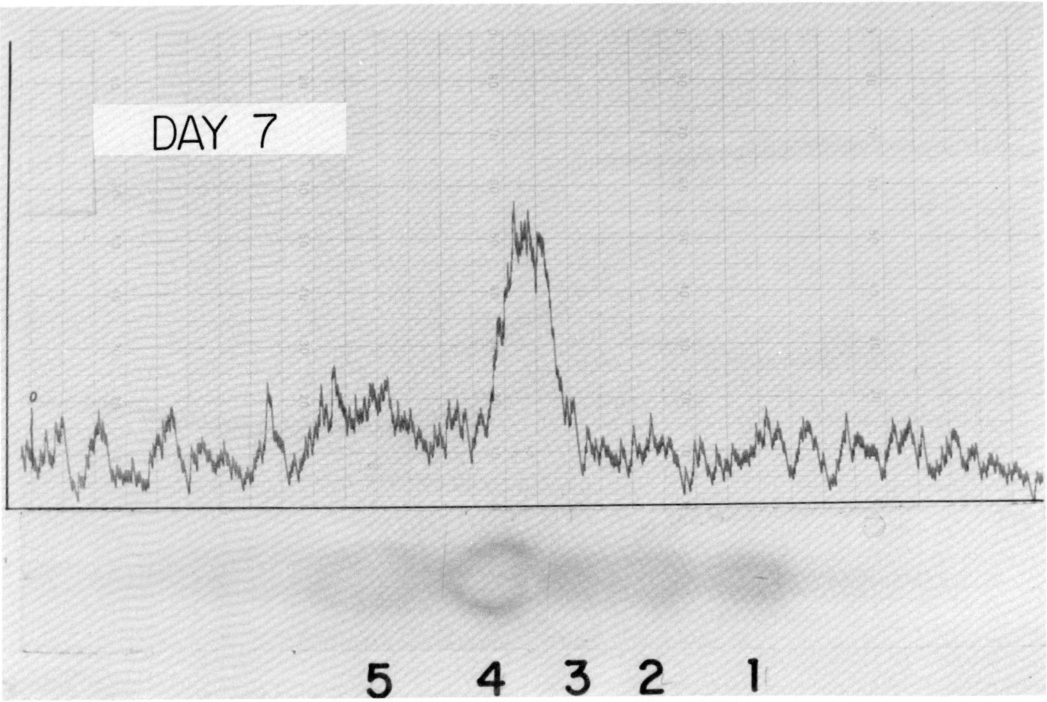

FIG. 4. *Radioactivity scan of a ninhydrin-treated B fraction of a 7-day sample, developed in propanol-pyridine-acetic acid-water. Left to right, Ninhydrin-positive components 5, 4 (^{32}P labeled), 3, 2, and 1.*

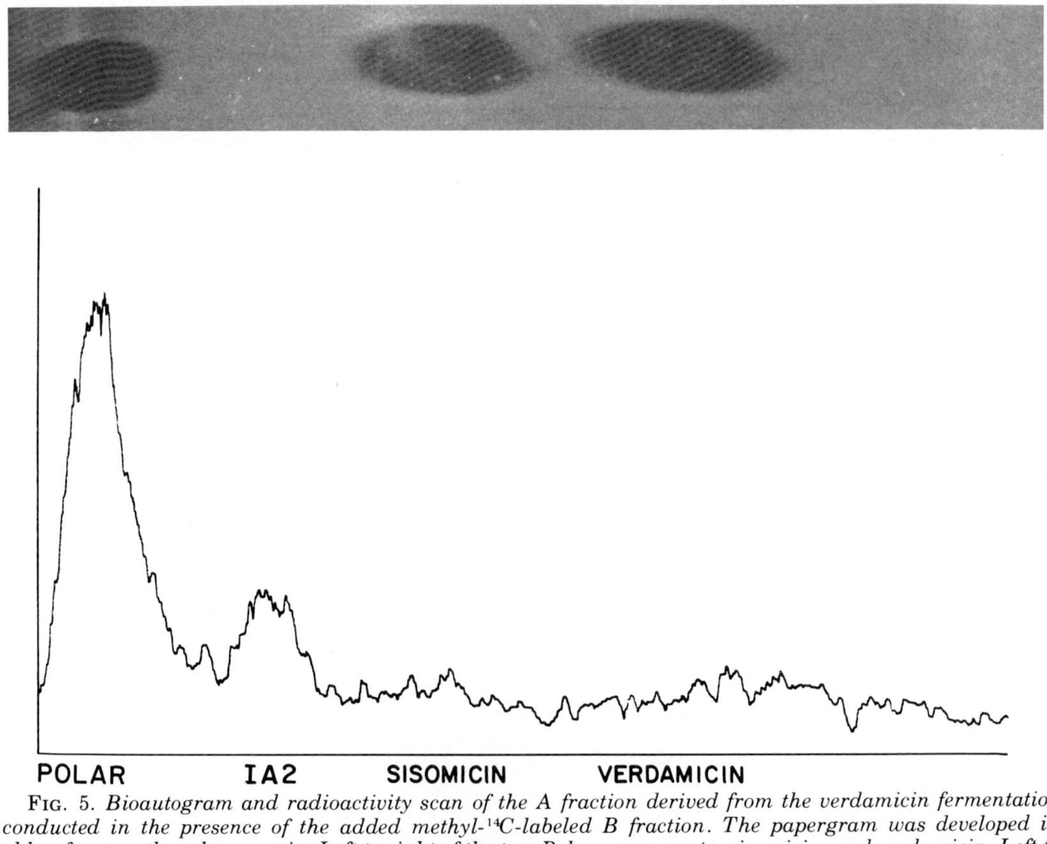

FIG. 5. *Bioautogram and radioactivity scan of the A fraction derived from the verdamicin fermentation conducted in the presence of the added methyl-^{14}C-labeled B fraction. The papergram was developed in chloroform-methanol-ammonia. Left to right of the top, Polar components, sisomicin, and verdamicin. Left to right of the bottom, Radioactive peaks corresponding to the polar components and the IA2 component. Note that no radioactive peaks representing sisomicin or verdamicin were found.*

ponents > sisomicin > verdamicin > the IA1 component > the IA2 component. At present, little is known about how these different methylated metabolites are involved in the biosynthesis of verdamicin.

The phosphorylated metabolite (component 4) present in the B fraction has not yet been characterized. Characterization of this metabolite will be very useful in learning the roles played by the substance on the biosynthesis of verdamicin.

ACKNOWLEDGMENTS

We wish to express gratitude to J. A. Marquez and R. Jaret for their criticisms and suggestions, and to D. Buffardi for typing the manuscript.

LITERATURE CITED

1. **Davis, D. H., D. Greeves, A. K. Mallams, J. B. Morton, and R. W. Tkach.** 1975. Structures of the aminoglycoside antibiotics 66-40B and 66-40D produced by *Micromonospora inyoensis*. J. Chem. Soc. Perkin Trans. 1:814–818.
2. **Lee, B. K., R. G. Condon, G. H. Wagman, and E. Katz.** 1975. *Micromonospora*-produced gentamicin components. Antimicrob. Agents Chemother. **9**:151–159.
3. **Lee, B. K., R. G. Condon, G. H. Wagman, K. Byrne, and C. Schaffner.** 1974. Incorporation of L-methionine-methyl-^{14}C into gentamicins. II. Large-scale preparation of methyl-^{14}C-gentamicins. J. Antibiot. **27**:822–825.
4. **Lee, B. K., R. T. Testa, G. H. Wagman, C. M. Liu, L. McDaniel, and C. P. Schaffner.** 1973. Incorporation of L-methionine-methyl-^{14}C into gentamicins. J. Antibiot. **26**:728–731.
5. **Miller, A. L., and J. B. Walker.** 1970. Accumulation of streptomycin-phosphate in cultures of streptomycin producers grown on a high phosphate medium. J. Bacteriol. **104**:8–12.
6. **Nomi, R., and O. Nimi.** 1959. Biosynthesis of streptomycin. VI. Chemical structure of a streptomycin precursor. Agric. Biol. Chem. **33**:1459–1463.
7. **Nomi, R., O. Nimi, T. Miyazaki, A. Matsuo, and H. Kiyohara.** 1966. Biosynthesis of streptomycin. II. Isolation of a natural precursor and an enzymatic substance transforming the precursor to streptomycin. Agric. Biol. Chem. **30**:1269–1276.
8. **Park, J. T.** 1952. Uridine-5′-pyrophosphate derivatives. I. Isolation from *Staphylococcus aureus*. J. Biol. Chem. **194**:877–884.
9. **Park, J. T.** 1952. Uridine-5′-pyrophosphate derivatives. II. A structure common to three derivatives. J. Biol. Chem. **194**:885–895.
10. **Park, J. T.** 1952. Uridine-5′-pyrophosphate derivatives. III. Amino acid-containing derivatives. J. Biol. Chem. **194**:897–904.
11. **Walker, J. B., and M. Skorvago.** 1973. Phosphorylation of streptomycin and dihydrostreptomycin by *Streptomyces*. J. Biol. Chem. **218**:2435–2440.
12. **Weinstein, M. J., G. H. Wagman, J. A. Marquez, R. T. Testa, and J. A. Waitz.** 1975. Verdamicin, a new broad spectrum aminoglycoside antibiotic. Antimicrob. Agents Chemother. **7**:246–249.

Antimicrobial Agents and Chemotherapy, Aug. 1976, p. 370-376
Vol. 10, No. 2

Printed in U.S.A.

In Vitro Susceptibility of Pathogenic *Naegleria* and *Acanthamoeba* Species to a Variety of Therapeutic Agents

RICHARD J. DUMA* AND RUTH FINLEY

Department of Medicine, Medical College of Virginia, Virginia Commonwealth University, Richmond, Virginia 23298

Received for publication 2 February 1976

Six pathogenic strains of *Naegleria fowleri*, two of *Acanthamoeba castellanii*, and three of *Acanthamoeba polyphaga* were tested in vitro for susceptibility to a variety of potentially useful therapeutic agents. Minimal motility inhibitory concentrations and minimal inhibitory concentrations were determined by a technique of subculturing pure clones of amoebae in plastic tissue culture chamber slides containing liquid axenic media and serially diluted drug, incubating at 30°C for *Acanthamoeba* and at 37°C for *Naegleria*, and observing on an inverted microscope at 6 h for inhibition of motility and at 24 and 48 h for inhibition of growth. Drug concentrations were selected on the basis of fluid levels achievable in humans. Amphotericin B, clotrimazole, and miconazole were the most effective drugs against *Naegleria*, whereas polymyxin B sulfate and pentamidine isethionate were somewhat effective against pathogenic *Acanthamoeba*. Our results suggest that amphotericin B is the most effective agent against *Naegleria*, but few agents are effective against *Acanthamoeba*.

Not until the 1960s was the pathogenicity of free-living amoebae fully appreciated, that is, when the disease primary amoebic meningoencephalitis (PAM), an acute, rapidly fatal infection occurring in otherwise healthy humans, was recognized (3, 15). In this disease victims are children or young adults who have been swimming in or exposed to fresh or brackish waters; the responsible pathogen is a free-living amoebo-flagellate belonging to the genus *Naegleria*, specifically, *Naegleria fowleri* (14). Amoebae enter the nose and during the subsequent 5 to 6 days migrate through submucosal structures and nerves, ultimately invading the subarachnoid space and brain substance beneath the cribriform plate. Within 72 h rapid deterioration of the patient ensues, resulting in coma and death. An almost identical disease may be produced experimentally in mice by intranasal instillation of these same amoebae (20).

In addition to *Naegleria*, within the last few years, amoebae of the genera *Acanthamoeba* and *Hartmannella* also are being increasingly incriminated as a cause of meningoencephalitis (14, 16, 23) and, in addition, as a cause of nonfatal infections, such as ophthalmitis (21; D. B. Jones, G. S. Visvesvara, and N. M. Robinson, Oxford Ophthalmological Congress, Oxford, England, 1975) and otitis (17). Experimental infections in mice with *Acanthamoeba-Hartmannella* spp. can also be produced (8, 10, 19); however, in contrast to *Naegleria*, when *Acanthamoeba* sp. are instilled intranasally, pneumonia is often the principal disease, and an incubation period longer than 7 days is usually present (19). Spread to the central nervous system occurs principally via the blood stream and generally has resulted in chronic (occasionally granulomatous) encephalitis and minimal, if any, meningitis.

Because of the serious nature of both *Naegleria* and *Acanthamoeba-Hartmannella* infections in humans and because of an almost complete lack of therapeutic agents available against these pathogens, a variety of drugs reported or demonstrated to have antiprotozoan activity was examined.

MATERIALS AND METHODS

Pure clones of six strains of pathogenic *Naegleria* and five strains of *Acanthamoeba* were studied (Table 1). All strains of *Naegleria* were identified as *N. fowleri* and were from fatal cases of human PAM, and all were capable of producing 70 to 100% mortality in mice when approximately 10^4 organisms were instilled intranasally. Three isolates (L.L., T.Y., and W.M.) were obtained from patients seen in 1967 and 1969 at the Medical College of Virginia Hospitals (13); two (F-66 and F-69) were from patients seen in Australia in 1966 and 1969 (5), courtesy of Rodney F. Carter; and one (G.J.) was from a 23-month-old child who died in Florida in 1973, courtesy of Eugene Meagor and Shih L. Chang. Of the five strains of *Acanthamoeba*, two were *Acantha-*

TABLE 1. *Strains of free-living amoebae studied*

Strain	Source	Year of isolation	Investigators
N. fowleri, F-66	Human PAM, Australia	1966	Fowler and Carter
N. fowleri, F-69	Human PAM, Australia	1969	Fowler and Carter
N. fowleri, W.M.	Human PAM, Virginia	1969	Duma and Nelson
N. fowleri,L.L.	Human PAM, Virginia	1968	Duma and Nelson
N. fowleri, T.Y.	Human PAM, Virginia	1969	Duma and Nelson
N. fowleri, G.J.	Human PAM, Florida	1973	Meager and Chang
A. castellanii, Gresham	Ocular infection, England	1974	Nagington
A. castellanii, CH-6	Fresh water, Kentucky	1969	Chang
A. polyphaga, Garcia	Ocular infection, Texas	1974	Jones
A. polyphaga, CH-5	Tissue culture	1972	Wang and Chang
A. polyphaga, P-6	Fresh water, United States	?	Page

moeba castellanii. (The Gresham strain was from a human ocular infection [21], courtesy of J. Nagington and Frederick Page, Cambridge, England; the CH-6 strain was from a freshwater lake in Kentucky, courtesy of Shih L. Chang; it was capable of producing up to 60% mortality in mice inoculated intranasally with 10^4 organisms [9].) Three strains were *A. polyphaga*. (The Garcia strain was from a human ocular infection [Jones et al., Oxford Ophthalmological Congress, 1975], courtesy of Daniel B. Jones; the CH-5 strain was a contaminant of tissue culture, courtesy of Dr. Chang; and the P-6 strain was found in a series of freshwater isolates collected in the United States by Frederick Page.)

The therapeutic agents tested were as follows: amphotericin B (E.R. Squibb & Sons, Inc., Princeton, N.J.) dissolved in dimethyl sulfoxide (range, maximum of 3.4% for 50 μg/ml to 0.006% for 0.098 μg/ml); clotrimazole or Bay 5097 (Delbay Pharmaceuticals, Inc., Bloomfield, N.J.) dissolved in dimethyl sulfoxide (range, maximum 2% for 100 μg/ml to 0.004% for 0.195 μg/ml); metronidazole (Searle & Co., San Juan, Puerto Rico) dissolved in *N,N*-dimethyl formamide (highest concentration, 0.120%); sulfamethoxazole (Hoffmann-La Roche, Inc., Nutley, N. J.) dissolved in 0.1 N sodium hydroxide (highest concentration, 0.01%); trimethoprim (Burroughs-Wellcome, Research Triangle Park, N.C.) dissolved in 0.1 N hydrochloric acid (highest concentration, 0.01%); a 20:1 mixture of sulfamethoxazole and trimethoprim; miconazole (Janssen R & D, Inc., New Brunswick, N.J.) plus miconazole placebo (0.115 ml of polyethoxylated castor oil, 0.5 mg of sodium bisulfite, and 1.62 mg of methylparaben per 1 ml); polymyxin B sulfate (Pfizer Laboratories, New York, N.Y.); pentamidine isethionate (Center for Disease Control, Atlanta, Ga.); paramomycin sulfate (Parke, Davis & Co., Detroit, Mich.); G-418 (Schering Corp., Bloomfield, N.J.); 5-fluorocytosine (Hoffmann-La Roche, Inc., Nutley, N.J.); and clindamycin hydrochloride, as well as its derivative U34728E (The Upjohn Co., Kalamazoo, Mich.), all dissolved in sterile distilled water. The top concentration of metronidazole was 250 μg/ml; for amphotericin B, 50 μg/ml; and for all other agents, 100 μg/ml. All tests were conducted in triplicate.

To test drug susceptibility, a liquid, bacteria-free (axenic) in vitro test system was developed and utilized (Fig. 1). Agents to be studied were solubilized in stock solutions from which maximum concentrations and subsequent twofold dilutions were made in modified Nelson's axenic liquid nutrient medium (22). The pH of this medium with and without drugs was between 7.2 and 7.4. Using an automatic non-electric pipette (BBL 60422), 0.4 ml of each drug concentration (obtained by making twofold serial dilutions of the drug in axenic media) was placed in chambers of an eight-chambered Lab-Tek tissue culture chamber/slide (Miles Laboratories, no. 4808). Again, using the automatic non-electric pipette, 0.1-ml suspensions containing 10^3 trophozoites from 48- to 72-h 37°C liquid axenic cultures of *Naegleria* or from 30°C liquid axenic cultures of *Acanthamoeba* were added to each chamber. (The decision to use 10^3 amoebae/0.1 ml was made to provide microscopic fields of approximately 25 to 40 organisms when a 25× ocular and 10× objective of an inverted, American Optical, ordinary light microscope were used.) To one chamber, as appropriate controls, amoebae were added to axenic media, containing, if necessary, a concentration of solvent equivalent to that used in the maximum drug concentration studied.

After incubation at either 37 or 30°C (depending on the species of amoeba being studied) for 6 h, minimal motility inhibition concentrations (MMIC) were determined by microscopic examination and comparison with controls. Immobilization of trophozoites was generally accompanied by certain morphological changes, as described previously (12): diminution in size, rounding up, watery ectoplasm, increase in granulation, and/or complete disintegration of amoebae. The MMIC was defined as the lowest concentration of drug at which no active pseudopodial activity was seen as compared with controls. After reincubation of the chamber slide for 24 h and again for a total of 48 h, the minimal inhibitory concentration (MIC) of growth was determined. The MIC was defined as the lowest concentration of drug at which growth was 50% less than that of the control, as determined visually on the inverted microscope (Fig. 2).

All susceptibility tests were run in triplicate (with one exception), and geometric means were calculated for the MMIC and 24- and 48-h MICs against each strain for every drug.

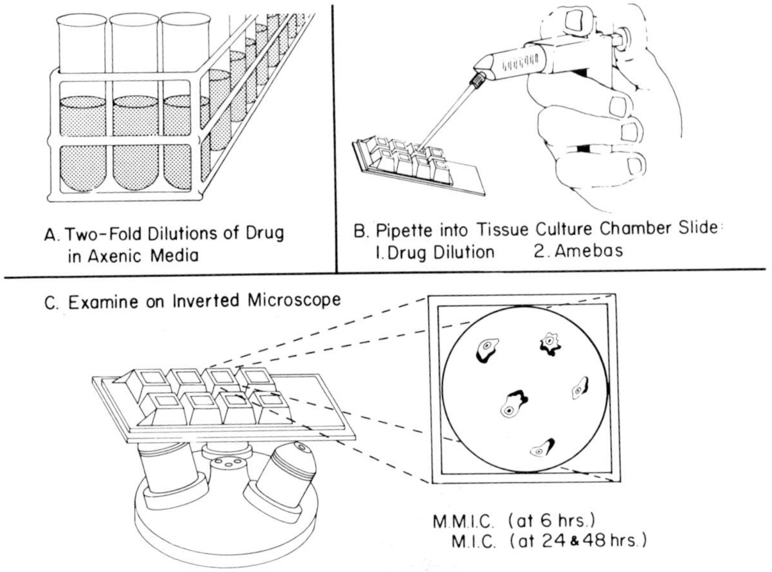

FIG. 1. *Schematic representation of in vitro technique utilized for antiamoebic susceptibility testing (see Materials and Methods for explanation).*

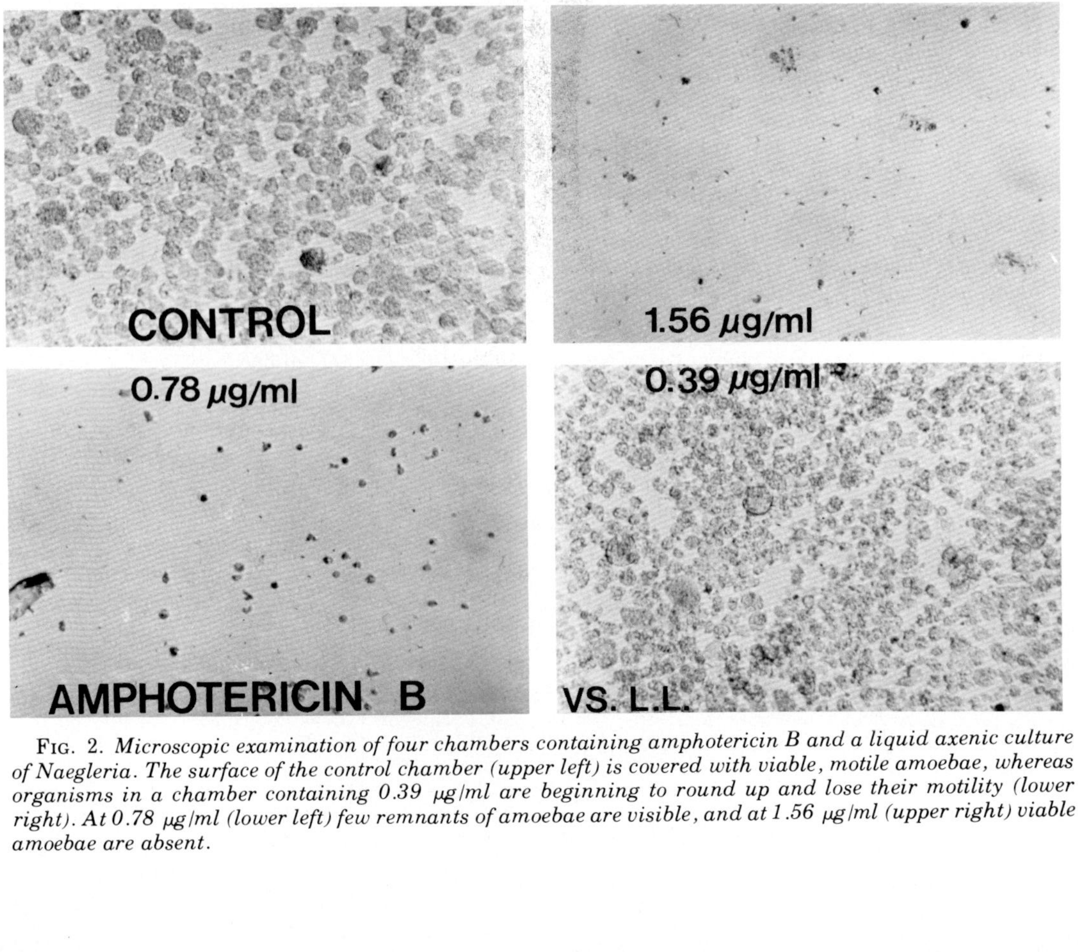

FIG. 2. *Microscopic examination of four chambers containing amphotericin B and a liquid axenic culture of Naegleria. The surface of the control chamber (upper left) is covered with viable, motile amoebae, whereas organisms in a chamber containing 0.39 μg/ml are beginning to round up and lose their motility (lower right). At 0.78 μg/ml (lower left) few remnants of amoebae are visible, and at 1.56 μg/ml (upper right) viable amoebae are absent.*

RESULTS

The results of this investigation confirmed earlier observations utilizing monaxenic cultures (containing *Enterobacter* as the sole source of nutrient for amoebae) that amphotericin B is still the most effective drug currently available against *Naegleria*. Mean MMICs (Table 2) against the six strains ranged from 0.98 to 1.97 μg/ml, with a mean MMIC for the group of 1.39 μg/ml, whereas mean MICs at 24 h ranged from 0.39 to 1.24 μg/ml, with a mean MIC for the group of 0.62 μg/ml. Mean MICs of amphotericin B at 48 h against these same six strains ranged from ≤0.15 to 0.39 μg/ml, with a mean for the total of ≤0.26 μg/ml. Differences in experimental results against any one strain never exceeded two dilutions of drug and were within one dilution in every instance but one. It was noted for amphotericin B that the 6-h MMIC values predicted 24- and 48-h growth inhibitory activity (MIC) in every instance.

Clotrimazole and miconazole were also effective against *Naegleria*, but their effect was not as rapid as was that of amphotericin B. For example, mean MMICs determined 6 h after exposure to clotrimazole were 50 μg/ml against all six strains. In addition, concentrations required to inhibit growth varied considerably from strain to strain, as mean 24-h MICs of clotrimazole against these same strains ranged from ≤0.39 μg/ml to as high as 39.69 μg/ml (Table 2). Similar results were observed for miconazole, as mean MMICs were always above 39.69 μg/ml, whereas mean 24-h MICs ranged from 0.78 to 25 μg/ml. Mean 48-h MICs for both clotrimazole and miconazole fell below those values observed at 24 h, ranging from <0.39 to ≤1.57 μg/ml and 0.98 to 1.97 μg/ml, respectively. In contrast to amphotericin B, 6-h MMICs of clotrimazole or miconazole did not often help in predicting which *Naegleria* strain would be inhibited. Again, with the test system used, triplicate determinations of 24- or 48-h MICs were in almost every instance within two dilutions (or not statistically significant).

No other therapeutic agents tested showed any inhibition of either motility or growth of *Naegleria* in the concentrations tested.

With strains of *Acanthamoeba*, of all agents tested, only polymyxin B and pentamidine isethionate appeared to be effective (Table 3), but only slightly so, with 6-h MMICs ranging from 50 to ≥100 μg/ml (mean, ≥60.15) and from 35.36 to ≥70.71 μg/ml (mean, ≥54.27), respectively. MICs of polymyxin B at 24 h were 50 to ≥100 ug/ml (mean, ≥72.36), and at 48 h they were 79.37 to ≥100 μg/ml (mean, ≥87.06). MICs for pentamidine at 24 h ranged from 35.36 to ≥100 μg/ml (mean, ≥45.85), and at 48 h they were from 12.5 to 50 μg/ml (mean, 22.93).

DISCUSSION

Based on this study and on prior in vitro data (4, 9, 12, 24), amphotericin B still appears to be the most reliable and effective agent against pathogenic strains of *Naegleria*. In this study, mean MMICs ranged from 0.98 to 1.97 μg/ml for the six pathogenic strains tested, and 24- and 48-h MICs ranged from 0.39 to 1.24 and from ≤0.15 to 0.39 μg/ml, respectively. Earlier observations in this laboratory, utilizing crude monaxenic cultures of five strains of pathogenic *Naegleria* grown with *Enterobacter aerogenes* as the sole source of nutrient, indicated that amphotericin B inhibited motility at 6 h at a concentration of ≤0.625 μg/ml and was amebicidal at concentrations of ≤0.078 μg/ml (12). Such figures were in general agreement with studies by Carter (4), who used agar plate assays and monaxenic techniques with *Escherichia coli* as the sole source of nutrient. Monaxenic techniques, especially using agar surfaces to cultivate amoebae, have lent themselves poorly to quantitation and to microscopic examination for motility. In addition, the presence of bacteria has added a variable whose

TABLE 2. *MMIC and 24- and 48-h MICs of amphotericin B, clotrimazole, and miconazole against Naegleria*[a]

Strain	Amphotericin B			Clotrimazole			Miconazole		
	MMIC (μg/ml)	MIC (μg/ml)		MMIC (μg/ml)	MIC (μg/ml)		MMIC (μg/ml)	MIC (μg/ml)	
		24 h	48 h		24 h	48 h		24 h	48 h
F-66	0.98	0.62	≤0.15	50	39.69	≤1.57	≥79.37	25	1.97
F-69	1.56	0.39	≤0.19	50	7.94	0.62	≥63	15.74	0.98
W.M.	1.56	0.78	0.25	50	≤0.62	≤0.50	39.69	1.56	1.24
L.L.	1.97	1.24	0.39	50	≤0.39	≤0.50	≥63	1.24	1.24
T.Y.	0.98	0.39	0.39	50	≤0.39	≤0.39	50	0.78	1.24
G.J.	1.56	0.62	0.31	50	≤0.39	≤0.50	≥63	1.56	1.24

[a] Numbers represent geometric mean of three experiments.

TABLE 3. *MMIC and 24- and 48-h MICs of polymyxin B sulfate and pentamidine isethionate against Acanthamoeba*

Strain	Polymyxin B sulfate[a]			Pentamidine isethionate[b]		
	MMIC (μg/ml)	MIC (μg/ml)		MMIC (μg/ml)	MIC (μg/ml)	
		24 h	48 h		24 h	48 h
CH-6	63	63	79.37	≥70.71	≥100	50
CH-5	50	50	79.37	70.71	35.36	12.5
Garcia	50	79.37	≥79.37	35.36	35.36	25
P6	50	79.37	≥100	50	35.36	17.68
Gresham	≥100	≥100	≥100			

[a] Numbers represent geometric mean of three experiments.
[b] Numbers represent geometric mean of only two experiments.

effect has been difficult to predict; i.e., too many bacteria may create an anaerobic environment, which may be inhibitory to amoebae, or too few may create a nutrient deficiency problem that may be misinterpreted as a direct inhibitory effect of the drug being tested, or the presence of bacteria or their by-products may possibly degrade or alter the test drugs being examined. However, perhaps most importantly, the presence of bacteria as a nutrient source is not comparable to the bacteria-free environment associated with the diseases produced by these organisms.

In vivo studies in mice also have indicated that amphotericin B administered in therapeutically acceptable quantities is effective in preventing PAM (4, 11). More importantly, however, studies in humans with PAM, from whom the responsible pathogen has been isolated and known to be *Naegleria,* have also indicated that amphotericin B in therapeutic doses may be rapidly effective (24 to 48 h) in sterilizing the central nervous system of infecting amoebae (13). In addition, the only cases of survival (2, 6) from culturally proven cases of PAM have been attributed to amphotericin B, the remarkable aspects of these cases being no apparent sequelae.

The precise mechanism of action of amphotericin B on *Naegleria* is not known; however, as a polyene, amphotericin B binds to sterols in the membrane, preferentially to ergosterol and cholesterol (1). Schuster and Rechthand have recently shown that amphotericin B is amebicidal when used during the lag phase of amoebic growth but mainly inhibitory when used during the log phase of growth (24). Ultrastructural changes that they observed were distortions of nuclear shape, increase in cytoplasmic membranes (both rough and smooth endoplasmic reticulum), decrease in food vacuoles, absence of pseudopods, abnormal mitochondria, increase in autophagic vacuoles, and blebbing of the plasma membrane. These investigators also observed that, with increased time of exposure to amphotericin B, these abnormalities increased, a finding supported by our studies, namely, that growth-inhibiting activity was greater after 48 h of exposure to amphotericin B than after 24 h of exposure. Also, by using time-lapse cinematography studies of pathogenic *Naegleria* exposed to lethal concentrations of amphotericin B, we have observed, over a period of less than 1 h, sequential rounding up (loss of pseudopods), increase in number and size of vacuoles (coalescing), development of watery cytoplasm, increased size of organisms, increased visibility of granules, and, eventually, rupturing or disintegration of the trophozoite with complete loss of contents (unpublished data).

It has been suggested in the literature that clotrimazole or some of its analogues might be used to treat PAM due to *Naegleria* (18). Jamieson and Anderson, in studying a New Zealand strain of pathogenic *Naegleria,* observed that amebostatic activity of clotrimazole lay in the range of 0.06 to 0.12 μg/ml, and amebicidal activity is in the range of 0.12 to 1.0 μg/ml (18). Although they studied 16 human pathogens and observed a uniform amebicidal concentration of 0.15 μg/ml for an inoculum size of 730 amoebae, they also observed that such a concentration failed to prevent growth when the inoculum size was increased to 7,300 amoebae. Although we also observed that clotrimazole and miconazole inhibited growth of pathogenic *Naegleria* after 24 to 48 h of exposure (Table 2), these agents did so less rapidly and with less predictability than did amphotericin B. For example, in our test system the 24-h growth of W.M., L.L., T.Y., and G.J. was inhibited in low concentrations by both clotrimazole and miconazole, but the two Australian strains (F-66 and F-69) were not. However, after 48 h of exposure to clotrimazole or miconazole, the two Australian strains finally demonstrated susceptibility. Thus, the length of time that was required for inhibition of amoebic growth by both these agents render them of less therapeutic value than amphotericin B. PAM is a disease in which rapid and, if possible, complete effect (less than 24 h) of therapeutic agents used must occur or the patient will probably die or suffer irreversible neurological sequelae. In addition, if the results reported by Jamieson and Anderson (18) of an adverse effect of inoculum size are correct, since studies of the number of amoebae that may be present in the cerebrospinal fluid of infected patients may be in excess of 150,000 trophozoites in the subarachnoid space alone (13), clotrimazole and miconazole would not appear to be indicated to treat this disease.

In general, in vitro studies on motility inhibition (MMIC) of amoebae may be a quick and simple method of suggesting the capability of an agent not only to inhibit the growth of amoebae but, more importantly, to destroy them rapidly (12). Amoebae depend on pseudopodial activity and motility for feeding. Such tests can be performed in any laboratory in 4 to 6 h and can offer the clinician treating the disease valuable guidance early in the course of therapy. By studying motility 6 h after exposure, MMICs of amphotericin B appeared to reliably predict rapid cidal activity and growth inhibition. On the other hand, such studies with miconazole, because of poor motility inhibition, suggested that rapid killing did not occur, even though eventually (by 24 h) inhibition of growth was demonstrated. All other agents tested did not affect motility, and, predictably, they did not inhibit growth.

The lack of or poor susceptibility of pathogenic *Acanthamoeba* species to all agents tested was disturbing. Only polymyxin B and pentamidine isethionate appeared to be slightly effective, but only in concentrations that would probably be unattainable in the subarachnoid space or brain substance unless introduced intrathecally. Although the two ocular pathogens (Gresham and Garcia) demonstrated the highest resistance, it is possible that in such infections (from which these strains were isolated), ophthalmic solutions could contain concentrations approaching the 24- and 48-h MICs. It is noteworthy that amphotericin B, clotrimazole, and miconazole, although effective against *Naegleria*, were ineffective against *Acanthamoebae*. The reason(s) for this is obscure, but for amphotericin B it probably relates to differing concentrations and availability of various sterols and lipids in the membranes of such species.

The lack of susceptibility of *Acanthamoeba* sp. to 5-fluorocytosine is in contrast to studies by Stevens and O'Dell (25) and Casemore (7). Their investigations found 5-fluorocytosine to be inhibitory in a range of 12.5 (7) to >40 μg/ml (25); however, Stevens and O'Dell noted that virulent *Acanthamoeba* sp. were more resistant than avirulent ones (25) and were susceptible only at concentrations exceeding 40 μg/ml. The explanation for resistance of our strains of *Acanthamoeba* to 5-fluorocytosine is unknown but could have been: (i) due to the enriched media used by us, which probably contained small quantities of competing pyrimidines, e.g., cytosine; (ii) because most of our strains were highly pathogenic and thus inherently more resistant; or (iii) simply due to variations in technique (e.g., solvents, solubility of agents tested, dilutions, media, etc.).

LITERATURE CITED

1. **Andreoli, T. E.** 1974. The structure and function of amphotericin B-cholesterol pores in lipid bilayer membranes. Ann. N.Y. Acad. Sci. **235**:448–468.
2. **Apley, J., S. K. R. Clarke, A. P. C. H. Roome, S. A. Sandry, G. Sazgi, B. Silk, and D. C. Warhurst.** 1970. Primary amoebic meningoencaphalitis in Britain. Br. Med. J. **1**:596–599.
3. **Butt, C. G.** 1966. Primary amebic meningoencephalitis. N. Engl. J. Med. **274**:1473–1476.
4. **Carter, R. F.** 1969. Sensitivity to amphotericin B of a *Naegleria* sp. isolated from a case of primary amoebic meningoencephalitis. J. Clin. Pathol. **22**:470–474.
5. **Carter, R. F.** 1970. Description of a *Naegleria* species isolated from two cases of primary amoebic meningoencephalitis and of the experimental pathological changes induced by it. J. Pathol. **100**:217–244.
6. **Carter, R. F.** 1972. Primary amoebic meningoencephalitis. An appraisal of present knowledge. Trans. R. Soc. Trop. Med. Hyg. **66**:193–213.
7. **Casemore, D. P.** 1970. Sensitivity of *Hartmannella (Acanthamoeba)* to 5-fluorocytosine, hydroxystilbamidine, and other substances. J. Clin. Pathol. **23**:649–652.
8. **Cerva, L.** 1967. Intranasal, intrapulmonary, and intracardiac inoculation of experimental animals with *Hartmannella castellanii*. Folia Parasitol. (Prague) **14**:207–215.
9. **Cerva, L.** 1972. *In vitro* drug resistance of pathogenic *Naegleria fowleri* strains, p. 431–432. *In* M. Hepžlar, M. Semonský, and S. Masák (ed.), Advances in antimicrobial and antineoplastic chemotherapy, vol. I. University Park Press, Baltimore.
10. **Culbertson, C. G., J. C. Smith, H. Cohen, and J. Minner.** 1959. Experimental infection of mice and monkeys by *Acanthamoeba*. Am. J. Pathol. **35**:185–197.
11. **Das, S. R.** 1971. Chemotherapy of experimental amoebic meningoencephalitis in mice infected with *Naegleria aerobia*. Trans. R. Soc. Trop. Med. Hyg. **65**:106–107.
12. **Duma, R. J.** 1971. In vitro susceptibility of pathogenic *Naegleria gruberi* to amphotericin B, p. 109–111. Antimicrob. Agents Chemother. 1970.
13. **Duma, R. J., W. Rosenblum, R. F. McGehee, M. Jones, and E. C. Nelson.** 1971. Primary amebic encephalitis caused by *Naegleria*. Two new cases, responses to amphotericin B and a review. Ann. Intern. Med. **24**:923–931.
14. **Duma, R. J.** 1972. Primary amebic meningoencephalitis. CRC Rev. Clin. Lab. Sci. **3**:163–192.
15. **Fowler, M., and R. F. Carter.** 1965. Acute pyogenic meningitis probably due to *Acanthamoeba sp*: a pre-

liminary report. Br. Med. J. 2:740–742.
16. **Jager, B. V., and W. P. Stamm.** 1972. Brain abscesses caused by free-living amoebas probably of the genus *Hartmannella* in a patient with Hodgkin's Disease. Lancet **ii**:1343–1345.
17. **Jakovljevich, R., and B. Talis.** 1969. Recovery of a hartmannellid ameba in the purulent discharge from a human ear. J. Protozool. **16**(Suppl.):36.
18. **Jamieson, A., and K. Anderson.** 1974. Primary amoebic meningoencephalitis. Lancet **i**:261.
19. **Martinez, A. J., S. M. Markowitz, and R. J. Duma.** 1975. Experimental pneumonitis and encephalitis caused by *Acanthamoeba* in mice: pathogenic and ultrastructural features. J. Infect. Dis. **131**:692–699.
20. **Martinez, A. J., E. C. Nelson, and R. J. Duma.** 1973. Animal model: primary amebic (Naegleria) meningoencephalitis in mice. Am. J. Pathol. **73**:545–548.
21. **Nagington, J., P. G. Watson, T. J. Playfair, J. McGill, B. R. Jones, and A. D. McG. Steele.** 1974. Amoebic infection of the eye. Lancet **ii**:1537–1540.
22. **Nelson, E. C., and M. Jones.** 1971. Culture isolation of agents of primary amebic meningoencephalitis. J. Parasitol. **56**:248.
23. **Robert, V. B., and L. B. Rorke.** 1973. Primary amebic encephalitis, probably from *Acanthamoeba*. Ann. Intern. Med. **79**:174–179.
24. **Schuster, F. L., and E. Rechthand.** 1975. In vitro effects of amphotericin B on growth and ultrastructure of the ameboflagellates *Naegleria gruberi* and *Naegleria fowleri*. Antimicrob. Agents Chemother. **8**:591–605.
25. **Stevens, A. R., and W. D. O'Dell.** 1974. In vitro and in vivo activity of 5-fluorocytosine on *Acanthamoeba*. Antimicrob. Agents Chemother. **6**:282–289.

ANTIMICROBIAL AGENTS AND CHEMOTHERAPY, Aug. 1976, p. 377-379
Vol. 10, No. 2

NOTES

Genotypic Stability of Methicillin Resistance in *Staphylococcus aureus* at Supraoptimal Temperature

FERENC ROZGONYI

Institute of Microbiology, University Medical School of Debrecen, H-4012 Debrecen, Hungary

Received for publication 15 December 1975

Methicillin resistance in a highly resistant mutant of *Staphylococcus aureus* could not be diminished by elevated temperature. After 100 subcultures at 43°C the resistance to methicillin was retained when determined at 37°C.

It was shown that the susceptibility of the methicillin-resistant (MR) strains of *Staphylococcus aureus* to methicillin was directly related to temperature and increased markedly with it (2, 5, 9). The phenotypic expression of the resistance, however, was suppressed by supraoptimal temperatures (2, 9). Subsequently, Al Salihy and James (1) reported that cells of the MR strain 13136 irreversibly lost their methicillin resistance after 35 subcultures at 43°C. This finding has suggested a reexamination of the question in as clear a system as possible.

Most of the naturally occurring MR strains of *S. aureus* have appeared to consist of mixed populations in which the majority of the cells are susceptible to methicillin and only a small minority are highly resistant (3–10, 12, 14, 15). Therefore, the results of experiments with such strains reflect the major susceptible fraction of the cell population rather than the really MR ones.

To avoid this ambiguity I have separated the methicillin-susceptible (MS) fraction of the population from the highly MR one of the same isolate. For this purpose the naturally occurring MR *S. aureus* strain 5814/1966 was used. This strain had been isolated from pus, produced coagulase, and consisted of a heteroresistant population (10).

The MS substrain was obtained as follows. A 24-h culture of the parent strain was diluted up to 10^{-7} with isotonic NaCl solution, pH 7.2, and 0.1-ml portions of the diluted culture were plated onto methicillin-free blood agar plates to obtain discrete colonies. Incubation lasted for 24 h at 37°C. Each colony was tested for methicillin susceptibility. Tube susceptibility tests were carried out using twofold dilutions of the drug from 16 to 0.5 μg/ml in Difco Casitone broth (16), pH 7.2, containing 1% glucose. Tubes were inoculated with 0.1 ml of a 1:100 dilution of a 24-h broth culture of the colony incubated in the same medium. This test was done in duplicate. Cultures inhibited by 8 μg of methicillin per ml or less after incubation at 37°C for 48 h were considered susceptible.

For selection of the MR mutant the Casitone broth containing 500 μg of methicillin per ml was seeded with an appropriate dilution of a 24-h culture of the parent strain so that the final inoculum amounted to 10^6 organisms/ml. After a 48-h incubation at 37°C the culture was subcultured on a blood agar plate free of the antibiotic. The subculture was tested for methicillin resistance by the tube dilution technique mentioned above.

A population analysis was also carried out and for the MR 5814R mutant 70% of the population has been able to grow in the presence of 500 μg of methicillin per ml and 55% in the presence of 800 μg of methicillin per ml on nutrient agar at 37°C (11). This mutant has maintained these levels of methicillin resistance since 1968.

The effect of elevated temperature on methicillin resistance was studied on this MR mutant. For comparison, the MS substrain 5814S was used. This strain was fully inhibited by 4 μg of methicillin per ml at 37°C after 2 days of incubation as tested by the tube dilution technique. The whole population of the strain proved also to be susceptible when it was cultured at 30°C on nutrient agar plates containing increasing concentrations of methicillin. After seeding each plate with 1.8×10^8 organisms and after incubation for 2 days, many discrete colonies were visible at 3 μg of methicillin per ml but none at 6 and 12 μg/ml. The biological, biochemical probes usually tested in the diagnostic laboratory appeared to be identical to those of the 5814R, and both substrains

TABLE 1. *Effect of elevated temperature on the methicillin susceptibility of the MS substrain 5814S and that of the MR mutant 5814R derived from the naturally occurring heteroresistant strain Staphylococcus aureus 5814/1966*

Temp of repeated growth (°C)	Test temp- (°C)	5814S (MIC, μg/ml)			5814R (MIC, μg/ml)		
		0.8	1.6	3.12	<12.5	1,600	3,200
37	37			+[a]			+
	43		+		+		
43	37			+			+
(9 subcultures)	43		+		+		
43	37			+		+	
(27 subcultures)	43		+		+		
43	37		+				+
(40 subcultures)	43	+			+		
43	37		+				+
(50 subcultures)	43	+			+		
43	37			+			+
(80 subcultures)	43	+			+		
43	37		+				+
(100 subcultures)	43	+			+		

[a] + indicates inhibition.

were identical in phage type to one another and to the parent strain. All of them were lysed by phage 77 only at 100 times the routine test dilution of the phages.

The effect of elevated temperature on the methicillin susceptibility of the MS substrain 5814S and that of the MR mutant 5914R is shown in Table 1.

The cells of both the substrain 5814S and the mutant 5814R in parallel were subcultured repeatedly in Difco broth (16) in the absence of the antibiotic at 37 and 43°C. After a number of subcultures at a given temperature the susceptibility to methicillin was determined at each of the two temperatures by the method described. Cells of the MS substrain 5814S grown repeatedly at 43°C retained a minimal inhibitory concentration (MIC) of 3.12 μg of methicillin per ml at 37°C and an MIC of 1.6 μg/ml at 43°C through 27 subcultures. Further repeated growth at 43°C generally lowered the 37°C MIC value to 1.6 μg of methicillin per ml and the 43°C MIC value to 0.8 μg/ml.

The behavior of cells of the MR mutant 5814R grown repeatedly at 43°C differed considerably. When the MIC of methicillin for mutant 5814R was tested at 43°C for 48 h, the cells appeared to be susceptible to methicillin regardless of the previous subculturing temperatures. On the contrary, on determining the MIC at 37°C, the MR mutant proved to be as resistant to methicillin after 100 subcultures at 43°C as it had been before the beginning of the passage. Neither the antibiotic susceptibility pattern nor the phage type of the strains changed during the subculturing at 43°C.

In conclusion, a supraoptimal growth temperature does not abolish the genotype of methicillin resistance but rather suppresses the phenotypic expression of this genetic property. The phenomenon seems likely to be similar to the finding of Sabath et al. (13), who demonstrated that acidification of the test medium resulted in a significant decrease in the level of methicillin resistance in *S. aureus*. This was also only a suppression and not a loss of methicillin resistance.

The reason why Al Salihy and James (1) obtained irreversible loss of resistance might derive from two facts. On the one hand, the strain 13136 has been shown to have only a few highly MR cells in its population (5, 8). Secondly, the highly MR cells are thought to have a longer generation time than the MS cells (6–10, 14, 15). Therefore, if such a heteroresistant strain is subcultured at an elevated temperature, which is not favorable for growth of the MR cells, the major MS fraction of the population will overgrow the minor MR fraction, and consequently the proportion of MR cells will decrease in parallel with the extent of the subculturing. After a sufficient number of passages the MR portion of the population will be reduced to the extent that it may be easily lost upon further dilution of the culture.

I am indebted to Katalin Szitha for her skilled technical assistance.

LITERATURE CITED

1. **Al Salihy, S. M., and A. M. James.** 1972. Loss of methicillin-resistance from resistant strains of *Staphylococcus aureus*. Lancet 2:331–332.
2. **Annear, D. I.** 1968. The effect of temperature on resistance of *Staphylococcus aureus* to methicillin and some other antibiotics. Med. J. Aust. 1:444–446.
3. **Barrett, F. F., R. F. McGehee, Jr., and M. Finland.** 1968. Methicillin-resistant *Staphylococcus aureus* at

Boston City Hospital: bacteriologic and epidemiologic observations. N. Engl. J. Med. 279:441–448.

4. **Chabbert, Y. A., J. G. Baudens, J. F. Acar, and G. R. Gerbaud.** 1965. La résistance naturelle des *Staphylococues* a la méthicilline et l'oxacilline. Rev. Fr. Etud. Clin. Biol. 10:495–506.
5. **Dyke, K. G. H.** 1969. Penicillinase production and intrinsic resistance to penicillins in methicillin-resistant cultures of *Staphylococcus aureus*. J. Med. Microbiol. 2:261–278.
6. **Gravenkemper, C. F., J. L. Brodie, and W. M. M. Kirby.** 1965. Resistance of coagulase-positive staphylococci to methicillin and oxacillin. J. Bacteriol. 89:1005–1010.
7. **Kayser, F. H., E. J. Benner, R. Troy, and P. D. Hoeprich.** 1971. Mode of resistance against β-lactam antibiotics in staphylococci. Ann. N.Y. Acad. Sci. 182:106–117.
8. **Knox, R.** 1961. Celbenin-resistant staphylococci. Br. Med. J. 1:126.
9. **Parker, M. T., and J. H. Hewitt.** 1970. Methicillin resistance in *Staphylococcus aureus*. Lancet 1:800–804.
10. **Rozgonyi, F., M. Illés, and I. Rédai.** 1968. Incidence and biological properties of methicillin and oxacillin resistant *Staphylococcus aureus* strains. Acta Microbiol. Acad. Sci. Hung. 15:245–252.
11. **Rozgonyi, F., and I. Rédai.** 1970. The effect of lysozyme and methicillin on the growth of methicillin resistant and sensitive *Staphylococcus aureus* strains. Acta Microbiol. Acad. Sci. Hung. 17:95–103.
12. **Sabath, L. D., F. F. Barrett, C. Wilcox, D. A. Gerstein, and M. Finland.** 1969. Methicillin resistance of *Staphylococcus aureus* and *Staphylococcus epidermidis*, p. 302–306. Antimicrob. Agents Chemother. 1968.
13. **Sabath, L. D., S. J. Wallace, and D. A. Gerstein.** 1972. Suppression of intrinsic resistance to methicillin and other penicillins in *Staphylococcus aureus*. Antimicrob. Agents Chemother. 2:350–355.
14. **Seligman, S. J.** 1966. Methicillin-resistant staphylococci: genetics of the minority population. J. Gen. Microbiol. 42:315–322.
15. **Sutherland, R., and G. N. Rolinson.** 1964. Characteristics of methicillin-resistant staphylococci. J. Bacteriol. 87:887–899.
16. **Váczi, L., J. K. Makleit, A. Réthy, and I. Rédai.** 1964. Studies on lipids in Pseudomonas pyocyanea. Acta Microbiol. Acad. Sci. Hung. 11:383–390.

ANTIMICROBIAL AGENTS AND CHEMOTHERAPY, Aug. 1976, p. 380-381 Vol. 10, No. 2

Change in Susceptibility of Group B Streptococci to Penicillin G from 1968 Through 1975

M. J. SEVERIN* AND J. L. WILEY

Creighton University, School of Medicine, Omaha, Nebraska 68178, and Omaha-Douglas County Health Department, Omaha, Nebraska 68105*

Received for publication 5 March 1976

This report describes a study of 212 isolates of group B streptococci from sore throats over an 8-year period. A small but increasing percentage showed increased resistance to penicillin G when tested in an in vitro system.

In 1938, Fry reported that group B, beta-hemolytic streptococci were causative agents of human disease (1). Subsequently, the syndromes of neonatal sepsis (5) and neonatal meningitis (4) due to group B streptococci were characterized.

During the evaluation of a throat culture program serving physicians and dentists in our community, it was apparent that non-group A streptococci were being isolated from throat swabs of clinically ill individuals on a constant basis. Dacron swabs received from clinicians were routinely processed by culturing them on blood agar plates containing 5% sheep erythrocytes. After overnight incubation at 35°C in an atmosphere of 5% CO_2, these plates were examined for streptococcal colonies demonstrating beta-hemolysis. All such isolates were screened by the fluorescent antibody technique (3) to identify group A streptococci. Non-group A isolates were examined by precipitin testing methods (2) to determine the isolates of groups B, C, D, and G. Isolates identified as group B streptococci, which by colony count appeared to represent at least 25% of the throat flora, were suspended in 0.5 ml of sterile sheep erythrocytes. These suspensions were stored at −20°C until antibiotic susceptibility tests could be performed. Before freezing, one of every 10 isolates was tested against penicillin G to determine a preliminary minimal inhibitory concentration (MIC). Representative isolates of group A streptococci (one per month) and group D streptococci (one per month) were similarly isolated, identified, tested, and stored. Later comparison with these preliminary MICs enabled us to determine the effects of time and freezing on the stored streptococci.

Streptococcal isolates were tested against penicillin G in a twofold dilution series using Todd-Hewitt broth as the antibiotic diluent. The concentrations of penicillin G prepared ranged from 2.50 to 0.009 units/ml. The MIC for each isolate was measured in duplicate with the same lot number of culture medium and antibiotic. Each series was inoculated with a suspension of 10^4 colony-forming units of test isolate per ml. All cultures were incubated at 35°C in an atmosphere of 5% CO_2. Results were read after 24 h of incubation. When a duplicate series differed from the original, the isolate was restudied to establish the true MIC. Streptococci isolated during the years 1968 through 1973 were evaluated in an initial study. A second study evaluated the isolates of 1974 and 1975.

A total of 212 group B streptococci isolates were studied during an 8-year period. The range of susceptibility to penicillin G was 0.62 to 0.009 unit/ml or below (Table 1). All the isolates obtained in years 1968 through 1971 were susceptible to 0.009 unit or less per ml. For some of the isolates obtained in years 1972 through 1975, the MIC was at least fourfold above the 0.009-unit/ml level (Table 2). In 1972, the MIC for 10% of the group B streptococcal isolates were 0.075 unit or greater per ml. During 1973 this figure rose to 21%, and in 1975 it was 24%. During this same 4-year period, 6% of group B streptococci were not susceptible to 0.15 unit/ml, and 3% were not susceptible to 0.3 unit/ml.

Each of the 96 group A control isolates was inhibited by MICs at or below 0.009 unit/ml.

TABLE 1. *Range of susceptibility of group B streptococci to penicillin G-212 isolates (1968–1975)*

MIC (U/ml)	No. of isolates
0.009	108
0.018	37
0.037	31
0.075	10
0.150	8
0.310	12
0.620	6

TABLE 2. *Change in susceptibility of group B streptococcal isolates to penicillin G (1968–1975)*

Year	No. of isolates	% Requiring for inhibition MIC > 0.075 U/ml
1968	15	0
1969	15	0
1970	17	0
1971	18	0
1972	30	10
1973	37	21.6
1974	39	17.6
1975	41	24

The MIC levels for the group D controls varied widely and are not included. There were no detectable differences in the susceptibility before and after freezing and storage.

This preliminary report of group B streptococci isolated from human sore throats indicates that a small but significant percentage of streptococci showed increased resistance to penicillin G. We cannot be sure that this same pattern will apply to group B streptococci from vaginal cultures.

LITERATURE CITED

1. **Fry, R. M.** 1938. Fatal infections by hemolytic streptococcus Group B. Lancet 1:199–201.
2. **Lancefield, R. C.** 1933. A serological differentiation of human and other groups of hemolytic streptococci. J. Exp. Med. 57:571–595.
3. **Moody, M. D., A. C. Siegel, B. Pittman, and C. C. Winter.** 1963. Fluorescent antibody identification of Group A streptococci from throat swabs. Am. J. Public Health 53:1083–1092.
4. **Rantz, L. A.** 1942. Streptococcus meningitis. Ann. Intern. Med. 16:716–726.
5. **Rantz, L. A., and W. M. Kirby.** 1942. Hemolytic streptococcus bacteremia. N. Engl. J. Med. 227:730–733.

ANTIMICROBIAL AGENTS AND CHEMOTHERAPY, Aug. 1976, p. 382-383
Vol. 10, No. 2
Printed in U.S.A.

Comparative In Vitro Activity of Sch 20656, Netilmicin, Gentamicin, and Tobramycin

CHATRCHAI WATANAKUNAKORN

Department of Internal Medicine, University of Cincinnati College of Medicine, Cincinnati, Ohio 45267

Received for publication 3 May 1976

Sch 20656 and netilmicin (Sch 20569), two new semisynthetic aminoglycosides, were as active as gentamicin and tobramycin against *Enterobacteriaceae*. Against *Pseudomonas aeruginosa*, Sch 20656 was the least active, whereas netilmicin was active against many highly gentamicin-resistant isolates.

Due to the marked increase in the prevalence of serious infections caused by gram-negative bacilli in the past decade, the clinical use of aminoglycoside antibiotics has become widespread, resulting in steady increases in the number of gram-negative bacilli resistant to clinically available aminoglycosides. Continued efforts have been made by pharmaceutical manufacturers to develop new aminoglycosides effective against resistant gram-negative bacilli and with less toxic potentials.

Sch 20656 and netilmicin (Sch 20569) are two new semisynthetic aminoglycosides structurally similar to the gentamicin complex. In this study, the in vitro activity of Sch 20656 and netilmicin was compared with that of gentamicin and tobramycin against *Pseudomonas aeruginosa* and members of the family *Enterobacteriaceae*. A total of 337 clinical isolates were obtained from the Clinical Microbiology Laboratories of the Cincinnati General Hospital and the Cincinnati Veterans Administration Hospital. These consisted of *P. aeruginosa* (140 isolates), *Escherichia coli* (72 isolates), *Klebsiella* sp. (36 isolates), *Enterobacter* sp. (18 isolates), *Serratia* sp. (18 isolates), *Proteus mirabilis* (41 isolates), and indole-positive *Proteus* sp. (12 isolates). Many of the *P. aeruginosa* isolates were known to be resistant to gentamicin but susceptible to tobramycin (4).

The minimal inhibitory concentration (MIC) of Sch 20656, netilmicin, gentamicin, and tobramycin was determined by the agar dilution method recommended by the WHO International Collaborative Study on antimicrobial susceptibility testing (1). Mueller-Hinton agar (Difco Laboratories, Detroit, Mich.) was used. The inoculum was 0.002 ml of a 10^{-2} dilution of an 18-h culture (approximately 10^3 to 10^4 organisms), delivered by a Steers replicator (3). For a given clinical isolate, the MIC of the four aminoglycosides was determined simultaneously by using the same inoculum.

The cumulative percent susceptibility of the organisms to the four aminoglycosides is listed in Table 1. Against *P. aeruginosa*, Sch 20656 was the least active, whereas netilmicin was less effective overall than gentamicin or tobramycin. However, at 32 μg/ml, more isolates (81.4%) were susceptible to netilmicin than to gentamicin (62.1%), and at 64 μg/ml the percent susceptible was almost the same for netilmicin (93.6%) and tobramycin (98.6%). Of the 45 isolates with an MIC >64 μg of gentamicin per ml, the MIC of netilmicin was >64 μg/ml for 6, 64 μg/ml for 11, 32 μg/ml for 19, and 16 μg/ml for 9 isolates. The four aminoglycosides appeared to be equally effective against members of *Enterobacteriaceae* tested.

This study was supported by a grant from Schering Corp., Bloomfield, N.J., and by the Morton Hamburger Memorial Fund.

I thank Thomas Bannister for excellent technical assistance.

LITERATURE CITED

1. **Ericsson, H. M., and J. C. Sherris.** 1971. Antibiotic sensitivity testing: report of an international collaborative study. Acta Pathol. Microbiol. Scand. Sect. B **217**(Suppl):1/90.
2. **Schering Corporation.** 1975. Informational material for the investigational drug Sch 20569. Schering Corp., Bloomfield, N.J.
3. **Steers, E., E. L. Foltz, and B. S. Graves.** 1959. An inocula replicating apparatus for routine testing of bacterial susceptibility to antibiotics. Antibiot. Chemother. **9**:307-311.
4. **Watanakunakorn, C., and T. Bannister.** 1975. In vitro activity of tobramycin and gentamicin against *Enterobacteriaceae* and gentamicin-resistant, carbenicillin-resistant *Pseudomonas aeruginosa*. Curr. Ther. Res. **17**:488-496.

Table 1. *Comparative in vitro susceptibility of P. aeruginosa and Enterobacteriaceae to four aminoglycoside antibiotics*

Determinants	No. tested	Cumulative % susceptibility at increasing concn (μg/ml)								
		0.5	1	2	4	8	16	32	64	>64
P. aeruginosa	140									
Tobramycin		1.4	7.9	44.3	70.7	86.4	90.0	96.4	98.6	100
Gentamicin		0	0.7	0.7	12.9	45.7	58.6	62.1	67.9	100
Sch 20656		0.7	0.7	1.4	1.4	3.6	11.4	47.9	87.1	100
Netilmicin		0.7	0.7	1.4	2.9	11.4	45.0	81.4	93.6	100
E. coli	72									
Tobramycin		1.4	38.9	80.6	91.7	91.7	94.4	98.6	98.6	100
Gentamicin		2.8	45.8	75.0	91.7	94.4	95.8	98.6	98.6	100
Sch 20656		0	19.4	69.4	93.1	95.8	98.6	98.6	98.6	100
Netilmicin		0	23.6	72.2	93.1	95.8	98.6	98.6	98.6	100
Klebsiella	36									
Tobramycin		2.8	83.3	91.7	94.4	97.2	97.2	97.2	100	100
Gentamicin		5.6	86.1	91.7	94.4	97.2	97.2	97.2	100	100
Sch 20656		2.8	83.3	91.7	94.4	97.2	97.2	100	100	100
Netilmicin		2.8	80.6	91.7	97.2	97.2	97.2	100	100	100
Enterobacter	18									
Tobramycin		11.1	77.8	88.9	100	100	100	100	100	100
Gentamicin		22.2	88.9	94.4	94.4	100	100	100	100	100
Sch 20656		0	50.0	94.4	100	100	100	100	100	100
Netilmicin		0	77.8	88.9	100	100	100	100	100	100
Serratia	18									
Tobramycin		0	0	55.6	88.9	94.4	100	100	100	100
Gentamicin		11.1	77.8	83.3	94.4	100	100	100	100	100
Sch 20656		0	72.2	83.3	94.4	100	100	100	100	100
Netilmicin		0	0	61.1	94.4	100	100	100	100	100
P. mirabilis	41									
Tobramycin		0	22.0	78.0	90.2	95.1	95.1	97.6	97.6	100
Gentamicin		0	24.4	68.3	90.2	95.1	97.6	100	100	100
Sch 20656		0	0	19.5	80.5	92.7	97.6	97.6	100	100
Netilmicin		0	0	17.1	90.2	95.1	97.6	100	100	100
Other *Proteus* sp.	12									
Tobramycin		0	8.3	33.3	83.3	83.3	83.3	91.7	91.7	100
Gentamicin		0	8.3	33.3	66.7	75.0	91.7	91.7	91.7	100
Sch 20656		0	8.3	50.0	66.7	75.0	83.3	91.7	91.7	100
Netilmicin		0	0	8.3	41.7	75.0	83.3	83.3	91.7	100

ANTIMICROBIAL AGENTS AND CHEMOTHERAPY, Aug. 1976, p. 384-386 Vol. 10, No. 2

Printed in U.S.A.

Comparison of Activity of Sisomicin and Gentamicin in Mouse Protection Tests with Gram-Negative Bacilli

BURT R. MEYERS AND SHALOM Z. HIRSCHMAN*

Division of Infectious Diseases, Department of Medicine, Mt. Sinai School of Medicine of the City University of New York, New York, New York 10029

Received for publication 3 January 1976

The efficacy of sisomicin and gentamicin was compared in mouse protection studies against strains of *Escherichia coli*, *Klebsiella* sp., *Enterobacter aerogenes*, *Serratia marcescens*, *Proteus mirabilis*, and *Pseudomonas aeruginosa*. There was no significant difference in mortality of the mice in any of the protocol groups when five different dosages of sisomicin and gentamicin given by three separate schedules were compared for each bacterial inoculum in each antibiotic protocol. The mean protective dose values of sisomicin were at least one-half those of gentamicin for each protocol against *Pseudomonas aeruginosa*.

The overall spectrum of antimicrobial activity in vitro of the new aminoglycoside antibiotic sisomicin (10) is similar to that of gentamicin, although sisomicin has been reported to show somewhat greater activity against *Pseudomonas aeruginosa*, *Klebsiella* sp., and indole-positive *Proteus* (2, 4, 6, 9, 11). In this study we compared the activity of sisomicin and gentamicin in mouse protection tests against six clinical gram-negative isolates, including one strain each of *Klebsiella* sp., *Escherichia coli*, *Enterobacter aerogenes*, *Serratia marscens*, *Proteus mirabilis*, and *Pseudomonas aeruginosa*. The minimal inhibitory and minimal bactericidal concentrations of sisomicin and gentamicin for these strains, determined by methods previously described (6), were in general quite similar (Table 1), so that susceptibility to the antibiotics in vitro was not a factor in this study.

The bacterial isolates were maintained on antibiotic seed agar and grown in tryptose phosphate broth (Difco). Both bacteria and antibiotics were diluted in normal saline. Bacterial inocula were chosen to achieve 100% mortality by 48 h after infection; animals inoculated with the strain of *Klebsiella* sp., however, died within 96 h of infection. The total bacterial inoculum in a volume of 0.25 ml was injected intraperitoneally into male CF1 mice (Carworth). The inocula used were 2×10^9 colony-forming units (CFU) for the strain of *Klebsiella* sp., 4×10^9 CFU for *E. coli*, 1.5×10^9 CFU for *E. aerogenes*, 1.3×10^9 CFU for *S. marcescens*, 1.65×10^9 CFU for *P. mirabilis*, and 1.5×10^9 CFU for *P. aeruginosa*.

The antibiotic doses used for both sisomicin and gentamicin were 2.5, 5, 10, 25, and 50 mg/kg. The antibiotics were administered according to several protocols. In protocol I, groups of 70 mice were injected intraperitoneally with one of the gram-negative bacterial strains. One hour later two sets of five groups of seven mice each were given subcutaneous injections of the five different doses of sisomicin and gentamicin. In protocol II the antibiotics were administered 2 h after bacterial inoculation. In protocol III, one-half of the doses given above for sisomicin and gentamicin were injected into the animals 0.5 h before bacterial inoculation. Four hours after bacterial inoculation the other one-half dose of antibiotic was given. For protocol IV, only the bacterial inocula, but no antibiotics, were administered to this group of mice. In protocol V, these mice did not receive a bacterial inoculum, but were injected with 50 mg of sisomicin or gentamicin per kg. In protocol VI, these animals were injected only with saline and consisted of six groups of seven animals each to serve as litter controls. The animals were examined at 24, 48, and 96 h.

The mean protective dose (PD_{50}) (milligram/kilogram) of each antibiotic against each bacterial isolate was determined by probit analysis (7). The mortality of the sets of mice receiving all the five doses of sisomicin and gentamicin for each bacterial isolate was compared by the chi-square test. In addition, the mortality at each dose of sisomicin and gentamicin for each bacterial isolate was analyzed by the chi-square method using the Yates correction (X^2_c) of the fourfold table (1).

There was no significant difference in mortality of mice inoculated with *Klebsiella* sp., *P. mirabilis*, *E. coli*, and *S. marcescens* treated with either sisomicin or gentamicin, whether the mortality of the sets of animals receiving the five doses of each antibiotic in each protocol was compared or the mortality of animals was compared separately for each dose of antibiotic (Table 1). There also was no significant difference in mortality of animals infected with *E. aerogenes* or *P. aeruginosa* and treated with sisomicin or gentamicin when the mortality of the sets of animals receiving the five doses of antibiotic was compared for each of the protocols. However, when the mortality of animals was compared for each dose separately, it was found that gentamicin gave significantly greater protection against *E. aerogenes* at a dose of 5 mg/kg when antibiotic was administered 1 h after bacterial infection (protocol I; $X^2_c = 6.4, P < 0.025$) and at a dose of 2.5 mg/kg when one-half the dose was given 0.5 h before bacterial inoculation and the other one-half dose was given 4 h after inoculation (protocol III; $X^2_c = 6.4, P < 0.025$) (Table 1). In contrast, when the mortality was compared for each dose separately in animals inoculated with *P. aeruginosa*, it was found that sisomicin gave significantly greater protection at a dose of 10 mg/kg when administered 1 h after infection (protocol I; $X^2_c = 4.57, P < 0.05$) and at 2 h after bacterial inoculation (protocol II; $X^2_c = 4.98, P < 0.05$) (Table 1). However, it should be cautioned that the number of animals tested at each dose was too small to establish real importance for these observations.

The PD_{50} of gentamicin was one-fourth that of sisomicin against *E. aerogenes* when the antibiotic was administered 1 h after bacterial inoculation (protocol I) (Table 2). The PD_{50} of sisomicin was lower than that of gentamicin, by at least one-half against *P. aeruginosa* for

TABLE 1. *Comparison of mortality of mice inoculated with gram-negative bacteria and treated with sisomicin (S) or gentamicin (G)*

Bacterium	MIC:MBC[a] (μg/ml)	Protocol I Dose (mg/kg)					Protocol II Dose (mg/kg)					Protocol III Dose (mg/kg)					IV
		2.5	5	10	25	50	2.5	5	10	25	50	2.5	5	10	25	50	
Klebsiella sp.	S 1.56:1.56	1[b]	2	1	1	0	2	5	5	5	3	1	1	1	0	1	7
	G 0.39:0.39	0	0	0	2	2	6	5	2	4	4	2	0	1	0	0	
Proteus mirabilis	S 3.13:3.13	1	1	0	0	0	2	6	2	3	1	0	0	0	0	0	7
	G 3.13:3.13	2	1	0	0	0	6	4	0	2	0	1	2	1	0	0	
Enterobacter aerogenes	S 0.78:1.56	5[c]	5[c, d]	0	1[c]	0[c]	5[c]	5[c]	2	0[c]	0[c]	5[c, d]	1[c]	2	0[c]	0[c]	6
	G 0.78:0.78	1[c]	0[c]	0[c]	0[c]	0[c]	4[c]	3[c]	0	2[c]	0[c]	0[c]	0[c]	0	0[c]	0[c]	
Escherichia coli	S 0.78:1.56	2	1	0	1	1	2	3	4	2	5	1	0	0	0	0	6
	G 0.39:0.78	3	1	1		3	4	4	2	2	2	1	0	0	0	0	
Pseudomonas aeruginosa	S 0.39:0.78	7	3	1[e]	1	0	7	6	3	0	0[e]	7	5	4	1	1	7
	G 0.39:0.78	7	7	6	4	1	6	7	6	4	5	7	6	7	3	1	
Serratia marcescens	S 0.39:1.56	1	1	0	1	0	6	6	3	1	1	0	0	0	0	0	7
	G 0.39:3.13	2	0	1	0	0	6	6	6	5	1	4	1	1	0	0	

[a] MIC, Minimal inhibitory concentration; MBC, minimal bactericidal concentration.
[b] Number of animals dead; seven animals were inoculated unless otherwise stated.
[c] Five animals were inoculated.
[d] $P < 0.025$.
[e] $P < 0.05$.

TABLE 2. *Comparison of PD_{50} (milligrams/kilogram) values of sisomicin (S) and gentamicin (G) against infection with gram-negative bacteria*

Bacterium	Protocol I		Protocol II		Protocol III	
	S	G	S	G	S	G
Klebsiella sp.	2.5	2.5	40	25	2.5	2.5
Proteus mirabilis	1	1.5	15	7.5	2.5	2.5
Enterobacter aerogenes	10	2.5	10	7.5	2.5	2.5
Escherichia coli	1.5	2			2.5	2.5
Pseudomonas aeruginosa	7.5	25	10	25	12.5	25
Serratia marcescens	2.5	2.5	10	30	2.5	3

each of the three protocols (Table 2). However, the PD_{50} values of sisomicin and gentamicin were quite similar against the other bacterial isolates.

The differences in mortality observed at several specific doses of the antibiotics and PD_{50} values against *P. aeruginosa* are of dubious clinical import. We chose an inoculum size that would result in 100% mortality; apparently, there is no consensus as to the optimum bacterial inoculum to be used in mouse protection tests (3). Although the pharmacokinetics of sisomicin and gentamicin administered either intramuscularly or intravenously are quite similar (5, 8), in mouse protection studies the drugs are usually injected subcutaneously. Furthermore, the range of PD_{50} values of aminoglycoside antibiotics derived from mouse protection studies against bacteria susceptible in vitro is very large (3, 9). Although mouse protection tests would appear to be useful guides to possible clinical efficacy of an antimicrobial agent when graded inocula and different antibiotic schedules, including repeated dosages, are used, such tests cannot substitute for clinical experience.

LITERATURE CITED

1. **Armitage, P.** 1971. Statistical methods in medical research, p. 313–335. John Wiley and Sons, New York.
2. **Crowe, C. C., and E. Sanders.** 1973. Sisomicin: evaluation in vitro and comparison with gentamicin and tobramycin. Antimicrob. Agents Chemother. 3:24–28.
3. **Davis, S. D.** 1975. Activity of gentamicin, tobramycin, polymyxin B, and colistimethate in mouse protection tests with *Pseudomonas aeruginosa*. Antimicrob. Agents Chemother. 8:50–53.
4. **Hyams, P. J., M. S. Simberkoff, and J. J. Rahal.** 1973. In vitro bactericidal effectiveness of four aminoglycoside antibiotics. Antimicrob. Agents Chemother. 3:87–94.
5. **Lode, H., B. Kemmerich, and P. Koeppe.** 1975. Comparative clinical pharmacology of gentamicin, sisomicin, and tobramycin. Antimicrob. Agents Chemother. 8:396–401.
6. **Meyers, B. R., B. Leng, and S. Z. Hirschman.** 1975. Comparison of the antibacterial activities of sisomicin and gentamicin against gram-negative bacteria. Antimicrob. Agents Chemother. 8:757–758.
7. **Miller, L. C., and M. L. Tainter.** 1944. Estimation of the ED_{50} and its error by means of logarithmic-probit graph paper. Proc. Soc. Exp. Biol. Med. 57:261–274.
8. **Rodriguez, V., G. P. Bodey, M. Valdivieso, and R. Feld.** 1975. Clinical pharmacology of sisomicin. Antimicrob. Agents Chemother. 7:38–41.
9. **Waitz, J. A., E. L. Moss, Jr., C. G. Drube, and M. J. Weinstein.** 1972. Comparative activity of sisomicin, gentamicin, kanamycin, and tobramycin. Antimicrob. Agents Chemother. 2:431–437.
10. **Weinstein, M. J., J. A. Marquez, R. T. Testa, G. H. Wagman, E. M. Oden, and J. A. Waitz.** 1970. Antibiotic 6640, a new micromonospora-produced aminoglycoside antibiotic. J. Antibiot. 23:551–554.
11. **Young, L. S., and W. L. Hewitt.** 1973. Activity of five aminoglycoside antibiotics in vitro against gram-negative bacilli and *Staphylococcus aureus*. Antimicrob. Agents Chemother. 4:617–625.

Antimicrobial Agents and Chemotherapy, Sept. 1976, p. 387-394
Vol. 10, No. 3
Printed in U.S.A.

Antimicrobial Susceptibility of *Propionibacterium acnes* and Related Microbial Species

U. HOEFFLER, H. L. KO, and G. PULVERER*

Institute of Hygiene, University of Cologne, Cologne, Germany

Received for publication 18 March 1976

The minimal inhibitory concentrations of 32 antimicrobial agents were established for 73 strains of *Propionibacterium acnes* and four related species (*P. granulosum, P. avidum, Corynebacterium minutissimum,* and *C. parvum*). Most strains showed good susceptibility to those agents usually considered active against gram-positive organisms. With the exception of *C. minutissimum,* the strains tested revealed more or less identical susceptibility ranges. The lowest minimal inhibitory concentrations were observed with benzylpenicillin, ampicillin, cephalothin, rifampin, erythromycin, clindamycin, and minocycline. *C. minutissimum* was more susceptible to gentamicin, sisomicin, tobramycin, and fusidic acid but more resistant to most other drugs than were the other species examined.

Microaerophilic propionibacteria may be regarded not only as normal inhabitants of the skin but also as facultative, pathogenic organisms. *Propionibacterium acnes* can regularly be isolated from acne vulgaris lesions (14) and frequently from actinomycotic (9) or nonspecific anaerobic infectious processes (13). There seems to be strong evidence that *P. acnes* is an important etiological factor in acne vulgaris because of the release of large amounts of free fatty acids from sebum triglycerides (16). Furthermore, in acne vulgaris only those antimicrobial agents that are able to attack *P. acnes* appear to be therapeutic (6). For this reason, information about the antibiotic susceptibility of *P. acnes* is needed, yet few reports have appeared to date (2, 3, 7, 8, 15). The present study was undertaken, therefore, to evaluate the susceptibility of 73 strains of *P. acnes* and related organisms to 32 antimicrobial drugs.

MATERIALS AND METHODS

Bacterial strains. A total of 73 well-defined strains of microaerophilic propionibacteria and corynebacteria were examined. These strains belonged to the following species.

(i) *P. acnes* (38 strains). Twenty strains of *P. acnes* were received from abroad: American Type Culture Collection (ATCC), strains 6919, 6921, 6922, 6923, and 11827; V. R. Dowell, Jr., Center for Disease Control, Atlanta, Ga., strains 5159, 6949, 6981, 6994, and 7010; J. G. Voss, The Proctor & Gamble Co., Cincinnati, Ohio, strains MC, A, A3, C45, C55, 174V, 0391, and UCLA18; C. S. Cummins, Anaerobe Laboratory, Virginia Polytechnic Institute and State University, Blacksburg, strains 0162 and 3706. Eighteen strains of *P. acnes* were isolated in our own laboratory from human hair or from infectious processes.

(ii) *P. granulosum* (15 strains). Ten strains of *P. granulosum* were cultivated in our institute and five strains were received from J. G. Voss (strains C51, D21, D34, and V1) or from C. S. Cummins (strain 0507).

(iii) *P. avidum* (16 strains). In Cologne we isolated 14 strains of *P. avidum*. Two additional strains were supplied by C. S. Cummins (strains 0575 and 0589).

(iv) *Corynebacterium minutissimum* (3 strains). Strains 22347, 22348, and 22349 were from ATCC.

(v) *C. parvum* (one strain). The only *C. parvum* strain tested was the ATCC strain 11829.

All strains were differentiated according to *Bergey's Manual of Determinative Bacteriology* (1); most had been used in previous published studies (4, 11, 12).

Media. For primary isolation, agar containing 0.43 M glycerol was used (5). Further cultivation was done on A-agar medium, the contents of which have been described by Jong et al. (4). Bacterial suspensions were prepared in Mueller-Hinton broth (Difco), and the antimicrobial drugs tested were added to Mueller-Hinton medium (Difco, pH 7.2).

Preparation of inocula. Cells from 48-h-old cultures on A-agar medium were added to Mueller-Hinton broth, carefully shaken to establish a homogeneous suspension, and brought to an extinction of 0.8 (measured at 540 nm against Mueller-Hinton broth using the Beckman photometer 1211). One drop (Pasteur pipettes) of each suspension was used as the inoculum. Based on the counts of the colony-forming units (CFU) that were done at least twice with one strain of each species, the following final inocula were calculated to be: *P. acnes* = 4×10^6 CFU, *P. granulosum* = 1×10^7 CFU, *P. avidum* = 3.1×10^7 CFU, *C. minutissimum* = 1.2×10^7 CFU, and *C. parvum* = 7×10^6 CFU.

For trimethoprim, sulfamethoxazole, and the combination of these two drugs (1 + 19 parts), subculturing was done on Mueller-Hinton medium. The strain suspension of *P. avidum* and of the remaining strains was diluted 1:100 and 1:10, respectively, in distilled water.

Antimicrobial agents. A total of 33 preparations of 32 drugs were used for the antimicrobial agents. Potassium benzylpenicillin, sodium oxacillin, sodium dicloxacillin, sodium ampicillin, disodium carbenicillin, streptomycin monosulfate, sisomicin sulfate, and chloramphenicol were supplied by Bayer AG, Leverkusen; sodium cephalothin, cephalexin monohydrate, sodium cefazolin, and tobramycin sulfate were from Eli Lilly GmbH, Giessen; kanamycin monosulfate, colistin methanesulfonate sodium, and tyrothricin were from Gruenenthal GmbH, Stolberg; gentamicin sulfate was from Merck, Darmstadt; tetracycline hydrochloride, rolitetracycline, lincomycin hydrochloride-monohydrate, and sodium novobiocin were from Hoechst AG, Frankfurt; oxytetracycline hydrochloride and doxycycline were supplied by Pfizer GmbH, Karlsruhe; chlortetracycline hydrochloride and minocycline monohydrochloride were from Lederle-Cyanamid GmbH, Munich; clindamycin hydrochloride was from Upjohn GmbH, Heppenheim; erythromycin glucoheptonate was from Schering AG, Berlin; fusidic acid was from Thomae GmbH, Biberach; sodium rifampin was from Ciba-Geigy AG, Wehr; bacitracin was from Dieckmann GmbH, Bielefeld; neomycin B hydrochloride was from Troponwerke, Cologne; and trimethoprim and sodium sulfamethoxazole were from Hoffmann-LaRoche AG, Grenzach.

All products were of known potencies and were dissolved and diluted according to the manufacturers' instructions.

Susceptibility tests. Minimal inhibitory concentrations (MICs) were determined using an agar dilution technique. Freshly prepared drug-Mueller-Hinton agar mixtures were poured into petri dishes. After solidification, the plates were dried for 3 h at 37°C and then inoculated immediately. Plates were incubated for 48 h at 37°C using the Heraeus anaerobic incubator VT/N_2 (95% N_2 and 5% CO_2 at normal atmospheric pressure), and the results were read immediately thereafter. The MIC was considered to be the lowest drug concentration in which no visible growth occurred. Antimicrobial activity controls with *Staphylococcus aureus* (strain SG 511-Jena) as well as growth controls of the strains tested, on drug-free medium, were included with each assay.

RESULTS

In Table 1 the MICs of eight β-lactam antibiotics are shown. Benzylpenicillin was the most active drug, and at 0.1 μg/ml it inhibited 70 of the 73 strains tested. Cephalothin proved to be the best cephalosporin and compared favorably with ampicillin. The three *C. minutissimum* strains showed the least susceptibility to the penicillins, but this was not the case with the cephalosporins. Nevertheless, it can be stated that all the organisms tested were more or less penicillin- and cephalosporin-susceptible.

The activity range of six aminoglycosides examined is summarized in Table 2. Gentamicin showed the best MIC values, whereas kanamycin was the least active aminoglycoside tested. The observation was made that the three *C. minutissimum* strains tested were highly susceptible to some of these agents.

In Table 3 the MICs of six tetracyclines are shown. Some differences in the susceptibility of the 73 strains studied were noted. Chlortetracycline was the least effective in vitro, whereas minocycline was the most active. The MICs of the others were fairly comparable.

Of the antibiotics presented in Table 4, erythromycin and clindamycin exhibited the best activity. The activity of lincomycin was clearly inferior to that of clindamycin, as can be seen best with the *C. minutissimum* strains tested. Novobiocin and fusidic acid were able to attack *P. acnes* strains, too, but their activity range was poor. It is of interest that the three *C. minutissimum* strains examined were particularly susceptible to fusidic acid.

The results in Table 5 show that all strains tested were susceptible to chloramphenicol and bacitracin and resistant to colistin. Rifampin attracts attention because of its high activity against *P. acnes*, *P. granulosum*, *P. avidum*, and *C. parvum*; on the other hand, all three *C. minutissimum* strains showed marked resistance to rifampin. The activity of sulfamethoxazole was poor but, in combination with subinhibitory amounts of trimethoprim, greater activity seemed apparent. Although *P. acnes*, *P. avidum*, and the single *C. parvum* strain tested were susceptible to 5% trimethoprim plus 95% sulfamethoxazole, the activity of this drug combination towards *P. granulosum* and *C. minutissimum* was low.

DISCUSSION

Little information about the antibiotic susceptibility of *P. acnes* was found in previous publications. In 1942 Craddock (3) stated that the "acne bacillus" was less susceptible to penicillin than *S. albus*. It is not only difficult to compare the results reported by Craddock with our own observations, but also the present resistance pattern of *S. epidermidis* is quite different (10). Smith and Waterworth (15) reported the MICs of benzylpenicillin and tetracycline against 32 *P. acnes* strains; all strains were inhibited by 0.4 μg of benzylpenicillin per ml and 94% were inhibited by 1.6 μg of tetracy-

TABLE 1. *Susceptibility of P. acnes and related species to β-lactam antibiotics (absolute numbers, 73 strains examined)*

Antibiotic	Species	No. of strains inhibited at an MIC (μg/ml) of:									
		12.5	6.25	3.1	1.6	0.8	0.4	0.2	0.1	0.04	≤0.02
Benzylpenicillin	*P. acnes*	—	—	—	—	—	—	—	—	35	3
	P. granulosum	—	—	—	—	—	—	—	6	9	—
	P. avidum	—	—	—	—	—	—	—	4	12	—
	C. minutissimum	—	—	—	—	—	2	1	—	—	—
	C. parvum	—	—	—	—	—	—	—	—	1	—
Oxacillin	*P. acnes*	—	—	—	—	1	15	17	5	—	—
	P. granulosum	—	—	—	—	7	8	—	—	—	—
	P. avidum	—	—	—	—	5	8	3	—	—	—
	C. minutissimum	—	—	3	—	—	—	—	—	—	—
	C. parvum	—	—	—	—	—	—	1	—	—	—
Dicloxacillin	*P. acnes*	—	—	—	—	1	10	24	3	—	—
	P. granulosum	—	—	—	6	9	—	—	—	—	—
	P. avidum	—	—	—	6	7	2	1	—	—	—
	C. minutissimum	—	3	—	—	—	—	—	—	—	—
	C. parvum	—	—	—	—	1	—	—	—	—	—
Ampicillin	*P. acnes*	—	—	—	—	—	—	1	25	10	2
	P. granulosum	—	—	—	—	—	—	—	15	—	—
	P. avidum	—	—	—	—	—	—	3	11	2	—
	C. minutissimum	—	—	—	—	3	—	—	—	—	—
	C. parvum	—	—	—	—	—	—	—	1	—	—
Carbenicillin	*P. acnes*	—	—	—	—	7	26	5	—	—	—
	P. granulosum	—	—	—	12	3	—	—	—	—	—
	P. avidum	—	—	—	6	8	2	—	—	—	—
	C. minutissimum	—	3	—	—	—	—	—	—	—	—
	C. parvum	—	—	—	—	1	—	—	—	—	—
Cephalothin	*P. acnes*	—	—	—	—	—	—	2	35	1	—
	P. granulosum	—	—	—	—	1	1	8	5	—	—
	P. avidum	—	—	—	—	—	5	7	4	—	—
	C. minutissimum	—	—	—	—	—	—	3	—	—	—
	C. parvum	—	—	—	—	1	—	—	—	—	—
Cephalexin	*P. acnes*	—	—	—	—	10	25	3	—	—	—
	P. granulosum	1	2	6	5	1	—	—	—	—	—
	P. avidum	1	—	—	—	11	4	—	—	—	—
	C. minutissimum	—	—	—	—	3	—	—	—	—	—
	C. parvum	—	1	—	—	—	—	—	—	—	—
Cefazolin	*P. acnes*	—	—	—	—	—	5	30	3	—	—
	P. granulosum	—	—	—	12	3	—	—	—	—	—
	P. avidum	—	—	—	—	1	13	2	—	—	—
	C. minutissimum	—	—	—	—	—	3	—	—	—	—
	C. parvum	—	—	—	1	—	—	—	—	—	—

TABLE 2. *Susceptibility of P. acnes and related species to aminoglycoside antibiotics (absolute numbers, 73 strains examined)*

Antibiotic	Species	No. of strains inhibited at an MIC (μg/ml) of:									
		≥100.0	50.0	25.0	12.5	6.25	3.1	1.6	0.8	0.4	0.2
Streptomycin	*P. acnes*	–	–	–	14	23	1	–	–	–	–
	P. granulosum	–	–	–	–	9	6	–	–	–	–
	P. avidum	–	–	–	2	14	–	–	–	–	–
	C. minutissimum	–	–	–	–	3	–	–	–	–	–
	C. parvum	–	–	–	–	1	–	–	–	–	–
Kanamycin	*P. acnes*	2	10	22	4	–	–	–	–	–	–
	P. granulosum	1	3	11	–	–	–	–	–	–	–
	P. avidum	16	–	–	–	–	–	–	–	–	–
	C. minutissimum	–	–	3	–	–	–	–	–	–	–
	C. parvum	–	–	1	–	–	–	–	–	–	–
Neomycin	*P. acnes*	–	–	22	12	4	–	–	–	–	–
	P. granulosum	–	–	7	1	4	2	1	–	–	–
	P. avidum	–	–	16	–	–	–	–	–	–	–
	C. minutissimum	–	–	–	3	–	–	–	–	–	–
	C. parvum	–	–	1	–	–	–	–	–	–	–
Gentamicin	*P. acnes*	–	–	–	–	3	24	11	–	–	–
	P. granulosum	–	–	–	–	–	–	4	7	4	–
	P. avidum	–	–	–	–	2	14	–	–	–	–
	C. minutissimum	–	–	–	–	–	–	–	–	3	–
	C. parvum	–	–	–	–	–	–	–	1	–	–
Tobramycin	*P. acnes*	–	–	1	7	–	29	1	–	–	–
	P. granulosum	–	–	–	1	–	11	2	1	–	–
	P. avidum	–	15	1	–	–	–	–	–	–	–
	C. minutissimum	–	–	–	–	–	–	–	2	1	–
	C. parvum	–	–	–	–	1	–	–	–	–	–
Sisomicin	*P. acnes*	–	–	13	19	2	4	–	–	–	–
	P. granulosum	–	9	5	–	–	1	–	–	–	–
	P. avidum	–	1	13	1	1	–	–	–	–	–
	C. minutissimum	–	–	–	–	–	–	–	–	–	3
	C. parvum	–	–	1	–	–	–	–	–	–	–

TABLE 3. *Susceptibility of P. acnes and related species to tetracyclines (absolute numbers, 73 strains examined)*

Antibiotic	Species	No. of strains inhibited at an MIC (μg/ml) of:									
		12.5	6.25	3.1	1.6	0.8	0.4	0.2	0.1	0.4	≤0.02
Tetracycline	*P. acnes*	—	—	9	13	12	2	1	1	—	—
	P. granulosum	—	1	—	5	8	1	—	—	—	—
	P. avidum	1	1	5	9	—	—	—	—	—	—
	C. minutissimum	—	—	—	3	—	—	—	—	—	—
	C. parvum	—	—	—	1	—	—	—	—	—	—
Oxytetracycline	*P. acnes*	—	—	8	30	—	—	—	—	—	—
	P. granulosum	—	—	—	6	6	3	—	—	—	—
	P. avidum	—	—	5	11	—	—	—	—	—	—
	C. minutissimum	—	—	—	—	3	—	—	—	—	—
	C. parvum	—	—	—	—	1	—	—	—	—	—
Chlortetracycline	*P. acnes*	—	9	7	13	4	4	1	—	—	—
	P. granulosum	—	—	4	6	1	1	1	2	—	—
	P. avidum	1	12	3	—	—	—	—	—	—	—
	C. minutissimum	—	3	—	—	—	—	—	—	—	—
	C. parvum	—	—	—	1	—	—	—	—	—	—
Rolitetracycline	*P. acnes*	—	—	—	1	19	18	—	—	—	—
	P. granulosum	—	—	—	—	12	3	—	—	—	—
	P. avidum	—	—	—	5	9	2	—	—	—	—
	C. minutissimum	—	—	—	—	3	—	—	—	—	—
	C. parvum	—	—	—	—	1	—	—	—	—	—
Doxycycline	*P. acnes*	—	—	1	27	10	—	—	—	—	—
	P. granulosum	—	—	3	4	6	2	—	—	—	—
	P. avidum	—	—	—	3	13	—	—	—	—	—
	C. minutissimum	—	—	—	—	3	—	—	—	—	—
	C. parvum	—	—	—	—	1	—	—	—	—	—
Minocycline	*P. acnes*	—	—	—	—	—	8	22	5	3	—
	P. granulosum	—	—	—	—	—	—	7	6	1	1
	P. avidum	—	—	—	—	—	14	2	—	—	—
	C. minutissimum	—	—	—	—	—	3	—	—	—	—
	C. parvum	—	—	—	—	—	—	1	—	—	—

TABLE 4. *Susceptibility of P. acnes and related species to lincomycin, novobiocin, erythromycin, and fusidic acid (absolute numbers, 73 strains examined)*

Antibiotic	Species	No. of strains inhibited at an MIC (μg/ml) of:								
		6.25	3.1	1.6	0.8	0.4	0.2	0.1	0.4	≤0.02
Lincomycin	*P. acnes*	—	—	—	1	10	25	2	—	—
	P. granulosum	1	—	—	—	3	8	3	—	—
	P. avidum	—	—	—	—	9	7	—	—	—
	C. minutissimum	3	—	—	—	—	—	—	—	—
	C. parvum	—	—	—	—	—	1	—	—	—
Clindamycin	*P. acnes*	—	—	—	—	2	3	20	13	—
	P. granulosum	—	—	—	—	—	1	1	12	1
	P. avidum	—	—	—	—	3	2	2	9	—
	C. minutissimum	—	—	—	—	—	3	—	—	—
	C. parvum	—	—	—	—	—	1	—	—	—
Novobiocin	*P. acnes*	—	17	15	6	—	—	—	—	—
	P. granulosum	3	8	2	2	—	—	—	—	—
	P. avidum	4	1	5	3	3	—	—	—	—
	C. minutissimum	—	3	—	—	—	—	—	—	—
	C. parvum	1	—	—	—	—	—	—	—	—
Erythromycin	*P. acnes*	—	—	—	—	—	—	2	22	14
	P. granulosum	—	—	—	—	—	—	—	—	15
	P. avidum	—	—	—	—	—	—	—	16	—
	C. minutissimum	—	—	—	—	1	2	—	—	—
	C. parvum	—	—	—	—	—	—	—	—	1
Fusidic acid	*P. acnes*	2	33	3	—	—	—	—	—	—
	P. granulosum	—	2	12	1	—	—	—	—	—
	P. avidum	1	15	—	—	—	—	—	—	—
	C. minutissimum	—	—	—	—	—	—	1	2	—
	C. parvum	—	—	—	1	—	—	—	—	—

TABLE 5. *Susceptibility of P. acnes and related species to miscellaneous antibiotics (absolute numbers, 73 strains examined)*

Antibiotic	Species	No. of strains inhibited at an MIC (μg/ml) of:													
		>100.0	100.0	50.0	25.0	12.5	6.25	3.1	1.6	0.8	0.4	0.2	0.1	0.04	≤0.02
Chloramphenicol	*P. acnes*	–	–	–	–	–	–	1	33	4	–	–	–	–	–
	P. granulosum	–	–	–	–	–	–	–	3	9	3	–	–	–	–
	P. avidum	–	–	–	–	–	–	1	15	–	–	–	–	–	–
	C. minutissimum	–	–	–	–	–	3	–	–	–	–	–	–	–	–
	C. parvum	–	–	–	–	–	–	–	–	–	1	–	–	–	–
Colistin	*P. acnes*	–	1	22	15	–	–	–	–	–	–	–	–	–	–
	P. granulosum	–	–	–	6	9	–	–	–	–	–	–	–	–	–
	P. avidum	–	14	2	–	–	–	–	–	–	–	–	–	–	–
	C. minutissimum	–	3	–	–	–	–	–	–	–	–	–	–	–	–
	C. parvum	–	–	–	–	1	–	–	–	–	–	–	–	–	–
Rifampin	*P. acnes*	–	–	–	–	–	–	–	–	–	–	1	–	10	27
	P. granulosum	–	–	–	–	–	–	–	–	–	–	–	–	–	15
	P. avidum	–	–	–	–	–	–	–	–	–	–	–	–	–	16
	C. minutissimum	1	1	1	–	–	–	–	–	–	–	–	–	–	–
	C. parvum	–	–	–	–	–	–	–	–	–	–	–	–	–	1
Bacitracin	*P. acnes*	–	–	–	–	–	–	–	–	–	12	25	1	–	–
	P. granulosum	–	–	–	–	–	–	–	–	–	7	6	1	1	–
	P. avidum	–	–	–	–	–	–	10	6	–	–	–	–	–	–
	C. minutissimum	–	–	–	–	–	–	–	–	–	3	–	–	–	–
	C. parvum	–	–	–	–	–	–	–	–	–	–	1	–	–	–
Tyrothricin	*P. acnes*	–	–	–	–	–	–	18	16	4	–	–	–	–	–
	P. granulosum	–	–	–	–	4	4	7	–	–	–	–	–	–	–
	P. avidum	–	–	–	4	9	3	–	–	–	–	–	–	–	–
	C. minutissimum	–	–	–	3	–	–	–	–	–	–	–	–	–	–
	C. parvum	–	–	–	1	–	–	–	–	–	–	–	–	–	–
Trimethoprim	*P. acnes*	–	–	–	–	–	–	–	–	18	18	2	–	–	–
	P. granulosum	–	–	–	–	1	4	4	4	–	–	2	–	–	–
	P. avidum	–	–	–	–	–	–	2	3	9	2	–	–	–	–
	C. minutissimum	–	–	2	–	1	–	–	–	–	–	–	–	–	–
	C. parvum	–	–	–	–	–	–	–	–	–	1	–	–	–	–
Sulfamethoxazole	*P. acnes*	38	–	–	–	–	–	–	–	–	–	–	–	–	–
	P. granulosum	14	–	1	–	–	–	–	–	–	–	–	–	–	–
	P. avidum	–	–	1	1	2	4	8	–	–	–	–	–	–	–
	C. minutissimum	3	–	–	–	–	–	–	–	–	–	–	–	–	–
	C. parvum	1	–	–	–	–	–	–	–	–	–	–	–	–	–
5% Trimethoprim-95% sulfamethoxazole	*P. acnes*	–	–	–	–	–	–	–	–	9	24	5	–	–	–
	P. granulosum	–	–	–	–	3	1	6	4	1	–	–	–	–	–
	P. avidum	–	–	–	–	–	–	–	3	6	7	–	–	–	–
	C. minutissimum	–	–	1	–	2	–	–	–	–	–	–	–	–	–
	C. parvum	–	–	–	–	–	–	–	–	–	–	1	–	–	–

cline per ml. Pochi and Strauss (8) examined 12 *P. acnes* strains and found benzylpenicillin, tetracycline, oxy- and chlortetracycline, novobiocin, erythromycin, and chloramphenicol to be very active, but only 17% of the strains were inhibited by 100.0 μg of neomycin per ml. Bordáčová and Výmola (2) performed susceptibility studies with seven antibiotics. All *P. acnes* strains tested were inhibited by 0.8 μg of ampicillin per ml, 1.6 μg of erythromycin per ml, and 0.2 μg of bacitracin per ml, but only 13% were inhibited by 3.1 μg of oxytetracycline per ml and 73% were inhibited by 6.2 μg of chloramphenicol per ml. Martin et al. (7) established in 1972 MICs of 10 antibiotics against 16 *P. acnes* strains and found that benzylpenicillin, cephalothin, tetracycline, chloramphenicol, erythromycin, rifampin, and lincomycin were highly active but that the aminoglycoside antibiotics were only poorly active. Our data confirm and extend these observations.

The results of our study with 32 drugs demonstrate that these drugs offer a broader spectrum of activity against *P. acnes* and the related species tested than was ever observed with previously tested drugs. This fact should be taken into consideration when chemotherapy of infections with these organisms must be planned.

LITERATURE CITED

1. **Bergey, D. H., R. E. Buchanan, and N. E. Gibbons.** 1974. Bergey's manual of determinative bacteriology, 8th ed. Williams and Wilkins Co., Baltimore.
2. **Bordáčová, J., and F. Výmola.** 1969. Die Empfindlichkeit von Corynebacterium acnes gegen Antibiotika. Drug Res. **19**:386–388.
3. **Craddock, S.** 1942. Use of penicillin in cultivation of the acne bacillus. Lancet **1**:558–559.
4. **Jong, E. C., H. L. Ko, and G. Pulverer.** 1975. Studies on bacteriophages of *Propionibacterium acnes*. Med. Microbiol. Immunol. **161**:263–271.
5. **Lentze, F. A.** 1950. Zur Bakteriologie und Serologie des sog. "Acne-Bacillus" sive Bacterium renale cuniculi (Manteufel u. Herzberg) – der A. B. als Luftkeim eine gefährliche Fehlerquelle der bakteriologisch-serologischen Technik. Zentralbl. Bakteriol. Parasitenkd. Infektionskr. Hyg. Abt. I Orig. **155**:290–294.
6. **Marples, R. R., D. T. Downing, and A. M. Kligman.** 1971. Control of free fatty acids in human surface lipids by *Corynebacterium acnes*. J. Invest. Dermatol. **56**:127–131.
7. **Martin, W. J., M. Gardener, and J. A. Washington II.** 1972. In vitro antimicrobial susceptibility of anaerobic bacteria isolated from clinical specimens. Antimicrob. Agents Chemother. **1**:148–158.
8. **Pochi, P. E., and J. S. Strauss.** 1961. Antibiotic sensitivity of *Corynebacterium acnes* (*Propionibacterium acnes*). J. Invest. Dermatol. **36**:423–429.
9. **Pulverer, G.** 1974. Problems of human actinomycosis. Postepy Hig. Med. Dosw. **28**:253–260.
10. **Pulverer, G., G. Damen, and M. Neugebauer.** 1972. Antibiotic resistance of *Staphylococcus albus*. Med. Microbiol. Immunol. **158**:32–43.
11. **Pulverer, G., and H. L. Ko.** 1973. Fermentative and serological studies on *Propionibacterium acnes*. Appl. Microbiol. **25**:222–229.
12. **Pulverer, G., W. Sorgo, and H. L. Ko.** 1973. Bakteriophagen von *Propionibacterium acnes*. Zentralbl. Bakteriol. Parasitenkd. Infektionskr. Hyg. Abt. I Orig. Reihe A **225**:353–363.
13. **Schaal, K. P.** 1974. Natürliches Vorkommen und klinische Bedeutung grampositiver, nicht sporenbildender Anaerobier. Zentralbl. Bakteriol. Parasitenkd. Infektionskr. Hyg. Abt. I Orig. Reihe A **228**:56–62.
14. **Shehadeh, N. H., and A. M. Kligman.** 1963. The bacteriology of acne. Arch. Dermatol. **88**:829–831.
15. **Smith, M. A., and P. M. Waterworth.** 1961. The bacteriology of acne vulgaris in relation to its treatment with antibiotics. Br. J. Dermatol. **73**:152–159.
16. **Voss, J. G.** 1974. Acne vulgaris and free fatty acids. A review and criticism. Arch. Dermatol. **109**:894–898.

ANTIMICROBIAL AGENTS AND CHEMOTHERAPY, Sept. 1976, p. 395-398
Vol. 10, No. 3
Printed in U.S.A.

Pharmacological Study of Cefazolin During Intermittent and Continuous Infusion: a Crossover Investigation in Humans

J. P. THYS,* B. VANDERKELEN, AND J. KLASTERSKY

Unité de Réanimation Médicale et Clinique Neuro-Chirurgicale, Hôpital Saint-Pierre, and Service de Médecine Interne, Institut Jules Bordet, Brussels, Belgium*

Received for publication 12 April 1976

Levels of cefazolin were determined in plasma, urine, bile, and cerebrospinal fluid in humans after a bolus intravenous injection and during a controlled, continuous intravenous infusion. All the patients were studied in a steady-state and crossover fashion. In plasma, the mean peak level after bolus injection (1.5 g) studied in 12 patients was 206.5 μg/ml; during continuous infusion (6 g daily), the mean level remained stable at 52.6 μg/ml. With bolus injection and continuous infusion, respectively, 89.7 and 86.3% of the administered dose of cefazolin were excreted in the urine of nine patients over the 6-h period considered. The levels of cefazolin in common bile duct bile were studied in six cholecystectomized patients. In bile collected during the two 3-h periods of the experiment, the mean concentration of the drug in the bile after bolus injection was 66.9 and 22.0 μg/ml, respectively; during continuous infusion, the corresponding biliary levels were 50.7 and 51.3 μg/ml, respectively. In four neurosurgical patients with an intraventricular catheter, neither bolus injection nor continuous infusion resulted in a demonstrable concentration of cefazolin in the cerebrospinal fluid. The continuous intravenous administration of cefazolin might have some advantage over the intravenous bolus intermittent injections. In plasma, the area under the curve is greater with continuous infusion than with bolus injection. In bile, the levels of cefazolin are more sustained with continuous infusion than with bolus injection. This approach to intravenous administration of cefazolin deserves more pharmacological and clinical trials.

To rapidly achieve an optimal concentration of antibiotics in infected sites, large doses of these drugs are frequently administered by the intravenous route. The mode of administration is either the intravenous bolus injection, which provides "peak" and "valley" blood levels, or continuous intravenous infusion, which produces sustained but relatively low concentrations of antibiotics in the blood. Whether one of these techniques of injection should be preferred in order to obtain optimal clinical results is still a matter of controversy.

This investigation was carried out to determine the levels of cefazolin, a relatively new cephalosporin, in various body fluids (plasma, urine, bile, and cerebrospinal fluid [CSF]) after a bolus intravenous injection and during a continuous intravenous perfusion.

(This paper was presented at the 9th International Congress of Chemotherapy, London, 1975.)

MATERIALS AND METHODS

The patients, with the exception of those in whom the biliary concentration of cefazolin was studied, were hospitalized in a neurosurgical unit at the Institut Jules Bordet. All had a normal renal function as determined by the creatinine clearance. The daily dose of cefazolin was 6 g. For intermittent administration, 1.5 g (dissolved in 9 ml of 5% dextrose in water) was injected over a 3-min period four times during a 24-h period. In the other experiment, the same amount of cefazolin (6 g) was dissolved in 1,000 ml of 5% dextrose in water and was given as a continuous intravenous infusion using an automated infusion device (Automated Infusion Unit, Decca, London) to strictly control the rate of administration. All the patients studied here received cefazolin by the two techniques of administration on 2 consecutive days.

The samples of the various fluids to be studied were obtained between h 18 and 24 of each experiment, a period that we have considered to represent a steady state. Samples of heparinized blood were obtained at various intervals of time after the bolus injection: 2 min after the end of the injection (thus, 5 min after its onset), and 10 and 30 min and 1, 2, 3, 4, and 6 h after the injection. During the 6-h period of the continuous infusion, blood samples were taken at 0, 1.30, 3, 4.30, and 6 h. Urine was obtained during this time as two 3-h collections through an indwelling catheter. The patients included in the study of the biliary levels of cefazolin provided urine by spontaneous voiding at the end of each 3-h period. These patients had been cholecystectomized for cholelithiasis or a nonfunctioning gall bladder between 5 and 14 days prior to the study. Samples of common bile duct bile were obtained through a T-tube over two 3-h periods.

To study the penetration of cefazolin in the CSF, four patients with no meningeal inflammation who were undergoing a monitoring of their intracranial pressure through an intraventricular catheter were investigated. The catheter allowed the collection of CSF simultaneously to the collection of blood samples.

All samples of plasma, urine, bile, and CSF were stored at −20°C until assayed. The assay of cefazolin in these various fluids was performed as described by Bennett and co-workers (3), using *Bacillus subtilis* (Subtilis spore suspension, Difco, Detroit, Mich.) as the test organism. Each assay was made in quadruplicate. To dilute the clinical fluid to be assayed and to prepare the reference curves, we used human plasma for plasma assays and human common bile duct bile (without any spontaneous antibacterial activity) for bile assays; for urine and CSF, phosphate buffer was employed.

RESULTS

Levels in plasma. After the bolus injection, the mean peak plasma level in 12 patients was 206.5 ± 10.9 μg/ml (mean ± standard error of the mean); after 3 and 6 h, the mean plasma levels were 29.1 ± 5.2 and 13.5 ± 3.3 μg/ml, respectively, as shown in Fig. 1. During the continuous infusion, the mean plasma level remained stable at 52.6 ± 6.5 μg/ml. Based on these data, the area under the curve associated with the continuous infusion was greater by 24.2% than that associated with the bolus injection.

Levels in urine. The urinary excretion of cefazolin was studied in nine patients. As indicated in Fig. 2, the bolus injection resulted, during the first 3 h after the injection, in a mean concentration of cefazolin of 7,320 ± 1,498 μg/ml and, over this period of time, 1,034 ± 95 mg was excreted. In the urine obtained during the next 3-h period, the mean concentration of cefazolin was 2,348 ± 528 μg/ml, and 311.2 ± 58 mg was excreted. During the continuous infusion the corresponding urinary levels of cefazolin were 5,099 ± 945 and 5,370 ± 830 μg/ml, respectively; the amounts of cefazolin excreted were 661.3 ± 38 and 634 ± 36 mg, respectively, indicating that during the continuous infusion the rate of the urinary excretion of cefazolin was constant.

With the bolus injection and the continuous infusion, respectively, 89.7 and 86.3% of the administered doses of cefazolin were excreted in the urine over the 6-h period considered.

Levels in common bile duct bile. The levels of cefazolin in common bile duct bile were studied in six patients (Table 1). After the bolus injection, the mean concentration in the bile obtained during the first 3-h period was 66.9 ± 36.7 μg/ml; it was 22.0 ± 12.7 μg/ml in the bile that was collected during the last 3 h of the experiment. During the continuous infusion, the corresponding biliary levels of cefazolin were 50.7 ± 21.1 and 51.3 ± 21.1 μg/ml, respectively. Patient 3, who presented no biliary tract obstruction, excreted very high levels of cefazolin into the common bile duct bile. In patients 4, 5, and 6, relatively lower levels of cefazolin

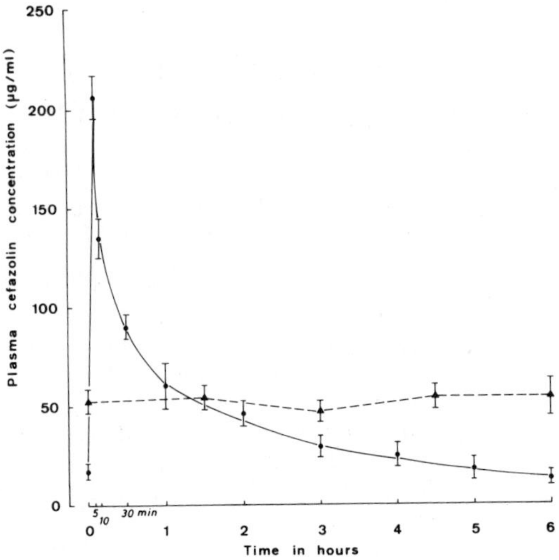

FIG. 1. *Plasma cefazolin levels after bolus injection (●) and during continuous infusion (▲).*

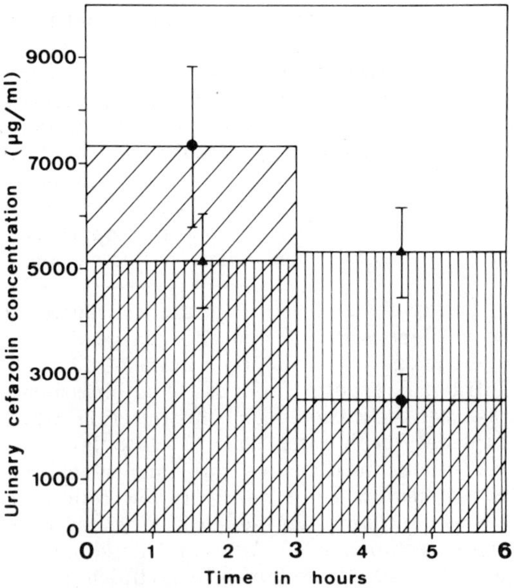

FIG. 2. *Urinary cefazolin concentrations after bolus injection (●, ▨) and during continuous infusion (▲, ▥).*

TABLE 1. *Concentrations of cefazolin in common bile duct bile*

Patient no.	Concn of cefazolin (μg/ml) after:			
	Bolus injection		Continuous infusion	
	0–3 h	3–6 h	0–3 h	3–6 h
1	9.7	5.2	16.8	17.0
2	4.4	1.0	11.5	12.5
3	245.0	84.0	150.0	148.0
4	41.5	16.3	35.0	34.5
5	57.5	17.2	60.0	69.5
6	43.0	8.5	31.0	26.0
Mean ± SEM[a]	66.9 ± 36.7	22.0 ± 12.7	50.7 ± 21.1	51.3 ± 21.1

[a] SEM, Standard error of the mean.

were found in the bile; patient 4 and patient 5 presented signs of biliary tract obstruction, but patient 6 had no such signs. In patients 1 and 2 only very low biliary cefazolin levels were observed; patient 1 had a slight cholostasis, but patient 2 had normal liver function.

Levels in CSF. In four patients with an intraventricular catheter, neither the bolus injection nor the continuous infusion of cefazolin resulted in a demonstrable concentration of the antibiotic in ventricular CSF.

DISCUSSION

The plasma levels of cefazolin obtained here with the intravenous bolus injection are comparable to those obtained by other investigators (5, 8, 16). The shape of the curve of the plasma levels after the bolus injection is also similar to that observed by others (9, 20). Very few authors, however, have studied the plasma levels of cefazolin during a continuous infusion. With a loading dose of 250 mg followed by a continuous infusion of 100 mg/h during 2 h, Kirby and Regamey (10) obtained a steady plasma level at 28.6 μg/ml. Simon et al. (20), with a daily dose of 4 g given as a continuous perfusion, observed a constant blood level of 25.1 μg/ml. With a daily dosage of 6 g, we obtained a constant plasma level of 52.6 μg/ml, which is similar to that observed by Reller et al. (18) during a steady state obtained by a continuous infusion of 240 mg/h (i.e., 6 g/24 h). The urinary excretion of cefazolin observed in our study was slightly higher than that found by other workers. (5, 8).

In the bile from the common bile duct, the concentration of cefazolin in our patients appeared to be adequate after intermittent and during continuous intravenous administration. At the dosage used in this study, the biliary levels of cefazolin were adequate against most clinical pathogens. Other authors stressed the good biliary levels of this cephalosporin (4, 11, 15, 17): the concentrations of cefazolin in the common bile duct bile were usually found to be equal to or higher than the blood level (4, 15, 17). However, for cefazolin, as for other antibiotics, the biliary concentration is variable from patient to patient, especially if obstruction is present; in this latter condition, the concentrations of antibiotic in the bile are usually extremely low. The biliary levels found in our patients were variable; however, the relationship between cholestasis and the levels of cefazolin in the common bile duct bile did not appear clearly.

We could not find any demonstrable cefazolin in the CSF of four patients without meningeal inflammation. This very poor diffusion of cefazolin through the blood-brain barrier has already been observed by other investigators (1; L. H. Baker, D. R. Hinthorn, D. A. Romig, and C. Liu, Abstr. Clin. Res. **XXII**:613A, 1974); thus, cefazolin should not be used to treat bacterial meningitis (12).

The basic problem of the respective effectiveness of intermittent or continuous administration of antibiotics has not yet stimulated many experimental and clinical investigations, and this question is still unsolved. Eagle et al. (6) noted that the total time during which penicillin has to be provided at effective levels is largely independent of the method of administration, provided the interval between successive injections would be short enough as not to allow the multiplication of the surviving bacteria. However, in the experiments of Eagle et al., it was not absolutely necessary to continuously maintain effective levels of penicillin to achieve cure. However, these studies suggested that the most effective form of treatment is the one that provides antibiotics continuously, in excess of the effective levels, so both the drug and the defenses of the host are continuously operative. On the other hand, Schmidt and Walley (19), using an experimental model of pneumonia in rats, concluded that relatively long intervals between successive administrations of penicillin were more effective than shorter ones. Similarly, in an experimental wound infection model, Ehrlich and co-workers (7) have found that the concentration of cephaloridine in the wound was greater with a bolus injection than with a continuous infusion. In a recent study, Barza and co-workers (2) demonstrated that the accumulation of penicillins and cephalosporins in experimental fibrin clots was greater with repetitive bolus injections than with continuous infusions. These findings appear to be explained by the higher peak concentration in the serum after the bolus injection and by the longer half-life of the antibiotic in the fibrin clots than in the serum. Thus, these observations suggest that an intermittent antibiotic therapy might be more effective than a continuous one.

The major aim of this study was to compare the levels of cefazolin in various sites after direct intravenous injection and during continuous infusion. By comparing the areas under the curves, plasma bioavailability of cefazolin appeared to be greater with continuous infusion than with intermittent injection. In addition, the concentration of cefazolin in common bile duct bile could be maintained at an adequate level with the continuous infusion only.

We also tried to compare the consequences of the two modes of intravenous administration on the CSF cefazolin levels; unfortunately, the very poor penetration of cefazolin through the normal meninges made this comparison impossible. However, experimental data in dogs suggest that the continuous infusion of antibiotics might be more effective in achieving adequate CSF levels than successive bolus injections (14).

We have attempted to study the penetration of cefazolin within the bronchial secretions: the levels of cefazolin in the bronchial purulent secretions of seven tracheotomized patients seemed to be very low. However, we found it difficult to assay accurately cefazolin in bronchial secretions, owing to a slight spontaneous antimicrobial activity of most specimens. Pennington and Reynolds (13) observed, with gentamicin in dogs, that the penetration into the bronchial fluid was relatively poor. In addition, a rapid intravenous injection of gentamicin produced a high but transient level in the bronchial secretions, but, on the other hand, intramuscular injection resulted in lower levels that were more sustained.

The basic question that we raise in the present study remains largely unsolved since the penetration of cefazolin through the two biological membranes that we planned to study, the meninges and the bronchial wall, was very poor. Nevertheless, we believe that the optimal way to administer antibiotics deserves further pharmacological and clinical studies.

ACKNOWLEDGMENTS

We thank A. Bremer and J. Brihaye (Université Libre de Bruxelles) for allowing us to study their patients.

The present study was supported by a grant from Bristol Laboratories, Benelux.

We thank H. Soep (Bristol Laboratories) for his helpful suggestions, and we are indebted to L. Vandenborre for her technical assistance.

LITERATURE CITED

1. **Armengaud, M., J. C. Auvergnat, and A. Gleises.** 1975. Diffusion de la céfazoline dans le liquide céphalo-rachidien (L.C.R.) en fonction du mode d'administration. Données cliniques humaines et expérimentales animales. Nouv. Presse Med. 4:668.
2. **Barza, M., J. Brusch, M. G. Bergeron, and L. Weinstein.** 1974. Penetration of antibiotics into fibrin loci in vivo. III. Intermittent vs. continuous infusion and the effect of probenecid. J. Infect. Dis. 129:73–78.
3. **Bennett, J. V., J. L. Brodie, E. J. Benner, and W. M. M. Kirby.** 1966. Simplified, accurate method for antibiotic assay of clinical specimens. Appl. Microbiol. 14:170–177.
4. **Brogard, J. M., M. Dorner, M. Pinget, M. Adloff, and J. Lavillaureix.** 1975. The biliary excretion of cefazolin. J. Infect. Dis. 131:625–633.
5. **Cahn, M. M., E. J. Levy, P. Actor, and J. F. Pauls.** 1974. Comparative serum levels and urinary recovery of cefazolin, cephaloridine, and cephalothin in man. J. Clin. Pharmacol. 14:61–66.
6. **Eagle, A., R. Fleischman, and M. Levy.** 1953. "Continuous" vs. "discontinuous" therapy with penicillin. The effect of the interval between injections on therapeutic efficacy. N. Engl. J. Med. 248:481–488.
7. **Ehrlich, H. P., V. Licko, and T. K. Hunt.** 1973. Kinetics of cephaloridine in experimental wounds. Am. J. Med. Sci. 265:33–44.
8. **Gold, J. A., J. J. Mc Kee, and D. S. Ziv.** 1973. Experience with cefazolin: an overall summary of pharmacologic and clinical trials in man. J. Infect. Dis. 128:(Suppl.):415–421.
9. **Hodges, G. R., and S. Saslaw.** 1973. Experiences with cefazolin: a new cephalosporin antibiotic. Am. J. Med. Sci. 265:23–32.
10. **Kirby, W. M. M., and C. Regamey.** 1973. Pharmacokinetics of cefazolin compared with four other cephalosporins. J. Infect. Dis. 128(Suppl.):341–346.
11. **Knothe, H., B. W. Lauer, and W. Hartel.** 1974. Die Gallenausscheidung von Cefazolin. Infection II(Suppl. 1):54–59.
12. **Lorber, B., J. Santoro, and R. M. Swenson.** 1975. Listeria meningitis during cefazolin therapy. Ann. Intern. Med. 82:226.
13. **Pennington, J. E., and H. Y. Reynolds.** 1975. Pharmacokinetics of gentamicin sulfate in bronchial secretions. J. Infect. Dis. 131:158–162.
14. **Plorde, J. J., M. Garcia, and R. G. Petersdorf.** 1964. Studies on the pathogenesis of meningitis. IV. Penicillin levels in the cerebrospinal fluid in experimental meningitis. J. Lab. Clin. Med. 64:960–969.
15. **Ram, M. D., and S. Watanatittan.** 1973. Levels of cefazolin in human bile. J. Infect. Dis. 128(Suppl.):361–363.
16. **Rattie, E. S., and L. J. Ravin.** 1975. Pharmacokinetic interpretation of blood levels and urinary excretion data for cefazolin and cephalothin after intravenous and intramuscular administration in humans. Antimicrob. Agents Chemother. 7:606–613.
17. **Ratzan, K. R., C. Ruiz, and G. L. Irvin III.** 1974. Biliary tract excretion of cefazolin, cephalothin, and cephaloridine in the presence of biliary tract disease. Antimicrob. Agents Chemother. 6:426–431.
18. **Reller, L. B., W. W. Karney, H. N. Beaty, K. K. Holmes, and M. Turck.** 1973. Evaluation of cefazolin, a new cephalosporin antibiotic. Antimicrob. Agents Chemother. 3:488–497.
19. **Schmidt, L. H., and A. Walley.** 1951. The influence of the dosage regimen on the therapeutic effectiveness of penicillin G in experimental lobar pneumonia. J. Pharmacol. Exp. Ther. 103:479–488.
20. **Simon, C., V. Malerczyk, E. Brahmstaedt, and W. Toeller.** 1973. Cefazolin, ein neues Breitspektrum-Antibiotikum. Dtsch. Med. Wochenschr. 98:2448–2450.

ANTIMICROBIAL AGENTS AND CHEMOTHERAPY, Sept. 1976, p. 399-401

Vol. 10, No. 3
Printed in U.S.A.

Activity of Newer Aminoglycosides and Carbenicillin, Alone and in Combination, Against Gentamicin-Resistant *Pseudomonas aeruginosa*

M. I. MARKS,* S. HAMMERBERG, G. GREENSTONE, AND BARRY SILVER

Departments of Pediatrics, Microbiology, and Immunology, McGill University-Montreal Children's Hospital Research Institute, Montreal, Quebec, Canada

Received for publication 28 April 1976

The in vitro activity of the aminoglycoside antibiotics tobramycin, sisomicin, amikacin, gentamicin, and netilmicin (SCH 20569) were compared against 26 gentamicin-resistant isolates of *Pseudomonas aeruginosa* cultured from hospitalized children. Tobramycin had the greatest activity on a weight basis, followed by sisomicin, gentamicin, amikacin, and netilmicin. All isolates were resistant to achievable concentrations of netilmicin and gentamicin, but 23% were inhibited by achievable concentrations of tobramycin, 8% by amikacin, and 4% by sisomicin. The combinations carbenicillin/tobramycin, carbenicillin/sisomicin, and carbenicillin/amikacin were synergistic for 92% of strains; antagonism was not encountered. These in vitro results suggest that tobramycin, sisomicin, or amikacin in combination with carbenicillin would be the safest initial regimen in the therapy of gentamicin-resistant *Pseudomonas* infections pending susceptibility studies.

Pseudomonas aeruginosa resistant to currently available antibiotics, including gentamicin, are becoming more prevalent. A study was undertaken to investigate the activity of several new aminoglycosides against a population of gentamicin-resistant *P. aeruginosa* to determine the extent of cross-resistance between tobramycin, sisomicin, amikacin, netilmicin (SCH 20569), and gentamicin. The possibility of carbenicillin/aminoglycoside synergism against this resistant population of *P. aeruginosa* was also examined.

MATERIALS AND METHODS

Twenty-six strains of *P. aeruginosa* were isolated from 23 patients at the Montreal Children's Hospital and identified by using standard microbiological techniques. At least 14 different types of *Pseudomonas* were represented among the isolates studied, as determined by serological and phage-typing methods (kindly performed by N. Hinton, Toronto). All strains were screened for resistance to gentamicin by a standardized disk diffusion test (16) and were considered resistant if the zone diameter was <13 mm and the agar dilution minimum inhibitory concentration (MIC) was ≥6.25 μg/ml. Bacteria were stored in sheep blood at −20°C until tested.

Tobramycin sulfate was supplied as a solution of 1,000 μg/ml and was stored at 4°C. Gentamicin, sisomicin, amikacin, netilmicin, and carbenicillin were supplied as dry powders and were reconstituted immediately before use. Agar dilution MICs were performed according to the method of Steers et al. (19) using Mueller-Hinton agar (Ca^{2+}, 7 mg/100 ml, Mg^{2+}, 3.6 mg/100 ml) and an inoculum of 10^6 to 10^7 bacteria/ml. The MIC was defined as the lowest concentration of drug allowing no colonial growth on the surface of the agar.

Plates for single antibiotic agar dilution studies were prepared 48 h in advance and stored at 4°C. Plates for combination studies were prepared 2 h before use. Synergism was tested by adding either 25 or 50 μg of carbenicillin per ml to each dilution of four of the aminoglycosides listed above. The combination was considered synergistic if there was a decrease of four double dilutions or greater in the aminoglycoside MIC and antagonistic if an increase of four double dilutions or greater in MIC was noted.

RESULTS

Susceptibilities of the 26 isolates of gentamicin-resistant *P. aeruginosa* are plotted in Fig. 1. At a concentration of ≤3.12 μg/ml, tobramycin inhibited 23% of all isolates, versus 4% for sisomicin and 0 for gentamicin, amikacin, and netilmicin. At ≤12.5 μg/ml (a readily achievable serum concentration), amikacin inhibited 8% of isolates. Ninety-two percent of isolates were inhibited by ≥50 μg of carbenicillin per ml.

The results of adding 25 or 50 μg of carbenicillin per ml to each concentration of four of the aminoglycosides are summarized in Table 1. Eighty-one percent of the organisms were susceptible to the combination of tobramycin and

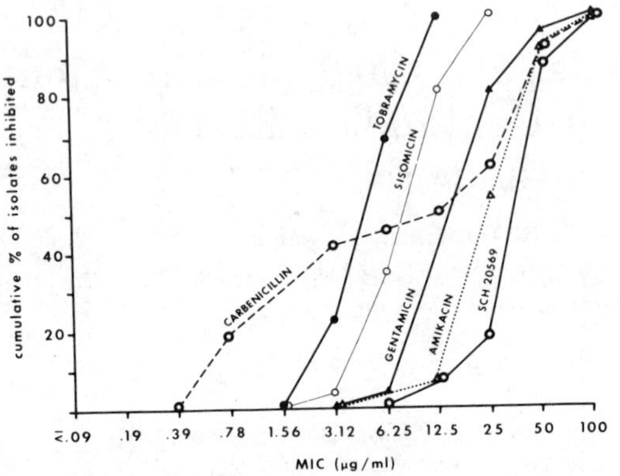

FIG. 1. *Activity of five aminoglycosides and carbenicillin against 26 recent clinical isolates of gentamicin-resistant P. aeruginosa (agar dilution method, 10^6 to 10^7-colony-forming units/ml inoculum). Sch 20569 is netilmicin.*

TABLE 1. *Effect of carbenicillin on the antipseudomonas activity of four aminoglycosides*

Antibiotic	% of strains inhibited: 25 μg of carbenicillin per ml	% of strains inhibited: 50 μg of carbenicillin per ml
Tobramycin	81	92
Sisomicin	77	92
Gentamicin	73	88
Amikacin	85	92

25 μg of carbenicillin per ml (Fig. 2). Seventy-seven percent of the organisms were susceptible to the sisomicin/carbenicillin combination, 85% to amikacin/carbenicillin, and 73% to gentamicin/carbenicillin combinations (Fig. 3). Synergy was more marked (88 to 92%) when 50 μg of carbenicillin per ml was added (Table 1). When the 15 highly gentamicin-resistant isolates (MIC >25 μg/ml) were considered, synergy was demonstrated against 87% with each of tobramycin, amikacin, gentamicin, and sisomicin combined with carbenicillin. Antagonism was not demonstrable between any of the four aminoglycosides and carbenicillin.

DISCUSSION

This study evaluated the susceptibility of a population of gentamicin-resistant strains of *P. aeruginosa* to tobramycin, sisomicin, gentamicin, amikacin, netilmicin, and carbenicillin. Tobramycin exhibited the greatest activity against *Pseudomonas,* as previously reported (8, 9, 12, 13, 15, 21). Sisomicin was active against gentamicin-resistant *Pseudomonas* but to a lesser degree than tobramycin (20). There was complete cross-resistance between amikacin, netilmicin, and gentamicin on a weight comparison basis but higher concentrations of amikacin were achievable in serum. Nevertheless, only 8% of the isolates were inhibited by ≥12.5 μg of amikacin per ml. This agrees with previous reports of tobramycin, gentamicin, and amikacin in vitro anti-*Pseudomonas* activity (14, 18, 20, 21). Two studies, using broth dilution methods, have reported higher amikacin activity against these strains (4, 11). The lack of complete cross-resistance between tobramycin and gentamicin is in accord with previous reports (3, 5–7, 12).

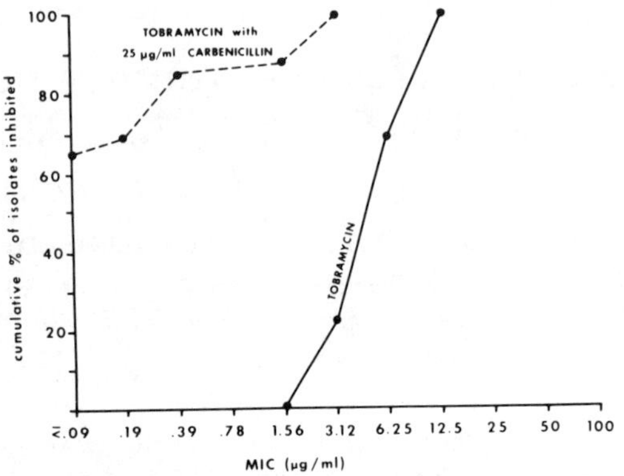

FIG. 2. *Effect of adding 25 μg of carbenicillin per ml on the activity of tobramycin against 26 recent clinical isolates of gentamicin-resistant P. aeruginosa (method as in Fig. 1).*

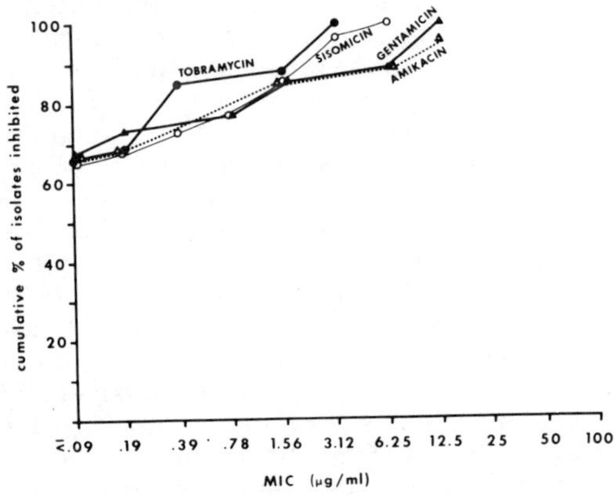

FIG. 3. *Effect of adding 25 μg of carbenicillin per ml on activity of four aminoglycosides against 26 recent clinical isolates of gentamicin-resistant P. aeruginosa (method as in Fig. 1).*

Although many strains of *Pseudomonas* are susceptible to achievable concentrations of carbenicillin, emergence of resistance is a limiting factor to the use of carbenicillin alone in the treatment of *Pseudomonas* infections. Synergism against *Pseudomonas* has been reported previously with combinations of tobramycin/carbenicillin (1, 9–11), gentamicin/carbenicillin (1, 9–11, 15, 17), amikacin/carbenicillin (10, 11), and sisomicin/carbenicillin (10). In this study, 73 to 92% of strains exhibited some potential for synergism when tobramycin was combined with 25 or 50 μg of carbenicillin per ml; however, no antagonism was noted. Kluge et al. (11) reported that highly gentamicin-resistant *Pseudomonas* were not inhibited by combinations of tobramycin or gentamicin with carbenicillin. As recently reported by Anderson et al. (1), however, we found that synergism could not be predicted by the degree of gentamicin resistance. Differences in methods (Kluge et al. [11] used Trypticase soy agar broth in microtiter; Anderson and our studies used Mueller-Hinton agar dilution) may be responsible.

ACKNOWLEDGMENTS

The assistance of N. Hinton and S. Sorger and the support of Eli Lilly, Schering Corp., and Bristol Labs are gratefully acknowledged.

LITERATURE CITED

1. **Anderson, E. L., P. K. Gramling, P. R. Vestal, and W. E. Farrar, Jr.** 1975. Susceptibility of *Pseudomonas aeruginosa* to tobramycin or gentamicin alone and combined with carbenicillin. Antimicrob. Agents Chemother. 8:300–304.
2. **Andriole, V. T.** 1974. Antibiotic synergy in experimental infection with Pseudomonas. II. The effect of carbenicillin, cephalothin, or cephanone combined with tobramycin or gentamicin. J. Infect. Dis. **129**:124–133.
3. **Black, H. R., and R. S. Griffith.** 1971. Preliminary studies with nebramycin factor 6, p. 314–321. Antimicrob. Agents Chemother. 1970.
4. **Bodey, G. P., and D. Stewart.** 1973. In vitro studies of BB-K8, a new aminoglycoside antibiotic. Antimicrob. Agents Chemother. 4:186–192.
5. **Brusch, J. L., M. Barza, M. G. Bergeron, and L. Weinstein.** 1972. Cross-resistance of *Pseudomonas* to gentamicin and tobramycin. Antimicrob. Agents Chemother. 1:280–281.
6. **Crowe, C. C., and E. Sanders.** 1972. Is there complete cross-resistance of gram-negative bacilli to gentamicin and tobramycin? Antimicrob. Agents Chemother. 2:415–416.
7. **Jedlickova, Z., and M. Ryc.** 1974. Tobramycin: comparative *in vitro* susceptibility studies. Chemotherapy **20**:303–314.
8. **Klastersky, J., D. Daneau, and V. de Maertelaer.** 1973. Comparative study of tobramycin and gentamicin with special reference to their anti-pseudomonas activity. Clin. Pharmacol. Ther. **14**:104–111.
9. **Klastersky, J., A. Henri, and L. Vandenborre.** 1973. Antimicrobial activity of tobramycin and gentamicin used in combination with cephalothin and carbenicillin. Am. J. Med. Sci. **266**:13–21.
10. **Klastersky, J., B. Nyamubeya, and L. Vandenborre.** 1974. Antimicrobial effectiveness of kanamycin, aminosidin, BB-K8, sisomicin, gentamicin and tobramycin combined with carbenicillin or cephalothin against gram-negative rods. J. Med. Microbiol. 7:465–72.
11. **Kluge, R. M., H. C. Standiford, B. Tatem, V. M. Young, W. H. Greene, S. C. Schimpff, F. M. Calia, and R. B Hornick.** 1974. Comparative activity of tobramycin, amikacin, and gentamicin alone and with carbenicillin against *Pseudomonas aeruginosa*. Antimicrob. Agents Chemother. **6**:442–446.
12. **Laxer, R. M., E. MacKay, and M. I. Marks.** 1975. Antibacterial activity of tobramycin against gram-negative bacteria and the combination of ampicillin/tobramycin against *E. coli*. Chemotherapy **21**:90–98.
13. **Levison, M. E., R. Knight, and D. Kaye.** 1972. In vitro evaluation of tobramycin, a new aminoglycoside antibiotic. Antimicrob. Agents Chemother. **1**:381–384.
14. **Marks, M. I.** 1975. *In vitro* antibacterial activity of amikacin, a new aminoglycoside, against clinical bacterial isolates from children. J. Clin. Pharmacol. **15**:246–251.
15. **Meyer, R. D., L. S. Young, and D. Armstrong.** 1971. Tobramycin (nebramycin factor 6): in vitro activity against *Pseudomonas aeruginosa*. Appl. Microbiol. **22**:1147–1151.
16. **National Committee for Clinical Laboratory Standards.** 1974. Revised tentative standard (August 1974). Performance standards for antimicrobial disc susceptibility tests. National Committee for Clinical Laboratory Standards, Philadelphia.
17. **Phair, J. P., C. Watanakunakorn, and T. Bannister.** 1969. In vitro susceptibility of *Pseudomonas aeruginosa* to carbenicillin and the combination of carbenicillin and gentamicin. Appl. Microbiol. **18**:303–306.
18. **Price, K. E., T. A. Pursiano, M. D. DeFuria, and G. E. Wright.** 1974. Activity of BB-K8 (amikacin) against clinical isolates resistant to one or more aminoglycoside antibiotics. Antimicrob. Agents Chemother. **5**:143–152.
19. **Steers, E., E. L. Foltz, and B. S. Graves.** 1959. An inocula-replicating apparatus for routine testing of bacterial susceptibility of antibiotics. Antibiot. Chemother. **9**:307–311.
20. **Stewart, D., and G. P. Bodey.** 1975. *In vitro* activity of sisomicin, an aminoglycoside antibiotic, against clinical isolates. J. Antibiot. **28**:149–155.
21. **Yourassowsky, E., E. Shoutens, and M. P. Vanderlinder.** 1975. Comparison of the *in vitro* activities of BB-K8 and three other aminoglycosides against 215 strains of pseudomonas and enterobacteriaceae with variable sensitivity to kanamycin and gentamicin. Chemotherapy **21**:45–51.

ANTIMICROBIAL AGENTS AND CHEMOTHERAPY, Sept. 1976, p. 402-410 Vol. 10, No. 3

Printed in U.S.A.

Inhibition of the Apparent Rate of Synthesis of the Vacuolar Glycoprotein Carboxypeptidase Y and Its Protein Antigen by Tunicamycin in *Saccharomyces cerevisiae*

ANDREJ HASILIK AND WIDMAR TANNER*

University of Regensburg, 84 Regensburg, West Germany

Received for publication 14 April 1976

Carboxypeptidase Y from *Saccharomyces cerevisiae* contains 14% mannose, the only neutral sugar present. An antiserum can be raised in rabbits which reacts with both the protein and the sugar moieties of the enzyme. This antiserum also precipitates yeast invertase and yeast cell wall mannan. Thus carboxypeptidase Y, which is known to be localized in yeast vacuoles, is very probably a mannoprotein. Tunicamycin inhibits the apparent formation of carboxypeptidase Y to a similar extent as that of the externally localized mannoprotein, invertase. No accumulation of an inactive nonglycosylated or partly glycosylated carboxypeptidase Y occurs as determined by the immunoprecipitation technique. Tunicamycin also inhibits the apparent formation of proteinase A, whereas it does not affect the increase in the activities of a number of other enzymes. It is suggested that in the synthesis of glycoproteins there exists a regulatory link between the synthesis of their polypeptide chains and the reactions involved in their glycosylation.

Carbohydrate moieties of glycoproteins are synthesized from sugar nucleotides. The reactions involved occur in tight association with membranes and proceed in part via lipid intermediates (4, 13, 21). This has been shown in a variety of organisms, including yeasts (20, 34). Transfer of *N*-acetylglucosamine to lipid is sensitive to tunicamycin (6, 38, 39), an antibiotic from *Streptomyces lysosuperificus* (37). In yeast protoplasts, tunicamycin has been shown to inhibit mannan synthesis and secretion of invertase and of acid phosphatase (18).

Carboxypeptidase Y is located in the vacuole (10, 22). It had been first purified and characterized as a glycoprotein by Hata and co-workers (11). Its carbohydrate moiety has been shown to constitute about 15% of the enzyme by weight and to be composed largely of a neutral sugar, with a smaller amount of *N*-acetylglucosamine (1, 12, 17). It has attracted the interest of several laboratories due to its low specificity and other unique catalytic properties (3, 14, 23) and has also become the object of several studies concerned with the physiology of yeast proteinases (15).

In the present paper, the effect of tunicamycin on the formation of carboxypeptidase Y has been investigated to see whether the formation of intracellular glycoproteins is also affected by this antibiotic.

The immunoprecipitation technique was used to differentiate between possible effects of the antibiotic on the changes in the activity of the glycoprotein and on its total concentration. Since this enzyme proved to have a complex antigenic activity, the precipitation characteristics of the antisera raised against it and used throughout this study are also described in some detail.

MATERIALS AND METHODS

Organism, cultivation, and harvesting. The diploid yeast *Saccharomyces cerevisiae* X2180, isolated by R. K. Mortimer (25), was used throughout this study. The culture was maintained on YPD agar slants consisting of 2% D-glucose, 2% peptone (Difco Laboratories, Detroit, Mich.), 1% yeast extract (Merck, Darmstadt), and 2% agar-agar (Merck, Darmstadt); all values represent weight per volume. Primary cultures were grown up to the stationary phase on YPD/2 medium containing 2% D-glucose, 1% peptone, and 0.5% yeast extract at 30°C and were stored in the same way as the slants at 4°C. The cultivations were performed in conic flasks, filled 10 to 20% with the medium, on a reciprocal shaker at 80 strokes/min. Main cultures were prepared by inoculating YPD/2 medium with 0.1 to 0.5% (by volume) of the primary cultures. Tunicamycin used in the inhibition studies was kindly provided by G. Tamura of the University of Tokyo.

Growth was followed by determining either the wet weight of harvested yeast or the optical density at 578 nm in 1-cm cuvettes in an Eppendorf photometer model 1101M (Eppendorf, Hamburg). For this latter purpose, the cultures were diluted to optical density values not exceeding 0.2.

The harvested cells were washed once with cold 50 mM potassium phosphate buffer, pH 7.0. Wet weight of the yeast was determined directly by differential weighing.

Homogenization. The yeast pellet was mixed with the cold potassium phosphate buffer, 2.5 ml/g (wet weight), and the suspension was homogenized by being passed twice through a 3/8-inch (ca. 1.0-cm) French pressure cell (Aminco, Silver Spring, Md.) at 10,000 lb/in^2. The homogenate was centrifuged for 10 min at 12,000 × *g*. The supernate obtained was referred to as crude extract.

Protein concentration in the crude extracts was determined according to Lowry et al. (24) in a total volume of 1.2 ml, using bovine serum albumin (Behringwerke, Marburg) as standard. The maximum yield of protein in the crude extracts per gram (wet weight) of harvested yeast was 60 mg.

Enzyme assays. Enzyme activities were determined by spectrophotometric methods, using a Gilford spectrophotometer model 240 (Gilford Instruments, Oberlin, Ohio). All the enzyme reactions were performed with crude extracts at 25°C unless stated otherwise. The activities of alcohol dehydrogenase and aconitase were determined according to previously described methods (5, 28). The method of Halvorson and Elias was used to determine α-glucosidase activity (9), except that the assay was performed at pH 7.0. Malate dehydrogenase was determined with 67 mM L-malate in reaction conditions given by Williamson and Corkey (41). The activities of proteinases were determined in activated crude extracts (31). For this purpose, the crude extracts were dialyzed against a 200-fold volume of distilled water in Visking dialysis tubes for 3 h at room temperature with one change of water. The dialyzed samples were buffered to pH 5.0 with 1 M sodium acetate buffer (final concentration, 40 mM), preserved with a mixture of antibiotics (10) and sodium azide (0.2 mg/ml), and incubated at 25°C. At intervals, proteinases were assayed and the maximum activities, usually found after 36 to 72 h, were determined. The activities of proteinases A and B were determined with acid-denatured hemoglobin and Azocoll, respectively. The methods and definition of activity units have been presented in detail elsewhere (30, 32). Carboxypeptidase Y was assayed according to Matern et al. (26), with *N*-acetyl-L-tyrosine ethyl ester as substrate. Triton X-100 (0.27%, reagent grade; Serva, Heidelberg) was also present. It lowered turbidity due to crude enzyme samples and also increased the esterase activity. The activity of purified carboxypeptidase Y was increased by 20% in the presence of Triton X-100. Since with the crude extracts the relationship between the reaction rate and the sample volume was not linear, activity was determined with sample volumes giving an absorbance change (ΔA) of 0.02 to 0.03/min at 340 nm. The esterase activity was calculated as micromoles of *N*-acetyl-L-tyrosine ethyl ester hydrolyzed per minute at 25°C. The contribution of proteinase B, about 10% of the total, was subtracted from the total esterase activity. It was calculated from the Azocoll hydrolyzing activity by using a ratio of 0.8 esterase unit per Azocoll unit (units/ΔA_{520}), found previously for purified proteinase B with a specific activity of 18 ΔA_{520}/min per mg (A. Hasilik, Ph.D. thesis, University of Freiburg, Freiburg, Germany, 1974).

To obtain activities of the above enzymes per milliliter of culture, the corresponding specific activities were multiplied by the maximum yield of the crude extract protein mentioned above and by the concentration of the cells in culture (grams [wet weight] per milliliter).

Invertase activity was determined with either 0.1 ml of cell suspension (this was referred to as the external activity) or with 5 μl of homogenate (uncentrifuged) to obtain the total activity. In the former case, the culture samples were centrifuged, the supernates were discarded, and the pellets were washed with 0.5 ml of 50 mM sodium acetate buffer, pH 5.0. The activity itself was measured according to Smith and Ballou (35), but the volumes were scaled down to 70% of the original ones. In one of two parallel samples, the reaction was stopped immediately by adding the reagent 3,5-dinitrosalicylate; in the other, it was stopped after a 15-min incubation with substrate at 37°C. The samples were then incubated for 5 min at 95°C and centrifuged. The ΔA_{520} values, as found between the supernate of the incubated sample and that of the control, were used to calculate the activity, which was expressed as micromoles of sucrose hydrolyzed per minute at 37°C. Both the external and total activities were calculated per milliliter of culture. In the latter case, the activity per milliliter of homogenate was multiplied by a factor of 3.42 ml/g, representing the volume of the homogenate obtained from 1 g of cells and by the wet weight (in grams) of cells harvested per 1 ml of culture.

Preparation of antisera. The antigen carboxypeptidase Y was purified to a specific activity of 120 U/mg. The purification procedure, which was analogous to that originally developed by Hata et al. (1, 11), consisted of acetone precipitation of an activated extract from baker's yeast, chromatography on hydroxyapatite and diethylaminoethyl Sephadex A-50, and gel filtration on Bio-Gel P-150. The enzyme solution containing 10 mM imidazole chloride buffer, pH 7.0, was stored at −30°C either frozen or in a solution made 50% in glycerol. The final preparation was homogeneous by the criteria of polyacrylamide disc gel electrophoresis and sodium dodecyl sulfate-polyacrylamide gel electrophoresis. The content and identity of neutral hexoses present in carboxypeptidase Y were determined by gas chromatography, using xylose as the inner standard, by Inge Fromme, Max Planck Institute of Immunobiology, Freiburg. The total content of neutral hexoses was also determined by the anthrone method (36), using mannose as standard.

For immunization, the antigen was diluted with 0.9% sodium chloride to a concentration of 1.85 mg of protein per ml and emulsified with complete Freund adjuvant (Behringwerke, Marburg). Two brown male rabbits were immunized on their backs with 220 μg of protein each; about two-thirds of each dose was injected intracutaneously; the rest was injected subcutaneously. One rabbit received the antigen that was stored in 50% glycerol (the final concentration of glycerol in the emulsion was 5.5%), and the other one received the antigen that was stored in the absence of glycerol. Each rabbit received an additional 200, 200, and 360 μg of protein in weekly injections of emulsions prepared as above, except that complete Freund adjuvant was replaced by incomplete adjuvant. About 40 ml of blood was collected from an ear vein on the 6th, 8th, and 10th days after the last injection. A booster injection of 0.5 mg of protein was repeated 3 weeks after the last injection of the first series, and blood was collected as before. The serum obtained from the rabbit immunized with the antigen containing glycerol was termed antiserum I. There was little variation in its titer for the purified carboxypeptidase Y among the portions collected at various times (48 μg/ml of serum, on the average), and its specificity did not vary. The same was true for antiserum II, obtained from the rabbit that was immunized with the antigen without glycerol. Here the average titer was 120 μg/ml. As shown in Results, the two antisera differed in their specificity very markedly. This is why the details of the immunization procedure are presented, although we do not know whether there is any causal relationship between the mode of immunization and the specificity of the antiserum obtained. No immunoprecipitation was observed with control sera collected before immunization.

Immunoprecipitation. Antigen solution adjusted to pH 7.0 to 7.5 was mixed with 50 mM tris(hydroxymethyl)aminomethane-chloride buffer, pH 7.5, containing 2 M KCl and 2% Triton X-100 and with antiserum at a volume ratio of 1:2:1 in capped plastic vessels and was kept for 14 to 20 h at 4°C. The vessels were then centrifuged for 4 min at 12,000 × *g*. The sediments were washed three times as described by Roberts and Roberts (29). The amount of protein in the immunoprecipitate was measured by the method of Lowry et al. (24), scaled down to a total volume of 1.2 ml.

To characterize the antisera, 50-μl aliquots were tested with various antigens. A crude extract was prepared from commercial baker's yeast as described above. Yeast cell wall mannan (fraction A), isolated according to Sentandreu and Northcote (33), was kindly provided by L. Lehle. The lyophilized preparation was extracted with 0.1 M potassium phosphate buffer, pH 7.0, and the 12,000 × *g* supernatant fraction was used. Protein measurement performed as mentioned above was used to determine the concentration of mannan in the extract. Yeast invertase, the grade "standardized, analytical grade," was purchased from Serva, Heidelberg.

To determine the concentration of carboxypeptidase Y in crude extracts, the precipitation was performed with an enriched gamma globulin fraction from antiserum I. It was obtained by precipitation of the antiserum with ammonium sulfate (2 M, pH 7.0) and gel filtration of the dialyzed precipitate on a Sephadex G-200 column equilibrated with 0.5 M glycine-0.2 M tris(hydroxymethyl)aminomethane-chloride (pH 7.6)-0.01% sodium azide. The pooled active fractions were concentrated on a PM30 ultrafilter (Amicon, Lexington, Mass.) to a titer of 0.1 mg of carboxypeptidase Y (as protein) per ml. The enriched gamma globulin fraction was used in an at least twofold excess over the antigen. A calibration curve was used to quantitate the enzyme in the immunoprecipitate.

Concentration of soluble mannan in the crude extracts was determined by immunoprecipitation with 0.2 ml of antiserum II. The amount of protein in the immunoprecipitate was determined as above and calculated per milliliter of culture in the same way as enzyme activity.

RESULTS

Antigenic properties of carboxypeptidase Y. Two rabbits were immunized with purified carboxypeptidase Y. The two antisera obtained, I and II, showed typical precipitation curves with one maximum each when used to precipitate the purified carboxypeptidase Y (Fig. 1). Such a curve was also observed with the crude extract when the extract was precipitated with the antiserum I. An additional peak of precipitation was seen, however, when antiserum II was used to precipitate the crude extract (Fig. 2). Whereas the main peak of precipitation corresponded well to the amount of carboxypeptidase Y in the crude extract (about 40 μg/ml) as inferred from the esterase activity, the additional peak occurred at much lower amounts of the crude extract.

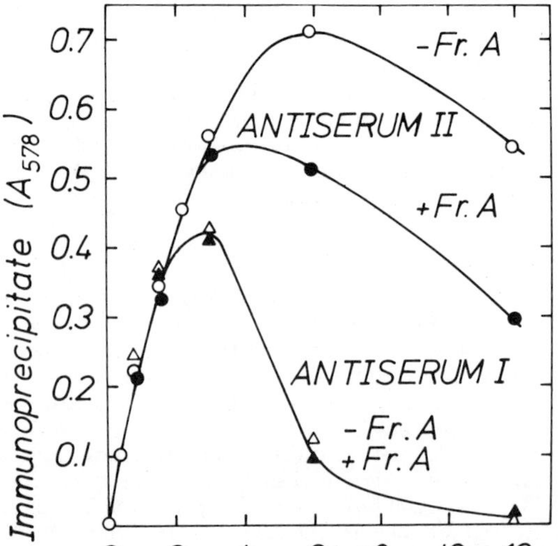

FIG. 1. *Immunoprecipitation of purified carboxypeptidase Y by rabbit antisera. The tests were performed with 50 μl of antiserum I in the absence (△) or presence (▲) of mannan fraction A (3.4 μg as protein), or with 50 μl of antiserum II in the absence (○) or presence of 3.4 μg of mannan fraction A (●).*

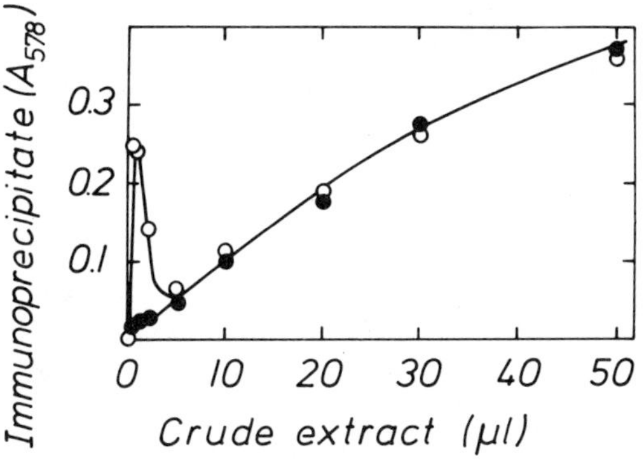

FIG. 2. *Immunoprecipitation of the crude yeast extract with rabbit antiserum prepared against carboxypeptidase Y. The tests were performed with 50 μl of antiserum II in the absence (○) or presence of 3.4 μg of mannan fraction A (●).*

Carboxypeptidase Y has been shown to contain about 3% *N*-acetylglucosamine and 14% neutral sugar (1, 11, 12, 17). Our preparation of the enzyme contained a similar amount of neutral sugar. Essentially all of it was identified as mannose by gas chromatography. A rather limited fraction of it appeared to be β-eliminable (Table 1).

Thus, carboxypeptidase Y seems to be a mannoprotein. The possibility has been considered, therefore, that antiserum II reacts with both the protein and the carbohydrate moieties of carboxypeptidase Y. In this case, it would be expected that the precipitation peak at low volumes of the crude extract obtained with antiserum II should be abolished by an excess of yeast mannan and that the titer of this antiserum for purified carboxypeptidase Y should be lowered in the presence of yeast mannan. In addition, one would predict that any other mannan- or mannoprotein-containing carbohydrate antigenic groups similar to those of carboxypeptidase Y should be precipitated by antiserum II. Indeed, the data shown in Fig. 1 and 2 demonstrate that yeast cell wall mannan, fraction A prepared according to Sentandreu and Northcote (33), suppressed the double specificity of antiserum II. Fraction A lowered the titer of this antiserum for the purified carboxypeptidase Y by about 30%, whereas it had no significant effect on the titer of antiserum I. The latter antiserum precipitated only carboxypeptidase Y, whereas antiserum II also precipitated fraction A cell wall mannan and invertase. Table 2 presents quantitative data on the maximum formation of precipitate and on the titers of the two antisera for different antigens. It can also be seen that excess of carboxypeptidase Y prevented the precipitation of either

TABLE 1. *Neutral sugar content of carboxypeptidase Y*[a]

Prepn	Sugar content	
	Anthrone[b]	Gas chromatography
Untreated	14.0[c]	13.5[d]
β-eliminated:		
Non-dialyzable		11.8[d]
Dialyzable	1.2	

[a] For β-elimination, the sample was treated with 0.1 N NaOH for 24 h at 25°C.

[b] Method used.

[c] Results expressed as percentage of mannose equivalents.

[d] Results expressed as percentage of mannose. Besides mannose, about 0.1% of a pentose, possibly ribose, and traces of glucose and a heptose were found. The amounts corresponded to much less than one residue of any of these sugars per molecule of carboxypeptidase Y.

fraction A mannan or invertase by antiserum II. No invertase was precipitated by this antiserum when fraction A mannan was present in excessive amounts as expected from the antigenic similarity of their sugar components, which has been observed by Smith and Ballou (35).

Antiserum II could be rendered specific for the protein moiety of carboxypeptidase Y by precipitating its antimannan components, for example, by proper amounts of the crude extract. Antiserum II pretreated in this way had a correspondingly lower titer for the purified carboxypeptidase Y (Table 2) and showed a single-peak precipitation curve with the crude extract (not shown) that mimicked the one obtained with the untreated antiserum II in the presence of fraction A mannan (Fig. 2).

Effect of tunicamycin on the apparent rate of synthesis of carboxypeptidase Y. It has been reported that the activities of yeast proteinases including carboxypeptidase Y are higher in cells growing on minimum medium as compared with a complex one and that in both cases an increase takes place in these activities as the culture approaches the stationary phase (31). The effect of tunicamycin has been studied, therefore, in cultures that undergo transition from fermentative to oxidative metabolism. Under these conditions, a number of enzymes known or believed to be subject to catabolite repression are actively synthesized. The activities of several of these were followed to see whether the effect of tunicamycin is selective.

The limited growth of the cultures studied was little affected by tunicamycin at a concen-

TABLE 2. *Immunoprecipitation of carboxypeptidase Y, yeast cell wall mannan fraction A, and invertase by two different antisera, I and II, raised against carboxypeptidase Y*

Antigen	Addition	Antiserum I		Antiserum II	
		Titer[a]	A_{578} max[b]	Titer[a]	A_{578} max[b]
Carboxypeptidase Y	None	3	0.42	6	0.71
	None			3[c]	0.46[c]
	3.4 μg of mannan	3	0.40	4	0.55
Mannan fraction A	None	≤0.01	≤0.01	0.2	0.24
	44 μg of carboxypeptidase Y			≤0.02	≤0.02
	3.8 μg of invertase			≤0.02	≤0.02
Invertase	None	≤0.02	≤0.01	0.25	0.13
	None			≤0.04[c]	≤0.02[c]
	44 μg of carboxypeptidase Y			≤0.04	≤0.02
	3.4 μg of mannan			≤0.04	≤0.02

[a] Expressed as micrograms of antigen at the equivalence point in the precipitation test with 50 μl of antiserum.

[b] Maximum absorbance at 578 nm in the assay of the immunoprecipitated protein.

[c] Precipitation was performed with supernatant fractions of the antisera precipitated with a crude extract from commercial baker's yeast (44 mg of protein per ml of crude extract, 25 μl of crude extract per ml of antiserum).

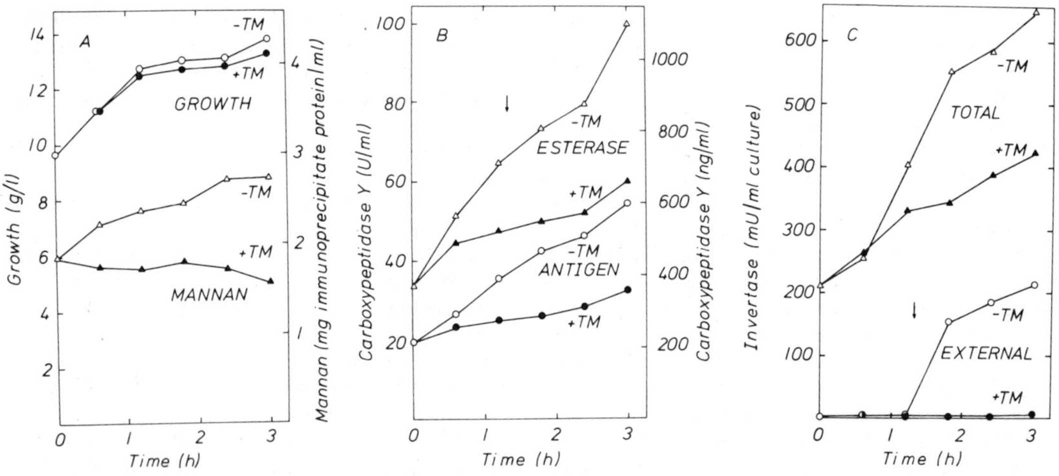

FIG. 3. *Effect of tunicamycin on the apparent synthesis of mannan and on that of several enzymes in growing yeast. Tunicamycin (6 μg/ml) was added to one aliquot of the culture at zero time. The arrow in the figure indicates the time of glucose exhaustion. The open symbols represent controls. The closed symbols show the data obtained with the culture aliquot treated with the antibiotic. (A) Growth (○, ●), and relative concentration of soluble mannan (△, ▲); (B) esterase activity of carboxypeptidase Y (△, ▲) and concentration of carboxypeptidase Y as determined by immunoprecipitation with a gamma globulin preparation specific for the protein moiety of the enzyme (○, ●); (C) external invertase (○, ●) and total invertase (△, ▲).*

tration of 6 μg/ml (Fig. 3A). The formation of mannan, immunoprecipitable from the crude extract by the double-specific antiserum II, was inhibited, however, by more than 90%. Tunicamycin also inhibited the apparent formation of carboxypeptidase Y (Fig. 3B). The inhibition of the increase in esterase activity of the enzyme was closely paralleled by that of the increase in the level of the proteinaceous antigens of this glycoprotein. It appears that there is no accumulation of carboxypeptidase Y molecules lacking the esterase activity and yet reacting with the antiserum specific for the protein moiety of this glycoprotein. Tunicamycin further caused a partial inhibition of the increase in total invertase activity, as determined with the crude cell homogenate, and a nearly complete inhibition of the development of external invertase activity, as determined with whole cells (Fig. 3C).

In Fig. 4, cumulative increases in the activities of various enzymes expressed as percentages of the controls are compared with the cumulative increase in the wet weight of the cells. The apparent synthesis of proteinase A was inhibited to the same extent as that of carboxypeptidase Y. Like carboxypeptidase Y, proteinase A is a glycoprotein (11) and is located in the vacuole (10, 22). Interestingly, the effect of tunicamycin could be noticed already during the activation of the proteinases in the dialyzed crude extracts. The extracts were rendered turbid by adjusting their pH to 5.0 and became more or less clear during subsequent incubation at 25°C. This clearing was much less extensive in the samples from early growth stages than in those from the later stages, just as expected from their proteinase contents. It also proceeded much more slowly in the samples from tunicamycin-treated cells as compared with the corresponding controls.

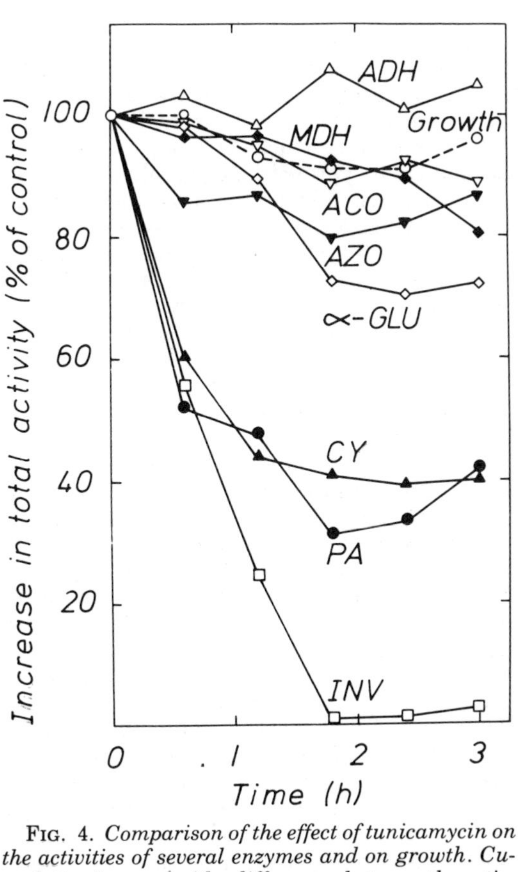

FIG. 4. *Comparison of the effect of tunicamycin on the activities of several enzymes and on growth. Cumulative increases (the differences between the activities at the times indicated on the abscissa and those at time zero) in the total activities in the inhibited culture shown are expressed as percentage of control. The data presented have been obtained in the same experiment as shown in Fig. 3. Symbols: Growth (○); alcohol dehydrogenase (△); malate dehydrogenase (◆); aconitase (▽); α-glucosidase (◇); carboxypeptidase Y esterase activity (▲); proteinase A (●); external invertase (□); proteinase B (▼).*

In contrast to carboxypeptidase Y and proteinase A, the change in the activity of proteinase B, another vacuolar hydrolase (10, 22), was not affected by tunicamycin. The appearance of the maximum proteinase B activity during activation of crude extracts, however, was delayed. This is in agreement with the mechanism proposed for activation of proteinase B in the crude extracts according to which proteinase A inactivates the inhibitor of proteinase B (32). Evidence exists that proteinase B is also a glycoprotein, but its sugar moiety seems to be built differently from that of carboxypeptidase Y (A. Hasilik, unpublished data).

There are a number of enzymes, however, the activities of which developed more or less unaffected by tunicamycin: malate dehydrogenase, aconitase, α-glucosidase, and alcohol dehydrogenase (Fig. 4). The small apparent increase in the rate of synthesis of alcohol dehydrogenase due to tunicamycin was observed in all experiments carried out.

In the presence of tunicamycin, the apparent rate of synthesis of the external invertase was considerably more inhibited than that of carboxypeptidase Y (Fig. 3). The following facts, however, have to be pointed out. In the control, the activity of carboxypeptidase Y increased steadily in the course of the experiment, whereas the formation of the external invertase was initiated only after glucose was used up. Then its activity rose very rapidly, reaching a maximum of about 15 U per g of cells in about 1 h. In the culture treated with tunicamycin the appearance of this activity was delayed for several hours, although glucose was consumed by essentially the same time as in the control. Later on, the activity started to increase slowly, reaching nearly 13 U per g of cells 8 h after the addition of the antibiotic (not shown). By varying the time of the addition of the antibiotic, the degree of the inhibition of the synthesis of external invertase was greatly changed, however. The inhibition was even less than 50% when tunicamycin was added 10 min after the initiation of the synthesis. It could also be shown that the difference in the degree of inhibition of the two enzymes is fairly small under certain conditions (Table 3). In this case, cells growing exponentially on medium YPD/2 were transferred into a similar but rather diluted medium. Within 15 min after the shift,

TABLE 3. *Effect of tunicamycin on the apparent rate of formation of the external invertase, of the esterase activity, and of the protein antigen of carboxypeptidase Y*[a]

Tunicamycin concn (μg/ml)	Rate of formation				Growth (g/liter)	
	Carboxypeptidase Y		Invertase (mU/h per ml)	Malate dehydrogenase (mU/h per ml)	Initial	After 2.5 h
	Esterase (mU/h per ml)	Protein antigen (ng/h per ml)				
0	14	150	55	90	9.3	12.3
6	8.4	84	13.6	90	9.3	12.2
	(60)	(56)	(75)	(0)		(3)

[a] The cells were grown in 2 liters of YPD/2 medium up to an optical density of 2.2, spun down, and resuspended in 0.5 liter of medium containing, per liter: 0.25 g of yeast extract, 0.5 g of peptone, 2.5 g of D-glucose, and 2 g of maltose monohydrate. Thirty minutes later, tunicamycin was added to one part of this culture. The cultures were sampled immediately before the addition of the inhibitor and then every 30 min for estimation of the external invertase activity and for preparation of crude extracts. All the activities shown changed in a nearly linear fashion over 2.5 h studied, and therefore average rates are presented. The numbers in parentheses indicate percentage of inhibition.

glucose was used up and little additional growth occurred. By this time the cells started to synthesize external invertase. Its activity increased rather slowly as compared with the experiment shown in Fig. 3. The increase was nearly linear and paralleled that in the activity of carboxypeptidase Y and malate dehydrogenase. One-half hour after the shift, tunicamycin was added to an aliquot of the culture, i.e., to cells that were actively synthesizing both carboxypeptidase Y and external invertase. Under these conditions, the synthesis of external invertase was inhibited by 75% and that of carboxypeptidase Y was inhibited by 60%.

DISCUSSION

Both the composition and the structure of the sugar moiety of the vacuolar enzyme carboxypeptidase Y resemble those of the components of the yeast cell wall. Like invertase and cell wall mannan, carboxypeptidase Y contains glucosamine and mannose, most of which is not β-eliminable. Based on a molecular weight of 61,000 to 62,000, about eight residues of glucosamine per molecule have been found (1, 17). The non-β-eliminable mannose content of 11.8% corresponds to 40 mol of mannose per mol of enzyme. It can be suggested that one molecule of carboxypeptidase Y contains four asparagine-linked oligosaccharide chains of an average composition $(N\text{-acetylglucosamine})_2$- $(\text{mannose})_{10}$. This formula resembles that of the inner core of the yeast cell wall mannan as proposed by Nakajima and Ballou (27). The analogy is also indicated by the antigenic similarity of the carbohydrate moieties of wall mannan and carboxypeptidase Y.

Sugars bound to polyprenylphosphates of the dolichol type have been shown to be intermediates in the glycosylation of glycoproteins in a number of eukaryotic cells (4, 13, 21). This is true for the formation of *N*-glycosidically (4, 16, 20, 21, 40) and *O*-glycosidically (2, 34) linked carbohydrate moieties. It is still a matter of debate, however, which class of glycoproteins is formed via polyprenols, i.e., whether these are constituents of membranes or are secretory proteins, or both. Evidence for the second possibility has come from the observation that unglycosylated protein moieties of defined glycoproteins could serve as artificial acceptors of sugars from dolichylphosphate sugars. This has been observed for the biosynthesis of immunoglobulin light chains (7) and for the yeast cell wall mannan (L. Lehle, P. Babczinski, and W. Tanner, in preparation).

Experiments by Kuo and Lampen on the inhibition by tunicamycin of the formation of external glycoproteins in yeast protoplasts (18) are pertinent to the same problem. Since it has been shown recently that in various systems the transfer of *N*-acetylglucosamine from uridine-5′-diphosphate-*N*-acetylglucosamine to the polyprenylphosphate acceptors is inhibited by tunicamycin (6, 38, 39), it is very probable that in yeast, *N*-acetylglucosamine linked to dolichylphosphate acts as an intermediate in the synthesis of external glycoproteins. Similarly, the results shown in the present paper indicate that this polyprenol derivative is involved in the synthesis of vacuolar glycoproteins as well.

It is possible that there are more similarities in the genesis of external and of vacuolar glycoproteins. In both cases it is required that a membrane be traversed by a macromolecule. Most likely this transport of macromolecules takes place at rough endoplasmic reticulum membranes and is closely associated with, and perhaps driven by, the processes participating in the synthesis of these macromolecules (19). It has also been suggested that the syntheses of secretory and of lysosomal glycoproteins in animal cells share a number of common features (8).

Kuo and Lampen have observed that although the secretion of invertase by yeast protoplasts is stopped in the presence of tunicamycin, the activity of internal invertase does not accumulate (18). Accumulation of an inactive enzyme within the cells, however, has not been excluded in their experiments. The observation that in the case of carboxypeptidase Y, not only the increase in activity but also the apparent formation of the protein antigen is inhibited by the antibiotic (Fig. 3B and Table 3) strongly suggests that the synthesis of the protein moiety of this glycoprotein is retarded unless the glycosylation can proceed normally. It is not excluded, however, that the synthesis of the protein moiety continues unaffectedly, even if the glycosylation reactions are inhibited, and that the incompletely glycosylated glycoprotein thus formed is rapidly degraded.

ACKNOWLEDGMENTS

We are indebted to G. Tamura for the supply of tunicamycin and to Inge Fromme for gas chromatographic analysis of neutral hexoses in carboxypeptidase Y. Thanks are also due to R. Leonhart for technical assistance and to L. Lehle for a sample of yeast cell wall mannan fraction A. The help of W. Kohlert and O. Muise in the preparation of the manuscript is acknowledged.

This work was supported by Deutsche Forschungsgemeinschaft.

LITERATURE CITED

1. **Aibara, S., R. Hayashi, and T. Hata.** 1971. Physical and chemical properties of yeast proteinase C. Agric. Biol. Chem. **35**:658–666.
2. **Babczinski, P., and W. Tanner.** 1973. Involvement of dolicholmonophosphate in the formation of specific mannosyl-linkages in yeast glycoproteins. Biochem. Biophys. Res. Commun. **54**:1119–1124.
3. **Bai, Y., and R. Hayashi.** 1975. A possible role for a single cysteine residue in carboxypeptidase Y. FEBS Lett. **56**:43–45.
4. **Behrens, N. H.** 1974. Polyprenol sugars and glycoprotein synthesis, p. 159–180. *In* E. Y. C. Lee and E. E. Smith (ed.), Biology and chemistry of eukaryotic cell surfaces. Academic Press Inc., New York.
5. **Bergmeyer, H. U., K. Gawehn, and M. Grassl.** 1974. Enzyme als biochemische Reagenzien, p. 454–558. *In* H. U. Bergmeyer (ed.), Methoden der enzymatischen Analyse. Verlag Chemie, Weinheim.
6. **Bettinger, G. E., and F. E. Young.** 1975. Tunicamycin, an inhibitor of Bacillus peptidoglycan synthesis: a new site of inhibition. Biochem. Biophys. Res. Commun. **67**:16–21.
7. **Eagon, P. K., A. F. Hsu, and E. C. Heath.** 1975. Role of dolichol intermediates in the glycosylation of endogenous and exogenous proteins. Fed. Proc. **34**:678.
8. **Goldstone, A., and H. Koening.** 1973. Physicochemical modifications of lysosomal hydrolases during intracellular transport. Biochem. J. **132**:267–282.
9. **Halvorson, H., and L. Elias.** 1958. The purification and properties of an α-glucosidase of *Saccharomyces italicus* Y1225. Biochim. Biophys. Acta **30**:28–40.
10. **Hasilik, A., H. Müller, and H. Holzer.** 1974. Compartmentation of the trytophan-synthase-proteolyzing system in *Saccharomyces cerevisiae*. Eur. J. Biochem. **48**:111–117.
11. **Hata, T., R. Hayashi, and E. Doi.** 1967. Purification of yeast proteinases. Part III. Isolation and physicochemical properties of yeast proteinase A and C. Agric. Biol. Chem. **31**:357–367.
12. **Hayashi, R., S. Moore, and W. H. Stein.** 1973. Carboxypeptidase from yeast. Large scale preparation and the application to COOH-terminal analysis of peptides and proteins. J. Biol. Chem. **248**:2296–2302.
13. **Hemming, F. W.** 1973. Lipids in glycan biosynthesis, p. 39–97. *In* T. W. Goodwin (ed.), Biochemistry, ser. 1, vol. 4, Biochemistry of lipids. University Park Press, Baltimore.
14. **Hermondson, M. A., R. W. Kuhn, K. A. Walsh, and H. Neurath.** 1972. Amino acid sequence of monkey amyloid protein A. Biochemistry **11**:2934–2938.
15. **Holzer, H., H. Betz, and E. Ebner.** 1975. Intracellular proteinases in microorganisms. Curr. Top. Cell. Regul. **9**:103–156.
16. **Hsu, A. F., J. W. Baynes, and E. C. Heath.** 1974. The role of a dolichol-oligosaccharide as an intermediate in glycoprotein biosynthesis. Proc. Natl. Acad. Sci. U.S.A. **71**:2391–2395.
17. **Kuhn, R. W., K. A. Walsh, and H. Neurath.** 1974. Isolation and partial characterization of an acid carboxypeptidase from yeast. Biochemistry **13**:3871–3877.
18. **Kuo, S.-C., and J. O. Lampen.** 1974. Tunicamycin—an inhibitor of yeast glycoprotein synthesis. Biochem. Biophys. Res. Commun. **58**:287–295.
19. **Lampen, J. O.** 1974. Movement of extracellular enzymes across cell membranes, p. 351–374. *In* Transport at the cellular level, 28th Symp. Soc. Exp. Biol. University Press, Cambridge.
20. **Lehle, L., and W. Tanner.** 1975. Formation of lipid-bound oligosaccharides in yeast. Biochim. Biophys. Acta **399**:364–374.
21. **Lennarz, W. J.** 1975. Lipid linked sugars in glycoprotein synthesis. Science **188**:986–991.
22. **Lenney, J. F., Ph. Matile, A. Wiemken, M. Schellenberg, and J. Meyer.** 1974. Activities and cellular localization of yeast proteases and their inhibitors. Biochem. Biophys. Res. Commun. **60**:1378–1383.
23. **Lerch, K., and E. H. Fischer.** 1975. Amino acid sequence of two functional sites in yeast glycogen phosphorylase. Biochemistry **14**:2009–2014.
24. **Lowry, O. H., N. J. Rosebrough, A. L. Farr, and R. J. Randall.** 1951. Protein measurement with the Folin phenol reagent. J. Biol. Chem. **193**:265–275.
25. **Manney, T. R.** 1968. Regulation of factors that influence the *in vitro* stability of tryptophan synthetase from yeast. J. Bacteriol. **96**:403–408.
26. **Matern, H., H. Betz, and H. Holzer.** 1974. Compartmentation of inhibitors of proteinases A and B and carboxypeptidase Y in yeast. Biochem. Biophys. Res. Commun. **60**:1051–1057.
27. **Nakajima, T., and C. E. Ballou.** 1975. Microheterogeneity of the inner core region of yeast manno-protein. Biochem. Biophys. Res. Commun. **66**:870–879.
28. **Racker, E.** 1950. Spectrophotometric measurements of the enzymatic formation of fumaric and cis-aconitic acids. Biochim. Biophys. Acta **4**:211–214.
29. **Roberts, J. W., and C. W. Roberts.** 1975. Proteolytic cleavage of bacteriophage lambda repressor in induction. Proc. Natl. Acad. Sci. U.S.A. **72**:147–151.
30. **Saheki, T., and H. Holzer.** 1974. Comparisons of the trytophan synthase inactivating enzymes with proteinases from yeast. Eur. J. Biochem. **42**:621–626.

31. **Saheki, T., and H. Holzer.** 1975. Proteolytic activities in yeast. Biochim. Biophys. Acta **384**:203–214.
32. **Saheki, T., Y. Matsuda, and H. Holzer.** 1974. Purification and characterization of macromolecular inhibitors of proteinase A from yeast. Eur. J. Biochem. **47**:325–332.
33. **Sentandreu, R., and D. H. Northcote.** 1968. The structure of a glycopeptide isolated from the yeast cell wall. Biochem. J. **109**:419–432.
34. **Sharma, C. B., P. Babczinski, L. Lehle, and W. Tanner.** 1974. The role of dolicholmonophosphate in glycoprotein biosynthesis in *Saccharomyces cerevisiae*. Eur. J. Biochem. **46**:35–41.
35. **Smith, W. L., and C. E. Ballou.** 1974. Immunochemical characterization of the mannan component of the external invertase (β-fructofuranosidase) of *Saccharomyces cerevisiae*. Biochemistry **13**:355–361.
36. **Spiro, R. G.** 1966. Analysis of sugars found in glycoproteins, p. 3–26. *In* E. F. Neufeld and V. Ginsburg (ed.), Methods in enzymology, vol. 8. Academic Press Inc., New York.
37. **Takatsuki, A., K. Arima, and G. Tamura.** 1971. Tunicamycin, a new antibiotic. I. Isolation and characterization of tunicamycin. J. Antibiot. (Tokyo) **24**:215–223.
38. **Takatsuki, A., K. Kohno, and G. Tamura.** 1975. Inhibition of biosynthesis of polyisoprenol sugars in chick embryo microsomes by tunicamycin. Agric. Biol. Chem. **39**:2089–2091.
39. **Tkacz, J. S., and J. O. Lampen.** 1975. Tunicamycin inhibition of polyisoprenyl N-acetylglucosaminyl pyrophosphate formation in calf-liver microsomes. Biochem. Biophys. Res. Commun. **65**:248–257.
40. **Wedgwood, J. F., C. D. Warren, R. W. Jeanloz, and J. C. Strominger.** 1974. Enzymatic utilization of P^1-di-N-acetylchitobiosyl-P^2-dolichyl pyrophosphate and its chemical synthesis. Proc. Natl. Acad. Sci. U.S.A. **71**:5022–5026.
41. **Williamson, J. R., and B. E. Corkey.** 1969. Assay of intermediates of the citric acid cycle and related compounds by fluorometric enzyme methods, p. 434–513. *In* J. M. Lowenstein (ed.), Methods in enzymology, vol. 13. Academic Press Inc., New York.

ANTIMICROBIAL AGENTS AND CHEMOTHERAPY, Sept. 1976, p. 411-416 Vol. 10, No. 3

Printed in U.S.A.

Mutants of *Pseudomonas aeruginosa* That Show Specific Hypersensitivity to Aminoglycosides

B. J. MILLS AND B. W. HOLLOWAY*

Department of Genetics, Monash University, Clayton, Victoria 3168, Australia

Received for publication 26 April 1976

A class of mutants in *Pseudomonas aeruginosa* have been found that are tolerant to aeruginocin 41 and also hypersensitive to aminoglycosides. They do not show any changes in susceptibility to a wide range of other toxic agents, including antibiotics and surfactants. This *tol* locus, *tolA*, has been mapped at 10 min from the FP2 origin and linked to *carA* (carbamyl phosphate synthetase) by transduction and conjugation. By selecting for revertants of the hypersensitivity phenotype, revertants to tol^+ were found, indicating that it is the *tolA* locus that is responsible for this specific hypersensitivity. The results indicate that a specific mechanism exists for the intrinsic resistance of *P. aeruginosa* to aminoglycosides.

Pseudomonas aeruginosa has a natural resistance to many of the commonly used antibiotics. The genetic basis of this resistance is not yet well understood, except in the cases in which resistance is due to R factor-mediated enzymatic modification of the antibiotic (3, 10, 13). Where there is no R factor present, it has recently been suggested that resistance to aminoglycosides may not be enzymatic and is, instead, a function of the cell envelope (20). This paper describes the isolation and characterization of two mutants in which the level of intrinsic resistance of *P. aeruginosa* to aminoglycosides is altered. We have looked for these mutants on the assumption that the antibiotic resistance would be lost, and hence we needed to find mutants hypersensitive to antibiotics. The nature of these mutants supports the view that the native resistance of *P. aeruginosa* to this class of antibiotic may be structural rather than metabolic.

MATERIALS AND METHODS

Bacterial strains and R factors. The bacterial strains and R factors are listed in Table 1.

Media. Media were as described previously from this laboratory (19): minimal medium, nutrient yeast broth (NYB), and nutrient agar (NA).

Antibiotics used were carbenicillin (Pyopen) from Beecham; streptomycin, kanamycin (739 U/mg), neomycin, and tetracycline from Sigma; paromomycin, sisomycin, lividomycin, butirosin, and tobramycin, which were kindly provided by J. Davies, Madison, Wis.; spectinomycin from Upjohn; kasugamycin from Boehringer Mannheim GmbH; gentamicin from Essex; and erythromycin from Abbotts, Australia.

Chemical reagents used were mercuric chloride from Ajax Chemicals Ltd.; ethylenediaminetetraacetic acid, sodium deoxycholate, Triton X-100, and sodium lauryl sulfate from BDH Chemicals; and ethyl methane sulfonate from Eastman.

2.5-Diphenyloxazole was from Packard. [^{3}H]dihydrostreptomycin sesquisulfate (3 Ci/mmol) was from the Radiochemical Centre, Amersham. Aeruginocin 41 (AR) was prepared as described previously (9).

Identification of *tol* mutants. Strains to be tested for susceptibility to AR were streaked onto Na plates that had been spread with 0.3 ml of AR (NA/AR). To distinguish AR tolerance from resistance, the strain being tested was streaked onto an NA/AR plate and grown overnight, and the growth was exposed to chloroform for 20 min at room temperature. The plate was then overlaid with soft agar seeded with PAO1 at about 10^7 cells/ml obtained from an exponential-phase culture. PAO1 is susceptible to AR and therefore is unable to grow. If the mutant is tolerant, it will adsorb AR and prevent it from killing PAO1. If it is resistant, it will not adsorb AR and hence growth of PAO1 will be inhibited. Thus, tolerant strains have an area of PAO1 growth above them, whereas resistant strains do not.

Mutant isolation. Ethyl methane sulfonate (0.1 ml) was added to 10 ml of an exponential-phase culture of bacteria in NYB. This was shaken vigorously and allowed to stand for 60 min at 37°C. The culture was then diluted 1:10 into fresh NYB and incubated overnight at 37°C to allow the expression of mutations. The cells were plated onto NA/AR to select for AR-insensitive mutants. The survivors (about 10^{-3} of the plated cells) were scored for antibiotic susceptibility by replica plating onto NA plates supplemented with the appropriate agent (streptomycin, 500 μg/ml; tetracycline, 250 μg/ml; kanamycin, 300 μg/ml; carbenicillin, 400 μg/ml).

Antibiotic susceptibility tests. The minimal inhibitory concentration (MIC) in each case was ob-

TABLE 1. *P. aeruginosa strains and R factors*

Strain	Genotype	R factor[a]	Reference/ source
PAO222	*ilv-226, his-4, lys-12, met-28, pro-82, trp-6*		21
PAO850	*pur-66, his-151, pyr-21, thi-1, car-160*[b] *ese-14*		This laboratory
PAO1670	*ade-136, leu-8, rif-1*		
PAO1670	*ade-136, leu-8, rif-1*	R38 (SM TC $HgCl_2$)	11
PAO1670	*ade-136, leu-8, rif-1*	R2 (SM CB NM/ KM)	11
PAO1670	*ade-136, leu-8, rif-1*	pMG2 (SM GM Su $HgCl_2$)	10
PAO1670	*ade-136, leu-8, rif-1*	RMS148 (SM)	Jacoby, in press
PAO1699	*ade-136, leu-8, rif-1, str-A55*		This paper
PAO1710	*ade-136, leu-8, tol-9, rif-1*	R38	This paper
PAO1712	*ade-136, leu-8, tol-12, rif-1*	R2	This paper
PAO1715	*ade-136, leu-8, tol-12, rif-1*		This paper
PAO1716	*ade-136, leu-8, tol-12*$^+$*, rif-1*		This paper
PAO1717	*ade-136, leu-8, str-A56, tol-12, rif-1*		This paper

[a] SM, Streptomycin; TC, tetracycline; CB, carbenicillin; NM, neomycin; KM, kanamycin; GM, gentamicin; Su, sulfonamide.

[b] *car-160* was formerly *arg-160* and has been renamed because the arginine requirement is due to a defect in carbamyl phosphate synthetase (T. Leisinger, personal communication).

tained by spotting 0.01 ml of a 10^{-5} dilution in NYB of an overnight culture onto NA plates supplemented with varying amounts of antibiotics. The MIC was defined as the highest concentration of antibiotic that permitted >90% cell survival.

For less accurate testing, an NA plate was spread with a lawn of bacteria, and a Multodisk (Oxoid Ltd.) was placed on top. The zone of inhibition of growth around each disk was then measured after overnight growth at 37°C.

Conjugation and transduction. Conjugation and transduction were carried out as described previously (19).

R factor transfer. R factor transfer was carried out as described previously (4).

Uptake of [^{3}H]streptomycin. Cells were grown in NYB to exponential phase. [^{3}H]streptomycin (0.1 mCi/ml, 0.02 ml) was added to 2 ml of the culture to give 0.5 μg of streptomycin per ml. To give 200 μg of streptomycin per ml, [^{3}H]streptomycin (1.0 mCi/ml, 0.02 ml) plus nonlabeled streptomycin (2×10^3 μg/ml, 0.2 ml) was added to 1.8 ml of the culture. This was incubated at 37°C with shaking for up to 40 min. Portions (0.1 ml) were taken at intervals, and the cells were collected on a membrane filter (Millipore; pore size, 0.45 μm). The filter was rinsed with 30 ml of minimal medium at pH 7.0 and dried. The filter was placed in a vial with 1 ml of Soluene 350 (Packard) and left at 43°C overnight to solubilize the cells. Scintillation fluid (10 ml of toluene plus 0.25% 2,5-diphenyloxazole) was added, and the radioactivity was counted in a Packard model 3320 liquid scintillation counter with an efficiency of 15%.

RESULTS

Mutant isolation. It has been demonstrated previously that bacteriocin-tolerant mutants show alterations in cell envelope structure and function (6, 9). It seemed a profitable hypothesis to assume that mutants affecting resistance levels would be found among such mutants. It was also felt that the levels of resistance conferred by plasmids might make the isolation of hypersensitive mutants easier. AR-insensitive mutants of strains PAO1670 (R2) and PAO1670 (R38) were isolated as described above. They were then screened for any alterations in the drug resistance properties of the R factor carried by each strain. Out of 1,000 mutants that survived in the presence of AR41 screened for each strain, about 1% showed an increase in susceptibility to some antibiotics, but not to others. For the mutants carrying R2, changes occurred for streptomycin and kanamycin, but not for carbenicillin. For the mutants carrying R38, the effect was found for streptomycin, but not for tetracycline or mercuric chloride. One mutant of each type was selected for further analysis and designated PAO1710 (R38) and PAO1712 (R2).

Resistance to antibiotics. The alteration in resistance of the mutants to various antibiotics was determined more accurately by comparing the MICs for the parental and mutant strains (Table 2). When the R factor codes for resistance to an aminoglycoside, such as streptomycin, kanamycin, or spectinomycin, the mutant is between 5 and 20 times less resistant to the drug than is the parent. For resistance to other antibacterial agents, specifically carbenicillin, tetracycline, and mercuric chloride, no differ-

TABLE 2. *Comparative resistance of the mutant and parent strains to antibiotics*

Strain	R factor[a]	MIC (μg/ml)						
		Tol	SM	KM	SPC[b]	CB	TC	$HgCl_2$
PAO1670	R2	+[c]	5,000	300	–	2,000	–	–
PAO1712	R2	–	500	50	–	2,000	–	–
PAO1670	R38	+	7,500	–	>5,000	–	400	250
PAO1710	R38	–	400	–	1,000	–	400	250

[a] R2 confers resistance to SM, KM and CB. R38 confers resistance to SM, SPC, TC, and $HgCl_2$.

[b] SPC, Spectinomycin. Other abbreviations are the same as those given in footnote *a* to Table 1.

[c] Tol^+, AR sensitive; Tol^-, AR tolerant.

ence could be detected in the MIC for the mutant and the parent.

To examine the effect of these mutations affecting plasmid-coded resistance on intrinsic resistance levels, it was necessary to cure the mutants of their R factors. In the case of R2, a high rate of spontaneous loss of the whole plasmid was found when the strain was propagated at 43°C. This is similar to the curing of F in *Escherichia coli* K-12 described by Stadler and Adelberg (18). When an R2-carrying strain is grown in NYB at 43°C with cell numbers kept low enough to prevent reinfection of the R factor, i.e., from 10^2 to 10^7 cells/ml, about 50% of the resulting cells are found to have lost R2. The "cured" lines have lost all three antibiotic resistances of R2 and have also lost the entry exclusion and incompatibility properties of R2 because they can readily be reinfected with the R factor. A cured derivative of PAO1712 (R2) was isolated in this way and named PAO1715.

The susceptibility of PAO1715 to various antibiotics, as compared with that of the parent PAO1670, is shown in Table 3. The results indicate that the observed effects on aminoglycoside resistance are not restricted to antibiotic resistance coded for by the plasmid. The MIC of PAO1715 was at least five times lower than that of PAO1670 for a range of aminoglycosides. Of more importance is the specificity of the mutation. PAO1715 showed increased susceptibility towards all the aminoglycosidic drugs tested, but no change towards other inhibitory agents, including ampicillin, cephaloridine, oleandomycin, erythromycin, lincomycin, naladixic acid, sulfonamide, novobiocin, and furoxone. There was also no change in susceptibility towards surfactants such as ethylenediaminetetraacetic acid, sodium deoxycholate, and polymixin or towards the detergent Triton X-100.

In the case of the other mutant strain, PAO1710 (R38), it was not possible to cure the R factor either by growth at 43°C or by the use of sodium lauryl sulfate. However, this mutant showed MIC levels for the various antibiotics that were identical to those of PAO1715 (except of course for the R38-coded resistances) (data not shown). Thus, the mutation in PAO1710 (R38) appears also to be specific for aminoglycoside hypersensitivity.

TABLE 3. *Pleiotropic effects of the tol⁻ mutation*[a]

Aminoglycoside	Other agent	MIC (μg/ml)		
		PAO1670 (tol⁺)	PAO1715 (tol⁻)	PAO1716 (tol⁺)
SM		25	5	25
KM		75	5	75
SPC		500	100	500
PM		100	25	100
GM		3	0.5	3
NM		25	5	25
TB		3	<1	3
SIS		3	<1	3
LV		25	<10	25
KAS		250	50	250
BUT		10	3	10
	CB	100	100	100
	TC	50	50	50
	$HgCl_2$	1	1	1
	EDTA	200	200	200
	EM	200	200	200

[a] Sodium deoxycholate, Triton X-100, chloramphenicol, polymixin, furoxone, ampicillin, cephaloridine, oleandomycin, lincomycin, nalidixic acid, sulfonamide, and novobiocin were tested by the disk method. PAO1715 did not show altered resistance to any of these compounds. SPC, Spectinomycin; PM, paromomycin; TB, tobramycin; SIS, sisomycin; LV, lividomycin; KAS, Kasugamycin; BUT, butirosin; EDTA, ethylenediaminetetraacetic acid; EM, erythromycin. Other abbreviations are the same as those given in footnote *a* to Table 1.

Effect of the mutation on high-level drug resistance. Once the R2-cured derivative of PAO1712 had been isolated, it was possible to transfer other R factors into it and determine the levels of R factor-mediated drug resistance (Table 4). The MICs for the aminoglycosides were lower than those of the R⁺ parent, whereas the levels of resistance to other antibiotics coded for by the R factors were unaffected in the mutant (data not given).

It was also possible to determine the effect of the mutation on high-level chromosomal streptomycin resistance. PAO1699 (= PAO1670 *str*ʳ) was selected on NA containing 500 μg of streptomycin per ml; PAO1717 (= PAO1715 *str*ʳ) was selected on NA containing 100 μg of streptomy-

TABLE 4. *Effect of tol on R factor-mediated drug resistance*

Strain	R factor[a]	Tol	MIC (μg/ml)	
			SM[b]	GM
PAO1670	pMG2	+	2,000	25
PAO1715	pMG2	−	250	<10
PAO1670	RMS148	+	2,000	−
PAO1715	RMS148	−	250	−
PAO1670	−	+	25	3

[a] pMG2 codes for gentamicin acetyltransferase (10). RMS148 codes for streptomycin adenylase or phosphorylase (11).

[b] Abbreviations are the same as those given in footnote *a* of Table 1.

cin per ml. The MIC of PAO1699 for streptomycin is >15,000 μg/ml, and the MIC of PAO1717 is between 7,500 and 10,000 μg/ml.

These results support the view that the mutation specifically affects aminoglycoside resistance levels and that this effect is independent of the genetic basis of the resistance.

AR tolerance. There was no detectable killing of either mutant by AR41, whereas the two parental strains showed a reduction of 10^{-5} in viable count on an NA/AR plate. The survival of both mutants was shown to be due to tolerance, rather than to resistance (see above).

A range of tolerant mutants has previously been isolated in *P. aeruginosa* (9). Several of the mutants were found to have altered sensitivity to phages and to membrane-active agents and to have altered colonial and cellular morphology. Such changes were thought to be the results of an altered envelope structure in these mutants. The two tolerant mutants described here do not show this sort of pleiotropy; colonial and cellular morphology were found to be normal, and there was no change in response to 30 selected bacteriophages. Also, there was no generalized change in susceptibility to surfactants (Table 3). An examination of the cell envelope has been made by polyacrylamide gel electrophoresis, but so far no major differences between the parental and mutant strains with respect to envelope proteins have been demonstrated.

Mapping of the *tol* mutations. The phenotypes of PAO1710 and PAO1712 are very similar; both show the same level of AR tolerance and the same increase in susceptibility to aminoglycosides. The genetic relationship of the two mutants was therefore investigated.

In the conjugation experiment shown in Table 5, the *tol* allele in both PAO1710 and PAO1712 showed high linkage to early markers in the multiply marked recipient PAO222. The highest linkage was seen when *ilv-226*$^+$ at 8 min and *his-4*$^+$ at 16 min were coselected; this implies that *tol*$^-$ is located between these two markers. This was confirmed by transduction with phage F116L. The *tol* marker in PAO1710 showed 95% cotransduction with *car-160* in PAO850, and the *tol* marker in PAO1712 showed 90% cotransduction with *car-160*. The *car* marker is at about 10 min on the PAO map (D. Haas, personal communication). Thus, the two mutations are either in very closely linked genes or they are in the same gene. This question cannot be resolved completely, due to the absence of a complementation system in *P. aeruginosa*.

Selection of revertant strains. To investigate the relationship of the Tol phenotype to

TABLE 5. *Conjugational mapping*

Selected markers[a]	Map position (min)	Coinheritance of *tol*$^-$ (%)	
		Cross (a)[b]	Cross (b)[c]
ilv-226$^+$	8	63	51
his-4$^+$	16	45	50
lys-12$^+$	19	30	28
met-28$^+$	29	17	5
trp-6$^+$	34	7	12
pro-82$^+$	45	12	6
ilv-226$^+$, *his-4*$^+$	8–16	87	85
his-4$^+$, *lys-12*$^+$	16–19	33	52
lys-12$^+$, *met-28*$^+$	19–29	37	33

[a] A total of 100 recombinants for each selected marker were scored for coinheritance of *tol*$^+$ by streaking onto NA/AR.

[b] Cross (a): PAO1710 (FP2) × PAO222.

[c] Cross (b): PAO1712 (FP2) × PAO222.

the aminoglycoside-hypersensitive phenotype, i.e., to find out whether they were a result of the same mutational event, it was necessary to isolate a revertant of one of the phenotypes. Tol$^+$ revertants cannot, of course, be selected directly. Therefore, a revertant of the hypersensitive phenotype was selected by plating PAO1715 in the presence of streptomycin at 10 μg/ml and scoring the resistant survivors for susceptibility to AR41 (as described in Materials and Methods). Of 250 candidate clones tested, 2 had become Tol$^+$; one strain was chosen for further study and designated PAO1716.

The phenotype of PAO1716 could have been due to the reversion of the *tol* allele to *tol*$^+$ or to suppression of the Tol$^-$ phenotype by a second mutation at another site. If the latter were the case, the *tol* allele would still be present in PAO1716, and it would be possible to transfer it into another strain by transduction. Phage F116L was therefore grown on PAO1716 and, using PAO850 as recipient, selection was made for *car*$^+$ transductants that were scored for susceptibility to AR41. Out of 200 transductants tested, none was Tol$^-$. Since the *tol* site is known to be about 90% cotransducible with the *car*$^+$ marker, this lack of recovery of the *tol*$^-$ allele strongly supports the view that PAO1716 is a true *tol*$^+$ revertant.

The other streptomycin-resistant survivors that remained Tol$^-$ are believed to be due to chromosomal mutations for low-level streptomycin resistance, as described in *E. coli* (12, 17) and *Salmonella typhimurium* (22). They show levels of resistance that are similar to that of the wild type PAO1670, and 48% show cross-resistance to the other aminoglycosides. Presumably the drug resistance levels of such double mutants result from epistasis of the hypersensitive phenotype and the low-level resistance phenotype of these mutations.

As shown in Table 3, PAO1716 has regained the wild-type level of resistance to aminoglycosides. Thus, Tol and hypersensitivity are corevertible and, hence, probably result from the same mutational event.

Uptake of streptomycin. Radioactive streptomycin was used to determine whether the hypersensitivity of the mutants could be correlated with increased uptake of an aminoglycoside. In experiments comparing the uptake of [^{3}H]streptomycin by the wild-type strain PAO1670 and the mutant PAO1715, a level of 0.5 μg of streptomycin per ml was used; this did not inhibit the growth of either strain. The rate of uptake was 2.5 times higher for the mutant than for the parent strain. This result indicates that the mutant has increased permeability for the drug and that this is the cause of the hypersensitive phenotype. However, even though the level of streptomycin was too low to affect the viable count of the mutant during this experiment, the possibility remained that the drug was still affecting protein synthesis to some degree. The increased rate of uptake may therefore have been due to some consequence of this, for example, a slightly defective membrane structure.

The two strains were therefore mutated to high-level streptomycin resistance. This is a low-frequency mutational event that leads to decreased affinity of the ribosomes for streptomycin (7), similar to the *strA* mutation in *E. coli* (16). PAO1699 and PAO1717 were isolated as described above. The rate of uptake of [^{3}H]streptomycin was still 2.5 times higher in the mutant than in the parent strain when the streptomycin-resistant derivatives were tested (Fig. 1), even though the drug could no longer be expected to have any effect on protein synthesis. Again, the growth rates of the two strains were virtually identical; therefore, cell number was not influencing the increased uptake rate.

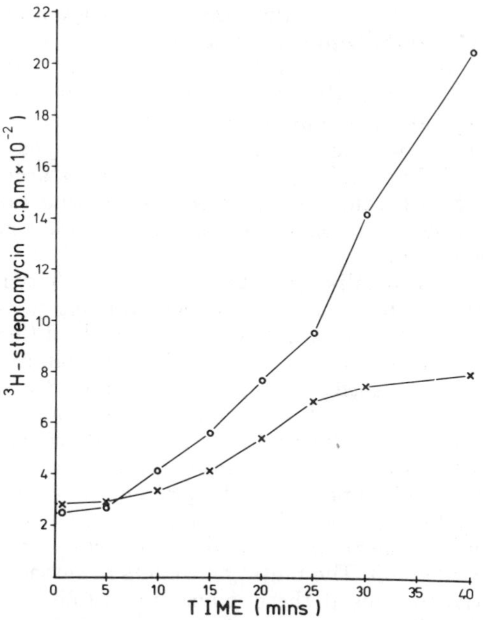

FIG. 1. *Uptake of [^{3}H]streptomycin by tolA$^+$ and tolA strains at a streptomycin concentration of 200 μg/ml. Symbols: ×, PAO1699; ○, PAO1717.*

DISCUSSION

In the studies reported here, we have identified a genetic locus that determines native specific resistance to aminoglycosides in strain PAO. Low-level resistance to many antimicrobial agents is common in hospital isolates of *P. aeruginosa* and is often referred to as intrinsic (or innate) resistance. It has not previously been clear whether this type of resistance was due to some property of *Pseudomonas* cells that conferred resistance to many agents in a nonspecific way or whether separate mechanisms were involved for each type of agent. It now appears that for the group of antibiotics listed in Table 3 and broadly classified as aminoglycosides low-level resistance can be specifically conferred.

Two mutants in which low-level resistance was lost have been studied. Independently isolated, the two mutations map very closely together and may indeed be in the same gene, but this cannot be precisely determined. In each case the mutation also confers tolerance to an AR. Tolerant mutants are blocked in some step subsequent to the binding of the bacteriocin to its receptor site on the cell surface (8, 15). The step may be involved in the transport of the bacteriocin to its target (1, 2) or in the transmission of a bacteriocin-induced message to the target (5, 15). Many tolerant mutants show an altered susceptibility to certain antibiotics and detergents, which presumably reflects the extent of cell envelope changes in the mutants (6, 9). The mutants described here do not show a general increase in susceptibility to antibiotics, surfactants, or phage; i.e., any change in envelope structure has not affected the general permeability of the cells.

The hypersensitivity to aminoglycosides appears to be due to increased permeability of the mutant for these antibiotics, since the mutant accumulates [^{3}H]streptomycin at a faster rate than does the parent. The major objection to this hypothesis is that the increased uptake might be the secondary result of another event, i.e., membrane damage caused by streptomycin. However, this is unlikely, since mutation to high-level streptomycin resistance does not alter the uptake rate of the drug. In this type of mutant the binding of streptomycin to its target in the ribosome is prevented, so the drug can have no effect on the synthesis of membrane components.

It is also unlikely that the hypersensitivity is due to a change in the ribosome, the antibiotic target site, because it is known that the different aminoglycosides have different binding sites in the ribosome and different modes of action in the cell. For example, streptomycin binds to the S12 protein in the 30S subunit and causes low-level misreading of the genetic code, kanamycin binds to the S6 protein and causes high-level misreading, and spectinomycin binds to the S5 protein and does not cause misreading (15). The mutation confers hypersensitivity towards all these compounds (Table 3).

Finally, the mutation affects R factor-coded aminoglycoside resistance (see Tables 2 and 3). The MIC for aminoglycosides when the mutant carries an R factor is in between those for the parental R^+ strain and the parental R^- strain; thus R factor-mediated resistance is reduced, but is still detectable, in the mutant. In two cases this resistance is known to be due to drug-modifying enzymes: RMS 148 codes for a streptomycin adenylase or phosphorylase and pMG2 codes for a gentamycin acetyltransferase (10; G. A. Jacoby, *in* D. Schlessinger, ed., *Microbiology—1976,* in press).

The possession of this intrinsic resistance to aminoglycosides may reflect evolutionary selection in an environment containing aminoglycosides, possibly soil. However, it is also possible that other types of selection may have occurred. To date we have only used hypersensitivity to antibiotics as an indication of this phenotype. We propose to measure permeability of other, nontoxic agents into *tolA* strains in the hope that the chemical structure of any such agents showing higher penetrability as compared with *tolA*$^+$ may help in determining the evolutionary origins of intrinsic resistance.

ACKNOWLEDGMENT

This work was supported by the Australian Research Grants Committee.

LITERATURE CITED

1. **Boon, T.** 1971. Inactivation of ribosomes *in vitro* by colicin E3. Proc. Natl. Acad. Sci. U.S.A. **68:**2421–2425.
2. **Bowman, C. M., J. E. Dahlberg, T. Ikemura, J. Konisky, and M. Nomura.** 1971. Specific inactivation of 16S ribosomal RNA induced by colicin E3 *in vivo*. Proc. Natl. Acad. Sci. U.S.A. **68:**964–968.
3. **Bryan, L. E., H. M. Van Den Elzen, and J. T. Tseng.** 1972. Transferable drug resistance in *Pseudomonas aeruginosa*. Antimicrob. Agents Chemother. **1:**22–29.
4. **Chandler, P. M., and V. Krishnapillai.** 1974. Phenotypic properties of R factors of *Pseudomonas aeruginosa:* R factors readily transferable between *Pseudomonas* and the *Enterobacteriaceae*. Genet. Res. **23:**239–250.
5. **Changeux, J. P., and J. Thiery.** 1967. On the mode of action of colicins: a model of regulation at the membrane level. J. Theor. Biol. **17:**315–318.
6. **Davies, J. K., and P. Reeves.** 1975. Genetics of resistance to colicins in *Escherichia coli* K-12: cross-resistance among colicins of group A. J. Bacteriol. **123:**102–117.
7. **Dunn, N. W., and B. W. Holloway.** 1971. Pleiotropy of p-FPA-resistant and antibiotic hypersensitive mutants of *Pseudomonas aeruginosa*. Genet. Res. **18:**185–197.
8. **Hill, C., and I. B. Holland.** 1967. Genetic basis of colicin E susceptibility in *Escherichia coli*. J. Bacteriol. **94:**677–686.
9. **Holloway, B. W., H. Rossiter, D. Burgess, and J. Dodge.** 1973. Aeruginocin tolerant mutants of *Pseudomonas aeruginosa*. Genet. Res. **22:**239–253.
10. **Jacoby, G. A.** 1974. Properties of R plasmids determining gentamicin resistance by acetylation in *Pseudomonas aeruginosa*. Antimicrob. Agents Chemother. **6:**239–252.
11. **Kawakami, Y., F. Mikoshiba, S. Nagasaki, H. Matsumoto, and T. Tazaki.** 1972. Prevalence of *Pseudomonas aeruginosa* strains possessing R factors in a hospital. J. Antibiot. **25:**607–609.
12. **Lundbäck, A. K., and K. Nordström.** 1974. Mutations in *Escherichia coli* K-12 decreasing the rate of streptomycin uptake. Antimicrob. Agents Chemother. **5:**500–507.
13. **Mitsuhashi, S., F. Kobayashi, and M. Yamaguchi.** 1971. Enzymatic inactivation of gentamycin C components by cell-free extract from *Pseudomonas aeruginosa*. J. Antibiot. **24:**400–401.
14. **Nomura, M., A. Tissières, and P. Lengyel.** 1974. Ribosomes. Cold Spring Harbor monograph series. Cold Spring Harbor Laboratory, Cold Spring Harbor, N.Y.
15. **Nomura, M., and C. Witten.** 1967. Interaction of colicins with bacterial cells. III. Colicin-tolerant mutations in *Escherichia coli*. J. Bacteriol. **94:**1093–1111.
16. **Ozaki, M., S. Mizushima, and M. Nomura.** 1969. Identification and functional characterization of the protein controlled by the streptomycin-resistant locus in *E. coli*. Nature (London) **222:**333–339.
17. **Roberts, L. M., and E. C. R. Reeve.** 1970. Two mutations giving low-level streptomycin resistance in *Escherichia coli* K12. Genet. Res. **16:**359–365.
18. **Stadler, J., and E. A. Adelberg.** 1972. Temperature dependence of sex-factor maintenance in *Escherichia coli* K-12. J. Bacteriol. **109:**447–449.
19. **Stanisich, V., and B. W. Holloway.** 1969. Conjugation in *Pseudomonas aeruginosa*. Genetics **61:**327–339.
20. **Tseng, J. T., and L. E. Bryan.** 1974. The effect of complement and other cell wall reagents on tetracycline and streptomycin resistance in *Pseudomonas aeruginosa*. Can. J. Microbiol. **20:**1101–1107.
21. **Watson, J. M., and B. W. Holloway.** 1976. Suppressor mutations in *Pseudomonas aeruginosa*. J. Bacteriol. **125:**780–786.
22. **Yamada, T., and J. Davies.** 1970. A genetic and biochemical study of streptomycin- and spectinomycin-resistance in *Salmonella typhimurium*. Mol. Gen. Genet. **110:**199–210.

ANTIMICROBIAL AGENTS AND CHEMOTHERAPY, Sept. 1976, p. 417-420 Vol. 10, No. 3

Printed in U.S.A.

Bacteriocin Production by *Neisseria gonorrhoeae*

WILLIAM D. LAWTON,* MARY ANN BELLINGER, MARION SCHLING, AND HASSAN A. GAAFAR

Division of Laboratories and Research, New York State Department of Health, Albany, New York 12201

Received for publication 18 April 1976

Seventeen apparently unrelated isolates of *Neisseria gonorrhoeae* out of 2,123 tested produced a diffusible growth-inhibitory substance against other gonococci. The inhibitor was destroyed by trypsin, not blocked by bovine serum albumin, and not soluble in chloroform-methanol; each isolate was resistant to the inhibitor it produced. Thus, the substance differs from previously described gonococcal inhibitors, and since it fits the description of a bacteriocin we designated it gonocin. The use of gonocin for typing was complicated by the observation that susceptibility to gonocin appears to depend on the gonococcal colony type.

Bacteriocins are antibacterial proteins that are produced by bacteria and act against others of the same or related species (8). Since typing schemes are limited for *Neisseria gonorrhoeae* and since bacteriocin typing has been used to classify various microorganisms (2, 8), we and others have investigated the possibility of bacteriocin production by *N. gonorrhoeae*. Flynn and McEntegart (3) reported that 75 of 100 gonococcal isolates tested produced bacteriocins, but Walstad et al. (9) were unable to confirm their observation. The latter authors found that *N. gonorrhoeae* produce inhibitory fatty acids and lysophosphatidylethanolamine but not true bacteriocins. Knapp et al. (7) also found a nonspecific inhibitor but no bacteriocins produced by *N. gonorrhoeae*. Kingsbury (6) reported on bacteriocin production in the closely related *Neisseria meningitidis*. This report details our observations on gonococcal bacteriocin production.

MATERIALS AND METHODS

Microorganisms and media. All of the isolates of *N. gonorrhoeae* used were received as patient specimens on Gonogrow transport medium (1) and were characterized as oxidase-positive, gram-negative diplococci that fermented glucose but not maltose. Cultures were stored at −70°C in GC broth containing IsoVitaleX (BBL) and 10% dimethyl sulfoxide. GC broth was made according to the formula for Difco GC base, except the agar was omitted. Although Difco GC base plus IsoVitaleX could be used for gonocin typing, clearer results were obtained with GC broth plus IsoVitaleX and 1% Difco purified agar.

Gonocin assays. Isolates of *N. gonorrhoeae* to be tested for gonocin production were suspended in GC broth plus IsoVitaleX at approximately 10^8 cells/ml. A replicator with metal prongs was used to inoculate up to 28 spots from the suspensions, each 5 mm in diameter, on the surface of a 1% agar plate. After incubation for 1 day at 36°C in a 5% CO_2 atmosphere, the spots were overlayered with 7 ml of soft agar (GC broth plus IsoVitaleX and 0.5% agar [Difco]) seeded with approximately 10^7 cells of an isolate to be tested for susceptibility to gonocin per ml. We found it unnecessary to treat the gonococcal spots with chloroform before pouring the soft-agar overlayer. The plates were reincubated overnight, and production of gonocin was measured as a clear zone extending approximately 5 to 8 mm from the edge of the gonocin-producing spot in the turbid lawn.

Gonocin extracted from cells was assayed by pouring a seeded soft-agar layer on an uninoculated plate, allowing it to harden, and then placing a drop of the material to be tested on the surface and incubating the plate overnight at 36°C in a 5% CO_2 atmosphere. Inhibition was shown, as above, by a clear zone on the turbid lawn.

Production of gonocin. Each gonocin-producing isolate of *N. gonorrhoeae* was inoculated into a 2-liter flask containing a 300-ml base layer of Difco GC base with 2% agar (Difco) and a 200-ml top layer of GC broth plus IsoVitaleX. The flask was then shaken in a 5% CO_2 atmosphere on a rotary shaker at 100 rpm at 36°C for 24 h. The cells were sedimented by centrifugation at 16,000 × g for 10 min, and the supernatant was dialyzed overnight against distilled water and lyophilized.

Trypsin and albumin treatment. Lyophilized gonocin was concentrated 10 times by resuspending at 50 mg/ml of 0.1 M sodium phosphate buffer, pH 6.2. For trypsin treatment, 0.5 ml of this suspension and 0.1 ml of Sigma type III trypsin (0.8 mg/ml) were incubated together at 36°C for 3 h. To determine the effect of bovine serum albumin, the same procedure was used with 0.1 ml of 20% bovine serum albumin (Pentex) in place of trypsin.

RESULTS

Initial screening. Each of 18 *N. gonorrhoeae* isolates was spotted on 18 agar plates and incubated overnight. Each isolate was then used in a soft-agar overlay on one plate of each set. Thus, each isolate was tested for both production of gonocin and susceptibility to gonocin with itself and 17 other isolates. This procedure was later repeated with another group of 72 isolates, for a total of 90 different gonococcal isolates.

Only one isolate produced a large clear zone of inhibition in the indicator lawns of most of the other isolates tested (Fig. 1). This was isolate 16765, to which 62 (86%) of the isolates in the second group were susceptible. To determine if the inhibitor produced by 16765 is specific to *N. gonorrhoeae,* we tested it with a variety of microorganisms. One of these, *Moraxella osloensis* 33413, showed a zone of inhibition larger than the zones seen in gonococcal indicator lawns. We therefore included *M. osloensis* 33413 as an indicator in our subsequent search for additional gonocin producers.

Mass screening for gonocin producers. Two especially susceptible indicators, *N. gonorrhoeae* 8109 and *M. osloensis* 33413, were used to screen gonococcal isolates for their ability to produce gonocin. A total of 2,123 isolates of *N. gonorrhoeae* were tested over a period of a year, and 22 of these produced clear zones of inhibition with both indicators. A few of these 22 isolates were taken from the same patient a few weeks apart (treatment failures), and a few were from admitted sex contacts. When these duplications were omitted, we had 17 apparently unrelated gonococcal isolates that produced gonocin, or 0.8% of all the isolates tested.

Differential production of gonocin by gonococci types 1 and 4. All of 14 single type 1 colonies (5) from isolate 16765 produced less gonocin than did 16 single type 4 colonies (5) from the same isolate. Three other gonocin producers were tested and behaved the same, but the demonstration of this was inconsistent, varying on different batches of medium. Type 1 cells shift rapidly to type 4 in vitro and, even when a single type 1 colony is used to make a spot of growth for testing gonocin production, the spot contains some type 4 cells. For this reason the finding remains uncertain. Type 1 cells may sometimes produce less gonocin than do type 4 cells; or, alternatively, type-1 cells may produce no gonocin, and the activity may result from the presence of a few type 4 cells in the type 1 colony.

Large-scale production of crude gonocin. Isolate 16765, type 4, was used in an attempt at large-scale production of gonocin. Athough this isolate grew well in a biphasic GC broth medium (several 2,000-ml batches were produced), the supernatant did not contain enough gono-

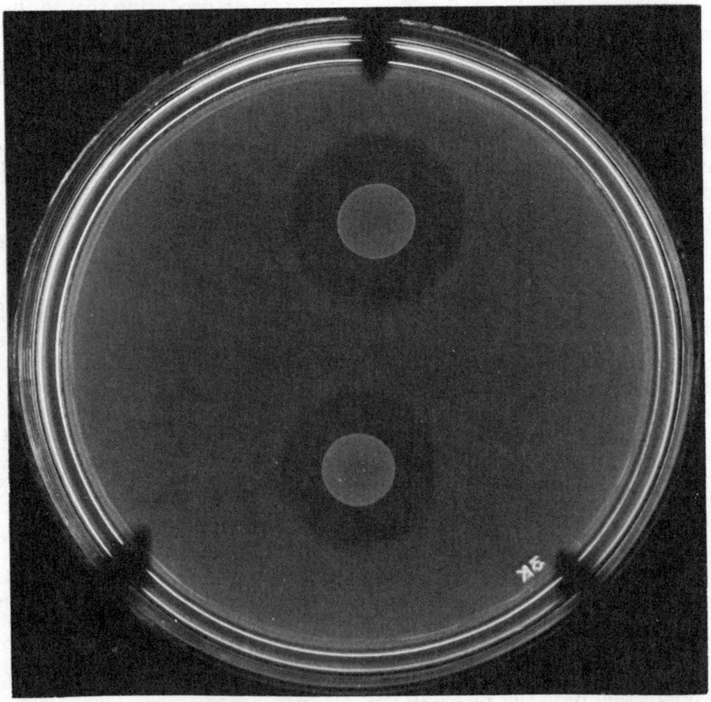

FIG. 1. *Inhibition zones surrounding two spots of N. gonorrhoeae 16765 in a lawn seeded with N. gonorrhoeae 903966.*

cin to assay. To achieve a 10-fold concentration, the supernatant was dialyzed overnight against distilled water, lyophilized, and resuspended at 50 mg/ml in distilled water. This material produced a clear zone of inhibition. An identical preparation from a non-gonocin-producing isolate showed no inhibitory zones in the indicator lawn.

Attempts to obtain greater quantities of gonocin after rupturing the cells by freeze-thawing, sonication, or 5% chloroform treatment were unsuccessful. We also failed to obtain significant yields of gonocin after growing a confluent lawn of strain 16765 on GC agar and extracting the agar with water, pH 6.2 buffer, or chloroform-methanol or by testing the fluid expressed from such agar after a freeze-thaw cycle.

Since the production of bacteriocins can often be increased by induction (6, 8), we made several attempts to increase the yield of gonocin by use of mitomycin C. Three different gonocin-producing isolates were tested, with mitomycin C concentrations of 0.1 to 10 μg/ml added at different stages of the growth curve, but no evidence was obtained to indicate a greater production of gonocin than was obtained from control cultures without mitomycin C.

Evidence for true gonocin. Since other workers (7, 9) have reported on inhibitory activity in *N. gonorrhoeae* but showed that the activity was not related to bacteriocins, we tested our crude gonocin extract from two isolates in several ways to demonstrate that it was different from the previously reported inhibitors (see Discussion). When 10-fold concentrated supernatants from gonocin-producing isolates 16765 and 82792 were treated with trypsin, the inhibitory activity disappeared, but treatment with 3% bovine serum albumin did not affect their activity (Fig. 2). Extraction of crude gonocin with chloroform-methanol (4) did not yield gonocin activity in the solvent. Removal of essentially all of the microorganisms from a spot of growth of isolate 16765 before adding an indicator lawn did not influence the zone of inhibition.

Use of gonocin for typing. All 17 gonocin-producing isolates were investigated to determine whether susceptibility to gonocin could be used to type various *N. gonorrhoeae* isolates. Twelve of the gonocin producers appeared to give different typing patterns, and subsequent testing was concentrated on them.

Our initial results with these 12 isolates were erratic, but when 15 isolates to be tested were

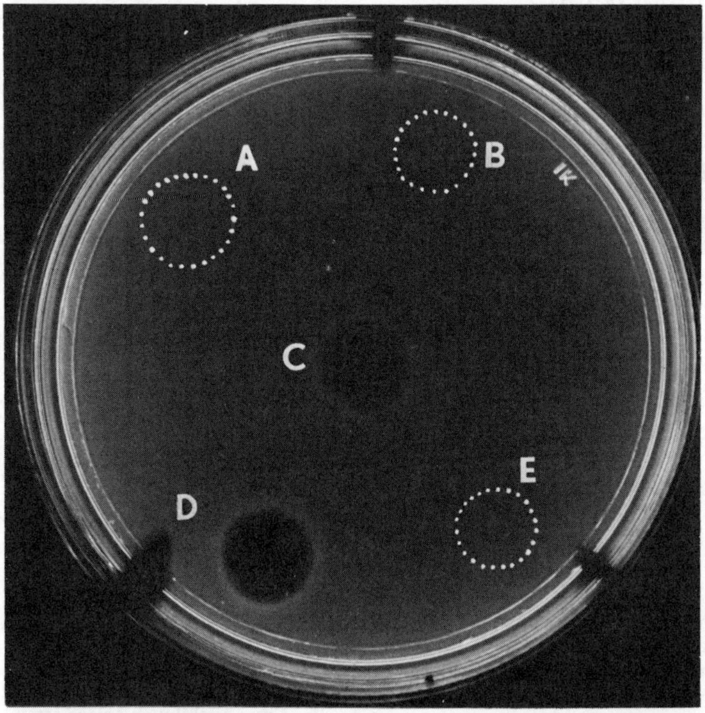

FIG. 2. *Effect of trypsin and bovine serum albumin (BSA) on activity of crude gonocin extract from N. gonorrhoeae 82792. The five spots on Difco GC base plus IsoVitaleX are: (A) trypsin plus buffer; (B) trypsin plus gonocin; (C) buffer plus gonocin; (D) BSA plus gonocin; (E) BSA plus buffer.*

separated into T1 and T4 populations (5) reproducible patterns emerged. All 15 T1 isolates, but only 4 T4 isolates, were susceptible to all 12 gonocin producers. The remaining 11 T4 isolates were sensitive to one group of six producers and resistant to the other six. The resistance patterns were clearly reproducible, and our attempts to type other gonococcal isolates focused on T4 only.

Typing with 60 T4 isolates indicated that at least two different gonocins were being produced and that the responses were as follows: (i) 36 test isolates were resistant to gonocin A and susceptible to gonocin B; (ii) 19 were susceptible to both gonocins; (iii) 1 was susceptible to gonocin A and resistant to gonocin B; and (iv) 4 were resistant to both gonocins. The gonocin A-producing strain was resistant to gonocin A but not to gonocin B; the gonocin B-producing strain was resistant to both gonocins.

Both of the isolates used to demonstrate trypsin susceptibility produce gonocin A. As soon as our typing results indicated that at least two different inhibitors were produced, we used isolate 69992 to demonstrate that gonocin B was also destroyed by trypsin but unaffected by bovine serum albumin.

DISCUSSION

The search for bacteriocin activity in *N. gonorrhoeae* is complicated by the fact that all isolates appear to produce a substance with growth-inhibitory activity against other gonococci. This substance was shown by Walstad et al. (9) to be lysophosphatidylethanolamine and free fatty acids and is probably the same inhibitor subsequently described by Knapp et al. (7). We have observed this type of inhibitory activity with many of our gonococcal isolates, regardless of whether they produce gonocin.

The inhibitor that we describe as gonocin differs from the previously described inhibitors in several ways. Most important, our inhibitor was destroyed by trypsin, indicating its protein nature. As expected with bacteriocins, no gonocin-producing strain was susceptible to its own gonocin when tested with a standard (50 mg/ml) preparation of gonocin. Whereas the fatty acid inhibitor described by Walstad et al. (9) was completely blocked by addition of 2% bovine serum albumin, gonocin was unaffected. That inhibitor was also soluble in chloroform-methanol; gonocin was not. The inhibitor described by Knapp et al. (7) was inhibited by serum; gonocin was not. Its activity caused irregular inhibition zones from 1 to 3 mm beyond the spot and was dependent on the presence of growth of the producing strains. In contrast, gonocin-producing isolates created zones extending 5 to 8 mm beyond the spot, and the zone of inhibition did not depend on the continued presence of the producing spot of growth. The "bacteriocin-like" inhibition described by Flynn and McEntegart (3) was not substantiated by Walstad et al. (9), and Knapp et al. (7) suggested that the non-bacteriocin inhibitor described by them accounted for the observation of Flynn and McEntegart. For these reasons, we believe that we have demonstrated true bacteriocin (gonocin) production in *N. gonorrhoeae* for the first time.

The usefulness of gonocin for typing gonococcal isolates remains in question. Only 0.8% of the strains tested produced gonocin, so typing isolates by their ability to produce gonocin would not be worthwhile. Typing by determining susceptibility to gonocin may be developed into a useful technique, but it is complicated by the fact that the susceptibility of an isolate can depend on its colonial type. Even when 60 type 4 isolates were selected (to obtain maximum differentiation by resistance patterns to two gonocins), 92% of the strains fell into only two groups. However, the technique could become more useful if more than two different gonocins were identified.

ACKNOWLEDGMENT

We thank Isobel DeForge for technical assistance in screening cultures for gonocin production.

LITERATURE CITED

1. **Chen, N. C., S. S. Hipp, W. D. Lawton, and H. A. Gaafar.** 1974. Gonogrow, an improved, selective medium for the isolation of *Neisseria gonorrhoeae*. Health Lab. Sci. **11**:173–177.
2. **Counts, G. W., L. Seeley, and H. N. Beaty.** 1971. Identification of an epidemic strain of *Neisseria meningitidis* by bacteriocin typing. J. Infect. Dis. **124**:26–32.
3. **Flynn, J., and M. G. McEntegart.** 1972. Bacteriocins from *Neisseria gonorrhoeae* and their possible role in epidemiological studies. J. Clin. Pathol. **25**:60–61.
4. **Garbus, J., H. F. DeLuca, M. E. Loomans, and F. M. Strong.** 1963. The rapid incorporation of phosphate into mitochondrial lipids. J. Biol. Chem. **238**:59–63.
5. **Kellogg, D. S., Jr., W. L. Peacock, Jr., W. E. Deacon, L. Brown, and C. L. Pirkle.** 1963. *Neisseria gonorrhoeae*. I. Virulence genetically linked to clonal variation. J. Bacteriol. **85**:1274–1279.
6. **Kingsbury, D. T.** 1966. Bacteriocin production by strains of *Neisseria meningitidis*. J. Bacteriol. **91**:1696–1699.
7. **Knapp, J. S., S. Falkow, and K. K. Holmes.** 1975. Reevaluation of bacteriocinogeny in *Neisseria gonorrhoeae*. J. Clin. Pathol. **28**:274–278.
8. **Reeves, P.** 1965. The bacteriocins. Bacteriol. Rev. **29**:24–45.
9. **Walstad, D. L., R. C. Reitz, and P. F. Sparling.** 1974. Growth inhibition among strains of *Neisseria gonorrhoeae* due to production of inhibitory free fatty acids and lysophosphatidylethanolamine: absence of bacteriocins. Infect. Immun. **10**:481–488.

ANTIMICROBIAL AGENTS AND CHEMOTHERAPY, Sept. 1976, p. 421-425 Vol. 10, No. 3

Printed in U.S.A.

Comparative Pharmacokinetics of Cefamandole, Cephapirin, and Cephalothin in Healthy Subjects and Effect of Repeated Dosing

MICHAEL BARZA,* SRIKUMARAN MELETHIL,[1] STEPHEN BERGER,[2] AND E. CHAIM ERNST[3]

Department of Medicine (Infectious Disease Service), Tufts-New England Medical Center Hospital, Boston, Massachusetts 02111, and North Dakota State University, College of Pharmacy, Fargo, North Dakota 58102*

Received for publication 26 April 1976

Cefamandole nafate, cephapirin, and cephalothin were administered intravenously in crossover fashion to 12 volunteers, in dosages of 2 g every 6 h for 16 doses. Mean peak levels of cefamandole were approximately 50% higher than those of the other agents. The serum concentration curves appeared to decline bi-exponentially, suggesting that a two-compartment model was most applicable for pharmacokinetic analysis; accordingly, the $t_{1/2}$ of cefamandole was significantly longer when the serum peak was omitted from the analysis (0.86 versus 0.73 h, $P < 0.05$). The half-lives of cephalothin and cephapirin, 0.34 and 0.36 h, respectively, were probably underestimates reflecting the inclusion of distribution-phase values in the calculation. Repeated dosing had no effect on the peak serum levels, half-life, serum clearance, or apparent volume of distribution with one exception: peak serum levels of cephapirin were significantly lower after the sixteenth than after the first dose. Marked variations within a given subject were noted in the half-life and apparent volume of distribution of cefamandole in several instances. Renal clearances of cefamandole exhibited saturation kinetics similar to those of penicillin G.

Cefamandole is a new cephalosporin with an extended spectrum against gram-negative bacilli (4). Recently, some aspects of its pharmacology have been reported; these suggest that it produces serum levels slightly higher than those of cephalothin, possesses a half-life similar to that of cephalothin, and displays the kinetics of a one-compartment model (5, 9, 12). The pharmacological behavior of cephapirin, while not extensively studied, appears to be similar to that of cephalothin; however, direct crossover comparisons of the two drugs are lacking (1, 10).

The present investigation was carried out as part of an examination of the comparative phlebitogenic potential of cefamandole, cephapirin, and cephalothin in healthy volunteers (3). The design of the study afforded an opportunity to compare the pharmacokinetics of the three drugs after single and multiple doses, the extent of intra-subject variability in these parameters, and the applicability of a one-compartment model to the kinetic analysis. In addition, the findings emphasize the effect of the serum level of cefamandole on its apparent renal clearance.

[1] Present address: College of Pharmacy, North Dakota State University, Fargo, N.D. 58102.

[2] Present address: New York Veterans' Administration Hospital, New York, N.Y. 10010.

[3] Present address: Sheeba Medical Center, Tel-Hashomer, Israel.

MATERIALS AND METHODS

The design of the present study, which was carried out during an investigation of the phlebitogenic potential of these cephalosporins, has been described (3). Briefly, 12 healthy volunteers were given cefamandole nafate, sodium cephapirin, or buffered sodium cephalothin in a dosage of 2 g every 6 h for 4 days; the drugs were administered intravenously over 30 min using an infusion pump. Each subject, with two exceptions, received all three drugs in randomized crossover fashion with a 24-h lapse between courses of therapy. Specimens of blood were obtained at 0.5 (peak), 1.5, 2.5, 4.5, and 6 h after the beginning of the first and last (sixteenth) infusions of each agent. Corresponding urine specimens were collected from 0 to 2 and 2 to 6 h after the onset of the infusion.

Assays for antibiotic content were done by an agar-diffusion bioassay using Trypticase soy agar plates seeded with *Bacillus subtilis* ATCC 6633 (2). Laboratory standard powders, furnished by Eli Lilly and Co. (sodium cephalothin and lithium cefamandole) and Bristol Laboratories (sodium cephapirin), were dissolved in pooled human serum and phosphate-buffered saline for the assay of serum and urine specimens, respectively. Samples containing high concentrations of drug were diluted appropriately. The assay had an accuracy of ±10% and a sensitivity of 0.3 μg/ml in serum.

The serum protein binding of cefamandole was measured by equilibrium dialysis at an initial antibiotic concentration of 20 μg/ml (2).

Pharmacokinetic analyses. Serum concentrations were plotted on semilogarithmic coordinates, and the first-order elimination rate constants (K) were determined from the slope of the least-squares linear regression line. Because of the apparent biphasic slopes of the curves, K values for cefamandole were determined with and without the 0.5-h value; however, for cephalothin and cephapirin, which were often undetectable in the serum at 4.5 h, the 0.5-h measurement had to be included in all calculations of K. The elimination half-life ($t_{1/2}$) was computed according to the usual equation: $t_{1/2} = \ln 2/K = 0.693/K$. Serum clearance and apparent volume of distribution (AVD) were estimated using the formulas: serum clearance = dose/AUC, and AVD = serum clearance/K, where AUC represents the total area under the serum concentration-time curve, calculated using the trapezoidal rule.

Renal clearance was determined from the usual formula, UV/P, where U and V represent urinary concentration and volume, respectively, and P is the midpoint serum level of drug. For the 0- to 2- and 2- to 6-h urine collections, the values for P at 1 and 4 h were approximated by linear interpolation at appropriate intervals in the individual plots of serum concentration. Measurements of serum and urine creatinine concentration were made by Autoanalyzer.

Statistical analyses were done by the paired t test, using only those values for which both members of the pair were available.

RESULTS

Serum concentration. A semilogarithmic plot of the mean serum levels of each drug at various intervals after the first and sixteenth doses suggested a biphasic curve (Fig. 1 and 2). A similar bi-exponential decline was noted when the values for individual subjects were plotted. The mean and standard error of the peak levels after the first and sixteenth doses were: cefamandole, 147 ± 16 and 157 ± 23 μg/ml; cephapirin, 127 ± 17 and 92 ± 11 μg/ml; and cephalothin, 96 ± 13 and 79 ± 12 μg/ml. The differences between values for the first and last doses were significant for cephapirin ($P < 0.01$). Levels of cefamandole were significantly higher than those of cephalothin after the first dose and higher than those of both cephalothin and cephapirin after the sixteenth dose ($P < 0.05$ in each instance). In addition to the marked inter-individual variations that are evident from the standard error, differences between values for the first and last doses within the same subject were sometimes striking.

Serum half-life. There were no significant changes in half-life values between the first

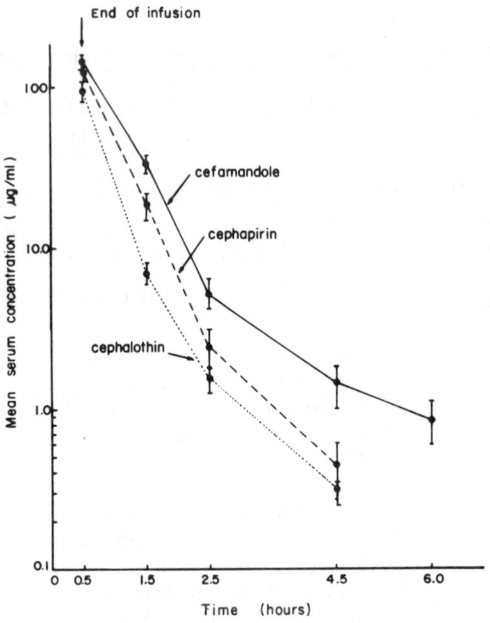

FIG. 1. *Semilogarithmic plot of mean serum concentrations of antibiotic at various intervals after the first dose of drug. Vertical bars represent standard error.*

and last doses for any of the agents (Table 1). When the data for each drug were pooled, the overall half-life values (mean ± standard deviation) were: cefamandole, 0.86 ± 0.25 h; cephapirin, 0.36 ± 0.08 h; and cephalothin, 0.34 ± 0.06 h. Inclusion of the levels at 0.5 h in the calculation for cefamandole shortened the overall half-life significantly (0.86 versus 0.73 h, $P < 0.05$). The resultant value was still substantially longer than the half-life of either cephalothin or cephapirin.

Intra-subject variations in the half-life of cephalothin or cephapirin were small (Table 1). In contrast, differences approaching twofold were noted in subjects 3 and 4 for cefamandole.

Serum clearance, renal clearance, and AVD of cefamandole. There was no difference between values for the first and sixteenth doses in terms of serum clearance, AVD, or renal clearance of cefamandole (Table 2). These parameters could not reliably be measured for cephalothin and cephapirin because the rapid elimination of these drugs afforded only a limited number of serum levels. Overall measurements (mean ± standard deviation) of the serum clearance and AVD of cefamandole were 230 ± 99 ml/min per 1.73 m^2 and 17.9 ± 8.4 liters, respectively. The AVD ranged from 10 to 67% of body weight, with most values falling between 20 and 30%. There was no significant correla-

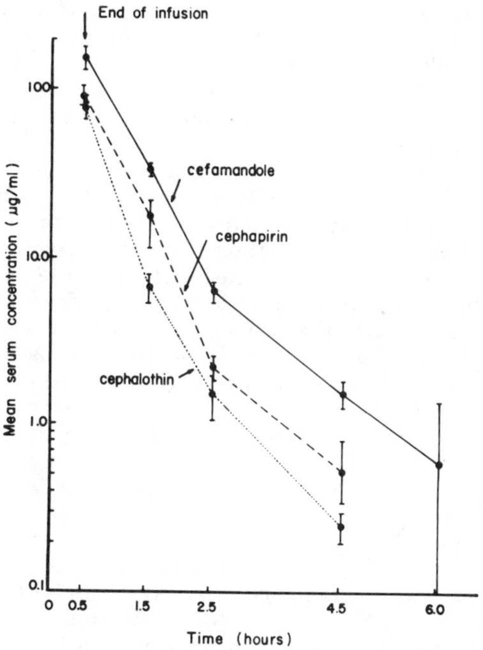

FIG. 2. *Semilogarithmic plot of mean serum concentrations of antibiotic at various intervals after the last dose of drug. Vertical bars represent standard error.*

TABLE 1. *Serum half-life (hours) after first and sixteenth doses of three cephalosporins*[a]

Subject	Cefamandole		Cephapirin		Cephalothin	
	1st dose	16th dose	1st dose	16th dose	1st dose	16th dose
1	0.72	0.84	0.37	0.35	0.33	0.39
2	1.0	0.81	0.40		0.28	0.28
3	1.8	0.92	0.35	0.29	0.34	
4	0.49	0.82	0.27		0.29	
5	0.79	0.78		0.30	0.26	0.26
6	1.1	0.71	0.33	0.37	0.47	0.37
7	0.79	0.74	0.37	0.41		0.36
8	0.68	0.88	0.29		0.34	0.38
9	0.89	0.80	0.23	0.35	0.34	0.35
10	0.89		0.33	0.36		
11			0.63	0.40	0.38	
12	0.72	0.89		0.40		0.44
Mean	0.90	0.82	0.36	0.36	0.34	0.35
SD[b]	0.34	0.07	0.11	0.04	0.06	0.06

[a] Values for cefamandole were computed from serum levels at 1.5, 2.5, 4.5, and 6 h; for cephalothin and cephapirin, data for 0.5, 1.5, 2.5, and (where detectable) 4.5 h were used.

[b] SD, Standard deviation.

tion between AVD and body weight. Intra-subject variations in serum clearance and in AVD were striking in a number of instances (Table 2).

When the renal clearances of cefamandole

TABLE 2. *Serum clearance and AVD after the first and sixteenth doses of cefamandole*

Subject	Serum clearance (ml/min per 1.73 m²)		AVD (liters)	
	1st dose	16th dose	1st dose	16th dose
1	182	193	11.4	14.1
2	329	389	30.6	29.3
3	250	134	40.1	11.0
4	531	117	24.1	8.9
5	197	285	13.1	18.7
6	260	166	21.7	9.0
7	266	268	20.8	19.7
8	196	276	14.4	26.3
9	192	167	17.6	13.7
10	120		9.2	
12	132	181	7.5	15.3
Mean	241	218	19.1	16.6
SD[a]	114	84	9.8	6.9

[a] SD, Standard deviation.

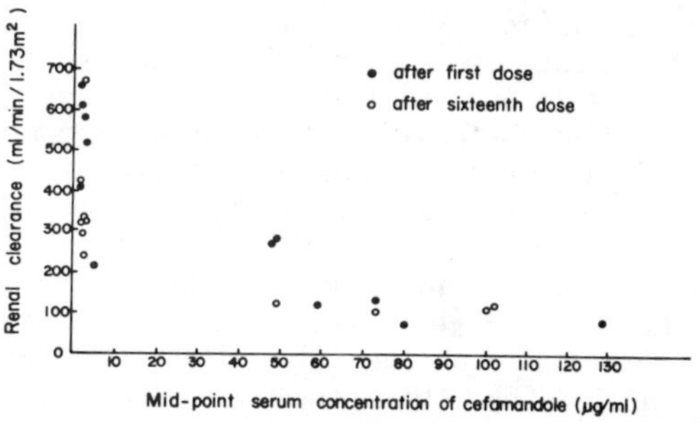

FIG. 3. *Relation between the renal clearance of cefamandole, as determined from the formula UV/P, and the midpoint serum concentration of antibiotic.*

were plotted against midpoint serum concentrations (P), the data fell into two groups: those obtained at 0 to 2 h (serum levels of 48 to 128 μg/ml) and those obtained at 2 to 6 h (serum levels of ≤5 μg/ml; Fig. 3). With two exceptions, clearance values at the higher serum concentrations were close to 100 ml/min per 1.73 m², whereas those at lower concentrations ranged from 220 to 670 ml/min per 1.73 m².

Serum protein binding. The mean value in 13 chambers was 67% (standard deviation, 2%), with a range of 56 to 78%.

DISCUSSION

The results of this study indicate that cefamandole produces higher levels of drug in the serum than those found after an equivalent dose of cephalothin or cephapirin. Its degree of serum protein binding is similar to that of cephalothin (5) and slightly higher than the 44 to 54% reported for cephapirin (7). Higher levels of cefamandole than of cephalothin have been reported by Fong et al. (5), and indirect comparisons of the serum levels of cephalothin and cephapirin are in agreement with the findings in the present study (1, 10). Because serum was not obtained during the infusion phase in the present study, the pharmacokinetic analysis slightly underestimates the AUC value and therefore overestimates that of serum clearance and AVD. Nevertheless, the serum clearances of cefamandole are in excellent agreement with those reported by Fong et al. (5). Values previously reported for the AVD of cefamandole include 17.1 liters (24% of body weight) and 12.8 liters/1.73 m^2 (5, 9), which are similar to our results obtained in the postdistribution phase.

The pharmacokinetic analysis is complicated somewhat by the biotransformation undergone by all threee agents. Cefamandole nafate is hydrolyzed in vivo to the active drug, cefamandole. Because of the rapidity of this process ($t_{1/2}$ about 13 min; J. S. Wold, R. R. Joost, and J. M. Indelicato, Prog. Abstr. Intersci. Conf. Antimicrob. Agents Chemother., 15th, Washington, D.C., Abstr. 82, 1975), it is unlikely that it appreciably affected the pharmacokinetic measurements. Cefamandole itself appears not to be metabolized as indicated by the extent of its urinary recovery (9) and by the similarity of its renal and serum clearance rates (5). Both cephalothin and cephapirin are metabolized to the less active *o*-desacetyl derivative, which comprises 33 and 41%, respectively, of the antibiotic found in the urine (10). Data from our own laboratory for cephalothin (unpublished data) and from Bristol Laboratories for both drugs (B. E. Cabana, unpublished data) indicate that in healthy individuals, levels of the desacetyl derivatives are only 5 to 15% of the concentrations of the parent substance in serum. Since the metabolite is one-fifth as active against the test organism (*B. subtilis*) as is cephalothin (8) or cephapirin (Bristol Laboratories, unpublished data), its presence appears unlikely to have interfered with the assay of the parent compound.

The rapid elimination of the cephalosporins would suggest that their peak serum levels and other pharmacokinetic characteristics should not be affected by repeated dosing (10). In one study of cefazolin, however, a reduction in the half-life was noted after multiple injections (13). In the present study, repeated administration did not influence the peak serum levels or half-life of these cephalosporins, or the serum clearance or AVD of cefamandole. One unexpected exception was cephapirin, for which peak serum levels were slightly, but significantly, lower after the sixteenth than after the first dose. We have no explanation for this observation; moreover, no such difference was apparent at the 1.5-h (18.6 versus 17.8 μg/ml) and 2.5-h (2.4 versus 2.2 μg/ml) intervals after the first and last doses of cephapirin. In any event, the extent of the decrease appears unlikely to be of clinical importance.

Except for the peak serum levels of cephapirin, there was no significant overall change in any of the pharmacokinetic measurements with repeated dosing; thus, it was of interest to examine the extent of variations in these parameters between the first and the last doses in the same individual. The serum half-lives of cephalothin and cephapirin were quite consistent for a given subject; in contrast, the half-life of cefamandole showed marked variations (twofold) in two recipients. The same individuals exhibited similar discrepancies in the serum clearance of this agent, and four volunteers displayed striking changes in the AVD of cefamandole.

Many authors have used a one-compartment model to analyze the pharmacokinetics of cephalosporins. Nightingale et al. have emphasized the problems of this approach which, by including the early, short-lived "distribution" phase, results in an artificially short serum half-life (10). They have noted that the kinetics of most cephalosporins best fit a two-compartment model. Figures 1 and 2 support the notion that the serum levels of these drugs exhibit a biphasic decline. For cefamandole, the distributive phase, during which serum levels declined very rapidly, lasted about 2 h; thereafter, levels decreased more slowly. Accordingly, exclusion of the 0.5-h serum level from the calculation resulted in a significant increase in the half-life (0.86 versus 0.73 h, $P < 0.05$), approximating more closely the β-phase half-life of the drug. Recently, Fong et al. reported that the elimination kinetics of cefamandole appeared to fit a one-compartment model (5); however, they examined the kinetics after infusion to steady state in one group (an approach that may have impaired the ability to discern the two-compartment characteristics of the drug [6]) and excluded serum levels obtained 30 to 45 min postinfusion in the other (5). The half-life of cefamandole in that study (0.56 h) was substantially shorter than our value; one possible explanation is that the higher dose of drug used in the present investigation saturated the renal clearance mechanisms, resulting in a longer $t_{1/2}$. In addition, inter-subject variations may have played a role in the difference.

It should be noted that the half-lives of cephalothin and cephapirin measured in this study were largely based upon the 0.5-, 1.5-, and 2.5-h serum levels and therefore probably include an appreciable contribution of the distributive phase. A more accurate measurement of the elimination rate of these rapidly excreted agents might better be made after infusion to equilibrium. Although the importance of these distinctions might not appear great, their influence on measurements of AVD and absorption and elimination rate constants is substantial (10), especially since the discrepancy between distributional and elimination-phase half-lives for cephalosporins is typically about fivefold.

A marked effect of serum level on the apparent clearance rate of cefamandole was noted (Fig. 3). This result was not surprising and simply reflects the saturability of the transport pump for organic anions of the proximal renal tubule (11). Although the lack of data in the middle range of serum concentrations precludes precise definition of the T_m of cefamandole, the shape of the curve suggests a value similar to that for penicillin G (11). This phenomenon probably also contributes to the divergent results reported by various investigators for the renal clearance of beta-lactam antibiotics.

ACKNOWLEDGMENTS

This work was supported by a grant from Eli Lilly and Co., Indianapolis, Ind. We also wish to thank William Shelver for assistance in writing the computer programs for pharmacokinetic and statistical analysis of the data.

LITERATURE CITED

1. **Axelrod, J., B. R. Meyers, and S. Z. Hirschman.** 1972. Cephapirin: pharmacology in normal human volunteers. J. Clin. Pharmacol. 12:84–88.
2. **Barza, M., T. Samuelson, and L. Weinstein.** 1974. Penetration of antibiotics into fibrin loci *in vivo*. II. Comparison of nine antibiotics: effect of dose and degree of protein binding. J. Infect. Dis. 129:66–72.
3. **Berger, S., E. C. Ernst, and M. Barza.** 1976. The comparative incidence of phlebitis due to buffered cephalothin, cephapirin, and cefamandole. Antimicrob. Agents Chemother. 9:646–648.
4. **Ernst, E. C., S. Berger, M. Barza, N. V. Jacobus, and F. P. Tally.** 1976. Activity of cefamandole and other cephalosporins against aerobic and anaerobic bacteria. Antimicrob. Agents Chemother. 9:852–858.
5. **Fong, I. W., E. D. Ralph, E. R. Engelking, and W. M. M. Kirby.** 1976. Clinical pharmacology of cefamandole as compared with cephalothin. Antimicrob. Agents Chemother. 9:65–69.
6. **Gibaldi, M., and D. Perrier.** 1975. Multicompartment models, p. 75–77. *In* J. Swarbrick (ed.), Drugs and the pharmaceutical sciences, vol. 1, Pharmacokinetics. Marcel Dekker, New York.
7. **Hottendorf, G. H., K. E. Price, and D. R. van Harken.** 1975. Comparative plasma bactericidal activity of cephapirin and cefazolin. Curr. Ther. Res. 18:364–370.
8. **Kirby, W. M. M., J. B. DeMaine, and W. S. Serrill.** 1971. Pharmacokinetics of the cephalosporins in healthy volunteers and uremic patients. Postgrad. Med. J. 47(Suppl.):41–46.
9. **Meyers, B. R., B. Ribner, S. Yancovitz, and S. Z. Hirschman.** 1976. Pharmacological studies with cefamandole in human volunteers. Antimicrob. Agents Chemother. 9:140–144.
10. **Nightingale, C. H., D. S. Greene, and R. Quintiliani.** 1975. Pharmacokinetics and clinical use of cephalosporin antibiotics. J. Pharm. Sci. 64:1899–1927.
11. **Pers, M.** 1954. Penicillin clearance as kidney function test, determinations with and without collection of urine. Scand. J. Clin. Lab. Sci. 6:341–348.
12. **Shemonsky, N. K., J. Carrizosa, and M. E. Levison.** 1975. In vitro activity and pharmacokinetics of cefamandole, a new cephalosporin antibiotic. Antimicrob. Agents Chemother. 8:679–683.
13. **Welling, P. G., W. A. Craig, G. L. Amidon, and C. M. Kunin.** 1974. Pharmacokinetics of cefazolin in normal and uremic subjects. Clin. Pharmacol. Ther. 15:344–353.

ANTIMICROBIAL AGENTS AND CHEMOTHERAPY, Sept. 1976, p. 426-435 Vol. 10, No. 3

Printed in U.S.A.

Laboratory Evaluation of BL-S786, a Cephalosporin with Broad-Spectrum Antibacterial Activity

F. LEITNER,* M. MISIEK, T. A. PURSIANO, R. E. BUCK, D. R. CHISHOLM, R. G. DEREGIS, Y. H. TSAI, AND K. E. PRICE

Department of Microbiological Research, Bristol Laboratories, Syracuse, New York 13201

Received for publication 3 May 1976

Biological and physicochemical properties of BL-S786 were compared with those of cephalothin, cephaloridine, and cefazolin. With few exceptions, BL-S786 was more active than the reference compounds against major gram-negative pathogenic species and its antibacterial spectrum was broader than that of cephalosporins currently available for clinical use. Although BL-S786 was generally less active than the control cephalosporins against gram-positive pathogens, it inhibited their growth at concentrations that should readily be achieved in humans after standard parenteral dosage. *Streptococcus faecalis,* a species relatively unsusceptible to cephalosporins in general, was an exception. BL-S786 was an effective bactericidal agent for strains of various gram-negative organisms. After intramuscular administration to mice, BL-S786 achieved high concentrations in blood, and its biological half-life was longer than that of the other three cephalosporins.

BL-S786 (Fig. 1) is a new semisynthetic cephalosporin with a broad spectrum of antibacterial activity. The following is a report on biological and physicochemical properties of BL-S786 in comparison with those of cephalothin, cephaloridine, and cefazolin, three cephalosporins widely used clinically in the United States and abroad.

MATERIALS AND METHODS

Cephalosporins. BL-S786, 7-[α-(2-aminomethylphenyl)acetamido]-3-[(1-carboxymethyltetrazol-5-ylthio)methyl]-3-cephem-4-carboxylic acid, was synthesized by members of the Product Development Department, Bristol Laboratories (W. J. Gottstein, M. A. Kaplan, J. A. Cooper, V. H. Silver, S. J. Nachfolger, and A. P. Granatek, submitted for publication). Cephalothin and cephaloridine were products of Eli Lilly and Co.; cefazolin was obtained from Fujisawa Pharmaceutical Co. and Smith Kline and French Laboratories.

Bacteria. The organisms, preponderantly of recent clinical origin, were obtained from numerous sources of broad geographical distribution. Obligate anaerobes were maintained in egg meat medium (Difco); *Mycobacterium* was stored on Lowenstein medium (Jensen modification; Difco). The techniques of storing all other organisms have been described previously (1).

Antibiotic spectrum. The growth-inhibitory activity of BL-S786 and the control compounds was determined by the antibiotic dilution technique. Procedures were as follows.

(i) Aerobic organisms (excluding *Mycobacterium*). Except for *Haemophilus* and *Neisseria,* the assay was performed in Mueller-Hinton medium (Difco). For fastidious organisms, i.e., *Streptococcus, Listeria, Pasteurella, Bordetella,* and *Vibrio,* the medium was supplemented with 4% defibrinated sheep blood. The antibiotic susceptibility of *Haemophilus* and *Neisseria* was determined in GC medium base (BBL) supplemented with 1% hemoglobin (BBL) and 1% IsoVitaleX (BBL).

Overnight broth cultures or an exponentially growing culture (*Neisseria*) served as the source of inoculum. A volume of approximately 0.003 ml of the undiluted or diluted culture was applied to the surface of the antibiotic-containing agar plates with the inoculator of Steers et al. (5). Cultures of *Neisseria, Streptococcus pneumoniae, S. viridans,* and *S. pyogenes* were used without dilution; those of all other organisms were diluted 100-fold. The inoculum contained about 10^3 viable cells for *Neisseria,* 10^5 for *S. pneumoniae* and *S. pyogenes,* 10^6 for *S. viridans,* and 10^4 for all other species. The culture plates were incubated at 37°C either overnight or for 24 h (*Haemophilus*), and the minimum inhibitory concentration, i.e., the lowest concentration of antibiotic that prevents visible growth, was recorded.

(ii) *Mycobacterium tuberculosis*. Antimycobacterial activity was assayed in Dubos liquid medium (Difco). To 1 ml of antibiotic-containing medium, 3 ml of a 50-fold diluted, 10-day-old culture was added. Minimum inhibitory concentration values were determined after further incubation at 37°C for 10 days.

(iii) Obligate anaerobes. The assay was performed on solid medium, consisting of brain heart infusion broth (BBL) supplemented with 5% defibrinated sheep blood and 1% Ionagar (Colab). A volume of approximately 0.003 ml of a cell suspension, con-

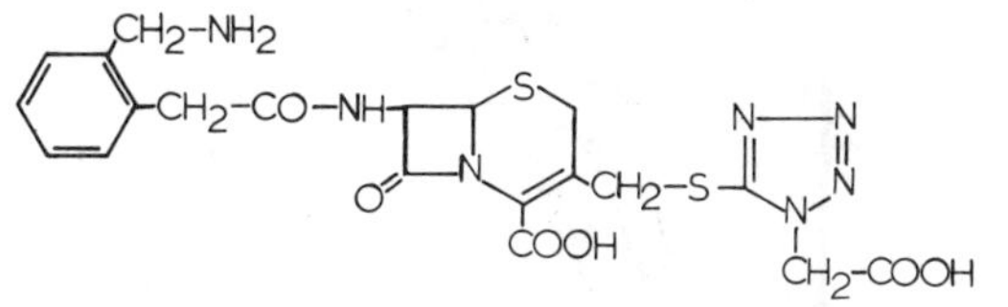

FIG. 1. *Structure of BL-S786.*

taining 10^4 viable cells, was applied to the surface of the medicated agar plates with the inoculator of Steers et al. (5). The plates were incubated at 37°C for 48 h under the oxygen-free conditions attained with a GasPak (BBL) brewer jar system.

Binding to serum proteins. The degree of binding to human serum proteins was estimated by means of the antibiotic diffusion technique of Scholtan and Schmid (4). The assays were performed in 95% pooled human serum. The range of cephalosporin concentrations was as follows: 3 to 20 μg/ml for BL-S786; 1 to 20 μg/ml for cephalothin; 0.5 to 5 μg/ml for cephaloridine; and 4 to 100 μg/ml for cefazolin.

Stability in solution. Stability in solution was determined at 37°C in 0.005 M phosphate buffer, pH 7.4. The initial antibiotic concentration was 0.2 mg/ml for cephalothin, 0.6 mg/ml for BL-S786 and cefazolin, and 2 mg/ml for cephaloridine. Residual antibiotic activity was determined periodically over a 24-h period by a turbidimetric assay procedure or by an antibiotic diffusion technique (cephalothin).

Antibiotic concentration in blood. Male Swiss-Webster mice, weighing 19 to 22 g, were given 0.2 ml of antibiotic solutions at appropriate concentrations by intramuscular injection. The vehicle was 0.01% phosphate buffer at pH 7.0. Eight animals were used for each dose level (5, 10, 20, and 40 mg/kg). Blood samples (0.03 ml) were obtained from the orbital sinuses by means of heparinized capillary tubes (Clay Adams) at 0.25, 0.5, 1, and 1.5 h after administration of the compound. Paper disks, 6.35 mm in diameter, were impregnated with the blood, and the antibiotic activity was assayed by the diffusion technique using seed agar (BBL) inoculated with *Bacillus subtilis* ATCC 6633. A standard line relating the diameter of the inhibition zone to drug concentration was obtained by assaying the compounds at known concentrations in heparinized mouse blood.

Recovery in urine. Male Sprague-Dawley rats, weighing 180 to 220 g, received a dose of 10 mg of antibiotic per kg in 0.4 ml of 0.01% phosphate buffer, pH 7.0, by intramuscular injection. Depending on the experiment, 4, 5, or 10 rats were used per compound. The animals were hydrated with 5 ml of water 0, 3, and 6 h after dosing. The rats were housed individually in metabolism cages, and urine specimens were collected over dry ice during intervals of 0 to 6 and 6 to 24 h after administration. Samples (0.03 ml) of appropriate dilutions of urine were placed on paper disks (6.35 mm in diameter), and the antibiotic activity was assayed by the diffusion technique on seed agar inoculated with *B. subtilis* ATCC 6633. A standard line relating the diameter of the inhibition zone to drug concentration was obtained by assaying the compounds at known concentrations in urine collected from untreated control animals.

Treatment of systemically infected mice. The procedures were identical to those published previously (2) except that: (i) the hog gastric mucin used in infections with *Staphylococcus aureus* no. 2 was purchased from American Laboratories, Inc., Omaha, Neb. (lot no 154163), and (ii) the medium used to suspend all other organisms contained 3% (rather than 4%) hog gastric mucin (type 1701W, Wilson Laboratories, Inc., Park Forest South, Ill.).

Miscellaneous. Methods for determining bactericidal activity and susceptibility to cell-free β-lactamase were those previously used (1).

RESULTS

Properties in vitro. (i) Antibiotic spectrum. The growth-inhibitory activity of BL-S786 and the three control cephalosporins is illustrated in Fig. 2 to 4 and Tables 1 and 2.

BL-S786 was from 2 to 16 times more active than the reference cephalosporins against *Escherichia coli, Klebsiella pneumoniae, Proteus mirabilis, Proteus vulgaris, Salmonella* sp., *Shigella* sp., and *Neisseria meningitidis* (Fig. 2 and 3). BL-S786 was also the most active of the four cephalosporins against a small number of strains of *Edwardsiella tarda, Arizona hinshawii,* and *Erwinia* sp. (Table 1). Ninety-eight percent of the *Providencia stuartii* and 78% of the *Proteus rettgeri* strains were inhibited by BL-S786 at a concentration of 16 μg/ml. At the same concentration, cefazolin inhibited 23% and 44% of the strains, respectively, whereas the percentage of strains inhibited 23 and 44% of the strains, respecnegligible for both species. Against *Enterobacter* sp. and *Citrobacter* sp., BL-S786 alone was active. Against *Haemophilus influenzae,* including nine ampicillin-resistant strains, BL-S786, cephaloridine, and cefazolin were about equally active, whereas cephalothin was more than twice as active as the other cephalosporins. *Neisseria gonorrhoeae* was equally susceptible to BL-S786, cephalothin, and cefazolin. Five strains of *Alcaligenes* sp. were susceptible and six were resistant to the four cephalosporins. *Pasteurella multocida* was highly susceptible, whereas *Proteus morganii, Serratia marcescans, Pseudomonas aeruginosa,* and *Bacteroides fragilis* were resistant to all of the cephalosporins.

BL-S786 was generally less active than the control compounds against staphylococci, streptococci, *Listeria monocytogenes,* and *Clostridium* sp. (Fig. 4 and Table 2). Nevertheless, BL-S786, at 4 μg/ml, inhibited 62 strains and, at 8 μg/ml, all 63 strains of *S. aureus*. Furthermore, BL-S786 inhibited all strains of *S. pneu-*

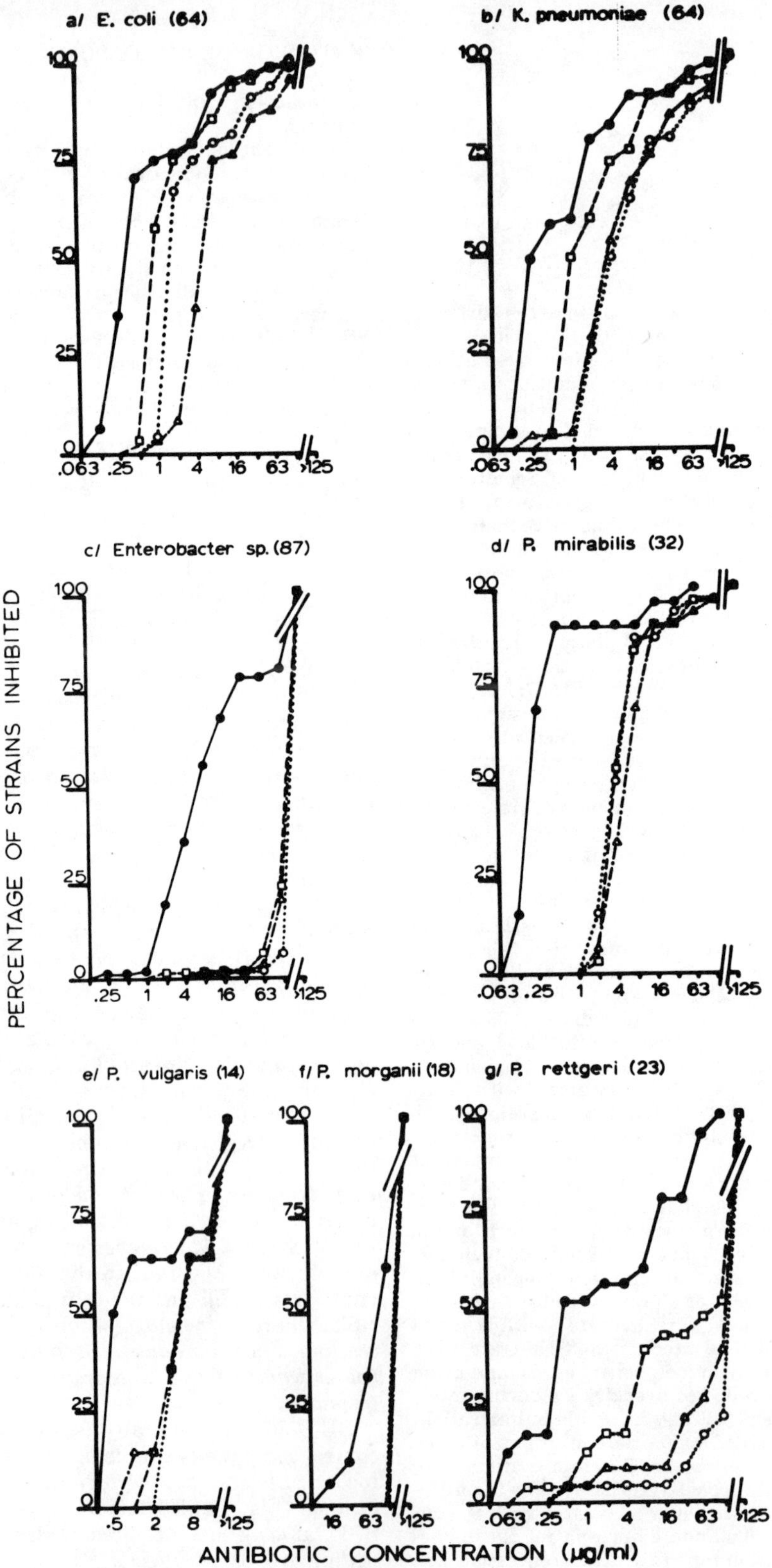

FIG. 2. *Growth-inhibitory activity of BL-S786 (●), cephalothin (△), cephaloridine (○), and cefazolin (□) against strains of various Enterobacteriaceae. The numeral in parentheses indicates the number of strains.*

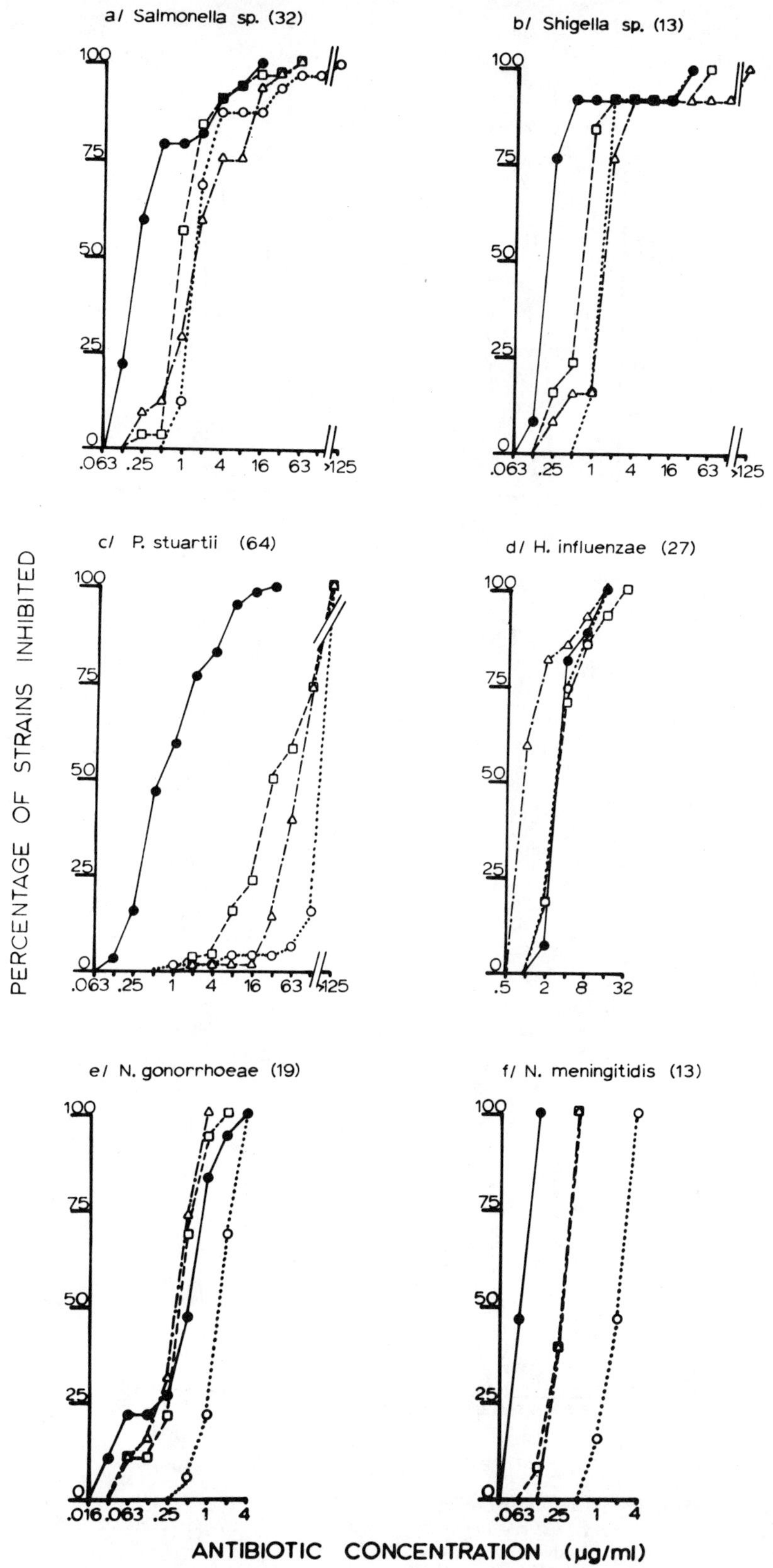

FIG. 3. *Growth-inhibitory activity of BL-S786 (●), cephalothin (△), cephaloridine (○), and cefazolin (□) against strains of various gram-negative organisms. The numeral in parentheses indicates the number of strains.*

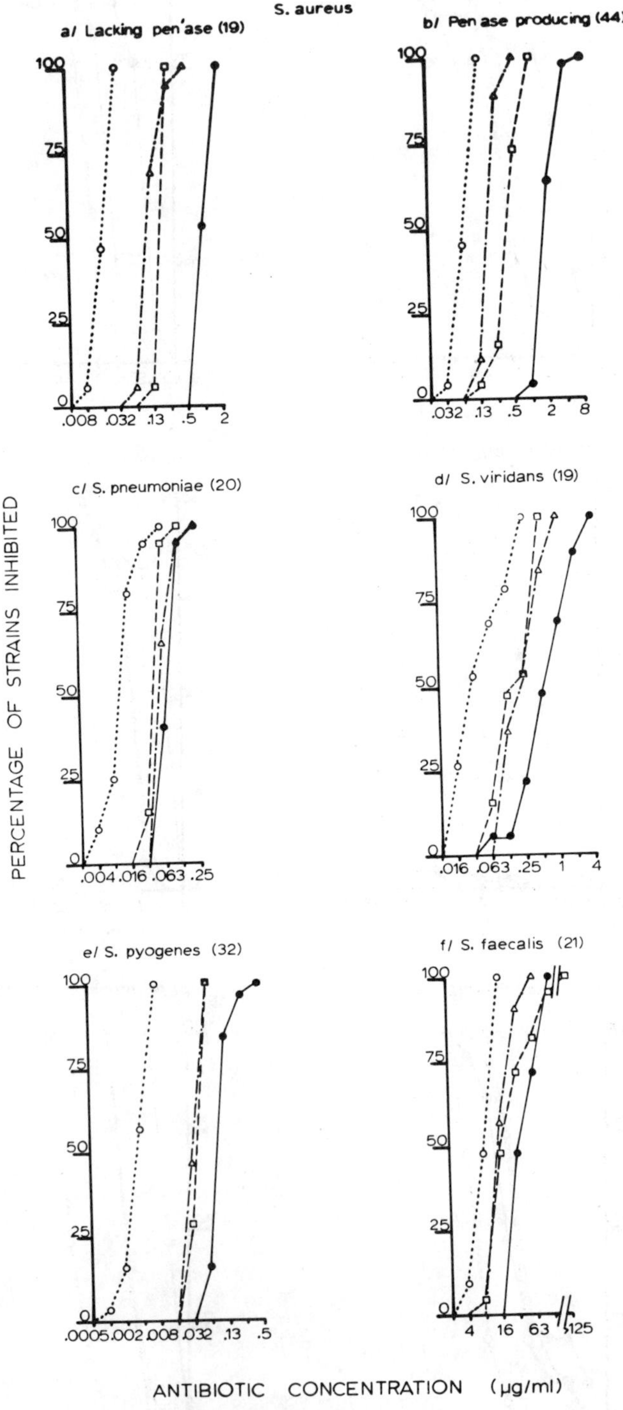

FIG. 4. *Growth-inhibitory activity of BL-S786 (●), cephalothin (△), cephaloridine (○), and cefazolin (□) against strains of various gram-positive organisms. The numeral in parentheses indicates the number of strains.*

TABLE 1. *Growth-inhibitory activity against strains of miscellaneous gram-negative organisms*

Organism	No. of strains	Minimum inhibitory concn[a] (μg/ml)			
		BL-S786	Cephalothin	Cephaloridine	Cefazolin
Edwardsiella tarda	2	0.13	1	1	0.71
Arizona hinshawii	2	0.13	2.8	2	1
Citrobacter sp.	4	1	63	>125	75
Citrobacter sp.	1	125	>125	>125	>125
Serratia marcescens	15	>125	>125	>125	>125
Erwinia sp.	5	0.66	5.3	2	1.5
Vibrio cholerae	1	4	1	16	4
Pasteurella multocida	2	0.25	0.09	0.5	0.5
Pseudomonas aeruginosa	16	>125	>125	>125	>125
Alcaligenes sp.	5	2.6	1.3	6.1	4.6
Alcaligenes sp.	2	63	>125	>125	>125
Alcaligenes sp.	4	>125	>105	>125	>105
Bordetella bronchiseptica	1	125	8	32	125
Bacteroides fragilis	3	100	125	79	50

[a] Geometric mean when applicable.

TABLE 2. *Growth-inhibitory activity against strains of miscellaneous gram-positive organisms*

Organism	No. of strains	Minimum inhibitory concn[a] (μg/ml)			
		BL-S786	Cephalothin	Cephaloridine	Cefazolin
Listeria monocytogenes	7	10.8	2	0.91	1.2
Clostridium sp.	3	2	0.5	0.63	0.4
Mycobacterium tuberculosis[b]	2	4	63	16	125
Mycobacterium tuberculosis[c]	1	16	250	63	250

[a] Geometric mean when applicable.
[b] Strain H37Rv: parent and streptomycin-resistant mutant.
[c] Strain H37Rv: isoniazid-resistant mutant.

moniae at 0.25 μg/ml, all strains of *S. pyogenes* at 0.5 μg/ml, and all strains of *S. viridans* at 4 μg/ml. The three strains of *Clostridium* sp. were inhibited at 2 μg/ml. BL-S786 was 4 to 32 times more active than the control compounds against *M. tuberculosis* H37Rv. *S. faecalis* was resistant to BL-S786.

(ii) Effect of inoculum size. A variation in the initial cell concentration of *Enterobacteriaceae* affected in a similar fashion the growth-inhibitory activity of BL-S786 and of the control compounds (Table 3). Thus, with few exceptions, the activity of all compounds declined sharply (from 16- to more than 1,000-fold) against strains of *Enterobacter cloacae*, *E. aerogenes*, and *P. rettgeri* but only moderately (from 2- to 8-fold) against strains of *E. coli*, *K. pneumoniae*, *P. mirabilis*, and *P. vulgaris* when the inoculum was increased from 10^2 to 10^6 organisms.

The effect of inoculum on the susceptibility of staphylococci to cephalosporins is illustrated in Table 4. The susceptibility of strains that lack penicillinase varied little with initial cell concentration. With penicillinase-producing strains, cell concentration affected only slightly the growth-inhibitory activity of BL-S786 and cephalothin, moderately that of cefazolin, and sharply that of cephaloridine.

(iii) Bactericidal activity. BL-S786 and the control compounds were effective bactericidal agents for strains of *E. coli*, *K. pneumoniae*, *P. mirabilis*, and *P. vulgaris* (Table 5). For most strains of *Enterobacter*, BL-S786 alone was significantly bactericidal. One strain of *P. rettgeri* was susceptible and the other was largely resistant to the bactericidal action of the cephalosporins.

(iv) Susceptibility to β-lactamase. Susceptibility to enzymatic hydrolysis was assessed by determining relative rates of hydrolysis by cell-free preparations of various β-lactamases (Table 6). BL-S786 was slightly to markedly less susceptible than the other cephalosporins to hydrolysis by β-lactamases of types Ia, Ib, IIIa, and IVa. All cephalosporins were poor substrates for type IIa and staphylococcal β-lactamases. The four cephalosporins were hydrolyzed at similar rates by the type IVb enzyme.

(v) Binding to serum proteins. In 95% human serum, BL-S786 and cephalothin were 67%, cephaloridine was 30%, and cefazolin was 76% protein bound.

(vi) Stability in solution. At pH 7.4 and 37°C, the half-life of BL-S786 and the control cephalosporins was greater than 24 h.

Properties in vivo. (i) Concentration in murine blood. Peak antibiotic concentrations of BL-S786 and the three control compounds were observed 0.25 h after intramuscular adminis-

TABLE 3. *Effect of inoculum size on the susceptibility of Enterobacteriaceae*

Organism	Strain	Minimum inhibitory concn (μg/ml)[a]							
		BL-S786		Cephalothin		Cephaloridine		Cefazolin	
		A	B	A	B	A	B	A	B
Escherichia coli	1	0.5	2	8	32	2	8	1	4
	3	0.25	1	4	16	2	4	1	2
	4	0.5	2	4	32	2	4	1	2
	5	1	2	4	32	4	8	1	2
	6	0.5	2	8	16	2	8	1	2
	7	0.25	2	1	8	2	4	1	2
	2	4	32	16	32	4	16	2	16
Klebsiella pneumoniae	1	0.5	1	2	8	2	4	1	2
	2	0.25	2	2	32	2	8	1	4
	3	0.5	4	2	16	2	16	1	4
	4	0.5	4	2	8	2	8	1	4
	5	0.5	2	2	32	2	16	1	4
	6	0.25	4	1	16	2	16	1	32
Enterobacter cloacae	1	1	>250	8	>250	4	>250	2	>250
	2	1	>250	16	>250	125	>250	32	>250
	3	2	>250	16	250	16	250	8	250
	4	2	>250	32	>250	>250	>250	63	>250
	5	8	250	16	250	63	>250	8	>250
Enterobacter aerogenes	1	1	>250	32	>250	63	>250	16	>250
Proteus mirabilis	1	0.5	2	8	16	4	16	4	8
	2	0.5	4	4	32	8	16	4	16
	3	0.5	2	16	32	8	32	8	32
	4	0.5	2	8	32	4	32	4	32
	5	0.5	4	8	32	4	16	4	16
Proteus vulgaris	1	1	4	1	4	4	16	4	250
	4	1	8	16	16	8	16	8	32
	2	1	8	8	125	8	250	8	32
Proteus rettgeri	1	0.13	125	0.25	250	4	250	0.5	>250
	2	0.13	63	0.25	>250	0.25	>250	0.25	>250
	3	0.25	>250	32	>250	16	>250	2	>250

[a] A, Inoculum of 10^2 organisms; B, inoculum of 10^6 organisms.

TABLE 4. *Effect of inoculum size on the susceptibility of S. aureus*

Organism type	No. of strains	MIC (μg/ml)[a]								MIC_B/MIC_A[b]			
		BL-S786		Cephalothin		Cephaloridine		Cefazolin		BL-S786	Cephalothin	Cephaloridine	Cefazolin
		A	B	A	B	A	B	A	B				
Lacking penicillinase	3	1.6	2.5	0.13	0.13	0.025	0.039	0.13	0.20	1.6	1.0	1.6	1.6
Penicillinase producer	26	3.8	5.7	0.20	0.44	0.077	1.6	0.22	0.79	1.5	2.2	20	3.6

[a] A, Inoculum of 10^2 organisms; B, inoculum of 10^6 organisms. The values are geometric means.
[b] MIC_A, Minimum inhibitory concentration with an inoculum of 10^2 organisms; MIC_B, minimum inhibitory concentration with an inoculum of 10^6 organisms.

tration. This is illustrated in Fig. 5 (left panel) for a dose of 20 mg/kg. At this dose, BL-S786 reached a peak concentration of 36 μg/ml, compared to 31 μg/ml for cefazolin, 23 μg/ml for cephaloridine, and 17 μg/ml for cephalothin. The concentration of BL-S786 in the blood declined at a slower rate ($t_{1/2}$ of 33 min) than that of the control cephalosporins ($t_{1/2}$ of 11 min for cephalothin, 22 min for cephaloridine, and 25 min for cefazolin). With all compounds, peak concentrations were essentially proportional to dose in the range tested (Fig. 5, right panel).

(ii) Recovery in rat urine. Rats, receiving intramuscularly 10 mg of BL-S786 per kg of body weight, excreted an average of 65% of the administered dose in urine. Comparable fractions of the dose were recovered when cephaloridine or cefazolin was given (59 and 75% of the dose, respectively). By contrast, only 22% of the cephalothin dose was accounted for in the urine. With all cephalosporins, over 96% of the recoverable dose was excreted within 6 h of administration.

(iii) Treatment of systemically infected mice. Against infections with *E. coli* and *K. pneumoniae* (Table 7), BL-S786, given intramuscularly, was either more active than the control cephalosporins (*E. coli* 1, *K. pneumoniae* 1) or at least as active as the most active of these compounds (*E. coli* 8 and 9, *K. pneumoniae* 7). In the treatment of infections with *P. mirabilis, P. vulgaris, P. morganii, P. rettgeri, Citrobacter* sp., and *P. stuartii,* BL-S786 was more active than the control cephalosporins. Against infections with *E. cloacae,* BL-S786 alone was effective.

In the treatment of streptococcal infections, BL-S786 was generally more active than cepha-

TABLE 5. *Minimum growth-inhibitory and bactericidal concentrations for Enterobacteriaceae*[a]

Organism	Strain	BL-S786		Cephalothin		Cephaloridine		Cefazolin	
		MIC	MBC	MIC	MBC	MIC	MBC	MIC	MBC
Escherichia coli	1	0.5	0.5	8	16	4	4	2	2
	3	0.25	0.5	4	8	2	2	2	2
	4	0.5	0.5	8	16	4	4	1	2
	5	1	1	16	16	4	4	2	2
	6	1	1	16	16	4	8	2	4
	2	16	16	32	32	16	16	8	16
Klebsiella pneumoniae	1	0.25	0.25	2	2	2	4	2	2
	2	0.25	0.25	4	8	4	4	1	2
	3	0.25	0.25	2	4	2	2	1	2
	4	0.5	0.5	4	4	4	4	2	4
	5	0.5	0.5	8	8	8	8	2	2
	6	0.5	1	2	2	2	2	2	4
Enterobacter cloacae	3	4	8	32	63	16	16	4	8
	4	8	63	250	>250	>250	>250	250	>250
	8	63	63	>250	>250	>250	>250	>250	>250
Enterobacter aerogenes	1	2	2	125	250	>250	>250	32	125
	2	2	2	125	>250	250	>250	63	>250
	3	8	16	250	>250	250	250	63	250
Proteus mirabilis	1	0.5	1	8	32	8	16	4	8
	2	0.5	0.5	8	32	8	8	8	16
	3	0.5	0.5	8	8	8	8	8	8
	4	0.25	0.5	4	8	8	8	4	8
	5	0.5	0.5	8	16	4	8	8	8
Proteus vulgaris	1	0.5	1	1	2	8	8	4	4
	4	0.5	1	8	16	8	16	8	16
	2	0.5	0.5	8	16	8	16	8	16
Proteus rettgeri	2	0.063	0.13	1	2	0.5	0.5	0.25	0.5
	3	0.25	63	125	250	32	>250	4	>250

[a] MIC, Minimum growth-inhibitory concentration; MBC, minimum bactericidal concentration; expressed as micrograms per milliliter. The inoculum was 10^4 cells.

TABLE 6. *Relative susceptibility to hydrolysis by β-lactamase in cell-free extracts*

Enzyme[a] Class	Enzyme[a] Type	Organism	Strain	Relative rate of hydrolysis (benzylpenicillin = 100): BL-S786	Cephalothin	Cephaloridine	Cefazolin
I	a	*Enterobacter cloacae*	214	700	2,100	7,900	10,000
	b	*Escherichia coli*	719	170	480	370	760
II	a	*Proteus mirabilis*	1266	<1	<1	2	<1
III	a	*Escherichia coli*	TEM	2	9	93	12
IV	a	*Klebsiella pneumoniae*	53	5	8	100	12
	b	*Klebsiella pneumoniae*	1169	27	43	50	31
		Staphylococcus aureus	A9606	<0.5	<0.5	<0.5	<0.5

[a] Enzyme classification according to Richmond and Sykes (3).

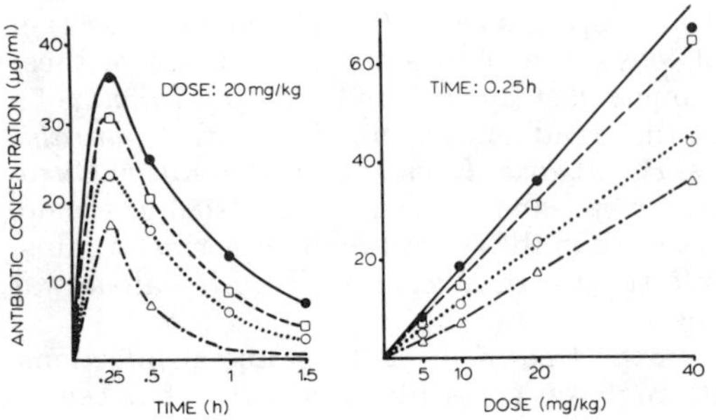

FIG. 5. *Antibiotic concentration in blood after intramuscular administration to mice. Symbols: ●, BL-S786; △, cephalothin; ○, cephaloridine; □, cefazolin.*

lothin but less active than cephaloridine and cefazolin (Table 8). Against staphylococcal infections, there was no well-defined efficacy pattern, but BL-S786 was at least as active as cephalothin.

DISCUSSION

BL-S786 compared favorably with cephalothin, cephaloridine, and cefazolin in activity and bioavailability. The compound had a broader spectrum of antibacterial activity than cephalosporins currently available for clinical use. Thus, it was active against the majority of strains of *Enterobacter* sp., *P. rettgeri*, *P.*

TABLE 7. *Efficacy of the intramuscular treatment of mice systemically infected with gram-negative organisms*[a]

Organism	Strain	Challenge (no. of organisms)	PD$_{50}$/treatment (mg/kg)[b] BL-S786	Cephalothin	Cephaloridine	Cefazolin
Escherichia coli	1	2×10^5	0.37	42	2.6	1.9
	8	6×10^5–4×10^6	1.5	97	2.2	4.9
	9	7×10^3–2×10^4	2.2	180	13	5.3
Klebsiella pneumoniae	1	4×10^4–5×10^4	2	94	8	16
	7	9×10^2–1×10^3	22	>380	41	94
Proteus mirabilis	1	7×10^6–9×10^6	1.4	41	19	16
	5	9×10^5–3×10^6	0.62	11	4	6.2
	8	6×10^5–4×10^6	0.59	14	5.5	6.5
Proteus vulgaris	1	1×10^6–2×10^6	1.8	11	6.4	11
	3	4×10^5	2.5	17	10	8
Proteus morganii	1	1×10^5–4×10^5	19	>350	180	62
	2	2×10^6–3×10^6	39	>400	230	140
Proteus rettgeri	4	2×10^6–3×10^6	2.4	140	66	9.5
Citrobacter sp.	1	5×10^6–2×10^7	3.5	>340	36	110
Providencia stuartii	2	1×10^6–5×10^6	5.9	>380	180	50
	3	2×10^7	8	160	150	70
Enterobacter cloacae	9	2×10^5–4×10^5	1.9	>400	200	170
	10	2×10^6–3×10^6	8.6	>400	>400	>400
	7	4×10^4–3×10^5	13	>400	>400	>370

[a] Animals were treated twice: 1 and 3.5 h after infection.
[b] PD$_{50}$, 50% protective dose.

TABLE 8. *Efficacy of intramuscular treatment of mice systemically infected with gram-positive organisms*[a]

Organism	Strain	Challenge (no. of organisms)	PD$_{50}$/treatment (mg/kg)[b] BL-S786	Cephalothin	Cephaloridine	Cefazolin
Streptococcus pneumoniae	1	2×10^3–9×10^3	0.52	4	0.1	0.39
	2	1×10^4–3×10^4	1.6	19	0.26	0.57
Streptococcus pyogenes	1	2×10^3–6×10^3	2.9	4.5	0.06	0.57
	2	1×10^4–5×10^4	0.93	2.7	0.02	0.27
Staphylococcus aureus	1	2×10^5–3×10^5	0.3	0.3	0.01	0.09
	2	1×10^9	5.4	9.3	3.2	5
	3	5×10^8–7×10^9	10	32	3.3	23

[a] Animals infected with penicillinase-producing staphylococcal strains (no. 2 and 3) were treated 0 and 2 h after infection; the others were treated 1 and 3.5 h after infection.
[b] PD$_{50}$, 50% protective dose.

stuartii, and *Citrobacter* sp., organisms typically resistant to the other cephalosporins. With few exceptions (*H. influenzae, N. gonorrhoeae*), BL-S786 was more active in vitro against major gram-negative pathogenic species than any of the three control cephalosporins. This advantage of BL-S786 was borne out in vivo. Although BL-S786 was generally less active than the reference compounds against gram-positive pathogens, it inhibited their growth at concentrations that should readily be achieved in humans after standard parenteral dosage. *S. faecalis,* a species relatively unsusceptible to cephalosporins in general, was an exception. BL-S786 was an effective bactericidal agent for strains of various gram-negative species, including *E. cloacae* and *E. aerogenes*. When given intramuscularly to mice, BL-S786 achieved high concentrations in blood and its biological half-life was longer than that of the other three cephalosporins. Two-thirds of the dose administered intramuscularly to rats was recovered in urine.

BL-S786 is to be subjected to clinical trials in the near future.

ACKNOWLEDGMENTS

We are indebted to the following for devoted technical assistance: M. Christine Arnold, Eileen W. Chaplinsky, Kenneth L. Den Bleyker, Kathlyn F. Frenette, Richard A. Goodhines, Thomas B. Hallett, Angela M. Hill, Thomas Ingram, Peter A Kresel, Antoinette C. Nutting, Christian E. Thater, Martha C. Thiesing, Jacqueline A. Randolph, Erwin B. Williams, and Ellen M. Yastrib. We also acknowledge the excellent clerical assistance of Evelyn Barenholtz and Maxine C. Postle.

LITERATURE CITED

1. **Leitner, F., R. E. Buck, M. Misiek, T. A. Pursiano, and K. E. Price.** 1975. BL-S640, a cephalosporin with a broad spectrum of antibacterial activity: properties in vitro. Antimicrob. Agents Chemother. **7**:298–305.
2. **Leitner, F., D. R. Chisholm, Y. H. Tsai, G. E. Wright, R. G. DeRegis, and K. E. Price.** 1975. BL-S640, a cephalosporin with a broad spectrum of antibacterial activity: bioavailability and therapeutic properties in rodents. Antimicrob. Agents Chemother. **7**:306–310.
3. **Richmond, M. H., and R. B. Sykes.** 1973. The β-lactamases of gram-negative bacteria and their possible physiological role. Adv. Microb. Physiol. **9**:31–88.
4. **Scholtan, W., and J. Schmid.** 1962. Die Bindung der Penicilline an die Eiweisskörper des Serums und des Gewebes. Arzneim. Forsch. **12**:741–750.
5. **Steers, E., E. L. Foltz, and B. S. Graves.** 1959. An inocula replicating apparatus for routine testing of bacterial susceptibility to antibiotics. Antibiot. Chemother. **9**:307–311.

ANTIMICROBIAL AGENTS AND CHEMOTHERAPY, Sept. 1976, p. 436-440 Vol. 10, No. 3
 Printed in U.S.A.

Reproducibility of Control Strains for Antibiotic Susceptibility Testing

MARIE B. COYLE,* MARY F. LAMPE, CONNIE L. AITKEN, POLLY FEIGL, AND JOHN C. SHERRIS

Departments of Microbiology and Immunology, Laboratory Medicine, and Biostatistics, School of Medicine, University of Washington, Seattle, Washington 98195*

Received for publication 18 May 1976

Inter- and intralaboratory reproducibility of susceptibility testing requires stable control strains. The Food and Drug Administration diffusion procedure recommends the Seattle strains of *Staphylococcus aureus* (ATCC 25923) and *Escherichia coli* (ATCC 25922) for this purpose. It was of interest to determine the present reproducibility of control cultures maintained in various laboratories over several years. Fifteen cultures each of *S. aureus* and *E. coli* were obtained from laboratories in different parts of the country. Their performance was compared with strains directly derived from ATCC. Diffusion susceptibility tests using a modified overlay technique were made with four replicates. Seven of the eight statistically significant differences in responses of the staphylococci were to penicillin, methicillin, or cephalothin. One culture was a penicillinase producer with a zone 15 mm less than the standard strain. Eleven of the 15 cultures showed no significant deviations or differences greater than 2 mm from the results with the strain derived directly from ATCC. All except the penicillinase producer were of identical phage type. Among 150 organism-antibiotic combinations tested with *E. coli*, all but one reading were within 2 mm of the standard. Four of the six statistically significant differences were in a culture from one laboratory. The stability of the cultures appears to have been influenced by the method of storage. Cultures that were kept frozen during extended storage were remarkably stable. Significant differences were found in cultures from four of five laboratories that maintained cultures in refrigerators or at ambient temperature.

Recommended quality control procedures for antimicrobial disk susceptibility tests require daily testing of *Escherichia coli* (ATCC 25922) and *Staphylococcus aureus* (ATCC 25923) (3, 4). These strains, originally isolated and used for quality control purposes in the University of Washington Hospital Clinical Laboratories, have now been maintained in many different laboratories for up to 7 years. This has raised the possibility that contamination or genetic drift may have occurred in some clones similar to that which was shown with the Oxford *Staphylococcus* by Oeding and Östervold (5). A study was therefore designed to determine whether any differences could be detected in control strains used routinely in clinical laboratories.

Laboratories in different parts of the country were requested to send working cultures of their control strains with information on their original source, the date obtained, and maintenance procedures used. These cultures were then compared with strains derived directly from the American Type Culture Collection using a closely standardized agar overlay diffusion procedure.

MATERIALS AND METHODS

Cultures. Cultures of *E. coli* and *S. aureus* submitted by 15 laboratories were tested. All were said to be derived from *E. coli* (ATCC 25922) and *S. aureus* (ATCC 25923) or from the "Seattle" control strains, which were the original source of the ATCC strains. The standard strains from the American Type Culture Collection with which all other cultures were compared had been subcultured only twice prior to the study.

Storage. The cultures from participating laboratories were streaked immediately upon receipt onto a blood agar plate and incubated overnight. One colony was inoculated into 3 ml of Trypticase soy broth supplemented with 1% yeast extract (TSY) and incubated until turbid. Blood agar plates were streaked from the broth and incubated overnight, and the growth was used to prepare a heavy suspension in a mixture of 50% TSY broth and 50% heat-inactivated fetal calf serum. A few drops of the suspension were added to 2-dram (ca. 3.55-g) vials containing glass beads and shaken to ensure that the beads were coated. Vials were stored at −70°C.

Susceptibility testing. Vials of the organisms to be tested were transferred from the −70°C freezer to a dry ice-ethanol bath, and single glass beads were removed and inoculated into 3 ml of TSY broth for overnight incubation. The resulting broth cultures were streaked onto blood agar plates and incubated overnight. Five colonies were inoculated into 3 ml of TSY and incubated for 2 to 4 h, and the optical density was adjusted with TSY broth to 0.14 ± 0.01 at 580 nm in a Bausch & Lomb Spectronic 20 spectrophotometer. A 0.1-ml amount of the standardized suspension was then added to each of two tubes containing 8 ml of aqueous 1.5% agar at 45°C, and duplicate 150-mm plates of Mueller-Hinton agar (Difco) containing 60 ml of medium were overlaid evenly with the agar suspension. Antibiotic disks were applied within 15 min and the plates were incubated overnight. Zone diameters were measured with calipers on the surface of the plates. All cultures of either *S. aureus* or *E. coli* were tested at the same time on two different occasions and read independently by two readers. Thus, there were four plates for each culture and a total of eight measurements.

Antibiotics. Disks (BBL) of the same lot number for each antibiotic were used throughout. Their content was that recommended by the Food and Drug Administration (FDA) (3) and the National Committee for Clinical Laboratory Standards (NCCLS) (4). The antibiotics tested were those indicated in Tables 2 and 4.

Phage typing of *S. aureus* strains. All cultures of *S. aureus* were typed with the following phages: 3A, 3C, 6, 29, 42D, 42E, 47, 52, 52A, 53, 54, 55, 71, 75, 77, 80, 81, 83A, 84, 85, 94, 187, and D11.

Biotyping of *E. coli* cultures. *E. coli* cultures were tested for the biochemical reactions listed in Table 31 of Edwards and Ewing (2) with the omission of KCN, gelatin, and cellobiose and the addition of nitrate, esculin, and trehalose. Reactions were read daily for 3 days.

Statistical analysis. An analysis of variance was performed on the *S. aureus* and *E. coli* data for each drug under study. The primary purpose was to estimate the variability associated with the mean response to each drug, where response was measured as the diameter of the zone of inhibition in millimeters. Components of variability associated with differences among laboratories, between readers, and between days were separated. Using the standard deviation estimated from the analysis of variance, Dunnett's t test for comparing multiple means to a control mean was performed to determine, separately for each drug, which laboratory means differed from the standard ATCC control strain (1).

RESULTS

***S. aureus* cultures.** All cultures were phage type 29/52/80/81+, except culture 3 which was untypable. The susceptibility test results are summarized in Table 1, which lists all mean zone diameters that differed from the ATCC standard by more than 1 mm and identifies all statistically significant differences. The culture from laboratory 3 was not *S. aureus* ATCC 25923, as evidenced by its penicillin resistance and phage type. With the exception of one erythromycin zone, differences of >1 mm were only found with the penicillins and cephalothin. Cultures from laboratories 5, 9, and 20 showed zone sizes that were significantly different from the standard strain. Six of the 15 cultures did not differ from the standard strain by more than 1 mm with any antibiotic tested.

The mean zones of the standard strain and the ranges of the mean zone sizes for all 16 cultures of *S. aureus,* including the standard strain, are shown in Table 2. The mean zone diameters are not comparable to control values recommended by FDA and NCCLS (3, 4) because a different technique was used which involved a heavier inoculum. Penicillin and cephalothin zones had the largest ranges. The right column lists the ranges for the 11 cultures that did not differ significantly (Table 1) from the standard. Reproducibility with these was excellent: only the mean penicillin zone sizes ranged more than 2 mm.

***E. coli* cultures.** Twelve of the *E. coli* cultures showed identical reactions with the 30 biochemical tests. Three cultures (11, 20, and 22) differed in one reaction, and culture 5 differed in three reactions. The results of the susceptibility tests are summarized in Table 3. Five cultures gave mean zone diameters differing from the standard strain by more than 1

TABLE 1. *Differences of >1 mm in mean zone diameters of S. aureus cultures from the standard ATCC 25923*

Laboratory of origin	Differences of >1 mm in mean zone diameter[a]			
	Penicillin	Oxacillin	Cephalothin	Erythromycin
2	−1.5			
3	−15.3[b]		−2.2	
4	−1.9		−1.2	
5	+4.4[b]		+3.9[c]	
8	−1.9		−1.1	
9	+3.6[b]	+2.5[c]	+1.5	+1.9[c]
11	−1.4			
18	+1.4		−1.1	
20	+7.1[b]	+1.9	+6.6[b]	

[a] No difference of >1 mm with tetracycline, chloramphenicol, clindamycin, kanamycin, streptomycin, or cultures from laboratories 1, 12, 15, 19, 21, and 22.

[b] Significance of mean difference from standard strain by Dunnett's test: $P < 0.01$.

[c] Significance of mean difference from standard strain by Dunnett's test: $P < 0.05$.

mm. Three of these, including culture 5, yielded results that were significantly different. Culture 11 showed four significant differences, and the others showed one each. Five other strains with statistically significant differences in ampicillin zones were not included in this table because the differences were 1 mm or less. This reflected a very narrow range of ampicillin readings as well as the fact that the ampicillin zones of the standard strain were larger than those of the other 15 cultures.

Table 4 lists the mean zones of the standard strain and the ranges of the mean zone sizes of all cultures. Results with cultures from laboratories 5 and 11 are excluded from the ranges listed in the right column. The other 13 cultures performed very closely to the standard.

Relationship of method of storage to performance. It appears that the method of storage influenced the stability of the cultures. Table 5 correlates methods and duration of extended storage with performance of the *S. aureus* cultures. None of the eight cultures that had been stored at −70°C showed any significant differences from the standard strain. One purporting to be of commercial origin was that which differed in phage type and penicillin susceptibility from the others. This was probably a case of contamination or error after receipt from the manufacturer, because FDA diffuson tests (3, 4) of four other *S. aureus* cultures from the same manufacturer indicated that they were satisfactory. Three of the five cultures stored in the refrigerator or at room temperature were found to show significant differences from the standard.

Table 6 presents the correlation of methods and duration of storage with the performance of the *E. coli* cultures. Significant differences greater than 1.2 mm from the standard strains were found with two of the four cultures of *E.*

TABLE 2. *Ranges (maximum − minimum) of mean zone diameters with 16 cultures of S. aureus ATCC 25923 from different sources*

Drug	Mean zone[a] of standard ATCC strain (mm)	Range of all 16 cultures (mm)	Range excluding laboratories 3, 5, 9, and 20
Penicillin	27.4	22.5	2.4
Oxacillin	18.9	2.8	1.3
Cephalothin	27.6	8.7	1.3
Tetracycline	22.6	1.5	0.7
Chloramphenicol	19.8	1.8	1.0
Clindamycin	21.6	1.8	1.2
Erythromycin	21.4	2.4	1.2
Kanamycin	19.3	1.0	1.0
Streptomycin	15.2	0.9	0.8

[a] The mean zone diameters are not comparable to control values recommended by FDA (3) and NCCLS (4) because a different technique was used involving a heavier inoculum.

TABLE 4. *Ranges (maximum − minimum) of mean zone diameters with 16 cultures of E. coli ATCC 25922 from different sources*

Drug	Mean zone[a] of standard ATCC strain (mm)	Range of all 16 cultures (mm)	Range excluding laboratories 5 and 11 (mm)
Ampicillin	16.5	1.2	1.8
Carbenicillin	20.2	3.3	1.5
Cephalothin	15.2	2.2	1.2
Tetracycline	21.5	2.2	0.8
Chloramphenicol	21.1	1.9	1.2
Gentamicin	16.6	1.7	1.0
Kanamycin	16.8	2.2	1.1
Streptomycin	13.1	1.7	0.5
Polymyxin	12.9	0.7	0.6
Nitrofurantoin	20.3	1.1	1.1

[a] The mean zone diameters are not comparable to control values recommended by FDA (3) and NCCLS (4) because a different technique was used involving a heavier inoculum.

TABLE 3. *Differences of >1 mm in mean zone diameters of E. coli cultures from the standard ATCC 25922*

Laboratory	Differences of >1 mm in mean zone diameter[a]								
	Ampicillin[b]	Carbenicillin	Cephalothin	Tetracycline	Chloramphenicol	Gentamicin	Kanamycin	Streptomycin	Nitrofurantoin
1							−1.1		−1.1
3	−1.2[c]								
4									−1.1
5		+1.8[d]	−2.0						
11		+2.6[c]		+1.3[c]	+1.3	−1.1	−1.6[c]	−1.1[d]	

[a] No difference of >1 mm with polymyxin B or cultures 2, 8, 9, 12, 15, 18, 19, 20, 21, and 22.

[b] The mean ampicillin zones from five additional cultures differed significantly from the standard, but since these differences were 1 mm or less they are regarded as clinically not of interest.

[c] $P < 0.01$.

[d] $P < 0.05$.

TABLE 5. *Correlation of method of storage with significant differences from standard S. aureus ATCC 25923*

Method of storage	Mean duration of storage (mo)	Total no. of laboratories	No. of cultures with statistically significant differences	Antibiotics
Frozen	33	8	0	
Commercial	7	2	1	Penicillin
Refrigerated	48	1	1	Penicillin, cephalothin
Room temp	31	2	1	Penicillin, cephalothin
Room temp under oil	31	2	1	Penicillin, oxacillin, erythromycin

TABLE 6. *Correlation of method of storage with significant differences of >1.2 mm[a] from standard E. coli ATCC 25922*

Method of storage	Mean duration of storage (mo)	Total no. of laboratories	No. of cultures with statistically significant differences	Antibiotics
Frozen	33	8	0	
Commercial	7	2	0	
Refrigerated	48	1	0	
Room temp	31	2	1	Carbenicillin
Room temp under oil	31	2	1	Carbenicillin, kanamycin, tetracycline

[a] The mean ampicillin zones from six cultures differed significantly from the standard, but since these differences were less than 1.2 mm they are regarded as clinically not of interest.

coli that had been stored at room temperature.

There was no evidence of a relationship between duration of storage and stability of the cultures.

FDA diffusion tests. The 15 *E. coli* cultures and the standard were tested against the antibiotics listed above by the FDA diffusion test procedures (3, 4). Four of 144 tests were outside FDA limits. On repeat tests all were within limits, except culture 5, which was again out of control with chloramphenicol. One result that was in control on the first test was 1 mm below the FDA limit for cephalothin on the repeat test. Results with carbenicillin, for which there are no FDA limits, were compared with the limits recommended by NCCLS. In the two series of tests, 9 of 32 carbenicillin zones were 1 to 2 mm below the recommended control values of 24 to 29 mm. The ATCC strain gave a mean value of 24.5 mm, and the overall mean of results from all strains was 24.2 mm. This suggests that the NCCLS limit may need revision.

The *S. aureus* cultures were also tested by the FDA diffusion test procedure. With the exception of culture 3, which was the penicillinase producer, all cultures were within the FDA recommended control limits. Since no limits have been established for oxacillin, we calculated the limits to be 19 to 23 mm, based on over 200 measurements from the routine quality control procedures in our laboratory. Only culture 9 was out of control, having an oxacillin zone of 24 mm. On a repeat test, this culture was in control.

DISCUSSION

Quality control of antibiotic susceptibility testing presumes the stability of standard organisms. When inhibitory zone diameters are outside the limits of FDA or NCCLS recommendations, the sources of error will first be sought in media production or in technique. The results from this study, which used a highly reproducible diffusion procedure, indicate that there are detectable differences in the performance of standard *E. coli* and *S. aureus* cultures from different laboratories. With the exception of the penicillin-resistant culture, however, none of the *S. aureus* cultures was found to yield a zone diameter outside the FDA ranges when tested by the routine standardized diffusion test. Most of the significant changes in susceptibilities of the *Staphylococcus* were with the penicillins and cephalothin. This was especially evident when the data were expressed as ranges of mean zone diameters. However, cultures from 11 of the 15 laboratories showed no significant deviations from the results with the strain derived directly from ATCC.

In the case of *E. coli* cultures, four of the six significant differences were with a culture from one laboratory. When this culture and culture 5, which had a different biotype, are excluded, the ranges of the zone diameters did not exceed 1.6 mm with any antibiotic tested. Only culture 5 was outside the FDA limits on both the initial and repeat tests using the standardized diffusion procedure. This culture had a light inner zone around the chloramphenicol disk that was not detected by the overlay procedure.

The method of storage appears to have influenced the stability of the strains. Disregarding the very small differences found with ampicillin and *E. coli*, none of the cultures that were kept frozen during extended storage showed significant differences from the standard strains. In contrast, 5 of the 10 cultures from laboratories that stored their strains in the refrigerator or at ambient temperature showed significantly different zone diameters from the ATCC strains. All of these cultures had been maintained for over 2 years.

These results show that 2 of the 30 cultures received were of different origin to the ATCC strains and unsuitable for control purposes. There was evidence of some genetic shift in cultures received from laboratories that stored them under conditions in which some growth as well as cell death could occur. Fortunately, this did not appear to have taken them outside the recommended FDA control limits, although the possibility of further shift exists. Excellent stability can be anticipated if basic stocks are maintained under nonmetabolizing conditions such as frozen or lyophilized. Replacement of working stock cultures from frozen portions on a weekly or monthly basis appears to be a satisfactory procedure.

LITERATURE CITED

1. **Dunnett, C. W.** 1964. New tables for multiple comparisons with a control. Biometrics **20**:482–491.
2. **Edwards, P. R., and W. H. Ewing.** 1972. Identification of *Enterobacteriaceae,* 3rd ed. Burgess Publishing Co., Minneapolis, Minn.
3. **Federal Register.** 1972. Rules and regulations. Antibiotic susceptibility discs. Fed. Regist. **37**:20525–20529.
4. **National Committee for Clinical Laboratory Standards.** 1975. Performance standards for antimicrobial disc susceptibility tests. National Committee for Clinical Laboratory Standards, Villanova, Pa.
5. **Oeding, P., and B. Østervold.** 1959. The stability of Oxford staphylococcus H and other penicillin reference strains. Acta Pathol. Microbiol. Scand. **46**:149–155.

Antimicrobial Agents and Chemotherapy, Sept. 1976, p. 441-446 Vol. 10, No. 3

Printed in U.S.A.

Active Metabolites of Isoxazolylpenicillins in Humans

H. H. W. THIJSSEN* and H. MATTIE

Departments of Clinical Pharmacology and Infectious Diseases and Department of Pharmacology, University Hospital, University of Leiden, Leiden, The Netherlands*

Received for publication 5 February 1976

Metabolites of the isoxazolylpenicillins that still possessed antibacterial activity were shown to be present in urine and serum. In healthy subjects, the amounts excreted in urine were low; 10 to 23% of the excreted penicillin activities represented the metabolites. The highest amount of metabolite in urine was found for oxacillin, and the lowest was found for flucloxacillin. No extreme differences in the amounts of metabolite excreted were observed when the compounds were administered orally or intravenously. In one healthy subject metabolite levels were estimated for cloxacillin in serum. Very low levels were found, i.e., about 9% of the activity. In subjects with highly impaired renal function, the metabolite may represent up to 50% of the total level of penicillin in serum. The antibacterial activities of the different metabolites were of the same order of magnitude as those of the respective parent compounds. Also, the activity against benzylpenicillin-resistant staphylococci was retained. It is not likely that the formation of the active metabolites should influence therapeutic results.

During their passage through animals and humans, penicillins, like other drugs and xenobiotics, are subject to biomodification. Cleavage of the β-lactam ring, resulting in the formation of the corresponding inactive penicilloic acids, seems to be the main route by which the penicillins are metabolized (4, 6, 7, 13). In addition, as the result of other metabolic pathways, metabolites of penicillins are formed that are still active as antimicrobials. For instance, the *para*-hydroxy derivative of phenoxymethylpenicillin is known (15), and of dicloxacillin the 5-hydroxymethyl derivative is the active metabolite (16). Also, active metabolites are formed out of oxacillin and cloxacillin (12). Nishida et al. described the formation of an active transformation product of ampicillin (10). The role of drug-metabolizing systems in its formation, however, is questionable, since this metabolite is also formed during incubation of ampicillin with urine and/or serum (10).

In view of the scanty qualitative and semiquantitative data on this topic, it seemed worthwhile to investigate the formation of active metabolites of penicillins in more detail because the formation of these metabolites might influence the correct estimation of relevant pharmacokinetic parameters as suggested by Nauta and Mattie (9) or, in case of differences in activity between parent compound and metabolite, because they might influence therapeutic results.

Data concerning the metabolic disposition of the isoxazolylpenicillins are described in the present paper. Aspects of the nature of the metabolites will be discussed elsewhere.

MATERIALS AND METHODS

Subjects and dosages. The isoxazolylpenicillins used are commercial preparations; oxacillin (Pentastapho) and dicloxacillin (Diclocil) were kindly provided by Bristol (The Netherlands), and cloxacillin (Orbenin) and flucloxacillin (Floxapen) were provided by Beecham Research Laboratories (The Netherlands). The compounds were administered to healthy volunteers, who were 21 to 39 years of age, either orally (2 g in capsules of either 250 or 500 mg, 0.5 h before breakfast) or by intravenous (i.v.) injection. Urine was pooled over a period of 7 to 8 h after oral administration and over a period of 5 h after i.v. administration. From one subject venous blood samples were drawn after i.v. administration of 2 g of cloxacillin. Venous blood samples from two patients undergoing chronic intermittent hemodialysis, who were under therapy with cloxacillin and flucloxacillin, respectively, were obtained from the hemodialysis department of the University Hospital, Leiden.

Assays. Total penicillin concentrations in urine and serum were measured by agar diffusion techniques, using *Sarcina lutea* (ATCC 9341) as the test organism. Reference curves were made by diluting the respective analytical grade penicillin either in saline (for urine assays) or in plasma (serum assays).

Separation and determination of metabolite and parent compound. Despite examples given in the literature (5, 8, 14), separation of closely related penicillins (i.e., isoxazolylpenicillins) could not be achieved by thin-layer adsorption chromatography. Separation of these substances has been accomplished by reversed-phase chromatography (1, 2, 11). Silanized silica gel F254 thin-layer chromatographic plates (Merck, Darmstadt) were used throughout the experiments.

Depending on the concentration of the penicillin in the urine, the latter was applied to the thin-layer chromatographic plate either directly or after extraction with an organic solvent. Extraction was performed with ether at pH 2. After evaporation of the ether extract, the residue was dissolved in the appropriate volume of phosphate buffer, pH 7. To determine the amount of metabolite in the serum, the following extraction procedure was employed: to 2.5 ml of serum, 0.1 ml of n-propanol was added and the mixture was heated at 60°C for 10 min. The mixture was acidified to pH 2 and extracted three times with 6-ml portions of n-hexane–i-butanol (vol/vol, 3:2). The combined organic layers were evaporated to dryness, and the residue was dissolved in the appropriate volume of ethylacetate.

From the respective samples 10 μl was spotted onto the plate. Four standards (10 μl of four dilutions of the analytical grade penicillin in 0.2 M NaCl) were chromatographed simultaneously on each plate. Prior to chromatography, the spots originating from aqueous samples were subjected to spot chromatography by applying 5 μl of acetone at their centers. Thus, tailing because of overloading of the plate was avoided. The chromatogram was developed at room temperature with a mixture of 0.3 M NaCl in 0.05 M potassium phosphate buffer (pH 5.6)-acetone (vol/vol, 2:1). After chromatography the substances were located by fluorescence quenching at 254 nm.

The parent compound, the metabolite, and the standards were recovered by scraping the spots from the plate and extracting with 0.4 to 0.5 ml of water saturated with methylethylketone. After centrifugation the amount of penicillin in the supernatant was estimated by means of the agar cup diffusion technique, using a susceptible microorganism (commonly *S. lutea* ATCC 9341) as the test organism. From the standards, reference curves were made. The recovery from the silica gel by this procedure was about 85 to 90% for dicloxacillin and flucloxacillin and about 90 to 95% for cloxacillin and oxacillin. The recovery as established from the simultaneously chromatographed references was not significantly different from 100%. The lowest amount of penicillin that could be determined accurately in this way was 0.3 μg for oxacillin, 0.6 μg for dicloxacillin, and 1 μg for cloxacillin and flucloxacillin.

The precision of the procedure was 10 ± 4%, as estimated from eight different samples; each sample was estimated four times.

The method implies that the metabolites are estimated in equivalents of parent compound activity. Therefore, it was preferable to express the amount of metabolite as the percentage of the estimated total amount of penicillin in the respective biological fluid.

The renal clearance was calculated from: urinary excretion rate $\left(\frac{dQ}{dt}\right)$ = renal clearance (Cl) × plasma concentration (Cp).

Antibacterial activity. Since the metabolites have not been isolated as the pure substances, a direct measurement of their actual antibacterial activity was not possible. Chromatography in combination with a spot test was used to approximate the concentration of a metabolite in a solution. Solutions of the metabolites were obtained by extracting the silica gel layer of a chromatogram obtained from 0.5 to 1 ml of urine. The urine sample was applied onto the thin layer in a stroke. Of these extracts dilutions were prepared in ratios of 2:3. Of the parent compound dilutions were also prepared in ratios of 2:3 starting from 20 μg/ml. Six successive dilutions of the parent compound and six successive dilutions of its metabolite were spotted onto a plate (20 by 20 cm) in 5-μl amounts. After development, the plate was placed in a tank saturated with ammonia vapor for 15 min, dried, and sprayed with a 0.5% starch solution and then with a solution of 1% sodium azide in 0.002 N iodine (2, 11). The compounds appeared as white spots on a blue background. The dilutions of the parent compound and metabolite that could not be visualized any more were supposed to be equal in concentration. As little as 20 ng of the penicillins could be detected. The amount of metabolite found in this way was compared with the amount of parent compound equivalents, as estimated by the agar cup diffusion technique.

Antibacterial spectrum. The relative susceptibilities of different strains of bacteria to the metabolites were established as follows. A solution of a metabolite was estimated for its parent compound equivalent by using the agar cup diffusion technique. Standard curves (log [micrograms per milliliter] versus zone diameter) were constructed for each of the isoxazolylpenicillins and each of the microorganisms. The amount of metabolite (micrograms per milliliter of parent compound activity) as estimated by *S. lutea* was put to unity.

RESULTS

Figure 1a shows an example of a reversed-phase chromatogram of oxacillin, cloxacillin, and dicloxacillin. Their R_f values are inversely correlated to their lipophilicity. In this chromatographic system flucloxacillin will run in between cloxacillin and dicloxacillin. Figure 1a also shows the chromatogram of an ether extract of a urine sample after the oral administration of 2 g of cloxacillin. The distribution of the antibacterial activity in this urine, expressed as the diameter of the zone of inhibition, is depicted in Fig. 1b, which clearly shows the existence of two additional antibacterial compounds. The active substance with the highest migration rate ($R_f \approx 0.64$) turned out to be a contamination (about 1 to 2% of the activity) of the cloxacillin preparations. Of the other isoxazolylpenicillins no such contaminations were detected. The compound migrating with $R_f \approx 0.50$, which was only found after passage through the body, is a metabolite of cloxacillin. After the administration of oxacillin, dicloxacillin, and flucloxacillin, chromatography of the respective urines resulted in similar chromatographic patterns.

An example of the estimation of the amount of metabolite in a urine specimen is given in Table 1 for dicloxacillin. When estimated with *S. lutea* as the test organism, the active metabolite of dicloxacillin represented 18.5% of the total antibacterial activity. When estimated with *Bacillus subtilis,* higher amounts of the metabolite were found (26.4%), indicating a higher susceptibility of this organism to the metabolite. The fact that, within the limits of error of the bioassay, the arithmetic summation of the estimated amounts of parent compound and metabolite fairly agrees with the estimated total activity indicates that no other antibacterial substances were present in substantial amounts.

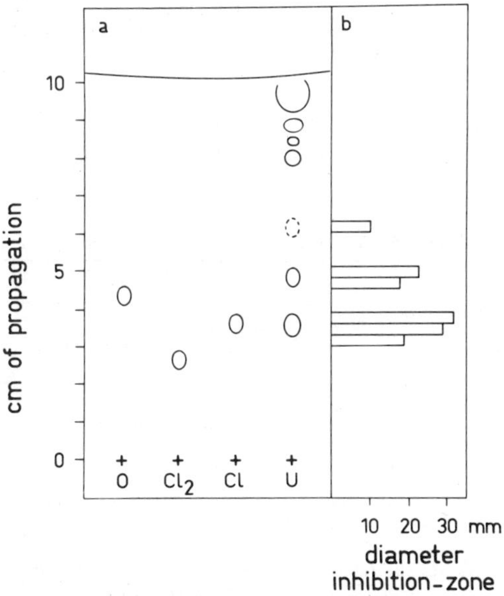

FIG. 1. *(a) Reversed-phase chromatogram of oxacillin (O), dicloxacillin (Cl_2), cloxacillin (Cl), and an ether extract of a urine specimen after oral administration of cloxacillin (U). (b) Distribution of antibacterial activity, expressed as the diameter of the zone of inhibition, over the chromatogram of U.*

Quantitative data concerning the amounts of metabolite excreted after oral administration are given in Table 2. The results indicate that, on an average, about 21% of the excreted oxacillin activity in urine, as measured by *S. lutea,* is due to an active metabolite. For cloxacillin and dicloxacillin this is about 14%, and for flucloxacillin it is about 10%. Roughly the same values for cloxacillin and dicloxacillin were obtained after i.v. administration: 13.5% for cloxacillin, 1 g i.v., subject HT; 12.5% for dicloxacillin, 1 g i.v., subject EN.

TABLE 2. *Active metabolites in 8-h urine after an oral dose of 2 g of the corresponding penicillin in capsules, as estimated by S. lutea*

Subject	Metabolite (% of total activity) of[a]:			
	O	Cl	Cl_2	FCl
RB		11		8
YL	18			
JM			12.5	8.5
WD	16	10	18.5	9.6
HT	23.4	15	12	13
DW	25.4	21	19	12.5
EN	21	14	13.5	10
Mean	20.7	14	15	10.2

[a] O, Oxacillin; Cl, cloxacillin; Cl_2, dicloxacillin; FCl, flucloxacillin.

TABLE 1. *Active metabolite in 8-h urine[a] after oral administration of 2 g of dicloxacillin in capsules (subject WD), estimated by S. lutea and B. subtilis, respectively (expressed as percentage of the total antibacterial activity)*

	Dicloxacillin equivalents (μg/ml) in urine[a] and/or extract[b] estimated by:							
	S. lutea				*B. subtilis*			
	Urine		Extract		Urine		Extract	
Dicloxacillin	1,050	1,200	1,100	1,100	1,100	1,100	1,000	1,075
Metabolite	220	250	275	270	410	350	365	415
Metabolite %	17.3	17.2	20	19.7	27.1	24.1	26.7	27.8
Mean	18.5				26.4			

[a] The total concentration in the urine as estimated by a bioassay using *S. lutea* was 1,430 μg/ml.

[b] An ether extract of the urine; after evaporation of the extract, the residue was dissolved in phosphate buffer up to the original volume.

The course of the concentrations of cloxacillin and its metabolite in serum and the renal excretion rates of cloxacillin and its metabolite after i.v. injection of 2 g of the penicillin are shown in Fig. 2. The metabolite represented only a small fraction of the total activity in the serum: 9% of the cloxacillin activity at 90 min after administration. In urine, on the other hand, the metabolite represented about 20% of the antibacterial activity at 90 min after injection. The renal clearance at 90 min, estimated from the respective serum and urine data, was about 110 ml/min for cloxacillin and 270 ml/min for the metabolite.

Enhanced levels of metabolite in serum were observed in subjects with highly impaired renal function. Table 3 summarizes the data on the metabolite content in the serum of two patients on chronic intermittent hemodialysis, who were being treated with cloxacillin and flucloxacillin, respectively. As can be seen, in both cases the amount of active metabolite steadily increased and may represent 40 to 50% of the penicillin activity.

In Table 4 the amount of metabolite in a solution as estimated by bioassay (parent compound equivalents) is compared with the amount as estimated by iodine titration (micrograms per milliliter). As can be seen, the outcomes of the different methods do not differ

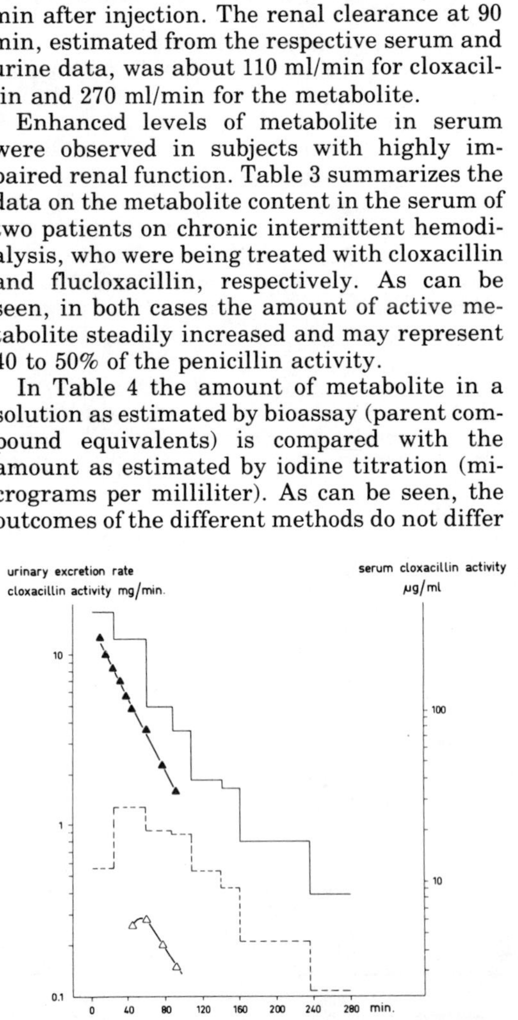

FIG. 2. *Urinary excretion rate and the concentration of cloxacillin and its metabolite in the serum versus time after an i.v. injection of 2 g of cloxacillin. Symbols:* ▲, *concentrations of cloxacillin in serum (micrograms per milliliter);* △, *concentrations of the metabolite in serum (micrograms per milliliter of cloxacillin activity);* —, *urinary excretion rate of cloxacillin (milligrams per minute);* - - -, *urinary excretion rate of the metabolite (milligrams per minute of cloxacillin activity).*

for the metabolites of cloxacillin and flucloxacillin, indicating that for *S. lutea* the antibacterial activities of these metabolites approximate the activities of the respective parent compounds. The metabolites of oxacillin and dicloxacillin, on the other hand, appeared to be less potent. Table 5 shows the susceptibilities, relative to *S. lutea,* of different bacterial

TABLE 3. *Metabolite content in the serum of subjects on chronic intermittent hemodialysis, after oral administration of 1 g of cloxacillin and/or flucloxacillin*

Penicillin	Metabolite (% of total activity) at time (h) after administration:			
	1	2	3	5
Cloxacillin (subject RH)	15	22		44
Flucloxacillin (subject JW)	16		41	

TABLE 4. *Amount of metabolite in a sample*

Metabolite of:	Amt of metabolite as:	
	Parent compound equivalents (µg/ml)[a]	Concn (µg/ml)
Oxacillin	8.3 ± 0.6 (n = 7)	14.5 ± 4.3 (n = 6)
Cloxacillin	22.1 ± 2.9 (n = 6)	20.6 ± 3.6 (n = 4)
Dicloxacillin	9.1 ± 1.0 (n = 5)	18.8 ± 4.0 (n = 5)
Flucloxacillin	15.5 ± 2.2 (n = 6)	13.8 ± 2.5 (n = 4)

[a] Parent compound equivalents were estimated, using *S. lutea* as the test organism.

TABLE 5. *Relative susceptibilities of different bacterial strains to the metabolites of isoxazolylpenicillins*

Organism	MIC[a] (µg/ml) for benzylpenicillin	Metabolite of[b]:			
		O	Cl	Cl_2	FCl
S. lutea		1	1	1	1
B. subtilis		1.7	1.1	2.3	1.2
S. aureus A55		1.1	0.5	1.5	0.6
S. aureus 6538		1.2	0.6	1.2	0.8
S. aureus NCTC 6571		0.5	0.6	1	0.5
Clinical isolates:					
Staphylococcus 39883	<0.075	0.8	0.6	1.6	1
Staphylococcus 39885	<0.075	0.9	0.8	0.8	0.8
Staphylococcus 39835	>10	0.6	0.8	1.3	1
Staphylococcus 39977	>10	1	0.7	1.4	1
Staphylococcus 40153	>10	0.75	0.8	1.6	0.8

[a] MIC, Minimal inhibitory concentration.
[b] Abbreviations are those given in footnote *a* of Table 2.

strains to the metabolites. The results indicate that, in comparison with the parent compound, the metabolite may differ two- to threefold in activity for the different strains. For instance, the relative susceptibilities to the oxacillin metabolite are between 0.5 (*Staphylococcus aureus* NCTC 6571) and 1.7 (*B. subtilis*). Of the different strains tested, *B. subtilis* proved to be the most susceptible to the metabolites. The benzylpenicillin-resistant strains of the *Staphylococcus* species (minimal inhibitory concentration > 10 μg/ml) appeared not to differ from the penicillin-susceptible strains (minimal inhibitory concentration < 0.075 μg/ml) in their susceptibility to the metabolites (Table 5).

If the antibacterial activities of the different metabolites against *S. lutea* (Table 4) are taken into account, it can be deduced from the relative susceptibilities that for most of the bacterial strains tested the activities of the cloxacillin and flucloxacillin metabolites approximate those of the parent compounds. The metabolites of oxacillin and dicloxacillin, in general, are somewhat less potent.

DISCUSSION

Analysis of body fluids (serum and urine) after oral or i.v. administration of the isoxazolylpenicillins revealed the presence of biologically active metabolites of these compounds. The existence of biologically active metabolites of oxacillin, cloxacillin, and dicloxacillin has been described in previous literature (12, 16), but no metabolite of flucloxacillin has been reported. The existence of an active metabolite of cloxacillin has been questioned in a recent study by Hellström et al. (6). However, the use of adsorption chromatography may explain why this metabolite of cloxacillin was not observed (6). In the reversed-phase system, the metabolites run ahead of the respective parent compounds, indicating that the metabolites are more hydrophilic (Fig. 1).

An approximation of the antibacterial activity of the metabolites could be assessed by titration on a chromatogram (Table 4). However, since the estimation of the metabolites was performed by bioassay, using the parent compound as the reference, the amount of metabolite in a biological fluid was expressed in terms of parent compound equivalents, i.e., as a fraction of the total antibacterial activity. Accordingly, the results are dependent on the microorganism used in the bioassay (Table 1).

After oral administration, oxacillin resulted in the highest amount of metabolite excreted in urine (21% of the total activity), and flucloxacillin resulted in the lowest (10%). Cloxacillin and dicloxacillin are in between (Table 2). However, correcting these figures for the observed antibacterial activity against *S. lutea* (Table 4), the actual amounts of the oxacillin and dicloxacillin metabolites excreted were about 31 and 26%, respectively. From these data no definite conclusions can be made about the extent of biomodification into active metabolites, since nothing is known about the pharmacokinetic features (e.g., inactivation) of these compounds. Cole et al. have shown that the extent of penicilloic acid formation, which apparently occurs in the liver, seems to be related to the water solubility of the penicillins (4). This would mean that the metabolites are more susceptible to biodegradation than are the parent compounds and that the metabolite of oxacillin will be most subject to degradation.

Levels of the metabolite of cloxacillin in the serum in a healthy subject appeared to be low: about 9% of the cloxacillin activity. The enhanced clearance of the metabolite (270 versus 110 ml/min) may be due to its greater water solubility and, related to the latter, its poorer protein binding, through which the glomerular filtration as well as the tubular secretion will be enhanced (3). Although data concerning the amounts of metabolites excreted in urine after i.v. administration were collected for only two penicillins (cloxacillin and dicloxacillin), the results suggest that there were no exceptional differences in the amounts metabolized. Thus, the isoxazolylpenicillins appear not to be liable to a so-called first-pass effect, a phenomenon that was suggested as a possible explanation for the observed discrepancies between resorption estimated from urine and serum data (9). Indeed, other phenomena, such as dose-dependent kinetics, may be the explanation for that observation (E. H. Nauta, Ph.D. thesis, Univ. of Leiden, Leiden, The Netherlands, 1975).

In impaired renal function, there is an accumulation of the active metabolite; hence, a much larger fraction of the isoxazolylpenicillin activity in the serum has to be ascribed to the metabolite (Table 3).

On the whole, the antibacterial activities of the metabolites do not differ extremely from those of the parent compounds. This especially holds true for the metabolites of cloxacillin and flucloxacillin (Tables 4 and 5). The metabolites of oxacillin and dicloxacillin, in general, are somewhat less potent. Dependent upon the microorganism, shifts to higher or lower potencies can be seen. All metabolites retained activity against benzylpenicillin-resistant staphylococci (Table 5).

In conclusion, since the formation of active metabolites of the isoxazolylpenicillins, regardless of the method of administration, is small and their antibacterial activities are of the same order of magnitude as the parent compounds, it is not to be expected that their formation will have any influence, either negative or positive, on the outcome of therapy. It is also unlikely that the presence of these metabolites should lead to grossly incorrect estimations of concentrations in the serum and/or urine. In subjects with impaired kidney function, however, more elevated concentrations of the metabolites in the serum are obtained. Theoretically this might influence therapy, for instance, when the distribution of the metabolite is different and/or when the activity of the metabolite against the particular pathogenic organism is much different.

ACKNOWLEDGMENTS

We wish to thank the volunteers and patients for their cooperation, W. Dusoswa for his skillful assistance, E. Noach, Pharmacology Department, and R. V. Furth, Department of Infectious Diseases, for their interest, and Gist Brocades (The Netherlands) who made available technical assistance and laboratory equipment.

LITERATURE CITED

1. **Biagi, G. L., A. M. Barbaro, M. F. Gamba, and M. C. Guerra.** 1969. Partition data of penicillins determined by means of reversed-phase thin-layer chromatography. J. Chromatogr. **41**:371–379.
2. **Bird, A. E., and A. C. Marshall.** 1971. Reversed-phase thin-layer chromatography and partition coefficients of penicillins. J. Chromatogr. **63**:313–319.
3. **Bowman, R. H.** 1975. Renal secretion of ^{35}S-furosemide and its depression by albumin binding. Am. J. Physiol. **229**:93–98.
4. **Cole, M., M. D. Kenig, and V. A. Hewitt.** 1973. Metabolism of penicillins to penicilloic acid and 6-aminopenicillanic acid in man and its significance in assessing penicillin absorption. Antimicrob. Agents Chemother. **3**:463–468.
5. **Hellberg, H.** 1968. Separation of penicillins by paper and thin-layer chromatography. J. Assoc. Off. Anal. Chem. **51**:552–557.
6. **Hellström, K., A. Rósen, and Å. Swahn.** 1974. Fate of oral ^{35}S-cloxacillin in man. Eur. J. Clin. Pharmacol. **7**:125–131.
7. **Hellstöm, K., A. Rośen, and Å. Swahn.** 1974. Absorption and decomposition of potassium-^{35}S-phenoxymethylpenicillin. Clin. Pharmacol. Ther. **16**:826–833.
8. **McGilveray, I. J., and R. D. Strickland.** 1967. Detection and separation of penicillins by thin-layer chromatography. J. Pharm. Sci. **56**:77–79.
9. **Nauta, E. H., and H. Mattie.** 1975. Pharmacokinetics of flucloxacillin and cloxacillin in healthy subjects and patients on chronic intermittent haemodialysis. Br. J. Clin. Pharmacol. **2**:111–121.
10. **Nishida, M., T. Murakawa, Y. Mine, S. Fukada, Y. Kono, and Y. Sueda.** 1971. Studies on the formation and the activity of the transformation product of ampicillin. J. Antibiot. **24**:641–646.
11. **Overvliet, G. M., H. M. Vos, and H. M. Smits.** 1974. Dunnelaagchromatografie van een aantal penicillinen en cephalosporinen op gesilaneerde silicagel. Pharm. Weekbl. **109**:537–542.
12. **Rolinson, G. N., and R. F. Batchelor.** 1963. Penicillin metabolites, p. 654–660. Antimicrob. Agents Chemother. 1962.
13. **Swahn, Å.** 1974. On the absorption and metabolism of some penicillins in man. Litopress, Stockholm.
14. **Vandamme, E. J., and J. P. Voets.** 1972. Separation and detection of degradation products of penicillins and cephalosporins by means of thin-layer chromatography. J. Chromatogr. **71**:141–148.
15. **Vanderhaeghe, H., G. Parmentier, and E. Evrard.** 1963. Identification of *p*-hydroxyphenoxymethylpenicillin as a metabolite of phenoxymethylpenicillin. Nature (London) **200**:891.
16. **van Harken, D. R., C. W. Dixon, and J. M. Essery.** 1970. An active metabolite of dicloxacillin. Pharmacologist **12**:220.

ANTIMICROBIAL AGENTS AND CHEMOTHERAPY, Sept. 1976, p. 447-449 Vol. 10, No. 3

Printed in U.S.A.

Reversible Thrombocytosis and Anemia Due to Miconazole Therapy

LEROY C. MARMION, KENNETH B. DESSER,* RALPH B. LILLY, AND DAVID A. STEVENS

The Department of Neurology and The Institute for Cardiovascular Diseases, Good Samaritan Hospital, Phoenix, Arizona 85062, and Division of Infectious Diseases, Department of Medicine, Santa Clara Valley Medical Center, San Jose, California 95128*

Received for publication 23 March 1976

Miconazole was administered intravenously in six consecutive patients with active coccidioidal infection. Such treatment was associated with progressive anemia and thrombocytosis. The hematological abnormalities appeared to be dose related and potentially reversible. Bone marrow studies demonstrated erythroid hypoplasia and increased or active platelet production in three subjects. No hemorrhagic or thrombotic episodes were identified. It is suggested that careful hematological monitoring be performed in subjects undergoing systemic miconazole therapy.

Miconazole has been administered systemically for the treatment of various fungal diseases in a limited number of patients. Available experimental and clinical data indicate that this agent has substantial antifungal activity and no major toxic effects (2, 3, 5, 11; D. A. Stevens, H. B. Levine, and S. C. Deresinski, Am. Rev. Respir. Dis. **111**:950, 1975).

We report here miconazole-induced anemia and thrombocytosis in six consecutive patients.

MATERIALS AND METHODS

Six consecutive patients with active coccidioidomycosis comprised the study group. There were six males and one female whose ages ranged from 15 to 72, with a mean of 45 years. Each subject had previously received systemic amphotericin B therapy with resultant toxicity or treatment failure, and the latter medication was discontinued before miconazole administration. Informed consent was obtained in each case as part of a protocol for the study of this drug. Miconazole was given in either a 5% dextrose or 5% dextrose and 0.9 NaCl solution via a central venous catheter. Three separate lots of the drug were utilized. A 500-ml solution was administered over a 60-min period every 8 h, with stepwise increments in the dosage of miconazole to a maximum of 1 g/infusion. The colloidal dispersion of miconazole in water was buffered and stabilized with the detergent Cremophor EL (polyethoxylated castor oil: a mixture of ricinoleic acid, polyglycol ester, glycerol polyglycol ethers, and polyglycols). Complete blood counts and platelet counts were determined before the induction of therapy and every other day during the course of miconazole administration.

RESULTS

Table 1 summarizes the diagnoses, drug dosages, and pertinent hematological data for the study group. Control values for hemoglobin level and platelet count, along with the maximal changes observed during and after stopping miconazole therapy, are presented. All subjects developed significant normocytic, normochromic anemia and progressive thrombocytosis with increasing doses of miconazole. Total amounts of the drug (in grams) given before the initial observed changes ranged from 1.8 to 12.6. The greatest degree of anemia developed at the time of maximal thrombocytosis after a period ranging from 5 to 23 days of miconazole administration in the six patients. Peripheral blood smears showed increased platelets of normal size. Bone marrow studies demonstrated adequate iron stores, erythroid hypoplasia, and increased or active platelet production in the three cases in which such aspiration was performed. Bleeding times, clotting times, and clot retraction were normal in all, except for an unexplained Lee-White clotting time of 20 min in patient no. 1, on repeated determinations. Moderate to marked rouleaux formation was observed in patient no. 2 during miconazole therapy. Stool guaiac study, reticulocyte count, plasma-free hemoglobin, direct and indirect Coombs tests, serum lactic dehydrogenase, urinalysis, serum bilirubin, and fibrin split products were obtained in each subject and did not indicate underlying blood loss or hemolysis. Prothrombin and partial thromboplastin times were likewise normal. No thrombotic or hemorrhagic complications were noted.

Development of an allergic rash in patient no. 1 prompted transient discontinuation of intravenous miconazole and afforded an opportunity to evaluate reproducibility of the observed

TABLE 1. *Summary of clinical diagnoses, drug dosages and hematological changes*

Patient	Age	Diagnosis	Total miconazole dose (g)	Hemoglobin (g/dl)			Platelet count/mm³		
				Control	During therapy	After therapy	Control	During therapy	After therapy
1	42	Coccidioidal meningitis	63.6	14.3	9.5	10.5	260,000	800,000	380,000
2	72	Pulmonary coccidioidomycosis	21.4	12.3	9.6	9.4	195,000	515,000	300,000
3	53	Coccidioidal meningitis	54.6	10.9	8.2	10.0	180,000	720,000	188,000
4	15	Coccidioidal meningitis	74.0	10.3	7.8	9.4	300,000	776,000	400,000
5	53	Coccidioidal meningitis	48.0	14.9	8.4	10.9	250,000	710,000	500,000
6	37	Coccidioidal meningitis	30.0	9.3	7.8	9.9	610,000	990,000	600,000

hematological changes. On day 10 of therapy, allopurinol was administered to this patient because of a serum uric acid of 10.8 mg/dl. Two days later, a generalized polymorphic pruritic rash appeared and all medications were withdrawn. The patient's hemoglobin had fallen from 14.3 to 10 g/dl, and the platelet count had increased from 260,000 to 460,000/mm^3. Forty-eight hours after drug withdrawal the dermatitis abated, and at that time the hemoglobin was 11.5 g/dl and the platelet count was 310,000/mm^3. Reinstitution of miconazole resulted in a progressive anemia (9.5 g/dl) and a rise in platelet count (800,000/min^3).

DISCUSSION

Studies in the six patients presented here demonstrated an impressive thrombocytosis in response to systemic miconazole administration. The development of a normochromic, normocytic anemia has been noted (11; Stevens et al., Am. Rev. Respir. Dis. 111:950, 1975), during the course of imidazole therapy for systemic mycoses, but to our knowledge an increased platelet count has not been previously reported. Neither the anemia nor thrombocytosis could be ascribed to amphotericin B (1), which had been discontinued before the institution of intravenous miconazole.

The bone marrow and peripheral blood studies described here are consistent with a direct or indirect stimulatory effect of miconazole on platelet production by megakaryocytes. There was no evidence of blood loss, hemolysis, hyposplenism, bone fracture, or malignant neoplasm, which might have resulted in reactive thrombocytosis. The temporal association of thrombocytosis with miconazole administration was amply demonstrated in case 1, where transient withdrawal of the drug effected a decline in the platelet count. Reinstitution of the drug in this patient was associated with substantial thrombocytosis. The potential reversibility of some of the observed changes was amply demonstrated in all cases, where termination of miconazole therapy was associated with a return of the thrombocyte count to normal and a rise of hemoglobin level in five of six subjects.

This reaction to miconazole administration may be similar to that described after the administration of vinca alkaloids in experimental animals or in humans (4, 6–8, 10). It is possible that the impressive increase of peripheral platelets was related to mobilization of splenic thrombocytes, but such a mechanism remains speculative. Alternatively, it is possible that miconazole prolonged the platelet life span.

The thrombocytosis observed in these patients may have been related to the particular drug lot or liquid vehicle (9) provided for miconazole therapy. Various buffers and carrier agents have been utilized in an attempt to diminish the phlebitis attendant to intravenous administration of the drug. The fact that three separate lots of miconazole were utilized in the six consecutive patients described here who developed increased platelet counts militates against a specific drug lot as an evoking agent in the production of thrombocytosis. It is possible that the carrier agent Cremophor EL was responsible for the thrombocytosis, but there are no data available on the influence of this detergent on erythrocyte or platelet production. Systematic hematological monitoring during oral miconazole therapy represents a possible approach for discerning whether or not the combination of miconazole and Cremophor EL or miconazole alone produced thrombocytosis. Unfortunately, oral miconazole therapy is usually started during intravenous administration of the drug-carrier combination or shortly thereafter. Prospective and serial study of blood counts and platelet levels are warranted in those subjects receiving isolated oral miconazole therapy.

The clinical significance of miconazole-induced thrombocytosis is not apparent. Clot retraction and bleeding times were normal, and no patient manifested clinical evidence of a thrombotic or hemorrhagic state. More sophisticated studies, including platelet factor 3 assay, isotopic platelet survival determination, and other tests of platelet adhesiveness, agglutination, and aggregation, will be necessary to ascertain whether or not thrombocyte function is normal in this setting. If such study indicates no adverse influence of miconazole or Cremophor EL on platelet function, then investigation of the influence of these agents on experimental thrombocytopenic states is warranted.

In conclusion, hematological monitoring should be undertaken in patients undergoing systemic miconazole therapy.

ACKNOWLEDGMENTS

We wish to acknowledge the technical assistance of Jeanette R. Goff.

The miconazole was supplied by Janssen R. and D., Inc., New Brunswick, N.J.

This work was supported by the E. Nichols and Kim Sigsworth Memorial Funds and The Institute for Cardiovascular Diseases, Inc.

LITERATURE CITED

1. **Brandriss, M. W., S. M. Wolff, R. Moores, and F. Stohlman, Jr.** 1964. Anemia induced by amphotericin B. J. Am. Med. Assoc. **189**:663–666.
2. **Daneels, R., R. Demeyere, L. Eggers, P. Lust, H. van Landuyt, and J. Symoens.** 1974. Zur Behandlung systemischer Candidiasis mit Micronazol. Med. Welt **25**:428–429.
3. **Hoeprich, P. D., and E. Goldstein.** 1974. Miconazole therapy for coccidioidomycosis. J. Am. Med. Assoc. **230**:1153–1157.
4. **Klener, P., L. Donner, V. Hyncica, and D. Safrankova.** 1974. Possible mechanism of vinblastine-induced thrombocytosis. Scand. J. Haematol. **12**:179–184.
5. **Levine, H. B., D. A. Stevens, J. M. Cobb, and A. E. Gebhardt.** 1975. Miconazole in coccidioidomycosis. I. Assays of activity in mice and in vitro. J. Infect. Dis. **132**:407–414.
6. **Robertson, J. H., E. H. Crozier, and B. E. Woodend.** 1970. The effect of vincristine on the platelet count in rats. Br. J. Haematol. **19**:331–337.
7. **Robertson, J. H., E. H. Crozier, and B. E. Woodend.** 1972. Vincristine-induced thrombocytosis studied with ^{75}Se selenomethionine. Acta Haematol. **47**:356–360.
8. **Robertson, J. H., and G. M. McCarthy.** 1969. Periwinkle alkaloids and the platelet-count. Lancet **2**:353–355.
9. **Savage, T. M., E. I. Foely, and B. R. Simpson.** 1973. Some cardiorespiratory effects of Cremophor EL in man. Br. J. Anaesth. **45**:515–516.
10. **Soppitt, G. D., and J. R. A. Mitchell.** 1969. Periwinkle alkaloids and platelets. Lancet **2**:539. (Letter)
11. **Stevens, D. A., H. B. Levine, and S. C. Deresinski.** 1976. Miconazole in coccidioidomycosis. II. Therapeutic and pharmacologic studies in man. Am. J. Med. **60**:191–202.

ANTIMICROBIAL AGENTS AND CHEMOTHERAPY, Sept. 1976, p. 450-456 Vol. 10, No. 3
 Printed in U.S.A.

Comparative Pharmacology of Josamycin and Erythromycin Stearate

LARRY J. STRAUSBAUGH, W. KLINE BOLTON, JOHN A. DILWORTH, RICHARD L. GUERRANT, AND MERLE A. SANDE*

Department of Internal Medicine, University of Virginia School of Medicine, Charlottesville, Virginia 22901

Received for publication 1 April 1976

Two macrolide antibiotics, josamycin and erythromycin stearate, were administered orally to healthy, adult male volunteers for a comparative study of their pharmacological properties. In comparable doses, josamycin and erythromycin produced similar plasma concentrations, with similar half-lives and elimination constants. An initial loading dose of 1.5 g of josamycin produced greater peak concentrations of antibiotic throughout a 10-day period with a regimen of every 6 h. In addition, josamycin tended to reach higher peak and trough concentrations after regimens of every 6 or 8 h were maintained for 2 days. Josamycin penetrated into saliva, sweat, and tears, and it was better tolerated in fasting subjects than was erythromycin stearate.

Josamycin is a macrolide antibiotic produced by *Streptomyces narbonensis* subsp. *josamyceticus*. Its spectrum of bacteriostatic activity is similar to that of erythromycin. Concentrations of 0.5 μg/ml inhibit most strains of *Mycoplasma pneumoniae, Streptococcus pneumoniae*, and *S. pyogenes* in vitro (6, 7). *Corynebacterium diphtheriae, Neisseria meningitidis, N. gonorrheae*, and *Bordetella pertussis* appear to be equally susceptible (6). A number of anaerobic bacteria, including *Bacteroides fragilis*, are susceptible to concentrations of 2 μg/ml (6, 7). Most strains of *Staphylococcus aureus* are also susceptible to concentrations of 2 μg/ml (6, 7). Josamycin inhibits most erythromycin-resistant staphylococci and, unlike erythromycin, it does not induce macrolide resistance in these strains (6).

Clinical trials with josamycin were initiated by Japanese investigators in 1967. The results of therapy in 785 patients with various infections have been reported (6). Josamycin was considered to be effective therapy in 82% of these patients, and on clinical grounds it was judged to have the same efficacy as erythromycin. Josamycin therapy was not associated with hematological, renal, hepatic, or other definable toxicity. Side effects were infrequent. Mild gastrointestinal disturbances such as anorexia and epigastric distress or nausea were noted by 4% of the treated patients, but discontinuation of josamycin was seldom required.

In spite of these favorable reports from Japan, the position of josamycin among the macrolide antibiotics has not been established, nor have the advantages that josamycin may offer over erythromycin been identified. The present study was designed to: (i) compare the pharmacokinetics, toxicity, and tolerance of orally administered josamycin and erythromycin stearate in 21 healthy, young male adults during a 4-day multidose cross-over trial; (ii) examine serum concentrations, toxicity, and tolerance in four subjects during a 10-day course of josamycin preceded by a loading dose, and (iii) determine the penetration of josamycin into urine, saliva, sweat, and tears.

MATERIALS AND METHODS

Antibiotics. Josamycin and erythromycin stearate were supplied by Endo Laboratories Inc., Garden City, N.Y.

Human volunteers. Twenty-one healthy men aged 23 to 35 years volunteered to participate in this study. Informed written consent was obtained. Their weights ranged from 71.8 to 89.1 kg. All subjects had normal creatinine clearances. None of the volunteers were taking any other antimicrobial agents during the investigational period.

Procedure. In the first part of this study, 21 subjects were randomly divided into groups of seven. Each group was then assigned to a different sequence of three antibiotic regimens to be taken during three dosing periods. Each period was 4 days in length, and there were 10 days between each period. During each of the three periods, one group was receiving 500 mg of josamycin orally every 8 h, one group was receiving 500 mg of josamycin orally every 6 h, and one group was receiving 500 mg of erythromycin orally every 6 h or 250 mg orally every 6 h. Because adverse gastrointestinal side effects during the first dosing period prompted two of seven subjects receiving 500 mg of erythromycin orally every 6 h to discontinue therapy, the dosage was decreased for the other two groups during the subsequent periods. One subject failed to conform to the dosage time schedule while on 500 mg of josamycin every 6 h and, therefore, his plasma concentrations were not included in the final analysis. Compliance was otherwise good. One subject inadvertently omitted one dose of josamycin during both the 6-h and 8-h schedules, and two subjects missed the final 1.5 days of the 250-mg erythromycin trial.

All subjects fasted for 12 h before each dosing period. A control venous blood sample was drawn prior to the first dose; no antibiotic activity was detectable in the 0-h bloods of any subject during the three dosing periods. After the first dose, all subjects fasted for 2 h before and after each subsequent dose. Venous blood samples for assay of plasma antibiotic concentration were obtained at 0.5, 1, 2, 3, 4.5, 6, 8, 12, 24, 48, 48.5, 49, 50, 51, 52.5, 54, 55, 56, 57, 58.5, 60, 72, 84, and 96 h. Plasma samples were frozen to −70°C. Antibiotic assays were performed (within 2 weeks). This method of storage did not affect the drug concentrations in the samples.

The following tests for possible adverse effects were performed twice before and once after each dosing period: hemoglobin, hematocrit, leukocyte count and differential, platelet estimation, urinalysis, serum glutamic oxaloacetic acid transaminase, serum glutamic pyruvic transaminase, alkaline phosphatase, total bilirubin, lactate dehydrogenase, blood urea nitrogen, fasting glucose, sodium, potassium, chloride, CO_2 combining power total protein, albumin, cholesterol, triglycerides, thyroxine, and electrocardiogram. In addition, the blood pressure and pulse were checked twice daily during each dosing period. All subjects were questioned daily during therapy.

In the second phase of this study four subjects received a 1,500-mg loading dose and then 500 mg orally every 6 h to complete a 10-day course. Subjects fasted 2 h before and 2 h after each dose. One subject withdrew from the study on day 9 because of gastrointestinal symptoms. Plasma samples were collected, at 0.33, 0.5, 0.67, 1, 2, 3, 4.5, 6, 8, 12, 24, 24.5, 25, 26, 30, 30.5, 31, 32, 54, 72, 72.5, 73, 74, 78, 78.5, 79, 80, 96, 168, 168.5, 170, 174, 174.5, 175, 176, 192, 198, 216, 216.5, 217, 218, 222, 222.5, 223, 224, and 240 h. A 24-h urine was collected between 0 and 24 h and between 168 and 192 h for determination of the josamycin concentration. Ten samples of saliva, seven samples of sweat, and six samples of tears were obtained at random from the four subjects during the 10 days of therapy for determination of josamycin concentration. Saliva was expectorated into sterile cups; in some cases salivation was stimulated by the chewing of paraffin. Sweat was collected with an ionphoresis analyzer. Tearing was induced with chemical and mechanical stimuli, and tears were then collected with a sterile tuberculin syringe. These four subjects were monitored for toxicity and side effects as in the previous study.

Antibiotic assays. The concentrations of josamycin or erythromycin were determined by an agar well diffusion technique, using *Sarcina lutea* ATCC 9341 as the test organism and antibiotic medium no. 11 (Difco). Reference standards were diluted in pooled human plasma for plasma assays, potassium phosphate buffer (pH 8) for urine assays, human saliva for saliva assays, and normal saline for sweat and tear assays. Urine samples were diluted in potassium phosphate buffer and adjusted to pH 8. All samples and standards were tested in triplicate. Assay plates were incubated at 37°C for 18 h. Zones of inhibition were measured with a Fisher Lilly zone reader. Antibiotic concentrations were computed by comparing the mean zone of inhibition for each sample with the curve constructed from the zone sizes of the standard dilutions.

Calculation of plasma half-life. Mean plasma concentrations obtained between 0 to 8 h and 48 to 56 h were plotted on semilog graph paper versus time. The half-life ($t_{1/2}$) was determined from the best-fit line through the points during the decline of blood levels, using the method of least squares.

The elimination rate constant (Kd) was determined from the formula: $Kd = 0.693/t_{1/2}$.

RESULTS

Josamycin and erythromycin stearate pharmacokinetics. The plasma concentration of josamycin usually peaked within 1 h after dosing and declined steadily over the next 5 h (Tables 1 and 2). At 1 h after the first 500-mg tablet, plasma concentrations for the two josamycin groups ranged between 0 and 1.43 μg/ml, with means of 0.71 and 0.61 μg/ml. After 6 h josamycin was not detectable in the plasma of most subjects. Higher plasma concentrations were observed on day 3. At 49 h the plasma concentrations in the 8-h group varied between 0 and 4.69 μg/ml, with a mean of 1.64 μg/ml, and in the 6-h group the concentrations ranged between 0.18 and 6.66 μg/ml, with a mean value of 2.31 μg/ml. The trough concentrations also increased during the first 2 days of therapy. At 48 h the mean concentration was 0.09 μg/ml in the 8-h group and 0.34 μg/ml in the 6-h group. This gradual increase in trough plasma concentrations leveled off after 54 h. With the 6-h schedule mean plasma concentrations were 0.45 μg/ml at 60 h, 0.46 μg/ml at 72 h, 0.40 μg/ml at 84 h, and 0.48 μg/ml at 96 h.

Plasma concentrations of erythromycin stearate were maximal between 1 and 3 h after each dose (Tables 3 and 4). At 2 h the 250-mg group had concentrations between 0 and 5.49 μg/ml, with a mean of 0.76 μg/ml. At 3 h the 500-mg group demonstrated plasma concentrations between 0.72 and 1.70 μg/ml, with a mean of 1.18 μg/ml. After 6 h the mean concentration was 0.14 μg/ml in the 250-mg group and 0.30 μg/ml in the 500-mg group. Plasma concentrations of erythromycin also increased slightly over the first 2 days. At 50 h the mean plasma concentration varied between 0 and 5.0 μg/ml, with a mean of 1.50 μg/ml in the 250-mg group,

TABLE 1. *Josamycin plasma concentrations in 21 subjects (500 mg every 8 h)*

Subject no.	Plasma concn (μg/ml) on day 1 at h:					Plasma concn (μg/ml) on day 3 at h:								
	0.5	1	2	3	4.5	48	48.5	49	50	51	52.5	54	55	56
1	0.73	0.92	0.53	0.34	0	0	0.34	0.82	0.60	0.31	0.23	0	0	0
2	1.32	0.56	0.35	0	0	0	0.79	1.11	0.78	0.47	0.28	0.24	0	0
3	0	1.43	0.46	0.38	0	0.17	0.76	2.90	0.73	0.96	0.53	0.46	0.35	0.30
4	0.83	0.87	0.36	0.30	0	0	0	0	0.35	0.42	0.25	0	0	0
5	0.58	0.98	0.45	0.51	0	0	0.40	1.42	1.06	0.45	0.25	0	0	0
6	0	0	0.28	0.27	NS[a]	0.30	0.44	1.50	1.25	1.17	0.53	0.54	0.46	0.35
7	0.28	0.79	0.31	0	0	0	1.67	1.25	0.52	0.22	0	0	NS	0
8	0	0.78	0.64	0.24	0.14	0.20	0.31	2.51	1.49	1.53	0.60	0.62	0.50	0.43
9	0.46	0.64	0.45	0.46	0	0.42	1.08	2.97	3.59	0.80	0.48	0.38	0.28	0.29
10	NS	1.10	0.36	0.33	0	0.37	4.75	3.18	2.26	0.67	0.45	0.32	0.28	0.28
11	0.65	0.36	0.29	0.36	0	0	1.58	4.69	0.76	0.61	0.34	0.24	0	0
12	0	0.53	0.36	0.26	0	0	0	1.54	0.93	0.68	0.35	0.32	0.27	0
13	1.38	0.53	0.35	0.27	0	0	0.37	0.40	0.32	0.29	0.23	0	0	0
14	0.56	0.73	0.36	0.25	0	0	0	0	0	0	0	0	0	0
15	0.21	0.22	0.25	0.27	0	0	0	1.79	0.90	0.58	0.30	0.25	0	0
16	0.67	0.40	0.31	0	0	0	0.39	2.79	2.18	0.82	0.48	0.32	0.28	0.27
17	0.61	0.95	0.56	0.52	0.18	0.31	1.69	2.32	1.40	1.45	0.67	0.65	0.55	0.41
18	0	0.26	0.23	0	0	0	0	0.39	1.24	0.44	0.38	0.20	0	0
19	1.79	0.84	0.39	0.26	0	0	0.60	1.51	0.79	0.45	0.23	0	0	0
20	0.28	0.62	0.28	0.25	0	0	0.79	0.96	0.52	0.48	0.24	0	0	0
21	1.47	1.38	0.56	0.37	0.25	NS	0.50	0.35	0.35	0.17	0	0	NS	0
Mean	0.59	0.71	0.39	0.27	0.03	0.09	0.78	1.64	1.04	0.62	0.32	0.22	0.16	0.11

[a] NS, No sample.

TABLE 2. *Josamycin plasma concentrations in 20 subjects (500 mg every 6 h)*

Subject no.	Plasma concn (μg/ml) on day 1 at h:						Plasma concn (μg/ml) on day 3 at h:						
	0.5	1	2	3	4.5	6	48	48.5	49	50	51	52.5	54
1	0	1.23	0.48	0.33	0	0	0.15	1.76	2.18	0.73	0.69	0.26	0.21
2	0.79	0.53	0.31	0	0	0	0.39	1.54	2.28	2.07	0.64	0.44	0.36
3	0	1.20	0.54	0.32	0.28	0	0.41	0.55	1.76	1.43	1.06	0.78	0.51
4	0.72	0.26	0.25	0.28	0	0	0.58	0.76	1.14	0.80	0.97	0.51	0.41
5	0.63	0.38	0.27	0	0	0	0	1.39	0.56	0.31	0.14	0	0
6	0	0.82	0.75	0.44	0.41	0	0.79	0.76	3.19	2.50	1.62	0.98	1.28
7	0	0	0	0	0	0	0	1.36	1.40	1.04	0.35	0.25	0
8	1.41	0.76	0.48	0.36	0	0	0.50	0.55	3.05	4.58	1.06	0.94	0.46
9	0.23	0.41	0.45	0.19	0	0	0.37	1.05	2.68	1.57	1.16	0.71	0.50
11	0.60	0.34	0.29	0.18	0	0	0.27	0.37	1.57	0.98	0.85	0.81	0.42
12	0	0.68	0.38	0	0	0	0.46	0.93	5.73	2.50	1.03	0.53	0.41
13	0.35	0.22	0	0	0	0	0.24	0.35	0.45	0.41	0.27	0	0.98
14	1.50	0.58	0.31	0.31	0	0	0	0	0.18	0.80	0.47	0.29	0.33
15	0.64	0.39	0.34	0.31	0	0	0.35	0.27	2.72	1.47	0.47	0.32	0.26
16	0.32	0.43	0.40	0.25	0	NS[a]	0.48	1.84	1.73	1.50	1.09	0.95	0.46
17	1.27	1.12	0.69	0.56	0.33	0.17	0.71	1.43	3.30	2.72	1.36	1.04	1.02
18	0.95	0.46	0.29	0.40	0	0	0	3.84	2.34	0.51	0.42	0	0
19	0.66	0.20	0.44	0.31	0	0	0.22	0.27	1.68	1.43	0.95	0.47	0.40
20	0	1.21	0.36	0.35	0	0	0	0.32	1.52	1.93	0.66	0.37	0.37
21	0.31	1.00	0.74	0.47	0.41	0	0.90	1.48	6.66	5.30	1.02	0.59	0.86
Mean	0.52	0.61	0.39	0.25	0.07	0.01	0.34	1.04	2.31	1.73	0.81	0.51	0.46

[a] NS, No sample.

and at 51 h in the 500-mg group the plasma concentrations were between 0.61 and 3.57 μg/ml, with a mean of 1.44 μg/ml. At 54 h the mean plasma levels had declined to 0.24 μg/ml in the 250-mg group and 0.56 μg/ml in the 500-mg group. Plasma concentrations at 60, 72, 84, and 96 h were comparable to those at 54 h.

The decline in mean plasma concentrations

TABLE 3. *Erythromycin plasma concentrations in 14 subjects (250 mg of erythromycin stearate every 6 h)*

Subject no.	Plasma concn (μg/ml) on day 1 at h:						Plasma concn (μg/ml) on day 3 at h:						
	0.5	1	2	3	4.5	6	48	48.5	49	50	51	52.5	54
1	0	0.68	0.97	NS[a]	0.26	0.05	0.06	0.39	0.55	1.37	0.89	0.15	0.13
2	0	0	0.19	0.13	0.06	0.04	0.05	0	0.26	0.62	0.53	0.23	0.08
5	0	0.10	0	1.76	0.29	0.20	0.03	0.10	0.43	1.82	1.74	0.12	0.06
6	0	0.55	0.20	1.15	0.36	0.26	0.68	0.46	0.66	0.83	1.31	1.37	0.87
7	0	0	1.40	0.48	0.09	0.17	0	0.05	0	4.07	0.32	0.13	0.07
9	0.04	0.10	0.61	0.31	0.18	0.10	0.13	0.11	0.80	1.40	1.27	0.95	0.74
10	0	0.12	5.49	0.65	0.15	0.26	0.03	0.04	0.13	2.37	0.27	0.09	0.07
12	0	0	0	0.22	0.22	0.12	0.20	0.15	0.43	0.46	0.74	0.52	0.43
14	0	0	0.17	0.22	0	0	0.03	0.04	0	0	0.09	0.07	0.04
15	0	0.24	0.05	0.35	0.16	0.10	0.07	0.06	0.44	0.34	0.81	0.40	0.12
16	0.04	0.70	0.45	0.34	0.12	0.08	0.13	0.11	0.16	0.36	1.54	0.67	0.26
18	0	0.13	0.37	0.28	0.17	0.24	0.12	0.12	0.38	1.56	0.40	0.13	0.08
19	0.05	0.13	0.42	0.59	0.33	0.14	0.08	0.07	0.80	0.74	0.64	0.35	0.12
21	0	0.34	0.33	0.71	0.12	0.13	0.83	0.65	2.46	5.00	0.82	0.44	0.28
Mean	0.009	0.22	0.76	0.55	0.18	0.14	0.17	0.17	0.54	1.50	0.81	0.40	0.24

[a] NS, No sample.

TABLE 4. *Erythromycin plasma concentrations in seven subjects (500 mg of erythromycin stearate every 6 h)*

Subject no.	Plasma concn (μg/ml) on day 1 at h:						Plasma concn (μg/ml) on day 3 at h:						
	0.5	1	2	3	4.5	6	48	48.5	49	50	51	52.5	54
3	0.24	1.05	1.93	1.70	1.14	0.74	0.16	0.31	0.99	2.51	0.79	1.03	0.85
4	0	0.38	0.75	1.17	0.30	0.12	1.97	0.76	2.26	2.10	1.74	1.07	0.53
8	0	1.02	0.67	0.92	0.28	0.14	NS[a]	NS	NS	NS	NS	NS	NS
11	0.03	0.14	0.72	0.72	0.21	0.08	0.37	0.47	0.43	0.75	0.61	1.21	0.39
13	0	0.38	0.81	0.98	0.47	0.25	0.26	0.54	0.65	1.13	0.93	1.13	0.44
17	0.22	0.86	1.81	1.14	0.70	0.28	0.73	0.71	1.16	1.15	3.57	1.54	0.87
20	0	0.24	0.94	1.61	0.81	0.48	0.27	0.27	0.40	0.41	0.97	0.59	0.29
Mean	0.07	0.58	1.09	1.18	0.56	0.30	0.63	0.51	0.98	1.34	1.44	1.10	0.56

[a] NS, No sample.

for each dosage group between 0 to 6 or 8 h and 48 to 54 or 56 h was used to determine the plasma half-life (Table 5). The plasma half-life determinations ranged between 1.34 and 1.56 h for josamycin and between 1.42 and 1.89 h for erythromycin. The elimination constant or the fraction of drug eliminated each hour varied between 0.45 and 0.52/h for josamycin and between 0.37 and 0.49/h for erythromycin.

The addition of a 1.5-g loading dose increased the peak and trough plasma concentrations of josamycin (Table 6). Plasma concentrations at 1 h on day 1 of therapy ranged between 3.94 and 6.47 μg/ml, with a mean of 5.06 μg/ml. Although the peak plasma concentrations were not as high on subsequent days, they tended to exceed those obtained in the 6-h josamycin group without a loading dose (mean, 2.31 μg/ml at 1 h on day 3). With the loading dose, the mean plasma concentration at 1 h was 3.18 μg/ml on day 2, 2.73 μg/ml on day 4, 3.62 μg/ml on day 3, and 2.61 μg/ml on day 10. The trough concentrations obtained at 0 and 6 h also tended to be higher after a loading dose. The mean trough plasma concentrations varied between 0.45 and 1.04 μg/ml during the 10 days of ther-

TABLE 5. *Plasma half-life and elimination constant for josamycin and erythromycin*

Drug	Dosage schedule	Observation period (h)	Plasma half-life (h)	Elimination constant/h
Josamycin	500 mg every 8 h	0–8	1.48	0.47
		48–56	1.53	0.45
Josamycin	500 mg every 6 h	0–6	1.56	0.45
		48–54	1.34	0.52
Erythromycin	250 mg every 6 h	0–6	1.55	0.45
		48–56	1.72	0.40
Erythromycin	500 mg every 6 h	0–6	1.42	0.49
		48–54	1.89	0.37

TABLE 6. *Josamycin plasma concentrations during a 10-day trial*[a]

Day of therapy	Subject no.	Plasma concn (μg/ml) at time (h) after first morning dose: 0	0.5	1	2	6
1	101	0	NS[b]	6.47	5.23	0.90
	102	0	NS	4.97	4.89	1.26
	103	0	2.25	3.94	3.71	0.65
	104	0	3.64	4.86	1.98	0.43
Mean			2.94	5.06	3.95	0.81
2	101	0.45	0.88	3.53	1.73	0.51
	102	0.72	1.52	4.25	2.65	1.06
	103	0.52	0.76	3.35	2.71	0.80
	104	0.10	1.81	1.58	0.68	0.21
Mean		0.45	1.24	3.18	1.94	0.64
4	101	1.23	NS	3.22	2.53	1.26
	102	1.47	NS	3.46	2.63	1.57
	103	0.76	3.02	2.37	1.70	0.56
	104	0.40	1.66	1.87	1.10	0.35
Mean		0.96	2.34	2.73	1.99	0.94
8	101	1.06	2.86	5.11	2.06	1.24
	102	1.14	4.57	4.67	2.08	1.14
	103	0.90	2.17	2.70	2.04	0.74
	104	0.26	2.84	1.98	1.01	0.37
Mean		0.84	3.11	3.62	1.80	0.87
10	101	2.00	2.19	3.20	2.48	1.11
	102	1.19	2.21	3.56	2.79	1.22
	103	0.82	0.60	1.08	2.42	0.79
Mean		1.00	1.67	2.61	2.56	1.04

[a] The initial dose was 1.50 g and then 0.5 g every 6 h for 10 days.

[b] NS, No sample.

apy in the four subjects who received a loading dose. In the 6-h josamycin group without a loading dose the mean concentrations at 0 and 6 h after day 2 ranged between 0.34 and 0.48 μg/ml. The higher mean peak and trough concentrations obtained with a loading dose were not due to subject variation. Three subjects participated in both studies (no. 3 = no. 102; no. 11 = no. 103; and no. 7 = no. 104). Their peak and trough plasma concentrations were consistently higher with the regimen that included a loading dose.

Josamycin concentration in urine, saliva, sweat, and tears. Mean concentrations in 24-h urine collections ranged between 195 and 465 μg/ml (Table 7). The urine recovery of an administered dose varied between 4.4 and 14.3% during the first 24 h. Between 168 and 192 h, the urinary recovery tended to be higher, ranging from 14.8 to 17.5%.

The concentration of josamycin in saliva, sweat, and tears was less than the mean peak plasma concentration, but it frequently exceeded the mean trough level (Table 8). Josamycin concentrations were highest in tear fluid, averaging 2.62 μg/ml. The mean concentration of josamycin was 1.03 μg/ml in saliva and 0.95 μg/ml in sweat.

Adverse reactions. No acute hematological, renal, or hepatic toxicity was observed with josamycin or erythromycin. There was no change in blood pressure or pulse determinations during therapy, and the miscellaneous blood chemistries were not influenced by either drug. Eosinophilia did develop in two subjects after 10 days of therapy with josamycin. The percentages of eosinophils after therapy were 7 and 8. A third subject started the 10-day study with 10% eosinophils and finished with 19% eosinophils. No other evidence of hypersensitivity was found in these subjects. Two had received josamycin before without developing eosinophilia.

Josamycin produced fewer side effects than did erythromycin stearate (Table 9). Only gastrointestinal side effects were recognized. Complaints of anorexia, mild epigastric discomfort relieved by food, or a change in stool characteristics was regarded as "mild" because it was not necessary to discontinue the study drug. Nausea with vomiting and diarrhea with abdominal cramps were considered to be "severe" side

TABLE 7. *Urinary excretion of josamycin*

Subject no.	Mean urine concn (μg/ml) at: 0–24 h	168–192 h	Urine recovery of administered dose (%) at: 0–24 h	168–192 h
101	465	410	7.4	17.1
102	293	370	14.3	17.5
103	276	380	7.3	14.8
104	195		4.4	

TABLE 8. *Josamycin concentration in saliva, sweat, and tears*

Fluid	No. of samples	Josamycin concn (μg/ml): Mean ± standard deviation	Range
Saliva	10	1.03 ± 0.43	0.54–1.8
Sweat	7	0.95 ± 0.30	0.57–1.3
Tears	6	2.62 ± 0.72	1.8–3.6

TABLE 9. *Gastrointestinal side effects of josamycin and erythromycin therapy*

Drug	Regimen	No. of subjects	Dosage days	Dosage days with gastrointestinal complaints (%)		
				None	Mild[a]	Severe[b]
Josamycin	500 mg every 6 h × 4 days	21	84	92	8	0
Josamycin	500 mg every 8 h × 4 days	21	84	95	5	0
Josamycin	500 mg every 6 h[c] × 10 days	4	39	95	5	0
Erythromycin stearate	500 mg every 6 h × 4 days	7	24	50	29	21
Erythromycin stearate	250 mg every 6 h × 4 days	14	53	77	23	0

[a] Mild: anorexia, mild epigastric discomfort relieved by food, or change in stool characteristics.
[b] Severe: nausea with vomiting and/or diarrhea with abdominal cramps.
[c] Initial loading dose, 1.5 g.

effects, since withdrawal of the study drug was necessary. None of the subjects treated with josamycin had severe side effects. Only 5 of the 21 subjects in the 6-h josamycin group had mild gastrointestinal complaints, and these involved 8% of the dosage days. With the other two josamycin dosage schedules side effects were noted on only 5% of the dosage days. One subject in the 10-day study discontinued josamycin on day 9 because of malaise, abdominal cramps, and loose stools. These symptoms may not have been related to the drug, since the patient's wife and daughter had similar symptoms at that time. In contrast, the percentage of complaint days during the 4-day trials was significantly higher for the erythromycin groups than for the two josamycin groups ($P < 0.05$ by chi-square analysis). The 500-mg erythromycin stearate group experienced severe side effects on 21% of the dosage days and mild side effects on 29% of the dosage days. Five of the seven subjects in this group had complaints, and two were forced to stop therapy because of vomiting (one case) and diarrhea (one case). The 250-mg dose of erythromycin produced mild gastrointestinal side effects in 6 of the 14 subjects on 23% of the dosage days. One subject in this group stopped therapy on day 3 because of abdominal discomfort and borborygmus.

DISCUSSION

In general, josamycin compares favorably with erythromycin. It has a similar spectrum of bacteriostatic activity in vitro; however, josamycin is less potent by weight against most susceptible organisms. Concentrations of 0.5 μg/ml are effective in inhibiting all strains of *M. pneumoniae*, *S. pneumoniae*, *S. pyogenes*, and *N. meningitidis* (6, 7). A 2-μg/ml amount is required to inhibit the majority of strains of *S. aureus* and *B. fragilis* (6, 7).

In this study, the ranges of plasma concentrations of josamycin and erythromycin after equivalent oral dosages were similar. Subjects receiving erythromycin reached peak concentrations that were considerably higher than those of josamycin after the first dose (mean, 1.18 versus 0.61 μg/ml). However, the josamycin levels increased over the 4-day period, and mean concentrations on day 3 were higher than those achieved with erythromycin (2.31 versus 1.44 μg/ml). The tendency of josamycin to accumulate over the first 48-h of administration was also reflected in the trough levels. After an initial dose of 500 mg, the mean concentrations were 0.01 μg/ml at 6 h and 0 μg/ml at 8 h. However, trough concentrations after 48 h of drug administration reached a plateau of 0.34 μg/ml with the 6-h schedule and 0.09 μg/ml with the 8-h schedule. The gradual accumulation during the first 2 days of therapy prompted the second study in which a loading dose was used. The addition of the 1.5-g loading dose produced higher peak and trough plasma concentrations from the first dose onward.

Josamycin, like the other macrolide antibiotics, is metabolized rapidly in the liver to an inactive form and excreted primarily in the bile (6). Urinary excretion accounts for less than 20% of the elimination of the active form, but urine concentrations are high (200 to 400 μg/ml). The josamycin assay measured only biologically active drug and may not have detected inactive metabolites. In spite of these high urine levels, josamycin would probably not be of value for urinary tract infections since the vast majority of enterobacteriaceae are highly resistant to josamycin.

Josamycin was also detected in other body fluids in concentrations similar to those achieved in plasma. The concentration in sweat (mean, 0.95 μg/ml) and saliva (mean, 1.03 μg/ml) corresponded to plasma trough levels, and those in tears (mean, 2.62 μg/ml) corresponded to plasma peak levels. The levels in tears and saliva are considerably higher than those reported by Hoeprich (5) and others (3) with erythromycin. Hoeprich reported undetectable concentrations in saliva and 1 to 2 μg of drug per ml in tears (5). Concentrations of josamycin achieved in these secretions may, therefore, make it of value in the chemoprophylaxis of the meningococcal carrier state.

Josamycin was better tolerated in this study than was erythromycin stearate. At the higher dosage of erythromycin (500 mg every 6 h), five of seven subjects developed gastrointestinal symptoms, and it was necessary to stop the drug in two. This incidence of side effects was higher than that reported in previous studies (1, 2, 4), in which the drug was administered in lower dosages and usually not in a strictly fasting state. In the present study with the lower dosage of erythromycin stearate (250 mg every 6 h), complaints were milder but were still experienced in 23% of the dosage days. In contrast, josamycin produced mild side effects on only 5 to 8% of the dosage days. Therefore, it appears that josamycin was well tolerated, even in high dosages in a strictly fasting state. The comparison with erythromycin, however, must be interpreted with caution because the drugs were not administered in a blind fashion. No attempt was made to determine the influence of psychological factors on subjective complaints.

In conclusion, this new macrolide antibiotic provides comparable blood and urine concentrations to its analogue, erythromycin. Because it is well tolerated and it demonstrably penetrates into saliva, sweat, and tears, josamycin should be further studied to define its value in the therapy of clinical infections caused by *M. pneumoniae*, streptococci, staphylococci, and perhaps *Neisseria* species.

LITERATURE CITED

1. **Alberti, R. L., J. W. Hamman, J. C. Sylvester, and G. H. Berryman.** 1965. Infections in office patients. Clin. Med. 72:1965–1974.
2. **Billow, B. W., E. A. Thompson, A. Stern, and A. Florio.** 1964. A clinical study of erythromycin: a comparative evaluation of several salts. Curr. Ther. Res. Clin. Exp. 6:381–384.
3. **Devine, L. F., R. C. Knowles, W. E. Pierce, R. O. Peckinpaugh, C. R. Hagerman, and R. I. Lytle.** 1968. Proposed model for screening antimicrobial agents for potential use in eliminating meningococci from the nasopharynx of healthy carriers. Antimicrob. Agents Chemother. 8:307–314.
4. **General Practitioner Research Group.** 1974. Antimicrobial efficacy of erythromycin stearate—a report from the General Practitioner Research Group. Practitioner 212:120–122.
5. **Hoeprich, P. D.** 1971. Prediction of antimeningococcic chemoprophylactic efficacy. J. Infect. Dis. 123:125–133.
6. **Mitsuhashi, S. (ed.).** 1971. Drug action and drug resistance in bacteria. University Park Press, Tokyo.
7. **Strausbaugh, L. J., J. A. Dilworth, J. M. Gwaltney, Jr., and M. A. Sande.** 1976. In vitro susceptibility studies with josamycin and erythromycin. Antimicrob. Agents Chemother. 9:546–548.

ANTIMICROBIAL AGENTS AND CHEMOTHERAPY, Sept. 1976, p. 457-461
Vol. 10, No. 3

Pharmacokinetics of Cefamandole in Patients Undergoing Hemodialysis and Peritoneal Dialysis

MARY JEAN AHERN, FREDERIC O. FINKELSTEIN, AND VINCENT T. ANDRIOLE*

Department of Internal Medicine, Yale University School of Medicine, New Haven, Connecticut 06510

Received for publication 18 March 1976

The pharmacokinetics of cefamandole nafate, a new parenteral cephalosporin derivative, were evaluated in 11 patients with chronic renal failure (creatinine clearance less than 5 ml/min), including five patients during hemodialysis, four patients during routine peritoneal dialysis, and two patients during the interdialytic period. Peak serum levels of cefamandole were comparable to those observed in patients with normal renal function. Clearance of the drug during the interdialytic period and during hemodialysis and peritoneal dialysis was minimal, with a resultant significant prolongation of serum half-life. The nondialyzability of cefamandole is in contrast with reported studies of cephalothin, where significant reduction of the serum half-life was achieved during hemodialysis but not peritoneal dialysis. The concentration of cefamandole in the peritoneal dialysate after parenteral administration was observed to be bactericidal for many gram-negative pathogens and, with the exception of *Streptococcus faecalis*, most gram-positive organisms found in bacterial peritonitis in patients with severe renal failure. The present data suggest that if stable bactericidal serum levels of cefamandole are to be maintained during hemodialysis and peritoneal dialysis, a parenteral loading dose must be administered followed by one-half the loading dose every half-life.

Cefamandole nafate is a new parenteral cephalosporin active against a wide variety of gram-positive and gram-negative organisms including cephalothin-resistant *Enterobacter* species, indole-positive *Proteus* species resistant to cephalothin, and particularly *Haemophilus influenzae* isolates (2, 9–11). In previous studies, the pharmacokinetics of cefamandole have been studied in normal volunteers, but no studies have been done in patients with chronic renal failure who are not being dialyzed or in patients undergoing hemodialysis or peritoneal dialysis. Therefore, it is the purpose of this investigation to evaluate the pharmacokinetics of this agent during the course of routine hemodialysis and peritoneal dialysis and during interdialytic periods.

MATERIALS AND METHODS

Patients. Eleven chronic dialysis patients with chronic renal failure (creatinine clearance <5 ml/min) were studied. Two chronic hemodialysis patients were studied during the interdialytic period, five patients during the course of a routine hemodialysis, and four patients during the course of a routine peritoneal dialysis. No patient was septic, nor had any received antibiotics for at least 2 weeks before the study. Informed consent was obtained from each patient.

Dialysis. (i) Peritoneal. All patients studied had indwelling Tenckhoff catheters in place. Dialysis solutions (1.5% dextrose) were prewarmed to a temperature of 37°C and instilled into the peritoneal cavity over a 10-min period. Dwell time in the peritoneal cavity was limited to 20 min, and dialysate was drained over a 30-min period. Heparin was not added to the dialysate. The overall flow rate was 2 liters/h.

(ii) Hemodialysis. Patients underwent dialysis for 6 h with a recirculating single-pass delivery system using extracorporeal Ex-23 coils. An initial loading dose of heparin, 1 mg/kg of body weight, was given followed by hourly injections of 1,000 U of heparin through the 4th hour of dialysis.

Study protocol. Control serum samples were taken from all patients just before administration of the antibiotic as well as before institution of dialysis for those patients being studied during dialysis. One gram of cefamandole nafate (supplied by Eli Lilly and Co.) was then administered intramuscularly. The time of the injection of the antibiotic was considered to be time zero. In patients studied during hemodialysis, dialysis was begun at time zero, and arterial (coil inflow) bloods were obtained from these patients at 0.5, 1, 2, 3, 4, 5, and 6 h. Concomitant venous (coil outflow) bloods were obtained at 2, 4, and 6 h. Patients who were studied while not being dialyzed had venous samples drawn at 0.5, 1, 2, 3, 4, 5, and 6 h. The patients being evaluated during peritoneal dialysis had blood drawn at 0.5 and 1 h after the injection of cefamandole, and dialysis was begun immediately after the 1-h sample was obtained. Thereafter, samples were obtained at the following intervals: 1.5 h after time zero (0.5 h after institution of dialysis) and 2.5, 6.5, 7.5, and 12.5 h after time zero. Aliquots of the outflow dialysate fluid were obtained from exchanges one, two, three, four, five, six, seven, and twelve at the start of the drainage period. Both serum and dialysate samples were either assayed immediately or stored for no longer than 48 h at −4°C before assay.

Antibiotic assay. The cefamandole standard was supplied by Eli Lilly and Co., Indianapolis, Ind., as cefamandole lithium. The standard was dissolved in sterile distilled water just before use. The assay used in the study is based on the procedure for gentamicin determination initially described by Winters et al. (12), utilizing *Bacillus globigii* as the test organism, and modified in our laboratory as previously described (8). All serum and dialysate assays were done in duplicate in each plate to verify reproducibility. Each plate contained, in duplicate, cefamandole standards of 20, 10, 5, 2.5, 1.25, and 0.625 μg/ml.

Data analysis. (i) Serum and peritoneal dialysate antibiotic levels. The values for each patient and standards were determined by linear regression analysis on a Monroe 1930 statistical calculator.

(ii) Clearance. The mean peritoneal clearance of the administered antibiotic, urea, and creatinine was calculated by the equation $C = (D \times V)/S \times t$, where C is the clearance in milliliters per minute; D is the mean dialysate concentration (antibiotic in micrograms per milliliter, creatinine or urea in milligrams per 100 ml); S is the mean serum concentration (micrograms per milliliter or milligrams per 100 ml as above); V is the volume of dialysate (in milliliters); and t is the time in minutes (60).

(iii) Amount of antibiotic removed. The total antibiotic removed per exchange over the 12 h of peritoneal dialysis was calculated by the equation $V \times D = A$, where V is the volume of dialysate (in milliliters); D is the dialysate antibiotic concentration (in micrograms per milliliter); and A is the amount of antibiotic removed per exchange.

The total antibiotic extracted over the 6 h of hemodialysis was calculated by the equation $S_1 - S_2 = A$, where S_1 is the peak arterial serum antibiotic concentration (in micrograms per milliliter); S_2 is the venous serum antibiotic concentration at 6 h (in micrograms per milliliter); and A is the total antibiotic extracted (in micrograms per milliliter).

(iv) Extraction ratio. The extraction ratio of the antibiotic and creatinine on the hemodialysis patients was determined at the end of the 2nd, 4th, and 6th hours and was calculated by the equation $ER = [(A - V)/A] \times 100$ (7), where ER is the extraction ratio; A is the arterial serum antibiotic concentration (in milligrams per milliliter) or arterial creatinine concentration (in milligrams per 100 ml); and V is the venous serum antibiotic concentration (micrograms per milliliter) or venous creatinine concentration (in milligrams per 100 ml). Extraction ratios for antibiotic and creatinine were then compared by the formula $(A/B) \times 100 = C$, where A is the extraction ratio of antibiotic; B is the extraction ratio of creatinine; and C is the ratio of the percentage of antibiotic extracted to the percentage of creatinine extracted at each time interval measured.

(v) Half-life. The kinetics of the present study are characterized by a monoexponential decay curve. Thus, the half-life of the antibiotic was determined by the method of least squares using the slope (m) as calculated from the formula (6):

$$m = \frac{N\Sigma(x \log y) - (\Sigma x)(\Sigma \log y)}{N\Sigma x^2 - (\Sigma x)^2}$$

$$\text{half-life} = \frac{\log 2}{m}$$

where x is the time in hours; y is the concentration of antibiotic in serum; and N is the number of observations.

RESULTS

Hemodialysis. In the five patients studied, the 1-h peak arterial concentration (Table 1, Fig. 1) was 27.85 μg/ml (range: 20.38 to 37.07). After 6 h of dialysis, the mean arterial concentration fell to 16.03 μg/ml (range: 11.72 to 24.84). The mean amount of antibiotic extracted over the 6-h dialysis was 13.27 μg/ml (range: 8.75 to 17.38). Extraction ratios calculated on each patient at 2, 4, and 6 h were

TABLE 1. *Half-life and serum concentration of cefamandole in patients undergoing hemodialysis*

Patient no.	Serum concn (μg/ml)										Half-life[a]
	0.5 h[b] (arterial)	1 h (arterial)	2 h		3 h (arterial)	4 h		6 h			
			Arterial	Venous		Arterial	Venous	Arterial	Venous		
1	35.686	37.068	32.248	30.655	29.327	28.605	26.879	22.298	19.685		7.243
2	34.041	32.380	32.245	31.062	27.422	26.79	25.795	24.836	21.341		11.578
3	19.135	23.832	23.270	22.407	21.038	19.598	18.418	14.359	12.674		6.743
4	17.971	25.579	24.077	22.612	20.193	16.655	12.956	11.715	9.219		4.738
5	13.330	20.380	19.711	18.754	17.622	16.536	14.959	12.082	11.634		6.567
Mean concn	24.033	27.848	26.310		23.120	21.636		16.033			6.61

[a] See text; each half-life determined by using monoexponential decay calculated from peak serum value of each patient.

[b] Time postinfusion.

variable with a mean of 8.8 ± 1.6 standard error. Comparison of the extraction of cefamandole with the extraction of creatinine at the above times was again variable, with a mean of 24.7 ± 8.3 standard error. The mean half-life determined by monoexponential decay was 6.61 h (range: 11.58 to 4.74).

Peritoneal dialysis. In the four patients studied, the observed mean peak serum concentration was 25.4 μg/ml (range: 19.5 to 33.96) 1.5 h after the intramuscular injection. The level fell to 8.71 μg/ml (range: 6.85 to 12.26) (Table 2, Fig. 2) 12.5 h after the injection (11.5 h after dialysis was begun). The mean peritoneal dialysate concentration (Table 3) was 5.79 μg/ml (range: 4.01 to 8.52). The mean quantity of antibiotic removed per exchange over the 12 h was 11.56 mg/h (range: 8.02 to 17.04). Total mean amount of drug removed was 139.2 mg, or 3.9% of the initial 1-g dose.

The mean clearance of cefamandole per exchange and the mean over 12 h are listed in Table 3. The mean was 10.22 ml/min, with a range of 8.25 to 11.64. The mean half-life (Table 2) calculated by monoexponential decay was 7.15 h (range: 5.68 to 8.67).

Chronic renal patients: interdialytic period. In the two patients studied, the mean peak serum concentration was 24.63 μg/ml 1 h after intramuscular injection of 1 g of cefamandole. Six hours after injection, the mean serum concentration was 20.21 μg/ml. The half-life of cefamandole in patient 1, calculated from antibiotic concentrations at 1, 2, 3, 4, 5, and 6 h, was 8.4 h. The half-life in patient 2, similarly calculated, was 9.24 h. The mean half-life was 8.84 h.

DISCUSSION

In an earlier study of the pharmacokinetics of cefamandole in patients with normal renal

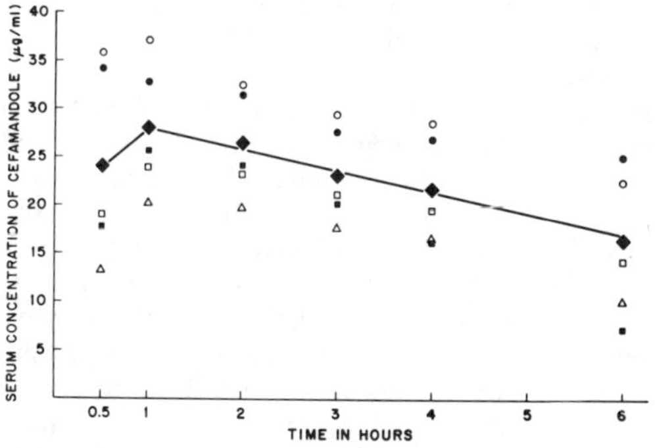

FIG. 1. *Serum concentrations of cefamandole in patients undergoing hemodialysis. Symbols: (○, ●, □, ■, △) Patients 1 through 5, respectively; ◆, mean.*

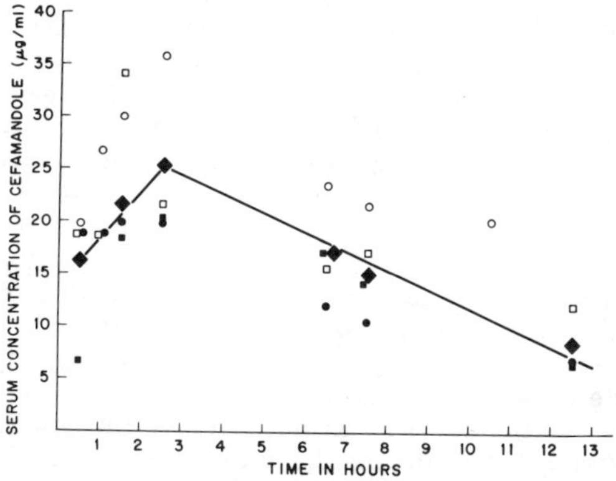

FIG. 2. *Serum concentrations of cefamandole in patients undergoing peritoneal dialysis. Symbols: (○, ●, □, ■) Patients 1 through 4, respectively; ◆, mean.*

TABLE 3. *Mean clearance and amount of cefamandole removed during peritoneal dialysis in four patients*

Time (h)	Mean clearance (ml/min)	Dialysate concn (μg/ml)	Total amt removed/exchange (mg/h)
1	11.18	8.52	17.04
2	9.26	6.78	13.56
3	8.25	5.69	11.14
4	9.60	6.19	12.38
5	10.32	4.57	9.14
6	10.73	5.47	10.94
7	10.83	5.15	10.3
12	11.64	4.01	8.02
Mean	10.22	5.79	11.56

TABLE 2. *Half-life and serum concentration of cefamandole of patients undergoing peritoneal dialysis*

Patient no.	Serum concn (μg/ml)							Half-life[a]
	0.5 h[b]	1.0 h	1.5 h	2.5 h	6.5 h	7.5 h	12.5 h	
1	19.74	26.699	29.82	35.769	23.39	21.50	20.22[c]	8.67
2	18.822	18.822	19.502	19.502	11.902	10.602	7.008	6.296
3	18.70	18.70	33.96	21.81	15.63	16.99	12.26	7.949
4	6.71		18.38	20.50	17.16	14.35	6.85	5.680
Mean	15.99	21.4	25.4	24.39	17.0	15.85	8.706	7.15

[a,b] See Table 1.
[c] Specimen taken at 10.5 h.

function (creatinine, 0.8 to 1.7 mg/100 ml; creatinine clearances, 31 to 123 ml/min), Shemonsky et al. (11) observed that doses of 6 to 11 mg/kg (comparable to a dose of 500 mg) given by intramuscular injection resulted in a mean peak serum concentration of 13.7 ± 3 μg/ml at 1.5 h and ≤1.0 μg/ml at 6 h. In the same study, with doses in the 11- to 17-mg/kg range (approximating the 1-g intramuscular dose used in the present study), the mean peak serum concentrations were observed to be 31.0 ± 17.8 μg/ml at 0.5 h and 1.7 ± 0.7 μg/ml 6 h after cefamandole administration. The calculated half-life in their study ranged from 49 to 129 min. In a similar study in normal volunteers given a 1-g intramuscular injection, the mean peak serum concentration was 21 μg/ml (3). In the same study (3), a 1-g intravenous dose of cefamandole given to normal volunteers resulted in a $t_{1/2}$ of 0.5 h. These workers (3) observed that cefamandole was 74% bound to serum protein and had a volume of distribution of 12.8 liters/1.73 m^2. The data observed in the present study, which were obtained from two patients with chronic renal failure who were studied during the interdialytic period, indicated a mean peak serum concentration of 24.63 μg/ml at 1 h after the injection of 1 g of cefamandole and were comparable to the results observed in normal patients (3, 11). However, the 6-h mean serum concentration in our patients was 20.21 μg/ml, and the calculated $t_{1/2}$ was 8.8 h. The striking contrast in serum levels in patients with chronic renal failure as compared with patients with normal renal function reflects the significant clearance of cefamandole by renal mechanisms.

The four patients in the present report who were studied on peritoneal dialysis again demonstrated peak serum levels comparable to those of normals, with a mean of 25.4 μg/ml. The 12.5-h postinjection mean level of 8.71 μg/ml suggests that cefamandole is not effectively removed by peritoneal dialysis. This statement is supported by our observations that approximately 130 mg of cefamandole, or 13% of the initial 1-g dose, was found in the dialysate over the 12-h period of dialysis. The present study also indicates that the mean half-life of cefamandole is prolonged in patients undergoing peritoneal dialysis, i.e., 7.5 h as compared with 30 min in patients with normal renal function.

Similarly, in our patients undergoing hemodialysis, the mean peak serum concentration of cefamandole was observed to be 27.85 μg/ml. Thus, mean peak serum concentrations of the antibiotic, after intramuscular injection of 1 g, appear comparable regardless of renal status. In contrast to the rapid excretion of cefamandole over 6 h in patients with normal renal function, however, the patients undergoing hemodialysis had an observed mean serum concentration of 16.03 μg/ml at 6 h. The calculated half-life was 6.61 h, similar to the value obtained for the peritoneal dialysis study group.

The pharmacokinetics of cefamandole in renal failure and dialysis differ in certain aspects from previous data derived from cephalothin studies in patients with renal failure. Kabins and Cohen (4) studied 12 azotemic patients (creatinine clearance <5 ml/min) given 1 g of cephalothin intravenously and observed that the peak serum concentrations 15 to 30 min postinjection ranged from 32 to 64 μg/ml. At 6 h, serum cephalothin values in the azotemic patients were in the range of 16 μg/ml as compared with undetectable levels in patients with creatinine clearances greater than 30 ml/min per 1.73 m^2. The half-life of cephalothin in these azotemic patients was increased over the normal $t_{1/2}$ of 0.5 h and was biphasic, i.e., 2.8 h over the first 8 h and 12 ± 4 and 19 h over 8 to 24 h and 24 to 48 h, respectively, reflecting the different urine excretion rates of cephalothin and its metabolite *o*-desacetyl cephalothin (4). An initial half-life value for cephalothin of 2.9 h has also been reported by Kunin and Atuk in patients with renal failure (5).

Yamasaku et al. (13) also studied cephalosporins, but not cefamandole, in patients with renal failure undergoing dialysis and found that the half-life for cephalothin was prolonged in uremic patients. These workers observed cephalothin half-life values of 4.6 h over the first 9 h and 15.9 h over the subsequent 72 h. However, half-life values were reduced to 2.3 h by hemodialysis on a coil dialyzer and to 2.6 h on the Kiil dialyzer. Cephalothin did not appear to be removed by peritoneal dialysis since the average half-life in six patients in this study was 5.1 h. Thus, both cephalothin and cefamandole have prolonged half-lives in patients with severe chronic renal insufficiency, and neither cephalothin nor cefamandole is effectively removed by peritoneal dialysis, whereas cephalothin, but not cefamandole, is significantly removed from the serum during hemodialysis.

We have no obvious explanation for the nondialyzability of cefamandole, or for the difference between the dialyzability of cefamandole and cephalothin during hemodialysis. Both cephalothin and cefamandole are similarly protein bound (70 and 74%, respectively) and have similar half-lives (30 and 34 min, respectively) as well as similar volumes of distribution (18.5 and 12.8 liters/1.73 m^2, respectively) and molecular weights (418 and 512, respectively) (3).

Even though cefamandole is not significantly removed from the serum during hemodialysis or peritoneal dialysis, our observations indicate that the concentration of cefamandole in the peritoneal dialysis fluid ranged from 8.52 μg/ml at 1 h to 4.02 μg/ml at 12 h, with a mean of 5.79 μg/ml. On the basis of these data, it appears that intramuscular cefamandole alone, without similar intraperitoneal instillation, should give sufficiently elevated peritoneal levels to be bactericidal for many gram-negative pathogens and, except for *Streptococcus faecalis,* most gram-positive organisms found in bacterial peritonitis (11).

Since the results of the present study indicate that the clearance of cefamandole during hemodialysis and peritoneal dialysis is minimal and that the half-life is significantly prolonged (greater than six times) in patients undergoing dialysis, the following dose recommendations can be calculated according to the formula $(Pk)(Vd)$ = dose in milligrams per square meter, where Pk is the peak serum antibiotic level felt to give adequate therapeutic levels = 25 μg/ml (11) and Vd is volume of distribution of the drug (12.8 liters/1.73 m^2) (3) = 7.45 liters/m^2. Substituting values, one gets the following: dosage (in milligrams per square meter) = $(25 \times 10^{-3}$ mg/ml$)$ $(7.45 \times 10^3$ ml/$m^2)$ = 186 mg/m^2. Therefore, patients with severe renal failure, regardless of whether they are undergoing hemodialysis or peritoneal dialysis, should receive a loading dose of cefamandole based on the above calculation, followed by one-half this loading dose every half-life (7.5 h during peritoneal dialysis and 6.6 h during hemodialysis). This method of administration has been shown to provide more stable drug levels (1).

ACKNOWLEDGMENTS

We wish to thank Susan Proto and Alan Siniscalchi for their technical assistance.

This investigation was supported in part by a grant from the American Heart Association.

LITERATURE CITED

1. **Cutler, R. E., A. M. Gyselynck, P. Fleet, and A. W. Forrey.** 1972. Correlation of serum creatinine concentration and gentamicin half-life. J. Am. Med. Assoc. **219:**1037–1041.
2. **Eykeyn, S., C. Jenkins, and A. King.** 1973. Antibacterial activity of cefamandole, a new cephalosporin antibiotic, compared with that of cephaloridine, cephalothin, and cephalexin. Antimicrob. Agents Chemother. **3:**657–661.
3. **Fong, I. W., E. D. Ralph, and W. M. M. Kirby.** 1976. Clinical pharmacology of cefamandole as compared to cephalothin. Antimicrob. Agents Chemother. **9:**65–69.
4. **Kabins, S. A., and S. Cohen.** 1965. Cephalothin serum levels in the azotemic patient, p. 207–219. Antimicrob. Agents Chemother. 1964.
5. **Kunin, C. M., and N. Atuk.** 1966. Excretion of cephaloridine and cephalothin in patients with renal impairment. N. Engl. J. Med. **274:**654–655.
6. **Kunin, C. M., and M. Finland.** 1958. A new tetracycline antibiotic that yields greater and more sustained antibacterial activity. N. Engl. J. Med. **259:**999–1005.
7. **Kunin, C. M., S. B. Rees, J. P. Merrill, and M. Finland.** 1959. Persistence of antibiotics in blood of patients with acute renal failure. I. Tetracycline and chlortetracycline. J. Clin. Invest. **38:**1487–1519.
8. **Malacoff, R. F., F. Finkelstein, and V. T. Andriole.** 1975. Effect of peritoneal dialysis on serum levels of tobramycin and clindamycin. Antimicrob. Agents Chemother. **8:**574–580.
9. **Myers, B. R., B. Leng, and S. Hirschman.** 1975. Cefamandole: antimicrobial activity in vitro of a new cephalosporin. Antimicrob. Agents Chemother. **8:**737–741.
10. **Neu, H. C.** 1974. Cefamandole, a cephalosporin antibiotic with an unusual wide spectrum of activity. Antimicrob. Agents Chemother. **6:**177–182.
11. **Shemonsky, N. K., J. Carrizosa, and M. Levison.** 1975. In vitro activity and pharmacokinetics in patients of cefamandole, a new cephalosporin antibiotic. Antimicrob. Agents Chemother. **8:**679–683.
12. **Winters, R. E., K. D. Litwack, and W. C. Hewitt.** 1971. Relation between dose and levels of gentamicin in blood. J. Infect. Dis. **124S:**90–95.
13. **Yamasaku, F., R. Tsuchida, and Y. Usuda.** 1970. A study of the kinetics of cephalosporins in renal failure. J. Postgrad. Med. **46S:**57–59.

ANTIMICROBIAL AGENTS AND CHEMOTHERAPY, Sept. 1976, p. 462-463
Vol. 10, No. 3

Printed in U.S.A.

Concentrations of Trimethoprim-Sulfamethoxazole in Blood After a Single, Large Oral Dose

THOMAS T. YOSHIKAWA* AND LUCIEN B. GUZE

Department of Medicine, Harbor General Hospital, Torrance, California 90509; Research and Medical Services, Wadsworth Hospital, Veterans Administration Center, Los Angeles, California 90073; and Department of Medicine, UCLA School of Medicine, Los Angeles, California 90024*

Received for publication 12 April 1976

Concentrations of trimethoprim (TMP) and sulfamethoxazole (SMZ) in blood were determined in seven healthy volunteers after ingestion of 720 mg of TMP and 3,600 mg of SMZ (nine tablets of TMP-SMZ, 1:5 ratio) as a single oral dose. The mean levels of drug in blood achieved during the first 8 h after drug administration ranged from 6.12 to 8.32 μg/ml for TMP and 98 to 120 μg/ml for SMZ. These concentrations easily exceeded the previously reported minimal inhibitory concentrations for clinical isolates of *Neisseria gonorrhoeae*. The combination of TMP-SMZ given as a single, large oral dose may be a useful therapeutic regimen for patients with uncomplicated gonorrhea and susceptible microorganisms.

Trimethoprim-sulfamethoxazole (TMP-SMZ) has been used to treat uncomplicated gonorrhea (1, 2, 4, 7-9, 11, 12). However, the cure rate has been somewhat variable, ranging from 62 to 98%. The treatment schedules instituted in these studies varied from a single-dose regimen for 1 to 5 days to multiple doses for several successive days. Although levels of TMP and SMZ were not determined, it would be anticipated that achievable concentrations of these drugs in blood would significantly differ depending on which treatment regimen was utilized. This, in part, may explain differences in therapeutic outcome.

To evaluate the potential usefulness of a single, large-dose regimen of TMP-SMZ for treatment of uncomplicated gonorrhea, preliminary studies were performed in healthy volunteers by administering 720 mg of TMP and 3,600 mg of SMZ. Serial blood concentrations of TMP and SMZ were determined at appropriate intervals. The data from this investigation are presented in this report.

EXPERIMENTAL

Seven healthy male and female volunteers between the ages of 24 and 34 years received a single oral dose of nine TMP-SMZ tablets (each tablet consisting of 80 mg of TMP and 400 mg of SMZ; courtesy of Hoffmann-La Roche, Inc., Nutley, N.J.). The medication was taken with 8 to 10 oz (ca. 0.24 to 0.3 liter)) of water in the morning after an overnight fast. Food was not eaten until 5 h after ingestion of drugs. Thereafter, food and fluids were not restricted.

A total of 10 ml of oxalated blood was drawn at 0 (before drug administration), 2, 4, 6, 8, and 24 h. Serum samples were immediately frozen for subsequent analysis. The determination of TMP and SMZ concentrations in blood was performed through the courtesy of Robert Weinfeld, Hoffmann-La Roche, Inc., Nutley, N.J., by previously described methods (5, 10).

RESULTS AND DISCUSSION

Levels of TMP and SMZ in blood from the seven volunteers are presented in Fig. 1 and 2, respectively. The mean blood concentrations of the drugs during the first 8 h after their administration ranged from 6.12 to 8.32 μg/ml (TMP) and 98 to 128 μg/ml (SMZ). At 24 h, the average levels of TMP and SMZ in blood were 2.16 and 31.7 μg/ml, respectively. The dose regimen was satisfactorily tolerated by most individuals, with two persons experiencing transient nausea.

Previous studies determining levels of TMP and SMZ in blood were performed in normal volunteers receiving relatively small, single oral doses of these drugs. One study administered 240 mg of TMP and 1,200 mg of SMZ and achieved average peak levels for TMP and SMZ of 3.0 and 65 μg/ml, respectively (3). Investigations by Kaplan et al. (6) in 24 healthy male volunteers after ingestion of a higher dose of the drugs, 400 mg of TMP and 2,000 mg of SMZ (five tablets of TMP-SMZ), revealed similar mean peak concentrations. However, in the present study after administration of nine tablets of trimethoprim-sulfamethoxazole, the mean peak concentrations achieved in the blood for TMP and SMZ were more than double

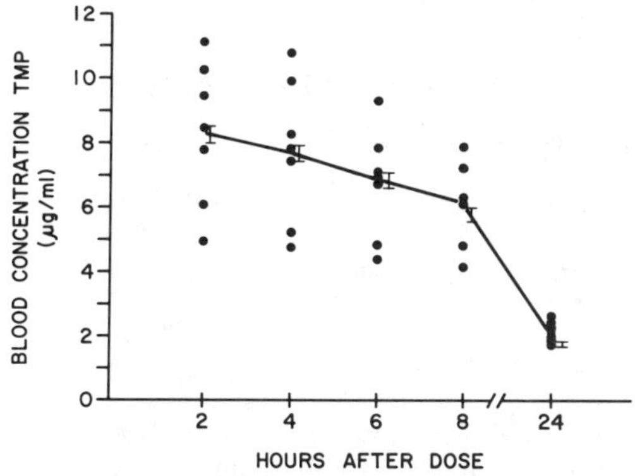

FIG. 1. *Distribution and mean levels of trimethoprim (micrograms per milliliter) in the blood of seven volunteers after a single oral dose of nine tablets of trimethoprim-sulfamethoxazole (±1 standard error of the mean represented by vertical bars).*

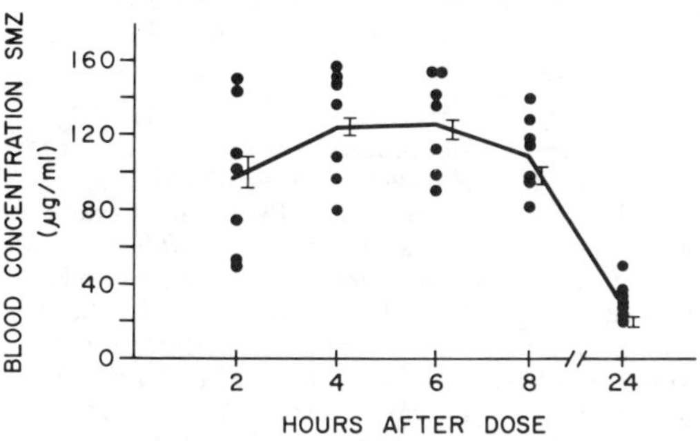

FIG. 2. *Distribution and mean levels of sulfamethoxazole (micrograms per milliliter) in the blood of seven volunteers after a single oral dose of nine tablets of trimethoprim-sulfamethoxazole (±1 standard error of the mean represented by vertical bars).*

the previously reported levels and persisted during the first 8 h after ingestion of the drug.

A recent in vitro investigation has demonstrated that 90 to 95% of clinical isolates of *Neisseria gonorrhoeae* are susceptible to TMP and SMZ at concentrations of 2.5 and 47.5 μg/ml, respectively (13). The present regimen of a single oral dose of nine tablets of TMP-SMZ achieved levels in the blood that easily exceeded these minimal inhibitory concentrations.

It would then appear that a treatment schedule of nine tablets of TMP-SMZ as a single oral dose may be a useful therapeutic regimen for patients with uncomplicated gonorrhea and susceptible microorganisms. Moreover, this would be especially important in individuals allergic to penicillin, tetracycline, or spectinomycin or in those who are treatment failures with these standard forms of therapy. Recently, there has been reported a clinical trial of nine tablets of TMP-SMZ as a single oral dose in males with gonococcal urethritis (W. C. Elliott, M. F. Rein, G. H. Reynolds, C. Thornsberry, H. W. Jaffe, and J. H. Armstrong, Prog. Abstr. Intersci. Conf. Antimicrob. Agents Chemother., 15th, Washington, D.C., Abstr. 391, 1975). In this study, there was an inordinately high failure rate of 25% with this TMP-SMZ regimen. Additional clinical trials will obviously be necessary to confirm these results. Furthermore, studies in women with uncomplicated gonorrhea using this TMP-SMZ dose schedule are lacking and need to be pursued.

ACKNOWLEDGMENT

We express our appreciation to Adrienne Bigcas for preparation of this manuscript.

LITERATURE CITED

1. **Arya, O. P., C. H. Pearson, and R. Blowers.** 1970. Treatment of gonorrhoea with trimethoprim-sulfamethoxazole in Uganda. Br. J. Vener. Dis. **46**:214–216.
2. **Austin, T. W., G. F. Brooks, M. Bethel, F. L. Roberts, M. Turck, and K. K. Holmes.** 1973. Trimethoprim-sulfamethoxazole in the treatment of gonococcal urethritis; clinical and laboratory correlates. J. Infect. Dis. **128**(Suppl.):S666–S672.
3. **Brumfitt, W., and R. Pursell.** 1973. Trimethoprim-sulfamethoxazole in the treatment of bacteriuria in women. J. Infect. Dis. **128**(Suppl.):S657–S663.
4. **Csonka, G. W., and G. J. Knight.** 1967. Therapeutic trial of trimethoprim as a potentiator of sulphonamides in gonorrhoea. Br. J. Vener. Dis. **43**:161–165.
5. **Kaplan, S. A., R. E. Weinfeld, and C. W. Abruzzo.** 1970. Biological availability and biological equivalence. Adv. Automated Analyses **2**:405–411.
6. **Kaplan, S. A., R. E. Weinfeld, C. W. Abruzzo, K. McFaden, M. L. Jack, and L. Weissman.** 1973. Pharmacokinetic profile of trimethoprim-sulfamethoxazole in man. J. Infect. Dis. **128**(Suppl.):S547–S566.
7. **Lawrence, A., I. Phillips, and C. Nicol.** 1973. Various regimens of trimethoprim-sulfamethoxazole used in the treatment of gonorrhea. J. Infect. Dis. **128**(Suppl.):S673–S678.
8. **Mahony, J. D. H., J. S. McCann, and J. R. W. Harris.** 1973. Comparison of trimethoprim-sulphamethoxazole and penicillin in the treatment of gonorrhoea. Br. J. Vener. Dis. **49**:517–520.
9. **Schofield, C. B. S., G. Masterton, M. Moffett, and M. I. McGill.** 1971. Gonorrhea in women: treatment with sulfamethoxazole and trimethoprim. J. Infect. Dis. **124**:533–538.
10. **Schwartz, D. E., B. A. Koechlin, and R. E. Weinfeld.** 1969. Spectrofluorimetric method for the determination of trimethoprim in body fluids. Chemotherapy **14**(Suppl.):22–29.
11. **Ullman, S., A. M. Niordson, and H. Zachariac.** 1971. Trimethoprim-sulphamethoxazole in gonorrhoea. Acta Dermato-Venerol. **51**:394–396.
12. **Wright, D. J. M., and A. S. Grimble.** 1970. Sulphamethoxazole combined with 2-4-diaminopyrimidines in the treatment of gonorrhoea. Br. J. Vener. Dis. **46**:34–36.
13. **Yoshikawa, T. T., S. Miyamoto, and L. B. Guze.** 1975. Comparison of in vitro susceptibility of *Neisseria gonorrhoeae* to trimethoprim-sulfamethoxazole on three different media. Antimicrob. Agents Chemother. **8**:515–517.

ANTIMICROBIAL AGENTS AND CHEMOTHERAPY, Sept 1976, p. 464-466

Vol. 10, No. 3
Printed in U.S.A.

Effect of Renal Failure and Dialysis on the Serum Concentration of the Aminoglycoside Amikacin

T. MADHAVAN,* K. YAREMCHUK, N. LEVIN, D. POHLOD, K. BURCH, E. FISHER, F. COX, AND E. L. QUINN

Division of Infectious Disease and Division of Nephrology, Henry Ford Hospital, Detroit, Michigan 48202, and University of Michigan, Ann Arbor, Michigan 48104*

Received for publication 12 January 1976

Serum and dialysate levels of amikacin were determined at appropriate intervals after a 300-mg intravenous dose as a continuous infusion in six patients with end-stage renal failure undergoing hemodialysis and in three patients on peritoneal dialysis. The mean serum half-life of amikacin was 3.75 h during (or after) hemodialysis and 29 h during (or after) peritoneal dialysis. Although not on hemodialysis in the same six patients, the serum half-life was 28 h. The results indicate that the maintenance dose of amikacin should be markedly decreased in patients with severe renal failure even if they are treated with peritoneal dialysis, and that serial serum antibiotic concentrations are essential to prevent cumulative toxicity of the drug.

Amikacin is a new aminoglycoside antibiotic with an antibacterial spectrum comparable to gentamicin and tobramycin (3, 4). Since aminoglycosides are excreted mainly through the kidney and not metabolized in the body, their toxic effects are increased in renal failure. However, these antibiotics may be the only available agents to treat life-threatening infections. It, therefore, is important to know how renal failure and renal dialysis effect the pharmacology of amikacin. We accordingly determined the serum concentration, half-life, and dialysate concentration of amikacin in patients with renal failure who were being dialyzed, and the results are the subject of this report.

MATERIALS AND METHODS

Patient selection. Studies were performed in six patients undergoing a 4-h hemodialysis using two Cordis-Dow model no. 4 hollow fiber kidneys. Blood flow during dialysis was approximately 200 ml/min, and dialysate flow was 500 ml/min. Three patients who were being treated with peritoneal dialysis using Impersol solution run at 2 liters/h for 48 h were studied. The patients had stable creatinine clearance values below 10 mg/min.

Patients with congestive heart failure, concurrent hepatic disease, and acute blood loss were excluded from this study. The age, sex, body weight, serum creatinine, total protein, and serum albumin levels in six patients with end-stage renal disease on hemodialysis are summarized in Table 1. All patients were evaluated before and 1 week after amikacin administration for adverse effects, and no changes were found in the histories and physical examinations, blood count, urinalysis, bilirubin, serum glutamic oxalacetic transaminase, alkaline phosphatase, serum protein, serum albumin, creatinine, blood urea nitrogen, and serum electrolytes.

Collection of specimens. Patients on hemodialysis. A single dose of 300 mg of amikacin was administered intravenously (i.v.) over a period of 60 min starting 75 min before the onset of dialysis. Blood samples were drawn at the beginning of dialysis and thereafter at 5, 30, 90, 210, and 270 min and 12 and 24 h. The dialysate was collected and pooled. Volumes were measured, and a 20-ml sample was taken for antibiotic assay and then frozen immediately. The same dose of amikacin was given 10 to 14 days later to the same six patients on a day when the patient was not on dialysis, and serial blood samples were collected for antibiotic assay.

Patients on peritoneal dialysis. Three patients were given a single 300-mg dose of amikacin over a period of 60 min starting 75 min before the initiation of peritoneal dialysis. Venous and arterial blood samples were drawn at 1, 2, 4, 6, 24, 30, and 48 h after the antibiotic infusion. The dialysate was pooled every 12 h through the 48th h. Total volume was measured, and 20-ml portions from each pool were frozen for subsequent antibiotic assay.

Determination of amikacin levels. Levels of amikacin were assayed by the modified cup plate method using *Bacillus subtilis* as the test organism (2). The regression lines of the logarithms of serum concentrations of amikacin versus time were calculated by the method of least squares to obtain the half-life in each patient, and their correlation coefficients (r) were determined.

RESULTS

Patients on hemodialysis. The mean serum concentrations after i.v. administration of a single dose of 300 mg of amikacin to six patients on hemodialysis are shown in Fig. 1. The mean

TABLE 1. *Patient data (hemodialysis)*

Patient	Age	Sex	Body wt (pounds)	Serum creatinine (mg%)	Serum protein concn	
					Total	Albumin
E.D.	53	M	153 (ca. 69.5 kg)	12.9	12.9	4.0
S.R.	29	F	138 (ca. 62.5 kg)	15.5	6.5	3.8
D.S.	53	F	152 (ca. 68.8 kg)	16	6.2	3.0
J.M.	42	M	157 (ca. 71.0 kg)	19.2	6.9	3.4
R.S.	44	M	139 (ca. 62.9 kg)	15.2	7.1	3.5
G.A.	54	F	138 (ca. 62.5 kg)	11.3	ND[a]	ND

[a] ND, Not done.

serum concentration obtained 0.5 h after the end of infusion (after equilibration) was 13.8 μg/ml. The mean serum concentrations at 3.5 and 4 h were 7.9 and 7.8 μg/ml, respectively. The serum half-life was 3 h and 45 min.

The average concentration of amikacin in the dialysate was 1.2 μg/ml (0.74 to 2.2 μg/ml), and the average recovery of amikacin in 4 h in the dialysate fluid was 158 mg (87.0 to 243 mg), or 53% of the administered dose (29 to 81%).

The same six patients were given 300 mg of amikacin i.v. 10 to 14 days after the initial determinations while not on dialysis, and the results are shown in Fig. 2. The mean serum concentration obtained was 15.8 μg/ml 0.5 h after the end of infusion. A mean serum concentration of 15.4 μg/ml was found at 3.5 h. The calculated half-life was 28 h.

Patients on peritoneal dialysis. Patients were given a single 300-mg dose of amikacin just before the beginning of peritoneal dialysis. At 1 and 4 h, the mean serum concentrations were 17.2 and 14.3 μg/ml (equilibration having occurred), respectively. The concentration then gradually fell to 7.3 μg/ml at 24 h, 6.8 μg/ml at 30 h, and 4.5 μg/ml at 48 h (Fig. 3). The serum half-life was 29 h. The dialysate contained from 0.7 to 4.98 μg of amikacin per ml. An average of 20% of the administered dose was recovered in the first 12 h of dialysis, and 57% was recovered in 48 h.

DISCUSSION

Bodey et al. determined the serum amikacin concentrations in normal human volunteers after intramuscular and i.v. administration of a single dose of 300 mg of amikacin per m^2 (1). The highest mean serum concentration after intramuscular administration was 25.4 μg/ml, obtained at 30 min. The serum half-life was 2.8

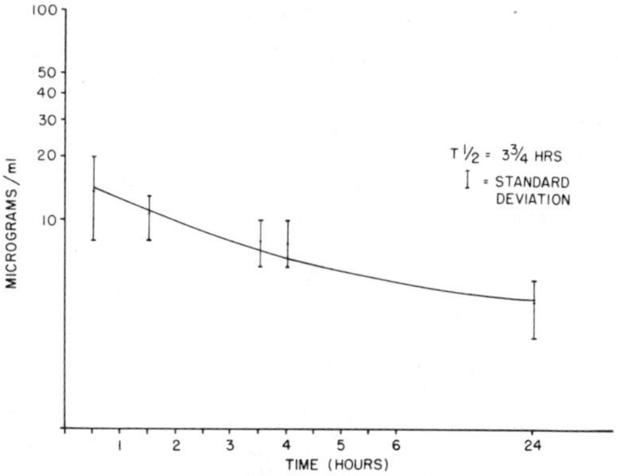

FIG. 1. *The mean serum concentrations and serum half-life (T-1/2) of amikacin after i.v. administration of a single dose of 300 mg to six patients on hemodialysis.*

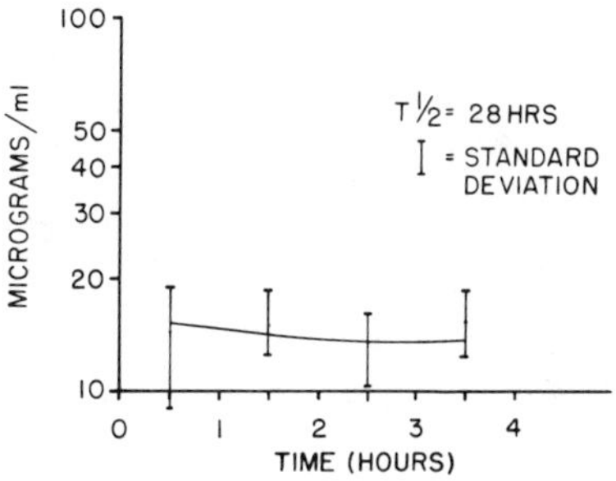

FIG. 2. *The mean serum concentrations and serum half-life of amikacin after i.v. administration of a single dose of 300 mg in the same six patients while not on hemodialysis.*

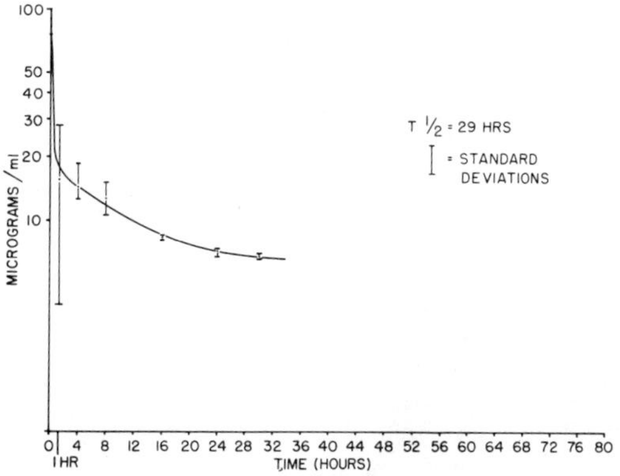

FIG. 3. *The mean serum concentration and serum half-life of amikacin after i.v. administration of a single dose of 300 mg to four patients on peritoneal dialysis.*

h. After a 15-min i.v. infusion of a similar dose, the peak concentration was 52.4 μg/ml at the end of infusion. The serum half-life was 2 h. Multiple doses of 150 mg of amikacin per m^2 every 6 h administered as a 30-min i.v. infusion yielded a mean peak serum concentration of 18.3 μg/ml on day 3 of therapy. The serum half-life was 1.7 h.

The present study revealed that in patients with severe renal failure (creatinine clearance less than 10 ml/min) given a single dose of amikacin, the serum concentration was similar to those with normal renal function. However, as expected, the half-life was prolonged to 28 h in these patients. Hemodialysis significantly reduced the half-life to 3 h and 45 min. On the other hand, peritoneal dialysis had little effect. Since the range of amikacin clearance varied from 29 to 81% of the administered dose, accurate predictions of serum levels in patients on hemodialysis are difficult, and monitoring the serum levels of aminoglycosides in critically ill patients is required to prevent cumulative toxicity of the drug.

ACKNOWLEDGMENTS

The study was supported by grants-in-aid from Bristol Laboratories.

LITERATURE CITED

1. **Bodey, G. P., M. Valdivieso, R. Feld, and V. Rodriquez.** 1974. Pharmacology of amikacin in humans. Antimicrob. Agents Chemother. 5:508–512.
2. **Grove, D., and W. Randall.** 1955. Assay methods of antibiotics: a laboratory manual p. 34–36. Antibiotics monograph no. 2. Med Encyclopedia, Inc., New York.
3. **Kawaguichi, H., T. Naito, S. Nakagawa, and K. Fujisawa.** 1972. BB-K8, a new semisynthetic aminoglycoside antibiotic. J. Antibiot. 25:695–708.
4. **Price, K. E., D. R. Chisholm, M. Misiek, F. Leitner, and Y. H. Tsai.** 1972. Microbiological evaluation of BB-K8, a new semi-synthetic aminoglycoside. J. Antibiot. 25:709–731.

Antimicrobial Agents and Chemotherapy, Sept. 1976, p. 467-469 Vol. 10, No. 3

Printed in U.S.A.

Comparison of Thrombophlebitis Associated with Three Cephalosporin Antibiotics

W. T. SIEBERT,[1]* E. L. WESTERMAN, J. D. SMILACK, M. W. BRADSHAW, and T. W. WILLIAMS, JR.

Department of Medicine, Baylor College of Medicine and The Methodist Hospital, Houston, Texas 77030

Received for publication 4 March 1976

A double-blind study with volunteers was performed to determine the incidence and severity of thrombophlebitis associated with cephalothin, cephapirin, cefamandole, and a water control. Although there were no statistical differences in the incidence of thrombophlebitis, cephalothin resulted in significantly more severe thrombophlebitis compared with the other agents.

The intravenous administration of cephalothin is associated with a high incidence of thrombophlebitis (7, 8). Cephapirin is a newer cephalosporin similar in bacterial spectrum to cephalothin (1). In single-blind studies, investigators found that cephapirin caused less thrombophlebitis than that reported for cephalothin (2, 5). In two reported double-blind studies, Inagaki and Bodey found a significant reduction in thrombophlebitis with cephapirin; however, this could not be substantiated by Carrizosa et al. (3, 4). The inability to perform a truly controlled study in patients because of the need for other intravenous medications perhaps contributed to these conflicting data. Cefamandole is a new cephalosporin with a somewhat broader gram-negative spectrum than that of cephalothin (6). There are no studies comparing the incidence of thrombophlebitis with cefamandole to other cephalosporin antibiotics. We undertook a double-blind study in normal volunteers to determine the incidence and severity of thrombophlebitis associated with the administration of cephalothin, cephapirin, cefamandole, and a vehicle control.

MATERIALS AND METHODS

Prior to performance, the study was reviewed and approved by four experimentation committees. After a detailed explanation, informed consent was obtained from 16 male volunteers with a negative history of penicillin and cephalosporin hypersensitivity. A continuous infusion of 5% dextrose and 0.2% sodium chloride at 1,000 ml/day was started in each volunteer via a 21-gauge "scalp vein" needle. Each volunteer served as his own control and received three cephalosporin antibiotics and a control vehicle in a sequential, randomized manner. The medications and dosages administered were: (i) cephalothin, 2 g every 6 h; (ii) cephapirin, 2 g every 6 h; (iii) cefamandole, 2 g every 6 h; and (iv) sterile water control, 20 ml every 6 h. The medications were given intravenously via Soluset in a total volume of 100 ml over a 30-min period. A 2-day rest period separated each 5-day infusion period.

The infusion site was examined and scored twice daily by two independent observers without knowledge of the medication received or the other observers' score. Thrombophlebitis was graded from 0 to +4 according to the following scale: 0, no evidence of thrombophlebitis; +1, erythema and tenderness along the vein less than 2.5 cm above the infusion site; +2, erythema and mild tenderness along the vein more than 2.5 cm above the infusion site; +3, erythema and moderate discomfort along the vein more than 2.5 cm above the infusion site; and +4, erythema and severe discomfort along the vein more than 2.5 cm above the infusion site. When a +4 score was rendered, the intravenous infusion was stopped, and hot soaks and elevation were applied to the affected arm. In all cases, the discomfort and inflammation abated within 24 h. If infiltration of fluids into subcutaneous tissue occurred, the infusion site was changed to the opposite arm.

RESULTS

Each volunteer received a morning and evening thrombophlebitis score for a total of 5 days. If +4 thrombophlebitis was graded, a +4 score was given for all subsequent grades. Only 3 of 16 volunteers receiving cephapirin and water, 1 of 16 receiving cephalothin, and 0 of 16 receiving cefamandole had no thrombophlebitis. Table 1 shows the mean thrombophlebits score for the three cephalosporins and water for each day of the study. The results were analyzed by the Friedman descriptive two-way analysis of variance by ranks. There were no statistical differences in the first 3 days of therapy, but by day 4 cephalothin reached a significantly higher mean of thrombophlebitis ($P < 0.01$),

[1] Address reprint requests to: W. T. Siebert, 6516 Bertner Blvd., Houston, TX 77030.

TABLE 1. *Descriptive statistics and results of the Friedman two-way analysis of variance by ranks*

Treatment	Severity score on day:									High[a]	Count[b]
	1 (p.m.)	2 (a.m.)	2 (p.m.)	3 (a.m.)	3 (p.m.)	4 (a.m.)	4 (p.m.)	5 (a.m.)	5 (p.m.)		
Cefamandole											
Mean	0.13	0.31	0.31	0.69	0.19	0.56	0.31	0.25	0.31	1.69	2.13
SD[c]	0.50	0.60	0.60	1.14	0.40	0.89	0.60	0.58	0.60	0.79	1.31
n	16	16	16	16	16	16	16	16	16	16	16
Cephapirin											
Mean	0.06	0.31	0.50	0.31	0.69	0.63	0.81	0.69	1.13	1.56	3.06
SD	0.25	0.60	0.73	0.60	0.95	1.09	1.17	1.20	1.54	1.36	2.84
n	16	16	16	16	16	16	16	16	16	16	16
Cephalothin											
Mean	0.06	0.44	0.88	1.38	1.25	2.06	2.44	2.56	2.63	2.94	5.19
SD	0.25	0.81	1.02	1.41	1.44	1.69	1.63	1.67	1.59	1.29	2.48
n	16	16	16	16	16	16	16	16	16	16	16
"Water"											
Mean	0.00	0.63	0.25	0.56	0.50	0.38	0.44	0.38	0.31	1.31	2.69
SD	0.00	0.81	0.58	0.81	0.63	0.62	0.73	0.50	0.60	0.79	2.21
n	16	16	16	16	16	16	16	16	16	16	16
Friedman two-way ANOVA[d]											
Result	0.11	0.69	2.87	5.31	4.86	5.32	12.94	10.99	13.63	8.23	9.81
Significance	0.99	0.87	0.41	0.15	0.18	0.15	<0.01	0.01	<0.01	0.04	0.02

[a] High, The highest score each patient received during a treatment period.
[b] Count, The number of non-zero severity score periods; total of +1 → +4 scores.
[c] SD, Standard deviation.
[d] ANOVA, Analysis of variance.

which was maintained throughout the duration of the study.

Infiltration of intravenous fluid was not a significant problem. Of the infusions that needed to be restarted, equal numbers appeared in the cephalothin, cephapirin, cefamandole, and water groups.

DISCUSSION

Although there were no significant differences in the incidence of thrombophlebitis resulting from infusion of water, cephapirin, cefamandole, and cephalothin, there was a statistically significant difference in the severity of thrombophlebitis. Cephalothin produced more severe thrombophlebitis than cephapirin, cefamandole, or water. There were no statistical differences in the severity of thrombophlebitis caused by cephapirin, cefamandole, and water.

Disadvantages of previously reported thrombophlebitis studies have been lack of control to assess incidence and severity of thrombophlebitis from the infusion vehicle alone (3–5) and inability to use each patient as his own control (4). The administration of water and each cephalosporin to all volunteers in the study circumvented these difficulties. The almost uniform need for other intravenous medications, the presence of other diseases, and the inability to assess the contribution of the vehicle alone restrict a controlled study to a volunteer population.

Our results are in agreement with those of Lane et al. (5) and Inagaki and Bodey (4) but in contrast with those of Carrizosa et al. (3). The most likely explanation for the difference is the duration of the study. Following the example of Lane et al. (5), we used a 5-day infusion period. In our experience, significant cephalothin thrombophlebitis occurred only at 72 h or later. Since Carrizosa stopped his study at 48 h, this may have been too short a time for the development of full cephalothin thrombophlebitis. There do not appear to be any major differences in the severity of thrombophlebitis caused by water, cephapirin, and cefamandole.

Our current study demonstrates that cephapirin and cefamandole produce less severe inflammation than cephalothin when evaluated in a 5-day infusion period. If pharmacological and microbiological parameters prove to be equal, it would appear that cephapirin and cefamandole are more desirable intravenous cephalosporins than cephalothin.

ACKNOWLEDGMENTS

This work was supported by grant RR-00350 from the General Clinical Research Centers Program of the Division of Research Resources, and Eli Lilly and Co., Indianapolis.

We are indebted to the nursing staff of the General Clinical Research Center, and to D. Kirkpatrick, Director of Treatment, C. Jeffries, Warden L. Beaird, and Medical Officer D. G. Donnell of the Texas Department of Corrections for their technical assistance. The volunteers are to be commended for their participation in the research program. We are grateful for the technical assistance of R. L. Brunelle in performing the statistical evaluation, and for the help, in manuscript preparation, of Donnadel DeClaris and Thelma Armstrong.

LITERATURE CITED

1. **Axelrod, J., B. R. Meyers, and S. Z. Hirschman.** 1971. Cephapirin: in vitro antibacterial spectrum. Appl. Microbiol. **22**:904–908.
2. **Bran, J. L., M. E. Levison, and D. Kaye.** 1972. Clinical and in vitro evaluation of cephapirin: a new cephalosporin antibiotic. Antimicrob. Agents Chemother. **1**:35–40.
3. **Carrizosa, J., M. E. Levison, and D. Kaye.** 1972. Double-blind controlled comparison of phlebitis produced by cephapirin and cephalothin. Antimicrob. Agents Chemother. **3**:306–307.
4. **Inagaki, J., and G. P. Bodey.** 1973. Phlebitis associated with cephalosporins: cephapirin versus cephalothin. Curr. Ther. Res. **15**:37–43.
5. **Lane, A. Z., J. G. Taggart, and R. L. Iles.** 1972. Relative incidence of phlebitis caused by continuous intravenous infusion of cephapirin and cephalothin. Antimicrob. Agents Chemother. **2**:234–235.
6. **Neu, H. C.** 1974. Cefamandole, a new cephalosporin antibiotic with an unusually wide spectrum of activity. Antimicrob. Agents Chemother. **6**:177–182.
7. **Perkins, R. L., and S. Saslaw.** 1966. Experiences with cephalothin. Ann. Intern. Med. **64**:13–24.
8. **Storey, G.** 1971. Clinical manifestations of chancroid. Br. J. Urol. **42**:738.

ANTIMICROBIAL AGENTS AND CHEMOTHERAPY, Sept. 1976, p. 470-475
Vol. 10, No. 3

Substrate Inhibition of Beta-Lactamases, a Method for Predicting Enzymatic Stability of Cephalosporins

DAVID F. MAHONEY, G. A. KOPPEL, AND J. R. TURNER*

Lilly Research Laboratories, Eli Lilly & Co., Indianapolis, Indiana 46206

Received for publication 28 April 1976

Selected cephalosporins, including cefamandole, cephaloridine, cephaloglycin, and cefoxitin, were examined for their ability to inhibit the enzymatic activity of and act as substrates for beta-lactamases produced by *Enterobacter cloacae* and *Staphylococcus aureus*. Enzyme inhibition was determined by Michaelis-Menten kinetic measurements and by a spot plate assay using a chromogenic substrate (Glaxo compound 87/312). These two methods provide comparable estimates of kinetic parameters. Inhibition of beta-lactamase, as measured by these two methods, was generally found to correlate with resistance to hydrolysis and is proposed as a preliminary method of assessing susceptibility of cephalosporins to beta-lactamase hydrolysis. Four 7-αOCH_3, 7-αH cephalosporin analogue pairs were also examined. The presence of the 7-αOCH_3 substituent invariably resulted in reduced susceptibility to enzymatic hydrolysis, regardless of the other C7 substituent. The 7-αOCH_3 compounds were also better inhibitors than were their 7-αH analogues, with the exception that 7-αOCH_3 compounds having C7 adipic acid substituents were less inhibitory to the *S. aureus* enzyme than were the corresponding 7-αH analogues. Response of these two enzymes to 7-αOCH_3 and 7-αH cephalosporins suggests that beta-lactamase hydrolysis of these compounds involves attack at the alpha side of the beta-lactam ring.

Two naturally occurring 7-α-methoxycephalosporins, 7-α-methoxycephalosporin C and deacetyl-3-*O*-carbamoyl-7-α-methoxycephalosporin C, were originally isolated from two species of *Streptomyces* by Nagarajan et al. (9). Both antibiotics exhibited greater activity against gram-negative organisms than did cephalosporin C or deacetyl-3-*O*-carbamoylcephalosporin C, their 7-hydrogen analogues, and the carbamoyloxymethyl derivative was reported (18) to be more active against gram-negative than gram-positive bacteria. Cefoxitin, a thienylacetyl derivative of deacetyl-3-*O*-carbamoyl-7-α-methoxycephalosporin C, has been reported to have activity against gram-positive and gram-negative organisms (21). This 7-methoxylated cephalosporin generally showed resistance to the action of beta-lactamases from both gram-positive and gram-negative bacteria (14), and it was suggested that this characteristic contributed to the broad antimicrobial spectrum observed. There is considerable disagreement as to the relative importance of beta-lactamases in bacterial resistance to beta-lactam antibiotics (20). Because of the lack of uniform correlation between in vitro minimal inhibitory concentration values and lability of these compounds to enzymatic hydrolysis (1, 10, 11), this lability, by itself, is not sufficient evidence to predict bacterial susceptibility. Despite this, it is probable that the action of these enzymes does contribute to resistance although not always as the limiting factor. Given this assumption, the affinity of a beta-lactamase for a given cephalosporin should play a role in overall resistance of a beta-lactamase-producing organism. The affinity (K_m) can be measured directly by using the compound as substrate or alternatively can be estimated from the K_i as determined from inhibition studies. Estimation of affinity by the latter method is particularly useful with beta-lactamases because many interesting cephalosporins are hydrolyzed at such low rates that accurate measurement of K_m values is not possible. The discovery of a chromogenic substrate for beta-lactamase (12), compound 87/312, has made this type of evaluation relatively straightforward since hydrolysis of 87/312 can be followed spectrophotometrically and is a good substrate for essentially all beta-lactamases.

This report describes a spot plate assay for beta-lactamase inhibition and shows a comparison of the results to standard kinetic inhibitor studies. Data are also presented that show some effects of the 7-α-OCH_3 substituent in cephalosporins on their stability and capacity to inhibit beta-lactamases.

(This report was presented in part at the 15th Interscience Conference on Antimicrobial Agents and Chemotherapy, Washington, D.C., 24–26 September 1975.)

MATERIALS AND METHODS

Organisms. *Enterobacter cloacae* 265A was obtained from the culture collection of Lilly Research Laboratories. The beta-lactamase-producing, methicillin-resistant *Staphylococcus aureus* 13136 was provided by M. Richmond and is a type A variant (16). Both organisms were maintained on Trypticase soy agar (BBL). Cultures for preparation of beta-lactamase were grown at 37°C in Trypticase soy broth (BBL).

Antibiotics. Cephaloridine, cephaloglycin, cefamandole, D-*O*-formyl cefamandole, L-*O*-formyl cefamandole, and compounds II (3-carbamoyloxymethyl-7-[2-(thienyl)acetamido]-3-cephem-4-carboxylic acid), III (7-[2-carboxy-2-phenylacetamido]-7-α-methoxycephalosporanic acid), and IV (7-[2-carboxy-2-phenylacetamido]cephalosporanic acid) were supplied by Lilly Research Laboratories. Cefoxitin (compound I) was obtained from Merck Sharp & Dohme, West Point, Pa. Cephalosporin C (compound VI) and compounds V (7-α-methoxycephalosporin C), VIII (deacetyl-3-*O*-carbamoylcephalosporin C), and VII were derived from or are fermentation products isolated at Lilly Research Laboratories. The chromogenic cephalosporin substrate compound 87/312 was obtained from Glaxo Research Ltd., Greenford, Middlesex, England.

Beta-lactamase purification. The beta-lactamase (Richmond type I) from *E. cloacae* 265A was purified in a manner similar to that described for *E. cloacae* P99 (17), except that chromatography was performed on diethylaminoethyl-Sephadex (Pharmacia Fine Chemicals, Inc., Piscataway, N.J.), pH 7.5, instead of QAE-Sephadex. The *S. aureus* 13136 beta-lactamase was purified according to a modification of a previous method (15). The modification consisted of the induction of midlog-phase cells with 1 mg of penicillin G (Eli Lilly & Co., Indianapolis, Ind.) per ml for 2.5 h at 37°C, adsorption of the 13136 enzyme on cellulose phosphate (grade P-11, Whatman), and subsequent elution with 2 M tris(hydroxymethyl)aminomethane-hydrochloride (Sigma Chemical Co., St. Louis, Mo.) buffer, pH 7.5. Fractions with detectable beta-lactamase activity were pooled, and bovine serum albumin (Calbiochem, Los Angeles, Calif.) was added to 0.07 mg of protein per ml. The 13136 enzyme was immediately dialyzed overnight (with one change) against 0.1 M sodium acetate buffer, pH 5.9. Portions (1 ml) were frozen and stored under liquid nitrogen.

Protein determination. Protein was determined by the method of Lowry et al. (8).

Enzymatic hydrolysis of cephalosporins. Hydrolysis rates of cephalosporins for both enzymes were determined by monitoring the optical density at the wavelength associated with maximum absorption of the beta-lactam ring (13). The maximum absorption varied slightly among the compounds examined, but all were within the range from 260 to 270 nm. The relative hydrolysis rate (RHR) is the rate as a percentage of the cephaloridine rate.

The reaction mixture for determination of the hydrolysis rate consisted of 0.4 ml of bovine serum albumin (0.5 mg of protein per ml of solution in 0.05 M $NaPO_4$, pH 7.0), 0.15 mg of substrate (dissolved in 0.05 M $NaPO_4$, pH 7.0), an appropriate amount of enzyme to give linear rates, and sufficient 0.05 M $NaPO_4$ buffer, pH 7.0, to give a total volume of 3.0 ml. The reaction mixture was placed in a 3-ml (1-cm light path) cuvette, and the optical density was monitored in a Gilford recording spectrophotometer equipped with thermal spacers to maintain temperature at 37°C. Hydrolysis rates were determined from the decrease in optical density that occurred during the first 5 min of the reaction.

Kinetic measurements. Determination of K_i for the various cephalosporins was made by assessing the ability of these antibiotics to inhibit the hydrolysis of compound 87/312. Reaction mixtures identical to that described above were used, except that 87/312 was used as the substrate and the optical density was measured at 482 nm. Inhibition constants (K_i) were determined from either Lineweaver-Burk (7) or Dixon plots (2).

Spot plate assay for determination of inhibition. Utilizing 87/312 as substrate, a spot plate assay was developed for the identification of cephalosporins that inhibit beta-lactamases. The assay is based on visual observation of the extent of hydrolysis of the chromogenic substrate 87/312 in the presence of a decreasing concentration of the putative inhibitor. Spot tests with 87/312 have previously been employed solely for the detection and quantitation of beta-lactamase activity (6, 12).

Cephalosporin solutions were prepared at concentrations of 2 mg/ml (or greater) in 0.05 M $NaPO_4$, pH 7.0, buffer. A portion (100 μl) of this solution was placed in a well of a spot plate (model 96U-WS; Linbro Chemical Co., Inc., New Haven, Conn.), and the cephalosporin concentration was serially diluted 1:5 by the sequential transfer, with an Eppendorf pipette, of 20 μl of solution to wells containing 80 μl of 0.05 M $NaPO_4$ buffer, pH 7.0. Enzyme (0.005 U) was then added to each well and mixed, and the mixture was incubated for 10 min at room temperature. One unit is the amount of enzyme required to hydrolyze 1 μmol of 87/312 in 1 min at 37°C and pH 7.0. A 20-μl amount of the chromogenic substrate 87/312 (0.516 mg/ml in 0.05 M $NaPO_4$, pH 7.0) was then added to each well and incubation was continued at room temperature. The final volume in each well was 120 μl. The end point for inhibition was read at 5 min after the addition of 87/312 and is defined as the highest concentration of the inhibitor that had no observable effect on the hydrolysis of 87/312. These end points are quite stable after a 5-min incubation period. To aid in end point determination, control wells that did not contain enzyme or inhibitor were included, and these were compared with test wells.

RESULTS

Substrate and inhibitor specificity. Since 87/312 plays an important role in the determination of K_i, as well as end point, the kinetic constants (K_m and V_{max}) for this compound are given in Table 1. The beta-lactamase from *S. aureus* that normally does not hydrolyze cephalosporins very rapidly can hydrolyze 87/312 at a relatively rapid rate. This substrate appears to be hydrolyzed at rates in excess of most cephalosporins that we have examined.

The beta-lactamases from *E. cloacae* 265A and *S. aureus* 13136 were characterized by their substrate specificity and inhibition, by assay against a selected group of cephalosporins (Table 2). End points obtained from the spot plate assay were compared with K_i values determined by kinetic measurements. The spot plate end points and K_i values are expressed as 10^{-6} M for each enzyme. End point and K_i values for the *E. cloacae* 265A and *S. aureus* 13136 enzymes were either very close or within fourfold of each other for a given compound. Since serial 1:5 dilutions of the inhibitors were used, this correlation is well within the resolution of the spot plate assay and shows good agreement between the spot plate and kinetic measurements.

Significant quantitative differences in inhibition between the two enzymes were observed in the presence of some compounds. Cephaloridine and cefamandole are potent inhibitors of the 13136 enzyme as judged by low end point and K_i values, although cephaloridine is a relatively poor inhibitor of the 265A enzyme, with an end point of 6.37×10^{-4} M and a K_i value of 9.68×10^{-4} M. The D and L isomers of *O*-formyl cefamandole did not show large differences in ability to inhibit the 13136 enzyme although a fivefold difference in end point appears for the 265A enzyme, indicating that a change in configuration from L to D has a slightly greater effect on the 265A enzyme. Cephaloglycin, which is quite resistant to enzymatic hydrolysis, shows the lowest affinity for the 13136 enzyme while having a similar affinity for the 265A enzyme as do three other compounds in this group.

TABLE 1. *Kinetics of hydrolysis of 87/312 by β-lactamases from strains 265A and 13136*

Source of β-lactamase	K_m (μM)	V_{max}[a]
E. cloacae 265A	195	170
S. aureus 13136	5.68	0.13

[a] Micromoles per minute per milligram of protein.

The inhibition of these two enzymes is also qualitatively different. The 13136 enzyme was competitively inhibited by all the cephalosporins in this group. The 265A enzyme, however, showed competitive inhibition only by cephaloridine, whereas the other four compounds acted as noncompetitive inhibitors.

Since all of these compounds show some degree of affinity for beta-lactamases, one might be able to predict beta-lactamase stability of beta-lactams by measuring their ability to inhibit these enzymes. In Table 2, the RHRs are given for these cephalosporins. For comparison, the hydrolysis rates were normalized to the hydrolysis rate of cephaloridine. There is a good correlation between the ability of a compound to inhibit the 265A enzyme and the lability of that compound to hydrolysis. That is, those compounds that are good substrates, such as cephaloridine and D-*O*-formyl cefamandole, tend to be poor inhibitors as judged by high K_i values and high spot plate end points, whereas cephaloglycin, cefamandole, and L-*O*-formyl cefamandole are poor substrates but good inhibitors. This correlation does not appear to hold in all instances for the 13136 enzyme. For example, the data show approximately equal RHRs for cephaloridine and D-*O*-formyl cefamandole, although the K_i values are 100-fold different. We do not have sufficient data as yet to know whether this is a general characteristic of the 13136 enzyme.

Stability studies of 7-αOCH_3 cephalosporins. The usefulness of determining hydrolysis rates and kinetic parameters in the study of the interaction between beta-lactamases and beta-

TABLE 2. *Comparison of spot plate end points, K_i, and RHR*

Compound	*E. cloacae* 265A			*S. aureus* 13136		
	End point (μM)	K_i (μM)	RHR	End point (μM)	K_i (μM)	RHR
Cephaloridine	637	968	100[a]	0.20	0.14	100[a]
Cephaloglycin	5.25	5.35	4	131	39.1	0
Cefamandole	4.55	4.40	1	0.91	0.25	23
D-*O*-formyl cefamandole	20.8	10.3	13	4.16	14.8	71
L-*O*-formyl cefamandole	4.16	4.41	0	4.16	6.33	21

[a] Micromoles per minute per milligram of protein relative to the rate obtained with cephaloridine.

lactam antibiotics is shown in Table 3. The structure of each cephalosporin is given in Fig. 1. The results (Table 3) show the effect of the 7-αOCH_3 group on hydrolysis by and inhibition of the beta-lactamases from strains 265A and 13136. Each 7-αOCH_3 cephalosporin is paired with its 7-αH analogue. As seen before, spot plate end points correlated well with K_i values obtained for the 265A enzyme and reasonably well with the 13136 enzyme. The 7-αOCH_3 cephalosporins, compounds V and VII, are weak inhibitors of the 13136 enzyme, whereas the 265A enzyme was inhibited by both compounds, with K_i values of 1.54×10^{-4} and 1.21×10^{-4} M, respectively. The 7-αH analogues, compounds VI (cephalosporin C) and VIII, are essentially ineffective inhibitors of the 13136 enzyme (K_i values could not be determined), with end point values of 1.61×10^{-2} M as opposed to end point values of about 6×10^{-4} M for their 7-αOCH_3 analogues, compounds V and VII. Following the pattern set by the other compounds, K_i values for compounds VI (cephalosporin C) and VIII were expected to be up to fivefold greater than their end point values, but could not be determined due to the insensitivity of the 13136 enzyme to these compounds. A K_i value for compound III could not be determined due to the limited solubility of the compound.

Substitution of -αOCH_3 for -αH in this group of compounds results in an increased affinity for the 265A enzyme. The magnitude of this change varies from 100-fold for compound I (cefoxitin) and its 7-αH analogue (compound II) to

TABLE 3. *Comparison of spot plate end points, K_i, and RHR, of 7-methoxycephalosporins and their 7-hydrogen analogues*

Compound	*E. cloacae* 265A			*S. aureus* 13136		
	End point (μM)	K_i (μM)	RHR	End point (μM)	K_i (μM)	RHR
I. 7-αOCH_3	0.95	0.52	0.3[a]	0.95	9.84	0[a]
II. 7-αH	25.4	75.0	287	<0.04	0.49	71
III. 7-αOCH_3	<0.04	0.01	0	22.9	ID[b]	0
IV. 7-αH	0.04	0.13	0.02	0.20	3.65	26
V. 7-αOCH_3	120	154	37	599	2,489	0
VI. 7-αH	129	359	180	16,103	ND[c]	79
VII. 7-αOCH_3	120	121	24	598	2,192	0
VIII. 7-αH	128	268	154	16,064	ND	92

[a] Micromoles per minute per milligram of protein relative to the rate obtained with cephaloridine (100).
[b] ID, Indeterminate (see text).
[c] ND, Not determined.

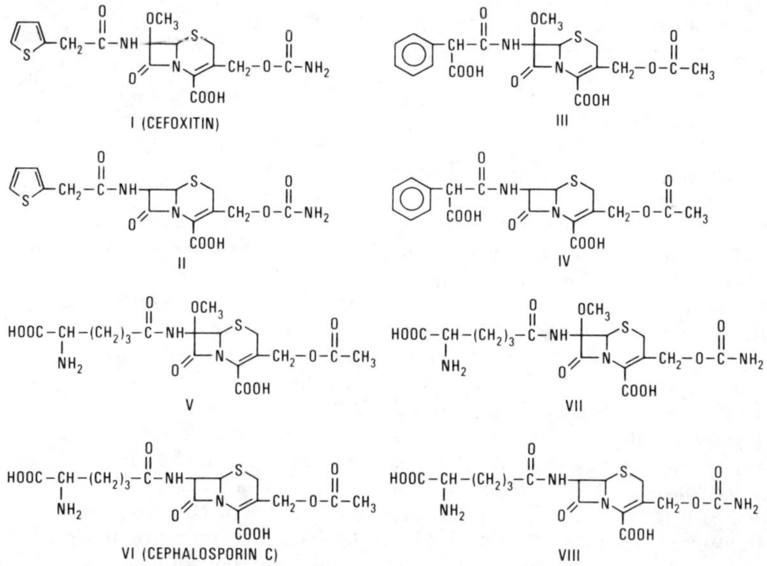

FIG. 1. *Structure of the 7-α-methoxycephalosporins and their 7-α-hydrogen analogues.*

about 2-fold for the compounds containing an adipic acid side chain. A similar increased affinity for the 13136 enzyme is seen with 7-αOCH_3-substituted compounds, providing that the adipic acid chain is also present. Affinity for the 13136 enzyme is reduced by the -αOCH_3 group when substituted on compounds having side chains other than adipic acid, that is, compounds I (cefoxitin) and III.

As opposed to the mixed response toward affinity caused by the substitution of 7-αH with 7-αOCH_3, the effect of this change on hydrolysis appears to be straightforward. In all cases, the compound containing the 7-αOCH_3 group is more resistant to hydrolysis than is its 7-αH analogue.

The type of inhibition found for both enzymes differs for this group of compounds (Table 4). For the first two analogue pairs, the 7-αH analogues (compounds II and IV) showed noncompetitive inhibition of the 265A enzyme and competitive inhibition of the 13136 enzyme. Compound I (cefoxitin) showed competitive inhibition with both enzymes. Unfortunately, the 7-αOCH_3 analogue of the second pair (compound III) could not be classified because of a nonlinear reaction rate in the presence of this compound. With the weaker inhibitors, i.e., the third and fourth analogue pairs, both 7-αOCH_3 and 7-αH compounds (compounds V through VIII) were competitive inhibitors of the 265A enzyme, whereas the 7-αOCH_3 analogues (compounds V and VII) showed noncompetitive inhibition of the 13136 enzyme. Inhibition of the 13136 enzyme by the 7-αH analogues of these two pairs (compounds VI and VIII) could not be classified because of the low affinity of these two compounds for the enzyme, as shown by the spot plate end points in Table 3.

TABLE 4. *Inhibition of 265A and 13136 β-lactamases by 7-αOCH₃ cephalosporins and their 7-αH analogues*

Compound	Type of inhibition	
	E. cloacae 265A	*S. aureus* 13136
I. 7-αOCH_3	Competitive	Competitive
II. 7-αH	Noncompetitive	Competitive
III. 7-αOCH_3	Non-Michaelis-Menten	ID[a]
IV. 7-αH	Noncompetitive	Competitive
V. 7-αOCH_3	Competitive	Noncompetitive
VI. 7-αH	Competitive	ND[b]
VII. 7-αOCH_3	Competitive	Noncompetitive
VIII. 7-αH	Competitive	ND

[a] ID, Indeterminate (see text).
[b] ND, Not determined.

DISCUSSION

As a preliminary step in the analysis of a new group of cephalosporins, the spot plate assay appears useful for predicting beta-lactamase stability since those compounds that were good inhibitors generally were stable to enzymatic hydrolysis. Exceptions to this were the responses of both enzymes to compound V and compound VII, where the K_i or end point (when K_i could not be determined) indicated weak inhibition ($\geqq 10^{-4}$ M) while the relative hydrolysis indicated good stability (<50% of cephaloridine). Another exception was found with both enzymes to compound II, where the K_i indicated good inhibition, but RHRs were high. Two other compounds, cephaloridine and D-*O*-formyl cefamandole, showed the same response to the 13136 enzyme, that is, good inhibition but relatively high hydrolysis rates. Overall, the hydrolysis rates for 10 of the 13 compounds correlated with affinity for the 265A enzyme, whereas hydrolysis rates for 8 of 13 compounds correlated with affinity for the 13136 enzyme. There is, of course, no a priori reason for a slow reaction velocity to be correlated with high affinity or vice versa. However, within the context of this study and generally with respect to the examination of beta-lactamases in which the numbers of potential substrates and enzymes are great, the observation that high affinity is generally associated with resistance to hydrolysis allows one to use a qualitative assay for inhibition to predict hydrolysis.

The reaction velocities and affinities found for the *Enterobacter* enzyme are in good agreement with preliminary studies of other gram-negative enzymes (D. Mahoney, unpublished data). The generally low activity of *S. aureus* enzymes against cephalosporins (12) probably is responsible for the slightly poorer correlation between affinity and reaction velocities found with this enzyme.

Substitution of 7-αH with 7-αOCH_3 in the cephalosporins examined here has a direct and unequivocal effect on enzymatic hydrolysis in that the 7-αOCH_3 analogue was always more resistant to enzymatic degradation. However, studies on the chemical hydrolysis of these compounds show that addition of a 7-αOCH_3 group has no effect on the stability of cephalosporins to nucleophiles because the beta-face of the beta-lactam ring remains open to attack (5). In contrast, the addition of a 6-αOCH_3 group to a penicillin results in chemical stability since both faces of the ring are then blocked. Since the rate of enzymatic hydrolysis is severely reduced by the addition of 7-αOCH_3 to cephalosporins, it seems reasonable that enzymatic attack may originate from the α-face rather than the beta-face of the beta-lactam ring and further that the beta-face may be inaccessible when the compound is bound to the enzyme.

Other related reports (3, 4) show that 7-αOCH_3-substituted cephalosporins are 10-fold better inhibitors of *Escherichia coli* transpeptidase than are their 7-αH analogues. The finding in this study that 7-αOCH_3-substituted cephalosporins invariably have greater affinity for the *Enterobacter* beta-lactamase and usually have greater affinity for the *S. aureus* beta-lactamase suggests again (19) the possibility that active centers on transpeptidase and beta-lactamase enzymes may share similar configurations. Therefore, a study of the mechanism by which compounds inhibit beta-lactamases may provide important information on the capability of these compounds to inhibit the activity of transpeptidases.

ACKNOWLEDGMENTS

We wish to thank Joseph M. Indelicato for his helpful discussions during preparation of this manuscript.

LITERATURE CITED

1. **Cornelis, G.** 1975. Distribution of β-lactamases A and B in some groups of *Yersinia enterocolitica* and their role in resistance. J. Gen. Microbiol. **91**:391–402.
2. **Dixon, M.** 1953. The determination of enzyme inhibitor constants. Biochem. J. **55**:170–171.
3. **Ho, P. P. K., R. D. Towner, J. M. Indelicato, W. A. Spitzer, and G. A. Koppel.** 1972. Biochemical and microbiological studies on 6-substituted penicillins. J. Antibiot. **25**:627–628.
4. **Ho, P. P. K., R. D. Towner, J. M. Indelicato, W. L. Wilham, W. A. Spitzer, and G. A. Koppel.** 1973. Biochemical and microbiological studies on 7-methoxycephalosporins. J. Antibiot. **26**:313–314.
5. **Indelicato, J. M., and W. L. Wilham.** 1974. Effect of 6-α substitution in penicillins and 7-α substitution in cephalosporins upon β-lactam reactivity. J. Med. Chem. **17**:528–529.
6. **Kammer, R. B., D. A. Preston, J. R. Turner, and L. C. Hawley.** 1975. Rapid detection of ampicillin-resistant *Haemophilus influenzae* and their susceptibility to sixteen antibiotics. Antimicrob. Agents Chemother. **8**:91–94.
7. **Lineweaver, H., and D. Burk.** 1934. The determination of enzyme dissociation constants. J. Am. Chem. Soc. **56**:658–666.
8. **Lowry, O. H., N. J. Rosebrough, A. L. Farr, and R. J. Randall.** 1951. Protein measurement with the Folin phenol reagent. J. Biol. Chem. **193**:265–275.
9. **Nagarajan, R., L. D. Boeck, M. Gorman, R. L. Hamill, C. E. Higgens, M. M. Hoehn, W. M. Stark, and J. G. Whitney.** 1971. β-Lactam antibiotics from *Streptomyces*. J. Am. Chem. Soc. **93**:2308–2310.
10. **Neu, H. C.** 1974. Cefoxitin, a semisynthetic cephamycin antibiotic: antibacterial spectrum and resistance to hydrolysis by gram-negative beta-lactamases. Antimicrob. Agents Chemother. **6**:170–176.
11. **Neu, H. C.** 1974. Cefamandole, a cephalosporin antibiotic with an unusually wide spectrum of activity. Antimicrob. Agents Chemother. **6**:177–182.
12. **O'Callaghan, C. H., A. Morris, S. M. Kirby, and A. H. Shingler.** 1972. Novel method for detection of β-lactamases by using a chromogenic cephalosporin substrate. Antimicrob. Agents Chemother. **1**:283–288.
13. **O'Callaghan, C. H., P. W. Muggleton, and G. W. Ross.** 1969. Effects of β-lactamase from gram-negative organisms on cephalosporins and penicillins, p. 57–63. Antimicrob. Agents Chemother. 1968.
14. **Onishi, H. R., D. R. Daonst, S. B. Zimmerman, D. Hendlin, and E. O. Stapley.** 1974. Cefoxitin, a semisynthetic cephamycin antibiotic: resistance to beta-lactamase inactivation. Antimicrob. Agents Chemother. **5**:38–48.
15. **Richmond, M. H.** 1963. Purification and properties of the exopenicillinase from *Staphylococcus aureus*. Biochem. J. **88**:452–459.
16. **Richmond, M. H.** 1965. Wild-type variants of exopenicillinase from *Staphylococcus aureus*. Biochem. J. **94**:584–593.
17. **Ross, G. W., and M. G. Boulton.** 1973. Purification of β-lactamases on QAE-Sephadex. Biochim. Biophys. Acta **309**:430–439.
18. **Stapley, E. O., M. Jackson, S. Hernandez, S. B. Zimmerman, S. A. Currie, S. Mochales, J. M. Mata, H. B. Woodruff, and D. Hendlin.** 1972. Cephamycins, a new family of β-lactam antibiotics. I. Production by Actinomyces, including *Streptomyces lactamdurans* sp. n. Antimicrob. Agents Chemother. **2**:122–131.
19. **Tipper, D. J., and J. L. Strominger.** 1965. Mechanism of action of penicillins: a proposal based on their structural similarity to acyl-D-alanyl-D-alanine. Proc. Natl. Acad. Sci. U.S.A. **54**:1133–1141.
20. **Tsang, J. C., G. A. Sansing, and M. A. Miller.** 1975. Relation of beta-lactamase activity to antimicrobial susceptibility in *Serratia marcescens*. Antimicrob. Agents Chemother. **8**:277–281.
21. **Wallick, H., and D. Hendlin.** 1974. Cefoxitin, a semisynthetic cephamycin antibiotic: susceptibility studies. Antimicrob. Agents Chemother. **5**:25–32.

ANTIMICROBIAL AGENTS AND CHEMOTHERAPY, Sept. 1976, p. 476-482
Vol. 10, No. 3

Antitrichomonad Action, Mutagenicity, and Reduction of Metronidazole and Other Nitroimidazoles

DONALD G. LINDMARK* AND MIKLÓS MÜLLER

The Rockefeller University, New York, New York 10021

Received for publication 26 May 1976

Twelve 4- and 5-nitroimidazole derivatives, including metronidazole and two of its metabolites, tinidazole, dimetridazole, and nimorazole, were tested for antitrichomonad action on *Tritrichomonas foetus* (KV_1) and *Trichomonas vaginalis* (ATCC 30001) for mutagenicity on a nitroreductase-positive (TA 100) and a nitroreductase-deficient (TA 100-FR_1) strain of *Salmonella typhimurium*, as well as for the reducibility of the nitro group by *T. foetus* homogenates. Compounds with activity <1% of that of metronidazole are regarded as inactive. All antitrichomonad compounds induce mutations and can be reduced. *S. typhimurium* TA 100 gave mutations under both aerobiosis and anaerobiosis; TA 100-FR_1, however, gave mutations only under anaerobiosis. Certain compounds that are reducible, and the nonreducible derivatives, were inactive. Metronidazole and its inactive 4-nitro analogue were reduced in a four-electron process in ferredoxin- or methyl viologen-mediated reactions with the same velocity. The results underscore the role of the reduction of the nitro group in the antitrichomonad and in the mutagenic activity of nitroimidazoles.

Metronidazole [Flagyl; 1-(2-hydroxyethyl)-2-methyl-5-nitroimidazole] and other derivatives of nitroimidazole are used extensively to treat infections due to anaerobic protozoa and bacteria (13). The main properties of these compounds that account for their therapeutic success are their selective uptake by and cytotoxic action on anaerobic organisms (9–11, 15, 29, 39). Their toxicity for aerobic microorganisms and for mammals is low (8, 10, 11, 40). However, recent studies have demonstrated that these drugs induce mutations in bacteria resistant to their killing activity (18, 19, 25, 32, 35, 42).

The mechanism of the cytotoxic and mutagenic action of nitroimidazoles on microorganisms is not well understood. It is assumed that derivatives arising by the reduction of the nitro group are responsible for the observed activities (4, 9, 15, 30). The products of reduction are not known but are assumed to be highly reactive and toxic for microorganisms, possibly by binding to deoxyribonucleic acid and other biopolymers (15, 43). In anaerobes, extensive transformation decreases the intracellular concentration of the unchanged drug and thus creates a gradient driving the uptake (15, 29).

The specificity of nitroimidazoles may be due to the occurrence of different redox processes in anaerobes and aerobes. In anaerobes low-redox potential reactions involving ferredoxin- or flavodoxin-type electron transport proteins are important (28). Such reactions are either nonexistent or, at best, insignificant in the metabolism of aerobes. It has been suggested that ferredoxin mediates the reduction of the nitro group of nitroimidazoles in susceptible anaerobes (4, 9, 15, 30).

In this paper we demonstrate a parallelism in the action of 12 nitroimidazole derivatives on two trichomonad species and in their mutagenic action in the *Salmonella* test. The nitro group of all active compounds was shown to be reduced by chemically or biologically reduced ferredoxin or methyl viologen. The reduction process involves the transfer of four electrons to metronidazole. Some of the results were previously presented at meetings (21; M. Müller, D. G. Lindmark, and J. McLaughlin, *in* H. van den Bossche [ed.], *Biochemistry of Parasites and Host-Parasite Relationships*, in press).

MATERIALS AND METHODS

Organisms. Two species of trichomonad flagellates were used: the human parasite *Trichomonas vaginalis* ATCC 30001, obtained from the American Type Culture Collection (Bethesda, Md.) and the cattle parasite *Tritrichomonas foetus*, KV_1 strain, obtained from B. M. Honigberg (Amherst, Mass.). Two strains of *Salmonella typhimurium* were used: the nitroreductase-positive histidine auxotroph strain TA 100 (26), obtained from B. N. Ames (Berkeley, Calif.), and its nitroreductase-deficient mutant TA 100-FR_1 (32), obtained from H. S. Rosenkranz (Valhalla, N.Y.). *T. vaginalis* was cultured in Diamond's TYM medium (6), pH 6.0, with 10% heat-inactivated horse serum, and *T. foetus* was cultured in the same medium without agar, pH 7.3, with 10% calf serum. The *S. typhimurium* strains were grown in Columbia broth (Baltimore Biological Laboratories, Cockeysville, Md.). All cultures were incubated at 37°C.

Growth inhibition tests. In most experiments, a single-layer agar plate technique was used (33). For the two trichomonad species, 0.1 ml of a 24-h culture of the test organism was mixed with 12 ml of plate medium (TYM medium of appropriate pH containing 0.8% agar and 10% serum) and poured into a petri dish of 100-mm diameter. Aqueous solutions (up to 500 μg/ml) of the compounds to be tested were added in a 20-μl volume to 6.35-mm sterile filter-paper disks (no. 1599-33, Difco Laboratories, Detroit, Mich.). The disks were placed on the plates, which were incubated for 48 h at 37°C in anaerobic jars (GasPak anaerobic system; BBL) containing an H_2 and CO_2 atmosphere (generated by GasPak no. 70304 disposable gas generator envelopes). The diameter of the clear zone around the disks was measured to the nearest millimeter.

The action of metronidazole was also tested in liquid cultures to obtain absolute values of its minimum inhibitory concentration for the microorganisms used in this study. Metronidazole was added to the media (TYM for trichomonads and Columbia broth for *S. typhimurium*) at concentrations ranging from 0.1 to 500 μg/ml for trichomonads and from 10 to 500 μg/ml for *S. typhimurium*. Tubes with trichomonads were incubated under the conditions used for the plates. Tubes with *S. typhimurium* were incubated both aerobically and anaerobically. After 48 h the minimum inhibitory concentration was recorded as the lowest concentration yielding no visible growth. Certain compounds that were not inhibitory in the plate assay were also tested in liquid cultures of *T. foetus* in concentrations ranging from 0.1 to 250 μg/ml to determine whether lack of effect was due to slow diffusion of the compounds in the agar.

Mutagenicity tests. Assays using *S. typhimurium* TA 100 and TA 100 FR_1 were carried out according to the method of Ames and co-workers (1) by incorporating the bacterium and the tested compound into an agar overlay. The plates were incubated at 37°C for 46 h aerobically or for 16 h in an anaerobic jar followed by 30 h of aerobic incubation (32). Revertants to histidine independence were enumerated after incubation.

Trichomonad homogenates. *T. foetus* and *T. vaginalis* cells were harvested from mass cultures (about 1,000 ml) by centrifugation, washed in 250 mM sucrose, resuspended in deaerated 250 mM sucrose containing 1 mM mercaptoethanol, and homogenized with a Teflon tissue homogenizer. The homogenization was performed, and the homogenate was kept under anaerobic conditions. Details of these procedures were published earlier (20).

Spectrophotometric tests. All solutions used were degased by boiling or by flushing with argon and were subsequently kept under this gas. The necessary amount of buffer or diluted homogenate was placed in semimicro spectrophotometric cells with stoppers (0.7-ml volume, 5-mm optical path; type 29, Precision Cells, Inc., Hicksville, N.Y.) that were closed with soft sleeve-type rubber stoppers (5 by 9 mm; no. 8826, A.M. Thomas Co., Philadelphia, Pa.) and were flushed with argon, using 26-gauge hypodermic needles as gas inlet and vent. Additions were made through the stopper with microliter syringes (Hamilton Co., Reno, Nev.). Changes in absorbance were followed at 25°C in a recording spectrophotometer. The following molar absorbance values (M^{-1} cm^{-1}) were used: ferredoxin (reduced minus oxidized) ϵ_{390}, 17,300 (21); methyl viologen (reduced) ϵ_{600}, 6,300 (20); metronidazole (no. 8) ϵ_{320}, 9,310 (43).

Compounds tested. The nitroimidazole derivatives used in this work are listed in Table 1. Compounds 1, 2, and 4 through 7 were synthetized by J. E. Stambaugh, Department of Pharmacology, Jefferson Medical College, Philadelphia, Pa., and were received from H. S. Rosenkranz, Department of Microbiology, New York Medical College, Valhalla, N.Y.; compounds 3 and 8 through 10 were from E. Kreider, Searle Laboratories, Chicago, Ill.; compound 11 was from J. E. Jefferis and N. Belcher, Central Research of Pfizer Inc., Groton, Conn.; and compound 12 was from J. Orizaga, Carlo Erba de Mexico, Mexico City, Mexico.

Other reagents. Reagents used in this work were obtained from Sigma Chemical Co., St. Louis, Mo. (methyl viologen, ferredoxin type IV from *Clostridium pasteurianum*), and from Matheson Coleman and Bell, East Rutherford, N.J. (sodium dithionite). All other reagents used were of analytical grade.

RESULTS

Table 1 summarizes our results obtained with 12 nitroimidazole derivatives. Inhibitory activity on trichomonads and mutagenic activity in the *S. typhimurium* test are expressed as relative values; effectiveness of metronidazole (no. 8) used is expressed as 100%. Comparison was done on a weight basis. Any compound with an activity of less than 1% of metronidazole is regarded as inactive. The results show that both trichomonads were strongly inhibited by metronidazole but that there were marked differences in the activity of the other compounds. There was a definite mutagenicity in *S. typhimurium* TA 100, both under aerobic and anaerobic conditions, and in TA 100 FR_1 under anaerobiosis for metronidazole and some of the other compounds. None of the compounds induced mutations in TA 100 FR_1 under aerobic conditions. Metronidazole, used in concentrations up to 500 μg/ml, did not affect either aerobic or anaerobic growth of either *S. typhimurium* strain.

The results also indicate that for any given compound the effects on different biological systems, i.e., killing of two eukaryotic anaerobic microorganisms and induction of mutations in two strains of *S. typhimurium*, have similar relative values.

In an anaerobic chemical system, metronidazole (no. 8) and its 4-nitro analogue (no. 3) are able to oxidize methyl viologen or ferredoxin that had been reduced with dithionite (Fig. 1). The oxidation of ferredoxin, as expressed by change in absorbance, is proportional to the amount of nitroimidazole added. Similar proportionality is seen if methyl viologen is used, except that initial additions of small amounts of nitroimidazoles do not produce a change. The cause of this "lag" is not yet understood. Such an effect could occur if methyl viologen contained an impurity, not absorbing at 600 nm, that was preferentially reoxidized by the first additions of metronidazole. The reaction between the reduced methyl viologen or ferredoxin and nitroimidazole is complete within the time limitations of the procedure; i.e., it lasts less than a few seconds. No difference was found between metronidazole and its 4-nitro analogue. From the amounts of compound added and the extent of absorbance change one can calculate that four electrons are transferred to each nitroimidazole molecule.

As described earlier (20), homogenates of trichomonads transfer electrons from pyruvate to ferredoxin or methyl viologen in a reaction catalyzed by an anaerobic pyruvate dehydrogenase (pyruvate synthase). This reaction can be followed spectrophotometrically (Fig. 2). If metronidazole is added to this system, the reaction proceeds at the same ratio as in the absence of the drug after a brief delay period. The duration of this delay is proportional to the amount of metronidazole added. The results suggest that metronidazole does not inhibit the dehydrogenase activity but serves rather as an electron acceptor, thus keeping the methyl viologen oxidized. From the rate of the dehydrogenase

TABLE 1. *Activity of nitroimidazole derivatives on trichomonads and on S. typhimurium as well as their reducibility in the methyl viologen-mediated in vitro assay*[a]

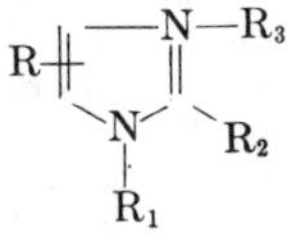

Compound no.	R	R_1	R_2	R_3	Nonproprietary name	Reference	Relative inhibition of growth[b]: *T. foetus*	Relative inhibition of growth[b]: *T. vaginalis*	Relative mutagenesis in *S. typhimurium*[c]: TA 100 Aerobic	TA 100 Anaerobic	TA 100 FR_1 Anaerobic	Reduction in the in vitro assay
1	4 (5)-NO_2	H	H			37	0	0	0	0	0	+
2	4 (5)-NO_2	H	CH_3			2, 37	0	0	0	0	0	+
3	4-NO_2	CH_2CH_2OH	CH_3			16, 37	0[d]	0[d]	0	0	0	+
4	4-NO_2	CH_3	H	CH_3		38	0	0	0	0	0	−
5	4-NO_2	CH_3	CH_3	CH_3		38	0	0	0	0	0	−
6	5-NO_2	CH_3	H			2, 5, 37	270	220	60	80	50	+
7	5-NO_2	CH_3	CH_3		Dimetridazole	2, 5, 37	300	310	200	160	150	+
8	5-NO_2	CH_2CH_2OH	CH_3		Metronidazole	2, 5, 16, 31, 37	100[d]	100[d]	100	100	100	+
9	5-NO_2	CH_2CH_2OH	CH_2OH			31, 36, 37	30[d]	20[d]	30	20	20	+
10	5-NO_2	CH_2COOH	CH_3			31, 36, 37	0[d]	0[d]	0	0	0	+
11	5-NO_2	$CH_2CH_2SO_2CH_2 \cdot CH_3$	CH_3		Tinidazole	4, 27	50	60	110	140	120	+
12	5-NO_2	$CH_2CH_2N\langle\ \rangle O$ (morpholine ring)	H		Nimorazole	3, 12	100	100	40	30	30	+

[a] Activities are expressed relative to metronidazole (no. 8).

[b] Minimum inhibitory concentration values for metronidazole: on *T. foetus*, 0.9 μg/ml; on *T. vaginalis*, 0.4 μg/ml.

[c] Mutagenetic effect of metronidazole, expressed as histidine revertants per microgram of drug, is 6.0 for aerobic TA 100, 7.8 for anaerobic TA 100, and 3.6 for anaerobic TA 100 FR_1.

[d] Confirmed in minimum inhibitory concentration test in liquid medium.

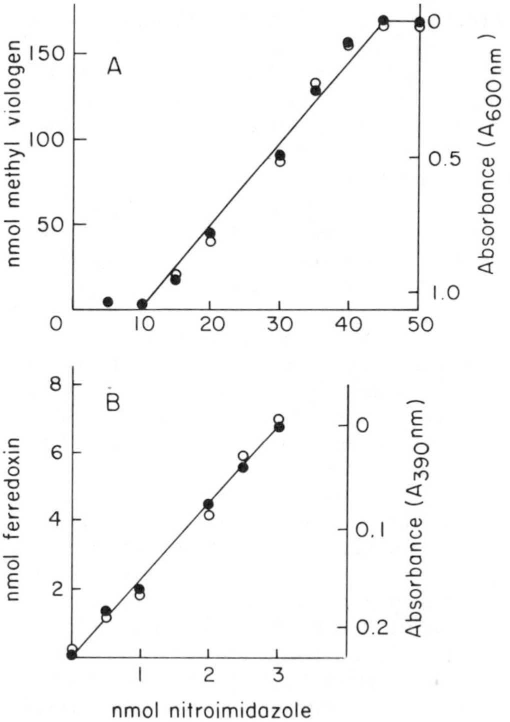

FIG. 1. *Oxidation of electron transport compounds by nitroimidazoles at 25°C. Symbols:* ●, *metronidazole (no. 8);* ○, *1-(2-hydroxyethyl)-2-methyl-4-nitroimidazole (no. 3). Cell contained, in 500 μl of 100 mM potassium phosphate buffer, pH 7.0, 175 nmol of methyl viologen (A) or 15 nmol of ferredoxin from C. pasteurianum (B). Ordinates, absorbance change and amount of compound oxidized; abscissa, amount of nitroimidazole added.*

reaction, length of delay, and amount of drug added, it can be calculated that four reducing equivalents were accepted by the drug.

All compounds studied were also tested in the pyruvate dehydrogenase assay (Table 1). With the exception of compounds 4 and 5, all interfered in the same way and to the same extent with the reduction of methyl viologen, indicating reduction of the compound in this system.

The reduction of metronidazole can be followed directly by the decrease in its absorbance at 320 nm. Homogenates of *T. foetus* are able to perform this reaction under anaerobic conditions if pyruvate is used as substrate (Fig. 3). The specific activity observed in the absence of exogenous electron transfer compounds was 47 nmol of nitroimidazole reduced/min per μg of protein. This value was markedly increased by the addition of ferredoxin from *C. pasteurianum* (120 nmol/min per μg of protein) or of methyl viologen (150 nmol/min per μg of protein). The latter values are close to those observed for pyruvate dehydrogenase of *T. foetus* with ferredoxin or methyl viologen (20). Experiments with *T. vaginalis* gave similar results.

DISCUSSION

In this study we compared the antitrichomonad activity and mutagenicity of 12 nitroimidazole derivatives. The results demonstrate that compounds with antitrichomonad activity are also able to induce mutations in *S. typhimurium,* whereas compounds inactive against trichomonads are not mutagenic. Although the mechanisms whereby nitroimidazoles kill anaerobes and induce mutations are unclear, our results suggest that both of these effects depend

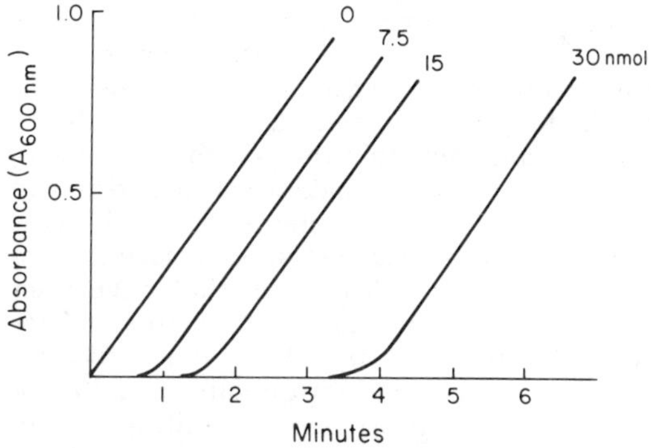

FIG. 2. *Effect of metronidazole on the reduction of methyl viologen by an anaerobic homogenate of T. foetus, with pyruvate as substrate (20). Reaction was started with simultaneous anaerobic addition of 2 μmol of methyl viologen and metronidazole in the stated amounts. The cells contained 200 μg of homogenate protein in a total volume of 500 μl.*

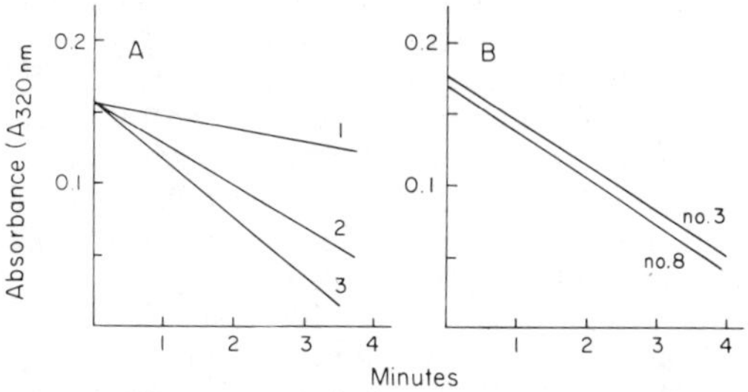

FIG. 3. *Reduction of nitroimidazoles by an anaerobic extract of T. foetus, with pyruvate as substrate (20). (A) Reduction of metronidazole (no. 8) without added electron transport compound (1) or with 50 nmol of ferredoxin (2) or 200 nmol of methyl viologen (3) added. Cells contained 21 μg of homogenate protein and 100 nmol of metronidazole. (B) Reduction of metronidazole (no. 8) and of 1-(2-hydroxyethyl)-2-methyl-4-nitroimidazole (no. 3). Cell contained 28 μg of homogenate protein and 100 nmol of nitroimidazole. Sample volume, 500 μl.*

on similar chemical properties of the compounds.

Clearly the activity observed in a given assay system depends not only on the compound tested, but also on the assay used. Thus, the use of other strains of organisms or other methods would likely give different results. Therefore, we wish to emphasize the overall results and not the relatively small numerical differences among the different drugs tested. Nevertheless, data obtained with the different compounds are usually in agreement with published results.

As expected, all nitroimidazoles currently used in human or veterinary medicine, as well as 1-methyl-5-nitroimidazole (no. 6), are highly active against trichomonads with minimum inhibitory concentration values below 1 μg/ml. The inactivity of the 4-nitro analogue of metronidazole (no. 3) is in agreement both with the findings of Kajfež et al. (16) and with the general conclusion that the 5-nitro compound is the more active of any pair of 4-nitro and 5-nitro derivatives (5, 17). Of interest is the observation that the major metabolic derivatives of metronidazole (no. 9 and 10) that have been demonstrated in the urine of humans and rodents (36) are less active than the parent compound, in agreement with published data (16, 31). Methyl substitution on both nitrogens (no. 4 and 5) abolishes the activity.

Metronidazole and several other compounds tested at very high concentrations did not inhibit growth of *S. typhimurium* under aerobic or anaerobic conditions. This confirms reports of the resistance by different *Enterobacteriaceae* to nitroimidazole derivatives (10, 11). All compounds active against trichomonads were found, however, to be mutagenic in the *S. typhimurium* tests. The mutagenicity of several nitroimidazoles has been reported (18, 19, 25, 32, 35, 42). As confirmed in this paper, all these compounds are weak mutagens, producing about one revertant or less per nanomole of compound in the *S. typhimurium* test (25). Similar results were obtained for several compounds in the aerobic TA 100 test (H. S. Rosenkranz, W. T. Speck, and J. E. Stambaugh, Jr., Mutat. Res., in press). We found the two major urinary metabolites (no. 9 and 10) of metronidazole less mutagenic than the parent compound, showing a parallelism to the antitrichomonad activities. On this basis, the urine of patients treated with metronidazole is expected to be mutagenic (35), but less so than the drug itself. Other workers, using another strain (TA 1535), reported, however, that the urine was more mutagenic and attributed this finding to the metabolic activation of metronidazole in the whole organism (18, 19). The presence in urine of compound 9, an oxidative metabolite of metronidazole, was assumed to be responsible for this effect. On TA 1535 this compound is indeed more active than metronidazole (19). The contradiction with our findings can be resolved if all data are converted to absolute values. Although compound 9 induces the same number of revertants in TA 100 and TA 1535, metronidazole is much less active in TA 1535 than in TA 100. The reason for this strain difference is not clear, but it seems that the effect is due to a low susceptibility of TA 1535 to metronidazole.

It has been repeatedly suggested that the reduction of the nitro group is an essential step in the antimicrobial action of nitroimidazole derivatives on anaerobes (4, 9, 15, 30). Our results suggest that reduction of the nitro group is also necessary for their mutagenic activity. The employed tester strain TA 100 has an active aerobic nitroreductase (23), as do most strains of *S. typhimurium*. Thus it is conceivable, as has been suggested previously (24, 32), that this enzyme converts nitro compounds into active reduced derivatives. The nitroreductase-deficient tester strain TA 100-FR_1, when exposed to nitroimidazoles, gives no revertants under aerobic conditions, extending the results of a previous report (32). Under anaerobic conditions, however, the same strain gives revertants when exposed to the same compounds, suggesting that TA 100-FR_1 has other reducing systems capable of activating nitroimidazoles in the absence of oxygen. Ferredoxin has been found in anaerobically grown *Escherichia coli* (41), and thus its occurrence in *S. typhimurium* seems to be likely. These findings suggest that the mutagenic action of nitroimidazoles is also due to certain reduced metabolites.

With the exception of those carrying methyl groups on both nitrogens, all compounds tested were reduced to the same extent and with similar kinetics in an in vitro enzymatic assay system. Thus, all active compounds are reducible, supporting the idea that reductive biotransformation is an essential component of the mechanism of action. Since the reducible compounds show different levels of activity, other properties of the molecules must also play a major role, possibly determining the interaction of the reduced products with cell components.

It is generally assumed that the reduction of nitroimidazoles is mediated by a ferredoxin- or flavodoxin-type electron transport protein (4, 9, 15, 30). In these studies, we found that metronidazole can be reduced in a non-enzymatic reaction by chemically reduced ferredoxin or methyl viologen, as shown by the oxidation of these electron donors.

These data are compatible with theoretical considerations. The possibility of a redox reaction between ferredoxin and nitroimidazole derivatives has been postulated on the basis of the redox potentials of the reactants (9, 15, 30). Because their reduction is irreversible, nitroimidazoles do not form redox couples, so polarographic data have to be used to characterize their reducibility. It has been shown that at pH 7 most 5-nitroimidazole derivatives have a half-wave potential ($E_{1/2}$) of about −450 mV and that the 4-nitro analogue of metronidazole has an $E_{1/2}$ of about −550 mV (7, 30, 34). Since the $E_{1/2}$ values of ferredoxins from *C. pasteurianum* and spinach chloroplasts are somewhat more negative (Y. W. Chien, J. Pharm. Sci., in press), they are suitable reductants for nitroimidazoles.

Anaerobic homogenates of *T. vaginalis* and *T. foetus* reduce metronidazole and other nitroimidazoles if pyruvate is provided as electron donor, and the reduction is much faster if exogenous ferredoxin or methyl viologen are also added to the system. Similar results have been obtained using different *Clostridium* species (4, 9, 30). These results are in agreement with the known properties of trichomonad homogenates, which contain oxidoreductases that can use ferredoxin or methyl viologen as electron acceptor (20, 22). Accordingly, these acceptors are first reduced by the substrates in enzymatic reactions and then in turn reduce the nitroimidazoles in non-enzymatic reactions.

An easy way to test nitroimidazole reduction in biological systems, a method used for all compounds, is to see whether any of the compounds interferes with the anaerobic pyruvate dehydrogenase assay. As long as reducible nitroimidazoles are present, they will act as terminal electron acceptors and will keep the methyl viologen reduced, i.e., colorless.

The number of electrons transferred to metronidazole during in vitro reduction was determined in several experimental systems, including experiments with ferredoxin, the assumed natural electron donor, reduced by dithionite or by anaerobic cell homogenates. The calculated number was four in all cases, which is in agreement with results obtained on *C. pasteurianum* homogenates (G. Coombs, personal communication). However, these results are at variance with a published work using different methods suggesting a six-electron transfer (30). These experiments utilized purified *C. pasteurianum* hydrogenase supplied with benzyl viologen or crude extracts of *C. acetobutilicum* supplemented with pyruvate and methyl viologen and measured H_2 uptake or decrease in H_2 production, respectively (30). The reason for this difference is not clear. A four-electron reduction is observed in the chemical titration of metronidazole where about 2 mol of dithionite are oxidized by 1 mol of drug and dithionite in excess remains unchanged (9, 43; M. Tomasz, personal communication). Direct current polarographic measurements at pH values below 10.0 show a complex wave pattern, in which the first wave corresponds to a four-electron reaction (7). Alternating current polarography at pH 6.0 also gives a current height corresponding to the same degree of reduction, as determined by the use of model compounds (Y. W. Chien, personal communication). These results suggest that the major reduction products correspond to the reduction level of a hydroxylamine derivative. Since these products have not been isolated, their chemical nature remains conjecture. It seems reasonably certain, however, that in ferredoxin-mediated reactions no further reduction occurs. The fact that both dithionite and reduced methyl viologen transfer the same number of electrons as does ferredoxin suggests that these compounds may be used in model experiments, which can contribute to understanding the mechanism of action of nitroimidazoles on susceptible anaerobes. Since the interaction of nitroimidazoles with nitroreductases of unsusceptible bacteria and the products of this interaction have not been studied, the significance of the above results in understanding the mutagenic action remains to be elucidated.

ACKNOWLEDGMENTS

We express our thanks to B. N. Ames, B. Honigberg, and H. S. Rosenkranz for providing the strains of microorganisms used; to N. Belcher, J. E. Jefferis, E. Kreider, J. Orizaga, and H. S. Rosenkranz for the nitroimidazoles tested; to Y. W. Chien, G. Coombs, H. S. Rosenkranz, and M. Tomasz for permission to quote material unpublished at the time this paper was written; to C. de Duve, J. S. Keithly, N. La Russo, J. McLaughlin, and H. S. Rosenkranz for criticism; and to C. Ward for conscientious assistance.

Figures 1B and 3A are reproduced from M. Müller, D. G. Lindmark, and J. McLaughlin, *in* H. van den Bossche (ed.), *Biochemistry of Parasites and Host-Parasite Relationships*, in press. Permission granted by the copyright owner, North-Holland Publishers, Amsterdam, is gratefully acknowledged.

This work was supported by Public Health Service grant AI-11942 from the National Institute of Allergy and Infectious Diseases.

LITERATURE CITED

1. **Ames, B. N., J. McCann, and E. Yamasaki.** 1975. Methods for detecting carcinogens and mutagens with the salmonella/mammalian-microsome mutagenicity test. Mutat. Res. 31:347–364.
2. **Butler, K., H. L. Howes, J. E. Lynch, and D. K. Pirie.** 1967. Nitroimidazole derivatives. Relationship between structure and antitrichomonal activity. J. Med. Chem. 10:891–897.
3. **Cavier, R., and J. Cénac.** 1972. Contribution a l'étude des propriétés trichomonacides du nimorazole. Therapeutique 48:391–394.

4. **Coombs, G. H.** 1973. Some studies on the biochemistry of action of Flagyl. J. Protozool. **20**:524–525.
5. **Cosar, C., C. Crisan, R. Horclois, R. M. Jacob, J. Robert, S. Tchelitcheff, and R. Vaupré.** 1966. Nitroimidazoles–préparation et activité chimiothérapeutique. Arzneim. Forsch. **16**:23–29.
6. **Diamond, L. S.** 1957. The establishment of various trichomonads of animals and man in axenic cultures. J. Parasitol. **43**:488–490.
7. **Dumanović, D., J. Volke, and V. Vajgand.** 1966. Simultaneous polarographic determination of 1-(2-hydroxyethyl)-2-methyl-5-nitroimidazole, 1-(2-hydroxyethyl)-2-methyl-4-nitroimidazole and 2-methyl-5-nitroimidazole. J. Pharm. Pharmacol. **18**:507–512.
8. **Eakins, M. N., P. J. Conroy, A. J. Searle, T. F. Slater, and R. L. Willson.** 1976. Metronidazole (Flagyl), a radiosensitiser of possible clinical use in cancer chemotherapy: some biochemical and pharmacological considerations. Biochem. Pharmacol. **25**:1151–1156.
9. **Edwards, D. I., M. Dye, and H. Carne.** 1973. The selective toxicity of antimicrobial nitroheterocyclic drugs. J. Gen. Microbiol. **76**:135–145.
10. **Füzi, M., and Z. Csukás.** 1970. Das antibakterielle Wirkungsspektrum des Metronidazols. Zentralbl. Bakteriol. Parasitenkd. Infektionskr. Hyg. Abt. 1 Orig. **213**:258–262.
11. **Füzi, M., and Z. Csukás.** 1972. A metronidazol selectiv antibacterialis hatása. Selektive antibakterielle Wirkung des Metronidazols. Kiserl. Orvostud. **24**:233–236. (In Hungarian, summary in German.)
12. **Giraldi, P. N., V. Mariotti, G. Nannini, G. P. Tosolini, E. Dradi, W. Logemann, I. de Carneri, and G. Monti.** 1970. Studies on antiprotozoans. Part II. Synthesis and biological activity of some N-alkylamino-nitroimidazoles. Arzneim. Forsch. **20**:52–55.
13. **Grunberg, E., and E. Titsworth.** 1974. Chemotherapeutic properties of heterocyclic compounds: monocyclic compounds with five membered rings. Annu. Rev. Microbiol. **27**:317–347.
14. **Howes, H. L., Jr., J. E. Lynch, and J. L. Kivlin.** 1970. Tinidazole, a new antiprotozoal agent: effect on *Trichomonas* and other protozoa, p. 261–266. Antimicrob. Agents Chemother. 1969.
15. **Ings, R. M. J., J. A. McFadzean, and W. E. Ormerod.** 1974. The mode of action of metronidazole in *Trichomonas vaginalis* and other microorganisms. Biochem. Pharmacol. **23**:1421–1429.
16. **Kajfež, F., V. Šunjić, D. Kolbah, T. Fajdiga, and M. Oklobdžija.** 1968. 1-Substitution in 2-methyl-4(5)-nitroimidazole. I. Synthesis of compounds with potential antitrichomonal activity. J. Med. Chem. **11**:167–169.
17. **Lancini, G. C., E. Lazzari, V. Arioli, and P. Bellani.** 1969. Synthesis and relationship between structure and activity of 2-nitroimidazole derivatives. J. Med. Chem. **12**:755–780.
18. **Legator, M. S., T. H. Connor, and M. Stoeckel.** 1975. Detection of mutagenic activity of metronidazole and niridazole in body fluids of humans and mice. Science **188**:1118–1119.
19. **Legator, M. S., T. Connor, and M. Stoeckel.** 1975. The detection of mutagenic substances in the urine and blood of man. Ann. N.Y. Acad. Sci. **269**:16–20.
20. **Lindmark, D. G., and M. Müller.** 1973. Hydrogenosome, a cytoplasmic organelle of the anaerobic flagellate *Tritrichomonas foetus* and its role in pyruvate metabolism. J. Biol. Chem. **248**:7724–7728.
21. **Lindmark, D. G., and M. Müller.** 1974. Reduction of metronidazole by homogenates of trichomonad flagellates. J. Protozool. **21**:436.
22. **Lindmark, D. G., M. Müller, and H. Shio.** 1975. Hydrogenosomes in *Trichomonas vaginalis*. J. Parasitol. **61**:552–554.
23. **McCalla, D. R., A. Reuvers, and C. Kaiser.** 1970. Mode of action of nitrofurazone. J. Bacteriol. **104**:1126–1134.
24. **McCalla, D. R., and D. Voutsinos.** 1974. On the mutagenicity of nitrofurans. Mutat. Res. **26**:3–16.
25. **McCann, J., E. Choi, E. Yamasaki, and B. N. Ames.** 1975. Detection of carcinogens as mutagens in the *Salmonella*/microsome test: assay of 300 chemicals. Proc. Natl. Acad. Sci. U.S.A. **72**:5135–5139.
26. **McCann, J., N. E. Spingarn, J. Kobori, and B. N. Ames.** 1975. Detection of carcinogens as mutagens: bacterial tester strains with R factor plasmids. Proc. Natl. Acad. Sci. U.S.A. **72**:979–983.
27. **Miller, M. W., H. L. Howes, and A. R. English.** 1970. Tinidazole, a potent new antiprotozoal agent, p. 257–260. Antimicrob. Agents Chemother. 1969.
28. **Mortenson, L. E., and G. Nakos.** 1973. Bacterial ferredoxins and/or iron-sulfur proteins as electron carriers, p. 37–60. *In* W. Lovenberg (ed.), Iron-sulfur proteins, vol. 1. Academic Press Inc., New York.
29. **Müller, M., and D. G. Lindmark.** 1976. Uptake of metronidazole and its effect on viability in trichomonads and *Entamoeba invadens* under anaerobic and aerobic conditions. Antimicrob. Agents Chemother. **9**:696–700.
30. **O'Brien, R. W., and J. G. Morris.** 1972. Effect of metronidazole on hydrogen production by *Clostridium acetobutylicum*. Arch. Mikrobiol. **81**:225–233.
31. **Ralph, E. D., and W. M. M. Kirby.** 1975. Bioassay of metronidazole with either anaerobic or aerobic incubation. J. Infect. Dis. **132**:587–591.
32. **Rosenkranz, H. S., and W. T. Speck.** 1975. Mutagenicity of metronidazole: activation by mammalian liver microsomes. Biochem. Biophys. Res. Commun. **66**:520–525.
33. **Samuels, R., and D. J. Stouder.** 1962. Disc testing of drugs against plated *Trichomonas vaginalis*. J. Protozool. **9**:249–254.
34. **Slamnik, M., F., Kajfež, and V. Šunjić.** 1967. Polarographic examination of N^1-substituted-2-methyl-4(5)-nitroimidazoles. J. Polarogr. Soc. **13**:83–85.
35. **Speck, W. T., A. B. Stein, and H. S. Rosenkranz.** 1976. Mutagenicity of metronidazole: presence of several active metabolites in human urine. J. Natl. Cancer Inst. **56**:283–284.
36. **Stambaugh, J. E., L. G. Feo, and R. W. Manthei.** 1968. The isolation and identification of the urinary oxidative metabolites of metronidazole in man. J. Pharmacol. Exp. Ther. **161**:373–381.
37. **Stambaugh, J. E., and R. W. Manthei.** 1967. The characterization of substituted nitroimidazoles on paper and thin layer chromatography by colorimetric reactions. J. Chromatogr. **31**:128–136.
38. **Stambaugh, J. E., and R. W. Manthei.** 1968. The infrared and nuclear magnetic resonance spectra of some 5-nitroimidazoles. Can. Spectrosc. **13**:134–138.
39. **Tanowitz, H. B., M. Wittner, R. M. Rosenbaum, and Y. Kress.** 1975. In vitro studies on the differential toxicity of metronidazole in protozoa and mammalian cells. Ann. Trop. Med. Parasitol. **69**:19–28.
40. **Urtasun, R. C., J. Sturmwind, H. Rabin, P. R. Band, and J. D. Chapman.** 1974. "High-dose" metronidazole: a preliminary pharmacological study prior to its investigational use in clinical radiotherapy trials. Br. J. Radiol. **47**:297–299.
41. **Vetter, H., Jr., and J. Knappe.** 1971. Flavodoxin and ferredoxin of *Escherichia coli*. Hoppe-Seyler's Z. Physiol. Chem. **352**:433–446.
42. **Voogd, C. E., J. J. Van Der Stel, and J. J. J. A. A. Jacobs.** 1974. The mutagenic action of nitroimidazoles. I. Metronidazole, nimorazole, dimetridazole and ronidazole. Mutat. Res. **26**:483–490.
43. **Willson, R. L., W. A. Cramp, and R. M. J. Ings.** 1974. Metronidazole ('Flagyl'): mechanism of radiosensitization. Int. J. Radiat. Biol. **26**:557–569.

Antimicrobial Agents and Chemotherapy, Sept. 1976, p. 483-490 Vol. 10, No. 3

Printed in U.S.A.

Basis for the Design of Anticandidal Agents from Studies of Peptide Utilization in *Candida albicans*

WAYNE D. LICHLITER, FRED NAIDER, and JEFFREY M. BECKER*

Department of Microbiology, University of Tennessee, Knoxville, Tennessee 37916, and Department of Chemistry, Richmond College of the City University of New York, Staten Island, New York 10301*

Received for publication 14 April 1976

The growth of *Candida albicans* WD 18-4, a methionine and lysine double auxotroph, on a variety of methionine- and lysine-containing peptides was determined. This yeast does not excrete extracellular peptidases. Thus, the growth response to peptides containing the required amino acid is a measure of peptide transport. A variety of methionine-containing peptides such as Met-Met, Met-Met-Met, and Met-Met-Met-Met-Met are transported. Acylation of the N-terminus of transported peptides does not affect their transport, but derivitization of the C-terminus prevents peptide uptake. In contrast, all lysine-containing peptides tested, except Lys-Gly, were not growth substrates. The inability of a peptide to substitute for the requisite amino acid was not due to the absence of cellular peptidases or to toxicity of the nonutilized peptides. Several potentially toxic amino acids were carried into *Candida* as a component of transported peptides. This establishes the peptide transport system as a possible tool for the design of antibiotics for *Candida albicans*.

The existence of peptide transport systems in a variety of cell types is an established fact. The great majority of studies were carried out using *Escherichia coli* and the mammalian gut as test systems (2). In addition, reports appeared concerning peptide transport in a number of other bacteria (1, 2, 5), in *Saccharomyces cerevisiae* (4, 13), and in *Neurospora crassa* (18–20). Most of these studies dealt with the characterization of the structural specificity of the peptide transport systems. In *E. coli*, in particular, numerous details are known about the molecular features of the peptide that are important for recognition by the oligopeptide permease (Opp) in this bacterium (2, 14).

Knowledge of the structural specificity of the peptide transport system in *E. coli* was used by several workers to attach normally impermeant molecules to peptides, which then carried these molecules into the cell (1, 7). This phenomenon, termed "illicit transport" (1), has far-reaching implications for the rational design of toxic compounds specifically active against one type of microorganism. The application of this concept, however, requires a detailed knowledge about the structural specificities of peptide transport systems in a great variety of cells in order that any striking differences can be incorporated into the design.

During our studies on the yeast *S. cerevisiae* we found that this microorganism could utilize peptides that were acylated on the amino terminus (13). Recently we have observed that radioactively labeled Ac-Met-Met-Met is accumulated by *S. cerevisiae* (unpublished data). These findings contrast strikingly with the fact that acylation of peptides completely prevents their transport into *E. coli* (2), *S. typhimurium* (M. B. Jackson, J. M. Becker, A. Steinfeld, and F. Naider, J. Biol. Chem., in press), mammalian intestine (15), and *N. crassa* (18). We decided to see whether the different structural specificities between *S. cerevisiae* and other cell types could also apply to a pathogenic yeast. In this study, we report on the structural specificity of peptide utilization in a methionine-lysine auxotroph of *Candida albicans*.

MATERIALS AND METHODS

Yeast strain, growth, and growth inhibition conditions. The yeast strain used throughout this report was *C. albicans* WD 18-4, a methionine-lysine double auxotroph kindly supplied by Alvin Sarachek, Wichita State University. The culture was maintained on agar slants containing 1% yeast extract, 2% peptone (Difco), and 2% glucose (wt/vol).

The minimal growth medium for all experiments contained yeast nitrogen base (Difco) (1%) and glucose (2%), supplemented by amino acids or peptides where indicated. The yeast nitrogen base was filter-sterilized (strength 10×) as suggested by the manufacturer. The glucose solutions (20%, wt/vol) were autoclaved separately at 121°C for 15 min, and solutions of peptides were filter-sterilized to prevent degradation during autoclaving. At the initiation of any growth experiment, all ingredients were added aseptically to presterilized flasks containing sterile distilled water.

For growth studies the yeast was inoculated into 5.0 ml of minimal medium with the required amino acids and grown overnight. In early experiments, 0.5 ml of this log-phase culture was used to inoculate 24.5 ml of minimal medium supplemented with the desired amino acid or peptide and contained in a 500-ml Erlenmeyer flask fitted with a side arm. The flask was placed in a reciprocating water bath kept at 37°C. In later experiments, 0.1 ml of the overnight culture was used to inoculate 4.9 ml of the complete medium contained in Klett tubes and incubated at 37°C in a rotary shaker. Comparable results were obtained using either procedure. Growth was determined by the increase in turbidity at 400 to 420 nm (blue filter) with a Klett-Summerson photoelectric colorimeter. Revertants of the *Candida* strains to prototrophy and possible contamination of growth flasks were checked periodically by streaking out 0.1 ml of the final culture on minimal agar plates supplemented with methionine or lysine, both of the amino acids, or no required supplements.

Chemicals. (L-Met), D-Met, and Met-Met were purchased from Sigma Chemical Co., St. Louis, Mo. Met-Gly, Gly-Met, Met-Met-Met, Met-Gly-Met, Gly-Met-Gly, and Met-Gly-Met-Met were purchased from Schwarz/Mann, Orangeburg, N.Y. Lysine, Lys-Lys, $(Lys)_3$, Lys-Gly, Gly-Lys, and the polylysines were purchased from Miles Laboratories, Elkhart, Ind. $(Lys)_4$ and $(Lys)_7$ were the gift of A. Yaron, Weizmann Institute, Rehovot, Israel. All other peptides were synthesized according to techniques published elsewhere (13). All peptides were homogeneous on thin-layer chromatograms in several solvent systems and on high-voltage paper electrophoresis.

Cell extract. Cells (1 liter) were harvested at the late logarithmic phase of growth (200 to 300 Klett units), washed twice with distilled water, and resuspended in 30 ml of 0.1 M phosphate buffer (pH 6.5). The cell suspension and glass beads (60 g; Sigma Chemical Co.; diameter, 75 to 150 μm) were added to the 50-ml size Omnimixer stainless steel cup (Ivan Sorvall, Inc., Norwalk, Conn.). The suspension was kept on ice and homogenized at top speed for two 5-min periods. The glass beads, unbroken cells, and cell debris were removed by centrifugation (2,000 × *g*, 10 min). The supernatant was dialyzed against 0.1 M phosphate buffer (pH 6.5) at 4°C, and the resulting solution was used as the cell extract. Protein determinations on the dialyzed extract were carried out by the Lowry technique using bovine serum albumin as the standard (11). The protein content of the extract was 1.1 mg/ml.

Peptidase assay. A portion of the cell extract (100 μl) was incubated at 37°C with an equal volume of various peptide solutions (1 or 2 mg/ml in distilled water). At various time intervals portions of the reaction mixture were removed (2 to 4 μl) and applied to a cellulose thin layer (Eastman Kodak Co., Rochester, N.Y.; 250 μm). The chromatograms were developed with 2-propanol–methyl ethyl ketone–1 N HCl (60:15:25). Plates were allowed to develop to 13 cm (about 2.5 h) by the method of Haworth and Heathcote (10). The plates were dried under infrared heat for about 5 min, and the chromatograms were sprayed with a ninhydrin reagent (Gelman Instrument Co., Ann Arbor, Mich.) and placed in a drying oven.

RESULTS

Growth of *C. albicans* WD 18-4 on peptides and peptide derivative. The growth response of *C. albicans* WD 18-4 to various concentrations of L-Met is represented in Fig. 1. The minimum amount of amino acid yielding maximum growth was 4 μg/ml. When the medium was supplemented with more than 4 μg/ml, no significant change in generation time or increase in cell crop was obtained. The complete lack of growth without L-methionine supplementation shows the absolute requirement of this mutant strain for this amino acid. Similar results were obtained when growth of the yeast was measured against lysine.

Various peptides were tested to see whether they could satisfy the amino acid requirements of strain WD 18-4. In all cases, the medium was supplemented with either L-methionine plus a lysine-containing peptide or L-lysine plus a methionine-containing peptide. Peptides were added to the growth medium so as to supply 4 μg of the required amino acid per ml in each growth flask. The data in Fig. 2 and Table 1

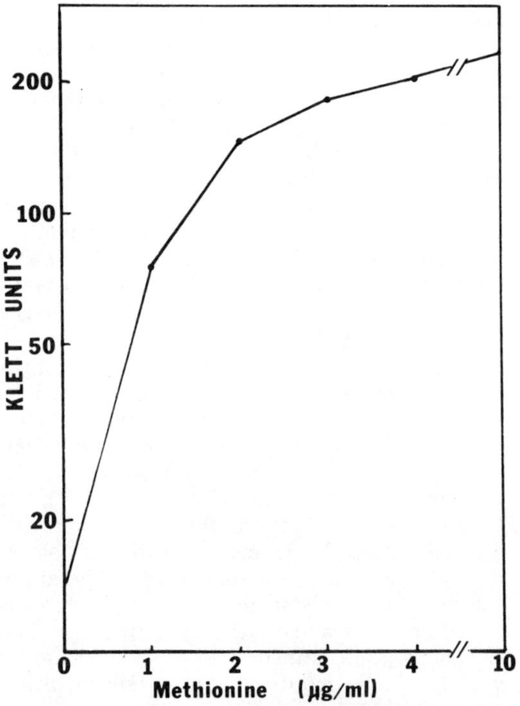

FIG. 1. *Growth response of C. albicans WD 18-4 to methionine. Minimal medium was supplemented with lysine (4 μg/ml) and methionine as indicated in the figure. Turbidity after 30 h at 37°C is shown on the ordinate.*

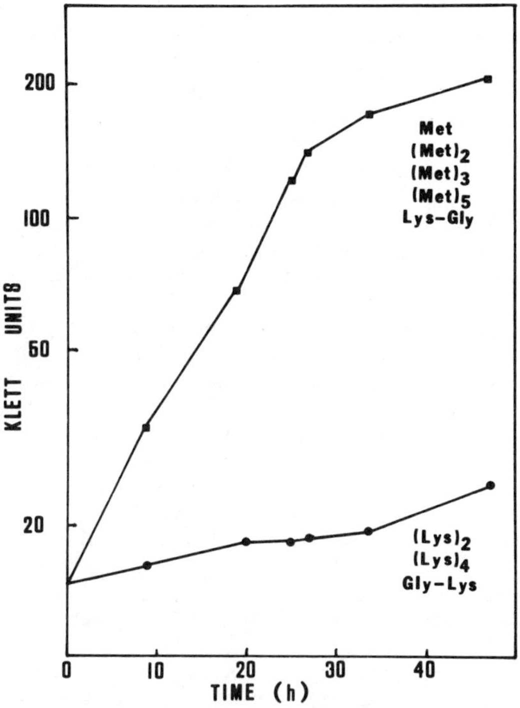

FIG. 2. *Growth response to various methionine- or lysine-containing peptides. Minimal medium was supplemented with lysine and methionine, lysine and (Met)$_2$, lysine and (Met)$_3$, lysine and (Met)$_5$, or methionine and Lys-Gly, (■); methionine and (Lys)$_2$, methionine and (Lys)$_4$, or methionine and Gly-Lys, (●). All peptides were added so that the final concentration of required amino acid was 4 μg/ml.*

summarize the growth responses to a number of peptides containing methionine or lysine residues. We found that pentamethionine as well as a number of di-, tri-, and tetrapeptides containing methionine all served as sources for methionine. In all cases growth was essentially equal to that on the free amino acid. It is of particular interest that two peptides (Met-Met-Eth and Met-Met-Norleu) which contain potentially toxic amino acids were utilized by strain WD 18-4. This result indicates that such amino acids can be tolerated by a peptide transport system in *Candida*. The lack of toxicity in the present study is most likely a result of the presence of methionine in the peptide. It is known that the often observed toxic effect of ethionine and norleucine is a consequence of their replacement of methionine in cellular proteins (8). This replacement is expected to be diminished when methionine is also present in the cytoplasm. In contrast, of all the lysine peptides examined, only Lys-Gly satisfied the nutritional requirement of strain WD 18-4 for L-lysine. Many of these findings are consistent with the growth response of auxotrophs of *S. cerevisiae* to various peptides and will be discussed in a later section.

The ability of several stereoisomers of trimethionine to serve as growth sources was examined. Preliminary experiments indicated that *C. albicans* WD 18-4 could grow on D-methionine. In the stereoisomer utilization experiments we supplemented the medium so that equivalent concentrations (micrograms per milliliter), of methionyl residues were present in each growth flask. Our results show that the methionine auxotroph grew well on either L-Met-L-Met-L-Met or D-Met-L-Met-L-Met (Fig.

TABLE 1. *Growth response of C. albicans WD 18-4 to peptides containing methionine or lysine*

Peptide[a]	Growth response[b]
Methionine-containing	
Dipeptides	
(Met)$_2$	+
Met-Gly	+
Met-Ala	+
Ala-Met	+
Val-Met	+
Phe-Met	+
Met-Phe	+
Tripeptides	
(Met)$_3$	+
Met-Gly-Met	+
Gly-Met-Gly	+
Gly-Met-Met	+
Met-Met-Gly	+
Met-Ala-Met	+
Met-Met-Eth	+
Met-Met-Nor	+
Other oligopeptides	
Met-Gly-Met-Met	+
Met-Met-Gly-Met	+
Met-Met-Gly-Gly	+
Met-Met-Met-Gly	+
(Met)$_5$	+
Lysine-containing	
Dipeptides	
(Lys)$_2$	−
Lys-Gly	+
Gly-Lys	−
Oligopeptides	
(Lys)$_3$	−
(Lys)$_4$	−
(Lys)$_7$	−
(Lys)$_n$[c]	−

[a] All peptides were supplemented so that each growth flask contained 4 μg of the required amino acid per ml. All residues are in the L-configuration.

[b] (+) denotes growth equal to that on the free amino acid, whereas (−) denotes no growth.

[c] Varous polylysines were used, with average molecular weights from 2×10^3 to 1×10^5.

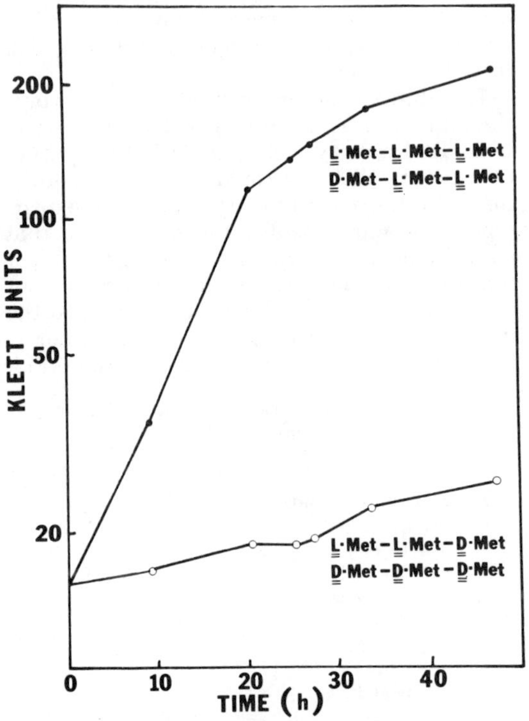

FIG. 3. *Growth response to various methionine-containing tripeptide stereoisomers. Medium was supplemented with lysine (4 μg/ml) and L-L-L or D-L-L,(●); lysine (4 μg/ml) and L-L-D, D-D-D, (○).*

3). The mutant was not able to utilize either L-Met-L-Met-D-Met, L-Val-L-Met-D-Met, or D-Met-D-Met-D-Met as methionine sources. The difference between L-Met-L-Met-D-Met and D-Met-L-Met-L-Met is particularly interesting as data to be shown later indicate that both of these peptides are rapidly broken down to the free amino acids by intracellular peptidases.

Strain WD 18-4 was able to utilize several acylated peptides as sources of methionine (Fig. 4). Acetyl trimethionine was as good a growth substrate as the free amino acid. In addition, two tripeptides containing a bulky tert-butyloxy-carbonyl blocking group (Boc-Met-Met-Gly and Boc-Gly-Met-Met) were efficient growth substrates. In contrast to the amino terminal derivatives, several peptide esters, L-Met-L-Met-L-Met-OMe, D-Met-L-Met-L-Met-OMe, $(Met)_4$-OMe, and $(Met)_5$-OMe, failed to serve as sources of L-methionine (Fig. 4). It is important to note that in each case the corresponding free peptide was a good source of methionine. None of the peptides or peptide derivatives that were not growth substrates was toxic to the yeast. Addition of a nonutilized peptide to growth flasks containing lysine and methionine did not affect the generation time or cell yield.

Peptidase activity of *C. albicans* WD 18-4. The inability of a cell to utilize a peptide as a source for an amino acid can result from the failure of the peptide to enter the cell or the absence of the necessary peptidase activity. Our studies showed that strain WD 18-4 contained the necessary peptidase activity to release the required amino acids from virtually all of the peptides used in the growth experiments. Most important we found that L-Met-L-Met-D-Met and L-Met-L-Met-L-Met were both rapidly cleaved to methionine during a 90-min incubation with a cell extract of WD 18-4. (Fig. 5). That the cleavage was enzymatic is attested to by our observation that boiling the extract for 1 min prior to incubation with the peptide resulted in the complete absence of peptide hydrolysis. In addition to the hydrolysis of the above stereoisomers of $(Met)_3$, we observed that L-Met-L-Met-L-Met-OMe was hydrolyzed to free methionine (Fig. 6). In other experiments we observed similar results with D-Met-L-Met-L-Met, $(Met)_4$-OMe, and $(Met)_5$-OMe. In contrast, D-Met-D-Met-D-Met was resistant to hydrolysis by the cell extract. Finally, the cell extract also contained the enzyme activity to release L-lysine from the lysine-containing peptides. The data in Fig. 7 show that both Lys-Gly and Gly-

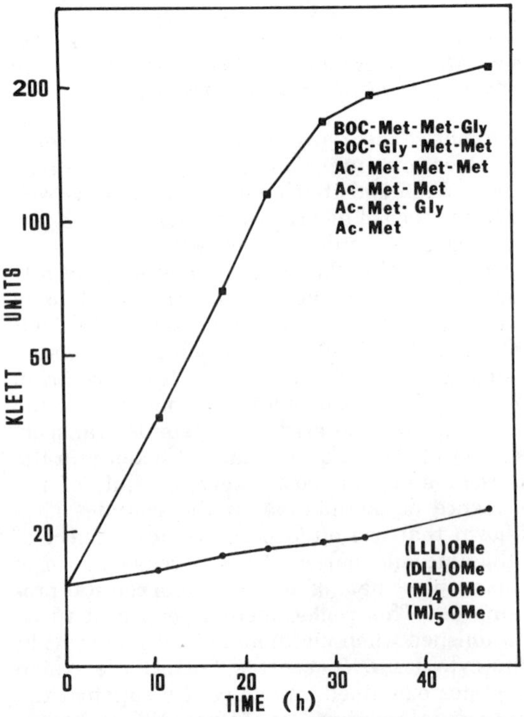

FIG. 4. *Growth response to various blocked methionine-containing peptides.*

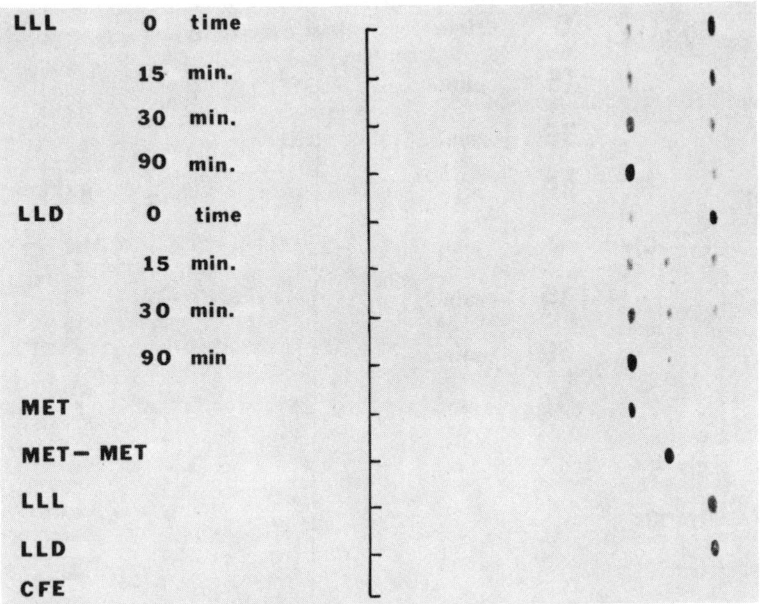

FIG. 5. *Thin-layer chromatogram of L-Met-L-Met-L-Met and L-Met-L-Met-D-Met at various time intervals after incubation with cell extract from C. albicans WD 18-4. The markers are methionine, (Met)$_2$, L-L-L, and L-L-D. CFE, Cell-free extract that gave no ninhydrin-positive spots after chromatography.*

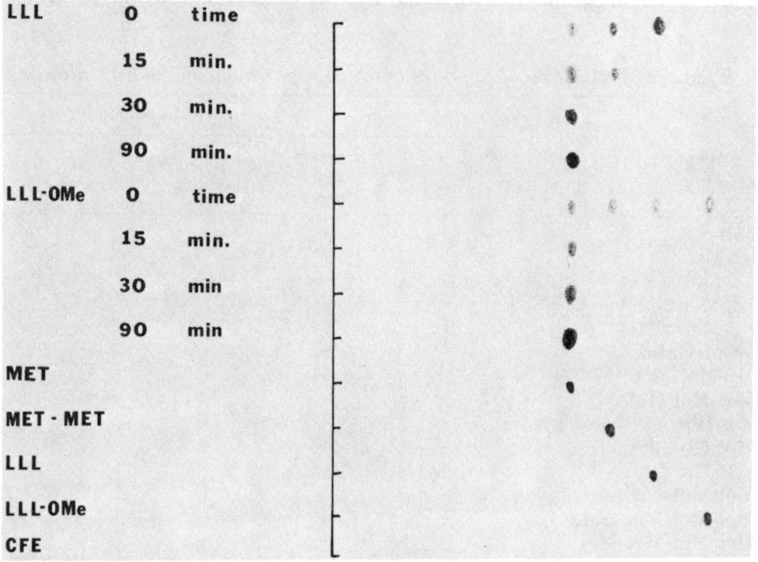

FIG. 6. *Thin-layer chromatogram of L-Met-L-Met-L-Met and L-Met-L-Met-L-Met-OMe at various time intervals after incubation with cell extract.*

Lys were rapidly and completely cleaved to glycine and lysine during a 90-min incubation with the cell extract. In similar experiments we observed that $(Lys)_2$, $(Lys)_3$, $(Lys)_4$, and polylysine also were hydrolyzed rapidly.

DISCUSSION

The measurement of the growth response of an amino acid auxotroph to peptides containing the required amino acid has been widely utilized to study peptide transport systems in microorganisms (2, 14). This method is an indirect way of measuring peptide transport and gives little information about the kinetics of peptide uptake. Nevertheless, auxotrophic growth of a microorganism allows one to gather considerable information about the structural specificity of the peptide transport system. The applica-

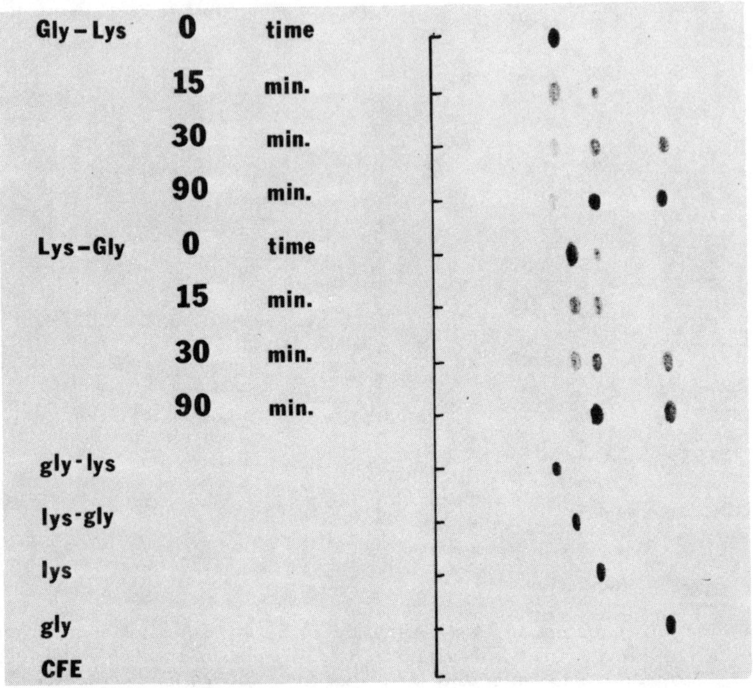

FIG. 7. *Thin-layer chromatogram of Gly-Lys and Lys-Gly at various time intervals after incubation with cell extract.*

TABLE 2. *Utilization of Peptides by E. coli, S. cerevisiae, and C. albicans*

Peptide	Growth response[a]				
	E. coli (*met*⁻)[b]	*S. cerevisiae* (*met*⁻)[c]	*C. albicans* (*met*⁻ *lys*⁻)[d]	*E. coli* (*lys*⁻)[e]	*S. cerevisiae* (*lys*⁻)[f]
Met-Met	+	+	+		
Ac-Met-Met	−	+	+		
L-Met-L-Met-L-Met	+	+	+		
D-Met-L-Met-L-Met	+	+	+		
L-Met-L-Met-D-Met	+	+	−		
Ac-Met-Met-Met	−	+	+		
Boc-Gly-Met-Met	−	+	+		
Met-Met-Met-OMe	+	+	−		
Gly-Met-Gly	+	−	+		
Met-Met-Gly-Met	+	+	+		
Met-Met-Gly-Gly	+	−	+		
Met-Met-Met-Gly	+	−	+		
Met-Met-Met-Met-OMe	+	+	−		
Met-Met-Met-Met-Met	−	+	+		
Lys-Lys			−	+	−
Lys-Gly			+	ND	+
Gly-Lys			−	ND	−
Lys-Lys-Lys			−	+	−

[a] (+) indicates that the peptide substitutes for the required amino acid. (−) indicates that the peptide is not a growth substrate. ND, Not done.

[b] See references 3 and 12.

[c] See references 4 and 13.

[d] This paper.

[e] See reference 9.

[f] See reference 4.

tion of this procedure to the study of peptide transport, however, requires that the species under test does not excrete extracellular peptidases. Previous studies on *S. cerevisiae* led to the conclusion that no extracellular peptidases toward methionine- or lysine-containing peptides were proliferated by this yeast (4, 13).

In the present work we found no evidence of peptidase activity in spent medium from *C. albicans* WD 18-4. Moreover, the failure of *C. albicans* WD 18-4 to utilize a number of peptides and peptide derivatives, despite the fact that these same compounds were rapidly hydrolyzed to the free amino acids by cell extracts of the mutant, gives additional evidence that peptidases are not extracellular. The specificity and array of peptidases in *C. albicans* is not well defined. Data in the literature, however, provide evidence that many dipeptidases and aminopeptidases have relatively broad specificity (6, 17). We believe that it is likely that L-Met-L-Met-L-Met and L-Met-L-Met-D-Met are hydrolyzed by the same peptidase activities. Similarly, Lys-Gly and Gly-Lys are probably hydrolyzed by the same enzyme. Since in each case the former compound is a growth substrate whereas the latter is not, one would have to argue that only those peptidases which cleave growth substrates are located extracellularly. We believe that this argument is tenuous and that the existence of nonutilized peptides which are stucturally similar to growth substrates provides strong evidence for the absence of extracellular peptidases in *C. albicans* WD 18-4. It is reasonable to assume, therefore, that a positive growth response is indicative of the transport of the intact peptide into the mutant.

Data presented in this manuscript show that *C. albicans* can utilize di-, tri-, and tetrapeptides as sources of methionine. In addition, pentamethionine and D-Met-L-Met-L-Met are good growth substrates, whereas L-Met-L-Met-D-Met, D-Met-D-Met-D-Met, and all peptide methyl esters that we examined failed to serve the nutritional requirement of WD 18-4 for methionine. Many of these results are consistent with those of analogous studies on a methionine auxotroph of *S. cerevisiae* G1333 (4, 13) (Table 2). We did observe, however, marked differences in the nature of the growth responses of these yeasts. The growth curve for *S. cerevisiae* was quite sensitive to the composition and sequence of the peptide under investigation. Seven tripeptides composed of methionine and glycine, for example, resulted in different growth responses (13). Those tripeptides having glycine at the carboxyl terminus were significantly poorer growth substrates, and Gly-Met-Gly was not utilized. In *C. albicans* WD 18-4 we did not observe any correlation between the peptide structure and the nature or the growth response. For the most part, the peptide was either a good growth substrate or it was not utilized at all. Three peptides that were not growth substrates for *S. cerevisiae* G1333 (Gly-Met-Gly, Met-Met-Gly-Gly, and Met-Met-Met-Gly) all satisfied the methionine requirement of *C. albicans*. It is not clear, at present, what these differences represent. We have observed recently that other auxotrophs of *S. cerevisiae* do have structural specificities which differ somewhat from those of strain G1333 (unpublished data).

The ability of *C. albicans* to discriminate between various diastereomers of trimethionine suggests that the peptide transport system in this yeast is stereospecific. It is especially of interest that strain WD 18-4 can utilize D-Met-L-Met-L-Met, whereas it fails to utilize L-Met-L-Met-D-Met (Fig. 3). Both of these diastereomers are rapidly hydrolyzed by cell extracts, and the different growth response is evidently a consequence of the failure of the latter compound to enter the yeast. We should note, however, that *C. albicans* is a eucaryotic microorganism containing many intracellular organelles. At present we are not certain of the exact location of the intracellular peptidases. It is possible that the discrimination between the L-Met-L-Met-D-Met and D-Met-L-Met-L-Met occurs not at the cytoplasmic membrane but at some secondary barrier such as the vacuolar membrane. It is likely that D-Met-D-Met-D-Met also fails to enter *C. albicans*. The resistance of this peptide to hydrolysis by cell extracts makes it impossible to rule out by growth response the possibility that this peptide enters the cell but remains unhydrolyzed. There are few reports in the literature on the stereospecificities of peptide transport systems. L-Met-L-Met-D-Met and D-Met-L-Met-L-Met were both observed to support the growth of methionine auxotrophs of *E. coli* (3). L-Val-L-Val-D-Val was taken up by *Pediococcus cerevisiae* (16).

Despite the growth of strain WD 18-4 on methionine-containing peptides, this auxotroph was unable to utilize most of the lysine-containing peptides tested as growth substrates (Table 1). Again all of the nonutilized peptides were rapidly cleaved to component amino acids during incubation with cell extracts of *C. albicans* WD 18-4, and none of the lysine peptides was toxic. The failure to utilize the lysine-containing peptides is thus a consequence of the failure of these peptides to reach the site of the peptidase activity. The finding that *C. albicans* readily utilized methionine peptides but fails to utilize lysine peptides is analogous to results of similar studies on *S. cerevisiae* (Table 2). Recently we found that a leucine-lysine auxotroph of *S. cerevisiae*, strain Z1-2D, can utilize leucine-containing peptides but does not grow on most lysine-containing peptides (unpublished data). In agreement with the present work, *S. cerevisiae* Z1-2D was unable to utilize Gly-Lys although it utilized Lys-Gly. The inability to transport lysine-containing peptides occurs in a number of mutants of *S. cerevisiae* and in *C. albicans* and may be a general feature of the peptide transport phenomenon in yeasts.

As mentioned previously, a rational drug design requires knowledge of the ability of peptide derivatives to enter microorganisms. Previous studies with *E. coli* showed that although modification of the carboxyl end of the oligopeptide could be tolerated by the peptide transport system, acylation of a peptide rendered it untransportable (14; Table 2). We found just the opposite to be true with *C. albicans* (Table 2). The fact that yeast can take up acylated peptides can be readily incorporated into the design of toxic peptides which could only enter yeast but which would not permeate into bacterial or mammalian cells. As part of the strategy, one must consider the failure of strain WD 18-4 to utilize peptide esters and a peptide with an L-L-D configuration. We are currently involved in efforts that will attempt to apply these concepts to the rational design of agents that will be toxic specifically toward *C. albicans*.

ACKNOWLEDGMENTS

This investigation was supported by grant CH-12 from the American Cancer Society. J.M.B. and F.N. are Career Development Awardees of Public Health Service grants GM-00094 and GM-00025, respectively, from the National Institute of General Medical Sciences.

LITERATURE CITED

1. **Ames, B. N., G. F.-L. Ames, J. D. Young, D. Tsuchiya, and J. Lecocq.** 1973. Illicit transport: the oligopeptide permease. Proc. Natl. Acad. Sci. U.S.A. **70**:456–458.
2. **Barak, Z., and C. Gilvarg.** 1975. Peptide transport, p. 167-218. *In* H. Eisenberg, E. Katchalski-Katzir, and L. A. Manson (ed.), Biomembranes, vol. 7, Plenum Press, New York.
3. **Becker, J. M., and F. Naider.** 1974. Stereospecificity of tripeptide utilization in a methionine auxotroph of *Escherichia coli* K-12. J. Bacteriol. **120**:191–196.
4. **Becker, J. M., F. Naider, and E. Katchalski.** 1973. Peptide utilization in yeast: studies on methionine and lysine auxotrophs of *Saccharomyces cerevisiae*. Biochim. Biophys. Acta **291**:388–397.
5. **Cascieri, T., Jr., and M. F. Mallette.** 1976. Peptide utilization by *Pseudomonas putida* and *Pseudomonas maltophilia*. *J. Gen. Microbiol.* **92**:283–295.
6. **DeLange, R. J., and E. L. Smith.** 1971. Leucine aminopeptidase and other N-terminal exopeptidases, p. 43–57. *In* P. D. Boyer (ed.), The enzymes, vol. 3. Academic Press Inc., New York.
7. **Fickel, T. E., and C. Gilvarg.** 1973. Transport of impermeant substances in *E. coli* by way of oligopeptide permease. Nature (London) New Biol. **241**:161–163.
8. **Fowden, L., D. Lewis, and H. Tristam.** 1967. Toxic amino acids: their action as antimetabolites. Adv. Enzymol. Relat. Areas Mol. Biol. **29**:89–163.
9. **Gilvarg, C., and E. Katchalski.** 1965. Peptide utilization in *Escherichia coli*. J. Biol. Chem. **240**:3093–3098.
10. **Haworth, C., and J. G. Heathcote.** 1969. An improved technique for the analysis of amino acids and related compounds on thin layers of cellulose. Part I. Qualitative separation. J. Chromatogr. **14**:380–385.
11. **Lowry, O. H., N. J. Rosebrough, A. L. Farr, and R. J. Randall.** 1951. Protein measurement with the Folin phenol reagent. J. Biol. Chem. **193**:265–275.
12. **Naider, F., and J. M. Becker.** 1975. Multiplicity of oligopeptide transport systems in *Escherichia coli*. J. Bacteriol. **122**:1208–1215.
13. **Naider, F., J. M. Becker, and E. Katchalski.** 1974. Utilization of methionine-containing peptides and their derivatives by a methionine requiring auxotroph of *Saccharomyces cerevisiae*. J. Biol. Chem. **249**:9–20.
14. **Payne, J. W., and C. Gilvarg.** 1971. Peptide transport. Adv. Enzymol. Relat. Areas Mol. Biol. **35**:187–244.
15. **Rubino, A., M. Field, and H. Shwachman.** 1971. Intestinal transport of amino acid residues of dipeptides. I. Influx of the glycine residue of glycyl-L-proline across mucosal border. J. Biol. Chem. **246**:3542–3548.
16. **Shankman, S., V. Gold, S. Higa, and R. Squires.** 1962. On the mode of action of a peptide inhibitor of growth in *P. cerevisiae*. Biochem. Biophys. Res. Commun. **9**:25–31.
17. **Simmonds, S.** 1972. Peptidase activity and peptide metabolism in *Escherichia coli*. *In* K. Elliot and M. O'Conner (ed.), Ciba Foundation Symposium on Peptide Transport in Bacteria and the Mammalian Gut. Elsevier, New York.
18. **Wolfinbarger, L., Jr., and G. A. Marzluf.** 1974. Peptide utilization by amino acid auxotrophs of *Neurospora crassa*. J. Bacteriol. **119**:371–378.
19. **Wolfinbarger, L., Jr., and G. A. Marzluf.** 1975. Specificity and regulation of peptide transport in *Neurospora crassa*. Arch. Biochem. Biophys. **171**:637–644.
20. **Wolfinbarger, L., Jr., and G. A. Marzluf.** 1975. Size restriction on utilization of peptides by amino acid auxotrophs of *Neurospora crassa*. J. Bacteriol. **122**: 949–956.

ANTIMICROBIAL AGENTS AND CHEMOTHERAPY, Sept. 1976, p. 491-497 Vol. 10, No. 3

Pirbenicillin: Pharmacokinetic Parameters in Mice

ARTHUR R. ENGLISH,* DENNIS GIRARD, AND JAMES A. RETSEMA
Central Research, Pfizer, Inc., Groton, Connecticut 06340

Received for publication 13 May 1976

The rapid intravenous administration to mice of pirbenicillin, carbenicillin, and ampicillin produced biexponential blood concentration-time curves when assessed by frequent blood samplings at short intervals. The pharmacokinetic behavior of pirbenicillin and the other penicillins was analyzed by the two-compartment open model. This is thought to be the first study giving detailed pharmacokinetic values of penicillins in mice. Some significant differences were noted between the pharmacokinetic values of pirbenicillin, ampicillin, and carbenicillin. These values suggest that the interchange of pirbenicillin between the central and peripheral body compartments of the mouse was slower than that of either carbenicillin or ampicillin and indicated that a greater fraction of the pirbenicillin than the ampicillin dose reached the peripheral compartment.

Pirbenicillin (former designation, CP-33,994), a new broad-spectrum, semisynthetic penicillin, has demonstrated two to four times greater activity than carbenicillin against several experimental infections in mice (12a). In vivo effectiveness of an antibiotic results from the complex interdependence of antibacterial activity at the site(s) of infection and pharmacokinetic processes. In addition to drug concentration in blood and urine, the processes that characterize and regulate the movement of a drug through the body are represented by its biological half-life, apparent volume of distribution, various distribution and elimination rate constants, and serum-tissue drug ratios. Usually these detailed pharmacokinetic parameters are determined in the late stages of antibiotic evaluation by studies in large animals or in man. However, as mice are routinely used in the early stages of antibiotic evaluation, it was of interest to determine these properties of pirbenicillin in this species.

MATERIALS AND METHODS

Pirbenicillin (sodium salt), ampicillin (trihydrate), and carbenicillin (disodium salt) were obtained from members of Chemical Research, Pfizer, Inc. Dosage forms were prepared as solutions in physiological saline.

Mice averaging 25 g were purchased from Blue Spruce Farms, Altamont, N. Y. After a single intravenous injection of 10 mg of drug per kg, whole blood samples were obtained from the orbital sinus of mice by using heparinized hemocrit tubes (14). Each mouse had an identification mark to insure bleeding in the same sequence at sampling times. A second group of 10 mice were maintained in a plastic metabolism cage to insure collection of feces-free urine. These mice were used only in the urine excretion study. Urine was collected in a tube packed in ice.

Antibiotic in mouse whole blood and urine was assayed using filter-paper disks (6.5 mm) moistened with 0.025 ml of sample placed on seed agar (Baltimore Biological Laboratories) in large plates. Two or three disks were prepared from each mouse at each time sample. Standard curves, as well as necessary sample dilution, were prepared in the respective fluid from normal mice. *Micrococcus luteus*, ATCC 9341, was used as the assay organism for pirbenicillin and ampicillin. The Ellsworth strain of *Pseudomonas aeruginosa*, NCTC 10490, was used to assay carbenicillin.

The mouse data at each time interval represent the mean value of samples from 15 to 20 individual mice, which were used during three to four individual experiments. Mean values and the standard error of the mean were calculated on a programmable desk-type calculator (Monroe 1860). In some instances, the significance of differences between mean values of the pharmacokinetic parameters of the antibiotics was determined by the t-test.

RESULTS

The calculated pharmacokinetic values presented are independent of dose; values obtained with dosages of 5 mg of pirbenicillin and ampicillin per kg and 20 mg of carbenicillin per kg agreed well with those presented for the 10-mg/kg dosage.

Semilog plots of mean whole blood concentrations of pirbenicillin, carbenicillin, and ampicillin after a 10-mg/kg intravenous injection versus time are presented in Table 1 and Fig. 1A, B, and C. The plots consist of two segments: (i) the first segment, or "α-phase" (distribution phase), which results primarily from rapid distribution of the drug between blood and the extravascular tissue compartment; and (ii) a

TABLE 1. *Pirbenicillin, carbenicillin, and ampicillin in mice: mean whole blood concentrations in mice (10 mg/kg, intravenous)*

Sample time (min)	Mean concn (μg/ml) with SEM[a]		
	Pirbenicillin	Carbenicillin	Ampicillin
1	18.20 ± 0.86 (18.20)[b]	16.6 ± 1.78 (17.7)[b]	18.70 ± 0.97 (20.4)[b]
3	9.40 ± 0.56 (9.51)	7.40 ± 0.54 (6.9)	10.60 ± 0.43 (10.15)
5	6.00 ± 0.36 (5.90)	4.67 ± 0.28 (4.70)	7.98 ± 0.34 (7.72)
10	3.65 ± 0.25 (3.37)	3.37 ± 0.17 (3.62)	6.36 ± 0.25 (6.24)
15	2.75 ± 0.21 (2.74)		5.20 ± 0.20 (5.38)
20		2.47 ± 0.04 (2.20)	
30	1.59 ± 0.25 (1.74)	1.82 ± 0.05 (1.84)	3.27 ± 0.28 (3.47)
45		1.37 ± 0.03 (1.11)	
60	0.64 ± 0.17 (0.72)	0.78 ± 0.01 (0.67)	1.58 ± 0.23 (1.45)
90	0.28 ± 0.09 (0.30)		0.58 ± 0.09 (0.60)
120	0.14 ± 0.05 (0.12)		0.26 ± 0.05 (0.25)

[a] SEM, Standard error of the mean.

[b] The numbers within parentheses were calculated using the biexponential equation of $C_p = Ae^{-\alpha t} + Be^{-\beta t}$. We thank J. Taylor of Pfizer, Inc. for these computer simulations.

straight segment, or "β-phase," the slope of which is determined by the rates of distribution, excretion, and/or metabolism of the drug. The decline in whole blood concentrations of pirbenicillin and the other penicillins occurs in a biexponential manner that can be mathematically fitted to a two-compartment open model (13):

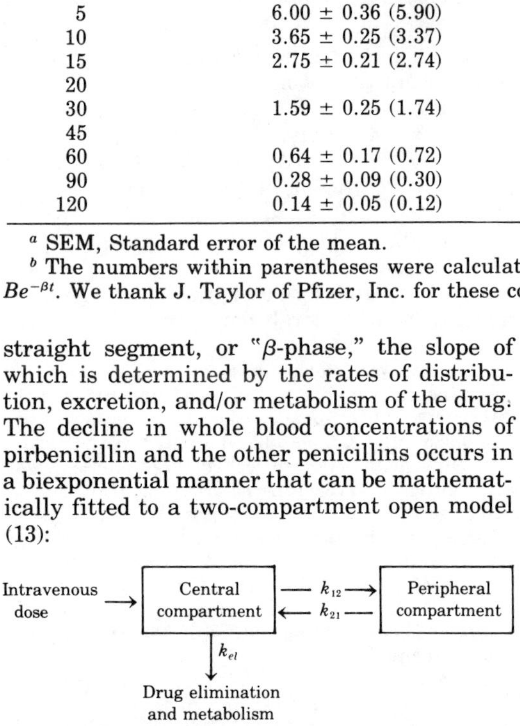

Solution of the differential equations resulting from this model yield the biexponential equation, $C_p = Ae^{-\alpha t} + Be^{-\beta t}$. C_p is the drug concentration in the blood at time t; A and B are the intercepts on the ordinate axis. At zero time, $C_p = A_0 + B_0$ (2, 7). The first-order distribution rate constants k_{12} and k_{21} control the movement of drug between the two compartments; k_{e1} is the sum of the first-order constants relevant to metabolism and excretion. These various parameters were determined by plotting the data on semilogarithmic paper and subsequent regression analysis by the method of least squares. A linear regression, constructed from the β-phase, was extrapolated to the ordinate. The importance of drug elimination that occurs in the very early stages after intravenous administration was considered in that the extrapolated β-phase values were subtracted from the observed α-phase values to give the residual lines shown in Fig. 1A, B, and C (7, 10). A_0 and α are the intercept and rate constant, respectively, of the residual α-phase line; B_0 and β are the intercept and rate constant, respectively, of the β-phase line. Biological half-life of each segment of the distribution-elimination curve is related to the slope of the segment and was calculated as $T1/2 = 0.693/\text{rate constant}$ (7). Values of A_0, B_0, α, and β for pirbenicillin, carbenicillin, and ampicillin are presented in Table 2. Also presented is the area under the concentration curve ($AUC_{0\rightarrow\infty}$) expressed as μg·ml/min as determined by the trapezoidal rule (11). That the blood concentration-time curves are well described by the use of the above-mentioned values in the biexponential equation is shown by the similarity of the calculated data points to observed points, which are presented in Table 1.

The individual rate constants in the two-compartment model were calculated following the detailed mathematical procedures described by Gillette (7). The first-order rate constant, k_{21}, for the passage of the drug from the peripheral to the central compartment was calculated as $k_{21} = (A_0 \cdot \beta + B_0 \cdot \alpha)/(A_0 + B_0)$; the first-order rate constant, k_{e1}, of the elimination of drug from the central compartment was calculated as $k_{e1} = \alpha \cdot \beta / k_{21}$; the first-order rate constant, k_{12}, for the passage of the drug from the central compartment to the peripheral compartment was calculated as

$$k_{12} = (\alpha + \beta) - (k_{21} + k_{e1})$$

A summary of these individual rate constants for pirbenicillin and the other penicillins is presented in Table 3.

Each antibiotic left the vascular system rapidly and penetrated the tissue compartment (Table 2). However, based on the half-life values of the α-phase (distribution), pirbenicillin did distribute more slowly than did either carbenicillin or ampicillin: 1.90 min compared

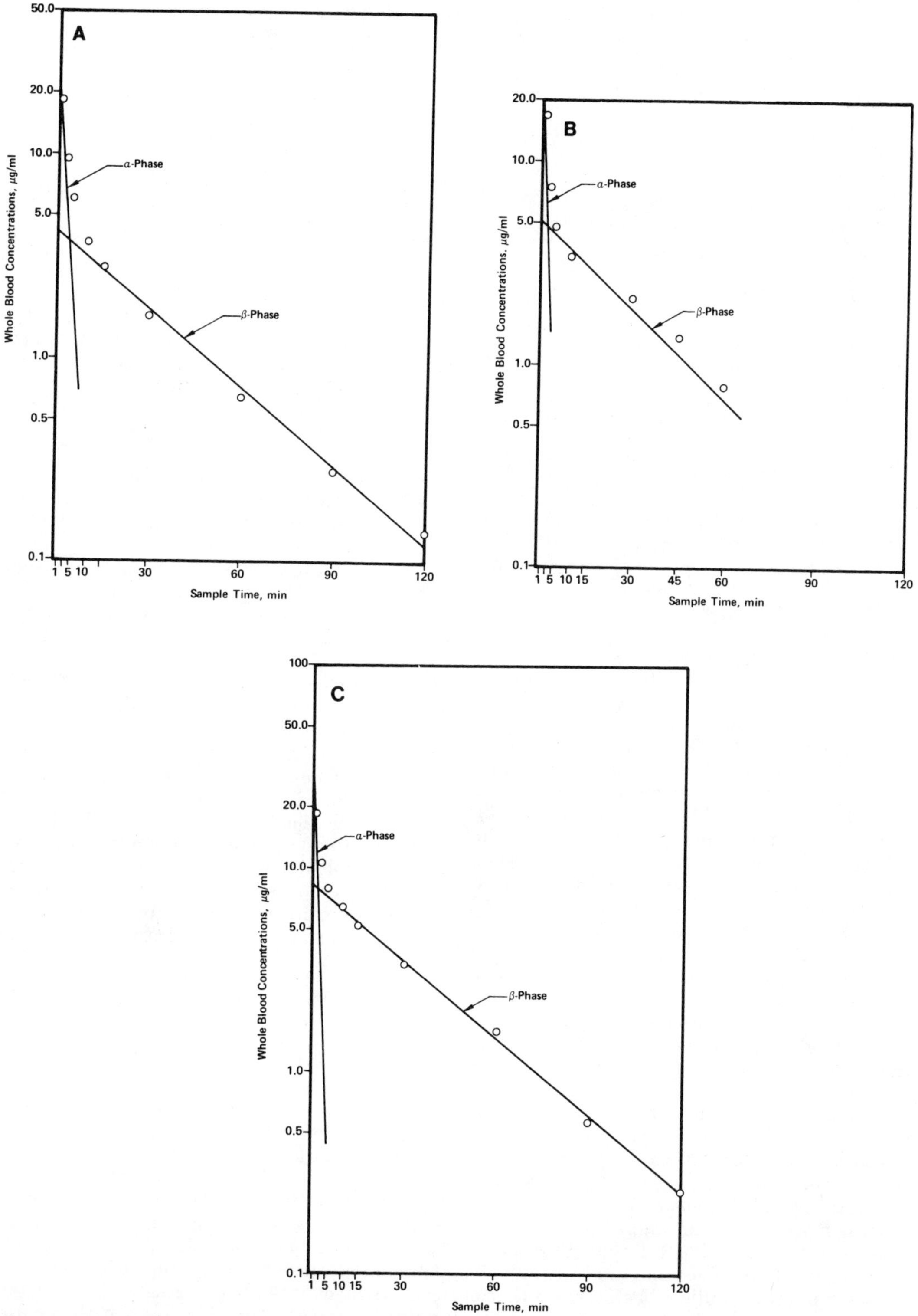

FIG. 1. *(A) Pirbenicillin; (B) carbenicillin; (C) ampicillin. Concentrations in mouse whole blood after a 10-mg/kg intravenous dosage. Constructed α- and β-phase lines.*

TABLE 2. *Pirbenicillin, carbenicillin, and ampicillin in mice: intravenous administration (10 mg/kg) – pharmacokinetic parameters of α- and β-phases*

Antibiotics	Pharmacokinetic parameters of:						AUC[a] curve ($\mu g \cdot ml/min$) $0 \rightarrow \infty$
	α-Phase			β-Phase			
	A_0 ($\mu g/ml$)	α[b]	Half-life (min)	B_0 ($\mu g/ml$)	β[b]	Half-life (min)	
Pirbenicillin	19.50 ± 2.49[c]	−0.389 ± 0.031	1.90 ± 0.17	4.33 ± 0.31	−0.032 ± 0.002	22.20 ± 1.68	178.89 ± 20.23
Carbenicillin	28.50 ± 3.49	−0.817 ± 0.072	0.93 ± 0.11	5.04 ± 0.29	−0.033 ± 0.002	21.27 ± 0.88	153.15 ± 4.90
Ampicillin	20.50 ± 3.38	−0.633 ± 0.059	1.18 ± 0.11	8.50 ± 0.25	−0.031 ± 0.001	23.20 ± 0.40	296.82 ± 23.44

[a] AUC, Areas under concentration.
[b] Rate constant of decline.
[c] Standard error of the mean.

TABLE 3. *Pirbenicillin, carbenicillin, and ampicillin in mice: intravenous administration (10 mg/kg) – elimination rate constants*

Antibiotics (10 mg/kg, i.v.)	Elimination rate constants		
	k_{12} (blood → periphery)	k_{21} (min^{-1}) (periphery → blood)	k_{e1} (min^{-1}) (elimination from blood)
Pirbenicillin	0.197 ± 0.026[a]	0.095 ± 0.004	0.129 ± 0.007
Carbenicillin	0.516 ± 0.061	0.156 ± 0.011	0.177 ± 0.017
Ampicillin	0.359 ± 0.051	0.213 ± 0.016	0.092 ± 0.008

[a] Standard error of the mean.

with 0.93 and 1.18 min. The difference between pirbenicillin and carbenicillin was significant (t-test) at $P = 0.005$; the difference between pirbenicillin and ampicillin, $P = 0.001$.

Relatively short half-lives in the distribution phase are seen also in larger animals; for example, for ampicillin the distribution half-lives are 4.8 min in beagles and 15.6 min in man (3, 10). Similarly, k_{12}, the rate constant describing the distribution of pirbenicillin from the blood to the peripheral compartment, was only one-third that of carbenicillin (t-test: $P = >0.001$) and one-half that of ampicillin (t-test: $P = 0.02$) (Table 3). Riegelman et al. have pointed out that the rate of uptake of a compound into tissues is controlled by several factors, including the rate of blood flow through the tissue, the mass or volume of the tissue, and the partition characteristics of the compound between plasma and the tissues (13). As the first two factors are common to all the antibiotics in these mouse studies, the partition characteristics may account for the observed differences in the distribution phase. Other studies have shown that in a butanol-water system, pirbenicillin is more polar than ampicillin but is less polar than carbenicillin (R. Rosati, Pfizer, Inc., unpublished data). Thus one might expect the k_{12} value of pirbenicillin to be between that of ampicillin and carbenicillin. Because it is substantially less than the k_{12} value for both ampicillin and carbenicillin, some other unknown factor may play an important role.

Relevant to the elimination phase, pirbenicillin appears more similar to carbenicillin than to ampicillin. The extrapolated value of B_0 (Table 2) in the elimination phase of pirbenicillin is similar to that of carbenicillin and only one-half that of ampicillin (t-test: $P = <0.001$). However, β, the rate constant of the decline in the second phase of pirbenicillin, is very similar to that of ampicillin and carbenicillin. All three penicillins have similar half-life values in the elimination phase (Table 2). The rate constant, k_{21}, describing the movement of drug from periphery to blood is about two times smaller for pirbenicillin than for carbenicillin (t-test: $P = <0.001$) and ampicillin (t-test: P = 0.01) (Table 3). The hybrid rate constant, k_{e1}, for both pirbenicillin and ampicillin is similar and smaller than that for carbenicillin.

The whole blood-peripheral distribution of pirbenicillin and the other penicillins was estimated by calculating the fraction of the administered dose in the extravascular peripheral and central compartments using average data for all mice and the analysis described by Rattie and Ravin (12):

$$A_{\text{tissue}} = \frac{k_{12}}{\alpha - \beta}\left(e^{-\beta t} - e^{-\alpha t}\right) \text{ and}$$

$$A_{\substack{\text{central}\\ \text{compartment}}} = \left[\left(\frac{\alpha - k_{21}}{\alpha - \beta}\right) e^{-\alpha t} + \left(\frac{k_{21} - \beta}{\alpha - \beta}\right) e^{-\beta t}\right]$$

Figure 2A presents the percentage of pirbenicillin dose estimated in the peripheral compartment and in the central compartment. Similar plots for carbenicillin and ampicillin are presented in Fig. 2B and C. The amount of pirbenicillin in the tissue compartment peaked at about 45% of the administered dose at 5 min, after which time the percentage of dose in this compartment was always greater than in the central compartment. The peak carbenicillin

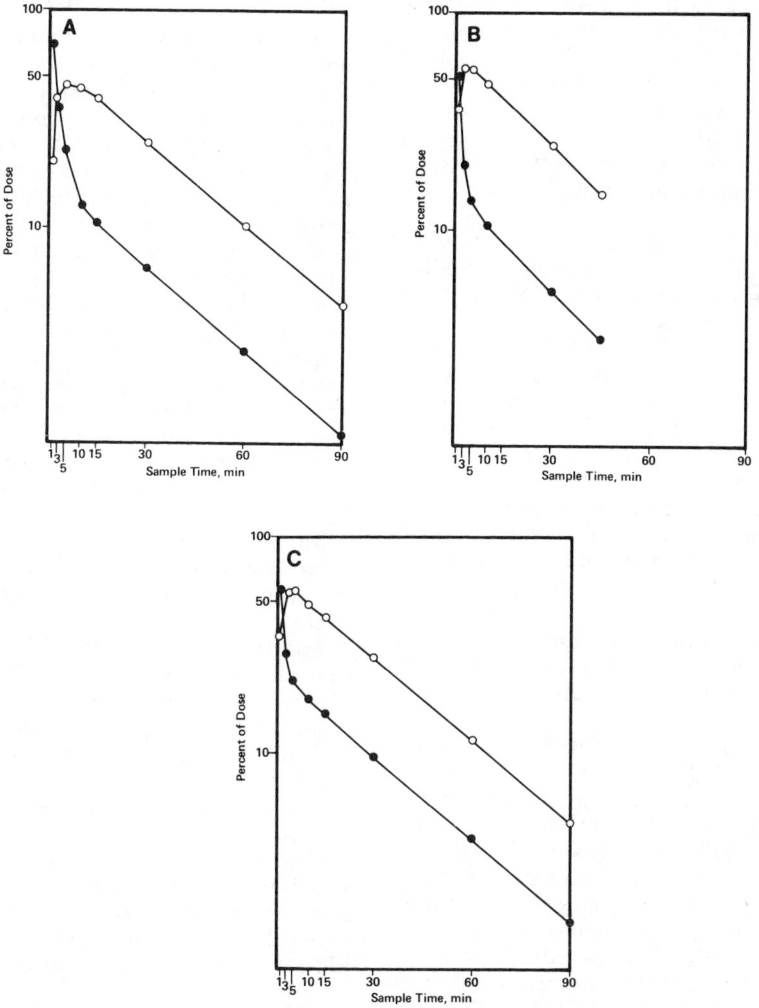

FIG. 2. *(A) Pirbenicillin; (B) carbenicillin; (C) ampicillin. Percentage of intravenous dose in mice (10 mg/kg) in peripheral (●) and central compartments (○).*

and ampicillin percentage of dose in the tissue compartment was about 55% after 3 to 5 min postinjection. As was true with pirbenicillin, subsequent decreases in both tissue and blood compartments were parallel. Again, the percentage of the dose in the tissue compartment after peaking was always greater than in the blood compartment. This has been observed in man with both penicillins and cephalosporins (5, 12).

The kinetic volume of distribution of the entire body was calculated from the parameters of the two-compartment model as follows:

$$V_{d(k)} = \frac{\text{dose } (T1/2 \text{ of } \beta\text{-phase})}{A_{a(0)} \cdot (T1/2 \text{ of } \alpha\text{-phase}) + B_{a(0)} \cdot (T1/2 \text{ of } \beta\text{-phase})} \quad (7)$$

Values for V_p were calculated by dividing the dose by C_p^0, the whole blood concentration at zero time ($A_0 + B_0$). Values for V_t were calculated by the relationship:

$$V_t = V_p \cdot \frac{k_{12}}{k_{21}} \quad (8)$$

In addition, the fraction V_t/V_p is equivalent to the ratio of the amount of drug in the extravascular tissue compartment to the amount of drug in the central compartment. These values are presented in Table 4.

The kinetic volume of distribution of ampicillin approximated the volume of the mouse; however, those of pirbenicillin and carbenicillin were greater than the mouse volume. The

$V_{d(k)}$ value of pirbenicillin was significantly greater than those of carbenicillin (t-test: P = 0.05) and ampicillin (P = 0.001). The apparent volume of the central compartment of pirbenicillin also was significantly greater than that of carbenicillin (t-test: P = 0.025) and, in addition, the V_t value of pirbenicillin was greater than that of ampicillin (t-test: P = 0.001) (Table 4).

Volumes of distribution values in mice and rabbits for antibiotics in addition to penicillins, i.e., tetracyclines, streptomycin, and macrolides, have been found greater than body volume (9, 15; A.R.E., unpublished data). Localization in a body tissue or fluid has been suggested as a possible explanation (1, 9). Also, serum binding is an important determinant in drug distribution and activity. It is generally agreed that only free drug can distribute into tissues because drug-protein complexes cannot penetrate cell membranes (6). However, as indicated in Table 5, serum binding to mouse serum proteins by pirbenicillin, carbenicillin, and ampicillin were nearly equivalent. It is likely, therefore, that the contribution of serum binding to the observed differences in distribution volumes was minimal.

Total clearance rates (TCR) were evaluated as TCR = $k_{e1} \cdot V_p$ (12). The TCR value for pirbenicillin was similar to that of carbenicillin. Both were greater than that for ampicillin (t-test: P = 0.001) (Table 6). It should be recalled that this is a measure of elimination by all processes and is always greater than elimination as a result of renal function only. Renal clearance rates (RCR) were calculated by using the fraction (f) of the dose recovered in the urine multiplied by TCR: RCR = TCR$\cdot f$ (12).

These data are presented in Table 6. The RCR of pirbenicillin and ampicillin were quite similar; both were higher than that of carbenicillin. Percentage of urinary recovery of the administered dose during a 24-h period for pirbenicillin, carbenicillin, and ampicillin, respectively, amounted to 43.2 ± 0.85%, 38.4 ± 0.25%, and 69.8 ± 1.9%.

DISCUSSION

The rapid intravenous administration of pirbenicillin, carbenicillin, and ampicillin to mice produced biexponential blood concentration-time curves when assessed by frequent blood samplings at short intervals (Table 1; Fig. 1A, B, and C). The two-compartment open model and the graphical technique for measuring the various parameters were adequate to interpret the pharmacokinetic behavior of pirbenicillin and the other penicillins studied in mice. The present study is thought to be the first giving detailed pharamacokinetic values for penicillins, or any other antibiotic, in mice. The biexponential curve is typical of penicillins, other antibiotics, and other therapeutic agents in man and larger animals (3–5).

The pharmacokinetic values of pirbenicillin, in a number of instances, were significantly different from those of carbenicillin and ampicillin, e.g., volume of distribution values, k_{12}, k_{21}, and α-phase half-life. Generally, the pharmacokinetic values suggest that the interchange between the central and peripheral compartments for pirbenicillin is slower than that of the other penicillins. The V_t/V_p ratio (fraction of the dose in the peripheral compartment) suggests that a greater fraction of the pirbenicillin dose than the ampicillin dose reaches the peripheral compartment; the values of both these antibiotics are smaller than that for carbenicillin.

Urinary recovery of pirbenicillin (43.2%) was intermediate between ampicillin (69.8%) and carbenicillin (38.4%). The difference between TCR and RCR suggests either considerable non-renal elimination or urinary excretion

TABLE 5. *Pirbenicillin, carbenicillin, and ampicillin serum binding[a] in mouse serum*

Penicillins	Mouse serum
Pirbenicillin	24.2% ± 1.2[b]
Carbenicillin	22.6% ± 1.9
Ampicillin	23.2% ± 0.0

[a] As determined by an ultrafiltration procedure.
[b] Standard error of the mean.

TABLE 4. *Pirbenicillin, carbenicillin, and ampicillin in mice: intravenous administration (10 mg/kg)—volume distribution values*

Antibiotics	Apparent vol of: Distribution V_{dk} (ml)	Central compartment V_p (ml)	Extravascular compartment V_t (ml)	V_t/V_p ratio
Pirbenicillin	46.93 ± 2.47[a]	12.60 ± 1.36	34.33 ± 2.07	3.03 ± 0.39
Carbenicillin	39.49 ± 2.30	8.20 ± 1.21	31.29 ± 2.02	4.39 ± 0.53
Ampicillin	27.25 ± 0.77	9.63 ± 0.89	17.62 ± 1.04	2.10 ± 0.37

[a] Standard error of the mean.

TABLE 6. *Pirbenicillin, carbenicillin, and ampicillin in mice: intravenous administration (10 mg/kg)–TCR and RCR rates*

Antibiotics	TCR[a]	RCR[a]
Pirbenicillin	1.60 ± 0.16[b]	0.60
Carbenicillin	1.43 ± 0.07	0.49
Ampicillin	0.83 ± 0.05	0.56

[a] TCR, Total clearance rate; RCR, renal clearance rate (milliliters per minute).
[b] Standard error of the mean.

of a biologically less active material for pirbenicillin, carbenicillin, and, to a lesser extent, ampicillin in the mouse.

Pharmacokinetic parameters represent important processes that characterize and regulate the movement of a drug through the body. However, overall assessment of efficacy of antibiotic against infections involve the above plus the further complexity and interplay or relative bacteriostatic and/or bactericidal activity at the site(s) of infection. In this regard, pirbenicillin has been shown previously to have greater antibacterial activity in vitro than carbenicillin, and this potency advantage was also observed in murine protection models with *Pseudomonas*, *Serratia*, and *Escherichia coli* (12a).

LITERATURE CITED

1. **Barza, M., and L. Weinstein.** 1974. Some determinants of the distribution of penicillins and cephalosporins in the body. Practical and theoretical considerations. Ann. N. Y. Acad. Sci. **235**:613–619.
2. **Benner, J.** 1971. Cephalosporin antibiotics: therapeutic discussions and future. Postgrad. Med. J. **47**(Suppl.): 135–142.
3. **Cabana, B. E., L. E. Willhite, and M. E. Bierwagen.** 1970. Pharmacokinetic evaluation of the oral absorption of different ampicillin preparations in beagle dogs, p. 35–41. Antimicrob. Agents Chemother. 1969.
4. **Davis, L. E., C. A. Nell, J. D. Baggot, and T. E. Powers.** 1971. Pharmacokinetics of chloramphenicol in domesticated animals. Am. J. Vet. Res. **33**:2259–2265.
5. **Dittert, L. W., W. O. Griffen, Jr., J. C. LaPiana, F. J. Shainfeld, and J. T. Doluisio.** 1970. Pharmacokinetic interpretation of penicillin levels in serum and urine after intravenous administration, p. 42–48. Antimicrob. Agents Chemother. 1969.
6. **Feldman, S.** 1974. Symposium on individualization of drug therapy. Drug distribution. Med. Clin. North Am. **58**:917–926.
7. **Gillette, J. R.** 1973. The importance of tissue distribution in pharmacokinetics. J. Pharmacokinet. Biopharm. **1**:497–520.
8. **Greenblatt, D. J., and J. Koch-Weser.** 1975. Drug therapy. Clinical pharmacokinetics. N. Engl. J. Med. **293**:702–705.
9. **Kuch, N. A., and G. S. Redin.** 1960. Comparison of demethylchlortetracycline with tetracycline in the control of experimental infections in mice. J. Pharmacol. Exp. Ther. **129**:350–355.
10. **MacLeod, C., H. Rabin, R. Ogilvie, J. Ruedy, M. Caron, D. Zarowny, and R. O. Davies.** 1974. Practical concepts of drug absorption, distribution and loss. Can. Med. Assoc. J. **111**:341–346.
11. **Notari, R. E.** 1971. Biopharmaceutics and pharmacokinetics, an introduction, p. 239–240. Marcel Dekker, Inc., New York.
12. **Rattie, E. S., and L. J. Ravin.** 1975. Pharmacokinetic interpretation of blood levels and urinary excretion data for cefazolin and cephalothin after intravenous and intramuscular administration in humans. Antimicrob. Agents Chemother. **7**:606–613.

12a. **Retsema, J. A., A. R. English, and J. E. Lynch.** 1976. Laboratory studies with a new broad-spectrum penicillin, pirbenicillin. Antimicrob. Agents Chemother. **9**:975–982.

13. **Riegelman, S., J. C. K. Loo, and M. Rowland.** 1968. Shortcomings in pharmacokinetic analysis by conceiving the body to exhibit properties of a single compartent. J. Pharm. Sci. **57**:117–123.
14. **Salem, H., M. H. Grossman, and D. L. J. Bilbey.** 1963. Micromethod for intravenous injection and blood sampling. J. Pharm. Sci. **52**:794–795.
15. **Spitzy, K. H., and G. Hitzenberger.** 1958. The distribution volume of some antibiotics. Antibiot. Ann. **1957–1958**:996–1003.

ANTIMICROBIAL AGENTS AND CHEMOTHERAPY, Sept. 1976, p. 498–502

Vol. 10, No. 3
Printed in U.S.A.

Chemical Nature of Agrocin 84 and Its Effect on a Virulent Strain of *Agrobacterium tumefaciens*

BARBARA A. McCARDELL AND C. F. POOTJES*
Department of Microbiology, The Pennsylvania State University, University Park, Pennsylvania 16802

Received for publication 19 April 1976

Agrocin 84, produced by *Agrobacterium radiobacter* K84, inhibited ribonucleic acid, deoxyribonucleic acid, and protein synthesis and amino acid transport in a susceptible, virulent strain of *A. tumefaciens* H-38-9. Cell motility was immediately stopped by action of the agrocin, 50% of the cells were killed within 15 min of contact, and the remainder were inhibited. Agrocin 84 is trypsin and pepsin resistant, but chemical analysis indicated a small peptide with a molecular weight of 2,500 containing six different amino acids, including nine molecules of glutamine or glutamic acid and seven molecules of serine.

Crown-gall is a neoplastic disease in plants produced by the bacterium *Agrobacterium tumefaciens*. Usually, two conditions must be met before the disease can be initiated: the plant must be wounded and the living virulent bacterial cells must come in direct contact with the dividing plant cells (for review see reference 10).

Htay and Kerr have shown that crown gall disease in plants can be controlled by the inhibitory action of an agrocin produced by *A. radiobacter* K84 upon the virulent *A. tumefaciens* strain (5). Some strains of *A. tumefaciens* are able to initiate tumors, and other closely related strains are unable to cause tumor production in plants. Recent work has shown this ability to be correlated with the presence of a large plasmid in the virulent strain. This plasmid in some strains not only codes for virulence but also codes for sensitivity to the agrocin produced by *A. radiobacter* K84 (15).

In this paper the action of agrocin 84 upon a susceptible, virulent strain of *A. tumefaciens* in regard to deoxyribonucleic acid, ribonucleic acid, and protein synthesis, amino acid transport, viability, and motility is described as well as the biochemical nature of agrocin 84.

MATERIALS AND METHODS

Bacterial strains. *A. radiobacter* K84, the agrocin 84-producing strain isolated by A. Kerr, was obtained from R. Hamilton, The Pennsylvania State University. The agrocin-susceptible, virulent strain of *A. tumefaciens* H-38-9 and the agrocin-resistant, avirulent strain of *A. tumefaciens* H-38-7 were derived from *A. tumefaciens* C-58 by R. Hamilton (4).

Media. Stock cultures of *A. radiobacter* K84 were maintained on AB agar, which contains K_2HPO_4, 3.0 g; NaH_2PO_4, 1.0 g; NH_4Cl, 1.0 g; $MgSO_4 \cdot 7H_2O$, 0.3 g; KCl, 0.15 g; $CaCl_2$, 0.01 g; $FeSO_4 \cdot 7H_2O$, 2.5 mg; glucose, 5.0 g (sterilized separately); agar, 15 g; and 1 liter of distilled water (2). *A. tumefaciens* H-38-9 and H-38-7 were grown on tryptic soy agar slants. All experiments were carried out in AB medium. For production of agrocin, AB broth was supplemented with 0.5% sodium glutamate. The cells were incubated for 3 days on a rotary shaker at 27°C. Upon centrifugation the agrocin was found in the supernatant fraction.

Agrocin 84 assay. Agrocin 84 activity was measured by the paper disk assay. A 30-ml portion of AB agar in a 15-cm petri dish was overlayed with 5 ml of AB 0.9% agar inoculated with a 0.5-ml suspension of *A. tumefaciens* H-38-9 from an overnight culture, which had been centrifuged and resuspended in AB broth to 3.0×10^9 cells/ml (30 Klett units, red filter).

A 60-μl portion of agrocin 84 was added to sterile 12.7-mm paper assay disks (Schleicher & Schuell Co.). The disks were dried and then placed on the surface of the agar overlay. After 24 h of incubation at 27°C, the zone of inhibition was measured from the edge of the disk to the edge of the zone. One arbitrary unit (AU) was defined as 1 mm of inhibition. The dose response was linear in the range of 16 to 133 AU/ml when tested at the appropriate dilution.

Isotopic labeling and radioactivity determination. Two 125-ml side-arm flasks containing 20 ml of AB broth were inoculated with 10^7 to 2×10^7 colony-forming units of of *A. tumefaciens* H-38-9 per ml and incubated on a rotary shaker at 27°C for 2 h. Agrocin at a final concentration of 8 AU/ml or an equal volume of AB broth was added, and immediately afterward ^{14}C-labeled mixed L-amino acids (NEC-445) or [^{14}C]uracil, to a final concentration of 0.5 μCi/ml, were added to both flasks (isotopes from New England Nuclear). Samples (50 μl) were pipetted onto 1-inch (ca. 2.5 cm) filter paper squares, dried, washed two times with cold 5% trichloroacetic acid and once with cold ethanol, dried, and counted in a Packard scintillation counter (8).

Transport of amino acids was measured in a similar manner, except that chloramphenicol (100 μg/

ml) was added to inhibit protein synthesis 30 min prior to the addition of ^{14}C-labeled mixed amino acids (0.5 μCi/ml). Cells were collected from 1.0-ml samples on a 0.22-μm membrane filter (Millipore Corp.), washed two times with 0.1 M phosphate buffer, pH 7.0, dried, and counted (8).

Motility was observed directly using a Zeiss phase contrast microscope. A drop of agrocin 84 was added to a wet mount of an overnight culture of *A. tumefaciens* H-38-9.

Cell killing was measured by the addition of agrocin 84 to 20 ml of a 2-h AB broth culture of *A. tumefaciens* and removing 0.1-ml samples at stated intervals for plating on AB agar.

Specificity of adsorption. Approximately 6 × 10^{10} *A. tumefaciens* H-38-9 or H-38-7 cells were mixed with 3 ml of agrocin 84, and at 0, 10, and 20 min 1-ml samples were filtered through a 0.22-μm membrane filter (Millipore Corp.) and assayed for biological activity.

Enzyme susceptibility. A 1-ml portion of agrocin 84 was incubated at 37°C for 2 h with 1 ml of Pronase (2 mg/ml) self-predigested for 2 h at 37°C (Sigma Chemical Co.) or trypsin (Sigma Chemical Co.) in 10 mM tris(hydroxymethyl)aminomethane buffer (pH 7.4) and then assayed for agrocin 84 activity by the paper disk assay. Pepsin was tested at pH 4.2.

Purification and molecular weight determination. The AB broth supernate was concentrated using an Amicon ultrafilter. The supernatant fluid was first passed through a XM300 membrane, which retains particles larger than 300,000 daltons. The filtrate was then passed through a UM10 membrane, which retains molecules larger than 10,000 daltons, and finally concentrated using a UM2 membrane, which retains molecules larger than 1,000 daltons and which, consequently, retained the agrocin. A 1-ml sample of this concentrated agrocin was then layered onto a G-25 Sephadex column (Pharmacia Fine Chemicals; bed size, 1.6 by 50 cm), equilibrated with 10 mM tris(hydroxymethyl)aminomethane buffer, pH 7.5. Fractions (0.5 ml) were collected with a Gilson automatic fraction collector, the adsorbance of each fraction was read at 260 nm, and the fractions were tested for biological activity by the paper disk assay. The molecular weight was determined from a standard curve prepared using oxytocin (Sigma Chemical Co.), glucagon (Sigma Chemical Co.), and bacitracin (Sigma Chemical Co.) as reference proteins (1). The amino acid analysis and molecular weight determination were made using the fraction from the G-25 column showing maximum biological activity, and the fractions collected before and after were used as controls.

RESULTS

Effect on *A. tumefaciens* H-38-9 cells. Protein synthesis, as measured by incorporation of ^{14}C-labeled amino acids, was almost completely inhibited within 10 min by the addition of agrocin 84. A similar pattern of inhibition occurred in DNA synthesis as measured by incorporation of [^{3}H]thymidine. The inhibitory effect on RNA synthesis was not apparent until 20 min after the addition of agrocin 84 and resulted in a 50% reduction of incorporation of [^{14}C]uracil when compared to the control cells (Fig. 1).

The transport of amino acids across the cell membrane was immediately stopped by the ad-

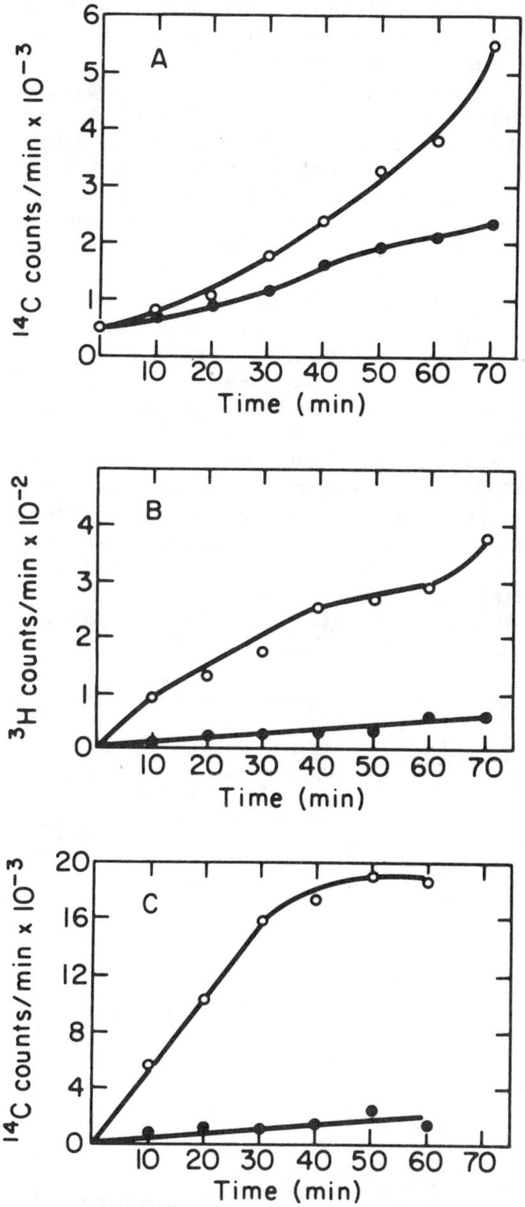

FIG. 1. *Effect of agrocin 84 on synthesis in A. tumefaciens H-38-9 agrocin added at zero time. (A) Ribonucleic acid synthesis at zero time. [^{14}C]uracil was added. (B) Deoxyribonucleic synthesis at zero time. [^{3}H]thymidine was added. (C) Protein synthesis at zero time. ^{14}C-labeled mixed amino acids were added. Symbols:* ●, *agrocin 84;* ○, *control.*

dition of agrocin to the cells, which correlates with the lack of incorporation of the ^{14}C-labeled amino acids into cell protein (Fig. 2).

The energy relationship of the effects of agrocin 84 on the susceptible cells was observed by the almost immediate cessation of motion, which occurred upon addition of agrocin 84 to a highly motile culture. The cells spun in place and then stopped entirely within 90 s.

Addition of agrocin 84 to an early-log-phase culture of *A. tumefaciens* H-38-9 resulted in the killing of between 40 and 50% of the cells within 15 min after addition of agrocin 84. No further reduction of colony-forming units occurred, but the remainder of the cells were inhibited, as the turbidity of the culture remained constant for 24 h.

Agrocin 84 did not adsorb to *A. tumefaciens* H-38-7, which is avirulent to plants but which does adsorb to the virulent, susceptible strain *A. tumefaciens* H-38-9 (Table 1). After 10 min of contact with the cells, 50% of the agrocin 84 was adsorbed.

Synthesis and characterization of agrocin 84. Maximum production of agrocin 84 occurred in AB medium supplemented with 0.5% sodium glutamate after 3 days of incubation at 27°C, when the *A. radiobacter* K84 culture was in stationary phase. No agrocin 84 was produced when the cells were grown in a complex medium containing peptone. Yields of agrocin 84 were less if the temperature of growth was 25 or 30°C rather than 27°C. The agrocin 84 was stable at room temperature, and no activity was lost after storage at 4°C for 6 months; however, boiling for 10 min caused complete inactivation. Treatment of the agrocin 84 with pepsin, trypsin, or Pronase did not reduce the biological activity.

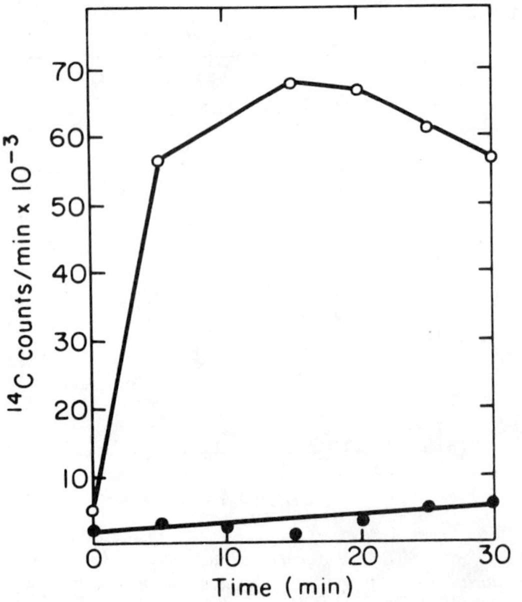

FIG. 2. *Effect of agrocin 84 on amino acid transport in A. tumefaciens H-38-9. Symbols:* ●, *agrocin 84;* ○, *control.*

TABLE 1. *Adsorption of agrocin 84*

Time (min)	Residual activity in filtrate (AU/ml)	
	H-38-9 (virulent)[a]	H-38-7 (avirulent)[a]
0	109	118
10	51	109
20	58	118

[a] *A. tumefaciens* strain used.

An estimate of the molecular weight of agrocin 84 was made by gel filtration on a Sephadex G-25 column. Agrocin 84 readily passes through a cellulose dialysis membrane, so the crude material was filtered through an Amicon ultra filter. The agrocin 84 passed through a UM10 membrane, which retains molecules larger than 10,000 daltons, but was retained by a UM2 membrane, which retains molecules larger than 1,000 daltons. When the filtrate was passed through a Sephadex G-25 column, the biological activity was located in a single peak, which also showed a slight absorbance at 260 nm (Fig. 3A). From a standard curve the molecular weight was estimated to be 2,450 (Fig. 3B).

Amino acid analysis of the fraction giving maximum biological activity demonstrated six different amino acids in the following proportions: arginine, 1; aspartic or asparagine, 1.7; serine, 6.9; glutamic or glutamine, 9; glycine, 3.1; and alanine residues, 3. On the basis of the amino acid analysis, the molecular weight estimate is 2,558 (Table 2).

DISCUSSION

The agrocin 84 produced by *A. radiobacter* K84 interacts specifically with the cell wall of the virulent strain of *A. tumefaciens* H-38-9 and does not adsorb onto the surface of the avirulent strain that was originally derived from the same parent strain, indicating that the receptor site on one strain is missing on the other strain. This reflects an alteration of a surface component coded for by the virulence plasmid. The bacterial cell surface is an important factor in virulence, as has been suggested by Lippincott and Lippincott (9). They postulate a specific receptor on the bacterial surface that interacts with a specific site on the plant

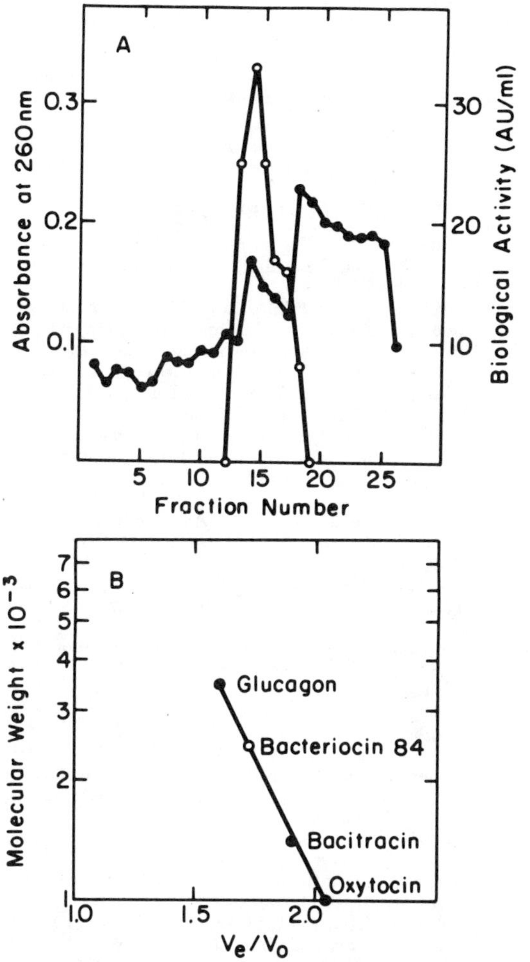

FIG. 3. *(A) Elution profile of agrocin 84 from a Sephadex G-25 column eluted with 10 mM tris(hydroxymethyl)aminomethane buffer, pH 7.5; 0.5-ml samples were collected. Symbols: ○, biological activity (AU/ml); ●, adsorbance at 260 nm. (B) Apparent molecular weight of agrocin 84 based upon elution from a Sephadex G-25 column. The void volume (V_0) was determined using blue dextran (2 mg/ml). To determine molecular weight, elution volume (V_e) divided by V_0 was plotted versus log_{10} of the molecular weight (1), using indicated marker proteins (●) and agrocin (○).*

cell wall to initiate crown gall disease. In competition experiments they demonstrate that virulent and avirulent strains compete for these sites. Kerr and Htay, however, demonstrated that an apparent competition between the virulent and avirulent strains could be the result of agrocin 84 produced by an avirulent strain that inhibited or killed the virulent strains (6). Both these mechanisms may be operative depending upon the strains involved in the competition.

The action of agrocin 84 is more than just the masking of a receptor site on the surface of the cell. The results show extensive inhibition of the susceptible strain by agrocin 84. The most immediate effect is loss of energy, as demonstrated by the abrupt loss of motility after contact with the agrocin. This reflects an influence upon the cell membrane, where the energy-generating reactions occur. Also, the transport of amino acids across the cell membrane was inhibited by the action of agrocin 84, again demonstrating an effect on the integrity of the membrane and associated transport functions.

A secondary effect on the cell was shown by the inhibition of deoxyribonucleic acid, ribonucleic acid, and protein synthesis, which ultimately led to the killing of half the cells, as measured by the ability to form colonies. The remainder of the cells, although still able to produce colonies, were inhibited from dividing in the presence of agrocin 84. On the susceptible cells, agrocin 84 has a very pronounced effect, similar to that shown by colicins K and E_1 on sensitive *Escherichia coli* cells (11, 12).

Agrocin 84 is, however, much smaller in size than the colicins. Most of the colicins have a

TABLE 2. *Amino acid analysis of agrocin fractions from a Sephadex G-25 column*[a]

Amino Acid	Preceding fraction (25 AU/ml)	Peak fraction (83 AU/ml)		Post-peak fraction (0 AU/ml)	Mol wt of amino acids
		Total	Ratio		
Lys		T			
Arg		73	1 (1)		156
Asp		127	1.7 (2)	113	230
Thr					
Ser		506	6.9 (7)	35	609
Glu	163	659	9.02 (9)	215	1161
Gly	54	230	3.1 (3)	250	171
Ala		220	3.0 (3)	91	213
Val					
Met					
Ile					
Leu					
Tyr					
Phe	X	X		X	
Water					18
Total mol wt					2558

[a] Values are expressed as picomoles per sample. Tryptophan, histidine, and proline are not detectable by the *O*-phthaladehyde method used (2). X indicates massive peak coming off in position of phenylalanine. The ratio represents the residues present calculated from the values obtained for the total amount. The numbers in parentheses indicate the theoretical content for each amino acid. Total number of residues was 25. T, Trace.

molecular weight of 50,000 or larger (7). Even the smaller bacteriocins such as streptocin A have a molecular weight of about 8,000 (14). Agrocin 84 has a molecular weight of 2,500, which is closer in size to the protein antibiotics such as gramicidin. The chemical analysis indicates agrocin 84 is a low-molecular-weight peptide composed of at least six different amino acids, predominated by serine and glutamine. The insensitivity of the molecule to trypsin indicates that the molecule lacks a peptide bond, in which the carbonyl function is donated by either a lysine or arginine residue, and resistance to pepsin shows lack of peptide bonds, in which the amino function is contributed by phenylalanine, tryosine, and tryptophan, as well as leucine and acidic amino acids (9). The amino acid analysis shows a lack of some of these amino acids, but it does contain the acidic amino acids aspartic and glutamic acid. Its resistance to Pronase suggests that it may have an unusual structure and be a circular polypeptide such as gramicidin or that it contains D- rather than L-amino acids.

Agrocin 84 is similar in some aspects to the agrocin produced by *A. tumefaciens* H100 and T37, first reported by Stonier (13). This agrocin was found to pass through a dialysis membrane and to be inhibited by the presence of peptone in the medium. Agrocin 84 is also not produced in a peptone-containing medium and does not show activity against cells growing in a complex medium. Different metabolic pathways are operative in a complex medium than in a defined medium, and either the agrocin 84 is not produced, or after production it is inactivated by combination with the ingredients in the complex medium.

The exact chemical nature of agrocin 84 and the receptor site on the bacterial cell surface are still unknown and remain for further study. This report shows the effect of agrocin 84 upon susceptible cells, separation of agrocin from the medium, and the chemical nature of this substance. Agrocin 84 should be a useful tool to identify exactly how the chemical structure of the cell surface of virulent cells differs from that of avirulent cells and provide a key to the interaction of the bacterial cell with the plant cell.

ACKNOWLEDGMENTS

We are grateful to T. M. Joys for performing the amino acid analysis and to R. H. Hamilton and V. A. Jedege for helpful discussions and comments.

This research was supported by project no. 2079 of The Pennsylvania Agricultural Experiment Station.

LITERATURE CITED

1. **Andrews, P.** 1965. The gel filtration of proteins related to their molecular weight over a wide range. Biochem. J. **96**:595–606.
2. **Benson, J. R., and P. E. Hare.** 1975. O-phthaldehyde: fluorogenic detection of primary amines in the picomole range. Comparison with fluorescamine and ninhydrin. Proc. Natl. Acad. Sci. U.S.A. **72**:619–622.
3. **Chilton, M. D., T. Currie, S. K. Farrand, A. J. Bendich, M. P. Gordon, and E. W. Nester.** 1974. *Agrobacterium tumefaciens* DNA and PS8 bacteriophage DNA not detected in crown gall tumors. Proc. Natl. Acad. Sci. U.S.A. **71**:3672–3676.
4. **Hamilton, R. H., and M. Z. Fall.** 1971. The loss of tumor-initiating ability in *Agrobacterium tumefaciens* by incubation at high temperature. Experientia **27**:229–230.
5. **Htay, K., and A. Kerr.** 1974. Biological control of crown gall: seed and root inoculation. J. Appl. Bacteriol. **37**:525–530.
6. **Kerr, A., and K. Htay.** 1974. Biological control of crown gall through bacteriocin production. Physiol. Plant Pathol. **4**:37–44.
7. **Konisky, J.** 1973. Chemistry of colicins, p. 42–58. *In* L. Hager (ed.), Chemistry and functions of colicins. Academic Press Inc., New York.
8. **Kramer, J., and H. Brandis.** 1975. Mode of action of *Streptococcus faecium* bacteriocins. Antimicrob. Agents Chemother. **7**:117–120.
9. **Lippincott, B. B., and J. A. Lippincott.** 1969. Bacterial attachment to a specific wound site as an essential stage in tumor initiation by *Agrobacterium tumefaciens*. J. Bacteriol. **97**:620–628.
10. **Lippincott, J. A., and B. B. Lippincott.** 1975. The genus *Agrobacterium* and plant tumorigenesis. Annu. Rev. Microbiol. **29**:377–405.
11. **Luria, S. E., and K. Fields.** 1969. Effects of colicins E1 and K on cellular metabolism. J. Bacteriol. **97**:64–77.
12. **Luria, S. E., J. Lusk, and C. A. Plate.** 1973. Colicins, p. 1–14. *In* L. Hager (ed.), Chemistry and functions of colicins. Academic Press Inc., New York.
13. **Stonier, T.** 1960. *Agrobacterium tumefaciens* Conn. II. Production of an antibiotic substance. J. Bacteriol. **79**:889–898.
14. **Tagg, J. R., A. S. Dajani, L. W. Wannamaker, and E. D. Gray.** 1972. Group A streptococcal bacteriocin: production, purification, and mode of action. J. Exp. Med. **138**:1168–1183.
15. **VanLarebeke, N., C. Genetello, J. Schell, R. A. Schilperoort, A. K. Hermans, J. P. Hernalsteens, and M. VanMontague.** 1975. Acquisition of tumor-inducing ability by non-onocogenic agrobacteria as a result of plasmid transfer. Nature (London) **255**:742–743.

ANTIMICROBIAL AGENTS AND CHEMOTHERAPY, Sept. 1976, p. 503-506 Vol. 10, No. 3

Printed in U.S.A.

Effect of Organic Mercurials and Sulfhydryl Compounds on the Urease Activity of *Proteus*: Inhibition by Urine and Ascorbic Acid

CALVIN M. KUNIN

Department of Medicine, Veterans Administration Hospital and University of Wisconsin School of Medicine, Madison, Wisconsin 53705*

Received for publication 5 May 1976

Meralluride, mercaptomerin, ethacrynic acid, and penicillamine inhibited urease activity of *Proteus mirabilis*. The activity of the organic mercurials and ethacrynic acid was markedly inhibited by human and dog urine. Antiurease activity could not be detected in the urine of a human and a dog given meralluride by injection. Urine from patients receiving penicillamine also failed to inhibit urease activity. Ascorbic acid inhibited, whereas dehydroascorbic acid enhanced, the activity of the mercurials, but neither agent altered the inhibitory effect of urine. The lethal effect of meralluride against *Proteus* occurred at the same concentration at which urease activity was inhibited, but penicillamine inhibited the enzymatic activity without affecting viability of the organism. The data suggest that these sulfhydryl-reactive compounds will not be useful against *Proteus* infections of the urinary tract.

The pathogenesis of *Proteus* infections of the urinary tract appears to be related, in part, to the generation of ammonia from urea catalyzed by bacterial urease. Several studies have demonstrated that invasion of the kidney and production of renal damage are associated with ammonia production (2, 9). In addition, the ability of *Proteus* to produce an alkaline urine favors the development of urinary stones and complicates the use of otherwise effective antimicrobial agents (9). A number of agents are known to interfere with urease activity, including acetohydroxamic acid and related compounds (1, 8), thiourea (2), hydroxyurea (2), suramin (14), and heavy metals such as mercury, copper, and zinc (10).

The lack of availability for clinical use of effective urease inhibitors led us to reexamine the observations of Seneca and Lattimer and their colleagues (6, 11, 12) on the ability of organic mercurials to inhibit bacterial urease. In addition, it seemed reasonable to explore the potential value of other agents with sulfhydryl activity since urease is known to be rich in sulfhydryl groups and activity might be blocked by the formation of disulfides (10).

This report confirms the findings of Seneca and co-workers that organic mercurial diuretics inhibit urease activity in *Proteus* and also appear to have a lethal effect against the organisms. In addition, other sulfhydryl-containing agents such as penicillamine and ethacrynic acid exhibit antiurease activity. Unfortunately, these agents are inhibited by human urine or require very high concentrations to be effective. The mechanism by which urine inhibits the mercurials is unclear, but may be related to the presence of antoxidants such as ascorbic acid.

MATERIALS AND METHODS

A strain of *P. mirabilis* recovered from a patient with a urinary tract infection was used as the assay organism. This strain readily generated ammonia in urea broth (Difco), resulting in a rise in pH from 7.0 to 9.2 after overnight culture at 37°C. Two other clinical isolates of *P. mirabilis* and two of *P. rettgeri* were also tested for susceptibility to meralluride as described below. Organisms were maintained by serial passage in tryptic soy broth (Difco). In individual experiments, the culture was grown overnight at 37°C and then diluted in physiological saline to the desired inoculum size. This was about 10^5 viable colonies per ml unless otherwise stated. Experimental end points were established by observing a color change in the urea broth medium, by direct measurement of pH using a Beckman model S53 meter and by quantitative pour plate cultures.

Compounds tested. The following chemical compounds were used in various experiments: meralluride (Mercuhydrin, Lakeside Laboratories, Inc.), mercaptomerin (Thiomerin, Wyeth Laboratories), ethacrynic acid (Edecrin, Merck, Sharpe & Dohme), D-penicillamine (Sigma Chemical Co.), acetozolamide (American Cyanamid Co., Lederle Laboratories Div.), furosemide (Hoechst Pharmaceuticals, Inc.), ascorbic acid (Cevalin, Eli Lilly & Co.), dehydroascorbic acid (K & K Laboratories, Inc.), cysteine (Mann Research Laboratories, Inc.), cystine (Mann

Research Laboratories, Inc.), and methionine (Calbiochem). All of the compounds were diluted initially in sterile water and then added to the test medium prior to use. All values for activity are expressed as the highest effective final concentration of the compound. In individual tests, 1.0 ml of each compound to be tested was dissolved in the appropriate diluent (urea broth, tryptic soy broth, or urine), mixed with 0.1 ml of the bacterial inoculum, and incubated overnight at 37°C. When compounds were mixed, equal volumes of serial dilutions of each compound were added to each other (1 ml each), and the inoculum was added as described above.

In vitro and in vivo studies of human and dog urine. Urine was freshly obtained from four normal human subjects and one dog. In addition, a 20-kg dog was given 125 mg of meralluride intramuscularly, and serial half-hour urine specimens were collected for 4 h. A 50-year-old man, weighing 114 kg, with congestive heart failure, was given 250 mg of meralluride intramuscularly, and urine specimens were collected at hourly intervals for 4 h. Four patients with rheumatoid arthritis treated with penicillamine were studied. Urine was obtained 2 and 4 h after the last oral dose (500 mg in three and 250 mg in one patient). Urine specimens collected from the patients and the dogs were adjusted to pH 7.0, and 0.1 ml of a 1:100 dilution of an overnight culture of *P. mirabilis* was added to 1 ml of urine. The specimens were incubated overnight at 37°C and tested for inhibition of growth and antiurease activity (e.g., block of a rise in pH above the initial value of the medium and of an uninoculated, sterile, control specimen).

Urease activity of acetone-killed organisms. *P. mirabilis* was grown overnight on a tryptic soy agar surface in bottle cultures and was harvested by a wash with 10 ml of sterile water. The fluid contained 3×10^9 colony-forming units per ml. The suspension was centrifuged, the supernatant was removed, and the sediment was washed three times with 10 ml of acetone and allowed to air dry. The sediment was then taken up in 10 ml of urea broth. All culture preparation was under sterile conditions.

RESULTS

Effect of various compounds in inhibiting pH change by *P. mirabilis* in urea broth. Meralluride blocked a change in pH in urea broth (i.e., it maintained the pH at 7.0 compared to 9.2 observed with uninhibited growth of *Proteus*) at concentrations ranging from 5 to 80 μg/ml depending on an inoculum size of 10^4 to 10^7 viable cell units per ml. All pH end points paralleled the bactericidal concentrations; i.e., the drug simultaneously killed the organisms and interfered with ammonia production. Meralluride exhibited the same effect with two other strains of *P. mirabilis* and *P. rettgeri*. Mercaptomerin was less active against the test strain of *Proteus,* requiring 50 to 400 μg/ml depending on inoculum size. Ethacrynic acid was bactericidal and blocked urease activity when tested in one experiment at 32 μg/ml and in another at 125 μg/ml. Penicillamine differed from the other compounds in being able to inhibit urease activity at concentrations of 400 to 500 μg/ml but failed to inhibit growth of the organism. A representative experiment is presented in Table 1.

Effect of meralluride in inhibiting bacterial urease. In view of the observation that the mercurial compounds killed the *Proteus* strain at the same concentration as that which inhibited a rise in pH in urea broth, it was important to determine whether the effect of the drug was directed primarily against the organism rather than urease activity. To test this point, meralluride was added, in serial dilution, to a preparation of acetone-killed organisms in urea broth and incubated overnight at 37°C together with control samples, which did not contain the drug. Urease activity was inhibited completely (i.e., no change of pH from 7.0 to 9.2) by drug concentrations of 40 μg or more per ml. In contrast, the pH of control tubes containing no mercurial rose to 9.2 after overnight incubation. In a parallel experiment, 40 μg of drug per ml sterilized a urea broth culture of about 10^5 viable *P. mirabilis* per ml.

Inhibitory effect of urine on activity of sulfhydryl-reactive compounds. Urine specimens were obtained from four normal subjects. Osmolalities varied from 232 to 1,078 with a mean of 641 mosmol/kg. The pH of each specimen was adjusted to 7.0 (pH of 5.5 or less inhibits this strain of *Proteus*). Sixteen- to 64-fold more meralluride was required to inhibit the organism in urine than in broth. In addition, the urine of one subject was diluted serially in urea broth and tested for activity of meralluride

TABLE 1. *Effect of sulfhydryl-reactive compounds on growth and urease activity of P. mirabilis in urea broth and human urine*[a]

Agent	Minimun concn that blocks pH rise (μg/ml): Urea broth	Minimun concn that blocks pH rise (μg/ml): Urine[b]	Minimun bactericidal concn (μg/ml): urea broth
Meralluride	5	80–160	5
Mercaptomerin	100	1,600–6,300	100
Ethacrynic acid	32	500	32
Penicillamine	500	1,000	>2,000

[a] Inoculum size, about 10^5 colony-forming units per ml. Diuretic and sulfhydryl compounds showing no activity at 500 to 1,000 μg/ml include cysteine, cystine, methionine, furosemide, and acetazolamide.

[b] Depending upon subject.

against the *Proteus* strain. Even when the urine was diluted 1:32, it required twofold more drug to inhibit the organism than in urea broth. A similar inhibitory effect of urine was observed with mercaptomerin and ethacrynic acid. Urine was also inhibitory to penicillamine, reducing activity at least twofold (Table 1).

Urine from a dog (pH 7.8) completely inhibited the activity of 6,300 μg of meralluride or mercaptomerin per ml. Undiluted specimens of urine collected in serial half-hour or sequential hourly volumes over a 4-h period from a dog and from a human given 125 and 250 mg of meralluride intramuscularly, respectively, failed to inhibit the growth of *Proteus* or prevent a rise in urinary pH. Urine from four patients receiving 250 to 500 mg of penicillamine orally was also ineffective.

Effect of ascorbic and dehydroascorbic acids on the inhibitory effect of meralluride against *Proteus*. Since the oxidation-reduction of sulfhydryl groups is known to affect their biological activity, ascorbic acid, a reducing compound, and dehydroascorbic acid, an oxidant, were examined for their ability to alter the action of meralluride on urease activity. The results of box titration experiments of the effect of ascorbic and dehydroascorbic acids on the action of meralluride against *Proteus* in urea broth are shown in Fig. 1. Ascorbic acid at 2,500 μg/ml had no effect against the organism, but dehydroascorbic acid was inhibitory at concentrations of 625 μg or more per ml. Ascorbic acid demonstrated a marked inhibitory effect on the activity of the mercurial at concentrations as low as 79 μg/ml, whereas dehydroascorbic acid markedly enhanced the activity at 20 μg or more per ml. Addition of dehydroascorbic acid to human urine obtained from two healthy volunteers, however, failed to enhance the antibacterial activity of the mercurial.

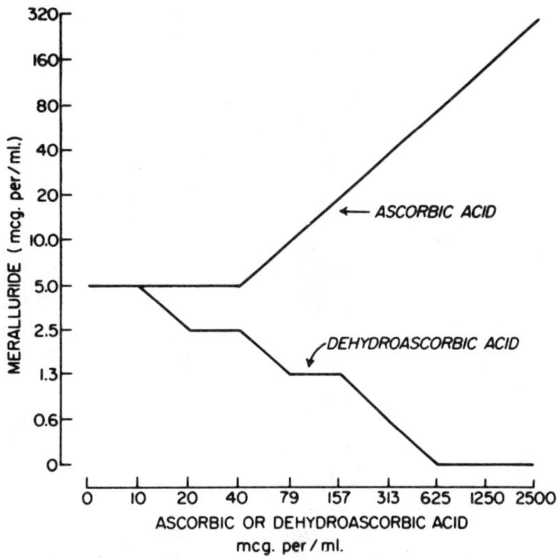

FIG. 1. *Effect of ascorbic acid and dehydroascorbic acid on the activity of meralluride in inhibiting growth and ammonia production by P. mirabilis in urea broth. The minimal inhibitory concentration of meralluride (ordinate) was influenced markedly by the concentration of ascorbic acid or dehydroascorbic acid (abscissa) added to the medium.*

DISCUSSION

Ureases obtained from a wide variety of species have been shown to be rich in sulfhydryl groups and to be inhibited by heavy metals such as mercury, copper, and zinc (10). The observations of Seneca and co-workers (6, 11, 12) on the activity of mercurial diuretics on inhibition of urease activity of *Proteus* and the critical role of ammonia production in urinary infections produced by this group of bacteria stimulated us to reevaluate their potential use.

The current results document the activity of some organic mercurial diuretics and sulfhydryl-reactive compounds such as ethacrynic acid and penicillamine against *Proteus*. The mercurials appear to kill *Proteus* at the same concentration at which they inhibit the urease activity of nonviable organisms, but these probably are unrelated effects since urease is not required for cell growth (1, 2, 8, 9). Penicillamine, as for acetohydroxamic acids (1, 8), inhibited urease activity without affecting bacterial growth. Unfortunately, the organic mercurials and ethacrynic acid show little promise for clinical use in inhibiting urease formation in urinary infections since their activity is inhibited markedly by urine. This effect did not appear to be related directly to osmolality, since it was observed in human urines widely varying in concentration and even in diluted urine. The nature of the urinary inhibitory substance is unknown. It may be due to interference by disulfides or other products of sulfhydryl metabolism reacting with the mercurials. Cysteine, for example, is known to reverse the inhibition of urease by mercurials (11).

Ascorbic acid inhibited, whereas dehydroascorbic acid augmented, the activity of meralluride against *Proteus*. These compounds were studied because of the known reactivity of sulfhydryl groups to conditions of oxidation and reduction (4, 5). The mechanism by which ascorbic acid inhibited the action of the mercurial is not entirely clear since the system contained whole, growing bacteria rather than purified urease. One possibility is that ascorbic acid tends to interfere with binding of the enzyme to mercury by maintaining the sulfhydryl groups in the reduced state. The activity of copper in inhibiting urease was studied by Mapson (7). He demonstrated that ascorbic acid enhanced inhibition of urease by copper by reducing Cu^{2+} to Cu^{+} ions. In contrast, antiurease activity of Hg^{2+} salts was decreased by ascorbic acid, in accord with the present findings. That diets are rich in ascorbic acid, which is excreted readily into the urine, may account, in part, for the inhibitory effect of urine against mercurials.

The major excretory product of common organic mercurials is the cysteine complex (13) rather than the free drug. The activity of the complex against urease was not studied; however, the urine of a dog and a human subject given meralluride by injection failed to inhibit *Proteus* either because of inactivation of the mercurial by urine or because of the formation of the complex, or both.

This study supports, in part, the demonstration by Seneca and co-workers (6, 12) that organic mercurials inhibit *Proteus* and its urease activity. Inactivation by urine, however, may explain the minimal efficacy of mercurials in treatment of urinary tract infections reported by this group.

Penicillamine, although active in vitro, requires relatively large amounts to inhibit urease and does not affect bacterial growth, and its activity is decreased in urine. The drug is excreted rapidly in the urine as a mixture of free penicillamine and penicillamine-cysteine disulfide. About 50% of the dose is excreted in the first 7 h; 73% is excreted by 24 h (3). No antiurease activity could be detected in urine of four patients receiving the drug.

Although these results make it unlikely that the sulfhydryl-active compounds examined in this study will prove to be useful in treatment of *Proteus* infections of the urinary tract, it is still possible that they may be effective in renal tissue, where *Proteus* produces damage, and that other related compounds will be found to be more active.

LITERATURE CITED

1. **Andersen, J. A.** 1975. Benurestat, a urease inhibitor for the therapy of infected ureolysis. Invest. Urol. 12:381–386.
2. **Aronson, M., D. Medalia, and B. Griffel.** 1974. Prevention of ascending pyelonephritis in mice by urease inhibitors. Nephron 12:94–104.
3. **Gibbs, K., and J. M. Walshe.** 1971. Studies with S^{35}-labelled DL-penicillamine in patients with Wilson's disease. Q. J. Med. 40:275–287.
4. **Jocelyn, P. C.** 1972. Biochemistry of the SH group. Academic Press Inc., London.
5. **King, C. G.** 1968. Present knowledge of ascorbic acid (vitamin C). Nutr. Rev. 26:33–36.
6. **Lattimer, J. K., H. Seneca, H. H. Zinsser, and J. T. Donovan.** 1961. Drug resistant bacteria made drug susceptible by enzyme inhibitors. J. Am. Med. Assoc. 178:764–766.
7. **Mapson, L. W.** 1946. Inhibition of urease by copper salts in the presence of ascorbic acid and related substances. Biochem. J. 40:240–247.
8. **Musher, D. M., D. P. Griffith, M. Tyler, and A. Woelfel.** 1974. Potentiation of the antibacterial effect of methenamine by acetohydroxamic acid. Antimicrob. Agents Chemother. 5:101–105.
9. **Musher, D. M., D. P. Griffith, D. Yawn, and R. U. Rossen.** 1975. Role of urease in pyelonephritis resulting from urinary tract infection with *Proteus*. J. Infect. Dis. 131:177–181.
10. **Reithel, F. J.** 1971. Ureases, p. 1–20. *In* P. D. Boyer (ed.), The enzymes, 3rd. ed., vol. 4. Academic Press Inc., New York.
11. **Seneca, H.** 1964. Enzyme profiles of microorganisms and urease inhibitors in chemotherapy of infections, p. 347–372. *In* R. S. Schnitzer and F. Hawking (ed.), Experimental chemotherapy, vol. 3. Academic Press Inc., New York.
12. **Seneca, H., J. K. Lattimer, and H. H. Zinsser.** 1960. Chemotherapy of urease and citrase producing bacteria of the urinary tract. Ann. Intern. Med. 53:468–474.
13. **Weiner, I. M., and O. H. Muller.** 1955. A polarigraphic study of mersalyl (salyrgan)—thio complexes and of the excreted products of mersalyl. J. Pharmacol. Exp. Ther. 113:241–249.
14. **Wills, E. D., and A. Wormall.** 1950. Studies on suramin 9. The action of the drug on some enzymes. Biochemistry 47:158–170.

ANTIMICROBIAL AGENTS AND CHEMOTHERAPY, Sept. 1976, p. 507-510
Vol. 10, No. 3

Comparison of the In Vitro Activity of Several Cephalosporin Antibiotics Against Gram-Negative and Gram-Positive Bacteria Resistant to Cephaloridine

ALEXANDER L. KISCH* AND LUANNA BARTHOLOMEW

Department of Medicine, School of Medicine, The University of New Mexico, Albuquerque, New Mexico 87131

Received for publication 9 February 1976

The in vitro activity of each of two oral [cefatrizine (BL-S640), cephalexin] and three parenteral (cefamandole, cefazolin, cephapirin) cephalosporin antibiotics was compared with that of cephalothin against 168 clinical isolates of gram-negative and gram-positive bacteria selected as resistant to 20 μg of cephaloridine per ml on the basis of agar dilution susceptibility test data. Each of the five other cephalosporins inhibited a greater percentage of gram-negative bacillary isolates than did cephalothin or cephaloridine, with minimal inhibitory concentration values ranging 2- to 50-fold lower. Significant differences between minimal inhibitory concentrations of the compounds tested were also observed in tests against strains of *Streptococcus faecalis* and of methicillin-resistant *Staphylococcus aureus*. Potential advantages of including more than a single cephalosporin antibiotic in the panel of antibiotics used for routine susceptibility testing, suggested by these observations, are discussed.

The number of semisynthetic cephalosporin antibiotics approved or under development for use in clinical therapeutics continues to increase. Thus, chemical modification of the nucleus of cephalosporin C, 7-aminocephalosporanic acid, has yielded a family of potent antibacterial agents differing somewhat from each other with respect to certain clinically relevant properties such as potential local and systemic toxicity, pharmacokinetic characteristics, cost, and, to a lesser extent, antibacterial spectrum. However, with the possible exception of the nephrotoxicity of cephaloridine at doses above 4 g daily (3, 9), no generally accepted rationale exists at present that constitutes a compelling basis for the preferential selection of any of the existing compounds over the others. Indeed, no cephalosporin antibiotic is currently the drug of choice for any infection (7). The generally broad and apparently quite similar spectra of antimicrobial activity of the cephalosporanic acid derivatives that have been studied form the basis for the recommendation that, except under unusual circumstances, only a single cephalosporin, usually cephalothin, need be used in routine susceptibility testing procedures (2). In some laboratories cephaloridine is used for this purpose because of its greater chemical stability.

We report here data that suggest that the simultaneous use of more than one cephalosporanic acid derivative in routine clinical antimicrobial susceptibility testing may result in more appropriate selection from among available antibiotics of a cephalosporin having potentially greater effectiveness for treatment of selected gram-negative or gram-positive bacterial infections.

MATERIALS AND METHODS

Bacteria. One hundred forty-nine isolates of gram-negative bacteria and 13 isolates of *Streptococcus faecalis* recently obtained from clinical specimens submitted to the routine clinical bacteriology laboratory of the Bernalillo County Medical Center were collected, using resistance to at least 20 μg of cephaloridine per ml in a standard agar dilution assay (6) as the criterion of selection. Seventy-eight strains of *Escherichia coli*, 47 of *Enterobacter*, 16 of *Klebsiella*, 6 of *Shigella*, and 2 of *Salmonella* comprised the gram-negative strains. All isolates were identified according to standard criteria (4) by or under the supervision of John A. Ulrich. Additionally, 8 strains of *S. aureus*, resistant to 12.5 μg of methicillin/ml, collected from patients during an outbreak of surgical wound infections produced by this organism (8) were also included in these tests.

Antibiotic susceptibility tests. The minimal inhibitory concentration (MIC) of each antibiotic tested for each bacterial strain was determined by the agar dilution method recommended by the International Collaborative Study (6). Mueller-Hinton agar (Difco Laboratories, Detroit, Mich.) was the bacteriological medium used. The inoculum was 0.002 ml of an overnight broth culture containing approximately 10^5 organisms delivered by means of a Steers replicator (10) (Melrose Machine Shop, Woodlyn, Pa.).

The antibiotics used were obtained as standard powders from their manufacturers: sodium cephalothin, cefamandole naphtate, cephalexin monohydrate, and sodium cefazolin from Eli Lilly and Co., Indianapolis, Ind.; and sodium cephapirin and cefatrizine (BL S640) from Bristol Laboratories, Syracuse, N.Y. The powders were stored at 4°C and diluted just before use in appropriate phosphate buffers before being added to the agar medium.

Except as indicated below, bacterial strains were defined as susceptible to a given concentration of antibiotic when fewer than 12 colonies were apparent after overnight (18 h, 35°C) incubation of the standard 0.002-ml inoculum. An identical simultaneous control inoculum included in each test for comparison yielded confluent bacterial growth.

RESULTS

The inhibitory activity of each of the cephalosporins tested against 78 strains of *E. coli* is shown in Fig. 1. Only 8% of the strains tested were susceptible to 25 μg of cephalothin per ml and none was inhibited by lower concentrations. All other cephalosporins tested, except cephapirin, inhibited significantly larger percentages of *E. coli* strains. Cephalothin also exhibited considerably less inhibitory activity against the *Enterobacter* and *Klebsiella* strains tested than did the other cephalosporins (Fig. 2, 3). Cefamandole inhibited 79% of *Enterobacter* strains and 76% of *Klebsiella* strains at a concentration of 25 μg or less per ml. A similar percentage of *Klebsiella* strains was also inhibited by 25 μg or less of cefatrizine (75%) or cephalexin (76%) per ml. The latter drug alone of the compounds tested also inhibited all of six *Shigella* strains at a concentration of 12.5 μg or less per ml; only one of these was susceptible to 12.5 μg of cefatrizine, and another to 1.56 μg of cefamandole per ml. Neither of the two cephalothin-resistant *Salmonella* strains tested was inhibited by less than 25 μg of any other cepha-

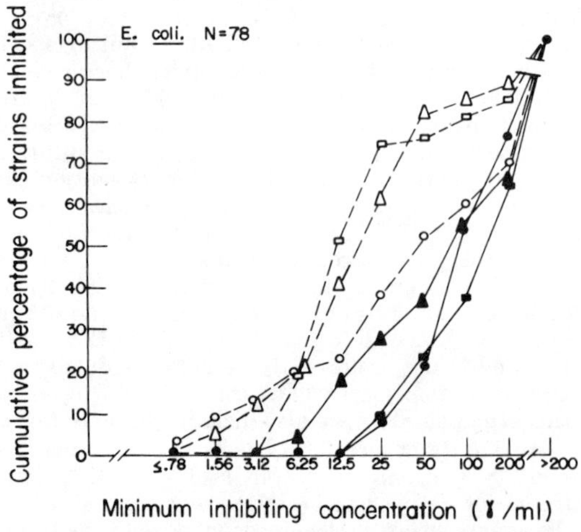

FIG. 1. *Minimum inhibitory concentrations (micrograms per milliliter) of six cephalosporin antibiotics for 78 clinical isolates of E. coli. Symbols:* ●, *cephalothin;* ○, *cefamandole;* ▲, *cefatrizine (BL-S640);* △, *cefazolin;* ■, *cephapirin;* □, *cephalexin.*

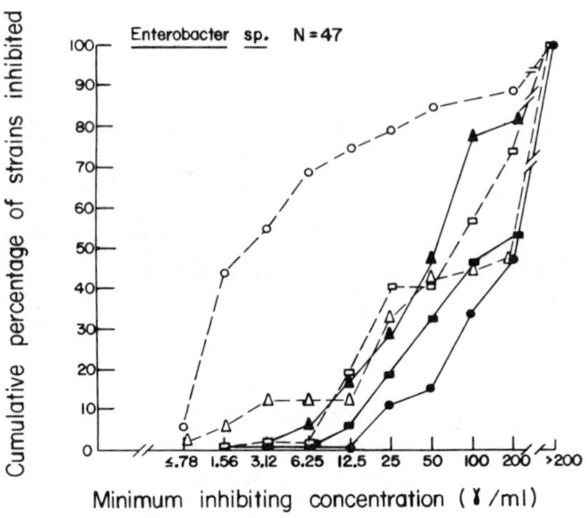

FIG. 2. *Minimum inhibitory concentrations (micrograms per milliliter) of six cephalosporin antibiotics for 47 clinical isolates of Enterobacter species. Symbols:* ●, *cephalothin;* ○, *cefamandole;* ▲, *cefatrizine (BL-S640);* △, *cefazolin;* ■, *cephapirin;* □, *cephalexin.*

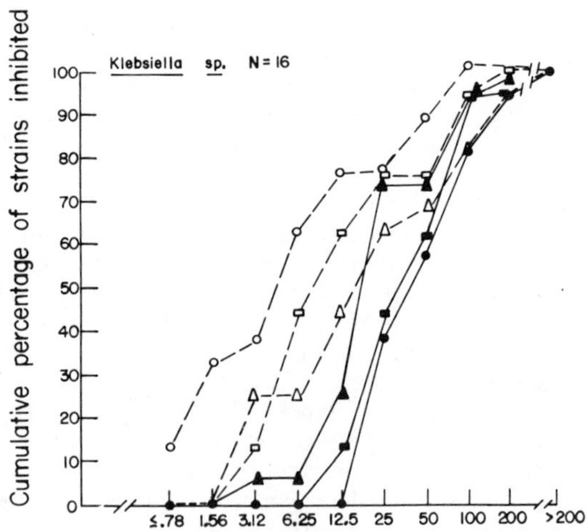

FIG. 3. *Minimum inhibitory concentrations (micrograms per milliliter) of six cephalosporin antibiotics for 16 clinical isolates of Klebsiella species. Symbols:* ●, *cephalothin;* ○, *cefamandole;* ▲, *cefatrizine (BL-S640);* △, *cefazolin;* ■, *cephapirin;* □, *cephalexin.*

losporin tested per ml, with the exception of the strain which was inhibited by 6.25 μg of cephalexin per ml. Though none of the 13 *S. faecalis* strains that had been identified as resistant to 20 μg of cephaloridine per ml was inhibited by 25 μg or less of either cephalexin or cefatrizine per ml, 92 and 85% of these strains were inhibited by 25 μg or less of cephalothin and cefamandole per ml, respectively, and all were susceptible to 25 μg or less of cefazolin or cephapirin per ml (Fig. 4).

By the standard definition of antibiotic susceptibility used in these studies and stated above, none of six strains of *S. aureus,* all of which were resistant to 12.5 μg of methicillin per ml, was identified as resistant to 12.5 μg of either cephalothin, cephapirin, or cefamandole per ml; four of six appeared resistant to cefazolin and five of six to both cefatrizine and cephalexin. Using a more stringent criterion of susceptibility, i.e., no detectable growth whatsoever after 24 h of incubation at 37°C, all six strains were identified as resistant to cefatrizine and cephalexin; all six appeared susceptible to cefamandole and cephapirin, five of six appeared susceptible to cephalothin, and two of six appeared susceptible to cefazolin.

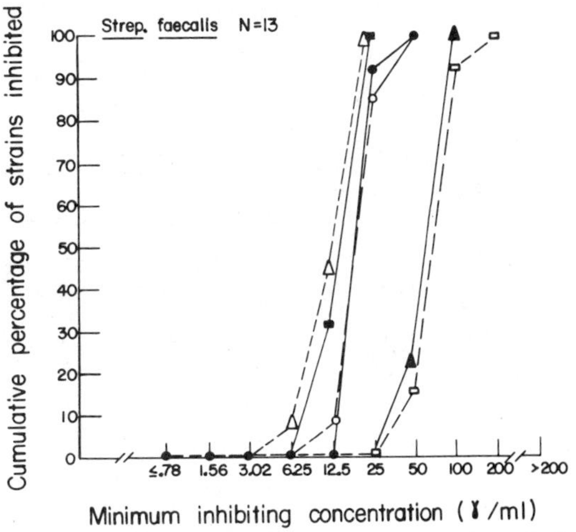

FIG. 4. *Minimum inhibitory concentrations (micrograms per milliliter) of six cephalosporin antibiotics for 13 clinical isolates of S. faecalis. Symbols:* ●, *cephalothin;* ○, *cefamandole;* ▲, *cefatrizine (BL-S640);* △, *cefazolin;* ■, *cephapirin;* □, *cephalexin.*

TABLE 1. *Percentage of strains inhibited by 25 μg of antibiotic per ml*

Antibiotic	*E. coli* (78)[a]	*Enterobacter* (47)	*Klebsiella* (16)	*S. faecalis* (13)
Cephalothin	8	11	38	92
Cefamandole	39	79	76	85
Cefatrizine (BL S640)	27	28	75	0
Cefazolin	61	33	63	100
Cephapirin	9	19	44	100
Cephalexin	75	40	76	0

[a] Number of strains tested.

DISCUSSION

The data presented here indicate that a substantial percentage of clinically isolated strains of gram-negative and gram-positive bacteria that are resistant in vitro to concentrations of cephaloridine and of cephalothin ordinarily achieved in the serum of patients receiving recommended dosages of these antibiotics may be susceptible, under identical in vitro test conditions, to concentrations of other cephalosporins that are readily attainable in the urine and in the serum of patients after administration of commonly used dosage schedules. Thus, for example, nearly 80% of 47 *Enterobacter* strains resistant to 12.5 μg of cephalothin per ml were susceptible to 12.5 μg or less of cefamandole per ml, and 75% of 16 similarly resistant *Klebsiella* strains were inhibited by the cephalosporin compound cefatrizine at similar concentrations. Table 1 presents a summary of the comparative data obtained. The magnitude of the observed MIC differences among the compounds tested varied widely over a range of 2- to 50-fold. Susceptibility differences of this magnitude possess obvious potential relevance to the design of clinical antimicrobial therapy of infections due to organisms designated "resistant" on the basis of routine antimicrobial susceptibility testing by the agar dilution technique using cephalothin or cephaloridine as the only prototype cephalosporin compound tested.

The significance of the apparent differences between cephalosporin MICs for the strains of methicillin-resistant *S. aureus* tested is uncertain. That these bacteria may appear falsely susceptible to cephalosporin antibiotics when standard in vitro susceptibility test procedures are used is well known in the case of cephalothin and cephaloridine (1, 5), and the therapeutic use of cephalosporins for the treatment of infections caused by methicillin-resistant *S. aureus* strains is not warranted.

ACKNOWLEDGMENTS

We wish to thank John A. Ulrich for providing the bacterial strains used in these studies and for their identification.

This investigation was supported in part by grants-in-aid from Eli Lilly and Co., Indianapolis, Ind., and from Bristol Laboratories, Syracuse, N. Y.

LITERATURE CITED

1. **Acar, J. F., P. Courvalin, and Y. A. Chabbert.** 1971. Methicillin-resistant staphylococcemia: bacteriological failure of treatment with cephalosporins. Antimicrob. Agents Chemother. **10**:280–285.
2. **Balows, A. (ed.).** 1974. Current techniques for antibiotic susceptibility testing, p. 140. Charles C Thomas, Publisher, Springfield, Ill.
3. **Benner, E. J.** 1970. Cephaloridine and the kidneys. J. Infect. Dis. **122**:104–105.
4. **Buchanan, R. E., and N. E. Gibbons (ed.).** 1974. Bergey's manual of determinative bacteriology, 8th ed. Williams and Wilkins Co., Baltimore, Md.
5. **Chabbert, Y. A.** 1967. Behaviour of methicillin heteroresistant staphylococci to cephaloridine. Postgrad. Med. J. 43(Suppl):40–42.
6. **Ericsson, H. M., and J. C. Sherris.** 1971. Antibiotic sensitivity testing. Report of an international collaborative study. Acta Pathol. Microbiol. Scand. Sect. B Suppl. 117, p. 1–90.
7. **Hamilton-Miller, J. M. T., and W. Brumfitt.** 1974. Whither the cephalosporins? J. Infect. Dis. **130**:81–84.
8. **Kisch, A. L., E. Stark, J. Strathman, L. Bartholomew, N. H. Berg, and U. G. Hodgin.** 1976. An outbreak of lethal infections due to methicillin-resistant Staphylococcus aureus complicating cardiac surgery. Clin. Res. **24**:152A.
9. **Mandell, G. L.** 1973. Cephaloridine. Ann. Intern. Med. **79**:561–565.
10. **Steers, E., E. L. Foltz, and B. S. Graves.** 1959. An inocula replicating apparatus for routine testing of bacterial susceptibility to antibiotics. Antibiot. Chemother. **9**:307–311.

ANTIMICROBIAL AGENTS AND CHEMOTHERAPY, Sept. 1976, p. 511-518 Vol. 10, No. 3

Printed in U.S.A.

In Vitro Synergistic Effect of Netilmicin, a New Aminoglycoside Antibiotic

KWUNG P. FU AND HAROLD C. NEU*

Department of Medicine and Department of Pharmacology, College of Physicians and Surgeons, Columbia University, New York, New York 10032*

Received for publication 19 May 1976

The combination of netilmicin (Sch 20569) with carbenicillin, cefazolin, chloramphenicol, and clindamycin was evaluated by in vitro tests against 91 clinical isolates of *Pseudomonas*, *Klebsiella*, and *Escherichia coli*. Combinations were considered to show synergy if there was a fourfold or greater reduction in minimal inhibitory concentration values of both antibiotics when combined. Synergy of netilmicin with carbenicillin could be demonstrated against 21 of 46 *Pseudomonas* isolates. Comparison of the synergy of carbenicillin with netilmicin or gentamicin showed that netilmicin was less active than gentamicin against *Pseudomonas aeruginosa*. However, at therapeutic concentrations of the antibiotics, significant differences were not observed. Synergy of netilmicin and cefazolin was demonstrated against only 1 of 21 *Klebsiella* strains tested, but partial synergy was found for 12 of 20 isolates. Synergy and antagonism were uncommon with the netilmicin-chloramphenicol and netilmicin-clindamycin combinations against *E. coli* and *Pseudomonas*.

Infections produced by gram-negative organisms have been associated with a continued high mortality in spite of the development of new antibiotics (13). Evidence of a synergistic effect has been well documented in vitro against *Pseudomonas aeruginosa* with the combination of aminoglycosides and carbenicillin (1, 5-7, 10). Netilmicin (Sch 20569), an ethyl derivative of dehydrogenated C_{1a} gentamicin, is active against many gentamicin-resistant members of the *Enterobacteriaceae* (14; K. P. Fu and H. C. Neu, submitted for publication). In vitro synergy studies were undertaken with this agent to determine if it showed in vitro synergy when combined with agents with which it would be used in clinical settings. It is necessary to clarify if in vitro antagonism would result from the combination of netilmicin and clindamycin or netilmicin and chloramphenicol. Netilmicin is the most active aminoglycoside against both susceptible and resistant *Escherichia coli* and *Klebsiella* (Fu and Neu, submitted for publication). This agent might be used to treat surgical infections in which antibiotics active against anaerobic bacteria are routinely employed because of the mixed bacterial population. We also wished to compare the synergistic activity of netilmicin and gentamicin when combined with carbenicillin, since netilmicin is less active in vitro against *Pseudomonas* than is gentamicin.

MATERIALS AND METHODS

Netilmicin and gentamicin were supplied by Schering Corporation. Carbenicillin was a gift from Beecham Laboratories. Chloramphenicol, clindamycin, and cefazolin were obtained from Parke, Davis & Co., Upjohn Company, and Eli Lilly & Company, respectively. All bacterial isolates, from blood, urine, sputum, and wounds, were from patients hospitalized at the Columbia Presbyterian Medical Center in the past 2 years.

Susceptibility test methods. Minimal inhibitory concentration (MIC) was determined by a standard twofold agar dilution method using Mueller-Hinton agar (BBL) and with a broth dilution method in Mueller-Hinton broth (BBL) as described previously (6).

Detection of β-lactamase. Penicillinase production was tested by agar plate iodometric assay as described by Workman and Farrar (17). Overnight incubations of isolates tested were streaked onto nutrient agar plates containing 0.2% soluble starch. These plates were then flooded with 3 ml of freshly prepared phosphate-buffered saline (pH 6.4) containing iodine (3 mg/ml), potassium iodine (15 mg/ml), and aqueous penicillin G (50 mg/ml) and observed for 30 min. Penicillinase-producing isolates became rapidly decolorized and surrounded by a transparent colorless zone.

Test for synergy. Synergy was defined according to the following criteria: (i) a reduction of the MIC values of both antibiotics by fourfold or more (5); (ii) any definite concavity of the isobologram obtained by graphing the data (7); (iii) a decrease of 1 log or more in viable cell count occurring at the end of 4 h with the antibiotic combination compared with that obtained with the most active single antibiotic (9, 12). Partial synergy was defined as a fourfold or greater reduction in MIC values of one compound but less than fourfold reduction in the MIC value of the second compound. Indifference was either no reduction in MIC values or only twofold. Antagonism was defined as fourfold reduction in MIC of either compound.

Tests for synergy were done with antibiotics combined in equal concentrations or at ratios similar to those that would be obtained in the blood after intravenous administration. Checkerboard patterns were used to provide isobolograms.

Killing curves. Bacterial killing studies were carried out in Mueller-Hinton broth with the concentration of one-fourth of the MIC of netilmicin alone and in combination with one-fourth of the MICs of other antibiotics studied. The initial concentration of organisms was approximately 10^5 viable cells in the early logarithmic growth. Bacterial cultures were placed in Erlenmeyer flasks in a rotary shaker incubator at 37°C. Samples were removed and immediately plated at multiple dilutions on Mueller-Hinton agar to determine viable cell counts.

RESULTS

Synergistic effect of netilmicin with carbenicillin. The isobologram data of the combination of netilmicin and carbenicillin tested in a checkerboard method are given in Fig. 1. Synergy of the combined antibiotics against three *P. aeruginosa* strains one *Pseudomonas maltophilia* strain as indicated by the reduction in MIC values is shown. This synergy of carbenicillin and netilmicin could be further demonstrated for *P. aeruginosa* 2960 using a killing curve method (Fig. 2). The addition of one-fourth of the MIC concentration of both netilmicin (5 μg/ml) and carbenicillin (100 μg/ml) resulted in more than 2-log decrease in viable bacteria compared to the number of colony-forming units when either agent was used alone.

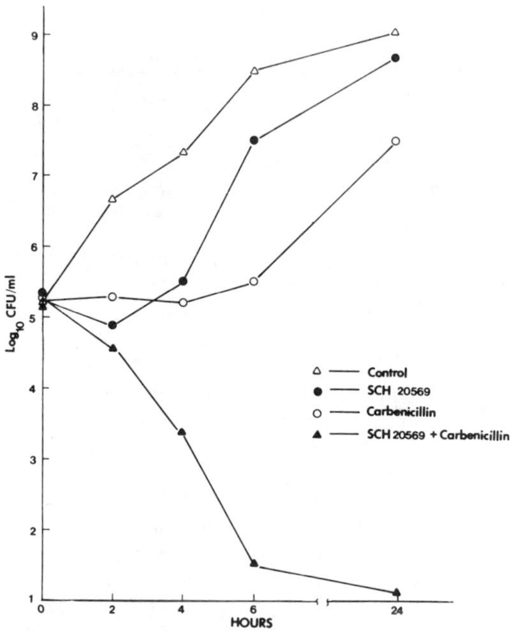

FIG. 2. *Bactericidal effect showing synergy of netilmicin (Sch 20569) and carbenicillin against P. aeruginosa 2960. Carbenicillin concentration was 25 μg/ml, and netilmicin concentration was 1.25 μg/ml.*

The overall effect of the combination of netilmicin and carbenicillin against 46 *P. aeruginosa* isolates is given in Table 1. There was true synergy in 21 instances and indifference in 17 when the comparison was made in agar.

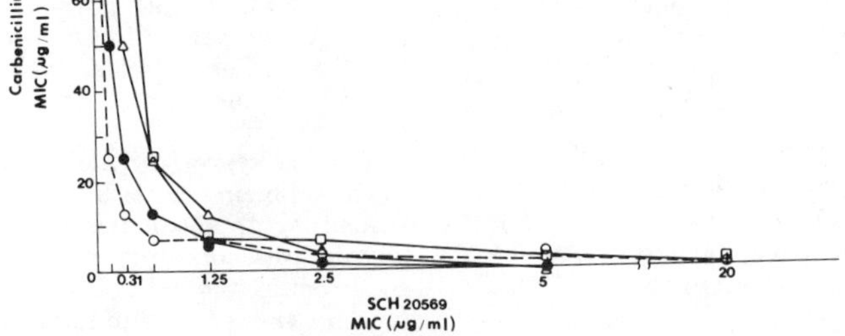

FIG. 1. *Isobolograms showing synergy of netilmicin (Sch 20569) and carbenicillin.*

Since the combination of an aminoglycoside and carbenicillin is often selected before the results of blood cultures are available, we determined the effect of the combination of netilmicin and carbenicillin against other species (Table 2). Included are examples of the actual results obtained for *Pseudomonas*. We did not find true synergy for the combination against three *E. coli,* two *Serratia,* one *Providencia,* one *Klebsiella*, or three enterococcal isolates. In no instance was antagonism encountered.

Comparative susceptibility of *P. aeruginosa* to netilmicin and gentamicin with varying concentrations of carbenicillin is shown in Fig. 3 and 4. Gentamicin was threefold more active against *Pseudomonas* than was netilmicin (Fu and Neu, submitted for publication), even in the presence of carbenicillin (1.6 to 12.5 μg/ml). A significant increase in the susceptibility of *P. aeruginosa* to netilmicin and gentamicin was produced in the presence of increasing concentrations of carbenicillin. But in the presence of 12.5 μg or less of carbenicillin per ml, the gentamicin MIC value was always threefold less than the netilmicin MIC value. The activity of netilmicin or gentamicin against netilmicin-resistant and gentamicin-resistant isolates (MIC > 5 μg/ml) is also shown in Fig. 3 and 4. At low levels of carbenicillin (12.5 μg/ml or less) the percentage of netilmicin-resistant isolates ranged from 22 to 60%, whereas at the same concentration the percentage of gentamicin-resistant isolates was 15 to 35%. It is clear that only at a concentration higher than 12.5 μg of carbenicillin per ml was there a significant difference in gentamicin or Sch 20569 activity against *Pseudomonas* isolates. Figure 5 compares the MIC values of netilmicin and gentamicin against each *P. aeruginosa* isolate tested in the presence of one-fourth of the MIC value of carbenicillin. Of six isolates with MIC ≥ 200 μg of carbenicillin per ml, only in one instance

TABLE 1. *Synergistic effect of netilmicin*[a]

Antibiotic combined	Organism	Synergy	Partial synergy	Indifferent
Carbenicillin	*P. aeruginosa* (46)[b]	21[c]	8	17
Cefazolin	*K. pneumoniae* (20)	1	21	7
Chloramphenicol	*E. coli* (25)	3	7	14
Clindamycin	*E. coli* (21)	3	4	12
Clindamycin	*P. aeruginosa* (13)	0	3	9

[a] MIC values were determined by the agar dilution method in Mueller-Hinton agar which had a 1.58 mM calcium content and 0.73 mM magnesium content.
[b] Total number of isolates tested.
[c] Number of isolates affected by netilmicin in combination with another antibiotic.

TABLE 2. *MICs of netilmicin and carbenicillin alone and in combination*[a]

Organism		MIC (μg/ml)			Synergy test[b]
		Netilmicin	Netilmicin + carbenicillin	Carbenicillin	
E. coli	2938	2.5	1.25–400	400	I
	2939	2.5	1.25–50	400	PS
	2969	0.31	0.16–200	400	I
Klebsiella	2864	2.5	0.31–25	200	S
Serratia	2967	20	10–100	400	PS
	2955	80	40–100	400	PS
Providencia	2943	20	10–200	400	I
P. aeruginosa	2956	40	2.5–0.8	6.3	S
	2963	2.5	2.5–6.25	6.3	I
	2134	40	10–25	100	S
	2912	5	1.25–12.5	25	PS
	2923	20	10–25	100	PS
	2560	20	20–400	400	I
P. maltophilia	2941	80	5–12.5	100	S
	2975	80	5–25	100	S
Enterococci	2555	5	0.16–1.6	3.1	PS
	2546	5	0.63–25	50	PS
	2547	5	0.31–25	50	PS

[a] MIC values were determined by the agar dilution method with Mueller-Hinton agar.
[b] Abbreviations: I, Indifference; PS, partial synergy; S, synergy.

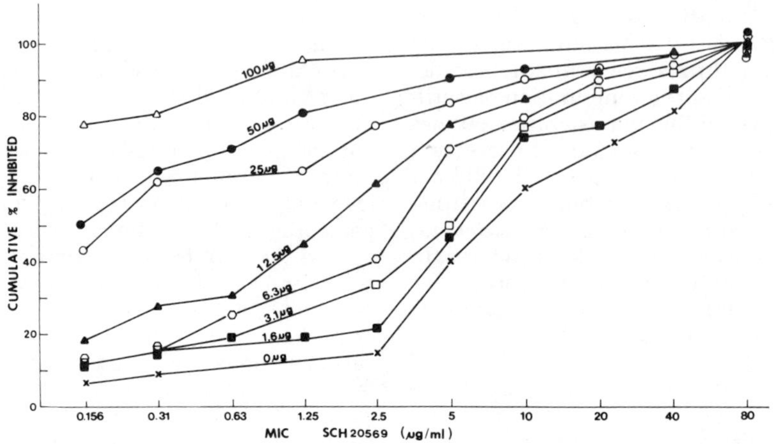

FIG. 3. *Activity of netilmicin (Sch 20569) in combination with various concentrations of carbenicillin as shown against P. aeruginosa.*

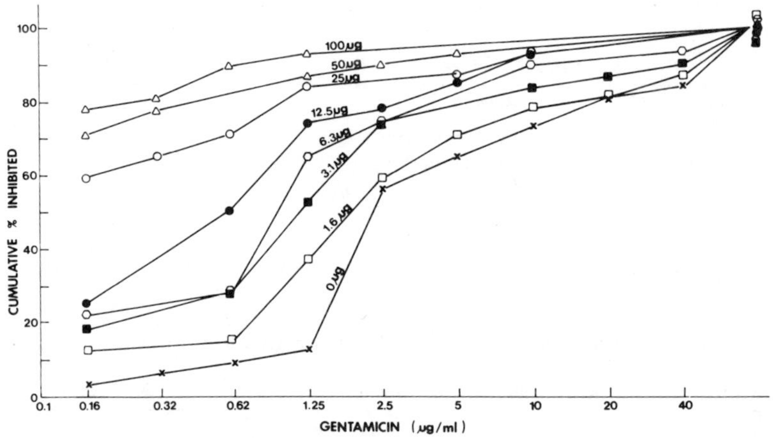

FIG. 4. *Activity of gentamicin in combination with various concentrations of carbenicillin as shown against P. aeruginosa.*

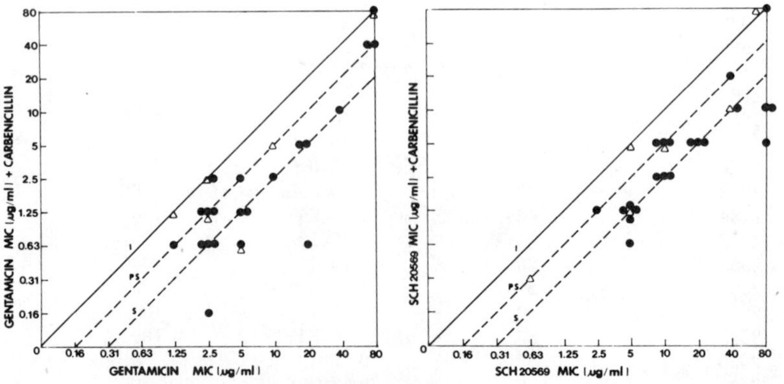

FIG. 5. *Comparative activity of netilmicin (Sch 20569) alone and with one-fourth of the MIC values of carbenicillin and the activity of gentamicin alone and with one-fourth of the MIC values of carbenicillin against P. aeruginosa. Symbols: (△) MIC ≥ 200 µg/ml; (●) MIC ≤ 100 µg of carbenicillin per ml. Abbreviations: I, Indifference; PS, partial synergy; S, synergy.*

could synergy be demonstrated. Partial synergy against two isolates and indifference with three was found with the combination of gentamicin and carbenicillin, whereas the carbenicillin and Sch 20569 combination yielded synergy against two, partial synergy against two, and indifference against two. When tested against *Pseudomonas* isolates with carbenicillin MIC values ≤100 μg/ml, the combination of carbenicillin and netilmicin was synergistic against 15, whereas carbenicillin-gentamicin was synergistic against 12. Five of 10 *Pseudomonas* with an MIC >5 μg of gentamicin per ml and 11 of 18 isolates with a netilmicin MIC >5 μg/ml were synergistically inhibited by the combination of the aminoglycoside with carbenicillin. It is also evident from Fig. 5 that gentamicin is more active than netilmicin even when combined at the concentration of one-fourth of the MIC of carbenicillin.

Synergy of netilmicin with cefazolin. Table 1 shows that only one isolate of the 20 *Klebsiella pneumoniae* tested was synergistically inhibited with the netilmicin and cefazolin combination. An isobologram for this organism is shown in Fig. 6. The MIC values of netilmicin and cefazolin alone and in combination are shown in Table 3. Although true synergy was uncommon, there was a fourfold or more decrease in MIC values against five isolates resistant to cefazolin. The MIC levels were those achievable in man with current dosage systems. The combination of netilmicin with cefazolin at the concentration of one-fourth of the MIC values of each antibiotic showed more than 1-log killing against *Klebsiella* after 4 h of incubation (Fig. 7).

Synergistic effect of netilmicin and chloramphenicol. The combination of netilmicin and chloramphenicol tested against *E. coli* is shown in Fig. 8. All of the *E. coli* isolates were sensitive to netilmicin (0.16 to 2.5 μg/ml). The combination of netilmicin and chloramphenicol was synergistic against three *E. coli* isolates with chloramphenicol MIC values greater than 100 μg (Fig. 8) but not against four of the isolates with MIC values greater than 100 μg. Although no synergistic effect was demonstrated in these isolates, more than a 16-fold reduction of MIC values of chloramphenicol was achieved. Antagonism was observed with one isolate that was sensitive to both chloramphenicol and netilmicin. Figure 6 illustrates the isobologram data when netilmicin and chloramphenicol are combined against *E. coli*. There was an eightfold reduction of MIC values of chloramphenicol in the presence of 0.08 μg of netilmicin per ml and a 32-fold reduction of the MIC value of netilmicin.

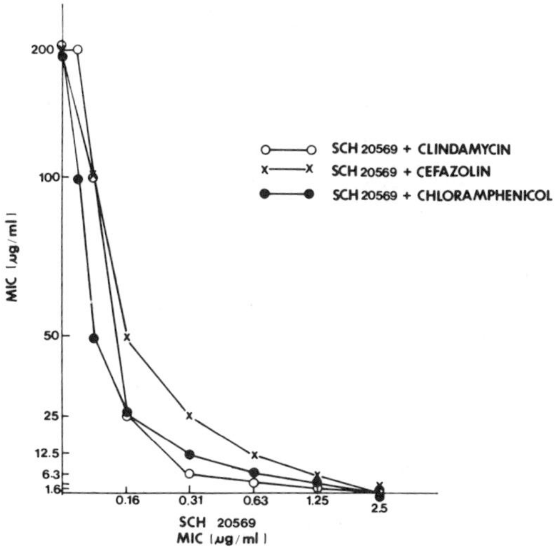

FIG. 6. *Isobolograms showing synergy of netilmicin (Sch 20569) with cefazolin, chloramphenicol, and clindamycin. Symbols:* (○) *E. coli 3003;* (×) *K. pneumoniae;* (●) *E. coli 2990.*

Synergistic effect of netilmicin with clindamycin. An isobologram plot (Fig. 6) of MIC values for an *E. coli* isolate shows the synergistic inhibition of *E. coli* by netilmicin and clindamycin. All *E. coli* isolates tested were sensitive to netilmicin (Fig. 9) but resistant to clindamycin (MIC ≥ 100 μg/ml). The netilmicin and clindamycin combination showed indifference or antagonism in most instances. In comparison, the combination of gentamicin and clindamycin produced no synergy, 1 antagonism, 5 partial synergies, and 14 indifferences against *E. coli*. No synergy could be demonstrated with a netilmicin-clindamycin (Fig. 9) or gentamicin-clindamycin combination against *P. aeruginosa*. All *P. aeruginosa* isolates had clindamycin MIC values higher than 200 μg and gentamicin MIC values between 0.3 to 5 μg/ml. One isolate showed an antagonistic effect of netilmicin-clindamycin, but no antagonism was seen with the gentamicin-clindamycin combination.

Relation of synergism to production of inactivating enzymes. Table 4 demonstrates that the presence or absence of β-lactamase did not determine whether synergy would result when netilmicin was combined with a β-lactam antibiotic such as carbenicillin or cefazolin. However, 20 of 41 strains that lacked a β-lactamase showed synergy versus 6 of 25 which contained a demonstrable β-lactamase.

DISCUSSION

The in vitro synergy of aminoglycosides with carbenicillin has been reported by many groups

TABLE 3. *Synergy of netilmicin and cefazolin against K. pneumoniae*

K. pneumoniae strain	MIC (μg/ml)			Synergy test[a]
	Cefazolin	Cefazolin + netilmicin	Netilmicin	
2986	6.3	3.1–0.16	0.63	PS
3001	25	6.3–0.31	1.25	S
3005	50	12.5–0.63	1.25	PS
3011	3.1	1.6–0.08	1.25	PS
2984	25	12.5–0.63	1.25	PS
3002	200	12.5–0.63	0.63	I
2987	>200	12.5–0.63	1.25	PS
2864	200	6.25–0.31	0.63	PS
2940	6.3	3.1–0.16	1.25	PS
2968	100	12.5–0.63	0.63	I
2954	100	12.5–0.63	1.25	PS
2842	1.6	0.8–0.04	0.31	PS
2945	3.1	3.1–0.16	0.63	I
2920	1.6	0.8–0.04	0.63	PS
2903	1.6	1.6–0.08	0.63	I
2556	50	25–1.25	1.25	I
2422	1.6	0.8–0.04	0.63	PS
2107	1.6	3.1–0.16	1.25	I
2807	12.5	12.5–0.63	2.5	I
1402	1.6	0.8–0.04	0.63	PS

[a] Abbreviations: PS, Partial synergy; S, synergy; I, indifference.

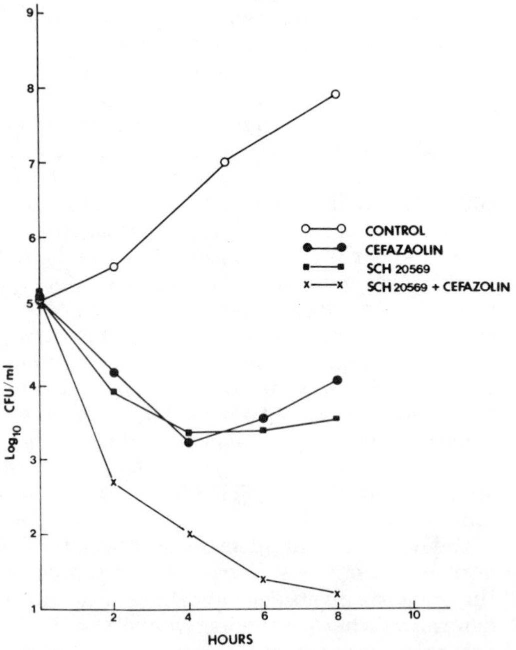

FIG. 7. *Bactericidal effect showing synergy of netilmicin (Sch 20569) and cefazolin against K. pneumoniae 3001. Cefazolin concentration was 6.3 μg/ml, and netilmicin concentration was 0.31 μg/ml.*

(1, 6, 7, 10, 12, 16). This in vitro synergistic effect has also been shown to be effective in prolonged survival of leukopenic animals (2, 11). The present study showed that netilmicin, like other aminoglycosides (10), when combined with carbenicillin, had a synergistic effect against *P. aeruginosa*. At therapeutic concentrations, the combination of netilmicin and carbenicillin synergistically inhibited more than 90% of the *P. aeruginosa* strains tested. The synergy studied in this investigation can be confirmed by three criteria; however, not all the isolates against which the combination showed synergy could be confirmed by the kill-

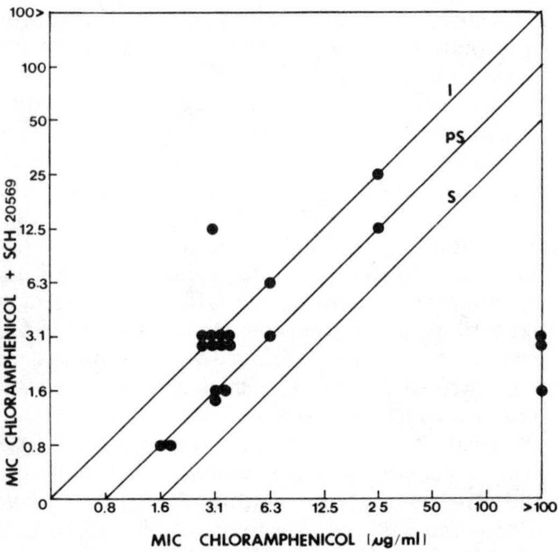

FIG. 8. *Comparative activity of chloramphenicol alone and with one-fourth of the MIC values of netilmicin (Sch 20569) against E. coli.*

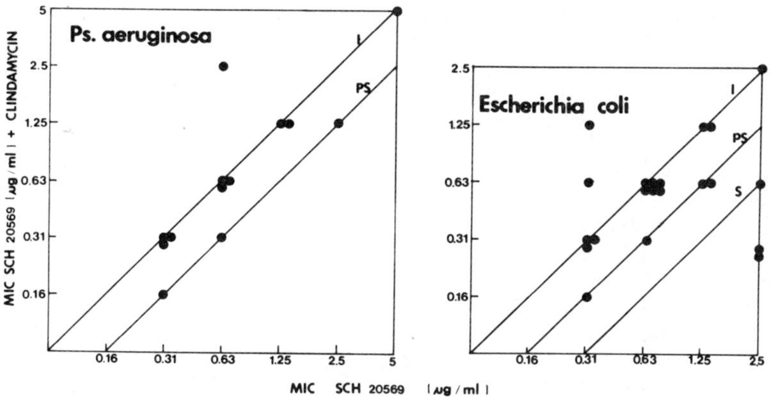

FIG. 9. *Comparative activity of netilmicin (Sch 20569) alone and with one-fourth of the MIC values of clindamycin.*

TABLE 4. *Relation of synergistic effect of netilmicin on β-lactamase production*

Antibiotic combined	Organism	β-Lactamase present	No. of isolates affected by synergism
Carbenicillin	*P. aeruginosa* (8)[a]	+	3
	P. aeruginosa (38)	−	18
	P. maltophilia (1)	+	1
	P. maltophilia (2)	−	2
	E. coli (3)	+	0
	Klebsiella (1)	+	1
	Serratia (2)	+	0
	Providencia (1)	+	0
Cefazolin	*Klebsiella* (9)	+	1

[a] Total number of isolates tested.

ing curve method, which is in agreement with other workers (7, 12).

Weinstein et al. (16) showed that amikacin demonstrated synergy against a greater percentage of isolates of *Pseudomonas* than did gentamicin when combined with carbenicillin. They also found that when analyzed in terms of the percentage of *Pseudomonas* isolates susceptible to each of the three drug combinations, no significant differences were seen. The netilnicin-carbenicillin combination showed synergy against more *Pseudomonas* isolates than did gentamicin-carbenicillin. However, susceptibility tests show that on the equal weight base the gentamicin-carbenicillin combination is more active at low carbenicillin concentrations (1.6 to 12.5 µg) than is the netilmicin-carbenicillin combination. At a concentration of 25 µg or greater of carbenicillin, attainable in humans, no significant difference could be seen between the two combinations. This study (Fig. 5) showed that 11 isolates of moderately and highly netilmicin-resistant *Pseudomonas* strains were synergistically inhibited compared to only 5 gentamicin-resistant isolates that were synergistically inhibited by gentamicin-carbenicillin. This suggests that netilmicin-carbenicillin may have a distinct advantage for isolates highly or moderately resistant to netilmicin.

The results here suggest that there are many variations in the response of synergy within the same strains, even isolates with the same MIC values. It is difficult to predict synergistic response from MIC values of the antibiotic. However, *P. aeruginosa* isolates with carbenicillin MIC values higher than 200 µg rarely were synergistically inhibited by the addition of netilmicin or gentamicin. Studies of the β-lactamase production of each *Pseudomonas* isolate revealed no correlation of its production with synergy (Table 4). Synergy of netilmicin with cefazolin, clindamycin, and chloramphenicol was seldom observed. Synergy of netilmicin with chloramphenicol was not related to susceptibility of *E. coli* to chloramphenicol, since isolates resistant to chloramphenicol show either synergistic effects or indifference. No distinct pattern of synergy was observed with the netilmicin-cefazolin combination against *K. pneumoniae*. It is possible that the higher susceptibility of *E. coli* and *Klebsiella* to netilmicin may account for the rare occurrence of synergy.

Clindamycin has been shown to act synergistically with gentamicin against 90% of *E. coli* and no *P. aeruginosa* isolates (8). The present results showed that the netilmicin-clindamycin combination was synergistic against only 29% of *E. coli* and against no *P. aeruginosa*. Like the gentamicin-clindamycin combination, synergism was observed only at concentrations of the agents which were not obtainable in man even though significant decreases of the MIC values of clindamycin were observed. Of importance is the fact that antagonism is not common, since this new agent will undoubtedly be used in combination with agents such as clindamycin and chloramphenicol to treat abdominal infections which are produced by a mixed population of aerobic and anaerobic bacteria.

The trimethoprim-sulfamethoxazole combination is the best model of synergistic action of antimicrobial agents. It blocks two successive steps of folic acid biosynthesis and acts synergistically against many organisms (3, 4). Unlike this combination, the synergistic effect of netilmicin varies not only with the antibiotics used in combination but also is more selective.

It is postulated that the mechanism of the synergy of the aminoglycoside with a penicillin such as carbenicillin is a result of partial disruption of the cell wall (12, 19). The presence of β-lactamase activity in *E. coli, Klebsiella, Providencia, Serratia,* and *Pseudomonas* did not determine whether a drug showed synergy, indifference, or antagonism (Table 4). The same was true concerning the presence of aminoglycoside inactivating enzymes. But if both inactivating mechanisms are present, such as was encountered in some *P. aeruginosa, P. maltophilia,* and *Providencia stuarti*, indifference was routinely seen.

Although these studies clearly demonstrated synergy of netilmicin with agents with which it would be used clinically, it is not clear that the reduction in MIC values would be of significance, and this must be evaluated in animal models and in clinical studies.

LITERATURE CITED

1. **Anderson, E. L., P. K. Gramling, P. R. Vestal, and W. E. Farrar, Jr.** 1975. Susceptibility of *Pseudomonas aeruginosa* to tobramycin or gentamicin alone and combined with carbenicillin. Antimicrob. Agents Chemother. 8:300–304.
2. **Andriole, V. T.** 1971. Synergy of carbenicillin and gentamicin in experimental infection with *Pseudomonas*. J. Infect. Dis. 124:S46–55.
3. **Bach, M. C., M. Finland, O. Gold, and C. Wilcox.** 1973. Susceptibility of recently isolated pathogenic bacteria to trimethoprim and sulfamethoxazole, separately and combined. J. Infect. Dis. 128:S508–S533.
4. **Brumfitt, W., J. M. T. Hamilton-Miller, and J. Kosmidis.** 1973. Trimethoprim-sulfamethoxazole: the present position. J. Infect. Dis. 128:S778–791.
5. **Brumfitt, W. A., A. Percival, and D. A. Leigh.** 1967. Clinical and laboratory studies with carbenicillin: a new penicillin active against *Pseudomonas pyocyanea*. Lancet 1:1289–1293.
6. **Dienstag, J., and H. C. Neu.** 1972. In vitro studies of tobramycin, an aminoglycoside antibiotic. Antimicrob. Agents Chemother. 1:41–45.
7. **Eickhoff, T. C.** 1969. In vitro effects of carbenicillin combined with gentamicin or polymyxin B against *Pseudomonas aeruginosa*. Appl. Microbiol. 18:469–473.
8. **Fass, R. J., C. A. Rotilie, and R. B. Prior.** 1974. Interaction of clindamycin and gentamicin in vitro. Antimicrob. Agents Chemother. 6:582–587.
9. **Jawetz, E.** 1968. The use of combination of antimicrobial drugs, p. 151–170. *In* H. W. Elliott, W. C. Cutting, and R. H. Dreisbach (ed.), Annual review of pharmacology, vol. 8. Annual Reviews, Palo Alto, Calif.
10. **Kluge, R. M., H. C. Standiford, B. Tatem, V. M. Young, W. H. Greene, S. C. Schmipff, F. M. Calia, and R. B. Hornick.** 1974. Comparative activity of tobramycin, amikacin, and gentamicin alone and with carbenicillin against *Pseudomonas aeruginosa*. Antimicrob. Agents Chemother. 6:442–446.
11. **Konickova, L., and W. Pratt.** 1971. Effect of carbenicillin, gentamicin and their combination on experimental *Pseudomonas aeruginosa* urinary infection. J. Clin. Pathol. 24:113–116.
12. **Libke, R. D., C. Regamey, J. T. Clark, and W. M. M. Kirby.** 1973. Synergism of carbenicillin and gentamicin against enterococci. Antimicrob. Agents Chemother. 4:564–568.
13. **Myerourtz, R. L., A. A. Medeiros, and T. F. Obrin.** 1971. Recent experience with bacilliemia due to gram-negative organisms. J. Infect. Dis. 124:239–246.
14. **Rahal, J. J., Jr., M. S. Simberkoff, K. Kagan, and N. H. Moldover.** 1976. Bactericidal efficacy of Sch 20569 and amikacin against gentamicin-sensitive and -resistant organisms. Antimicrob. Agents Chemother. 9:595–599.
15. **Smith, C. B., P. E. Dans, J. N. Wilfert, and M. Finland.** 1969. Use of gentamicin in combination with other antibiotics. J. Infect. Dis. 119:370–377.
16. **Weinstein, R. J., L. S. Young, and W. L. Hewitt.** 1975. Comparison of methods for assessing *in vitro* antibiotic synergism against *Pseudomonas* and *Serratia*. J. Lab. Clin. Med. 86:853–862.
17. **Workman, R. G., and W. E. Farrar, Jr.** 1970. Activity of penicillinase in *Staphylococcus aureus* as studied by the iodometric method. J. Infect. Dis. 121:433–437.
18. **Zimmerman, R. A., R. C. Moellering, Jr., and A. N. Weinberg.** 1971. Mechanism of resistance to antibiotic synergism of enterococci. J. Bacteriol. 105:873–879.

ANTIMICROBIAL AGENTS AND CHEMOTHERAPY, Sept. 1976, p. 519-525
Vol. 10, No. 3

Selection and Characterization of Strains of *Staphylococcus aureus* Displaying Unusual Resistance to Aminoglycosides

STEPHEN G. WILSON* AND CHRISTINE C. SANDERS

Department of Medical Microbiology, Creighton University School of Medicine, Omaha, Nebraska 68178

Received for publication 23 March 1976

Susceptibility tests with aminoglycosides against *Staphylococcus aureus* have revealed discrepancies between the minimal inhibitory concentrations and the minimal bactericidal concentrations. To further evaluate these discrepancies, kill curves were performed against a susceptible strain of *S. aureus* with five different aminoglycosides (amikacin, kanamycin, tobramycin, gentamicin, sisomicin) at concentrations up to 16-fold above the minimal inhibitory concentration. Results revealed the presence of small subpopulations of cells capable of growth within 24 h in concentrations of aminoglycoside up to eightfold above the minimal inhibitory concentration for the parent strain. These subpopulations occurred at a frequency of $\geq 10^{-7}$ parent cells, were not physiologically different from the susceptible parent strains, and were present in approximately one-half of 30 strains of *S. aureus* tested. The resistance of these subpopulations was approximately eightfold higher than that of the parent for all five aminoglycosides and was independent of concentration or type of aminoglycoside used to select them. This resistance was not due to extracellular degradation of drug and was stable over eight transfers in drug-free medium, except when selected by gentamicin or sisomicin.

Studies concerning the effects of procedural variations on the activity of aminoglycosides have revealed that a single procedural change can significantly alter results, particularly in tests with *Staphylcoccus aureus* (14). Variations in such factors as inoculum and type of medium used may at times also alter the clinical interpretation of results, and significant discrepancies between the minimal inhibitory concentrations (MICs) and minimal bactericidal concentrations (MBCs) of aminoglycosides have been observed (5, 9, 12, 16). These observations suggest the presence of a small subpopulation of cells within the susceptible parent strain which are more resistant to the effects of the aminoglycoside. Therefore, the purpose of this study was to (i) evaluate the bactericidal activity of aminoglycosides against *S. aureus* by the use of kill curves, (ii) characterize the more resistant cells selected from strains of *S. aureus* which appeared to be susceptible to aminoglycosides by MIC determinations, and (iii) determine the prevalence of strains containing these more resistant cells.

MATERIALS AND METHODS

Isolates. All isolates of *S. aureus* were obtained from clinical sources (Shand's Teaching Hospital and Clinic, Gainesville, Fla.; and Creighton Memorial St. Joseph's Hospital, Omaha, Neb.).

Antibiotics. Gentamicin, sisomicin (Schering Corp., Bloomfield, N.J.), kanamycin (Bristol Laboratories, Syracuse, N.Y.), and tobramycin (Eli Lilly and Co., Indianapolis, Ind.) were used in the form of sulfates; amikacin (Bristol Laboratories, Syracuse, N.Y.) was used as the base. Stock solutions of 1,000 μg/ml were prepared in sterile distilled water (weight corrected for potency) and then sterilized by membrane filtration (pore size, 0.45-μm; Millipore Corp., Bedford, Mass.). Appropriate dilutions were made in sterile Mueller-Hinton broth (MHB; Baltimore Biological Laboratories) to yield 100 μg of each drug per ml.

Broth dilution susceptibility tests. Serial twofold tube dilution tests were performed in MHB in a volume of 3 ml per tube. Dilutions of an 18-h broth culture were made to produce a final bacterial population in each tube of 10^4 to 5×10^4 colony-forming units (CFU) per ml. MIC was defined as the lowest concentration of drug that prevented macroscopic growth after incubation for 18 to 24 h at 37°C. MBCs were determined by subculturing 0.01 ml (calibrated loop) from each clear tube onto a blood agar plate. The MBC was defined as the lowest concentration of drug that prevented all growth on subculture. Dilution susceptibility tests were performed simultaneously with all five aminoglycosides against each strain. All subsequent references to MICs or MBCs, unless otherwise stated, pertain to results derived from broth dilution susceptibility tests. Since stationary-phase cells were used in these assays, all further studies were also performed with stationary-phase cells for consistency.

Kill curves. Flasks containing aminoglycoside in MHB were inoculated with an appropriate dilution of an 18-h culture of *S. aureus* to produce a final bacterial population of approximately 10^5 CFU/ml. Samples were removed at 0, 0.5, 1, 2, 4, 6, 8, 24, and 48 h of incubation, and the number of viable cell units was counted using a standard agar dilution, pour-plate technique in Mueller-Hinton agar (MHA). Colony counts were based on counts on duplicate plates. Kill curves were performed on each strain simultaneously with all five aminoglycosides.

Antibiotic inactivation tests. MHB containing aminoglycoside was inoculated with approximately 10^5 CFU/ml and incubated for 24 h at 37°C. All bacteria were removed by membrane filtration (Millipore Corp.). Arithmetic dilutions of the filtrates were made, and 0.02 ml of each was added to a sterile 7-mm paper disk. These disks were then tested for activity against a laboratory stock strain of *S. aureus* using the procedure described by Bauer and associates (1). Activity was determined by comparison of zone sizes with those produced by aminoglycoside in MHB freshly prepared. For controls, this assay was performed on filtrates from 24-h MHB cultures without aminoglycoside and uninoculated MHB with aminoglycoside incubated for 24 h.

Frequency of resistant cells. An inoculum of bacterial cells (10^8 CFU/ml) was placed into MHA containing concentrations of aminoglycoside 2-, 4-, 8-, and 16-fold above the MIC determined in broth tests. The frequency of cells capable of growing in concentrations above the MIC was calculated by dividing the number of colonies growing in drug-containing agar (resistant subpopulations) by the total number of cells in the original inoculum (parent population).

Physiological comparisons. Both parent and resistant subpopulations were compared for ability to ferment glucose, mannitol (Fisher Scientific Co., Fairlawn, N.J.), sucrose, and lactose (BBL) in purple broth base plus 1% Trypticase (BBL). Coagulase and deoxyribonuclease (DNase) production were determined by standard agar diffusion procedures, using coagulase plasma (BBL) and DNase agar (Difco).

Stability of resistance. Each strain was subcultured daily on drug-free blood agar plates. The susceptibility of each subculture to all five aminoglycosides was determined simultaneously by an agar dilution procedure. Organisms (approximately 5×10^4 CFU) were placed onto the surface of each plate with a multiple inoculator device (15). The MIC was defined as the lowest concentration of drug inhibiting all growth after incubation for 24 h at 37°C in air.

RESULTS

Kinetics of the bactericidal activity of aminoglcyosides against *S. aureus*. To more closely examine the discrepancies seen between the MICs and MBCs of aminoglycosides for *S. aureus*, the kinetics of bactericidal activity were studied by the use of kill curves. Various concentrations of each aminoglycoside above the MIC were used in these tests. As shown in Fig. 1, amikacin at two- to eightfold above the MIC caused a decrease in viable cell counts for the first 7 h of incubation. This was followed over the next 17 h by a significant increase in the number of viable cells. The magnitude of the initial drop in viability increased with each increase in aminoglycoside concentration. However, complete killing without significant growth after 7 h was observed only with concentrations 16-fold above the MIC. Similar results were obtained with kanamycin, tobramycin, and gentamicin. An initial drop in viable cell counts followed by a significant increase in viable cells was also observed with sisomicin at two- and fourfold above the MIC (Fig. 2). Although viable cells were recoverable after 7 h with sisomicin at a concentration eightfold above the MIC, their numbers did not reach levels that could be counted with accuracy (≥30 CFU/ml). No viable cells were detectable between 7 and 24 h of incubation with sisomicin at concentrations 16-fold above the MIC.

The frequency of cells in the parent strain

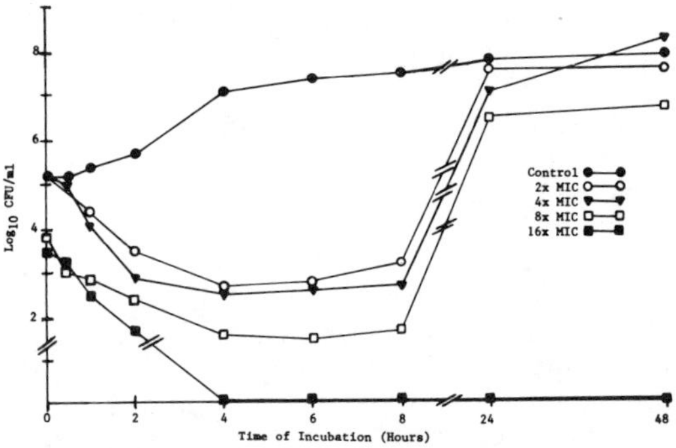

FIG. 1. *Bactericidal activity of amikacin against Staphylococcus aureus in various concentrations above the MIC (0.8 μg/ml).*

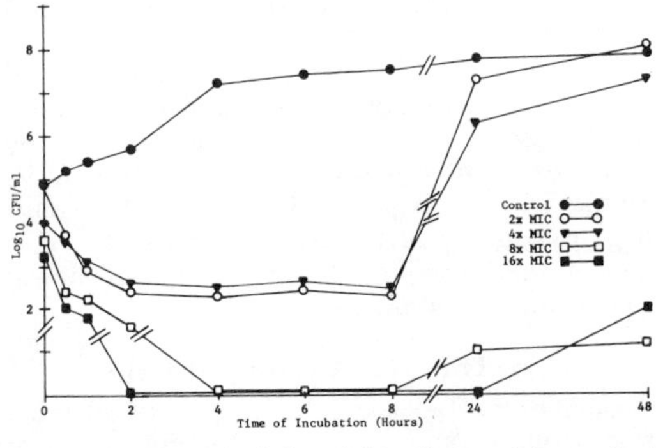

FIG. 2. *Bactericidal activity of sisomicin against Staphylococcus aureus in various concentrations above the MIC (0.2 μg/ml).*

that were capable of growing in concentrations of aminoglycoside above the MIC (superinhibitory concentrations) was determined in agar tests (Table 1). The frequencies of cells capable of growing in drug-containing agar decreased progressively one log per twofold increase in amikacin, kanamycin, and tobramycin. At eightfold above the MIC for the parent strain (8-MIC_p), the frequency was 10^{-7} or greater. The frequency of cells capable of growing in gentamicin dropped two logs between two- and fourfold above the MIC, but was also 10^{-7} at 8-MIC_p. For sisomicin, the frequency dropped one log per twofold increase in concentration, but the frequency at 8-MIC_p was less than 10^{-7}.

The growth observed in the kill curves after 7 h in superinhibitory amounts of aminoglycoside suggested the presence of a more resistant cell population. Therefore, the cells recovered at 24 h were tested for their susceptibility to the aminoglycoside which had been used in the kill curve and compared to that of the parent strain (Table 2). For each aminoglycoside, the increase in MIC for these cells above that for the parent strain was similar regardless of the concentration used in the kill curve. Furthermore, every increase observed was fourfold or greater. The increase in MBCs for these cells above that for the parent strain showed no consistent pattern like that seen for the MICs. Since the increases in MICs were similar regardless of the concentration used to select the cells, further studies were performed only on cells recovered at 24 h in 8-MIC_p of aminoglycoside (R8 cells).

Further studies on R8 cells. R8 cells were next tested for cross-resistance to aminoglycosides not used in their selection. MICs and MBCs of all five aminoglycosides were determined simultaneously. Regardless of aminoglycoside used to select the R8 cells, an increased resistance to all five aminoglycosides was observed. MICs of amikacin, kanamycin, and tobramycin against the R8 cells selected by amikacin, kanamycin, or tobramycin increased eightfold above the MIC for the parent strain; the MICs of gentamicin and sisomicin increased only fourfold. MICs for the R8 cells selected by gentamicin and sisomicin increased eightfold above the MIC of the parent for all five aminoglycosides. Furthermore, the size of the increases in MIC corresponded closely to the size of the discrepancies seen between the MICs and MBCs of the parent strain with each of the five aminoglycosides. However, as before, increases in MBC for the R8 cells showed no consistent pattern. Since MBCs for the R8 cells also increased in some instances, discrepancies between MIC and MBC were not always eliminated (Table 3). Discrepancies between MICs and MBCs did not occur in every test with tobramycin or sisomicin, and when they occurred, they were not as large as those observed with R8 cells selected by the other three aminoglycosides.

TABLE 1. *Frequency of cells within parent strain capable of growth in agar containing superinhibitory concentrations of aminoglycoside*

Aminoglycoside	Multiple above MIC against parent			
	2×	4×	8×	16×
Amikacin	10^{-4}[a]	10^{-5}	10^{-6}	10^{-7}
Kanamycin	10^{-4}	10^{-5}	10^{-6}	10^{-7}
Tobramycin	10^{-5}	10^{-6}	10^{-7}	10^{-8}
Gentamicin	10^{-4}	10^{-6}	10^{-7}	10^{-8}
Sisomicin	10^{-6}	10^{-7}	10^{-8}	10^{-8}

[a] Number of cells growing in drug-containing agar/total number of cells in original inoculum.

TABLE 2. *Activity of aminoglycosides against cells selected with superinhibitory concentrations of drug*

Aminoglycoside used	Parent strain	Cells selected with aminoglycoside above the MIC for parent		
		2×	4×	8×
Amikacin	0.8/6.5[a]	12.5/50	12.5/12.5	6.3/200
Kanamycin	0.8/12.5	25/100	12.5/25	6.3/200
Tobramycin	0.2/1.6	0.8/1.6	1.6/3.1	1.6/6.3
Gentamicin	0.2/1.6	1.6/3.1	0.8/1.6	1.6/12.5
Sisomicin	0.2/0.8	0.8/0.8	1.6/6.3	1.6/1.6

[a] MIC/MBC in micrograms per milliliter.

Since the R8 cells selected with amikacin had large discrepancies between MICs and MBCs, tests were performed to determine if these R8 cells contained even more highly resistant cells. These R8 cells were placed in broth containing a concentration of amikacin eightfold above the MIC for the R8 cells. The cells that were recovered in 24 h were then tested for their susceptibility to all five aminoglycosides. The MIC of all five aminoglycosides for these cells was increased to the level of the MBC for the R8 cells, and the MBCs for these cells did not increase. Thus, the discrepancies between MICs and MBCs were eliminated.

Kill curves were repeated to compare the R8 cells to the parent strain relative to (i) bactericidal activity of aminoglycosides and (ii) their normal growth rates. A single concentration of 8-MIC_p was used in these tests. As shown in Fig. 3, the viability of the parent strain dropped initially as before with amikacin, kanamycin, tobramycin, and gentamicin, with growth occurring after 7 h. No significant growth was observed in sisomicin between 7 and 24 h. In tests with the R8 cells, amikacin slowed the growth rate of the R8 cells, but growth continued steadily until, at 24 h, it was equivalent to the two controls (Fig. 3A). Kanamycin also slowed the growth rate of the R8 cells to the extent that at 24 h the number of viable cells was one log lower than both controls (Fig. 3B). Tobramycin produced a bacteriostatic effect on the R8 cells, whereas both controls were equivalent (Fig. 3C). Gentamicin produced little effect on the growth rate of the R8 cells; however, the growth rate of the R8 control was somewhat slower than that of the parent control (Fig. 3D).

TABLE 3. *Relationship between MBCs and MICs of aminoglycosides for Staphylococcus aureus parent strain and R8[a] cells*

Aminoglycoside	Parent strain	Cells selected with:				
		Amikacin	Kanamycin	Tobramycin	Gentamicin	Sisomicin
Amikacin	8[b]	32	16	32	64	16
Kanamycin	16	8	32	64	32	16
Tobramycin	8	2	1	4	4	4
Gentamicin	8	8	8	16	8	2
Sisomicin	4	2	2	4	1	1

[a] Cells growing in 8-MIC_p in 24 h.
[b] Ratio MBC/MIC.

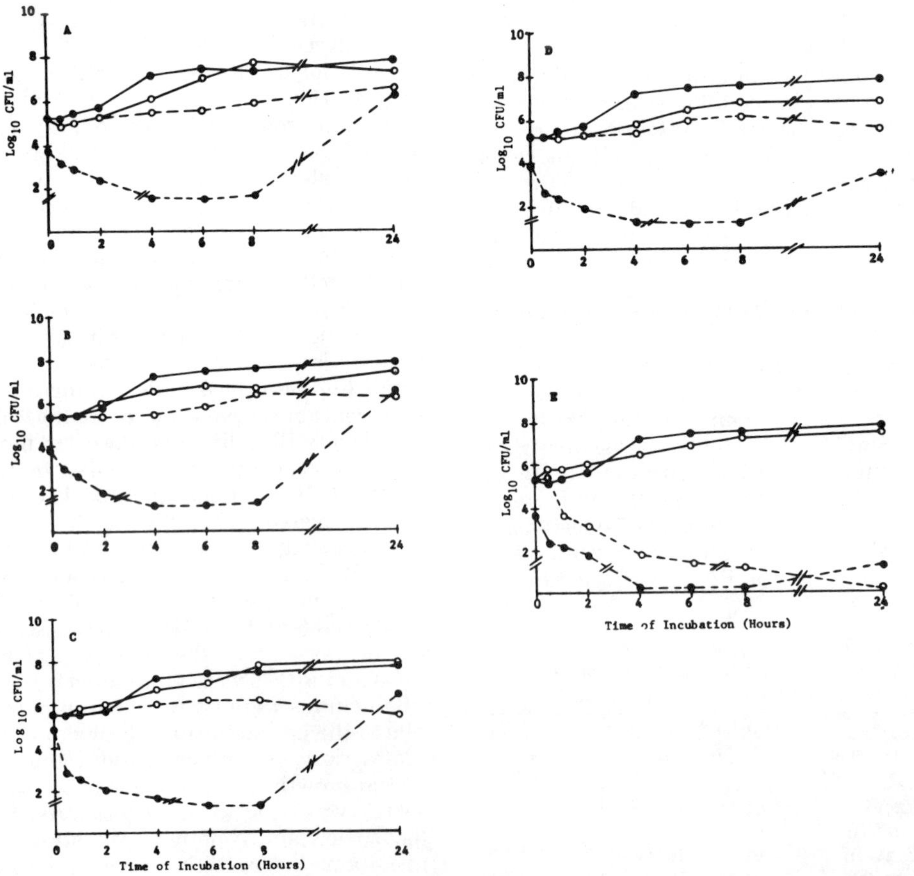

FIG. 3. *Activity of (A) amikacin, (B) kanamycin, (C) tobramycin, (D) gentamicin, and (E) sisomicin against R8 cells (○) and parent strain (●). Concentration of each drug was eightfold above the MIC for the parent (MICs: amikacin and kanamycin [0.8 μg/ml], tobramycin, gentamicin, and sisomicin [0.2 μg/ml]). Test, dashed lines; control, solid lines.*

Sisomicin produced a drop in the viable cell count of both parent and R8 cells, and no significant growth occurred after 7 h. The parent and R8 cell controls were equivalent (Fig. 3E). The changes observed in the kill curves with the R8 cells further substantiated the presence of a subpopulation of more resistant cells within the parent strain.

Prevalence of R8 cells in clinical isolates of *S. aureus*. Concentrations of aminoglycoside, 8-MIC_p, appeared to be the maximum concentration in broth for the selection of R8 cells. Therefore, 30 different clinical isolates of *S. aureus* were examined for the presence of R8 cells (Table 4). Of 30 strains tested, the percentage of strains containing R8 cells was 73% for amikacin, 77% for kanamycin, 93% for tobramycin, 83% for gentamicin, and 87% for sisomicin.

These 30 strains were next screened for the presence of cells capable of growing in agar containing aminoglycoside at 8-MIC_p and occurring at a frequency of 10^{-7} parent cells or more. The percentage of the 30 strains containing such cells was 53% for amikacin, 43% for kanamycin, 60% for tobramycin, 53% for gentamicin, and 47% for sisomicin. The percentage of the 30 strains that contained the more resistant cells in both the broth and agar tests was 43% for amikacin, 36% for kanamycin, 53% for tobramycin, 43% for gentamicin, and 40% for sisomicin. The limiting factor of this evaluation was the frequency of 10^{-7} since several of the strains demonstrated R8 cells in broth tests, but agar tests showed the more resistant cells occurred at a frequency less than 10^{-7}. A resistant subpopulation was thus defined as cells within a parent strain of *S. aureus* (i) occurring at a frequency of at least 1 in 10^7 parent cells and (ii) capable of growing in concentrations of aminoglycoside 8-MIC_p within 24 h.

Characterization of the resistance. The resistant subpopulations were characterized with regard to stability of resistance, extracellular degradation of drug, and physiological similarity to the parent strain. To determine the stability of this resistance, each subpopulation was transferred daily for 8 days in drug-free media and retested for its susceptibility to aminoglycosides. Those subpopulations selected by gentamicin and sisomicin reverted to the parent sensitivity to all five aminoglycosides after two transfers. The subpopulations selected by amikacin, kanamycin, and tobramycin maintained their resistance to all five aminoglycosides after eight transfers. Tests for bioactive drug were performed on cell-free filtrates made from 24-h subpopulation cultures, growing in concentrations of aminoglycoside 8-MIC_p. The tests revealed that these filtrates contained as much active antibiotic as fresh drug and drug incubated in sterile broth. To determine their physiological similarity to the parent strain, resistant subpopulations were tested for the ability to ferment glucose, sucrose, mannitol, and lactose, and for the ability to produce coagulase and DNase. The tests revealed no physiological differences between the parent strain and subpopulations.

TABLE 4. *Percentage of strains of Staphylococcus aureus containing cells capable of growth in concentrations of aminoglycoside 8-MIC_p*

Aminoglycoside	In broth	In agar at frequency of 10^{-7} parent cells	Both in broth and in agar at frequency of 10^{-7} parent cells
Amikacin	22(73%)[a]	16(53%)	13(43%)
Kanamycin	23(77%)	13(43%)	11(36%)
Tobramycin	28(93%)	18(60%)	16(53%)
Gentamicin	25(83%)	16(53%)	13(43%)
Sisomicin	26(87%)	14(47%)	12(40%)

[a] Number of strains (percentage of total 30 strains).

DISCUSSION

The results of this study indicated that the discrepancies observed between the MICs and MBCs of aminoglycosides against *S. aureus* were due to the presence of small subpopulations of cells more resistant to the bactericidal effects of aminoglycosides than the parent strain. These subpopulations were selected by a single exposure to superinhibitory concentrations of aminoglycoside. Kill curves performed with the subpopulations in concentrations of aminoglycoside 8-MIC_p showed no decreased viability (except with sisomicin), but did suggest some bacteriostatic effect, particularly with tobramycin. The drop in the viability of the sisomicin-selected subpopulations in sisomicin may have been due to reversion to parent strain susceptibility since sisomicin-selected subpopulations were unstable. The resistant subpopulations selected by each of the five aminoglycosides were physiologically similar to the parent strain, and those subpopulations selected by amikacin, kanamycin, and tobramycin were stable upon transfer to drug-free medium.

The resistant subpopulations that were selected with amikacin, kanamycin, and tobramycin in this study have somewhat different characteristics than the resistant cells described by Price et al. (12) and by Weinstein et al. (18). In those studies the resistant cells were selected in vitro by multiple transfer in subinhibitory amounts of aminoglycoside. Although the cells showed cross-resistance to the other aminoglycosides, they reverted rapidly to susceptibility, grew more slowly than the parent strain, were nutritionally dependent, and lacked virulence. The results of this study are most similar to those described in studies with the penicillin, BL-P1654 and *Pseudomonas* (7, 14). As in this study, large discrepancies had been observed between MICs and MBCs of BL-P1654 against *Pseudomonas*. Strains of *Pseudomonas* were shown to contain small subpopulations of cells 4- to 32-fold more resistant to BL-P1654 than the parent *Pseudomonas* strain. Those subpopulations were selected by a single exposure to superinhibitory concentrations of drug and were stable upon transfer in drug-free media. The presence of those subpopulations explained the significant discrepancies observed between the MIC and MBC of BL-P1654.

Determination of the precise mechanism of resistance of the subpopulations was beyond the scope of this study. However, physiological similarities of the subpopulations to the parent strain as demonstrated by growth curves in drug-free media and biochemical tests, and the cross-resistance to the other aminoglycosides, suggested the production of an inactivating enzyme. Since no extracellular inactivation of the aminoglycoside was observed, enzyme inactivation, if it is responsible for the resistance, must occur within or at the surface of the cell. The only known enzyme capable of inactivating all five of the aminoglycosides used in this study is kanamycin acetyltransferase, which has not been demonstrated in *S. aureus* (2, 16, 20). The frequency of these subpopulations (10^{-7} parent cells) is approximately that of spontaneous mutation which produces ribosomal resistance (8, 19). However, ribosomal resistance usually confers a high level of resistance (MIC ≥ 250 μg/ml), higher than that of the subpopulations, and it has not been demonstrated to confer cross-resistance to other aminoglycosides (4). The only other known mechanism of resistance to aminoglycosides is cellular impermeability. This mechanism has been shown to be responsible for the cation-dependent resistance of *Pseudomonas* (21) and the intrinsic resistance of enterococci (11) to aminoglycosides. Although cellular impermeability to methicillin has been suggested in strains of methicillin-resistant *S. aureus* (3), impermeability to aminoglycosides has not been reported to date.

The presence of such subpopulations in a high percentage of clinical isolates of *S. aureus* may be of clinical importance. The physiological similarity of the subpopulations to the parent strain suggests that they may also have equivalent pathogenic capabilities. Thus, they may be responsible for some of the staphylococcal complications observed during therapy with aminoglycosides. The most frequently observed complication is that of staphylococcal superinfection during aminoglycoside therapy for gram-negative infections (6, 10). In certain instances, these superinfections may arise from in vivo selection of resistant subpopulations since the concentration of aminoglycoside required to kill the subpopulations in vitro were at or above levels that can be achieved with safety in man. Similar studies with staphylococci isolated from patients with superinfections should be performed to directly determine the role of such subpopulations in this complication of aminoglycoside therapy.

ACKNOWLEDGMENTS

We express our sincere appreciation to Cynthia A. Walker and Dean Watt for their professional assistance.

This work was supported in part by General Research Support grant no. 5 S01 RR05390. Antibiotic powders and disks were kindly supplied by Schering Corp., Bristol Laboratories, and Eli Lilly and Co.

LITERATURE CITED

1. **Bauer, A. W., W. M. M. Kirby, J. C. Sherris, and M. Turck.** 1966. Antibiotic susceptibility testing by a standardized single disk method. Am. J. Clin. Pathol. **45**:493–496.
2. **Benveniste, R., and J. Davies.** 1971. Enzyme acetylation of aminoglycoside antibiotics by *Escherichia coli* carrying an R factor. Biochemistry **10**:1787–1796.
3. **Benveniste, R., and J. Davies.** 1973. Mechanisms of antibiotic resistance in bacteria. Annu. Rev. Biochem. **42**:471–506.
4. **Davies, J.** 1971. Bacterial resistance to aminoglycoside antibiotics. J. Infect. Dis. **124**(Suppl.):S7–S10.
5. **Heifetz, C. L., M. W. Fisher, J. A. Chodubski, and M. O. DeCarlo.** 1972. Butirosin, a new aminoglycosidic antibiotic complex: antibacterial activity in vitro and in mice. Antimicrob. Agents Chemother. **2**:89–94.
6. **Jaffe, G., W. Ravreby, B. R. Meyers, and S. Z. Hirschman.** 1974. Clinical study of the use of the new aminoglycoside tobramycin for therapy of infections due to gram-negative bacteria. Antimicrob. Agents Chemother. **5**:75–81.
7. **Kurtz, S., K. Holmes, and M. Turck.** 1975. Disparity between inhibitory and killing effects of BL-P1654. Antimicrob. Agents Chemother. **7**:215–218.
8. **Lederburg, J., and E. M. Lederburg.** 1952. Replica plating and indirect selection of bacterial mutants. J. Bacteriol. **63**:399–406.
9. **Levison, M. E., R. Knight, and D. Kaye.** 1972. In vitro evaluation of tobramycin, a new aminoglycoside antibiotic. Antimicrob. Agents Chemother. **1**:381–384.
10. **Macmillan, B. G.** 1971. Ecology of bacteria colonizing the burned patient given topical and systemic gentamicin therapy: a five-year study. J. Infect. Dis. **124**(Suppl.):S278–S286.
11. **Moellering, R., A. Weinberg, R. Zimmerman, and C. Wennersten.** 1970. Antibiotic synergism against group D streptococci. Clin. Res. **18**:445.
12. **Price, K. E., D. R. Chisholm, M. Misiek, F. Leitner, and Y. H. Tsai.** 1972. Microbiological evaluation of BB-K8 a new semisynthetic aminoglycoside. J. Antibiot. **25**:709–731.
13. **Sanders, C. C., and W. E. Sanders, Jr.** 1975. BL-P1654: a bacteriostatic penicillin? Antimicrob. Agents

Chemother. 7:435–440.

14. **Sanders, C. C., and W. E. Sanders, Jr.** 1975. Effects of procedural variations on the activity of aminoglycosides in vitro. Am. J. Clin. Pathol. **63**:438–445.
15. **Steers, E., E. L. Foltz, and B. S. Graves.** 1959. Inocula replicating apparatus for routine testing of bacterial susceptibility to antibiotics. Antibiot. Chemother. **9**:307–311.
16. **Umezawa, H., M. Okanishi, R. Utahara, K. Maeda, and S. Kondo.** 1967. Isolation and structure of kanamycin inactivated by a cell-free system of kanamycin-resistant *E. coli*. J. Antibiot. Ser. A **20**:136–141.
17. **Waitz, J. A., E. L. Moss, Jr., E. M. Oden, and M. J. Weinstein.** 1970. Biological studies with antibiotic 6640, a new broad-spectrum aminoglycoside antibiotic. J. Antibiot. (Tokyo) **23**:559–565.
18. **Weinstein, M. J., C. G. Drube, E. L. Moss, Jr., and A. Waitz.** 1971. Microbiologic studies related to bacterial resistance to gentamicin. J. Infect. Dis. **124**(Suppl.):S11–S17.
19. **Weisblum, B., and J. Davies.** 1968. Antibiotic inhibitors of the bacterial ribosome. Bacteriol. Rev. **32**:493–528.
20. **Yamamoto, H., M. Yagisawa, H. Naganawa, S. Kondo, T. Takeuchi, and H. Umezawa.** 1972. Kanamycin 6′-acetate and ribostamycin 6′-acetate, enzymatically inactivated products by *Pseudomonas aeruginosa*. J. Antibiot. **25**:746–747.
21. **Zimelis, V. M., and G. G. Jackson.** 1973. Activity of aminoglycoside antibiotics against *Pseudomonas aeruginosa*: specificity and site of calcium and magnesium antagonism. J. Infect. Dis. **127**:663–669.

ANTIMICROBIAL AGENTS AND CHEMOTHERAPY, Sept. 1976, p. 526-534 Vol. 10, No. 3

In Vitro Study of Netilmicin Compared with Other Aminoglycosides

KWUNG P. FU AND HAROLD C. NEU*

Department of Medicine and Department of Pharmacology, College of Physicians and Surgeons, Columbia University, New York, New York 10032*

Received for publication 7 May 1976

Netilmicin (Sch 20569) is an ethyl derivative of gentamicin C_{1a} that is active against most *Enterobacteriaceae*, *Pseudomonas aeruginosa*, and *Staphylococcus aureus* isolates. Among 342 clinical isolates tested, all staphylococci, 92% of *Escherichia coli*, 93% of *Klebsiella pneumoniae*, and 92% of *Enterobacter* were inhibited by 0.8 μg or less of netilmicin per ml, but only 78% of *P. aeruginosa* were inhibited by 3.1 μg or less per ml. Most clinical isolates of enterococci, *Serratia marcescens*, and *Providencia* were not inhibited by 3.1 μg of netilmicin per ml. Like other aminoglycosides, the netilmicin in vitro activity was markedly influenced by the growth medium used, with activity decreased by sodium, calcium, and magnesium. Netilmicin was more active at alkaline pH. Addition of magnesium to *Pseudomonas* or *Serratia* pretreated with netilmicin produced inhibition of killing. Netilmicin was more active than gentamicin, sisomicin, tobramycin, or amikacin against *E. coli* and *K. pneumoniae*. Netilmicin inhibited growth of all gentamicin-resistant isolates of *Klebsiella* and *Citrobacter* tested, but only 73% of *E. coli; Pseudomonas* and *Providencia* were resistant to netilmicin. Most *Serratia* (95%) and indole-positive *Proteus* (83%) isolates were resistant to netilmicin but were inhibited by amikacin.

Serious infections caused by gram-negative microorganisms resistant to many of the currently available antibiotics have continued to increase (11, 12, 15). Although gentamicin has remained a highly effective antibiotic, the sporadic occurrence of strains of *Enterobacteriaceae* or *Pseudomonas* resistant to the gentamicin complex prompted us to evaluate the antimicrobial activity of netilmicin (Sch 20569), 1-*N*-ethyl sisomicin, a new semisynthetic aminoglycoside antibiotic produced by *Micromonospora inyoensis*. This compound closely resembles the C_{1a} component of the gentamicin complex.

The purpose of this study was to assess the in vitro activity of netilmicin against recent clinical, bacterial isolates, to compare the activity of netilmicin with sisomicin, gentamicin, tobramycin, and amikacin, and to determine the activity of netilmicin against clinical isolates that were resistant to gentamicin.

MATERIALS AND METHODS

Antibiotics. Netilmicin, sisomicin, and gentamicin were supplied by Schering Corp. Tobramycin was a gift from Eli Lilly & Co., and amikacin was a gift from Bristol Laboratories. Fresh dilutions of all the aminoglycoside antibiotics were prepared daily in sterile medium or distilled water. Bacterial isolates were obtained from patients hospitalized at the Columbia Presbyterian Medical Center during the past 2 years. The isolates came from sputum, blood, and urine specimens and did not represent the same strains insofar as could be determined by general antibiograms and bacteriocin typing.

Susceptibility tests. The antimicrobial activity was measured by the broth dilution method as previously described (6). Serial twofold dilutions of antibiotics in Mueller-Hinton broth (BBL) were used. An inoculum of 0.5 ml containing 10^5 cells (colony-forming units [CFU]) from a diluted overnight culture was added to 0.5 ml of antibiotic solution. Cultures were incubated at 35°C for 18 h. The minimal inhibitory concentration (MIC) was defined as the lowest concentration that inhibited development of visible turbidity. The minimum bactericidal concentration (MBC) was determined by plating 0.01 ml from clear tubes onto agar. MIC values were also determined by the agar dilution method (6). A 100-fold dilution of an overnight culture was applied with an inocula replicator. The MIC was taken as the highest concentration of antibiotic on which there was no visible growth or less than five colonies.

The effect of growth medium on the activity of netilmicin was determined with Trypticase soy (BBL), brain heart infusion (BBL), and nutrient broth (BBL). Concentrations of ions were determined by standard chemical assays, using flame photometry and/or atomic absorption spectrophotometry.

RESULTS

Antimicrobial activity of netilmicin. The in vitro activity of netilmicin against 342 gram-positive and gram-negative organisms is summarized in Table 1. All isolates of *Citrobacter* and *Staphylococcus aureus* were inhibited at a concentration of 0.8 μg of netilmicin per ml. Of the *Escherichia coli, Klebsiella, Enterobacter*, and *Salmonella* isolates tested, more than 90% were inhibited by 0.8 μg/ml. At a concentration of 3.1 μg/ml, 91% of *Proteus mirabilis*, 81% of indole-positive *Proteus*, and 75% of *Acinetobacter* were inhibited. There were 51% of the strains of *P. aeruginosa* inhibited by 0.8 μg of netilmicin per ml and 78% inhibited by 3.1 μg/ml. Markedly resistant strains (≥12.5 μg/ml) were rare. A number of *Serratia marcescens*, *Providencia*, and enterococcal isolates had netilmicin MIC values above 6.3 μg/ml.

Effect of growth medium. The size of the initial inoculum of most organisms tested had little effect on the netilmicin MIC values determined by the broth dilution method (Table 2). However, *Serratia* isolates showed a two- to eightfold increase in MIC values when the inoculum size was increased from 10^3 to 10^7 CFU.

The effect of different medium and pH of the medium used to determine the activity of netilmicin is shown in Table 3. The netilmicin MIC values determined for *Pseudomonas, E. coli, Klebsiella,* and *Serratia* were lowest in nutrient broth among the four media tested. Netilmicin was also more active at pH 8 than at pH 6 regardless of the medium used.

A comparison of MIC and MBC values of netilmicin showed that the MBC values were only slightly higher than its MIC. MIC values determined by both agar dilution and broth dilution were similar, except for *Pseudomonas* and *Serratia* isolates (Table 4). A 2- to 16-fold increase in MIC value was observed in Mueller-Hinton agar as compared with that in Mueller-Hinton broth for 13 of 22 strains of *P. aeruginosa* tested. The MIC values of netilmicin were significantly higher in nutrient broth with added cations than those in nutrient broth, even at the physiological concentration of calcium, magnesium, and sodium (Table 5). Magnesium had the greatest inhibitory effects at an equimolar concentration among the cations tested. This is also illustrated in Fig. 1. At the concentration of 2 mM magnesium, the netilmicin inhibition of *Serratia* could be reversed within 1 h, whereas it took 10 mM calcium to

TABLE 2. *Effect of inoculum size on the activity of netilmicin (Sch 20569)*[a]

Organism	MIC (μg/ml) at:		
	10^3 CFU	10^5 CFU	10^7 CFU
E. coli 2826	0.8	3.1	3.1
E. coli 2175	1.6	3.1	3.1
P. aeruginosa 2182	0.2	0.4	0.4
P. aeruginosa 2716	0.2	0.2	0.4
P. aeruginosa 2699	0.4	0.8	1.6
P. aeruginosa 2632	1.6	1.6	1.6
P. aeruginosa 2139	1.6	1.6	3.1
K. pneumoniae 2920	0.2	0.4	0.8
K. pneumoniae 2933	0.1	0.2	0.4
S. marcescens 2944	3.1	3.1	6.3
S. marcescens 2744	25	25	100
S. marcescens 2569	12.5	25	25
S. marcescens 2327	1.6	1.6	6.3

[a] Mueller-Hinton broth was used to determine MIC.

TABLE 1. *Cumulative percentage of isolates susceptible to netilmicin (Sch 20569)*[a]

Organism	No. of isolates	Susceptible isolates (%) at an MIC (μg/ml) of:												
		0.025	0.05	0.1	0.2	0.4	0.8	1.6	3.1	6.3	12.5	25	50	100
S. aureus	20		4	40	68		100							
Enterococci	32								12	62	88	100		
E. coli	27				26	81	92			100				
Shigella	14				12		78	100						
K. pneumoniae	29				63	89	93		96	100				
Enterobacter	25				28	80	92		96	100				
S. marcescens	29					4		10	17	27	64	78	92	100
Salmonella	25				8	72	96	100						
Citrobacter	20	15			35	60	100							
Proteus, indole positive	26				18	73		76	81	92	100			
P. mirabilis	29				3	21	31	68	91			95	100	
Providencia	15					7		13	26	86	93	100		
P. aeruginosa	41				10	32	51	74	78	87	96		100	
Acinetobacter	10				10	30	40	70		80		90	100	

[a] MICs were determined in Mueller-Hinton agar.

TABLE 3. *Effect of medium and its pH on the activity of netilmicin (Sch 20569)*

Organism	MIC and MBC (μg/ml)[a]											
	Brain heart infusion			Mueller-Hinton broth			Trypticase soy broth			Nutrient broth		
	pH 6	pH 7	pH 8	pH 6	pH 7	pH 8	pH 6	pH 7	pH 8	pH 6	pH 7	pH 8
E. coli 2826	3.1 (3.1)	3.1 (3.1)	0.8 (3.1)	3.1 (3.1)	0.8 (3.1)	0.4 (0.4)	3.1 (3.1)	3.1 (6.3)	0.2 (0.2)	0.025 (0.025)	0.025 (0.025)	<0.025 (<0.025)
P. aeruginosa 2182	0.8 (3.1)	0.8 (0.8)	0.8 (1.6)	0.4 (0.8)	0.4 (0.4)	0.4 (0.8)	1.6 (3.1)	1.6 (3.1)	0.8 (0.8)	0.05 (0.05)	0.05 (0.05)	<0.025 (0.025)
K. pneumoniae 2920	1.6 (3.1)	0.8 (0.8)	0.8 (0.8)	1.6 (1.6)	0.4 (0.4)	0.2 (0.2)	3.1 (3.1)	6.3 (6.3)	0.4 (0.8)	<0.025 (<0.025)	<0.025 (0.025)	<0.025 (0.025)
S. marcescens 2744	50 (50)	50 (100)	50 (50)	100 (100)	25 (50)	25 (100)	25 (100)	25 (25)	25 (100)	3.1 (3.1)	0.8 (3.1)	0.4 (0.8)

[a] Numbers in parentheses indicate MBCs.

TABLE 4. *Effect of broth dilution and agar dilution method on the activity of netilmicin (Sch 20569)*

Organism	MIC (μg/ml) in Mueller-Hinton agar	Mueller-Hinton broth	
		MIC (μg/ml)	MBC (μg/ml)
E. coli 2826	1.6	1.6	3.1
E. coli 2938	6.3	6.3	12.5
E. coli 2939	6.3	3.1	3.1
K. pneumoniae 2933	0.2	0.1	
K. pneumoniae 2920	0.8	0.2	0.4
K. pneumoniae 2940	0.4	0.2	
S. marcescens 2744	25	12.5	25
S. marcescens 2944	25	6.3	
P. vulgaris 2924	0.4	0.4	
P. mirabilis 2339	12.5	12.5	
P. aeruginosa 2182	0.8	0.2	0.8
P. aeruginosa 2923	12.5	3.1	12.5
P. aeruginosa 2968	6.3	6.3	25
P. aeruginosa 2142	12.5	3.1	3.1
P. alcaligenes 2942	50	50	50
P. maltophilia 2941	12.5	12.5	25
P. maltophilia 2975	50	25	50

antagonize netilmicin growth inhibition of *Serratia*. The addition of calcium or magnesium within 1 h to cells of *Pseudomonas* or *Serratia* pretreated with netilmicin would halt normal killing and allow regrowth. The addition of horse blood had little effect on the activity of netilmicin against *P. aeruginosa*, *K. pneumoniae*, and *E. coli* (Table 6).

Comparative activity of netilmicin with gentamicin, sisomicin, tobramycin, and amikacin. The comparative in vitro activity of netilmicin, amikacin, sisomicin, tobramycin, and gentamicin against 342 clinical isolates determined by the agar dilution method is shown in Fig. 2 through 7. The activity of netilmicin closely paralleled that of gentamicin, sisomicin, and tobramycin. Netilmicin was the most active of the aminoglycosides tested against *Klebsiella* and *E. coli*. Netilmicin was twofold more active against *E. coli* than were gentamicin and sisomicin, which were in turn more active than tobramycin and amikacin. Sisomicin, tobramycin, and gentamicin were equally

TABLE 5. *Effect of cations on the activity of netilmicin (Sch 20569)*

Cation[a]	Concn of added salt (mM)	MIC (μg/ml)[b]			
		P. aeruginosa	*K. pneumoniae*	*S. marcescens*	*E. coli*
Calcium	0	0.06	0.03	0.5	0.03
	0.025	0.06	0.03	1	0.06
	0.5	0.06	0.03	1	0.06
	1.0	0.25	0.03	2	0.12
	2.0	1	0.03	4	0.12
Magnesium	0.1	0.06	0.03	0.25	1
	1	1	0.12	1	8
	2	4	1	8	64
Sodium	2	0.06	0.03	0.03	0.5
	10	0.06	0.06	0.12	2.0
	50	0.06	0.25	0.5	8.0
	100	0.12	0.5	1	64

[a] Calcium was added as $CaCl_2$, magnesium as $MgSO_4$, and sodium as NaCl.
[b] MIC values were determined in nutrient broth that has an Mg^{2+} of 0.18 mM, a Ca^{2+} of 0.02 mM, and an Na^+ of 9.8 mM.

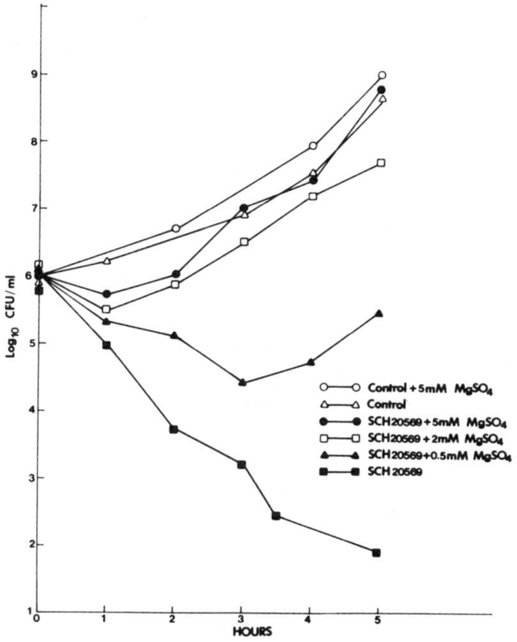

FIG. 1. *Rate of killing of S. marcescens 2944 in nutrient broth (BBL) containing 2 μg of netilmicin (Sch 20569) per ml and $MgSO_4$ at the concentration shown.*

TABLE 6. *Effect of horse blood on the activity of netilmicin (Sch 20569)*[a]

Organism	No. of isolates	Horse blood added (%)	MIC (μg/ml)	
			Range	Median
E. coli	24	0	0.31–2.5	0.47
		1	0.31–2.5	0.40
		5	0.31–2.5	0.46
		10	0.31–2.5	0.32
K. pneumoniae	20	0	0.31–2.5	0.62
		1	0.31–2.5	0.70
		5	0.31–2.5	0.45
		10	0.31–2.5	0.45
P. aeruginosa	22	0	1.25–40	10.10
		1	1.25–40	7.50
		5	1.25–50	7.50
		10	1.25–40	9.0

[a] MICs were determined by agar dilution method on Mueller-Hinton agar containing horse blood as noted.

active against *Klebsiella* and less active than netilmicin, which in turn was about threefold more active than amikacin at lower concentrations. On the other hand, netilmicin was the least active against *Providencia*. Amikacin was consistently the least active agent against aminoglycoside-susceptible isolates, although it was most active against *Providencia* and *Serratia*. Tobramycin was slightly more active than

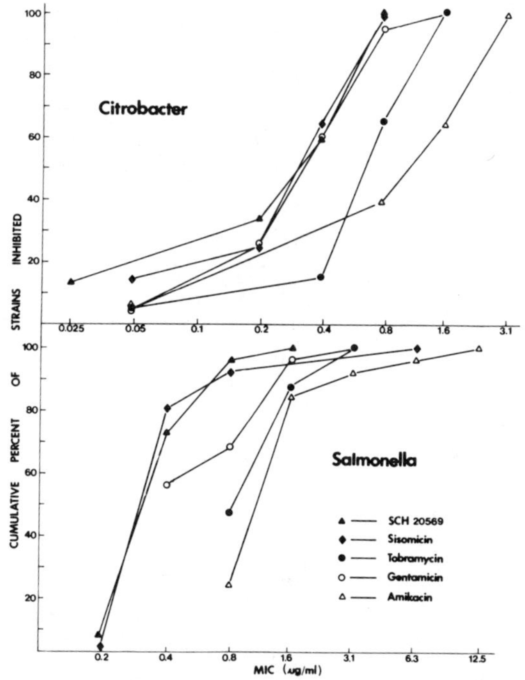

FIG. 2. *Comparative activity of aminoglycoside antibiotics against Citrobacter (20 isolates) and Salmonella (25 isolates). Tested by agar dilution method. Scale is logarithmic. Sch 20569, Netilmicin.*

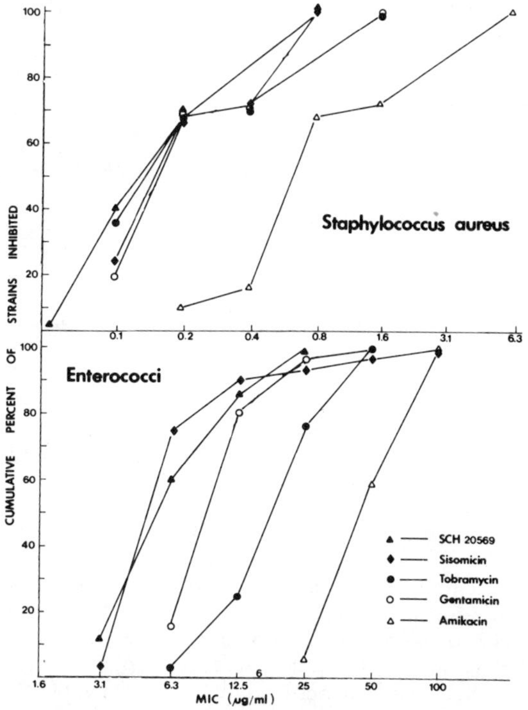

FIG. 3. *Comparative activity of aminoglycoside antibiotics against S. aureus (20 isolates) and enterococci (32 isolates). Sch 20569, Netilmicin.*

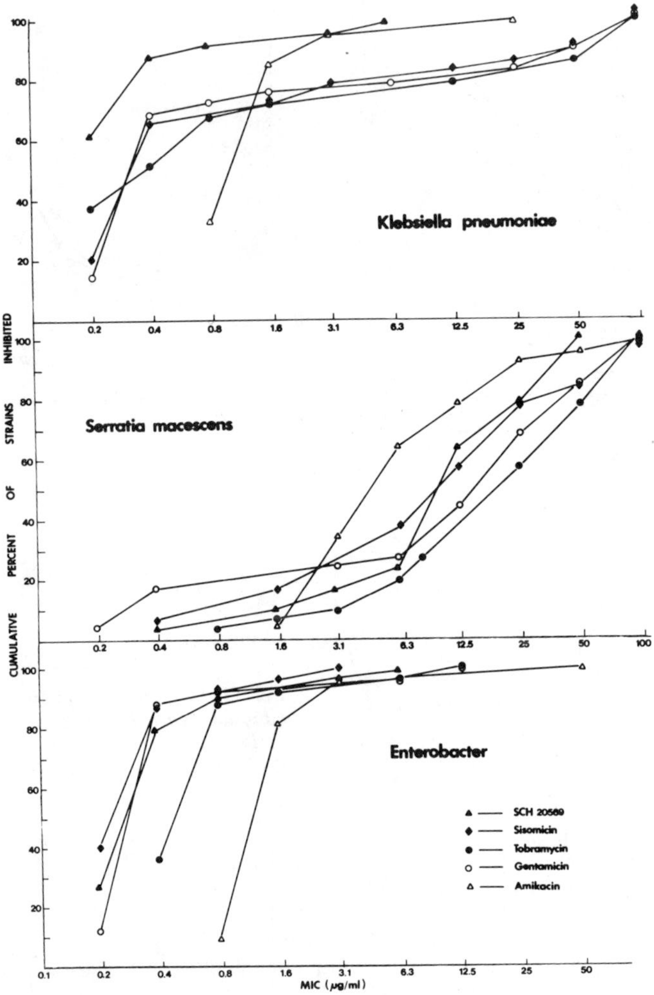

FIG. 4. *Comparative activity of aminoglycoside antibiotics against Enterobacter (25 isolates), S. marcescens (29 isolates), and K. pneumoniae (29 isolates). Sch 20569, Netilmicin.*

sisomicin and two- to fourfold more active than gentamicin against *Pseudomonas*. Netilmicin was much less active against *Pseudomonas* than the aforementioned agents, but more active than amikacin.

Activity of netilmicin against gentamicin-resistant isolates. Table 7 enumerates the activity of netilmicin against 68 gentamicin-resistant isolates. The majority of isolates of *E. coli*, *Klebsiella*, *Enterobacter*, and *Citrobacter* that had gentamicin MIC values of 12.5 μg or greater per ml were susceptible to 3.1 μg or less of netilmicin per ml. Most gentamicin-resistant *S. marcescens*, *Providencia*, *P. rettgeri*, and *P. aeruginosa* had netilmicin MIC values of 12.5 μg or greater per ml.

A comparison of the activity of gentamicin, netilmicin, tobramycin, sisomicin, and amikacin demonstrated that gentamicin-resistant *S. marcescens* were also resistant to tobramycin and sisomicin, whereas all but one were susceptible to concentrations of amikacin that could be achieved in humans. Gentamicin-resistant *K. pneumoniae* were resistant to sisomicin and tobramycin, but very susceptible to netilmicin, which is three times more active than amikacin. *Enterobacter* resistant to gentamicin were usually resistant to tobramycin and sisomicin, with rare exceptions. A similar situation was encountered with *E. coli*. Some gentamicin-resistant *P. aeruginosa* isolates were susceptible to tobramycin and to sisomicin, and all but

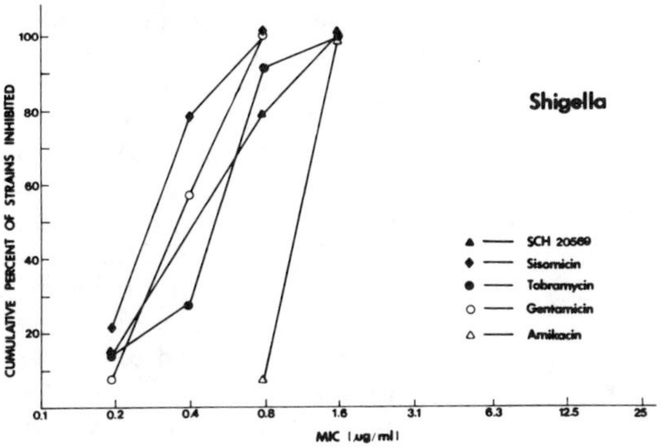

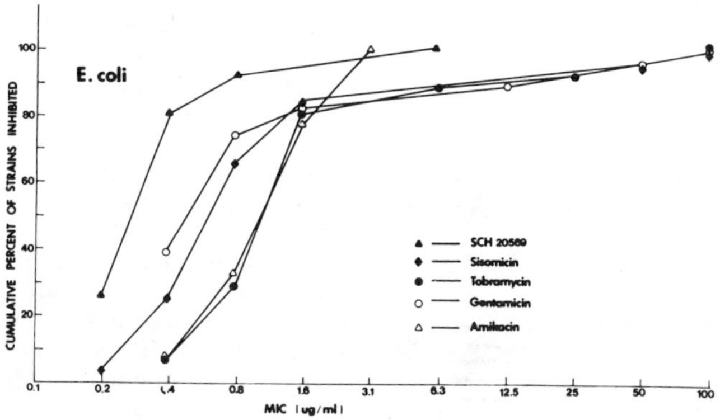

FIG. 5. *Comparative activity of aminoglycoside antibiotics against Shigella (14 isolates) and E. coli (27 isolates). Sch 20569, Netilmicin.*

TABLE 7. *Comparative activity of netilmicin (Sch 20569), amikacin, sisomicin, and tobramycin against gentamicin-resistant organisms*

Organism	No. of strains	MIC (μg/ml)									
		Gentamicin		Netilmicin		Tobramycin		Sisomicin		Amikacin	
		Range	Median	Range	Median	Range	Median	Range	Median	Range	Median
S. marcescens	22	6.3->100	37.5	3.1->100	32.5	1.6->100	40	0.4->100	21.3	3.1-50	10
K. pneumoniae	11	25->100	65	0.2-6.3	0.8	3.1->100	50	12.5->100	60	1.6-6.3	2.6
Providencia 2943		12.5		25		6.3		3.1		1.6	
Providencia 748	2	6.3		12.5		6.3		3.1		1.6	
Enterobacter	3	6.3-50	16.5	3.1-12.5	6.3	6.3-50	16.5	1.6-50	16.5	0.8-50	6.3
Citrobacter 3007	1	50		0.4		50		50		1.6	
P. mirabilis 2576	1	50		50		50		50		50	
P. rettgeri	4	6.3-12.5	7.8	3.1-25	12.5	3.1-6.3	4.7	1.6-6.3	3.1	0.8-1.6	1
P. morganii	1	6.3		6.3		12.5		6.3		1.6	
P. vulgaris	1	6.3		25		12.5		6.3		3.1	
E. coli	11	12.5->100	40	0.4-12.5	4.2	1.6->100	40	0.8->100	35	0.4-12.5	2.1
P. aeruginosa	6	6.3->100	18.8	12.5-50	8.1	0.8->100	8.1	1.6-50	4.6	1.6-50	9.3
P. maltophilia	4	12.5-50	37.5	25-50	31.3	12.5-50	31.3	1.6-50	18.8	50-50	50
P. alcaligenes	1	100		>100		12.5		50		50	

one were susceptible to amikacin. Amikacin was the agent active against the largest number of gentamicin-resistant isolates of all organisms tested.

DISCUSSION

Netilmicin, an ethyl derivative of gentamicin C_{1a}, has excellent activity against the majority

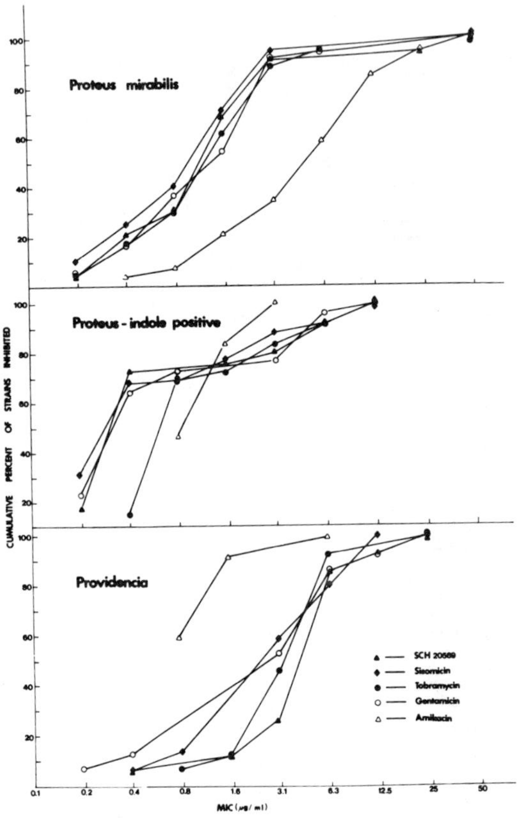

FIG. 6. *Comparative activity of aminoglycoside antibiotics against P. mirabilis (29 isolates), indole-positive Proteus (26 isolates), and Providencia (15 isolates). Sch 20569, Netilmicin.*

of gram-negative bacteria and *S. aureus*. Most of the isolates tested were inhibited by netilmicin at the concentration achievable in human blood (S. Sate, personal communication). Several reports have documented that factors such as inoculum size (6), presence of serum (5), and different medium and the pH of the medium (6), as well as cation content of the medium, greatly influence the activity of aminoglycoside antibiotics (7, 10, 14). These factors were shown to affect the MIC values of netilmicin.

Netilmicin was most active in nutrient broth which contains less magnesium and calcium than that encountered in the physiological situation. Netilmicin, like most other aminoglycosides, was more active in an alkaline medium (6, 16). The low MIC of netilmicin in nutrient and alkaline medium may be due to more active netilmicin accumulation in cells by active transport (2). Zimelis and Jackson (18) showed that the calcium and magnesium antagonism is species specific against *P. aeruginosa*. In this investigation, we observed significant changes in the MIC of netilmicin not only against *P. aeruginosa* but also against *Klebsiella*, *E. coli*, and *S. marcescens* brought about by calcium and magnesium. The reason may be due to the different medium utilized.

In agreement with other reports (3, 9), tobramycin was found to be the most active aminoglycoside against *P. aeruginosa*, and amikacin was constantly the least active aminoglycoside on a basis of micrograms per milliliter. Netilmicin was threefold less active than gentamicin against *Pseudomonas* isolates. Rahal et al. (13) recently found that netilmicin, gentamicin, and amikacin exhibited similar activity against *Pseudomonas*, in contrast to the data of this paper. Our median MIC values of netilmicin, amikacin, and gentamicin are 0.9, 2.25, and 0.38 µg/ml, respectively. The difference in results may be caused by the more resistant organisms in the Rahal et al. (13) study. Furthermore, in contrast to the data of Rahal et al. (13), we found that *Citrobacter* were equally susceptible to gentamicin, sisomicin, and netilmicin. The reason for the difference in our results may be that we have not encountered significant aminoglycoside resistance in our institution.

Amikacin was the most active agent against gentamicin-resistant *S. marcescens*. The mean MIC values against seven gentamicin-susceptible *Serratia* strains were 1.14 µg of gentamicin per ml, 4.95 µg of sisomicin per ml, 34.5 µg of netilmicin per ml, 7.36 µg of amikacin per ml, and 23.3 µg of tobramycin per ml. Netilmicin was active against *E. coli*, *Klebsiella*, and *Enterobacter* which were resistant to gentamicin. This was also true of amikacin but not of sisomicin and tobramycin.

The in vitro disadvantage of amikacin as compared with the other amino-glycoside antibiotics appears to be offset by the evidence that it achieves significantly higher serum levels in animals and humans (4) and it was active against netilmicin-resistant or other aminoglycoside-resistant organisms, as shown in this study which was in agreement with other reports (12, 13, 17).

Aminoglycoside resistance mediated by enzymatic acetylation, adenylylation, and phosphorylation has been well documented (1, 8) and undoubtedly explains the resistance of isolates to netilmicin. We currently are determining the enzymatic inactivating patterns of the organisms that are resistant to netilmicin.

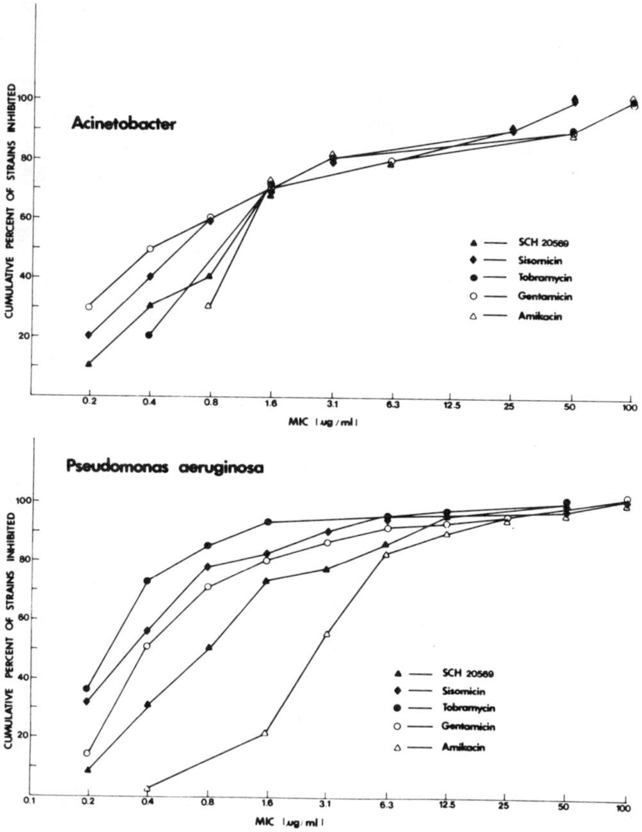

FIG. 7. *Comparative activity of aminoglycoside antibiotics against Acinetobacter (10 isolates) and P. aeruginosa (41 isolates). Sch 20569, Netilmicin.*

LITERATURE CITED

1. **Benveniste, R., and J. Davis.** 1973. Mechanism of antibiotic resistance in bacteria. Annu. Rev. Biochem. 42:471–506.
2. **Bryan, L. E., and H. M. Van Der Elzen.** 1975. Gentamicin accumulation by sensitive strains of *Escherichia coli* and *Pseudomonas aeruginosa*. J. Antibiot. 27:696–703.
3. **Burger, L. M., J. P. Sanford, and T. Zweighaft.** 1973. Tobramycin: biological evaluation. Am. J. Med. Sci. 265:135–142.
4. **Cabana, B. E., and J. A. Taggart.** 1973. Comparative pharmacokinetics of BB-K8 and kanamycin in dogs and humans. Antimicrob. Agents Chemother. 3:478–483.
5. **Crowe, C. C., and E. Sanders.** 1973. Sisomicin: evaluation in vitro and comparison with gentamicin and tobramycin. Antimicrob. Agents Chemother. 3:24–28.
6. **Dienstag, J., and H. C. Neu.** 1972. In vitro studies of tobramycin, an aminoglycoside antibiotic. Antimicrob. Agents Chemother. 1:41–45.
7. **Gilbert, D. N., E. Kutsher, P. Ireland, J. A. Barnett, and J. P. Sanford.** 1971. Effect of the concentrations of magnesium and calcium on the in vitro susceptibility of *Pseudomonas aeruginosa* to gentamicin. J. Infect. Dis. 124(Suppl.):37–45.
8. **Kawabe, H., T. Naito, and S. Mitsuhashi.** 1975. Acetylation of amikacin, a new semisynthetic antibiotic, by *Pseudomonas aeruginosa* carrying an R factor. Antimicrob. Agents Chemother. 7:50–54.
9. **Levison, M. E., and D. Kaye.** 1974. In vitro comparison of four aminoglycoside antibiotics: sisomicin, gentamicin, tobramycin, and BB-K8. Antimicrob. Agents Chemother. 5:667–669.
10. **Medeiros, A. A., T. F. O'Brien, W. E. C. Wacken, and N. F. Yulung.** 1971. Effect of salt concentration on the apparent *in vitro* susceptibility of *Pseudomonas aeruginosa* and other gram-negative Bacilli to gentamicin. J. Infect. Dis. 124(Suppl.):59–64.
11. **Noriega, E. R., R. Leibowitz, A. S. Richmond, E. Rubinstein, S. Schaefler, M. S. Simberkoff, and J. J. Rahal, Jr.** 1975. Nosocomial infection caused by gentamicin-resistant, streptomycin-sensitive Klebsiella. J. Infect. Dis. 131(Suppl.):45–50.
12. **Price, K. E., T. A. Pursiano, M. D. Defuria, and G. E. Wright.** 1974. Activity of BB-K8 (amikacin) against clinical isolates resistant to one or more aminoglycoside antibiotics. Antimicrob. Agents Chemother. 5:143–152.
13. **Rahal, Jr., J. J., M. S. Simberkoff, K. Kagan, and N. H. Moldover.** 1976. Bactericidal efficacy of Sch 20569 and amikacin against gentamicin-sensitive and resistant organisms. Antimicrob. Agents Chemother. 9:595–599.
14. **Reller, L. B., F. D. Schoenknecht, M. A. Kenny, and J. C. Sherris.** 1974. Antibiotic susceptibility testing on

Pseudomonas aeruginosa: selection of a control strain and criteria for magnesium and calcium content in media. J. Infect. Dis. 130:454–463.
15. **Snelling, C. F. T., A. R. Ronald, C. Y. Cates, and W. C. Forsythe.** 1971. Resistance of gram-negative Bacilli to gentamicin. J. Infect. Dis. 124(Suppl.):264–270.
16. **Stewart, D., and G. P. Bodey.** 1975. *In vitro* activity of sisomicin, an aminoglycoside antibiotic, against clinical isolates. J. Antibiot. 28:149–155.
17. **Young, L. S., and W. L. Hewitt.** 1973. Activity of five aminoglycoside antibiotics *in vitro* against gram-negative bacilli and *Staphylococcus aureus*. Antimicrob. Agents Chemother. 4:617–625.
18. **Zimelis, V. M., and G. G. Jackson.** 1973. Activity of aminoglycoside antibiotics against *Pseudomonas aeruginosa*: specificity and site of calcium and magnesium antagonism. J. Infect. Dis. 127:663–669.

ANTIMICROBIAL AGENTS AND CHEMOTHERAPY, Sept. 1976, p. 535-542

Vol. 10, No. 3
Printed in U.S.A.

Synergy of Mecillinam, a Beta-Amidinopenicillanic Acid Derivative, Combined with Beta-Lactam Antibiotics

HAROLD C. NEU

Department of Medicine and Department of Pharmacology, College of Physicians and Surgeons, Columbia University, New York, New York 10032*

Received for publication 2 June 1976

Mecillinam, a β-amidinopenicillanic acid derivative, was combined with ampicillin, amoxicillin, carbenicillin, cephalothin, cefamandole, and cefoxitin and tested against most members of the *Enterobacteriaceae* and *Pseudomonas*. Synergy was demonstrated with selected isolates of most of the organisms tested. Isolates highly susceptible to mecillinam (minimum inhibitory concentration, <0.8 μg/ml) were not synergistically inhibited by addition of another β-lactam antibiotic. Synergy of mecillinam and a β-lactamase-resistant penicillin, cloxacillin, was demonstrated. In media of osmolality >10 mOsm or of conductivity >6 mS, mecillinam and β-lactam antibiotics showed synergy in most instances, whereas at low osmolality and conductivity the activity of mecillinam is so great that synergy cannot be demonstrated. The proportion of mecillinam to β-lactam antibiotic that will be synergistic ranged from 100:1 to 1:1 to 1:100. Mecillinam did not increase the activity, minimum inhibitory concentration or minimum bactericidal concentration values, of β-lactam compounds against streptococci, staphylococci, clostridia, listeria, or bacteroides. Synergy was not demonstrated with combinations of mecillinam and aminoglycosides (kanamycin, gentamicin, tobramycin, amikacin), chloramphenicol, tetracycline, or polymyxins.

The increasing incidence of resistance of members of the *Enterobacteriaceae* to penicillin, cephalosporins, and aminoglycoside antibiotics has prompted a search for agents that might overcome resistance through structural modification of the antimicrobial agent (14). In 1972 Lund and Tybring (10) reported on the synthesis of a new class of penicillanic acid derivatives, the β-amidinopenicillanic acids. One of these compounds, a 6β-hexahydro-1-H-azepin-1-ly-methyleneamino penicillanic acid, mecillinam (formerly called FL 1060), was shown to be unusually active against certain gram-negative bacilli, particularly *Escherichia coli* (22). Studies in several laboratories showed that mecillinam produced a swelling of bacteria so that they became spherical (12). This was different from the morphological changes produced by benzylpenicillin or ampicillin. Park and Burman (17) noted that the mecillinam did not inhibit murein transpeptidase. James et al. (7), using *E. coli* B/r in exponential and synchronous cultures, showed that mecillinam blocked an event occurring early in the cell cycle essential for normal cell elongation. Spratt (21) subsequently showed that mecillinam bound preferentially to one of the penicillin-binding proteins, namely, protein two, which is involved in the shape of bacilli, rather than to the proteins involved in elongation or septum formation.

These observations suggested to us that mecillinam might act in a synergistic manner with other β-lactam compounds that act on the cell proteins that are involved with elongation or septum formation. We performed a systematic investigation of the combined antimicrobial activity of mecillinam with antibiotics that inhibit cell wall formation, those that bind to the bacterial cytoplasmic membrane, and those whose entry into the bacterial cell has been facilitated by previous exposure to penicillins.

(This material was presented at the 15th Interscience Conference on Antimicrobial Agents and Chemotherapy, Washington, D.C., on 24 September 1975.)

MATERIALS AND METHODS

Bacteria. Bacteria were isolates collected over a period of several years from patients hospitalized at the Columbia Presbyterian Medical Center. They had been maintained on Trypticase soy agar (BBL) slants and were grown up freshly in the particular medium used for the synergy test just before the test.

Antibiotics. Mecillinam was used as a hydrochloride dihydrate provided by C. Demos of Roche Diagnostics. Ampicillin, amoxicillin, and carbenicillin were gifts of Beecham Pharmaceuticals. Cephalothin, cefazolin, and cefamandole were gifts from Eli Lilly & Co.. Cefoxitin was a gift from Merck & Co., Inc. All antibiotics were stored in refrigerated desiccators and were prepared fresh daily in the particular medium used for assay.

Medium. A medium previously described (13) was used, with the osmolality adjusted between 185 and 400 mOsm and conductivity between 6 and 15 mS. The pH was 6.7 to 6.9 and incubation was at 35°C.

Tests for synergy. There were four methods used to test for synergy. The first used a checkerboard arrangement of tubes, with the concentration of antibiotic varying twofold in both directions from 0 to 400 μg/ml. An overnight culture of organisms was diluted in fresh medium to provide a final inoculum of 5×10^4 colony-forming units. The second method used was an agar method similar to the broth dilution method. With a replicating device, 10^5 colony-forming units were applied to the antibiotic-containing plates, which were incubated at 35°C for 16 h. The minimum inhibitory concentration (MIC) was the lowest concentration that inhibited visible growth in broth or visible growth or <5 colonies in agar. Bactericidal levels (minimum bactericidal concentration [MBC]) were determined by the broth dilution method by plating clear tubes to agar that did not contain antibiotic. The third method of testing for synergy was an agar method in which the concentration of one agent was varied twofold, from 400 μg/ml to 0 μg, while the concentration of the second agent, mecillinam, was kept constant at a level fourfold below the MIC of mecillinam in agar for the organism being tested. The final method was one in which fixed ratios of both antibiotics were used beginning at 1,000:1, drug A to B. Ratios of 1,000:1, 100:1, 10:1, 5:1, 1:1, 1:5, 1:10, etc. were run in twofold dilution steps in broth. The MIC and MBC were determined as noted above.

Synergy was defined as a fourfold or greater reduction of the MIC of both compounds compared to the MIC of each antibiotic alone. Activity was considered partially synergistic when the MIC of one drug in the combination was at least four times as effective as the MIC of that drug alone and the MIC of the second drug was only twice as effective as it was alone. The activity was considered indifferent if both agents were only twice as effective as when used alone and antagonistic when an agent was four times less effective than either agent used alone.

β-Lactamase activity was determined by previously described methods (15). Specific conductivity was measured with a model 31 (Yellow Springs Instrument Co.) conductivity bridge, and osmolality was measured by the cryostatic method, using an osmometer.

RESULTS

A typical isobologram is shown in Fig. 1 for amoxicillin and mecillinam and caphalothin and mecillinam. In both examples, marked synergy is shown by the combination of the antibiotics. Table 1 illustrates the type of synergy seen with amoxicillin and mecillinam for a number of different organisms. Synergy can be demonstrated for both amoxicillin-susceptible and -resistant *E. coli*. Organisms completely resistant to both compounds, such as *Proteus morganii, Serratia marcescens,* and some *Klebsiella* and *Enterobacter*, cannot be synergistically inhibited by the two compounds. A killing curve technique (Fig. 2) demonstrated that an *E. coli* strain can grow in the presence of either compound alone, but in the presence of both agents at 1/1,000 the concentration of ampicillin and 1/10 the concentration of mecillinam growth is inhibited. In Fig. 3 is shown the effect of the combination of mecillinam and ampicillin against a *Shigella sonnei* strain that had a mecillinam MIC value of 0.8 μg/ml but

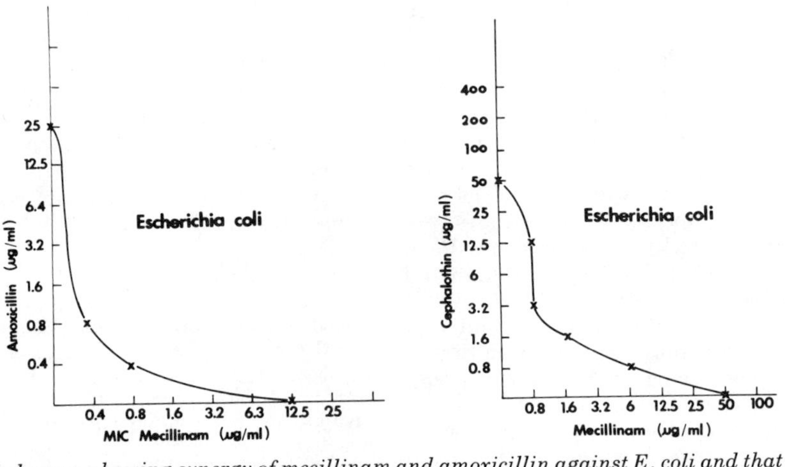

FIG. 1. *Isobologram showing synergy of mecillinam and amoxicillin against E. coli and that of mecillinam and cephalothin against E. coli.*

TABLE 1. *Synergy of mecillinam and amoxicillin*[a]

Organism	MIC (μg/ml)			
	Amoxicillin	Mecillinam	Amoxicillin +	mecillinam
E. coli 1	500	125	12	12
E. coli 2	125	31	6	6
E. coli 3	8	2	0.4	0.4
Klebsiella A	125	250	12.5	12.5
Klebsiella B	125	31	<0.2	<0.2
Enterobacter	250	31	<0.2	1.0
Citrobacter	125	250	8	1.6
P. morganii	500	>500	250	50
Serratia	>250	>250	>125	>125
Enterobacter	>500	250	250	125
Klebsiella	>500	250	50	250

[a] Assays were performed in NIH broth of 6 mS and 185 mOsm.

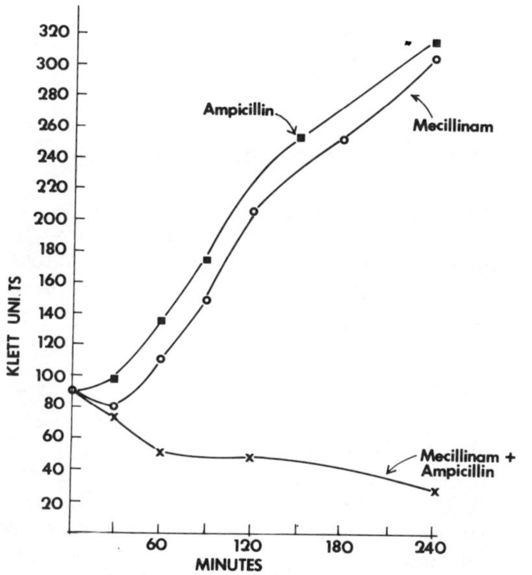

FIG. 2. *Killing curve of mecillinam and ampicillin against E. coli.*

an MBC value of 25 μg/ml. Regrowth had begun at 8 h in the presence of mecillinam alone, but not in the presence of the combination of drugs.

Table 2 shows the various penicillin and cephalosporin derivatives that showed complete synergy, a fourfold reduction in MIC of both compounds, when tested against different *Enterobacteriaceae* and *Pseudomonas*. Of particular significance is the fact that the isolates selected were those that produced β-lactamase of either a penicillin or cephalosporin preference, which accounted for their resistance to the penicillin or cephalosporin. Although there is a higher percentage of synergy seen with the cephalosporins, this is artificial. The large number of *E. coli* and *Klebsiella pneumoniae* tested were so susceptible to mecillinam that although the MIC was lowered from 200 to 25 μg/ml, there was only a twofold reduction in the mecillinam MIC value, from 0.8 to 0.4 μg/ml, which I consider partial synergy.

This is better illustrated in Table 3, in which it is shown that highly susceptible strains of *E. coli*, *Klebsiella*, *Citrobacter*, *Enterobacter*, and *Shigella* are not synergistically inhibited if only the MIC is considered; however, if one looks at the MBC values of the combination, since, as we have previously shown (13), there is often a marked discrepancy of MIC and MBC values for mecillinam, synergy is shown. For example, a *Klebsiella* strain for which the MIC of mecillinam was 0.5 μg/ml and that of ampicillin was 125 μg/ml required for inhibition MIC values of 0.25 μg/ml when both agents were combined. The mecillinam MBC value was 8 μg/ml, but the combined MBC values were 1 μg of mecillinam and 0.1 μg of ampicillin per ml. All of the *E. coli* in Table 3 are β-lactamase producing (Richmond type 3 enzyme) (6) and resistant to >1,000 μg of ampicillin per ml.

The effect of varying the ratio of mecillinam and the other β-lactam antibiotic was explored. Table 4 is an example of the combination of carbenicillin and mecillinam tested against

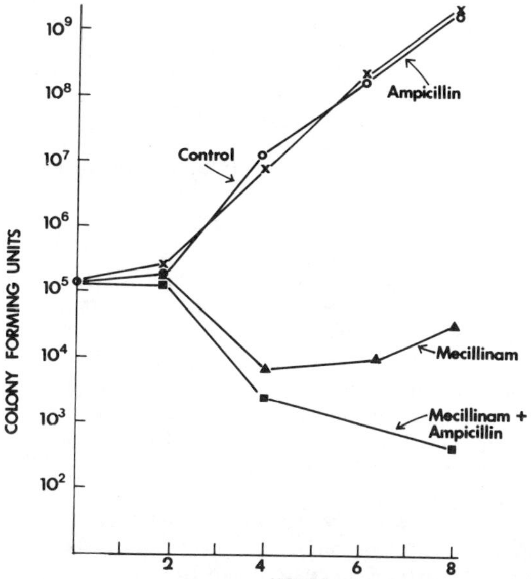

FIG. 3. *Killing curve of mecillinam and ampicillin against an S. sonnei strain with a mecillinam MIC of 0.8 μg/ml and MBC of 25 μg/ml. Ampicillin alone, 100 μg/ml; mecillinam alone, 0.8 μg/ml; ampicillin and mecillinam, 0.8 + 4 μg/ml.*

TABLE 2. *Synergy of mecillinam with β-lactam antibiotics*[a]

Organism	No. showing synergy with:					
	Ampicillin	Amoxicillin	Carbenicillin	Cephalothin	Cefamandole	Cefoxitin
E. coli	18/24[b]	8/9		2/3		
K. pneumoniae	13/20	4/5	1/1	1/2		
E. cloacae	3/3	2/3	1/1	2/2	1/1	3/3
C. freundii	7/10			1/1	1/1	
S. marcescens	3/4			1/1		
S. sonnei	4/4		2/2	1/1		
S. typhimurium	2/2					
P. vulgaris	1/5	0/1			2/2	1/1
P. morganii	2/8		0/1			
P. rettgeri	1/1					1/1
P. aeruginosa	2/9		3/5			
Acinetobacter	2/2	1/1			1/1	1/1
P. mirabilis	6/6					
Providencia	0/2	1/1				
% Synergy	58	80	70	80	100	100

[a] Agar dilution method using a checkboard arrangement of antibiotics.
[b] Number showing synergy/number tested.

TABLE 3. *Correlation of susceptibility of organisms to mecillinam with synergy*[a]

Organisms	No. tested	No. with:		
		MIC <0.8 μg/ml	MIC >1.6 μg/ml	MIC <0.8 μg/ml, MBC >3.2 μg/ml
E. coli	5	0	5	5
K. pneumoniae	5	0	5	5
C. freundii	3	0	3	3
E. cloacae	5	0	5	5
S. sonnei	3	0	3	3

[a] Studies performed in NIH broth and plated by MBC values.

Pseudomonas aeruginosa. Synergy is present when 1 part of mecillinam is combined with 100 parts of carbenicillin but is not present when the reverse is done. Synergy was not usually present above the 10:1 ratio of mecillinam to other antibiotics, whereas it was seen at a 100:1 ratio of penicillin or cephalosporin to mecillinam. Of 17 organisms tested by this method, 13 were synergistically inhibited at a ratio of 100 parts of carbenicillin, amoxicillin, ampicillin, cephalothin, or cefoxitin to 1 part of mecillinam. Only one isolate was inhibited at a ratio of 100 parts of mecillinam to 1 part of the other agent. All were both inhibited and killed at a ratio of 5 parts of mecillinam to 1 part of the other agent. Optimal MBC values were obtained at a 5:1 or 1:1 ratio of drugs in combination with either agent in excess.

A plot of the combination of ampicillin and mecillinam tested in agar against 50 organisms is given in Fig. 4. The x axis reflects the MIC of ampicillin alone, and the y axis reflects the ampicillin MIC in the presence of one-fourth the mecillinam MIC. The combination shows indifference for 13 organisms, partial synergy for four, and synergy for the remainder. Indole-positive *Proteus* (*P. morganii*, *P. vulgaris*) and *S. marcescens* were least likely to show synergy by this technique. All of these organisms had mecillinam MIC values >3.2 μg/ml.

Since I had previously shown that the marked difference between MIC and MBC values of mecillinam was in part due to destruction of the antibiotic by β-lactamase (13), I combined mecillinam with cloxacillin. Table 5 shows that addition of cloxacillin could reduce the mecillinam MIC and MBC values against

TABLE 4. *Effect of varying concentrations of mecillinam and carbenicillin against P. aeruginosa*

Ratio		MIC (μg/ml)		MBC (μg/ml)	
Carbenicillin	Mecillinam	Carbenicillin	Mecillinam	Carbenicillin	Mecillinam
	None	250		500	
100	1	16	0.16	500	1
10	1	4	0.4	8	8
5	1	8	1.6	125	25
1	1	1.6	1.6	6	6
1	5	6.2	31	12.4	62
1	10	6.2	62	25	250
1	100	2.5	250	0.5	500
None			>500		>500

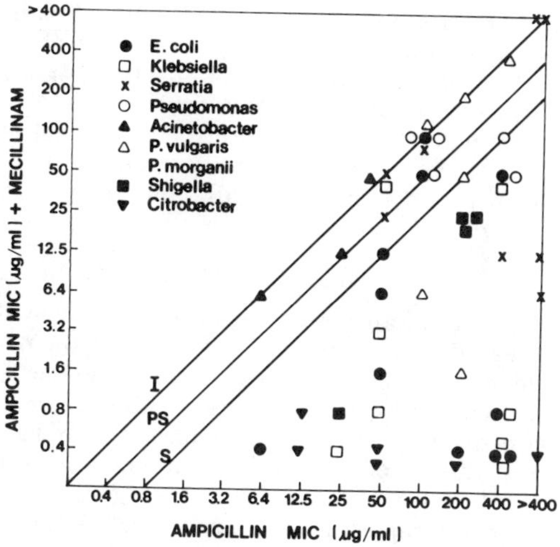

FIG. 4. *Plot of MICs, determined in agar, of the organisms listed. The x axis is the ampicillin MIC; the y axis is the ampicillin MIC in the presence of one-fourth the mecillinam MIC. I, Indifference; PS, partial synergy; S, synergy.*

TABLE 5. *Synergy of mecillinam and cloxacillin*[a]

Organism	Mecillinam		Cloxacillin		Mecillinam and cloxacillin	
	MIC[b]	MBC[b]	MIC	MBC	MIC	MBC
E. cloacae	8	125	125	500	0.5	8
E. coli	16	>500	500	>500	4	31
S. sonnei	1.6	100	500	>500	0.4	3.2

[a] In equal parts in broth assay system using NIH broth.
[b] MICs and MBCs are given in micrograms per milliliter.

Enterobacter cloaceae (Richmond type I β-lactamase), *E. coli* (type III β-lactamase), and *S. sonnei* (type III β-lactamase).

In contrast to the foregoing examples of synergy, Table 6 demonstrates that although there was synergy in terms of MIC values when *P. mirabilis* was studied, there was no synergy when the MBC values were considered. This is in contrast to the situation with other organisms. It is not due to destruction of ampicillin or mecillinam by the *P. mirabilis* strains, since these lacked β-lactamase.

Mecillinam failed to show synergy against group D streptococci, *Listeria*, *Staphylococcus aureus*, *Bacteroides fragilis*, *Clostridium*, or *Pasteurella* when combined with amoxicillin (Table 7). Furthermore, there was no reduction in the ampicillin, amoxicillin, and cephalothin MBC values against *Listeria monocytogenes* and the enterococci *Streptococcus faecalis* and *S. durans*. For example, the amoxicillin MBC of the *S. durans* in Table 7 was 1.6 µg/ml and the MBC, when combined with mecillinam, was 1.6 µg/ml. The same was true for the *Listeria* strains; the MBC was 12.5 µg/ml for amoxicillin alone and 12.5 µg/ml for amoxicillin combined with mecillinam. Of note was the fact that the ampicillin MIC with several enterococci was actually one tube or twofold greater when mecillinam was present. This was not a universal finding, however.

Although mecillinam showed synergy with all of the β-lactam antibiotics tested, it did not show synergy when combined with aminoglycosides, chloramphenicol, polymyxin B, or clindamycin (Table 8). Organisms susceptible and resistant to the aminoglycosides were tested. In only two instances was antagonism seen. This was with tetracycline and chloramphenicol in which cases the mecillinam MIC was increased. The organisms susceptible to mecillinam (MIC, 0.4 µg), such as a kanamycin-resistant (MIC, 50 µg/ml) *E. coli*, had the same mecillinam MIC (0.4 µg/ml).

TABLE 6. *Failure of mecillinam and ampicillin to demonstrate synergy in terms of MBC values*[a]

P. mirabilis strain:	Ampicillin		Ampicillin + mecillinam[b]	
	MIC	MBC	MIC	MBC
2639	0.61	1.25	0.15	1.25
2385	1.25	1.25	0.3	0.3
2868	1.25	2.5	0.3	1.25
2386	1.25	2.5	0.3	1.25
2313	1.25	1.25	0.3	1.25

[a] MICs and MBCs are given in micrograms per milliliter.
[b] Mecillinam MIC values for all five isolates, >100 µg/ml.

TABLE 7. *Failure of mecillinam to show synergy*

Organism	MIC (µg/ml)		
	Amoxicillin	Mecillinam	Both (1:1)[a]
S. fecium	0.2	>25	0.2
S. faecalis	0.2	>25	0.4
S. durans	0.4	>25	0.4
S. faecalis	0.4	>25	0.2
S. bovis	0.2	>25	0.2
L. monocytogenes	0.1	>25	0.2
L. monocytogenes	0.1	>25	0.2
S. aureus	0.005	>10	0.0025
S. aureus	0.08	>10	0.08
S. viridans	0.05	>10	0.05
B. fragilis	6.2	400	6.2
B. fragilis	50	400	50
Clostridium perfringens	0.2	200	0.1
Peptococcus	0.2	12.5	0.1
Pasteurella multocida	0.2	12.5	0.1

[a] Combined at a 1:1 ratio and tested in NIH broth.

Effect of medium upon synergy. Previous work from my laboratory has shown the effect of osmolality and cation content on the mecillinam MIC (13). I determined the effect of sodium and osmolality on synergy. The results are shown in Table 9. In a medium of low conductivity (<6 mS), there is no demonstrable synergy when the MIC values are considered. However, if the MBC values are used, there is definite synergy. This was also true for the mecillinam-cephalothin combination when tested against *Klebsiella* strain 2557.

When studies of synergy were performed in nutrient broth with an inoculum of 10^4 colony-forming units or less, it was not possible to show synergy between mecillinam and ampicillin against most *E. coli*, *K. pneumoniae*, *Citrobacter freundii*, and *E. cloacae*, since their mecillinam MIC values were 0.4 μg/ml or less in this medium, which has an osmolality of 38 mOsm and conductivity of 1.5 mS. In contrast, in Trypticase soy broth, Mueller-Hinton broth, or brain heart infusion broth, in which the conductivity is ≥10 mS, synergy was routinely demonstrated since the mecillinam MIC values are high.

TABLE 8. *Combination of mecillinam and non-β-lactam antibiotics*

Antibiotic	Organism	No. tested	No. showing: Synergy	No. showing: Antagonism
Kanamycin	*E. coli* susceptible	3	0	
	E. coli resistant	2	0	
Gentamicin	*E. coli*	2	0	
	Serratia	1	0	
	Acinetobacter	1	0	
	Pseudomonas	2	0	
	Enterococci	2		
Tobramycin	*Serratia*	1	0	
	Pseudomonas	1	0	
Amikacin	*E. coli*	1	0	
	Pseudomonas	1	0	
Chloramphenicol	*Klebsiella*	1	0	1
	E. coli	2	0	1
Tetracycline	*E. coli*	1	0	1
	P. mirabilis	1	0	
Polymyxin B	*Klebsiella*	1	0	
	P. vulgaris	1	0	
	Serratia	1	0	
	P. mirabilis	1	0	

DISCUSSION

Synergy of antibiotics has become a topic of increased interest in recent years with the development of multiply resistant enteric bacteria. Reviews by Jawetz (8) and Lacey (9) have defined synergism as the enhanced rate of bacterial killing of a two-drug combination over the rate of killing seen with either agent alone. Other techniques used to demonstrate synergy have been the use of a "checkerboard" arrangement of tubes (19) or a combination of antibiotics in agar.

Previous studies of synergy have concentrated upon use of compounds that affect two points in a biochemical pathway, such as is seen with the trimethoprim-sulfamethoxazole combination (2). Other approaches have involved a combination of antibiotics of the same class, in which one agent prevents the inactivation of the other antibiotic. This approach has been used with β-lactam antibiotics such as ampicillin and cloxacillin (16, 19). A third approach is that of combining carbenicillin and amino-glycosides to effect killing of *Pseudomonas* (3, 20) or combining cephalosporins with aminoglycosides to react against indole-positive *Proteus* (5). The mechanism used to explain this synergy is the increased entry of the aminoglycoside to reach its receptor site.

The β-amidinopenicillin mecillinam appeared not to inhibit murein transpeptidase (11), but rather seemed to bind to a protein involved in cell elongation (7, 17, 21). Thus, I was prompted to see if this agent would act in a synergistic fashion with β-lactam compounds that are thought to be involved in elongation and septum formation. These studies have

TABLE 9. *Effect of osmolality and ion content upon synergy of mecillinam*

Organism	Osmolality (mOsm)	Conductivity (mS)	MIC (μg/ml): Amoxicillin	MIC (μg/ml): Mecillinam	MBC (μg/ml): Amoxicillin	MBC (μg/ml): Mecillinam	Both drugs (1:1): MIC	Both drugs (1:1): MBC
Klebsiella 2551	185	5.8	62	0.4	500	250	0.2	6
	402	12	62	250	125	>500	0.8	6
Klebsiella 2557	185	5.8	125	0.2	125	8	0.2	0.5
	402	12	125	31	500	125	0.2	3
Citrobacter	185	5.8	125	0.8	125	250	0.4	0.8
	402	12	125	250	250	500	6	6

demonstrated that mecillinam shows synergy with ampicillin, amoxicillin, carbenicillin, cephalothin, cefazolin, cefoxitin, and cefamandole. Many members of the *Enterobacteriaceae*, *P. aeruginosa*, and *Acinetobacter* are inhibited in a synergistic manner. However, this inhibition is not universal for the members of a group nor will all β-lactam antibiotics show the same effect against a particular organism. Thus, mecillinam may show synergy with amoxicillin against a *Klebsiella* strain and not show synergy when combined with cephalothin or cefoxitin against the same strain. Organisms highly susceptible to inhibition by mecillinam do not show synergy if MIC data is considered. However, there is often a wide difference between the mecillinam MIC and the MBC even in media of low conductivity (<6 mS) and low osmolality (200 mOsm) (13). Synergy is demonstrated when MBC values are used. In media of low osmolality and low conductivity, most *E. coli*, *Klebsiella*, *Enterobacter*, *Shigella*, and *Salmonella* are so susceptible to mecillinam that synergy cannot be demonstrated. When conditions are such that an organism can resist the lytic action of mecillinam, synergy with penicillins or cephalosporins will result.

Mecillinam is destroyed by Richmond type III β-lactamases (6, 13), but this can be prevented by cloxacillin. Studies are underway to determine if a combination of three agents would inhibit organisms resistant to mecillinam plus ampicillin.

The failure of mecillinam to show synergy with aminoglycosides against gram-positive organisms such as *S. faecalis* and *L. monocytogenes* is in keeping with its poor activity against gram-positive coccal and bacillary forms (13). Antagonism could be demonstrated, with increased mecillinam MIC, when mecillinam was combined with chloramphenicol or tetracycline, and this is comparable to the situation seen with benzyl penicillin.

These findings, along with the animal experiments of Grunberg et al. (4), suggest that the combination of mecillinam with β-lactam antibiotics may be extremely useful. Studies by Baltimore et al. (1) and Tybring and Melchior (23) also have shown synergy against selected *Proteus*, *E. coli*, and *Klebsiella* strains. The observation of this study that the ratio of other β-lactam antibiotics to mecillinam shows synergy from 100:1 to 1:1 indicates that even small amounts of mecillinam may prove beneficial. In contrast to the situation with trimethoprim-sulfamethoxazole, there is not a small range in proportion of one antibiotic to the other. Further animal and clinical studies are indicated, since preliminary studies of the human pharmacology indicate that it yields adequate urine and blood levels (18).

ACKNOWLEDGMENTS

I wish to acknowledge the technical assistance of Lourdes Sainz and typing of the manuscript by Iris Rivera.

These studies were supported by a grant from Roche Laboratories.

LITERATURE CITED

1. **Baltimore, R. S., J. O. Klein, C. Wilcox, and M. Finland.** 1976. Synergy of mecillinam (FL 1060) with penicillins and cephalosporins against *Proteus* and *Klebsiella* with observations on combinations with other antibiotics and against other bacterial species. Antimicrob. Agents Chemother. **9**:701–705.
2. **Bushby, S. R. M., and G. H. Hitchings.** 1968. Trimethoprim, a sulphonamide potentiator. Br. J. Pharmacol. Chemother. **33**:72.
3. **Dienstag, J., and H. C. Neu.** 1972. In vitro studies of tobramycin, an aminoglycoside antibiotic. Antimicrob. Agents Chemother. **1**:41–45.
4. **Grunberg, E., R. Cleeland, G. Beskind, and W. F. DeLorenzo.** 1976. In vivo synergy between 6β-amidinopenicillanic acid derivatives and other antibiotics. Antimicrob. Agents Chemother. **9**:589–594.
5. **Hyams, P. J., M. S. Simberkoff, and J. J. Rahal, Jr.** 1974. Synergy between cephalosporin and aminoglycoside antibiotics effective against *Providencia* and *Proteus*. Antimicrob. Agents Chemother. **5**:571–577.
6. **Jack, G. W., and M. H. Richmond.** 1970. A comparative study of eight distinct β-lactamases synthesized by gram-negative bacteria. J. Gen. Microbiol. **61**:43–61.
7. **James, R., J. Y. Haga, and A. B. Pardee.** 1975. Inhibition of an early event in the cell division cycle of *Escherichia coli* by FL 1060, an amidinopenicillanic acid. J. Bacteriol. **122**:1283–1292.
8. **Jawetz, E.** 1968. The use of combinations of antimicrobial drugs. Annu. Rev. Pharmacol. **8**:151–170.
9. **Lacey, B. W.** 1958. Mechanisms of chemotherapeutic synergy. Symp. Soc. Gen. Microbiol. **8**:247–288.
10. **Lund, F., and F. Tybring.** 1972. 6β-amidinopenicillanic acids—a new group of antibiotics. Nature (London) New Biol. **236**:135–137.
11. **Matsuhashi, T., T. Kamiryo, P. M. Blumberg, P. Linett, E. Willoughby, and J. L. Strominger.** 1974. Mechanism of action and development of resistance to a new amidino penicillin. J. Bacteriol. **117**:578–587.
12. **Melchior, N. J., J. Blom, L. Tybring, and A. Birch-Andersen.** 1973. Light and electron microscopy of the early response of *Escherichia coli* to a 6-β-amidinopenicillanic acid (FL 1060). Acta Pathol. Microbiol. Scand. Sect. B **81**:339–407.
13. **Neu, H. C.** 1976. Mecillinam, a novel penicillanic acid derivative with unusual activity against gram-negative bacteria. Antimicrob. Agents Chemother. **9**:793–799.
14. **Neu, H. C.** 1976. Molecular modifications of antimicrobial agents to overcome drug resistance, p 87–111. *In* F. E. Hahn (ed.), Antibiotics and chemotherapy, vol. 20. S. Karger, Basel.
15. **Neu, H. C., and E. B. Winshell.** 1970. Purification and characterization of penicillinases from *Salmonella typhimurium* and *Escherichia coli*. Arch. Biochem. Biophys. **139**:278–290.
16. **Neu, H. C., and E. B. Winshell.** 1971. In vitro antimicrobial activity of 6[D(−)α-amino-*p*-hydroxyphenylacetamido] penicillanic acid, a new semisynthetic penicillin, p. 407–410. Antimicrob. Agents Chemother. 1970.

17. **Park, J. T., and L. Burman.** 1973. FL 1060, a new penicillin with a unique mode of action. Biochem. Biophys. Res. Commun. 51:863-869.
18. **Roholt, K., B. Nielsen, and E. Kristensen.** 1975. Pharmacokinetic studies with mecillinam and pivmecillinam. Chemotherapy (Basel) 21:146-166.
19. **Sabath, L. D., C. E. McCall, N. H. Steigbigel, and M. Finland.** 1967. Synergistic penicillin combinations for treatment of human urinary-tract infections, p 149-155. Antimicrob. Agents Chemother. 1966.
20. **Sonne, M., and M. Jawetz.** 1969. Combined action of carbenicillin and gentamicin on *Pseudomonas aeruginosa* in vitro. Appl. Microbiol. 17:893-896.
21. **Spratt, B. G.** 1975. Distinct penicillin binding proteins involved in the division, elongation and shape of *Escherichia coli* K12. Proc. Natl. Acad. Sci. U. S. A. 72:2999-3003.
22. **Tybring, L.** 1975. Mecillinam (FL 1060), a 6β-amidinopenicillanic acid derivative: in vitro evaluation. Antimicrob. Agents Chemother. 8:266-270.
23. **Tybring, L., and N. H. Melchior.** 1975. Mecillinam (FL 1060), a 6β-amidinopenicillanic acid derivative: bactericidal action and synergy in vitro. Antimicrob. Agents Chemother. 8:271-276.

ANTIMICROBIAL AGENTS AND CHEMOTHERAPY, Sept. 1976, p. 543-548
Vol. 10, No. 3

5″-Amino-5″-Deoxybutirosin, a Semisynthetic Analogue of Butirosin A: Antibacterial Activity In Vitro and in Mice

C. L. HEIFETZ,* C. A. FREY, I. A. PEARSON, AND J. C. SESNIE

Biological Research and Development Department, Research and Medical Affairs Division, Parke, Davis & Company, Detroit, Michigan 48232

Received for publication 21 May 1976

Aminodeoxybutirosin (AD-BTN), the 5″-amino-5″-deoxy derivative of butirosin (BTN), was synthesized to improve on the antibacterial activity of BTN by preventing bacterial enzymatic phosphorylation at the 5″ position. AD-BTN possesses the spectrum characteristic of BTN and gentamicin (GTM) and was active at low levels in vitro against a wide variety of gram-negative species including *Pseudomonas aeruginosa*, indole-positive *Proteus* and *Serratia marcescens;* its action was bactericidal against both light and heavy inocula, and it was not antagonized by human serum. AD-BTN was as active as GTM against GTM-sensitive *P. aeruginosa* in vitro and in mice, and was markedly improved over BTN. AD-BTN retained the good activity of the parent compound against other gram-negative pathogens. Whereas GTM minimal inhibitory concentrations were elevated 35-fold against GTM-resistant *P. aeruginosa* in vitro, the minimal inhibitory concentration of AD-BTN was only doubled. At 6.3 μg/ml, AD-BTN inhibited 68% of 82 isolates insusceptible to that concentration of GTM. In murine toxicity tests AD-BTN was about one-third to one-half as toxic as GTM.

Culbertson, Watson, and Haskell synthesized 5″-amino-5″-deoxybutirosin as a means of preventing the enzymatic phosphorylation of the 5″ position of butirosin, and its inactivation, by resistant bacteria (1). Reported herein are studies regarding the in vitro and mouse-protective antibacterial activities of this semisynthetic butirosin analogue.

MATERIALS AND METHODS

The antibiotics were handled, evaluated, and reported in terms of base content. We used butirosin sulfate (BTN) containing 710 μg of base per mg and gentamicin sulfate (GTM) containing 561 μg of base per mg. The latter was obtained through the generosity of Marvin J. Weinstein of the Schering Corp. The 5″-amino-5″-deoxybutirosin sulfate (AD-BTN), containing 688 μg of base per mg, was derived from the A component of butirosin, because the B component derivative was found to be less active (1).

Minimal inhibitory concentrations (MICs) were determined by previously published procedures (5). Agar dilution in standardized Mueller-Hinton agar (MHA) was performed according to the recommendations of the international collaborative study (2). Approximately 10^4 colony-forming units of bacteria were applied to the surface of a plate with a Steers replicator (9). Trypticase soy broth (TSB) or TSB with 10% bovine serum were used in the microtitration procedure (7); inocula contained approximately 2,000 colony-forming units in 0.05-ml volumes. For *Mycobacterium tuberculosis*, a tube dilution method with a synthetic TB medium was used (3). All incubations were aerobic at 37°C for 16 to 18 h (except *M. tuberculosis* which was incubated for 2 weeks). Bacteria manifesting MICs of BTN >25 μg/ml or MICs of GTM >6.3 μg/ml were classified as resistant (5).

To determine minimal bactericidal concentrations (MBCs), a microtitration procedure was used (4). After microtitration MICs were determined the presence of residual viable bacteria in the antibiotic-containing wells was assessed by subculturing 0.05-ml volumes onto MHA plates, using microtiter loops for sampling.

Tests in vivo were done in 18- to 20-g female CD-1 mice (Charles River). They received mouse laboratory chow (Purina) and water ad libitum. Subcutaneous (SC) injections were in 0.5-ml volumes of physiological saline and intravenous doses were 0.25 ml in distilled water.

To determine acute drug toxicities in mice, single 1.5-fold graded doses of compound were administered SC and intravenously to groups of 10 mice. The subacute toxicity of AD-BTN in mice was ascertained by injecting 1.5-fold graded doses of SC twice daily for 5 days. Because no deaths occurred after the second day, the tests were not extended for an additional 5 days as had been done previously with BTN and GTM (5). The median lethal doses (LD_{50}'s) were estimated by log-probit analysis (8), using pooled percent mortality data from at least two tests.

Protective activities of AD-BTN, BTN, and GTM were compared in standard acute mouse protection tests (5). Single SC doses in twofold rising incremental series were administered concurrently with bacterial challenge. Challenges were accomplished by the intraperitoneal injection of an estimated 100 LD_{50} suspended in 0.4 ml of 5% hog gastric mucin or 0.5 ml of TSB (*Klebsiella* only). Generally ≥90% of the untreated controls died within 48 to 72 h. Final survival percentages, obtained after 7 days of observation among groups of 8 to 15 mice, were pooled and used to estimate median protective doses (PD_{50}) by the log-probit method (8).

RESULTS

The antibacterial spectrum of AD-BTN in vitro is delineated in Table 1. The antibiotic was active at low levels against a wide variety of clinically important gram-negative species including *Pseudomonas aeruginosa* and indole-positive *Proteus* species (*P. morganii*, *P. rettgeri*, *P. vulgaris*, and *Providencia*). Also susceptible were *Enterobacter cloacae*, *Escherichia coli*, *Klebsiella pneumoniae*, *Protus mirabilis*, various *Salmonellae* and *Shigellae*, and *Serratia marcescens*.

Activity against other species were variable. Although inhibitory against *M. tuberculosis*, *Staphylococcus epidermidis*, and strains of *S. aureus* with limited antibiotic resistance, AD-BTN was weak or inactive against pneumococci, streptococci, and multi-antibiotic resistant *S. aureus*.

The bacteriostatic and bactericidal activities of AD-BTN, BTN, and GTM versus light and heavy bacterial inocula of single strains of five bacterial species are compared in Table 2. With one exception, the MICs and MBCs of AD-BTN were equal. This finding indicates a possible superiority in bactericidal potency over the parent compound for which the MBCs were twice the MICs against heavy inocula. A 1,000-fold increase in inocula generally produced only a doubling of MICs and MBCs of AD-BTN.

None of the compounds was appreciably antagonized by serum. In the presence of 25% human serum in TSB, microtitration MICs of AD-BTN, BTN, and GTM were the same or 1 dilution lower than the MICs in serum-free

TABLE 1. *Antibacterial spectrum of aminodeoxybutirosin*

Species	No. of strains tested	Test method[a]	MIC (μg/ml)	
			Range	Geometric mean
Enterobacter cloacae	5	MHA	1.6	1.6
Escherichia coli	9	MHA	1.6–3.1	2.0
Klebsiella pneumoniae	10	MHA	0.4–1.6	0.9
Proteus mirabilis	2	MHA	3.1–12.5	6.3
P. morganii	1	MHA	1.6	1.6
P. rettgeri	2	MHA	1.6–3.1	2.2
P. vulgaris	2	MHA	6.3	6.3
Providencia sp.	6	MHA	1.6–25	14.7
Pseudomonas aeruginosa	47	MHA	0.8–12.5	3.8
Salmonella enteritidis	2	MHA	1.6	1.6
S. minnesota	1	MHA	1.6	1.6
S. paratyphi	1	MHA	0.4	0.4
S. typhimurium	1	MHA	3.1	3.1
S. typhosa	4	TSB	1.6–6.3	5.2
Serratia marcescens	6	MHA	1.6–12.5	3.5
Shigella dysenteriae	2	MHA	3.1–6.3	4.4
S. flexneri	4	MHA	3.1–6.3	5.3
S. sonnei	3	MHA	1.6–3.1	2.5
Staphylococcus aureus				
Antibiotic sensitive	1	TSB	0.8	0.8
Limited resistance[b]	2	TSB	12.5–25	17.7
Macrolide resistant	1	TSB	0.8	0.8
Methicillin resistant	1	TSB	1.6	1.6
Multiresistant	1	TSB	50	50
S. epidermidis	2	TSB	0.8–1.6	1.3
Streptococcus faecalis	1	TSB + S	>100	>100
S. pneumoniae	1	TSB + S	100	100
S. pyogenes	1	TSB + S	50	50
Mycobacterium tuberculosis	1	TB	5	5

[a] TSB and TSB + S, Microtitration dilution in TSB and TSB with 10% bovine serum; TB, tube dilution in synthetic TB medium.

[b] Phage type 80/81 strains resistant to penicillin and streptomycin, and susceptible to neomycin, kanamycin, and paromomycin.

broth, when tested against *P. aeruginosa* (strain no. 28) and *S. aureus* (strain UC-76).

Antibacterial spectrums of AD-BTN, BTN, and GTM against several GTM-sensitive bacteria (GTM MIC <6.3 μg/ml) are compared in Table 3. The results demonstrate that AD-BTN possesses the spectrum characteristic of the structurally similar antibiotics. The most striking difference between AD-BTN and BTN was the improved activity of the former against *P. aeruginosa*. A comparison of geometric mean MICs revealed that the analogue was about four times as active as the parent compound against *P. aeruginosa* and, further, was almost as active as GTM against these GTM-sensitive isolates. In the case of *S. marcescens*, AD-BTN was two to three times more potent than BTN, bridging the activity gap between that antibiotic and GTM. AD-BTN and BTN were equipotent against *S. aureus* and the remaining *Enterobacteriaceae*.

Table 4 compares the relative antibacterial activities in vitro of the three aminoglycosides against gentamicin-susceptible and -insusceptible isolates of *P. aeruginosa*. As noted before, against GTM-susceptible members of that species AD-BTN was almost as active as GTM and several times more potent than BTN. The geometric mean MIC of GTM against pseudomonads resistant to that antibiotic was found to be approximately 35-fold higher than the MIC attained against susceptible isolates. In contrast, there was only an approximate twofold elevation of the MICs of AD-BTN and BTN. At 6.3

TABLE 2. *Comparative bacteriostatic and bactericidal activities of aminodeoxybutirosin, butirosin, and gentamicin versus light and heavy inocula in vitro*

Test organism	Inoculum size (approx. no. of cells)	Aminodeoxybutirosin		Butirosin		Gentamicin	
		MIC[a]	MBC	MIC	MBC	MIC	MBC
Enterobacter cloaceae IMM-50	10^2	6.3	6.3	6.3	6.3	3.1	3.1
	10^5	12.5	25	12.5	12.5	6.3	6.3
Klebsiella pneumoniae MGH-1	10^2	6.3	6.3	3.1	3.1	1.6	1.6
	10^5	25	25	25	50	6.3	6.3
Pseudomonas aeruginosa 28	10^2	6.3	6.3	25	25	3.1	6.3
	10^5	12.5	12.5	50	200	6.3	6.3
P. aeruginosa 733	10^2	3.1	3.1	12.5	12.5	6.3	6.3
	10^5	6.3	6.3	25	50	6.3	6.3
Serratia marcescens IMM-5	10^2	3.1	3.1	12.5	12.5	6.3	6.3
	10^5	6.3	6.3	25	50	6.3	6.3

[a] MIC was determined by microtitration dilution in terms of micrograms of salt per milliliter run in TSB.

TABLE 3. *Comparative antibacterial spectrums of aminodeoxybutirosin, butirosin, and gentamicin in vitro*

Test organism	No. of susceptible[a] isolates	Geometric mean MIC[b] (μg/ml)		
		Aminodeoxybutirosin	Butirosin	Gentamicin
Enterobacter cloacae	5	1.6	1.6	0.5
Escherichia coli	9	2.0	2.0	0.7
Klebsiella pneumoniae	10	0.9	1.1	0.8
Proteus mirabilis	2	6.2	12.5	1.6
Proteus, indole positive[c]	5	3.2	2.4	0.6
Pseudomonas aeruginosa	45	3.3	13.9	2.3
Salmonella spp.[d]	5	1.4	2.1	0.3
Serratia marcescens	6	3.5	8.9	1.1
Shigella spp.[e]	8	3.7	2.9	0.9
Staphylococcus aureus	2	0.6	1.1	0.1

[a] Selected for presentation because of inhibition by ≤25 μg of butirosin and ≤6.3 μg of gentamicin per ml.
[b] MIC, determined by agar dilution in MHA; compounds were handled in terms of base (assay) content.
[c] One isolate of *P. morganii* and two each of *P. rettgeri* and *P. vulgaris*.
[d] Two isolates of *S. enteritidis* and one each of *S. minnesota*, *S. paratyphi* A, and *S. typhimurium*.
[e] Two isolates of *S. dysenteriae*, four of *S. flexneri*, and three of *S. sonnei*.

TABLE 4. *Antibacterial activity of aminodeoxybutirosin, butirosin, and gentamicin versus gentamicin-susceptible and -insusceptible P. aeruginosa in vitro*

MIC[a]	Cumulative % of isolates susceptible[b]					
	Gentamicin susceptible (50)[c]			Gentamicin insusceptible (82)		
	AD-BTN	BTN	GTM	AD-BTN	BTN	GTM
0.8	8	0	20	2	0	0
1.6	30	0	40	17	0	0
3.1	64	8	86	56	2	0
6.3	84	28	100	68	13	0
12.5	96	40		80	43	12
25	96	90[d]		87	66	17
50	96	96[d]		98	77	39
100	100	100		99	84	56
>100				100	100	100
Geometric mean MIC	3.8	16.3	2.3	6	27.7	83

[a] MIC was determined by agar dilution in MHA; results expressed in micrograms of base per milliliter.
[b] Gentamicin-susceptible isolates were inhibited by ≤6.3 μg of that antibiotic.
[c] Number of isolates in parentheses.
[d] Three GTM-susceptible isolates insusceptible to BTN included.

μg/ml, AD-BTN inhibited 56 of 82 isolates of *P. aeruginosa* insusceptible to that concentration of GTM. Again, against the GTM-susceptible isolates, the aminodeoxy derivative proved markedly more potent than the parent compound, BTN, versus *P. aeruginosa*.

Drug toxicity tests in mice comparing AD-BTN, BTN, and GTM are summarized in Table 5. In all three categories (acute IV and acute and subacute SC), AD-BTN fell in between the other two compounds and was about one-third to one-half as toxic as GTM.

Comparisons of MICs in vitro and of mouse protective activities of single SC doses of AD-BTN, BTN, and GTM versus *Enterobacteriaceae* are summarized in Table 6. Similar data derived with isolates of *P. aeruginosa* are given in Table 7. In both tables, the isolates are arrayed in order of decreasing in vitro susceptibilities to BTN, since an effort was made to include as many mouse-virulent BTN-resistant (MIC >25 μg/ml) organisms as possible in this comparison.

With the exception of *S. marcescens*, AD-BTN and BTN possessed approximately equivalent mouse-protective activities against BTN-susceptible *Enterobacteriaceae*. As expected, the PD_{50}'s of BTN were much higher against BTN-resistant isolates; AD-BTN was several times more potent than BTN against these bacteria. Against the two strains resistant to BTN but sensitive to GTM in vitro, AD-BTN was at least as effective as the latter in mice. However, against strains resistant to both BTN and GTM in vitro, the latter was more effective

TABLE 5. *Comparative mouse toxicities of aminodeoxybutirosin, butirosin, and gentamicin*

Toxicity test	LD_{50} ± 95% confidence limits (mg of base/kg)		
	Amino-deoxy-butirosin	Butirosin	Gentamicin
Single intravenous dose	126 ± 7	460 ± 14	50 ± 6
Single SC dose	1420 ± 158	6000 ± 470	410 ± 12
Subacute SC dose	770 ± 118	4260 ± 422	340 ± 89

than AD-BTN in five of eight instances. The geometric mean PD_{50}'s of AD-BTN and GTM versus all BTN-resistant *Enterobacteriaceae* were 50 and 26 mg of base per kg, respectively.

Among isolates of *P. aeruginosa*, the relationships between in vitro susceptibilities and responses in mouse protection tests were unpredictable. This finding may have derived from the fact that many of the bacteria lie on the borderline between in vitro susceptibility and resistance to BTN and/or GTM. However, some generalizations may be drawn. Against apparently BTN-susceptible strains, the aminodeoxy derivative was three to four times more active than the parent compound and was equally as effective as GTM. The geometric mean PD_{50}'s of AD-BTN, BTN, and GTM were 23, 76, and 21 mg of base per kg, respectively, against these 14 *P. aeruginosa* strains. Against the 8 BTN-resistant varieties, the same general relationship existed between the three antibiotics, at an approximate sevenfold diminished level of activity. Thus, the geometric mean PD_{50}'s of

AD-BTN, BTN, and GTM, respectively, were 158, 519, and 157 mg of base per kg.

DISCUSSION

By preparing the 5″-amino-5″-deoxy derivative, Culbertson, Watson, and Haskell (1) attempted to improve upon the antibacterial activity of BTN, a compound noted for its low toxicity and for its activity against approximately half of the GTM-resistant isolates against which it had been tested (5, 6). They attempted to accomplish such improvement by preventing enzymatic phosphorylation at the 5″ position of BTN.

TABLE 6. *Comparative in vitro and mouse-protective activities of aminodeoxybutirosin, butirosin, and gentamicin versus Enterobacteriaceae*

Test organism	Aminodeoxybutirosin		Butirosin		Gentamicin	
	MIC (μg/ml)	PD_{50} (mg/kg)	MIC (μg/ml)	PD_{50} (mg/kg)	MIC (μg/ml)	PD_{50} (mg/kg)
Enterobacter cloacae IMM-11	1.6	2.7	1.6	2.7	0.8	1.5
Klebsiella pneumoniae MGH-2	1.6	4.1	1.6	5.9	0.8	1.9
Proteus vulgaris UC-232	6.3	4.3	3.1	6.8	1.6	1.7
Serratia marcescens IMM-5	3.1	25	6.3	100	0.4	5.4
Providencia sp. D 288 (BTN-R)[a]	1.6	22	50	174	3.1	46
Enterobacter sp. B 2716 (BTN/GTM-R)	50	85	100	220	12.5	0.6
Providencia sp. 2328 (BTN-R)	6.3	19	>100	213	6.3	17
Providencia sp. C482 (BTN/GTM-R)	25	27	>100	>710	25	39
K. pneumoniae B 1447 (BTN/GTM-R)	50	80	>100	263	25	35
K. pneumoniae D 1013 (BTN/GTM-R)	100	75	>100	355	25	22
P. morganii C 558 (BTN/GTM-R)	25	100	>100	>710	25	56
P. rettgeri B1796 (BTN/GTM-R)	12.5	49	>100	375	12.5	59
P. rettgeri B 2038 (BTN/GTM-R)	12.5	100	>100	994	12.5	67
P. rettgeri C 941 (BTN/GTM-R)	6.3	35	>100	852	12.5	40

[a] BTN-R, Butirosin resistant; GTM-R, gentamicin resistant; BTN/GTM-R, resistant to both.

TABLE 7. *Comparative in vitro and mouse-protective activities of aminodeoxybutirosin, butirosin, and gentamicin versus P. aeruginosa*

P. aeruginosa isolate	Aminodeoxybutirosin		Butirosin		Gentamicin	
	MIC (μg/ml)	PD_{50} (mg/kg)	MIC (μg/ml)	PD_{50} (mg/kg)	MIC (μg/ml)	PD_{50} (mg/kg)
Bernardi	0.8	18	3.1	18	0.8	8
SD-1C	0.8	6	3.1	9	0.8	2.7
SD-5C	0.8	18	3.1	57	0.8	7
Siebart	1.6	62	3.1	87	0.8	17
SD-4B	1.6	36	6.3	82	0.8	22
SD-4C	0.8	31	6.3	53	1.6	13
SD-7A	0.8	37	6.3	74	1.6	18
SD-7B	0.8	18	6.3	85	1.6	13
72 (GTM-R)[a]	3.1	11	12.5	43	25	84
Assemany	3.1	40	25	89	3.1	32
SD-3B	1.6	31	25	>710	0.8	15
UI-18	3.1	27	25	65	3.1	32
VAD-12-7-7	3.1	30	25	82	1.6	23
G 75 (GTM-R)	12.5	110	25	362	200	>280
1174 (BTN-R)	12.5	210	50	568	6.3	163
71 (BTN/GTM-R)	12.5	100	50	376	100	>280
G 30 (BTN/GTM-R)	6.3	135	50	259	200	>280
G76 (BTN/GTM-R)	12.5	92	50	259	200	>280
PIU PMG 5 (BTN-R)	100	>344	100	>710	1.6	12
Moeller 13485 (BTN/GTM-R)	6.3	34	100	128	25	12
Bold 6-22 (BTN/GTM-R)	50	88	>100	>710	50	170
Jenkins (BTN/GTM-R)	50	>355	>100	>710	50	>266

[a] BTN-R, Butirosin resistant; GTM-R, gentamicin resistant; BTN/GTM-R, resistant to both.

AD-BTN demonstrated some superiority over BTN with respect to relative bactericidal to bacteriostatic potency against heavy inocula. Both in vitro and in mice, this analogue was clearly more potent than BTN against *P. aeruginosa* and *S. marcescens*, whereas it retained the good activity of BTN against other gram-negative bacterial pathogens. AD-BTN was almost as active as GTM against GTM-sensitive isolates of *P. aeruginosa* and was active against a majority of GTM-resistant strains of *P. aeruginosa*.

As often appears to be the case with aminoglycoside antibiotics, the price of improved antibacterial potency was increased toxicity. Thus, AD-BTN was found to be about four times as toxic as BTN in acute intravenous and SC tests in mice, and about 5.5 times as toxic in subacute SC tests. How these observations relate to more pertinent chronic renal and ototoxicity in other species or possible tolerated doses in man has not been determined.

LITERATURE CITED

1. **Culbertson, T. P., D. R. Watson, and T. H. Haskell.** 1973. 5″-Amino-5″-deoxybutirosin, a new semi-synthetic aminoglycoside antibiotic. J. Antibiot. **26**:790–793.
2. **Ericsson, H., and J. C Sherris.** 1971. Antibiotic sensitivity testing. Report of an international collaborative study. Acta Pathol. Microbiol. Scand. **217** (Suppl.):64–73.
3. **Fisher, M. W., M. C. Manning, L. A. Gagliard, M. R. Gaetz, and A. L. Erlandson.** 1960. Paromomycin: experimental antibacterial activity. Antibiot. Annu. 1959–1960, p. 293–303.
4. **Harwick, H. J., P. Weiss, and F. R. Fekety, Jr.** 1968. Application of microtitration techniques to bacteriostatic and bactericidal antibiotic susceptibility testing. J. Lab. Clin. Med. **72**:511–516.
5. **Heifetz, C. L., J. A. Chodubski, I. A. Pearson, C. A. Silverman, and M. W. Fisher.** 1974. Butirosin compared with gentamicin in vitro and in vivo. Antimicrob. Agents Chemother. **6**:124–135.
6. **Heifetz, C. L., M. W. Fisher, J. A. Chodubski, and M. O. DeCarlo.** 1972. Butirosin, a new aminoglycoside antibiotic complex: antibacterial activity in vitro and in mice. Antimicrob. Agents Chemother. **2**:89–94.
7. **Marymont, J. H., Jr., and R. M. Wentz.** 1966. Serial dilution antibiotic sensitivity testing with the microtitrator system. Am. J. Clin. Pathol. **45**:548–551.
8. **Miller, L. C., and M. L. Tainter.** 1944. Estimation of the ED_{50} and its error by means of logarithmic-probit graph paper. Proc. Soc. Exp. Biol. Med. **57**:261–274.
9. **Steers, E., E. L. Foltz, and B. S. Graves.** 1959. An inocula replicating apparatus for routine testing of bacterial susceptibility of antibiotics. Antibiot. Chemother. **9**:307–311.

Antimicrobial Agents and Chemotherapy, Sept 1976, p. 549-554
Vol. 10, No. 3

Therapeutic Effects of Ribavirin Given by the Intraperitoneal or Aerosol Route Against Influenza Virus Infections in Mice

E. L. STEPHEN,* J. W. DOMINIK, J. B. MOE, and J. S. WALKER

United States Army Medical Research Institute of Infectious Diseases, Fort Detrick, Frederick, Maryland 21701

Received for publication 29 March 1976

Ribavirin (1-β-D-ribofuranosyl-1,2,4-triazole-3-carboxamide) is an effective antiviral agent against type A influenza infection of mice. Therapy was most effective when administered as a small-particle aerosol early in the infection. Treatment was also effective by either the intraperitoneal or aerosol route in mice with histological evidence of pneumonia. Ribavirin increased the percent survival, lowered lung virus titers, and decreased the development of lung pathology when therapy was initiated at 6 h as a small-particle aerosol. There was no evidence of pulmonary toxicity or immunosuppressive effects.

Virus diseases of man and animals represent an important group of disease entities. Notwithstanding the influenza pandemic of 1918 to 1919, which was accompanied by great loss of life, influenza, like most virus diseases, is usually self-limiting and not associated with high mortality unless complicated by bacterial pneumonia. In 1957, Horsfall estimated that man suffers with viral diseases for 7 years of a 70-year life span (5). Loosli has stated that influenza is the major incapacitating viral disease not adequately controlled by vaccines (9).

Ribavirin has antiviral activity against both ribonucleic and deoxyribonucleic acid viruses (6, 13, 17). The demonstration that small-particle aerosols containing rimantadine or amantadine-hydrochloride were effective for the treatment of influenza virus-infected mice (15, 16) and the reported efficacy of parenterally injected ribavirin against lethal influenza infections in mice (1, 7) suggested that aerosols of ribavirin might be useful for the treatment of influenza. This report describes the therapeutic efficacy of ribavirin given in small-particle aerosols to treat experimental influenza virus infection in mice.

MATERIALS AND METHODS

Mice. Five-week-old outbred, female mice, Tac:(SW)fBR, were used for all experiments. Upon arrival, mice were housed 15 to a cage in random order. Each group of mice contained a separate subgroup destined for the same treatment, but reserved for serial sacrifice studies in addition to those recorded for survival. Groups contained 55 mice except that continuously treated groups contained 40 mice.

Virus. The mouse-adapted variant of the A/Aichi/2/68 (H3N2) strain of influenza virus used to infect the mice has been previously described (12, 15).

Lung virus titers. Lung samples were homogenized in 4.5 ml of heart infusion broth and assayed in 10- to 12-day-old embryonated eggs (15). Lung titers, expressed as the mean egg infective dose per lung, are the geometric mean of three individual mouse lungs at the indicated times postexposure. When no virus was detected in a lung sample, a value of 1.0 was assigned to calculate the geometric mean titer.

Aerosol sampling and dissemination system. The dissemination system used to infect the mice and for intermittent therapy has been previously described (15). The aerosols for continuous therapy were generated by a modified Collison system developed in our laboratory. The particles generated by this system have a mass median diameter of 1.4 μm, with 95% less than 5.2 μm (unpublished data, our laboratory). The relative humidity in the exposure chamber prior to treatment was 56.8 ± 1.9% standard error of the mean. After exposure, the relative humidity increased to 65.3 ± 1.7% for the intermittent method and approximately 70.0% for the continuous method.

Aerosol samples were collected for virus assay and quantitative analysis of ribavirin (15). The concentration of ribavirin per milliliter of collecting fluid in the glass impingers was determined by ultraviolet spectroscopy at a wavelength of 205 nm with a Beckman model DBG spectrophotometer. A standard curve was prepared by measuring the absorbance of known quantities of ribavirin.

Drug and treatment schedules. Ribavirin, obtained from the Nucleic Acid Research Institute of ICN Pharmaceuticals, Inc., Irvine, Calif., was dissolved in sterile triple-distilled water before aerosol or intraperitoneal (i.p.) administration. Injections (i.p.) were given once each day at a dose of 16 mg/kg per day. Aerosol treatments were either intermittent (80 min/day) or continuous (22 h/day). The dosage of the two aerosol methods of treatment was adjusted by using a spray suspension containing either 100 or 20 mg of ribavirin per ml for the intermittent and continuous methods, respectively. The retained aerosol dose (50% of presented dose) for intermittent aerosol (80 min/day) was 21.5 mg/kg per day, whereas that for the continuously disseminated aerosol was 58 mg/kg per day, based on the calculated inhaled dose (14) and the retention properties of small-particle aerosols (4). Virus control mice were sham treated with sterile triple-distilled water for 80 min/day.

Two treatment schedules were followed. In one, therapy was initiated at 6 h postexposure to the virus and continued through 4 days. The second schedule involved initiation of therapy 3 days postexposure to the virus and continued through 7 days.

Gross lung lesion scores and histopathology. Five mice were killed on days 1, 2, 4, 6, 7, and 9 postinfection; the lungs were examined for gross lesions. The degree of pathological change was scored by the method of Fazekas de St. Groth and Donnelley (2) with the modification that dead animals were not included. Complete lung consolidation was scored as a 4 under this system. The values plotted represent the mean lung lesion scores of five mice from each group for each day.

Three mice were killed from each group 7, 14, and 21 days postexposure for histological examination. The lungs were fixed and processed as previously described (15).

Data. The percentage of survival was based on deaths occurring on days 5 through 21 after aerosol exposure to the virus. Mice used for survival data were separate from those used for virus titers or pathology examination. Intergroup comparisons were made using chi-square analysis for survival and one-way analysis of variance and Fisher's protected least significant difference test (13) for time to death. The mean time of death was calculated using only mice dying during the observation period. Survivors were not included in the calculations. Survival and time-to-death data from two replicate experiments were not statistically different and were combined.

RESULTS

Survival and MTD. Significant increases in percent survival ($P < 0.005$) occurred in all groups of mice given ribavirin regardless of the method of treatment or time of initial treatment (Table 1). There was no difference between the percentage of the survival of mice treated with continuous or intermittent small-particle aerosols when treatment was initiated at 6 h. Both aerosol methods of treatment resulted in significantly greater survival ($P < 0.005$) than the i.p. method of treatment. When treatment was initiated at 3 days, survival following all methods of therapy was significantly greater than that of the sham-treated virus control mice ($P < 0.005$). The aerosol methods were not superior to i.p. treatment when therapy was initiated on day 3. Treatment initiated at 6 h resulted in significantly greater percent survival ($P < 0.005$, by analysis of variance) than the same method of treatment initiated at 3 days.

Treatment (i.p.) initiated at 6 h did not significantly affect the mean time-to-death (Table 1). However, the time-to-death of mice treated from days 3 through 7 was significantly greater ($P < 0.01$) than for sham-treated virus control mice regardless of the method of treatment.

Virus titers. When therapy was initiated at 6 h, the peak lung virus titer of mice treated with continuously disseminated aerosols was significantly lower ($P < 0.05$) than the peak virus titer of sham-treated virus control mice at 48 h (Fig. 1, top). At 96 and 144 h, both intermittent and continuous aerosol methods of treatment resulted in significantly lowered lung virus ti-

TABLE 1. *Effect of ribavirin on survival and time-to-death of mice challenged with influenza virus by the aerosol route*[a]

Therapy route	Regimen	Survival		Mean time to death ± SEM[b] (days)
		Survivors/total	%	
Treated 6 h to 4 days				
Sham treated	80 min/day	27/109	24	7.6 ± 0.2
i.p.	1/day	62/110	56[c]	8.3 ± 0.3
Aerosol	80 min/day	105/110	95[c,d]	11.0 ± 1.4[e]
Aerosol	22 h/day	76/79	96[c,d]	11.3 ± 1.5[e]
Treated 3 to 7 days				
Sham treated	80 min/day	19/110	17	7.2 ± 0.1
i.p.	1/day	46/110	41[c]	8.8 ± 0.3[c]
Aerosol	80 min/day	59/110	53[c]	9.6 ± 0.5[c]
Aerosol	22 h/day	38/79	48[c]	9.4 ± 0.6[c]

[a] Challenge dose (mean egg infective dose per mouse) was $10^{4.8 \pm 0.06}$ mean egg infective doses/mouse.
[b] SEM, Standard error of the mean.
[c] $P < 0.005$ versus sham treated.
[d] $P < 0.005$ versus i.p.
[e] $P < 0.01$ versus sham treated.

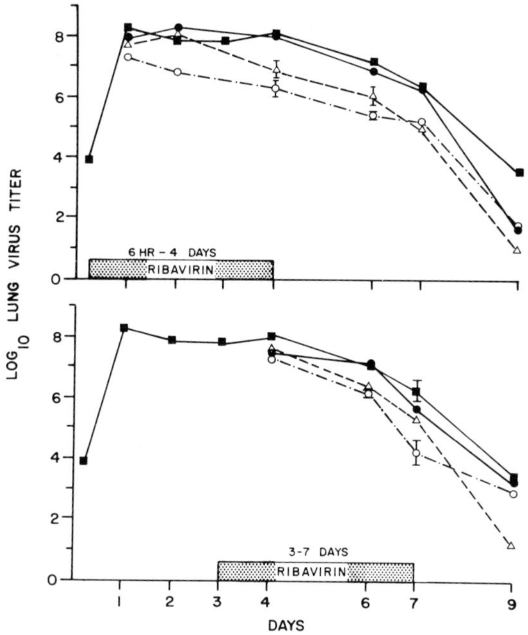

FIG. 1. *Effect of ribavirin on lung virus titers in influenza-infected mice. (Top) Therapy initiated 6 h postexposure to the virus and continued for 4 days. (Bottom) Therapy initiated 3 days postexposure and continued for 4 days. Symbols: sham-treated virus control (■); i.p.-treated (●); aerosol-treated, 80 min/day (△); continuous aerosol-treated (○).*

ters ($P < 0.025$ and $P < 0.005$, respectively) compared with titers from sham-treated virus control mice. The i.p. therapy had no effect on titers of these time periods. When treatment was from 3 through 7 days, only continuously administered aerosols resulted in significantly ($P < 0.05$) lower lung virus titers at 6 and 7 days (Fig. 1, bottom).

Serology. Serum was collected from surviving mice at 42 days after infection to gain insight into the effect ribavirin might have on the immune system. Hemagglutination-inhibition titers of surviving sham-treated virus control mice (Table 2) were equivalent to those of surviving treated mice.

Pathology. By day 3 sham-treated virus control mice had bronchopneumonia with an accompanying bronchial hyperplasia (Fig. 2). The effects of ribavirin treatment initiated 6 h after infection on gross pathology are shown in Fig. 3. Gross lung changes were evident in the sham-treated infected control mice 24 h after histopathological evidence of pneumonia. The lungs of sham-treated control mice were totally consolidated by day 6. Gross lung lesions in mice treated i.p. with ribavirin initially at 6 h were not different from those observed in control mice (Fig. 3). When the compound was administered by aerosol, marked reduction in gross pathology was evident.

Similar reductions in pathology were noted by histological examination at 7, 14, and 21 days. Representative sections of lungs 21 days after infection from each of the four groups of mice initially treated at 6 h are shown in Fig. 4. The sections from the lungs of aerosol-treated mice are essentially normal. Aerosol-treated mice (Fig. 4C and D) did not have bronchial hyperplasia. Bronchial hyperplasia was seen in both the sham-treated control mice (Fig. 4A) and to a lesser extent in i.p.-treated mice (Fig. 4B). Alveolar fetalization was noted in the i.p.-treated groups, but not in aerosol-treated groups. The alveolar fetalization and bronchopneumonia seen at 21 days in the i.p.-treated mice were less than those observed in the sham-treated controls.

DISCUSSION

We have previously reported that rimantadine, amantadine, and ribavirin are therapeutically effective against influenza infection

TABLE 2. *Effect of ribavirin treatment on 42-day-serum hemagglutination-inhibition influenza titers*

Duration of therapy	Route of therapy (geometric mean reciprocal titer)			
	Sham-treated virus control (n = 5)	i.p. treatment (n = 10)	Aerosol 80 min (n = 10)	Aerosol continuous (n = 10)
6 h to 4 days	139 (121,160)[a]	242 (184,320)	160 (138,185)	80 (63,101)
3 to 7 days	127 (101,160)	118 (104,133)	187 (169,207)	139 (109,179)

[a] ± Standard error of geometric mean.

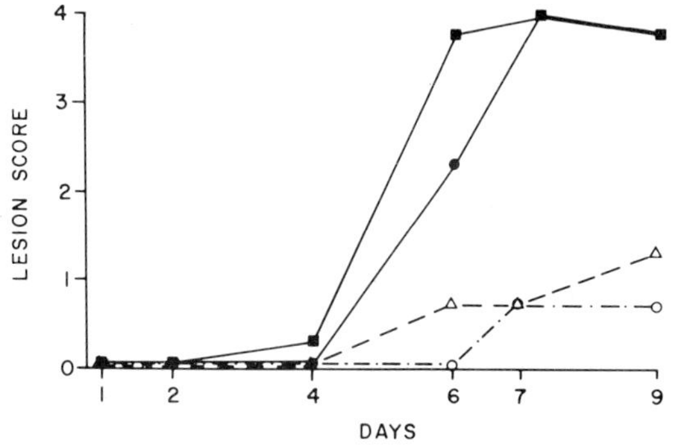

FIG. 3. *Effect of ribavirin on the development of gross lung lesions in influenza-infected mice. Therapy was initiated 6 h postexposure and continued for 4 days. Symbols: sham-treated control (■); i.p.-treated (●); aerosol-treated, 80 min/day (△); continuous aerosol-treated (○).*

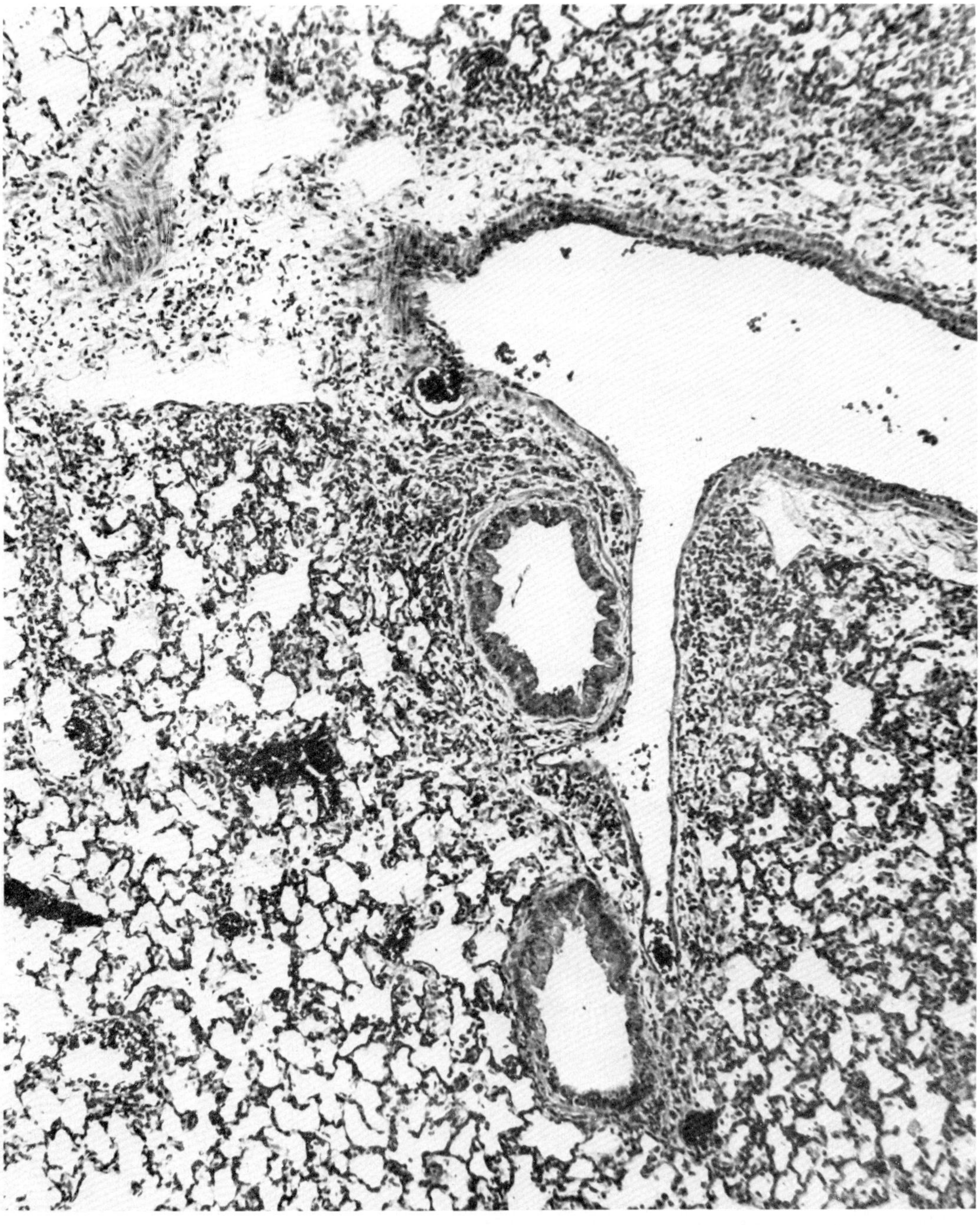

FIG. 2. *Histological changes observed in mouse lungs 3 days postexposure to the virus. Note evidence of bronchopneumonia and bronchial hyperplasia with initial alveolar changes in alveoli closely associated with the bronchi.*

when administered as small-particle aerosols (15, 16). Amantadine was ineffective when given i.p., but resulted in significantly increased survival rates when administered as a small-particle aerosol. Although rimantadine was therapeutically effective both by the aerosol and i.p. routes, it was most effective as continuously administered aerosol for 4 days. Rimantadine did not affect either the concentration of virus or the development of lesions in

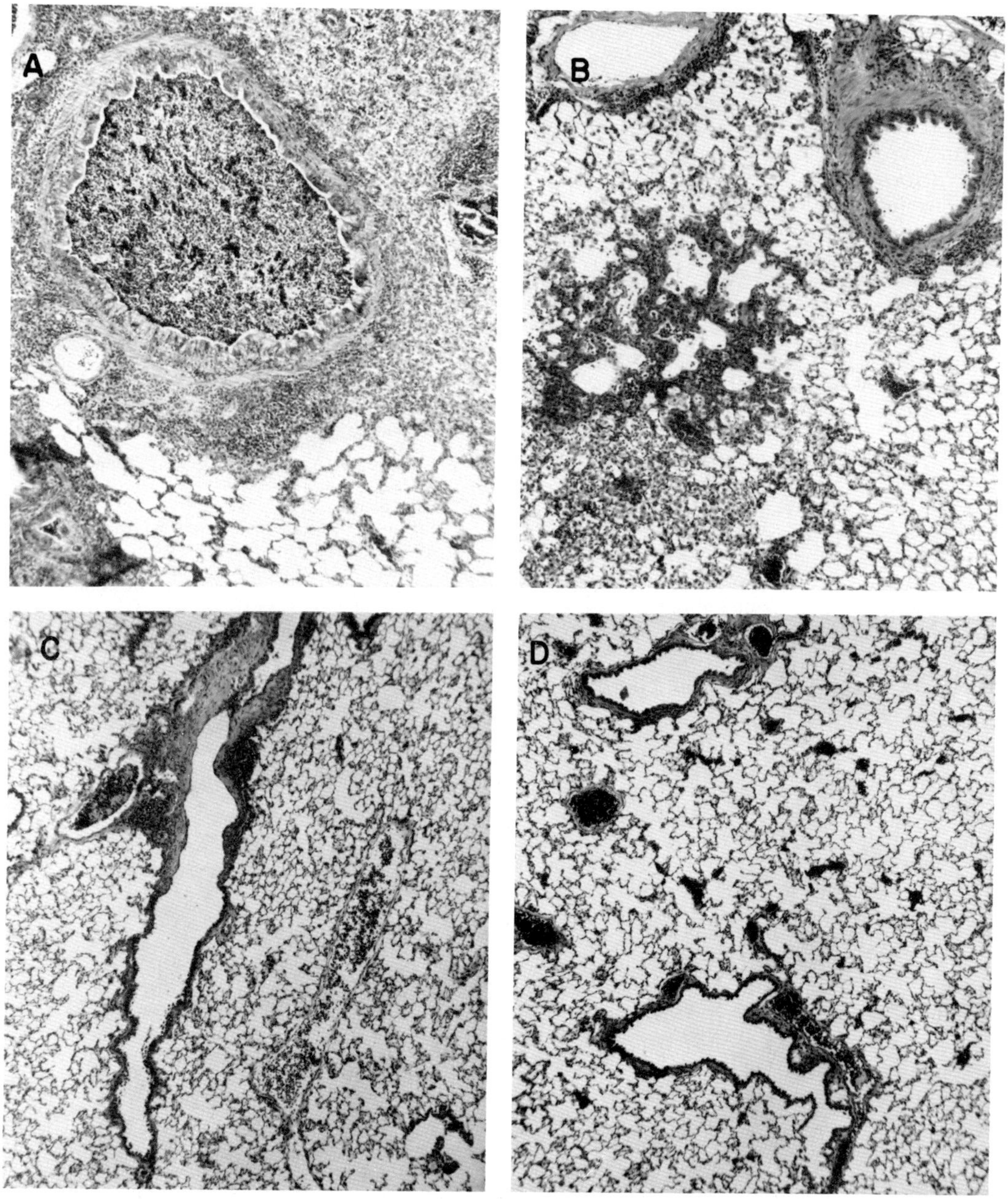

FIG. 4. *Histological differences 21 days postinfection in the lungs of untreated and ribavirin-treated mice when therapy was initiated 6 h postexposure to influenza virus. (A) Lung section from a sham-treated virus control mouse showing severe bronchopneumonia, bronchial hyperplasia, and alveolar fetalization. (B) Section from a mouse treated i.p. showing some bronchopneumonia, alveolar fetalization, and a microabscess. (C) Normal-appearing section from a mouse treated with small-particle aerosols of ribavirin 80 min/day for 4 days. Note normal-appearing bronchial mucosa. (D) Lung section from a mouse treated with continuous aerosols of ribavirin. Note the lack of bronchial hyperplasia and the normal-appearing alveolar duct.*

the lungs regardless of method or schedule of administration. The effect of aerosols of amantadine was similar to that of rimantadine when therapy was initiated at 6 h; however, when therapy was initiated 3 days postinfection, it appeared to reduce the development of lesions and concentration of virus in the lungs (16). In contrast, ribavirin appeared to affect virus titers and the extent of lesions when administered as an aerosol (16).

Our present study has confirmed previous findings with ribavirin and provided detailed information on the extent to which ribavirin affects virus titers and prevents the development of lung lesions when administered at 6 h as an aerosol. After i.p. administration, however, survival was significantly increased, but the development of lesions and virus titers in the lungs were unaffected. Aerosols of ribavirin were most effective when therapy was initiated at 6 h, but therapy initiated at day 3 also significantly increased the percent survival and lowered virus titers. Less extensive development of lung lesions occurred when the drug was administered at 6 h than at 3 days. By day 3 the pathological process was established and, therefore, therapy initiated at 3 days had the effect of expediting resolution rather than preventing lesion development.

We have stated as a hypothesis that the administration of an effective antiviral compound such as ribavirin directly to the surface mucosa of the respiratory tract would be the most efficacious method of administering the drug for the treatment of respiratory infections (16). The present findings confirm this hypothesis and emphasize the beneficial effect of aerosol treatment.

The mode of action of ribavirin is different from that of rimantadine and amantadine. Ribavirin administered as a small-particle aerosol is clearly antiviral in influenza virus-infected mice, whereas rimantadine and amantadine do not consistently lower virus titers in the lungs or affect the pulmonary pathology observed (15, 16). Our observation that ribavirin is effective therapeutically at 3 days, at a time when virus titers have reached a peak in the lungs and pneumonia exists, does not support the suggestion that ribavirin is effective because it prevents virus titers from exceeding critical levels (1). Ribavirin is highly effective after lung virus titers have reached their peak, suggesting that the therapeutic effect of ribavirin involves more than a simple antiviral effect. The dramatic effect of ribavirin in inhibiting developing lung pathology suggests that an "anti-inflammatory" effect may be an important facet of its activity. There is evidence that other drugs effective against influenza may also work in a similar fashion (3).

Ribavirin is an effective antiviral drug for treatment of influenza. It not only increases survival but lowers virus titers and greatly modifies the development of histological lesions in the lungs when administered as a small-particle aerosol. The most efficacious method of administering ribavirin is as a small-particle aerosol (<5 μm), and systems are available to do this (8). Strict attention must be given to the control of particle size of the aerosol and the dosage delivered.

LITERATURE CITED

1. **Durr, F. E., H. F. Lindh, and M. Forbes.** 1975. Efficacy of 1-β-D-ribofuranosyl-1,2,4-triazole-3-carboxamide against influenza virus infections in mice. Antimicrob. Agents Chemother. **7**:582–586.
2. **Fazekas de St. Groth, S., and M. Donnelley.** 1950. Studies in experimental immunology of influenza. IV. The protective value of active immunization. Aust. J. Exp. Biol. Med. Sci. **28**:61–75.
3. **Fujita, H., Y. Seto, and S. Toyoshima.** 1975. Mechanism of action of anti-influenza benzamidine derivatives. Antimicrob. Agents Chemother. **7**:426–430.
4. **Hatch, T. F., and P. Gross.** 1964. Pulmonary deposition and retention of inhaled aerosols, p. 65–67. Academic Press Inc., New York.
5. **Horsfall, F. L.** 1957. Midcentury inventory. Public Health Rep. **72**:905–906.
6. **Huffman, J. H., R. W. Sidwell, G. P. Khare, J. T. Witkowski, L. B. Allen, and R. K. Robins.** 1973. In vitro effect of 1-β-D-ribofuranosyl-1,2,4-triazole-3-carboxamide (Virazole, ICN 1229) on deoxyribonucleic acid and ribonucleic acid viruses. Antimicrob. Agents Chemother. **3**:235–241.
7. **Khare, G. P., R. W. Sidwell, J. T. Witkowski, L. N. Simon, and R. K. Robins.** 1973. Suppression by 1-β-D-ribofuranosyl-1,2,4-triazole-3-carboxamide (Virazole, ICN 1229) of influenza virus-induced infections in mice. Antimicrob. Agents Chemother. **3**:517–522.
8. **Larson, E. W., H. W. Young, and J. S. Walker.** 1976. Aerosol evaluations of the DeVilbiss no. 40 and Vaponefrin nebulizers. Appl. Environ. Microbiol. **31**:150–151.
9. **Loosli, C. G.** 1974. Influenza virus epidemics: a continuing problem. Geriatrics **29**:103–120.
10. **May, K. R.** 1973. The Collison nebulizer: description, performance and application. Aerosol Sci. **4**:235–243.
11. **Roessler, W. G., and D. A. Kautter.** 1962. Modifications to the Henderson apparatus for studying air-borne infections. Evaluations using aerosols of *Listeria monocytogenes*. J. Infect. Dis. **100**:17–22.
12. **Scott, G. H., and R. J. Sydiskis.** 1976. Responses of mice immunized with influenza virus by aerosol and parenteral routes. Infect. Immun. **13**:696–703.
13. **Sidwell, R. W., L. B. Allen, G. P. Khare, J. H. Huffman, J. T. Witkowski, L. N. Simon, and R. K. Robins.** 1973. Effect of 1-β-D-ribofuranosyl-1,2,4-triazole-3-carboxamide (Virazole, ICN 1229) on herpes and vaccinia keratitis and encephalitis in laboratory animals. Antimicrob. Agents Chemother. **3**:242–246.
14. **Steel, R. G. D., and J. H. Torrie.** 1960. Principles and procedures of statistics. McGraw-Hill Book Co., Inc., New York.
15. **Stephen, E. L., J. W. Dominik, J. B. Moe, R. O. Spertzel, and J. S. Walker.** 1975. Treatment of influenza infection of mice by using rimantadine hydrochlorides by the aerosol and intraperitoneal routes. Antimicrob. Agents Chemother. **8**:154–158.
16. **Walker, J. S., E. L. Stephen, and R. O. Spertzel.** 1976. The use of small-particle aerosols of antiviral compounds for the treatment of type A influenza pneumonia in animal models. J. Infect. Dis. **133**(Suppl): A140–A144.
17. **Witkowski, J. T., R. K. Robins, R. W. Sidwell, and L. N. Simon.** 1972. The design synthesis and broad spectrum antiviral activity of 1-β-D-ribofuranosyl-1,2,4-triazole-3-carboxamide and related nucleosides. J. Med. Chem. **15**:1150–1154.

ANTIMICROBIAL AGENTS AND CHEMOTHERAPY, Sept. 1976, p. 555-563 Vol. 10, No. 3

Printed in U.S.A.

Can Mannitol Reduce Amphotericin B Nephrotoxicity? Double-Blind Study and Description of a New Vascular Lesion in Kidneys

WARD E. BULLOCK,* ROBERT G. LUKE, CHARLES E. NUTTALL, AND DINYAR BHATHENA

Divisions of Infectious Disease and Nephrology, Departments of Medicine and Pathology, University of Kentucky College of Medicine, Lexington, Kentucky 40506*

Received for publication 16 March 1976

Eleven patients with systemic mycotic infections were treated with amphotericin B, 1 mg/kg, on alternate days. Five patients also received mannitol (M), 1 g/kg, in the amphotericin infusion, while six served as controls (C). Renal function studies prior to therapy were repeated at a total cumulative amphotericin B dosage of 25 mg/kg; renal biopsies were obtained from 10 patients. Inulin and creatinine clearances decreased in both the C and M groups, significantly so in the latter. Urinary concentrating ability of five patients (2C, 3M) decreased as did the capacity of three (1C, 2M) to acidify urine after an acid load. Neither the peak and valley levels of amphotericin B in serum nor the urinary excretion thereof differed between the C and M groups. Striking vacuolization of smooth muscle cells, previously unrecognized, was observed in the media of arterioles and arteries in all renal biopsies. Tubular calcification was present in both groups. In summary, M therapy (1 g/kg) did not protect against the nephrotoxicity of amphotericin B. A unique lesion of the renal vasculature secondary to amphotericin B is described.

Many of the side effects associated with amphotericin B therapy can be ameliorated by therapy every other day and by judicious cotherapy with such agents as heparin, corticosteroids, and antiemetics. Unfortunately, there has been little success in reducing the nephrotoxic effects that often restrict therapy. These include reduction in glomerular filtration rate (GFR) and renal blood flow (5, 24) and abnormalities of distal tubular function. The latter are manifested histologically by intratubular and interstitial calcium deposition (25) and functionally by impaired urinary concentrating ability (13), and by renal tubular acidosis with secondary potassium wasting (4, 5, 17).

Although individual susceptibility to the nephrotoxicity of amphotericin B appears to vary widely (18), the likelihood of at least transient renal impairment is high with the large dose (1.5 to 2.5 g) usually required to treat adequately many of the systemic mycotic infections (5). It has been suggested that alkali therapy might prevent some aspects of amphotericin B nephrotoxicity (17), and in an experimental rat model administration of bicarbonate during amphotericin therapy was shown to improve several measures of renal function (11). Unfortunately, similar studies in man are not available.

More recently, it has been reported that administration of an osmotic diuretic, mannitol, significantly reduces the nephrotoxicity of acute amphotericin B administration to dogs (12). Mannitol therapy appeared to prevent a rise in the blood urea nitrogen and serum creatinine (Cr) values as well as the degeneration of renal tubular epithelium that occurred when amphotericin B was administered alone. Clinically, mannitol has been employed extensively as cotherapy with amphotericin B, and protective effects on the kidney have been claimed in one small uncontrolled study (20). Because of widespread interest in the therapeutic potential of mannitol (3), we have conducted and here report the results of a double-blind controlled study designed to evaluate the capacity of this agent to diminish the nephrotoxicity of amphotericin B in man.

MATERIALS AND METHODS

Patient selection. Potential subjects for study were screened for suitability as participants by four criteria: (i) proof of active systemic mycotic infection; (ii) no prior amphotericin B therapy; (iii) normal renal function as judged by urinalysis and levels of blood urea nitrogen and serum creatinine; (iv) absence of diabetes mellitus and hypertension (diastolic pressure > 90 mm of Hg). Patients meeting these criteria were advised of the study verbally and in writing. Those giving informed consent were then entered into a treatment protocol approved by the

University of Kentucky Human Investigation and Studies Committee. Upon entry into the study, renal function of all patients was evaluated by measurement of inulin clearance (C_{In}), creatinine clearance (C_{Cr}), and urinary concentrating and acidifying ability. Serum electrolytes, calcium, phosphorus, and uric acid were measured, and urine cultures were performed. An intravenous pyelogram was normal in all patients.

Investigational protocol. After completion of renal function studies, amphotericin B (hereafter designated as A), supplied and labeled under a Food and Drug Administration investigational new drug number by E. R. Squibb & Co., was administered intravenously in three increasing doses until the full dosage schedule of 1 mg/kg of body weight, given every other day, was attained. Full doses were given in 500 ml of 5% dextrose in water over a 4-h period. Assignment of patients to a control (C) group receiving A therapy alone or to a mannitol (M) treatment group was made by a physician and a pharmacist not associated with the daily care of study patients. M was added without labeling to the A solution of patients chosen to receive M cotherapy so that the contents of an infusion, other than A concentration, were unknown to both the attending physicians and patients during the course of therapy. In all cases, the dose of M administered with A was 1 g/kg of body weight. This dose is in the range used to treat acute renal failure (16) but below that producing toxic effects (9). Attending physicians prescribed medications from a preselected panel of drugs when necessary for relief of various side effects caused by A. These included: (i) heparin, 1,000 U or less added to each 500 ml of infusion to control phlebitis; (ii) 20 mg of hydrocortisone or its equivalent delivered as an intravenous bolus immediately prior to each A infusion; (iii) Proclorperazine, 10 mg, orally, 0.5 h before infusion of A and every 8 h to a total of three doses; (iv) aspirin, 600 mg, orally, 0.5 h prior to infusion and every 6 h as needed for reduction of fever (>102°F) induced by therapy; (v) $NaHCO_3$ for replacement of bicarbonate when serum CO_2 fell to 18 meq/liter; (vi) KCl, 1 g, orally three times daily, as needed for serum potassium levels less than 3.8 meq/liter.

Criteria for the removal of a patient from study were: (i) interruption of A therapy as the result of noncompliance, (ii) nephrotoxicity sufficient to elevate Cr to 3.5 mg/100 ml, or (iii) to decrease the C_{Cr} to 25% or less of the pretreatment control value. In fact, no patient was dropped from the study for these reasons.

In addition to clinical assessment of patients, mandatory clinical studies at weekly intervals included weighing, 24-h urine collection, complete blood count, urinalysis, and measurement of serum electrolytes, Cr, blood urea nitrogen, and erythrocyte sedimentation rate. At intervals of 2 weeks to 1 month, appropriate X-ray studies, fungal cultures, and fungal serologies were repeated. At a total cumulative A dosage of 25 mg/kg of body weight, all renal function studies were repeated. In addition, percutaneous renal biopsy was performed under fluoroscopic guidance in 10 patients, all of whom gave informed consent. Biopsy was not carried out in one patient (no. 8) because of severe kyphosis. After biopsy, the course of A was completed to a total mean dosage of 43 mg/kg of body weight in 10 patients. One patient failed to return after receiving 1.7 g.

Assay of A in blood and urine. After the third administration of A at full daily dosage (1 mg/kg of body weight), serum and urine specimen were collected for assay at weekly intervals from all patients. Blood for peak A levels was drawn within 30 min after completion of the infusion. For assay of valley levels, blood was drawn just prior to the next infusion 48 h later. Twenty-four-hour urine collections were started at the beginning of an infusion. During collection, urine was kept at 4°C, after which a 10-ml portion was removed and, along with serum, frozen at −60°C until assayed. The remaining urine was assayed for creatinine as a check on adequacy of collection. Serum and urinary concentrations of A were measured on coded specimens through the courtesy of the Squibb Institute of Medical Research, New Brunswick, N.J. Levels were determined by bioassay using the *Paecilomyces varioti* small-plate agar diffusion assay (21).

Renal function studies. All renal studies and renal biopsies were performed at least 24 h after an infusion of A on the "off" day of therapy. Inulin clearance studies were performed in the morning after a light breakfast. Two sequential hourly urine collections were taken during a modest water diuresis (100 ml/h), and the average value was used; a bladder catheter was employed for two patients. Inulin was measured by the method of Kulka (14). Serum and urinary creatinine were measured by an autoanalyzer (Technicon). Serum electrolytes, uric acid, calcium, and phosphorus were measured by the clinical laboratory. To measure urine concentrating ability, 5 U of pitressin tannate in oil (Parke, Davis & Co.) was given intramuscularly after voiding at 10 p.m. The osmolality of the next three voided urine specimens was measured by an advanced osmometer, and the highest value was selected. The "short" ammonium chloride loading test was performed by the method of Wrong and Davies (26); fresh urine was collected under mineral oil, and urinary pH was measured by a Beckman pH meter.

Histological methods. Light, electron, and fluorescence microscopy of renal biopsies was carried out by one of us (D.B.) without knowledge of which patients received M. For light microscopy studies, serial sections (1 to 2 μm thick) were made of formalin-fixed tissue and stained by hematoxylin and eosin, periodic acid Schiff, periodic acid silver methenamine-Masson trichrome, and von Kossa methods. For electron microscopy, 1-mm tissue cubes were fixed in 3.5% buffered glutaraldehyde, postfixed in 1% osmium tetroxide for 1 h, embedded in epon, and sectioned with subsequent double staining by lead citrate-uranyl acetate. For immunofluorescence studies, sections of snap-frozen tissue were stained by the direct technique with fluorescein-conjugated goat antisera to human immunoglobulins G, A, and M, βIC, and fibrin.

Statistical methods. In most instances, the significance of differences between group data was determined by the Student *t* test (paired if appropriate). Serum levels and urinary excretion of A were analyzed by means of a split plot design (22). Urinary pH measurements were corrected to whole numbers for calculation of mean and standard error of the mean.

RESULTS

General clinical features. All 11 patients who volunteered for study were Caucasians and ranged in age from 19 to 75 years. The infecting organism in each patient is listed in Table 1. Fungus could not be isolated from a lung biopsy of one patient. However, the pathology and a complement-fixing antibody titer of 1:256 against yeast and mycelial-phase antigens of *Histoplasma capsulatum* were regarded as diagnostic of histoplasmosis. The M-treated (n = 6) and C groups (n = 5) differed in two respects (Table 1): (i) the average age of the M group (58 ± 4.7 years) was greater than that of the C (48.4 ± 8.8 years) ($P > 0.1$); (ii) one of six patients in the M group was female, whereas of five in the C group three were females.

The clinical response to A therapy was favorable among patients of both groups (Table 1). Five of six patients in the M group were considered to be clinically arrested at the termination of therapy and at followup checks ranging from 12 weeks to 2 years post-treatment. Likewise, infection was cured or arrested in four of five in the C group. Arrest was defined by four criteria: (i) clinical well being; (ii) failure to isolate the infecting fungus from sputum or other sites; (iii) stabilization or improvement in X-ray findings; and (iv) decrease of complement-fixing antibody titer to *H. capsulatum* in patients with histoplasmosis. Patient no. 2 relapsed 8 months post-treatment as judged by a marked rise in complement-fixing antibody titer and weight loss; sputum cultures did not give fungal growth. Side effects attributable to A infusion were witnessed with equal frequency in the M and C groups; these included nausea, chills, fever, and malaise.

Renal function. In the overall group of 11 patients studied prior to therapy, the C_{In} was 113 ± 9 ml/min per 1.73 m^2 (mean ± standard error of mean), the C_{Cr} was 86 ± 7 ml/min per 1.73 m^2, and the Cr was 0.9 ± 0.04 mg/100 ml. The mean urinary osmolality (U_{osm}) after pitressin was 659 ± 79 mosm/kg (excluding patient no. 4 with a normal inulin clearance but who failed to concentrate in association with a persistent urinary tract infection secondary to an indwelling catheter necessitated by her neurological state). The mean minimum urinary pH after NH_4Cl was 5.2 (patient no. 4 excluded).

At the "target" dose of 25 mg/kg of A, there was a considerable drop in the inulin and creatinine clearance of both the C and M groups (Fig. 1; Table 2). Of interest, two patients in the C group showed very little change in GFR during A treatment (Fig. 1, no. 2 and 4). The mean xenith level of Cr during A therapy in the C group was 1.8 ± 0.3 mg/100 ml and 1.5 ± 0.2 mg/100 ml in the M group ($P < 0.1$). Overall, older patients appeared to have a less marked drop in GFR. Thus, in patients over 60 years of age from both groups (n = 5), the mean drop in C_{Cr} was 10 ± 4 ml/min as compared to 55 ± 3 ml/min in patients less than 60 years of age (n = 6) of both groups ($P < 0.001$).

Five patients (2C, 3M) showed a drop in concentrating ability, and three (1C, 2M) showed a drop in minimum hydrogen ion concentration after ammonium chloride loading (Table 3; Fig. 2 and 3). Signs of sodium depletion were carefully sought, but not found, in any patient.

TABLE 1. *Clinical features of 11 patients*

Group	Patient no.	Age (yr)	Sex	Wt (kg)	Treatment	Pathogen[a]	Site	Total A dosage (g)	Result
Control	1	19	F	53	C	B	Disseminated	2.5	Arrested[b]
Control	2	61	M	50	C	H	Lung, cavitary	2.3	Relapse
Control	3	50	F	54	C	B	Lung	2.4	Arrested
Control	4	70	F	50	C	C	Meninges	2.4	Cure
Control	5	42	M	70	C	H	Lung, cavitary	2.6	Arrested
Mannitol	6	41	M	91	M	B	Disseminated	2.5	Arrested
Mannitol	7	58	M	59	M	H	Lung, cavitary	2.5	Arrested
Mannitol	8	75	M	43	M	B	Disseminated	2.0	Arrested
Mannitol	9	50	M	42	M	H	Lung, cavitary	1.7[c]	Improved
Mannitol	10	62	F	53	M	H ?	Lung	2.0	Arrested
Mannitol	11	62	M	42	M	H	Lung, cavitary	1.8	Arrested

[a] Abbreviations: B, *Blastomyces dermatitidus*; H, *Histoplasma capsulatum*; C, *Cryptococcus neoformans*.
[b] See text for definition.
[c] Failed to complete therapy.

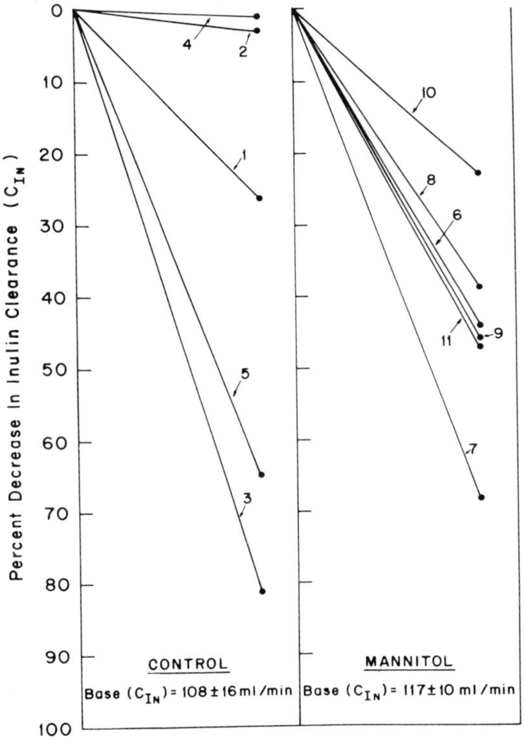

FIG. 1. *Change in GFR at a cumulative A dosage of 25 mg/kg. Data presented for patients no. 6 and no. 11 based on C_{Cr} values.*

All but one patient (no. 6) required supplemental potassium, and the nadir levels of serum potassium were not different beween the two groups (3.4 ± 0.2 meq/liter in C and 3.1 ± 0.2 meq/liter in M). Sodium bicarbonate therapy was not required in any patient; the mean nadir serum bicarbonate was 22.6 ± 0.5 meq/liter in the C group and 22.8 ± 0.5 meq/liter in the M group. The lowest serum bicarbonate observed was 19 meq/liter in patient no. 11. Urinary casts, mainly of the hyaline type, were seen frequently in four of five in the C group and in one of six in the M group. After completion of therapy, no casts were detected. Proteinuria was not detected by routine urinalysis in any patient during the study.

If the group of 11 patients is considered as a whole, a significant deterioration in GFR, urinary concentrating ability, and urinary acidification after an acid load was observed (Table 4).

Renal biopsies. At least 10 nonsclerosed glomeruli/biopsy were seen. By light microscopy, no specific glomerular lesion was found, and immunofluorescence studies were negative. Since 9 of the 10 patients were over 40 years of age, it is not surprising that arterial and arteriolar sclerotic changes were common. Tubular calcification was scored by an arbitrary scale on which 1+ signified minimal calcification (1 calcified focus/10 high-power fields). Extensive calcification (more than one focus/high-power

TABLE 2. *Changes in GFR during A therapy*

Patient no.	C_{In} (ml/min per 1.73 m²)[a]			C_{Cr} (ml/min per 1.73 m²)			Cr (mg/100 ml)		
	Base	Target	Δ	Base	Target	Δ	Base	Target	Δ
C group									
1	70	52	−18	76	24	−52	1.0	1.9	+0.9
2	120	117	−3	75	74	−1	1.1	1.0	−0.1
3	91	18	−73	96	36	−60	0.9	1.5	+0.6
4	95	94	−1	59	55	−4	0.8	0.9	+0.1
5	166	58	−108	128	68	−60	0.9	1.7	+0.8
	108 ± 16[b]	68 ± 17	−41 ± 21	87 ± 12	51 ± 10	−35 ± 14	0.9 ± 0.1	1.4 ± 0.2	0.5 ± 0.2
			NS[c]			$P < 0.10$[d]			$P < 0.10$
M group									
6	—	87	—	108	61	−47	1.1	1.7	+0.6
7	152	49	−103	107	60	−47	0.9	1.4	+0.5
8	125	76	−49	60	38	−22	0.8	1.1	+0.3
9	110	59	−51	96	36	−60	0.9	1.5	+0.6
10	93	71	−22	67	61	−6	0.7	0.8	+0.1
11	105	—	—	75	56	−19	1.0	1.0	0.0
	117 ± 10	68 ± 6	−56 ± 17 $P < 0.05$	86 ± 9	52 ± 5	−34 ± 9 $P < 0.02$	0.9 ± 0.1	1.3 ± 0.1	+0.3 ± 0.2 NS

[a] C_{In}, Inulin clearance.
[b] Mean ± standard error of mean.
[c] NS, Not significant.
[d] Probability (P) value for differences in GFR during A therapy as compared with pretreatment base-line values.

TABLE 3. *Changes in tubular function during A therapy*

Group	Pitressin test (U_{osm} [mosm/kg])			NH_4Cl load (urinary [H^+] $\times 10^{-7}$ eq [pH])		
	Base	Target	Δ	Base	Target	Δ
Controls ($n = 5$)	674 ± 110[a]	445 ± 50	−229 ± 80,[b] $P < 0.10$[c]	55 ± 20[a] (5.3)	41 ± 18 (5.4)	−14 ± 26, NS[d]
Mannitol ($n = 6$)	649 ± 118	516 ± 34	−132 ± 108, NS	64 ± 14 (5.2)	46 ± 16 (5.3)	−17 ± 17, NS

[a] Omits patient no. 4.
[b] Mean ± standard error of mean.
[c] Probability (P) value for differences in tubular function during A therapy as compared with pretreatment base-line values.
[d] NS, Not significant.

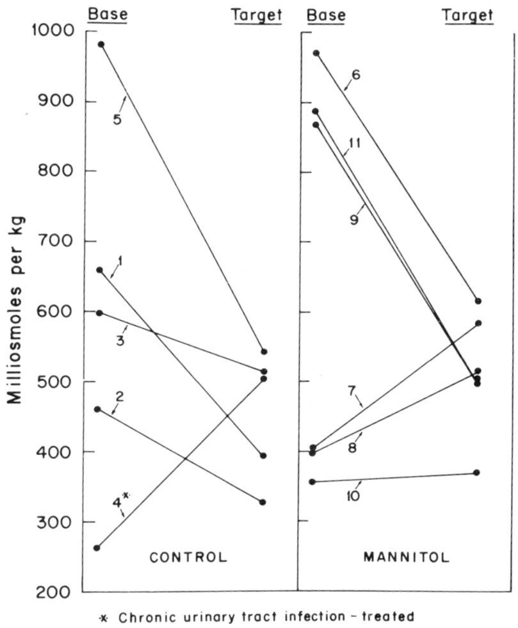

FIG. 2. *Change in urine concentration ability (pitressin test) at a cumulative A dosage of 25 mg/kg.*

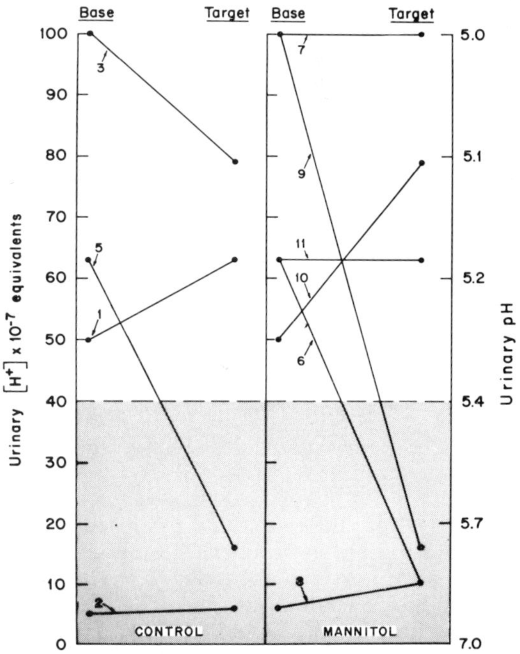

FIG. 3. *Change in urinary acidification ability at a cumulative A dosage of 25 mg/kg as determined by the short NH_4Cl loading test. Points falling within shaded area are below the normal range. Patient no. 4 excluded from figure.*

field) was scored as 3+ and intermediate calcification as 2+ (Table 5).

In varying degrees tubular calcification was observed in all but one patient (no. 4) and tended to be worse in the M group. There was, however, no correlation between tubular calcification and changes in glomerular and tubular function. There was no evidence of coagulation necrosis in the tubular lining cells, and there appeared to be no significant difference in the tubular cell cytoplasmic vacuolization between the M and C group.

A striking vacuolization in the media of small arterial and arteriolar profiles was seen in all biopsies (Fig. 4). The vacuolization was focal even in the most extensively affected biopsy specimens. Because of this, and the varying amounts of renal tissue sampled from case to case, qualitative assessment was necessarily arbitrary. Larger and frequently encountered lesions in small arteries and arterioles with relatively few uninvolved profiles were classed as 3+ (Table 5). Small vacuoles found in only an occasional vessel were classified as 1+ severity. Assessment of the severity of vacuolization was made "blindly" on two occasions by the same observer with good agreement.

There was no relationship between the degree of vacuolization and the arterial and arteriolar sclerotic changes. In ultramicroscopic studies of more severely involved biopsies, vacuoles were both more numerous as well as

TABLE 4. *Mean change of renal function in 11 patients during A therapy*

Renal function	C_{In} (ml/min per 1.73 m^2)[a]	C_{Cr} (ml/min per 1.73 m^2)	Cr (mg/100 ml)	Pitressin test (mosm/kg)	NH_4Cl load ($[H^+] \times 10^{-7}$ eq)
GFR	-48 ± 13.5[b] $P < 0.01$[c]	-35 ± 7.4 $P < 0.001$	0.4 ± 0.13 $P < 0.02$		
Tubular function				-171 ± 70 $P < 0.05$	-16 ± 6 $P < 0.05$

[a] C_{In}, Inulin clearance.
[b] Mean ± standard error of mean.
[c] Probability (*P*) values for differences in renal function during therapy as compared with pretreatment base-line values.

TABLE 5. *Histological changes in renal biopsy specimens*

Group	Patient no.	Tubular calcification	Medial vacuolization	Arteriosclerotic changes
Control	1	2+	1+	0
Control	2	2+	1+	2+
Control	3	1+	2+	3+
Control	4	0	2+	3+
Control	5	2+	1+	2+
Mannitol	6	3+	3+	2+
Mannitol	7	3+	2+	ND[a]
Mannitol	9	2+	2+	2+
Mannitol	10	2+	3+	2+
Mannitol	11	3+	3+	2+

[a] ND, Not determined. Larger arteries were not sampled.

larger, sometimes displacing the nucleus of the smooth muscle cells (Fig. 4B). Vacuoles appeared to evolve by fusion of dilated smooth and rough endoplasmic reticulum; in one instance, invaginating pinocytic vesicle formations suggested continuity with the peripheral plasma membrane of a medial cell. Vacuoles were more striking in arterioles than in the arteries, and occasionally they were seen in afferent arterioles. In general, changes were more marked in the M group (Table 5). To our knowledge, these changes have not been previously described as a consequence of A therapy.

Serum levels and urinary excretion of A. The peak and valley levels and urinary excretion of A were remarkably uniform for each patient during the course of therapy. Mean values for the C and M group are listed in Table 6 where it can be seen that there was no significant difference between the peak and valley levels of A measured in either group. Furthermore, there was no significant difference in the urinary excretion of A between the C and the M group, although excretion was slightly higher in the latter group.

DISCUSSION

Under conditions of this study, M in a dosage of 1 g/kg of body weight did not prevent the functional and histological manifestations of A nephrotoxicity. There was a significant and at least as great a fall in inulin and creatinine clearance within the M-treated group as in controls. Likewise, there was at least as much alteration of tubular function in the group treated with M as in the C group. Further, a newly recognized abnormality in the media of small arteries and arterioles appeared more severe in the M group.

A produces renal impairment by two substantially independent mechanisms. Firstly, an acute reduction in renal blood flow and GFR has been observed in man (2, 4, 5, 24), dogs (6), and rats (11). Infusion of the drug into the renal artery of a dog is associated with radiologically demonstrable intense vasoconstriction of small intrarenal blood vessels and cortical ischemia (6). Secondly, specific impairment of distal nephron functions, such as impaired concentrating ability (13), and distal renal tubular acidosis (4, 17), has been attributed to effects of the drug on tubular cell membranes; A interacts with membrane-bound sterols (1) to increase passive permeability to sodium, potassium, hydrogen ion, water, and low-molecular-weight solutes such as urea (1, 15, 23). In toad bladder studies, A increases membrane permeability only on the mucosal side of the membrane (15). Such effects on tubular cell membranes could explain potassium wasting and the inability to maintain a hydrogen ion and an osmotic gradient in the distal nephron.

Mannitol has both renal vasodilatory and "tubular flushing" effects (16) which might have been expected to influence favorably both of the nephrotoxic mechanisms associated with A therapy. In rats during renal hypoperfusion induced by aortic clamping (19), and after 2 h of complete obstruction of the renal artery (8), M can maintain glomerular filtration and urinary flow when infusion of saline cannot. There is also evidence in dogs of the ability of M to reduce renal vascular resistance in similar circumstances (7, 10). M increases medullary blood flow and reduces medullary hyperosmolality (9) and thus may diminish the levels of A

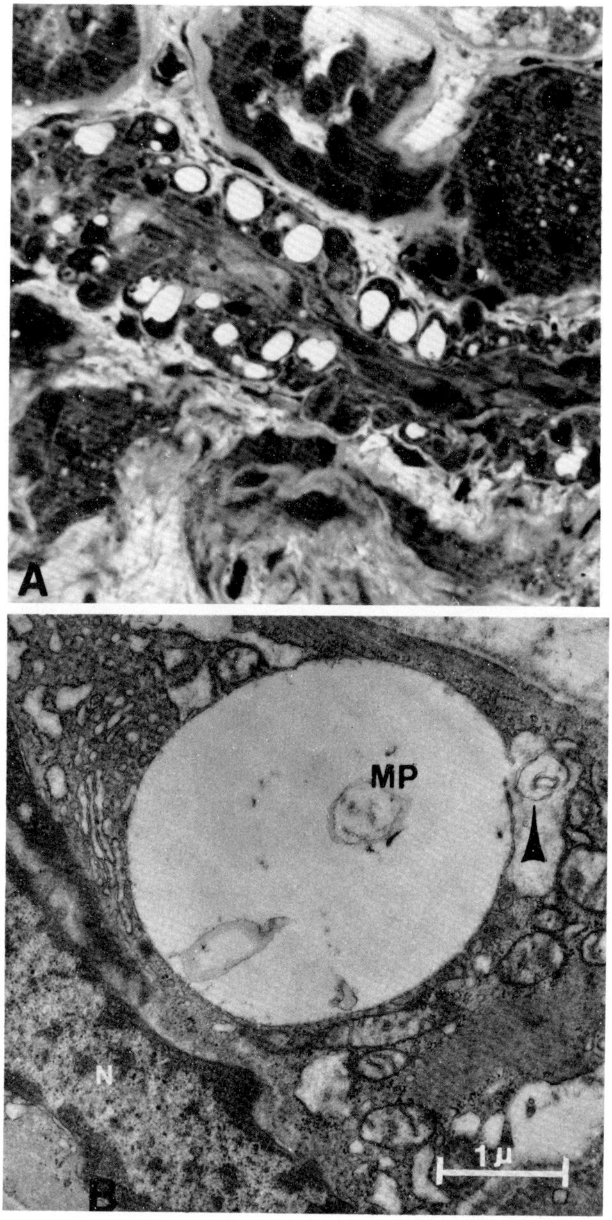

FIG. 4. *(A) Histological section of renal biopsy showing several vacuoles within the media of an arteriole. Epon-embedded, 1-μm section, using toluidine blue stain. ×160. (B) Electron micrograph of smooth muscle cell in the media of a renal arteriole. A large vacuole is situated centrally within the cell, near the nucleus (N). Membranes of the dilated rough endoplasmic reticulum (arrow) tend to break and form irregular membrane profiles (MP) suspended in the vacuolar lumen. ×9,500.*

in the vasa recta and, possibly, in the medullary interstitium itself. The osmotic diuresis induced by M infusion might be expected both to dilute A concentrations in the distal tubular lumina and to decrease luminal membrane contact time, especially if M also increased the GFR.

Despite the attractiveness of these hypothetically protective mechanisms and the previously reported protective effect in dogs (12), this controlled study has failed to confirm a beneficial effect of M. It is, of course, possible that a larger dose might have been protective, but the dose used (1 g/kg) was approximately twice that

TABLE 6. *Mean peak and valley serum levels and urinary excretion of A*

Group	No. of patients	No. of samples	Serum levels		Urinary excretion (mg/24 h)
			Peak (μg/ml)	Valley (μg/ml)	
Control	5	53	1.47 ± 0.05	0.36 ± 0.01	2.06 ± 0.27
Mannitol	6	58	1.60 ± 0.05[a]	0.42 ± 0.03[a]	2.20 ± 0.21[a]

[a] Differences from control values are not statistically significant.

used in the dog study (12) and in a report on the use of M in four patients (20). Further increase in M dosage might be hazardous for two reasons. Retention of M in the presence of a reduced GFR would tend to expand the extracellular fluid and cause hyponatremia; alternatively, osmotic diuresis may cause obligatory losses of sodium, water, and potassium which may be especially hazardous in patients receiving A. In addition, the histological and electron microscopic studies of renal biopsies from our patients suggest that a medial vacuolar lesion of arterioles and arteries may be more marked in patients receiving both A and M.

The vacuoles within renal vasculature appear to be made up of periodic acid Schiff stain-negative electron-lucent material which contains protoplasmic sap and some of the cytoplasmic organelles in varying stages of degeneration (Bhathena, D., W. E. Bullock, C. E. Nuttall, and R. G. Luke, submitted for publication). Continuity of vacuoles with the external cell membrane was suggested on electron microscopic study of at least one biopsy. It seems likely that these vacuoles are related to the increase in solute permeability of plasma membranes produced by A or to the intense renal vasoconstriction associated with administration of this drug or a combination of these effects. Whereas changes in membrane permeability appear to result from interactions of A with membrane-bound sterols to form pores (1), there is as yet no satisfactory explanation for the mechanism of vasoconstriction induced by A.

ACKNOWLEDGMENTS

We express appreciation to house staff members of the Department of Medicine at the University of Kentucky Medical Center for their outstanding care of the study patients and assistance with details of the treatment protocol. We wish also to thank the following: Peggy Herndon for assistance in preparation of infusion solutions, Marguerite Larsen for transport of specimens to the Squibb Laboratories for assay, Michael Kashgarian and Bernard Panner for helpful suggestions, and Catherine Fine for excellent editorial assistance.

This project was supported in part by a grant from E. R. Squibb & Sons, New York, N.Y. D.B. was supported in part by Public Health Service training grant AM 05701 from the National Institute of Arthritis, Metabolism, and Digestive Diseases.

LITERATURE CITED

1. **Andrioli, T. D.** 1973. On the anatomy of amphotericin B-cholesterol pores in lipid bilayer membranes. Kidney Int. **4**:337–345.
2. **Bell, N. H., V. T. Andriole, S. H. Sabesin, and J. P. Utz.** 1962. On the nephrotoxicity of amphotericin B in man. Am. J. Med. **33**:64–69.
3. **Bennett, J. E.** 1974. Chemotherapy of systemic mycoses. N. Engl. J. Med. **290**:30–32, 320–323.
4. **Burgess, J. L., and R. Birchall.** 1972. Nephrotoxicity of amphotericin B with emphasis on changes in tubular function. Am. J. Med. **53**:77–84.
5. **Butler, W. T., J. E. Bennett, D. W. Alling, P. T. Wertlake, J. P. Utz, and G. J. Hill II.** 1964. Nephrotoxicity of amphotericin B: early and late effects in 81 patients. Ann. Intern. Med. **61**:175–187.
6. **Butler, W. T., G. J. Hill, II, C. F. Szwed, and V. Knight.** 1964. Amphotericin B renal toxicity in the dog. J. Pharmacol. Exp. Ther. **143**:47–56.
7. **Camishion, R. C., R. W. Solit, J. Iida, and W. F. Ballinger, II.** 1966. The effect of mannitol on renal vascular resistance. Surgery **59**:1037–1042.
8. **Flores, J., D. R. DiBona, C. H. Beck, and A. Leaf.** 1972. The role of cell swelling in ischemic renal damage and the protective effect on hypertonic solute. J. Clin. Invest. **51**:118–126.
9. **Gennari, F. G., and J. P. Kassirer.** 1974. Osmotic diuresis. N. Engl. J. Med. **291**:714–720.
10. **Goldberg, A. H., and L. S. Lilienfield.** 1965. Effects of hypertonic mannitol on renal vascular resistance. Proc. Soc. Exp. Biol. Med. **119**:635–642.
11. **Gouge, T. H., and V. T. Andriole.** 1971. An experimental model of amphotericin B nephrotoxicity with renal tubular acidosis. J. Lab. Clin. Med. **78**:713–724.
12. **Hellebusch, A. A., F. Salama, and E. Eadie.** 1972. The use of mannitol to reduce the nephrotoxicity of amphotericin B. Surg. Gynecol. Obstet. **134**:241–243.
13. **Holeman, C. W., and H. Einstein.** 1963. The toxic effects of amphotericin B in man. Calif. Med. **99**:90.
14. **Kulka, R. G.** 1956. Colorimetric estimation of ketopentoses and ketohexoses. Biochem. J. **63**:542.
15. **Lichtenstein, N. S., and A. Leaf.** 1965. Effect of amphotericin B on the permeability of the toad bladder. J. Clin. Invest. **44**:1328–1342.
16. **Luke, R. G., and A. C. Kennedy.** 1967. Prevention and early management of acute renal failure. Postgrad. Med. J. **43**:280–289.
17. **McCurdy, D. K., M. Frederic, and J. R. Elkington.** 1968. Renal tubular acidosis due to amphotericin B. N. Engl. J. Med. **278**:124–131.
18. **Miller, R. P., and J. H. Bates.** 1969. Amphotericin B toxicity. Ann. Intern. Med. **71**:1089–1095.
19. **Morris, C. R., E. A. Alexander, F. J. Burns, and N. G. Levinsky.** 1972. Restoration and maintenance of glomerular filtration by mannitol during hypoperfusion of the kidney. J. Clin. Invest. **51**:1555–1564.
20. **Olivero, J. J., J. Lozano-Mendez, E. M. Ghafary, G. E. Knoyan, and W. N. Suki.** 1975. Mitigation of amphotericin B nephrotoxicity by mannitol. Br. Med. J. **I**:550–551.

21. **Shadomy, S., J. A. McCoy, and S. I. Schwartz.** 1969. Bioassay for hamycin and amphotericin B in serum and other biological fluids. Appl. Microbiol. **17**:497-503.
22. **Snedecor, G. W., and W. G. Cochran.** 1967. Statistical methods. Iowa University Press, Ames.
23. **Steinmetz, P. R., and L. R. Lawson.** 1970. Defect in urinary acidification induced *in vitro* by amphotericin B. J. Clin. Invest. **49**:596-601.
24. **Utz, J. P., J. E. Bennett, M. K. Brandriss, W. T. Butler, and G. J. Hill II.** 1964. NIH staff conference: amphotericin B toxicity. Ann. Intern. Med. **61**:340-343.
25. **Wertlake, P. T., W. T. butler, G. J. Hill II, and J. P. Utz.** 1963. Nephrotoxic tubular damage and calcium deposition following amphotericin B therapy. Am. J. Pathol. **43**:449-457.
26. **Wrong, O., and H. E. F. Davies.** 1959. The excretion of acid in renal disease. Q. J. Med. **28**:259-313.

Antimicrobial Agents and Chemotherapy, Sept. 1976, p. 564-566 Vol. 10, No. 3

Printed in U.S.A.

NOTES

New Method for Detecting In Vitro Inactivation of Penicillins by *Haemophilus influenzae* and *Staphylococcus aureus*

WIE-SHING LEE* AND LOUIS KOMARMY

Microbiology Laboratory, Children's Hospital, San Francisco, California 94119

Received for publication 17 February 1976

A new technique for detecting penicillinase production in *Haemophilus influenzae* and *Staphylococcus aureus* was compared with the capillary procedure for detecting beta-lactamase and the Bauer-Kirby disk susceptibility procedure. Isolates were classified similarly by all three procedures.

Ampicillin-resistant strains of *Haemophilus influenzae* have appeared with increasing frequency since reported by Thomas et al. in 1974 (13). Khan et al. (5) showed that these resistant strains produced beta-lactamase (penicillinase). Subsequently, a variety of assays for beta-lactamase have been used to detect ampicillin-resistant strains of *H. influenzae*. These assays have involved the use of an iodometric technique with a starch indicator (3, 8), chromogenic cephalosporin as the enzymatic substrate (4, 6), or other colorimetric methods (1, 11, 14).

We have developed a method to detect the ability of strains of *H. influenzae* and *Staphylococcus aureus* to neutralize penicillins. Isolates that neutralize penicillin as determined by our technique were also classified as penicillin resistant by the standard Bauer-Kirby antibiotic susceptibility procedure and had beta-lactamase detected by the capillary technique. Since our method does not require special reagents, it may be applicable in other laboratories required to test haemophilus isolates for penicillinase production.

Fifty-four isolates of *H. influenzae* from clinical specimens were studied. Additional verification of the new procedure was performed by testing 40 isolates of *S. aureus*.

Spore-seeded plates were prepared by a modification of the method of Sabath et al. (12). Five-milliliter portions of nutrient agar were distributed into screw-capped tubes. The caps were tightened and the tubes were stored in a refrigerator. To prepare the plates, stored agar was melted and cooled to about 57°C. One drop of Subtilis spores (Difco Laboratories, Detroit, Mich.) was added to the melted agar aseptically. The suspension was mixed thoroughly and poured onto the plate (100 by 15 mm).

The streak method was performed by using heavy inocula of the test organism picked from pure culture with a bacteriological loop. The streak patterns were made in two ways. (i) Unknown and non-penicillinase-producing control organisms were streaked in a cross pattern, but disconnected at the center to avoid contamination (Fig. 1A). (ii) Unknown and control organisms were streaked about 8 to 10 mm apart in a parallel line as shown in Fig. 1B. Antibiotic disks were placed as illustrated, and the plates were incubated at 37°C for 4 h or until growth was clearly visible. The inactivation of ampicillin was well demonstrated in cross-streaked patterns by inhibition zones that resembled a pair of kidney beans (Fig. 1A). The *Bacillus subtilis* grew along the streak of the resistant isolate due to the inactivation of ampicillin. On the other hand, if two isolates were streaked in parallel, the pattern illustrated in Fig. 1B appeared. The inhibition zone on the side of the resistant isolate was reduced noticeably.

The capillary technique for detecting beta-lactamase production (11, 14) and the Bauer-Kirby agar diffusion procedure (2) were used as reference methods. A slight modification of the Bauer-Kirby method was used for susceptibility tests of *H. influenzae* (15). Inocula were adjusted to contain 10^6 to 10^7 colony-forming units/ml. The medium was prepared from Mueller-Hinton agar with 5% chocolatized rabbit blood and 1% IsoVitaleX (Baltimore Biological Laboratory, Cockeysville, Md.).

The results of the classification of our isolates by the three test procedures are presented in Table 1.

All of the isolates that produced beta-lactamase as detected by the capillary tube method were demonstrated to neutralize penicillin by the use of our technique. These isolates were

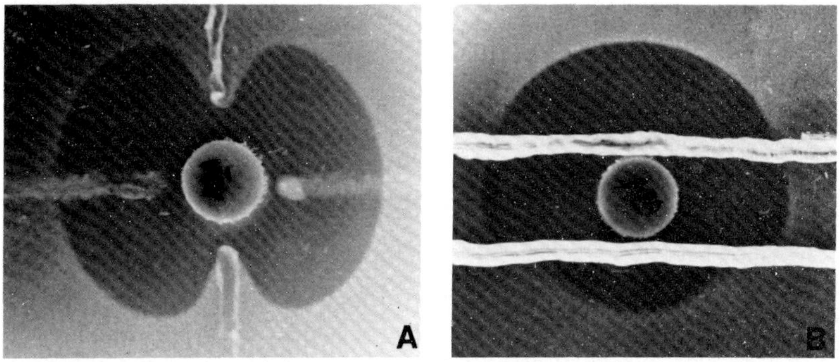

FIG. 1. *Patterns of the streak method illustrate the different effects of ampicillin-resistant and -susceptible H. influenzae isolates on inhibition zones. (A) Cross-streak pattern. The resistant isolate (upper-lower streak) caused distortion at the spherical inhibition zone, and the susceptible isolate (left-right streak) showed no effect on the zone. (B) Parallel streak pattern. The inhibition zone on the side of a resistant isolate (lower) was much smaller than the zone near the susceptible isolate (upper).*

TABLE 1. *Classification of isolates by Bauer-Kirby, capillary tube, and new streak methods*

Organism	Bauer-Kirby method	No. of isolates	Capillary tube method		Streak method	
			No. of beta-lactamase producers	No. of not beta-lactamase producers	No. of penicillinase producers	No. of not penicillinase producers
H. influenzae	Ampicillin resistant	13	13	0	13	0
(54 isolates)	Ampicillin susceptible	41	0	41	0	41
S. aureus	Penicillin resistant	21	21	0	0	0
(40 isolates)	Penicillin susceptible	19	0	19	0	19

also classified as penicillin resistant on the basis of the Bauer-Kirby technique. The classification of isolates that were not beta-lactamase producers was also consistent among the three techniques.

We believe our techniques have several useful features. The results are available more rapidly than are the Bauer-Kirby results. There is no need to purchase penicillin powder or prepare chromogenic cephalosporin powder, as is necessary for other methods (4, 14). Even when the tests are performed infrequently, preparation of spore-seeded plates from stored agar tubes can be completed quickly. Special antibiotic disks are not necessary for our technique because the method uses the same antibiotic disks as does the Bauer-Kirby procedure.

Since several antibiotic disks can be used on the same plate, it appears possible to test the inactivation of a variety of antibiotics. Previous studies have compared penicillinase production with resistance of gram-negative enteric organisms and *Bacteroides fragilis* (7, 9, 10). Preliminary tests have encouraged us to extend the use of our technique for studies of these other organisms as well.

Anthony Rooklin, Children's Hospital, Oakland, Calif., and Guido Controni, Children's Hospital, Wahington, D.C., kindly provided us with several test isolates. Doris Ceccotti provided valuable secretarial assistance.

LITERATURE CITED

1. **Adam, A. P., A. L. Barry, and E. J. Benner.** 1970. A simple rapid test to differentiate penicillin-susceptible from penicillin-resistant *Staphylococcus aureus*. J. Infect. Dis. 122:544–546.
2. **Bauer, A. W., W. M. M. Kirby, J. C. Sherris, and M. Turck.** 1966. Antibiotic susceptibility testing by a standardized single disc method. Am. J. Clin. Pathol. 45:493–496.
3. **Grove, D. C., and W. Randall.** 1955. Assay methods of antibiotics, p. 223–225. Medical Encyclopedia Inc., New York.
4. **Kammer, R. B., D. A. Preston, J. R. Turner, and L. C. Hawely.** 1975. Rapid detection of ampicillin-resistant *Haemophilus influenzae* and their susceptibility to sixteen antibiotics. Antimicrob. Agents Chemother. 8:91–94.
5. **Khan, W., S. Ross, W. Rodriguez, G. Controni, and A.**

K. Saz. 1974. *Haemophilus influenzae* type B resistant to ampicillin. A report of two cases. J. Am. Med. Assoc. 229:298–301.

6. **O'Callagham, C. H., A. Morris, S. M. Kirby, and A. H. Shindler.** 1972. Novel method for detection of β-lactamase by using a chromogenic cephalosporin substrate. Antimicrob. Agents Chemother. **1**:283–288.
7. **Percival, A., W. Brumfitt, and J. de Louvios.** 1963. The role of penicillinase in determining natural and acquired resistance of gram-negative bacteria to penicillins. J. Gen. Microbiol. **32**:77–89.
8. **Perrett, C. J.** 1954. Iodometric assay of penicillinase. Nature (London) **174**:1012–1013.
9. **Pincus, G., G. Veto, and A. I. Braude.** 1968. *Bacteriodes* penicillinase. J. Bacteriol. **96**:1437–1438.
10. **Richmond, M. H., and R. B. Sykes.** 1973. The β-lactamases of gram-negative bacteria and their possible physiological role. Adv. Microb. Physiol. **9**:31–88.
11. **Rosen, I. G., J. Jacobson, and R. Rudderman.** 1972. Rapid capillary tube method for detecting penicillin resistance in *Staphylococcus aureus*. Appl. Microbiol. **23**:649–650.
12. **Sabath, L. D., J. I. Casey, P. A. Ruch, L. L. Stumpf, and M. Finland.** 1971. Rapid microassay for circulating nephrotoxic antibiotics, p. 83–90. Antimicrob. Agents Chemother. 1970.
13. **Thomas, W. J., J. W. McReynolds, C. R. Mock, and D. W. Bailey.** 1974. Ampicillin-resistant *Haemophilus influenzae* meningitis. Lancet **1**:313.
14. **Thornsberry, C., and L. A. Kirven.** 1974. Ampicillin resistance in *Haemophilus influenzae* as determined by a rapid test for beta-lactamase production. Antimicrob. Agents Chemother. **6**:653–654.
15. **Thornsberry, C., and L. A. Kirven.** 1974. Antimicrobial susceptibility of *Haemophilus influenzae*. Antimicrob. Agents Chemother. **6**:620–624.

ANTIMICROBIAL AGENTS AND CHEMOTHERAPY, Sept. 1976, p. 567-568 Vol. 10, No. 3

Evolution of Transferable Antibiotic Resistance in Coliform Bacteria from Remote Environments

SHARON J. BURT AND D. R. WOODS*

Department of Microbiology, Rhodes University, Grahamstown, 6140, South Africa

Received for publication 24 May 1976

The influence of a mission hospital on the evolution of antibiotic resistance in coliform bacteria from a remote antibiotic-free Xhosa community and environment is described.

An initial study of the incidence of antibiotic resistance and R plasmids in urban and remote Xhosa communities and their environments was undertaken in 1973 (2). The study of the remote population and environment was initiated at a recently established mission hospital in a very remote area of the Transkei, East Coast, South Africa, among a Xhosa population and environment that had not previously been exposed to antibiotics. Since further investigations should provide a useful opportunity for the study of the evolution of resistance among populations and their environments, a second study of antibiotic resistance and R plasmids was carried out after 3 years among the same populations.

The urban population studied was a Xhosa community living in a crowded, modern township near East London, South Africa. These people have easy access to hospitals and doctors and are thus exposed to antibiotics. A total of 102 human stool specimens were obtained from hospitalized patients. The remote population was a Xhosa community from the Eastern Transkei. These rural people live in thatched mud huts that are clustered in groups of 5 to 10, each with its own cattle pen. This particular community is a "Red Blanket" community that is particularly reluctant to accept western customs and modern medicine. The isolated community is served by only one mission hospital, and the majority of the people have not been exposed to antibiotics. A total of 91 human stool specimens were obtained only from "first time" patients at the mission hospital, that is, those with no record of previous contact with a doctor or hospital. Forty-three environmental samples were obtained from the soil, dams, huts, cooking areas, and cattle pens.

The fecal and environmental samples were incubated in brilliant green bile broth (Difco) at 37°C before streaking on MacConkey purple agar. Isolated, yellow nonmucoid colonies, which were indole positive and formed gas in brilliant green bile lactose broth, were regarded as coliforms. The methods for determining antibiotic resistance and its transfer have been previously described (3).

During the 3 years between 1973 and 1976, the incidence of resistance to antibiotics of coliform bacteria from the remote community increased from 19 to 48%, but the transferable resistance remained the same (12 and 11%) (Table 1). The remote environment also showed an increase in resistance from 26 to 36% and a striking increase in transferable resistance from 0 to 7%. The urban population showed an increase in resistance from 69 to 83%, but a decrease in transferable resistance from 48 to 33%.

The difference in R plasmid-mediated resistance of the individual antibiotics in the remote population and environment over the 3 years is significant. In 1973 the transferable resistance of the remote population was due to ampicillin R plasmids, and no R plasmid strains were isolated from the environment. During the present study, strains harboring R plasmids for ampicillin, chloramphenicol, kanamycin, streptomycin, tetracycline, and septrin (23.5 μg of septrin-sulfamethoxazole plus 1.5 μg of trimethoprim) were isolated from the remote population. R plasmids for ampicillin, chloramphenicol, and tetracycline were isolated from coliform bacteria from the environment. Particularly interesting is the isolation from both the urban and remote populations of R plasmids for septrin, which has only been used over the last few years in South Africa. The highest degree of resistance in bacteria from both the urban and remote populations and the remote environment was for streptomycin, and the present study showed a marked increase in streptomycin resistance as compared with our 1973 results. Streptomycin is extensively used to combat the high incidence of tuberculosis among the Xhosa community.

The striking differences between the resist-

TABLE 1. *Resistance and transferable resistance in coliform bacteria from urban and remote communities*

Antibiotic	Urban population				Remote population				Remote environment			
	1973 study[a] (67)[b]		Present study (102)		1973 study (90)		Present study (91)		1973 study (51)		Present study (43)	
	R[c]	TR	R	TR	R	TR	R	TR	R	TR	R	TR
Ampicillin	49	45	62	25	7	17	8	7	4	0	3	5
Cephaloridine	7	0	2	0	6	0	11	0	16	0	8	0
Chloramphenicol	19	31	29	5	1	0	4	2	2	0	3	5
Kanamycin	18	42	24	13	0	0	1	1	0	0	0	0
Nalidixic acid	2	0	0	0	0	0	0	0	0	0	0	0
Nitrofurantoin	0	0	0	0	0	0	0	0	0	0	2	0
Streptomycin	46	10	81	18	11	0	38	7	6	0	12	0
Tetracycline	22	27	34	8	1	0	15	8	0	0	3	2
Septrin	9	0	22	8	0	0	10	1	0	0	1	0
Total[d]	69	48	83	33	19	12	48	11	26	0	36	7

[a] Results are from reference 2.
[b] Numbers in parentheses indicate the total number of strains.
[c] R, Percentage of resistant strains; TR, percentage of resistant strains that transfer resistance.
[d] Total of all the antibiotics studied.

ance in bacteria between the urban and remote communities demonstrate the selective force of antibiotics. The influence of the mission hospital and the selective force of antibiotics are further illustrated by the evolution of R plasmids in the remote population and environment.

We conclude that it is the influence of the use of antibiotics among the human population since there are no veterinary services in the area and the addition of antibiotics to animal feeds is not practiced (1). Continued monitoring of transferable drug resistance in these communities is important if the full benefit of modern antimicrobial therapy is to be derived.

D.R.W. acknowledges a grant from the South African Medical Research Council.

We thank S. Maarsingh, H. Bauer, and T. Botha for assistance with the collection of samples.

LITERATURE CITED

1. **Anderson, E. S.** 1965. Origin of transferable drug-resistance factors in the Enterobacteriaceae. Br. Med. J. 2:1289–1291.
2. **Marcos, D., and D. R. Woods.** 1973. Ecology of R factors: a study of urban and remote communities and their environments. S. Afr. Med. J. 47:340–341.
3. **Woods, D. R., D. Marcos, and D. A. Hendry.** 1972. The incidence of R factors among coliform bacteria. S. Afr. Med. J. **46**:189–191.

ANTIMICROBIAL AGENTS AND CHEMOTHERAPY, Sept. 1976, p. 569-570 Vol. 10, No. 3

Printed in U.S.A.

Inhibition of Antibiotic Activity In Vitro by Synthetic Melanin

MICHAEL BARZA,* JULES BAUM, AND ANNE KANE

Departments of Medicine and Ophthalmology, New England Medical Center Hospital and Tufts University School of Medicine, Boston, Massachusetts 02111*

Received for publication 12 April 1976

Synthetic melanin (100 to 1,000 μg/ml) markedly inhibited the in vitro activity of aminoglycosides and tetracyclines but did not affect the activity of beta-lactam antibiotics, erythromycin, or clindamycin.

In the course of studies of the penetration of antimicrobial agents into ocular tissues of rabbits, striking disparities in the concentrations of certain agents were noted between albino and pigmented rabbits (unpublished data). Since the only pertinent difference recognized between these species is the presence or absence of melanin, the following studies were undertaken to examine the effect of this pigment on antibacterial activity in vitro. To exclude the effect of other variables, a synthetic preparation of melanin was used.

Suspensions containing 100 and 1,000 μg of synthetic melanin (Sigma Chemical Co., St. Louis, Mo.) per ml of phosphate-buffered saline were distributed in test tubes. The following antibiotics were obtained as dry powders: sodium cephalothin, sodium cefazolin, potassium penicillin G, erythromycin gluceptate, and vancomycin hydrochloride (Eli Lilly and Co.), sodium oxacillin (Bristol Laboratories), clindamycin hydrochloride (Upjohn Co.), tetracycline hydrochloride (Lederle Laboratories), and streptomycin sulfate (Pfizer Laboratories). Gentamicin sulfate (Schering Corp.) and tobramycin sulfate (Eli Lilly and Co.) were obtained as injectable solutions. The antibiotics were dissolved in phosphate-buffered saline to concentrations of 1,000 and 100 μg/ml. One-fifth milliliter of antibiotic solution was added to 1.8 ml of melanin suspension; the combination was thoroughly mixed and assayed immediately and then stored at room temperature and assayed again 18 h later.

Antibiotic standards (100 to 3.1 μg/ml) were prepared in phosphate-buffered saline from the same parent solutions as those mixed with the pigment and were kept at room temperature together with the latter. Standards were always plated at the same time as specimens containing melanin, using a filter-paper disk modification of an agar diffusion bioassay (1). A strain of *Sarcina lutea* was used to assay clindamycin.

There was no effect of melanin on the antibacterial activity of penicillin G, oxacillin, cephalothin, cefazolin, erythromycin, or clindamycin when compared to the same concentration of antibiotic without the pigment. The results for the other five agents are shown in Table 1.

The activity of vancomycin was slightly reduced in the presence of melanin, whereas that of tetracycline and the aminoglycosides was strikingly decreased. With a few exceptions, the following generalizations appeared applicable regarding the inhibitory effect: (i) it was greater at the higher than at the lower concentration of melanin; (ii) it was evident immediately, but was slightly more pronounced after 18 h; (iii) at the lower concentration of pigment, inhibition was more striking in solutions containing 10 rather than 100 μg of antibiotic per ml. The last observation was not true of tetracycline or streptomycin after 18 h.

In tubes containing 100 μg of melanin and 100 μg of antibiotic per ml, a striking correlation was noted between the extent of inhibition of antibiotic activity and the formation of a dark-brown precipitate. The pH of the various solutions was 7.2 to 7.4 in each instance.

Synthetic melanin is a polymer of tyrosine of incompletely defined structure. The results of the present study indicate that melanin markedly inhibits the activity of aminoglycoside antibiotics and tetracycline, but not that of various other antimicrobial agents. Because polyvalent cations are known to interfere with the activity of tetracyclines and aminoglycosides, we determined the content of magnesium and calcium in the more concentrated suspension of pigment, using atomic absorption, and found these to be 0.3 and <0.1 mg/dl, respectively, levels that would be exceedingly unlikely to

TABLE 1. *Percentage of decrease in antibiotic activity after exposure to synthetic melanin suspension*

Antibiotic (μg/ml)	Concn of melanin (μg/ml)	% Decrease in activity	
		Immediate	After 18 h
Vancomycin[a]			
10	1,000	No effect	23 ± 2
100	1,000	No effect	31 ± 6
10	100	No effect	No effect
100	100	No effect	No effect
Tetracycline[b]			
10	1,000	26, 33	43, 48
100	1,000	25, 32	55, 58
10	100	No effect	No effect
100	100	No effect	20, 36
Gentamicin[a]			
10	1,000	66 ± 7	80 ± 2
100	1,000	74 ± 2	81 ± 4
10	100	21 ± 8	54 ± 5
100	100	9 ± 9	8 ± 12
Tobramycin[b]			
10	1,000	80, 82	88, 89
100	1,000	81, 82	88, 91
10	100	28, 35	65, 65
100	100	15, 16	5, 16
Streptomycin[b]			
10	1,000	26, 46	60, 78
100	1,000	19, 30	52, 63
10	100	12, 14	18, 44
100	100	0, 3	20, 22

[a] Mean ± standard deviation of three experiments.

[b] Data from two experiments.

inhibit the drugs. The effects of concentration and time on the interaction observed in these studies, as well as the correlation between inhibition and the formation of a visible precipitate, suggest that the phenomenon is due to a tight binding of antibiotic to the pigment.

Similar findings with regard to the aminoglycosides have been reported with a number of substances, including pus (2), feces (5), and tissue homogenates (3, 4). Kunin has suggested that binding of aminoglycosides may correlate with the number of free amino groups (4), and our data support this notion insofar as tobramycin possesses five, gentamicin three, and tetracycline one such structure, whereas streptomycin has two guanido groups. The structure of vancomycin is not known with certainty. The relevance of the present observations to the in vivo situation is not clear, especially since melanin is normally sequestered in intracellular organelles; however, it seems possible that this phenomenon could interfere with the assay of certain antibiotics in homogenates of melanin-containing tissues.

This study was supported by Public Health Service research grant EY01517 from the National Eye Institute.

We gratefully acknowledge the help of Eli Dubinsky in the measurements of calcium and magnesium.

LITERATURE CITED

1. **Barza, M., R. B. Brown, D. Shen, M. Gibaldi, and L. Weinstein.** 1975. Predictability of blood levels of gentamicin in man. J. Infect. Dis. **132**:165–174.
2. **Bryant, R. E., and D. Hammond.** 1974. Interaction of purulent material with antibiotics used to treat *Pseudomonas* infections. Antimicrob. Agents Chemother. **6**:702–707.
3. **Kaplan, J. M., G. H. McCracken, Jr., and E. Snyder.** 1973. Influence of methodology upon apparent concentrations of antibiotics in tissue. Antimicrob. Agents Chemother. **3**:143–146.
4. **Kunin, C. M.** 1970. Binding of antibiotics to tissue homogenates. J. Infect. Dis. **121**:55–63.
5. **Wagman, G. H., J. V. Bailey, and M. J. Weinstein.** 1974. Binding of aminoglycosides to feces. Antimicrob. Agents Chemother. **6**:415–417.

Antimicrobial Agents and Chemotherapy, Sept. 1976, p. 571-572
Vol. 10, No. 3

Antiviral Effects of Virazole in Chronic Hepatitis B Surface Antigen-Seropositive Chimpanzees

ALEXANDER E. DENES,* JAMES W. EBERT, KENNETH R. BERQUIST, BERT L. MURPHY, AND JAMES E. MAYNARD

Phoenix Laboratories Division, Center for Disease Control, Phoenix, Arizona 85014

Received for publication 17 May 1976

Virazole (Ribavirin, ICN 1229), a broad-spectrum, antiviral chemotherapeutic agent was used to treat two adult chronically hepatitis B surface antigen (HB_s Ag)-seropositive chimpanzees. No significant change in serum hepatitis B surface antigen was noted and no adverse reactions were observed. The role of viral replication in the chronic carrier state of hepatitis B is discussed.

Virazole (Ribavirin, ICN 1229, 1-β-D-ribofuranosyl-1,2,4-triazole-3-carboxamide) is a synthetic nucleoside with demonstrated activity against several ribonucleic acid and deoxyribonucleic acid viruses (8). The active metabolite, Virazole 5′-phosphate, is thought to inhibit guanosine 5′-phosphate biosynthesis in infected cells at the step involving the conversion of inosine 5′-phosphate to xanthosine 5′-phosphate and thus inhibit viral replication (9). In South America, preliminary clinical studies with the drug have been reported with encouraging results in acute hepatitis B as well as in chronic carriers of hepatitis B surface antigen (HB_s Ag) (5, 10, 11).

We treated two adult chronically HB_s Ag-seropositive chimpanzees with Virazole. Both animals were in good health and had no evidence of active liver disease either clinically or by liver biopsy. Virazole was given orally, as a liquid suspension, for 21 days. It was administered at 7 a.m. and 4 p.m. daily in 600-mg doses, with a total daily dose of 1,200 mg (ca. 20 mg/kg). Prior to initiation of the study, each animal had a complete blood count and automated chemistry profile (SMA-12), which includes the following serum chemistry determinations: calcium, phosphorus, urea nitrogen, glucose, uric acid, cholesterol, total proteins, albumin, total bilirubin, alkaline phosphatase, lactic dehydrogenase, and glutamic-oxaloacetic transaminase. These determinations, as well as a serum HB_s Ag determination, were performed twice a week during the period of drug administration and for 4 weeks thereafter. Liver biopsies were obtained weekly and examined after staining with hematoxylin and eosin and also by immunofluorescence for HB_s Ag and hepatitis B core antigen (HB_c Ag) (3). All serological determinations for HB_s Ag were by radioimmunoassay (Ausria II, Abbott Laboratories) (7).

No adverse reactions were noted. There were no significant changes in hematocrit, hemoglobin, or leukocyte counts. The only significant change in blood chemistry was a decrease in serum alkaline phosphatase in both animals, which returned to pretreatment values after the study was completed. Both animals remained highly seropositive for HB_s Ag during the investigation (Table 1). Serial dilutions of serum also did not demonstrate any significant decrease in the titer of HB_s Ag.

We were not able to show any beneficial effect of Virazole in our chronically HB_s Ag-seropositive animals. Although this study involved only two animals, our results suggest that Virazole may not be as effective in terminating the chronic HB_s Ag carrier state as has been reported (5). Although the results can be interpreted as demonstrating a lack of antiviral activity of this agent against the hepatitis B virus, they also raise an intriguing question about the role of viral replication in some chronically healthy carriers of HB_s Ag. Serial liver biopsies from both animals demonstrated cytoplasmic HB_s Ag by immunofluorescence prior to and after treament with Virazole but failed to show HB_c Ag in hepatocyte nuclei.

Table 1. *HB_s Ag content of Virazole-treated chimpanzees*

Animal no.	HB_s Ag content (SR units[a]) on day:							
	0	7	14	21	28	35	42	50
109	37	36	33	37	37	39	33	33
120	30	34	30	32	31	30	31	30

[a] Sample ratio (SR) units = counts per minute of test sample/counts per minute of control sample. Ratios above 2.6 were recorded as HB_s Ag positive. For titration purposes all specimens were assayed with one radioimmunoassay kit.

Early studies using immunofluorescence and immune electron microscopy demonstrated hepatitis B antigens in both cytoplasm and nuclei of hepatocytes (4, 6). The identification of the two antigens HB_s Ag and HB_c Ag resolved this problem (1). Subsequently, several investigators showed the exclusive localization of HB_c Ag in hepatocyte nuclei and its association with viral replication (2, 3). During acute hepatitis B virus infection, it is possible that a segment of the viral genome (a component of HB_c Ag) is integrated into the host's genome in much the same way that bacteriophages interact with lysogenic bacteria. Under certain circumstances, this interaction could result in the continuous cytoplasmic production of HB_s Ag without concurrent viral replication. In this situation, an agent such as Virazole would be without effect.

Virazole was supplied by ICN Pharmaceuticals, Irvine, Calif.

LITERATURE CITED

1. **Almeida, J. D., M. Rubenstein, and E. J. Scott.** 1971. New antigen-antibody system in Australia-antigen positive hepatitis. Lancet 2:1225–1227.
2. **Barker, L. F., F. U. Chisari, P. P. McGrath, D. W. Dalgart, R. L. Kirschstein, J. D. Almeida, T. S. Edgington, D. G. Sharp, and M. R. Peterson.** 1973. Transmission of type B viral hepatitis to Chimpanzees. J. Infect. Dis. 127:648–662.
3. **Berquist, K. R., J. M. Peterson, B. L. Murphy, J. W. Ebert, J. E. Maynard, and R. H. Purcell.** 1975. Hepatitis B antigens in serum and liver of chimpanzees acutely infected with hepatitis B virus. Infect. Immun. 12:602–605.
4. **Brzosko, W. D., K. Madalinski, K. Krawczynski, and A. Nowoslawski.** 1973. Duality of hepatitis B antigen and its antibody. I. Immunofluorescence studies. J. Infect. Dis. 127:424–428.
5. **Galvao, P. A. A., and I. O. Castro.** 1974. Treatment of acute viral hepatitis with a new antiviral compound. Rev. Bras. Clin. Ter. 3:221–228.
6. **Huang, S.-N., I. Millman, A. O'Connell, A. Aronoff, H. Gault, and B. S. Blumberg.** 1972. Virus-like particles in Australia antigen-associated hepatitis. Am. J. Pathol. 67:453–462.
7. **Ling, C., and L. Overby.** 1972. Prevalence of hepatitis B surface antigen as revealed by direct radioimmunoassay with ^{125}I-antibody. J. immunol. 109:834–841.
8. **Sidwell, R. W., J. H. Huffman, G. P. Khare, L. B. Allen, J. T. Witkowski, and R. K. Robins.** 1972. Broad spectrum antiviral activity of Virazole: 1-β-D-ribofuranosyl-1,2,4-triazole-3-carboxamide. Science 177:705–706.
9. **Streeter, D. G., J. T. Witkowski, P. K. Gyaneshwar, R. W. Sidwell, R. J. Bauer, R. K. Robins, and L. N. Simon.** 1973. Mechanism of action of 1-β-D-ribofuranosyl-1,2,4-triazole-3-carboxamide (Virazole), a new broad-spectrum antiviral agent. Proc. Natl. Acad. U.S.A. 70:1174–1178.
10. **Vilelea, M. P., W. A. Siqueira, S. H. S. Domingues, and F. S. Rodrigues.** 1974. Behaviour of Australia Antigen in cases of hepatitis treated with 1-beta-D-ribofuranosyl-1,2,4-triazole-3-carboxamide. Rev. Bras. Clin. Ter. 3:27–28.
11. **Zuniga, C. B., C. Almeida, A. C. S. Iervolino, I. O. Castro, and P. A. A. Galvao.** 1974. Action of 1-beta-D ribofuranosyl-1,2,4,-triazole-3-carboxamide (viramid, ICN 1229) in the treatment of acute viral hepatitis. Rev. Assn. Med. Brazil. 20:386–390.

ANTIMICROBIAL AGENTS AND CHEMOTHERAPY, Oct. 1976, p. 573-578 Vol. 10, No. 4

Printed in U.S.A.

Classification of R Plasmids by Incompatibility in *Pseudomonas aeruginosa*

H. SAGAI,* K. HASUDA, S. IYOBE, L. E. BRYAN, B. W. HOLLOWAY, AND S. MITSUHASHI

Department of Microbiology, School of Medicine, Gunma University, Maebashi, Japan; Department of Medical Bacteriology, University of Alberta, Edmonton, Canada; and Department of Genetics, Monash University, Clayton, Victoria 3168, Australia*

Received for publication 10 March 1976

R plasmids identified in *Pseudomonas aeruginosa* strains isolated in our laboratories were classified by their incompatibility characters by using intraspecies conjugation in *P. aeruginosa*. The fertility factor, FP2, was compatible with R plasmids belonging to all groups, and was classified in a new group. From these data, the plasmids examined have been placed into seven or eight incompatibility groups.

R plasmids in *Enterobacteriaceae* were originally classified by their *fi* character (18) or type of sex pili (14). More recently, the classification of R plasmids based on incompatibility has been generally used (4, 7), resulting in the recognition of more than 20 groups in the *Escherichia coli* system (9). In *Pseudomonas aeruginosa* strains, many R plasmids have been isolated (1, 2, 11-13, 15, 16), but almost all have been found to be either conjugally nontransferable or transferable at very low frequency to *E. coli* (1, 11, 16); therefore they cannot readily be classified in this system. Those few that are conjugally transferable to *E. coli* have been classified as P group (7) or C group (6, 13). Bryan et al. (1, 2, 17) proposed an incompatibility classification of plasmids detected in *P. aeruginosa* based on intraspecies conjugation in *Pseudomonas* and classified R plasmids into four incompatibility groups, P-1, P-2, P-3, and P-4. This paper deals with the classification of additional R plasmids from *P. aeruginosa* by incompatibility testing, using intraspecies conjugation in *Pseudomonas*.

MATERIALS AND METHODS

Bacterial strains. Two strains of *P. aeruginosa*, ML4262 (*trp⁻ his⁻ ilv⁻ met⁻ rif*ʳ) (*rif*ʳ indicates rifampin resistant) and ML4600 (*trp⁻ his⁻*), which are isogenic except for the characters given, and two independently isolated strains, *P. aeruginosa* 280 (*rif*ʳ *met⁻*) (1) and *P. aeruginosa* 5265 (1), were used as host strains for the R plasmids.

R plasmids. R plasmids and their resistance markers are shown in Table 1.

Drugs. Tetracycline (Tc), chloramphenicol (Cm), streptomycin (Sm), and sulfanilamide (Su) were kindly supplied by Japan Lederle Co., Sankyo Seiyaku Co., Kyowa Hakko Co., and the Dainihon Seiyaku Co., respectively. Carbenicillin (Cb), lividomycin (Lv), rifampin (Rp), and gentamicin C complex (Gm) were supplied by the Fujisawa Seiyaku Co., Kowa Co., Daiichi Seiyaku Co., and Shionogi Co., respectively. Mercuric chloride (Hg; Wako Jyunyaku) was obtained commercially.

Media. Nutrient broth and nutrient agar were used routinely. Nutrient broth consisted of 10 g of beef extract, 10 g of peptone, and 3 g of NaCl in 1,000 ml of distilled water. Nutrient agar consisted of nutrient broth supplemented with 1.5% agar. The transconjugants that had acquired drug resistance were selected on nutrient agar containing the appropriate selective drug together with Rp. For the assay of Su resistance or the selection of Su-resistant transconjugants, semisynthetic medium was used, which consisted of 1,000 ml of medium A (8) to which 2 g of Casamino Acids, 10 mg of tryptophan, 2 mg of nicotinic acid, 10 mg of thiamine, 2 g of glucose, and 15 g of agar were added. Medium A consisted of 8 g of $Na_2HPO_4 \cdot 12H_2O$, 2 g of KH_2PO_4, 0.4 g of sodium citrate, 0.1 g of $MgSO_4 \cdot 7H_2O$, and 1.0 g of $(NH_4)_2SO_4$ in 1,000 ml of distilled water.

Incompatibility experiments. Two milliliters of a culture of recipient cells (ML4262), either carrying or not carrying an R plasmid, and 0.5 ml of donor culture (ML4600 R^+) were mixed at early stationary phases of growth. The mixed culture was incubated with gentle shaking at 37°C for 2 h, and appropriate dilutions were then spread on selective plates. Five of the colonies that grew on the plates were cloned three times, using the same medium, and their drug resistance was examined. The stability of two R plasmids coexisting in the same cell was examined after subculture for at least 10 generations in nutrient broth containing no drug.

Transconjugants carrying two plasmids. When transconjugant cells were concluded to carry two R plasmids, 2 ml of recipient (ML4262) culture and 0.5 ml of donor (ML4600 R_1^+ R_2^+) culture were mixed and gently shaken for 2 h. Then appropriate dilutions of the mixed culture were plated on two plates, selecting for either R_1 or R_2, and the resistance patterns of the transconjugants that grew on each plate were examined. The percentage of transconjugants possessing only R_1 (or R_2) as a fraction of the total

TABLE 1. *R plasmids*

R plasmid	Drug resistance	Reference
Rms159	Tc.Cm.Sm.Hg	This paper
Rms161	Cm.Sm.Su.Km.Hg	This paper
Rms161-1[a]	Cm.Km.Hg	This paper
Rms164	Sm.Su.Gm.Hg.	This paper
Rms164-1[a]	Su.Gm.Hg	This paper
Rms178	Tc.Cm.Sm.Su.Cb	Iyobe et al. (11)
Rms163	Tc.Cm.Su	Iyobe et al. (11)
Rms176	Sm	Iyobe et al. (11)
Rms148	Sm	Sagai et al. (16)
Rms149	Sm.Su.Gm.Cb	Sagai et al. (16)
Rms149-1[a]	Su.Cb	Sagai et al. (16)
RP4	Tc.Km.Cb	Datta et al. (7)
R1b931	Tc.Sm.Hg	Bryan et al. (1)
R1b130	Sm.Su.Gm.Hg	Bryan et al. (1)
R1b151	Sm.Su.Gm.Cb	Bryan et al. (2)
R1b5265	Sm.Su	Shahrabadi et al. (17)
FP2	Hg	Holloway (10)

[a] Rms161-1, Rms164-1, and Rms149-1 are mutants that have lost one or more resistance markers.

number of the transconjugants obtained by selection for R_1 (or R_2) was calculated.

RESULTS

Classification of R plasmids by incompatibility tests. Incompatibility testing of R plasmids isolated from *P. aeruginosa* strains in Japan (11) and West Germany (16) and from RP4 (7) was performed. Rms159 was transferred to the recipient strain at a frequency of 10^{-2}, but its transfer frequency was decreased when the recipient strain carried Rms161, Rms161-1, Rms164, or Rms164-1 (Table 2). In these four cases, all resistances conferred by the resident R plasmids were eliminated from the transconjugants by the newly transferred Rms159. In reciprocal transfer experiments, the transfer of Rms164 or Rms164-1 was slightly reduced by Rms159, and neither plasmid could coexist with Rms159. When Rms159, Rms164, or Rms161 was transferred to the Rms178$^+$ recipient, Rms178 was eliminated by all three, although the transfer frequency of Rms159 or Rms164 was not reduced. In reciprocal transfers, Rms178 coexisted with Rms159 or Rms164 but not with Rms161, although the transfer frequency of Rms178 was reduced by the presence of either one of the three plasmids in the recipient (Table 2). If Rms178 coexists with either Rms159 or Rms164 separately in a cell, the two plasmids may be transferred independently from the transconjugant. But retransfer of R plasmids from five clones of ML4262 that had acquired the drug resistances of both Rms178 and Rms159 (or Rms164) showed that resistance markers specific for each of the plasmids did not subsequently segregate in 20 transconjugants, even when selected for either Cb, an Rms178 marker, or Hg, an Rms159 (or Rms164) marker. These data suggested that Rms159 or Rms164 coexisted with Rms178 after the formation of a recombinant between both plasmids. Therefore, we concluded that Rms178 did not coexist with Rms159 or Rms164 as an independent plasmid; i.e., it was not compatible with Rms159 or Rms164. On the other hand, Rms159 coexisted stably with each of three plasmids, Rms149, Rms163, and RP4, and Rms164-1 coexisted with Rms148 in the same host cell. Therefore, we concluded that Rms159, Rms161, Rms164, and Rms178 form a single incompatibility group, different from each of the plasmids Rms163, Rms149, Rms148, and RP4.

Rms163 was transferred to recipient cells carrying either Rms159, Rms164, Rms176, Rms149, Rms148, or RP4. In all cases except Rms176, the transfer frequency of Rms163 was not reduced by the resident R plasmid and Rms163 coexisted with the resident plasmid in the recipient. When Rms176 was transferred to a recipient carrying Rms163, the transfer frequency was reduced, and Rms163 was excluded by Rms176. Therefore, Rms163 and Rms176 form a single incompatibility group, different from the group of Rms159 and from each of the plasmids Rms148, Rms149, and RP4.

The transfer frequency of Rms149 was not reduced by the presence of Rms159, Rms163, or RP4 but was reduced slightly by Rms149-1, and Rms149 coexisted with each of the plasmids Rms159, Rms163, and RP4. When the transconjugants concluded to carry both Rms149 and Rms149-1 were examined by retransfer experiments, the resistance pattern of all transconjugants thus obtained was Sm.Su.Gm and Cb, and the markers of Rms149-1 (Su.Cb) were not obtained even when selection was made for Su or Cb. Therefore we concluded that Rms149 eliminated Rms149-1. Rms149-1 coexisted with Rms148. In reciprocal experiments, Rms148 coexisted with Rms164-1, Rms163, RP4, and Rms149-1, and RP4 coexisted stably with Rms159, Rms163, Rms149, and Rms148 (Table 2). In these cases, the transfer frequency of Rms148 or RP4 was not reduced by the resident R plasmid in the recipient strains. From the results described above, we therefore conclude that there are five groups, consisting of (i) Rms159, Rms161, Rms164, and Rms178, (ii) Rms163 and Rms176, (iii) Rms148, (iv) Rms149, and (v) RP4.

Retransfer of R plasmids from the transconjugants. Incompatibility testing was carried out to determine whether two plasmids coexisted in the same host. It is possible, however, that two incompatible R plasmids may appear to coexist in a cell after recombination

TABLE 2. *Incompatibility testing of R plasmids*[a]

Donor (ML4600) carrying:	Recipient (ML4262) carrying:	Selection	Frequency	Drug resistance of transconjugants	
				Ratio[b]	Possessing[a]:
Rms159		Tc	4.2×10^{-2}		
		Sm	4.1×10^{-2}		
		Hg	5.8×10^{-2}		
	Rms164	Tc	1.2×10^{-3}	5/5	Rms159 only
	Rms164-1	Tc	3.1×10^{-4}	5/5	Rms159 only
	Rms161	Tc	6.0×10^{-4}	5/5	Rms159 only
	Rms161-1	Sm	9.0×10^{-4}	5/5	Rms159 only
	Rms178	Hg	4.5×10^{-2}	5/5	Rms159 only
					Rms159 only
Rms164		Gm	2.2×10^{-1}		
	Rms159	Gm	2.1×10^{-2}	5/5	Rms164 only
	Rms161	Gm	1.3×10^{-3}	5/5	Rms164 only
	Rms178	Gm	1.7×10^{-1}	5/5	Rms164 only
Rms164-1		Gm	7.8×10^{-2}		
	Rms159	Gm	4.5×10^{-3}	5/5	Rms164-1 only
Rms161		Lv	9.3×10^{-3}		
	Rms164	Lv	2.3×10^{-7}	5/5	Rms161 only
	Rms178	Lv	7.8×10^{-6}	5/5	Rms161 only
Rms178		Tc	1.3×10^{-2}		
		Cb	1.0×10^{-2}		
	Rms159	Cb	1.7×10^{-4}	5/5	Both
	Rms164	Cb	1.2×10^{-6}	5/5	Both
	Rms161	Tc	4.0×10^{-6}	5/5	Rms178 only
Rms159	Rms163	Sm	6.1×10^{-2}	5/5	Both
	Rms149	Tc	3.7×10^{-2}	5/5	Both
	RP4	Sm	5.8×10^{-2}	5/5	Both
Rms164-1	Rms148	Gm	5.3×10^{-2}	5/5	Both
Rms163		Tc	3.8×10^{-2}		
		Su	8.2×10^{-2}		
	Rms159	Su	2.5×10^{-2}	5/5	Both
	Rms164	Tc	7.7×10^{-2}	5/5	Both
	Rms176	Tc	3.2×10^{-7}	5/5	Rms163 only
	Rms149	Tc	4.9×10^{-2}	5/5	Both
	Rms148	Tc	3.1×10^{-3}	5/5	Both
	RP4	Su	3.6×10^{-2}	5/5	Both
Rms176		Sm	1.1×10^{-2}		
	Rms164-1	Sm	2.6×10^{-2}	5/5	Both
	Rms163	Sm	6.2×10^{-6}	5/5	Rms176 only
Rms149		Gm	6.0×10^{-6}		
		Cb	4.0×10^{-6}		
	Rms159	Cb	2.9×10^{-6}	5/5	Both
	Rms163	Cb	5.4×10^{-6}	5/5	Both
	Rms149-1	Gm	3.2×10^{-7}		
	RP4	Gm	5.1×10^{-6}	5/5	Both
Rms149-1		Cb	5.2×10^{-6}		
	Rms148	Cb	5.1×10^{-6}	5/5	Both

TABLE 2—*Continued*

Donor (ML4600) carrying:	Recipient (ML4262) carrying:	Selection	Frequency	Drug resistance of transconjugants	
				Ratio[b]	Possessing[a]:
Rms148		Sm	1.7×10^{-3}		
	Rms164-1	Sm	4.7×10^{-3}	5/5	Both
	Rms163	Sm	2.1×10^{-3}	5/5	Both
	Rms149-1	Sm	1.4×10^{-3}	5/5	Both
	RP4	Sm	2.5×10^{-3}	5/5	Both
RP4		Lv	1.4×10^{-1}		
		Cb	1.3×10^{-1}		
	Rms159	Lv	1.2×10^{-1}	5/5	Both
	Rms163	Lv	7.7×10^{-2}	5/5	Both
	Rms149	Lv	6.3×10^{-2}	5/5	Both
	Rms148	Cb	2.1×10^{-1}	5/5	Both

[a] See text for details.
[b] Nominator, number of transconjugants possessing the indicated R plasmid(s); denominator, number of transconjugants examined.

between the plasmids, as was seen in the case of Rms159 and Rms178 and of Rms164 and Rms178. In these cases, the two original plasmids were not transferred separately from the transconjugants. Retransfer of plasmids from the transconjugants that were concluded to carry two plasmids was considered necessary to confirm the separate existence of both plasmids in the cell. The data of retransfer experiments are shown in Table 3.

In all combinations of the five groups, two plasmids were retransferred separately from the transconjugants, indicating that both plasmids existed separately in the transconjugants and thus confirming the five incompatibility groups of *P. aeruginosa* R plasmids.

Comparison of incompatibility groups with other plasmids. It was reported that Rlb130, Rlb931, and other plasmids form one incompatibility group, P-2 (1), and that Rlb151 belongs to a separate group, P-3 (2). The P-3 group was identical with the C group (17) that was classified in the *E. coli* system (6). We carried out further incompatibility testing of all plasmids that were classified by the tests described above, using Rlb130, Rlb931, Rlb151, and FP2. FP2 is an extrachromosomal and transferable genetic element in *P. aeruginosa* and has been used as a sex factor for genetic studies (10).

The transfer frequency of Rlb130 was reduced by the presence of Rms159 in the recipient but not by any other plasmid including FP2, and Rlb130 did not coexist with Rms159 (Table 4). Rlb931, a member of incompatibility group P-2, did not coexist with Rms164. Therefore it can be concluded that Rms159, Rms161, Rms164, and Rms178 belong to the P-2 group (Table 4).

TABLE 3. *Retransfer of the R plasmids from transconjugants*

Donor (ML4600) carrying both plasmids[a]		Selection for:		% of cells carrying only[b]:	
R_1	R_2	R_1 or R_2	Drug	R_1	R_2
Rms163	Rms164	R_1	Tc	80	
		R_2	Cm		93
Rms149	Rms159	R_1	Cb	10	
		R_2	Tc		100
Rms164-1	Rms148	R_1	Hg	100	
		R_2	Sm		100
Rms159	RP4	R_1	Sm	100	
		R_2	Cb		56
Rms163	Rms149	R_1	Tc	93	
		R_2	Sm		8
Rms148	Rms163	R_1	Sm	100	
		R_2	Tc		100
Rms163	RP4	R_1	Cm	100	
		R_2	Lv		100
Rms149-1	Rms148	R_1	Cb	5	
		R_2	Sm		100
Rms149	RP4	R_1	Sm	15	
		R_2	Tc		100
RP4	Rms148	R_1	Cb	100	
		R_2	Sm		100

[a] ML4262 was used as the recipient.
[b] Ratio of cells carrying only one type of R plasmid to total number of transconjugants obtained when selected for either R_1 or R_2.

The transfer frequency of Rlb151 was not affected by the presence of any of the resident plasmids, Rms159, Rms163, Rms149, Rms148, RP4, and FP2, in the recipient, and Rlb151 coexisted with Rms161-1, Rms163, Rms149-1, Rms148, RP4, and FP2 (Table 4). Retransfer experiments showed that all transconjugants that apparently carried two plasmids subse-

TABLE 4. *Incompatibility testing of R plasmids*

Donor (ML4600) carrying:	Recipient (ML4262) carrying:	Selection	Frequency	Drug resistance of transconjugants	
				Ratio	Possessing[a]:
Rlb130		Sm	9.2×10^{-1}		
		Gm	6.9×10^{-1}		
		Hg	7.0×10^{-1}		
	Rms159	Gm	1.2×10^{-3}	5/5	Rlb130 only
	Rms163	Sm	1.9×10^{-1}	5/5	Both
	Rms149	Hg	2.7×10^{-1}	5/5	Both
	Rms148	Gm	2.8×10^{-1}	5/5	Both
	RP4	Sm	1.7×10^{-1}	5/5	Both
	FP2	Sm	1.9×10^{-1}		
Rlb931		Tc	3.2×10^{-1}		
	Rms164	Tc	4.1×10^{-2}	5/5	Rlb931 only
Rlb151		Sm	2.8×10^{-1}		
		Gm	8.1×10^{-1}		
	Rms161-1	Gm	9.9×10^{-1}	5/5	Both
	Rms163	Sm	3.0×10^{-1}	5/5	Both
	Rms149-1	Sm	2.8×10^{-1}	5/5	Both[b]
	Rms148	Gm	7.8×10^{-1}	5/5	Both[c]
	RP4	Sm	3.2×10^{-1}	5/5	Both
	FP2	Sm	3.1×10^{-1}	5/5	Both
FP2		Hg	3.0×10^{-2}		
	Rms178	Hg	1.7×10^{-2}	5/5	Both
	Rms163	Hg	7.6×10^{-3}	5/5	Both
	Rms149	Hg	4.2×10^{-3}	5/5	Both
	Rms148	Hg	2.8×10^{-3}	5/5	Both
	RP4	Hg	3.1×10^{-3}	5/5	Both
	Rlb151	Hg	8.2×10^{-3}	5/5	Both

[a] See text.

[b] Incompatibility testing was done with Sm, Gm, and Cb resistance. Both R plasmids specify Cb resistance, but Rms149-1 specifies a higher level of Cb resistance (800 μg/ml) than Rlb151 (200 μg/ml) in ML4262.

[c] Both plasmids specify Sm resistance, but Rms148 specifies a higher level of resistance than Rlb151.

quently transferred each plasmid independently (Table 5), and Rlb151 was concluded to be compatible with each of Rms161-1, Rms163, Rms149-1, Rms148, RP4, and FP2.

Shahrabadi et al. (17) reported that Rlb5265 was compatible with the R plasmids that were classified into P-1, P-2, and P-3 groups and was assigned to the P-4 group. However, because Rlb5265 was not transferable to the test strains, ML4262 and ML4600, *P. aeruginosa* 280 (rif^r met^-) (1) was used as the recipient, and its incompatibility was tested by the method of Bryan et al. (1). The transfer frequency of Rlb5265 was not reduced by the resident plasmids, RP4, Rlb931, Rlb151, Rms163, Rms148, and FP2, and Rlb5265 coexisted stably with RP4, Rlb931, Rlb151, Rms163, and FP2. The coexistence of Rlb5265 and Rms148 could not be examined because the single resistance marker of Rms148 was masked by those of Rlb5265. The incompatibility testing of Rlb5265 and Rms149 was impossible due to nontransferability of Rms149 to 280 (rif^r met^-).

DISCUSSION

The data of the incompatibility groups are summarized in Table 6 and show additions to the classification of Bryan et al., (1). Rms148 and Rms149 are shown as P-7 and P-8 group plasmids, respectively, although we could not perform complete incompatibility testing because of nontransferability of Rms149 and

TABLE 5. *Retransfer of plasmids from transconjugants*

Donor (ML4600) carrying either[a]:		Selection for either:		% of cells carrying only[b]:	
R_1	R_2	R_1 or R_2	Drug	R_1	R_2
Rms161-1	Rlb151	R_1	Lv	77	
		R_2	Sm		100
Rms163	Rlb151	R_1	Tc	92	
		R_2	Sm		100
Rlb151	Rms149-1	R_1	Sm	100	
		R_2	Cb[c]		3
Rlb151	Rms148	R_1	Cb	100	
		R_2	Sm[d]		27
RP4	Rlb151	R_1	Tc	93	
		R_2	Sm		93
FP2	Rlb151	R_1	Hg	68	
		R_2	Sm		100
FP2	Rms178	R_1	Hg	86	
		R_2	Tc		100
FP2	Rms163	R_1	Hg	100	
		R_2	Tc		100
FP2	Rms149	R_1	Hg	100	
		R_2	Sm		100
FP2	Rms148[e]	R_1	Hg	1.5	
		R_2	Sm		100
FP2	RP4	R_1	Hg	100	
		R_2	Tc		100

[a] ML4262 was used as the recipient.

[b] Ratio of cells carrying only one type of R plasmid to total number of transconjugants obtained when selected for either R_1 or R_2.

[c] 300 μg of Cb per ml was used for selection of Rms149-1.

[d] 100 μg of Sm per ml was used for selection of Rms148.

[e] ML4262 was used as the host strain of R plasmids (see text).

TABLE 6. *Summarized data of the incompatibility grouping of R plasmids in P. aeruginosa*

Group	R plasmid
P-1	RP4
P-2	Rlb931, Rlb130, Rlb680, Rlb290, Rlb546, Rlb442, Rlb454, Rlb3108, Rlb55, Rlb13, Rsu38, Rms159, Rms161, Rms164, Rms178, Rms169, Rms170, Rms171, Rms172, Rms173, Rms174, Rms162, Rms146, Rms196, Rms197, Rms198, Rms199
P-3	Rlb151
P-4	Rlb5265
P-5	Rms163, Rms176
P-6	FP2
P-7	Rms148
P-8	Rms149

Rlb5265 and because of masking of Rms148-specified streptomycin resistance by Rlb5265.

Almost all of the R plasmids demonstrated from *P. aeruginosa* in Japan have been classified into the P-2 group (Table 6) except two plasmids, Rms163 and Rms176 (11). A similar prevalence of the P-2 group has been observed among R plasmids detected in isolates of *P. aeruginosa* in North America (2, 17). Transfer of P-2 group R plasmids by conjugation to *E. coli* strains has not been observed (1, 11, 17). These results suggest that the P-2 plasmids are representative of conjugative R plasmids in *P. aeruginosa* and that the origin of R plasmids in *P. aeruginosa* may be different from that of plasmids identified in species of the *Enterobacteriaceae*. The P-5 plasmids, Rms163 and Rms176, were detected in *P. aeruginosa* strains of the same clinic (11), and both P-7 and P-8 plasmids were isolated from the same strain in Germany (16). These groups are seen to be rare types in *P. aeruginosa*.

We are collecting many R plasmids in an attempt to extend the P-4, P-6, P-7, and P-8 incompatibility groups and to clarify the relationship between the P-4 and the P-7 and P-8 groups.

LITERATURE CITED

1. **Bryan, L. E., S. D. Semeka, M. H. Van Den Elzen, J. E. Kinnear, and R. E. S. Whitehouse.** 1973. Characteristics of R931 and other *Pseudomonas aeruginosa* R factors. Antimicrob. Agents Chemother. 3:625–637.
2. **Bryan, L. E., M. S. Shahrabadi, and H. M. Van Den Elzen.** 1974. Gentamicin resistance in *Pseudomonas aeruginosa* R-factor-mediated resistance. Antimicrob. Agents Chemother. 6:191–199.
3. **Coetzee, J. N., N. Datta, and R. W. Hedges.** 1972. R factors from *Proteus rettgeri*. J. Gen. Microbiol. 72:543–552.
4. **Datta, N.** 1974. Epidemiology and classification of plasmids, p. 9–15. *In* D. Schlessinger (ed.), Microbiology – 1974. American Society for Microbiology, Washington, D.C.
5. **Datta, N., and R. W. Hedges.** 1971. Compatibility groups among fi⁻ R factors. Nature (London) **234**:222–223.
6. **Datta, N., and R. W. Hedges.** 1972. R factors identified in Paris, some conferring gentamicin resistance, constitute a new compatibility group. Ann. Inst. Pasteur Paris **129**:849–852.
7. **Datta, N., R. W. Hedges, E. J. Shaw, R. B. Sykes, and M. H. Richmond.** 1971. Properties of an R factor from *Pseudomonas aeruginosa*. J. Bacteriol. **108**:1244–1249.
8. **Davis, B. D., and E. S. Mingioli.** 1960. Mutants of *Escherichia coli* requiring methionine or vitamin B12. J. Bacteriol. **60**:17–29.
9. **Hedges, R. W., V. Rodriguez-Lemoine, and N. Datta.** 1975. R factors from *Serratia marcescens*. J. Gen. Microbiol. **86**:88–92.
10. **Holloway, B. W.** 1969. Genetics of *Pseudomonas*. Bacteriol. Rev. **33**:419–443.
11. **Iyobe, S., K. Hasuda, A. Fuse, and S. Mitsuhashi.** 1974. Demonstration of R factors from *Pseudomonas aeruginosa*. Antimicrob. Agents Chemother. **5**:547–552.
12. **Kawakami, Y., F. Mikoshiba, S. Nagasaki, H. Matsumoto, and T. Tazaki.** 1972. Prevalence of *Pseudomonas aeruginosa* strains possessing R factor in a hospital. J. Antibiot. **25**:607–609.
13. **Kontomichalou, P., and E. Papachristou.** 1975. Multiresistance plasmids in *Pseudomonas aeruginosa* highly resistant to gentamicin, p. 329–348. *In* S. Mitsuhashi and H. Hashimoto (ed.), Microbial drug resistance. University of Tokyo Press, Tokyo.
14. **Lawn, A. M., G. G. Meynell, E. Meynell, and N. Datta.** 1967. Sex pili and the classification of sex factors in the *Enterobacteriaceae*. Nature (London) **216**:343–346.
15. **Roe, E., B. J. Jones, and E. J. L. Lowbury.** 1971. Transfer of antibiotic resistance between *Pseudomonas aeruginosa, Escherichia coli,* and other gram-negative bacilli in burns. Lancet **1**:149–152.
16. **Sagai, H., V. Krcmery, K. Hasuda, S. Iyobe, H. Knothe, and S. Mitsuhashi.** 1975. R factor mediated resistance to aminoglycoside antibiotics in *Pseudomonas aeruginosa*. Jpn. J. Microbiol. **19**:427–432.
17. **Shahrabadi, M. S., L. E. Bryan, and H. M. Van Den Elzen.** 1975. Further properties of P-2 R-factors of *Pseudomonas aeruginosa* and their relationship to other plasmids. Can. J. Microbiol. **21**:592–605.
18. **Watanabe, T., H. Nishida, C. Ogata, T. Arai, and S. Sato.** 1964. Episome-mediated transfer of drug resistance in *Enterobacteriaceae*. VII. Two types of naturally occurring R factors. J. Bacteriol. **88**:716–726.

Antimicrobial Agents and Chemotherapy, Oct. 1976, p. 579-591
Vol. 10, No. 4

Mode of Action of Penicillins In Vivo and In Vitro in *Bacillus megaterium*

TETSUO OKA

Tokyo Research Laboratory, Kyowa Hakko Co., Machidashi, Tokyo, Japan

Received for publication 10 February 1976

A new system in which the in vivo and in vitro formation of cross-links in the peptidoglycan of *Bacillus megaterium* can be compared directly has been developed. The method for the determination of the in vivo cross-linking consists of lysozyme digestion of acetylated [^{14}C]diaminopimelic acid-labeled cells and Bio-Gel P-6 gel filtration of the digest. The elution profile indicates the cell wall synthesized in vivo consists of highly cross-linked fractions (44%), bisdisaccharide peptide(s) (38%), and disaccharide peptide(s) (18%). The in vitro system showed a high synthetic activity of cross-linked peptidoglycan. The synthesis was inhibited completely by 83.3 μg of ristocetin or vancomycin per ml or 10^{-4} M *p*-chloromercuribenzoate and inhibited only partially by penicillins. The polymerization was stimulated by high concentrations of sucrose, glycerol, amino acids, or dimethyl sulfoxide. The formation of cross-links was inhibited 50% at 0.3 μg of dicloxacillin per ml and 90% at 0.5 μg or more. It was also stimulated by high concentrations of sucrose, glycerol, or dimethyl sulfoxide. Effective concentrations of dicloxacillin on the growth, viability, and morphology of *B. megaterium* were determined. Sharp inhibition of cross-linking occurred in vivo and in vitro at these effective concentrations, whereas the incorporation of [^{14}C]-diaminopimelate into bacterial cells was not affected at all. Cell-bound dicloxacillin reduced severely the degree of cross-linking in the cell wall synthesized after transfer to a dicloxacillin-free medium. Cell wall synthesized in the presence of dicloxacillin showed a higher rate of turnover than did the normal cell wall. Moreover, disaccharide peptide(s) was degraded faster than was bisdisaccharide peptide(s) in dicloxacillin-treated cells. From these observations, the primary target of penicillin action in *B. megaterium* is discussed in relation to the inhibition of cross-linking, penicillin-binding components, and cell lysis.

Although it has long been believed that penicillin interferes with the biosynthesis of the structural element of the bacterial cell wall, its exact target is still ambiguous. Most studies have been done with *Escherichia coli*, which is relatively insensitive to penicillins. Besides, it is increasingly clear that there is more than one target of penicillin action in it (2, 20), making the situation complex.

The other aspect of the problem is that there are quite a few systems in which exact comparison of in vivo and in vitro action of penicillin is possible. For example, although *E. coli* was the first organism to show penicillin-sensitive transpeptidation in vitro (7), penicillin did not affect the cross-linking in vivo (19). Although *Bacillus* are quite sensitive to penicillins and their in vitro cell wall-synthesizing system also catalyzes transpeptidation (26), it has only recently become possible to measure the extent of cross-linking of diaminopimelic acid (Dpm) in vivo (3).

A new system by which in vivo and in vitro cell wall synthesis and cross-linking are easily compared has been developed in this laboratory. In addition to fundamental properties of the system, the results of studies to answer the following questions will be presented in this paper. (i) Will penicillins inhibit in vivo cross-linking at concentrations effective in vitro? If so, to what extent and how? (ii) Will cell-bound penicillins inhibit the formation of cross-links during successive growth in a penicillin-free medium? (iii) What is the fate of the cell wall synthesized in the presence of penicillin after growth in a penicillin-free medium?

MATERIALS AND METHODS

Growth. *Bacillus megaterium* KM (17) was grown in a 30-liter jar fermenter with agitation (400 rpm) and aeration (20 liters/min) at 37°C. The fermenter contained 20 liters of a bouillon medium consisting of 2% dehydrated nutrient broth (Kyokuto, Tokyo) and 0.5% yeast extract (pH 7). Cells were harvested by centrifugation late in the logarithmic phase of growth, washed once with saline (0.8% NaCl in 0.01 M phosphate buffer, pH 7, containing 0.001 M $MgCl_2$), and stored frozen at −20°C.

Preparation of *B. megaterium* KM particulate. A total of 20 g of the frozen cells was mixed with the same amount of washed alumina powder (Merck, Darmstadt, Germany) and ground in a mortar with a pestle at 0°C for 20 min. A 30-ml amount of 0.05 M tris(hydroxymethyl)aminomethane (Tris)-hydrochloride buffer (pH 7.5) containing 10^{-3} M $MgCl_2$ and 10^{-3} M dithiothreitol was added to the homogenate, and the mixture was first centrifuged at 10,000 × *g* for 10 min and then centrifuged at 100,000 × *g* for 30 min. The precipitates were washed once by centrifugation and finally suspended in the same buffer at a protein concentration of 3 to 6 mg/ml, as measured by the method of Lowry et al. (8). They were dispensed in 200-μl quantities into small test tubes and were stored frozen at −20°C.

Assay of polymerization in vitro. The standard reaction mixture consisted of 0.167 M Tris-hydrochloride (pH 8.5), 0.0167 M $MgCl_2$, 10^{-3} M uridine diphosphate-*N*-acetylglucosamine (UDP-GlcNAc) (Sigma Chemical Co., St. Louis, Mo.), and 10^{-4} M UDP-*N*-acetylmuramyl-LAla-DGlu-[^{14}C or ^{3}H]*meso*-Dpm-DAla-DAla (UDP-MurNAc-pentapeptide). It was incubated at 25°C for 2 h unless otherwise stated. The reaction was stopped by applying 20 μl of the reaction mixture to Whatman 3 MM paper and drying quickly with a hair dryer. The paper was developed in a solvent system consisting of 5 volumes of isobutyric acid and 3 volumes of 1 N NH_4OH in a descending paper chromatographic apparatus. After developed overnight at 25°C, the chromatogram was air-dried and the origin corresponding to newly polymerized peptidoglycan was cut out for counting.

Assay of cross-linking in vitro. After areas corresponding to peptidoglycan were counted in a liquid scintillation counter, the radioactive strips were washed with toluene three times and once with ether and then air-dried. The strips were cut into pieces and incubated at 37°C for 15 to 24 h with 20 mg of egg-white lysozyme and a few milligrams of chloramphenicol in 2 ml of 0.1 M potassium phosphate buffer (pH 6.8). The digestion was stopped by addition of 0.5 ml of 25% trichloroacetic acid, and the precipitates were separated by centrifugation at 5,000 rpm. The supernatant was applied to a Bio-Gel P-6 column (1.5 by 120 cm) equilibrated and eluted with 0.05 M KCl. UDP-MurNAc-pentapeptide or -tripeptide was used as the internal standard. Fractions were collected (3 ml/tube) and counted. A typical elution profile from the column is shown in Fig. 5. The degree of cross-linking is expressed as the percentage of cross-linked disaccharide peptide monomer [percent cross-linked or BDP/(BDP + DP)], which was calculated as follows: [total counts in BDP/(total counts in BDP + total counts in DP)] × 100, where BDP is bisdisaccharide peptide (cross-linked) and DP is disaccharide peptide. When highly cross-linked fractions were significant, their total counts were combined with those of BDP.

Assay of cross-linking in vivo. For labeling experiments, cells were grown at 37°C overnight in a Monod tube containing 200 mg of dehydrated nutrient broth, 50 mg of yeast extract, 2 mg of L-lysine, and 0.25 mg of *meso*-rich Dpm (Kyowa Hakko Co., Tokyo) in 10 ml. The overnight culture (0.2 ml) was transferred to another tube containing the same medium, and the subsequent growth was followed turbidimetrically, using a Kotaki spectrophotometer (Tokyo Koden, Tokyo) equipped with a 660-μm filter. A 1-μCi amount of [1,7-^{14}C]Dpm was added to a tube at a cell density of 0.3 mg/ml, and the subsequent growth and incorporation were followed. At indicated times, cells were pipetted into tubes containing cold 10% trichloroacetic acid to give a final concentration of 5%.

To measure the extent of cross-linking, cells in 5% trichloroacetic acid were heated at 90°C for 20 min, and then the precipitates were collected on membrane filters (25-mm diameter, 0.45 μm; Millipore Corp.) by filtration. The precipitates were washed four times with 4 ml of 5% trichloroacetic acid and then three times with water. The precipitates on filters were then acetylated at 0°C overnight by the method of Araki et al. (1). This was done by placing filters upside down in vials for scintillation counting and adding 120 mg of $NaHCO_3$, 0.09 ml of acetic anhydride, and 1 ml of water. After acetylation, the pH was adjusted to around 6 by the addition of 1 ml of 0.1 M potassium phosphate buffer (pH 7) and a few crystals of $NaHCO_3$. Then the acetylated cell wall was digested with 20 mg of egg-white lysozyme and applied to the Bio-Gel P-6 column as described above.

Assay of D-alanine carboxypeptidase. [^{14}C]alanine-labeled UDP-MurNAc-pentapeptide (specific activity, 6.1 μCi/μmol; labeling pattern not known) was used as the substrate. The reaction mixture was the same as that for polymerization, except that UDP-GlcNAc was omitted. Separation of the product was done as described above. The chromatogram was placed in the dark in contact with X-ray film (Fuji Photo Film Co., Tokyo) for 10 to 14 days to locate D-alanine (R_f = 0.65).

Preparation of substrates. UDP-MurNAc-pentapeptide labeled with [^{3}H or ^{14}C]Dpm or [^{14}C]alanine was prepared by treating *B. cereus* T with 20 μg of ristocetin per ml as previously reported (17). Cells were grown in a bouillon medium containing 2% dehydrated nutrient broth, 0.5% yeast extract, 200 μg of L-lysine per ml, and 25 μg of *meso*-rich Dpm per ml. Cells were cultured overnight at 30°C in a Monod tube containing 10 ml of the medium and then transferred to 2-liter Erlenmeyer flasks containing 500 ml of the medium that were shaken at 400 rpm at 30°C. Cells were harvested at around 1 mg (dry weight)/ml and washed three times with 0.01 M potassium phosphate buffer (pH 7) containing 10^{-3} M $MgCl_2$, 0.8% NaCl, and 20 μg of chloramphenicol per ml. The washed cells were resuspended at 2 mg/ml in an "accumulation medium" containing glucose (10 g/liter), uracil (0.04 g/liter), L-glutamate (0.125 g/liter), $MgSO_4 \cdot 5H_2O$ (0.75 g/liter), chloramphenicol (0.025 g/liter), [^{3}H or ^{14}C]Dpm, or [^{14}C]alanine in 0.002 M potassium phosphate buffer (pH 7.5). Ristocetin was added at 20 μg/ml, and the suspension was shaken at 30°C for 20 min on a rotary shaker (400 rpm). Cells were harvested by centrifugation at 2°C and intracellular [^{3}H]- or [^{14}C]UDP-MurNAc-pentapeptide was extracted with cold 5% trichloroacetic acid twice and purified by Dowex 1 × 2 column chromatography (6) and paper chromatography (7). The specific activity of [^{3}H]Dpm-labeled UDP-MurNAc-pentapeptide was 12 to 15 μCi/μmol.

Preparation of peptidoglycan. Peptidoglycan of *B. megaterium* was obtained as follows. Cells (10 g) were sonically treated at 10 kc for 15 min in a Kubota ultrasonic generator KMS-250 (Kubotasei-sakusho, Tokyo), and unbroken cells were removed by centrifugation at 7,000 × *g* for 10 min. The supernatant solution was made 4% with sodium dodecyl sulfate (SDS) and heated at 100°C for 40 min. After cooling, peptidoglycan was obtained by centrifugation at 100,000 × *g* for 30 min and washed twice with water by centrifugation. The precipitates were suspended in 5% trichloroacetic acid and heated at 90°C for 20 min. The precipitates were collected and washed twice with water by centrifugation. The precipitates were then treated with Pronase AS (Kaken Chemicals; 250,000 tyrosine units/mg, 50 mg) at 37°C overnight in 0.1 M phosphate buffer (pH 7.5). The peptidoglycan was then recovered and washed with water twice by centrifugation at 15,000 × *g* for 10 min and lyophilized (250 mg). The purified peptidoglycan was acetylated prior to the lysozyme digestion or hydrolysis.

Determination of radioactivity. In the cases in which radioactivity was counted directly on paper, the relevant sections of the chromatogram were cut out, placed in vials covered with scintillation fluid {4 g of PPO [2,5-diphenyloxazole] and 100 mg of POPOP [2,2′-*p*-phenylene-bis-(5-phenyloxazole)] in 1 liter of toluene}. Samples in solution (up to 1 ml) were mixed with 10 ml of dioxane base scintillation fluid (100 g of naphthalene, 10 g of PPO, and 250 mg of POPOP in 1 liter of dioxane). Radioactive determinations were made using a Packard Tri-Carb liquid scintillation counter 3320. When necessary, the radioactivity of solid samples was measured by burning samples in an Aloka automatic sample combustion system ASC-112.

Materials. The following antibiotics were used: ampicillin (Beecham Research Laboratories), amoxicillin (Kyowa Hakko Co.), 6-aminopenicillanic acid (Sigma Chemical Co.), cephaloridine (Glaxo Laboratories Ltd.), cephamycin A (Merck, Sharp and Dohme), chloramphenicol (Kyowa Hakko Co.), dicloxacillin (Bristol Laboratories), mecillinam (FL-1060) (a kind gift from F. Lund [9], Leo Pharmaceuticals Co.), and ristocetin (Abbot Laboratories).

L-[U-^{14}C]alanine (130 mCi/mmol) was purchased from Daiichikagaku Co., Tokyo. [G-^{3}H]2,6-Dpm hydrochloride (300 mCi/mmol) was obtained from the Radiochemical Centre, Amersham, England. [1,7-^{14}C]2,6-Dpm (29.6 mCi/mmol) was the product of ICN Pharmaceuticals, Cleveland, Ohio. Benzyl-[^{14}C]penicillin (potassium 6-phenyl-[1-^{14}C]acetamidopenicillanate) was the product of the Radiochemical Centre (specific activity, 38.2 mCi/mmol). Egg-white lysozyme (6× crystallized) was obtained from Seikagaku Fine Chemicals, Tokyo. Reagents for scintillation counting were obtained from Nakarai Chemicals, Tokyo. Other chemicals were of reagent grade.

RESULTS

Properties of the system synthesizing cross-linked peptidoglycan in vitro. The particulate fraction from *B. megaterium* had a high activity for polymerization (20 to 40 nmol/mg of protein per h). The incorporation of radioactivity into peptidoglycan was completely dependent on the presence of UDP-GlcNAc (Table 1), with the reaction linear for at least 2 h and optimal at 30°C (Fig. 1). The effect of pH on polymerization and cross-linking was studied over the range of pH 7.5 to 8.5. It had little effect on either reaction. The polymerization had an optimum at around 0.02 M Mg^{2+} and was stimulated by 35% at 0.02 M, with the stimulation almost cancelled at 0.05 M.

The polymerization was accompanied by a penicillin-sensitive formation of cross-links. The degree of cross-linking varied from 46 to 54%, depending on the culture. However, preparations from the same batch of culture gave almost the same degree of cross-linking. Whereas the polymerization proceeded linearly, the degree of cross-linking increased gradually at 20 and 30°C (Fig. 2). This result is consistent with that obtained in vivo by Fordham and Gilvarg (3). Both polymerization and cross-linking were suppressed at 35°C.

Inhibitors. The presence of 83.3 μg of ristocetin or vancomycin per ml completely inhibited the polymerization. Dicloxacillin inhibited the polymerization only partially, even at higher concentrations (up to 100 μg/ml), and inhibited the formation of cross-links severely at 0.5 μg/ml (Fig. 3, Table 1). Nonidet P-40 and SDS were very inhibitory to the polymerization. *p*-Chloromercuribenzoate (*p*-CMB) inhibited the polymerization completely at 10^{-4} M. It did not affect the cross-linking at a concentration that inhibited the polymerization 54%. Iodoacetamide did not affect significantly either polymerization or cross-linking.

Stimulators. The effects of some organic solvents on polymerization are shown in Table 2. Dimethyl sulfoxide stimulated the reaction remarkably. The ratio of stimulation was around 3.8 between 20 and 31.5°C and 2.2 at 37°C. Since Me_2SO stimulated the reaction, the effects of some other aprotic polar solvents were studied (Table 2). Only dimethyl formamide stimulated the reaction 60 to 70% at 8.3% (vol/vol). Hexamethylphosphoric triamide, the most powerful aprotic polar solvent among solvents tested (27), was not effective at all. Me_2SO also stimu-

TABLE 1. *In vitro incorporation of radioactive UDP-MurNAc-pentapeptide into peptidoglycan under various conditions*[a]

Expt no.	Addition or omission	Amt	Incorporation (% of control)	Transpeptidation $\left(\% \frac{BDP}{BDP + DP}\right)$
2879-64	-UDP-GlcNAc		3.0 (2,286 cpm)	—[b] (51%)
	Vancomycin	83.3 μg/ml	4.0	—
	Ristocetin	10 μg/ml	43.8	—
		83.3 μg/ml	3.5	—
	Bacitracin	83.3 μg/ml	32.0	—
	Dicloxacillin	83.3 μg/ml	67.6	7.5
	Ampicillin	83.3 μg/ml	77.7	6.5
	Cephaloridine	83.3 μg/ml	62.2	—
3190-83	*p*-CMB	5×10^{-5} M	46.2 (2,503 cpm)	49.0 (48%)
		10^{-4} M	6.6	—
	Iodoacetamide	1.7×10^{-4} M	107	45.4
3057-14	SDS	0.001%	78.0 (1,435 cpm)	—
		0.01%	16.5	—
	Nonidet P-40	0.001%	45.5	—
		0.01%	38.0	—
3290-19	Diethyldithiocarbamate	10^{-3} M	75.6 (3,783 cpm)	50.0 (50%)
	o-Phenanthroline	10^{-3} M	105	49.7

[a] Assays were done under the standard conditions given. The figures given in parentheses show the incorporation and percent cross-linked in the control to each experiment.

[b] —, Not determined.

lated the formation of cross-links (Table 3). Stimulation of polymerization by Me_2SO was also observed with a particulate fraction from *E. coli* Y-10 (7) (data not shown) and from *Pseudomonas aeruginosa* (17).

To see the effect of high osmosis on the process, the effects of sucrose, glycerol, and NaCl were studied. Sucrose and glycerol at high concentrations stimulated both polymerization and cross-linking (Table 3). However, NaCl was inhibitory to the polymerization, which contradicts the explanation that the above effect is simply due to high osmosis. Amino acids also stimulated the polymerization. However, except for proline, they were inhibitory to the formation of cross-links, perhaps due to their incorporation to the terminal alanine of disaccharide peptide(s) (26).

Inhibition of cross-linking by amino acids. Wickus and Strominger (26) have reported the incorporation of [^{14}C]Dpm into peptidoglycan by a particulate fraction from *B. megaterium* QMB-1551. It was dependent on the synthesis of peptidoglycan and susceptible to penicillins. Our system also catalyzed the incorporation. However, it was only 1/10 or less of the incorporation of MurNAc-pentapeptide under conditions similar to those of Wickus and Strominger (data not shown). This is also reflected in the weak inhibition of cross-linking by Dpm at 5×10^{-4} M (Fig. 4). Thus, KM transpeptidase(s) has more rigid specificity toward Dpm in nascent disaccharidepeptide(s) than does QMB transpeptidase.

The inhibition of cross-linking by other amino acids, their derivatives, and dipeptides was studied (Table 4).Racemic or *meso*-rich Dpm, D-valine, glycine, and D-alanine markedly lowered the degree of cross-linking. These amino acids were still effective at 10^{-3} M (Fig. 4). D-Alanine (10^{-2} M) lowered the extent of cross-linking to 17.5%, whereas it was 42% in the presence of 10^{-2} M L-alanine. Modifications done at the carboxyl group of glycine or alanine always resulted in a decrease in the inhibition, whereas acetylation of the amino group completely abolished the inhibition by glycine or alanine. Homologous dipeptides of glycine or alanine were much less effective than their monomers.

Effects of β-lactam antibiotics on in vitro cell wall synthesis and cross-linking. The effects of penicillins and cephalosporins on the in vitro cell wall synthesis and cross-linking were measured as described above. A typical result is given in Fig. 5. Dicloxacillin inhibited the peptidoglycan synthesis up to 40%, and the inhibition was almost saturated at 1 μg/ml. At the

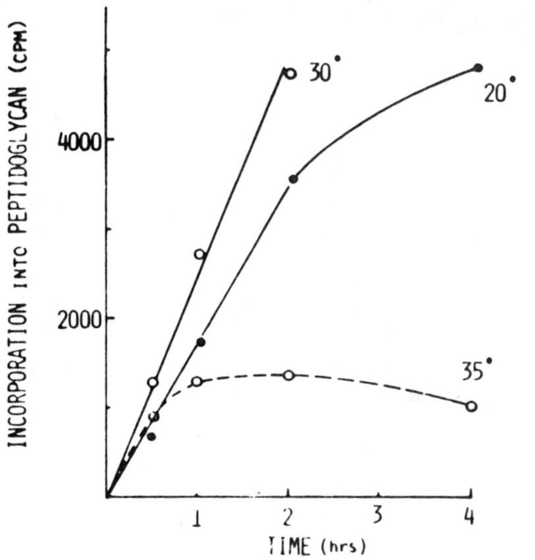

FIG. 1. *Time course of the incorporation of MurNAc-pentapeptide into peptidoglycan at 20, 30, and 35°C. A large-scale incubation mixture with the given composition was incubated at the indicated temperature. Samples (20 μl) were removed at intervals and spotted on Whatman 3 MM paper, and the products were separated by paper chromatography.*

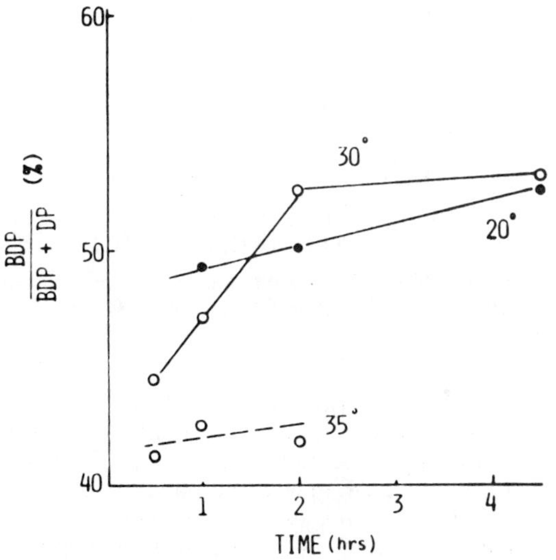

FIG. 2. *Time course of in vitro cross-linking at 20, 30, and 35°C (data are from the same experiment shown in Fig. 1).*

same time the degree of cross-linking was decreased from the normal 52% to around 10%. The inhibition of cross-linking was saturated at 0.5 μg/ml (Fig. 3). This concomitant inhibition of both reactions was observed with every β-lactam tested at their effective concentrations shown (Table 5), and the inhibition of polymerization was always partial (from 25 to 42%) even at higher concentrations.

As summarized in Table 5, the transpeptidase(s) in *B. megaterium* is quite susceptible to penicillins and cephalosporins. Even mecillinam, which was reported not to inhibit the transpeptidase in *E. coli* (14), inhibited the transpeptidation 50% at 30 μg/ml.

Estimation of the extent of cross-linking in vivo. To estimate the extent of cross-linking in vivo, [^{14}C]Dpm was added with or without β-lactam antibiotics to a growing culture of *B. megaterium*. The incorporation was stopped by the addition of cold trichloroacetic acid, and the acid precipitates were acetylated prior to lysozyme digestion. The digests were fractionated by a Bio-Gel P-6 column to measure the extent of cross-linking. Acetylation was necessary for complete digestion since bacilli may contain *N*-nonsubstituted glucosamine residues, which accounts for the resistance to lysozyme (1). In Fig. 6 a typical elution profile from the column is shown. There are differences in the profile of the digest between the cell wall synthesized in vivo and that synthesized in vitro. The higher molecular components are significant (44%) in the cell wall synthesized in vivo, whereas they are not so significant (at most 10%) in the cell wall synthesized in vitro (Fig. 5 and 6). These

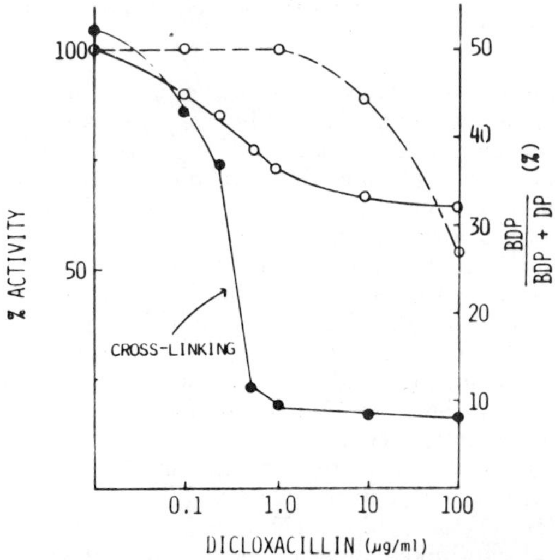

FIG. 3. *Effect of dicloxacillin on the in vitro incorporation of MurNAc-pentapeptide into peptidoglycan, cross-linking, and carboxypeptidation by a particulate fraction from B. megaterium. Symbols: ●—●—●, percent cross-linked; ○—○, incorporation into peptidoglycan; ○- - -○, carboxypeptidation. The incorporation in the control tube (no addition) was 5,232 cpm.*

TABLE 2. *Effects of solvents on the in vitro incorporation of labeled UDP-MurNAc-pentapeptide into peptidoglycan*

Solvent	Incorporation (% of control) into peptidoglycan at % (vol/vol)						Control (cpm)
	1.0	2.1	4.2	8.3	16.6	33.3	
Methanol		102	101	92.7			1,424
Acetone		107	90.8	64.8			1,424
Dimethyl sulfoxide			149	219	284	183	6,247
Dimethyl formamide			103	172	76.5		1,469
Dimethyl acetamide	104	103	97.2	58.0			1,469
Hexamethylphosphoric triamide			86.7	85.2	76.8		1,414

TABLE 3. *Effect of Me_2SO, sucrose, glycerol, NaCl, and amino acids on polymerization and cross-linking in vitro*

Compound	Concn	Polymerization (% of control)	Degree of cross-linking [% BDP/(BDP + DP)]
Me_2SO	16.6% (vol/vol)	364 (1,747)[a]	62.1 (47.7)[b]
Sucrose	20% (wt/wt)	142 (6,007)	52.2 (46.4)
	30% (wt/wt)	177 (6,007)	57.0 (46.4)
Glycerol	16.6% (vol/vol)	205 (2,717)	55.6 (50.3)
Glycine	10% (wt/wt)	135 (6,503)	2.7 (51.0)
	20% (wt/wt)	163 (6,503)	2.7 (51.0)
L-Alanine	20% (wt/wt)	179 (6,755)	8.6 (51.0)
L-Serine	20% (wt/wt)	158 (6,755)	3.5 (51.0)
L-Proline	20% (wt/wt)	177 (6,755)	57.3 (51.0)
NaCl	0.16 M	62.9 (2,219)	—[c]
	0.5 M	13.6 (2,219)	—

[a] Incorporation in counts per minute.
[b] Percent cross-linked in the control to each experiment.
[c] —, Not determined.

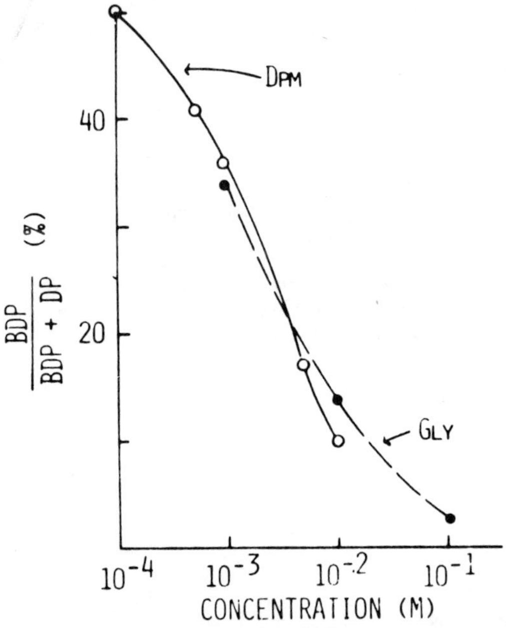

FIG. 4. *Effect of Dpm and glycine on cross-linking in vitro. Symbols: ○, effect of Dpm; ●, effect of glycine.*

fractions are believed to be disaccharide peptide trimer, tetramer, or highly cross-linked disaccharide peptide units, since repeated acetylation and lysozyme digestion did not degrade these fractions further. Besides, the β-elimination reaction (22) on this fraction did not give any fraction corresponding to un-cross-linked peptides (Fig. 7 and see below). The second peak is considered a bisdisaccharide peptide(s) by the following evidence. (i) It contains diaminopimelate and has the amino acid composition shown in Table 6. (ii) The result of the β-elimination reaction on this fraction indicates that there is no significant amount of tetrasaccharide peptide in this fraction. The β-elimination reaction will clearly discriminate between a glycan-linked dimer (a tetrasaccharide with a peptide linked to each MurNAc residue) and a peptide-linked dimer (bisdisaccharide peptide) since hydroxyl ions will only attack free reducing moieties of muramic acid to release lactyl peptides (Fig. 7). (iii) It was eluted from the column with an authentic bisdisaccharide peptide obtained from peptidoglycan synthesized in vitro (data not shown).

Dinitrophenylation of the ε-NH_2 group of Dpm in this fraction failed, probably due to the concomitant acetylation of the group. The third peak was assigned to be disaccharide peptide by the following evidences. (i) It contains diaminopimelate and has the amino acid composition shown. (ii) It was eluted from the Bio-Gel P-6 column with an authentic disaccharide peptide prepared from peptidoglycan synthesized in vitro (data not shown). (iii) It was eluted one tube (3 ml) behind an authentic UDP-MurNAc-pentapeptide (molecular weight, 1,193) and eluted together with an authentic UDP-MurNAc-tripeptide (molecular weight, 1,051) prepared from *B. cereus* T (data not shown).

The following results will also support the above assignment. (i) Lysozyme digest of Dpm-

TABLE 4. *Effect of glycine, alanine, and their derivatives on cross-linking in vitro*

Compounds (10^{-2} M)	Degree of cross-linking $\left(\% \frac{BDP}{BDP + DP}\right)$
Glycine	14.1
Glycinamide	22.3
Glycine methyl ester	32.5
N-acetylglycine	49.7
Glycylglycine	34.6
D-Alanine	17.5
L-Alanine	42.1
D-Alanine methyl ester	36.6
D-Alanine chloromethyl ketone	40.7
N-acetyl(D,L)alanine	49.0
D-Alanyl-D-alanine	48.0
D-Valine	8.4
Racemic-Dpm	9.4
meso-Rich Dpm	11.4
None	51.3

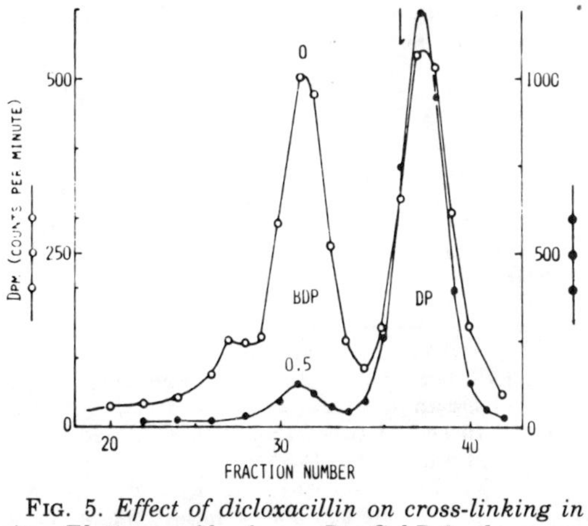

FIG. 5. *Effect of dicloxacillin on cross-linking in vitro. Elution profiles from a Bio-Gel P-6 column are shown. Peptidoglycan synthesized in the presence or absence of 0.5 μg of dicloxacillin was digested with lysozyme and applied to the column. Symbols:* ○, *peptidoglycan synthesized in the absence of dicloxacillin;* ●, *peptidoglycan synthesized in the presence of 0.5 μg of dicloxacillin per ml. BDP, bisdisaccharide peptide(s); DP, disaccharide peptide(s). The arrow indicates the position of an authentic UDP-MurNAc-pentapeptide.*

labeled *E. coli* K-12 (12) gave only two peaks in the chromatogram, one at the position of bisdisaccharide peptide and the other at the position of disaccharide peptide (data not shown). (ii) As shown in the next section, the presence of β-lactam antibiotics reduced the amount of peak 1 and 2 components, which indicates that these two are cross-linked.

Although a double auxotroph requiring lysine and diaminopimelate was not available in these experiments, the incorporation of [^{14}C]Dpm under the conditions given is a reliable measure of the cell wall synthesis in this strain of *B. megaterium* (Table 7). The result also indicates that the whole procedure (acetylation, lysozyme digestion, and gel filtration) is quite reproducible.

Effects of dicloxacillin on in vivo peptidoglycan synthesis and cross-linking. To determine the concentration to be used for in vivo experiments, the effects of dicloxacillin on the growth, viability, and morphology of *B. megaterium* were observed.

TABLE 5. *Effects of beta-lactam antibiotics on cross-linking in vitro*

Compound	Concn required for 50% inhibition (μg/ml): Peptidoglycan transpeptidase	Concn required for 50% inhibition (μg/ml): D-Alanine carboxypeptidase	Concn required for cell lysis (μg/ml)
Dicloxacillin	0.35	100	1-2
Ampicillin	0.2	–[a]	>5
Amoxicillin	0.2	–	>5
6-Aminopenicillanic acid	2.5	100	–
Mecillinam	30	>100	10-20
Cephaloridine	0.3	–	–
Cephamycin A	1.0	–	–

[a] –, Not determined.

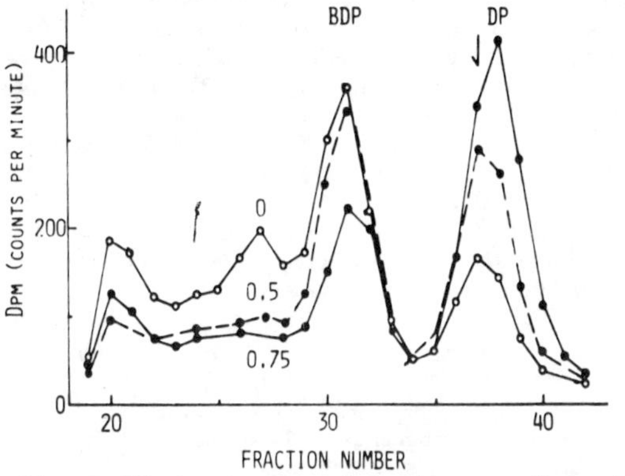

FIG. 6. *Elution profiles of the lysozyme-digested cell wall of B. megaterium from Bio-Gel P-6. The arrow indicates the position of an authentic UDP-MurNAc-pentapeptide. BDP, bisdisaccharide peptide(s); DP, disaccharide peptide(s). Each culture received dicloxacillin (amounts indicated by figures in micrograms per milliliter) together with 1 μCi of [^{14}C]Dpm and was incubated for 40 min at 37°C. The reaction was stopped by the addition of trichloroacetic acid, and the labeled precipitates were acetylated prior to lysozyme digestion as described above.*

The addition of 1 μg of dicloxacillin per ml to a growing culture of *B. megaterium* resulted in the formation of irregular forms of the cell, in which bulbous cells and club-shaped cells were dominant.

However, no significant change was observed within the first 1 h of addition. Few cells were elongated even at lower concentrations (down to 0.1 μg/ml).

Cells were lysed 1 h after the addition of 3 μg of dicloxacillin per ml and stopped growing 1 h after the addition of 1.5 μg/ml. Little effect on the growth rate was observed within the first 30 min of the addition of dicloxacillin to 0.5, 0.75, and 1 μg/ml. When these cells were transferred to a dicloxacillin-free medium, growth resumed immediately with diminished rates or with a lag time (Fig. 8B).

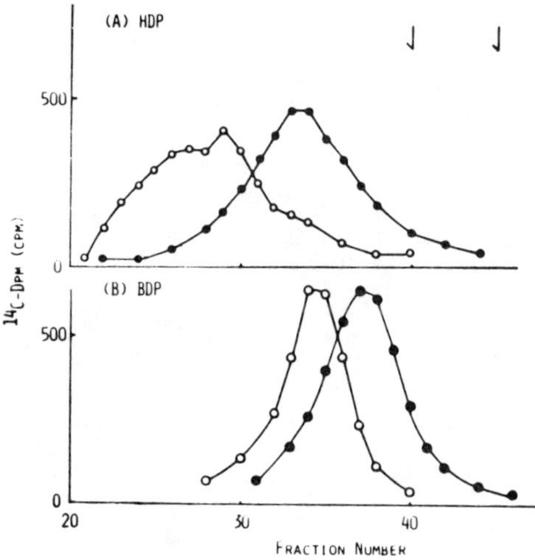

FIG. 7. *Bio-Gel P-6 elution profile of products of the beta-elimination reaction on HDP and BDP. The β-elimination reaction was done by incubating these fractions in 2 ml of 4 M NH_3 for 2 h at 37°C. After incubation, they were neutralized with 6 N HCl and applied to the Bio-Gel P-6 column described above. The arrows indicate the position of UDP-MurNAc-tripeptide (molecular weight, 1,051) and diacetyllysyl-DAla-DAla (molecular weight, 372), respectively (from left to right). The product of the β-elimination reaction on BDP ([14C]Dpm labeled) was co-chromatographed with the product from DP (synthesized in vitro and labeled with [3H]Dpm) in the column, and the separation was found to be complete (data not shown). Symbols: ○, before alkali treatment; ●, after the treatment.*

Cells started to lose the ability to form colonies 1 h after the addition of 0.25 μg/ml or immediately after the addition of 0.75 or 1.5 μg/ml.

From the results shown above, a concentration range of dicloxacillin from 0.25 to 1.5 μg/ml was judged to be appropriate to observe the effect. Dicloxacillin at 0.25 μg/ml affected exclusively the synthesis of the highly cross-linked fractions. With the increasing concentration, the synthesis of both bisdisaccharide peptide and disaccharide peptide was affected. The decrease in the amount of one component was always compensated for by the increase in the amount of disaccharide peptide (Table 7).

TABLE 6. *Amino acid composition of BDP and DP fractions from Bio-Gel P-6*[a]

Fraction	Molar ratio of: Dpm	Alanine	Glutamic acid
Purified peptidoglycan	1	2.11	1.11
BDP	1	2.11	1.11
DP	1	2.25	1.25

[a] The purified peptidoglycan of *B. megaterium* was acetylated prior to lysozyme digestion or acid hydrolysis. Samples were hydrolyzed with 6 N HCl at 110°C in sealed tubes and then analyzed in an amino acid analyzer JLC-5AH (Japan Electron Optics Lab., Tokyo). No other amino acids were detected in any of the samples. Amino acids account for around 50% of the total weight of the purified peptidoglycan. We are indebted to the analytical section of this laboratory for the data.

TABLE 7. *Effect of dicloxacillin on peptidoglycan synthesis and cross-linking in vivo*[a]

Concn of dicloxacillin (μg/ml)	Incorporation of [14C]Dpm (cpm of dry cells per mg for 40 min)	[14C]Dpm recovered after Bio-Gel P-6 gel filtration	Composition of cell wall: HDP (cpm)	BDP (cpm)	DP (cpm)	% (HDP + BDP)/(HDP + BDP + DP)[b]
0	191,800 (260,520)	168,660 (240,943)	1,233	1,069	509	81.9
0.25	181,866 (251,428)	148,114 (211,591)	581	1,072	939	63.8
0.5	187,760 (259,760)	161,940 (231,343)	699	840	1,157	57.1
0.75	190,040 (260,720)	157,500 (225,000)	603	705	1,317	49.8

[a] Numbers in parentheses show disintegrations per minute obtained by combusting labeled cells on membrane filters in a sample oxidizer and correcting by the external standardization method (data are from the same experiment as shown in Fig. 6). Values of each fraction were obtained by totaling the counts per minute under the corresponding peak in Bio-Gel P-6 chromatograms.

[b] HDP, Highly cross-linked disaccharide peptide units.

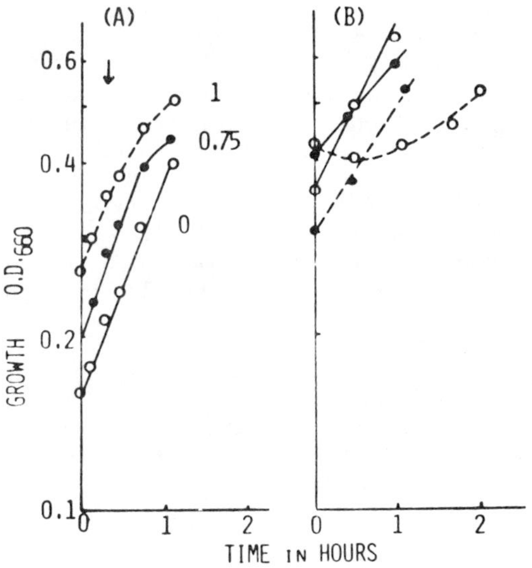

FIG. 8. *Effect of dicloxacillin on the growth and recovery of growth from the treatment. (A) Growth curve before and after the addition of dicloxacillin (indicated by the arrow); (B) growth curve of washed dicloxacillin-treated cells in dicloxacillin-free medium. Numbers indicate the amount of dicloxacillin (micrograms per milliliter) added to each culture. ●- - -● in (B) shows the growth of cells treated with 0.5 μg of dicloxacillin per ml. The growth curve of these cells in (A) was almost identical with that of the control. Cells were grown at 37°C in the bouillon medium containing 200 μg of L-lysine per ml and 25 μg of meso-rich Dpm per ml. After dicloxacillin treatment for 45 min, cells were washed by centrifugation three times and resuspended in the fresh medium without dicloxacillin.*

Thus, the effect of dicloxacillin on the in vivo peptidoglycan synthesis was negligible in the concentration range used in the experiment shown in Fig. 6, whereas the extent of cross-linking was decreased considerably (Table 7). Besides, the drastic decrease in the degree of cross-linking in vivo and in vitro was observed almost in the same concentration range (Fig. 9).

Effect of cell-bound dicloxacillin on the subsequent cell wall synthesis. If penicillin-binding components (2) are involved in cell wall synthesis, saturation of these components with penicillin will affect subsequent cell wall synthesis in a penicillin-free medium. Only two studies of limited scope have dealt with this question (15, 16, 19). Thus, we took advantage of this system to throw light on the problem. Dicloxacillin-treated cells were allowed to grow for an indicated length of time in a penicillin-free medium and were then transferred to test tubes containing both [^{14}C]Dpm and chloramphenicol to examine the cell wall being synthesized. Table 8 shows that cell-bound dicloxacillin inhibited the formation of cross-links almost to the same extent as did 0.75 μg of dicloxacillin per ml (Table 7). As cells grew, the inhibition was gradually decreased, probably due to de novo synthesis of transpeptidase(s) in the membrane. However, the inhibition was still dis-

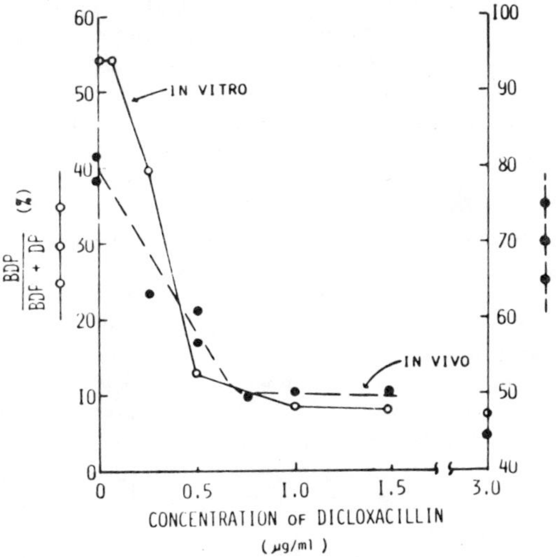

FIG. 9. *Effect of dicloxacillin on cross-linking in vivo and in vitro. Symbols: ○, cross-linking in vitro; ●, in vivo. Cross-linking data in Fig. 3 are replotted in the arithmetic scale instead of the logarithmic scale used in the original figure.*

TABLE 8. *Effect of cell-bound dicloxacillin on the subsequent formation of cross-links*[a]

Lapse of time in dicloxacillin-free medium (min)	Composition of cell wall (cpm)			% Cross-linked (HDP + BDP)/(HDP + BDP + DP)
	HDP	BDP	DP	
0	387	456	1,114	43.1
30	792	991	1,319	57.5
60	2,645	3,642	2,956	68.0

[a] Cells were grown in the presence of 0.75 μg of dicloxacillin per ml for 45 min at 37°C and then washed three times by centrifugation. The washed cells were resuspended in the fresh medium without dicloxacillin and incubated at 37°C. At intervals, samples (1 ml) were withdrawn into tubes containing 1 μCi of [^{14}C]Dpm (with or without 20 μg of chloramphenicol) and incubated at 37°C for 10 min. The reaction was stopped by the addition of 1 ml of 10% trichloroacetic acid, and the acid precipitates were treated as described above to obtain the percentage of cross-linking. Chloramphenicol was added to stop further protein synthesis. However, it did not affect peptidoglycan synthesis or cross-linking significantly (data not shown).

tinct, even after growth in the absence of the penicillin for 60 min.

Turnover of the cell wall synthesized in the presence of dicloxacillin. To measure the turnover, cells were labeled with [^{14}C]Dpm in the presence or absence of dicloxacillin. After repeated washings, cells were transferred to a dicloxacillin-free medium to follow changes in the total count and the extent of cross-linking. It was found that the normal cell wall turned over with a half-life of 170 min, whereas it was 85 min for the cell wall of dicloxacillin-treated cells (Fig. 10). Moreover, the elution profile from the Bio-Gel P-6 column changed from that typical of the dicloxacillin-treated cells to that of the normal cells during growth in the dicloxacillin-free medium. This change was not observed with the control culture. The result was unexpected and confirmed repeatedly (Table 9).

Effect of mecillinam on the in vivo and in vitro cross-linking in *B. megaterium*. A new amidinopenicillin, mecillinam (9), was reported not to inhibit any of the three penicillin-susceptible enzymes in *E. coli* (14). Unlike ordinary penicillins, it has more effect on gram-negative organisms than on gram-positive organisms. Thus, it is supposed that there must exist some other enzyme activity in gram-negative bacteria that is extremely susceptible to the amidinopenicillin (2).

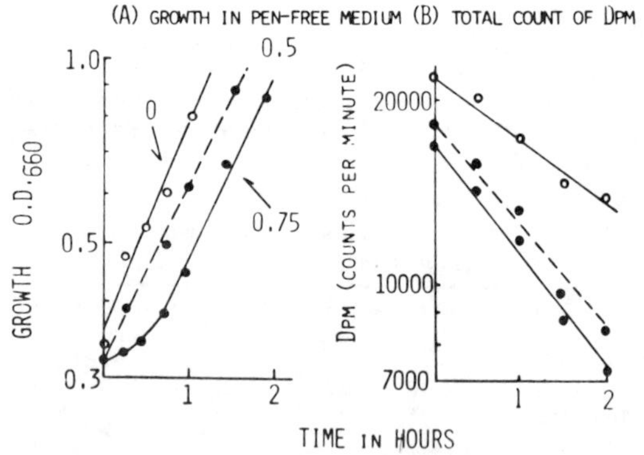

FIG. 10. *Turnover of the cell wall synthesized in the presence of dicloxacillin. Cells were grown in the bouillon medium containing 200 μg of L-lysine per ml and 25 μg of Dpm per ml. At a cell density of 0.3 mg/ml, 1 μCi of [^{14}C]Dpm was added together with varying amounts of dicloxacillin. Cells were grown at 37°C for an additional 35 min and then harvested and washed three times by centrifugation. Washed labeled cells were resuspended in the bouillon medium containing 200 μg of L-lysine per ml and 100 μg of meso-rich Dpm per ml and incubated at 37°C. Samples were taken into tubes containing 2 ml of 10% trichloroacetic acid to measure the remaining counts and the extent of cross-linking (see Table 9). (A) Growth curve of the washed labeled cells in dicloxacillin-free medium. Numbers show the amount of dicloxacillin received in the pretreatment in micrograms per milliliter; (B) total counts of Dpm in cells.*

The effect of mecillinam on the in vivo and in vitro cross-linking in *B. megaterium* was studied at concentrations effective in disturbing a growing culture, and it was found that the penicillin inhibited considerably the formation of cross-links (Fig. 11 and 12). Thus, although poor as an inhibitor of cross-linking, mecillinam interferes with the growth of *B. megaterium* by the same mechanism as that of other β-lactam antibiotics.

To confirm this, competitive binding of mecillinam with penicillin G was studied. Unlike in *E. coli* (10), mecillinam competed partially with penicillin G for binding sites in *B. megaterium* in prebound experiments (Table 10).

DISCUSSION

Inhibition of polymerization by penicillins. The high synthetic activity of the system permits the use of radioactive Dpm-labeled UDP-MurNAc-pentapeptide as the substrate, which is low in the specific activity but easy to prepare (12 to 15 μCi/μmol). This substrate gives correct amounts of synthesized peptidoglycan under various conditions that may affect remaining amounts of the terminal and penultimate D-alanine. Thus, it became possible to measure the exact effect of penicillins on peptidoglycan synthesis as well as that on transpeptidation. Two features of this experiment are worth mentioning. First, although small as compared with the marked inhibition of the transpeptidation, a partial inhibition of the polymerization was observed with every penicillin tested. Second, most of the inhibition occurred in the concentration range in which sharp inhibition of cross-linking was also observed.

Thus, both inhibition curves consist of two parts, the sensitive part and the less sensitive part. The curve is very similar to that of penicillin G on the in vivo cell wall synthesis in *E. coli* W173-25 (20). Mirelman et al. (11) also reported the inhibition of peptidoglycan synthesis by penicillins in a crude cell wall preparation from *Micrococcus luteus*. They assumed that the elongation of the peptidoglycan strand occurs by both transpeptidation and transglycosylation. Although this is an attractive hypothesis, we have not observed any consistent, dose-responsive inhibition of the in vivo cell wall synthesis by dicloxacillin in the concentration range effective in inhibiting the formation of cross-links.

Stimulation of peptidoglycan synthesis and cross-linking. Dimethyl sulfoxide, sucrose,

TABLE 9. *Changes in the degree of cross-linking in the cell wall synthesized in the presence of dicloxacillin after transfer to a dicloxacillin-free medium*[a]

Expt no.	Pretreatment concn of dicloxacillin (μg/ml)	Time after transfer (min)	Composition of the cell wall			
			HDP (cpm)	BDP (cpm)	DP (cpm)	Cross-linked (%)
3515-1	0	0	1,011	1,463	633	78.8[b]
		120	1,063	1,766	611	82.2
	0.75 (40 min)	0	1,298	1,055	2,090	53.1
		120	856	845	620	73.3
3515-15	0	0	3,319	3,482	1,809	77.1
		120	2,659	2,691	873	85.9
	0.75 (35 min)	0	1,141	2,316	3,236	51.6
		120	1,031	937	806	70.9
3515-54	0	0	1,233	1,069	509	81.9
		120	518	726	256	82.9
	0.75 (40 min)	0	603	705	1,317	49.8
		120	687	633	328	80.1

[a] Experimental details are given in the legend to Fig. 10. Values of each fraction were obtained by totaling the counts per minute under the corresponding peaks in Bio-Gel P-6 chromatograms.
[b] A part of this sample was lost during the preparation for Bio-Gel P-6 gel filtration.

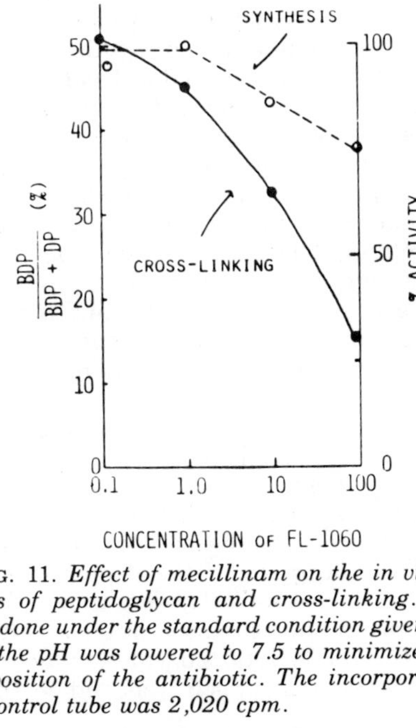

FIG. 11. *Effect of mecillinam on the in vitro synthesis of peptidoglycan and cross-linking. Assays were done under the standard condition given, except that the pH was lowered to 7.5 to minimize the decomposition of the antibiotic. The incorporation in the control tube was 2,020 cpm.*

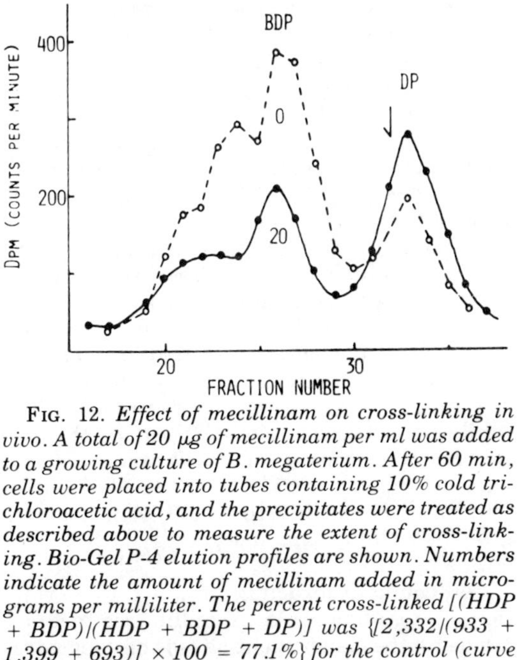

FIG. 12. *Effect of mecillinam on cross-linking in vivo. A total of 20 μg of mecillinam per ml was added to a growing culture of B. megaterium. After 60 min, cells were placed into tubes containing 10% cold trichloroacetic acid, and the precipitates were treated as described above to measure the extent of cross-linking. Bio-Gel P-4 elution profiles are shown. Numbers indicate the amount of mecillinam added in micrograms per milliliter. The percent cross-linked [(HDP + BDP)/(HDP + BDP + DP)] was {[2,332/(933 + 1,399 + 693)] × 100 = 77.1%} for the control (curve 0) and {[1,215/(341 + 874 + 1,052)] × 100 = 53.6%} in the presence of 20 μg of mecillinam per ml (curve 20).*

glycerol, and some amino acids stimulated the in vitro peptidoglycan synthesis remarkably. The rate-limiting step in the polymerization would be the translocation of carriers across the membrane, and these reagents may stimulate the reaction by affecting the particular microenvironments (13). In fact, Heydanek et al. (5) have reported a threefold stimulation of the transfer reaction (UDP-MurNAc-pentapeptide plus acceptor → acceptor-phosphoMurNAc-pentapeptide plus uridine 5′-monophosphate

TABLE 10. *Effect of mecillinam on the binding of penicillin G*[a]

Preincubation with:	[^{14}C]penicillin G binding: Total cpm	Inhibition of the binding (%)
None	650	0
Mecillinam (20 μg/ml)	460	41.9
Penicillin G (3 μg/ml)	197	100

[a] Preincubation was done in 0.03 M phosphate buffer (pH 6.8) containing 3 mg (dry weight) of *B. megaterium* cells and penicillins per ml at 25°C for 30 min. Cells were harvested and washed with 0.03 M phosphate buffer twice. Then they were suspended in the buffer containing 0.05 μCi of penicillin G per ml (0.049 μg/ml) and incubated at 25°C for 30 min. Cells were collected by filtration on membrane filters and counted.

[UMP]) and the biphasic stimulation inhibition of the reaction by detergents.

The stimulation of the cross-linking by these reagents will also be explained by the change in the polarity of the microenvironment in which the cross-linking takes place. Frére et al. (4) have reported that the portion of the activity of DD-carboxypeptidase-transpeptidase of *Streptomyces* R 61 that can be channeled in the transpeptidation and the hydrolytic pathways depends on the pH and the polarity of the environment. They found a 7.5-fold increase in the ratio of transpeptidation to hydrolysis in a medium containing water-ethylene glycol-glycerol (6:9:5, by volume), as compared with that observed in an aqueous environment.

Action of penicillins in vivo in *B. megaterium*. The in vivo and in vitro formation of cross-links was inhibited sharply within a narrow range of dicloxacillin concentration. Both inhibition curves are similar in shape (Fig. 9). Besides, the inhibition of cross-linking occurred both in vivo and in vitro at the low concentration of dicloxacillin that also affected the growth, viability, and morphology of *B. megaterium*.

Cell-bound dicloxacillin inhibited the formation of cross-links in a penicillin-free medium almost to the same extent as did the concentration of dicloxacillin used to equilibrate the cell. Even after growth in the absence of the penicillin for 60 min, the inhibition was still distinct. This means that penicillins inhibit the cross-linking by binding to cells and that most of the penicillin molecules, once bound, remain at their target. Recovery from the inhibition has to wait for de novo synthesis of transpeptidases, which will gradually bring the degree of cross-linking in the cell wall to the normal level.

As shown above, the cell wall synthesized in the presence of dicloxacillin showed a higher rate of turnover. This is probably due to the higher rate of degradation of less cross-linked parts of the cell wall, since disaccharide peptide(s) degraded more quickly than did bisdisaccharide peptide(s) or highly cross-linked disaccharide peptide units (Table 9). This phenomenon may be explained in other ways. For example, the increase in the degree of cross-linking is due to some kind of repair system that can correct defects in the cell wall, or the increase is a normal kinetics of transpeptidase as reported by Fordham and Gilvarg (3). However, these alternatives do not explain well the faster turnover of dicloxacillin cell wall. Besides, the amount of transpeptidase(s) involved would not be enough to explain the increase since most of the "older" transpeptidases were still penicillin bound under this condition. The higher turnover rate of dicloxacillin cell wall would be explained by the need to hydrolyze fewer bonds to release the same number of counts per minute and/or by the triggering of autolytic enzymes by penicillin (25).

Drugs that inhibit the biosynthesis or the normal assembly of bacterial cell walls are bacteriolytic. The involvement of cellular autolytic enzymes has been suggested and demonstrated (23, 24). According to these authors, lysis is a secondary phenomenon; it is the consequence of the uncoupling of the two processes, the activity of cellular lytic enzymes and the biosynthesis of cell wall polymers. If so, lysis will depend not only on the amount and nature of autolytic enzymes but also on the structural integrity of bacterial cell walls (Fig. 10 and Table 9).

In conclusion, the transpeptidase(s) in *B. megaterium* is the primary target of the penicillin action. Penicillins inhibit the enzyme by irreversibly binding to cells (penicillin-binding components). The inhibition of the enzyme results in the decrease in the degree of cross-linking in the cell wall. The less that cell wall is cross-linked, the more susceptible it is to the action of cellular lytic enzymes, which will ultimately bring about cell lysis and death.

ACKNOWLEDGMENTS

I wish to thank S. Kinoshita and N. Nakamizo for their interest and support of this work, K. Izaki, E. Ito, P. E. Reynolds, and F. Lund for providing bacterial strains and antibiotics, and F. Tomita for his critical reading of the manuscript.

LITERATURE CITED

1. **Araki, Y., T. Nakatani, K. Nakayama, and E. Ito.** 1972.

Occurrence of N-nonsubstituted glucosamine residues in peptidoglycan of lysozyme-resistant cell walls from *Bacillus cereus*. J. Biol. Chem. 247:6312–6322.

2. **Blumberg, P. M., and J. L. Strominger.** 1974. Interaction of penicillin with the bacterial cell: penicillin-binding proteins and penicillin-sensitive enzymes. Bacteriol. Rev. 38:291–335.
3. **Fordham, W. D., and C. Gilvarg.** 1974. Kinetics of cross-linking in peptidoglycan in *Bacillus megaterium*. J. Biol. Chem. 249:2478–2482.
4. **Frére, J-M., J-M. Ghyusen, H. Perkins, and M. Nieto.** 1973. Kinetics of concomitant transfer and hydrolysis reactions catalyzed by the exocellular DD-carboxypeptidase-transpeptidase of *Streptomyces* R 61. Biochem. J. 135:483–492.
5. **Heydanek, M. G., Jr., W. G. Struve, and F. C. Neuhaus.** 1969. On the initial stage in peptidoglycan synthesis. III. Kinetics and uncoupling of phospho-N-acetylmuramyl-pentapeptide translocase. Biochemistry 8:1214–1221.
6. **Ito, E., G. Nathenson, D. N. Dietzler, J. S. Anderson, and J. L. Strominger.** 1966. Formation of UDP-acetylmuramyl peptides, p. 324–337. *In* E. F. Neufeld and V. Ginsburg (ed.), Methods in enzymology, vol. VIII. Academic Press Inc., New York.
7. **Izaki, K., M. Matsuhashi, and J. L. Strominger.** 1968. Biosynthesis of the peptidoglycan of bacterial cell walls. XIII. Peptidoglycan transpeptidase and D-alanine carboxypeptidase. J. Biol. Chem. 243:3180–3192.
8. **Lowry, O. H., N. J. Rosebrough, A. L. Farr, and R. J. Randall.** 1951. Protein measurement with the Folin phenol reagent. J. Biol. Chem. 193:265–275.
9. **Lund, F., and L. Tybring.** 1972. 6-Beta-amidinopenicillanic acids – a new group of antibiotics. Nature (London) New Biol. 236:135–136.
10. **Matsuhashi, S., T. Kamiryo, P. M. Blumberg, P. Linnett, E. Willoughby, and J. L. Stominger.** 1974. Mechanism of action and development of resistance to a new amidinopenicillin. J. Bacteriol. 117:578–587.
11. **Mirelman, D., R. Bracha, and N. Sharon.** 1974. Studies on the elongation of bacterial cell wall peptidoglycan and its inhibition by penicillin. Ann. N.Y. Acad. Sci. 235:326–344.
12. **Nagai, K., and G. Tamura.** 1972. Mutant of *Escherichia coli* with thermosensitive protein in the process of cellular division. J. Bacteriol. 112:959–966.
13. **Neuhaus, F. C.** 1971. Initial translocation reaction in the biosynthesis of peptidoglycan by bacterial membranes. Acc. Chem. Res. 4:297–303.
14. **Park, J. T., and L. Burman.** 1973. A new penicillin with a unique mode of action. Biochem. Biophys. Res. Commun. 51:863–868.
15. **Park, J. T., J. R. Edwards, and E. M. Wise.** 1974. In vivo studies on the uptake and binding of β-lactam antibiotics in relation to inhibition of cell wall synthesis and cell death. Ann. N.Y. Acad. Sci. 235:300–309.
16. **Park, J. T., M. E. Griffith, and I. Stevenson.** 1971. Resistance to penicillin in mutants of a penicillinase-negative organism, *Staphylococcus aureus* H. J. Bacteriol. 108:1154–1160.
17. **Presslitz, J. E., and V. A. Ray.** 1975. DD-Carboxypeptidase and peptidoglycan transpeptidase from *Pseudomonas aeruginosa*. Antimicrob. Agents Chemother. 7:578–581.
18. **Reynolds, P. E.** 1971. Peptidoglycan synthesis in *Bacilli*. I. Effect of temperature on the in vitro system from *Bacillus megaterium* and *Bacillus stearothermophilus*. Biochim. Biophys. Acta 237:239–254.
19. **Rogers, H. J.** 1967. The inhibition of mucopeptide synthesis by benzylpenicillin in relation to irreversible fixation of the antibiotic by *Staphylococci*. Biochem. J. 103:90–102.
20. **Schwartz, U., A. Asmus, and H. Frank.** 1969. Autolytic enzymes and cell division of **E. coli**. J. Mol. Biol. 41:419–429.
21. **Spratt, B. G.** 1975. Distinct penicillin binding proteins involved in the division, elongation and shape of *Escherichia coli* K-12. Proc. Natl. Acad. Sci. U.S.A. 72:2999–3003.
22. **Tipper, D. J.** 1968. Alkali-catalyzed elinination of D-lactic acid from muramic acid and its derivatives and the determination of muramic acid. Biochemistry 7:1441–1449.
23. **Tomasz, A.** 1974. The role of autolysins in cell death. Ann. N.Y. Acad. Sci. 235:439–447.
24. **Tomasz, A., A. Albino, and E. Zanati.** 1970. Multiple antibiotic resistance in a bacterium with suppressed autolytic system. Nature (London) 227:138–140.
25. **Tomasz, A., and S. Waks.** 1975. Mechanism of action of penicillin: triggering of the pneumococcal autolytic enzyme by inhibitors of cell wall synthesis. Proc. Natl. Acad. Sci. U.S.A. 72:4162–4166.
26. **Wickus, G. G., and J. L. Strominger.** 1972. Penicillin-sensitive transpeptidation during peptidoglycan biosynthesis in cell-free preparations from *Bacillus megaterium*. J. Biol. Chem. 247:5307–5311.
27. **Yoshida, Z., and S. Yoneda.** 1971. Fundamental characters of polar solvents, p. 3–16. *In* R. Oda, N. Tokura, and Z. Yoshida (ed.), New organic synthesis using polar solvents, Kagaku special issue. Kagakudozin, Kyoto.

ANTIMICROBIAL AGENTS AND CHEMOTHERAPY, Oct. 1976, p. 592-597 Vol. 10, No. 4

Printed in U.S.A.

Comparative Activity of Netilmicin, Gentamicin, Amikacin, and Tobramycin Against *Pseudomonas aeruginosa* and *Enterobacteriaceae*

DALIUS J. BRIEDIS AND HUGH G. ROBSON*

Departments of Medicine and Microbiology, Royal Victoria Hospital and McGill University, Faculty of Medicine, Montreal, Quebec, H3A 2B4 Canada

Received for publication 11 June 1976

Netilmicin (Sch 20569), a semisynthetic aminoglycoside antibiotic, was compared with gentamicin, tobramycin, and amikacin against 242 clinical isolates of *Pseudomonas* and *Enterobacteriaceae*. The minimum inhibitory concentration (MIC) was determined in both solid and liquid media. Netilmicin exhibited typical aminoglycoside properties, such as little effect of inoculum size on MIC, relatively small gap between MIC and minimum bactericidal concentration, and potentiation of anti-*Pseudomonas* activity in the presence of carbenicillin. Netilmicin provided no advantage in antimicrobial activity over gentamicin for either *Pseudomonas* or *Enterobacteriaceae*. Nearly complete cross-resistance to netilmicin was encountered with isolates resistant to gentamicin in either solid or liquid media. Netilmicin was less active than gentamicin against isolates of *Pseudomonas* and *Providencia*. Major discrepancies between MIC values determined in agar as opposed to those determined in broth were encountered for most isolates of *Pseudomonas* but also, depending upon antibiotic tested, for between 15 and 40% of isolates of *Enterobacteriaceae*. This new aminoglycoside agent will be useful clinically only if it is shown to be significantly less toxic than presently available analogues.

Gentamicin, with or without the concomitant administration of carbenicillin, is widely used in the treatment of hospital-acquired, gram-negative bacillary infection, including those caused by *Pseudomonas aeruginosa*. Gentamicin is far from an ideal antimicrobial agent. Peak serum levels after administration of recommended doses may barely exceed the inhibitory concentrations for frequently isolated gram-negative bacilli, whereas the administration of larger doses may lead to significant toxicity. Further, the emergence of isolates with high-level resistance to gentamicin has been well documented (3).

Accordingly, the search continues for new aminoglycoside antibiotics that might exhibit greater antibacterial activity and less toxicity. Netilmicin (Sch 20569), an agent differing from sisomicin by the presence of an ethyl group at the 1-N position of the deoxystreptamine moiety, has recently been provided for in vitro work. Initial animal toxicity studies indicated that this agent may be less oto- and nephrotoxic than gentamicin (5). Our study compares the in vitro activity of netilmicin with those of gentamicin, tobramycin, and amikacin against recent isolates of *P. aeruginosa* and various *Enterobacteriaceae*. In addition, the potentiation of the activity of the four aminoglycosides against *P. aeruginosa* by carbenicillin was evaluated.

MATERIALS AND METHODS

Bacterial isolates. Two hundred and forty-two clinical isolates were obtained from the diagnostic microbiology laboratory of the Royal Victoria Hospital. These isolates included *Escherichia coli* (35), *Klebsiella pneumoniae* (36), *Enterobacter* (36), *Proteus mirabilis* (37), indole-positive *Proteus* (25), *Providencia stuartii* (10), and *P. aeruginosa* (63). The identity of all isolates was confirmed by standard methods. Not more than one isolate of a given species per patient was included.

Antibiotics. Gentamicin sulfate and netilmicin sulfate were supplied by the Schering Corp. Amikacin was supplied by Bristol Laboratories, tobramycin by Eli Lilly and Co., and carbenicillin disodium by Ayerst Laboratories. Antibiotic stock solutions were stored at −70°C.

Agar dilution susceptibility. Minimal inhibitory concentrations (MIC) were determined for all isolates by an agar dilution method in Mueller-Hinton agar. Parallel series of antibiotic-containing plates were inoculated for each antibiotic by a multiple inoculator apparatus (8) using both 10^{-4} and 10^{-2} dilutions of an overnight Mueller-Hinton broth

(MHB) culture. The Mueller-Hinton agar batch used had concentrations of calcium and magnesium of 9.1 and 4.25 mg/dl, respectively, as determined by atomic absorption (Perkin-Elmer atomic absorption spectrophotometer, model 303).

Broth dilution susceptibility. Twenty resistant or relatively resistant isolates each of *P. aeruginosa* and *Enterobacteriaceae*, as determined by agar dilution testing, were selected for broth dilution susceptibility testing. The aminoglycoside antibiotics were serially diluted in twofold steps in MHB (final volume, 2.0 ml). Each tube was then inoculated with 0.05 ml of a 10^{-2} dilution of an overnight MHB culture. The lowest concentration that inhibited visible growth after overnight incubation at 37°C was taken as the MIC. A sample (0.01 ml) of each clear tube was subcultured to antibiotic-free Mueller-Hinton agar, and the minimal bactericidal concentration (MBC) was taken to be the lowest antibiotic concentration to yield fewer than five colonies after overnight incubation at 37°C. The MHB contained 1.18 mg of calcium and 0.208 mg of magnesium per dl, again measured by atomic absorption.

Activity of aminoglycoside-carbenicillin combinations. The 20 isolates of *P. aeruginosa* selected for aminoglycoside susceptibility tests in MHB were also evaluated for susceptibility to aminoglycoside-carbenicillin combinations. To each tube in a twofold aminoglycoside dilution series in MHB a fixed amount of carbenicillin was added to give a final carbenicillin concentration of 50 μg/ml in a volume of 2.0 ml. Each tube was inoculated with 0.05 ml of a 10^{-2} dilution of an overnight MHB culture and incubated aerobically overnight at 37°C. The resulting MIC of each aminoglycoside for each isolate was compared in the presence and absence of carbenicillin.

RESULTS

Agar dilution MIC. Varying the inoculum size had relatively little effect on the results. In almost all instances increasing the inoculum 100-fold resulted in either no change in MIC or a twofold increase. Accordingly, the results presented are those obtained with the larger inoculum, as a similar inoculum was used in the subsequent broth dilution tests.

MICs of the four aminoglycosides tested against the large inocula of *E. coli*, *K. pneumoniae*, and *Enterobacter* are shown in Table 1. The in vitro activities of netilmicin and gentamicin were almost identical, inhibiting 90% or more of isolates at a concentration of 3.1 μg/ml. A small percentage of *K. pneumoniae* and *Enterobacter* (3 to 5%) had netilmicin or gentamicin MICs ≥ 12.5 μg/ml. Tobramycin inhibited all *E. coli* and *K. pneumoniae* at a concentration of 1.6 μg/ml, but about 3% of *Enterobacter* isolates had MICs ≥ 12.5 μg/ml. Amikacin inhibited all isolates at a concentration of 12.5 μg/ml or less.

The MIC values of the four agents for isolates of *P. mirabilis*, indole-positive *Proteus*, and *P. stuartii* are presented in Table 2. In each instance netilmicin and gentamicin demonstrated similar activity. Netilmicin inhibited 70.3% of *P. mirabilis* and 80% of indole-positive *Proteus* at a concentration of 3.1 μg/ml, compared to 78.4 and 76%, respectively, inhibited by gentamicin. Tobramycin showed greater activity, inhibiting 86.5% of *P. mirabilis* and 92.0% of indole-positive *Proteus* at a concentration of 3.1 μg/ml. None of these three agents showed significant activity against *P. stuartii*. Amikacin was highly active against these isolates, inhibiting 83.7% of *P. mirabilis*, 96% of indole-positive *Proteus*, and all *P. stuartii* at a concentration of 12.5 μg/ml.

Almost complete cross-resistance was exhibited to netilmicin by isolates of *Enterobacteriaceae* highly resistant to gentamicin (MIC ≥ 25 μg/ml). One of the 14 such isolates had a netilmicin MIC of 6.3 μg/ml; all other MIC values were ≥12.5 μg/ml (Table 3). Tobramycin also showed little activity against most gentamicin-resistant isolates but amikacin was

TABLE 1. *Agar dilution MIC of aminoglycoside antibiotics for E. coli, Klebsiella, and Enterobacter*

Organism (no. tested)	Antibiotic	Cumulative % isolates inhibited at (μg/ml):								
		0.2	0.4	0.8	1.6	3.1	6.3	12.5	25.0	50.0
E. coli (35)	Netilmicin	0	8.6	62.8	100.0					
	Gentamicin	0	2.9	74.3	97.2	100.0				
	Tobramycin	0	28.6	91.4	100.0					
	Amikacin	0	0	2.9	28.6	82.9	91.4	100.0		
K. pneumoniae (36)	Netilmicin	2.8	30.6	86.0	97.2	97.2	97.2	100.0		
	Gentamicin	5.6	38.9	83.2	97.2	97.2	97.2	97.2	100.0	
	Tobramycin	11.1	77.8	91.6	100.0					
	Amikacin	0	0	5.6	63.8	91.6	100.0			
Enterobacter (36)	Netilmicin	0	4.2	55.6	86.0	91.6	94.5	97.2	97.2	97.2
	Gentamicin	0	11.1	63.8	94.5	94.5	94.5	94.5	97.2	97.2
	Tobramycin	0	27.8	86.0	97.2	97.2	97.2	97.2	100.0	
	Amikacin	0	0	0	44.4	94.5	100.0			

TABLE 2. *Agar dilution MIC of aminoglycoside antibiotics for P. mirabilis, indole-positive Proteus, and P. stuartii*

Organism (no. tested)	Antibiotic	Cumulative % isolates inhibited at (μg/ml):								
		0.2	0.4	0.8	1.6	3.1	6.3	12.5	25.0	50.0
P. mirabilis (37)	Netilmicin	0	0	5.4	45.9	70.3	86.5	89.2	100.0	
	Gentamicin	0	0	29.7	54.1	78.4	86.5	89.2	97.3	100.0
	Tobramycin	0	21.6	67.6	81.1	86.5	89.2	89.2	89.2	100.0
	Amikacin	0	0	0	8.1	37.8	59.4	83.7	89.1	89.1
Indole-positive *Proteus* (25)	Netilmicin	0	4.0	36.0	60.0	80.0	92.0	92.0	96.0	100.0
	Gentamicin	0	8.0	28.0	60.0	76.0	88.0	88.0	100.0	
	Tobramycin	8.0	28.0	60.0	80.0	92.0	100.0			
	Amikacin	0	0	4.0	32.0	64.0	84.0	96.0	100.0	
P. stuartii (10)	Netilmicin	0	0	0	0	0	20.0	30.0	70.0	90.0
	Gentamicin	0	0	0	0	0	20.0	60.0	90.0	100.0
	Tobramycin	0	0	0	10.0	20.0	40.0	60.0	90.0	100.0
	Amikacin	0	0	10.0	60.0	90.0	100.0			

TABLE 3. *MIC by agar dilution of netilmicin, tobramycin, and amikacin for highly gentamicin-resistant Enterobacteriaceae (MIC ≥ 25 μg/ml)*

Organism (no. highly resistant/no. tested)	MIC (μg/ml)			
	Gentamicin	Netilmicin	Tobramycin	Amikacin
K. pneumoniae (1/36)	25	12.5	1.6	1.6
Enterobacter spp. (2/36)	>50	>50.0	25.0	3.1
	25	12.5	1.6	1.6
Indole-positive *Proteus* (3/25)	25	25.0	6.3	1.6
	25	50.0	3.1	1.6
	25	6.3	6.3	12.5
P. mirabilis (4/37)	50	25.0	50.0	>50.0
	25	25.0	50.0	>50.0
	25	25.0	50.0	>50.0
	25	25.0	50.0	>50.0
P. stuartii (4/10)	25	50.0	25.0	1.6
	25	50.0	25.0	1.6
	25	>50.0	50.0	6.3
	50	25.0	12.5	3.1

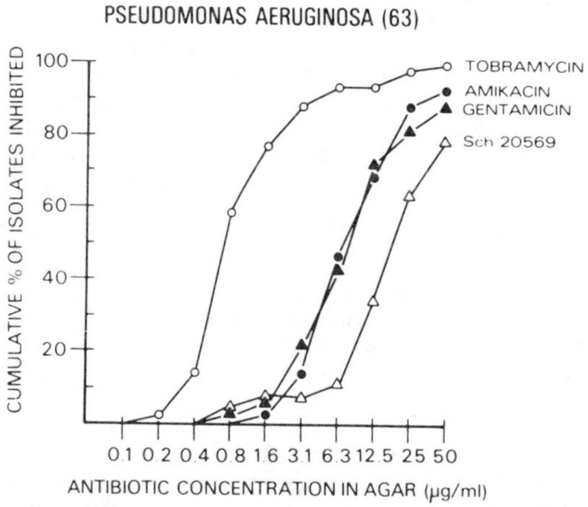

FIG. 1. *Antibiotic susceptibility pattern of P. aeruginosa. Netilmicin is designated as Sch 20569.*

highly active, inhibiting 10 isolates at a concentration of 12.5 μg/ml. The four amikacin-resistant *P. mirabilis* isolates were also resistant to the other agents tested by this method.

Netilmicin exhibited little activity against *P. aeruginosa* when tested by the agar dilution method, inhibiting only 7.9% of isolates at a concentration of 3.1 μg/ml compared to 22.2% inhibited by gentamicin (Fig. 1). Tobramycin was the most active anti-*Pseudomonas* agent; 87.3% of isolates had MICs of 3.1 μg/ml or less. Amikacin inhibited 68.3% of *P. aeruginosa* at a concentration of 12.5 μg/ml. Of 18 gentamicin-resistant *P. aeruginosa* (MIC ≥ 25 μg/ml), none had a netilmicin MIC lower than 25 μg/ml. In contrast, tobramycin inhibited 11 such isolates at 3.1 μg/ml. Only one gentamicin-resistant *P. aeruginosa* was inhibited by amikacin at a concentration of 12.5 μg/ml.

Broth dilution susceptibility tests. The MIC of the four aminoglycosides was determined in MHB for 20 isolates each of *Enterobacteriaceae* and *P. aeruginosa*. Eighteen of the 20 *Enterobacteriaceae* and all 20 *P. aeruginosa* selected had gentamicin MICs ≥ 12.5 μg/ml by the agar dilution method.

The correlations between MICs determined in agar or broth for *Enterobacteriaceae* are shown in Fig. 2. Broth dilution MIC values were one-quarter or less of those determined in agar for 8 of 20 isolates tested with netilmicin and gentamicin, 5 of 20 tested with tobramycin, and 3 of 20 tested with amikacin. Agar dilution MIC values of netilmicin for all 20 *Enterobacteriaceae* were ≥6.3 μg/ml; when retested in broth, only 8 showed MICs of 3.1 μg/ml or less. Three of the four *P. mirabilis* isolates that exhibited high-level resistance to the four antibiotics by the agar dilution method (Table 3) were tested by broth dilution. All had netilmicin, gentamicin, and tobramycin MICs ≤ 3.1 μg/ml and an amikacin MIC ≤ 12.5 μg/ml.

Twelve isolates of *Enterobacteriaceae* had gentamicin MICs ≥ 6.3 μg/ml by tube dilution (Table 4). Only one of these isolates had a netilmicin MIC < 6.3 μg/ml, and only two had a tobramycin MIC < 6.3 μg/ml. In contrast, the amikacin MIC of 10/12 gentamicin-resistant isolates was <12.5 μg/ml.

The relationships between the MIC of the agents determined by agar dilution and those determined by broth dilution for *P. aeruginosa* are shown in Fig. 3. In the great majority of

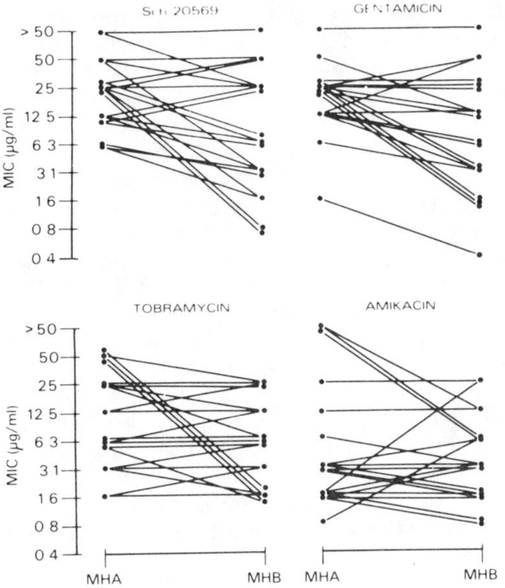

FIG. 2. *Comparison of MICs of antibiotics for Enterobacteriaceae as determined in Mueller-Hinton agar (MHA) and MHB. Each line represents a single isolate. Netilmicin is designated as Sch 20569.*

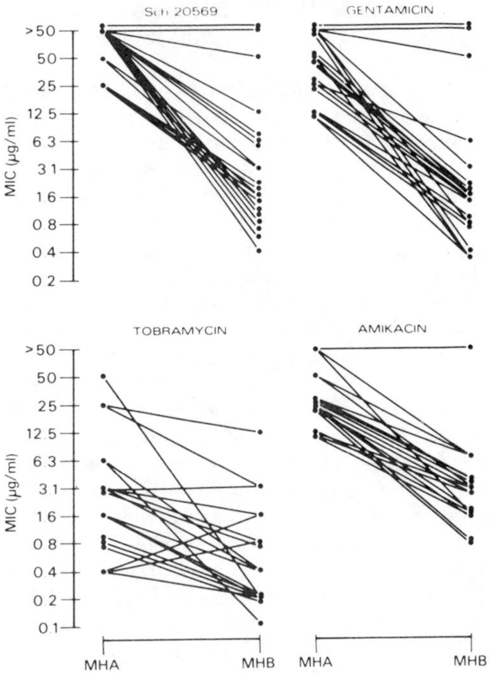

FIG. 3. *Comparison of MICs of antibiotics for P. aeruginosa as determined in Mueller-Hinton agar (MHA) and MHB. Each line represents a single isolate. Netilmicin is designated as Sch 20569.*

TABLE 4. *Activity of netilmicin, tobramycin, and amikacin in MHB against gentamicin-resistant[a] Enterobacteriaceae*

Isolate	Gentamicin		Netilmicin		Tobramycin		Amikacin	
	MIC[b]	MBC[b]	MIC	MBC	MIC	MBC	MIC	MBC
1. *Providencia*	12.5	50	25	100	25	50	0.8	1.6
2. *Providencia*	25.0	100	25	100	25	50	3.1	12.5
3. *Providencia*	25.0	100	50	50	25	50	3.1	12.5
4. *Providencia*	6.3	12.5	6.3	12.5	25	25	6.3	12.5
5. *Providencia*	50.0	100	50	>100	6.3	50	25.0	25.0
6. *Providencia*	12.5	100	25	100	12.5	50	1.6	12.5
7. *Providencia*	12.5	25	12.5	50	6.3	12.5	1.6	12.5
8. *Klebsiella*	50.0	50	25	50	3.1	6.3	1.6	1.6
9. *Enterobacter*	12.5	25	6.3	12.5	1.6	3.1	0.8	1.6
10. *Enterobacter*	>100.0	>100	100	>100	12.5	25	1.6	6.3
11. *P. mirabilis*	6.3	12.5	3.1	12.5	6.3	12.5	25.0	50.0
12. Indole-positive *Proteus*	25.0	100	50	100	12.5	25	1.6	6.3

[a] Gentamicin MIC >6.3 μg/ml in tube dilution test.
[b] MICs and MBCs are given in micrograms per milliliter.

cases, a fourfold or greater decrease in the MIC as determined in broth was noted: this occurred for netilmicin and gentamicin with 17 of 20 isolates, for tobramycin with 14 of 20 isolates, and for amikacin with 18 of 20 isolates. The numbers of isolates out of 20 tested with broth dilution MICs > 3.1 μg/ml for netilmicin, gentamicin, and tobramycin were 7, 4, and 1, respectively. Only 1 of the 20 isolates tested had an amikacin MIC > 6.3 μg/ml under the same conditions.

Comparison of MBC with MIC for the 40 isolates evaluated showed that in only three instances was there a greater than fourfold increase in MBC over MIC for netilmicin and gentamicin, whereas 7 of 40 isolates had tobramycin or amikacin MBCs fourfold or more greater than the corresponding MIC value.

Potentiation of aminoglycoside activity by carbenicillin. Eighteen of the 20 *P. aeruginosa* isolates whose MIC to the aminoglycosides had been determined by the tube dilution method were resistant to 50 μg of carbenicillin per ml alone in MHB. The effect of added carbenicillin (50 μg/ml) on the MICs of the four aminoglycosides for these 18 isolates is shown in Fig. 4.

Netilmicin and gentamicin MICs determined in the presence of carbenicillin were lowered to one-quarter or less of the value obtained in its absence for 15 of 18 isolates. The netilmicin MICs measured in the presence of carbenicillin were 3.1 μg/ml or less for 16 of 18 isolates; two remained resistant, with MICs of 50 and >100 μg/ml, respectively. Similar results were obtained with gentamicin; MICs of 15 of 18 isolates were <3.1 μg/ml. In no instance was there evidence of drug antagonism.

A similar fourfold or greater reduction of MIC was observed in 9 of 18 isolates for tobramycin and 16 of 18 isolates for amikacin.

DISCUSSION

In contrast to previously published data (5), we found netilmicin provided no advantage in antimicrobial activity over gentamicin for either *P. aeruginosa* or *Enterobacteriaceae*. Nearly complete cross-resistance to netilmicin was encountered with isolates resistant to gentamicin when tested in solid or liquid media. Netilmicin was less active than gentamicin against isolates of *P. aeruginosa* and *P. stuartii*. Netilmicin exhibits typical aminoglycoside characteristics, such as little effect of inoculum size on MIC, relatively small gap between MIC and MBC, and the potentiation of its anti-*Pseudomonas* activity when combined with carbenicillin. Major discrepancies between MIC values determined in agar as opposed to those determined in broth for *P. aeruginosa*, well described for other aminoglycosides, are also found with netilmicin. These discrepancies have been attributed in the case of *P. aeruginosa* to a cell wall-stabilizing effect of high concentrations of divalent cations, especially

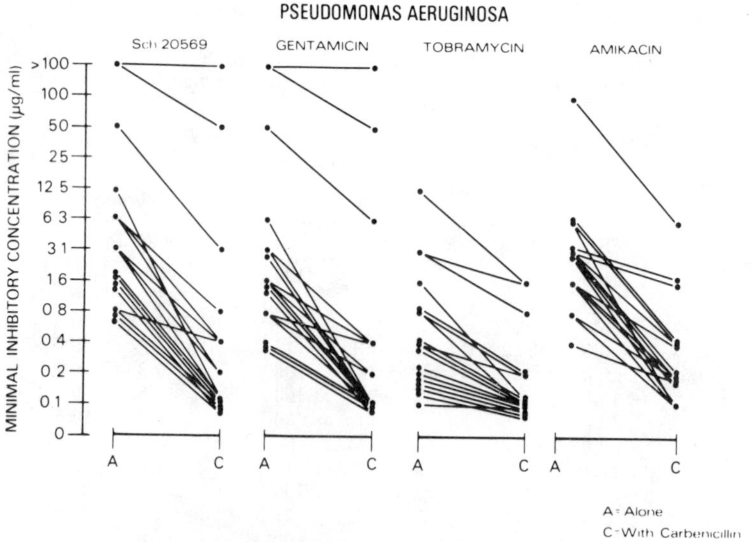

FIG. 4. *Comparison of MICs of four aminoglycoside antibiotics measured alone or in the presence of 50 μg of carbenicillin per ml for P. aeruginosa. Each line represents a single isolate. Netilmicin is designated as Sch 20569.*

Ca^{2+} and Mg^{2+}, which are usually present in the solid but not the liquid media (1, 2, 7). Supporting this is the fact that markedly increased binding and presumably cell wall penetration of ^{3}H-labeled gentamicin to *Pseudomonas* occurs in media with low divalent ion concentrations (6). In addition, the "protective" effect of high divalent cation concentrations is lost when the organism being tested is a carbenicillin-induced spheroplast in hypertonic medium (9). Previous investigators have concluded that the divalent cation concentration in the medium has little or no effect in susceptibility tests of *Enterobacteriaceae* (2, 4, 9). These conclusions, however, rest upon the testing of relatively small numbers of isolates. We found that, depending upon which aminoglycoside was used, between 15 and 40% of the isolates of *Enterobacteriaceae* exhibited fourfold or greater diminutions of MIC when tested in broth as compared to agar. For some *Enterobacteriaceae* differences in media may create as significant a problem in interpretation of in vitro susceptibility test results, as already exists for *P. aeruginosa*.

If further studies in experimental animals and humans demonstrate that netilmicin indeed possesses less toxic potential than other currently available aminoglycoside antibiotics, this agent may become a useful therapeutic tool.

ACKNOWLEDGMENTS

We thank Eva Hawkins and Fereshteh Ghadirian for technical assistance. This study was supported by a grant-in-aid from the Schering Corp.

LITERATURE CITED

1. **Garrod, L. P., and P. M. Waterworth.** 1969. Effect of medium composition on the apparent sensitivity of *Pseudomonas aeruginosa* to gentamicin. J. Clin. Pathol. **22**:534–538.
2. **Gilbert, D. N., E. Kutscher, P. Ireland, J. A. Barnett, and J. Sanford.** 1971. Effect of the concentrations of magnesium and calcium on the in vitro susceptibility of *Pseudomonas aeruginosa* to gentamicin. J. Infect. Dis. **124**(Suppl.):S37–S45.
3. **Greene, W. H., M. Moody, S. Schimpff, V. M. Young, and P. H. Wiernik.** 1973. *Pseudomonas aeruginosa* resistant to carbenicillin and gentamicin: epidemiologic and clinical aspects in a cancer center. Ann. Intern. Med. **79**:684–689.
4. **Medeiros, A. A., T. F. O'Brien, W. E. C. Wacker, and N. F. Yulug.** 1971. Effect of salt concentration on the in vitro susceptibility of *Pseudomonas* and other gram-negative bacilli to gentamicin. J. Infect. Dis. **124**(Suppl.):S59–S64.
5. **Rahal, J. J., M. S. Simberkoff, K. Kagan, and N. H. Moldover.** 1976. Bactericidal efficacy of Sch 20569 and amikacin against gentamicin-sensitive and -resistant organisms. Antimicrob. Agents Chemother. **9**:595–599.
6. **Ramirez-Ronda, C. H., R. K. Holmes, and J. P. Sanford.** 1975. Effects of divalent cations on binding of aminoglycoside antibiotics to human serum proteins and to bacteria. Antimicrob. Agents Chemother. **7**:239–245.
7. **Reller, L. B., F. D. Schoenknecht, M. A. Kenny, and J. C. Sherris.** 1974. Antibiotic susceptibility testing of *Pseudomonas aeruginosa:* selection of a control strain and criteria for magnesium and calcium content in media. J. Infect. Dis. **130**:454–463.
8. **Steers, E., E. L. Foltz, and B. S. Graves.** 1959. An inocula replicating apparatus for routine testing of bacterial susceptibility to antibiotics. Antibiot. Chemother. **9**:307–311.
9. **Zimelis, V. M., and G. G. Jackson.** 1973. Activity of aminoglycoside antibiotics against *Pseudomonas aeruginosa:* specificity and site of calcium and magnesium antagonism. J. Infect. Dis. **127**:663–669.

Antimicrobial Agents and Chemotherapy, Oct. 1976, p. 598-603 Vol. 10, No. 4

Antibiotic Resistance of Bacteria in Water Containing Ornamental Fishes

T. J. TRUST* and J. L. WHITBY

Departments of Bacteriology and Biochemistry, University of Victoria, Victoria, British Columbia, and Departments of Microbiology and Immunology, University of Western Ontario, London, Ontario, Canada*

Received for publication 26 May 1976

Water containing ornamental fishes was found to frequently contain countable numbers of bacteria that were resistant to one or more antibiotic or chemotherapeutic agents. The multidrug-resistant strains most commonly isolated were lactose-fermenting *Citrobacter freundii*. The overall resistance of these aquaria strains was greater than the previously described resistance of clinical isolates of *C. freundii*. Although the strains examined appeared to lack R-factors, this pool of resistant bacteria may have public health implications.

Large numbers of ornamental fish are cultured and shipped internationally to be offered for sale to the public. During culture and shipping, the water housing the fish is often treated with antibiotics or other chemotherapeutic compounds in an attempt to reduce fish mortality. The compounds commonly used include chloramphenicol (Cm), kanamycin (K), penicillin (P), sulfonamides, and tetracycline (Te) (9).

Aquaria containing these fish can be found in homes, school classrooms, medical and dental offices, eating establishments, department stores, nursing homes, and even in hospital wards. Fish in these aquaria can be further treated with antibacterial agents since products containing neomycin (Ne), nitrofurans, streptomycin (Sm), sulfonamides, and tetracycline can be purchased by the public. It was recently demonstrated that the dosage levels recommended for these treatments are likely to be subtherapeutic (8). Richmond (5) has shown that the use of antibiotics at subtherapeutic levels leads to an increase in the frequency of drug-resistant strains of bacteria. The presence of multidrug-resistant bacteria in aquaria has public health implications since Trust and Bartlett (7) have demonstrated that water containing ornamental fish contain bacteria that are potential pathogens of humans.

The present study was initiated to determine the extent to which drug-resistant bacteria are associated with the aquarium environment and to determine the patterns of resistance present. In addition, the opportunity was taken to more fully characterize those multidrug-resistant species of *Enterobacteriaceae* that were most commonly isolated from the aquarium environment.

MATERIALS AND METHODS

Water samples. Ornamental fish were purchased from 14 retail outlets in Victoria, British Columbia, Canada. The fish were supplied in plastic bags containing water taken from the aquaria in which the fish had been housed. The water in each container was sampled for bacteriological examination immediately upon arrival at the laboratory, and the fish were transferred to holding aquaria. There was a total of 40 water samples, each representing a single aquarium and including a single fish species. The number of fish purchased ranged from one to five and included neon tetras (*Hyphessobrycon innesi*), puffer fish (*Tetraodom fluviatilis*), white clouds (*Tanichthys albonubes*), guppies (*Lebistes reticulatus*), Jack Dempsey (*Cichlasoma biocellatum*), angels (*Pterophyllum eimekei*), zebras (*Brachydanio rerio*), catfish (*Corydoras aneus*), and common goldfish (*Carassius auratus*).

A population of the goldfish collected from the above sources was also maintained at the University of Victoria. Goldfish were transferred from the holding aquarium to test aquaria. These test aquaria were 6-liter, round glass jars, each containing 5 liters of distilled water (adjusted to pH 7 before the addition of fish). The jars were aerated at 1 liter/min and held at 22°C. Ten goldfish (mean weight, 1.2 g; range of weights, 0.9 to 1.6 g) were placed in each aquarium. The fish were held in the test aquaria for 72 h, at which time water samples were taken for bacteriological examination. The pH of the water in the aquaria was then between 6.5 and 6.8.

Antibacterial compounds. Chloramphenicol and kanamycin were purchased from Sigma Chemical Co., St. Louis, Mo., and potassium penicillin, neomycin sulfate, sodium sulfamerazine, sodium sulfamethazine, sodium sulfathiazole, streptomycin sulfate, and tetracycline hydrochloride were purchased from Nutritional Biochemicals Corp., Cleveland, Ohio. All solids were dried to a constant weight before use.

Quantitative bacteriological examination. Duplicate dilutions of the water samples were prepared in 0.1% (wt/vol) peptone water (pH 7.2), and the viable aerobic bacteria present were enumerated by the drop-plate method of Miles and Misra (3). Total counts were done on Mueller-Hinton agar (Baltimore Biological Laboratory, Cockeysville, Md.) or on this medium supplemented with one, two, or three antibacterial compounds. Counts of lactose-fermenting organisms were done on MacConkey agar or on this medium supplemented with antibacterial compounds. When added singly to Mueller-Hinton agar, the following concentrations (expressed as active ingredients) were used: neomycin, 120 μg/ml; penicillin, 300 U/ml; streptomycin, 40 μg/ml; sulfathiazole (Su), 300 μg/ml; triple sulfa (SSS), 300 μg/ml (100 μg each of sulfamerazine, sulfamethazine, and sulfathiazole per ml); and tetracycline, 30 μg/ml. Lower concentrations were generally employed in MacConkey agar due to the selective nature of this medium, and final concentrations for single antibacterials were: neomycin, 30 μg/ml; penicillin, 10 U/ml; triple sulfa, 30 μg/ml; sulfathiazole, 300 μg/ml; streptomycin, 10 μg/ml; and tetracycline, 30 μg/ml. Chloramphenicol and kanamycin were used only in combination with other antibacterials; in combination plates, a concentration of 30 μg of antibiotic per ml was used for all antibacterials, regardless of the medium employed.

Spectrum of drug resistance. Antibiotic-resistant strains were purified by subculture to antibiotic-free Mueller-Hinton agar and then grown overnight in Trypticase soy broth (BBL). Plates of Mueller-Hinton agar (BBL) were spread with 0.1 ml of overnight culture and overlaid with susceptibility disks (BBL) containing: ampicillin, 10 μg; chloramphenicol, 30 μg; kanamycin, 30 μg; neomycin, 30 μg; penicillin, 10 U; streptomycin, 10 μg; tetracycline, 30 μg; and triple sulfa, 250 μg.

Identification of isolates. All gram-negative, lactose-fermenting bacilli were identified by performing a series of 32 identification tests. Motility, lysine and ornithine decarboxylase, indole production, gluconate reduction, growth in KCN, oxidase, and O/F glucose were determined by standard methods. Carbohydrate fermentation tests, malonate utilization, urease, gelatinase, deoxyribonuclease, cephalosporinase, and phenylalanine deaminase were performed on solid media. Carbohydrate plates contained 1% (wt/vol) of the designated carbohydrate, which was sterilized separately and added to a basal medium of peptone water agar that was adjusted to pH 7.6 to 7.8 with an appropriate agar concentration to inhibit spreaders. Bromothymol blue (0.002%) was added as an indicator. The media were poured into conventional 8.5-cm, circular, disposable, plastic petri dishes and inoculated, using a replicator consisting of 37 flat-ended steel bars (3 mm in diameter and 12 mm apart; made by Biotech Co. of Canada and marketed by K.V.L. Laboratories, Cambridge, Ontario). Antibiotic susceptibility determinations were made using this same replicator, a standardized inoculum, and media into which the following concentrations of antibiotic were incorporated: penicillin, 0.06 μg; ampicillin, 8 μg; carbenicillin, 100 μg; tetracycline, 4 μg; kanamycin, 8 μg; gentamicin, 4 μg; polymyxin, 12.5 μg; nalidixic acid, 12.0 μg; nitrofurantoin, 30 μg; sulfonamide, 1 mg; trimethoprim, 10 μg; streptomycin, 16 μg; and chloramphenicol, 16 μg.

Experiments designed to demonstrate transmissible resistance were performed using *Escherichia coli* K-12 strain CSH 55 (F^- *lac*$^-$ *pro*$^-$ nalidixic acid resistant) and CSH 55 (F' *lac*$^+$ *pro*$^+$ nalidixic acid resistant); the latter strains were obtained from matings of CSH 55 with CSH 23 (F' *lac*$^+$ *pro*$^+$). CSH strains were initially obtained from Cold Spring Harbor Laboratory, Cold Spring Harbor, N.Y.

RESULTS

Table 1 shows that water samples from aquaria containing goldfish maintained at the University of Victoria contained 9.5×10^6 viable aerobic bacteria per ml, including 2.9×10^4 organisms able to ferment lactose during growth on MacConkey agar. Between 0.2% (Te_{30}) and 28.4% (P_{300}) of the bacteria present grew on media supplemented with a single antibiotic. Countable lactose-fermenting bacteria were not observed on the Ne_{30}-MacConkey medium, but between 3% (Sm_{10}) and 93% (P_{10}, Te_{30}) of the total lactose fermenters present in the water samples grew on MacConkey agar supplemented with a single antibiotic.

Water samples containing ornamental fishes purchased at retail outlets also contained bacteria capable of growth on media supplemented with antibiotics or chemotherapeutic agents. Table 2 shows that these water samples all contained from 10^2 to 10^4 viable aerobic bacteria per ml capable of growing on Mueller-Hinton agar supplemented with eight different combinations of two antibacterials and one medium supplemented with three antibacterials. These

TABLE 1. *Numbers of viable bacteria in aquarium water[a] capable of growth in the presence of single antibacterial compounds[b]*

Medium	Total viable aerobic counts/ml (mean)[c]	Medium	Total lactose-fermenting organisms/100 ml (mean)[c]
MH	9.5×10^6	Mc	2.9×10^6
MH + Ne_{120}	6.0×10^4	Mc + Ne_{30}	TFC
MH + P_{300}	2.7×10^6	Mc + P_{10}	2.7×10^6
MH + Su_{300}	9.1×10^5	Mc + Su_{300}	3.4×10^5
MH + SSS_{300}	1.4×10^5	Mc + SSS_{300}	3.4×10^5
MH + Sm_{40}	2.0×10^6	Mc + Sm_{10}	8.6×10^4
MH + Te_{30}	2.0×10^4	Mc + Te_{30}	2.7×10^6

[a] Aquaria maintained at the University of Victoria.
[b] Abbreviations: MH, Mueller-Hinton agar; Mc, MacConkey agar; TFC, too few organisms to count.
[c] Mean value from four samples.

values represent from 0.16 to 21.3% of the total aerobes present. Countable numbers of lactose fermenters were not found growing on MacConkey agar supplemented with $Cm_{30}Te_{30}$, $K_{30}Su_{30}$, $K_{30}Te_{30}$, or $Ne_{30}Te_{30}$, but between 4.7 and 53.1% of the total lactose-fermenting organisms present were able to grow on MacConkey agar supplemented with $Su_{30}Te_{30}$, $Sm_{30}Te_{30}$, or $Sm_{30}Te_{30}Su_{30}$.

The patterns of antibiotic resistance of strains isolated from the various antibacterial-containing media are shown in Table 3. Of the 415 strains tested, 198 were found to be non-lactose fermenters, which included 57 isolates identified as species of *Aeromonas*, 57 *Pseudomonas* isolates, and 51 *o*-nitrophenyl-β-D-galactopyranoside-positive strains of *Citrobacter*. Other strains included species of *Acinetobacter*, *Flavobacterium*, *Proteus*, *Providencia*, *Serratia*, *Staphylococcus*, and *Vibrio*. A total of 70 different patterns of resistance were demonstrated, with 47% of the isolates being resistant

TABLE 2. *Numbers of multidrug-resistant bacteria in water containing ornamental fishes purchased from retail outlets*[a]

No. of samples	Medium[b]	Total viable aerobic counts/ml (mean)	Medium[b]	Total lactose-fermenting organisms/100 ml (mean)
40	MH	3.8×10^5	Mc	1.6×10^5
13	MH + Cm Te	1.7×10^4	Mc + Cm Te	TFC
6	MH + K Su	6.4×10^2	Mc + K Su	TFC
13	MH + K Te	3.8×10^4	Mc + K Te	TFC
13	MH + Ne Te	4.8×10^4	Mc + Ne Te	TFC
13	MH + Su Te	8.1×10^4	Mc + Su Te	8.5×10^4
34	MH + Sm Te	3.5×10^3	Mc + Sm Te	7.5×10^3
13	MH + Sm Te Su	9.9×10^3	Mc + Sm Te Su	1.4×10^4

[a] Abbreviations: MH, Mueller-Hinton agar; Mc, MacConkey agar; TFC, too few organisms to count.
[b] Medium contained 30 μg of each antibacterial per ml.

TABLE 3. *Drug resistance patterns of resistant strains of bacteria isolated from water containing ornamental fishes*

Resistance pattern[a]	No. of lactose fermenters	No. of other species[b]	Resistance pattern	No. of lactose fermenters	No. of other species	Resistance pattern	No. of lactose fermenters	No. of other species
P Ne Cm Te K SSS Sm Am	7	6	Ne Te K SSS Sm		1	P Te K	1	
P Ne Cm Te K SSS Sm	21	2	P Cm Te Sm Am		1	P Te SSS	4	8
P Ne Cm Te SSS Sm Am	4	3	P Cm Te K SSS		1	Te SSS Sm	10	3
P Cm Te K SSS Sm Am		1	P Te K Sm	1		P Ne Am		1
P Ne Cm Te SSS Sm	25	4	Cm Te SSS Sm	4	3	Cm SSS Sm		1
P Ne Te K SSS Sm	13	1	P Te SSS Sm	16	10	K SSS Sm	7	2
P Ne Cm Te K SSS		1	P Cm K SSS	1	1	P Cm Sm		2
			P Ne Te K	1				
P Ne Te SSS Sm Am	3	1	P Ne Te SSS	4	1	P Cm SSS		1
P Ne K SSS Sm Am		1	P Cm SSS Sm	2	1	P K SSS		1
P Cm Te K SSS Sm	2		P Cm Te SSS	2	5	Cm Te SSS		2
P Cm Te K Sm Am		1	P Ne K SSS	1		Cm SSS Sm	3	3
P Cm Te SSS Sm Am	1	1	Ne Te SSS Sm	2	1	P SSS	1	5
P Cm Te SSS Am	2		P Te K SSS	1				
P Ne Cm Te SSS		2	P Te SSS Am	1		P Ne	1	
P Ne Te SSS Sm	26	1	P Cm Te Am		1	Te SSS		
P Ne Te Sm Am		1	P Ne Te Am		1	P Te	1	2
P Ne Te K SSS		1	P Ne SSS Sm		2	Te K		1
			P K SSS Sm	1				
P Ne K SSS Sm		1	Ne K SSS Sm		1	Cm Te		1
			Te K SSS Sm	1				
P Cm K SSS Sm	4	1	P K SSS Sm		1	P Sm		2
P Cm Te SSS Sm	9	14	P Te Sm	11		P Cm		1
P Te SSS Sm Am	6	2	P SSS Sm	6	22	SSS Sm	10	4
Ne Cm K SSS Sm	1	1	P Ne K	1		P K		1

[a] Penicillin, 10 U; neomycin, 30 μg; chloramphenicol, 30 μg; tetracycline, 30 μg; kanamycin, 30 μg; triple sulfa, 250 μg; streptomycin, 10 μg; ampicillin, 10 μg.
[b] Other species include *Acinetobacter* (2), *Aeromonas* (50), *Citrobacter* (45), *Flavobacterium* (12), *Proteus morganii* (2), *Providencia* (2), *P. fluorescens* (16), *Serratia* (3), *Staphylococcus* (2), and *Vibrio* (6).

to five or more of the antibacterials employed; the most frequent patterns of resistance common to both lactose-fermenting and non-lactose-fermenting isolates were P Te SSS Sm and P Cm Te SSS Sm. The most frequent patterns of resistance displayed by lactose-fermenting isolates were P Ne Te SSS Sm, P Ne Cm Te SSS Sm, and P Ne Cm Te K SSS Sm, whereas P SSS Sm was the most frequent pattern displayed by non-lactose-fermenting isolates.

The multidrug-resistant, lactose-fermenting isolates were subjected to an intensive biochemical characterization, and their resistance to a wide variety of antibacterials was confirmed by the agar dilution method. The biochemical tests employed and the number of strains positive in each test are shown in Table 4. All 218 strains were identified as *Citrobacter* species, and since none fermented adonitol they were considered to be *Citrobacter freundii*. The antibiotic resistances of the 218 *C. freundii* strains are given in Table 5. The majority of strains were resistant to penicillin, tetracycline, streptomycin, ampicillin, cephaloridine, sulfonamide, and kanamycin, but resistance to chloramphenicol, furadantin, and nalidixic acid was not uncommon. Resistance to carbenicillin and trimethoprim was rare, and resistance to gentamicin and polymyxin was not observed.

Since aquaria form a common adjunct to the domestic environment and are also commonly found as a decoration in public places, offices, and even pediatric wards in hospitals, it seemed important to attempt to determine whether the presence of plasmid-mediated resistance transfer factor could be detected in these highly antibiotic-resistant strains. For this purpose individual direct matings between 10 penicillin-, ampicillin-, cephalothin-, tetracycline-, streptomycin-, and kanamycin-resistant *C. freundii* strains representing five biotypes and a nalidixic acid-resistant strain of *E. coli* K-12 were attempted. In no experiment were any recombinants found. Attempts were also made to mobilize a citrobacter plasmid by an F plasmid using an F′ lac^+ pro^+ plasmid of *E. coli* K-12. The F′ lac^+ pro^+ *E. coli* K-12 was mixed with cells from the same 10 citrobacter strains, and after 9 min the F^- Nal^r *E. coli* K-12 was added. Again no recombinants were demonstrated, but it was not possible to prove that F had been transmitted to the *C. freundii* strains since the latter were all lac^+. In this respect the experiments were inconclusive, but they failed to demonstrate the presence of transferable resistance plasmids in the *C. freundii* strains. If transfer had occurred, it would have been detected at any frequency greater than 1 in 10^7 bacterial cells.

TABLE 4. *Biochemical characteristics of multidrug-resistant strains of C. freundii isolated from aquaria*

Test on substrate	No. of positive strains[a]	Positive (%)	Positive Ewing and Davis (1) series (%)
Glucose fermentation	218	100	100
H_2S production in TSI[b]	179	82.1	81.6
Indole	20	9.2	6.7
Motility	209	96.5	95.7
Gluconate	1	0.5	
Malonate	39	17.9	21.8
Citrate	194	89.0	90.4
Phenylalanine deaminase	0	0	
Urease	0	0	69.4
Gelatin	0	0	0
Deoxyribonuclease	0	0	
Oxidase	0	0	
Cephalosporinase	212	97.2	
Lysine decarboxylase	0	0	0
Ornithine decarboxylase	43	19.7	17.2
Lactose	217	99.5	39.4[c]
Sucrose	214	98.2	15.3
Mannitol	218	100	99.8
Dulcitol	65	29.8	59.8
Salicin	35	16.0	4.1
Adonitol	0	0	0
Inositol	0	0	3.3
Sorbitol	218	100	98.0
Arabinose	217	99.5	100
Raffinose	204	93.6	14.2
Rhamnose	218	100	99.4
Maltose	217	99.5	98.5
Xylose	213	97.7	99.8
Trehalose	218	100	100
Cellobiose	102	46.8	60.8
Glycerol	204	93.6	97.9
Esculin	35	16.0	0.9

[a] A total of 218 strains were tested.
[b] TSI, Triple sugar iron agar.
[c] An additional 58% were late lactose fermenters.

TABLE 5. *Antibiotic resistance of C. freundii strains isolated from aquaria*

Antibiotic	No. of strains resistant[a]	Resistant (%)
Penicillin	218	100
Ampicillin	155	71.1
Carbenicillin	10	4.5
Cephaloridine	140	64.2
Tetracycline	215	98.6
Kanamycin	123	56.4
Gentamicin	0	0
Polymyxin	0	0
Nalidixic acid	29	13.3
Nitrofurantoin	52	23.8
Sulfonamide	162	74.3
Trimethoprim	5	2.3
Streptomycin	172	78.9
Chloramphenicol	102	46.8

[a] A total of 218 strains were tested.

DISCUSSION

These data indicate that water containing ornamental fishes frequently contains bacteria that are resistant to more than one antibiotic or chemotherapeutic agent. The multidrug-resistant strains most commonly isolated from aquarium water in this study were identified as lactose-fermenting *C. freundii*. It is interesting to note that these drug-resistant strains of *Citrobacter* were isolated on the assumption that they were *E. coli*, but biochemical tests revealed that no isolations of *E. coli* were in fact obtained.

There is fairly close accord with the behavior of these strains of *C. freundii* and those reported by Ewing and Davis (1), with a few exceptions. Some differences require comment; the multiple-inoculation method we use for urease determination is only suitable for reading within 24 h of inoculation. *C. freundii* strains are not rapid urease producers and are almost always negative when tested by this method. The strains selected for examination had already been found to be lactose fermenters; therefore, comparison with Ewing and Davis is inappropriate for lactose fermentation. There is a notable difference in the high frequency of fermentation of sucrose and raffinose by our strains and of dulcitol by the "strains" of Ewing and Davis, which may reflect their different origins. Our strains were all isolated from aquaria, but 399 of the 616 isolates reported by Ewing and Davis were from human sources, whereas only 20 were from water and 37 were from foods and feeds.

According to Ewing and Davis, malonate utilization is a characteristic possessed by a minority of *C. freundii* strains. Our series contained 39 strains that were malonate positive, and of these 37 were ornithine decarboxylase positive, 33 were esculin positive, 33 were salicin positive, and 32 were glycerol negative. A positive result in malonate and ornithine decarboxylase tests would be typical of *C. diversus*, but the strains all failed to ferment adonitol and were indole negative. The KCN test was performed on all malonate-positive strains, and 18/39 were found to be positive, with some positive examples from all the observed biotypes. The KCN test does not distinguish between *C. freundii* and *Enterobacter cloacae*, and on the tests so far outlined the strains might have been gluconate-negative examples of *E. cloacae*, more particularly since the strains were also H_2S negative and esculin positive. The methyl red test was found to be positive for all 39 strains; thus it is likely that the 39 strains were examples of less usual biotypes of *C. freundii* and were not examples of *E. cloacae*.

Many of the multidrug-resistant species isolated in this study, such as *Pseudomonas fluorescens*, are probably naturally resistant to many of the antibiotic agents tested. *Citrobacter* strains from clinical isolates are not necessarily highly antibiotic resistant, and the overall resistance of these aquaria strains was greater than, for instance, that described by Lund et al. (2) for H_2S-negative strains of *C. freundii* and by Slifkin and Engwall (6) for *C. intermedium*. In particular, our strains were much more resistant to tetracycline, streptomycin, kanamycin, sulfonamides, and chloramphenicol, which are all antibiotics commonly used in the cultivation of ornamental fish. In contrast, no strains were found to be resistant to gentamicin or polymyxin, and few strains displayed resistance to carbenicillin or trimethoprim. These antibacterials are not used by fish growers and are not available to the public as aquarium medications. This may explain the low resistance of the *Citrobacter* strains to these antibacterials.

It seemed likely that some of this multidrug resistance would be mediated by resistance transfer factors since R-factors are considered to be the most important elements responsible for resistance to tetracycline, chloramphenicol, streptomycin, sulfanilamide, ampicillin, and kanamycin among most genera of *Enterobacteriaceae* (4). It is not clear at this time why the strains examined appeared to lack R-factors since other studies have shown that multidrug-resistant *Citrobacter* strains carry R-factors (4). The result may only indicate that the experimental conditions used or the recipient strains selected were not appropriate for the *Citrobacter* strains examined.

Regardless of the mechanism by which this multidrug resistance is mediated, this pool of resistant bacteria may have considerable public health significance since people can be exposed to aquarium-borne, drug-resistant bacteria in numerous situations inside and outside the home. This exposure can be by either direct contact with the water or indirect contact mediated by the spread of a bacterial aerosol formed by the action of the aquarium aerator. This exposure could present considerable clinical significance to individuals at risk, such as young children, persons with impaired immunological responses, persons undergoing antibiotic therapy, and debilitated individuals. It is in these persons that normally innocuous bacteria such as *C. freundii*, *P. fluorescens* and *Aeromonas hydrophila* can cause severe infections. Interestingly, the opportunity for acquiring infections often exists since aquaria are often used as ornamentation in areas for such people.

In addition to those multidrug-resistant strains that have been selected by the use of antibacterial agents during the culture and shipping of ornamental fishes, populations of drug-resistant bacteria may also be induced in home aquaria. The aquarium contains a mixed bacterial culture growing in a liquid menstruum, and it is in these conditions in which microorganisms of different species and strains coexist and multiply simultaneously that there is ample opportunity for the transfer of genetic information, including that concerned with drug resistance. The use of antibacterial products at subtherapeutic levels will certainly provide the selection pressures necessary to increase the numbers of these drug-resistant strains in aquaria and hence in the environment. Since the efficacy of these products in protecting fish health is not proven and since the incidence of human infections by drug-resistant bacteria is on the increase, the unrestricted availability of aquarium products containing antibacterials also used in human medicine is not warranted.

Compounds used in the therapy of fish diseases should not include antibiotics used in human medicine or those known to induce R-factors. Efforts should be made to find other drugs whose application can be restricted to fish culture. These measures should lead to a decrease in the numbers of multidrug-resistant bacteria in the environment, since experience has shown that withdrawal of an antibiotic commonly leads to a decrease in the number of resistant strains encountered.

ACKNOWLEDGMENTS

We thank Amin G. Khouri for his technical assistance.

This work was supported by a grant from the University of Victoria Research Leave and Travel Committee.

LITERATURE CITED

1. **Ewing, W. H., and B. R. Davis.** 1971. Biochemical characterization of *Citrobacter freundii* and *Citrobacter diversus*. Center for Disease Control, Atlanta.
2. **Lund, M. E., J. M. Matsen, and D. J. Blazevic.** 1974. Biochemical and antibiotic susceptibility studies of H_2S-negative *Citrobacter*. Appl. Microbiol. 28:22-25.
3. **Miles, A. A., and S. S. Misra.** 1938. The estimation of the bactericidal power of the blood. J. Hyg. 38:732-749.
4. **Mitsuhashi, S.** 1971. Epidemiology of R-factors, p. 25-38. *In* S. Mitsuhashi (ed.), Transferable drug resistance factor R. University Park Press, Baltimore, Md.
5. **Richmond, M. H.** 1972. Some environmental consequences of the use of the antibiotics: or "what goes up must come down." J. Appl. Bacteriol. 35:155-176.
6. **Slifkin, M., and C. Engwall.** 1967. The clinical significance of *Citrobacter intermedium*. Am. J. Clin. Pathol. 52;351-355.
7. **Trust, T. J., and K. H. Bartlett.** 1974. Occurrence of potential pathogens in water containing ornamental fishes. Appl. Microbiol. 28:35-40.
8. **Trust, T. J., and D. C. Chipman.** 1974. Evaluation of aquarium antibiotic formulations. Antimicrob. Agents Chemother. 6:379-386.
9. **Watanabe, T., T. Aotei, Ch. Yada, Y. Ogata, K. Sugawara, T. Saito, and S. Egusa.** 1971. Fish culturing and R factors, p. 131-142. *In* V. Krčméry, L. Rosival, and T. Watanabe (ed.), Bacterial plasmids and antibiotic resistance. Avicenum-Czechoslovak Medical Press, Prague.

Antimicrobial Agents and Chemotherapy, Oct. 1976, p. 604-609
Vol. 10, No. 4

Printed in U.S.A.

Kinetics of the Actions of Tetracyclines on *Escherichia coli* as Studied by Microcalorimetry

PER-ANDERS MÅRDH,* TORVALD RIPA, KARL-ERIK ANDERSSON, AND INGEMAR WADSÖ

Institute of Medical Microbiology, Thermochemistry Laboratory, Chemical Center, University of Lund, and Department of Clinical Pharmacology, University Hospital, S-223 62 Lund, Sweden*

Received for publication 26 April 1976

Microcalorimetry was used to study the kinetics of the actions of various tetracyclines on a strain of *Escherichia coli*. Differences in the capacity to suppress the metabolism of this bacterium were observed. When the antibiotic was present from the start of the experiment, a heat production of 2.0 μW/ml was registered after 12.5 h using minocycline; the corresponding figures for doxycycline, oxytetracycline, and tetracycline were 7.3, 6.6, and 4.5 h, respectively. In these experiments, equal concentrations, i.e., half the minimum inhibitory concentration (MIC), of each drug were used. The MIC for all the tetracyclines tested, determined by the broth dilution technique, was 0.8 μg/ml. In other experiments, the antibiotic (concentration, 1.6 μg/ml = 2× MIC) was introduced into the growth vessel during the logarithmic growth phase of the organism. The extent and duration of the inhibitory effect on the metabolism, as judged from the decrease in heat production, varied with the different tetracyclines. Immediately after introduction, minocycline, doxycycline, oxytetracycline, and tetracycline decreased the heat production in decreasing order of potency. With tetracycline, the heat production rose after about 1 h, and with minocycline it rose after about 9 h. The heat production remained at a low level for at least 19 h when using doxycycline and oxytetracycline. The results indicate that microcalorimetry offers a means for studies of the kinetics of the antibacterial actions of antibiotics and provides information that cannot be obtained by conventional bacteriological techniques. This information may be of use, in conjunction with pharmacokinetic data, in establishing optimum doses and dose intervals in antibiotic therapy.

Microcalorimetry provides a general analytical tool for characterization of microbial growth processes (for a recent review see reference 9), for identification of microorganisms (2, 6, 8; K. Ljungholm, I. Wadsö, and P.-A. Mårdh, J. Gen. Microbiol., in press), for susceptibility testing (1), and for evaluation of optimal growth media (T. Ripa, P.-A. Mårdh, B. Hovelius, and K. Ljungholm, manuscript in preparation). The heat produced by a bacterial culture can be continuously recorded as a "thermogram," without introducing any analytical factors into the culture system. The method has a low specificity but a high phenomenological resolution, which is of advantage in studies of complex biochemical systems such as bacterial broth cultures.

In the present investigation, the thermograms produced by a strain of *Escherichia coli*, cultured in the presence of doxycycline, minocycline, oxytetracycline, and tetracycline, were studied by means of batch and flow microcalorimeters of the heat conduction type. The various effects obtained by introducing these drugs in different concentrations at different stages of the growth cycle of the bacterium were investigated. The standardized test conditions used allowed comparative studies on the kinetics of the effects of the tetracyclines tested.

MATERIALS AND METHODS

Calorimeters. A batch twin microcalorimeter of the heat conduction type, a slightly modified version of an instrument recently described by Wadsö (10), was used. The samples were enclosed in stainless-steel ampoules (volume, 4 ml). The calorimeters were thermostated at 37.00°C. The voltage signal was amplified with a Keithley 150B microvolt Ammeter (10-, 30-, or 100-μV range) and was recorded by means of a Servogors RE541 recorder (100-mV range). The base-line stability for the instrument was 1.5 μW/24 h.

In other experiments, a flow microcalorimeter was used, which essentially was identical to that earlier described by Monk and Wadsö (5). The instrument was fitted with a flow-through cell consisting of a Teflon coil imbedded in Wood's metal in a thin-walled aluminum box. The volume of the cell was 0.70 ml.

Bacterium. A strain of *E. coli* was used as the test organism. The minimum inhibitory concentrations (MICs) for doxycycline, minocycline, oxytetracycline, and tetracycline, as determined by the broth dilution technique (13), were 0.8 μg/ml. The medium used in these determinations was the same as that used in the calorimetric experiments. In additional experiments, two other strains of *E. coli* were used; the MICs for these were 3.0 and 40 μg/ml, respectively. The three strains of *E. coli* were isolated from urine cultures from patients with acute infections of the urinary tract.

Culture media. Trypticase soy broth (BBL), pH 7.2, was used as test medium. In some experiments, the test organism was harvested from blood agar plates consisting of blood agar base no. 2 (Oxoid) with 4% defibrinated horse blood.

Antibiotics. Minocycline hydrochloride (Lederle), doxycycline hydrochloride, oxytetracycline hydrochloride, and tetracycline hydrochloride (Pfizer) were used. Stock solutions of the antibiotics (containing 1,000 μg/ml) were prepared in distilled water. Further dilutions were made in phosphate-buffered saline, pH 7.2. The final concentrations of the antibiotics (expressed in micrograms per milliliter) were based upon the active portion of the drugs.

Batch calorimetric measurements. The calorimetric ampoules were heat sterilized before they were charged with 3 ml of a broth culture of the test bacterium (test ampoule) and with sterile growth medium (reference ampoule). The gas phase (1 ml) in the ampoules was air. At the start of the experiments, the media in the ampoules were thermostated for 5 min at 37°C before being introduced into the calorimeter. They were equilibrated for 3 plus 7 min in the two heat-exchange positions and were then inserted into the ampoule holder in the thermopile zone.

In this type of experiment, the bacteria were grown in the broth medium and incubated at 37°C for 4 h. Thereafter, the culture was diluted with fresh medium to 10^6 bacteria/ml. From this medium, 0.03 ml was inoculated into the antibiotic-containing medium of the test ampoule, giving a final concentration of 10^4 bacteria/ml. The bacterial concentrations were estimated by optical density and controlled by viable counts. Non-antibiotic-containing cultures were tested for comparison.

Flow calorimetric measurements. In the flow calorimetric experiments, the broth culture, initially containing 10^4 bacteria/ml (enumerated as described above), was grown in an aerated growth vessel (a constant flow of air bubbling through the broth), which was kept in the thermostatic bath of the calorimeter. The bacteria used had been harvested from a blood agar plate and were suspended in Trypticase soy broth. The antibiotic was added to the broth culture when the thermogram indicated that the bacterial culture was in its logarithmic growth phase and at exactly the same heat production level (40 μW/ml) in each test of this type. During the experiment, the bacterial suspension was pumped through the calorimeter cell by aid of a peristaltic pump (LKB 10200) at a flow rate of 15 ml/h.

RESULTS

Heat effects produced by *E. coli* grown in the presence of tetracyclines: addition of drugs in the lag phase (batch calorimeter). Representative thermograms obtained when the test strain of *E. coli* was grown in the presence of minocycline, doxycycline, oxytetracycline, and tetracycline, 0.4 μg/ml (0.5× MIC), are shown in Fig. 1. In this test, the antibiotic was present from the start of the experiment, i.e., introduced during the lag phase of the culture. In the figure is also shown the thermogram from one of the control experiments in which no antibiotic was present.

The time interval between the start of the experiment and the ascending phase of the thermogram suggests that minocycline retarded bacterial growth longer than did the other tetracyclines tested (Fig. 1). The time for reaching a heat effect of 2.0 μW/ml was about 12.5 h for minocycline, 7.3 h for doxycycline, 6.6 h for oxytetracycline, and 4.5 h for tetracycline. The corresponding time for the non-antibiotic-containing culture was approximately 2.5 h.

The heat production, relative to the control, was reduced in the presence of all the tetracyclines (Fig. 1). The maximum heat effect was reached first by the culture containing tetracycline and then in those with oxytetracycline, doxycycline, and minocycline in that order.

Addition of drugs in the log phase (flow calorimeter). Figure 2 shows representative thermograms obtained when each of the four tetracyclines tested (concentration, 1.6 μg/ml; i.e., 2× MIC) was added to the growth vessel of the flow calorimeter. The drugs were added when the culture of the test strain of *E. coli* produced the same heat effect (40 μW/ml) during the logarithmic growth phase. The thermogram from a control experiment, where no antibiotic was added to the test ampoule, is also given (Fig. 2).

After the introduction of doxycycline (Fig. 2), the heat production decreased and remained without marked changes at a level between 30 and 60 μW/ml for at least 16 h. The heat production was less reduced by tetracycline and remained at a fairly constant level for about 1 h; then the heat production again increased. When using minocycline, the period of reduced and fairly constant heat production was about 9 h; then the heat effects increased rapidly. When oxytetracycline was tested, the heat production was reduced and remained so for at least 16 h.

Variation of the concentration of doxycycline. Figure 3 shows thermograms obtained when a culture of the test bacterium in the logarithmic growth phase was inoculated with

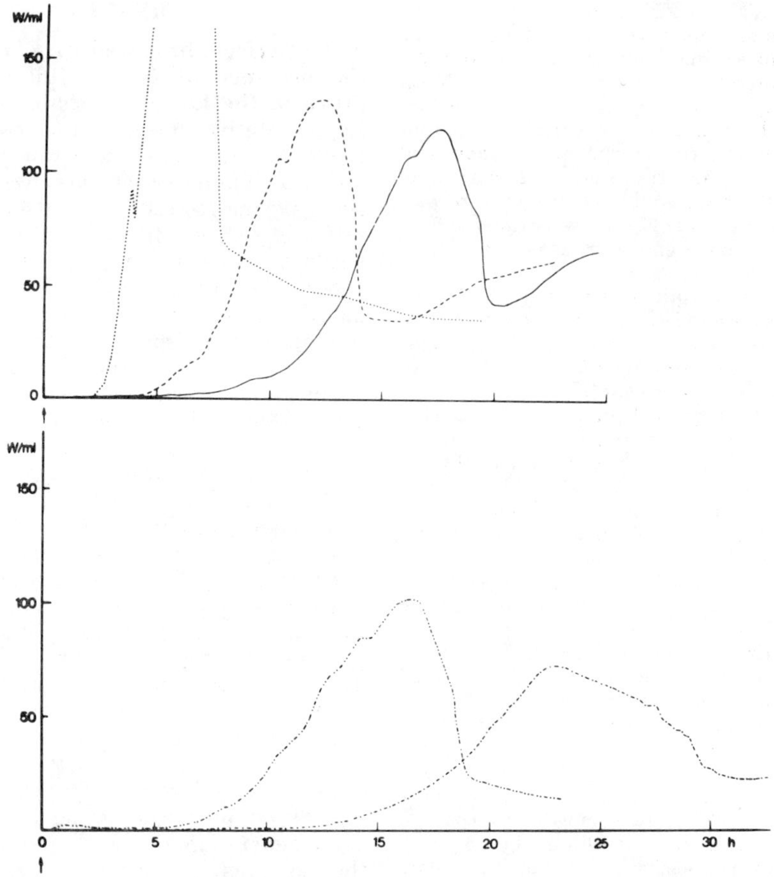

FIG. 1. *(Upper panel) Heat effects produced by E. coli cultured in the presence of tetracycline* (-----) *and doxycycline* (——). *For comparison, the thermogram of a non-antibiotic-containing culture is shown* (· · · · · ·). *(Lower panel) Heat effects produced by E. coli in the presence of oxytetracycline* (–··–··–··–) *and minocycline* (–·–·–·–). *The concentration of the antibiotics was 0.4 μg/ml (0.5× MIC). Arrows indicate introduction of drugs. The experiments were carried out in the batch calorimeter.*

concentrations of doxycycline corresponding to 0.5, 1, 2, and 10 times the MIC, i.e., 0.4, 0.8, 1.6, and 8.0 μg/ml. As can be seen, the depressing effect on the heat production was concentration dependent.

Viable counts and MIC determinations. The number of organisms in samples collected from the growth vessel 0.3, 1, and 9 h after the addition of minocycline did not differ according to viable-count determinations (Table 1). The MICs of the organisms isolated from the same specimens were equal and had not changed from the original, i.e., 0.8 μg/ml.

Strains with different MICs. Figure 4 shows the heat effects produced by three strains of *E. coli*. Their MICs were 0.8, 3.0, and 40 μg/ml. Doxycycline, in concentrations corresponding to 2× MIC (1.6, 6.0, and 80 μg/ml), suppressed the heat production for at least 19 h.

TABLE 1. *Number and MIC of organisms isolated from the growth vessel at different times after the addition of minocycline*

Sampling time (h) after introduction of minocycline	No. of organisms/ml	MIC (μg/ml)
0.3	0.6×10^7	0.8
1	1.0×10^7	0.8
9	0.2×10^7	0.8

DISCUSSION

Studies of antibiotics by conventional pharmacological and microbiological methods can provide information about absorption, concentrations attained in body fluids and tissues, binding to serum proteins and tissue constitu-

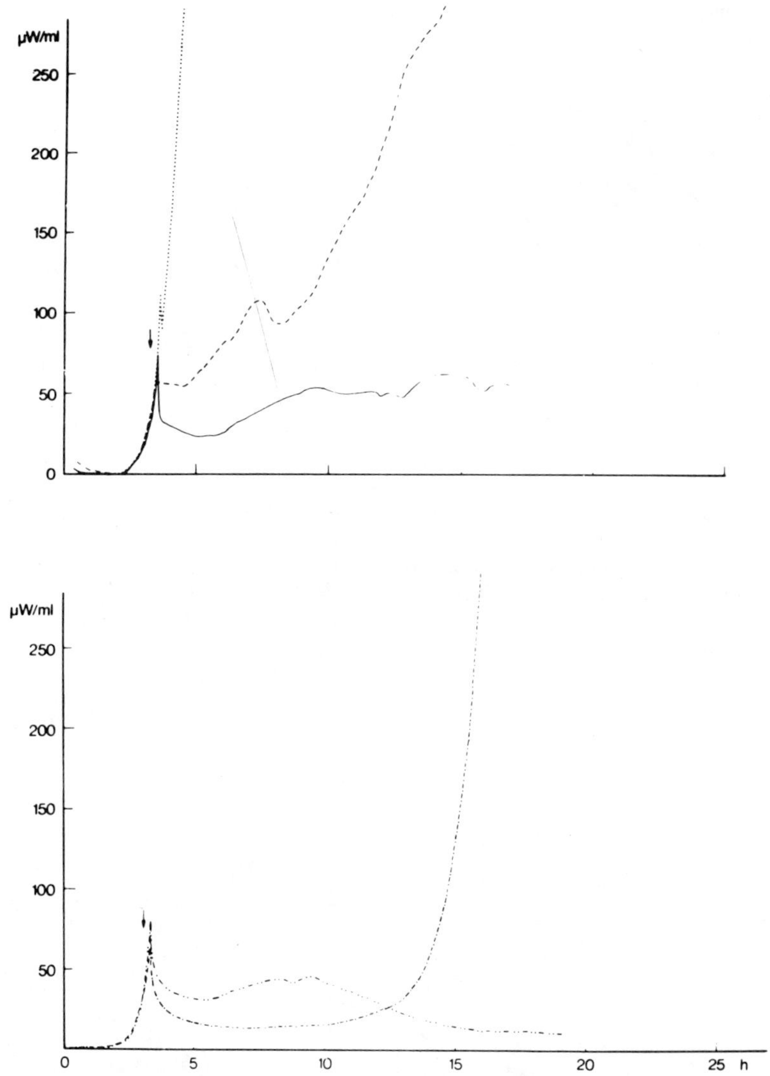

FIG. 2. *(Upper panel) Heat effects produced by E. coli cultured in the presence of tetracycline and doxycycline. The thermogram of a non-antibiotic-containing culture is included. (Lower panel) Heat effects produced by E. coli cultured in the presence of oxytetracycline and minocycline. The antibiotics were added (indicated by arrows) in the logarithmic growth phase at a heat production of 40 μW/ml. The concentration of the antibiotics was 1.6 μg/ml (2 × MIC). The experiments were carried out in the flow calorimeter. Symbols as in Fig. 1.*

ents, and metabolism and excretion of the drugs. The effects of antibiotics on bacteria are usually studied by the determination of the MIC, or minimum bactericidal concentration. Such studies do not make it possible to study the kinetics of the action of an antibiotic on a microorganism, the "target organ" of antimicrobial agents. However, by calorimetry, it is possible to study the time course of the events, as reflected by the changes in heat production, taking place when bacteria are exposed to antibiotics.

We have chosen to study herein the kinetics of the action of different tetracyclines. These antibiotics, with some exceptions (3, 7), are generally considered to be rather similar in their effects on bacteria, although their pharmacokinetic characteristics are known to differ. The present investigation showed that the kinetics of antibacterial action of the tetracy-

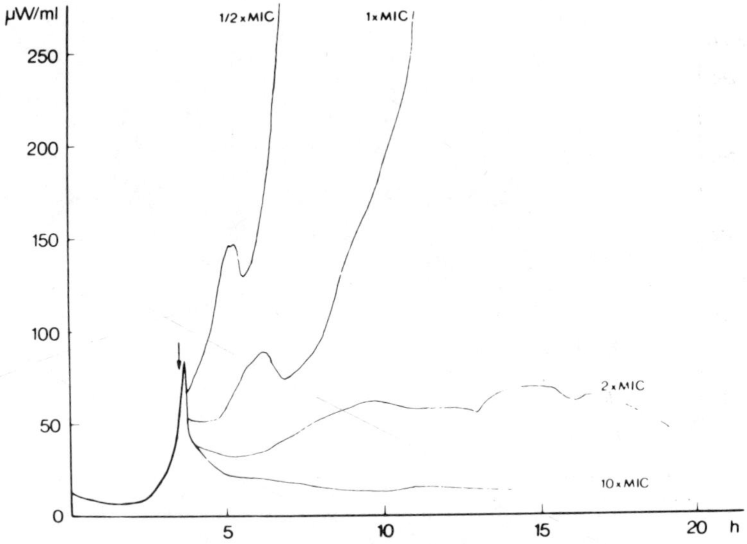

FIG. 3. *Heat effects of E. coli cultured in the presence of various concentrations of doxycycline, i.e., 0.4, 0.8, 1.6, and 8.0 µg/ml (0.5, 1, 2, and 10× MIC). Experiments performed as in Fig. 2.*

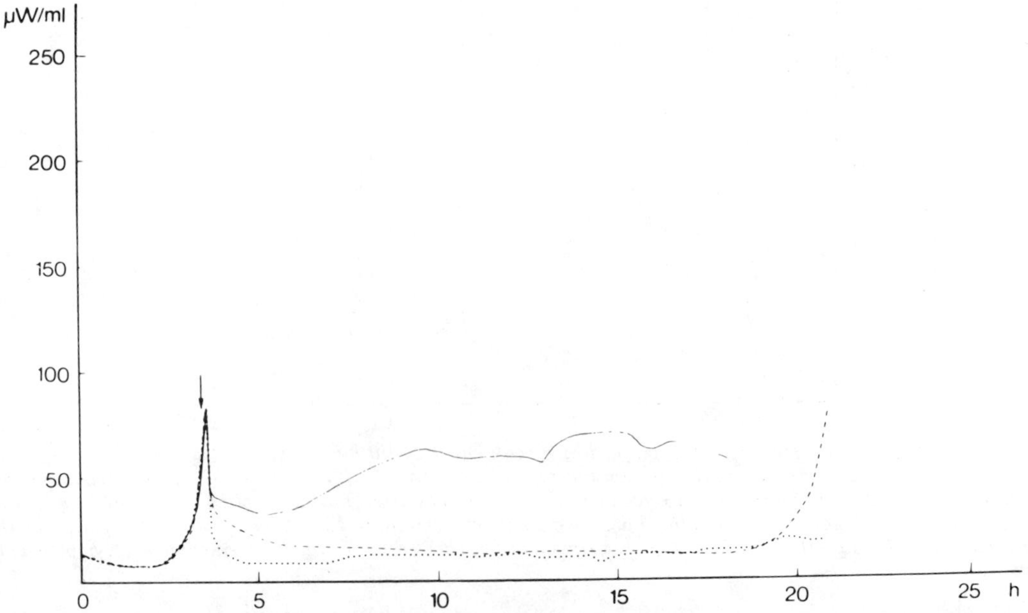

FIG. 4. *Heat effects produced by three strains of E. coli with different MICs. Doxycycline (concentration, 2× MIC) was added (indicated by arrow) in the logarithmic growth phase of the cultures at a heat production of 40 µW/ml. Symbols: MIC, 0.4 µg/ml (——); 3.0 µg/ml (-----); 40 µg/ml (· · · · · ·). The experiments were carried out in the flow calorimeter.*

clines tested, as reflected by changes in heat production, also differed. It should be noted that the MICs for the drugs against the strain of *E. coli* used throughout the experiments were the same.

There was a clear difference in the capacity of the tetracyclines to suppress the metabolism of the test organism as judged from the reduced heat effects. In this respect, minocycline was the most effective, followed by doxycycline, oxytetracycline, and tetracycline in that order. This was valid for concentrations below and above the MICs.

The duration of the inhibitory action on the

heat production exerted by the drugs differed notably in the present experiments. Thus, in cultures to which minocycline and tetracycline had been added in the lag phase, there was a time difference of about 8 h before a distinct heat effect (2.0 μW/ml) was obtained. It cannot be excluded that this reflects a difference of importance also for the bacteriostatic effect in vivo for the drugs tested. The experiments in the batch calorimeter started with aerobic conditions, but a shift to anaerobic metabolism of the bacteria tested cannot be excluded. In the flow calorimeter experiments the broth culture was oxygenated throughout the experimental period by continuous bubbling of air through the growth vessel, giving aerobic conditions for growth (4).

As shown by Eriksson and Wadsö (4), there are direct correlations between heat production, dry-weight determination, and glucose concentration in a growing culture of *E. coli*. Thus, the changes in heat production recorded in the bacterial cultures of the present study directly relate to changes in growth rate.

By using a flow calorimeter, the action of the antibiotics could be recorded with only a short delay, corresponding to the time needed for the medium to be pumped from the growth vessel to the flow cell. All the tetracyclines tested had an almost immediate effect on the test bacterium, as judged from the decrease in the heat production that could be observed when the drugs were added to the culture in the logarithmic growth phase.

In the presence of tetracycline and minocycline, there was a further increase in the heat production after about 1 and 9 h, respectively. Determinations of the MICs of bacteria recovered from samples taken from the growth vessel at various intervals during the experiment did not indicate that this increase in heat effects was due to selection of less susceptible mutants. There was no change in the number of organisms, as determined by viable counts, during the period of time from when the antibiotic was added until the heat effects increased again (Fig. 2 and Table 1).

ACKNOWLEDGMENTS

This work was supported by grants from the Swedish Board for Technical Development and the Swedish Medical Research Council (B76-16X-04509).

LITERATURE CITED

1. **Binford, J. S., L. F. Binford, and P. Adler.** 1973. A semiautomated microcalorimetric method of antibiotic sensitivity tests. Am. J. Clin. Pathol. 59:86–94.
2. **Boling, E. A., G. G. Blanchard, and W. J. Russel.** 1973. Bacterial identification by microcalorimetry. Nature (London) 241:472–473.
3. **Brogden, R. N., T. M. Speight, and G. S. Avery.** 1975. Minocycline: a review of its antibacterial and pharmacokinetic properties and therapeutic use. Drugs 9:251–291.
4. **Eriksson, R., and I. Wadsö.** 1971. Design and testing of a flow microcalorimeter for studies of aerobic bacterial growth, p. 319–327. *In* E. Broda, A. Locker, and H. Springer-Lederer (ed.), First European biophysics congress, proceedings, vol. IV. Vienna Academy of Medicine, Vienna.
5. **Monk, P., and I. Wadsö.** 1968. A flow micro reaction calorimeter. Acta Chem. Scand. 22:1842–1852.
6. **Monk, P., and I. Wadsö.** 1975. The use of microcalorimetry for bacterial classification. J. Appl. Biol. 38:71–74.
7. **Otten, H., M. Plempel, and W. Wiegenthaler (ed.).** 1975. Tetracycline, p. 319–336. *In* Antibiotika-Fibel, 4th ed. Thieme Verlag, Stuttgart.
8. **Russel, W. J., S. R. Farling, G. C. Blanchard, and E. A. Boling.** 1975. Interim review of microbial identification by microcalorimetry, p. 22–31. *In* D. Schlessinger (ed.), Microbiology—1975. American Society for Microbiology, Washington, D.C.
9. **Spink, C., and I. Wadsö.** 1976. Calorimetry as an analytical tool in biochemistry and biology, p. 1–159. *In* D. Glick (ed.), Methods in biochemical analysis, vol. 23. Wiley-Interscience, New York.
10. **Wadsö, I.** 1974. A microcalorimeter for biological analysis. Sci. Tools 21:18–21.
11. **Washington, J. A., II, and A. L. Barry.** 1974. Dilution test procedures, p. 410–417. *In* E. H. Lennette, E. H. Spaulding, and J. P. Truant (ed.), Manual of clinical microbiology, 2nd ed. American Society for Microbiology, Washington, D.C.

ANTIMICROBIAL AGENTS AND CHEMOTHERAPY, Oct. 1976, p. 610-612 Vol. 10, No. 4

Printed in U.S.A.

Effects of Doxycycline in Actively Purging Cholera Patients: a Double-Blind Clinical Trial

M. MUJIBUR RAHAMAN,* M. A. MAJID, A. K. M. JAMIUL ALAM, AND M. RAFIQUL ISLAM

Clinical Division, Cholera Research Laboratory, Dacca, Bangladesh

Received for publication 14 April 1976

In 51 actively purging cholera patients the efficacy of doxycycline, a long-acting tetracycline, was compared with a placebo and tetracycline hydrochloride. Seventeen patients who were given doxycycline at the recommended dose of 2 mg/kg at the beginning of the study, at 12 h, and at the repeated dose once daily purged a mean volume of 5.1 liters of stool and received an average of 5.7 liters of intravenous fluid. Nineteen patients receiving the placebo purged 10.1 liters of stool and received 9.7 liters of fluid. Fifteen patients given tetracycline hydrochloride at 6-h intervals passed 4.8 liters of stool and received 5.5 liters of fluid. The durations of diarrhea calculated in 8-h periods were 3.5, 8.0, and 4.1 h in the respective groups receiving doxycycline, placebo, and tetracycline. The differences between the doxycycline and placebo treatments and the tetracycline and placebo treatments were statistically significant. Those receiving doxycycline became vibrio-free in about 3 days as compared with 2 days for those receiving tetracycline; the group given the placebo were vibrio positive for the duration of their hospitalization. The results show that in the treatment of cholera the administration of doxycycline once daily has effects equal to those when tetracycline is administered at 6-h intervals. This is a distinct advantage because it decreases the demand on nursing personnel in epidemics. Also, doxycycline may be safely administered in cases of suspected renal failure from prolonged shock in cholera.

The rapid correction of dehydration and the replacement of electrolytes have been primarily responsible for the striking reduction in mortalities in cholera (2, 4, 5). Antibiotics are considered to be very useful adjuncts in cholera therapy because they bring about a significant reduction in the duration of diarrhea and the amount of intravenous (i.v.) fluid required. They also make the patients vibrio-free, which reduces the possibility of transmission. Tetracycline has been found to be the antibiotic of choice, except in small children and pregnant mothers where furazolidone may be substituted (1, 4, 6, 8). These antimicrobial agents, however, must be administered at 6-h intervals, which requires a considerable amount of nursing time.

A temporarily reduced urine output after prolonged dehydration and shock in cholera is not infrequent, particularly in patients who come to a treatment center from remote areas. Acute renal failure may develop in some of these patients. Toxic concentrations of drug in the serum may be produced in these patients if tetracycline hydrochloride is administered. Doxycycline, a tetracycline derivative with a long serum half-life requiring less frequent administration, has been used as a safe antibiotic in renal failure (3, 7).

Since doxycycline seemed to offer some distinct advantages over the short-acting tetracyclines for use in cholera, a therapeutic trial was carried out at the Cholera Research Laboratory during the 1974 to 1975 epidemic, wherein the efficacy of doxycycline was compared with a placebo as well as with tetracycline.

MATERIALS AND METHODS

Patients. Cases admitted with a short history of acute, watery diarrhea and with clinical signs of uncomplicated cholera were initially selected as prospective subjects for inclusion in the study. None were selected if they had been treated outside with antimicrobial agents. After admission, vital signs were recorded and a clinical assessment of dehydration was made. An i.v. infusion with Dacca solution, containing 133 meq of Na^+ per liter, 13 meq of K^+ per liter, 48 meq of HCO_3^- per liter, and 98 meq of Cl^- per liter (4), was used for the correction of dehydration and the replacement of electrolytes. The rate of initial rehydration was varied according to the degree of dehydration and the body weight of the patients. After the initial hydration was completed, which took between 2 and 3 h, the subsequent output of stool, urine, and vomitus, if any, was measured at 8-h intervals. This volume was matched by the subsequent administration of Dacca solution in the next 8-h interval. Rectal swabs were obtained on admission and cultured for *Vibrio cholerae*, using tellurite-taurocholate agar plates, and for *Shigella* and *Salmonella*, using *Salmonella-Shigella* and MacConkey agar media. Adults purging a volume of stool of 1 liter or more and children between 8 and 15 years passing 500 ml or more in an 8-h period after admission were classified as active purgers and were subjected to the clinical trial. The selection of patients into the placebo, doxycycline, and tetracycline groups was made by picking up cards arranged strictly in that order.

Doses. Doxycycline for oral use in 100-mg capsules and syrups containing 50 mg/teaspoon (5 ml) in coded forms was supplied with identical-looking placebos by the Pfizer Laboratories (Bangladesh) Ltd. The codes were held in a sealed envelope until the completion of the study by the principal investigator. A single, approximate dose of 2 mg of doxycycline per kg was administered at the beginning of the trial followed by another dose at 12 h. Capsules of 100 mg of doxycycline were given to adults above 15 years of age. For children, measured volumes were used according to body weight. The administration was repeated once every 24 h for a total of 4 days, or a course of five doses of capsules or syrup. Tetracycline hydrochloride (Dow Chemical Co., United States) in capsules and syrup was given in doses of 20 mg/kg per 24 h in divided doses at 6-h intervals for a 4-day period. There were no placebos for tetracycline.

Evaluation. Vital signs, the intake of fluid, and the output of stool, urine, and vomitus were recorded every 8 h during the period of diarrhea. Stool and urine were collected in separate containers.

Rectal swabs for culturing *V. cholerae* were taken daily from each patient.

RESULTS

A total of 190 patients were screened for the study; 51 were found to be active purgers and bacteriologically positive for *V. cholerae*. Of these, 19 belonged to the placebo group, 17 belonged to the doxycycline group, and 15 belonged to the tetracycline group. Table 1 shows the mean age, height, and weight of the patients. The mean stool volume passed and the i.v. fluid required before subjecting them to the trial are also shown in Table 1.

Stool volume, i.v. requirements, and duration of diarrhea. The mean volume of total stool passed after the beginning of the administration of antibiotics showed a reduction of 48 and 52% while the patients were treated with doxycycline and tetracycline, respectively, as compared with the placebo. Similarly, there was reduction of 41 and 43% in the requirement of the amount of i.v. fluids. As compared with 64 h as the mean duration of diarrhea while on the placebo, it was only 28 h with doxycycline, or a reduction of 56%, and 33 h with tetracycline, or a reduction of 49%. Table 2 shows the actual values. The differences between the placebo and doxycycline groups and the placebo and tetracycline groups were statistically significant. However, those between the doxycycline and tetracycline groups were not significant.

Duration of *Vibrio* excretion. *V. cholerae* were isolated daily from all patients in the placebo group. They were given tetracycline before discharge. The tetracycline group remained positive for *V. cholerae* for 1.8 ± 0.8 days, whereas the doxycycline group remained positive for 2.6 ± 0.7 days. The difference between the groups was statistically significant ($P < 0.01$).

None of the patients selected for the study developed complications. All patients, including those on the placebo, recovered within a period of 3 to 4 days. No side effects due either to the long-acting or to the short-acting tetracyclines were noted.

DISCUSSION

This study clearly showed that doxycycline, which requires less frequent administration, was as effective clinically as tetracycline, which requires more frequent administration. As much as 6 h of the time of one skilled nurse may be required for the routine administration of a single drug four times in 24 h in a ward with 50 patients. By using doxycycline, this could be reduced to one-third. It may, however, be argued that cholera patients require frequent observation for adjusting the intake of

TABLE 1. *Particulars of cholera patients in the clinical trial*

Group	No. of patients	Age (yr)		Height (cm)		Weight (kg)		Stool volume (liters)[a]		i.v. Given (liters)[a]	
		Mean	SD[b]	Mean	SD	Mean	SD	Mean	SD	Mean	SD
Placebo	19	23	18	147	24	33	13	2.0	1.1	5.2	2.0
Doxycycline	17	18	14	130	25	25	11	2.1	1.7	4.4	2.3
Tetracycline	15	22	16	138	28	30	13	2.0	1.7	4.2	2.2

[a] Before the administration of drugs.

[b] SD, Standard deviation.

TABLE 2. *Effects of the oral administration of placebo, doxycycline, and tetracycline in the treatment of cholera*

Group	Total stool volume (liters)		Total i.v. given (liters)		Duration of diarrhea in 8-h period		*Vibrio* positive (days)	
	Mean	SD[a]	Mean	SD	Mean	SD	Mean	SD
Placebo	10.0	6.0	9.7	4.8	8.0	3.2	All days	
Doxycycline	5.2[b]	4.0	5.7[b]	4.9	3.5[c]	2.1	2.6[b]	0.7
Tetracycline	4.8[b]	3.1	5.5[b]	3.9	4.1[c]	2.1	1.8[b]	0.8

[a] SD, Standard deviation.
[b] $P < 0.01$.
[c] $P < 0.001$.

fluid according to the rate of purging and that the administration of a drug would require a nurse to keep a more watchful eye over the patients.

The price of doxycycline per dose is considerably higher than that for ordinary tetracycline; however, the total cost for a course of therapy in cholera makes it only slightly more expensive than with ordinary tetracycline. The price of 5 gm of a local brand of tetracycline is $1.40, which may be compared with $1.75 for 600 mg of doxycycline. However, the cost of the antibiotic is only a fraction of the total cost in the management of cholera, where personnel and i.v. fluids are the more expensive items.

With the advent of modern replacement therapy, using balanced fluids in adequate quantities, acute renal shutdown after prolonged shock in cholera has become rather infrequent (9). Caution, however, has to be observed when a patient from a rural area arrives in a hospital after an interval of a number of days from the onset of acute diarrhea. These patients coming from rural areas are often treated at their home with an inadequate quantity of fluid. They may develop a prolonged, but frequently temporary, suppression of urine, correctable by adequate rehydration. As a precautionary measure, ordinary tetracycline is withheld from these patients until they have started to pass urine in adequate quantities. Doxycycline may be used to reduce the duration of diarrhea in these patients because this antibiotic has been found to be safe for use in renal failure (3, 7).

The marginal advantage of tetracycline over doxycycline in making a patient vibrio-free at an earlier time is probably due to its continued high concentration in the gut by frequent administration. Doxycycline, on the other hand, is quickly absorbed and slowly excreted (10). Cholera is known to shorten the mean transit time through the small intestine to as little as 40 min in some patients. This short transit time may not allow adequate time for the complete absorption of doxycycline. It is, however, reassuring to note that in spite of a known, short mean transit time in cholera and less frequent administration, the clinical effect of doxycycline was similar to that of tetracycline.

ACKNOWLEDGMENTS

We wish to thank the Pfizer Laboratories (Bangladesh) Ltd. for supplying us doxycycline and the placebos.

The Cholera Research Laboratory is supported by the governments of the People's Republic of Bangladesh, the United States, the United Kingdom, and Australia.

LITERATURE CITED

1. **Carpenter, C. C. J., D. Barua, R. B. Sack, C. K. Wallace, P. P. Mitra, S. R. Khanra, S. A. Wells, P. E. Dans, and R. N. Choudhuri.** 1966. Clinical studies in Asiatic cholera. IV. Antibiotic therapy in cholera. Bull. Johns Hopkins Hosp. 118:216–229.
2. **Carpenter, C. C. J., A. Mondal, R. B. Sack, P. P. Mitra, P. E. Dans, S. A. Wells, E. J. Hinman, and R. N. Choudhuri.** 1966. Clinical studies in Asiatic cholera. II. Development of 2:1 saline:lactate regimen. Comparison of this regimen with traditional methods of treatment. April and May, 1963. Bull. Johns Hopkins Hosp. 118:174–196.
3. **Curtis, J. R., K. G. Koutsaimanis, D. Buggey, and J. B. Eastwood.** 1974. Evaluation of doxycycline administration in patients with renal failure and in normal subjects. Opus. Med. Suppl. XXXIII:51–56.
4. **Greenough, W. B., III, I. S. Rosenberg, R. S. Gordon, and B. I. Davis.** 1964. Tetracycline in the treatment of cholera. Lancet I:355–357.
5. **Gutman, R. A., D. J. Drutz, G. E. Whalen, and R. H. Watten.** 1969. Double blind fluid therapy evaluation in pediatric cholera. Pediatrics 44:922–931.
6. **Karchmer, A. W., G. T., Curlin, M. I. Huq, and N. Hirschhorn.** 1970. Furazolidone in paediatric cholera. Bull. W.H.O. 43:373–378.
7. **Mahon, W. A., J. V. Wittenberg, and P. G. Tuffnel.** 1970. Studies on the absorption and distribution of doxycycline in normal patients and in patients with severely impaired renal function. Can. Med. Assoc. J. 103:1031–1034.
8. **Pierce, N. F., J. G. Banwell, R. C. Mitra, G. J. Caranasos, R. I. Keimowitz, J. Thomas, and A. Mondal.** 1968. Controlled comparison of tetracycline and furazolidone in cholera. Br. Med. J. 3:277–280.
9. **Rahman, A. S. M. M.** 1969. Experience in treating cholera at a rural hospital. J. Pak. Med. Assoc. 19:366–370.
10. **Wetterfors, J., and R. Sjodahl.** 1974. Doxycycline concentrations in certain tissues following intravenous and oral administration. Opus. Med. Suppl. XXXIII:64–67.

ANTIMICROBIAL AGENTS AND CHEMOTHERAPY, Oct. 1976, p. 613-617
Copyright © 1976 American Society for Microbiology
Vol. 10, No. 4
Printed in U.S.A.

Growth of *Physarum gyrosum* on Agar Plates and in Liquid Culture[1]

RICHARD L. TAYLOR AND M. F. MALLETTE*

Department of Biochemistry and Biophysics, Pennsylvania State University, University Park, Pennsylvania 16802

Received for publication 11 June 1976

The physical and nutritional requirements of the antibiotic-producing slime mold *Physarum gyrosum* were examined to develop a liquid medium for this myxomycete. Liquid culture is desired to expedite a useful scale of production of antibiotic materials for ease of isolation and structure study. Culture conditions were selected to favor antibiotic production rather than maximum growth. The medium devised consisted of 0.010 M potassium phosphate buffer (pH 6.0), 2% bakers' yeast, and 0.2% glucose and was supplemented with either 10^{-7} M hemoglobin (preferred) or 2.0 ml of live *Escherichia coli* per 100 ml of culture medium grown to a steady-state population in nutrient broth. The slime mold, which contained some *E. coli* carried along with the inoculum, was allowed to grow as a surface plasmodium at 20°C in the dark with weekly subculturing for stocks or for 10 days for antibiotic production. *P. gyrosum* produced the same antibiotic materials when grown in liquid medium as it did when grown on agar plates. A seeded plate disk assay against *Bacillus cereus* was employed to follow antibiotic activity.

Interest in slime molds has increased since the first liquid culture of *Physarum polycephalum* by Daniel and Rusch (5). Modification of their culture medium by Ross (12) enabled him to culture successfully *Physarum flavicomum*, *Physarella oblonga*, and the myxamoebae of *Badhamia curtisii*. Henney and Henney (8) reported different nutritional requirements for *Physarum rigidum* as did Schroeder et al. (14) for *Physarum gyrosum*. Although the basic nutritional requirements of these various slime molds are similar, their individual specific requirements must be satisfied for successful long-term culturing.

Locquin and Prevot (9) reported the presence of antibiotic materials in ethanolic extracts of several species of myxomycetes. Considine and Mallette (2) reported that *P. gyrosum* also produced antibiotic materials. To isolate and determine the chemical structures of the active materials, it would be desirable to grow *P. gyrosum* in liquid culture. Since initial attempts to do so by Schroeder et al. (14) were unsuccessful, further studies on nutritional requirements of *P. gyrosum* have been made in the hope that inocula could be transferred successfully from agar plates to liquid culture.

[1] Pennsylvania Agricultural Experiment Station publication no. 5090.

MATERIALS AND METHODS

Cultures. A two-member culture of *P. gyrosum* and *Escherichia coli* was established as described by Mayberry et al. (11). *P. gyrosum* was then grown on an agar medium developed by Schroeder et al. (14) made up of 2% agar (Difco), 0.025 M potassium phosphate buffer (pH 6.8), 2% bakers' yeast (Anheuser-Busch, Inc.), and 0.2% glucose. The medium was sterilized for 15 min at 15 lb/in^2 and 121°C. It was supplemented with approximately 0.1 g of autoclaved rolled oats per plate, finely ground in a Waring blender, and 2 ml of live *E. coli* grown in nutrient broth overnight at 37°C to a steady-state population. Stock plasmodium was allowed to grow in the dark at 20°C and was subcultured weekly.

Protein determination. Plasmodium grown on agar plates was scraped off the surface and homogenized with a known volume of water in a Potter-Elvehjem tissue homogenizer. After centrifugation at 570 × *g* at 25°C to remove particulate material, the supernatant was analyzed for protein by the method of Lowry et al. (10) using bovine serum albumin as the reference standard. Two 1-cm-diameter loops of surface plasmodium from liquid cultures were transferred to 10 ml of water and subjected to sonic oscillation for 1 min to disrupt the plasmodium, and the protein content was determined as above.

Dry weights. Growth of *P. gyrosum* in liquid culture was best followed by dry weight determination. Two loops (1-cm diameter) full of surface plasmodium were placed on a weighed watch glass. After drying for 24 h (to constant weight) in a vacuum desiccator over P_2O_5, the watch glass was reweighed.

Antibiotic assay. Antibiotic production was followed by a disk assay test against *Bacillus cereus*. A 1.0-ml portion of a 1:100 dilution of a 4-h culture of *B. cereus* grown in nutrient broth was used to inoculate a tube (10 ml) of 1% Noble agar (Difco) heated to 45°C. Two milliliters of this inoculated agar was spread over a 10-cm petri plate containing 25 ml of Difco nutrient agar preincubated to 37°C. After hardening for 30 min at room temperature, a paper assay disk (no. 740-E with a 12.7-mm diameter; Schleicher & Schuell Co.) containing the material to be tested and prepared according to Schroeder and Mallette (15) was placed on the test plate and moistened with approximately 0.1 ml of 0.1 M phosphate buffer (pH 7.0). Material under test was allowed to diffuse for 2 h at room temperature, and these assay plates were incubated for 4 h at 37°C before measuring zones of inhibition. All plates were reread at 24 h to confirm the zones of inhibition.

Antibiotic materials were isolated and fractionated according to Schroeder and Mallette (15) for plasmodia grown on agar plates. For plasmodia grown in liquid culture, the dialysis step was replaced by centrifugation at 10,000 × *g* for 20 min at 4°C. The supernatant was concentrated to 1% of the original volume by rotary evaporation at 40°C under reduced pressure and extracted with *n*-butanol as described earlier for the dialysate.

Weights of fractions to be tested for antibiotic activity were determined by drying in sample vials for 2 h at 56°C under vacuum against P_2O_5 in an Abderhalden drying pistol, cooling to room temperature in a desiccator over P_2O_5, and weighing.

RESULTS

Gray (6), working with *P. polycephalum*, found that his strain had an optimal pH range of 4 to 5 for growth using a 1:10 dilution of McIlvaine dibasic sodium phosphate-citric acid buffer. However, *P. gyrosum* failed to grow on agar using this buffer. Attempts to culture *P. gyrosum* on a 0.029 M citric acid-potassium phosphate buffer or 0.025 M potassium phosphate buffer were successful. Table 1 shows that best growth occurred with phosphate buffer at pH 6.0. Citrate was somewhat inhibitory, particularly at nonoptimal values of pH. Antibiotic materials were produced, at least over the optimum growth range of pH 5 to 6.8, as shown in Table 2. Cultures grown at pH 6.0 produced the greatest weight of antibiotic fraction Z.

Since variation in phosphate concentration might affect growth, four levels were employed in the experiment of Fig. 1 to show that the optimum concentration was about 0.025 M. Growth was inhibited with 0.1 M phosphate. Phosphate concentrations have been shown by Weinberg (16) to have a significant effect on the production of such secondary metabolites as antibiotics. Since Weinberg reported that secondary metabolite production is favored by phosphate concentrations below those for maximum rate of growth, 0.010 M phosphate buffer was chosen in the present study, because it offered good growth at lower phosphate concentration.

TABLE 1. *pH dependency of growth*[a]

Buffer	pH	Protein (mg/plate)
0.025 M potassium phosphate	3.0	5.4
	4.0	9.9
	5.0	13.6
	6.0	14.5
	6.8	7.1
	8.0	6.2
0.029 M citrate-phosphate	3.0	NG
	4.0	6.8
	5.0	7.6
	6.0	12.1
	6.8	NG
	8.0	NG

[a] *P. gyrosum* was grown on agar medium and supplemented with live *E. coli*. Incubation was at 25°C in the dark for 10 days, the time of maximum growth. NG, No growth.

TABLE 2. *Antibiotic production and pH*[a]

Buffer system	Dry wt (mg)		*B. cereus* zone (mm)	
	Total	Assayed	Test 1	Test 2
Citrate-phosphate, pH 5.0	24	3.0	23	24
Potassium phosphate, pH 6.0	37.5	3.0	24	24
Potassium phosphate, pH 6.8	22.5	3.0	24	24

[a] Antibiotic fraction Z, obtained according to the method of Schroeder and Mallette (15), was tested against *B. cereus* as described in Materials and Methods. Data in the right hand columns are from two different tests. The yield (column 2, total dry weight), is total of fraction Z material produced by five culture plates.

Figure 2 shows the effect of temperature on growth of *P. gyrosum*. A temperature of 30°C gave a poor response when measured as milligrams of protein per plate, whereas 20°C produced the best growth. In another experiment, growth was considerably less at 16°C than at 20°C and occurred at neither 37 nor 4°C. Table 3 shows that antibiotic production, as measured by dry weight, was favored by lower temperatures. The coupling of slow, steady growth with maximum antibiotic production has been reported in many cases. Weinberg (16), for example, observed that secondary metabolite production is best at temperatures below those for

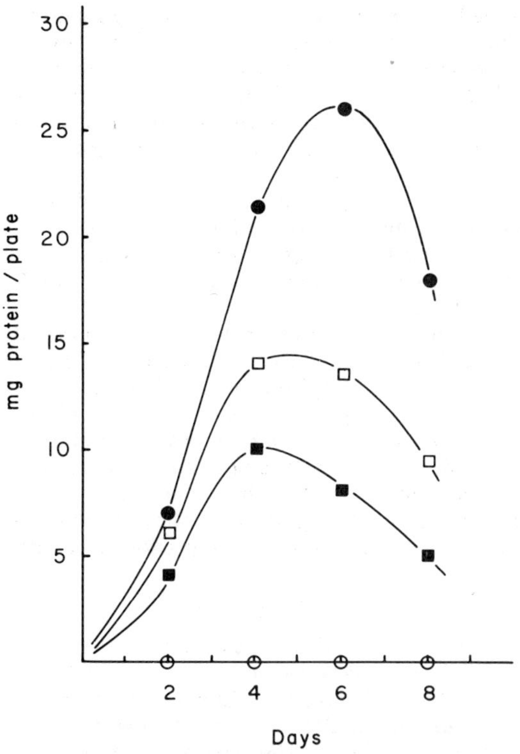

FIG. 1. *Effect of phosphate concentration on growth. P. gyrosum was grown in the dark at 25°C on agar medium made with potassium phosphate buffer (pH 6.0) at the concentrations indicated. Symbols: ○, 0.100 M; ●, 0.025 M; □, 0.010 M; ■, 0.001 M. No growth occurred at 0.100 M.*

maximum rate of growth. Since growth at 16°C was considerably slower than at 20°C and because the 20°C reading gave a somewhat better specific activity than either 16 or 25°C, 20°C was chosen.

Alternative carbon and nitrogen sources were tried with no success. Increasing the glucose concentration to 1% inhibited growth. No growth was observed when 0.05 M sodium acetate replaced glucose. Commercial growth supplements were also detrimental (e.g., tryptone [Difco] in 0.5, 1.0, 1.5, and 2.0% was toxic). 2% Hy-Case (Sheffield Chemical) and 1% yeast extract (Difco) inhibited growth. Similar results were reported by Scholes (13) for *Fuligo septica*.

After numerous and varied unsuccessful attempts, plasmodium was transferred from agar plates to liquid culture by intermediate growth on a sterile membrane filter (no. GSWP 142 00, 0.22-μm pores; Millipore Corp.) and placed on top of a standard agar culture plate (containing 2% Difco agar, 0.010 M potassium phosphate buffer [pH 6.0], 2% autoclaved bakers' yeast, and 0.2% glucose and supplemented with rolled oats and live *E. coli*). After the plasmodium had grown for 1 week, the filter and the myxomycete were placed in a sterile, 1-liter, cotton-plugged Erlenmeyer flask where it was supported on glass wool that was almost covered with liquid culture medium (see above). After several days in the dark at 20°C, small pieces of

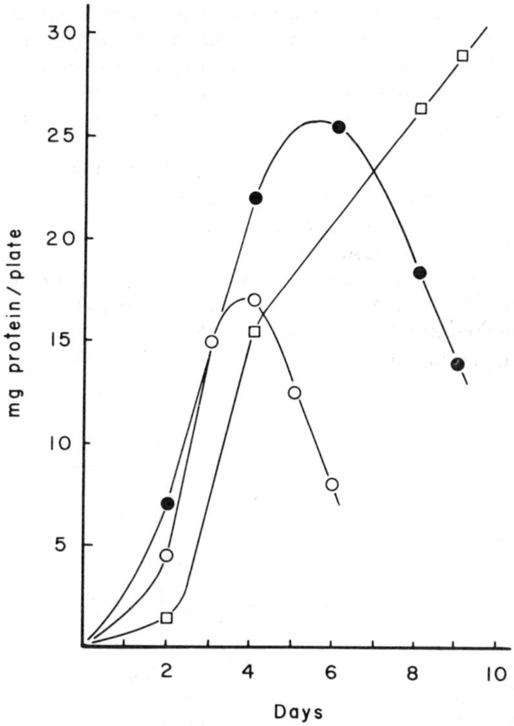

FIG. 2. *Effect of temperature on growth. P. gyrosum was grown in the dark on agar medium that was made with 0.025 M potassium phosphate buffer (pH 6.0) and supplemented with live E. coli. Symbols: ○, 30°C; ●, 25°C; □, 20°C.*

TABLE 3. *Antibiotic production at various temperatures*[a]

Temp	Dry wt (mg)		*B. cereus* zone (mm)	
	Total	Assayed	Test 1	Test 2
25°C	17	3.0	24	24
20°C	22	3.0	25	26
16°C	34	3.0	24	24

[a] Material assayed was a butanol extract of dialysate from culture plates (0.025 M potassium phosphate buffer [pH 6.8]), grown in the dark for 10 days and for 17 days for cultures grown at 16°C. For details of the activity see Materials and Methods. The yield (column 2, total dry weight) is the total butanol-extracted material produced by five culture plates.

plasmodium floated off onto the surface of the liquid medium. This culture fluid with plasmodium was then used to inoculate fresh medium not containing glass wool, and again plasmodium grew on the surface.

To confirm that the organism growing in these cultures was *P. gyrosum*, the culture was centrifuged at 250 × *g* for 5 min at 4°C in sterile, screw-capped conical centrifuge tubes. The pellet was transferred to an agar culture plate. After several days, a plasmodium typical of *P. gyrosum* was observed growing over the plate. Microscopic examination of liquid cultures showed microplasmodia similar to those reported by Guttes et al. (7) for *P. polycephalum*. Inoculation into nutrient broth tubes or onto nutrient agar plates and incubating at 37 or 25°C revealed *E. coli* as the only accompanying viable organism.

Figure 3 illustrates growth of *P. gyrosum* in liquid culture at 20°C. In most cases, growth peaked at 4 to 6 days when screw-capped Erlenmeyer culture flasks (250 ml) containing 125 ml of medium were used. Daniel et al. (4) reported that *P. polycephalum* required hematin or heme proteins for good growth. For *P. gyrosum* Fig. 3 shows that 10^{-7} M hemoglobin from acetone-extracted sheep erythrocytes could replace the associated live *E. coli*. Not adding either hemoglobin or *E. coli* resulted in reduced growth. A control culture of only *E. coli* showed no measurable growth under these conditions. See the control in Fig. 3. Figure 4 shows that protein production paralleled growth when followed by dry weight.

Antibiotic production of *P. gyrosum* in liquid culture is shown in Table 4. The fractions correspond to those of Schroeder and Mallette (15). When chromatographed on thin-layer plates according to the method of Schroeder and Mallette (15), C-1 gave one major active fraction (D-1). A comparison of these fractions to those from cultures grown on agar plates showed that the same antibiotic materials are produced in both cases.

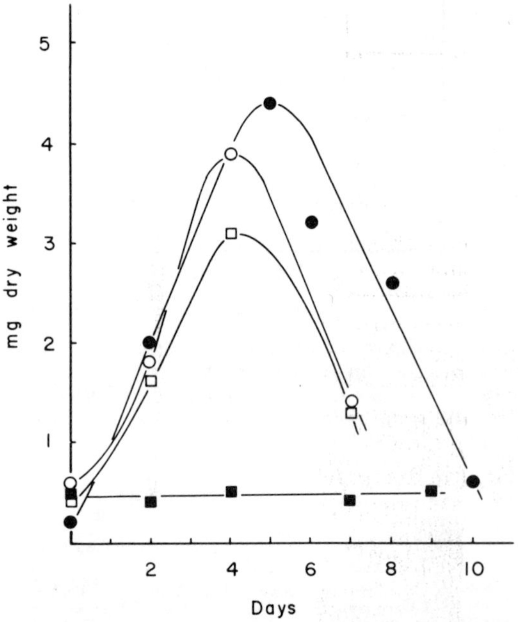

FIG. 3. *Growth of P. gyrosum in liquid culture. P. gyrosum was grown in culture medium containing 0.010 M potassium phosphate buffer (pH 6.0), 2% bakers' yeast, and 0.2% glucose that was either unsupplemented (□) or supplemented with 2.0 ml of live E. coli in nutrient broth (○) or with 10^{-7} M hemoglobin (●). A control (■) of culture medium supplemented with 2.0 ml of live E. coli in nutrient broth was also tested. Two 1-cm-diameter loops of surface plasmodium were removed from the cultures at the time indicated, and the dry weight was determined as described in Materials and Methods.*

DISCUSSION

P. gyrosum has different nutritional requirements than those reported by Daniel and Rusch (5) for *P. polycephalum*. Earlier attempts by Bohinski and Mallette (unpublished data) to grow *P. gyrosum* in the partially defined medium of Daniel and Rusch and in other media were unsuccessful. Apparently the inhibitory

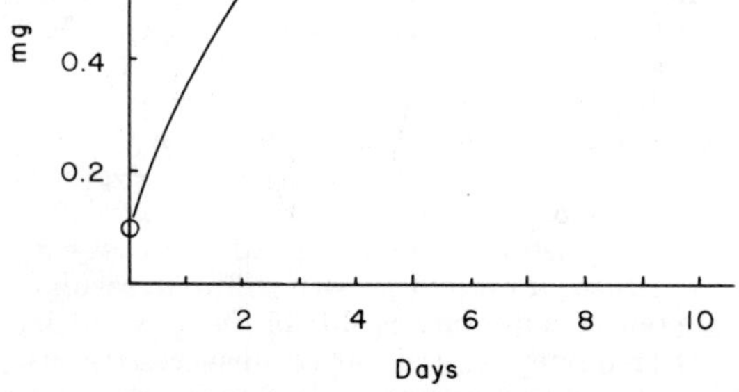

FIG. 4. *Protein production by P. gyrosum in liquid culture. P. gyrosum was grown in the liquid culture medium supplemented with 10^{-7} M hemoglobin as described in Fig. 3. Two 1-cm-diameter loops of surface plasmodium were removed from the cultures on the days indicated, and the protein content was determined as described in Materials and Methods.*

TABLE 4. *Antibiotic production in liquid culture*[a]

Material	Wt assayed (mg)	*B. cereus* zone (mm)	
		Test 1	Test 2
Butanol extract, lot-5	3.0	19	19
Butanol extract, lot-7	3.0	19	19
Fraction Z, lot-7	3.0	20	20
Fraction Z, lot-8	3.0	24	24
Fraction C-1, lot-8	2.0	17	17
Fraction C-1, pooled	2.0	16	17
Fraction C-2, pooled	2.0	19	19
Fraction C-3, pooled	2.0	17	17

[a] *P. gyrosum* was grown in a liquid culture medium consisting of 0.010 M potassium phosphate buffer (pH 6.0), 2% bakers' yeast, 0.2% glucose, and 10^{-7} M hemoglobin. For details of the activity assay see Materials and Methods. Fractions assayed are those using the method of Schroeder and Mallette (15).

effect of citrate and toxicity of yeast extract and tryptone were responsible in part. Additional attempts (14) to grow *P. gyrosum* in a defined medium of inorganic salts, vitamins, and amino acids of Daniel et al. (3) were equally unsuccessful. Based on our results, an effective liquid culture medium of the following composition was developed: 0.010 M potassium phosphate buffer (pH 6.0), 2% autoclaved bakers' yeast, 0.2% glucose, and 10^{-7} M hemoglobin. When incubated in the dark at 20°C, this medium successfully supported growth of *P. gyrosum* for 1 year with weekly subculturing by adding 25 ml of inoculum to 100 ml of fresh culture medium.

Other simpler media may support *P. gyrosum* for short periods of subculturing but may be unable to maintain cultures of *P. gyrosum* indefinitely. (For example, see Fig. 3, where failure to add extra live *E. coli* or hemoglobin resulted in reduced growth.) Many researchers have reported short-term (two to four) subculturing of various myxomycetes, but successful long-term culturing on defined or partially defined liquid media has been limited to only a few species.

The antibiotic materials isolated by Schroeder and Mallette (15) from *P. gyrosum* showed a broad spectrum of activity against both gram-positive and gram-negative bacteria as well as against yeasts, *Saccharomyces cerevisae* and *Torulopsis sphaerica*. The possibility that one antibiotic system could have such a broad spectrum of activity would be significant, since few useful antibiotic materials exhibit such capability. Purified antibiotic material has not been tested to determine if this material has the same broad spectrum of activity as the butanol extract, because sufficiently large quantities have not been available in the past. Production of antibiotic materials by *P. gyrosum* grown in liquid culture was comparable to growing the slime mold on agar plates, but the ease of extracting antibiotic materials from liquid medium makes it superior to plate cultures. In addition, this new medium could be adapted to a fermentation technique like that of Brewer et al. (1) for *P. polycephalum* if large-scale antibiotic production becomes desirable.

ACKNOWLEDGMENT

This work was supported in part by the Pennsylvania Agricultural Experiment Station.

LITERATURE CITED

1. **Brewer, E. N., S. Kuraishi, J. C. Garver, and F. M. Strong.** 1964. Mass culture of *Physarum polycephalum*. Appl. Microbiol. **12**:161–164.
2. **Considine, J. M., and M. F. Mallette.** 1965. Production and partial purification of antibiotic materials formed by *Physarum gyrosum*. Appl. Microbiol. **13**:464–468.
3. **Daniel, J. W., K. L. Babcock, A. H. Sievert, and H. P. Rusch.** 1963. Organic requirements and synthetic media for growth of the myxomycete of *Physarum polycephalum*. J. Bacteriol. **86**:324–331.
4. **Daniel, J. W., J. Kelley, and H. P. Rusch.** 1962. Hematin-requiring plasmodial myxomycete. J. Bacteriol. **84**:1104–1110.
5. **Daniel, J. W., And H. P. Rusch.** 1961. The pure culture of *Physarum polycephalum* on a partially defined soluble medium. J. Gen. Microbiol. **25**:47–59.
6. **Gray, W. D.** 1939. The relation of pH and temperature to the fruiting of *Physarum polycephalum*. Am. J. Bot. **26**:709–714.
7. **Guttes, E., S. Guttes, and H. P. Rusch.** 1961. Morphology of *Physarum polycephalum* grown in liquid culture. Dev. Biol. **3**:588–614.
8. **Henney, H. R., Jr., and M. R. Henney.** 1968. Nutritional requirements for the growth in pure culture of the myxomycete *Physarum rigidum* and related species. J. Gen. Microbiol. **53**:333–339.
9. **Locquin, M., and A. R. Prevot.** 1948. Etude de quelques antibiotiques produits par les myxomycetes. Ann. Inst. Pasteur Paris **75**:8–13.
10. **Lowry, O. H., N. J. Rosebrough, A. L. Farr, and R. J. Randall.** 1951. Protein measurement with the Folin phenol reagent. J. Biol. Chem. **193**:265–275.
11. **Mayberry, J. M., C. L. Fergus, and M. F. Mallette.** 1962. Pure culture of the slime mold *Physarum gyrosum*. Mycologia **54**:580–581.
12. **Ross, I. K.** 1964. Pure culture of some myxomycetes. Bull. Torrey Bot. Club **91**:23–31.
13. **Scholes, P. M.** 1962. Some observations on the cultivation, fruiting, and germination of *Fuligo septica*. J. Gen. Microbiol. **29**:137–148.
14. **Schroeder, H. R., C. L. Fergus, and M. F. Mallette.** 1974. Culture of *Physarum gyrosum*. Mycologia **66**:349–354.
15. **Schroeder, H. R., and M. F. Mallette.** 1973. Isolation and purification of antibiotic material from *Physarum gyrosum*. Antimicrob. Agents Chemother. **4**:160–166.
16. **Weinberg, E. D.** 1974. Secondary metabolism: control by temperature and inorganic phosphate. Dev. Ind. Microbiol. **15**:70–81.

ANTIMICROBIAL AGENTS AND CHEMOTHERAPY, Oct. 1976, p. 618-622
Vol. 10, No. 4

Tirandamycin, an Inhibitor of Bacterial Ribonucleic Acid Polymerase

FRITZ REUSSER

Research Laboratories, The Upjohn Company, Kalamazoo, Michigan 49001

Received for publication 28 June 1976

The antibiotic tirandamycin (a 3-acyltetramic acid structurally related to streptolydigin) specifically inhibits transcription by interfering with the function of bacterial ribonucleic acid polymerase. Ribonucleic acid polymerases from rat liver nuclei are not subject to tirandamycin inhibition. Qualitatively, the mode of action of the antibiotic is identical to that of streptolydigin in inhibiting chain initiation as well as chain elongation during the transcriptional process. However, tirandamycin is approximately 40 times less potent than streptolydigin. The structures of the 3-acyl groups of the two acyltetramic acid antibiotics tirandamycin and streptolydigin differ only slightly in the degree of oxidation of the terminal dioxabicyclo(3.1)nonane system and possess the same stereochemistry (D. J. Duchamp, A. R. Branfman, A. C. Button, and K. L. Rinehart, 1973). More significantly, major differences occur at the 1 and 5 positions of the tetramic acids. Tirandamycin contains no substituents; streptolydigin contains a substituted acetamide function at position 5 and a sugar moiety at position 1. The lack of substituents at the 1 and 5 positions of the tetramic acid portion in tirandamycin is probably responsible for the reduced biopotency of tirandamycin as compared with streptolydigin.

Tirandamycin, a new antibacterial agent, was isolated from the culture broth of *Streptomyces tirandis* sp. nov. (6; O. K. Sebek and C. E. Meyer, U.S. Patent 3,671,628, 1972). The compound was crystallized in the form of its sodium salt, which has a molecular weight of 439.

Structural studies indicated that tirandamycin is a 3-acyltetramic acid related to streptolydigin (5). The structural formulas for tirandamycin and streptolydigin are shown in Fig. 1.

Chemically, tirandamycin differs from streptolydigin in minor functional groups within the acyl substituent at position 3 of the tetramic acid, but more significantly lacks the substituents present at position 1 (sugar) and position 5 (substituted acetamide) of the tetramic acid in streptolydigin.

Tirandamycin is a moderately active growth inhibitor of a variety of gram-positive bacteria in vitro, but has proved ineffective for the systemic treatment of experimental bacterial infections in mice.

Investigations of the mode of action of tirandamycin have shown that the agent is an inhibitor of bacterial ribonucleic acid (RNA) polymerase in a manner similar to streptolydigin. A preliminary account of these studies has been presented (7).

MATERIALS AND METHODS

RNA polymerase was isolated from *Escherichia coli* and assayed as described previously (7). One RNA polymerase unit corresponds to 1 nmol of poly[d(A-T)]-directed adenosine 5'-triphosphate (ATP) incorporated per min.

The binding of *E. coli* RNA polymerase to template deoxyribonucleic acid (DNA) was assessed by the membrane (Millipore Corp.) filtration technique described by Jones and Berg (4).

Mammalian RNA polymerase was isolated from rat liver nuclei by the procedures of Roeder and Rutter (9). Fraction 4, containing the total nuclear RNA polymerases, was used as the enzyme source. Polymerase activity of this fraction was assayed as described by Chesterton and Green (2).

E. coli ^{14}C-labeled DNA (specific activity, 0.038 μCi/μg) and [γ-^{32}P]guanosine 5'-triphosphate (GTP) (specific activity, 1.51 Ci/mmol) were purchased from Amersham/Searle.

RESULTS

Effect of tirandamycin on *E. coli* RNA polymerase. Tirandamycin effectively inhibited the de novo synthesis of RNA catalyzed by RNA polymerase (Fig. 2). The concentration of antibiotic required to inhibit the reaction to the extent of 50% amounted to 0.8 mM, which suggests that tirandamycin is an inhibitor of moderate potency for RNA polymerase. For comparative purposes the results obtained with

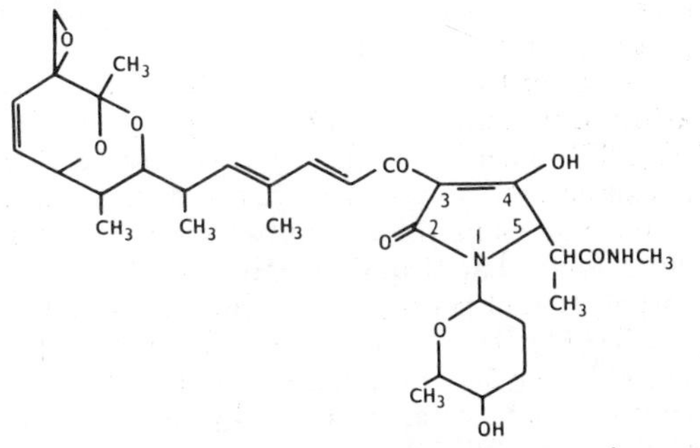

Streptolydigin (Rinehart et al., 1963)

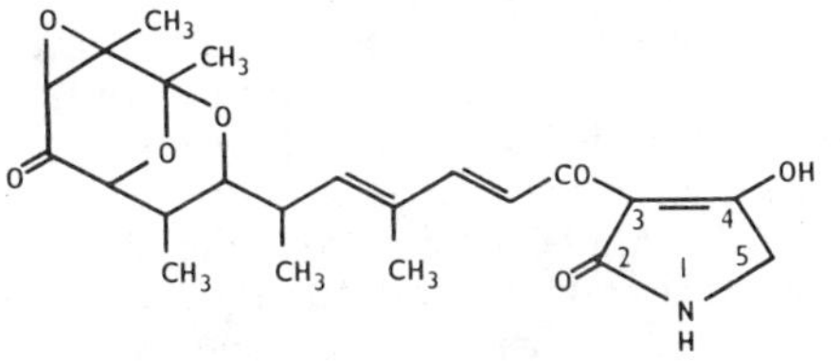

Tirandamycin (MacKellar et al., 1971)

FIG. 1. *Structural formulas for streptolydigin and tirandamycin.*

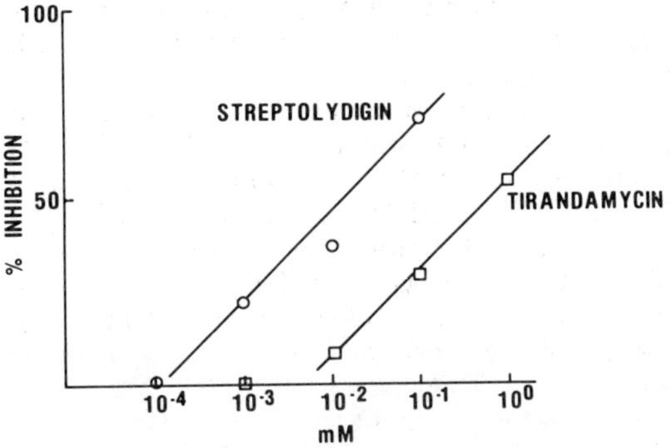

FIG. 2. *Effects of tirandamycin and streptolydigin on DNA-mediated E. coli RNA polymerase. The assay mixtures contained, in a total volume of 0.25 ml: tris(hydroxymethyl)aminomethane - hydrochloride buffer (pH 7.9), 5 μmol; $MgCl_2$, 1 μmol; mercaptoethanol, 3 μmol; $MnCl_2$, 0.25 μmol; GTP, UTP, and CTP, 0.1 μmol each; [8-^{14}C]ATP, 0.1 μmol, 0.05 μCi; poly[d(A-T)], 0.04 optical density at 260 nm units/ml; and polymerase, 0.5 U. Reactions were run at 30°C for 15 min and terminated by the addition of 3 ml of cold 3.5% perchloric acid per tube. The acid-insoluble product was collected on 0.45-μm membrane filter paper disks, washed, and assayed for radioactivity.*

streptolydigin assayed in the same system are also shown in Fig. 2. A streptolydigin concentration of approximately 0.02 mM sufficed to inhibit the reaction to the extent of 50%. Hence, in this cell-free system, using poly[d(A-T)] as a template, tirandamycin proved approximately 40 times less potent than streptolydigin.

Variation of template DNA or polymerase. An inhibitor of RNA polymerase usually exerts its action by specific interaction with either the polymerase or the template. Streptolydigin is known to interact with the polymerase per se (1, 11). The close chemical relationship between this antibiotic and tirandamycin led us to expect that tirandamycin should possess similar properties. This assumption proved to be correct, as shown in the following.

Increasing concentrations of DNA template in the reaction mixtures did not affect the extent of inhibition of RNA synthesis induced by tirandamycin (Table 1). Inhibitions of approximately 40 to 45% resulted in each case, regardless of the concentration of template present in the reaction mixtures. However, the addition of increasing amounts of RNA polymerase caused a gradual reversal of the inhibition induced by tirandamycin (Table 2). In the presence of 0.3 U of enzyme per sample, the reaction was inhibited to the extent of 62%; a fourfold increase in polymerase concentration caused only 40% inhibition of the same reaction. These data thus show that tirandamycin, analogous to strepto-

TABLE 1. *Variation of template poly[d(A-T)] concentrations on RNA polymerase activity*[a]

Concn of poly[d(A-T)] (OD_{260}[b] units/sample)	cpm/sample		Inhibition (%)
	Control	Tirandamycin	
0.1	15,200	6,080	40
0.05	10,390	4,570	44
0.02	6,700	2,640	39
0.01	4,180	1,920	46

[a] The experimental conditions were as described in the legend to Fig. 2. The tirandamycin concentration was 0.5 mM.

[b] OD_{260}, Optical density at 260 nm.

TABLE 2. *Reversal of tirandamycin inhibition by increasing concentrations of RNA polymerase*[a]

Polymerase (U/sample)	cpm/sample		Inhibition (%)
	Control	Tirandamycin	
0.3	3,530	1,410	60
0.6	5,370	2,510	53
0.9	6,440	3,480	46
1.2	6,560	3,820	42

[a] Reaction mixtures were as described in the legend to Fig. 2. The tirandamycin concentration was 0.5 mM.

lydigin, inhibits RNA synthesis by interacting with the polymerase per se rather than with the DNA template.

Effect of tirandamycin on the binding of polymerase to template DNA. The effect of tirandamycin on RNA polymerase binding to *E. coli* ^{14}C-labeled DNA was assessed by the membrane (Millipore Corp.) filtration technique (4). This assay is based on the observation that template DNA-RNA polymerase complexes are retained by these filters, whereas enzyme-free DNA passes through.

In a first experiment the effect of tirandamycin on the formation of DNA-RNA polymerase complexes was assessed (Table 3). The results show that tirandamycin did not interfere with the association of the complex, despite the presence of high concentrations of antibiotic. Congo red, a known inhibitor of this type of complex formation, proved highly inhibitory in our system.

If the DNA-RNA polymerase complex was allowed to form in the absence of tirandamycin and was then treated with the antibiotic, no dissociation of the preformed complex was observed (Table 4). Hence, tirandamycin does not interfere with the formation or stability of template-enzyme complexes.

Effect of tirandamycin on RNA chain initiation and elongation. The incorporation of [γ-^{32}P]GTP in conjunction with [^{14}C]uridine 5′-triphosphate (UTP) was used to assess chain initiation and elongation simultaneously. The results show that tirandamycin inhibited the incorporation of [γ-^{32}P]GTP to the same extent as [^{14}C]UTP with salmon sperm DNA as a template (Table 5). This suggests that both events, chain initiation (as reflected by the incorporation of [γ-^{32}P]GTP) and chain elongation (as reflected by [^{14}C]UTP incorporation) are equally inhibited by tirandamycin.

This conclusion was further substantiated with rifamycin, an inhibitor of chain initiation only. Rifamycin SV and tirandamycin were added to parallel reaction mixtures at 5 min after the initiation of the reaction (Fig. 3). The results show that in the mixtures containing rifamycin, RNA synthesis continued at a reduced rate for at least an additional 10 min after the addition of the antibiotic. Tirandamycin, on the other hand, caused immediate cessation of RNA synthesis upon the addition of the antibiotic. This indicates that tirandamycin, in contrast to rifamycin, inhibits RNA chain elongation as well as chain initiation.

TABLE 3. *Binding of RNA polymerase to E. coli DNA*[a]

Sample	Concn (mM)	^{14}C-labeled DNA retained (cpm/sample)	% of control
Control		5,860	100
No polymerase		900	15
Tirandamycin	1	5,330	90
Tirandamycin	0.1	5,900	100
Tirandamycin	0.01	5,940	101
Congo red	0.05	280	4

[a] Reaction mixtures contained in a total volume of 0.25 ml: tris(hydroxymethyl)aminomethane-hydrochloride, pH 7.9, 0.04 M; $MgCl_2$, 0.01 M; ethylenediaminetetraacetic acid, 0.1 mM; dithiothreitol, 0.1 mM; KCl, 0.15 mM; RNA polymerase, 0.4 U; *E. coli* ^{14}C-labeled DNA, 0.1 μg containing approximately 8,000 cpm. The reaction was initiated by the addition of RNA polymerase last. The samples were incubated for 5 min at 37°C.

TABLE 4. *Effect of tirandamycin on stability of DNA-RNA polymerase complex*[a]

Sample	Concn (mM)	^{14}C-labeled DNA retained (cpm/sample)	% of control
Control		6,820	100
No polymerase		770	11
Tirandamycin	1	6,610	96
	0.1	6,920	101
	0.01	6,700	98
Congo red	0.05	310	4

[a] Reaction mixtures were as described in the legend to Table 3. The DNA-polymerase complex was preformed by incubating the samples for 5 min at 37°C; tirandamycin was then added, and incubation was continued for an additional 5 min.

TABLE 5. *Effect of tirandamycin on [γ-^{32}P]GTP and [^{14}C]UTP incorporation*[a]

Sample	Concn (mM)	[^{14}C]UTP incorporation (cpm/sample)	Inhibition (%)	[γ-^{32}P]GTP incorporation (cpm/sample)	Inhibition (%)	Ratio of ^{32}P/^{14}C
Control		1,680	0	1,470	0	0.85
Tirandamycin	1	770	55	760	49	0.98
Tirandamycin	0.5	940	46	730	51	0.77
Tirandamycin	0.1	1,490	12	1,360	8	0.91

[a] Reaction mixtures were as described in the legend to Fig. 2, except: salmon sperm DNA, 10 μg/sample; [^{14}C]UTP, 0.05 μCi/sample; [γ-^{32}P]GTP, ~0.2 μCi/sample.

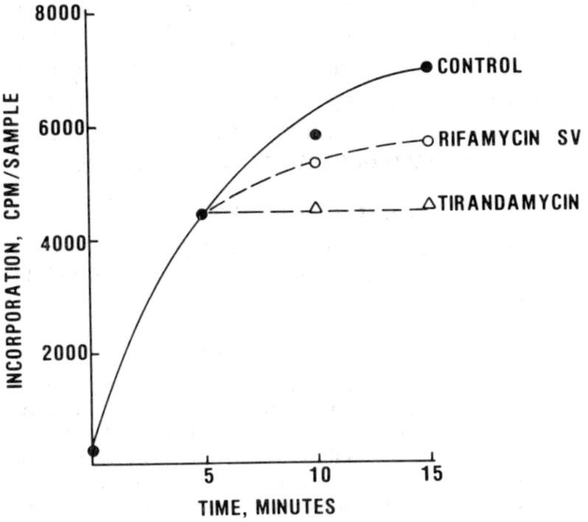

FIG. 3. *Effects of rifamycin SV and tirandamycin on RNA polymerase. Reaction mixtures were those described in the legend to Fig. 2. Rifamycin SV, 2 μg/ml; tirandamycin, 1 mM.*

Effect of tenuazonic acid. The fungal metabolite tenuazonic acid closely resembles the tetramic acid portions present in streptolydigin and tirandamycin, as shown in the structure below:

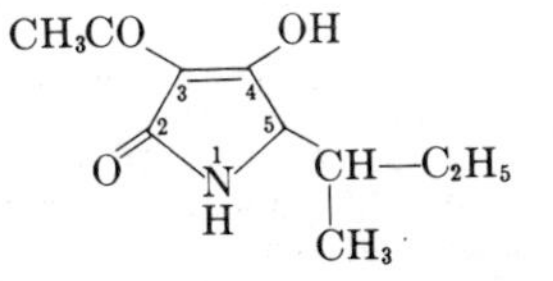

Interestingly, tenuazonic acid possesses essentially no antibacterial activity and is toxic in animals. In addition, it was reported that this acid acts as an inhibitor of protein synthesis in eucaryotic cells and cell-free systems (10). It appeared appropriate to test the effect of tenuazonic acid in our cell-free, bacterial RNA polymerase system. The results assembled in Table 6 show that tenuazonic acid had no effect on the activity of bacterial RNA polymerase.

Effect of tirandamycin on mammalian RNA polymerase. The effect of tirandamycin on RNA polymerase of animal origin was studied in a test system derived from rat liver. RNA polymerase was purified from isolated rat liver nuclei to the step prior to diethylaminoethylcellulose chromatography, as described by Roeder and Rutter (9). The preparation thus contained all of the nuclear polymerase species. Tirandamycin (or streptolydigin) did not inhibit RNA synthesis catalyzed by this enzyme preparation (Table 7). Hence, tirandamycin specifically inhibits the catalytic function of the bacterial RNA polymerase species and does not impair the function of the animal polymerases.

DISCUSSION

The data presented demonstrate that tirandamycin acts as a specific inhibitor of the bacterial enzyme RNA polymerase. RNA polymerases of mammalian origin are not inhibited by the antibiotic. Tirandamycin does not prevent the binding of RNA polymerase to its template DNA. The processes of chain initiation and chain elongation are both subject to inhibition by tirandamycin.

Chemically, tirandamycin closely resembles the antibiotic streptolydigin and differs from the latter, especially in that it lacks the sugar substituent at the *N* position and the adjacent substitution at the 5 position of the tetramic acid. The mode of action of tirandamycin is qualitatively identical with that of streptolydigin. However, on a molar basis streptolydigin proves approximately 40 times more potent than tirandamycin. The substituents at the 1 and 5 positions of the tetramic acid as present in streptolydigin are thus not essential for the interaction of the inhibitor with RNA polymerase, but impart a strong potentiating effect.

TABLE 6. *Effect of tenuazonic acid on RNA polymerase*[a]

Sample	Concn (mM)	Incorporation (cpm/sample)	Inhibition (%)
Control		5,120	0
Streptolydigin	0.1	1,680	68
Tirandamycin	0.1	2,970	42
Tenuazonic acid	0.5	4,870	5
Tenuazonic acid	0.1	4,620	10

[a] Reaction mixtures are described in the legend to Fig. 2.

TABLE 7. *Effect of tirandamycin on mammalian RNA polymerase*[a]

Sample	Concn (mM)	[^{14}C]UTP incorporation (cpm/sample)	% of control
Control		1,110	100
Tirandamycin	0.5	1,080	97
Tirandamycin	0.25	1,100	98
Streptolydigin	0.3	1,200	107
Streptolydigin	0.15	1,140	102

[a] Reaction mixtures contained in a total volume of 0.25 ml: tris(hydroxymethyl)aminomethane-hydrochloride, pH 7.9, 0.12 M; $(NH_4)_2SO_4$, 0.2 M; $MgCl_2$, 0.03 M; mercaptoethanol, 25 mM; salmon sperm DNA, 50 μg; ATP, GTP, CTP, 37 μg each; [^{14}C]UTP, 0.1 μCi. Polymerase (fraction 4), 0.1 ml; samples were incubated for 30 min at 37°C.

Further substantiation that streptolydigin and tirandamycin possess identical modes of action stems from the observation that both antibiotics inhibit the growth of *Staphylococcus aureus* mutant strains resistant to ansamycins. On the other hand, tirandamycin does not inhibit *S. aureus* strains resistant to streptolydigin (Reusser, unpublished data).

Neither tirandamycin nor streptolydigin impairs the function of bacterial RNA polymerase by sequestration of the tightly bound Zn^{2+} from the polymerase since the addition of Zn^{2+} to the reaction mixtures did not reverse the inhibitory activity exerted by these drugs (data not shown).

Lastly, I compared the structurally related compound tenuazonic acid with streptolydigin or tirandamycin. Tenuazonic acid is toxic in animals and does not inhibit bacterial RNA polymerase, but inhibits protein synthesis in higher organisms. Tirandamycin and streptolydigin, on the other hand, are not toxic in animals, but inhibit the growth of bacteria by the specific inhibition of the bacterial RNA polymerase species. Tenuazonic acid does not contain the complex substituents at position 3 [dioxabicyclo(3.1)nonane system and conjugated diene] present in streptolydigin and tirandamycin. This would suggest that the minimal active moiety essential for bacterial RNA polymerase inhibition resides within the complex 3-acyl groups of streptolydigin and tirandamycin.

However, recently a series of synthetic tetramic acids with various simple substituents at positions 1, 3, and 5 have been prepared, and some of these have shown inhibitory activity against bacterial RNA polymerase comparable in potency to tirandamycin and streptolydigin (V. J. Lee, K. L. Rinehart, and F. Reusser, Abstr. 170th Natl. Am. Chem. Soc. Meet. 1975, MEDI 7).

This negates the above conclusion and suggests that the tetramic acid moiety in conjunction with various substituents at positions 1, 3, and 5 is basically responsible for RNA polymerase inhibition. These substituents have to satisfy highly specific structural requirements to induce inhibition of bacterial RNA polymerase.

ACKNOWLEDGMENTS

I thank K. L. Rinehart, University of Illinois, for discussions. The technical assistance of J. L. Kay is gratefully acknowledged.

LITERATURE CITED

1. **Cassani, G., R. R. Burgess, H. M. Goodman, and L. Gold.** 1971. Inhibition of RNA polymerase by streptolydigin. Nature (London) New Biol. **230**:197–200.
2. **Chesterton, C. G., and M. H. Green.** 1968. Early-late transcription switch: isolation of a lambda DNA-RNA polymerase complex active in the synthesis of late RNA. Biochem. Biophys. Res. Commun. **31**:919–924.
3. **Duchamp, D. J., A. R. Branfman, A. C. Button, and K. L. Rinehart.** 1973. X-ray structure of tirandamycic acid p-bromophenyl ester. Complete stereochemical assignments of tirandamycin and streptolydigin. J. Am. Chem. Soc. **95**:4077–4078.
4. **Jones, O. W., and P. Berg.** 1966. Studies on the binding of RNA polymerase to polynucleotides. J. Mol. Biol. **22**:199–209.
5. **MacKellar, F. A., M. F. Grostic, E. C. Olson, R. J. Wnuk, A. R. Branfman, and K. L. Rinehart.** 1971. Tirandamycin. I. Structure assignment. J. Am. Chem. Soc. **93**:4943–4945.
6. **Meyer, C. E.** 1971. Tirandamycin, a new antibiotic: isolation and characterization. J. Antibiot. **24**:558–560.
7. **Reusser, F.** 1970. Tirandamycin: inhibition of ribonucleic acid polymerase. Infect. Immun. **2**:77–81.
8. **Rinehart, K. L., J. R. Beck, D. B. Borders, T. H. Kinstle, and D. Krauss.** 1963. Streptolydigin. III. Chromophore and structure. J. Am. Chem. Soc. **85**:4038–4039.
9. **Roeder, R. G., and W. J. Rutter.** 1970. Specific nucleolar and nucleoplasmic RNA polymerases. Proc. Natl. Acad. Sci. U.S.A. **65**:675–682.
10. **Shigeura, H. T.** 1967. Tenuazonic acid, p. 360–365. *In* D. Gottlieb and P. Shaw (ed.), Antibiotics. I. Mechanism of action. Springer Verlag, Berlin.
11. **Siddikol, C., J. W. Erbstoeszer, and B. Weisblum.** 1969. Mode of action of streptolydigin. J. Bacteriol. **99**:151–155.

ANTIMICROBIAL AGENTS AND CHEMOTHERAPY, Oct. 1976, p. 623-625
Vol. 10, No. 4

Printed in U.S.A.

Pharmacokinetics of Cefamandole in the Presence of Renal Failure and in Patients Undergoing Hemodialysis

GERALD B. APPEL, HAROLD C. NEU,* MICHAEL F. PARRY, MARK J. GOLDBERGER, AND GINETTE B. JACOB

Departments of Medicine and Pharmacology, College of Physicians and Surgeons, Columbia University, New York, New York 10032*

Received for publication 12 May 1976

The pharmacology of cefamandole in seven patients with stable renal insufficiency and in eight patients undergoing hemodialysis was determined. All patients had creatinine clearances less than 5 ml/min. The half-life of cefamandole in those patients with stable chronic renal failure was 7.7 ± 2.2 h. The mean venous level 1 h after intravenous injection of a 1-g dose was 85.3 ± 32.0 μg/ml. The mean venous half-life of cefamandole during hemodialysis was 6.1 h. The venous serum level after 5.5 of hemodialysis was 50.4 ± 20.8 μg/ml. The mean coefficient of extraction was 0.155, and the mean clearance was 34.7 ml/min. The time interval between doses of cefamandole administered intravenously should be lengthened to 24 h in the presence of stable renal failure. No major change in dosage schedule is necessary for patients undergoing dialysis.

Cefamandole, 7-D-mandelamido-3{[(1-methyl-1H-tetrazol-5-yl)thio]methyl}-3-cephem-4-carboxylic acid, is a new semisynthetic cephalosporin antibiotic with a broad spectrum of activity against most gram-positive and gram-negative bacteria (1, 6). It has greater in vitro activity than other commercially available cephalosporins against most strains of *Escherichia coli*, *Enterobacter*, *Klebsiella*, *Haemophilus*, *serratia*, and *Proteus* species (6). Preliminary data suggest that cefamandole is useful in the treatment of septicemia and serious infections of the respiratory tract, urinary tract, or soft tissues due to susceptible microorganisms (8; unpublished observations). Such infections occur frequently in patients with renal insufficiency, and many of these patients are managed by extracorporeal dialysis. Therefore, we wished to establish the pharmacokinetics of cefamandole in patients with severe renal impairment and in patients undergoing hemodialysis.

MATERIALS AND METHODS

Subjects for study included eight patients with stable chronic renal failure and creatinine clearance of 5 ml/min or less. The mean age was 44 years (range, 20 to 62 years). There were four male and four female patients. None of these patients were dehydrated or receiving other antibiotics at the time of the study. Each patient received 1 g of cefamandole nafate by intravenous (i.v.) infusion over a 5-min period. Venous blood samples were obtained at 1-, 2-, 4-, 6-, and 18-h intervals in most instances. No patient underwent dialysis during the interval of plasma sampling. Seven additional patients with stable chronic renal failure and creatinine clearance of less than 5 ml/min were studied during dialysis. The mean age was 48 years (range, 22 to 74 years). There were four male and three female patients. Each patient was maintained on thrice weekly chronic hemodialysis. Dialyses were performed using a twin-coil Travenol RSP dialyzer with an Ultra Flow II cuprophane membrane and lasted 5.5 h per session. Dialysate flow rates were constant at 600 ml/min and blood flow rates were maintained at 200 to 250 ml/min. At the beginning of dialysis each patient received 1 g of cefamandole nafate by i.v. injection over 5 min. Specimens of arterial and venous blood and dialysate were obtained at 15 min, at 1 h, 2 h, 3 h, and 4 h, and at the termination of dialysis.

Written, informed consent was obtained from all subjects prior to their participation in the study.

Blood samples were centrifuged 30 to 45 min after collection, and the serum was separated and stored at −20°C until assayed. Serum levels of cefamandole were determined using an agar well plate technique with *Bacillus subtilis* as the assay organism. Standards of cefamandole as a lithium salt were prepared with pooled human serum, and plasma samples were diluted in pooled human serum. Assays were run in quadruplicate using a Latin-square randomization technique.

Plots of the serum concentration of cefamandole versus time were constructed, and the half-life of the antibiotic was determined when the blood levels were declining exponentially during the elimination phase. The formula used for the half-life was $T_{1/2} = (\ln 2/K_e)$, where ln 2 is the natural logarithm of 2 and K_e is the slope of the regression line determined by method of least squares. The coefficients of extraction for cefamandole during hemodialysis were computed according to the formula:

$$E_c = (D_i - D_o)/D_i$$

where D_i is the concentration of cefamandole in arterial serum and D_o is the concentration of cefamandole in serum leaving the coil. Clearance during dialysis was calculated according to the formula:

$$C_d = Q_b(D_i - D_o)/D_k$$

where Q_b is the blood flow rate through the dialysis coil. Coefficients of extraction and clearances were calculated for each patient sample.

RESULTS

The peak serum levels and $T_{1/2}$ in the seven patients with chronic renal failure are given in Table 1. Venous serum levels at 1 h ranged from 45 to 150 μg/ml, with a mean of 85.3 ± 32 μg/ml. The correlation of the height of serum level with mean body surface area was fair for most patients.

The mean concentrations of cefamandole in arterial serum, venous serum, and dialysate for the eight hemodialyzed patients are listed in Table 2. Serum arterial and venous levels when plotted versus time on dialysis describe similar curves (Fig. 1). The mean half-life for arterial plasma was 5.9 h and for venous plasma 6.1 h. Mean arterial and venous serum levels at 1 h were 108.3 ± 32.0 and 94.4 ± 31.9 μg/ml, respectively. At termination of dialysis mean arterial and venous levels were 61.4 ± 23.3 and 50.4 ± 120.8 μg/ml, respectively. The mean coefficients of extraction and the mean clearance of cefamandole at 1, 2, 3, and 4 h are listed in Table 2. Based on the dialysate levels, there was 143.3 ± 58.9 mg of cefamandole recovered during the 5.5-h hemodialysis periods.

DISCUSSION

The pharmacokinetics of cefamandole in individuals with normal renal function are similar to those of cephalothin in normal individuals (5). The $T_{1/2}$ of cefamandole is 27 to 34 min, whereas the $T_{1/2}$'s for the other cephalosporins are: cephalothin, 30 to 50 min; cephaloridine, 66 to 90 min; cefazolin, 96 to 120 min; and cephalexin, 36 to 54 min (2, 4). Cefamandole is predominantly excreted by renal mechanisms. The

TABLE 1. *Data from dialysis and uremic studies*

Study	Patient	Age (yr)	Sex	Wt (kg)	Ht (cm)	Surface area (m²)	Diagnosis[a]	Peak serum level (μg/ml)	$T_{1/2}$ (h)
Dialysis	R.G.	48	F	43.8	165	1.42	Sarcoid-CRF	243	8.6
	M.S.	56	F	62.3	175	1.76	DM	105	4.7
	E.G.	74	M	62.8	168	1.73	CGN	270	5.2
	A.V.	46	M	66.0	188	1.89	CPN	103	9.0
	E.B.	64	F	72.8	160	1.77	DM	79	3.9
	O.E.	44	M	62.0	165	1.70	CGN	145	4.6
	J.P.	32	M	70.6	163	1.78	CGN	150	5.2
	J.C.	22	F	52.9	163	1.56	DM	124	3.7
Uremic	J.P.	32	M	60	163	1.66	CGN	120	5.5
	B.Mc	29	M	61	175	1.74	HRD	63	9.7
	M.D.	56	F	38.6	152	1.37	HRD	117	8.5
	B.R.	61	F	73.8	165	1.80	DM	70	5.0
	F.S.	46	M	89.0	180	2.10	DM	47	11.0
	M.C.	62	F	39.0	152	1.32	CPN	175	9.0
	M.W.	20	F	55.0	160	1.55	HRD	95	5.5

[a] Abbreviations: CRF, Chronic renal failure; DM, diabetes mellitus; CGN, chronic glomerulonephritis; CPN, chronic pyelonephritis; HRN, hypertensive renal disease.

TABLE 2. *Mean concentrations of cefamandole in arterial serum, venous serum, and dialysate, mean coefficients of extraction, and mean clearance after i.v. injection of 1.0 g*

Min after p̄ injection	Arterial plasma (μg/ml)	Venous plasma (μg/ml)	Dialysate (μg/ml)	Coefficients of extraction	Clearance
60	108.3 ± 32.0	94.4 ± 31.9	1.99 ± 1.40	0.140 ± .089	31.4 ± 20.0
120	95.9 ± 24.7	79.6 ± 28.8	1.11 ± 0.92	0.187 ± .109	42.0 ± 24.5
180	82.5 ± 28.7	70.4 ± 20.8	1.47 ± 0.92	0.127 ± .103	28.6 ± 22.9
240	75.4 ± 24.4	62.7 ± 26.3	0.70 ± 0.14	0.165 ± .172	37.0 ± 38.8
330	61.4 ± 23.3	50.4 ± 20.8	0.70 ± 0.40		

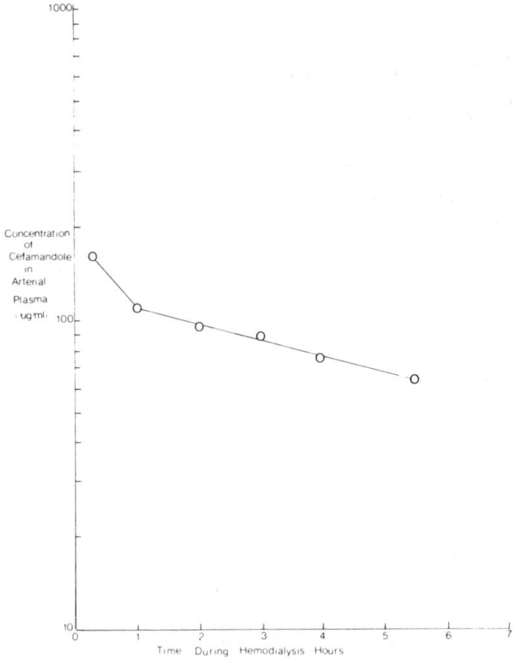

FIG. 1. *Mean artęrial plasma levels of cefamandole in the seven patients during dialysis.*

half-life of cefamandole is prolonged to 7.7 ± 2.2 h in patients with severe stable chronic renal failure. The $T_{1/2}$'s of the other cephalosporins in uremia are: cephalothin, 12 to 18 h; cephaloridine, 20 to 25 h; cefazolin, 35 to 56 h; and cephalexin, 14 to 20 h (5, 7). Hemodialysis with a Travenol RSP machine and a UF II coil reduces the half-life of cefamandole to approximately 6.0 h. Although the half-life is only moderately decreased, the antibiotic is removed, as demonstrated by the clearances (range, 28.6 to 42 ml/min) and by the amount of drug removed, based on dialysate levels (143.3 ± 58.9 mg, 14.3%). Nevertheless, serum levels at the end of 5.5 h of hemodialysis are still sufficiently high (mean venous serum level, 50.4 ± 20.8 μg/ml) to inhibit most strains of susceptible microorganisms if the cefamandole has been given by i.v. injection.

The serum levels after i.v. administration in the patients with $C_{cr} < 5$ ml/min are comparable to those achieved in normal volunteers (3). There appears to be a fair correlation of the height of the serum level with body surface area.

From these data, certain recommendations regarding the dosage of cefamandole in patients with renal dysfunction may be made. If a 1-g dose is given i.v. to a patient with normal renal function (every 4 h), this time interval should be extended in the face of severe renal failure. If a standard dose were given every three half-lives, the drug would be administered at 1 g every 23 h. For convenience of administration, this dose could be given every 24 h. If the patient is undergoing extracorporeal dialysis, a similar schedule is reasonable. An additional dose of cefamandole is not needed after hemodialysis if the patient has received a dose of the drug just prior to the institution of dialysis. These recommendations apply only to an i.v. administered drug, since the blood levels after intramuscular administration are considerably lower.

ACKNOWLEDGMENTS

We wish to thank the Nursing Staff of the Hemodialysis Unit of Columbia Presbyterian Medical Center for their cooperation during this study; Alice S. Appel for technical assistance in preparation of this paper; and Iris P. Rivera for typing preparation.

LITERATURE CITED

1. **Eykyn, S., C. Jenkins, A. King, and I. Phillips.** 1973. Antibacterial activity of cefamandole, a new cephalosporin antibiotic, compared with that of cephaloridine, cephalothin, and cephalexin. Antimicrob. Agents Chemother. **3**:657–661.
2. **Fong, I. W., E. D. Ralph, E. R. Engelking, and W. M. M. Kirby.** 1976. Clinical pharmacology of cefamandole as compared with cephalothin. Antimicrob. Agents Chemother. **9**:65–69.
3. **Meyers, B. R., R. Ribner, S. Yancovitz, and S. Z. Hirschman.** 1976. Pharmacological studies with cefamandole in human volunteers. Antimicrob. Agents Chemother. **9**:140–144.
4. **Moellering, R. C., and M. N. Swartz.** 1976. The newer cephalosporins. N. Engl. J. Med. **294**:24–28.
5. **Neu, H. C.** 1973. Guidelines to antibiotic therapy in renal failure. Med. Times **11**:47–53.
6. **Neu, H. C.** 1974. Cefamandole, a cephalosporin antibiotic with an unusually wide spectrum of activity. Antimicrob. Agents Chemother. **6**:177–182.
7. **Nightingale, C. H., D. S. Greene, and R. Quintiliani.** 1975. Pharmacokinetics and clinical use of cephalosporin antibiotics. J. Pharm. Sci. **64**:1899–1927.
8. **Shemonsky, N. K., J. Carrizosa, and M. E. Levison.** 1975. In vitro actiyity and pharmacokinetics in patients of cefamandole, a new cephalosporin antibiotic. Antimicrob. Agents Chemother. **8**:679–693.

ANTIMICROBIAL AGENTS AND CHEMOTHERAPY, Oct. 1976, p. 626-629 Vol. 10, No. 4

Nosocomial Infection with Gentamicin-Carbenicillin-Resistant *Pseudomonas aeruginosa*

IAN M. BAIRD,* JERRY M. SLEPACK,[1] CAROL A. KAUFFMAN, AND JOHN P. PHAIR

Infectious Disease Division, Department of Internal Medicine, University of Cincinnati College of Medicine, Cincinnati, Ohio 45267, and Medical Service, Cincinnati Veterans Administration Hospital, Cincinnati, Ohio 45220*

Received for publication 30 April 1976

Pseudomonas aeruginosa resistant to both gentamicin and carbenicillin was isolated with increasing frequency at the Cincinnati Veterans Administration Hospital during the period 1971 to 1974. A comparison of patients from whom *P. aeruginosa* was isolated during this period failed to reveal any significant clinical differences between the patients colonized or infected with resistant organisms and those colonized or infected with susceptible organisms. Overt clinical infection attributable to either organism was rare. The antibiotic-resistant organisms were isolated most frequently from urine. Isolation of the antibiotic-resistant organisms was more frequent from patients who had previously received gentamicin.

Recent reports in both the clinical and microbiological literature have described *Pseudomonas aeruginosa* strains resistant to both carbenicillin and gentamicin (2, 8, 9). Organisms with this resistance pattern have been isolated with increasing frequency at the Cincinnati Veterans Administration Hospital over the past several years. Previous reports from this institution have established that the antibiotic resistance of these strains of *P. aeruginosa* was R-factor mediated and that the responsible R-factor was of the P-2 group (10, 11). It has also been shown that the majority of these antibiotic-resistant organisms belonged to immunotype 7. Furthermore, this R-factor did not influence the organism as to immunotype, pyocin type, or virulence in rats and, although it readily transferred resistance to other *P. aeruginosa,* it did not transfer resistance to *Escherichia coli* or to *Proteus* species (10, 15). Since our clinical impression and reports of others (8) suggested that the resistant organisms rarely caused infection, a study was undertaken to determine the clinical significance of the isolation of resistant organisms as compared with the isolation of susceptible organisms.

MATERIALS AND METHODS

Susceptibility patterns of *P. aeruginosa* isolates at the Cincinnati Veterans Administration Hospital were determined by a disk diffusion method (1). Isolates obtained during December 1971, March, June, September, and December 1972 and 1973, and January and March 1974 were reviewed, and the incidence of gentamicin- and carbenicillin-resistant isolates of *P. aeruginosa* (G^RC^R) was determined. Clinical records of patients from whom *P. aeruginosa* was isolated during December 1972, June 1973, and January 1974 were analyzed in depth, with particular reference to the clinical significance of the isolation of *P. aeruginosa* and its role in causing infection. Parameters that were studied included the source of the bacterial isolate, the presence or absence of a urinary tract foriegn body and/or urinary tract obstruction, the presence or absence of underlying diseases, and the administration of antibiotics in the 7 days prior to the isolation of *P. aeruginosa*. The number of patients with leukopenia, who were immunosuppressed either by therapy or by virtue of their underlying diseases, was also recorded. The presence of fever, in addition to either chills, leukocytosis, or signs of infection at the anatomical site of isolation (e.g., pyuria and purulent drainage), was considered evidence of infection. The isolation of *P. aeruginosa* without clinical evidence of infection at the site of isolation was considered to represent bacterial colonization. The 3 months used for in-depth analysis were chosen as representative of months of low, intermediate, and high frequency of recovery of isolates of G^RC^R organisms. Statistical analysis was performed throughout, using the chi-square test with Yates correction.

RESULTS

During the 11 months selected for study, *P. aeruginosa* was isolated 564 times from 535 patients. Eighty-five of the patients were infected or colonized with G^RC^R, and 450 were infected or colonized with *P. aeruginosa* that was susceptible to both gentamicin and carbenicillin (G^SC^S). Figure 1 demonstrates that both the

[1] Present address: Permanente Clinic, Portland, OR 97217.

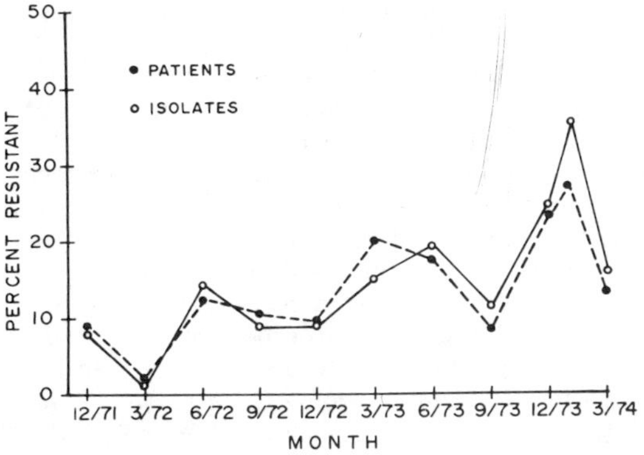

FIG. 1. *Increasing incidence of isolation of antibiotic-resistant P. aeruginosa between 1971 and 1974. Symbols:* ●, *percentage of all patients from whom P. aeruginosa was isolated in whom the isolate was resistant in vitro to gentamicin and carbenicillin;* ○, *percentage of all P. aeruginosa isolates that were resistant in vitro to gentamicin and carbenicillin.*

percentage of patients with G^RC^R and the percentage of all G^RC^R isolates increased from December 1971 through January 1974. Table 1 lists the medical services of the patients from whom the G^RC^R were isolated; most of these patients were located on the urology and medicine wards. A total of 79% of these organisms were isolated from the urine; in contrast, 40% of the 478 G^SC^S isolates were found in the urine. The increased frequency of isolation of G^RC^R organisms from urine cultures is statistically significant ($P < 0.001$). A total of 7% of G^RC^R and 33% of G^SC^S were recovered from the sputum, which is again a statistically significant difference ($P < 0.001$). The 289 urine cultures represented 51% of the 564 cultures, and 24% of the pseudomonas isolated from urine were of the G^RC^R resistance pattern. In contrast, only 3.5% of the 169 pseudomonas isolated from sputum had the G^RC^R pattern.

A review of the 106 clinical records of patients with *P. aeruginosa* isolates in December 1972, June 1973, and January 1974 revealed 78 patients from whom 115 G^SC^S were isolated and 28 from whom 51 G^RC^R were isolated (Table 2). There was no difference overall in the incidence of serious underlying disease in the two groups. Diabetes mellitus and hepatocellular disease were diagnosed with equal frequency in both groups, but there was significantly more renal disease among patients with G^RC^R ($P < 0.001$). As with the large group of patients described above, G^RC^R was isolated significantly more often from the urine, and G^SC^S was isolated more often from the sputum. The presence of a

TABLE 1. *Location of patients with P. aeruginosa isolates*[a]

Service	Ward	No. of patients with *P. aeruginosa* isolates	No. of patients with G^RC^R isolates	Total (%)
Surgery	4S	51	9	10.5
Surgery	4N	39	5	5.9
Neurology/neurosurgery	5S	40	4	4.7
Urology	5N	90	19	22.4
Medicine	6S	106	18	21.2
Medicine	6N	88	17	20.0
Other		121	13	15.3

[a] Selected months: December 1971 to March 1974.

TABLE 2. *Comparison of clinical findings in 106 patients with P. aeruginosa isolates*

Clinical finding	Patients with G^SC^S (total = 78)	Patients with G^RC^R (total = 28)	*P* value[a]
Underlying disease	74	27	NS[b]
Diabetes mellitus	14	7	NS
Hepatocellular disease	4	1	NS
Renal disease	14	15	<0.001
Urinary isolation	32	22	<0.01
Sputum isolation	32	4	<0.05
Infection	9	2	NS
Colonization	31	6	NS
Other infection[c]	38	20	NS
Previous antibiotics	45	21	NS
Previous gentamicin	10	15	<0.001
Previous broad-spectrum antibiotics	25	6	NS

[a] Determined by the chi-square test with Yates correction.
[b] NS, Not statistically significant.
[c] The patient did have clinical infection, but *P. aeruginosa* was not the etiological agent.

urinary tract foreign body or obstruction, however, was no more commonly noted in patients infected or colonized with G^RC^R. There were six patients with clinical conditions that were considered to increase the risk of infection; three had hematological malignancy, one had generalized sarcoidosis, one was receiving prednisone, and one was leukopenic (<3,000/mm^3). Two of the six were considered infected by *P. aeruginosa*, both with G^SC^S organisms. Two patients were colonized by G^SC^S and two were colonized by G^RC^R organisms.

An analysis of the clinical evidence for infection due to *P. aeruginosa* revealed that chills, fever, and leukocytosis occurred no more frequently in patients with G^RC^R than in patients with G^SC^S. When the patients with urinary isolates were considered, the incidence of pyuria did not differ significantly between those with G^RC^R (19 of 22) and those with G^SC^S (23 of 32) organisms ($P > 0.05$). Other localizing findings indicative of infection (wound drainage, pulmonary infiltrates, or pleural effusion) also occurred with equal frequency in both groups of patients.

Eleven patients were thought to be infected solely with *P. aeruginosa*, as evidenced by (i) the recovery of the organism from blood or a closed body cavity or (ii) the fact that *P. aeruginosa* was the only isolate in association with clinical signs of infection, and clinical improvement occurred after the institution of appropriate chemotherapy. Nine were infected with G^SC^S; two were infected with G^RC^R. This difference is not statistically significant. Only one of the 106 patients had *P. aeruginosa* bacteremia, and the isolate was susceptible to gentamicin and carbenicillin. An additional 58 patients (38 with G^SC^S and 20 with G^RC^R) had evidence of infection, but culture revealed multiple organisms, and a clinical response was attained with antibiotic therapy not specifically chosen to treat *P. aeruginosa* infection. The remaining 37 patients were considered colonized by *P. aeruginosa* since the isolation of the organism was not associated with signs of infection and antibiotic therapy was not instituted. There was no difference in the percentage of patients colonized by either G^RC^R or G^SC^S.

An analysis of the role of antibiotics in leading to infection or colonization revealed that 45 of 78 patients in the G^SC^S group and 21 of 28 patients in the G^RC^R group received antibiotics during the week before the isolation of the *P. aeruginosa*. This was not a significant difference ($P > 0.1$). However, when the prior administration of gentamicin (either alone or in combination with other antimicrobials) was considered, a significant difference was found. Ten patients in the G^SC^S group of 78 and 15 patients in the G^RC^R group of 28 had received gentamicin ($P < 0.001$). None of the patients whose charts were reviewed in detail had received carbenicillin prior to the isolation of *P. aeruginosa*.

DISCUSSION

The widespread distribution of *P. aeruginosa* in a hospital environment is well recognized (3), and its potential to cause infection has been emphasized. Earlier reports of *P. aeruginosa* infections, however, dealt with infection occurring in patients with impaired defense mechanisms. Such patients included those with extensive burns, leukemia, Hodgkin's disease and other lymphomas, and patients with widespread solid tumors who were receiving toxic antineoplastic agents (12, 14). Although reports in the recent literature have acknowledged the role of *P. aeruginosa* in nosocomial infections in general (4, 5), few have examined the extent of infection or colonization with antibiotic-susceptible or antibiotic-resistant *P. aeruginosa* in a general hospital, where only an occasional patient is immunosuppressed (7, 13). The 106 patients in this report did have underlying diseases, most frequently atherosclerotic heart disease, chronic pulmonary disease, and cerebrovascular or other neurological diseases. A few patients were in the postoperative period after abdominal surgery, and others had sustained second- and third-degree burns, but none had greater than 20% of the total body surface area involved. Only six patients could be considered immunosuppressed.

Despite an abundance of *P. aeruginosa* in the hospital environment (3), it can only rarely be directly incriminated as a cause of infection. One study of gentamicin- and carbenicillin-resistant strains of *P. aeruginosa* suggested that the antibiotic-resistant strains were less pathogenic than the antibiotic-susceptible strains (8). However, our investigation and another recent study (13) were unable to demonstrate either increased or decreased pathogenicity of the antibiotic-resistant strains.

When the records of 106 patients from whom *P. aeruginosa* had been isolated were reviewed, the only factor that significantly predisposed to the isolation of a gentamicin-carbenicillin-resistant strain was whether the patient had received parenteral gentamicin therapy during the 7-day period prior to the bacterial isolation. A higher percentage of the resistant isolates were recovered from the urinary tract, and a higher percentage of antibiotic-susceptible organisms were recovered from the respiratory tract. This probably does not represent any inherent difference between the two strains, but reflects the empiric administration of gentamicin in urinary tract infection. Possibly, the increasing prevalence of gentamicin-carbenicillin-resistant strains of *P. aeruginosa* during the study period is the result of the increasing usage of gentamicin (gentamicin usage at Cincinnati Veterans Administration Hospital doubled between 1971 and 1974) and the well-recognized phenomenon of antibiotic selection of hospital-acquired microbial flora (6).

There was no difference in the percentage of patients judged to be clinically infected by G^RC^R or G^SC^S pseudomonas. Both resistant and susceptible organisms were the sole cause of infection in 10% of the patients from whom pseudomonas was isolated. This finding correlates with another clinical report (13) and with animal studies that revealed no difference in mortality in animals infected with G^RC^R versus G^SC^S organisms (15).

In summary, from 1971 to 1974 increasing numbers of *P. aeruginosa* resistant gentamicin and carbenicillin were isolated from patients at the Cincinnati Veterans Administration Hospital. The majority of the resistant organisms were isolated from the urinary tract, and the majority of patients from whom such organisms were isolated had received gentamicin alone or in combination with other antibiotics in the 7-day period prior to isolation. *P. aeruginosa*, both with and without the R-factor-mediated G^RC^R resistance pattern, rarely caused infection in this general hospital population.

ACKNOWLEDGMENTS

This study was supported by Public Health Service grant AI 12309 from the National Institute of Allergy and Infectious Diseases, by V. A. research grant project no. 4834 (C. A. Kauffman), by a grant from the Merrell-National Laboratories, and by the Morton Hamburger Memorial Fund.

Both I. M. Baird and J. M. Slepack were Infectious Disease Fellows at the Cincinnati Veterans Administration Hospital.

We wish to thank Stanley Williams of the Microbiology Laboratory, Cincinnati Veterans Administration Hospital, for his cooperation.

LITERATURE CITED

1. **Barry, A. L., F. Garcia, and L. D. Thrupp.** 1970. An improved disc method for testing the antibiotic susceptibility of rapidly growing organisms. Am. J. Clin. Pathol. 53:149–158.
2. **Chadwick, P.** 1973. Resistance of *Pseudomonas aeruginosa* to gentamicin. Can. Med. Assoc. J. **109**:585–587.
3. **Farmer, J. J.** 1976. Pseudomonas in the hospital. Hosp. Pract. **11**:63–70.
4. **Feingold,** D. S. 1970. Hospital acquired infection. N. Engl. J. Med. **283**:1384–1391.
5. **Fekety, F. R.** 1971. Nosocomial infections. Postgrad. Med. **50**:115–117.
6. **Finland, M.** 1969. Changing pattern of susceptibility of common bacterial pathogens to antimicrobial agents. Ann. Intern. Med. **76**:1009–1036.
7. **Gaman, W., C. Cates, C. F. T. Snelling, B. Lank, and A. R. Ronald.** 1976. Emergence of gentamicin- and carbenicillin-resistant *Pseudomonas aeruginosa* in a hospital environment. Antimicrob. Agents Chemother. **9**:474–480.
8. **Greene, W. H., S. Moody, S. Schimpff, V. M. Young, and P. H. Wiernick.** 1973. *Pseudomonas aeruginosa* resistant to carbenicillin and gentamicin. Ann. Intern. Med. **79**:684–689.
9. **Knothe, H., V. Kiemery, W. Sietzen, and J. Barst.** 1973. Transfer of gentamicin resistance from *Pseudomonas aeruginosa* strains highly resistant to gentamicin and carbenicillin. Chemotherapy **18**:229–234.
10. **Korfhagen, T. R., and J. C. Loper.** 1975. RPL 11, an R factor of *Pseudomonas aeruginosa* determining carbenicillin and gentamicin resistance. Antimicrob. Agents Chemother. **7**:69–73.
11. **Korfhagen, T. R., J. C. Loper, and J. A. Ferrell.** 1975. *Pseudomonas aeruginosa* R factors determining gentamicin plus carbenicillin resistance from urinary tract colonization. Antimicrob. Agents Chemother. **7**:64–68.
12. **Levine, A. S., R. G. Graw, and R. C. Young.** 1972. Management of infection in patients with leukemia and lymphoma: current concepts and experimental approaches. Semin. Hematol. **9**:141–179.
13. **Meyer, R. D., R. P. Lewis, J. Halter, and M. White.** 1976. Gentamicin-resistant *Pseudomonas aeruginosa* and *Serratia marcescens* in a general hospital. Lancet **1**:580–583.
14. **Schimpff, S. C., V. M. Young, W. H. Greene, G. D. Vermuelen, M. R. Moody, and P. H. Wiernick.** 1972. Origin of infection in acute non-lymphocytic leukemia. Ann. Intern. Med. **77**:707–714.
15. **Slepack, J. M., T. Korfhagen, J. C. Loper, J. S. Tan, and J. P. Phair.** 1975. Virulence in rats of gentamicin-carbenicillin-resistant *Pseudomonas*. Antimicrob. Agents Chemother. **8**:513–514.

ANTIMICROBIAL AGENTS AND CHEMOTHERAPY, Oct. 1976, p. 630-638
Vol. 10, No. 4

Metabolism of [^{14}C]Cefaclor, a Cephalosporin Antibiotic, in Three Species of Laboratory Animals

HUGH R. SULLIVAN,* SUSAN L. DUE, DONALD L. K. KAU, JOHN F. QUAY, AND WARREN M. MILLER

The Lilly Research Laboratories, Indianapolis, Indiana 46206

Received for publication 7 May 1976

The metabolic fate of the orally effective cephalosporin antibiotic cefaclor (Lilly 99638) has been studied in rats, mice, and dogs. Cefaclor is efficiently absorbed from the gastrointestinal tract as the intact antibiotic. In rats and mice, cefaclor, for the most part, escapes metabolism in the body and is eliminated unchanged as unaltered antibiotic, primarily by renal excretion. In dogs, however, cefaclor is more labile to metabolism and only a portion of the administered antibiotic is eliminated unchanged via the kidney.

Cefaclor (see Fig. 1), 3-chloro-7-D-(2-phenylglycinamido)-3-cephem-4-carboxylic acid (Lilly 99638), is an orally effective, broad-spectrum antibiotic active against gram-positive cocci, including penicillin-resistant strains, as well as against many gram-negative organisms. Cefaclor is a cephalosporin antibiotic structurally related to orally active cephalexin [generic name given to 7-(D-2-amino-2-phenylacetamido)-3-methyl-3-cephem-4-carboxylic acid] (6). The study described below, which is patterned after earlier studies (1, 7-9), shows that cefaclor is well absorbed after oral administration and that this antibiotic is, like cephalexin, resistant to metabolic degradation or alteration. As in earlier studies on the in vivo fate of cephalosporin antibiotics from these laboratories, radiocarbon labeling was used to facilitate the present investigation.

MATERIALS AND METHODS

[^{14}C]cefaclor. D-[1-^{14}C]phenylglycine (1.59 mmol, 20.86 μCi/mg) was allowed to react with 2.06 mmol of methyl acetoacetate in a solution of 1.62 mmol of NaOH in 15 ml of methanol. After heating the reaction mixture for 1.5 h at reflux temperature, 15 ml of acetonitrile was added and heating was continued for 30 min. Methanol was removed by distillation and was replaced with an appropriate amount of acetonitrile. After cooling to room temperature, the precipitated methyl [1-^{14}C]3-(D-3-β-carboxybenzyl amino)crotonate sodium salt was collected by filtration, washed with acetonitrile, and dried in vacuo. The yield of product was 1.50 mmol.

Methyl chloroformate (1.58 mmol) was allowed to react with 1.50 mmol of methyl [1-^{14}C]3-(D-3-β-carboxybenzylamino)crotonate sodium salt in solution with 25 ml of dry dimethylformamide containing 1 drop of *N,N*-dibenzylamine at −40°C. After stirring the resulting solution for 30 min at this temperature, a solution of 1.40 mmol of *p*-nitrobenzyl-3-chloro-3-cephem-4-carboxylate in 5 ml of dimethylformamide was added rapidly with stirring. The resulting mixture was stirred at −40°C for 2.5 h and then was allowed to stand overnight at room temperature. Upon cooling the mixture to 0°C, water (0.5 ml) and then 0.9 ml of concentrated HCl was added dropwise. Zinc dust (5.46 mmol) was added to the reaction mixture over a period of 30 min, keeping the temperature between 0 and 5°C. After complete addition, the reaction mixture was stirred at 0°C for 2.5 h. Concentrated HCl (0.56 ml) was then added, and stirring was continued for 1 h. The pH of the reaction mixture was then adjusted from 1.6 to 3.5 with triethylamine and filtered. Semicarbazide·hydrochloride (1.44 mmol) was added portionwise to the filtrate over a period of 30 min, maintaining the pH at 3.5 with triethylamine. After complete addition, the pH of reaction solution was adjusted to 6.8 with stirring in an ice bath to facilitate precipitation. The crude product was collected by filtration, washed with dimethylformamide, and then dissolved in a solution containing 9.3 ml of water, 0.12 ml of concentrated HCl, and tetrasodium ethylenediaminetetraacetate dihydrate (0.022 mmol). After adding 0.02 g of decolorizing carbon, the solution was filtered, and the filtrate was adjusted to pH 4.6 with diluted NH_4OH. Acetonitrile (10 ml) was added, and the filtrate was cooled to induce precipitation. The purified product was collected by filtration, washed with 5 ml of water, and dried in vacuo at 40°C for 8 h. The yield of pure [^{14}C]cefaclor was 0.50 mmol (40%), with a specific radioactivity of 7.35 μCi/mg. Paper chromatography, followed by microbiological and radiological assay, showed the product to be pure.

Chromatographic methods. Paper chromatography was carried out on Whatman no. 1 paper and a butan-2-ol-acetic acid-water (3:1:1) solvent system was used for development. Areas of biological activity were located by a bioautographic technique described by Miller (5), using *Sarcina lutea*. The radioactive zones were located by means of a scanner (Vanguard 880 automatic chromatogram scanner).

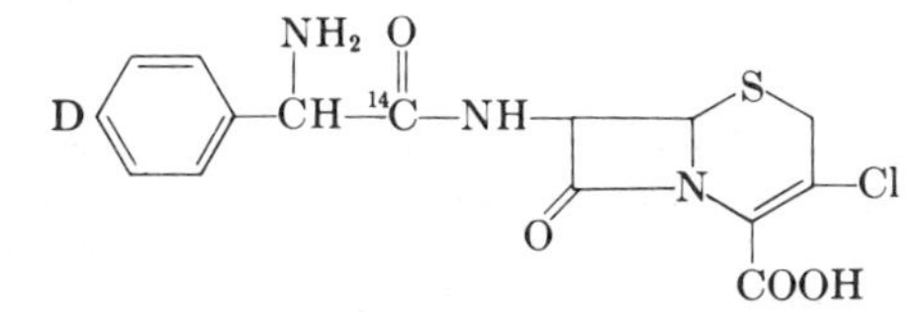

FIG. 1. *Structure of [14C]cefaclor.*

Sample preparation: microbiological assay. Urine and bile samples were acidified with glacial acetic acid immediately upon collection. Samples were diluted as required with pH 4.5 aqueous buffer containing, in millimoles per liter: Na^+, 160; PO_4^{3-}, 5; acetate, 12; Cl^-, 150. Standard solutions of cefaclor containing 0.025 to 1 μg/ml were prepared in the buffer on the day of the animal test.

Whole-blood samples were frozen and thawed to effect hemolysis. One part, by volume, of hemolyzed blood was diluted with 2 volumes of pH 6.0 buffer containing the ionic constituents listed above. Standard solutions of cefaclor were prepared on the day of animal test in a compound diluent composed of 1 volume of whole hemolyzed control blood and 2 volumes of buffer. When further dilutions of blood samples were required, the same compound diluent was used.

Samples of synovial fluid, cerebrospinal fluid, aqueous humor, and serum were diluted 1 part to 3, by volume, with pH 4.5 buffer. Standard solutions of cefaclor were prepared in control samples of these biological fluids diluted appropriately with buffer. All standard solutions were stored at 4°C until assayed.

Microbiological assay method. Antibiotic activity in unknown samples was compared to that in previously prepared standard solutions using a disk-plate agar diffusion test (*S. lutea* X-186: inoculum, 2.5%, by volume, of 53% light transmission stock culture; agar [BBL no. 6] at 20 g/liter, pH 6.6; pour volume, 6 ml/plate; disks, Schleicher & Schuell no. 740E, 6.35 mm). Internal variation in the assay was minimized by measuring 12 zone diameters for each sample and by controlling the significant factors identified by Davis and Stout (2, 3).

Elimination studies: rodents. A solution of [14C]cefaclor (4.25 mg/ml in 0.05 M sodium acetate buffer, pH 4.5) was administered orally (16.9 mg/kg, 46 μmol/kg) to groups of three fasted (24 h), 250-g, male Purdue-Wistar rats and eight male, 30-g, ICR (Cox) mice. Prior to antibiotic administration isotonic saline (20 ml/kg) was administered intraperitoneally to each animal. After antibiotic administration, animals were placed in stainless-steel metabolism cages. Urine samples were collected at 2, 4, 6, 8, and 24 h after administration, and feces samples were collected after 24 h. Immediately after each urine collection, isotonic saline was again administered intraperitoneally to each animal.

The radiocarbon content of each urine sample was determined by liquid scintillation counting. The nature of the radioactive urinary components was determined by paper chromatography. The biologically active metabolite was identified by comparison chromatography using an authentic sample of [14C]cefaclor. Quantitative determination of unaltered [14C]cefaclor in urine samples was accomplished by microbiological assay. Feces samples were dried, ground, and analyzed for radiocarbon content by combustion using a Packard Tri-Carb sample oxidizer.

For biliary elimination studies, three 200-g fasted male rats were anesthetized with ether and a cannula was placed into the common bile duct of each animal. After collection of a 2-h sample of normal bile fluid, [14C]cefaclor (16.9 mg/kg) in buffer solution was administered orally and bile fluid was collected for 24 h. Radiocarbon content was determined by liquid scintillation counting of a sample of the bile fluid. Unaltered antibiotic was again identified by comparison chromatography using an authentic sample of [14C]cefaclor. The levels of unaltered antibiotic present in the bile were quantitated by the microbiological assay method described above.

To determine whole body radiocarbon residues, each animal was sacrificed 24 h after administration of [14C]cefaclor, and the carcasses were dissolved in a solution of 56 g of KOH in 300 ml of ethanol (2 h). The resulting solution was diluted to 500 ml with ethanol. Three 1-ml samples of each solution were removed and dissolved in 10 ml of liquid scintillation counting medium (Isolab Inc.) for radiocarbon assay.

Rodent blood and tissue level studies. A solution of [14C]cefaclor (46 μmol/kg) in 0.05 M sodium acetate buffer (pH 4.5) was administered orally to a group of three 250-g fasted Purdue-Wistar rats. At given time intervals blood samples were removed from the tail vein. The samples, averaging 200 mg in weight, were processed for liquid scintillation counting using the wet-tissue digestion method of Mahin and Lofberg (4).

[14C]cefaclor, 46 μmol/kg, in sodium acetate buffer solution was administered by the oral route to 24 fasted male ICR (Cox) mice. At eight time intervals, three mice were sacrificed by decapitation, and total available blood was collected. Blood from each animal was sampled and processed for liquid scintillation counting by the wet-tissue digestion method.

For tissue level determinations, [14C]cefaclor (46 μmol/kg) in sodium acetate buffer solution (pH 4.5) was administered to 12 fasted male Purdue-Wistar rats (250 g) and to 12 fasted ICR (Cox) mice (30 g). One, four, six, and twenty-four hours after administration, a group of three animals was sacrificed by decapitation. The appropriate tissues and organs were removed and wet weights were recorded. Duplicate weighed samples of each tissue and organ were removed and prepared for liquid scintillation counting using the wet-tissue digestion method.

Metabolism studies in dogs. A solution of [14C]cefaclor (10.6 mg/ml) in pH 4.2 isotonic saline was administered orally (46 μmol/kg) to one fasted female mongrel dog, 15 kg, fitted with a urinary catheter. At specific times after administration, blood samples were removed from the front leg vein and urine samples were collected. Two portions of each blood and urine sample were taken and processed for liquid scintillation counting by the wet-tissue digestion method. Blood samples were then centrifuged at 1,000 × *g* for 10 min in heparinized tubes to separate the plasma and cellular fractions. Two portions (200 mg) of each plasma sample were processed for liquid scintillation counting in the same manner. The nature of the radioactivity in all plasma and urine samples was determined by comparison paper chromatographic analysis using an authentic sample of [14C]cefaclor. The quantitative determination of unaltered [14C]cefaclor concentrations in plasma and urine was accomplished using the microbiological method described above.

In another study, one female mongrel dog, 14.0 kg, was anesthetized with Seconal and the bile duct was cannulated. A solution of [14C]cefaclor (10.6 mg/ml) in pH 4.2 isotonic saline was administered intravenously via the femoral vein. At specified time intervals, urine, bile fluid, and blood samples were taken, with the latter being obtained from the femoral artery. Radioactivity in the blood, plasma, urine, and bile samples was determined by liquid scintillation counting. The nature of the radioactivity was determined by comparison paper chromatography, using an authentic sample of [14C]cefaclor.

For tissue level studies a solution of [14C]cefaclor (10.6 mg/ml) in pH 4.2 isotonic saline was administered by the oral route (46 μmol/kg) to one fasted female mongrel dog (10 kg), fitted with a urinary catheter. At a given time (90 min) after administration, the dog was anesthetized with Seconal and a sample of cerebral spinal fluid was drawn. The dog was sacrificed with a lethal dose of Seconal, and appropriate tissues and fluids were removed. A weighed sample each tissue and fluid was prepared for liquid scintillation counting using the wet-tissue digestion method. Samples of all fluids were quantitatively analyzed for unaltered [14C]cefaclor using the microbiological assay described above.

RESULTS

Elimination studies: rats. The recoveries of total radioactivity and of unaltered antibiotic in the urine of rats after oral administration of a single dose of [14C]cefaclor are shown in Fig. 2. Forty-four percent of the administered radiocarbon appeared in the urine after 2 h, 69% after 6 h, and 80.8% after 24 h. The recovery of unaltered [14C]cefaclor, determined by microbiological assay, was 38.6% after 2 h, 53.5% after 6 h, and 54.5% after 24 h. The feces collected during this 24-h period were found to contain no detectable quantity of radioactivity. Residual radiocarbon in the rats was found by whole body assay to account for 19.2% of the administered radioactive dose. Cannulation of the common duct of rats immediately prior to oral administration of a single dose of [14C]cefaclor showed that 32.8% of the administered radioactive dose was eliminated via biliary excretion (Fig. 2). The recovery of microbiologically active material in bile fluid was, however, quite low, 6.8%. This microbiological activity was found by radio- and bio-autography to be equally divided between unchanged [14C]cefaclor and a more polar unknown metabolite. No detectable quantity of this biologically active metabolite of [14C]cefaclor could be found in the urine of normal animals. Isolation studies indicated this metabolite to be relatively unstable when compared to the parent antibiotic.

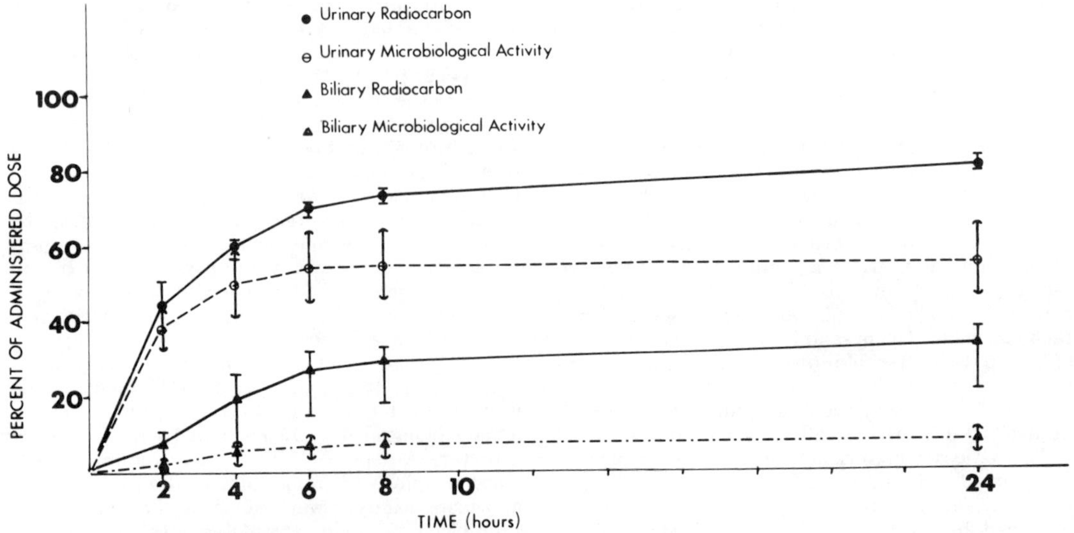

FIG. 2. *Renal and biliary elimination of radiocarbon and microbiological activity in rats (3) after oral administration of 46 μmol of [14C]cefaclor per kg.*

Elimination studies: mice. The oral administration of [14C]cefaclor to a group of ICR (Cox) mice resulted in elimination of a large percentage of administered radiocarbon via the kidney. Twenty-one percent of the administered radiocarbon appeared in the urine in 2 h, 49% in 4 h, 58% in 6 h, and 72% in 24 h. Microbiological assay of these urine samples showed the initial 2-h sample to contain essentially unchanged antibiotic. The recovery of unaltered [14C]cefaclor was 19% of the administered dose in 2 h, 37% in 4 h, 41% in 6 h, and 43% in 24 h. These results, like those with rats, show that initially unaltered antibiotic accounted for a major portion of eliminated radiocarbon. Later samples, however, were found to contain, for the most part, biologically inactive metabolic products. Unlike results found in rat studies, mouse fecal material was found to contain 15% of administered radiocarbon, thus implying biliary elimination and the lack of enterohepatic recirculation in mice. Residual radiocarbon in the mice 24 h after administration was found to represent 13% of the radioactive dose.

Elimination studies: dogs. Figure 3 shows the recoveries of total urinary radioactivity and of unaltered antibiotic in the urine of a dog after oral and intravenous administration of a single dose of [14C]cefaclor. After oral administration, 30% of the radioactive dose was recovered in the urine after 2 h, 57% after 6 h, and 65% after 24 h. The recovery of unaltered [14C]cefaclor after oral administration was considerably below these figures, with 15% being recovered unchanged in 2 h, 21% in 6 h, and 21.5% in 24 h. Six hours after intravenous administration, the recovery of total radiocarbon in the urine was 79%, whereas that in the bile fluid was 3.5%. Microbiological assays showed the urine to contain 47% unchanged antibiotic and the bile to contain 0.4%. It is apparent from these results that cefaclor, after oral administration, was considerably more labile to metabolic degradation in dogs than in the other species studied. The site of this degradation may well be the gastrointestinal tract as opposed to the liver.

Blood level studies. The radiocarbon blood level curve obtained after oral administration of 16.9 mg/kg (46 μmol/kg) of [14C]cefaclor to rats is shown in Fig. 4. A maximum level equivalent to 4.5 μg/ml was obtained 1 h after administration. The initial declining phase of the blood level curve indicated the apparent half-life of [14C]cefaclor in rats to be 2.5 h. These results can be seen to compare quite favorably to similar data obtained after oral administration of 46 μmol of [14C]cephalexin per kg to rats. A peak concentration of 3.8-μg equivalents was obtained in 30 min, and the blood level curve decayed with an apparent half-life of 1.5 h.

The radiocarbon blood level curve obtained after oral administration of 46 μmol of [14C]cefaclor per kg to mice showed that a peak level of 9.4-μg equivalents of [14C]cefaclor per ml was obtained at the first sample time, 15 min after administration. The blood level curve

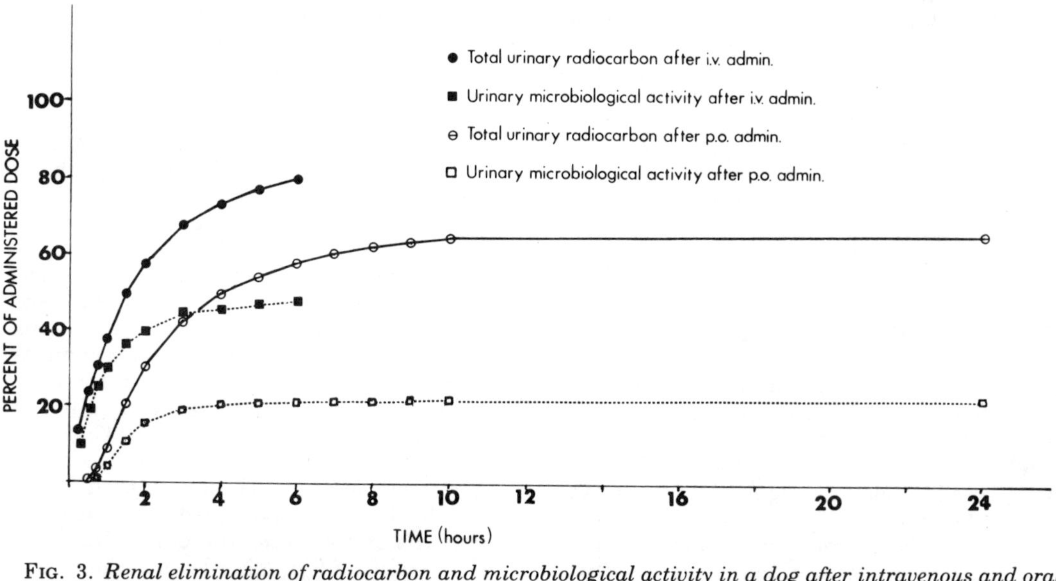

FIG. 3. *Renal elimination of radiocarbon and microbiological activity in a dog after intravenous and oral administration of 46 μmol of [14C]cefaclor per kg.*

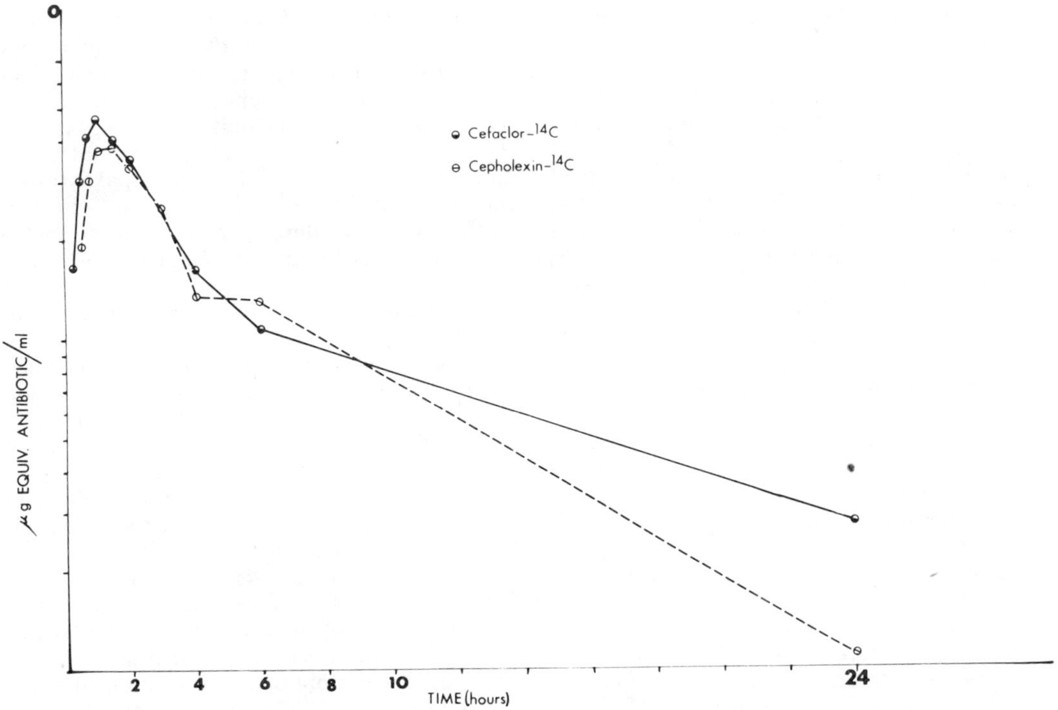

FIG. 4. *Average total radiocarbon blood levels in three rats after oral administration of 46 µmol of [14C]cefaclor and [14C]cephalexin per kg.*

itself was bimodal in character, with the apparent half-life of the initial phase being of the order of 1.5 h.

Blood samples were taken from dogs after oral and intravenous administration of 46 µmol of [^{14}C]cefaclor per kg. Radiocarbon and unaltered [^{14}C]cefaclor concentrations in each sample were determined. Results obtained from analysis of samples taken after oral administration are shown in Fig. 5. A maximum radiocarbon blood level equivalent to 17 µg of [^{14}C]cefaclor per ml was obtained 2 h after administration. The maximum blood level of unaltered antibiotic, determined by microbiological analysis, was 8 µg/ml at the same time. The initial decay phase of the radiocarbon blood level curve declined with an apparent half-life of 2.4 h, whereas the apparent half-life of [^{14}C]cefaclor was 1.9 h. Separation of blood samples into their cellular and plasma fraction, with subsequent radiocarbon and microbiological analysis, revealed that [^{14}C]cefaclor and its metabolites were preferentially concentrated in the plasma fraction by a factor of 1.5 to 1.6 over the cellular fraction.

The total radiocarbon and unaltered antibiotic blood level curves obtained after intravenous administration of 46 µmol of [^{14}C]cefaclor to a dog are shown in Fig. 6. Utilizing that portion of the curves between 30 and 360 min for computerized linear regression analysis, the half-life of total radiocarbon was 106 min, whereas that of unaltered antibiotic was 76 min. By mathematical comparison of the areas under the total radiocarbon blood level curves after oral and intravenous administration, a figure representing the degree of absorption of [^{14}C]cefaclor in dogs after oral administration was calculated to be 75%. By similar treatment of the areas under the unaltered antibiotic curves, the degree of bioavailability of [^{14}C]cefaclor in dogs after oral administration was calculated to be 60%.

Tissue level studies. [^{14}C]cefaclor (46 µmol/kg) was administered orally to rats and mice. The radiocarbon levels in tissue and organs were determined 1, 4, 6, and 24 h after administration. The levels of radiocarbon in these tissues are expressed as microgram equivalents of [^{14}C]cefaclor per gram of body tissue. The levels of radiocarbon found in various tissues of the rat are shown in Fig. 7. These results show that although all tissues examined contained concentrations of antibiotic, the only tissues possessing significantly higher levels than that in the blood were the kidney and the liver, organs

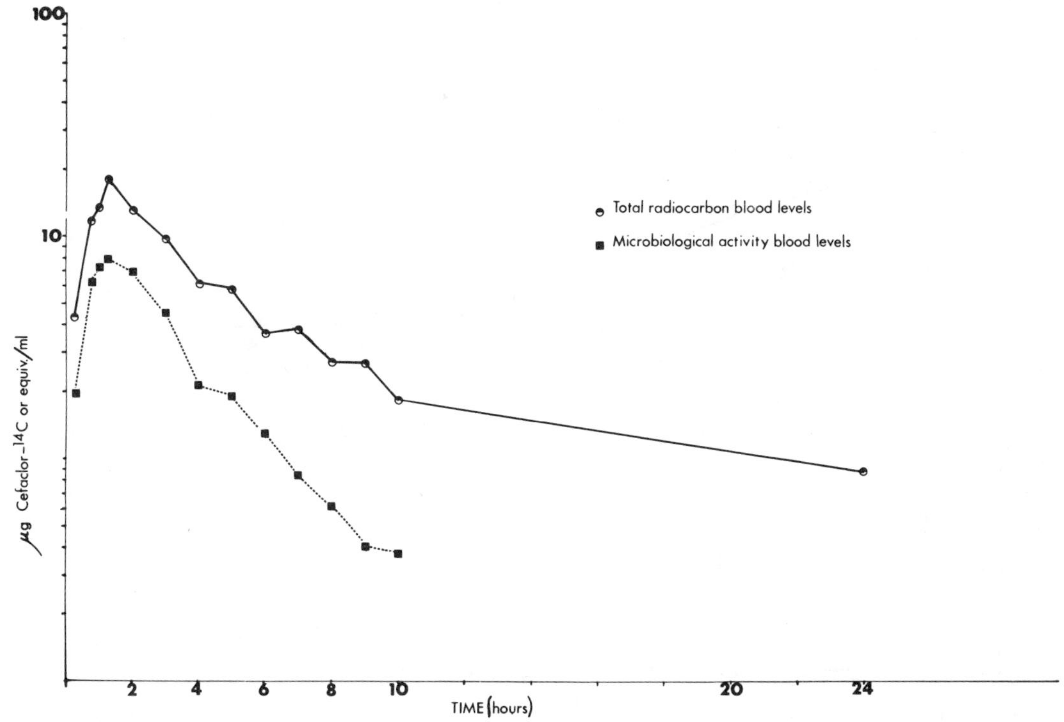

FIG. 5. *Total radiocarbon and microbiological activity blood levels in a dog after oral administration of 46 μmol of [^{14}C]cefaclor per kg.*

responsible for metabolism and elimination. Levels of radiocarbon in the brain were considerably lower than those found in other tissues. In general, the apparent half-life of the disappearance of radiocarbon from all tissues was of the same order and approximated that of the blood.

Radiocarbon tissue levels found in mice 1, 4, 6, and 24 h after oral administration of 46 μmol of [^{14}C]cefaclor per kg are shown in Fig. 8. Curves constructed from these data appeared to be bimodal in character. Tissues possessing levels significantly higher than those found in blood were, again, the kidney and liver. There appeared to be no abnormal deposition of radiocarbon in any one particular tissue. The half-life of radiocarbon in all tissues was quite similar to that determined for the blood level.

Radiocarbon levels and unaltered antibiotic levels were determined in various tissues and fluids of dogs 90 min after a single oral administration of 46 μmol of [^{14}C]cefaclor per kg. Table 1 shows the levels of total radiocarbon and unchanged [^{14}C]cefaclor in the various tissues and fluids. The only tissues having significantly higher radiocarbon levels than those found in blood were the liver and kidney. Hard bone was found, however, to possess radiocarbon levels comparable to the blood concentration. Appreciable levels were also found in bone marrow. High levels of radiocarbon and of unchanged antibiotic were also found in urine. Biliary elimination in dogs, like that in rats, was not an important route of elimination of radiocarbon or of unchanged antibiotic. Of the fluids examined other than the urine and bile, only the synovial fluid possessed levels of radiocarbon and of unchanged antibiotic comparable to blood levels.

DISCUSSION

Rats. Results, obtained from radiocarbon elimination studies in rats, showed cefaclor to be completely absorbed from the gastrointestinal tract after oral administration. The major, if not only, route of elimination of parent antibiotic and metabolites is via renal excretion. The finding that the major portion, 67%, of the urinary radiocarbon represented unchanged [^{14}C]cefaclor implied that the antibiotic is, for the most part, absorbed intact and argues for its in vivo stability to metabolism in this species. These results compare very favora-

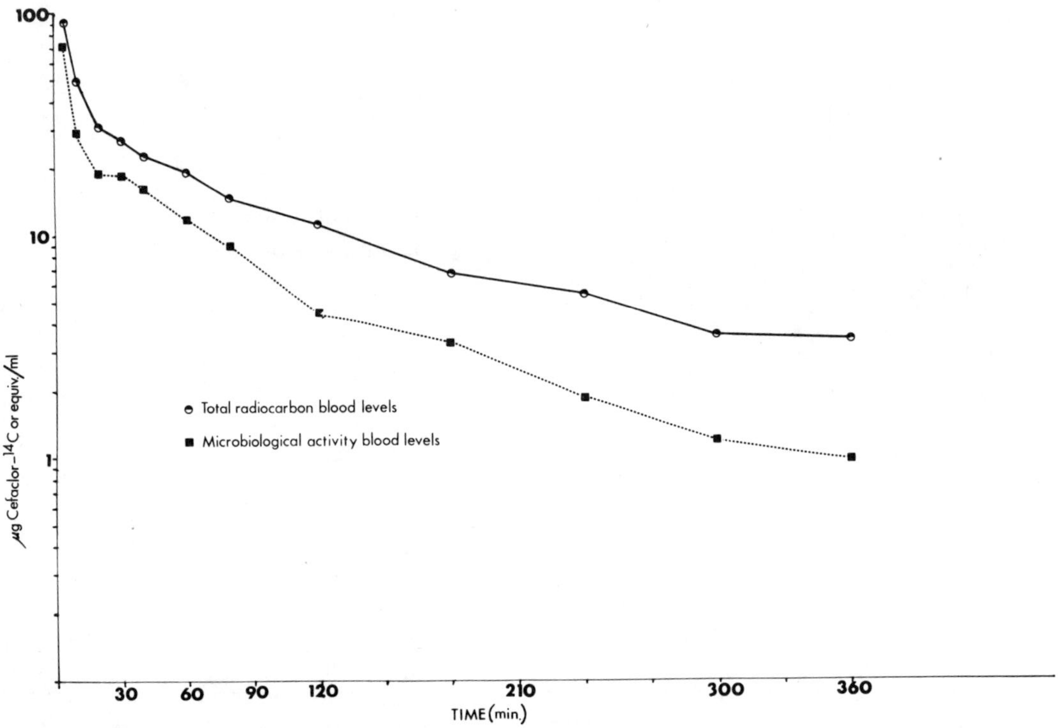

FIG. 6. *Total radiocarbon and microbiological activity blood levels in a dog after intravenous administration of 46 μmol of [14C]cefaclor per kg.*

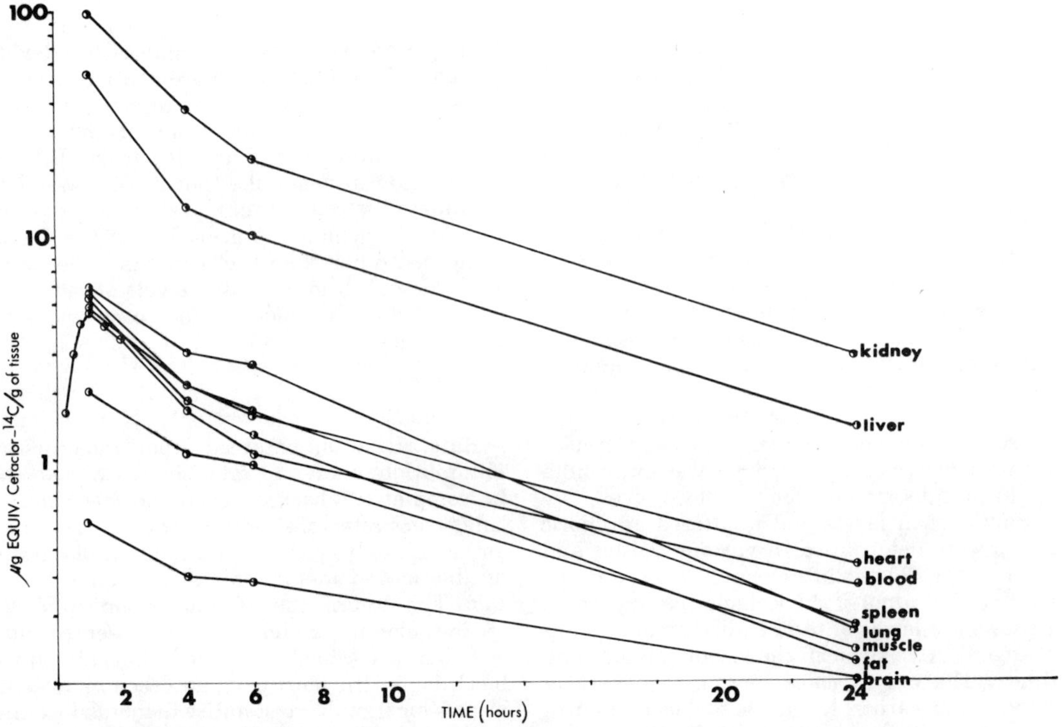

FIG. 7. *Average radiocarbon blood and tissue levels in three rats after oral administration of 46 μmol of [14C]cefaclor per kg.*

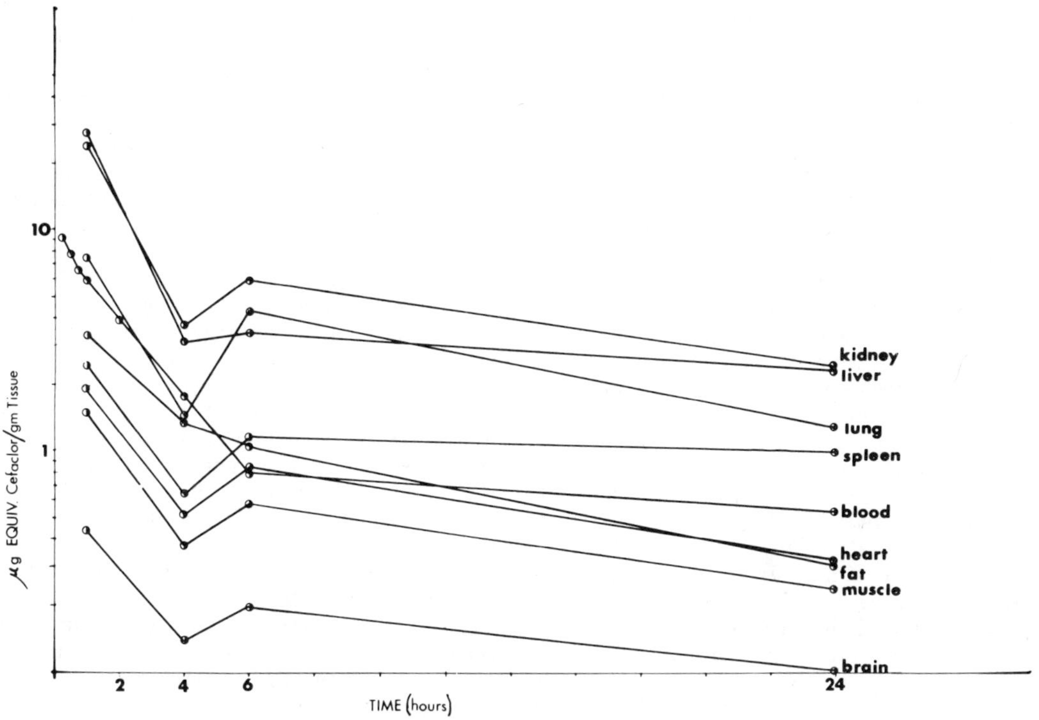

FIG. 8. *Average radiocarbon blood and tissue levels in three mice after oral administration of 46 μmol of [14C]cefaclor per kg.*

TABLE 1. *Total radiocarbon and unaltered [14C]-cefaclor tissue and fluid levels in dogs after oral administration of a single dose of [14C]-cefaclor (46 μmol/kg)*

Tissue or fluid	Radiocarbon levels (μg equivalents of cefaclor/g)	Unaltered antibiotic (μg/ml)
Blood	9.1	10.0
Liver	31.9	ND
Kidney	138.7	ND
Spleen	4.4	ND
Adrenal	5.3	ND
Bone marrow	4.1	ND
Hard bone	9.3	ND
Urine	2,082.0	1,275.0
Bile	127.3	25.0
Synovial	14.9	8.9
Cerebrospinal	0.2	0.3
Aqueous humor	0.7	0.8

[a] ND, Not determined.

bly with those obtained in a similar study after oral administration of [14C]cephalexin to rats (8). Similar studies in bile-cannulated animals show that biliary excretion was indeed involved in the metabolism of cefaclor. Therefore, in normal rats, enterohepatic recirculation is involved in the metabolism and ultimate renal elimination of cefaclor and its metabolites. The isolation of a microbiologically active metabolite from the bile and failure to confirm its presence in urine supports this supposition. The residual radiocarbon in rats 24 h after administration undoubtedly represents phenylglycine, produced by the enzymatic or hydrolytic cleavage of the amide bond of the parent antibiotic and its incorporation into the normal amino acid pools in this species.

Blood and tissue level studies only serve to confirm data obtained in the above studies. Peak radiocarbon levels were obtained in 1 h, indicating rapid absorption in rats. The total radiocarbon blood level curve obtained for [14C]cefaclor can be seen (Fig. 4) to be very similar to that obtained from an identical dose of [14C]cephalexin (9). Results of radiocarbon tissue level studies also show that the absorption of [14C]cefaclor after oral administration is quite rapid. No abnormal deposition of radiocarbon in any tissue was observed.

Mice. Metabolism studies in mice show [14C]cefaclor to be rapidly and completely absorbed from the gastrointestinal tract after oral administration. The major route of elimination of antibiotic and metabolite is by renal excretion. Unlike results observed in rats, however, biliary excretion does play a minor role in the elimination scheme, as implied by the recovery of 15% of administered radiocarbon in the feces. The recovery again of relatively large portions of administered antibiotic unchanged in the urine argues for its in vivo stability to metabolism. These results again closely parallel results obtained in a similar study of the metabolic fate of the structurally related antibiotic, cephalexin (8). In addition, the unknown microbiologically active metabolite, found only in the bile of cannulated rats, was found in the urine of mice. Its presence, although representing less than 2% of the dose, suggests that enterohepatic recirculation of the antibiotic and its metabolites does not occur in mice. Blood and tissue total radiocarbon level studies serve to confirm the rapid absorption of [^{14}C]cefaclor in mice after oral administration. No abnormal deposition of radioactivity in any tissue or organ was observed.

Dogs. Elimination and blood level studies in dogs after oral administration of [^{14}C]cefaclor indicate that the antibiotic was absorbed from the gastrointestinal tract but that it was considerably more labile to metabolism in dogs than in the other species investigated. Radiocarbon levels both in blood and urine were considerably higher than levels of unaltered antibiotic. Comparison of blood level data obtained after oral administration to that obtained after intravenous administration permitted the calculation of the degree of absorption and the bioavailability of [^{14}C]cefaclor after oral administration. These calculations show that approximately 75% of the oral dosage of [^{14}C]cefaclor was absorbed from the gastrointestinal tract and that the bioavailability of intact antibiotic was approximately 60%. In comparison with other species studied, a relatively small percentage of eliminated radiocarbon was associated with unchanged [^{14}C]cefaclor. As in other species investigated, biliary excretion plays a very minor to trace role in the elimination of parent antibiotic and metabolites. Tissue level studies in dogs 90 min after oral administration of [^{14}C]cefaclor show only the liver and kidney, tissues directly involved with metabolism and elimination, to possess radiocarbon levels greater than that found in the blood. Of the fluids examined, only synovial fluid was found to contain significant levels, comparable to those found in blood, of total radiocarbon and of unaltered antibiotic.

In summary, these metabolism studies show [^{14}C]cefaclor to be rapidly absorbed as the intact antibiotic from the gastrointestinal tract of dogs, rats, and mice after oral administration. In the latter two species the antibiotic, for the most part, is resistant to metabolism and is eliminated unchanged. In dogs, however, [^{14}C]cefaclor is labile to metabolism and only a minor fraction of the administered dose is eliminated unchanged. These results are of particular interest when compared with those obtained from studies of the metabolic fates of cephaloglycin [generic name given to 7-(D-2-amino-2-phenylacetamido)-3-acetoxymethyl-3-cephem-4-carboxylic acid] (7) and cephalexin (8), two closely related cephalosporin antibiotics, in rats and mice. Cephalexin, like cefaclor, is quantitatively absorbed in the gastrointestinal tract as the intact antibiotic. It is not metabolized and is eliminated unchanged via the kidney. Cephaloglycin, on the other hand, is not as efficiently absorbed and is rapidly metabolized in these species via two pathways: hydrolysis of the amide linkage to form D-2-phenylglycine and by deacetylation to form desacetylcephaloglycin. Thus, the substitution of a chlorine or methyl group for the acetoxymethyl moiety of cephaloglycin produces cephalosporin antibiotics, cefaclor and cephalexin, which are more readily absorbed from the gastrointestinal tract of rats and mice and are remarkably more resistant to metabolism.

ACKNOWLEDGMENTS

We wish to thank W. R. Brown and M. Clarkson for technical assistance in the microbiological assay procedure.

LITERATURE CITED

1. **Culp, H. W., F. J. Marshall, and R. E. McMahon.** 1964. Metabolism and absorption of 7-(phenylacetamido-*1-^{14}C*)-cephalosporanic acid, p. 243–246. Antimicrob. Agents Chemother. 1963.
2. **Davis, W. W., and T. R. Stout.** 1971. Disc plate method of microbiological antibiotic assay. I. Factors influencing variability and error. Appl. Microbiol. **22**:659–665.
3. **Davis, W. W., and T. R. Stout.** 1971. Disc plate method of microbiological antibiotic assay. II. Novel procedure offering improved accuracy. Appl. Microbiol. **22**:666–670.
4. **Mahin, D. T., and R. T. Lofberg.** 1966. A simplified method of sample preparation for determination of tritium, carbon-14 or sulfur-35 in blood or tissue by liquid scintillation counting. Anal. Biochem. **16**:500–509.
5. **Miller, R. P.** 1962. A paper chromatographic assay for cephalosporins. Antibiot. Chemother. **12**:689–693.
6. **Ryan, C. W., R. L. Simon, and E. M. Van Heyningen.** 1969. Chemistry of cephalosporin antibiotics. XIII. Desacetoxycephalosporin. The synthesis of cephalexin and some analogs. J. Med. Chem. **12**:310–313.
7. **Sullivan, H. R., R. E. Billings, and R. E. McMahon.** 1969. Metabolism of D-cephaloglycin-^{14}C and L-cephaloglycin-^{14}C in the rat. J. Antibiot. **22**:27–33.
8. **Sullivan, H. R., R. E. Billings, and R. E. McMahon.** 1969. Metabolism of cephalexin-^{14}C in mice and in rats. J. Antibiot. **22**:195–200.
9. **Sullivan, H. R., and R. E. McMahon.** 1967. Metabolism of oral cephalothin and related cephalosporins in the rat. Biochem. J. **102**:976–982.

Antimicrobial Agents and Chemotherapy, Oct. 1976, p. 639-645 Vol. 10, No. 4

Multiple Antibiotic Resistance in Clinical Strains of *Neisseria gonorrhoeae* Isolated in South Carolina

JAMES T. POWELL[1] AND JOHN H. BOND*

Department of Microbiology, Clemson University, Clemson, South Carolina 29632

Received for publication 1 March 1976

Minimal inhibitory concentration (MIC) values for penicillin G, tetracycline, amoxicillin, and actinomycin D were determined for 81 strains of *Neisseria gonorrhoeae* isolated from patients attending public health clinics in the Piedmont region of South Carolina. Gonococcal isolates were also screened for high-level resistance to streptomycin. Significant positive correlations ($r \geq 0.45$, $P \leq 0.01$) were found between all possible pairs of the antibiotics penicillin G, tetracycline, and amoxicillin. The MIC values of actinomycin D showed no significant positive correlations with the MIC values of the other antibiotics. Gonococcal strains that were resistant to streptomycin tended to be resistant to penicillin G, tetracycline, and amoxicillin. Of the 81 isolates, 18.5% were multiply resistant to penicillin G, tetracycline, amoxicillin, and streptomycin. Spontaneous mutants with reduced antibiotic susceptibility, selected for decreased susceptibility to penicillin G, displayed small decreases in susceptibility to tetracycline, amoxicillin, and actinomycin D. Spontaneous mutants selected for decreased susceptibility to actinomycin D displayed small losses in susceptibility to penicillin G. The results show that multiple antibiotic resistance occurs in clinically isolated gonococcal strains in South Carolina. The results further suggest the presence of a common genetic mechanism determining antibiotic resistance in *N. gonorrhoeae*.

The inherent ability of *Neisseria gonorrhoeae* to develop resistance to antibiotics is a major contributing factor to the continuing spread and marked increases in reported gonococcal infections in the past 20 years (20). Sensitivities of random isolates of *N. gonorrhoeae* to such clinical antibiotics as penicillin, tetracycline, and streptomycin have significantly decreased in many areas (9, 20, 24). In addition, several investigators have reported positive correlations between the susceptibilities of individual isolates of *N. gonorrhoeae* to a wide variety of antibiotics, including penicillin, tetracycline, erythromycin, streptomycin, spiramycin, and chloramphenicol (12, 14, 15). Multiply antibiotic-resistant gonococcal strains pose a serious problem in the treatment and control of gonorrhea. At this time, the underlying basis for multiple resistance has not been conclusively established. The current need for regional surveillance of gonococcal antibiotic susceptibility levels and regional analysis of levels of multiple antibiotic resistance has been pointed out by several investigators (3, 9, 12, 20, 24).

[1] Present address: Department of Immunology and Medical Microbiology, College of Medicine, Box J-266, JHM Health Center, University of Florida, Gainesville, FL 32610.

For the years 1972, 1973, and 1974, South Carolina has ranked first, third, and fifth, respectively, among states in the number of reported gonococcal infections per 100,000 population, and can be considered a problem area in terms of gonorrhea control (1, 2). In this investigation, we sought to measure the antibiotic susceptibility levels of random isolates of *N. gonorrhoeae* from a particular region of South Carolina and determine the extent to which these strains were multiply antibiotic resistant. The antibiotics used in this investigation were penicillin G, tetracycline, amoxicillin, streptomycin, and actinomycin D. These antibiotics were chosen for their chemical dissimilarity and their varying modes of action. In addition, multiply antibiotic-resistant mutants were isolated by specific selection for penicillin G and actinomycin D resistance. Our results provide evidence for a common mechanism for multiple antibiotic resistance in *N. gonorrhoeae*.

MATERIALS AND METHODS

Bacterial strains. Fifty-four randomly isolated strains of *N. gonorrhoeae* were collected in July and August 1974 at the Greenville County Public Health Department, Greenville, S.C. Twenty-seven additional strains were collected during the same period at the Anderson County Public Health Department, Anderson, S.C. The study population consisted of 81 symptomatic male patients. No further screening or treatment follow-up was done. Cultures were confirmed as *N. gonorrhoeae* by colonial morphology, Gram stain, positive oxidase reaction using *N*,*N*-dimethyl-*p*-phenylenediamine monohydrochloride (J. T. Baker Chemical Co.), degradation of glucose but not maltose, and failure to grow on nutrient agar. Three reference strains possessing known antibiotic susceptibilities were kindly provided by P. F. Sparling, University of North Carolina, Chapel Hill.

Culture media and growth. Primary isolation and purification of *N. gonorrhoeae* isolates were done on enriched chocolate agar (ECA), which consisted of GC medium base (Difco) containing 2% hemoglobin (Difco) and 1% Difco supplement C. Routine subculture and culture maintenance were done on GC medium base containing 1% concentrations of supplements 1 and 2 of White and Kellogg (23). Sugar degradations were performed by using cystine tryptic agar (Difco) to which 1% filter-sterilized (Morton filter) sugars were added. Broth dilutions were made in either tryptic soy broth (Difco) or GC base broth (proteose-peptone no. 3, 1.5 g; corn starch, 0.1 g; K_2HPO_4, 0.4 g; KH_2PO_4, 0.1 g; NaCl, 0.5 g; distilled water, 100 ml). All cultures were incubated at 36°C in a moist atmosphere of 5% CO_2 unless otherwise specified. Strains were stored at −70°C in tryptic soy broth (Difco) plus 20% glycerol.

Testing for susceptibility to antibiotics. The wells of a replicator-inoculating device, similar in design to a Steers replicator (21), were filled with standardized suspensions of gonococcal cells (approximately 10^6 colony-forming units [CFU]/ml). Approximately 10^3 CFU of each suspension was transferred with the replicator to a series of ECA plates containing doubling dilutions of antibiotic and at least three ECA control plates containing no antibiotic. The minimal inhibitory concentration (MIC) value was defined as the lowest concentration that prevented visible growth of more than one oxidase-positive colony after 24 h of incubation. All MIC determinations were performed in duplicate, and results were reproducible within twofold limits on replicate determinations. Gonococcal isolates were screened for high-level resistance to streptomycin by observing growth or no growth on an antibiotic plate containing 300 μg of streptomycin per ml. Three control strains possessing known antibiotic susceptibilities were included in each test.

Selection of antibiotic-resistant mutants. Multistep spontaneous antibiotic-resistant mutants of *N. gonorrhoeae* were obtained by subculturing on increasing concentrations of either penicillin G or actinomycin D. Cells were suspended in broth to a turbidity greater than 100 Klett units (Klett-Summerson colorimeter, no. 54), and 0.25-ml portions were spread onto a series of ECA plates containing doubling concentrations of the selected antibiotic. Selected colonies from the plate containing the highest concentration of antibiotic showing growth were subcultured to plates containing that concentration of antibiotic. The selection process was then repeated, using the selected mutant cultures, until a series of antibiotic-resistant mutants was obtained. Finally, MIC values for selected and nonselected antibiotics were determined for each antibiotic-resistant mutant.

Determination of cell survival on increasing concentrations of antibiotics. Gonococcal cells were suspended in broth and adjusted to a turbidity corresponding to 80 to 85 Klett units (approximately 3 × 10^8 CFU/ml). Suspensions were agitated using a Vortex mixer to minimize cell clumping. Suspensions were 10^{-5} diluted, and 0.1-ml portions were spread onto the surface of a series of ECA plates containing increasing concentrations of antibiotic and also onto control plates containing no antibiotic. All plating was done in duplicate, and survival determinations were repeated two or more times for each gonococcal strain.

Data analysis. The coefficient of correlation (r) was computed for each pair of antibiotics with the aid of a Monroe 1930 programed calculator, and t tests were used to determine which of the r values differed significantly from zero (19).

Antibiotics. Sources of antibiotics were: Lilly, penicillin G and streptomycin; Beecham-Massengill, amoxicillin; Lederle, tetracycline; and Merck Sharp & Dohme, actinomycin D.

RESULTS

Antibiotic susceptibility. The measured antibiotic susceptibilities to four antibiotics for 81 strains of *N. gonorrhoeae*, isolated in Greenville and Anderson, S.C., are shown in Fig. 1. Penicillin G MIC values ranged from very susceptible (0.004 μg/ml) to very resistant (2.0 μg/ml) and were unevenly distributed. Of the 81 isolates 32.1% were resistant to penicillin G (MIC > 0.3 μg/ml). Amoxicillin MIC values ranged from 0.015 to 1.0 μg/ml and showed an uneven distribution similar to that of penicillin G. Tetracycline MIC values showed a normal distribution and peaked in a range corresponding to tetracycline resistance (1.0 μg/ml). Of the isolates, 23.3% were highly resistant to tetracycline (MIC > 1.0 μg/ml). The range of actinomycin D MIC values was very narrow, with the majority of the gonococcal strains being inhibited by 2.0 μg/ml. Thirty-three (41%) of the 81 gonococcal isolates displayed high-level resistance to streptomycin (MIC > 300 μg/ml). Fifteen (18.5%) of the 81 isolates were multiply resistant to penicillin G (MIC > 0.3 μg/ml), tetracycline (MIC ≥ 1.0 μg/ml), amoxicillin (MIC ≥ 0.5 μg/ml), and streptomycin (MIC > 300 μg/ml.)

Correlations between MIC values. Significant positive correlations ($r \geq 0.45$, $P \leq 0.01$) were found between the susceptibilities of the 81 isolates of *N. gonorrhoeae* to all pairs of the antibiotics penicillin G, tetracycline, and

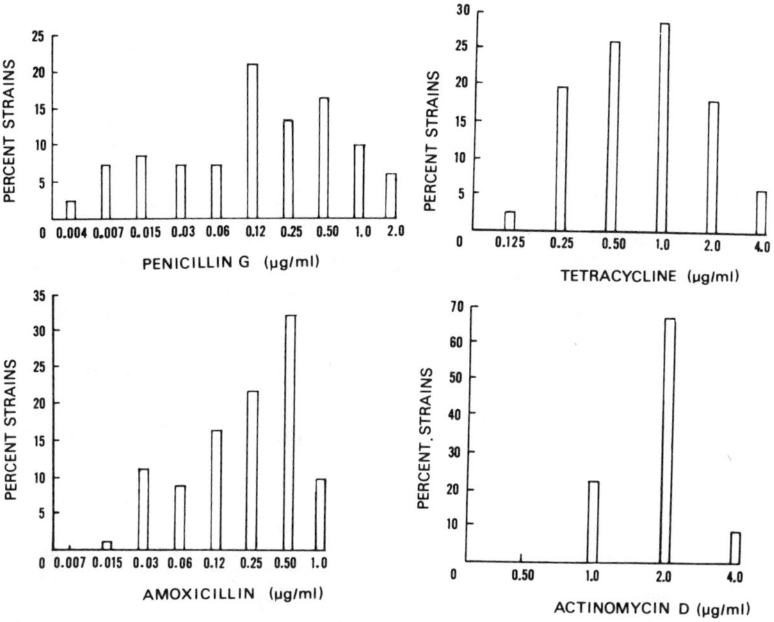

FIG. 1. *Distribution of penicillin G, amoxicillin, tetracycline, and actinomycin D MIC values for 81 random isolates of Neisseria gonorrhoeae.*

amoxicillin (Table 1). Representative scattergram plots of penicillin G versus tetracycline and penicillin G versus amoxicillin reveal roughly proportional and continuous relationships over the ranges of MIC values observed (Fig. 2 and 3). No significant positive correlations ($r < 0.28$, $P > 0.01$) were found between the susceptibilities to actinomycin D and penicillin G, amoxicillin, or tetracycline. The scattergram plot of penicillin G versus actinomycin D is representative and shows no proportional relationship (Fig. 4).

The percentage of streptomycin-resistant strains at each susceptibility level of penicillin G, amoxicillin, tetracycline, and actinomycin D is shown in Table 2. The results show that gonococcal strains that were less susceptible to either penicillin G, amoxicillin, or tetracycline tended to be resistant also to streptomycin. Roughly equal proportions of streptomycin-resistant strains were present at the lowest and highest levels of actinomycin D resistance. These results suggest that positive correlations exist between gonococcal susceptibilities to streptomycin and those to penicillin G, amoxicillin, and tetracycline. There is no apparent correlation, however, between streptomycin and actinomycin D susceptibilities in *N. gonorrhoeae*.

Spontaneous antibiotic-resistant mutants. The phenotypes of selected penicillin G and actinomycin D mutants are shown in Table 3.

TABLE 1. *Correlation coefficients (r values) for MIC values of the various pairs of antibiotics for 81 strains of Neisseria gonorrhoeae*

Antibiotic	Antibiotic[a] pen	tet	amx	act
pen		0.79	0.62	0.14[b]
tet	0.79		0.45	0.23[b]
amx	0.62	0.45		0.06[b]
act	0.14[b]	0.23[b]	0.06[b]	

[a] Abbreviations: pen, penicillin G; tet, tetracycline; amx, amoxicillin; act, actinomycin D.
[b] *r* values not significant ($P > 0.01$).

The results showed that decreasing the susceptibility to penicillin G 16-fold in vitro was sufficient to cause a concomitant fourfold decrease in amoxicillin susceptibility and a twofold decrease in tetracycline susceptibility. Decreased penicillin susceptibility did not change the MIC values for actinomycin D or result in a loss of streptomycin susceptibility. Fourfold decreases in resistance to actinomycin D did not alter the MIC values of penicillin G, tetracycline, or amoxicillin and did not cause a loss of susceptibility to streptomycin.

Survival on increasing concentrations of antibiotics. Survival of wild-type parent gonococcal isolate GV77 is compared with that of four GV77 less penicillin-susceptible mutants on increasing concentrations of actinomycin D in Fig. 5. At 0.75 μg of actinomycin D per ml,

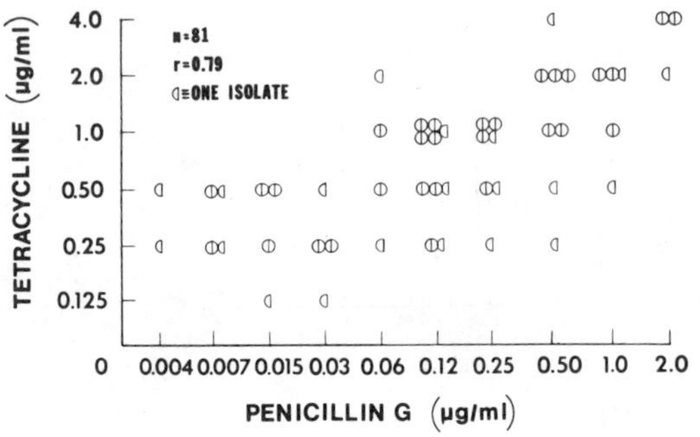

FIG. 2. *Scattergram of penicillin G versus tetracycline MIC values for 81 isolates of Neisseria gonorrhoeae.*

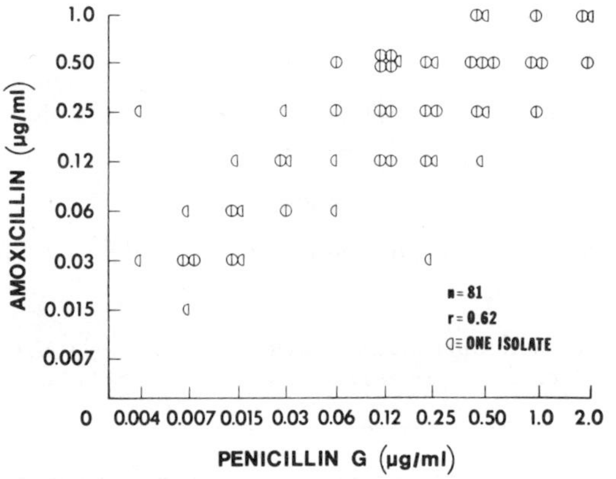

FIG. 3. *Scattergram of penicillin G versus amoxicillin MIC values for 81 isolates of Neisseria gonorrhoeae.*

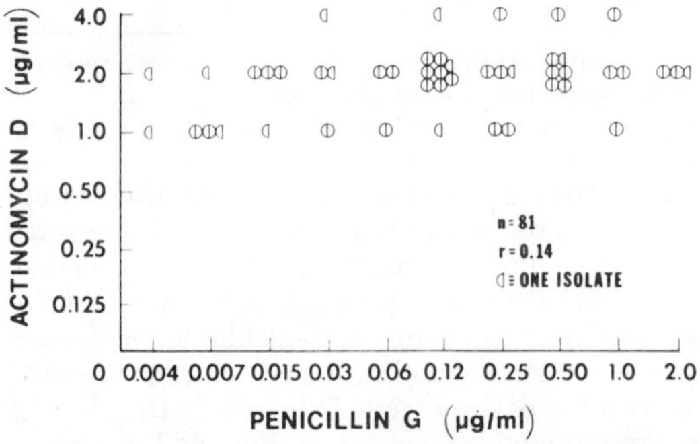

FIG. 4. *Scattergram of penicillin G versus actinomycin D MIC values for 81 isolates of Neisseria gonorrhoeae.*

less than 10% of the average number of CFU counted on control plates containing no antibiotics was present for wild-type strain GV77. At this same level, however, 30 to 35% of the less penicillin-susceptible mutants GV77Pen.03 (penicillin MIC + 0.03 µg/ml), GV77Pen.06, and GV77Pen.12 and 64% of GV77Pen.25 was present. At 1.0 µg of actinomycin D per ml, all strains were inhibited except GV77Pen.25, which showed 65% survival.

The survival, on increasing concentrations of penicillin G, of the GV77 wild-type strain and two less actinomycin D-susceptible mutants is shown in Fig. 6. At 0.0087 µg of penicillin G per ml, GV77Act4.0 (actinomycin D MIC + 4.0 µg/ml) showed 49% survival and GV77Act8.0 showed 83% survival. No colonies of the GV77 wild-type strain were observed at this level.

DISCUSSION

The ranges and distributions of gonococcal antibiotic susceptibilities found in this investi-

TABLE 2. *Streptomycin-resistant strains at each susceptibility level of penicillin G, amoxicillin, tetracycline, and actinomycin D*

MIC (µg/ml)	No. of strains	% Streptomycin resistant[a]
Penicillin		
0.004	2	0
0.007	6	0
0.015	7	0
0.03	6	16
0.06	6	50
0.12	17	53
0.25	11	57
0.50	13	54
1.0	8	63
2.0	5	100
Total	81	41
Tetracycline		
0.125	2	0
0.25	16	19
0.50	21	14
1.0	23	65
2.0	14	57
4.0	5	80
Total	81	41
Amoxicillin		
0.015	1	0
0.03	9	0
0.06	7	14
0.12	13	15
0.25	17	17
0.50	26	73
1.0	8	88
Total	81	41
Actinomycin D		
1.0	18	28
2.0	55	47
4.0	8	25
Total	81	41

[a] Streptomycin resistant = MIC > 300 µg/ml.

TABLE 3. *Phenotypes of selected antibiotic-resistant spontaneous mutants of Neisseria gonorrhoeae*

Strain	MIC (μg/ml)[a]				
	pen	tet	amx	act	str
GV77 wild type	0.015	0.25	2.0	≤300	
GV77Pen.03	0.03	0.25	2.0	≤300	
GV77Pen.06	0.06	0.25	2.0	≤300	
GV77Pen.12	0.12	0.25	2.0	≤300	
GV77Pen.25	0.25	0.50	2.0	≤300	
GV77Pen4.0	0.015	0.25	4.0	≤300	
GV77Pen8.0	0.015	0.25	8.0	≤300	

[a] Abbreviations: pen, penicillin G; tet, tetracycline; amx, amoxicillin; act, actinomycin D; str, streptomycin

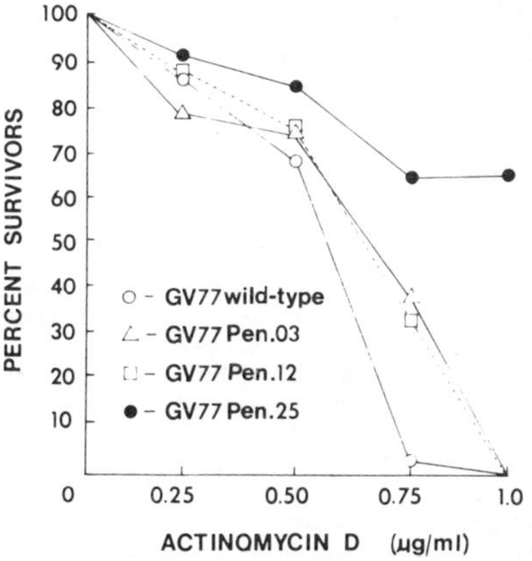

FIG. 5. *Survival of less penicillin G-susceptible mutants on increasing concentrations of actinomycin D. Approximately 300 CFU equals 100% survival.*

gation in the Piedmont region of South Carolina support previous observations by other investigators that regional variations in antibiotic susceptibilities do exist. The percentage of penicillin-resistant strains (MIC > 0.3 μg/ml) found in patients in the present study (32%) was significantly lower than the penicillin-resistant percentage of those tested in Philadelphia, Pa., in 1973 (54%) (11). However, the percentage of penicillin-resistant isolates was higher than the latest reported national averages (17.4%) (6). In addition, a higher percentage of penicillin-resistant strains was found in the Greenville-Anderson area than in any individual location examined by the cooperative national survey (6). The percentage of gonococcal isolates resistant to tetracycline (MIC > 1.0 μg/ml) in the present study (23%) was slightly higher than the latest reported national average (14.0%) (6). The percentage of tetracycline-resistant strains in the Greenville-Anderson area was also higher than those from the 1973 Philadelphia survey (7%) (11) and the 1972 Vermont state survey (0%) (4). On the basis of this study, the high reported gonorrhea case rate per 100,000 population for South Carolina, when compared with other states, does positively correlate with a higher percentage of penicillin- and tetracycline-resistant strains. However, a direct cause and effect relationship between antibiotic resistance and prevalence of gonococcal infection cannot be assumed on the basis of our data.

Amoxicillin in vitro activity was greater than penicillin G activity against the most penicillin-resistant gonococcal strains (Fig. 3). This effect has been observed with other broad-spectrum penicillins, especially ampicillin (12, 13).

Actinomycin D is not used to treat clinical infections due to its excessive toxicity. It was used in this study because of its chemical structure and mode of action, as well as its unique ability to provide a tool for studying the effects of an antibiotic to which the gonococci have never been previously exposed in vivo. There have been no previous reports of the susceptibility of *N. gonorrhoeae* to actinomycin D.

By plotting MIC values on scattergrams and calculating *r* values, we have shown significant positive correlations between antibiotic susceptibilities to penicillin G, tetracycline, and amoxicillin in natural isolates of *N. gonorrhoeae*. Our calculated coefficient of correlation for penicillin G versus tetracycline (r = 0.79) agrees with similar studies done by Maier et al. (12), who calculated an *r* value of 0.75 for their penicillin-versus-tetracycline MIC values. It is somewhat surprising that penicillin G MIC values correlated more closely with those of tetracycline (r = 0.79) than with those of amoxicillin (r = 0.62), since penicillin G and amoxicillin are structurally related. We cannot explain this

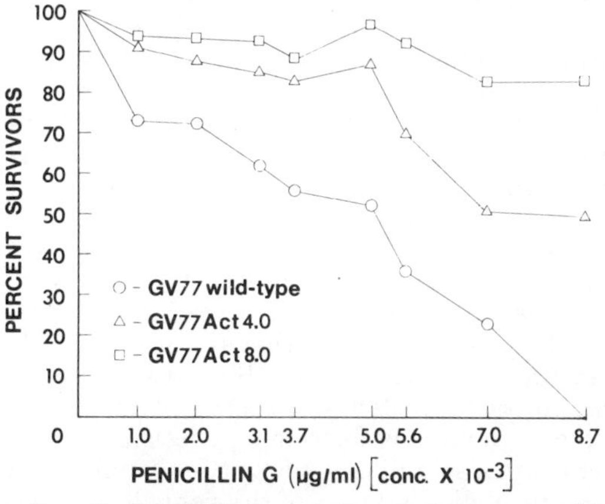

FIG. 6. *Survival of less actinomycin D-susceptible mutants on increasing concentrations of penicillin G. Approximately 300 CFU equals 100% survival.*

on the basis of our experiment other than to point out that gonococcal strains that showed the highest levels of observed resistance to any one of these three antibiotics were resistant to the others as well.

Our demonstration that spontaneous mutants, selected for decreased susceptibility to penicillin G, were less sensitive to tetracycline and amoxicillin agrees with similar studies by Maness and Sparling (14) and Maier et al. (12) and supports the hypothesis that resistance to dissimilar antibiotics may be under the control of a common genetic mechanism.

Our hypothesis that small decreases in actinomycin D susceptibility were occurring in conjunction with decreases in penicillin G susceptibility was demonstrated by observing differences in the average number of CFU observed as standard inocula of wild-type and mutant *N. gonorrhoeae* cells were spread on a series of plates containing increasing concentrations of a specific antibiotic (Fig. 5 and 6). The results suggest that simultaneous decreases in susceptibility to penicillin G and actinomycin D in *N. gonorrhoeae* can occur as a result of one or several spontaneous mutations. The increased survival capabilities probably reflect decreases in susceptibility to each antibiotic in the mutant cultures, resulting in less selective pressure from the restrictive antibiotic plates. These decreases in susceptibility were most likely small because no changes in susceptibility were detectable by standard MIC procedures.

The most likely mechanism for common resistance to these two antibiotics would be a mutation, or possibly several distinct mutations, that affects the permeability properties of the cell envelope. Several investigators have proposed that differences in cell envelope permeability were responsible for spontaneous losses in antibiotic susceptibility to penicillin G and several other antibiotics in *N. gonorrhoeae* (5, 12, 14). Also, bacterial resistance to actinomycin D has been found to result from differences in cell envelope permeability (7, 8, 10, 18). A cell envelope permeability hypothesis for antibiotic resistance is supported by the fact that no enzymes have been found that actively degrade actinomycin D in bacterial cells (22) and by the observation that the gonococci do not produce penicillinase (16). Alterations in specific target sites or transport systems as possible explanations for common resistance patterns are also unlikely due to the chemical and structural dissimilarity of the penicillin G and actinomycin D molecules. The lack of correlation between penicillin G and actinomycin D MIC values in clinical isolates is most likely due to the standard MIC procedure not being sufficiently sensitive to detect small changes in actinomycin D susceptibility. The results of the present study suggest that actinomycin D may be useful in the further study of multiple antibiotic resistance mechanisms in *N. gonorrhoeae*.

ACKNOWLEDGEMENT

Robert K. Shockley ably assisted with some of the work.

LITERATURE CITED

1. **Center for Disease Control.** 1972. Morbidity and Mortality Weekly Report, vol. 21, p. 13. United States Department of Health, Education, and Welfare, Atlanta, Ga.
2. **Center for Disease Control.** 1974. Morbidity and Mortality Weekly Report, vol. 23, p. 13. United States Department of Health, Education, and Welfare, Atlanta, Ga.
3. **Cornelius, C. E., III.** 1970. Six city study of treatment of gonorrhea in men using single oral doses of 1.5 and 3 g tetracycline hydrochloride. Br. J. Vener. Dis. 46:330–333.
4. **Gump, D. W., and P. T. Berry.** 1973. Increased susceptibility of *Neisseria gonorrhoeae* from a rural area. Antimicrob. Agents Chemother. 3:503–505.
5. **Guymon, L. F., and P. F. Sparling.** 1975. Altered crystal violet permeability and lytic behavior in antibiotic-resistant and -sensitive mutants of *Neisseria gonorrhoeae*. J. Bacteriol. 124:757–763.
6. **Jaffe, H. W., J. W. Biddle, C. Thornsberry, R. E. Johnson, R. E. Kaufman, G. G. Reynolds, P. J. Wiesner, and the Cooperative Study Group.** 1976. National gonorrhea therapy monitoring study: in vitro antibiotic susceptibility and its correlation with treatment results. N. Engl. J. Med. 294:5–9.
7. **Leive, L.** 1965. Release of lipopolysaccharide by EDTA treatment of *E. coli*. Biochem. Biophys. Res. Commun. 21:290–296.
8. **Leive, L.** 1968. Studies on the permeability change produced in coliform bacteria by ethylenediaminetetraacetate. J. Biol. Chem. 243:2373–2380.
9. **Lucas, J. B.** 1971. Gonococcal resistance to antibiotics. South. Med. Bull. 59:22–28.
10. **MacAlister, T. J., J. W. Costerton, and K. J. Cheng.** 1972. Effect on the removal of outer cell wall layer on the actinomycin susceptibility of a gram-negative bacterium. Antimicrob. Agents Chemother. 1:447–449.
11. **Maier, T. W., H. R. Bielstein, and L. Zubrzycki.** 1974. Antibiotic disk susceptibility tests with *Neisseria gonorrhoeae*. Antimicrob. Agents Chemother. 5:210–216.
12. **Maier, T. W., H. R. Bielstein, and L. Zubrzycki.** 1974. Multiple antibiotic resistance in *Neisseria gonorrhoeae*. Antimicrob. Agents Chemother. 6:22–28.
13. **Maier, T. W., L. Zubrzycki, and M. Coyle.** 1975. Genetic analysis of drug resistance in *Neisseria gonorrhoeae*: identification and linkage relationships of loci controlling drug resistance. Antimicrob. Agents Chemother. 7:676–681.
14. **Maness, M. J., and P. F. Sparling.** 1973. Multiple antibiotic resistance due to a single mutation in *Neisseria gonorrhoeae*. J. Infect. Dis. 128:321–330.
15. **Reyn, A., and M. W. Bentzon.** 1969. Relationships between the sensitivities in vitro of *Neisseria gonorrhoeae* to spiramycin, penicillin, tetracycline, and erythromycin. Br. J. Vener. Dis. 45:223–226.

16. **Rodriguez, W., A. K. Saz, and H. Schneider.** 1975. Possible mechanism of decreased susceptibility of *Neisseria gonorrhoeae* to penicillin. Antimicrob. Agents Chemother. **7**:788-792.
17. **Ronald, A. R., J. Eby, and J. C. Sherris.** 1969. Susceptibility of *Neisseria gonorrhoeae* to penicillin and tetracycline, p. 431-434. Antimicrob. Agents Chemother. 1968.
18. **Sekiguchi, M., and S. Lida.** 1967. Mutants of *Escherichia coli* permeable to actinomycin. Proc. Natl. Acad. Sci. U.S.A. **58**:2315-2320.
19. **Snedecor, G. W.** 1946. Statistical methods, 4th ed. Iowa State College Press, Ames.
20. **Sparling, P. F.** 1972. Antibiotic resistance in *Neisseria gonorrhoeae*. Med. Clin. N. Am. **56**:217-242.
21. **Steers, E., E. L. Foltz, and B. S. Graves.** 1959. An inocula replicating apparatus for routine testing of bacterial susceptibility to antibiotics. Antibiot. Chemother. **9**:307-311.
22. **Voll, M. J., and L. Leive.** 1970. Actinomycin resistance and actinomycin excretion in a mutant of *Escherichia coli*. J. Bacteriol. **102**:600-602.
23. **White, L. A., and D. S. Kellogg, Jr.** 1965. *Neisseria gonorrhoeae* identification in direct smears by a fluorescent antibody-counterstain method. Appl. Microbiol. **13**:171-174.
24. **Willcox, R. R.** 1970. A survey of problems in the antibiotic treatment of gonorrhea with special reference to south-east Asia. Br. J. Vener. Dis. **46**:217-236.

ANTIMICROBIAL AGENTS AND CHEMOTHERAPY, Oct. 1976, p. 646-651
Vol. 10, No. 4

Printed in U.S.A.

Synergistic Activity of Carbenicillin and Gentamicin in Experimental *Pseudomonas* Bacteremia in Neutropenic Rats

RITA E. SCOTT AND HUGH G. ROBSON*

Division of Infectious Diseases, Departments of Medicine and Microbiology, Royal Victoria Hospital, and Faculty of Medicine, McGill University, Montreal, Quebec, H3A 2B4 Canada*

Received for publication 26 May 1976

Rats made neutropenic with cyclophosphamide were infected intraperitoneally with *Pseudomonas aeruginosa*. The challenge organism was killed synergistically in vitro by the combination of gentamicin and carbenicillin. Untreated neutropenic rats infected with 3×10^6 *Pseudomonas* died between days 2 and 7, and the overall mortality was 70%. Groups of infected neutropenic rats were treated intramuscularly with 1.5 or 6 mg of gentamicin per kg per dose, 100 or 400 mg of carbenicillin per kg per dose, or 1.5 mg of gentamicin and 100 mg of carbenicillin per kg per dose. Treatment was begun at 2 h postinfection and was continued every 8 h for about 72 h. Cultures of blood and peritoneal washings were performed in control and treated rats at 1, 4, 24, 48, and 72 h postinfection. Gentamicin at either dose level was ineffective in preventing death, but mortality was significantly reduced by high-dose carbenicillin and low-dose combination therapy. In addition, the latter regimens sterilized the peritoneal fluid and blood. Carbenicillin and gentamicin showed in vivo synergy in the treatment of neutropenic *Pseudomonas*-infected rats.

Infections caused by *Pseudomonas aeruginosa* constitute a serious problem in patients with underlying neoplastic disease (26). The incidence of bacteremic *Pseudomonas* (refers throughout the text specifically to *P. aeruginosa*) infection has increased largely due to the aggressive use of potent antineoplastic chemotherapy that may result in prolonged periods of severe neutropenia. Patients colonized with *Pseudomonas* are at an increased risk of invasive infection during periods of drug-induced neutropenia (23, 24).

Antimicrobial therapy of *Pseudomonas* bacteremia has often proved unsuccessful, and few controlled comparative trials of therapy have been performed in humans (10). Although polymyxin B and sodium colistimethate exhibit in vitro activity against almost all strains of *Pseudomonas*, they are usually ineffective in the therapy of bacteremic infection, particularly in patients with unremitting neutropenia (26). Gentamicin, also active in vitro against most *Pseudomonas* isolates, may be similarly ineffective in the neutropenic host with bacteremic infection (4, 5, 21, 25). The introduction of carbenicillin was reported by Bodey et al. to have led to the increased survival of patients with *Pseudomonas* bacteremia; good results were noted even in patients with persisting neutropenia (6, 7). A 71% complete response rate was reported in a group of 38 patients treated with carbenicillin alone for bacteremic *Pseudomonas* infection (7).

Gentamicin and carbenicillin show antibiotic synergy in vitro against many strains of *Pseudomonas* (11, 19). This antibiotic combination is frequently employed in the therapy of proven *Pseudomonas* infection as well as empirically in febrile neutropenic patients prior to the availability of culture results (21). Despite the early institution of combined antibiotic regimens incorporating carbenicillin and gentamicin, the therapy of *Pseudomonas* bacteremia occurring in a neutropenic host may still fail, particularly if the underlying hematological disease cannot be controlled. In recent studies the successful control of *Pseudomonas* bacteremia with combination therapy has been reported variously in 33% (23), 60% (27), 62% (22), and 85% of cases (21).

Due to the difficulties involved in performing and interpreting trials of antibiotic efficacy in severely ill patients with varying types and degrees of underlying illness, the potential disparity between in vitro and in vivo results, and the potential emergence of *Pseudomonas* strains resistant to formerly effective agents (12), studies of therapy in appropriate animal models seem justified. Such animal experiments may generate significant data that may be impossible to obtain from studies in humans.

The present experiments were designed to

evaluate the therapeutic efficacy of gentamicin and carbenicillin alone and in combination in experimental *Pseudomonas* bacteremia in neutropenic rats. A model infection similar to that described by Andriole (1, 2) for nonneutropenic animals was employed; severe neutropenia was induced by the administration of cyclophosphamide. The *Pseudomonas* strain employed was killed synergistically in vitro by the combination of gentamicin and carbenicillin. Animals treated with a low-dose antibiotic combination showed significantly improved survival as compared with those treated with either gentamicin or carbenicillin in equivalent doses.

(This paper was presented in part at the 15th Interscience Conference on Antimicrobial Agents and Chemotherapy, Washington, D.C., 24–26 September 1975).

MATERIALS AND METHODS

Experimental animals. Female, pathogen-free, Sprague-Dawley CFE rats (Carworth Farms, Wilmington, Mass.) weighing 185 to 200 g were used.

Induction of neutropenia. Cyclophosphamide (Procytox; Frank W. Horner Ltd., Montreal, Quebec, Canada) was administered intraperitoneally in a dose of 120 mg/kg. The median leukocyte count on days 4 and 5 after cyclophosphamide was approximately 1,000 cells/mm^3; on the same days, median neutrophil counts were about 100/mm^3. Circulating leukocytes increased by day 6 and reached normal levels by day 10 after injection. No special precautions were taken with the rats during the period of neutropenia, and there were no deaths in neutropenic noninfected rats observed for 15 days. In subsequent experiments neutropenic rats were infected 96 h after the administration of cyclophosphamide.

Microorganism and in vitro susceptibility studies. *P. aeruginosa* 407 was provided by V. T. Andriole, New Haven, Conn. This strain is known to be inhibited synergistically by the combination of gentamicin and carbenicillin (1). The microorganism was lyophilized; for each experiment a fresh vial was used.

The synergistic bactericidal activity of the combination of gentamicin and carbenicillin against *Pseudomonas* 407 was determined in Trypticase soy broth. A 1-ml amount of an overnight broth culture of *Pseudomonas* 407 was added to 99 ml of broth to give a concentration of about 10^6 colony-forming units (CFU)/ml. Appropriate antibiotic solutions were added to a series of flasks to produce the following final concentrations (in micrograms per milliliter): gentamicin, 2 or 10; carbenicillin, 25 or 100; a combination of gentamicin, 2, plus carbenicillin, 25; or a combination of gentamicin, 2, plus carbenicillin, 100.

Flasks were incubated at 37°C without shaking; at various times after incubation 1-ml portions were removed, and the number of CFU of *Pseudomonas* was determined in agar pour plates. Synergistic bactericidal activity was defined as a 100-fold increase in killing by the combination as compared with the most effective single agent after 24 h of incubation.

Studies of lethality. Rats were infected intraperitoneally with graded 1.0-ml inocula containing *Pseudomonas* 407; deaths were scored daily and the animals were observed for 15 days. Commercially supplied gentamicin sulfate (Schering Corporation Ltd., Pointe Claire, Quebec, Canada) and disodium carbenicillin (Ayerst Laboratories, Montreal, Quebec, Canada) were dissolved in water to the required concentration immediately prior to injection. The amounts of drug administered are expressed in milligrams per kilogram per dose. Antibiotic doses were administered by the intramuscular route in volumes of 0.2 ml into the hind limb at 2, 10, 20, 28, 34, 44, 52, 58, and 68 h after bacterial challenge. Attempts were made to alternate injection sites. Doses of the antibiotic combination were administered concurrently, but each agent was injected into a different hind limb. The results were analyzed statistically for significance by the fourfold, chi-square contingency table method.

Quantitative bacteriology. Blood was obtained by cardiac puncture from groups of three rats in the different treatment groups at 1, 4, 24, 48, and 72 h after infection. The number of CFU per milliliter of *Pseudomonas* was determined by incorporating portions of 10-fold dilutions of blood in pour plates. Immediately after blood had been obtained for quantitative culture, the rats were sacrificed and the enumeration of *Pseudomonas* in the peritoneal cavity was carried out by using the method of Cohn (9).

RESULTS

Synergistic bactericidal activity in vitro of gentamicin and carbenicillin against *Pseudomonas* 407. Synergy in vitro was demonstrated for both combinations of gentamicin and carbenicillin against *Pseudomonas* 407. The flask containing the combination of 2 μg of gentamicin per ml and 100 μg of carbenicillin per ml contained no viable organisms at 24- and 48-h incubation periods (Fig. 1).

Virulence of *Pseudomonas* 407 for normal and neutropenic rats. A total of 15 of 20 normal rats infected with 3 × 10^8 bacteria died of infection (Fig. 2A). All deaths occurred within the first 24 h after bacterial challenge. Smaller inocula were nonlethal for normal rats.

Eighteen of twenty neutropenic rats challenged with 3 × 10^7 organisms died (Fig. 2B). Fourteen of twenty neutropenic rats infected with 3 × 10^6 *Pseudomonas* died; all deaths occurred between days 2 and 6 postinfection. One-half of the deaths occurred on day 2 postinfection. Only 3 of 20 animals infected with 3 × 10^5 bacteria died. At autopsy *Pseudomonas* was recovered from heart blood cultures. Pleural effusions were usually noted, and most spleens contained numerous abscesses of 2 to 3 mm in diameter that yielded *Pseudomonas* in pure culture.

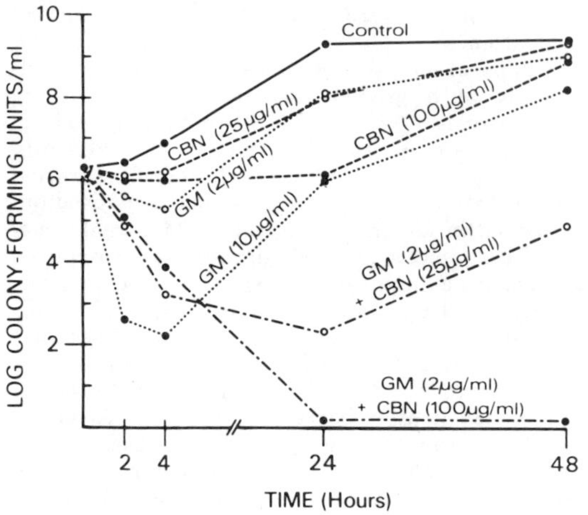

FIG. 1. *Effect of gentamicin, carbenicillin, and gentamicin-carbenicillin in combination against Pseudomonas 407. Abbreviations: CBN, carbenicillin; GM, gentamicin.*

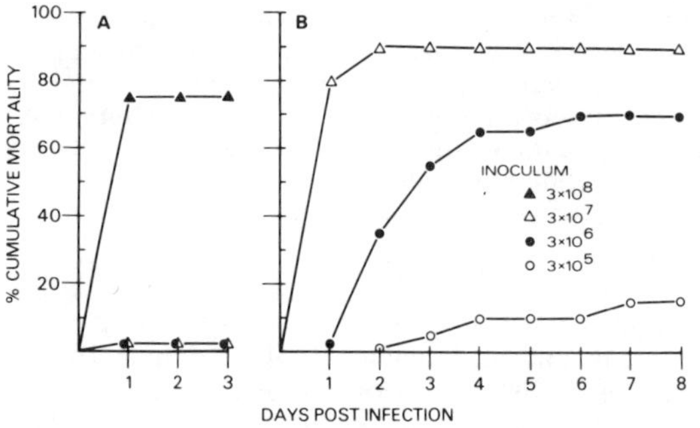

FIG. 2. *Cumulative mortality of rats infected intraperitoneally with graded inocula of Pseudomonas 407. Neutropenic rats were injected intraperitoneally 4 days prior to infection with 120 mg of cyclophosphamide per kg. (A) Normal rats; (B) neutropenic rats.*

The percent mortality of neutropenic rats infected with *Pseudomonas* was related to the number of organisms employed in the challenge. Neutropenia induced by cyclophosphamide greatly increased the susceptibility of rats to lethal infection. A challenge inoculum of 3×10^6 *Pseudomonas* was employed in the subsequent experiments.

Efficacy of antibiotic regimens in neutropenic infected rats. Groups of 30 neutropenic rats received either no therapy, 1.5 or 6 mg of gentamicin per kg, 100 or 400 mg of carbenicillin per kg, or a combination of 1.5 mg of gentamicin plus 100 mg of carbenicillin per kg.

Twenty-two of thirty neutropenic infected control rats (73%) died. Therapy with gentamicin alone was ineffective (Fig. 3A). A total of 24 of 30 animals (80%) treated with 1.5 mg of gentamicin per kg and 21 of 30 (70%) treated with 6 mg/kg died, although the deaths were delayed in the group that received high-dose gentamicin therapy. A total of 15 of 30 rats treated with 100 mg of carbenicillin per kg died (Fig. 3B). None of the animals in this treatment group died during the treatment period in the first 3 days after infection. Although the results suggested a beneficial effect of low-dose carbenicillin therapy, this regimen was not significantly better than the control ($\chi^2 = 3.45$; $0.1 > P > 0.05$). A total of 4 of 30 (13%) and 6 of 30 (20%), respectively, animals that received either high-dose carbenicillin or combined low-dose therapy died. Both of these forms of therapy were significantly better than the control ($P < 0.01$) and also were better than 100 mg of carbenicillin per kg ($P < 0.01$). No rat treated with high-dose carbenicillin or combined low-dose therapy died during the first 3 days after infection. The results indicate that the combination of carbenicillin and gentamicin exhibited antibiotic synergy both in vitro against *Pseudomonas* 407 and in vivo against infection caused by this organism in neutropenic animals.

Effect of antibiotic regimens on bacteremia and peritoneal lavage cultures. *Pseudomonas* was present in the blood of untreated animals at 1 h after infection, and the degree of bacteremia rose progressively over the first 24 h of infection (Fig. 4). Too few control animals survived past 24 h to allow later cultures. Bacteremia was detected at some time in all other treatment groups. At 48 and 72 h after infection, rats treated with 100 mg of carbenicillin per kg showed persistent bacteremia of 10^2 to

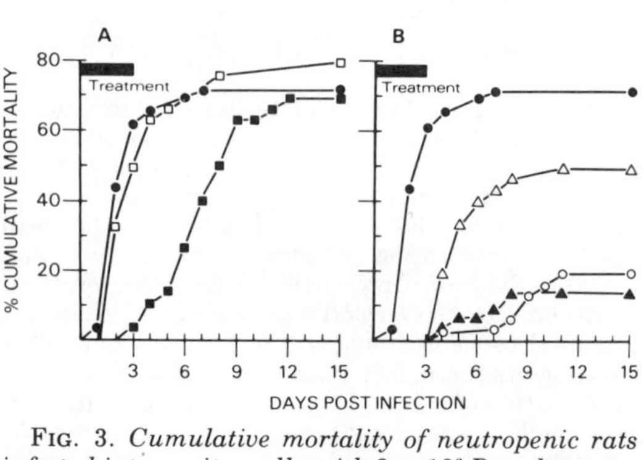

FIG. 3. *Cumulative mortality of neutropenic rats infected intraperitoneally with 3×10^6 Pseudomonas 407. (A) Treatment with: □, gentamicin, 1.5 mg/kg; ■, gentamicin, 6 mg/kg. (B) Treatment with: △, carbenicillin, 100 mg/kg; ▲, carbenicillin, 400 mg/kg; or ○, carbenicillin, 100 mg/kg, and gentamicin, 1.5 mg/kg. ●, Control untreated rats.*

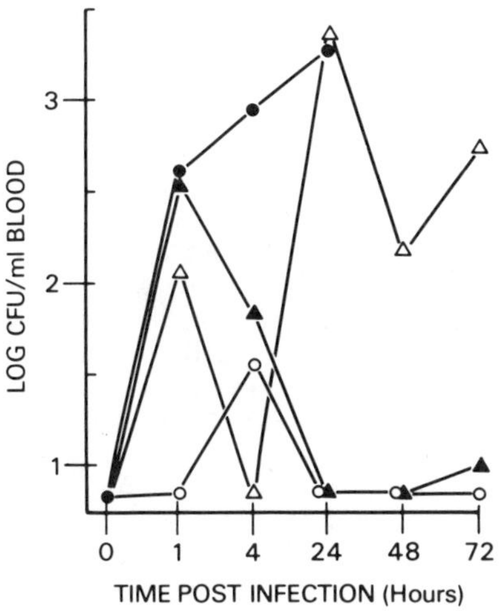

FIG. 4. *Quantitative blood cultures of neutropenic rats infected intraperitoneally with 3 × 10^6 Pseudomonas 407. Treatment groups included: ●, untreated control; △, carbenicillin, 100 mg/kg: ▲, carbenicillin, 400 mg/kg; ○, carbenicillin, 100 mg/kg, and gentamicin, 1.5 mg/kg. Values represent the mean of three animals.*

10^3 CFU/ml of blood. Blood cultures of rats treated with 400 mg of carbenicillin per kg were sterile at 24 and 48 h, although one of three treated with this dose was bacteremic at 72 h. All blood cultures of rats treated with combined carbenicillin and gentamicin were sterile at 24 h after infection and at later times.

Peritoneal lavage cultures correlated well with the degree and persistence of bacteremia (Fig. 5). The number of *Pseudomonas* present in the peritoneum at zero time (immediately after infection) has been plotted as a theoretic value, assuming complete recovery and viability of the inoculum in the washout fluid. The mean number of CFU recovered from the peritoneum of control rats rose between 4 and 24 h after infection to greater than 10^4. Peritoneal counts of *Pseudomonas* diminished progressively in rats treated with 100 mg of carbenicillin per kg, but organisms were recovered at all time intervals. Both 400 mg of carbenicillin per kg and combined carbenicillin-gentamicin regimens sterilized the peritoneal fluid. This effect was observed at 24 h after infection in rats treated with the antibiotic combination and at 48 h in rats treated with high-dose carbenicillin.

DISCUSSION

There are some important similarities between this model infection and *Pseudomonas* infection in a human neutropenic host. Normal rats are highly resistant to infection with *Pseudomonas* 407. In our hands an intraperitoneal inoculum of 3 × 10^8 organisms caused 70% mortality of control animals within 24 h, but smaller inocula were nonlethal. During the period of severe neutropenia 100-fold fewer organisms produced equivalent mortality. Quantitative bacteriological studies in neutropenic infected control rats showed increasing numbers of *Pseudomonas* in the peritoneum and blood between 4 and 24 h after infection, manifestations of uncontrolled sepsis. Splenic abscesses were noted, indicating the additional presence of multiple parenchymal foci of bacterial proliferation. Native resistance to *Pseudomonas* in healthy individuals, increased susceptibility during periods of granulocytopenia, and bacteremic infection with metastatic abscesses are features of the human interaction with this pathogen.

Antibiotic therapy was administered early (2 h) after the onset of infection, since protective effects had been previously shown when treatment was instituted at 2 h, but not when delayed to 6 h after *Pseudomonas* 407 infection of nonneutropenic rats (1). The critical importance of early antibiotic therapy to a successful outcome in infected neutropenic humans has been well documented (21).

Despite a prompt institution of therapy, gentamicin alone in doses of 1.5 or 6 mg/kg failed to

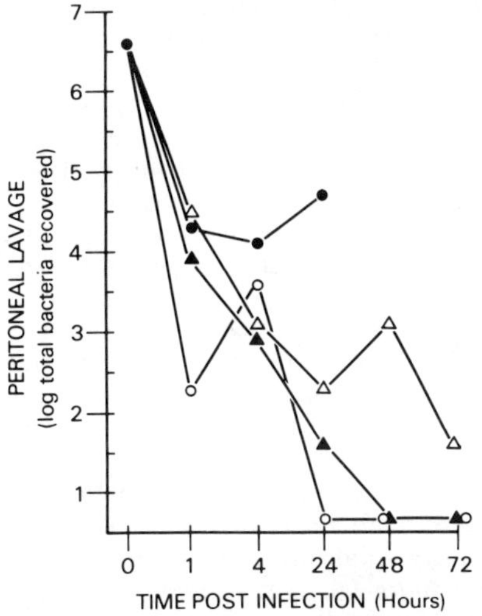

FIG. 5. *Quantitative cultures of peritoneal washout fluid of neutropenic rats infected intraperitoneally with 3 × 10^6 Pseudomonas 407. Treatment groups included: ●, untreated control; △, carbenicillin, 100 mg/kg; ▲, carbenicillin, 400 mg/kg; ○, carbenicillin, 100 mg/kg, and gentamicin, 1.5 mg/kg. Values represent the mean of three animals.*

improve the overall survival of neutropenic infected rats. Rats treated with high doses of gentamicin showed short-term benefit only, with no deaths observed during the treatment period, whereas the course of infection was completely unaffected by the lower dose. The reason for the lack of efficacy of gentamicin in the neutropenic rat is not entirely clear and requires further study; however, preliminary data suggest an important pharmacological reason for drug failure in this model. Infected neutropenic rats showed concentrations of detectable gentamicin in serum for only 1.5 to 2 h after an intramuscular dose of 6 mg/kg (R. E. Scott and H. G. Robson, unpublished data). Similar observations were reported by Luft and Kleit; gentamicin was barely detectable in rat sera at 3 h after a single subcutaneous injection of 10 mg/kg (17). The half-life of gentamicin in rat serum was estimated to be about 30 min (17). The failure of gentamicin to cure some patients with *Pseudomonas* sepsis has also been attributed to inadequate serum and tissue levels that may occur at various times after intermittent drug administration (13, 18). Shorter intervals between doses, larger doses, or the continuous administration of gentamicin as suggested by Bodey et al. (3) may provide improved therapeutic results; such approaches can be assessed using this model. Other factors may also be implicated, however, including antibiotic inactivation by purulent material (8) and deficient phagocytosis and intracellular killing of gentamicin-damaged microorganisms during neutropenia (13).

In contrast to gentamicin, carbenicillin in the large dose employed (400 mg/kg) was highly effective. Despite its short duration, this therapeutic regimen significantly reduced mortality, eradicated *Pseudomonas* from the original peritoneal site of infection, and sterilized the blood. Although the lower dose employed (100 mg/kg) did not significantly reduce eventual mortality, deaths were prevented during therapy, the number of viable *Pseudomonas* present in the peritoneum was reduced, and the magnitude of bacteremia did not increase between 24 and72 h of infection. The lack of overall benefit of this regimen may be attributable to the eventual multiplication of persisting *Pseudomonas* when treatment was discontinued, despite survival of the animals to the stage where return of neutrophils to the circulation could be predicted. The effect of more prolonged carbenicillin therapy at the 100-mg/kg dose level remains to be explored. A similar dose response relationship for nonneutropenic rats infected with *Pseudomonas* 407 has been observed (2).

Although low-dose gentamicin and carbenicillin regimens were largely ineffective when employed singly, the combination was highly active. We interpret this as evidence of in vivo drug synergy; this phenomenon has previously been documented in nonneutropenic rats (1, 2). Our finding is in agreement with the recent work of Lumish and Norden in a similar neutropenic rat model (Prog. Abstr. Intersci. Conf. Antimicrob. Agents Chemother., 15th, Washington, D.C., Abstr. 201, 1975). These authors also noted the lack of efficacy of gentamicin employed as the sole antimicrobial agent under similar conditions. In another study Saslaw et al. failed to show in vivo synergy in neutropenic monkeys infected with *Pseudomonas* (20).

An equivalent reduction in mortality was observed in rats treated with high-dose carbenicillin, but the effect of the antibiotic combination on bacteremia and peritoneal fluid cultures was even more striking; all cultures were sterile at 24 h and subsequent times. Recent studies by Klastersky et al. have shown that an improvement in response rates of gram-negative infection occurring in patients with neoplasia can be obtained with combinations of antibiotics when the causative agents can be shown to be synergistically inhibited in vitro (14). The number of severely neutropenic patients infected with *Pseudomonas* was small (14–16); improved survival of this subgroup treated with the carbenicillin-gentamicin combination as compared with either drug alone could not be demonstrated (16).

Our studies provide further evidence to support the view that the initial therapy of *Pseudomonas* sepsis in the neutropenic patient should include both carbenicillin and gentamicin. It will be important to extend these observations to infection in neutropenic rats caused by strains of *Pseudomonas* that show partial synergy or no synergy in vitro to the carbenicillin-gentamicin combination. The combination has previously been shown to be effective in vivo in nonneutropenic rats infected with a strain of *Pseudomonas* that showed only partial synergy in vitro (1). This model infection may also prove valuable in assessing the efficacy of agents such as tobramycin, amikacin, and ticarcillin in infections caused by *Pseudomonas* resistant to carbenicillin or gentamicin.

ACKNOWLEDGEMENT

We wish to thank Fereshteh Ghadirian and Eva Hawkins for their assistance.

This research ws supported by Ayerst Laboratories, Montreal, Quebec, Canada.

ADDENDUM

Since submission of this manuscript, the work of R. M. Lumish and C. W. Norden has been published (J. Infect. Dis. **133**:538-547, 1976).

LITERATURE CITED

1. **Andriole, V. T.** 1971. Synergy of carbenicillin and gentamicin in experimental infection with *Pseudomonas*. J. Infect. Dis. **124**(Suppl.):S46-S55.
2. **Andriole, V. T.** 1974. Antibiotic synergy in experimental infection with *Pseudomonas*. II. The effect of carbenicillin, cephalothin or cephanone combined with tobramycin or gentamicin. J. Infect. Dis. **129**:124-133.
3. **Bodey, G. P., H.-Y. Chang, V. Rodriguez, and D. Stewart.** 1975. Feasibility of administering aminoglycoside antibiotics by continuous intravenous infusion. Antimicrob. Agents Chemother. **8**:328-333.
4. **Bodey, G. P., E. Middleman, T. Umsawadi, and V. Rodriguez.** 1972. Infection in cancer patients. Results with gentamicin sulfate therapy. Cancer **29**:1697-1701.
5. **Bodey, G. P., and V. Rodriguez.** 1973. Advances in the management of *Pseudomonas aeruginosa* infections in cancer patients. Eur. J. Cancer **9**:435-441.
6. **Bodey, G. P., V. Rodriguez, and J. K. Luce.** 1969. Carbenicillin therapy of Gram-negative bacilli infections. Am. J. Med. Sci. **257**:408-414.
7. **Bodey, G. P., J. P. Whitecar, E. Middleman, and V. Rodriguez.** 1971. Carbenicillin therapy for *Pseudomonas* infections. J. Am. Med. Assoc. **218**:62-66.
8. **Bryant, R. E., and D. Hammond.** 1974. Interaction of purulent material with antibiotics used to treat *Pseudomonas* infections. Antimicrob. Agents Chemother. **6**:702-707.
9. **Cohn, Z. A.** 1962. Determinants of infection in the peritoneal cavity. Yale J. Biol. Med. **35**:12-28.
10. **Davis, S. D., A. Ianetta, and R. J. Wedgewood.** 1971. Antibiotics for *Pseudomonas aeruginosa* sepsis: inadequate proof of efficacy. (Editorial.) J. Infect. Dis. **124**:104-106.
11. **Eickhoff, T. C.** 1969. In vitro effects of carbenicillin combined with gentamicin or polymyxin B against *Pseudomonas aeruginosa*. Appl. Microbiol. **18**:469-473.
12. **Greene, W. H., M. Moody, S. Schimpff, V. M. Young, and P. H. Wiernik.** 1973. *Pseudomonas aeruginosa* resistant to carbenicillin and gentamicin. Epidemiologic and clinical aspects in a cancer center. Ann. Intern. Med. **79**:684-689.
13. **Jackson, G. G., and L. J. Riff.** 1971. *Pseudomonas* bacteremia: pharmacologic and other bases for failure of treatment with gentamicin. J. Infect. Dis. **124**(Suppl.):S185-S191.
14. **Klastersky, J., R. Cappel, and D. Daneau.** 1972. Clinical significance of in vitro synergism between antibiotics in gram-negative infections. Antimicrob. Agents Chemother. **2**:470-475.
15. **Klastersky, J., R. Cappel, and D. Daneau.** 1973. Therapy with carbenicillin and gentamicin for patients with cancer and severe infection caused by gram-negative rods. Cancer **31**:331-336.
16. **Klastersky, J., A. Henri, C. Hensgens, and D. Daneau.** 1974. Gram-negative infections in cancer. Study of empiric therapy comparing carbenicillin-cephalothin with and without gentamicin. J. Am. Med. Assoc. **227**:45-48.
17. **Luft, F. C., and S. A. Kleit.** 1974. Renal parenchymal accumulation of aminoglycoside antibiotics in rats. J. Infect. Dis. **130**:656-659.
18. **Pennington, J. E., D. C. Dale, H. Y. Reynolds, and J. D. MacLowry.** 1975. Gentamicin sulfate pharmacokinetics: lower levels of gentamicin in blood during fever. J. Infect. Dis. **132**:270-275.
19. **Phair, J. P., C. Watanakunakorn, and T. Bannister.** 1969. In vitro susceptibility of *Pseudomonas aeruginosa* to carbenicillin and the combination of carbenicillin and gentamicin. Appl. Microbiol. **18**:303-306.
20. **Saslaw, S., H. N. Carlisle, and M. Moheimani.** 1973. Comparison of gentamicin, carbenicillin and gentamicin, and carbenicillin in *Pseudomonas* sepsis in monkeys. Antimicrob. Agents Chemother. **3**:274-278.
21. **Schimpff, S., W. Satterlee, V. M. Young, and A. Serpick.** 1971. Empiric therapy with carbenicillin and gentamicin for febrile patients with cancer and granulocytopenia. N. Engl. J. Med. **284**:1061-1065.
22. **Schimpff, S. C., W. H. Greene, V. M. Young, and P. H. Wiernik.** 1973. Pseudomonas septicemia: incidence, epidemiology, prevention and therapy in patients with advanced cancer. Eur. J. Cancer **9**:449-455.
23. **Schimpff, S. C., W. H. Greene, V. M. Young, and P. H. Wiernik.** 1974. Significance of *Pseudomonas aeruginosa* in the patient with leukemia or lymphoma. J. Infect. Dis. **130**(Suppl):S24-S31.
24. **Schimpff, S. C., V. M. Young, W. H. Greene, G. D. Vermeulen, M. R. Moody, and P. H. Wiernik.** 1972. Origin of infection in acute non-lymphocytic leukemia. Ann. Intern. Med. **77**:707-714.
25. **Tapper, M. L., and D. Armstrong.** 1974. Bacteremia due to *Pseudomonas aeruginosa* complicating neoplastic disease: a progress report. J. Infect. Dis. **130**(Suppl.):S14-S23.
26. **Whitecar, J. P., Jr., M. Luna, and G. P. Bodey.** 1970. *Pseudomonas* bacteremia in patients with malignant disease. Am. J. Med. Sci. **260**:216-223.
27. **Young, L. S.** 1971. Gentamicin: clinical use with carbenicillin and in-vitro studies with recent isolates of *Pseudomonas aeruginosa*. J. Infect. Dis. **124**-(Suppl.):S202-S206.

Antimicrobial Agents and Chemotherapy, Oct. 1976, p. 652-656 Vol. 10, No. 4
 Printed in U.S.A.

Radioimmunoassay of Iodinated Tobramycin

ALAN BROUGHTON,* JAMES E. STRONG, LARRY K. PICKERING, AND GERALD P. BODEY

Department of Pathology and Program in Infectious Diseases, University of Texas Medical School, and Department of Developmental Therapeutics, University of Texas System Cancer Center, M.D. Anderson Hospital and Tumor Institute, Houston, Texas 77025*

Received for publication 1 June 1976

A radioimmunoassay for tobramycin was developed using antisera from rabbits injected with a tobramycin-bovine serum albumin conjugate. The antibody had a relatively high affinity for ^{125}I-labeled tobramycin (1.6×10^9 liters/mol), thus indicating little interference in immunoreactivity by iodination. The radioimmunoassay was highly specific, and only minor cross-reaction occurred with other aminoglycoside antibiotics. The radioimmunoassay was also more sensitive than previously published tobramycin assays (minimum sensitivity, 280 pg), and there was a significant correlation ($P < 0.05$) with both the radioenzymatic and microbiological assays.

Tobramycin, a new aminoglycoside antibiotic, was originally isolated as factor 6 from the nebramycin antibiotic complex produced by *Streptomyces tenebrarius* (1). This antibiotic displays greater antibacterial effect in vitro than gentamicin against isolates of *Pseudomonas aeruginosa* (2, 10). The therapeutic efficacy of tobramycin is similar to that of gentamicin, and the antibiotic exhibits a low therapeutic index, thus indicating a need for monitoring serum drug concentrations to achieve maximum chemotherapeutic efficacy and minimum toxicity.

Therapeutic drug monitoring is dependent upon the availability of sensitive, rapid, specific, and precise assay techniques. Tobramycin has been previously measured in biological fluids by both a radioenzymatic assay (17) and a microbiological assay (8). Radioimmunoassays offer definite advantages over microbiological assays especially regarding specificity and speed of assay. The use of a ^{125}I label in radioimmunoassay also eliminates the need for liquid scintillation counting required in radioenzymatic assays. We have previously reported radioimmunoassays for two other aminoglycoside antibiotics, sisomicin (5) and gentamicin (4). Using similar techniques, we now report the development of a radioimmunoassay for another aminoglycoside antibiotic, tobramycin, and compare this assay with a radioenzymatic and a microbiological assay.

MATERIALS AND METHODS

Haptene-protein conjugation. Tobramycin was conjugated to bovine serum albumin (Sigma) using 1-ethyl-3-(3-dimethyl aminopropyl) carbodiimide (Story). The procedure used for conjugation and purification was as follows. Bovine serum albumin (BSA) (100 mg) was dissolved in 1 ml of phosphate-buffered saline (PBS; 0.01 M phosphate, 0.15 M NaCl, 0.1% sodium azide, pH 7.5) and mixed with 5 ml of 40-mg/ml tobramycin reagent (Eli Lilly & Co., Indianapolis, Ind.). Ethyl carbodiimide (800 mg) was dissolved in 1 ml of PBS and added slowly to the BSA-tobramycin mixture with constant stirring. The mixture was stirred for 1 h at room temperature and incubated for 3 days at 4°C. After incubation, the conjugate was dialyzed for 16 h against PBS (2,000 ml) and chromatographically purified using a Sephadex G-25 column (0.9 by 25 cm).

Immunization. Two New Zealand white rabbits were immunized by monthly intramuscular injections of the conjugate emulsified in complete Freund adjuvant as described by Hurn and Landon (9). A primary injection was administered by injecting each of the limbs with 1 ml of a 0.5-mg/ml tobramycin-BSA conjugate emulsified in PBS-Freund adjuvant (1:3, vol/vol). Subsequent monthly booster injections were administered intramuscularly in either the hind or fore limbs. Sera, obtained from the ear vein 14 days after the third monthly injection, had a final titer of 1:10,000.

Iodination. The iodination procedure of Bolton and Hunter (3) was modified to produce ^{125}I-labeled tobramycin. The acylating agent, 3-(4-hydroxyphenyl) propionic acid-*N*-hydroxysuccinimide ester (Tagit, Calbiochem) was dissolved in benzene (0.2 mg/ml), and 10 μl of this solution (0.76 mM) was evaporated to dryness under nitrogen. This residue was treated with 1 mCi of high-specific-activity (100 mCi/ml), carrier-free ^{125}I (Amersham/Searle), 10 μl of chloramine-T (17.7 mM, 5 mg/ml of 0.2 M phosphate buffer, pH 7.5), 10 μl of sodium metabisulfite (63 mM, 12 mg/ml of 0.2 M phosphate buffer, pH 7.2), 10 μl of potassium iodide (0.12 M, 20 mg/ml of 0.2 M phosphate buffer, pH 7.5) and 10 μl of dimethylformamide. This mixture was extracted twice with 0.4-ml samples of benzene, and the benzene extracts were rapidly evaporated to dryness with nitrogen. Next, 50 μl of tobramycin (55 μg/ml of 0.1 M borate buffer, pH 8.5) was added to the evaporated extracts and incubated overnight at room temperature. The reaction was terminated by adding 0.2 ml of glycine (15 mg/ml of 0.1 M borate buffer). Iodinated tobramycin was isolated using a Sephadex G-10 column (0.9 by 30 cm) with PBS eluant.

Radioimmunoassay procedure. The tobramycin radioimmunoassay was performed using the following protocol. Each assay tube contained 500 μl of PBS, 100 μl of standard or unknown diluted in PBS to be within the range of the standard curve, 100 μl of ^{125}I-labeled tobramycin diluted in PBS to 40,000 cpm/100 μl, and 100 μl of antisera diluted 1:2,000 in 0.1% gelatin that had been suspended in PBS. After thorough mixing, the tubes were incubated 30 min at 37°C. A 200-μl sample of dextran-coated charcoal (2% Dextran T-70, Pharmacia, and 2% Norit, Fisher Scientific Co., in PBS) was added, and after brief incubation (10 min, 4°C) the assay tubes were centrifuged (1,500 × g, 10 min, 4°C). The supernatants were decanted, and radioactivity was measured in an automatic gamma counter (Nuclear-Chicago). Each standard or unknown sample was run in duplicate, and control tubes with samples of known concentration were included.

Radioenzymatic assay. Concentrations of tobramycin in serum were determined by the radioenzymatic method utilizing the enzyme gentamicin adenyl transferase with ^{14}C-labeled adenosine 5′-triphosphate as the substrate (15). This R factor-mediated enzyme was released from a mutant strain of *Escherichia coli* W677/HJR66 using osmotic disruption. The assay procedure was described previously (16).

Microbiological assay. The microbiological assay of tobramycin in serum was performed by an agar well diffusion method using *Bacillus globogii* as the test organism (8).

RESULTS

The standard curve depicted in Fig. 1 was linear on a logit-log plot. The assay sensitivity, defined as the least amount of tobramycin which can be significantly distinguished ($P <$ 0.05) from no drug, was 280 pg/tube. The assay precision was estimated by measuring nine aliquants of a serum specimen. The coefficient of variation for these samples was 7.6%, with a mean value of 22.2 ng/ml. Recovery experiments were also performed on 12 serum specimens ranging in concentrations from 2 to 8 μg/ml. The mean recovery was 97.9% ± 2.7% standard error of the mean.

Cross-reactivity of the tobramycin radioimmunoassay with other antibiotics was measured by determining the amount of drug necessary to produce 50% inhibition of antibody binding to [^{125}I]tobramycin. The efficiency of this inhibition was related to the amount of unlabeled tobramycin required and is expressed in Table 1 as the percentage of cross-

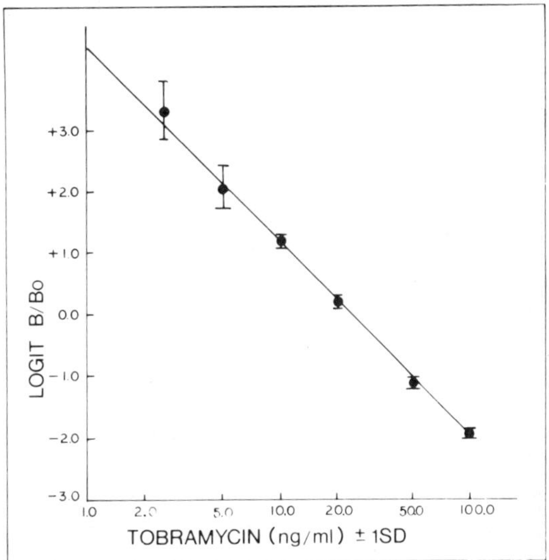

Fig. 1. *Standard curve for radioimmunoassay of tobramycin. Logit B/Bo is the logit (logit X = ln X/100-X) of the ratio of antibody-bound radioactivity to radioactivity bound at zero concentration of unlabeled tobramycin. Each point represents the mean ± standard deviation for six replicates.*

Table 1. *Tobramycin specificity*[a]

Drug	Concn for 50% B/Bo (ng/ml)	% Cross-reactivity
Tobramycin	28	100.0
Kanamycin	350	8.0
Gentamicin	1,900	1.5
Amikacin	3,500	0.8
Sisomicin	3,500	0.8

[a] The concentration for 50% B/Bo was the concentration of drug necessary to reduce binding of [^{125}I]-tobramycin by 50%. The percentage of cross-reactivity was the relative efficiency of competition by the other aminoglycoside drugs compared to tobramycin.

reactivity. Kanamycin that differs from tobramycin by one substituent group showed the greatest degree of cross-reactivity of all antibiotics tested (8.0%). Drugs not shown in Table 1 that produced less than 0.1% cross-reactivity were: streptomycin (Pfizer), chloramphenicol (Parke-Davis), neomycin (Upjohn), methicillin (Bristol), and carbenicillin (Beecham-Massengill).

The affinity of tobramycin antisera was measured by two different techniques. Figure 2 shows a Scatchard plot (13) and an equilibrium technique (14) that were used in measuring antibody avidity for [^{125}I]tobramycin. Both procedures resulted in estimating the affinity constant as 1.6 × 10^9 liters/mol. The specific activity of [^{125}I]tobramycin was approximately 47.5

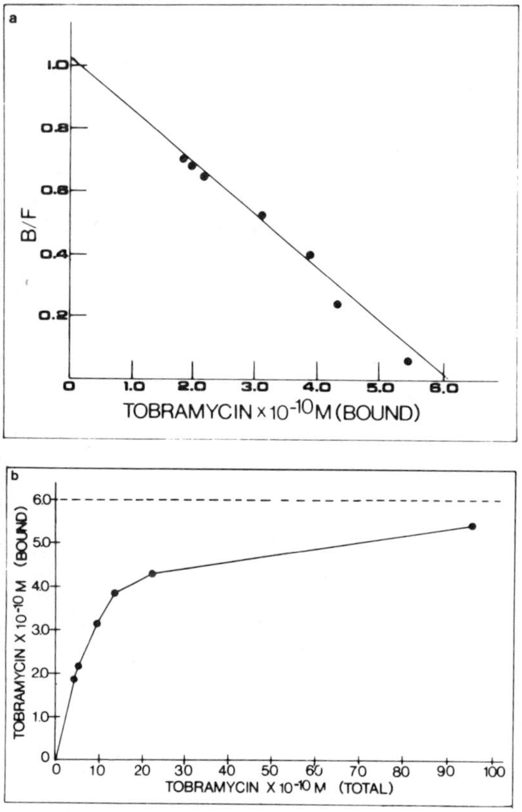

FIG. 2. *(a) Scatchard plot for antibody binding* ^{125}*I-labeled tobramycin. The ratio of bound to free labeled tobramycin is plotted against the concentration of labeled tobramycin bound by antibody. The slope of the linear regression* (-0.16) *indicated the affinity constant of this antisera to be* 1.6×10^9 *liters/mol. (b) Saturation curve of tobramycin antiserum. The concentration of free* ^{125}*I-labeled tobramycin at 50% antibody saturation is calculated from the difference between the concentrations of total and bound labeled tobramycin. The antibody saturation concentration was determined from the Scatchard plot estimation of the total number of antibody-binding sites (q). Since at 50% antibody saturation the affinity constant equals the reciprocal of the free antigen concentration, the resulting value for the affinity constant of* 1.6×10^9 *liters/mol was obtained.*

μCi/μg, with an incorporation of 12.1×10^{-3} atoms of ^{125}I per molecule of tobramycin.

Patient serum specimens were analyzed for tobramycin concentration by the radioimmunoassay, a microbiological assay, and a radioenzymatic assay. The results of each were compared, and the correlations are shown in Fig. 3. The best correlation was achieved between the radioimmunoassay and the radioenzymatic assay ($r = 0.954$, slope $= 1.055$). A good correlation was achieved between the microbiological assay and either the radioimmunoassay ($r = 0.970$, slope $= 0.774$) or the radioenzymatic assay ($r = 0.980$, slope $= 0.708$); however, the microbiological assay consistently measured tobramycin levels higher than the other two assays.

It has been reported that gentamicin is biologically and immunologically inactivated by incubation with carbenicillin in vitro (11, 18, 19). Therefore, experiments were designed to determine whether tobramycin, measured by radioimmunoassay, would decrease in immunoreactivity after incubation with carbenicillin or other antibiotics containing the β-lactam ring.

Tobramycin (4 μg/ml) was incubated at 37°C with carbenicillin (100 or 200 μg/ml) in normal donors' sera. Samples were removed and frozen after incubation for 0, 24, 48, and 72 h. The results of this incubation (Fig. 4) showed that the relative immunoreactivity of tobramycin decreased in the presence of carbenicillin and that the rate of decline was proportional to the concentration of carbenicillin. The ratio of carbenicillin to tobramycin also had an effect on tobramycin immunological inactivation since 10 μg of tobramycin per ml plus 100 μg of carbenicillin per ml produced little decrease in immunoreactivity after 48 h of incubation. Two other antibiotics containing the β-lactam ring moiety were incubated with tobramycin (10 μg/ml) but produced no significant decrease in immunoreactivity after 48 h of incubation (37°C). These antibiotics were methicillin (10 μg/ml) and cephaloridine (30 μg/ml).

DISCUSSION

Therapeutic monitoring of aminoglycoside antibiotics is well established and provides a means for increasing therapeutic efficacy and avoiding toxicity (6, 12). Each of the three methods available for measuring tobramycin has distinct advantages and disadvantages. The microbiological assays are relatively inexpensive and do not require specialized equipment or personnel. However, these assays require longer incubation and are subject to interference by other antimicrobial agents. An additional problem with microbiological assays is the difficulty of interpreting results especially when variations in support media or "double zoning" are encountered. The radioenzymatic assay is a rapid alternative to microbial assays and is specific for aminoglycoside antibiotics. In addition, radioenzymatic assays are highly versatile and can be used to measure different aminoglycoside antibiotics. The radioenzymatic assays require liquid scintillation counting equipment.

The radioimmunoassay for tobramycin de-

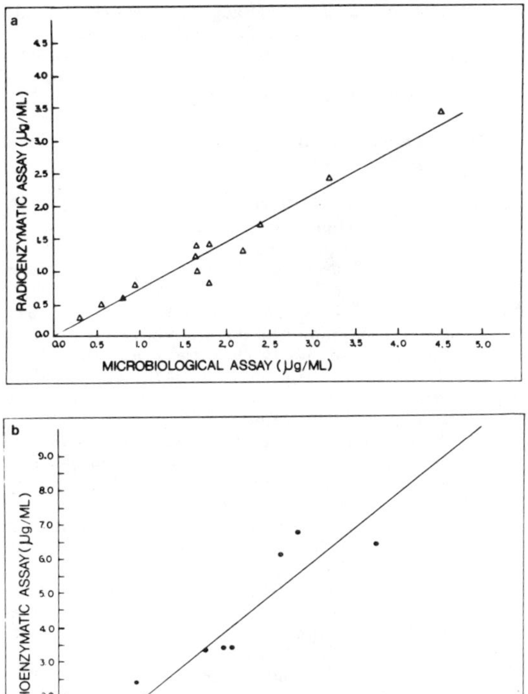

FIG. 3. *(a) Comparison of the tobramycin radioenzymatic assay and the microbiological assay. Patient specimens (13) were analyzed by both the radioenzymatic and microbiological assays, and the correlation coefficient (r) was 0.980. The slope of the linear regression was 0.708 and the intercept was 0.01. (b) Comparison of the tobramycin radioimmunoassay and the radioenzymatic assay. Patient serum specimens (20) were analyzed by both the radioimmunoassay and the radioenzymatic assay. The coefficient of correlation (r) was 0.954, with a linear regression of slope 1.055 and intercept −0.12. (c) Comparison of the tobramycin radioimmunoassay and the microbiological assay. Patient specimens (22) were analyzed by both assays and the correlation coefficient (r) was 0.970, with a linear regression slope equal to 0.774 and intercept 0.138.*

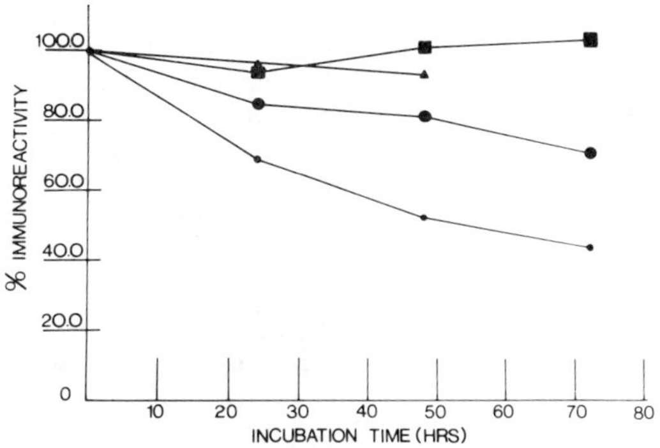

FIG. 4. *Inactivation of tobramycin immunoreactivity. Tobramycin was incubated in normal donor sera at 37°C with varying concentrations of carbenicillin. The percentage of immunoreactivity represents the concentration of tobramycin determined by radioimmunoassay expressed as the percentage of the concentration of tobramycin in the zero-hour sample. Tobramycin (4 μg/ml), ■; tobramycin (4 μg/ml) plus carbenicillin (100 μg/ml), ●; tobramycin (4 μg/ml) plus carbenicillin (200 μg/ml), ●; tobramycin (10 μg/ml) plus carbenicillin (100 μg/ml), ▲.*

scribed herein is more rapid than microbiological assays and is so specific that closely related aminoglycoside antibiotics do not significantly interfere. The tobramycin radioimmunoassay is more sensitive than either the microbial assay or the radioenzymatic assay. This sensitivity is not required for monitoring therapeutic concentrations of tobramycin in the blood but is useful for analyzing microliter blood samples. Another use for the sensitivity of radioimmunoassays is in monitoring pharmacokinetics of tobramycin. Gentamicin, a closely related aminoglycoside, exhibits a biphasic concentration-versus-time curve after bolus intravenous administration. However, the terminal phase of this curve is not evident until serum concentrations fall below the detection capabilities of microbial or radioenzymatic assays (W.J. Jusko, 2nd Annual Pine Mountain Conference on Therapeutic Drug Monitoring, Pine Mountain, Ga., 28 March–1 April 1976). This terminal elimination half-life may have clinical significance since those patients that exhibited oto or renal gentamicin toxicity had longer terminal half-lives than patients who did not develop sequelae. Disadvantages of the tobramycin radioimmunoassay include the necessity for specialized equipment and decreased stability of ^{125}I-labeled tobramycin compared with tritium-labeled acetyl coenzyme A or ^{14}C-labeled adenosine 5′-triphosphate. Thus, the radioimmunoassay for tobramycin offers certain advantages and disadvantages compared with the other two commonly used techniques for tobramycin measurement in blood and other body fluids. Since the correlation coefficient between the three methods was greater than 0.95, the choice of method depends upon personnel and facilities available.

LITERATURE CITED

1. **Black, H. R., and R. S. Griffith.** 1971. Preliminary studies with nebramycin factor 6, p. 314–321. Antimicrob. Agents Chemother. 1970.
2. **Bodey, G. P., and D. Stewart.** 1972. In vitro studies of tobramycin. Antimicrob. Agents Chemother. **2:**109–113.
3. **Bolton, A. E., and W. M. Hunter.** 1973. The labeling of proteins to high specific activity by conjugation to a ^{125}I-containing acylating agent. Biochem. J. **133:**529–539.
4. **Broughton, A., and J. E. Strong.** 1976. Radioimmunoassay of iodinated gentamicin. Clin. Chim. Acta **66:**125–129.
5. **Broughton, A., J. E. Strong, and G. P. Bodey.** 1976. Radioimmunoassay of sisomicin. Antimicrob. Agents Chemother. **9:**247–250.
6. **Dahlgren, J. G., E. T. Anderson, and W. L. Hewitt.** 1975. Gentamicin blood levels: a guide to nephrotoxicity. Antimicrob. Agents Chemother. **8:**58–62.
7. **Goodfriend, T. L., L. Levine, and G. D. Fasman.** 1964. Antibodies to bradykinen and angiotensin: a use of carbodiimides in immunology. Science **144:**1344–1346.
8. **Horikoshi, N., M. Valdivieso, and G. P. Bodey.** 1974. Clinical pharmacology of tobramycin. Am. J. Med. Sci. **266:**453–458.
9. **Hurn, B. A. L., and J. Landon.** 1971. *In* K. E. Kirkham and W. E. Hunter (ed.), Radioimmunoassay methods, p. 121–142, Churchill Livingstone, Edinburgh.
10. **Hyams, P. J., M. S. Simberkoff, and J. J. Rahal.** 1973. In vitro bactericidal effectiveness of four aminoglycoside antibiotics. Antimicrob. Agents Chemother. **2:**214–216.
11. **McLaughlin, J. E., and D. S. Reeves.** 1971. Clinical and laboratory evidence for inactivation of gentamicin. Lancet **1:**261–264.
12. **Noone, P., T. M. C. Parsons, J. R. Pattison, R. C. B. Slack, D. Garfield-Davies, and K. Hughes.** 1974. Experience in monitoring gentamicin therapy during treatment of serious gram-negative sepsis. Br. Med. J. **1:**477–481.
13. **Odell, W. D., G. Abraham, and H. R. Raud.** 1969. Influence of immunization procedures on the titer affinity, and specificity of antisera to glycopeptides. Acta Endocrinol. (Copenhagen) **142**(Suppl.)**:**54–70.
14. **Scatchard, G.** 1949. The attractions of proteins for small molecules and ions. Ann. N.Y. Acad. Sci. **51:**660–672.
15. **Smith, A. L., and D. H. Smith.** 1974. Gentamicin: adenine mononucleotide transferase: partial purification, characterization and use in the clinical quantitation of gentamicin. J. Infect. Dis. **129:**391–401.
16. **Smith, D. H., B. Van Otto, and A. L. Smith.** 1972. A rapid chemical assay for gentamicin. N. Engl. J. Med. **286:**583–586.
17. **Stevens, P., L. S. Young, and W. L. Hewitt.** 1975. Improved acylating radioenzymatic assay of amikacin, tobramicin, and sisomicin in serum. Antimicrob. Agents Chemother. **3:**374–376.
18. **Stevens, P., L. S. Young, and W. L. Hewitt.** 1975. Radioimmunoassay, acylating radio-enzymatic assay, and microbioassay of gentamicin: a comparative study. J. Lab. Clin. Med. **86:**349–359.
19. **Waitz, J. A., C. G. Drube, E. L. Moss, E. M. Oden, J. V. Bailey, G. H. Wagman, and M. J. Weinstein.** 1972. Biological aspects of the interaction between gentamicin and carbenicillin. J. Antibiot. **25:**219–225.

Antimicrobial Agents and Chemotherapy, Oct. 1976, p. 657-663
Vol. 10, No. 4

Comparison of the Antibacterial Activity of Nine Cephalosporins Against *Enterobacteriaceae* and Nonfermentative Gram-Negative Bacilli

LUDO VERBIST
Department of Microbiology, St. Rafaël University Hospital, Leuven, Belgium

Received for publication 19 July 1976

The in vitro antibacterial activity of nine cephalosporins (cephalothin, cephaloridine, cephalexin, cefazolin, cefamandole, cefuroxime, cefatrizine, cefoxitin, and cefazaflur) was determined against 344 strains of *Enterobacteriaceae* and 99 nonfermentative gram-negative bacilli. Cefamandole, cefazaflur, and cefuroxime were the most active cephalosporins against the *Enterobacteriaceae* (with the exception of *Serratia marcescens*). However, cefoxitin was the only cephalosporin that inhibited all 30 *S. marcescens* strains in a concentration of 16 μg/ml and was by far the most active compound against selected cephalothin-resistant strains of *Escherichia coli*, *Klebsiella*, and *Proteus mirabilis*. *Acinetobacter* spp. were inhibited best by cefuroxime, but none of the cephalosporins had appreciable activity against the *Pseudomonas* spp.

Infections with gram-negative bacilli constitute a major problem, especially among hospitalized patients. An increasing number of these organisms are resistant to most of the currently used antibiotics. Newly developed cephalosporins may offer a safe alternative treatment.

A serious drawback to the first clinically available cephalosporins, cephalothin, cephaloridine, cephalexin, and cefazolin, is that they have only slight activity against *Enterobacter* spp., *Providencia* spp., and indole-positive *Proteus* spp., and *Serratia marcescens* and *Pseudomonas aeruginosa* are completely resistant to these antibiotics. However, recently a number of new cephalosporins have been synthesized that seem to have a markedly broader spectrum against gram-negative bacilli. Among the most promising are cefamandole (2, 4, 5, 7, 10), cefuroxime (5, 11, 12), cefatrizine (6, 7, 13, 15), cefoxitin (3, 7-9, 11, 14), and cefazaflur (SKF 59962) (1).

In this study the antibacterial activities of these newer cephalosporins against clinical isolates of 344 *Enterobacteriaceae* and 99 nonfermentative gram-negative bacilli were compared with each other and with that of the older cephalosporins.

MATERIALS AND METHODS

Clinical isolates of *Enterobacteriaceae* and nonfermentative gram-negative bacilli were collected during a 2-month period in St. Raphaël, the teaching hospital of the University of Leuven. After identification by standard criteria the following numbers of strains were selected for study: 60 *Escherichia coli*, 55 *Klebsiella pneumoniae*, 16 *Klebsiella oxytoca*, 56 *Enterobacter* spp., 15 *Citrobacter freundii*, 10 *Citrobacter diversus*, 62 *Proteus mirabilis*, 30 *Proteus vulgaris*, 14 *Proteus morganii*, 11 *Proteus rettgeri*, 15 *Providencia* spp., 30 *S. marcescens*, 25 *Acinetobacter* spp., 67 *P. aeruginosa*, and 7 *Pseudomonas* spp. The susceptibility of the strains was determined by an agar dilution technique. Overnight cultures in Trypticase soy broth were diluted in sterile Trypticase soy broth and inoculated with an automatic multipoint inoculator (16) to deliver an inoculum of 10^4 to 10^5 colony-forming units.

Serial twofold dilutions of the cephalosporins were prepared in sterile distilled water. After the addition of one part of each dilution to nine parts of melted and cooled Diagnostic Sensitivity Test agar (DST Oxoid), the final concentration in the petri dishes ranged from 128 to 0.25 μg/ml. The plates were used on the day of preparation or within 24 h. Pure drugs were obtained from the manufacturers: cephalothin, cephaloridine, cefazolin, cephalexin, and cefamandole from Eli Lilly & Co.; cefuroxime from Glaxo; cefatrizine from Bristol Laboratories; cefoxitin from Merck, Sharp and Dohme; and cefazaflur (SKF 59962) from RIT (Belgium).

Control drug-free plates were similarly inoculated. For *Proteus* strains, *p*-nitrophenyl-β-D-glucoside in a final concentration of 50 μg/ml was added to the antibiotic plates and to control plates to avoid swarming. After incubation at 37°C for 18 h, the minimal inhibitory concentration (MIC) was recorded as the lowest concentration of antibiotic that completely inhibited growth; the presence of three or less colonies was disregarded.

Clinical susceptibility to an antibiotic was arbitrarily defined as inhibition of strains at or below half the peak levels of antibiotics achieved after the usual dose and way of administration in clinical use or in studies with volunteers. The following MICs were considered as limits of susceptibility: cephalothin, 8 μg/ml; cephaloridine, 16 μg/ml; cephalexin, 16 μg/ml; cefazolin, 16 μg/ml; cefamandole, 16 μg/ml; cefuroxime, 16 μg/ml; cefatrizine, 8 μg/ml; cefoxitin, 16 μg/ml; and cefazaflur, 16 μg/ml. For the calculation of the geometric means of inhibition, strains resistant to 128 μg/ml were considered as having an MIC of 256 μg/ml.

RESULTS

The percentage of strains susceptible to the different cephalosporins, according to the criteria defined above, is summarized in Table 1. The species have been divided into three groups based upon their susceptibility pattern to cephalothin and cephaloridine. Group 1 comprises the species of which the majority of isolates are susceptible to these antibiotics, namely, *Escherichia coli*, *Klebsiella* spp., *P. mirabilis*, and *C. diversus*. Group 2 contains the species with only a minority of isolates susceptible to cephalothin and cephaloridine, namely, *Enterobacter* spp., indole-positive *Proteus* spp., *Providencia* spp., *Acinetobacter* spp., and *C. freundii*. Group 3 includes *Pseudomonas* spp. and *S. marcescens*, which are uniformly and highly resistant to these drugs.

In group 1 there were only minor differences in the percentage of susceptibility to the different cephalosporins at the critical concentrations. Cefoxitin inhibited 99.5% of the strains at 16 μg/ml. Most other cephalosporins inhibited from 98.0 to 92.6% of the isolates, except cephaloridine (85.2%) and cephalothin (78.8%). The species of group 2 were clearly more susceptible to the newer cephalosporins than to cephalothin, cephaloridine, cephalexin, and cefazolin. The highest percentages of susceptibility were found toward cefamandole (83.1%), cefuroxime (74.7%), and cefazaflur (67.1%). Cefoxitin inhibited 55.4% of the strains and cefatrizine (42.2%) inhibited a percentage still substantially higher than that of the older cephalosporins (from 10.8 to 31.9%). Cefoxitin had a low score against *Enterobacter* spp. (18% susceptible) and against *C. freundii* (20%), but was the most active compound against the indole-positive *Proteus* and *Providencia* spp.

Cefazaflur and cefatrizine were only moderately active against the *Acinetobacter* spp. The *Pseudomonas* strains remained resistant to the newer cephalosporins. In contrast all 30 isolates of *S. marcescens* were susceptible to 16 μg of cefoxitin per ml, and 13 isolates were also susceptible to 16 μg of cefamandole per ml. A total

TABLE 1. *Susceptibility of gram-negative bacilli to different cephalosporins*

Species	No. tested	% of strains inhibited at an MIC (μg/ml) of at least:								
		8 (CLT[a])	16 (CLD)	16 (CLX)	16 (CZL)	16 (CMD)	16 (CFU)	8 (CTZ)	16 (CFO)	16 (CZF)
Group 1										
E. coli	60	73	90	93	98	100	95	90	98	92
K. pneumoniae	55	69	78	100	100	98	100	95	100	100
K. oxytoca	16	87	81	94	87	94	94	87	100	93
C. diversus	10	70	80	90	90	90	90	90	100	80
P. mirabilis	62	92	89	92	95	98	97	92	100	97
Total	203	78.8	85.2	94.6	96.6	98.0	96.6	92.6	99.5	96.6
Group 2										
Enterobacter spp.	56	11	16	25	37	95	86	54	18	74
C. freundii	15	7	7	7	47	80	93	53	20	80
P. vulgaris	30	10	10	37	23	77	43	37	100	80
P. rettgeri	11	18	27	27	27	91	55	36	64	55
P. morganii	14	0	7	7	7	100	86	64	100	50
Providencia spp.	15	13	13	33	53	100	100	47	100	93
Acinetobacter spp.	25	16	24	24	24	44	64	24	52	25
Total	166	10.8	15.1	24.7	31.9	83.1	74.7	45.2	55.4	67.1
Group 3										
S. marcescens	30	0	0	0	0	43	3	0	100	3
P. aeruginosa	67	0	0	0	0	0	0	0	0	0
Pseudomonas spp.	7	0	0	0	0	0	0	0	0	0

[a] CLT, Cephalothin; CLD, cephaloridine; CLX, cephalexin; CZL, cefazolin; CMD, cefamandole; CFU, cefuroxime; CTZ, cefatrizine; CFO, cefoxitin; CZF, cefazaflur.

of 18 of the 30 *S. marcescens* isolates were resistant to 100 μg of carbenicillin per ml. Cefamandole inhibited 10 of the 12 strains susceptible to carbenicillin, but only 3 of the 18 strains resistant to carbenicillin.

The distribution of the susceptibility to the different cephalosporins, expressed as the cumulative percentage of strains inhibited at increasing concentrations, is shown in Tables 2 and 3. Table 2 summarizes the susceptibility pattern of *E. coli*, *Klebsiella*, *P. mirabilis*, *Enterobacter* spp., and the indole-positive *Proteus* and *Providencia* spp. Cefamandole and cefazaflur inhibited a large percentage of the *E. coli*, *Klebsiella*, and *P. mirabilis* strains already at 0.25 and 0.5 μg/ml, but the remaining isolates were inhibited over a wide range of MIC values. Cefoxitin, in contrast, inhibited the strains from a concentration of 1 μg/ml, but generally over a shorter range of MIC values. Cefamandole and to a lesser extent cefazaflur also inhibited part of the strains of the *Enterobacter* spp. and the indole-positive *Proteus* spp. and *Providencia* spp. at the lowest concentrations.

Cefuroxime was the most active cephalosporin against the *Acinetobacter* spp., followed by cefoxitin and cefamandole (Table 3).

Cefoxitin was clearly the most active compound against *S. marcescens*, and cefamandole was active in part of these strains. However, against the *Pseudomonas* spp. there was scarcely any activity of the cephalosporins. Table 4 shows the geometric means of the MIC values of the different cephalosporins. The newer cephalosporins had clearly lower mean MICs than did the older ones. Against the species of group 1, the lowest mean MICs were obtained with cefamandole (0.8 μg/ml), cefazaflur (0.9 μg/ml), and cefuroxime (1.5 μg/ml). Against the species of group 2, the same cephalosporins had the lowest mean MIC values: cefamandole, 3.1 μg/ml; cefuroxime, 7.8 μg/ml; and cefazaflur, 10.1 μg/ml. Cefoxitin took only the fourth place as a whole (14.1 μg/ml) due to its weaker activity against *Enterobacter* spp. and *C. freundii*. However, against the indole-positive *Proteus* spp. and the *Providencia* spp., cefoxitin was the second best, with a mean MIC of 3.1 μg/ml, cefamandole being most effective with a mean MIC of 2.3 μg/ml. The activity of cefoxitin against *S. marcescens*, with a mean MIC of 10.4 μg/ml, was similar to the activity of this antibiotic against the species of group 2 (namely, 10.1 μg/ml). Since the activity of all cephalosporins was tested simultaneously on the same inoculum of each species, a direct comparison between the MICs of each cephalosporin and the MIC of cephalothin as a reference was possible for each isolate. Therefore, the linear regression lines of the log MICs between each cephalosporin and cephalothin were calculated for these species, whereby more than half of the isolates were at least susceptible to 128 μg of cephalothin per ml (resistance to 128 μg/ml was considered as susceptibility to 256 μg/ml for convenience in the calculations). In the other species, with more than half of the strains resistant to 128 μg of cephalothin per ml, the lack of an exact end point of inhibition made the calculation of regression lines less valuable.

Table 5 shows the correlation coefficients for *E. coli*, *Klebsiella* spp., *P. mirabilis*, *Enterobacter* spp., *C. freundii*, *P. vulgaris*, and *Providencia* spp. between the log MICs of each cephalosporin and cephalothin. A perfect correlation (coefficient $r = 1.0$) could not be expected. Therefore, the statistical difference was calculated between the observed r values and a correlation coefficient of at least 0.90.

The correlation coefficients of cephaloridine, cefazolin, cephalexin (with the exception of the *Klebsiella* spp.), and cefatrizine (except the *Enterobacter* spp.) toward cephalothin were not statistically different from $r = 0.90$. This means that higher or lower MIC values with one of these cephalosporins corresponded very well with higher or lower MICs with cephalothin.

In other words, isolates resistant to cephalothin were as a rule less susceptible or even resistant to these other cephalosporins. In contrast, especially cefoxitin and to a lesser extent cefuroxime had very poor correlation coefficients with cephalothin. Cefamandole took a place in between, and cefazaflur tended rather to a parallel susceptibility with cephalothin.

Table 6 shows the geometric mean MICs of the different cephalosporins according to the susceptibility of the isolates to cephalothin at a concentration of 16 μg/ml. The ratio between the geometric mean MIC of the susceptible isolates and of the cephalothin-resistant isolates reflects the degree of cross-resistance or cross-susceptibility with cephalothin. This ratio was 1:26 for cephalothin in the species of group 1 (*E. coli*, *Klebsiella* spp., and *P. mirabilis*). The ratios for cefazolin, cephaloridine, cefamandole, cefatrizine, and cefazaflur were very similar and varied from 1:15 to 1:28. In the species of group 2 (*Enterobacter*, *C. freundii*, indole-positive *Proteus*, *Providencia*, and *Acinetobacter*) the ratio between the geometric mean MIC of susceptible and resistant isolates was 1:15 for cephalothin and between 1:8 and 1:19 for cephalexin, cefazaflur, cephaloridine, cefatrizine, and cefazolin. The susceptibility to cefoxitin

TABLE 2. *Activity of different cephalosporins against E. coli, Klebsiella spp., P. mirabilis, Enterobacter spp., and indole-positive Proteus and Providencia spp.*

Determination	% of strains inhibited at an MIC (μg/ml) of:										
	0.25	0.5	1	2	4	8	16	32	64	128	>128
60 *E. coli*											
Cephalothin				3	45	73	90	90	93	93	100
Cephaloridine				58	70	83	90	92	97	100	
Cephalexin					48	85	93	93	93	93	100
Cefazolin			63	82	90	98	98	98	98	100	
Cefamandole	40	67	68	83	92	95	100				
Cefuroxime			5	65	88	93	95	100			
Cefatrizine		8	52	75	85	90	93	93	98	98	100
Cefoxitin			5	47	90	95	98	98	100		
Cefazaflur	35	61	78	86	88	92	92	94	98	100	
71 *Klebsiella* spp.											
Cephalothin			18	49	61	73	89	96	99	99	100
Cephaloridine				38	61	68	79	90	99	99	100
Cephalexin				17	85	99	99	99	100		
Cefazolin			48	59	75	93	97	99	99	99	100
Cefamandole	37	52	59	68	79	92	97	99	99	99	100
Cefuroxime		4	63	92	96	97	99	99	99	99	100
Cefatrizine		25	58	66	76	93	94	99	99	99	100
Cefoxitin			34	83	94	99	100				
Cefazaflur	43	62	70	75	90	95	98	98	98	100	
62 *P. mirabilis*											
Cephalothin			35	85	90	92	92	95	97	98	100
Cephaloridine			6	47	85	85	89	92	92	95	100
Cephalexin			2	15	65	90	92	97	97	98	100
Cefazolin			13	79	90	94	95	97	100		
Cefamandole	58	85	89	92	92	97	98	100			
Cefuroxime	18	77	92	92	95	97	97	97	97	97	100
Cefatrizine		15	85	90	92	92	95	95	95	95	100
Cefoxitin		2	61	97	100						
Cefazaflur	11	44	84	89	90	92	97	97	98	100	
56 *Enterobacter* spp.											
Cephalothin					4	11	25	32	45	54	100
Cephaloridine					5	14	16	21	27	30	100
Cephalexin					7	12	25	50	54	75	100
Cefazolin			4	16	20	21	37	43	50	57	100
Cefamandole	7	16	57	66	86	91	95	95	100		
Cefuroxime			2	18	54	77	86	89	98	100	
Cefatrizine			4	18	45	54	62	68	87	93	100
Cefoxitin				2	11	16	18	21	50	71	100
Cefazaflur		7	24	34	49	62	74	84	93	98	100
70 Indole-positive *Proteus* and *Providencia* spp.											
Cephalothin		3	3	4	6	10	14	23	36	37	100
Cephaloridine		3	3	6	6	7	13	16	23	66	100
Cephalexin				4	6	10	29	41	59	84	100
Cefazolin		6	7	10	10	16	27	44	61	91	100
Cefamandole	13	29	44	49	60	86	89	97	99	99	100
Cefuroxime	6	7	19	33	37	53	66	76	96	99	100
Cefatrizine		4	7	23	24	44	51	71	94	99	100
Cefoxitin		4	19	64	70	93	94	96	96	100	
Cefazaflur	4	11	19	34	41	53	73	84	90	97	100

TABLE 3. *Activity of different cephalosporins against Acinetobacter spp., S. marcescens, and Pseudomonas spp.*

Determination	% of strains inhibited at an MIC (μg/ml) of:								
	1	2	4	8	16	32	64	128	>128
25 *Acinetobacter*									
Cephalothin				16	20	24	24	40	100
Cephaloridine		16	20	24	24	40	52	64	100
Cephalexin			20	24	24	28	36	48	100
Cefazolin				20	24	28	36	52	100
Cefamandole		12	24	32	44	76	84	92	100
Cefuroxime	8	24	36	44	64	80	84	96	100
Cefatrizine	8	24	24	24	28	36	68	80	100
Cefoxitin		12	32	36	52	80	80	92	100
Cefazaflur			4	13	25	29	42	63	100
30 *S. marcescens*									
Cephalothin									100
Cephaloridine									100
Cephalexin						3	3	7	100
Cefazolin									100
Cefamandole	3	10	10	17	43	73	90	93	100
Cefuroxime				3	3	23	53	90	100
Cefatrizine						3	3	13	100
Cefoxitin	3	7	13	37	100				
Cefazaflur					3	3	7	10	100
74 *Pseudomonas* spp.									
Cephalothin									100
Cephaloridine						3	4	4	100
Cephalexin									100
Cefazolin									100
Cefamandole						1	1	3	100
Cefuroxime					3	4	4	8	100
Cefatrizine									100
Cefoxitin						1	1	12	100
Cefazaflur									100

was by far the most independent from resistance to cephalothin and was of an equal degree in the species of group 1 (ratio of 1:3) and those of group 2 (ratio of 1:2). Cefamandole showed a definite lowered activity against cephalothin-resistant isolates of the group 1 species (ratio of 1:25), but much less against those of group 2 (ratio of 1:4). Susceptibility to cefuroxime was relatively independent of resistance to cephalothin. This was somewhat more apparent among the species of group 2 (ratio of 1:5) than among those of group 1 (ratio of 1:11).

DISCUSSION

The comparative value of the nine cephalosporins simultaneously tested in vitro against the same clinical isolates of gram-negative bacilli may be evaluated according to two different criteria. A first criterion is based on the percentage of strains that have MIC values above a critical level that is achievable in vivo after the administration of the usual dose by the usual route of administration and above which the possibility of a therapeutic success becomes highly improbable. A second criterion is based on the geometric mean MIC of the different cephalosporins for a species or a group of species. It takes into account the entire range of individual MIC values from the very susceptible to the very resistant isolate within a species, and it accentuates more the therapeutic margin between the critical inhibition concentration and the mean MIC of the species or group of species.

With regard to the first criterion, the differences between the cephalosporins in the percentage of resistant isolates were rather small in the species of group 1, except for cephaloridine and cephalothin, but they were more pronounced in the species of group 2. As a whole cefamandole inhibited the highest number of isolates at the critical level, followed in decreasing order by cefazaflur < cefuroxime < cefoxitin < cefatrizine < cefazolin < cephalexin < cephaloridine < cephalothin.

TABLE 4. *Geometric mean MICs of different cephalosporins*

Species	No. tested	Geometric mean MIC (μg/ml) of:								
		CLT[a]	CLD	CLX	CZL	CMD	CFU	CTZ	CFO	CZF
Group 1										
E. coli	60	8.7	4.3	7.6	1.7	0.7	2.9	2.1	3.2	0.8
K. pneumoniae	55	4.6	6.6	4.3	2.2	1.5	1.3	1.9	2.1	0.8
K. oxytoca	16	4.2	5.7	3.5	4.2	1.2	1.9	1.9	1.2	0.7
C. diversus	10	7.5	6.5	6.5	3.5	1.5	3.5	2.6	2.5	1.5
P. mirabilis	62	2.2	4.2	5.5	2.5	0.5	0.7	1.2	1.3	1.0
Total	203	4.5	5.0	5.5	2.3	0.8	1.5	1.7	2.0	0.9
Group 2										
Enterobacter spp.	56	79.0	115.9	52.5	45.8	1.8	6.8	13.0	68.9	6.7
C. freundii	15	40.3	73.5	48.5	25.4	2.4	3.8	12.1	30.6	6.1
P. vulgaris	30	84.4	99.3	45.2	44.2	8.2	18.8	15.6	2.1	5.8
P. rettgeri	11	56.4	53.0	60.1	38.6	2.3	5.8	13.2	9.1	9.1
P. morganii	14	210.0	190.2	115.9	95.1	0.7	11.9	11.3	6.9	19.5
Providencia spp.	15	55.7	73.5	26.6	14.1	1.0	1.7	16.0	1.4	4.8
Acinetobacter spp.	25	108.4	48.5	73.5	84.4	20.5	12.5	33.8	17.9	76.1
Total	166	81.2	90.1	54.2	43.8	3.1	7.8	15.5	14.1	10.1
Group 3										
S. marcescens	30	>256	>256	233.4	>256	24.3	77.0	222.9	10.4	217.8
P. aeruginosa	67	>256	243.1	>256	>256	253.4	226.1	>256	240.9	>256
Pseudomonas spp.	7	>256	156.0	>256	>256	190.2	210.0	>256	128.0	>256

[a] Abbreviations are the same as those given in the footnote to Table 1.

TABLE 5. *Correlation coefficients of the linear regression between the log MICs of the different cephalosporins and the log MICs of cephalothin*

Species	No. tested	Correlation coefficients (r) with:							
		CLD[a]	CLX	CZL	CMD	CFU	CTZ	CFO	CZF
E. coli	60	0.87	0.88	0.89	0.79[b]	0.79[b]	0.95	0.70[b]	0.87
Klebsiella spp.	71	0.92	0.72[b]	0.90	0.91	0.69[b]	0.92	0.50[b]	0.92
P. mirabilis	62	0.92	0.83	0.92	0.93	0.88	0.93	0.42[b]	0.95
Enterobacter spp.	56		0.87	0.88	0.53[b]	0.44[b]	0.64[b]	0.18[b]	0.62[b]
C. freundii	15	0.77	0.84	0.91	0.73	0.49[b]	0.76	0.34[b]	0.84
P. vulgaris	30	0.90	0.83	0.87	0.43[b]	0.67[b]	0.82	0.14[b]	0.64[b]
Providencia spp.	15	0.83	0.92	0.97	0.10[b]	0.19[b]	0.92	0.02[b]	0.66

[a] Abbreviations are the same as those given in the footnote to Table 1.

[b] Correlation coefficient is statistically different from $r = 0.90$ at $P < 0.005$.

TABLE 6. *Geometric mean MIC of the different cephalosporins according to the susceptibility of group 1 and group 2 microbial species to cephalothin*

Susceptibility to 16 μg of cephalothin per ml	No.	Geometric mean MIC (μg/ml) of:								
		CLT[a]	CLD	CLX	CZL	CMD	CFU	CTZ	CFO	CZF
Species of group 1	203									
Susceptible	183	3.26	3.64	4.52	1.75	0.60	1.14	1.25	1.77	0.62
Resistant	20	84.44	90.50	31.99	25.99	14.92	12.55	31.99	5.27	17.21
Ratio		1:26	1:25	1:7	1:15	1:25	1:11	1:25	1:3	1:28
Species of group 2	166									
Susceptible	29	8.59	13.86	9.68	3.90	1.07	2.14	2.20	7.44	1.73
Resistant	137	130.60	133.94	77.95	73.08	3.89	10.23	23.48	16.14	14.65
Ratio		1:15	1:10	1:8	1:19	1:4	1:5	1:11	1:2	1:8

[a] Abbreviations are the same as those given in the footnote to Table 1.

With regard to the second criterion and ranged in the order of increasing geometric mean MICs, the classification was: cefamandole < cefazaflur and cefuroxime < cefatrizine and cefoxitin < cefazolin < cephalexin, cephalothin, and cephaloridine.

Cefoxitin is known to be less active against *Enterobacter* spp. than against the other *Enterobacteriaceae*, but one of the most active cephalosporins against *S. marcescens* (3, 7, 8, 14). In the present study an even 100% of the 30 isolates of *S. marcescens* were found susceptible to 16 μg of cefoxitin per ml. Furthermore, cefoxitin is a cephamycin structurally different from the other cephalosporins.

This chemical difference seems to be very important, as reflected by its lack of correlation with cephalothin susceptibility (cf. Table 5) and its high activity against cephalothin-resistant isolates in the species of group 1 that are as a group susceptible to the older cephalosporins. From the in vitro results of this study it may be concluded that the newer generation of cephalosporins has several advantages over the older ones.

First, they present a broader spectrum against gram-negative bacilli, extending the activity to indole-positive *Proteus* spp., *Providencia* spp., *Enterobacter* spp., and *C. freundii*. This is true especially for cefamandole, cefazaflur, cefuroxime, and cefoxitin (with the exception of *Enterobacter* spp. and *C. freundii*) but less for cefatrizine. Furthermore they inhibit gram-negative bacilli at appreciable lower MIC values, preserving activity against strains that have a low degree of resistance to the older cephalosporins. Finally, cefoxitin seems to open a new and independent class of cephalosporins that preserves largely its activity against isolates highly resistant to the other cephalosporins and that will be appreciated as a safe treatment for infection with *S. marcescens*.

ACKNOWLEDGMENT

The technical assistance of Jos Vandeven is gratefully acknowledged.

LITERATURE CITED

1. **Actor, P., J. V. Uri, J. R. Guarini, I. Zajac, L. Phillips, C. S. Sachs, R. M. Demarinis, J. R. E. Hoover, and J. A. Weisbach.** 1975. A new parenteral cephalosporin. SKF 59962: in vitro and in vivo antibacterial activity and serum levels in experimental animals. J. Antibiot. 28:471–476.
2. **Bodey, G. P., and S. Weaver.** 1976. In vitro studies of cefamandole. Antimicrob. Agents Chemother. 9:452–457.
3. **Brumfitt, W., J. Kosmidis, J. M. T. Hamilton-Miller, and J. N. G. Gilchrist.** 1974. Cefoxitin and cephalothin: antimicrobial activity, human pharmacokinetics, and toxicology. Antimicrob. Agents Chemother. 6:290–299.
4. **Eykyn, S., C. Jenkins, A. King, and I. Phillips.** 1973. Antibacterial activity of cefamandole, a new cephalosporin antibiotic compared with that of cepahloridine, cephalothin, and cephalexin. Antimicrob. Agents Chemother. 3:657–661.
5. **Eykyn, S., C. Jenkins, A. King, and I. Phillips.** 1976. Antibacterial activity of cefuroxime, a new cephalosporin antibiotic, compared with that of cephaloridine, cephalothin, and cefamandole. Antimicrob. Agents Chemother. 9:690–695.
6. **Leitner, F., R. E. Buck, M. Misiek, T. A. Pursiano, and E. Price.** 1975. BL-S 640, a cephalosporin with a broad spectrum of antibacterial activity: properties in vitro. Antimicrob. Agents Chemother. 7:298–305.
7. **Lewis, R. P., R. D. Meyer, and L. L. Kraus.** 1976. Antibacterial activity of selected beta-lactam and aminoglycoside antibiotics against cephalothin-resistant *Enterobacteriaceae*. Antimicrob. Agents Chemother. 9:780–786.
8. **Moellering, R. C., M. Dray, and L. J. Kunz.** 1974. Susceptibility of bacteria to cefoxitin and cephalothin. Antimicrob. Agents Chemother. 6:320–323.
9. **Neu, H. C.** 1974. Cefoxitin, a semisynthetic cephamycin antibiotic antibacterial spectrum and resistance to hydrolysis by gram-negative beta-lactamases. Antimicrob. Agents Chemother. 6:170–176.
10. **Neu, H. C.** 1974. Cefamandole, a cephalosporin antibiotic with an unusually wide spectrum of activity. Antimicrob. Agents Chemother. 6:177–182.
11. **Norrby, R., J. E. Brorsson, and S. Seeberg.** 1976. Comparative study of the in vitro antibacterial activity of cefoxitin, cefuroxime, and cephaloridine. Antimicrob. Agents Chemother. 9:506–510.
12. **O'Callaghan, C. H., R. B. Sykes, A. Griffiths, and J. E. Thornton.** 1976. Cefuroxime, a new cephalosporin antibiotic: activity in vitro. Antimicrob. Agents Chemother. 9:511–519.
13. **Overturf, G. D., R. L. Ressler, P. B. Marengo, and J. Wilkins.** 1975. In vitro evaluation of BL-S640, a new oral cephalosporin antibiotic. Antimicrob. Agents Chemother. 8:305–310.
14. **Wallick, H., and D. Hendlin.** 1974. Cefoxitin, a semisynthetic cephamycin antibiotic: susceptibility studies. Antimicrob. Agents Chemother. 5:25–32.
15. **Watanakunakorn, C., T. Bannister, and C. Glotzbecker.** 1975. Susceptibility of clinical isolates of *Enterobacteriaceae* to BL-S640, a new oral cephalosporin. Antimicrob. Agents Chemother. 7:381–385.
16. **Watt, P. R., L. Jeffries, and S. A. Price.** 1966. An automatic multipoint inoculator for Petri-dishes, p. 125–128. *In* B. M. Gibbs and F. A. Skinner (ed.), Identification methods for microbiologists, part A. Academic Press Inc., London.

ANTIMICROBIAL AGENTS AND CHEMOTHERAPY, Oct. 1976, p. 664-667
Vol. 10, No. 4
Printed in U.S.A.

Enzymatic Adenylylation by Aminoglycoside 4′-Adenylyltransferase and 2″-Adenylyltransferase as a Means of Determining Concentrations of Aminoglycoside Antibiotics in Serum

P. SANTANAM AND F. H. KAYSER*

Institute of Medical Microbiology, University of Zurich, CH-8028, Zurich, Switzerland

Received for publication 3 May 1976

A fast and accurate enzymatic estimation of the concentration of aminoglycoside antiobiotics in serum is given by aminoglycoside 4′-adenylyltransferase (synonym: tobramycin adenylyltransferase), a new enzyme recently found in tobramycin-resistant staphylococci (P. Santanam and F. H. Kayser, J. Infect. Dis. [Suppl.], in press). This enzyme is useful in assaying the kanamycins, the butirosins, amikacin, ribostamycin and, if required, the neomycins, tobramycin, and paromomycin. In combination with the assay using aminoglycoside 2″-adenylyltransferase (synonym: gentamicin adenylyltransferase) to determine the level of gentamicin, sisomicin, and tobramycin, a convenient method to estimate a wide range of aminoglycoside antibiotics in patients' sera is described.

Enzymatic adenylylation and acetylation have been used to estimate the concentration of aminoglycoside antibiotics in sera of patients undergoing treatment with these drugs (3, 5, 7–9, 14, 15, 17). The enzymatic assays are known to be fast and accurate and are valuable in the assessment for maintaining an effective and nontoxic serum level of the drugs. Aminoglycoside 3-*N*-acetyltransferase [AAC(3)] is used in assaying the gentamicin C antibiotics and sisomicin (18). Aminoglycoside 2″-adenylyltransferase [AAD(2″)] is used in assaying the C gentamicins, the kanamycins, sisomicin, and tobramycin (7, 9, 15). The aminoglycoside 6′-*N*-acetyltransferase [AAC(6′)], because of its broad substrate spectrum, is useful in assaying a wide range of aminoglycoside antibiotics (3, 8, 17). As an alternative to AAC(6′), we propose to use two adenylylating enzymes. With aminoglycoside 4′-adenylyltransferase [AAD(4′)], serum levels of the kanamycins, the butirosins, amikacin, ribostamycin, and, if required, the neomycins and paromomycin can be determined. With AAD(2″), the gentamicin C antibiotics, sisomicin, and tobramycin can be assayed.

MATERIALS AND METHODS

Antibiotics and chemicals. Tobramycin was supplied by Eli Lilly and Co. (Indianapolis, Ind.); the kanamycins, butirosins, and amikacin were supplied by Bristol laboratories (Syracuse, N.Y.); the neomycins were provided by Upjohn Co. (Kalamazoo, Mich.); paromomycin was supplied by Parke, Davis and Co. (Detroit, Mich.); the gentamicins and sisomicin were supplied by Schering Corp. (Bloomfield, N.J.).

Commercial samples of gentamicin C complex, kanamycin, and neomycin were provided by the hospital pharmacy of the University of Zurich.

Radioactive chemicals were supplied by the Radiochemical Centre (Amersham, England). Dithiothreitol and adenosine triphosphate (ATP) were supplied by Calbiochem (Los Angeles, Calif.). All other inorganic salts of analytical grade were supplied by E. Merck AG (Darmstadt, Germany).

Production of enzymes. AAD(4′) was extracted by the osmotic shock method from *Staphylococcus epidermidis* 109 (P. Santanam and F. H. Kayser, J. Infect. Dis. [Suppl.], in press). The procedure was slightly modified by using 20% sucrose in tris(hydroxymethyl)aminomethane (Tris)-hydrochloride buffer (pH 7.3) that contained 0.006 instead of 0.003 M ethylenediaminetetraacetic acid for suspending the cells before the shock step. The enzymatic extract obtained by osmotic shock is stable for several hours at room temperature, for 1 week at 4°C, and for several months at −40°C (Santanam and Kayser, in press). AAD(2″) was obtained by osmotic shock treatment of *Escherichea coli* W677/HJR66 as described elsewhere (7, 12).

Enzymatic assays. The methods used were described by Benveniste, Davies, and their associates (2, 6). Serum samples were kept for 5 min in a water bath at 60°C before use to inactivate any trace of adenosine triphosphatase.

To measure adenylylation of drugs by AAD(4′), the reaction mixture consisted of 1.5 μmol of Tris-hydrochloride buffer, 1 μmol of $MgCl_2$, 55 nmol of dithiothreitol, 20 nmol of [2-^{3}H]ATP (specific activity, 60 μCi/μmol), 10 μl of serum, and 25 μl of osmotic shockate, in a total volume of 60 μl. The pH of the buffer was adjusted to 8.3, found to be optimum for assaying the neomycins and paromomycin, and to 7.5, found to be optimum for assaying the rest, in the presence of serum. After incubation for 35 min at 35°C, 50-μl samples were pipetted onto 2-cm^2 phosphocellulose paper (Whatman P-81; Balsbone, Maidstone, U.K.), which was washed twice with distilled water, dried at 55°C, and counted for radioactivity in 10 ml of a toluene-based scintillation fluid. Reaction mixtures devoid of either the enzyme or the drug were used as controls for nonspecific binding of [2-^{3}H]ATP. The adenylylation of drugs by AAD(2") was examined by a slight modification of the procedure described by Furger et al. (7). The reaction mixture contained 1.5 μmol of Tris-hydrochloride buffer at pH 8.3, 1.0 μmol of $MgCl_2$, 55 nmol of dithiothreitol, 20 nmol of [2-^{3}H]ATP (specific activity, 60 μCi/μmol), 20 μl of serum containing the drug, and 25 μl of osmotic shockate. After 15 min of incubation at 35°C, 50-μl samples were pipetted onto 2-cm^2 phosphocellulose papers, which were washed, dried, and then counted for radioactivity as described above.

RESULTS

Standard solutions containing 20, 10, 5, and 2.5 μg of laboratory standard samples of amikacin, kanamycin, neomycin, paromomycin, and butirosin per ml were prepared by a twofold dilution in pooled human sera from stocks and assayed by AAD(4'). The degree of adenylylation of these antibiotics was found to be directly proportional to the drug between 2.5 and 20 μg/ml (Fig. 1). The high molar ratio of ATP to the drug (20 nmol of ATP to 0.34 to 0.68 nmol of drug) allowed the estimation of kanamycin, neomycin, and paromomycin also at serum concentrations between 20 and 40 μg/ml. Because of the slow adenylylation of amikacin and butirosin (Santanam and Kayser, in press), however, either the incubation time for assaying these drugs must be doubled or the serum sample must be appropriately diluted. Dilution to concentrations between 2.5 and 20 μg/ml was practical and gave reproducible and accurate results. The incubation time of 35 min at 35°C was necessary for completion of adenylylation in the presence of serum. The drugs, however, are not all adenylylated to the same extent, possibly because the end products differ in their ability to inhibit the enzymatic reaction. On the basis of known drug concentrations in pooled human sera and the concentrations assayed, it is possible to calculate the efficiency of assay (Table 1). The average adenylylation of amikacin, for example, was 96.3%, and the relative standard deviation was 5.5%. Similar data were obtained with the other drugs. Assays of 36 different human serum samples, containing either 5 or 10 μg of amikacin per ml, gave a relative standard deviation of 6% and 4%, respectively, which shows no significant variation between different serum samples.

Standards of commercially available gentamicin complex, tobramycin, and sisomicin were

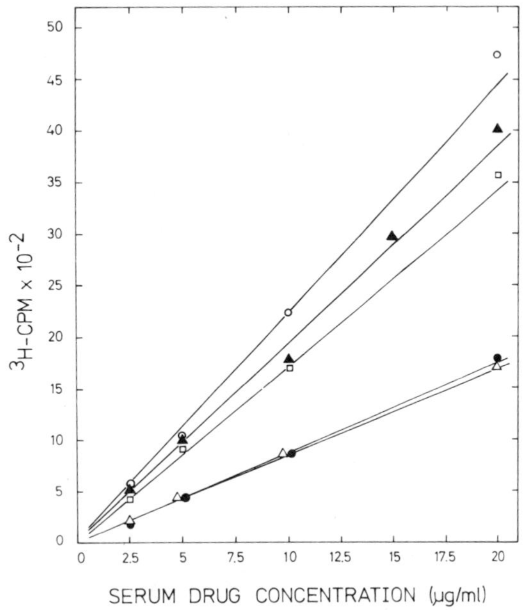

FIG. 1. *Enzymatic adenylylation by aminoglycoside 4'-adenylyltransferase of various aminoglycoside antibiotics in human blood sera (standard curves). Experimental details of the assay are given in the text. Count rates are corrected for background activity. Symbols: (●) amikacin, (□) kanamycin, (△) butirosin, (○) neomycin, (▲) paromomycin.*

TABLE 1. *Efficiency of the assay for amikacin*

Amikacin assayed (μg/ml)	Amt of amikacin in assay tubes (mmol × 10^{-8})	Amt of amikacin determined by enzymatic assay (mmol × 10^{-8})	Adenylylation[a] (%)
3	5.13	4.87	95
3.5	5.98	5.3	88.6
4	6 84	7.35	107.5
4.5	7.69	7.01	91.1
6	10.26	9.58	93.3
7	11.97	12.14	101.4
8	13.68	12.14	88.8
9	15.39	14.8	96.1
12	20.52	20.7	100.8
14	23.94	23.1	96.4
16	27.36	26.3	96.3
18	30.78	30.78	100

[a] The average adenylylation was 96.3%, and the standard deviation was 5.5%.

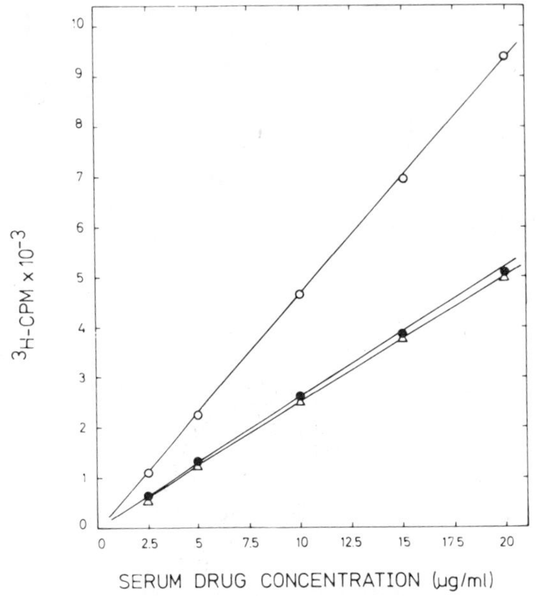

FIG. 2. *Enzymatic adenylylation by aminoglycoside 2'adenylyltransferase of different aminoglycoside antibiotics in human blood sera (standard curves). Experimental details of the assay are given in the text. Count rates are corrected for background activity. Symbols: (●) gentamicin, (△) tobramycin, (○) sisomicin.*

TABLE 2. *Efficiency of the assay for gentamicin*

Gentamicin assayed (µg/ml)	Amt of gentamicin in assay tubes (mmol × 10^{-7})	Amt of gentamicin determined by enzymatic assay (mmol × 10^{-7})	Adenylylation[a] (%)
0.25	0.09	0.08	88.9
0.4	0.15	0.16	106.6
0.7	0.26	0.22	88.0
1.4	0.52	0.44	84.6
2.1	0.77	0.7	91.0
2.8	1.03	0.92	89.3
3.5	1.29	1.24	96.1
4.2	1.55	1.47	94.8
5.6	2.06	2.09	101.4
6.2	2.28	2.39	104.8
6.8	2.51	2.43	96.8
7.5	2.76	2.77	100.3
8.4	3.09	3.06	99.0
10.2	3.75	3.68	98.1
12.4	4.56	4.52	99.1
15.0	5.5	5.32	96.7

[a] The average adenylylation was 96%, and the standard deviation was 6.2%.

prepared from 20-µg/ml stocks and assayed by AAD(2″) as described. The linear relationship between adenylylation and the amount of drug is demonstrated in Fig. 2. Table 2 summarizes efficiency of the assay for gentamicin. The average adenylylation was 96%, and the relative standard deviation was 6.2%.

DISCUSSION

In the last few years, a number of rapid methods have been developed for measuring the concentration of aminoglycoside antibiotics in serum and other body fluids. These methods include microbiological assays (1, 13), radioimmunoassays (4, 10), and enzymatic assays (3, 5, 7–10, 14–17). Each type of assay has its own advantages. Radioimmunoassays and enzymatic assays are highly specific and are useful in assaying aminoglycosides, particularly in the presence of other antibiotics. However, workers having experience with both assay systems prefer enzymatic assays to radioimmunoassays because the reagents are easier to prepare, the experimental protocols are somewhat simpler, and the results are less affected by minor variations in experimental procedures (10).

AAD(2″) was the first enzyme proposed for enzymatic determination of gentamicin (16). This enzyme has been satisfactorily used in our laboratory for more than 3 years. Because of production of new aminoglycoside antibiotics, which are not modified by this enzyme, and because of demands by clinicians to determine in certain patients concentrations of neomycin and paromomycin, the suitability of AAD(4′) was examined. The ability of AAD(4′) to adenylylate the aminoglycoside 4′-OH group and perhaps also the 4″-OH group, because 4′-deoxykanamycin was found to be a substrate but not 4′deoxybutirosin, makes it unique in having a very broad substrate spectrum (Santanam and Kayser, in press). It surpasses AAC(6′) in this respect and eliminates the requirement for [^{14}C]acetyl coenzyme A as a cosubstrate, thus reducing the cost per assay to less than half. It is also more stable at room temperature than AAC(6′) (8), and the activity does not appreciably change during storage at −40°C over a period of at least 2 months (Santanam and Kayser, in press). AAD(2″), on the other hand, adenylylates the three components of commercially available gentamicin, whereas AAC(6′) does not acetylate gentamicin C_1. Since this component is present in varying amounts from batch to batch (professional brochure, Schering Corp., 1974) and since gentamicin C_1 shows a somewhat different pharmacokinetic behavior than the gentamicin complex (11), it would be appropriate to use AAD(2″) for assaying gentamicin.

Thus, AAD(4′) in conjunction with AAD(2″)

is ideally suited to assay, with identical reagents, many of the aminoglycoside antibiotics that are used currently in chemotherapy. Both the enzymes are easily extractable in the form of osmotic shockate, which can be used directly without purification.

LITERATURE CITED

1. **Bennett, J. V., J. L. Brodie, E. J. Benner, and W. M. M. Kirby.** 1966. Simplified, accurate method for antibiotic assay of clinical specimens. Appl. Microbiol. 14:170–177.
2. **Benveniste, R., T. Yamada., and J. Davies.** 1970. Enzymatic adenylylation of streptomycin and spectinomycin by R-factor-resistant *Escherichia coli*. Infect. Immun. 1:109–119.
3. **Broughall, J. M., and S. S. Reeves.** 1975. Properties of the gentamicin acetyltransferase enzyme and application to the assay of aminoglycoside antibiotics. Antimicrob. Agents Chemother. 8:222–223.
4. **Broughton, A., and J. E. Strong.** 1976. Radioimmunoassay of antibiotics and chemotherapeutic agents. Clin. Chem. 22:726–732.
5. **Daignueault, R., M. Gagne, and M. Brazeau.** 1974. A comparison of two methods of gentamicin assay: an enzymatic procedure and an agar diffusion technique. J. Infect. Dis. 130:642–645.
6. **Davies, J., M. Brzezinska, and R. Benveniste.** 1971. R-factors: biochemical mechanisms of resistance to aminoglycoside antibiotics. Ann. N.Y. Acad. Sci. 182:494–499.
7. **Furger, F., A. Russi, and F. H. Kayser.** 1973. Schnellmethoden zur quantitativen Bestimmung von Aminoglykosid-Antibiotika. Schweiz. Med. Wochenschr. 103:779–782.
8. **Haas, M. J., and J. Davies.** 1973. Enzymatic acetylation as a means of determining serum aminoglycoside concentrations. Antimicrob. Agents Chemother. 4:497–499.
9. **Holmes, R. K., and J. P. Sanford.** 1974. Enzymatic assay for gentamicin and related aminoglycoside antibiotics. J. Infect. Dis. 129:519–527.
10. **Minshew, B. H., R. K. Holmes, and C. R. Baxter.** 1975. Comparison of a radioimmunoassay with an enzymatic assay for gentamicin. Antimicrob. Agents Chemother. 7:107–109.
11. **Mosegaard, A., P. G. Welling, and P. O. Madsen.** 1975. Gentamicin and gentamicin C_1 in the treatment of complicated urinary tract infections: comparative study of efficacy, tolerance, and pharmacokinetics. Antimicrob. Agents Chemother. 7:328–332.
12. **Neu, H. C., and L. A. Heppel.** 1965. The release of enzymes from *E. coli* by osmotic shock and during the formation of spheroplasts. J. Biol. Chem. 240:3685–3692.
13. **Noone, P., J. R. Pattison, and D. Samson.** 1971. Simple rapid method for assay of aminoglycoside antibiotics. Lancet ii:16–19.
14. **Shaw, W. V., J. Carter, and J. Sachs.** 1972. Enzymatic assay of gentamicin and kanamycin in body fluids. Clin. Res. 20:83.
15. **Smith, A. L., and D. H. Smith.** 1974. Gentamicin: adenine mononucleotide transferase: partial purification, characterization, and use in the clinical quantitation. J. Infect. Dis. 129:391–401.
16. **Smith, D. H., B. R. Otto, and A. L. Smith.** 1972. A rapid chemical assay for gentamicin. N. Engl. J. Med. 286:583–586.
17. **Stevens, P., L. S. Young, and W. L. Hewitt.** 1975. Improved acetylating radioenzymatic assay of amikacin, tobramycin, and sisomicin in serum. Antimicrob. Agents Chemother. 7:374–376.
18. **Williams, J. W., J. S. Langer, and D. B. Northrop.** 1975. A spectrophotometric assay for gentamicin. J. Antibiot. 28:982–987.

ANTIMICROBIAL AGENTS AND CHEMOTHERAPY, Oct. 1976, p. 668-676 Vol. 10, No. 4

Printed in U.S.A.

Effect of Treatment with Exogenous Interferon, Polyinosinic Acid-Polycytidylic Acid, or Polyinosinic Acid-Polycytidylic Acid-Poly-L-Lysine Complex on Encephalomyocarditis Virus Infections in Mice[1]

GREGG A. OLSEN,* EARL R. KERN, LOWELL A. GLASGOW, AND JAMES C. OVERALL, JR.

Departments of Pediatrics and Microbiology, University of Utah, College of Medicine, Salt Lake City, Utah 84132*

Received for publication 12 April 1976

The effect of treatment with exogenous interferon was compared with two interferon inducers, polyinosinic acid-polycytidylic acid [poly(I:C)] and [poly(I:C)]-poly-L-lysine complex (P-L-L complex), in two model encephalomyocarditis virus infections of mice. Although both inducers stimulated the production of interferon, the peak serum levels induced by P-L-L complex were five- to eightfold greater than those induced with poly(I:C). When encephalomyocarditis virus was inoculated by either the intraperitoneal or the intranasal route, interferon and both of the inducers protected mice against mortality and prolonged the mean day of death when the compounds were given prior to or immediately after viral challenge. In general, treatment with interferon was not as successful as treatment with poly(I:C) or P-L-L complex. In these infections, P-L-L complex appeared to be the most effective agent in that successful treatment resulted when drug therapy was initiated as late as 48 h after virus inoculation. An examination of the effect of treatment on the pathogenesis of the infection indicated that protection was associated with the prevention of viremia and subsequent seeding of target organs, particularly the central nervous system.

Enteroviruses are a frequent cause of human infections and result in a wide spectrum of disease, including nonspecific febrile illness, respiratory infections, aseptic meningitis, encephalitis, myocarditis, or pericarditis (16, 21, 23). The infection of mice with encephalomyocarditis (EMC) virus appears to simulate some human enterovirus infections in that EMC virus is a murine picornavirus, target organs are seeded by viremia, and death results primarily from the involvement of the central nervous system (25). This murine infection, therefore, provides a model for the evaluation of antiviral chemotherapeutic agents that may have potential for use in the treatment of human disease.

Interferon is thought to be an important component of host resistance to viral infections. Results from a number of laboratories have suggested that both interferon (9, 10, 18) and interferon inducers (2-4, 11, 14, 15) may be used successfully in the prevention or treatment of certain viral infections in experimental animals and in humans. Although exogenous interferon has been evaluated in several clinical trials in humans (6, 17, 19, 27), controlled studies in animals have been relatively limited. Because high-titered preparations of mouse interferon have recently become available, we compared the efficacy of interferon and interferon inducers against experimental EMC virus infections in this species. The most common interferon inducer used in murine viral infections, polyinosinic acid-polycytidic acid [poly-(I:C)], stimulates relatively low levels of interferon in humans, presumably because of the rapid hydrolysis that occurs when poly(I:C) is mixed with primate serum (24). A new interferon inducer, a complex of poly(I:C) with poly-L-lysine (P-L-L complex), is 5 to 10 times as resistant to this hydrolysis as poly(I:C) (22) and induces significant levels of interferon in the serum of monkeys under conditions when poly(I:C) does not. The purpose of this study was to compare the therapeutic efficacy of exogenous murine interferon with the two interferon inducers, poly(I:C) and P-L-L complex, in the treatment of two experimental EMC virus infections in mice. The effect of treatment was evaluated by determining the alteration of mortality, mean day of death, and pathogenesis of the infection.

[1] Publication no. 26 from the Cooperative Antiviral Testing Group National Institute of Allergy and Infectious Disease.

MATERIALS AND METHODS

Animals and experimental infections. Seven-week-old mice were obtained from Simonsen Laboratories, Gilroy, Calif. Animals were inoculated by either the intraperitoneal (i.p.) or intranasal route. Mice infected by the i.p. route were given approximately 50 plaque-forming units (PFU) (3 mean lethal doses [LD_{50}]) of EMC virus, which resulted in an 80 to 90% mortality. In the intranasal infection, ether-anesthetized mice were allowed to inhale 0.05 ml of a virus suspension containing approximately 2.7×10^4 PFU (3 LD_{50}), which resulted in a 75 to 85% mortality. All animals were observed for 21 days after virus inoculation.

Virus. The strain of EMC virus used in these studies was a large plaque variant originally obtained from K. K. Takemoto (National Institutes of Health, Bethesda, Md.). Virus pools were prepared by harvesting brains from infected suckling mice and titered 10^7 PFU/ml on L-cell fibroblast cultures. Vesicular stomatitis virus (VSV), Indiana strain, was obtained from the American Type Culture Collection (Rockville, Md.), and stock pools were prepared in primary chicken embryo cells as described previously (25).

Media, cell cultures, virus assays, and interferon assays. The media utilized, the maintenance of mouse L-cell (L-929) fibroblast cultures, and the assay for EMC virus have been described in a previous publication (25). Interferon was assayed by using a plaque reduction method with VSV as the challenge virus as described previously (20). A reference mouse serum interferon preparation was included in each assay.

Interferon and interferon inducers. All compounds being evaluated were provided by the Antiviral Substances Testing Program, National Institute of Allergy and Infectious Diseases, Bethesda, Md. Exogenous interferon was prepared in mouse L-929 cells either by Kurt Paucker at the Medical College of Pennsylvania, Philadelphia, Pa., or by Bionetics Laboratories, Kensington, Md. The interferon prepared by Dr. Paucker was received as a lyophilized powder and stored at −70°C (per his instructions) until diluted for use to an appropriate concentration with phosphate-buffered saline (PBS). Bionetics interferon was received as a frozen liquid at a concentration of 10^6 U/ml and stored at −30°C until use (per manufacturer's recommendation). Poly(I:C), prepared by P-L Biochemicals, Inc., Milwaukee, Wis., had a concentration of 1 mg/ml and was stored at −20°C until use. The P-L-L complex was prepared by H. B. Levy at the National Institute of Allergy and Infectious Diseases. Poly(I:C) (2 mg/ml) was complexed with poly-L-lysine (1.5 mg/ml) in 0.5% carboxymethyl cellulose in saline (22). This solution was stored at 4°C and diluted with an equal volume of PBS at the time of use. All drugs were administered in a 0.1-ml volume by the i.p. route. Virus control animals received 0.1 ml of PBS administered i.p. on the same treatment schedules.

Statistical evaluation. The differences in mortality between animals treated with drug and control animals receiving PBS were evaluated by chi-square analysis. To compare the mean day of death of drug-treated and PBS-treated control animals, the data were evaluated by the use of the Student *t* test. A *P* value of ≤ 0.05 was considered to be significant.

RESULTS

Interferon induction. The levels of interferon in the serum of mice after the injection of 100 μg of either poly(I:C) or P-L-L complex are shown in Table 1. Peak titers occurred 9 h after injection with both compounds. The response induced by P-L-L complex was approximately five times higher and lasted 24 h longer than that induced by poly(I:C).

Interferon induction after repeated injections. The levels of interferon in the serum of mice after multiple injections of 100 μg of either poly(I:C) or P-L-L complex administered according to the treatment schedules utilized in this series of experiments are shown in Table 2. Poly(I:C) induced a lower, but still substantial, level of serum interferon after the second injection, but with subsequent injections hyporeactivity of the interferon response occurred. In contrast, although P-L-L complex induced a greater serum interferon response than did poly(I:C) after the first injection, the second injection failed to induce more than 900 to 1,200 U of interferon per ml. The data in Table 2 demonstrate that the kinetics of the interferon response are not changed with multiple doses of either inducer.

Effect of treatment on mortality of mice inoculated i.p. with EMC virus. The effect of treatment with exogenous interferon, poly(I:C), or P-L-L complex on the mortality and mean day of death of mice infected i.p. with EMC virus is shown in Table 3. The results in the treated groups in separate experiments were compared with the results in control groups pooled from all experiments. The virus-infected control animals, treated with PBS i.p. twice

TABLE 1. *Titers of interferon in the serum of adult mice inoculated i.p. with poly(I:C) or P-L-L complex*

Time (h)	Titer[a] of interferon: Poly(I:C) (100 μg)	P-L-L complex (100 μg)
3	3,850	1,700
6	3,750	23,250
9	5,275	25,250
12	3,400	18,500
24	150	13,000
36	<50	980
48	<50	200

[a] Interferon titers are expressed as the reciprocal of the highest dilution that inhibited 50% of the VSV challenge.

TABLE 2. *Titers of interferon in the serum of adult mice repeatedly inoculated i.p. with poly(I:C) or P-L-L complex*

Inducer	Time (h)	Titer[a] of interferon on day after initiation of treatment:					
		0	1	2	3	4	6
Poly(I:C) given on days 0, 1, 3, 4, and 6	6	6,465	4,055		1,585	1,620	3,735
	12	5,000	830		1,245	NS[b]	2,810
	24	250	<50		168	95	120
P-L-L complex given on days 0, 2, 4, and 6	6	30,425		545		730	1,195
	12	24,330		870		NS	910
	24	27,765		345		1,005	495
	36	880		<50		130	80

[a] Interferon titers are expressed as the reciprocal of the highest dilution that inhibited 50% of the VSV challenge.
[b] NS, No sample.

TABLE 3. *Effect of treatment with exogenous interferon, poly(I:C), or P-L-L complex on the mortality and mean day of death in adult mice infected i.p. with EMC virus*

Treatment[a]	Mortality			Mean day of death	P value
	No.	%	P value		
None	33/40	83		5.7	
Exogenous interferon					
Expt 1[b]					
−3 h	1/15	7	≤0.001	8.0	
+1 h	1/14	7	≤0.001	8.8	
+24 h	9/15	60	NS[c]	5.6	NS
Drug control[b]	1/15	7		5.0	
Expt 2[d]					
−1 h	0/15	0	≤0.001		
+1 h	2/15	13	≤0.001	7.0	
+24 h	11/15	73	NS	5.5	NS
Drug control[d]	0/15	0			
Poly(I:C)[e]					
−6 h	1/25	4	≤0.001	8.0	
+1 h	1/24	4	≤0.001	10.0	
+24 h	10/25	40	≤0.01	6.1	NS
Drug control[e]	0/25	0			
P-L-L- complex[f]					
−24 h	1/25	4	≤0.001	14.0	
+1 h	8/25	32	≤0.001	7.8	≤0.01
+24 h	10/25	40	≤0.01	7.0	NS
Drug control[f]	0/25	0			

[a] Treatment was initiated at the indicated times prior to or after viral challenge.
[b] 20,000 U/mouse was given twice daily for 7 days (Paucker).
[c] NS, Not significant.
[d] 40,000 U/mouse was given twice daily for 7 days (Paucker).
[e] 100 μg/mouse was given on the basis of once daily for 2 consecutive days and then skipping a day, for 7 days.
[f] 100 μg/mouse was given once every other day for 7 days.

daily for 7 days, exhibited an 83% final mortality, with a mean day of death of 5.7 days. Infection was characterized by hunching and circling by day 3, hind limb paralysis by day 4, and death by day 5 to 7 after viral inoculation. In experiment 1 treatment consisted of 20,000 U of exogenous interferon administered twice daily for 7 days. Treatment initiated 3 h prior to or 1 h after viral inoculation reduced the final mortality to only 7% ($P \leq 0.001$). Therapeutic efficacy was lost when treatment was initiated 24 h after virus inoculation. In experiment 2 the dose was increased to 40,000 U of interferon given i.p. twice daily for 7 days. The results of therapy with this increased dose of interferon were similar to those of experiment 1 in that treatment was highly effective when initiated prior to or 1 h after, but not 24 h after, infection. Although repeated injections of poly(I:C) were shown to result in progressive hyporeactivity of the interferon response, previous data from our laboratory indicated that treatment of mice infected with EMC virus, utilizing multiple doses of poly(I:C), was more effective than a single dose (26). Based on these data, therapy consisted of six doses of 100 μg of poly(I:C) administered on days 0, 1, 3, 4, 6, and 7 of the infection. Because the serum interferon response to P-L-L complex reached higher levels and lasted longer, 100 μg was administered i.p. every other day for 7 days (a total of four doses). Treatment with either poly(I:C) or P-L-L complex resulted in a significant reduction in mortality, even when the initiation of therapy was delayed until 24 h after viral challenge.

Effect of treatment on mortality of mice inoculated intranasally with EMC virus. To approximate a more natural route of infection, mice were inoculated intranasally with EMC virus. This experimental infection was also characterized by hunching and hind limb paralysis by day 4, followed by death on days 5 to 7 of infection. The effect of exogenous interferon, poly(I:C), or P-L-L complex treatment on the mortality and mean day of death of mice infected intranasally with EMC virus is shown in Table 4. The same therapeutic regimens as described above were used for each compound and

TABLE 4. *Effect of treatment with exogenous interferon, poly(I:C), or P-L-L complex on the mortality and mean day of death in adult mice infected intranasally with EMC virus*

Treatment[a]	Mortality			Mean day of death	P value
	No.	%	P value		
None	32/40	80		5.3	
Exogenous interferon					
Expt 1[b]					
−3 h	1/10	10	≤0.001	6.0	
+1 h	1/10	10	≤0.001	7.0	
+24 h	2/10	20	≤0.001	7.0	
Drug control[b]	0/10	0			
Expt 2[c]					
+1 h	6/19	32	≤0.001	7.5	≤0.05
+24 h	6/10	60	NS[d]	6.8	≤0.05
+48 h	15/20	75	NS	5.5	NS
Drug control[c]	0/20	0			
Poly(I:C)[e]					
−6 h	0/10	0	≤0.001		
+1 h	1/20	5	≤0.001	9.0	
+24 h	6/20	30	≤0.001	7.2	NS
+48 h	7/10	70	NS	5.4	NS
Drug control[e]	0/20	0			
P-L-L complex[f]					
−24 h	0/10	0	≤0.001		
+1 h	6/29	21	≤0.001	7.0	≤0.01
+24 h	3/20	15	≤0.001	7.0	≤0.01
+48 h	9/20	45	≤0.001	6.6	≤0.01
Drug control[f]	0/20	0			

[a] Treatment was initiated at the indicated times prior to or after viral challenge.
[b] 40,000 U/mouse was given twice daily for 7 days (Paucker).
[c] 100,000 U/mouse was given twice daily for 7 days (Bionetics; see text).
[d] NS, Not significant.
[e] 100 μg/mouse was given on a basis of once daily on 2 consecutive days and then skipping a day, for 7 days.
[f] 100 μg/mouse was given once every other day for 7 days.

the results of separate experiments are presented. The control group represents data pooled from all of the experiments. The virus-infected control animals treated i.p. with PBS twice daily for 7 days exhibited an 80% final mortality (mean day of death, 5.3 days). In experiment 1 treatment with 40,000 U of interferon (Paucker) twice daily for 7 days beginning 3 h prior to infection resulted in a final mortality of 10% ($P \leq 0.001$) and mean day of death of 6.0 days. In contrast to the results of the treatment of the infection initiated by the i.p. route, therapy beginning either 1 or 24 h after viral inoculation were both highly effective in reducing mortality. To determine whether higher doses of interferon would increase efficacy, a dose of 100,000 U twice daily of interferon (Bionetics) was used in the second experiment. Initiation of therapy at 1 h after infection resulted in similar protection, whereas therapy started at either 24 or 48 h after infection did not significantly reduce the final mortality. Although both interferon preparations were effective when treatment was initiated at 1 h after infection, the Bionetics preparation was less effective with treatment beginning at 24 h. Even though the Bionetic interferon preparation titered approximately 10^6 U/ml at the beginning of the experiments, assays performed 15 weeks later, or 6 weeks after the completion of these studies, indicated that the titers had decreased 10- to 50-fold. Repeat titrations with the Paucker interferon revealed no deterioration in titer. Therapy with poly(I:C) initiated 6 h prior to infection completely protected all animals, and treatment initiated 1 or 24 h after infection significantly reduced the final mortality. Therapeutic efficacy was lost when treatment was begun 48 h after infection. Treatment with P-L-L complex begun either prior to or at 1 or 24 h after viral challenge afforded a similar degree of protection as did poly(I:C). In addition, treatment with P-L-L complex initiated as late as 48 h after infection significantly protected mice, as well as increased the mean day of death.

Effect of treatment on EMC virus pathogenesis. In an attempt to elucidate the mechanism of protection by interferon in EMC virus-infected mice, the effect of drug treatment on the pathogenesis of the infection was defined. In separate experiments, animals were infected intranasally and treated with exogenous interferon or P-L-L complex beginning either at 1 or 48 h after infection. Three individual mice from each group were sacrificed daily and bled by cardiac puncture, and the blood was homogenized undiluted. The lungs, liver, spleen, heart, and brain were removed and homogenized as 10% suspensions in minimal essential medium with 10% fetal bovine serum. Tissue homogenates from the individual animals were centrifuged, supernatants were collected, and all samples were stored at −70°C until assayed for virus.

The effect of 100,000 U of exogenous interferon (Bionetics) given twice daily for 5 days on the pathogenesis of EMC virus infection is summarized in Table 5. It should be noted that the death rate in a control group of mice followed for mortality was 90%, indicating that not all animals in each group became infected. No virus could be detected on day 1 of the infection in any of the control animals treated with PBS. By day 2 of the infection, 10^4 to 10^6 PFU of EMC virus per g were isolated from the lungs and heart, 10^3 to 10^4 PFU/g were isolated from the liver and spleen, and 10^2 to 10^4 PFU/ml were isolated from the blood in two animals. No virus was isolated from the third animal. On day 3, virus was detected at levels of 10^4 to 10^6 PFU/g in multiple tissues in one animal, but only in lung tissue in the second animal. Virus was not recovered from the third animal. On day 4, all animals were infected and titers of virus from 10^4 to 10^7 PFU/g were recovered from multiple tissues. In animals treated with interferon beginning at 1 h after infection, a marked reduction in the recovery of virus from tissues was observed. Only 4 of the 12 sampled animals demonstrated evidence of infection with EMC virus. The death rate in a companion group of animals treated with the same regimen and followed for mortality was 33%. When interferon therapy was begun at 48 h after viral inoculation, a time when the viremia had occurred and high titers of virus were already present in the organs of infected animals, the pathogenesis of infection was similar to that of PBS-treated control animals. The mortality was 80% in a companion group of animals treated with the same regimen. These data correlate with the protection against mortality observed when the treatment was initiated at 1 h after infection and with the absence of protection when the treatment was initiated at 48 h after infection.

The effect of 100 μg of P-L-L complex given once every other day for 5 days on the pathogenesis of intranasal EMC virus infection of mice is summarized in Table 6. In this experiment all three virus control animals demonstrated evidence of viral replication in lung tissue on day 1, and six of the nine control animals harvested on days 2, 3, and 4 were infected with virus. The death rate in a control group of animals was 80%, again indicating that not all animals in each group were infected. In contrast, in the group of animals in

TABLE 5. *Effect of treatment with exogenous interferon on the pathogenesis of intranasal EMC virus infection*

Tissue examined	Titer[a] of EMC virus on day:											
	1			2			3			4		
Virus control												
Blood	<1,	<1,	<1	<1,	2.8,	4.4	<1,	<1,	4.2	<1,	6.0,	<1
Brain	<2,	<2,	<2	<2,	<2,	<2	<2,	<2,	6.2	6.5,	7.6,	6.0
Heart	<2,	<2,	<2	<2,	5.0,	NS[b]	<2,	<2,	5.7	4.3,	6.0,	6.0
Lung	<2,	<2,	<2	<2,	6.3,	4.2	3.6,	<2,	4.3	4.9,	6.0,	5.8
Liver	<2,	<2,	<2	<2,	3.5,	3.9	<2,	<2,	3.5	<2,	5.4,	5.0
Spleen	<2,	<2,	<2	<2,	3.3,	4.4	<2,	<2,	4.0	5.2,	5.6,	4.1
Treatment initiated at 1 h[c]												
Blood	<1,	<1,	3.3	<1,	<1,	6.0	<1,	<1,	<1	<1,	<1,	<1
Brain	<2,	<2,	<2	<2,	<2,	<2	<2,	<2,	<2	<2,	<2,	<2
Heart	<2,	<2,	<2	<2,	<2,	6.0	<2,	<2,	<2	3.4,	3.3,	<2
Lung	<2,	<2,	5.4	<2,	<2,	6.0	<2,	<2,	<2	3.8,	3.8,	<2
Liver	<2,	<2,	<2	<2,	<2,	5.0	<2,	<2,	<2	4.0,	3.2,	<2
Spleen	<2,	<2,	<2	<2,	<2,	4.5	<2,	<2,	<2	4.3,	3.4,	<2
Treatment initiated at 48 h[c]												
Blood	<1,	2.9,	<1	<1,	<1,	3.4	4.3,	3.9,	<1	3.7,	3.6,	<1
Brain	<2,	<2,	<2	<2,	<2,	<2	NS,	5.9,	<2	5.6,	5.2,	<2
Heart	4.2,	5.7,	<2	4.4,	<2,	5.9	4.0,	4.2,	<2	6.3,	5.7,	3.5
Lung	6.2,	6.0,	5.3	6.1,	<2,	6.2	5.5,	3.4,	<2	5.7,	3.4,	4.1
Liver	<2,	3.2,	<2	<2,	<2,	3.4	<2,	2.9,	<2	3.4,	4.9,	<2
Spleen	2.4,	3.0,	<2	<2,	<2,	3.3	<2,	4.6,	<2	4.6,	4.3,	<2

[a] Titers of EMC virus in organs of animals from each group. Viral titers are expressed as $\log_{10}$ PFU per gram of tissue or $\log_{10}$ PFU per milliliter of blood. Each column indicates viral titers in organs of one animal.
[b] NS, No sample.
[c] 100,000 U/mouse was given twice daily for 5 days (Bionetics; see text).

TABLE 6. *Effect of treatment with P-L-L complex on the pathogenesis of intranasal EMC virus infection*

Tissue examined	Titer[a] of EMC virus on day:											
	1			2			3			4		
Virus control												
Blood	<1,	<1,	<1	1.4,	2.2,	<1	1.7,	<1,	<1	<1,	<1,	5.5
Brain	<2,	<2,	<2	4.4,	3.8,	<2	1.7,	<2,	<2	<2,	<2,	8.0
Heart	<2,	<2,	<2	4.1,	4.0,	<2	4.5,	<2,	<2	5.7,	2.6,	<2
Lung	3.9,	4.1,	3.2	4.1,	3.8,	<2	4.1,	<2,	<2	<2,	<2,	5.9
Liver	<2,	<2,	<2	<2,	<2,	<2	3.2,	<2,	<2	<2,	<2,	6.0
Spleen	<2,	<2,	<2	3.6,	2.9,	<2	<2,	<2,	<2	<2,	3.8,	6.0
Treatment initiated at 1 h[b]												
Blood	<1,	<1,	<1	<1,	<1,	<1	<1,	<1,	<1	<1,	<1,	<1
Brain	<2,	<2,	<2	<2,	<2,	<2	<2,	<2,	<2	<2,	<2,	<2
Heart	<2,	<2,	<2	<2,	<2,	<2	<2,	<2,	<2	<2,	<2,	<2
Lung	<2,	2.7,	2.4	3.2,	<2,	<2	<2,	<2,	<2	<2,	<2,	<2
Liver	<2,	<2,	<2	<2,	<2,	<2	<2,	<2,	<2	<2,	<2,	<2
Spleen	<2,	<2,	<2	<2,	<2,	<2	<2,	<2,	<2	<2,	<2,	<2
Treatment initiated at 48 h[b]												
Blood	<1,	<1,	<1	1.4,	4.2,	2.7	4.2,	<1,	<1	<1,	<1,	2.9
Brain	<2,	<2,	<2	<2,	<2,	<2	<2,	<2,	<2	<2,	<2,	7.5
Heart	<2,	<2,	<2	3.3,	4.1,	4.1	3.7,	<2,	<2	<2,	3.8,	5.6
Lung	<2,	5.2,	4.0	4.5,	4.1,	5.4	5.9,	3.5,	<2	<2,	4.9,	5.1
Liver	<2,	<2,	<2	3.0,	3.9,	<2	<2,	<2,	<2	<2,	2.7,	5.1
Spleen	<2,	<2,	<2	4.1,	4.1,	<2	<2,	<2,	<2	<2,	5.0,	4.1

[a] Titers of EMC virus in organs of animals from each group. Viral titers are expressed as $\log_{10}$ PFU per gram of tissue or $\log_{10}$ PFU per milliliter of blood. Each column indicates viral titers in organs of one animal.
[b] 100 μg/mouse was given once every other day for 5 days.

which therapy with P-L-L complex was begun at 1 h, viral replication was observed in only 3 of 12 animals. Only lung tissue appeared to be involved early in the course of the infection. The death rate in a companion group of animals treated with the same regimen and followed for mortality was 30%. In the group of mice that received treatment beginning at 48 h, three of the six animals examined on days 3 and 4 demonstrated either no virus in tissues or virus that was confined to lung tissue. In the remaining treated animals the virus titers in tissues were similar to those observed in the virus control group. Mortality was 50% in a companion group of animals treated with the same regimen. These data correlate with protection against mortality observed when the treatment was initiated at 1 h after infection and with the fact that approximately half of the mice were protected when P-L-L complex was initiated at 48 h after virus infection.

DISCUSSION

It has frequently been reported that the administration of exogenous interferon or interferon inducers can reduce the mortality of animals inoculated with viruses that infect the central nervous system (7, 9, 12, 13, 16, 25, 28). In general, these studies have also demonstrated that these compounds are most effective when administered prior to or immediately after inoculation of virus. With the recent availability of high-titered preparations of murine interferon and the development of P-L-L complex, an interferon inducer that stimulates higher serum levels of circulating interferon in mice and primates than poly(I:C) (22), we compared the antiviral effect of these compounds in experimental EMC virus infections of mice to determine whether the achievement of higher levels of interferon would result in increased therapeutic efficacy. In two model EMC virus infections, all three compounds (interferon, poly(I:C), and P-L-L complex) were effective in preventing mortality if treatment was begun at 1 h after viral challenge. Of the compounds evaluated in this study, P-L-L complex was the most effective in that treatment could be delayed until 48 h after intranasal inoculation, whereas efficacy was lost after 24 h with either exogenous interferon or poly(I:C). This increased effectiveness is likely due to the fact that P-L-L complex induces higher and longer lasting levels of serum interferon. Previous studies (3, 5, 12, 13, 28) of treatment with interferon or interferon inducers in EMC virus infections have not demonstrated as great a reduction in mortality as noted in the current study. This may reflect our use of a lower viral inoculum (3 LD_{50}), which resulted in only 80 to 90% mortality, and the employment of larger doses of interferon or interferon inducers.

Increasing the dose of exogenous interferon from 40,000 to 80,000 U a day did not significantly improve protection against i.p. challenge with EMC virus. There are several possible explanations for this observation. First, doubling the dose of interferon may not provide a significant increase in interferon levels within target organs and considerably larger doses may be required in order to further increase efficacy. Second, the possibility exists that there is a plateau beyond which increased concentrations of interferon do not give increased protection. Further studies are needed to determine which, if either, of these two possibilities are correct.

In these experiments we utilized two preparations of exogenous interferon which were produced by the same technique, but in two different laboratories. When treatment was initiated at 1 h after intranasal infection with EMC virus, there was no significant difference in the final mortality of mice that received 80,000 U daily of the Paucker preparation of interferon as compared with those that were given 200,000 U daily of Bionetics interferon. If therapy was initiated at 24 h after infection, however, daily treatment with 80,000 U of the Paucker preparation resulted in significant protection, whereas treatment with 200,000 U daily of Bionetics interferon did not. The reduced effect of the Bionetics preparation may have been due to the decrease in titer that we observed after the completion of these experiments. Although we adhered to the storage conditions recommended for both preparations of interferon, it is possible that the frozen liquid interferon provided by Bionetics was less stable than the lyophilized preparation from Dr. Pauker.

In an effort to elucidate the mechanisms of protection, the effect of therapy on the pathogenesis of the infection in individual animals was defined. In our previous studies of a systemic EMC virus infection in mice, it was demonstrated that protection due to treatment with poly(I:C) or tilorone hydrochloride correlated with the complete suppression of viremia and prevention of seeding of target organs (25, 26). In the present study utilizing an intranasal inoculation of EMC virus, replication occurred in the lungs by 24 to 48 h, and viremia and seeding of the brain, heart, liver, and spleen were detected by 48 h after the initiation of infection. The early presence of circulating interferon (1 h treatment), whether administered exogenously or induced by P-L-L complex, inhibited viral replication in the lungs and prevented the development of the subsequent viremia and seeding of target organs. This observation would agree with the evidence that protection due to circulating interferon is a result of the inhibition of viral replication at the initial site of infection (1, 7, 25, 26) and suggests that if sufficiently high levels of interferon are achieved virus replication in target organs can be completely inhibited. If therapy was not initiated until 48 h after infection, treatment with exogenous interferon was ineffective in preventing mortality. The greater efficacy of the P-L-L complex, which induced higher initial levels of interferon in the serum of mice, was evidenced by the capacity of this inducer to suppress replication of virus in the target organs of some animals in which treatment was initiated as late as 48 h. This observation correlates with the fact that about 50% of the animals in this group were protected. Our data concerning the pathogenesis of this infection suggest that the seeding of target organs occurs at approximately 48 h and, thus, it appears that the levels of circulating interferon initially induced by P-L-L complex were sufficient to prevent viral replication in the target organs of some animals. It appears, however, that in spite of the high initial levels of interferon induced by P-L-L complex, once the virus infection was established in the central nervous system therapy was ineffective. This interpretation further supports the conclusions of De-Clercq and Merigan (5) and Finter (8), who reported that once the central nervous system of mice had been seeded with VSV or Semliki forest virus, therapy with interferon inducers was ineffective in preventing mortality.

The results of this study suggest that the capacity of interferon or interferon inducers to modify a viral infection may be enhanced by producing higher levels of interferon in the infected host. On the other hand, once viral replication has become established in critical target organs, neither interferon inducers nor exogenous interferon appeared to exert beneficial antiviral effects. The data do suggest, however, that for either exogenous interferon or interferon inducers to be optimally effective, there is a need to further increase the capacity to administer, or induce, higher and more sustained levels of interferon.

ACKNOWLEDGMENTS

This work was supported by Public Health Service contract NOI-AI-42524 from the Antiviral Substances Program of the National Institutes of Allergy and Infectious Disease and by Public Health Service grant AI-10217 from the National Institute of Allergy and Infectious Disease.

James C. Overall, Jr., is an investigator of the Howard Hughes Medical Institute.

LITERATURE CITED

1. **Baron, S., C. E. Buckler, R. M. Friedman, and R. V. McCloskey.** 1966. Role of interferon during viremia. II. Protective action of circulating interferon. J. Immunol. **96**:17–24.
2. **Catalano, L. W., Jr., and S. Baron.** 1970. Protection against herpes virus and encephalomyocarditis virus encephalitis with a double-stranded RNA inducer of interferon. Proc. Soc. Exp. Biol. Med. **133**:684–687.
3. **Catalano, L. W., Jr., W. T. London, J. M. Rice, and J. C. Sever.** 1972. Prophylactic and therapeutic use of poly (I)·poly (C) (poly-D-lysine) against herpesvirus encephalitis in mice. Proc. Soc. Exp. Biol. Med. **140**:66–71.
4. **De Clercq, E., and P. De Somer.** 1971. Comparative study of the efficacy of different forms of interferon therapy in the treatment of mice challenged intranasally with Vesicular Stomatitis Virus. Proc. Soc. Exp. Biol. Med. **138**:301–307.
5. **De Clercq, E., and T. C. Merigan.** 1969. Local and systemic protection by synthetic polyanionic interferon inducers in mice against intranasal Vesicular Stomatitus Virus. J. Gen. Virol. **5**:359–368.
6. **Emodi, G., R. O'Reilly, A. Müller, L. K. Eberson, U. Binswanger, and M. Just.** 1976. The effect of human exogenous leukocyte interferon in cytomegalovirus infection. J. Infect. Dis.**133**(Suppl):A199–A204.
7. **Finter, N.** 1964. Protection of mice by interferon against systemic virus infections. Br. Med. J. **2**:981–985.
8. **Finter, N. B.** 1966. Interferon as an antiviral agent *in vivo:* quantitative and temporal aspects of the protection of mice against Semliki Forest virus. Br. J. Exp. Pathol. **47**:361–371.
9. **Finter, N. B.** 1966. Interferon in animals and man, p. 232–267. *In*. N. B. Finter (ed.), Interferons. North Holland Publishing Co. Amsterdam.
10. **Finter, N. B.** 1970. Exogenous interferon in animals and its clinical implications. Arch. Intern. Med. **126**:147–157.
11. **Gerone, P. J., D. A. Hill, L. H. Appell, and S. Baron.** 1971. Inhibition of respiratory virus infections of mice with aerosols of synthetic double-stranded ribonucleic acid. Infect. Immun. **3**:323–327.
12. **Gresser, I., C. Bourali, M. T. Thomas, and E. Falcoff.** 1968. Effect of repeated inoculation of interferon preparations on infection of mice with encephalomyocarditis virus. Proc. Soc. Exp. Biol. Med. **127**:491–496.
13. **Gresser, I., D. Fontaine-Brouty-Boye, C. Bourali, and M. T. Thomas.** 1969. A comparison of the efficacy of endogenous, exogenous, and combined endogenous-exogenous interferon in the treatment of mice infected with encephalomyocarditis virus. Proc. Soc. Exp. Biol. Med. **130**:236–242.
14. **Hilleman, M. R.** 1970. Double stranded RNA's (poly I:C) in the prevention of viral infections. Arch. Intern. Med. **126**:109–124.
15. **Hilleman, M. R.** 1970. Prospects for the use of double-stranded ribonucleic acid (poly I:C) inducers in man. J. Infect. Dis. **121**:196–211.
16. **Horstmann, D. M.** 1965. Enterovirus infections: etiologic, epidemiologic, and clinical aspects. Calif. Med. **103**:1–8.
17. **Jones, B. R., D. J. Coster, M. G. Falcon, and K. Cantell.** 1976. Clinical trials of topical interferon therapy of ulcerative viral keratitis. J. Infect. Dis. **133**(Suppl.):A169–A172.
18. **Jones, B. R., J. E. K. Galbraith, and M. K. Al-Hussaine.** 1962. Vaccinial keratitis treated with inter-

feron. Lancet 1:875–879.

19. **Kaufman, H. E., R. F. Meyer, P. R. Laibson, S. R. Waltman, A. B. Nesburn, and J. J. Shuster.** 1976. Human leukocyte interferon for the prevention of recurrences of herpetic keratitis. J. Infect. Dis. **133**(Suppl.):A165–A168.
20. **Kern, E. R., J. C. Overall, Jr., and L. A. Glasgow.** 1975. *Herpesvirus hominis* infection in newborn mice: treatment with interferon inducer polyinosinic-polycytidylic acid. Antimicrob. Agents Chemother. **7**:793–800.
21. **Kibrick, S.** 1964. Current status of Coxsackie and ECHO viruses in human disease. Prog. Med. Virol. **6**:27–70.
22. **Levy, H. B., G. Buer, S. Baron, C. E. Buckler, C. J. Gibbs, M. J. Iodarola, W. T. London, and J. Rice.** 1975. A modified polyribonosinic-polyribocytidylic acid complex that induces interferon in primates. J. Infect. Dis. **132**:434–439.
23. **McLean, D. M.** 1966. Coxsackieviruses and echoviruses. Am. J. Med. Sci. **251**:351–368.
24. **Nordlund, J. J., S. M. Wolff, and H. B. Levy.** 1970. Inhibition of biologic activity of poly I:poly C by human plasma. Proc. Soc. Exp. Biol. Med. **133**:439–444.
25. **Stringfellow, D. A., J. C. Overall, Jr., and L. A. Glasgow.** 1974. Interferon inducers in therapy of infection with encephalomyocarditis virus in mice. I. Effect of single doses of polyinosinic-polycytidylic acid and tilorone hydrochloride on viral pathogenesis. J. Infect. Dis. **130**:470–480.
26. **Stringfellow, D. A., J. C. Overall, Jr., and L. A. Glasgow.** 1974. Interferon inducers in therapy of infection with encephalomyocarditis virus in mice. II. Effect of multiple doses of polyriboinosinic-polyribocytidylic acid on viral pathogenesis. J. Infect. Dis. **130**:481–488.
27. **Sundmacher, R., D. Neumann-Haefelin, K. F. Manthey, and A. Müller.** 1976. Interferon in treatment of dendritic keratitis in humans: a preliminary report. J. Infect. Dis. **133**(Suppl.):A160–A164.
28. **Worthington, M., and S. Baron.** 1971. Late therapy with an interferon stimulator in an arbovirus encephalitis in mice. Proc. Soc. Exp. Biol. Med. **136**:323–327.

Antimicrobial Agents and Chemotherapy, Oct. 1976, p. 677-681 Vol. 10, No. 4

In Vitro Susceptibility of Gentamicin-Resistant *Enterobacteriaceae* and *Pseudomonas aeruginosa* to Netilmicin and Selected Aminoglycoside Antibiotics

RICHARD D. MEYER,* LINDA L. KRAUS, AND KAREN A. PASIECZNIK

Infectious Disease Section, Research and Medical Services, Veterans Administration, Wadsworth Hospital Center, Los Angeles, California 90073, and the Department of Medicine, UCLA School of Medicine, Los Angeles, California 90024*

Received for publication 14 June 1976

Netilmicin (Sch 20569), a semisynthetic aminoglycoside related to gentamicin C_{1a}, was evaluated in vitro in agar dilution testing against 224 different clinical isolates of gentamicin-resistant *Enterobacteriaceae* and *Pseudomonas aeruginosa* in parallel with amikacin, gentamicin, sisomicin, and tobramycin. Netilmicin showed a very high degree of activity against gentamicin-resistant organisms, but amikacin was more active in vitro, particularly against *Providencia stuartii* and *P. aeruginosa*. Sisomicin and tobramycin were consistently less active than either netilmicin or amikacin. Netilmicin was bactericidal in broth testing against *P. aeruginosa*. Netilmicin showed a greater difference between results with agar and broth dilution testing than did amikacin.

Resistance to aminoglycoside antibiotics has commonly followed clinical use of these agents (4). Resistance to gentamicin among the *Enterobacteriaceae* and *Pseudomonas aeruginosa* appears to be a problem of increasing importance (5, 12). At the Wadsworth VA Hospital amikacin was shown to be the most effective aminoglycoside in vitro against gentamicin-resistant *Enterobacteriaceae* and *P. aeruginosa* (8, 12). Likewise, it has been highly effective in treating infections caused by gentamicin-resistant, gram-negative bacilli (11).

Netilmicin (Sch 20569) is a new semisynthetic aminoglycoside related to sisomicin, a dehydrogenated analogue of gentamicin C_{1a}, but it contains an additional ethyl group on the central ring (15). Rahal et al. have compared netilmicin in vitro with amikacin and gentamicin against gentamicin-susceptible and gentamicin-resistant gram-negative bacilli and have shown considerable activity (15). Early clinical investigation with netilmicin indicates that the blood levels achieved are equal to or greater than those achieved with gentamicin, which it closely resembles pharmacologically (L. S. Young, personal communication, 1976). This study was designed to compare the in vitro effectiveness of netilmicin with other aminoglycosides currently licensed or under clinical investigation, i.e., amikacin (8, 9, 11, 12, 15, 19, 20), sisomicin (8, 9, 20), and tobramycin (8, 9, 13, 20). Two-hundred and twenty-four different recent clinical isolates of gentamicin-resistant *Enterobacteriaceae* and *P. aeruginosa* were available.

MATERIALS AND METHODS

Different clinical isolates of *Enterobacteriaceae* and *P. aeruginosa* resistant to gentamicin by standardized disk testing (1) in the Microbiology Laboratory of Wadsworth VA Hospital were collected from August 1974 to March 1976 and identified by standard criteria. All isolates within a genus were from different patients. *Serratia marcescens* was identified to species by the fermentation of arabinose. Organisms showing a zone size of ≤12 mm to a 10-μg gentamicin disk on subsequent standardized disk testing (1) as recommended for *P. aeruginosa* (18) were tested by the agar plate dilution method (3) recommended by the International Collaborative Study of the World Health Organization. Approximately 10^4 organisms grown overnight at 37°C in Mueller-Hinton broth culture were inoculated with a replicating device (17) onto media prepared from Mueller-Hinton broth solidified with 1.5% agar (Difco) and 5% defibrinated sheep blood prepared to contain amikacin, gentamicin, netilmicin, sisomicin, or tobramycin in twofold dilutions from 128 to 1 μg/ml. Plates identical except for lack of antibiotic were used as controls. Amikacin sulfate was supplied by E. Yevak of Bristol Laboratories, and tobramycin base was supplied by R. S. Griffith of Eli Lilly & Co. Gentamicin sulfate, netilmicin, and sisomicin sulfate were gifts of George Hough of the Schering Corporation. A single lot of Mueller-Hinton broth was utilized because of the effect of varied cation activity on aminoglycoside testing (6, 10). Freeze-thaw extraction of the agar media was performed. The magnesium content of the liquid extracted from the media, which was repeatedly frozen and thawed, was from 0.71 to 1.54 mg/100 ml (mean, 1.23 mg/100 ml on three determinations) as measured by atomic absorption spectrophotometry; these results are similar to previous measurements (12). The minimal inhibitory concentration (MIC) was recorded as the lowest concentration of antibiotic showing only a haze, one colony, or no growth after overnight incubation (3). Reference strains of *Staphylococcus aureus* ATCC 25923 and *Escherichia coli* ATCC 25922 were included in parallel tests. All determinations were made in duplicate or triplicate, and the MICs were expressed as averages. Only organisms with a gentamicin MIC ≥ 16 μg/ml in agar dilution testing or ≥ 8 μg/ml in broth dilution testing were included. Two hundred and twenty-four isolates fulfilled these criteria.

Because of the known effect of cation concentration and especially magnesium (6, 10; K. P. Fu and H. C. Neu, Abstr. Annu. Meet. Am. Soc. Microbiol. 1976, A30, p. 6) on susceptibility testing of aminoglycosides with *P. aeruginosa,* as well as our initial results of higher MICs to netilmicin with *P. aeruginosa* than with *Enterobacteriaceae,* broth dilution testing was performed in parallel with netilmicin, amikacin, and gentamicin. MICs in broth were performed as outlined (3) with an inoculum of approximately 5×10^5 organisms/ml. Minimal bactericidal concentrations were performed by inoculating approximately 0.01 ml from tubes showing no turbidity onto antibiotic-free agar plates and recording the concentration of antibiotic at which five or fewer colonies grew after overnight incubation. This corresponds to 99.9% or greater killing. The magnesium content of the broth was 0.35 to 0.53 mg/100 ml (mean, 0.42 mg/100 ml on 11 determinations).

RESULTS

P. aeruginosa. Amikacin showed the greatest degree of in vitro activity in agar testing (Fig. 1). Gentamicin and the two most active agents in agar testing, amikacin and netilmicin, were also utilized in broth dilution testing (Fig. 2). A greater difference between agar and broth MICs was seen with netilmicin than with either amikacin or gentamicin (Fig. 2). Netilmicin broth MICs ranged from 2 to 16 times lower than agar MICs, but a smaller range was seen with amikacin. Various *P. aeruginosa* isolates that required 32 to 128 μg of netilmicin per ml for inhibition in broth were inhibited by relatively lower concentrations of amikacin (≤ 16 μg/ml), but cross-resistance was noted in some strains. Conversely, no isolate of *P. aeruginosa* resistant to amikacin in broth (MIC ≥ 32 μg/ml) was inhibited by netilmicin at a concentration of ≤ 16 μg/ml, and almost all of these organisms were inhibited by netilmicin only at a concentration of 64 to 128 μg/ml.

S. marcescens. Both netilmicin and amikacin were highly effective in vitro. Sisomicin and tobramycin were considerably less active (Fig. 3).

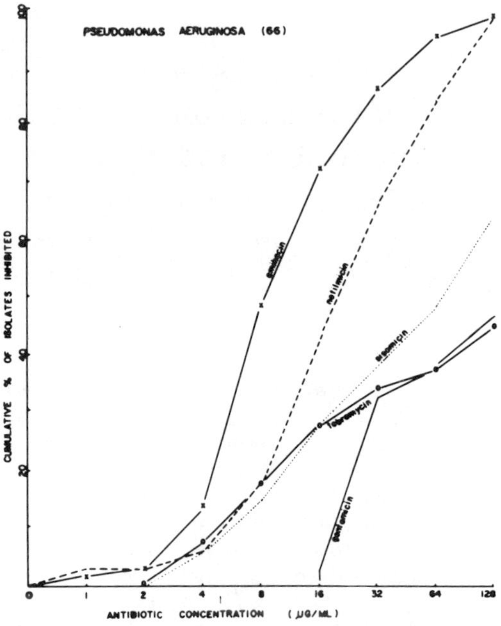

FIG. 1. *Antibiotic susceptibility patterns of 66 different clinical isolates of gentamicin-resistant P. aeruginosa in agar dilution testing.*

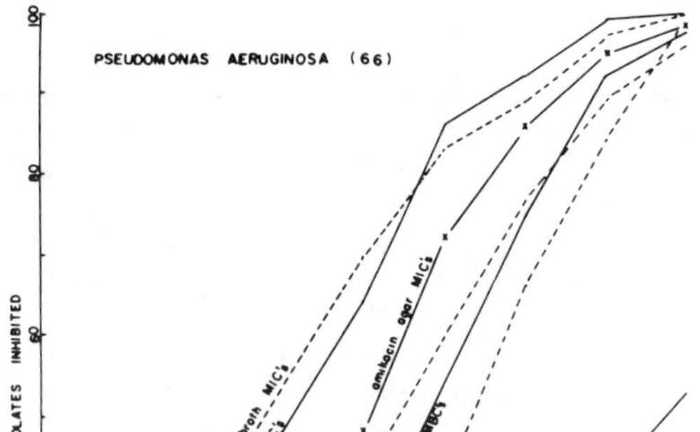

FIG. 2. *Comparison of agar MICs, broth MICs, and broth minimal bactericidal concentrations (MBCs) of 66 different clinical isolates of gentamicin-resistant P. aeruginosa with amikacin, gentamicin, and netilmicin.*

Klebsiella pneumoniae. As with *S. marcescens*, netilmicin and amikacin were the most active agents in vitro (Fig. 4).

Providencia stuartii. Amikacin was the most active agent. Netilmicin and sisomicin showed less activity than amikacin but were similar to each other (Fig. 5).

***Enterobacter* sp.** Netilmicin and amikacin were both highly active in vitro. Sisomicin was less active; tobramycin results were generally parallel to gentamicin (Fig. 6).

E. coli. Netilmicin was the most active agent in vitro. Amikacin was also highly effective, but sisomicin and tobramycin again were less active (Fig. 7).

Indole-positive *Proteus* sp. Amikacin was the most effective in vitro agent (Fig. 8). All five strains of *P. morganii* were inhibited by 2 μg or less of netilmicin per ml, but three strains of *P. rettgeri* required high levels of netilmicin for inhibition while showing inhibition at low levels of amikacin.

DISCUSSION

Our results show that netilmicin is highly active in vitro against almost all strains of gentamicin-resistant *Enterobacteriaceae*, with the exception of *P. stuartii*. It is bactericidal against *P. aeruginosa* in broth testing, but the medium affects results markedly. Agar dilution testing with netilmicin certainly appears suitable for gram-negative bacilli other than *P. aeruginosa*. The marked differences, however, between agar and broth MICs in netilmicin testing with *P. aeruginosa* indicate that more information is required before either agar or broth dilution testing with netilmicin can be

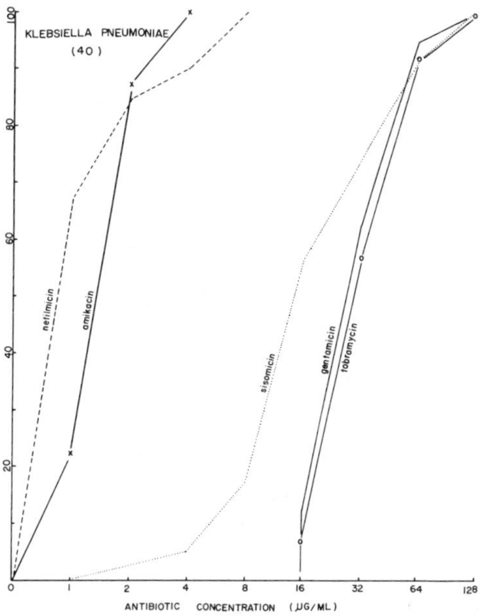

FIG. 4. *Antibiotic susceptibility patterns of 40 different clinical isolates of gentamicin-resistant Klebsiella pneumoniae in agar dilution testing.*

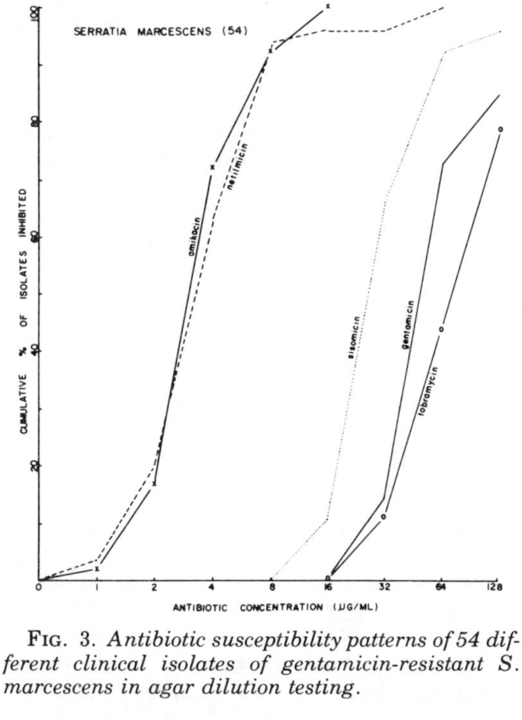

FIG. 3. *Antibiotic susceptibility patterns of 54 different clinical isolates of gentamicin-resistant S. marcescens in agar dilution testing.*

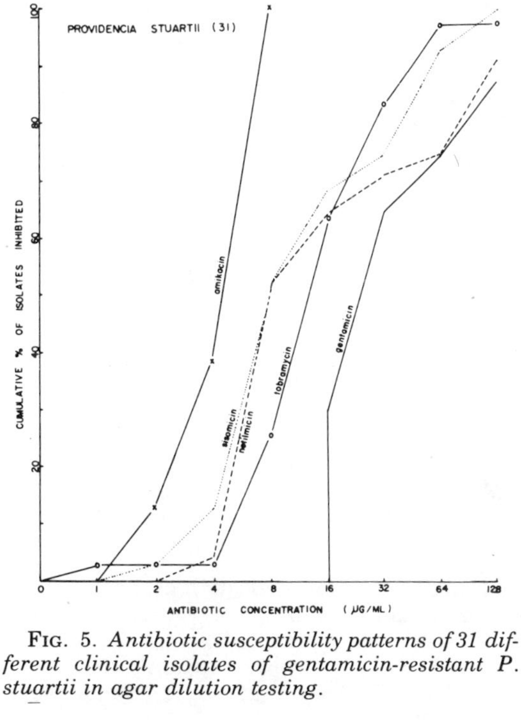

FIG. 5. *Antibiotic susceptibility patterns of 31 different clinical isolates of gentamicin-resistant P. stuartii in agar dilution testing.*

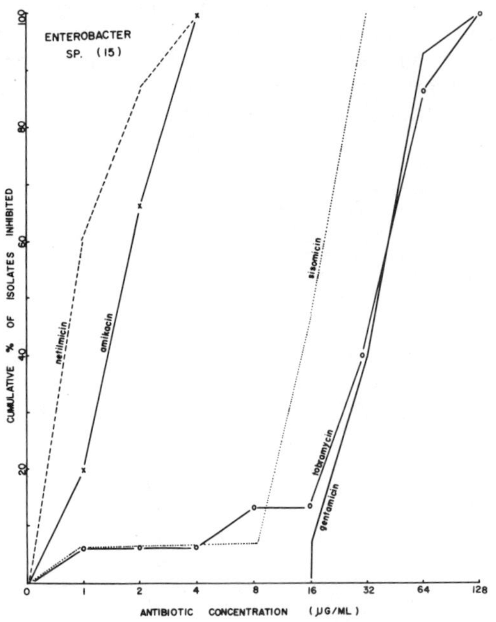

FIG. 6. *Antibiotic susceptibility patterns of 15 different clinical isolates of gentamicin-resistant Enterobacter sp. in agar dilution testing.*

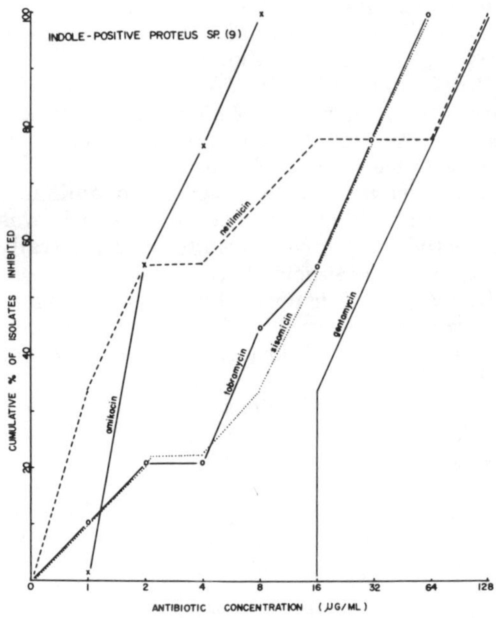

FIG. 8. *Antibiotic susceptibility patterns of nine different clinical isolates of gentamicin-resistant, indole-positive Proteus sp. in agar dilution testing.*

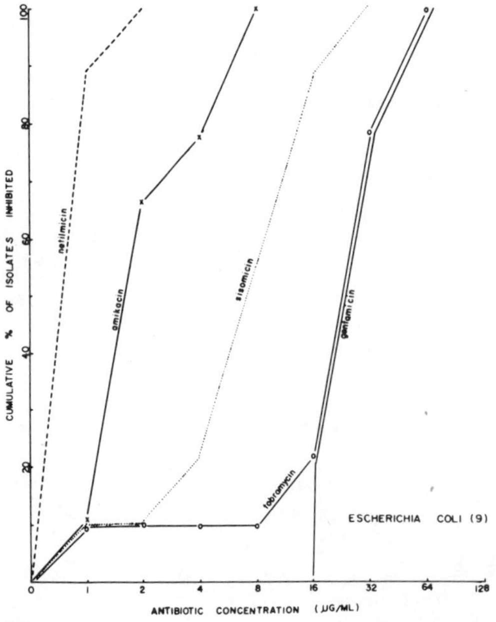

FIG. 7. *Antibiotic susceptibility patterns of nine different clinical isolates of gentamicin-resistant E. coli in agar dilution testing.*

recommended. Standardization of media, more in vitro data, and clinical correlation of in vitro test results with serum levels and therapeutic responses will be of value. Certainly the differences between agar and broth results were more noteworthy with netilmicin than those with amikacin or gentamicin. The disparity between results with agar and broth testing with *P. aeruginosa* with netilmicin has been noted by others (L. S. Young, personal communication, 1976). Although calcium content of the media, which also has been shown to affect in vitro results (16), was not measured, magnesium concentrations of our media from a single lot were similar. Magnesium content has been noted to affect in vitro testing with netilmicin more than other ions (Fu and Neu, Abstr. Annu. Meet. Am. Soc. Microbiol. 1976, A30, p. 6). Our results agree with those of Rahal et al., who found amikacin to be the most active agent against *Providencia* and found a high degree of activity of both netilmicin and amikacin against gentamicin-resistant *E. coli, Klebsiella,* and *Enterobacter* sp. (15). The findings of Rahal et al. (15) *Serratia* and indole-positive *Proteus* sp. with cross-resistance between netilmicin and amikacin differ from ours in that all of our gentamicin-resistant isolates of these genera were susceptible to amikacin, but not all were susceptible to netilmicin.

Our results also differ from those of Rahal et al. (15), who demonstrated similar activity with netilmicin and amikacin against *P. aeruginosa* in broth testing. Our results show amikacin to be the most active against gentamicin-resistant *P. aeruginosa* when the anticipated blood levels are considered. Our previous studies showed a mean 1-h peak blood level of 27.6 μg/ml with amikacin (11). On comparison on a weight basis, however, our results with *P. aeruginosa* are similar to those of Rahal et al. (15) in showing that netilmicin is the most active agent until the higher concentrations, when amikacin appears so.

The high degree of in vitro activity of amikacin against gentamicin-resistant *Enterobacteriaceae* and *P. aeruginosa* agrees with our previous findings reported in a smaller number of different clinical isolates (8, 12). Although gentamicin and tobramycin are active against some strains of *Providencia* (7), our experience agrees with that of Overturf et al., who found gentamicin-resistant strains that were susceptible to amikacin (14).

The wider range of amikacin than netilmicin against gentamicin-resistant organisms may be due to either permeability factors or to resistance to inactivation by enzymes produced by R-factors. Amikacin is inactivated only by kanamycin acetyltransferase (2), which is also known as aminoglycoside acetyltransferase (6′). Netilmicin is inactivated not only by aminoglycoside acetyltransferase (6′) but also by aminoglycoside acetyltransferase (2′) and by aminoglycoside acetyltransferase (3′)-II (Kenneth E. Price, personal communication, 1976). These observations may explain the patterns of resistance noted in our isolates, although assays for specific enzymes have not been performed.

Netilmicin has a wide range of activity in vitro against gentamicin-resistant *Enterobacteriaceae* and *P. aeruginosa*. Amikacin, however, remains the currently available agent that has the widest range of activity against these gentamicin-resistant organisms. Clinical studies with netilmicin are merited; studies of efficacy and toxicity comparing it to amikacin and other aminoglycosides are needed to determine its exact role.

ACKNOWLEDGMENTS

This work was supported by a grant from the Schering Corporation, Bloomfield, N.J.

We thank Jack Coburn for the magnesium determinations.

LITERATURE CITED

1. **Bauer, A. W., W. M. M. Kirby, J. C. Sherris, and M. Turck.** 1966. Antibiotic susceptibility testing by a standardized single disk method. Am. J. Clin. Pathol. **45**:493–496.
2. **Benveniste, R., and J. Davies.** 1973. Mechanisms of antibiotic resistance in bacteria. Annu. Rev. Biochem. **42**:471–506.
3. **Ericsson, H. M., and J. C. Sherris.** 1971. Antibiotic sensitivity testing: report of an international collaborative study. Acta. Pathol. Microbiol. Scand. Sect. B Suppl. **217**:9–87.
4. **Finland, M.** 1972. Changing patterns of susceptibility of common bacterial pathogens to antimicrobial agents. Ann. Intern. Med. **76**:1009–1036.
5. **Gaman, W., C. Cates, C. F. T. Snelling, B. Lank, and A. R. Ronald.** 1976. Emergence of gentamicin- and carbenicillin-resistant *Pseudomonas aeruginosa* in a hospital environment. Antimicrob. Agents Chemother. **9**:474–480.
6. **Garrod, L. P., and P. M. Waterworth.** 1969. Effect of medium composition on the apparent sensitivity of *Pseudomonas aeruginosa* to gentamicin. J. Clin. Pathol. **22**:534–538.
7. **Klastersky, J., A.-M. Bogaerts, J. Noterman, E. Van Laer, D. Daneau, and E. Mouawd.** 1974. Infections caused by Providence bacilli. Scand. J. Infect. Dis. **6**:153–160.
8. **Lewis, R. P., R. D. Meyer, and L. L. Kraus.** 1976. Antibacterial activity of selected beta-lactam and aminoglycoside antibiotics against cephalothin-resistant *Enterobacteriaceae*. Antimicrob. Agents Chemother. **9**:780–786.
9. **McGowan, J. E., C. Garner, C. Wilcox, and M. Finland.** 1974. Antibiotic susceptibility of Gram-negative bacilli isolated from blood cultures. Am. J. Med. **57**:225–238.
10. **Medieros, A. A., T. F. O'Brien, W. E. C. Wacker, and N. F. Yulag.** 1971. Effect of salt concentration on the apparent *in vitro* susceptibility of *Pseudomonas* and other Gram-negative bacilli to gentamicin. J. Infect. Dis. **124**:S59–S64.
11. **Meyer, R. D., R. P. Lewis, E. D. Carmalt, and S. M. Finegold.** 1975. Amikacin therapy for serious Gram-negative bacillary infections. Ann. Intern. Med. **83**:790–800.
12. **Meyer, R. D., R. P. Lewis, J. Halter, and M. White.** 1976. Gentamicin-resistant *Pseudomonas aeruginosa* and *Serratia marcescens* in a general hospital. Lancet **1**:580–583.
13. **Meyer, R. D., L. S. Young, and D. Armstrong.** 1971. Tobramycin (nebramycin factor VI): in vitro activity against *Pseudomonas aeruginosa*. Appl. Microbiol. **22**:1147–1151.
14. **Overturf, G. D., J. Wilkins, and R. Ressler.** 1974. Emergence of resistance of *Providencia stuartii* to multiple antibiotics: speciation and biochemical characterization of *Providencia*. J. Infect. Dis. **129**:353–357.
15. **Rahal, J. J., Jr., M. S. Simberkoff, K. Kagan, and N. H. Moldover.** 1976. Bactericidal efficacy of Sch 20569 and amikacin against gentamicin-sensitive and -resistant organisms. Antimicrob. Agents Chemother. **9**:595–599.
16. **Reller, L. B., F. D. Schoenknecht, M. A. Kenny, and J. C. Sherris.** 1974. Antibiotic susceptibility testing of *Pseudomonas aeruginosa*: selection of a control strain and criteria for magnesium and calcium content in media. J. Infect. Dis. **130**:454–463.
17. **Steers, E., E. L. Foltz, and B. S. Graves.** 1959. An inocula replicating apparatus for routine testing of bacterial susceptibility to antibiotics. Antibiot. Chemother. **9**:307–311.
18. **Traub, W. H.** 1970. Susceptibility of *Pseudomonas aeruginosa* to gentamicin sulfate in vitro: lack of correlation between disc diffusion and broth dilution sensitivity data. Appl. Microbiol. **20**:98–102.
19. **Weinstein, R. J., L. S. Young, and W. L. Hewitt.** 1975. Activity of three aminoglycosides and two penicillins against four species of gram-negative bacilli. Antimicrob. Agents Chemother. **7**:172–178.
20. **Young, L. S., and W. L. Hewitt.** 1973. Activity of five aminoglycoside antibiotics in vitro against gram-negative bacilli and *Staphylococcus aureus*. Antimicrob. Agents Chemother. **4**:617–625.

ANTIMICROBIAL AGENTS AND CHEMOTHERAPY, Oct. 1976, p. 682-686 Vol. 10, No. 4

Differential Effects of 5-Methylmercapto-2′-Deoxyuridine on the Replication of Herpes Simplex Virus Type 1 in Two Cell Systems

ROBERT HARDI, R. G. HUGHES, JR.,* Y. K. HO, K. C. CHADHA, AND T. J. BARDOS

*Department of Medicinal Chemistry, State University of New York at Buffalo, Buffalo, New York 14214, and Department of Medical Viral Oncology, Roswell Park Memorial Institute, Buffalo, New York 14263**

Received for publication 19 April 1976

5-Methylmercapto-2′-deoxyuridine (MeMUdR), a structural analogue of thymidine (TdR), inhibits herpes simplex virus type 1 production in mouse L (Lb) cells at concentrations that are not inhibitory to viral growth in monkey kidney (CV-1) cells. It is moderately toxic to Lb cells but not to CV-1 cells at a concentration that causes 95% inhibition of viral replication in Lb cells. MeMUdR is incorporated into cellular and viral deoxyribonucleic acid (DNA) in both systems, but to a significantly higher level (compared with thymidine) in Lb cells. These results indicate that MeMUdR is a substrate for enzymes leading to DNA synthesis and suggest that the biological function of herpes simplex virus type 1 DNA is impaired only when the incorporation of MeMUdR into the DNA reaches a relatively high level.

Nucleoside analogues represent an important family of antiviral agents (7). A member of this family, 5-methylmercapto-2′-deoxyuridine (MeMUdR) was first synthesized by Kotick et al. (3). The structure of this compound is shown in Fig. 1. It was stated by Stout and Robins (6) that MeMUdR showed significant inhibition of type 1 herpes simplex (HSV-1) in their antiviral screen, but the cell system used was not described. The present report shows that the compound has a differential effect on HSV-1 replication in two cell-virus systems, with replication in mouse L (Lb) cells being more sensitive to inhibition than replication in monkey kidney CV-1 cells. We also show that the compound is incorporated into viral and cellular deoxyribonucleic acid (DNA) in both cell-virus systems.

MATERIALS AND METHODS

Cells and virus. The sources of CV-1 monkey kidney fibroblasts and Lb mouse fibroblasts have been described (1, 5). These cells were maintained in a modified Eagle medium (1), supplemented with nonessential amino acids and 5% calf serum (EM5C). The source of HSV-1, strain KOS (HSV-1, KOS 1.1), has also been described (1).

MeMUdR was prepared according to Kotick et al (3). [^{3}H]methyl-labeled MeMUdR was synthesized via selective S-methylation of 5-mercapto-2′-deoxyuridine (MUdR) with [^{3}H]MeI (manuscript in preparation).

Virus inhibition assay. Cells were grown to confluency in plastic tissue culture dishes (Lux Scientific Corp.) and were infected at a multiplicity of infection of 5 plaque-forming units per cell. Virus was adsorbed for 1 h at 37°C, and the cultures were washed twice with medium and then incubated in medium containing MeMUdR. Cells were scraped into the medium 24 h postinfection, frozen, and then thawed before titrations were carried out as previously described (1).

Cytotoxicity assay. Cells were seeded in 60-mm dishes at 10^5 cells per dish and, after attachment, were cultured in medium containing the drug. Dishes, in triplicate, were trypsinized and counted each day for 5 days.

Preparation and separation of cellular and viral DNA. Cells were grown in 75-cm^2 plastic tissue culture flasks (Lux Scientific Corp.) and were infected at 10 plaque-forming units per cell. Virus was adsorbed for 1 h at 37°C. Cultures were then washed twice with EM5C, and 10 ml of EM5C was replaced. Label was added 6 h postinfection {[^{3}H]thymidine (TdR), 333 μCi/μmol, 10^{-5} M final concentration; [^{3}H]MeMUdR, 100 μCi/μmol, 10^{-5} M final concentration}.

Cells were scraped off 24 h postinfection. A 1-ml sample was frozen and later titrated to verify productive infection. Nucleic acids were extracted by a slightly modified procedure of the method of Kraiselburd et al. (4). Cells were suspended in 0.02 M tris(hydroxymethyl)aminomethane - hydrochloride (pH 8), containing 0.01 M ethylenediaminetetraacetic acid, 1 mg of Pronase per ml, and 0.5% sodium dodecyl sulfate, and incubated overnight at 37°C. Extraction was done with phenol-chloroform (1:1), and nucleic acids were precipitated with cold ethanol. The precipitate was dissolved in 0.1× SSC (0.15 M NaCl plus 0.015 sodium citrate) and dialyzed over-

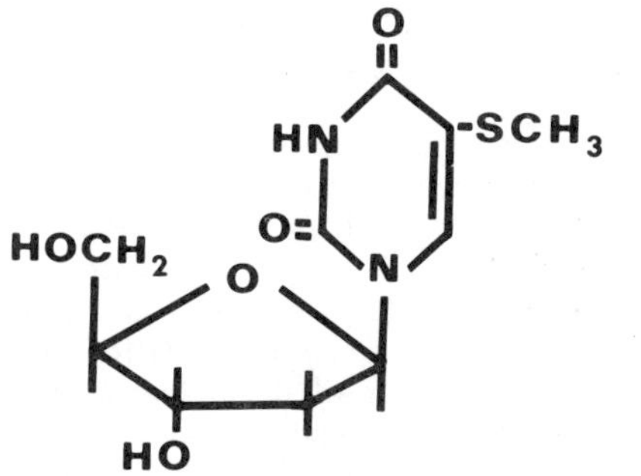

FIG. 1. *The structure of 5-methylmercapto-2'-deoxyuridine.*

night against the same buffer. Two optical density units of nucleic acid in 0.7 ml of solution were layered on top of 10 ml of CsCl. Samples were centrifuged for 72 h at 50,000 rpm at 25°C in a Beckman 65 rotor. Fractions were collected and measured for absorbance at 260 nm and for radioactivity.

Identification of MeMUdR in DNA. The enzymes used for the digestion of DNA were deoxyribonuclease from beef pancreas (3,000 units/mg), venom phosphodiesterase (20 units/mg), and alkaline phosphatase from *Escherichia coli* (34 units/mg). Enzymes were purchased from Worthington Biochemical Corp., Freehold, N.J.

A solution in a final volume of 2 ml containing 70 μg of MeMUdR-labeled DNA isolated from Lb cells infected with HSV-1 (3×10^3 cpm/μg), 40 μg of deoxyribonuclease, 30 mM $MgCl_2$, 250 mM acetate buffer, pH 6.6, and two drops of $CHCl_3$ was incubated at 37°C for 48 h. Subsequently, 1 ml of ammonium acetate buffer (200 mM, pH 9.2) was added followed by 0.1 ml of venom phosphodiesterase (1 mg/ml). The reaction mixture was incubated at 37°C for 6 h after which 0.1 ml of alkaline phosphatase (0.22 mg/ml) was introduced, and incubation was continued for another 20 h. The digested mixture was purified on a Sephadex G-10 column and analyzed by thin-layer chromatography. Separation was carried out on Eastman sheet, 13254 cellulose, with two solvent systems: A, *n*-butanol-ammonium hydroxide-water (86:5:14); and B, ammonium hydroxide (1.5 M)-2-ethoxyethanol-*n*-butanol (3:2:1).

RESULTS

Inhibition of viral replication. The results in Table 1 show that in the presence of 10^{-5} M MeMUdR, HSV-1 production in Lb cells was inhibited by about 95%, whereas in CV-1 cells at this drug concentration little, if any, inhibition was observed. Thus, at the given concentration, MeMUdR can almost completely block virus replication in Lb cells and, since the same effect is not observed in CV-1 cells even though all viral-specific processes are presumably the same in permissive cells, this effect must be exerted through some cellular process.

MeMUdR bears a structural resemblance to TdR and, as data in the next section will show, is incorporated into DNA. Therefore, it was of interest to see if TdR could reverse the inhibitory effect of MeMUdR. TdR at 10^{-4} M inhibited virus growth by 38% relative to virus growth in its absence. However, virus growth was inhibited by only 16% in a mixture of 10^{-4} M TdR and 10^{-5} M MeMUdR relative to virus growth in 10^{-4} M TdR alone (Table 1). These data indicate that MeMUdR acts as an antimetabolite of TdR and that it effectively competes with the latter at less than a 1:1 ratio. No studies were carried out on the effect of MeMUdR on ribonucleic acid metabolism.

The cytotoxicity of MeMUdR, although lower, paralleled its antiviral activity. As Fig. 2 shows, 10^{-5} M MeMUdR inhibited the growth of Lb cells by about 60%, but had no effect on the rate of growth of CV-1 cells. These results suggest that the cellular process that results in MeMUdR being actively antiviral in Lb cells also results in the compound being cytotoxic for the same cells.

Incorporation of MeMUdR into viral and cellular DNA. Figures 3 and 4 show the results of CsCl equilibrium density gradient centrifugation of DNA extracted from HSV-1-infected CV-1 and Lb cells cultured in [^{3}H]MeMUdR or [^{3}H]TdR. These data show that [^{3}H]MeMUdR was incorporated both into HSV-1 DNA (den-

TABLE 1. *Inhibition by MeMUdR of the replication of HSV-1 and its reversal by TdR*[a]

Concn (M) of compound:		HSV-1 titer (PFU/ml × 10^{-7}) in:	
MeMUdR	TdR	Lb cells	CV-1 cells
0	0	7.3	42.0
10^{-6}	0	4.4	58.0
10^{-5}	0	0.36	36.0
10^{-5}	10^{-6}	1.8	42.0
10^{-5}	10^{-5}	2.4	32.0
10^{-5}	10^{-4}	3.8	28.0
	10^{-4}	4.5	22.0

[a] Lb or CV-1 cells were infected with HSV-1 at 5 plaque-forming units (PFU)/cell. After 1 h at 37°C, cell layers were washed, medium containing the indicated concentrations of compounds was added, and the cultures were reincubated at 37°C. Compounds were added simultaneously where mixtures are indicated. Some cultures were harvested at 6 h postinfection as eclipse samples. The virus titers of these samples are near the minimum of the HSV-1 growth cycle. Values in excess of the eclipse values at later times in the growth cycle indicate the production of new infectious virus by the infected cells. Eclipse samples were taken in the presence of 10^{-5} M MeMUdR; Lb cells, 5×10^5 PFU/ml; CV-1 cells, 1.3×10^6 PFU/ml. The samples whose titers are given in the table were harvested 24 h postinfection.

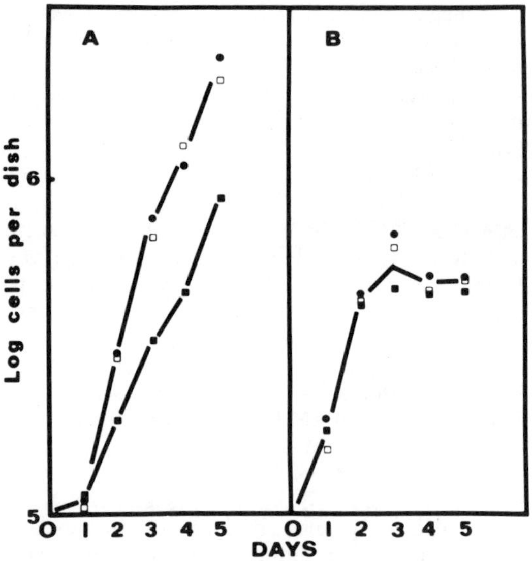

FIG. 2. *Cytotoxicity of MeMUdR. (A) Lb cells; (B) CV-1 cells. Symbols: ●, control; □, 10^{-6} M MeMUdR; ■, 10^{-5} M MeMUdR.*

sity, approximately 1.71 g/cm³) and cellular DNA in infected Lb and CV-1 cells. Since TdR nucleotide pool sizes were not known in the infected cells, the amounts of incorporation reflect the numbers of nucleoside residues incorporated from the TdR or MeMUdR in the medium and may represent less than the true values of TdR or MeMUdR incorporation due to dilution by the endogenous TdR nucleotide pools. However, if the TdR nucleotide pools in a given infected cell type do not differ in cells exposed to MeMUdR from those exposed to TdR, the relative numbers of TdR or MeMUdR residues incorporated per unit of viral DNA can be compared. Although there was no difference in the incorporation of [³H]MeMUdR and [³H]TdR in infected CV-1 cells (Fig. 4), in Lb cells [³H]MeMUdR was incorporated to a greater extent than [³H]TdR (Fig. 3). These data indicate that the number of MeMUdR residues per viral DNA molecule, i.e., the extent of modification of the viral DNA, is higher in the Lb cells than in CV-1 cells.

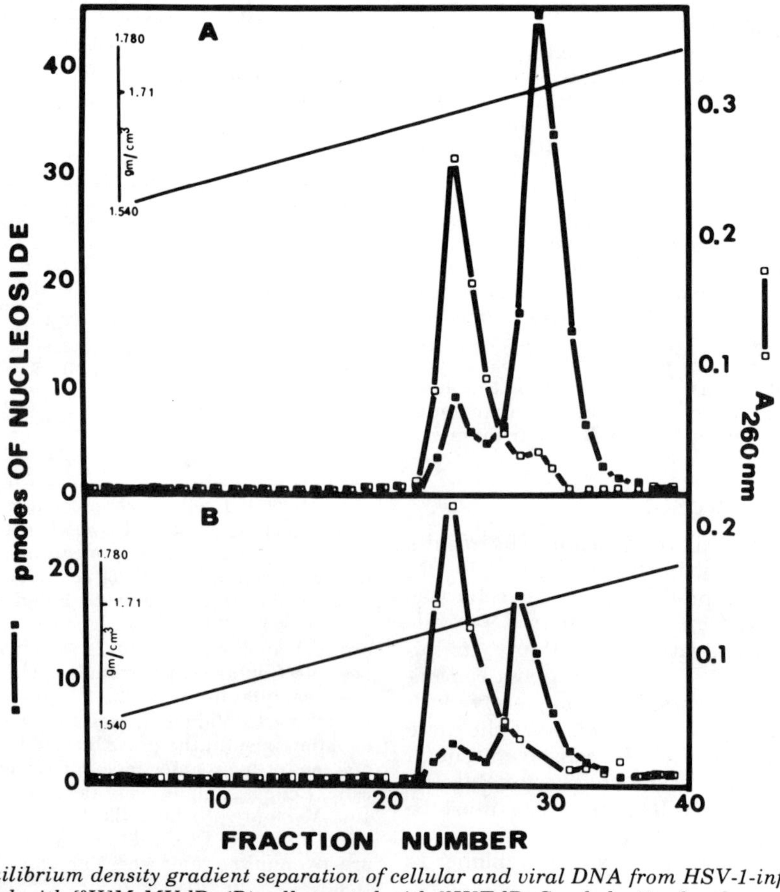

FIG. 3. *Equilibrium density gradient separation of cellular and viral DNA from HSV-1-infected Lb cells. (A) cells treated with [³H]MeMUdR; (B) cells treated with [³H]TdR. Symbols: □, absorbancy at 260 nm; ■, picomoles of ³H-labeled nucleoside residues in DNA.*

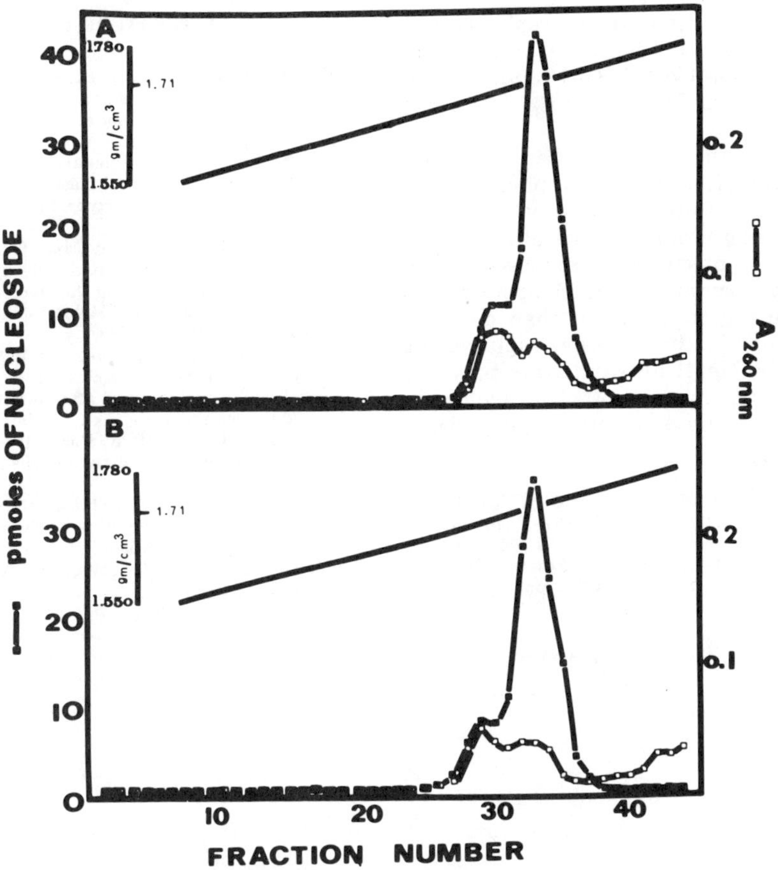

FIG. 4. *Equilibrium density gradient separation of cellular and viral DNA from HSV-1-infected CV-1 cells. (A) Cells treated with [^{3}H]MeMUdR; (B) cells treated with [^{3}H]TdR. Symbols:* □, *absorbancy at 260 nm;* ■, *picomoles of ^{3}H-labeled nucleoside residues in DNA.*

To obtain direct evidence for the incorporation of MeMUdR into the DNA of cells infected with HSV-1, radioactive DNA was isolated from infected Lb cells which had been cultured in the presence of MeMUdR. This DNA was digested enzymatically, and the nucleosides obtained were separated by thin-layer chromatography. Only one radioactive peak was observed in each case with an R_f value identical to that of an authentic sample of MeMUdR. The R_f of MeMUdR in solvent system A was 0.33, and in solvent system B the R_f was 0.85. These data indicate that MeMUdR was incorporated intact into the DNA.

DISCUSSION

MeMUdR inhibits HSV-1 production in Lb cells, but at the same concentration has no inhibitory effect on the replication of the virus in CV-1 cells. As expected on the basis of its structure and as shown by the data in Table 1, MeMUdR acts as a TdR analogue. Because it appears in both viral and cellular DNA, MeMUdR and its intermediate metabolites, respectively, must be substrates in all of the enzymatic steps of the pathway leading from TdR to DNA. The higher level of incorporation into viral DNA in infected Lb cells suggests that one of these cellular enzymes in Lb cells recognizes MeMUdR (or its appropriate metabolic derivatives) as a better substrate than TdR (or the corresponding metabolic derivative of TdR). This enzyme is probably not the cellular TdR kinase, since MeMUdR was as effective in inhibiting virus replication in Ltk$^-$ cells, a line of L cells lacking TdR kinase (2), as it was in Lb cells (data not shown). As an alternative explanation, one should consider the possibility that the pool size of one of the intermediate metabolites of TdR might be altered by MeMUdR to a different degree in Lb cells than it is in CV-1 cells. If such were the case, this too could account for both the differential incorporation and differential inhibitory effects of MeMUdR in the two cell systems.

The difference in susceptibility to the inhibitory effect of MeMUdR on HSV-1 replication in CV-1 and Lb cells is not absolute. In the presence of 10^{-4} M MeMUdR, HSV-1 replication in CV-1 cells was inhibited by 97% (data not shown).

In summary, the data indicate that MeMUdR is an inhibitor of HSV-1 replication and that it behaves as an analogue of TdR. The compound is incorporated into viral and cellular DNA both in infected CV-1 and Lb cells. Lb cells seem to incorporate the compound into viral DNA to a greater extent than do CV-1 cells, and it may be the excessive replacement of thymidine by MeMUdR residues in the viral DNA that results in the loss of its biological function in producing infectious progeny virus.

ACKNOWLEDGMENTS

This work was supported by Public Health Service grants CA-13114, CA-14801, and CA-06695 from the National Cancer Institute and by grant CH-20C from the American Cancer Society. Y.K.H. was a Research Fellow of the National Cancer Institute (IF22 CA02065).

LITERATURE CITED

1. **Hughes, R. G., Jr., and W. H. Munyon.** 1975. Temperature-sensitive mutants of herpes simplex virus type 1 defective in lysis but not in transformation. J. Virol. **16**:275–283.
2. **Kit, S., D. Dubbs, L. Piekarski, and T. Hsu.** 1963. Deletion of thymidine kinase activity from L cells resistant to bromodeoxyuridine. Exp. Cell Res. **31**:297–312.
3. **Kotick, M. P., C. Szantay, and T. J. Bardos.** 1969. Synthesis of 5-S-substituted 2'-deoxyuridines. Study of the factors influencing the stereoselectivity of the silyl modification of the Helbert-Johnson reaction. J. Org. Chem. **34**:3806–3813.
4. **Kraiselburd, E., L. P. Gage, and A. Weissbach.** 1975. Presence of a herpes simplex virus DNA fragment in an L cell clone obtained after infection with irradiated herpes simplex virus 1. J. Mol. Biol. **97**:533–542.
5. **Sanford, K. K., and W. R. Earle.** 1948. The growth in vitro of single isolated tissue cells. J. Natl. Cancer Inst. **9**:229–246.
6. **Stout, M. G., and R. K. Robins.** 1972. The synthesis of some 5-methoxypyrimidine nucleosides. J. Heterocycl. Chem. **913**:545–550.
7. **Tilles, J. G.** 1974. Antiviral agents. Annu. Rev. Pharmacol. **14**:469–489.

ANTIMICROBIAL AGENTS AND CHEMOTHERAPY, Oct. 1976, p. 687-690 Vol. 10, No. 4
 Printed in U.S.A.

Comparative Toxicological Studies of Amphotericin B Methyl Ester and Amphotericin B in Mice, Rats, and Dogs

G. R. KEIM, JR.,* P. L. SIBLEY, Y. H. YOON, J. S. KULESZA, I. H. ZAIDI, M. M. MILLER, AND J. W. POUTSIAKA

Departments of Toxicology and Pathology, The Squibb Institute for Medical Research, New Brunswick, New Jersey 08903*

Received for publication 16 June 1976

In acute and subacute toxicological studies, amphotericin B methyl ester was shown to be much less toxic than the parent antibiotic. As a single intravenous dose in mice, the methyl ester was approximately 20 times less toxic than amphotericin B. Also, the acute toxicity of the methyl ester in mice was not enhanced by the presence of chemically induced hepatic or renal damage or by the concurrent administration of amphotericin B or flucytosine. In a 1-month intraperitoneal study in rats, the methyl ester was about one-fourth as nephrotoxic as amphotericin B. In a 1-month intravenous study in dogs, the methyl ester was about one-eighth as nephrotoxic and one-fourth to one-half as hepatotoxic as the parent compound. In addition, the methyl ester, unlike amphotericin B, produced minimal renal effects, which did not increase in severity with increasing dosage. Based on the results of these studies, it is concluded that amphotericin B methyl ester has the potential for an improved therapeutic ratio in the treatment of systemic mycoses.

Intravenously administered amphotericin B is the most effective agent currently available for the treatment of many systemic fungal infections. This drug is therapeutically active in a number of mycoses that, prior to its availability, were invariably fatal. The use of amphotericin B for the treatment of systemic disease, however, is associated with toxic side effects; the most common of these is nephrotoxicity. Over 80% of patients given intravenous amphotericin B develop decreased renal function and abnormal urine sediment, and it is often the degree of kidney malfunction, and not the patient's therapeutic response, that determines the duration of drug administration (1, 11).

Amphotericin B methyl ester (AME) is a water-soluble derivative of amphotericin B that was developed by Mechlinski and Schaffner (8, 10). Both in vitro and in vivo studies have demonstrated that AME possesses significant antifungal activity (2, 4, 5, 7). Also, based on single-dose parenteral experiments in mice and dogs, AME was shown to be much less toxic than amphotericin B (6). The initial studies were conducted with the hydrochloride salt of AME, which proved to be unstable. Subsequently, the free base of AME was found to be stable (3). This report presents toxicological data from repeat-dose studies in which AME free base was compared to amphotericin B. Results from additional single-dose tests are also summarized.

MATERIALS AND METHODS

Drugs. AME (batch NN009NB) with a bioassay potency of 1,210 μg/mg was stored at −20°C. A 1% solution of the antibiotic in 0.2% ascorbic acid was prepared immediately prior to use. This procedure resulted in the formation of AME ascorbate in situ. Amphotericin B for injection, USP (Fungizone Intravenous, lots 5B530 and 5D573, E. R. Squibb and Sons, Inc., Princeton, N.J.) was reconstituted according to the manufacturer's instructions. Another antifungal compound, flucytosine (Ancobon, 250-mg capsules, lot 0005-05163, Roche Laboratories, Nutley, N.J.), was tested in a single acute experiment.

Acute toxicity in mice. Male Charles River CD-1 outbred albino mice, weighing 19.0 to 22.5 g, were used in these studies. The animals were fasted for 1 h prior to treatment. Individual doses were administered to groups of 15 or 20 mice. The intravenous injection rate was 0.1 ml/5 s. Mean lethal dose (LD_{50}) values were calculated by the method of Miller and Tainter (9), based on 7- to 10-day mortality data. LD_2 values were estimated graphically.

In one study, AME and amphotericin B were administered intravenously as single doses of 12.5, 25, 35, 50, 70, 100, and 140 mg/kg (AME) or 3, 4, 6, 9, and 12 mg/kg (amphotericin B). In another study, liver or kidney damage was produced in mice by pretreatment with either oral doses of carbon tetrachloride (5.6 ml/kg) or intravenous doses of uranyl nitrate (7.1 mg/kg), respectively. After 1 day in carbon tetrachloride-treated animals or 4 days in uranyl nitrate-treated mice, AME was given intravenously as single doses of 50, 70, 100, or 140 mg/kg.

In a third study, different intravenous doses of AME (41, 57, 80, or 110 mg/kg) were given concurrently with single intravenous doses of amphotericin B (either one-half of the LD_{50} [3.1 mg/kg] or the estimated LD_2 [2.2 mg/kg]). In a fourth study, a single oral dose of flucytosine (the estimated LD_2 [2,670 mg/kg]) was administered 3 h prior to the same graded doses of AME.

One-month intraperitoneal toxicity in rats. Groups of five male and five female Charles River CD outbred albino rats were used in this study. They were housed individually in stainless-steel cages in a room with constant temperature and humidity that was illuminated 12 h daily. The animals were offered commercial pelleted laboratory chow and tap water ad libitum. The rats were started on test at 5 weeks of age when the males weighed 123 to 158 g and the females weighed 114 to 137 g.

AME was administered intraperitoneally to three groups once daily, 7 days a week, for 1 month at doses of 10, 20, and 40 mg/kg per day. Amphotericin B was given intraperitoneally to one group on the same schedule at a daily dose of 10 mg/kg. A fifth group of rats that was given 4 ml of 0.2% ascorbic acid/kg daily served as control. Criteria for evaluation included survival, body-weight changes, food and water consumptions, behavior, physical condition, ophthalmoscopy, hematology, serum chemistry, urinalysis, and gross and histopathology.

One-month intravenous toxicity in dogs. Groups of two male and two female immunized and deparasitized young-adult purebred beagles were used in this study. They were housed individually in stainless-steel metabolism cages in a room with constant temperature that was illuminated 12 h daily. The animals were offered tap water ad libitum and a daily ration of commercial dog meal. The dogs weighed 7.9 to 10.5 kg at the start of the study.

AME was administered intravenously to three groups once daily, 7 days a week, for 1 month at doses of 2.5, 5, and 10 mg/kg per day. Amphotericin B was given intravenously to another three groups on the same schedule at daily doses of 0.625, 1.25, and 2.5 mg/kg. A group of six dogs that was given 1 ml of 0.2% ascorbic acid/kg daily served as control. Criteria for evaluation were the same as in the rat study but in addition included electrocardiography and electrolyte analyses.

RESULTS

Acute toxicity in mice. The results of acute toxicity studies in mice are summarized in Table 1. The intravenous LD_{50} values for AME and amphotericin B were 85 and 6 mg/kg, respectively; the LD_2 values were 53 and 2 mg/kg, respectively.

In mice with hepatic or renal damage induced experimentally, the acute intravenous toxicity of AME was not significantly different from that obtained in normal animals.

The concurrent administration of AME with amphotericin B or AME with flucytosine resulted in lethality values for AME that were not significantly different from the values obtained when AME was given alone.

TABLE 1. *Acute toxicity in mice*

Study	Intravenous lethal doses (mg/kg)	
	LD_{50}	LD_2
Amphotericin B alone in normal mice	6	2
AME alone in normal mice	85	53
AME in mice with hepatic damage	98	45
AME in mice with renal damage	82	51
AME when given with one-half LD_{50} of amphotericin B	76	37
AME when given with LD_2 of amphotericin B	80	40
AME when given with LD_2 of flucytosine	98	60

One-month intraperitoneal toxicity in rats. The results of the 1-month intraperitoneal toxicological study in rats are summarized in Table 2. The administration of both AME and amphotericin B resulted in retardation of body-weight gain that was associated with reduced food consumption and decreased efficiency of food utilization. Males given AME showed a dose-related retardation of weight gain, but females exhibited this change only at the high dose. Males given amphotericin B (10 mg/kg) showed a retardation of gain that was comparable to that observed in males of the group that received 20 mg of AME/kg.

Renal dysfunction, as evidenced by increases in serum urea nitrogen and water intake and decreases in urinary specific gravity, was produced by the administration of both compounds. Serum urea nitrogen was elevated only in the groups that received 40 mg of AME/kg and 10 mg of amphotericin B/kg; the mean values for these two groups were identical. Male rats given AME showed a dose-related increase in water consumption, but females had increased intake only at the high dose. In the group that received amphotericin B, water consumption for both sexes was greater than that recorded for the AME high-dose animals. Urinary specific gravity was moderately decreased in rats of the AME high-dose and amphotericin B groups. This parameter was also slightly decreased by the intermediate dose of AME.

The intraperitoneal administration of both antibiotics produced chronic peritonitis as a result of the chemical-irritant effect of these agents. Leukocytosis was observed and was considered to be secondary to the peritonitis. Group means for weights of uterus, prostate gland, and seminal vesicles from all test groups were lower than controls, but no histological abnormalities were seen in these organs.

One-month intravenous toxicity in dogs. All of the doses of AME (2.5 to 10 mg/kg) and the low dose of amphotericin B (0.625 mg/kg) were tolerated. Only slight or moderate decreases in body weight and food consumption were observed in two or three dogs of each AME group. The highest dose of amphotericin B (2.5 mg/kg) was not tolerated, and all of the dogs in this group were sacrificed in very poor physical condition during the second or third week of the test. Prior to necropsy, these animals showed marked decreases in body weight and food consumption, dehydration, and bloody feces. The dogs that received 1.25 mg of amphotericin B/kg per day also had marked weight loss and were dehydrated; however, they completed the scheduled 1-month study.

AME produced minimal renal changes, which did not increase in severity with increasing dosage. In contrast, the administration of amphotericin B resulted in dose-related nephrotoxicity that was severe in the animals given the two higher doses of this compound. A summary of the renal effects of the two compounds is presented in Table 3. Serum urea nitrogen and creatinine were normal in dogs that received 2.5 mg of AME/kg, slightly elevated in those that received 5 and 10 mg of AME/kg and 0.625 mg of amphotericin B/kg, and moderately to markedly elevated in those that received 1.25 and 2.5 mg of amphotericin B/kg. Hypokalemia was seen only in the amphotericin B high-dose group. Increased water intake and urine output and decreased urinary specific gravity were observed to similar degrees in all test animals. Glucosuria was evident only during the first week in dogs treated with either compound. Morphological evidence of kidney damage, most significantly focal tubular necrosis and calcification, was present in all animals given amphotericin B. These changes were slight at the low dose and marked at the two higher doses. In the AME groups, although most dogs showed histopathological alterations, these changes were always slight and consisted primarily of tubular atrophy rather than necrosis and calcification.

Both compounds produced mild hepatotoxicity; the data are summarized in Table 4. Changes in serum activities of glutamate pyruvate transaminase and alkaline phosphatase were associated with hydropic degeneration of hepatocytes. A dose-response relationship for the morphological change was observed for both antibiotics; however, the biochemical data did not show such a relationship and did not correlate well with the histopathological alterations. AME was less toxic to the liver than amphotericin B, since higher doses of the former antibiotic were required to produce comparable morphological changes.

TABLE 2. *One-month intraperitoneal toxicological study of AME and amphotericin B (AMB) in rats* [a]

Group	Body weight (g)		Serum urea nitrogen (mg/100 ml)	Water intake (ml/kg/24 h)		Urinary specific gravity
	Males	Females		Males	Females	
AME (40 mg/kg)	216 ± 11	179 ± 10	34 ± 2	216 ± 20	226 ± 17	1.019 ± 0.001
AME (20 mg/kg)	245 ± 6	197 ± 5	19 ± 1	179 ± 11	167 ± 14	1.028 ± 0.003
AME (10 mg/kg)	283 ± 13	209 ± 6	18 ± 1	165 ± 8	185 ± 8	1.040 ± 0.002
AMB (10 mg/kg)	259 ± 12	193 ± 11	34 ± 3	232 ± 17	260 ± 16	1.018 ± 0.002
Control	303 ± 9	203 ± 6	16 ± 1	134 ± 7	178 ± 9	1.040 ± 0.004

[a] Data are presented as group means ± standard error for analyses made at the end of the study.

TABLE 3. *Comparison of nephrotoxicity of AME and amphotericin B (AMB) in 1-month intravenous toxicological study in dogs*

Group	Serum chemistry[a] (mg/100 ml)				Renal tubular histopathology[b]		
	Urea nitrogen		Creatinine		Focal necrosis, calcification	Dilation	Atrophy
	Week 2	Week 4	Week 2	Week 4			
AME (10 mg/kg)	30 ± 3	44 ± 3	1.4 ± 0.03	1.6 ± 0.08	1/4, slight	0/4	4/4, slight
AME (5 mg/kg)	30 ± 5	44 ± 5	1.2 ± 0.15	1.6 ± 0.09	1/4, slight	3/4, slight	4/4, slight
AME (2.5 mg/kg)	18 ± 1	22 ± 2	1.0 ± 0.08	1.2 ± 0.05	0/4	0/4	2/4, slight
AMB (2.5 mg/kg)	140 ± 21		4.6 ± 0.82		4/4, marked	4/4, marked	4/4, slight
AMB (1.25 mg/kg)	82 ± 2	74 ± 8	2.7 ± 0.28	3.2 ± 0.32	4/4, marked	4/4, marked	3/4, moderate
AMB (0.625 mg/kg)	37 ± 4	32 ± 3	1.3 ± 0.11	1.5 ± 0.13	4/4, slight	4/4, slight	4/4, slight
Control	17 ± 2	18 ± 1	1.0 ± 0.06	1.2 ± 0.02	0/6	0/6	0/6

[a] Data are presented as group means ± standard error for analyses made during week 2 and week 4 of the study.
[b] Data are presented as incidence and severity of change.

TABLE 4. *Comparison of hepatotoxicity of AME and amphotericin B (AMB) in 1-month intravenous toxicological study in dogs*

Group	Serum chemistry[a]				Liver histopathology-hydropic degeneration of hepatocytes	
	Glutamate pyruvate transaminase (IU/liter)		Alkaline phosphatase (B-L-B units)			
	Week 2	Week 4	Week 2	Week 4	Incidence	Severity
AME (10 mg/kg)	38 ± 6	192 ± 102	3.2 ± 0.6	3.4 ± 0.8	4/4	Marked
AME (5 mg/kg)	124 ± 71	199 ± 83	10.7 ± 8.9	13.2 ± 9.8	4/4	Moderate
AME (2.5 mg/kg)	42 ± 13	108 ± 43	1.6 ± 0.4	2.7 ± 0.7	4/4	Slight
AMB (2.5 mg/kg)	215 ± 64		5.8 ± 0.9		3/4	Marked
AMB (1.25 mg/kg)	24 ± 2	83 ± 36	2.2 ± 0.2	2.0 ± 0.3	2/4	Moderate
AMB (0.625 mg/kg)	27 ± 3	24 ± 3	2.6 ± 0.2	2.7 ± 0.6	1/4	Slight
Control	21 ± 1	24 ± 2	1.5 ± 0.3	1.6 ± 0.2	0/6	

[a] Data are presented as group means ± standard error for analyses made during week 2 and week 4 of the study.

DISCUSSION

The results of these studies clearly indicate that AME is much less toxic than amphotericin B. As a single intravenous dose in mice, AME was approximately 20 times less toxic than the parent antibiotic. Also, the acute toxicity of AME in mice was not enhanced by the presence of hepatic or renal damage or by the concurrent administration of amphotericin B or flucytosine.

In the repeat-dose studies, relative toxicity was determined by comparing minimal doses of AME and amphotericin B that produced specific changes. By the intraperitoneal route in rats, AME was about one-fourth as nephrotoxic as amphotericin B. By the intravenous route in dogs, AME was approximately one-eighth as nephrotoxic and one-fourth to one-half as hepatotoxic as amphotericin B.

These results agree well with our initial report (6) on the comparative acute toxicities in mice and dogs of AME hydrochloride and amphotericin B. In those studies, the difference in mice between the two compounds was also about 20-fold; the difference in renal dysfunction in dogs that received single doses of the compounds was also about 8-fold. Based only on histological evaluation, Bonner et al. (4) reported that AME was one-tenth as nephrotoxic as amphotericin B in a 3-week intraperitoneal study in mice with experimental fungal infections.

The therapeutic utility of AME can only be assessed after careful clinical study. Even if it proves to be less active against pathogenic fungi than amphotericin B, AME may still have a greater therapeutic ratio because our studies suggest that comparatively large doses of AME could be given without producing nephrotoxicity. Moreover, AME may not have the potential to produce more than only mild renal dysfunction at any dose, since it did not cause an increase in severity of renal effects with increasing dosage as did amphotericin B. It is conceivable, therefore, that therapeutically active doses of AME could be given without the occurrence of significant nephrotoxicity.

ACKNOWLEDGMENTS

We thank G. J. Lockwood, C. K. Parekh, D. W. Rothermal, R. J. Shuren, and T. L. Szepsy for their technical assistance.

LITERATURE CITED

1. **Bennett, J. E.** 1974. Chemotherapy of systemic mycoses. N. Engl. J. Med. 290:30–32.
2. **Bonner, D. P., W. Mechlinski, and C. P. Schaffner.** 1972. Polyene macrolide derivatives. III. Biological properties of polyene macrolide ester salts. J. Antibiot. 25:261–262.
3. **Bonner, D. P., W. Mechlinski, and C. P. Schaffner.** 1975. Stability studies with amphotericin B and amphotericin B methyl ester. J. Antibiot. 28:132–135.
4. **Bonner, D. P., R. P. Tewari, M. Solotorovsky, W. Mechlinski, and C. P. Schaffner.** 1975. Comparative chemotherapeutic activity of amphotericin B and amphotericin B methyl ester. Antimicrob. Agents Chemother. 7:724–729.
5. **Howarth, W. R., R. P. Tewari, and M. Solotorovsky.** 1975. Comparative in vitro antifungal activity of amphotericin B and amphotericin B methyl ester. Antimicrob. Agents Chemother. 7:58–63.
6. **Keim, G. R., J. W. Poutsiaka, J. Kirpan, and C. H. Keysser.** 1973. Amphotericin B methyl ester hydrochloride and amphotericin B: comparative acute toxicity. Science 179:584–585.
7. **Lawrence, R. M., and P. D. Hoeprich.** 1975. Treatment of experimental coccidioidomycosis with amphotericin B methyl ester. Clin. Res. 23:416.
8. **Mechlinski, W., and C. P. Schaffner.** 1972. Polyene macrolide derivatives. I. N-acylation and esterification reactions with amphotericin B. J. Antibiot. 25:256–258.
9. **Miller, L. C., and M. L. Tainter.** 1944. Estimation of the ED_{50} and its error by means of logarithmic-probit graph paper. Proc. Soc. Exp. Biol. Med. 57:261–264.
10. **Schaffner, C. P., and W. Mechlinski.** 1972. Polyene macrolide derivatives. II. Physical-chemical properties of polyene macrolide esters and their water-soluble salts. J. Antibiot. 25:259–260.
11. **Weinstein, L.** 1975. Antifungal agents, p. 1236–1238. *In* L. S. Goodman and A. Gilman (ed.), The pharmacological basis of therapeutics, 5th ed. Macmillan Publishing Co., Inc., New York.

ANTIMICROBIAL AGENTS AND CHEMOTHERAPY, Oct. 1976, p. 691-696
Vol. 10, No. 4
Printed in U.S.A.

Antiviral Activity of BL-3849A, a Low-Molecular-Weight Oral Interferon Inducer[1]

EARL R. KERN,* JOHN R. HAMILTON, JAMES C. OVERALL, JR., AND LOWELL A. GLASGOW

Departments of Pediatrics and Microbiology, University of Utah College of Medicine, Salt Lake City, Utah 84132*

Received for publication 13 July 1976

Oral administration of BL-3849A to adult mice resulted in peak serum interferon titers of 4,000 units from 15 to 30 h after administration, with detectable levels persisting until 48 h. After intraperitoneal (i.p.) inoculation, peak serum interferon titers of 1,000 to 3,000 units were noted between 9 and 18 h. Multiple injections of the inducer by either route resulted in a marked decrease in the interferon response with each successive dose. In mice infected intranasally with the Rochester mouse virus strain of encephalomyocarditis virus, oral treatment with BL-3849A reduced mortality when initiated either 18 h before or 1 h after infection. In contrast, administration of drug by the i.p. route decreased mortality only if begun before infection. In mice inoculated i.p. with encephalomyocarditis virus, treatment by both the oral and the i.p. route decreased the mortality whether initiated 18 h before or 1 h after infection. Treatment by the oral, but not the i.p., route reduced mortality of mice inoculated i.p. with Semliki forest virus or *Herpesvirus hominis* type 2. BL-3849A appeared to be as effective as tilorone hydrochloride, but less effective than polyriboinosinic-polyribocytidylic acid, in the treatment of these viral infections of mice.

One limitation to the use of interferon inducers as antiviral chemotherapeutic agents is the production of toxic side effects in the host. In recent years there has been considerable interest in the development of nontoxic, low-molecular-weight compounds that induce the production of interferon in vivo. A number of natural or synthetic compounds of this type, including 9-methylstreptimidone (12), CP-20,961 (3), 10-carboxymethyl-9-acridanone (7), quinacrine (2), MA-56 (15), tilorone hydrochloride (8, 17), 2-amino-5-bromo-6-methyl-4-pyrimidinol (U-25,166) (10), and BL-20803 (14), have been reported to induce interferon and have antiviral activity in a variety of experimental viral infections. Of particular interest are the compounds quinacrine, MA-56, tilorone, U-25,166, and BL-20803, which induce high levels of interferon after oral administration. BL-3849A, the structure of which is shown in Fig. 1, is a 7-methyl derivative of BL-20803 (14). The purpose of this paper is to describe the interferon-inducing capacity of this compound and its antiviral activity in a number of experimental viral infections in mice.

[1] Publication no. 27 from the Cooperative Antiviral Testing Group of the National Institute of Allergy and Infectious Diseases, Bethesda, Md.

MATERIALS AND METHODS

Animals. Adult (7 to 9 weeks old), female Swiss Webster mice and newborn (5 to 7 days old) mice were obtained from Simonsen Laboratories, Gilroy, Calif. They were housed under conditions of constant temperature and a 12-h light cycle, with food and water provided as needed.

Viruses. Rochester mouse virus (RMV) is a large-plaque variant of encephalomyocarditis (EMC) virus which will infect mice when administered by the intranasal route. The isolation and characterization of this virus has been described previously (16). Virus pools were prepared as suspensions of suckling mouse brains. The strain of EMC virus used to inoculate mice by the intraperitoneal (i.p.) route was originally obtained from K. Takemoto, National Institutes of Health (NIH), Bethesda, Md. Virus pools were also prepared as suckling mouse brain suspensions. The type 2 MS strain of *Herpesvirus hominis* utilized in these studies was obtained from A. Nahmias, Emory University, Atlanta, Ga. The virus pool used was propagated in secondary rabbit kidney cells. The strain of Semliki forest virus (SFV) used was obtained from S. Baron, NIH, and stock pools were prepared as suspensions of suckling mouse brain. Vesicular stomatitis virus, Indiana strain, was obtained from the American Type Culture Collection, Rockville, Md., and virus pools were propagated in primary chicken embryo cells.

Media, cell cultures. Eagle minimal essential medium containing 5% fetal bovine serum, 100 U of

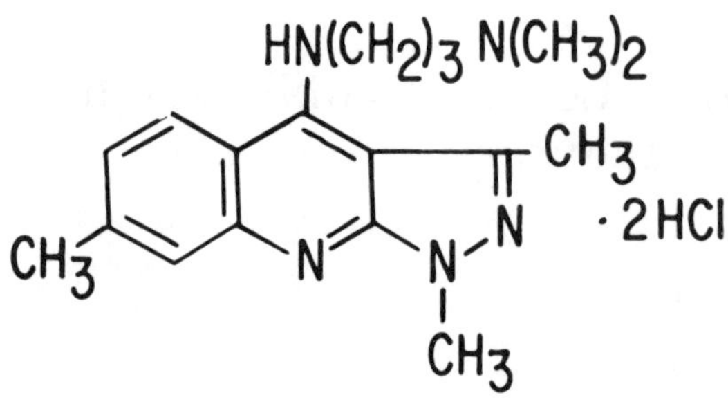

FIG. 1. *Structure of BL-3849A. (Provided to the Antiviral Substances Program, courtesy of Bristol Laboratories, Syracuse, N.Y.)*

penicillin per ml, and 50 μg of streptomycin per ml was used to propagate and maintain a continuous line of mouse L-cell fibroblasts (L-929) obtained from the American Type Culture Collection.

Interferon induction and assay. BL-3849A was prepared by Bristol Laboratories, Syracuse, N.Y., and was provided to us through the Antiviral Substances Program, NIH. The drug was stored as a powder at room temperature until used. For oral or i.p. administration, the drug was dissolved in phosphate-buffered saline (PBS) at appropriate concentrations to give a volume of 0.1 ml/mouse. Oral administration of drug was accomplished by using an infant feeding tube (size, 5 French; Pharmaseal Laboratories, Glendale, Calif.) attached to a 1-ml syringe. Polyriboinosinic-polyribocytidylic acid [poly(I:C)] was prepared by P-L Laboratories, Milwaukee, Wis., and was provided to us through the Antiviral Substances Program, NIH. It was supplied as a solution at a concentration of 1 mg/ml and stored at −20°C until used. Tilorone hydrochloride was kindly furnished by G. D. Mayer, Merrell-National Laboratories, Cincinnati, Ohio, and was stored as a powder at 4°C until used. It was dissolved in PBS just before use and was administered orally with the infant feeding tube.

Interferon in mouse serum was assayed using confluent L-cell monolayer cultures in 35-mm plastic petri dishes. The plaque reduction assay, using vesicular stomatitis virus as the challenge virus, has been described previously (6, 17). An internal laboratory reference interferon standard was included with each assay, and the sensitivity of our assay was compared with the interferon standard obtained from NIH. In our assay system, the NIH standard had a titer of approximately 5,000 units in comparison with its accepted titer of 6,500 units.

Statistical evaluation. To compare the final mortality of untreated and drug-treated mice, the data were evaluated by the Fisher exact test. To evaluate the differences in the mean day of death (MDD) between untreated and treated animals, the data were compared by the Mann-Whitney U test. A P value of <0.05 was considered to be significant.

RESULTS

Kinetics of interferon response induced by BL-3849A. The serum interferon response induced by BL-3849A in adult and newborn mice is illustrated in Fig. 2. BL-3849A was administered to adult mice by either the oral (300 mg/kg) or the i.p. route (100 mg/kg). Newborn mice were given BL-3849A by the i.p. route at a concentration of 100 mg/kg. At each of the indicated times after injection of the inducers, four mice were bled, and the serum was collected, pooled, and assayed for interferon. The results are plotted as a mean of two separate experiments. After i.p. administration to adult mice, a peak serum interferon titer of 3,000 units was observed at 18 h, with a gradual decline to undetectable levels by 36 h. The serum interferon levels were above 1,000 units between 9 and 18 h. After oral administration of BL-3849A to adult mice, a plateau in the interferon response of approximately 4,000 units was observed between 15 and 30 h. Detectable levels of interferon persisted until 48 h after administration of the inducer. Newborn mice exhibited a marked decrease in the interferon response after i.p. injection as compared with adult mice. A maximum titer of only 300 units occurred at about 18 h and gradually declined to undetectable levels at 36 h. The interferon response to oral administration of tilorone and to i.p. injection of poly(I:C) in adult mice was also examined (data not shown) and shown to be similar to that published previously (4a, 17). Peak serum levels of 3,000 to 5,000 units were observed 6 to 9 h after injection of poly(I:C), and levels of 4,000 to 8,000 units were observed 18 to 24 h after tilorone administration.

Hyporeactivity to interferon induction. One potential limitation to the use of interferon inducers as chemotherapeutic agents is hyporeactivity or the progressive reduction in the magnitude of the interferon response that develops with multiple doses of the inducer (4a, 6, 17). To determine if multiple injections of BL-3849A resulted in the development of a hyporeactive interferon response, groups of mice were inoculated with 300 mg/kg orally or 100 mg/kg i.p. every 48 h. Serum samples were collected from

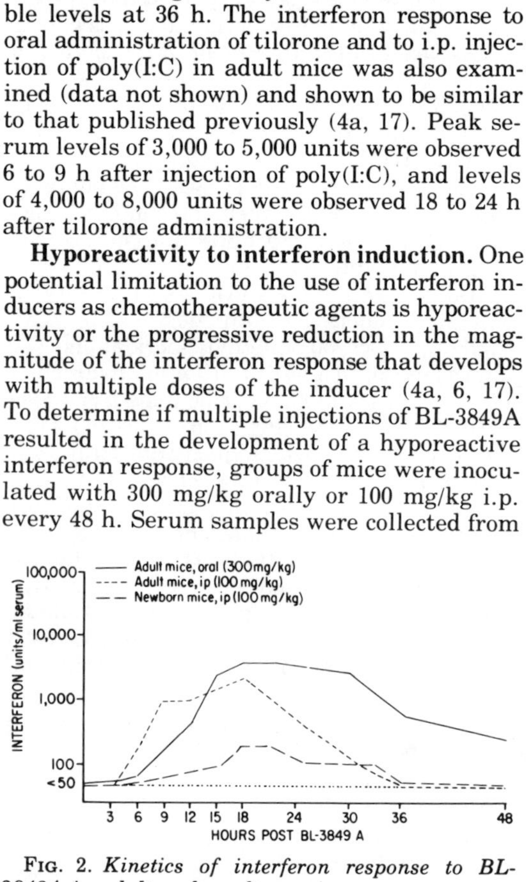

FIG. 2. *Kinetics of interferon response to BL-3849A in adult and newborn mice.*

one group of four mice 18 h after each injection and assayed for interferon. The mean interferon titers from two experiments are summarized in Table 1. After the initial injection of BL-3849A, 4,300 and 3,800 units of interferon were induced by oral and i.p. administration, respectively. After the second injection of the inducer, the interferon response was reduced to 10 to 20% of that with a single dose. After the fourth dose by either route, the serum interferon levels decreased to 3% of the response with a single injection.

Treatment of mice inoculated intranasally with RMV. Adult mice were infected by the intranasal route with 0.03 ml, containing 10^5 plaque-forming units, of RMV by applying the inoculum to the external nares through a 26-gauge needle. The animals exhibited ruffled fur and hunching by day 3 after inoculation, followed by paralysis and death on days 4 to 7. The pathogenesis of this experimental infection is illustrated in Fig. 3. After intranasal inoculation, initial viral replication occurred in the lung. A viremia was first detected at 12 to 24 h after inoculation, with seeding of the heart and lungs by 36 h. Virus was first detectable in brain tissue at 48 h; replication to high titers was observed until the death of the mice. The results of treatment with BL-3849A on this experimental infection are summarized in Table 2. The untreated control group of mice had a final mortality of 80%, with a MDD of 4.6 days. Animals that received BL-3849A orally either 18 h before or 1 h after RMV inoculation had a significant reduction in final mortality and an increased MDD. Initiation of treatment 24 h after viral inoculation failed to significantly alter final mortality or the MDD. Administration, i.p., of BL-3849A 18 h before RMV inoculation also significantly reduced final mortality. Treatment initiated i.p. 1 or 24 h after infection, however, was not effective.

Treatment of mice inoculated i.p. with EMC virus. To determine the effectiveness of treatment of BL-3849A on an EMC virus infection initiated systemically, adult mice were inoculated by the i.p. route with approximately 10 plaque-forming units of EMC virus. The pathogenesis of this model infection has been published previously (9) and is characterized by a viremia, followed by spread of virus to visceral target organs and to the brain. The animals exhibit fur ruffling and hunching on days 4 to 6, followed by paralysis and death on days 6 to 8. The effect of treatment on EMC virus infection of mice is shown in Table 3. For purposes of comparison, similar groups of animals were treated with tilorone by the oral route or with poly(I:C) administered i.p. The virus control group that received PBS on the same schedule as the drug-treated groups had a final mortality of 80% and a MDD of 6.4 days. BL-3849A administered orally 18 h before infection was highly effective in reducing final mortality and increasing the MDD. Treatment initiated after infection was less effective. Similar results were observed with oral tilorone therapy. BL-3849A given by the i.p. route either 18 h before or 1 h after viral inoculation also significantly reduced final mortality. If treatment was initiated 24 h after infection, no effect on mortality was observed, but the MDD was significantly increased. Poly(I:C) treatment i.p. was more effective than BL-3849A in that therapy could be initiated as late as 24 h after infection and still significantly reduce mortality and increase the MDD.

TABLE 1. *Hyporeactivity of interferon response in adult mice after multiple doses of BL-3849A*

Day drug was administered[a]	Serum interferon levels (units) 18 h after drug administration	
	i.p.	Oral
0	3,800	4,300
0, 2	850	500
0, 2, 4	400	300
0, 2, 4, 6	125	150

[a] Dosing of drug every 48 h: 100 mg/kg i.p.; 300 mg/kg orally.

Treatment of mice inoculated i.p. with SFV. To evaluate the efficacy of BL-3849A on another ribonucleic acid virus infection, adult mice were infected by the i.p. route with approximately 10 plaque-forming units of SFV. In this infection, animals became paralyzed and died 6 to 8 days after inoculation. The virus control group treated with PBS had a final mortality of 80% and a MDD of 6.6 days (Table 4). Treatment with BL-3849A orally, initiated either 18 h before or 1 h after SFV inoculation, significantly reduced final mortality and increased the MDD. When treatment was initiated 24 h after infection, no effect was observed. Administration of drug i.p. failed to alter final mortality or MDD, regardless of the time treatment was initiated.

Treatment of adult mice inoculated i.p. with *H. hominis* type 2. Adult mice inoculated by the i.p. route with 10^5 plaque-forming units of *H. hominis* type 2 developed paralysis and died between days 8 and 12 after infection. Virus could be detected in the brain on day 6, with low levels of *H. hominis* in visceral organs. Results of treatment of this infection with BL-3849A by either the oral or i.p. route are summarized in Table 5. For purposes of comparison,

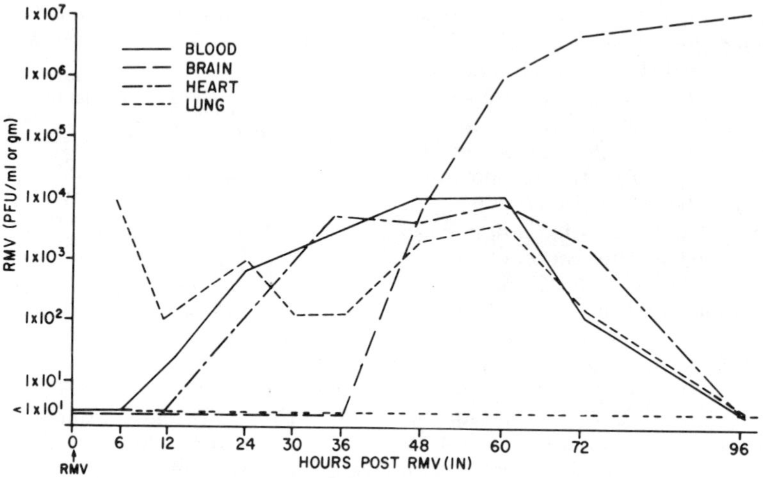

FIG. 3. *Pathogenesis of intranasal RMV infection in adult mice.*

TABLE 2. *Effect of treatment with BL-3849A on the mortality of adult mice infected intranasally with RMV*

Treatment[a]	Mortality		P	MDD	P
	No.	%			
Untreated control	24/30	80		4.6	
BL-3849A, oral					
−18 h	5/30	16	<0.001	6.2	<0.05
+1 h	13/30	43	<0.01	7.0	<0.05
+24 h	25/30	83	NS[b]	4.5	NS
BL-3849A, i.p.					
−18 h	10/30	33	<0.001	4.9	NS
+1 h	24/30	79	NS	5.4	NS
+24 h	27/30	90	NS	5.0	NS

[a] BL-3849A was administered at the indicated times before or after viral challenge at 300 mg/kg orally and 100 mg/kg i.p. every 48 h; total of three doses.
[b] NS, Not significant.

TABLE 3. *Effect of treatment with BL-3849A, tilorone, and poly(I:C) on the mortality of adult mice inoculated i.p. with EMC virus*

Treatment	Mortality		P	MDD	P
	No.	%			
PBS i.p.	12/15	80		6.4	
BL-3849A,[a] oral					
−18 h	2/15	13	<0.001	11.0	<0.05
+1 h	8/15	53	NS[b]	7.9	<0.01
+24 h	5/15	33	<0.05	8.6	NS
BL-3849A,[c] i.p.					
−18 h	1/15	7	<0.001	3.0	
+1 h	3/15	20	<0.01	7.7	NS
+24 h	9/15	60	NS	9.4	<0.001
Tilorone,[d] oral					
−18 h	3/15	20	<0.01	10.3	<0.01
+1 h	6/15	40	NS	9.7	<0.01
+24 h	5/14	43	NS	9.4	NS
Poly(I:C),[e] i.p.					
−18 h	0/15	0	<0.001		
+1 h	3/15	20	<0.01	9.0	<0.01
+24 h	2/15	13	<0.001	15.6	<0.05

[a] 300 mg/kg once every other day for 8 days.
[b] NS, Not significant.
[c] 100 mg/kg once every other day for 8 days.
[d] 250 mg/kg once every other day for 8 days.
[e] 100 μg/mouse once every other day for 8 days.

groups of mice were also treated with tilorone orally or with poly(I:C) i.p. In the virus control group treated with PBS, the mice had a final mortality of 93% and a MDD of 11.3 days. When BL-3849A was administered orally, only those mice that received the drug 18 h before infection had a reduced final mortality. A similar result was noted in the tilorone-treated mice. No significant effect was noted when BL-3849A was given by the i.p. route. In contrast, treatment with poly(I:C) by the i.p. route was very effective in reducing final mortality, even when therapy was initiated 24 h after infection.

DISCUSSION

BL-3849A is a new low-molecular-weight compound which induces high levels of circulating interferon after either oral or i.p. administration. The onset of the interferon response after oral treatment was delayed as compared with i.p. administration. This suggests that there is a period of time necessary for absorption of the drug from the gastrointestinal tract and distribution to the interferon-producing cells. Although the peak levels of interferon in the serum were noted 18 h after administration by either route, serum levels were higher and persisted for a longer period of time after oral administration. The fact that newborn mice produced only 10% as much interferon as adult mice suggested that a process of maturation was necessary either in the absorption and metabolism of the compound or in the cells that produce interferon, perhaps certain cells of the reticuloendothelial system.

Multiple injections of BL-3849A resulted in a marked hyporeactivity on the part of the host to produce interferon. This is not unusual in that every inducer we have tested has also resulted in hyporeactivity of interferon induction after the second or third injection (4a, 6, 11, 17). Although there is evidence to suggest that the antiviral state induced by interferon production in vivo may persist in spite of decreasing levels of serum interferon (1, 13, 19), this potential limitation to the use of interferon inducers and its relationship to antiviral effect need to be further investigated.

Oral treatment with BL-3849A of mice inoculated with RMV, EMC virus, SFV, or *H. hominis* was successful only if treatment was initiated before or shortly after infection. Although studies of the alteration of the pathogenesis of the RMV and EMC virus infections by BL-3849A therapy were not performed as part of these experiments, it is likely that early induction of interferon (onset of the response either before or within 10 to 15 h after viral challenge) was necessary to inhibit the development of viremia and subsequent seeding of target organs. This requirement for early induction of interferon for successful treatment of EMC virus infections with poly(I:C) or poly(I:C)-poly-L-lysine has been described previously (11, 18). In no case was therapy effective if initiated 24 h after infection. The lack of efficacy at this time period appears to be due to the amount of time required for the induction of interferon by BL-3849A. By the time circulating interferon was detectable, viremia had already developed and target organs were being seeded. The reasons why i.p. therapy with BL-3849A was less successful than oral treatment in the infections with RMV, SFV, and *H. hominis* are not completely explained. It may be that the lower levels and shorter duration of the interferon response associated with the i.p. route of inoculation played a role.

BL-3849A is a new, relatively nontoxic interferon inducer that induces high levels of interferon in mice when administered by either the oral or i.p. route and has antiviral activity against both ribonucleic acid and deoxyribonucleic acid viral infections of mice. When administered by the oral route the effectiveness was similar to that of tilorone, but when injected by the i.p. route it was less effective than poly(I:C). The possibility that BL-3849A will offer the advantages of an oral interferon inducer and also be less toxic suggests that further evaluation of this compound is warranted. It should be noted, however, that tilorone hydrochloride, another low-molecular-weight compound which also induces interferon by the oral route in mice, is not an effective inducer in humans (4). This observation suggests that BL-3849A should be studied in other animal species, including primates and humans, before its full potential as an antiviral agent can be determined.

TABLE 4. *Effect of treatment with BL-3849A on the mortality of adult mice inoculated i.p. with SFV*

Treatment	Mortality		P	MDD	P
	No.	%			
PBS, i.p.	12/15	80		6.6	
BL-3849A,[a] oral					
−18 h	3/15	20	<0.01	12.7	<0.01
+1 h	3/15	20	<0.01	8.7	<0.05
+24 h	11/15	73	NS[b]	7.4	NS
BL-3849A,[c] i.p.					
−18 h	10/15	67	NS	7.7	NS
+1 h	10/15	67	NS	6.8	NS
+24 h	10/15	67	NS	7.8	NS

[a] 300 mg/kg once every other day for 8 days.
[b] NS, Not significant.
[c] 100 mg/kg once every other day for 8 days.

TABLE 5. *Effect of treatment with BL-3849A, tilorone, and poly(I:C) on the mortality of adult mice infected i.p. with H. hominis type 2*

Treatment	Mortality		P	MDD	P
	No.	%			
PBS	14/15	93		11.3	
BL-3849A,[a] oral					
−18 h	4/15	27	<0.001	11.5	NS[b]
+1 h	13/15	87	NS	10.9	NS
+24 h	12/15	80	NS	10.9	NS
BL-3849A,[c] i.p.					
−18 h	9/15	60	NS	10.2	NS
+1 h	11/15	73	NS	10.6	NS
+24 h	11/15	73	NS	10.6	NS
Tilorone,[d] oral					
−18 h	2/15	13	<0.001	14.5	
+1 h	13/15	87	NS	10.9	NS
+24 h	12/15	80	NS	10.6	NS
Poly(I:C),[e] i.p.					
−18 h	1/15	7	<0.001	14.0	
+1 h	5/15	33	<0.001	12.6	NS
+24 h	8/15	53	<0.05	12.3	NS

[a] 300 mg/kg every other day for 8 days.
[b] NS, Not significant.
[c] 100 mg/kg every other day for 8 days.
[d] 250 mg/kg every other day for 8 days.
[e] 100 μg/mouse every other day for 8 days.

ACKNOWLEDGMENTS

This work was supported by Public Health Service contract no. NOI-AI-42524 from the Antiviral Substances Program of the National Institute of Allergy and Infectious Diseases and by Public Health Service grant no. AI-10217 from the National Institute of Allergy and Infectious Diseases.

We wish to thank James T. Richards for excellent technical assistance. J.C.O. is an investigator, Howard Hughes Medical Institute.

LITERATURE CITED

1. **DeClercq, E.** 1972. Hyporeactivity to interferon production by double-stranded RNA associated with hyporeactivity to antiviral protection and hyporeactivity to toxicity. Proc. Soc. Exp. Biol. Med. **141**:340-345.
2. **Glaz, E. T., E. Szolgay, I. Stoger, and M. Talas.** 1973. Antiviral activity and induction of interferon-like substance by quinacrine and acranil. Antimicrob. Agents Chemother. **3**:537-541.
3. **Hoffman, W. W., J. J. Korst, J. F. Niblack, and T. H. Cronin.** 1973. *N,N*-dioctadecyl-*N,N'*-bis (2-hydroxyethyl) propanediamine: antiviral activity and interferon stimulation in mice. Antimicrob. Agents Chemother. **3**:498-502.
4. **Kaufman, H. E., Y. M. Centifanto, E. D. Ellison, and D. C. Brown.** 1971. Tilorone hydrochloride: human toxicity and interferon stimulation. Proc. Soc. Exp. Biol. Med. **137**:357-360.

4a. **Kern, E. R., L. A. Glasgow, and J. C. Overall, Jr.** 1976. Antiviral activity of an extract of *Brucella abortus*: induction of interferon and immunopotentiation of host resistance. Proc. Soc. Exp. Biol. Med. **152**:372-376.

5. **Kern, E. R., J. C. Overall, Jr., and L. A. Glasgow.** 1973. Herpesvirus hominis infection in newborn mice. I. An experimental model and therapy with iododeoxyuridine. J. Infect. Dis. **128**:290-299.
6. **Kern, E. R., J. C. Overall, Jr., and L. A. Glasgow.** 1975. *Herpesvirus hominis* infection of newborn mice: treatment with interferon inducer polyinosinic-polycytidylic acid. Antimicrob. Agents Chemother. **7**:793-800.
7. **Kramer, M. J., R. Cleeland, and E. Grunberg.** 1976. Antiviral activity of 10-carboxymethyl-9-acridanone. Antimicrob. Agents Chemother. **9**:233-238.
8. **Krueger, R. F., and G. D. Mayer.** 1970. Tilorone hydrochloride: an orally active antiviral agent. Science **169**:1213-1214.
9. **Murphy, B. R., and L. A. Glasgow.** 1968. Factors modifying host resistance to viral infection. III. Effect of whole body x-irradiation on experimental encephalomyocarditis virus infection in mice. J. Exp. Med. **127**:1035-1052.
10. **Nichol, F. R., S. D. Weed, and G. E. Underwood.** 1976. Stimulation of murine interferon by a substituted pyrimidine. Antimicrob. Agents Chemother. **9**:433-439.
11. **Olsen, G. A., E. R. Kern, L. A. Glasgow, and J. C. Overall, Jr.** 1976. Effect of treatment with exogenous interferon, polyinosinic acid-polycytidylic acid, or polyinosinic acid-polycytidylic acid-poly-L-lysine complex on encephalomyocarditis virus infections in mice. Antimicrob. Agents Chemother. **10**:668-676.
12. **Saito, N., F. Suzuki, K. Sasaki, and N. Ishida.** 1976. Antiviral and interferon-inducing activity of a new glutarimide antibiotic, 9-methylstreptimidone. Antimicrob. Agents Chemother. **10**:14-19.
13. **Sharpe, T. J., P. J. Birch, and D. N. Planterose.** 1971. Resistance to virus infection during the hyporeactive state of interferon induction. J. Gen. Virol. **12**:331-333.
14. **Siminoff, P., A. M. Bernard, V. S. Hursky, and K. E. Price.** 1973. BL-20803, a new, low-molecular-weight interferon inducer. Antimicrob. Agents Chemother. **3**:742-743.
15. **Soehner, R. L., M. M. Gambardella, and E. F. Hou.** 1974. Oral induction of interferon by a low-molecular weight compound. Proc. Soc. Exp. Biol. Med. **145**:1114-1119.
16. **Stringfellow, D. A., and L. A. Glasgow.** 1972. Hyporeactivity of infection: potential limitation to therapeutic use of interferon-inducing agents. Infect. Immun. **6**:743-747.
17. **Stringfellow, D. A., and L. A. Glasgow.** 1972. Tilorone hydrochloride: an oral interferon-inducing agent. Antimicrob. Agents Chemother. **2**:73-78.
18. **Stringfellow, D. A., J. C. Overall, Jr., and L. A. Glasgow.** 1974. Interferon inducers in therapy of infection with encephalomyocarditis virus in mice. I. Effect of single doses of polyriboinosinic-polyribocytidylic acid and tilorone hydrochloride on viral pathogenesis. J. Infect. Dis. **130**:470-480.
19. **Stringfellow, D. A., J. C. Overall, Jr., and L. A. Glasgow.** 1974. Interferon inducers in therapy of infection with encephalomyocarditis virus in mice. II. Effect of multiple doses of polyriboinosinic-polyribocytidylic acid on viral pathogenesis. J. Infect. Dis. **130**:481-488.

ANTIMICROBIAL AGENTS AND CHEMOTHERAPY, Oct. 1976, p. 697-706

Vol. 10, No. 4
Printed in U.S.A.

Suppression of the Lytic and Bactericidal Effects of Cell Wall-Inhibitory Antibiotics

RUBEN LOPEZ, CONCHITA RONDA-LAIN, ALFONSO TAPIA, SUSAN B. WAKS, AND ALEXANDER TOMASZ*

*Instituto di Immunolgia y Biologia Microbiana, Madrid, Spain, and The Rockefeller University, New York, New York 10071**

Received for publication 10 June 1976

The bacteriolytic effect of beta-lactam antibiotics on *Bacillus subtilis* and on *Streptococcus pneumoniae* was found to be a function of the pH; lysis was suppressed if the pH of the pneumococcal culture was below 6.0 during penicillin treatment. In the case of *B. subtilis,* growth at pH 6.6 prevented penicillin-induced lysis. In pneumococci, the addition of trypsin to the growth medium also protected against lysis. The pH-dependent protection phenomenon resembled in several respects the antibiotic "tolerance" of pneumococci with a defective autolytic system. (i) At the pH nonpermissive for lysis, the bacteria retained their normal sensitivity to beta-lactam and to other cell wall inhibitors; however, instead of lysis, the drug-treated bacteria simply stopped growing. Loss of viability of the cells was also greatly reduced. (ii) Protection against lysis was independent of the dose and chemical nature of the cell wall inhibitors. (iii) The protection effect was reversible; lysis and loss of viability could be triggered by a postincubation of the drug-treated bacteria at the pH permissive for lysis.

The beta-lactams, D-cycloserine and beta-halogeno-D-alanine, can inhibit specific enzymatic reactions in the cell wall metabolism of bacteria. In most bacteria treatment with these antibiotics results in a rapid loss of viability, and in many species the treated cells actually disintegrate (lyse).

How inhibition of the antibiotic-sensitive enzymatic reactions may lead to the important antimicrobial effects of these drugs (namely, to the killing and lysis of the bacteria) is not well understood. The possible involvement of cell wall-hydrolyzing enzymes (autolysins) in penicillin-induced lysis has been considered repeatedly in the literature (12, 14, 21). More recently, direct experimental evidence for such a role has been obtained in pneumococci. In studies reported previously (17, 18), suppression of the activity of the *N*-acetylmuramic acid-L-alanine amidase resulted in a striking change in the response of this bacterium to penicillin and other cell wall inhibitors; although the drug-treated bacteria stopped growing, they no longer lysed and the rate of loss of cellular viability was greatly reduced. Such a "tolerant" response to cell wall inhibitors was subsequently also observed in lysis-defective mutants of *Bacillus licheniformis* (13).

In this communication, we describe growth conditions that can produce antibiotic tolerance in pneumococci and in *Bacillus subtilis.* We have observed that a suitable choice of pH in the growth media can dramatically change the response of these bacteria to cell wall inhibitors from lysis to simple growth inhibition; the same conditions also cause a substantial reduction in the rate of loss of viability. In pneumococci, addition of trypsin to the growth medium also has a similar effect. We suggest that the mechanism of these protective phenomena involves the suppression of the activity (or inactivation) of an autolysin that catalyzes the antibiotic-induced lysis of the bacterial cells.

MATERIALS AND METHODS

Bacterial strains. Two bacterial strains were used: *Streptococcus pneumoniae* strain R36A (Rockefeller University laboratory stock) and *B. subtilis* 168 (obtained from Leonard Mindich of the Public Health Research Institute, New York, N.Y.).

Antibiotics. Amidino penicillin FL 1060 (mecillinam) was obtained from Leo Co., Ballerup, Denmark. D-Cycloserine (Merck) and benzylpenicillin (Squibb) were commercial products; sodium dicloxacillin was obtained from Wyeth Labs, Inc., Philadelphia, Pa.; cephalothin was a gift of Kenneth Price of Bristol Laboratories, Syracuse, N.Y.; and beta-chloro-D-alanine was kindly supplied by James Manning of The Rockefeller University, New York, N.Y. Trypsin (2× recrystallized, Worthington Biochemicals Corp., Freehold, N.J.) and all other reagents and medium components were reagent-grade, commercially available products.

Growth media. A synthetic medium containing

acid-hydrolyzed casein (7a, 16; C-medium) was used with both pneumococci and *B. subtilis* in all the experiments illustrated in the figures. In the case of *B. subtilis*, the pH of the medium was set by potassium phosphate buffers (at pH values of 8.0 or 6.6) at a final concentration of 0.1 M (3). Cultures of *B. subtilis* were grown aerobically in a shaker bath at about 60 strokes per min (Gyrotory water bath shaker model G76, New Brunswick Corp.).

Pneumococci were cultured in glass test tubes, without shaking, in C-medium containing potassium phosphate buffers at a final concentration of 0.05 M and with initial pH values of 8.0 or 6.6.

Occasionally, *B. subtilis* cultures were also grown in the medium of Anagnostopoulos and Spizizen (1) buffered at pH 8.0 or 6.6. In a few experiments with *B. subtilis*, the pH 8 phosphate buffer of the C-medium was replaced by 0.1 M tris(hydroxymethyl)aminomethane (Tris), pH 8 (potassium phosphate was added to such media to give a concentration of 0.02 M). The effects of culture pH on lysis sensitivity were reproduced with these media. However, only experiments with phosphate-buffered media are illustrated in figures.

The sharp pH dependence of some of thephenomena to be described in this paper made it necessary to monitor changes in the pH of cultures as a function of bacterial growth. In the case of *B. subtilis* cultures grown with aeration and with buffer concentrations of 0.1 M, there was relatively little change in the culture pH during the experiments. As the cell concentration of the cultures reached the range of 10^7 to 10^8 viable cells per ml, the pH of the phosphate-buffered media was found to shift from the initial 8.0 to about 7.5 and from the initial pH of 6.6 to about 6.0; with the Tris buffer the pH changed from 8.0 to about 7.8 only.

In contrast to the *B. subtilis* cultures, the phosphate-buffered pneumococcal cultures underwent more substantial changes in the medium pH during growth, presumably due to the production of lactic acid. With buffer concentrations of 0.05 M, the pH values of cultures were found to change in a characteristic manner during bacterial growth (for details, see Fig. 9). At a cell concentration of 5×10^7 viable units per ml, the pH of cultures containing pH 6.6 buffers had shifted to about 5.8 and the pH had further dropped to 4.5 to 4.8 in the stationary phase of growth. The pH of cultures with pH 8 buffers had dropped to about 6.9 when the cell concentration reached 5×10^7 viable units per ml (corresponding to the light-scattering value of N = 200 on the Coleman nephocolorimeter used to monitor bacterial growth), and the pH value stabilized at 6.5 to 6.6 in the stationary phase of growth.

Growth of the cultures was measured by monitoring the light scattering of the suspensions using a Coleman nephocolorimeter (16). The arbitrary "nephelometric (N) units" of the instrument were calibrated by determining the corresponding colony-forming units of the bacteria. Viability was determined by the routine agar plating methods (1, 16). Antibiotics were "removed" before plating by dilution to levels that had no detectable effect on bacterial growth in liquid culture or in agar medium. Growth media were used as diluents.

To avoid the activation of the lytic response on the agar plates, the antibiotic-treated bacteria (such as the ones titrated in Fig. 4 through 6 and Table 1) were plated on agar media whose pH had been adjusted to values that protect against lysis in liquid cultures (i.e., 0.1 M phosphate at pH 6.6 for *B. subtilis* and 0.05 M phosphate for pneumococci).

Assay of autolysis. The bacterial suspensions or debris were incubated in the appropriate buffers at 37°C and at intervals the turbidities were determined using a Zeiss spectrophotometer (optical density at 660 nm) (22).

Assay of radioactive material secreted into the medium. Radioactive choline ([*methyl*-^{3}H]choline, 0.5 Ci/mmol, 2 μCi and 5 μg/ml of medium) was added to the medium of exponentially growing pneumococci at a cell concentration of about 5×10^7 viable units per ml. Incorporation of the isotope into total macromolecular material secreted into the medium was determined by a published procedure (20), the essential features of which are as follows: 100-μl portions of the suspension were removed and treated with cold 10% trichloroacetic acid for 15 min; the precipitated material was collected on to glass-fiber filter disks (GFA) under vacuum. After drying at 100°C for 10 min, the disks were transferred to scintillation vials and the amounts of radioactivity were determined by using toluene-based cocktail with 2,5-diphenyl-oxazole (PPO) and a scintillation spectrometer (Mark II, Nuclear-Chicago Corp.).

Material secreted into the medium was first separated from the bacteria by centrifugation: 500-μl portions of the cultures were centrifuged for 10 min in an Eppendorf microcentrifuge (Brinkman Co.), and 100-μl portions of the supernatant solutions were assayed as described above.

RESULTS

Protection against antibiotic-induced lysis in *B. subtilis* cultures grown at pH 6.6. Figure 1 demonstrates the strikingly different response of *B. subtilis* cultures to four cell wall-inhibiting antibiotics, dependent upon the pH of the growth medium. In contrast to the behavior of cultures at pH 8.0, the low-pH cultures were not lysed but only inhibited by the antibiotic treatments. Several additional conclusions may also be drawn from the figure: (i) the dose responses of the high- and low-pH cultures to the various antibiotics were similar in spite of the fact that the antibiotics had a bacteriolytic effect at the high pH, whereas at the lower pH they only acted as bacteriostatic agents; (ii) the antibiotic tolerance at low pH did not seem to depend on the antibiotic dose, since lysis did not occur even at very high doses of the antibiotics (e.g., treatment with 500 times the minimal inhibitory concentration of cloxacillin for 5 h); and (iii) the antibiotic tolerance was independent of the chemical nature of the drug and did not depend on the inhibition of a specific enzymatic reaction, since a low pH was found to protect equally well against lysis by beta-lactams and by D-cycloserine.

Reversibility of the tolerant response. Figures 2 and 3 demonstrate the reversibility of the pH-dependent antibiotic tolerance. In these experiments, bacterial cultures were first treated with the four different antibiotics at the low pH. After the cultures had stopped growing, the bacteria were centrifuged, washed, and resuspended in fresh, antibiotic-free growth media at two different pH values corresponding to the lysis-permissive (pH 8.0) and lysis-nonpermissive (pH 6.6) conditions. The lytic response of the bacteria could be reactivated by the postincubation at the permissive pH. However, the degree of clearing of the cultures (as registered by the light scattering) seemed less extensive than the lysis observed during incubation in a single, lysis-permissive medium. The causes of this discrepancy are not known.

These experiments suggest that: (i) the primary (growth-inhibitory) effect of the antibiotics may be experimentally separated, in time, from the secondary (lytic) effect; and (ii) during treatment at the low pH, the antibiotics reach their normal specific inhibitory targets, since the "normal" (i.e., lytic) response can be reactivated in the absence of added antibiotics after pretreatment at the low pH.

Protection against the cytocidal effect of antibiotics. The low pH also gave a dramatic protection against the killing effects of cloxacillin and mecillinam (Fig. 4 and 5). This protection effect was reversible; after pretreatment of the bacteria with cloxacillin at the low pH, one could trigger the killing effect by a postincubation at the high pH in the absence of the antibiotic (Fig. 6).

pH dependence of autolysis in *B. subtilis*. In an attempt to better characterize the biochemical nature of the process inactivated at the low pH, we determined the pH dependence of autolysis in *B. subtilis*. Figure 7 shows the effect of pH on the rate of lysis of mechanically disrupted bacteria (i.e., the washed, crude debris obtained after brief [2-min] sonication of the cells in a Raytheon sonicator) (22). In Fig. 8 intact exponentially growing bacteria were suspended in 0.1 M Tris-maleate buffers of various pH values and were incubated at 37°C. Apparently, cells were unstable under these conditions and autolyzed. With both the disrupted and the intact cells, the rate of autolysis increased with the pH up to about pH 8.5. Autolysis was substantially slower below pH 7.0. These findings suggest that the autolytic processes are catalyzed by the *B. subtilis* amidase (*N*-acetylmuramic acid-L-alanine amidase); the purified amidase has a pH optimum at 8.5 (4).

Antibiotic tolerance of pneumococci grown at low pH. It was important to test the possible applicability of the pH-dependent antibiotic tolerance in pneumococci, since the mechanism of antibiotic-induced lysis and killing has been most extensively studied in this microorganism (17–20). The tolerant response to benzylpenicillin, mecillinam, and cephalothin could also be invoked in pneumococci by the suitable choice of pH. Pneumococcal cultures grew with comparable growth rates in media with initial pH values of 8.0 and 6.6. On the other hand, lysis by benzylpenicillin only occurred at the higher pH (Fig. 9). The pH changed in a reproducible manner during culture growth (as a function of cell concentration) in these media (see also Materials and Methods). Lysis occurred if the culture pH was in the vicinity of 7 during penicillin treatment (see figure). Lysis was inhibited if the pH was below 6.0 during drug treatment (see figure) or if it was above 8.0 (not shown). The rapid loss of viability observable during beta-lactam treatment of cultures growing at the higher pH was also dramatically slowed down at the lower pH (Table 1).

The tolerant response of pneumococci could also be reversed (by shifting the pH of the antibiotic-treated culture to the pH permissive for lysis; data not shown) in a manner exactly analogous to that of the *B. subtilis* cultures.

Secretion of a choline-containing autolysin inhibitor during treatment of pneumococci with penicillin under conditions nonpermissive for lysis. Leakage of a choline-containing macromolecular autolysin inhibitor into the growth medium has been observed during treatment of autolysin-defective mutant pneumococci with cell wall inhibitors (20). A similar leakage of macromolecular choline compounds occurred during penicillin treatment of a wild-type pneumococcus growing under conditions nonpermissive for lysis (pH 5.8) (Fig. 10).

Protection against lysis by trypsin. Lysis of pneumococci (growing in the medium with initial pH of 8.0) by D-cycloserine or benzylpenicillin could also be inhibited by the addition of trypsin or Pronase to the growth medium (Fig. 11). Heat-denatured trypsin or serum albumin (bovine serum albumin, Armour fraction V) added at the same concentration (500 μg/ml) had no protective effect. Even the spontaneous lysis characteristic of late-stationary-phase cultures of pneumococci was inhibited in the presence of the proteolytic enzyme (Fig. 11).

DISCUSSION

Disintegration (lysis) of bacteria upon treatment with antibiotics involves damage to both structural components of the cells, the cell

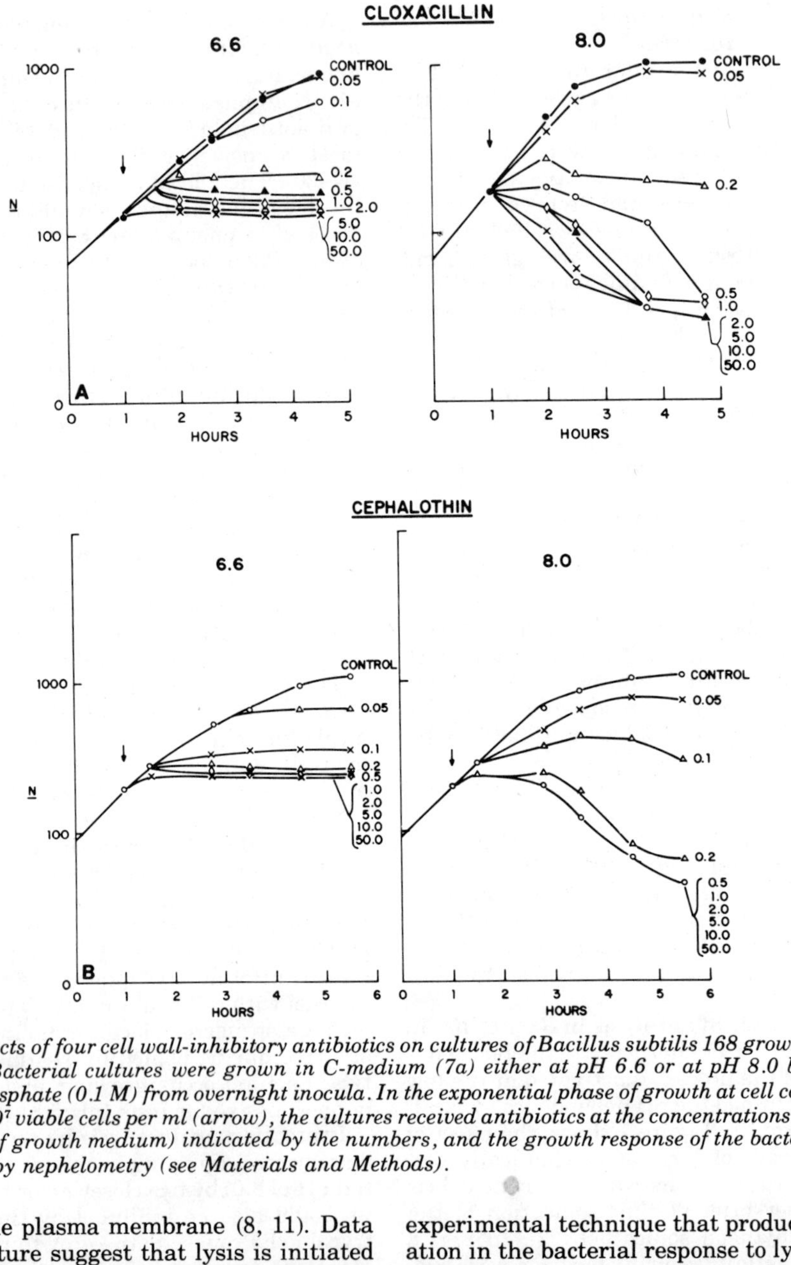

FIG. 1. *Effects of four cell wall-inhibitory antibiotics on cultures of Bacillus subtilis 168 growing at pH 6.6 and pH 8.0. Bacterial cultures were grown in C-medium (7a) either at pH 6.6 or at pH 8.0 buffered with potassium phosphate (0.1 M) from overnight inocula. In the exponential phase of growth at cell concentrations of about 5 × 10^7 viable cells per ml (arrow), the cultures received antibiotics at the concentrations (micrograms per milliliter of growth medium) indicated by the numbers, and the growth response of the bacterial cultures was followed by nephelometry (see Materials and Methods).*

walls and the plasma membrane (8, 11). Data in the literature suggest that lysis is initiated by damage to the cell wall. In pneumococci, the agent responsible for this damage is the *N*-acetylmuramic acid-L-alanine amidase (17). Participation of autolysins in penicillin-induced lysis has also been confirmed in *B. licheniformis* (13).

Until now, the mechanism of lytic phenomena could only be investigated through the use of lytic mutants or, in the case of pneumococci, by the use of ethanolamine-grown bacteria (15). In this communication we describe a simple experimental technique that produces an alteration in the bacterial response to lytic antibiotics exactly analogous to that of the lytic-defective mutants. Both in pneumococci and in *B. subtilis,* appropriate modulation of the pH of the growth medium produces the typical features of antibiotic tolerance. (i) The cellular response to lytic antibiotics changes from lysis to bacteriostasis, while the cells retain their normal sensitivity (dose response) to the drugs. (ii) The cells become tolerant not only to penicillin but also against drugs inhibiting "early" steps of wall synthesis. However, one should add at

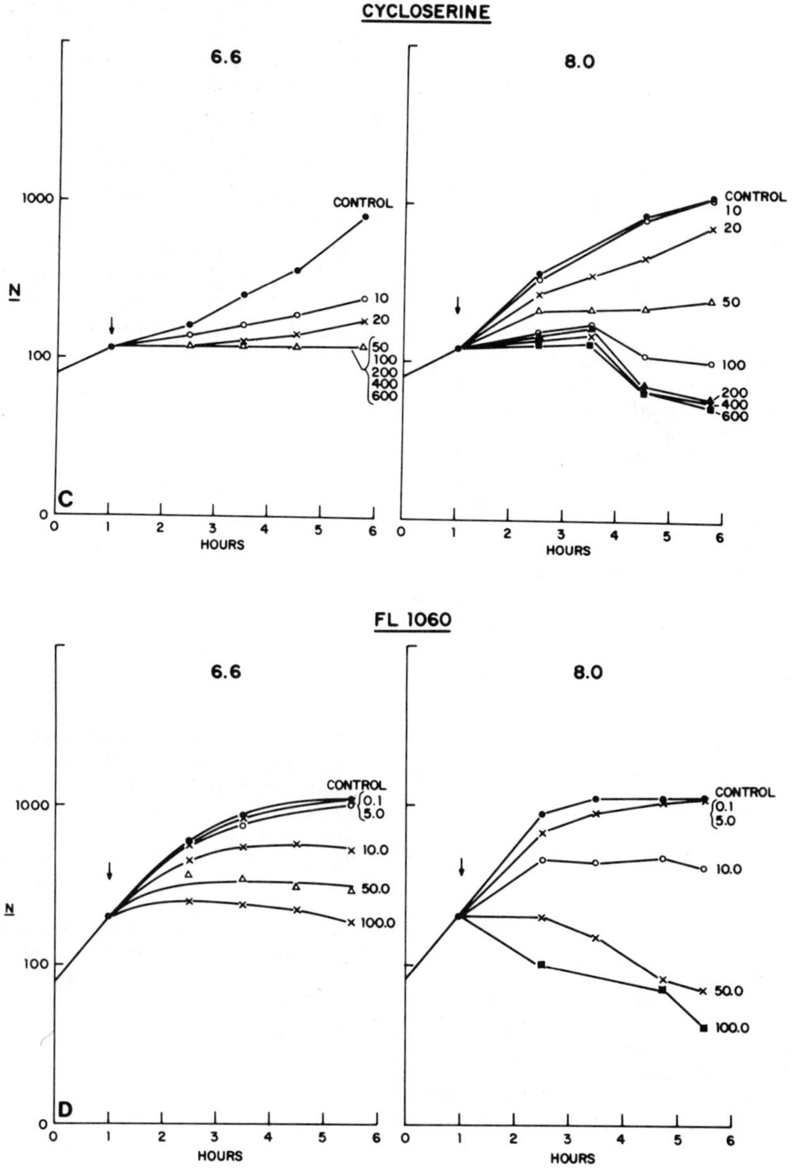

FIG. 1. C, D

this point that D-cycloserine-induced lysis (as determined by the light-scattering method; see Fig. 1C and 3) has always been less extensive than lysis by the beta-lactams. The reasons for this discrepancy are not understood at the present time. (iii) The tolerant phenotype is reversible. (iv) In both species, the conditions nonpermissive for lysis also provide a substantial protection against loss of viability.

The growth rates of cultures are similar if not identical under the lytic and tolerant conditions. Furthermore, the antibiotics seem to reach their "normal" enzymatic targets in the cells growing under the tolerant condition, since (i) the dose responses under lytic and tolerant conditions are similar and (ii) it is possible to invoke the lytic response by the following sequence of treatments: exposure of cells to penicillin under tolerant conditions, followed by removal of penicillin (by penicillinase) and, finally, transfer of cells to fresh growth medium with the pH optimal for lysis.

It therefore appears that there exist two kinds of growth conditions for these bacteria:

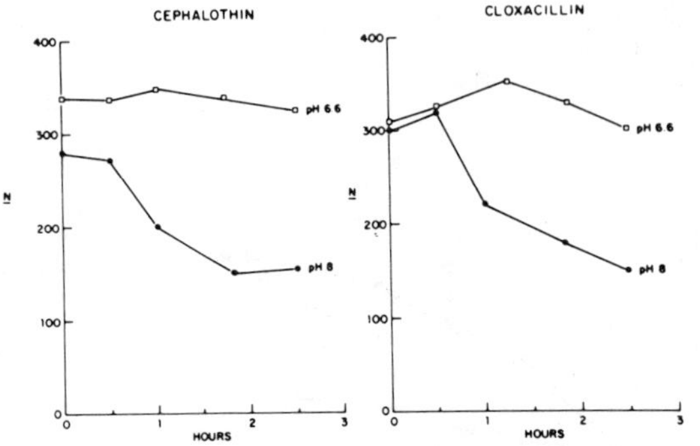

FIG. 2. *Reactivation of the lytic response of B. subtilis to cephalothin and cloxacillin. Bacterial cultures were treated with cephalothin (0.5 μg/ml) and cloxacillin (0.2 μg/ml), respectively, for 2 h in growth media at pH 6.6. The cultures were next centrifuged, washed with buffer-free medium, and resuspended each in two different media, one at pH 6.6 and the other at pH 8.0. Both media were free of antibiotics The change of light scattering of these suspensions was followed (nephelometry) during incubation at 37°C. Note that the light-scattering data are plotted on a linear scale (unlike the log scales in Fig. 1).*

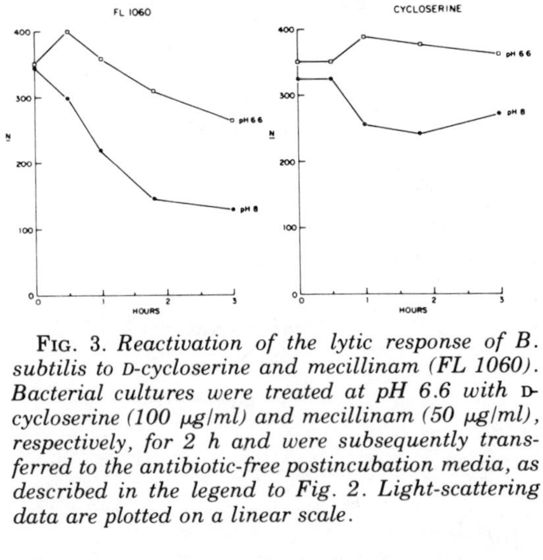

FIG. 3. *Reactivation of the lytic response of B. subtilis to* D*-cycloserine and mecillinam (FL 1060). Bacterial cultures were treated at pH 6.6 with* D*-cycloserine (100 μg/ml) and mecillinam (50 μg/ml), respectively, for 2 h and were subsequently transferred to the antibiotic-free postincubation media, as described in the legend to Fig. 2. Light-scattering data are plotted on a linear scale.*

one permissive and another nonpermissive for lysis. In pneumococci the permissive pH was found to be in the vicinity of pH 7.0; cultures kept at a pH less than 6.0 showed inhibition of lysis, and lysis was also suppressed at pH 8 and above (data not shown). In *B. subtilis* the permissive pH was around and above 8; pH values below 6.6 were inhibitory for lysis. Although the absolute pH values permissive for lysis are different in the two organisms, in each case they correspond to the in vitro pH optima of the activity of the major murein hydrolases (*N*-acetyl-muramic acid-L-alanine amidase) (4, 6). The pneumococcal enzyme has about 30% of its maximal activity (at the pH optimum of 6.9) at pH 6.0 and about 20% of maximal activity at pH 8 (6). These observations suggest that in *B. subtilis* as in pneumococci, the murein hydrolase responsible for the antibiotic-induced cell lysis is the amidase (rather than the muramidase [2] that has also been detected in this bacterium).

Although bacteria are known to regulate their intracellular pH, it seems likely that the activity of enzymes located on the outer surface of the plasma membrane or in the periplasmic

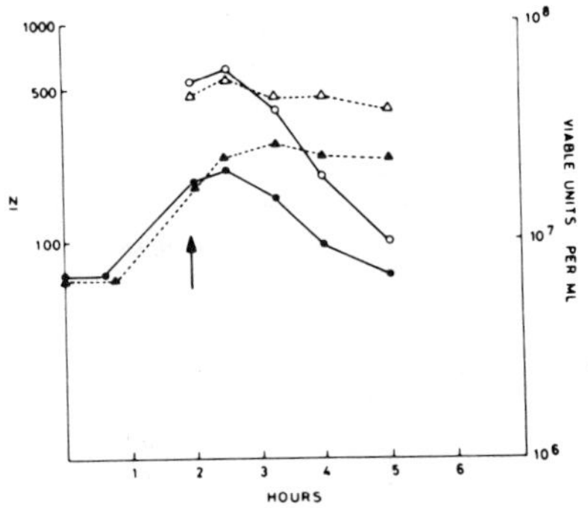

FIG. 4. *Protection against cloxacillin-induced loss of viability at low pH. Bacillus subtilis cultures, growing at pH 6.6 and pH 8.0, respectively, received cloxacillin (0.2 μg/ml) at the time indicated by the arrow, and the rate of loss of viable bacteria in the cultures was followed by agar plating, during incubation with the antibiotic. Open symbols indicate viable units per milliliter; closed symbols represent growth measured by nephelometry. Viability at pH 6.6 (△, dashed line); growth at pH 6.6 (▲, dashed line); viability at pH 8.0 (○, solid line); growth at pH 8.0 (●, solid line).*

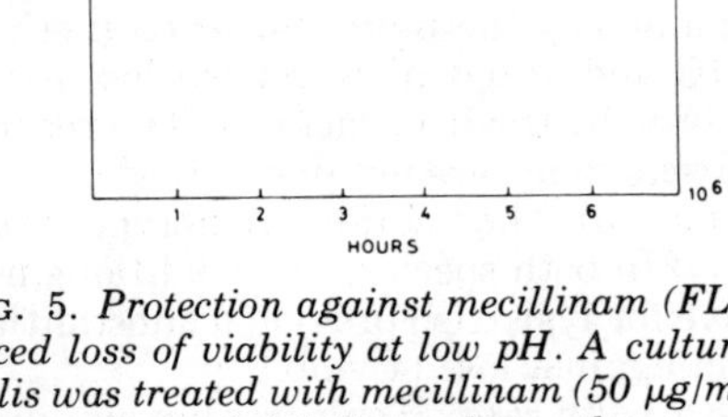

FIG. 5. *Protection against mecillinam (FL 1060)-induced loss of viability at low pH. A culture of B. subtilis was treated with mecillinam (50 μg/ml), and the rates of loss of viability and growth were assayed as described in the legend to Fig. 4. Symbols are the same as in Fig. 4.*

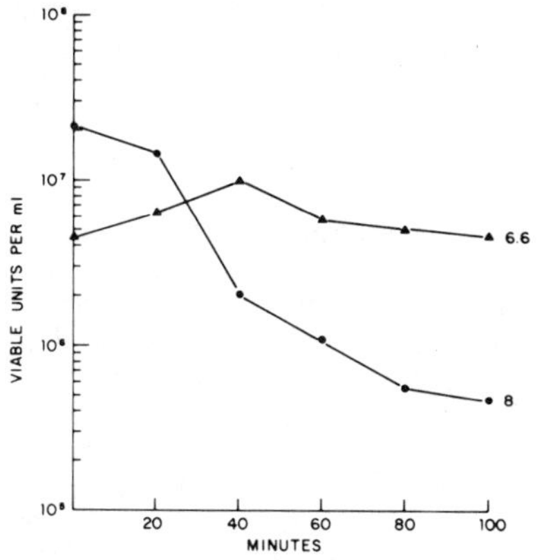

FIG. 6. *Reactivation of the killing effect of cloxacillin by postincubation at pH 8.0. A culture of B. subtilis was pretreated with cloxacillin (0.2 μg/ml) for 2 h at pH 6.6. The culture was divided into two parts; both were centrifuged, and the cells were washed with buffer-free media and resuspended in fresh, antibiotic-free media at pH 6.6 and pH 8.0, respectively. The two suspensions were incubated at 37°C, and samples were removed at intervals for the determination of the viable titer.*

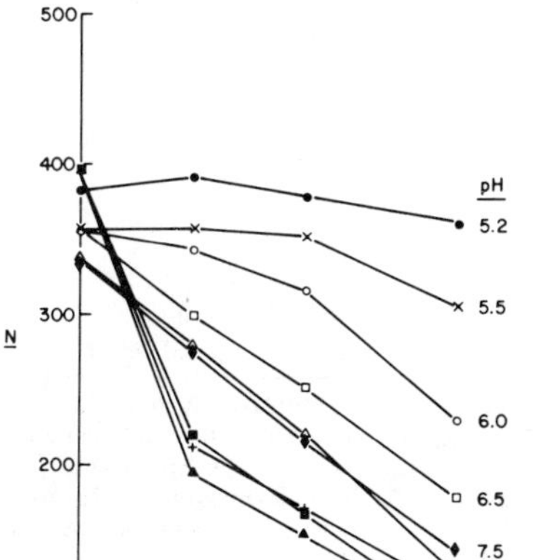

FIG. 7. *Autolysis of sonically disrupted Bacillus subtilis at different pH values. A 100-ml culture of B. subtilis growing exponentially at pH 8.0 was harvested by centrifugation at a cell concentration of 2 × 10⁸ viable cells per ml. The cells were resuspended in 10 ml of ice-cold 0.15 M saline and sonicated for 2 min in a Raytheon sonicator. Examination of the sonicated suspension by phase-contrast microscopy showed that over 90% of the cells had become "empty." The suspension was centrifuged, resuspended in 10 ml of fresh saline, and diluted 10-fold into test tubes containing Tris-maleate buffers (0.1 M) ranging in pH from 5.2 to 9.0. The rate of loss of turbidity (optical density at 660 nm) was followed during incubation at 37°C.*

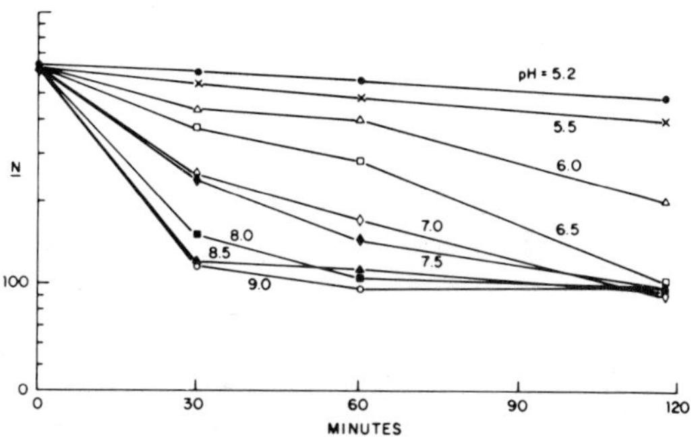

FIG. 8. *Autolysis of Bacillus subtilis suspensions in buffers of various pH values. An exponentially growing culture of B. subtilis (2×10^8 viable cells per ml) in pH 8.0 medium was centrifuged; the pelleted cells were rinsed with saline (0.15 M NaCl) and resuspended in saline at 10 times the original cell concentration. This stock suspension was then quickly diluted 10-fold into a series of test tubes, each containing 0.1 M Tris-maleate buffer at the pH values indicated by the numbers on the figure. The suspensions were incubated at 37°C, and the turbidity (optical density at 660 nm) change was monitored at intervals, using a Zeiss spectrophotometer.*

space would be accessible to manipulation by changes in the ionic milieu of the growth medium. The molecular sieve properties of the bacterial outer envelopes are known to allow the free penetration of molecules of substantial molecular weights (9). We suggest that pH values nonpermissive for antibiotic-induced lysis inhibit the endogenous activity of murein hydrolases which, under the permissive conditions, are responsible for the antibiotic-induced destruction of the bacteria.

The pH value of the bacterial growth medium is, of course, a major parameter of bacterial growth, and different pH values may cause complex physiological differences in the cells. For instance, bacteria are known to produce different phospholipids when shifted to subphysiological pH (7), and the plasma membrane of such bacteria may be more stable to osmotic lysis (10). We cannot exclude with certainty that such indirect changes in cellular physiology may not also contribute to the pH-dependent drug tolerance. However, the quick reversibility of bacteriostatic to lytic response and the remarkable similarity of the phenomenon to the well-documented cases of drug tolerance in lytic mutants suggest that in this case we may be observing direct and relatively simple consequences of the suppression of a surface-located enzyme activity. Additional evidence supporting this interpretation comes from the observation that pneumococci growing in a medium with a pH permissive for lysis can nevertheless be protected against lysis by the

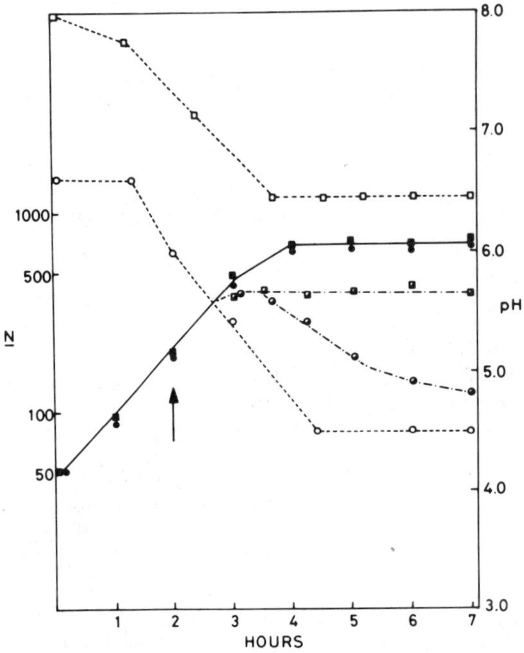

FIG. 9. *Protection of pneumococci against penicillin-induced lysis by growth at low pH. Two test tube cultures (A and B) of Streptococcus pneumoniae (20 ml each) were grown from small inocula (2 × 10^5 to 5 × 10^5 viable cells per ml) in C-medium (7a) containing potassium phosphate buffers (0.05 M) at pH 8.0 and pH 6.6. When the cell concentration had reached 5 × 10^7 viable cells per ml, each culture was divided in two (A1, A2, and B1, B2), and one of the cultures (A1 and B1) received benzylpenicillin (0.1 μg/ml) (see arrow in figure); the other two cultures (A2 and B2) served as controls. Growth and lysis were followed by nephelometry (N). Periodically, samples were removed for the determination of the culture pH, using a Beckman automatic pH meter equipped with class microelectrodes (Beckman model Zeromatic SS-3). The changes in the culture pH of culture A1 and A2 were found to be virtually identical. No significant differences were observed between the pH values of cultures B1 versus B2. Symbols: (——) Growth of the control cultures; (■) A2; (●) B2; (----) pH of the cultures; (□) A1 and A2; (○) B1 and B2; (-·-·) growth and lysis of penicillin-treated cultures; (◑) A1; (◪) B1.*

simple addition of trypsin to the growth medium. We interpret this observation as the proteolytic destruction of amidase molecules that are liberated into the periplasm or onto the surface of the cell wall and thus made accessible to trypsin. The pneumococcal autolysin is extremely sensitive to proteolysis. The relative resistance of the *B. subtilis* amidase to proteolytic enzymes (4) may be the reason for the failure of trypsin to protect *B. subtilis* against penicillin lysis.

The pH-dependent antibiotic tolerance described in this communication may have a general applicability, since closely similar effects have been observed in a number of species, such as *Escherichia coli*, staphylococci, and *Streptococcus faecium* (W. Goodell, R. Lopez, and A. Tomasz, submitted for publication). It is possible that in some species of bacteria additional unique properties of the murine hydrolases (such as salt sensitivity) could also be exploited for the selective suppression of the activity of these enzymes. Such studies may

TABLE 1. *Protection against the killing action of beta-lactams in the lysis-nonpermissive growth medium*[a]

Antibiotic (μg/ml)	Duration of treatment (min)	Antibiotic treatment in:[b]	
		Lysis-permissive medium	Lysis-nonpermissive medium
Benzylpenicillin (0.1)	0	5.0	5.0
	20	4.5	4.8
	40	0.8	2.0
	60	0.1	1.0
	120	0.0003	0.2
Cephalothin (5)	0	5.2	5.2
	20	0.5	1.0
	40	0.07	0.8
	60	0.04	0.6
	120	0.0001	0.3
Mecillinam (50)	0	5.4	5.4
	20	0.6	2.0
	40	0.4	1.0
	60	0.08	0.5
	120	0.0002	0.2

[a] Two pneumococcal cultures (A and B, 30 ml each) were grown from small inocula (5 × 10^5 viable cells per ml) in C-medium containing potassium phosphate buffers (0.05 M) at pH 8.0 (culture A, lysis-permissive medium) and pH 6.6 (culture B, lysis-nonpermissive medium). At a cell concentration of 5 × 10^7 viable bacteria per ml (corresponding to the light-scattering value of N = 200 on the nephelometer scale), each culture was divided into three portions; one pair of cultures (A1 and B1) received benzylpenicillin (0.1 μg/ml), and the second pair (A2, B2) received cephalothin (5 μg/ml); mecillinam (50 μg/ml) was added to the third pair (A3, B3). Just before the addition of drugs, samples were removed from A and B to determine the initial (0 min) titer of viable bacteria and to measure the pH. The pH values were 7.1 in culture A and 6.0 in culture B. The cultures were incubated at 37°C, and samples were removed at intervals to determine the viable titers. The pH values of the cultures were also determined after 60 and 120 min of incubation with the antibiotics. The pH of the A cultures was 6.8 at 60 min and 6.5 at 120 min. In the B cultures, the pH dropped to 5.6 at 60 min and to 5.0 at 120 min. There was virtually no difference between the pH values of cultures A1, A2, or A3. Similarly, the pH values of cultures B1, B2, and B3 were practically identical. Samples for the viable-titer determination were diluted in lysis-nonpermissive C-medium and plated in 1.0% agar-containing lysis-nonpermissive C-medium.

[b] Number of surviving viable cell per milliliter (×10^7).

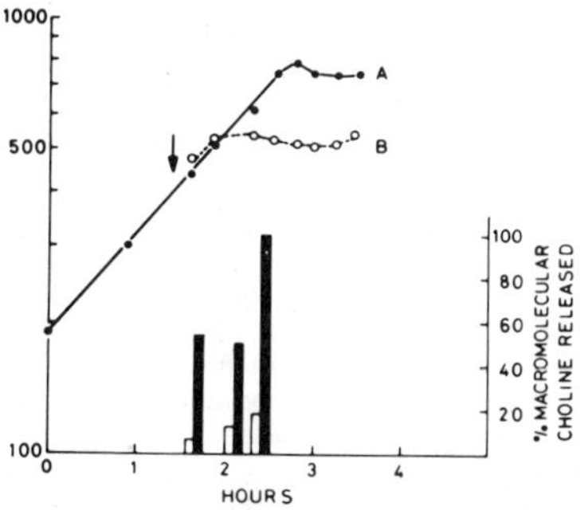

FIG. 10. *Secretion of choline-containing macromolecules during penicillin treatment of pneumococci at low pH. A pneumococcal culture was grown at pH 6.6. At the time indicated by the arrow, the culture was divided; one of the two cultures received benzylpenicillin (0.1 μg/ml), and the other served as control. Immediately after penicillin addition, both cultures received radioactive choline (1 μCi and 0.1 μg of [methyl-³H]choline per ml; specific radioactivity in the medium; 5.1 μg and 0.5 μCi/ml). The cultures were incubated at 37°C, growth was monitored by nephelometry, and at intervals aliquots were removed for the determination of the total isotope incorporated into macromolecular choline compounds and also for the quantitation of macromolecular choline label that had escaped into the culture medium (see text). (Curve A) Control; (curve B) penicillin-treated culture. The histogram indicates the percentage of macromolecular choline label that has escaped into the growth medium in the control (empty bars) and in the penicillin-treated (solid bars) cultures.*

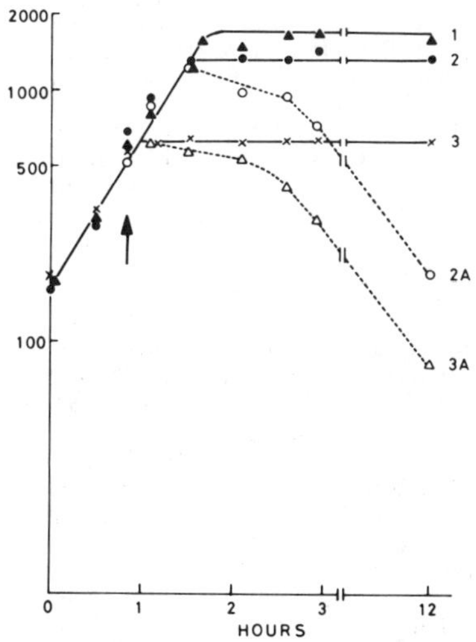

FIG. 11. *Protection of pneumococci against penicillin-induced lysis by trypsin added to the growth medium. Pneumococci growing in pH 8.0 culture medium were distributed to a number of culture tubes at the time indicated by the arrow. Cultures 1, 2, and 3 received trypsin (500 μg/ml); cultures 2 and 2A received D-cycloserine (100 μg/ml), and cultures 3 and 3A received benzylpenicillin (0.1 μg/ml). Incubation at 37°C continued, and growth and lysis were measured by nephelometry.*

provide simple experimental systems for the investigation of the mechanism of action of cell wall-inhibitory antibiotics.

An important conclusion emerging from these observations and from findings described earlier in the pneumococcal system concern the mechanism of action of penicillin and other cell wall inhibitors. We suggest that, contrary to the common notion, the direct primary effect of penicillins and cell wall inhibitors on bacteria is inhibition of growth. However, this primary effect can only be observed in bacteria with a suppressed autolytic system. The most important antimicrobial effects of these antibiotics (namely, lysis and killing) are indirect, secondary consequences of the inhibition of cell wall synthesis. Lysis and, at least in part, killing are caused by the uncontrolled activity of bacterial autolytic enzymes (murein hydrolases). Recent studies with pneumococci indicated that interruption of murein synthesis by cell wall inhibitors can cause a loss into the medium of a lipoteichoic acid-containing autolysin inhibitor (20). It has been suggested that such a loss of an endogenous inhibitor constitutes the direct cause of the triggering of the self-destructive activity of autolytic enzymes (19, 20).

The possible involvement of bacterial autolysins in the mode of action of penicillin and the indirect nature of the cytocidal and cytolytic action of this drug have been considered repeatedly in the literature (5, 8, 11, 12, 21), and the present studies provide further experimental evidence for these views. We are presently testing the possibility that, as in pneumococci and other bacteria too, the lytic and killing process triggered by cell wall inhibitors is accompanied by the leakage to the medium of lipopolysaccharide-like material.

ACKNOWLEDGMENTS

This investigation was supported in part by a grant from the National Institutes of Health (Biomedical Support Grant to The Rockefeller University) and by a grant from the National Science Foundation.

LITERATURE CITED

1. **Anagnostopoulos, C., and J. Spizizen.** 1961. Requirements for transformation in *Bacillus subtilis*. J. Bacteriol. 81:741–746.
2. **Brown, W. C., and F. E. Young.** 1970. Dynamic interactions between cell wall polymers, extracellular proteases and autolytic enzymes. Biochem. Biophys. Res. Commun. 38:564–568.
3. **Gomori, G.** 1955. Preparation of buffers for use in enzyme studies, p. 138–148. *In* S. P. Colowick and N. O.

Kaplan (ed.), Methods in enzymology, vol. 1 Academic Press Inc., New York.

4. **Herbold, D. R., and L. Glaser.** 1975. *Bacillus subtilis* N-acetylmuramic acid L-alanine amidase. J. Biol. Chem. **250**:1676–1682.
5. **Hobby, G. L., K. Meyer, and E. Chaffee.** 1942. Observations on the mechanism of action of penicillin. Proc. Soc. Exp. Biol. Med. **50**:281–285.
6. **Holtje, J. V., and A. Tomasz.** 1976. Purification of the pneumococcal N-acetyl-muramyl-L-alanine amidase to biochemical homogeneity. J. Biol. Chem. **251**:4199–4207.
7. **Houtsmuller, U., and L. van Deenan.** 1965. On the amino acid esters of phosphatidyl glycerol from bacteria. Biochim. Biophys. Acta **106**:564–576.

7a. **Locks, S., and R. D. Hotchkiss.** 1960. A study of the genetic material determining an enzyme activity in Pneumococcus. Biochim. Biophys. Acta **39**:508–517.

8. **Lederberg, J., and J. St. Clair.** 1958. Protoplasts and L-type growth of *Escherichia coli*. J. Bacteriol. **75**:143–160.
9. **Leive, L.** 1974. The barrier function of the gram-negative envelope. Ann. N. Y. Acad. Sci. **235**:109–127.
10. **Op den Kamp, J. A. F., W. van Iterson, and L. L. M. van Deenan.** 1967. Studies on the phospholipids and morphology of protoplasts of *Bacillus megaterium*. Biochim. Biophys. Acta **135**:862–884.
11. **Prestidge, L., and A. Pardee.** 1957. Induction of bacterial lysis by penicillin. J. Bacteriol. **74**:48–59.
12. **Rogers, H. J.** 1967. Killing of staphylococci by penicillins. Nature (London) **213**:31–33.
13. **Rogers, H. J., and C. W. Forsberg.** 1971. Role of autolysins in killing of bacteria by some bacterial antibiotics. J. Bacteriol. **108**:1235–1243.
14. **Schwarz, U., and W. Weidel.** 1965. Zum Wirkungsmechanismus von Penicillin. I. Isolierung und Charakterisierung 2.6.Diaminopimelinsäure enthaltender niedermolekularen Peptide aus Penicillinsphäroplasten von *Escherichia coli* B. Z. Naturforsch. **20b**:147–153.
15. **Tomasz, A.** 1968. Biological consequences of the replacement of choline by ethanolamine in the cell wall of pneumococcus: chain formation, loss of transformability and loss of autolysis. Proc. Natl. Acad. Sci. U.S.A. **59**:86–93.
16. **Tomasz, A.** 1970. Cellular metabolism in genetic transformation of pneumococci: requirement for protein synthesis during induction of competence. J. Bacteriol. **101**:860–871.
17. **Tomasz, A.** 1974. The role of autolysins in cell death. Ann. N.Y. Acad. Sci. **235**:439–448.
18. **Tomasz, A., A. Albino, and E. Zanati.** 1970. Multiple antibiotic resistance in a bacterium with suppressed autolytic system. Nature (London) **227**:138–140.
19. **Tomasz, A., and S. Waks.** 1975. Enzyme replacement in a bacterium: phenotypic correction by the experimental introduction of the wild type enzyme into a live enzyme defective mutant pneumococcus. Biochem. Biophys. Res. Commun. **65**:1311–1319.
20. **Tomasz, A., and S. Waks.** 1975. Mechanism of action of penicillin: triggering of the pneumococcal autolytic enzyme inhibitors of cell wall synthesis. Proc. Natl. Acad. Sci. U.S.A. **72**:4162–4166.
21. **Weidel, W., and H. Pelzer.** 1964. Bagshaped macromolecules—a new outlook on bacterial cell walls. Adv. Enzymol. **26**:193–232.
22. **Young, F. E.** 1966. Autolytic enzyme associated with cell walls of *Bacillus subtilis*. J. Biol. Chem. **241**:3462–3467.

Antimicrobial Agents and Chemotherapy, Oct. 1976, p. 707-712

Vol. 10, No. 4
Printed in U.S.A.

Variation in the Susceptibility of Strains of *Staphylococcus aureus* to Oxacillin, Cephalothin, and Gentamicin

C. G. MAYHALL, G. MEDOFF,[1]* and J. J. MARR

Divisions of Dermatology, Infectious Disease, and Laboratory Medicine, Departments of Medicine and Pathology, Washington University School of Medicine, and Barnes Hospital, St. Louis, Missouri 63110

Received for publication 10 June 1976

Three cases of staphylococcal bacteremia caused by organisms that were inhibited by low concentrations of oxacillin, but were resistant to the killing effects of oxacillin, stimulated us to screen 60 clinical isolates of *Staphylococcus aureus* for their susceptibility to oxacillin, cephalothin, and gentamicin. All 60 strains were inhibited by low concentrations of the antibiotics. The antibiotics were bactericidal against 27 of the 60 strains and only bacteriostatic against the other 33 after 24 h of incubation. However, after 48 h of incubation, the antibiotics were also bactericidal against the latter group.

The introduction of the penicillinase-resistant semisynthetic penicillins has resulted in a significant improvement in the therapy of severe staphylococcal infections. However, in spite of the use of these effective antibiotics, the mortality of staphylococcal bacteremia remains high, approaching 50% in some series (17). This high mortality cannot be attributed to drug resistance because, unlike the European experience (1, 7), reports of methicillin-resistant staphylococci have been few in number in the United States (2, 15).

We have encountered three patients with staphylococcal bacteremias over the past 3 years who failed to respond to adequate dosages of oxacillin despite evidence of the organisms' susceptibility to this drug and required the addition of gentamicin to control the infections. Tube dilution susceptibility tests revealed that the oxacillin had a low minimal inhibitory concentration (MIC) but a very high minimal bactericidal concentration (MBC) against these organisms. The three cases stimulated an investigation of the frequency of the occurrence of this phenomenon in a large number of clinical isolates of *Staphylococcus aureus* picked randomly from isolates in the Barnes Hospital Microbiology Laboratory. The results of these studies are the subject of this report.

CASE REPORTS

Case 1. An 18-year-old man was admitted to Barnes Hospital with a 3-day history of chills, fever, and right-sided pleuritic chest pain. He was a frequent user of heroin intravenously and had administered his last dose 1 week before admission. On examination, he had a rectal temperature of 105°F (40.6°C). He had a pleuritic rub heard at the base of his right lung. No heart murmur was noted. Chest X-ray showed scattered nodular lesions in both lung fields. He was started on 2 g of oxacillin, given intravenously, every 4 h. Four blood cultures drawn before initiation of therapy grew *S. aureus*. In spite of the oxacillin therapy, he remained febrile and one of four blood cultures was positive for *S. aureus* 48 h after initiation of therapy. The organism was susceptible to methicillin and oxacillin by the disk diffusion method (3). An oxacillin tube dilution susceptibility test, using Mueller-Hinton broth, showed an MIC of 0.20 μg/ml and an MBC of 50 μg/ml. A serum specimen taken 1 h after a dose of oxacillin was bacteriostatic against his organism at a 1:8 dilution but was not bactericidal. The organism was susceptible to gentamicin by the disk diffusion method, and tube dilution tests showed gentamicin to be bacteriostatic at 1.5 μg/ml and bactericidal at 3.0 μg/ml. Gentamicin was added to his therapy at a dosage of 1 mg/kg intravenously every 8 h, and he defervesced 12 h after gentamicin was started; subsequent blood cultures were negative. Serum specimens were bactericidal against his organism at a dilution of 1:8 while the patient was on both antibiotics. He was treated with oxacillin and gentamicin for 5 weeks and recovered. Tests for synergism of oxacillin and gentamicin showed that the MBC of the combination against his organism was 0.5 μg of oxacillin plus 0.25 μg of gentamicin.

Case 2. A 67-year-old man with lymphosarcoma developed chills, fever, and mental obtundation. Three of three blood cultures were positive for *S. aureus*, and the organism was susceptible by disk diffusion to oxacillin and gentamicin. He was given 2 g of oxacillin intravenously every 4 h, but his temperature remained elevated, and blood cultures were still positive over the next 48 h. His serum, drawn 1 h after a dose of oxacillin, inhibited growth of the staphylococcus at a dilution of 1:16 but was not bactericidal. Gentamicin was added to his therapy and he defervesced in about 24 h; blood cultures became negative. The MIC of oxacillin against his

[1] Present address: Division of Infectious Diseases, Medical College of Virginia, P.O. Box 92, Richmond, VA 23298.

organism was 0.20 μg/ml, and the MBC was 25 μg/ml. The MIC of gentamicin was 0.5 μg/ml, and the MBC was 4.0 μg/ml. The MBC of the combination was 0.5 μg of oxacillin per ml and 0.5 μg of gentamicin per ml.

Case 3. A 79-year-old man with cancer of the prostate and multiple metastatic lesions developed *S. aureus* bacteremia during his hospitalization. The organism was susceptible to oxacillin and gentamicin by disk. He failed to respond to 2 g of oxacillin intravenously every 4 h and remained febrile over the next 5 days. No follow-up blood cultures were drawn before 1 mg of gentamicin per kg every 8 h was added to his regimen. Twenty-four hours after gentamicin treatment was started he became afebrile and had negative blood cultures. The MIC of oxacillin against his organism was 0.20 μg/ml with an MBC of 25 μg/ml. The MIC of gentamicin was 1.5 μg/ml with an MBC of 6.0 μg/ml. The MBC of the combination was 1.0 μg of oxacillin per ml and 1 μg of gentamicin per ml.

MATERIALS AND METHODS

Bacteria. Sixty strains of *S. aureus* collected randomly from clinical specimens submitted to the Barnes Hospital Microbiology Laboratory over the period of 12 months were studied. All of the isolates were from different patients, and there was no consistent pattern of antibiotic susceptibility, except that all were penicillin resistant. All of the clinical isolates were identified as *S. aureus* on the basis of their gross and microscopic morphology, coagulase positivity, and ability to grow in 6.5% sodium chloride agar.

Antimicrobial agents. The following antimicrobial agents were tested: oxacillin, purchased as Prostaphlin from Bristol Laboratories; cephalothin, purchased as Keflin from Eli Lilly and Co.; and gentamicin, purchased as Garamycin from Schering Corp. All antibiotics were dissolved in sterile, distilled water and stock solutions were prepared at concentrations of 200 μg/ml and frozen at −10°C until used. All stock solutions were used within 1 month of preparation.

Antimicrobial susceptibility tests. Tube dilution susceptibility tests were performed on each organism in clear plastic tubes (22 by 77 mm) with Mueller-Hinton broth (Difco) prepared from the same batch of powder (603741). Antibiotic concentrations tested ranged from 0.1 to 100 μg/ml in a volume of 0.5 ml. Inocula were prepared from cultures on blood agar plates and transferred into tubes with 5 ml of broth. After incubation at 37°C for 18 h, turbidity was measured and the suspensions of organisms were diluted in broth to a concentration of 10^5/ml, and 0.5-ml portions were added to each tube containing the antibiotics. Control tubes without antibiotics were included in each series of dilutions; all tests were done in duplicate. After incubation for 18 to 20 h, the MIC, defined as the lowest concentration of antibiotic that prevented visible growth, was recorded. Broth was then removed from each clear tube by a calibrated platinum loop (0.03-ml) and streaked on blood agar plates. After overnight incubation, the MBC was determined; it was defined as the lowest concentration of antibiotic that resulted in less than two surviving colonies on the blood agar plates. This required a killing of 99.9% or greater of the initial inoculum by the bactericidal antibiotic. MICs were determined without shaking the tubes because our earlier studies had demonstrated that shaking caused significant numbers of organisms to be inoculated and to survive on the inside walls of the tubes above the incubation mixtures. Shaking the tubes when reading the MICs washed some of these viable organisms into the broth, and these grew on a subculture giving a spuriously high MBC.

Killing curves. Killing curves were performed in broth prepared from the same batch of powder as that used in the tube dilution susceptibility testing. Ten strains of *S. aureus* were chosen. Oxacillin had a high MBC against six strains and a low MBC against the other four strains. The effects of 25 μg of oxacillin per ml, 25 μg of cephalothin per ml and 6.25 μg of gentamicin per ml were measured on the colony counts of these organisms as a function of time. The appropriate dilution of each antibiotic, in Mueller-Hinton broth, was added to each tube in a volume of 2 ml. Inocula of 10^5 organisms/ml were prepared as described above, and 2 ml of each inoculum was added to each tube to bring the final volume to 4 ml.

The staphylococci were incubated with the antimicrobial agents at 37°C, and 0.5-ml portions were removed from each of the incubation mixtures at 4, 8, 12, 24, and 48 h. Several tests were performed at 30°C with comparable results. Each sample was carried through several 10-fold dilutions in sterile normal saline, and 0.1 ml of these dilutions was spread on the surface of blood agar plates with a glass rod. After incubation overnight, the colonies were counted and recorded. Killing studies were performed in duplicate on each organism.

RESULTS

Tube dilution susceptibility testing to oxacillin on the 60 strains of *S. aureus* revealed two distinct groups based on differences ($P < 0.001$) in the MBCs (Table 1). Oxacillin had similar MICs for both groups (0.33 ± 0.18 for group 1 and 0.30 ± 0.53 for group 2). For the organisms in group 2, the MBCs of oxacillin were close to

TABLE 1. *Minimal inhibitory and bactericidal concentrations (MIC, MBC) for the 60 isolates of Staphylococcus aureus*[a]

Isolates	Mean MIC (μg/ml)	MBC (μg/ml)
Group 1 (33)	0.33 ± 0.18[b]	>100[b]
	(0.1–0.80)[c]	(50–>100)[c]
Group 2 (27)	0.30 ± 0.53	2.2 ± 5.33
	(0.1–1.60)[c]	(0.20–12.5)[c]

[a] The values are the average of three tests run in duplicate.

[b] Standard deviation.

[c] Range.

the MICs and always at concentrations that were easily achievable in blood by normal therapeutic doses, 2.5 ± 5.33 μg/ml. The MBCs for group 1 (>100 μg/ml), however, were always markedly different from the MICs. The distribution of the MBCs of the organisms in both groups was clearly bimodal, with no overlap between the groups when 25 μg/ml was used as the division point. An MIC of 25 μg/ml has been the level usually used to differentiate methicillin-resistant and -sensitive strains (12).

There were 33 organisms in group 1 and 27 in group 2. Confluent growth was never seen on subcultures from the tubes with concentrations of oxacillin higher than the MICs of the organisms, and the survivors on subculture of the organisms in group 1 represented 0.1 to 10% of the initial inocula. In most strains, however (17 out of 33), survivors were approximately 1% of the initial inocula. Subcultures of the organisms in group 1, recovered from tubes with high concentrations of oxacillin, did not give rise to a homogeneous population of cells resistant to the bactericidal effects of oxacillin. On retesting, the bacteria derived from these subcultures behaved like the parent strains, with only a small percentage of the organisms resistant to killing by oxacillin. The ability of the group 1 strains to resist the oxacillin-induced killing was not influenced by inoculum size. Oxacillin was not bactericidal when 10^3 or 10^6 organisms per ml were used as the initial inoculum.

Ten organisms (six from group 1 and four from group 2, Table 2), were picked randomly from the two groups and the effects of oxacillin, cephalothin, and gentamicin on colony counts over a 48-h period were measured. Figure 1 shows the response of these 10 strains to 25 μg of oxacillin per ml. This concentration of oxacillin was used because it was the dividing point between the MBCs of group 1 and group 2 organisms (Table 1). At 24 h, oxacillin was bactericidal for the organisms in group 2, but only bacteriostatic for the organisms in group 1. The killing curves of the organisms in group 2 were steeper than the ones in group 1, and at every point measured, there was a statistically significant difference between the colony counts of the two groups ($P < 0.01$ by the analysis of variance). This confirmed our previous tube dilution studies on these organisms (Table 1). After 48 h of incubation, oxacillin became bactericidal for the organisms in group 1. It is also important to note that at 48 h of incubation, there was no regrowth of the organisms in group 2. In addition, growth rates of the organisms in group 1 were the same as those in group 2 (data not shown). Similar results were seen with 25 μg of cephalothin per ml (Fig. 2); there was a statistically significant difference between the killing curves and the colony counts of the organisms in groups 1 and 2 ($P < 0.01$, analysis of variance). Lower concentrations of oxacillin and cephalothin were bactericidal at 48 h for some of the organisms in group 1, but neither was effective below 10 μg/ml.

Figure 3 shows the responses of organisms in groups 1 and 2 to 6.25 μg of gentamicin per ml. This concentration of gentamicin was chosen

TABLE 2. *Characteristics of the 10 isolates on which the antibiotic bactericidal effects were analyzed*

Strains	MIC[b] (μg/ml)	MBC[b] (μg/ml)
Group 1		
WE 3395	0.80	>100
WE 3262	0.20	>100
3445	0.20	50
WE 185	0.40	>100
RE 658	0.80	>100
WE 409	0.20	>100
Group 2		
WE 3449	0.20	0.10
WE 3399	0.20	0.20
RE 966	0.40	0.40
RE 1532	0.20	0.20

[a] The values are the results of three tests run in duplicate.

[b] Oxacillin.

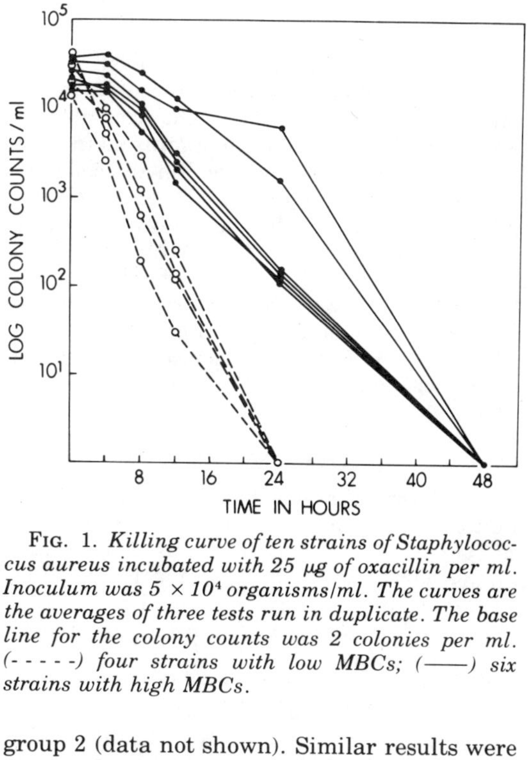

FIG. 1. *Killing curve of ten strains of Staphylococcus aureus incubated with 25 μg of oxacillin per ml. Inoculum was 5 × 10^4 organisms/ml. The curves are the averages of three tests run in duplicate. The base line for the colony counts was 2 colonies per ml. (- - - - -) four strains with low MBCs; (——) six strains with high MBCs.*

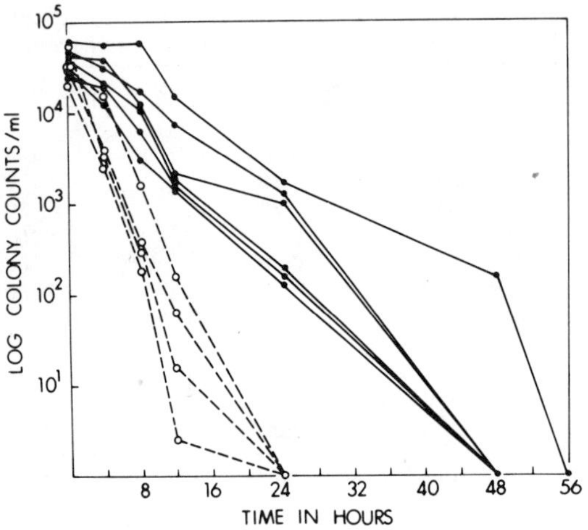

FIG. 2. *Same as Fig. 1. Incubation with 25 μg of cephalothin per ml.*

because it is a high therapeutic level of this drug and therefore comparable to the 25-μg/ml concentration of oxacillin and cephalothin used. Gentamicin killed the organisms in both groups more rapidly than oxacillin and cephalothin. Three of the organisms in group 2 were killed completely by 4 h, and one was killed by 8 h. It required 8 h to kill three of the organisms in group 1 and 12 h to kill the other three. Although there was some overlap in the responses of these organisms to gentamicin, the difference between the responses of the two groups was significant ($P < 0.01$, analysis of variance).

DISCUSSION

The observation that oxacillin was only inhibitory and not bactericidal for the three clinical isolates of *S. aureus* that caused the bacteremias which were unresponsive to oxacillin stimulated us to study the frequency of this susceptibility pattern in *S. aureus* isolated in Barnes Hospital.

All 60 of the strains selected at random from the Clinical Microbiology Laboratory were inhibited by low concentrations of oxacillin. This was not unexpected and was consistent with the susceptibility of the great majority of strains of *S. aureus* tested for susceptibility to methicillin and oxacillin at our hospital. Oxacillin had very high MBCs against 33 of the 60 strains, and these organisms resembled the strains isolated from our three patients. Only a small percentage of the staphylococci in cultures of these organisms resisted the killing effects of oxacillin and subcultures of these "resistant" bacteria behaved like the parent strains, with only a small percentage of cells resisting killing by oxacillin. In this respect, the pattern of resistance was similar to that found in true methicillin-resistant staphylococci (14).

The variability in response to the killing action of oxacillin that we have found confirms the report of a similar phenomenon described by Best et al. (5). The difference in the frequency of occurrence of relatively resistant organisms in their series and ours is probably due to differences in criteria for the MBC of oxacillin. In their study they defined a bactericidal effect of oxacillin as 99% killing, whereas we required 99.9% killing for our definition of a bactericidal effect.

When the time-dependent effects of the antibiotics at high therapeutic concentrations were studied, the organisms also segregated themselves into two distinct populations. It is clear that the responses to these concentrations of drugs were determined by the rates of bacterial killing. All of the organisms from group 2 were killed within 24 h by oxacillin, and the organisms from group 1 required 24 to 48 h of exposure to the drugs for complete killing to occur. Therefore, the organisms in group 1 were not truly oxacillin resistant.

Gentamicin killed all of the organisms more rapidly than oxacillin or cephalothin, but the organisms also segregated into two groups with the same populations in each on the basis of the rapidity of their response to the concentration of gentamicin used. Therefore, the differences in responses of group 1 and group 2 organisms were not specific to cell wall antibiotics. A very rapid killing effect of gentamicin compared

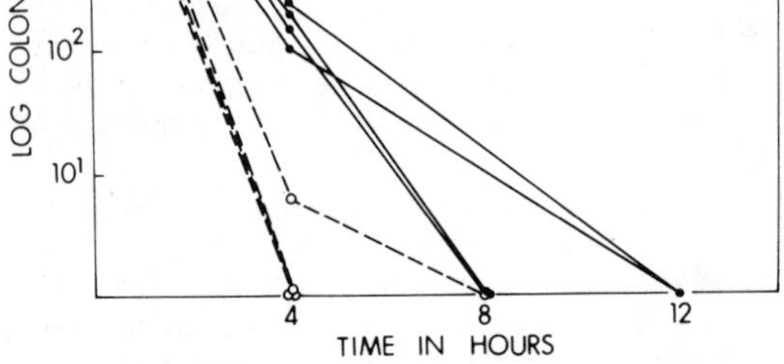

FIG. 3. *Same as Fig. 1. Incubation with 6.75 μg of gentamicin per ml.*

with penicillin has also been noted by others (13, 16), but in these studies there was eventual regrowth of the organisms after prolonged incubation with the drug. In our studies, regrowth was not seen. The difference between our results and others may be due to the lower initial inocula and higher gentamicin concentrations used in our studies.

The mechanism underlying the differences in the responses of the two groups of staphylococci to oxacillin, cephalothin, and gentamicin is unknown. There was no difference in growth rate of the two groups and the presence of L-forms or cell wall-deficient bacteria is unlikely because our media were not selective for L-forms and the response to gentamicin, an inhibitor of protein synthesis, was the same as the responses to the cell wall antibiotics. We did not perform phage typing of the organisms in groups 1 and 2, but antibiotic susceptibility patterns of the organisms within the groups were not uniform and there was no relationship between the antibiotic sensitivity patterns and the MBCs of oxacillin, cephalothin, and gentamicin.

Hobby et al. (11) have described so-called "bacterial persisters" in the presence of penicillin. Bigger (6) and Gunnison et al. (9) also carried out extensive studies on the action of penicillin on strains of *S. aureus* and observed that a small number of organisms survived incubation in bactericidal concentrations of penicillin for 24 or more h. They postulated that the persisting cells survived the action of penicillin because they were in a dormant state unable to initiate division or cell wall synthesis at the time of exposure to penicillin. More recently, Greenwood (8) has offered a hypothesis to explain the phenomenon of microbial persisters that is based on the observation of Hartmann et al. (10). The latter showed that in addition to its inhibitory effects on cell wall synthesis, penicillin also inhibited the action of two mucopeptide hydrolases in the cell wall of *Escherichia coli*. Greenwood has proposed that cells with complete cell envelopes at the time of penicillin exposure would remain intact because the penicillin would inhibit the activity of mucopeptide hydrolases. This hypothesis has received support from the studies of Best et al. (4), who noted a diminished level of cell wall autolysin activity of a tolerant strain of *S. aureus* when compared with a susceptible strain after exposure of both organisms to oxacillin. We cannot be certain, but we suspect, that our group 1 organisms are similar to the so-called bacterial persisters described by those previous workers. Further characterization of our organisms will have to be done to confirm this notion.

Any discussion of the clinical implications of our findings is speculative. Unfortunately, the organisms in our case reports were lost before killing curves could be performed so we do not know if they would have responded to oxacillin in a fashion identical to that of our group 1 organisms. The lack of clinical response of the patients to oxacillin is unusual in our experience, but the underlying disease in each of the patients may be responsible for this. At this point, we have no basis for stating that infections with group 1 organisms are more difficult to treat. Careful analysis of clinical cases of staphylococcal infection, their outcomes, and correlations with the MICs and MBCs of the organisms to the antibiotics used will have to be done before any such conclusions can be drawn.

ACKNOWLEDGMENTS

This investigation was supported, in part, by Public Health Service training grants NIAMD 05611 and AI 00459 from the National Institute of Arthritis, Metabolism, and Digestive Diseases and the National Institute of Allergy and Infectious Diseases, respectively, Public Health research grant AI 10622 from the National Institute of Allergy and Infectious Diseases, a grant from the John A. Hartford Foundation, and a grant from the National Science Foundation (BMS71-01597AO1).

LITERATURE CITED

1. **Barber, M.** 1964. Naturally occurring methicillin-resistant staphylococci. J. Gen. Microbiol. 35:183–190.
2. **Barrett, F. F., R. F. McFehee, Jr., and M. Finland.** 1968. Methicillin-resistant *Staphylococcus aureus* at Boston City Hospital. Bacteriologic and epidemiologic observations. N. Engl. J. Med. 279:441–448.
3. **Bauer, A. W., W. M. M. Kirby, J. C. Sherris, and M. Turck.** 1966. Antibiotic susceptibility testing by a standardized single disk method. Am. J. Clin. Pathol. 45:493–496.
4. **Best, G. K., N. H. Best, and A. V. Koval.** 1974. Evidence for participation of autolysins in bactericidal action of oxacillin on *Staphylococcus aureus*. Antimicrob. Agents Chemother. 6:825–830.
5. **Best, G. K., A. V. Koval, and N. H. Best.** 1965. Susceptibility of clinical isolates of *Staphylococcus aureus* to killing by oxacillin. Can. J. Microbiol. 21:1692–1697.
6. **Bigger, J. W.** 1944. The bactericidal action of penicillin on *Staphylococcus pyogenes*. Irish J. Med. Sci. 6:553–568, 585–595.
7. **Eriksen, K. R., and I. Erichsen.** 1964. Resistance to methicillin, isoxazolyl penicillins, and cephalothin in *Staphylococcus aureus*. Acta Pathol. Microbiol. Scand. 62:255–275.
8. **Greenwood, D.** 1972. Mucopeptide hydrolases and bacterial "persisters." Lancet 2:465.
9. **Gunnison, J. B., M. A. Fraher, and E. Jawetz.** 1964. Persistence of *Staphylococcus aureus* in penicillin *in vitro*. J. Gen. Microbiol. 35:335–349.
10. **Hartmann, R., J. Höltje, and U. Schwarz.** 1972. Targets of penicillin action in *Escherichia coli*. Nature (London) 235:426–429.
11. **Hobby, G. L., K. Meyer, and E. Chaffee.** 1942. Observations on the mechanism of action of penicillin. Proc. Soc. Exp. Biol. Med. 50:281–285.
12. **Sabath, L. D., C. D. Leaf, D. A. Gerstein, and M. Finland.** 1970. Altered cell walls of *Staphylococcus*

aureus resistant to methicillin. Nature (London) 225:1074.

13. **Sande, M. A., and M. L. Johnson.** 1975. Antimicrobial therapy of experimental endocarditis caused by *Staphylococcus aureus*. J. Infect. Dis. 131:367–375.
14. **Sutherland, R., and G. N. Rolinson.** 1964. Characteristics of methicillin-resistant staphylococci. J. Bacteriol. 87:887–899.
15. **Thornsberry, C., J. Q. Caruthers, and C. N. Baker.** 1973. Effect of temperature on the *in vitro* susceptibility of *Staphylococcus aureus* to penicillinase-resistant penicillins. Antimicrob. Agents Chemother. 4:263–269.
16. **Watanakunakorn, C., and C. Glotzbecker.** 1974. Enhancement of the effects of anti-staphylococcal antibiotics by aminoglycosides. Antimicrob. Agents Chemother. 6:802–806.
17. **Watanakunakorn, C., J. S. Tan, and J. P. Phair.** 1973. Some salient features of *Staphylococcus aureus* endocarditis. Am. J. Med. 54:473–481.

ANTIMICROBIAL AGENTS AND CHEMOTHERAPY, Oct. 1976, p. 713-720 Vol. 10, No. 4

Printed in U.S.A.

Susceptibility of Respiratory Tract Anaerobes to Orally Administered Penicillins and Cephalosporins

DAVID F. BUSCH, LUBNA AFZAL KURESHI, VERA L. SUTTER, AND SYDNEY M. FINEGOLD*

Medical and Research Services, Veterans Administration, Wadsworth Hospital Center, Los Angeles, California 90073, and Department of Medicine, UCLA School of Medicine, Los Angeles, California 90024*

Received for publication 13 July 1976

Anaerobic bacteria recovered from airway-related infections were tested by agar dilution against selected penicillins and cephalosporins available for oral administration. Against 136 isolates, penicillins G and V showed comparable activity, particularly when pharmacological differences were considered. Although many isolates were exquisitely susceptible to the penicillins, only 55% of the *Bacteroides* species and 72% of all isolates were inhibited at 0.5 μg of penicillin G per ml. Results for penicillin V at 1 μg/ml were similar (59 and 73%). The two cephalosporins were more active at achievable levels, inhibiting 94 to 95% of *Bacteroides* and 95 to 96% of all isolates at 8 μg/ml. These levels represent approximately 50% of the reported peak serum levels after oral administration of 625 mg of the penicillins and 500 mg of the cephalosporins. Dicloxacillin and nafcillin were tested against 50 isolates. The two were comparably active on a weight basis; dicloxacillin was more active when pharmacological differences were considered, but did not match the other penicillins or the cephalosporins.

The anaerobic bacteria that populate the oropharyngeal secretions in concentrations of approximately 10^8/mm^3 (18) participate in anaerobic pleuropulmonary infections and infections following human bites as well as in a variety of dental infections, other local infections of the oral cavity, and infections of the paranasal sinuses, middle ear, and facial structures. They may also participate in brain abscesses. Penicillin G is considered the antimicrobial agent of choice for the treatment of most infections due to these organisms (2, 5, 7). Although penicillin may be administered intravenously as the initial therapy for seriously ill patients with pulmonary infections, the course of treatment is often continued by the oral route, particularly in patients requiring long-term antimicrobial therapy of lung abscesses. Some infections associated with the oropharyngeal anaerobes are treated initially by the oral route. In cases in which *Staphylococcus aureus* is suspected or implicated, an orally administered penicillinase-resistant penicillin or cephalosporin may be prescribed. Tetracycline, although occasionally used in these situations, has been shown to be relatively inactive against a number of strains of both *S. aureus* (12) and anaerobic gram-positive cocci (17). Because of potential toxicities, chloramphenicol and clindamycin, although effective against these organisms, should be reserved for life-threatening situations or for those in which an acceptable alternative antibiotic is not available.

Although the in vitro activity of penicillin G, carbenicillin, and the parenteral cephalosporins against anaerobic bacteria has been extensively investigated (21, 24), there is limited published information describing the anti-anaerobic activity of the oral agents penicillin V, cephalexin, and cephradine or of the penicillinase-resistant penicillins. In previous testing in this laboratory, penicillin V, dicloxacillin, and nafcillin were found to be distinctly less active than penicillin G against isolates of *Bacteroides melaninogenicus* and anaerobic gram-positive cocci (4, 6; S. M. Finegold, P. T. Sugihara, and A. B. Miller, Bacteriol. Proc., p. 96, 1967). In another study, Tally et al. showed cephalexin to be the least active of four cephalosporins and the cephamycin cefoxitin tested against 155 clinical strains of anaerobic bacteria (24). In none of these investigations were organisms recovered from airway sources evaluated separately from those recovered from other sources.

We have studied the in vitro activity of the antibiotics penicillin G, penicillin V, cephalexin, cephradine, dicloxacillin, and nafcillin against anaerobic bacteria recovered from patients with airway-related infections.

(This paper will be presented in part at the 16th Interscience Conference on Antimicrobial Agents and Chemotherapy, Chicago, Illinois, 29 October 1976.)

MATERIALS AND METHODS

Bacteria. All strains tested were isolated between October 1974 and May 1976 from specimens collected from patients with airway-related infections. All patients were hospitalized at the Wadsworth Hospital Center, Veterans Administration, Los Angeles. Specimen sources included transtracheal aspirates (61 isolates), aspirates obtained through endotracheal or tracheostomy tubes or from bronchoscopy (23 isolates), pleural fluid aspirates (6 isolates), and aspirates of neck or oral wounds occurring in conjunction with major otolaryngological surgery or mandibular osteomyelitis (46 isolates). The isolates were identified by procedures described previously (23), using also criteria of the Virginia Polytechnic Institute and State University Anaerobe Laboratory (11).

The 64 *Bacteroides* species isolated included *B. melaninogenicus* (25 isolates). A total of 13 isolates were identified by the criteria used as *B. oralis* and 12 as *B. ruminicola*. Only two isolates of the *B. fragilis* group (one *B. fragilis* and one *B. thetaiotaomicron*) were recovered from airway-associated infections during this period. Both were isolated from a transtracheal aspirate from one patient. Other *Bacteroides* tested were *B. capillosus* (two isolates), *B. corrodens* (two isolates), *B. pneumosintes* (one isolate), and *Bacteroides* species (eight isolates).

Anaerobic cocci tested included *Peptococcus* species (13 isolates), *Peptostreptococcus* species (14 isolates), and *Veillonella* species (13 isolates). There were 19 gram-positive bacilli: *Eubacterium* species (5 isolates), *Lactobacillus* species (6 isolates), *Propionibacterium* species (5 isolates), and *Actinomyces* species (3 isolates). Thirteen isolates of *Fusobacterium* species completed the total of 136 strains tested against penicillin G, penicillin V, cephalexin, and cephradine.

Fifty of the 136 isolates were also tested against dicloxacillin and nafcillin. These strains included *B. melaninogenicus* (nine isolates), *B. oralis* (eight isolates), *B. ruminicola* (four isolates), and *Bacteroides* species (three isolates). Also tested were *Peptococcus* species (five isolates), *Peptostreptococcus* species (five isolates), *Veillonella* species (five isolates), *Eubacterium* species (two isolates), *Lactobacillus* species (two isolates), *Propionibacterium* species (two isolates), and *Fusobacterium* species (five isolates).

Antibiotics. Laboratory standard powders of penicillin G, penicillin V, and cephalexin were supplied by Lilly Research Laboratories, Indianapolis, Ind. Cephradine was supplied by the Squibb Institute for Medical Research, Princeton, N.J.; sodium dicloxacillin by Ayerst Laboratories, New York, N.Y.; and sodium nafcillin by Wyeth Laboratories, Philadelphia, Pa. Antibiotic stock solutions (1,280 μg/ml) were prepared, using phosphate-buffered saline, pH 6.0, for the initial dilution of dicloxacillin and penicillin V and sterile distilled water for the other antibiotics. Solutions were either prepared on the day of inoculation or stored at -20°C for a maximum of 30 days prior to use. All antibiotics were tested in concentrations from 64 to 0.125 μg/ml.

Antimicrobial susceptibility tests. Minimal inhibitory concentrations were determined by the agar dilution method as previously described (23). Rapidly growing strains were incubated for 4 to 6 h, and slowly growing strains were incubated for 18 to 24 h prior to inoculation. All cultures were adjusted to one-half the turbidity of the number 1 McFarland standard to give an inoculum of 10^5 to 10^6 colony-forming units when the organisms were inoculated by means of a Steers replicator (20).

RESULTS

Against the 64 *Bacteroides* species tested (Fig. 1), penicillin G and penicillin V showed equivalent activity on a weight basis. Only at $\geq$16 μg of either agent per ml were over 90% of the strains inhibited. Cephalexin and cephradine likewise showed comparable activity although >90% inhibition was achieved at 4 μg of cephradine per ml and 8 μg of cephalexin per ml. Both isolates of *B. fragilis* tested were resistant to both the penicillins and cephalosporins. Additionally, approximately one-third of the isolates of *B. melaninogenicus* and *Bacteroides* species were resistant to levels of penicillin G or penicillin V achievable after oral administration of these agents. At concentrations below 16 μg/ml, the penicillinase-resistant penicillins were distinctly less active than either the cephpalosporins or penicillin G or V.

Against *Fusobacterium* species, penicillin G was slightly more active than penicillin V at concentrations $\leq$0.5 μg/ml, but the two antibiotics were equivalent at higher levels (Fig. 2). The cephalosporins both inhibited all 13 strains tested at $\leq$2 μg/ml. Nafcillin showed more activity on a weight basis than did dicloxacillin against the five *Fusobacterium* isolates tested with these two agents.

Although penicillins G and V were inhibitory to the gram-positive anaerobic bacilli examined (Fig. 3) at lower levels than were the cephalosporins, >90% of these organisms were inhibited by readily achievable blood levels of all four agents. On a weight basis, nafcillin appeared slightly more active than dicloxacillin against these organisms.

The *Peptococcus* species and *Peptostreptococcus* species studied (Fig. 4) were again considerably more susceptible to penicillins G and V at low levels than to the cephalosporins at the same concentrations. In addition, the cephalosporins had minimal inhibitory concentrations of $\geq$32 μg/ml against three strains (one *Peptococcus variabilis*, one *P. asaccharolyticus*,

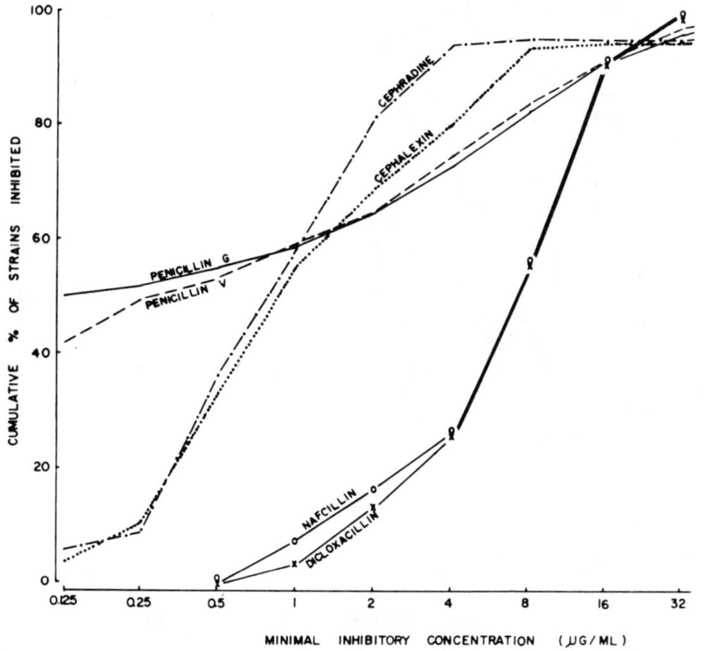

FIG. 1. *Antibiotic susceptibility patterns of Bacteroides species from airway-related infections (64 strains tested against penicillin G, penicillin V, cephalexin, and cephradine; 24 strains tested against dicloxacillin and nafcillin).*

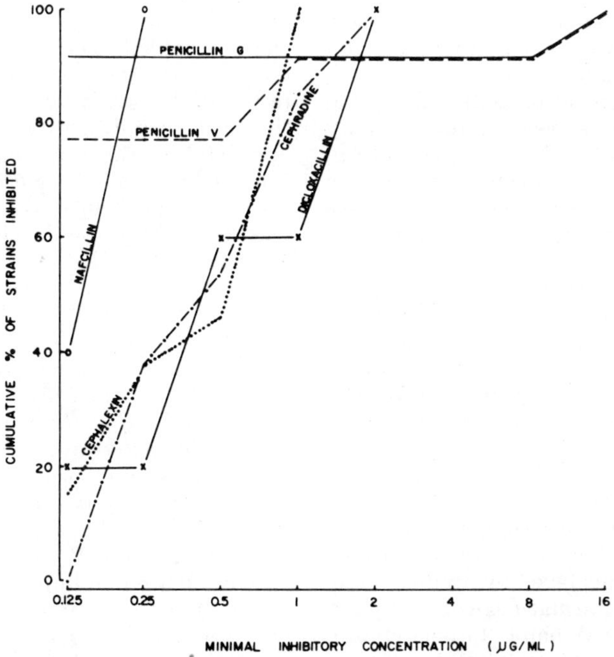

FIG. 2. *Antibiotic susceptibility patterns of Fusobacterium species from airway-related infections (13 strains tested against penicillin G, penicillin V, cephalexin, and cephradine; 5 strains tested against dicloxacillin and nafcillin).*

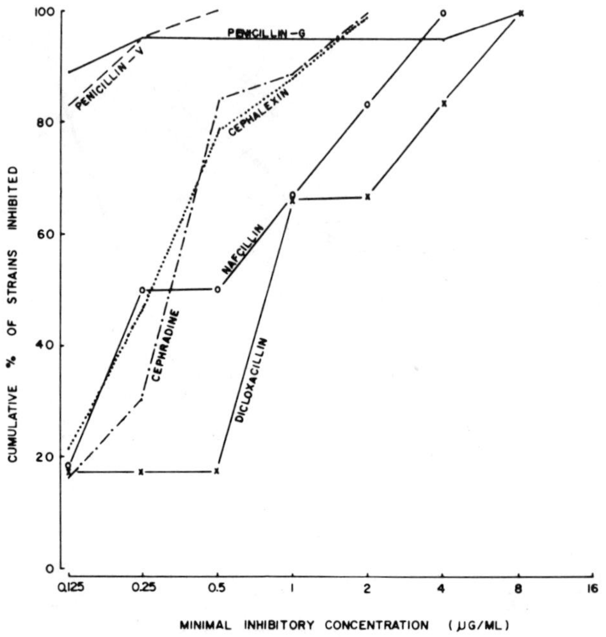

FIG. 3. *Antibiotic susceptibility patterns of anaerobic gram-positive bacilli from airway-related infections (19 strains tested against penicillin G, penicillin V, cephalexin, and cephradine; 6 strains tested against dicloxacillin and nafcillin).*

and one *Peptostreptococcus micros*). In testing against 10 of the anaerobic gram-positive cocci, the penicillinase-resistant penicillins demonstrated activity equivalent to or slightly better than that of the cephalosporins.

Equal concentrations of penicillin G, cephalexin, and cephradine showed similar activity against 13 isolates of *Veillonella* species (Fig. 5). Penicillin V was somewhat less active against these organisms. The five isolates tested against dicloxacillin and nafcillin were distinctly resistant to these antibiotics.

The pattern of activity of the six antibiotics tested against the entire panel of organisms (Fig. 6) indicates the general equivalence of penicillin G with penicillin V, of cephalexin with cephradine, and of nafcillin with dicloxacillin (when considered on a weight basis).

DISCUSSION

An interpretation of antimicrobial susceptibility test results requires comparison of the minimal inhibitory and/or minimal bactericidal concentrations achieved by an antimicrobial agent with the pharmacological characteristics of the drug. Break points for susceptibility are generally defined in relation to achievable serum levels of the agent tested. Although organisms inhibited by ≤ 0.25 μg of penicillin G per ml have been considered susceptible for purposes of oral therapy of mild infections (3), similar criteria have not been proposed for penicillin V, the orally administered cephalosporins, or penicillinase-resistant penicillins. Table 1 shows the inhibition of the anaerobes tested in this study by penicillins G and V and the oral cephalosporins at approximately 50 and 100% of the reported peak serum levels achieved after a 625-mg oral dose of the penicillins (14) or a 500-mg oral dose of the cephalosporins (10). At these levels, penicillin G was slightly more active than penicillin V against *Veillonella* species, but the two were otherwise equivalent. Even at peak levels, only 58 to 64% of all *Bacteroides* tested were inhibited by these antibiotics. In contrast, the cephalosporins inhibited 95% of the *Bacteroides* strains and all isolates of *Veillonella* at peak levels and were comparably active at 50% of the peak levels. At 16 μg/ml, the only isolates not inhibited by the cephalosporins were the two *B. fragilis* strains, one *B. oralis*, one *P. variabilis*, one *P. asaccharolyticus*, and one *P. micros*. The two cephalosporins showed no important differences in activity. Both were more active against the airway-associated anaerobes examined in this study than was cephalexin in testing against a panel of anaerobes isolated from all clinical sources by Tally et al. (24). This may be explained in part by the small numbers of *B.*

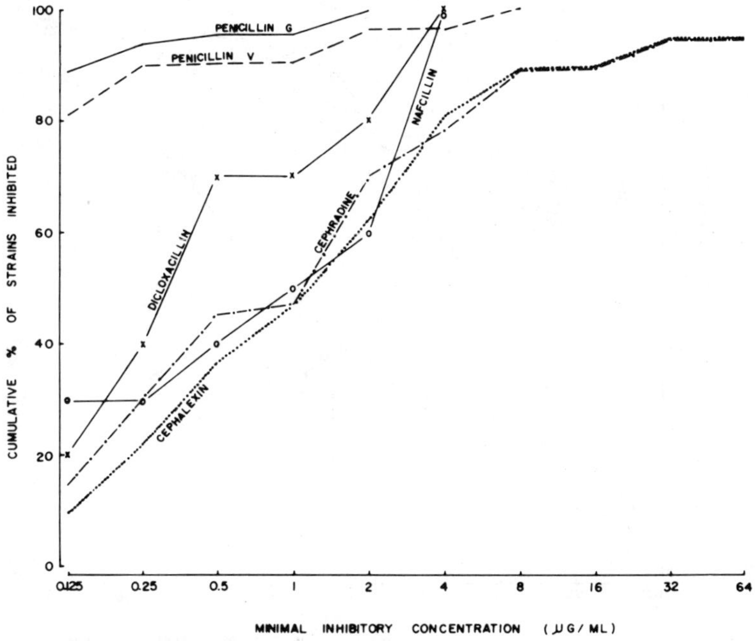

FIG. 4. *Antibiotic susceptibility patterns of anaerobic gram-positive cocci from airway-related infections (27 strains tested against penicillin G, penicillin V, cephalexin, and cephradine; 10 strains tested against dicloxacillin and nafcillin).*

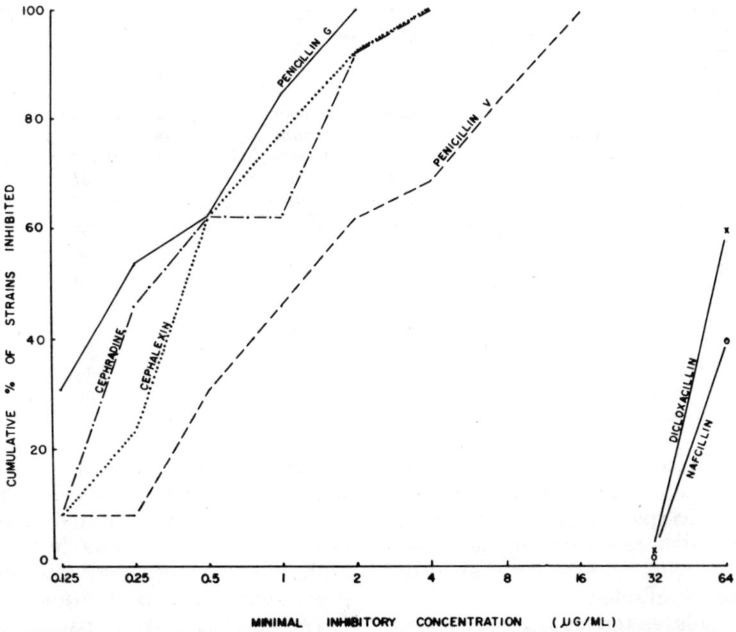

FIG. 5. *Antibiotic susceptibility patterns of Veillonella species from airway-related infections (13 strains tested against penicillin G, penicillin V, cephalexin, and cephradine; 5 strains tested against dicloxacillin and nafcillin).*

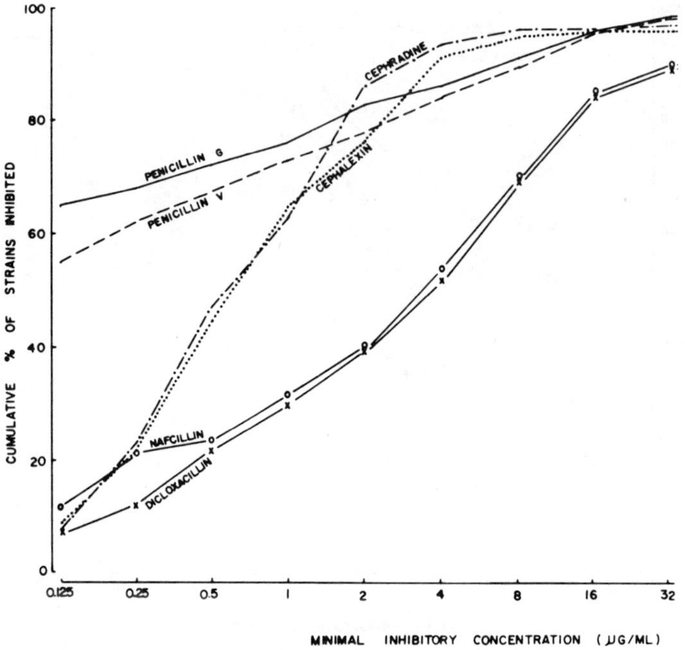

FIG. 6. *Composite antibiotic susceptibility patterns of anaerobic bacteria recovered from airway-related infections (136 strains tested against penicillin G, penicillin V, cephalexin, and cephradine; 50 strains tested against dicloxacillin and nafcillin).*

TABLE 1. *Antibiotic susceptibility of 136 anaerobic bacteria from airway-related infections to penicillins and cephalosporins at approximately 50 and 100% of the peak serum concentrations achieved after a 500-mg oral dose of cephalosporin or a 625-mg oral dose of penicillin given every 6 h (10, 14)*

Antibiotic	Peak serum level (μg/ml)	Level tested (μg/ml)	% of peak level	% Susceptible					
				Bacteroides species (64 strains)	*Fusobacterium* species (13 strains)	Anaerobic gram-positive bacilli (19 strains)	Anaerobic gram-positive cocci (27 strains)	*Veillonella* species (13 strains)	All organisms (136 strains)
Penicillin G	0.81	0.5	62	55	92	95	96	62	72
		1	123	58	92	95	96	85	76
Penicillin V	1.56	1	64	59	92	100	89	46	73
		2	128	64	92	100	96	62	78
Cephalexin	19.8	8	40	94	100	100	89	100	95
		16	81	95	100	100	89	100	96
Cephradine	19.2	8	42	95	100	100	89	100	96
		16	83	95	100	100	89	100	96

fragilis and the absence of *Clostridium* species in the present study. The possibility that strains of anaerobic species isolated from airway sources may be more susceptible to certain antibiotics than their counterparts at other sites has not been evaluated.

Data from 50 isolates tested against dicloxacillin and nafcillin (Table 2) show inferior activity of the latter antibiotic. Although nafcillin was generally as active as dicloxacillin on a weight basis, the lower peak levels reportedly achieved by orally administered nafcillin (even when given with probenecid) (8, 9) resulted in the lower activity of nafcillin recorded in this table. Dicloxacillin was less active than the cephalosporins against *Bacteroides* species and was inactive against *Veillonella* species.

The susceptibility to penicillin G of the *Bacteroides* species tested in this study is similar to that recorded by Staneck and Washington in 1974 (19). These strains are, however, more resistant than those tested by Finegold and

TABLE 2. *Antibiotic susceptibility of 50 anaerobic isolates from airway-related infections to dicloxacillin and nafcillin at approximately 50 and 100% of the peak serum concentrations achieved after a 500-mg oral dose given every 6 h (8, 9)*

Antibiotic	Peak serum level (μg/ml)	Serum level (μg/ml)	% of peak level	% Susceptible: *Bacteroides* species (24 strains)	*Fusobacterium* species (5 strains)	Anaerobic gram-positive bacilli (6 strains)	Anaerobic gram-positive cocci (10 strains)	*Veillonella* species (5 strains)	All organisms (50 strains)
Dicloxacillin	17	8	47	58	100	100	100	0	70
		16	94	92	100	100	100	0	86
Nafcillin[a]	0.8	0.5	62	0	100	50	40	0	24
		1.0	125	8	100	67	50	0	32

[a] Given with probenecid.

Sutter in 1972 (6); in that study, only 2 of 44 isolates of *B. melaninogenicus* and *B. oralis* were not inhibited by ≤0.8 μg of penicillin G per ml. As 92% of the 64 *Bacteroides* strains tested in the present study were inhibited by penicillin G at 16 μg/ml and only two strains were resistant at 32 μg/ml, this resistance should be considered relative; these levels can be effectively achieved in serum with the use of intermittently administered intravenous penicillin. Ampicillin, amoxicillin, and carbenicillin, although not tested in this study, have been shown to have activity generally comparable on a weight basis to that of penicillin G against anaerobic bacteria in general and *Bacteroides* species in particular (22). After the oral administration of 500 mg, the following approximate peak serum levels may be achieved: ampicillin, 4.5 μg/ml (16); amoxicillin, 9.3 μg/ml (16); and indanyl carbenicillin, 6 μg/ml (13). These are all levels considerably higher than those achieved by penicillins G or V after oral administration.

Penicillin G is currently the antibiotic of choice for pulmonary infections involving anaerobic bacteria. To date, this drug has been effective in the treatment of a limited number of anaerobic pulmonary infections, even when *B. fragilis* was isolated as part of a mixed flora (2). This organism, although not normally resident in the upper airway, has been recovered in 15 to 20% of the anaerobic pleuropulmonary infections in two series (1, 15) and is generally resistant to penicillin G. The importance of the increasingly resistant strains of other *Bacteroides* species in airway-associated infections has not yet been established. The presence of these organisms should be considered in patients not responding to low-dose parenteral or oral penicillin therapy given for anaerobic pleuropulmonary infections or other anaerobic infections associated with oropharyngeal flora. Other orally administered penicillins such as ampicillin, amoxicillin, or carbenicillin may be useful in these circumstances because of the higher serum levels achieved by these agents; however, there is at present little or no recorded clinical experience in treating anaerobic infections with amoxicillin or oral carbenicillin. The oral cephalosporins may provide another alternative to the institution of high-dose intravenous penicillin therapy or the use of a potentially more toxic antibiotic such as clindamycin or chloramphenicol. The cephalosporins may also be satisfactory agents for the therapy of certain mixed aerobic and anaerobic infections involving the oropharyngeal flora and, for example, *S. aureus*. They may also be considered in the initial treatment of these infections in selected penicillin-allergic patients.

ACKNOWLEDGMENTS

This work was supported by grants from Eli Lilly & Co., Indianapolis, Ind., and Wyeth Laboratories, Philadelphia, Pa.

LITERATURE CITED

1. **Bartlett, J. G., and S. M. Finegold.** 1974. Anaerobic infections of the lung and pleural space. Am. Rev. Respir. Dis. **110**:56–77.
2. **Bartlett, J. G., and S. L. Gorbach.** 1975. Treatment of aspiration pneumonia and primary lung abscess: penicillin G vs clindamycin. J. Am. Med. Assoc. **234**:935–937.
3. **Ericsson, H. M., and J. C. Sherris.** 1971. Antibiotic sensitivity testing: report of an international collaborative study. Acta Pathol. Microbiol. Scand. Sect. B Suppl. **217**:1–90.
4. **Finegold, S. M.** 1968. Infections due to anaerobes. Med. Times **96**:174–187.
5. **Finegold, S. M., J. G. Bartlett, A. W. Chow, D. J. Flora, S. L. Gorbach, E. J. Harder, and F. P. Tally.** 1975. Management of anaerobic infections. Ann. Intern. Med. **83**:375–389.
6. **Finegold, S. M., and V. L. Sutter.** 1972. Antimicrobial susceptibility of anaerobic gram-negative bacilli, p. 275–297. *In* T. MacPhee (ed.), Host resistance to commensal bacteria. Churchill Livingstone, Edinburgh.
7. **Gorbach, S. L., and J. G. Bartlett.** 1974. Anaerobic

infections. N. Engl. J. Med. 290:1177-1184, 1237-1245, 1289-1294.

8. **Gravenkemper, C. F., J. V. Bennett, J. L. Brodie, and W. M. M. Kirby.** 1965. Dicloxacillin: in vitro and pharmacologic comparisons with oxacillin and cloxacillin. Arch. Intern. Med. 116:340-345.
9. **Hartman, R. E., J. Carleton, A. Lustberg, and M. Hamburger.** 1967. Effect of dicloxacillin, oxacillin, and nafcillin upon staphylococcal population and rate of healing of soft-tissue lesions, p. 64-68. Antimicrob. Agents Chemother. 1966.
10. **Harvengt, C., P. De Schepper, F. Lamy, and J. Hansen.** 1973. Cephradine absorption and excretion in fasting and nonfasting volunteers. J. Clin. Pharmacol. 13:36-40.
11. **Holdeman, L. V., and W. E. C. Moore (ed.).** 1972. Anaerobe laboratory manual. Virginia Polytechnic Institute and State University Anaerobe Laboratory, Blacksburg, Va.
12. **Kayser, F. H.** 1975. Methicillin resistant staphylococci 1965-75. Lancet II:650-653.
13. **Knirsch, A. K., D. C. Hobbs, and J. J. Korst.** 1973. Pharmacokinetics, toleration, and safety of indanyl carbenicillin in man. J. Infect. Dis. 127(Suppl.):S105-S108.
14. **Linden, H., S. M. Finegold, and W. L. Hewitt.** 1956. Serum penicillin concentration following oral administration of penicillin V, p. 477-482. *In* Antibiotics annual 1955-1956. Medical Encyclopedia Inc., New York.
15. **Lorber, B., and R. M. Swenson.** 1974. Bacteriology of aspiration pneumonia: a prospective study of community- and hospital-acquired cases. Ann. Intern. Med. 81:329-331.
16. **Neu, H. C.** 1974. Antimicrobial activity and human pharmacology of amoxicillin. J. Infect. Dis. 129(Suppl.):S123-S131.
17. **Pien, F. D., R. L. Thompson, and W. J. Martin.** 1972. Clinical and bacteriologic studies of anaerobic gram-positive cocci. Mayo Clin. Proc. 47:251-257.
18. **Rosebury, T.** 1966. Microorganisms indigenous to man. McGraw-Hill Book Co., New York.
19. **Staneck, J. L., and J. A. Washington II.** 1974. Antimicrobial susceptibilities of anaerobic bacteria: recent clinical isolates. Antimicrob. Agents Chemother. 6:311-315.
20. **Steers, E., E. L. Foltz, and B. W. Graves.** 1959. An inocula replicating apparatus for routine testing of bacterial susceptibility to antibiotics. Antibiot. Chemother. 9:307-311.
21. **Sutter, V. L., and S. M. Finegold.** 1975. Susceptibility of anaerobic bacteria to carbenicillin, cefoxitin and related drugs. J. Infect. Dis. 131:417-422.
22. **Sutter, V. L., and S. M. Finegold.** 1976. Susceptibility of anaerobic bacteria to 23 antimicrobial agents. Antimicrob. Agents Chemother. 10:736-752.
23. **Sutter, V. L., V. L. Vargo, and S. M. Finegold.** 1975. Wadsworth anaerobic bacteriology manual, 2nd ed. University of California, Los Angeles, Extension Division, Los Angeles.
24. **Tally, F. P., N. V. Jacobus, J. G. Bartlett, and S. L. Gorbach.** 1975. Susceptibility of anaerobes to cefoxitin and other cephalosporins. Antimicrob. Agents Chemother. 7:128-132.

ANTIMICROBIAL AGENTS AND CHEMOTHERAPY, Oct. 1976, p. 721-726
Vol. 10, No. 4

Printed in U.S.A.

Antimicrobial Susceptibility Testing of Yeasts: a Turbidimetric Technique Independent of Inoculum Size

JOHN N. GALGIANI* AND DAVID A. STEVENS

Department of Medicine, Santa Clara Valley Medical Center, San Jose, California 95128, Department of Medicine, Stanford, California 94305*

Received for publication 23 April 1976

The current development of potent antifungal drugs necessitates reliable methods of in vitro susceptibility testing of clinical isolates. Other laboratories have noted with some antimicrobials that conventional tube dilution visual end points for determining minimal inhibitory concentrations (MIC) vary markedly with the inoculum. With seven isolates (four species) we compared the conventional method with one developed with a spectrophotometer. Yeasts were diluted to inocula of 10^2 to 10^5 cells/ml and incubated at 37°C with 5-fluorocytosine or miconazole or without drug in a synthetic defined medium. At frequent intervals MICs were determined by the lowest drug concentration without visible turbidity. Concurrently, the percent transmission of each tube was measured and an inhibitory concentration ($IC_{1/2}$) was calculated from the turbidimetric measurements. MICs of both drugs for all strains varied with the inoculum. Intrastrain differences averaged 128-fold for miconazole and greater than 8-fold with 5-fluorocytosine. This variability in MIC occurred when readings were made after 12 to 48 h of incubation. In contrast, $IC_{1/2}$ values of all isolates varied less than two-fold with the same range of inocula. Most isolates showed this independence when measured at 48 h. Fast-growing yeasts showed greater $IC_{1/2}$ variability unless the turbidimetric measurements were taken earlier while the drug-free growth was still in a rapid growth phase. This method is reproducible, inoculum independent, rapid, free from subjectivity and observer variability, and suitable for adaptation to a clinical setting.

Fungal infections are an increasing problem with the growing use of immunosuppressive therapy, valve prostheses, and intravenous and urinary catheters and with the increased survival of patients with congenital and acquired immunodeficiencies (6, 9). Potent antifungal agents, such as amphotericin B and 5-fluorocytosine (5-FC), are currently available, but their administration carries the risk of serious toxic reactions (2). Newer agents are being developed, and they will require careful clinical evaluation. Reliable and practical in vitro sensitivity testing is necessary to select appropriate therapy.

There is no standardized method of testing the susceptibility of yeasts to antifungal agents. Most commonly, broth dilutions of the antifungal agent are performed. The lowest drug concentration that allows no visible growth of some inoculum is used as an end point (termed the minimal inhibitory concentration [MIC]). This method has the advantage of simplicity and can be performed in any clinical laboratory. However, it is subject to observer variability. Furthermore, 5-FC MICs for cryptococci reportedly are influenced considerably by variations in the initial inoculum size (4). Inoculum size is not standardized between laboratories and often is not precisely standardized within the same laboratory (e.g., dilutions of an overnight broth culture).

We report here a method of susceptibility testing that employs turbidimetric techniques to measure growth inhibition. The lowest drug concentration that inhibits growth to a fraction of that in drug-free controls is determined. This method has the advantage of objective measurement, thus minimizing observer variability. In addition, it appears free from inoculum-dependent variability.

MATERIALS AND METHODS

Seven yeasts were studied: *Candida albicans* (two strains), *C. parapsilosis* (three strains), *C. tropicalis*, and *Torulopsis glabrata*. All isolates were from clinical specimens, except the *C. tropicalis* (laboratory reference strain). The yeasts were identified as to species by current standard methods (10) and were maintained on Sabouraud dextrose agar until tested.

All susceptibility testing was performed in a completely defined synthetic liquid medium (8), modified by the substitution of cysteine for cystine. This medium is free from known inhibitors of antifungal agents.

Miconazole (Janssen and Co., Beerse, Belgium) was stored as a solution, stable at room temperature. 5-FC (supplied as a powder by Hoffman-La Roche, Nutley, N.J.) was dissolved and frozen in portions until used.

Yeast inocula were prepared from 18- to 24-h cultures in liquid media. These were adjusted to 60% transmission (%T) at 540 nm (Coleman Junior spectrophotometer). A 1:100 dilution of this broth and subsequent 10-fold serial dilutions produced inocula of approximately 2 (range of 1.3 to 3.7) % 10^5, 2×10^4, 2×10^3, and 2×10^2 cells/ml by hemocytometer count.

For susceptibility studies, antifungal agents were diluted in media to 20 and 500 μg of miconazole and 5-FC, respectively, per ml, and then serial twofold dilutions were made. A 0.9-ml amount of drug suspension or drug-free media was combined with an equal volume of fungal suspension in sterile, disposable plastic tubes (12 by 75 mm) and placed at 37°C for stationary incubation. At the onset of incubation all tubes were completely clear. At intervals the tubes were inspected for turbidity. Simultaneously the %T of each tube was measured against a tube containing only medium.

Susceptibility was estimated by both a visual and a turbidimetric method. The visual MIC was read as the lowest drug concentration that remained clear. The inhibitory concentration (IC_n) was then calculated from the turbidimetric data as the lowest drug concentration that met the criterion $\%T \geq (\%T_{control} + n[100 - \%T_{control}])$, where %T = percent transmission, control = drug-free tube, and n = a selected fraction less than 1 (1/2, 3/4, or 7/8). This formula was constructed to define a fraction of inhibition (set by the value of n) as a function of the turbidity in the drug-free control tubes.

RESULTS

Variation in MIC (visual) end point with inocula. Seven isolates were tested against 5-FC and six were tested against miconazole at inocula of 10^5 to 10^2 cells/ml (Fig. 1 and 2). All isolates except one (Me strain against 5-FC) showed inocula-dependent variation, with more resistant MICs for higher inocula. The one isolate not showing this effect was resistant to >250 μg of 5-FC per ml at all inocula tested. The MIC of each of two isolates spanned the entire 11-tube range of miconazole concentrations tested (10 to 0.01 μg/ml). The mean difference between the highest and the lowest for the range of inocula tested was 128-fold for all strains tested against miconazole. 5-FC MIC variation with inoculum size was not as great, but still averaged more than eightfold.

Independence of the IC (densitometric) end point from inocula effects. In contrast to intrastrain MIC variability, there was remarkable intrastrain uniformity in ICs calculated from turbidimetric measurements. Values for the $IC_{1/2}$, $IC_{3/4}$, and $IC_{7/8}$ are shown compared with the concurrent MICs for several isolates against miconazole and 5-FC in Fig. 3 and 4, respectively. Although a variety of n values yield similarly uniform inoculum independence, we have chosen $IC_{1/2}$ values to be represented in further comparisons. For all strains tested against both drugs, variation in the $IC_{1/2}$ over the range of inocula was never greater than twofold.

Relationship of incubation time to MIC variability. The MICs shown in Fig. 1 and 2 were read at 48 h to allow the control growths with the smallest inocula to become turbid. However, repeated MIC determinations were performed on most isolates (four strains with 5-FC and five strains with miconazole) beginning at 12 h of incubation. The variability in MIC with inoculum size was observed at all observation times for each strain, with no apparent tendency toward convergence at either early or late readings. This is illustrated in the next section, which compares MIC as a function of increasing cell growth.

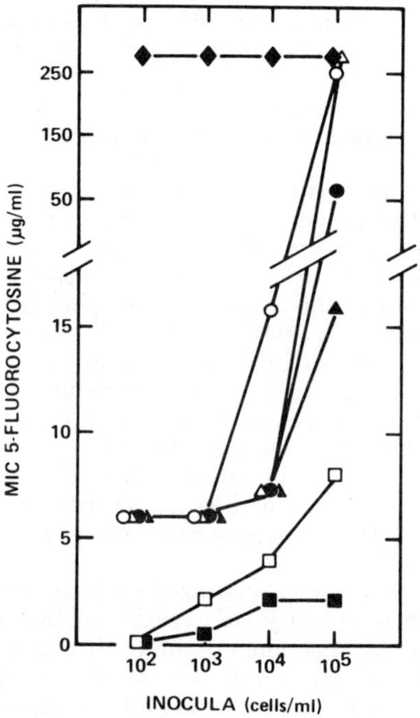

FIG. 1. *MIC of 5-FC at different inoculum sizes for several strains of yeast. Symbols:* ◆, *C. parapsilosis (Me strain);* ○, *C. albicans (St strain);* △, *C. albicans (Ba strain);* ●, *C. parapsilosis (Ba strain);* ▲, *C. parapsilosis (Wi strain);* □, *C. tropicalis (laboratory strain);* ■, *T. glabrata (Cu strain).*

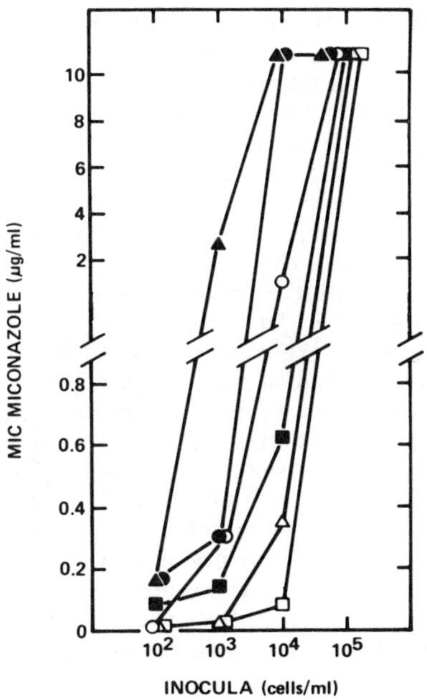

FIG. 2. *The MIC of miconazole at different inoculum sizes for several strains of yeast. Symbols are the same as those in Fig. 1.*

$IC_{1/2}$ dependence on control growth. During the course of our studies it was realized that faster-growing yeasts showed increased variation of $IC_{1/2}$ (i.e., four- to eightfold differences) over the inoculum range tested unless turbidimetric readings were taken earlier than 48 h. The time period during which $IC_{1/2}$ readings remained uniform was related to continued growth in the control tubes. Figure 5 demonstrates this relationship for one isolate whose growth in drug-free medium reached a "plateau" at 29%T (optical density, 0.53). The plateau is defined as the phase of the growth curve during which turbidity does not further increase with continued observation. As can be seen from this example, the $IC_{1/2}$ for various inocula showed no greater than twofold differences until the control tube approached the plateau. After a point, which could be defined as the lowest %T of control growth that gave an $IC_{1/2}$ variation of no more than twofold over the range of inocula tested, the $IC_{1/2}$ values increased and showed more variation over this inoculum range. For this isolate, the point is 50%T. Figure 6 represents the concurrent MIC determinations and illustrates that, even with the visual end point plotted as a function of

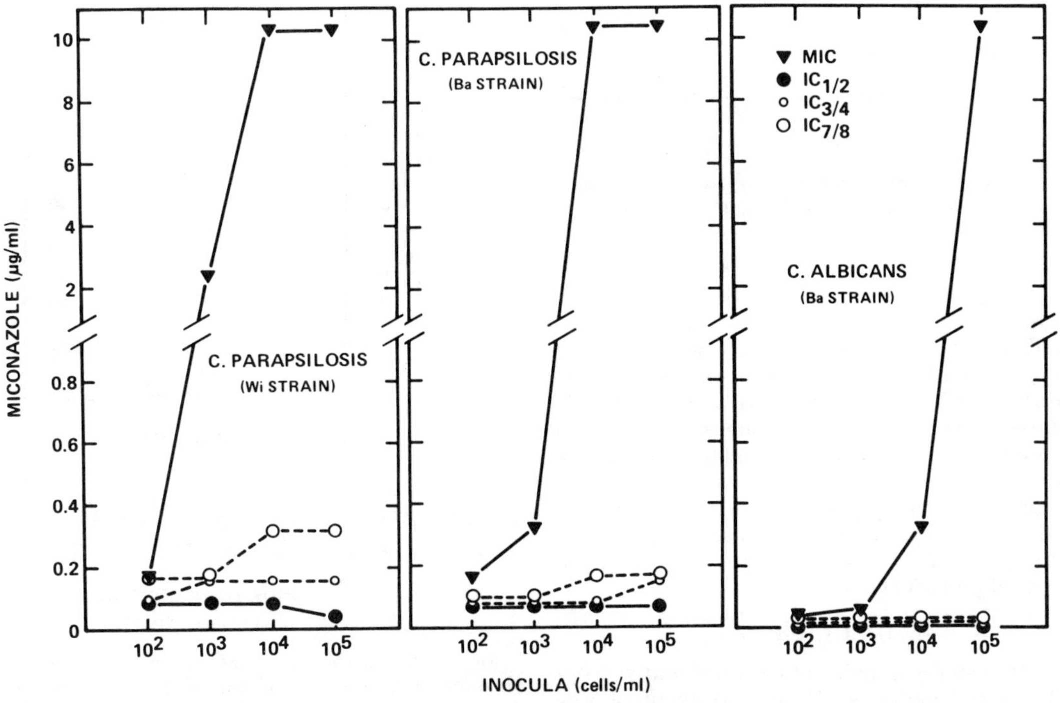

FIG. 3. *A comparison of the MIC and three calculated IC_n values for miconazole of three yeasts at different inoculum sizes.*

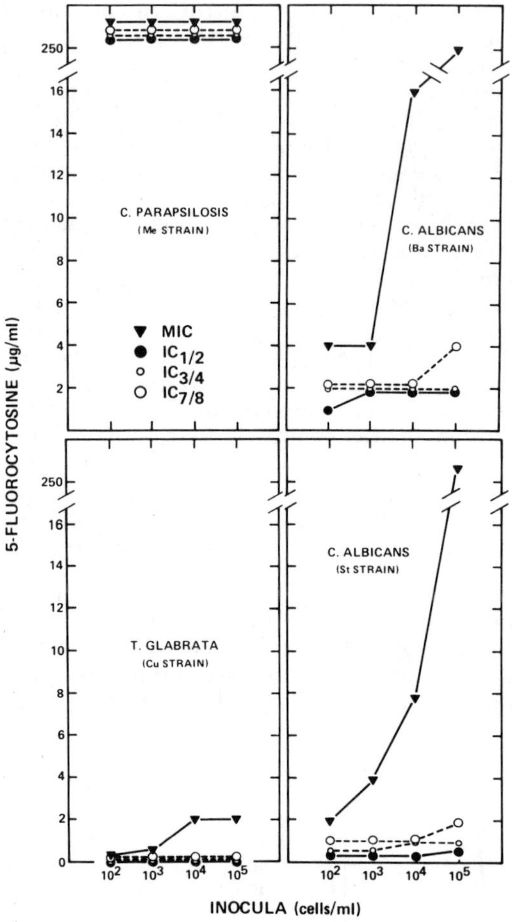

FIG. 4. *A comparison of the MIC and three calculated IC_n values of 5-FC of four yeasts at different inoculum sizes.*

control growth, variability with inoculum size persists.

Table 1, derived from serial observations of several strains in a manner similar to that illustrated in Fig. 5, shows the control growth plateau. The lowest %T consistent with no more than twofold variation in $IC_{1/2}$ is shown. Although this latter point varied for each strain, all of our isolates demonstrated minimal variation when the $IC_{1/2}$ was calculated before the control tube reached a turbidity of 50%T (optical density, 0.30).

DISCUSSION

The visual end point of conventional susceptibility test methods, although convenient, entails several serious problems. First, it clearly requires a subjective judgment concerning which drug concentration is the lowest that demonstrates "no growth." Neither variation between observers nor that which might occur between laboratories was examined in our studies, since all determinations were performed by the same investigator. However, variation would be expected to be maximal with an end point that attempted to distinguish "almost no growth" from "complete absence of growth." Second, the commonest criterion of no growth, no visible turbidity, assumes that very small changes in turbidity are always caused by cell growth. We also employed this criterion in the visual studies since it seemed the sharpest end point, but we are not convinced that the underlying assumption is always correct. In particular, suspensions that became minimally turbid during incubation with high concentrations of miconazole did not demonstrate significant increases in numbers of organisms (hemocytometer counts). It is possible that with some drugs and/or yeasts other events, such as increased adhesiveness with cell clumping or cell

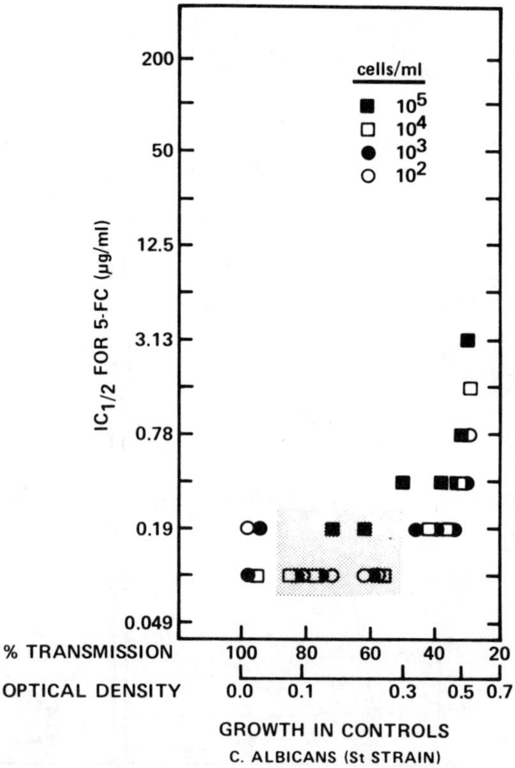

FIG. 5. *$IC_{1/2}$ values for 5-FC calculated from sequential measurements of four different inoculum sizes for one strain of yeast. Each point represents the $IC_{1/2}$ value for the inoculum as a function of the turbidity of the drug-free control. The shaded area is the range of least $IC_{1/2}$ variation.*

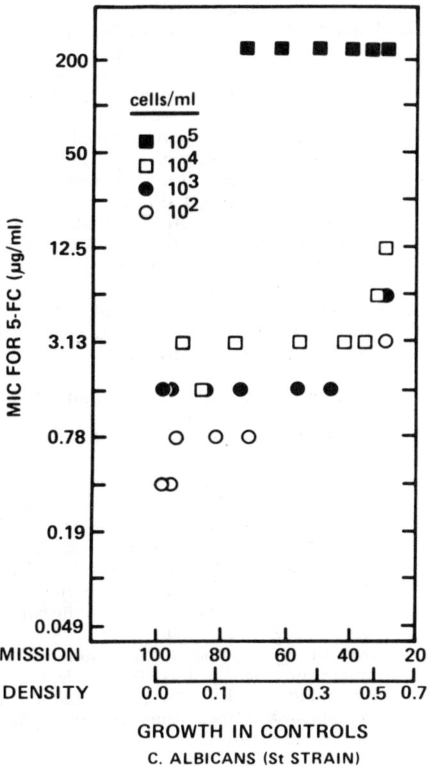

FIG. 6. *MIC values for 5-FC determined from sequential readings of four different inoculum sizes for the same yeast strain as shown in Fig. 5. Each point represents the MIC value for the inoculum as a function of the turbidity of the drug-free control.*

swelling (1), could account for minor changes in visual clarity independent of cell multiplication. It seems impossible to control for this with visual methods. A third drawback is inoculum dependence. Block et al. (4), for example, demonstrated this for cryptococcus against 5-FC. We have demonstrated this for several species for both 5-FC and miconazole. To make visual methods reproducible one must be careful to standardize inocula. Because of different growth characteristics of various yeasts, the practice of using a standard dilution of an overnight growth would not be sufficient. Furthermore, our results suggest that in comparing the relative sensitivity of strains between different inocula, even if standardized, results can be conflicting. Thus in Fig. 1 and 2 strains that appear to have different susceptibilities at 10^4 cells/ml have identical MICs at 10^3 cells/ml. Therefore, even with standardized inocula, visual MICs have serious limitations as an in vitro parameter to correlate with clinical events.

The turbidimetric method reported here avoids the problems just listed. Other authors have described similar turbidimetric assays and found them sensitive and reproducible (1, 7). The calculated value of $IC_{1/2}$ avoids a subjective end point. Furthermore, this turbidimetric end point is an objective measure of reduced growth. The $IC_{1/2}$ criterion obviates problems in discriminating between two similar tubes and in pondering the significance of minimal changes in tube clarity. Finally, we find that this criterion of sensitivity is free from the inoculum dependence seen with conventional methods. All of our initial inocula were below the visible range. However, Bennett, using slightly turbid suspensions and studying a narrower range of inocula, also showed inoculum independence with a similar method (1).

Other research techniques for susceptibility testing, such as killing curves constructed by colony or hemocytometer counts, may also avoid problems of the visual MIC determination. However, they require much more attention and materials. In contrast, this turbidimetric technique could readily be adapted to clinical use. Since results do not vary with inocula, a standard dilution of an overnight broth could be used. At times, for slower-growing isolates, a higher inoculum might be more convenient. The preparation of drug dilutions is identical with that used in visual techniques. We have purposely employed readily available plastic disposable tubes for incubation and have found their optical properties sufficiently uniform for the purposes of this technique. Similarly, the simple spectrophotometer used in this study is available in many clinical labs. With more sophisticated spectrophotometric equipment, this test could be automated. A few serial readings of the control tube should be performed to ensure that the drug-free mixture is

TABLE 1. *Turbidity of yeasts in drug-free medium at plateau and at limit of least $IC_{1/2}$ variation*

Species	%T at plateau	Lowest %T with intrastrain[a] $IC_{1/2}$ variation ≤ 2-fold	
		Miconazole	5-FC
C. albicans (St strain)	30	30	50
C. parapsilosis (Ba strain)	27	27	NT[b]
C. parapsilosis (Wi strain)	29	32	32
C. tropicalis (lab strain)	31	32	39
T. glabrata (Cu strain)	16	18	27

[a] Starting inocula of 10^2 to 10^5 cells/ml.
[b] NT, Not tested.

actively growing at the time of the $IC_{1/2}$ determination. It appears that most strains can be read at 24 to 48 h, with a variety of initial inocula. Repeated measurements of the drug tubes appear unnecessary.

The clinically important level of susceptibility is presently unknown. Turbidimetric methods will usually yield values below concurrent visual MICs although, as noted in Fig. 4 and 5, MICs with low initial inocula tend to approximate $IC_{1/2}$ values. As one example, fungal meningitis can respond to therapy despite very low levels of antifungal activity in the cerebrospinal fluid, i.e., drug concentrations below the MIC for the organism as determined by the visual method (3, 5). At present, it seems most important to utilize a method of susceptibility testing that is reliable, so that more firm correlations can be made with clinical efficacy.

ACKNOWLEDGMENTS

John N. Galgiani was supported by National Research Service Award no. 1 F32 AI05170-01 and the C. F. Aaron Endowment Fund.

LITERATURE CITED

1. **Bennett, J. E.** 1967. Susceptibility of *Cryptococcus neoformans* to amphotericin B, p. 405–410. Antimicrob. Agents Chemother. 1966.
2. **Bennett, J. E.** 1974. Chemotherapy of systemic mycoses. N. Engl. J. Med. 290:30–32.
3. **Bindschadler, D. D., and J. E. Bennett.** 1969. A pharmacologic guide to the clinical use of amphotericin B. J. Infect. Dis. 120:427–436.
4. **Block, E. R., A. E. Jennings, and J. E. Bennett.** 1973. Variables influencing susceptibility testing of *Cryptococcus neoformans* to 5-fluorocytosine. Antimicrob. Agents Chemother. 4:392–395.
5. **Deresinski, S. C., R. B. Lilly, H. B. Levine, J. N. Galgiani, and D. A. Stevens.** 1976. Treatment of fungal meningitis with miconazole. Am. Rev. Respir. Dis. 113(Suppl.):71.
6. **Frei, E., R. H. Levin, G. P. Bodey, E. E. Morse, and E. J. Freireich.** 1965. The nature and control of infections in patients with acute leukemia. Cancer Res. 25:1511–1515.
7. **Hamilton, J. D., and D. M. Elliot.** 1975. Combined activity of amphotericin B and 5-fluorocytosine against *Cryptococcus neoformans in vitro* and *in vivo* in mice. J. Infect. Dis. 131:129–137.
8. **Hoeprich, P. D., and P. D. Finn.** 1972. Obfuscation of the activity of antifungal antimicrobics by culture media. J. Infect. Dis. 126:353–361.
9. **Seelig, M. S., C. P. Speth, P. J. Kozinn, C. L. Taschdjian, E. F. Toni, and P. Goldberg.** 1974. Patterns of *Candida* endocarditis following surgery: importance of early diagnosis and therapy. Prog. Cardiovasc. Dis. 17:125–160.
10. **Silva-Hutner, M., and B. H. Cooper.** 1974. Medically important yeasts, p. 491–507. *In* E. H. Lennette, E. H. Spaulding, and J. P. Truant (ed.), Manual of clinical microbiology, 2nd ed. American Society for Microbiology, Washington, D.C.

ANTIMICROBIAL AGENTS AND CHEMOTHERAPY, Oct. 1976, p. 727-732 Vol. 10, No. 4

Aerobically Incubated Thioglycolate Broth Disk Method for Antibiotic Susceptibility Testing of Anaerobes

TERRENCE A. KURZYNSKI,* JOHN W. YRIOS, ARLAN G. HELSTAD, AND CHARLES R. FIELD

General Bacteriology Unit, Wisconsin State Laboratory of Hygiene, and Department of Preventive Medicine, University of Wisconsin, Madison, Wisconsin 53706

Received for publication 7 June 1976

The anaerobic broth disk (AnBD) method of Wilkins and Thiel and a new modification, designated the thioglycolate broth disk method, were compared with an agar dilution technique. The thioglycolate broth disk method was incubated aerobically (AeTBD) or anaerobically (AnTBD). One hundred anaerobic bacteria representing 15 species were tested with clindamycin, chloramphenicol, erythromycin, penicillin, and tetracycline. Agreement of results by the two methods with minimal inhibitory concentration determinations were: AnBD, 95.2%; AnTBD, 91.5%; AeTBD, 94.5%. With clindamycin, chloramphenicol, and penicillin, the agreement of the AeTBD and agar dilution results was 100%, 100%, and 95%, respectively. Using the AeTBD method, only 1.1% of all tests gave false susceptible readings, whereas 4.4% gave false resistant readings. All susceptibility testing errors occurred with tetracycline, erythromycin, and, to a lesser extent, penicillin. For each method, the changes in designation of bacteria as being susceptible or resistant to an antibiotic between trials primarily involved strains with minimal inhibitory concentrations which were ± one dilution of the respective breakpoint value. The same situation was true for most bacteria that yielded false resistant readings within each trial. False resistant readings with tetracycline were determined to be unrelated to excess cation content of test media. These results reaffirm the reliability of the AnBD method and indicate that the AeTBD modification is equally reliable. The greater convenience and lower cost of the AeTBD method should make possible more widespread performance of susceptibility testing for anaerobic bacteria in hospital laboratories.

In recent years, physicians and clinical microbiologists have become increasingly aware of the significance of anaerobic bacteria in a variety of infections. Specimen collection, transport, and culturing methods have been developed for the maximal recovery and quantitation of anaerobic bacteria from clinical specimens (12). As a consequence, there has been a demand by physicians for antibiotic susceptibility testing of anaerobes. Several investigators have described techniques for susceptibility tests using anaerobic incubation (5, 9, 10, 13, 15). Probably the most widely used of these is the broth disk method of Wilkins and Thiel (16), developed at the Virginia Polytechnic Institute. Wilkins and Thiel reported 97% agreement between their broth disk method and a broth dilution procedure. Unfortunately, the Wilkins and Thiel broth disk method is impractical for small laboratories since it requires the use of anaerobic grade CO_2, a gassing apparatus, and prereduced broth.

We have modified the Wilkins and Thiel method by substituting thioglycolate broth and the use of aerobic incubation. A comparison of antibiotic susceptibilities using the Wilkins and Thiel broth disk method, our aerobic thioglycolate modification, and an agar dilution method is presented.

MATERIALS AND METHODS

Bacterial strains. Anaerobic bacteria used were those that had been routinely submitted to the Wisconsin State Laboratory of Hygiene for isolation and/or identification. They were identified by methods developed by Holdeman and Moore (6) and then stored at −70°C in chopped meat glucose broth (CMG).

One hundred anaerobic bacteria representing 15 different species were studied. Identity of the bacteria and number of strains of each (in parentheses) were: *Bacteroides* sp. (4), *Bacteriodes fragilis* subsp. *fragilis* (38), *Bacteroides melaninogenicus* (7), *Bacteroides ruminicola* (1), *Fusobacterium nucleatum* (5), *Fusobacterium necrophorum* (2), *Fusobacterium mortiferum* (4), *Clostridium perfringens* (10), *Eubacterium lentum* (5), *Peptostreptococcus anaerobius* (8),

Peptostreptococcus intermedius (6), *Peptococcus prevotii* (1), *Peptococcus asaccharolyticus* (3), *Veillonella parvula* (3), and *Veillonella alcalescens* (3).

Media. All media were prepared in our laboratory and stored no longer than 2 weeks at room temperature. The medium used for the agar dilution method was prereduced and contained brain heart infusion (BHI broth, Difco), 2.5% agar, supplemented with 0.0005% hemin, 0.002% menadione, and 0.5% yeast extract (BHI-S). Prereduced BHI-S broth was used for the anaerobic broth disk (AnBD) method of Wilkins and Thiel (16).

For the thioglycolate broth disk (TBD) modification, thioglycolate broth (BBL no. 11720) was used in 5-ml quantities in screw-capped tubes (16 by 125 mm). Tubed media was stored in the dark at room temperature for up to 1 week, boiled for 10 min within 2 h before use, and cooled rapidly to room temperature in a water bath. For strains of *B. melaninogenicus,* a 0.5-ml supplement of 9 parts of rabbit serum plus 1 part of hemin-menadione stock solution (500 μg of hemin, 50 μg of menadione) was added to 4.5 ml of the cooled thioglycolate medium.

Antibiotics. Five reference standard antibiotic powders were used. Clindamycin (The Upjohn Co., Kalamazoo, Mich.) was initially dissolved in distilled water, chloramphenicol (Parke Davis and Co., Detroit, Mich.) in 95% ethanol, erythromycin (Eli Lilly and Co., Indianapolis, Ind.) in absolute methanol, tetracycline (Bristol Laboratories, Syracuse, N.Y.) in 0.01 N HCl, and potassium penicillin G (Bristol Laboratories, Syracuse, N.Y.) in 0.1 M phosphate buffer, pH 6.0 (8). Antibiotics were stored in sterile distilled water at 1,000 μg/ml (penicillin G at 1,000 units/ml) at −70°C for up to 4 months.

Antibiotic disks (Difco) were of the high concentration type. They were stored with a calcium chloride desiccant at 4°C in screw-capped bottles. Disk stability was determined by measuring zone sizes using the *Staphylococcus aureus* ATCC 25923 and *Escherichia coli* ATCC 25922 strains.

Determination of MICs. Minimal inhibitory concentration (MIC) determinations were determined for each antibiotic by an agar dilution method modified after Martin et al. (9). After thawing, organisms were inoculated into prereduced peptone yeast glucose broth, supplemented when necessary (e.g., *B. melaninogenicus*) with hemin and menadione, and incubated for 24 h at 37°C. The broth culture was diluted under 100% CO_2 to a turbidity equal to a no. 1 MacFarland standard, for inoculation by a Steers replicator. Serial twofold dilutions of antibiotics in 3 ml of distilled water were added into separate 27-ml amounts of molten (55°C) BHI-S agar, the contents were mixed well, and each was poured into a square Falcon "integrid" plastic dish (100 by 15 mm). Final antibiotic concentrations ranged from 0.1 to 50 μg/ml (penicillin in units/ml); for tetracycline the concentration ranged up to 100 μg/ml. Antibiotic dilutions and agar plates were prepared on the day of the test, and the plates were air dried for approximately 2 h before inoculation. An antibiotic-free control plate was inoculated at the beginning and end of the inoculation procedure. A control strain of *S. aureus* ATCC 25923 was included with each batch of cultures tested.

Inoculated plates were incubated in a GasPak (150) jar containing a tube of aqueous methylene blue. Anaerobic conditions were achieved by the evacuation replacement technique, using three consecutive evacuations and replacements with the gas combination 80% N_2, 10% CO_2, and 10% H_2. Plates were incubated at 37°C for 48 h except for slow growers such as *B. melaninogenicus,* which required 72 h.

The MIC was interpreted as the lowest antibiotic concentration that resulted in two or less tiny colonies or a faint haze.

AnBD method. In the Wilkins and Thiel AnBD method (16), high concentration commercial antibiotic disks are added to separate tubes containing 5 ml of prereduced BHI-S broth. The number of disks added per tube for each antibiotic is: clindamycin, four; chloramphenicol, two; erythromycin, one; penicillin, one; and tetracycline, one. This results in final test concentrations of 1.6 μg/ml for clindamycin, 12 μg/ml for chloramphenicol, 3 μg/ml for erythromycin, 2 units/ml for penicillin, and 6 μg/ml for tetracycline. These concentrations are considered to be easily achievable in blood under normal therapeutic regimens. Tubes are inoculated anaerobically with 1 drop of an overnight CMG culture, incubated overnight, and observed for turbidity. The majority of tests involve only a judgment of growth versus no growth, and resistance is indicated when the turbidity is 50% or greater than the control culture. Susceptibility is indicated when there is no turbidity or the turbidity is obviously less than 50% of that in the control tube. Results in which the turbidity is very close to 50% of that in the control tube are reported as indeterminate.

Thioglycolate broth disk (TBD) method. The Wilkins and Thiel (16) method was modified by substituting thioglycolate broth (BBL no. 11720) for BHI-S broth. The appropriate number of antibiotic disks were added into screw-capped tubes (16 by 125 mm) containing 5 ml of boiled and cooled thioglycolate broth. Uninoculated tubes were then kept at room temperature for 2 h to allow for diffusion of the antibiotics into the medium. This prediffusion step was used to overcome the diffusion inhibitory effect of the 0.07% agar present in thioglycolate broth (1), a step that is not necessary in the AnBD method. Preliminary data indicate that the prediffusion period must be at least 1 h to avoid some false resistant readings. Tubes were then inoculated with 2 drops of an overnight CMG culture using a Pasteur pipette, and the screw caps were tightened. The tubes were inverted twice and incubated at 37°C overnight. In our experience, this latter step resulted in more uniform bacterial growth and made the results easier to read.

With slow-growing organisms, incubation was extended to 48 h to achieve adequate growth. For the anaerobic TBD (AnTBD) method, screw caps were loosened, and tubes were incubated at 37°C in an anaerobic jar under 80% N_2, 10% CO_2, and 10% H_2 (evacuation replacement technique). For the aerobic

TBD (AeTBD) method, the cultures were tested by leaving the screw caps tight and incubating without an anaerobic atmosphere at 37°C. Interpretation of results for the AnTBD and the AeTBD methods was the same as for the AnBD method. For comparative purposes, indeterminate readings were recorded as resistant.

The agar dilution, AnBD, and AnTBD determinations were always run simultaneously on the same culture. The AeTBD determinations were run separately. In addition, all agar dilution, AnBD, and AnTBD tests were repeated once to determine reproducibility. Reproducibility was not determined for the AeTBD method since only one trial was made, but AeTBD results were compared separately to first and second trial agar dilution results.

RESULTS

Reproducibility of MICs. Table 1 lists the variation in MIC results that occurred with each antibiotic upon repeat testing. A fourfold variation in MIC values upon testing is considered acceptable (3). The percentage of determinations within the acceptable fourfold range varied from 87% with erythromycin to 98% for clindamycin. The cumulative data for all antibiotics shows that 93% of the determinations were within the acceptable limits of variation.

Of greater significance, however, is the reproducibility of the agar dilution method in designating strains as being susceptible or resistant. Table 1 shows that susceptibility designation reproducibility was 95% or greater for all antibiotics except tetracycline (87%). Eleven of 13 isolates whose reproducibility was unacceptable for tetracycline were *B. fragilis* subsp. *fragilis*. Overall, the susceptibility designations were acceptable in 96% of the repeat tests. Furthermore, if the latter figures are adjusted by accepting as being in agreement, the results for those strains having MICs within one dilution of the breakpoint value in both trials but opposite susceptibility designations, greater reproducibility is indicated. As a result, Table 1 shows that adjusted susceptibility reproducibility was 100% for all antibiotics except tetracycline (95%). Overall, the adjusted susceptibility designations were acceptable in 99% of the repeat tests.

Individual susceptibility patterns are not presented since no significant variation was noted from more extensive studies (9, 11).

Agreement of AnBD, AnTBD, and AeTBD methods results with MICs. The overall correlation of the AnBD method with simultaneous MIC determinations was 95.2% (Table 2). False resistant readings averaged 3.4%, whereas false susceptible readings averaged 1.4%. Furthermore, susceptibility designations of 14 out of 100 strains changed from the first to the second trial (data not shown), involving six strains for tetracycline, seven for erythromycin, and one for penicillin. Except for one strain tested with tetracycline, all bacteria involved in change in susceptibility designation between trials had MICs within ± one dilution of the breakpoint value. No such changes occurred with clindamycin or chloramphenicol.

The AnTBD method results (Table 2) were also shown to agree well with simultaneous MIC determinations, yielding an average correlation of 91.5%. False resistant readings and false susceptible readings averaged 7.6% and 0.9%, respectively, for this method. There were 34 instances of change of susceptibility designation between trials (data not shown); 23 of these occurred with erythromycin, seven with tetracycline, and four with penicillin. The number of strains involved in MIC changes that had MICs ± one dilution of the breakpoint value were 6 of 23 for erythromycin, 5 of 7 for tetracycline, and 1 of 4 for penicillin.

For the AeTBD method, 97 of the original 100 strains were retested once using aerobic incubation of tubes. As a result, the correlation of AeTBD results with MICs (Table 2) increased to 94.9% if compared with first trial MICs and

TABLE 1. *Reproducibility of agar dilution MICs and susceptibility designations determined in two trials*

Determinant	% Reproducibility for each antibiotic[a]					
	CC	C	E	Pen	Tet	All
Reproducibility of MICs within acceptable fourfold range	98	94	87	97	90	93
Reproducibility of susceptibility designations	100	100	95	99	87	96
Adjusted reproducibility of susceptibility designations[b]	100	100	100	100	95	99

[a] Abbreviations: CC, Clindamycin; C, chloramphenicol; E, erythromycin; P, penicillin; T, tetracycline; All, average for all antibiotics.

[b] Figures are adjusted by designating as being in agreement the results for those strains having MICs within a dilution of the breakpoint value in both trials but opposite susceptibility designations.

94.0% if compared with second trial MICs (average of 94.5%). False resistant readings dropped to an average of 4.4% as compared with 7.6% in the AnTBD method. The incidence of FSRs remained approximately the same as with the AnTBD method (1.1% versus 0.9%, respectively). Extent of growth in thioglycolate broth inoculated from CMG and incubated aerobically was very similar to that obtained in prereduced BHI-S broth, except for several strains of *Fusobacterium* species which obviously grew better in thioglycolate broth.

False susceptible readings are considerably more important clinically than are false resistant readings, but false susceptible readings were minimal and relatively similar for each method, ranging from a low of 0.9% (average) in the AnTBD method to a high of 1.4% (average) in the AnBD method.

For the AnBD and AnTBD methods, the percentage of agreement of results compared to MIC readings between trials (Table 2) varied less than 1%, indicating adequate reproducibility. Since the AeTBD method was only run once and the results were compared to MICs determined in two trials, the data is inadequate to establish reproducibility for the AeTBD method.

TABLE 2. *Agreement of broth disk method results with minimal inhibitory concentration (MIC) determinations and types of error*

Method	No. of strains	% Agreement with MIC[a]	Type of error: % False resistant readings[b]	% False susceptible readings
AnBD:[b]				
First trial	100	95.8	2.6	1.6
Second trial	99	94.6	4.2	1.2
Avg		95.2	3.4	1.4
AnTBD:[b]				
First trial	100	91.6	7.6	0.8
Second trial	99	91.4	7.6	1.0
Avg		91.5	7.6	0.9
AeTBD:[b]				
First trial	97	94.9	3.9	1.2
Second trial	97	94.0	5.0	1.0
Avg		94.5	4.4	1.1

[a] Total for five antibiotics.
[b] Abbreviations: AnBD, Anaerobic broth disk; AnTBD, anaerobic thioglycolate broth disk; and AeTBD, aerobic thioglycolate broth disk.

Distribution of errors. It is of interest to inspect the distribution of errors for each method according to antibiotic. Table 3 shows that with the AnBD method there were neither false resistant nor false susceptible readings to either clindamycin or chloramphenicol. False resistant readings were most common with tetracycline (totaling 24 for two trials), and 19 involved bacteria for which the MIC was ± one dilution of the breakpoint value. With erythromycin, three of six false resistant readings involved bacteria having MICs ± one dilution of the breakpoint value. This association was not observed for the four penicillin false resistant readings.

With the AnTBD method, Table 3 shows that there were only 1 and 2 false resistant readings for clindamycin and chloramphenicol, respectively, and no false susceptible readings for these two antibiotics. Again, false resistant readings were most common with tetracycline, totaling 38. Eighteen of these 38 false resistant readings involved bacteria having MICs ± one dilution of the breakpoint value. It is notable that a total of 26 false resistant readings occurred with erythromycin and only five of those involved bacteria having an MIC ± one dilution of the breakpoint value. With penicillin, one of nine false resistant readings had an MIC ± one dilution of the breakpoint value.

The noticeable improvement in AeTBD results as compared with AnTBD results was largely due to a decreased incidence of false resistant readings (Table 3). This is especially evident for erythromycin (total of 16 fewer false resistant readings in AeTBD method) and to a lesser extent for tetracycline (total of 11 fewer

TABLE 3. *Distribution of errors for broth disk methods according to antibiotic and the incidence of borderline MIC values among the errors*

Method	Ratio of no.[a] of false resistant readings for which MIC was within one dilution of breakpoint value to no.[a] of false resistant readings						Ratio of no. of false susceptible readings which MIC was within one dilution of breakpoint value to no. of false susceptible readings					
	CC[b]	C	E	P	T	All	CC	C	E	P	T	All
AnBD[c]	0/0	0/0	3/6	0/4	19/24	22/34	0/0	0/0	0/7	0/2	5/3	5/12
AnTBD[c]	0/1	0/2	5/26	1/9	18/38	24/76	0/0	0/0	2/3	1/2	1/4	4/9
AeTBD[c]	0/0	0/0	6/10	1/6	16/27	23/43	0/0	0/0	2/6	1/3	2/2	5/11

[a] Numbers are totals for two trials except for the AeTBD method which was run once and results compared separately to MICs from two trials.
[b] Abbreviations: see footnote, Table 1.
[c] Abbreviations: see footnote, Table 2.

false resistant readings). A total of three fewer false resistant readings occurred for penicillin with aerobic incubation. Strains with MIC values which were ± one dilution of the breakpoint values accounted for a total of 6 of 10 erythromycin false resistant readings, 1 of 6 penicillin false resistant readings, and 16 of 27 tetracycline false resistant readings in the AeTBD method.

The cumulative totals for all antibiotics (Table 3) show that the proportion of false resistant readings with MICs ± one dilution of the breakpoint values ranged from 31.6% (24 out of 76) of all false resistant readings in the AnTBD method to 64.7% (22 out of 34) of all false resistant readings in the AnBD method.

Table 3 shows that for all methods, some false susceptible readings were also associated with bacteria having MICs ± one dilution of the breakpoint values.

DISCUSSION

Agreement of the AnBD method and MIC results averaged 95.2%. This figure closely approximates those of Wilkins (16) and Blazevic (2) who obtained 97% and 95.6% correlations of the AnBD method results with MICs, respectively. In our experience, the AnBD method of Wilkins is a very reliable method of antibiotic susceptibility determination for the most commonly isolated anaerobes. Its major disadvantages are media expense and need for a gassing apparatus and anaerobic gas.

Results obtained with the AnTBD method approached the accuracy of AnBD results (average of 91.5% versus 95.2% agreement with MIC results, respectively). The data of Ingham et al. (7) and Eagle et al. (3) on the inactivation of erythromycin by CO_2-induced acidity suggested that fewer false resistant readings might be obtained by aerobic incubation of the tubes in the TBD method. Under anaerobic incubation, decreased activity of erythromycin was evident in the TBD method by the frequent observation of heavy bacterial growth at the top of the thioglycolate broth (where the pH could be assumed to be lowest due to dissolved CO_2) and no growth or diminished growth deep in the medium. As a result, this growth pattern was incorrectly recorded as indeterminate (resistant). This growth pattern only occurred in erythromycin tubes and only with strains of *B. fragilis* subsp. *fragilis* (11 total strains). Consequently, 97 of the original 100 strains were retested using the TBD method with incubation under aerobic conditions (AeTBD method). As a result, the correlation of AeTBD results with MICs increased to an average of 94.5% (Table 2). Surface growth was not observed with aerobic incubation, and the respective strains of *B. fragilis* subsp. *fragilis* were correctly recorded as being susceptible to erythromycin.

That CO_2 induced acidity did not appreciably decrease the activity of erythromycin in the AnBD method (despite the fact that the tubes were gassed with 100% CO_2) may be due to the absence of agar in the BHI-S broth and/or differences in buffering capacity of the two media. In thioglycolate broth, agar would have the effect of concentrating CO_2 in the uppermost portion of the medium therby appreciably lowering the pH in that restricted volume. In addition, the growth-enhancing effect of CO_2 may also contribute to enhanced surface growth in thioglycolate broth. In contrast, with BHI-S broth, convection currents in the fluid medium would more easily dilute the CO_2 and maintain a higher pH throughout. However, further work is necessary to test the validity of these speculations.

For each method, the changes in susceptibility designations between trials primarily involved strains having MICs which were ± one dilution of the breakpoint values. The same situation was true for most bacteria which yielded false resistant readings within each trial.

In this study, no explanation is apparent for the tetracycline, erythromycin, and penicillin false resistant readings which involved bacterial strains with MICs greater than ± one dilution of the breakpoint values. Consideration was made of inactivation of tetracycline through chelation by excess cation concentrations (14). Table 4 shows the concentration of Ca and Mg in the media used for each method studied. It is evident that BHI-S agar used for all MIC determinations had the highest Ca and Mg concentrations of all the media used. Consequently, MIC determinations with tetracycline should have been affected to a greater extent than the broth disk susceptibility determinations. Secondly, thioglycolate broth had a much higher Ca and Mg concentration than did BHI-S broth, yet the number of tetracycline false resistant readings obtained in both broths

TABLE 4. *Cation concentration of susceptibility test media as determined by atomic absorption spectrophotometry*

Cation	Cation concn (μg/ml)		
	BHI-S broth	BHI-S agar	Thioglycolate broth
Ca	1.80	44.1	39.2
Mg	2.43	39.6	34.2

by the respective methods was approximately the same (Table 3). Thus, the presence of excess cations in the test media was not associated with inactivation of tetracycline.

However, related to this problem is the report of Wilkins (16) that different batches of 30-μg tetracycline disks varied in content from 26.7 to 44.0 μg. This variation in disk content of antibiotic is great enough to lead to erroneous susceptibility determinations by any broth disk method when testing bacteria having MICs ± one dilution of the breakpoint value.

In summary, the AeTBD method was found to be a reliable method of antibiotic susceptibility testing for the most commonly isolated anaerobes from clinical specimens. With clindamycin, chloramphenicol, and penicillin, which are the three primary antibiotics used to treat anaerobic infections, the agreement of the AeTBD and agar dilution results was 100%, 100%, and 95%, respectively. The advantages of reliability, convenience (most hospital laboratories can easily prepare thioglycolate medium), and low cost make possible more widespread performance of susceptibility testing for anaerobic bacteria in hospital laboratories.

ACKNOWLEDGMENT

We wish to thank R. Zimmerman for determinations of cation concentrations.

LITERATURE CITED

1. **Alvarez, J. P.** 1955. A simplified sensitivity procedure for anaerobic micro-organisms. Am. J. Med. Technol. 21:249–253.
2. **Blazevic, D. J.** 1975. Evaluation of the modified broth-disk method for determining antibiotic susceptibilities of anaerobic bacteria. Antimicrob. Agents Chemother. 7:721–723.
3. **Eagle, H., M. Levy, and R. Fleischman.** 1952. The effect of the pH of the medium on the antibacterial action of penicillin, streptomycin, chloramphenicol, terramycin, and bacitracin. Antibiot. Chemother. 2:563–575.
4. **Ericsson, H. M., and J. C. Sherris.** 1971. Antibiotic sensitivity testing – report of an international collaborative study. Acta Pathol. Microbiol. Scand. Sect. B., Suppl. 217.
5. **Hauser, K. J., J. A. Johnston, and R. J. Zabransky.** 1975. Economical agar dilution technique for susceptibility testing of anaerobes. Antimicrob. Agents Chemother. 7:712–714.
6. **Holdeman, L. V., and W. E. C. Moore (ed).** 1972. Anaerobe laboratory manual. Virginia Polytechnic Institute Anaerobe Laboratory, Virginia Polytechnic Institute and State University, Blacksburg.
7. **Ingham, H. R., J. B. Selkon, A. A. Codd, and J. H. Hale.** 1970. The effect of carbon dioxide on the sensitivity of *Bacteroides fragilis* to certain antibiotics *in vitro*. J. Clin. Pathol. 23:254–258.
8. **MacLowry, J. D., M. J. Jaqua, and S. T. Selepak.** 1970. Detailed methodology and implementation of a semiautomated serial dilution microtechnique for antimicrobial susceptibility testing. Appl. Microbiol. **20:**46–53.
9. **Martin, W. J., M. Gardner, and J. A. Washington II.** 1972. In vitro antimicrobial susceptibility of anaerobic bacteria isolated from clinical specimens. Antimicrob. Agents Chemother. 1:148–158.
10. **Stalons, D. R., and C. Thornsberry.** 1975. Broth-dilution method for determining the antibiotic susceptibility of anaerobic bacteria. Antimicrob. Agents Chemother. 7:15–21.
11. **Staneck, J. L., and J. Washington II.** 1974. Antimicrobial susceptibilities of anaerobic bacteria: recent clinical isolates. Antimicrob. Agents Chemother. 6:311–315.
12. **Sutter, V. L., H. R. Attebery, J. E. Rosenblatt, K. S. Bricknell, and S. M. Finegold.** 1972. Anaerobic bacteriology manual. Wadsworth Hospital Center, Veterans Administration, Los Angeles, Calif.
13. **Sutter, V. L., Y. Y. Kwok, and S. M. Finegold.** 1972. Standardized antimicrobial disc susceptibility testing of anaerobic bacteria. I. Susceptibility of *Bacteroides fragilis* to tetracycline. Appl. Microbiol. 23:268–275.
14. **Washington, J. A., II.** 1974. The agar-dilution technique, p. 60. *In* A. Balows (ed.), Current techniques for antibiotic susceptibility testing. Charles C Thomas Publisher, Springfield, Ill.
15. **Wilkins, T. D., L. V. Holdeman, I. J. Abramson, and W. E. C. Moore.** 1972. Standardized single-disk method for antibiotic susceptibility testing of anaerobic bacteria. Antimicrob. Agents Chemother. 1:451–459.
16. **Wilkins, T. D., and T. Thiel.** 1973. Modified broth-disk method for testing the antibiotic susceptibility of anaerobic susceptibility of anaerobic bacteria. Antimicrob. Agents Chemother. 3:350–356.

ANTIMICROBIAL AGENTS AND CHEMOTHERAPY, Oct. 1976, p. 733–735
Vol. 10, No. 4
Printed in U.S.A.

Concentration of Cefamandole in Serum Interstitial Fluid, Bile, and Urine

N. G. WATERMAN,* H. U. EICKENBERG, AND L. SCHARFENBERGER

Price Institute of Surgical Research, and the Department of Surgery, University of Louisville School of Medicine, Health Sciences Center, Louisville, Kentucky 40201*

Received for publication 2 June 1976

Cefamandole readily diffuses from the serum into soft tissue interstitial fluid. The rate of diffusion differs little from that of cephalothin. The concentrations of antibiotic were greater in bile and urine during the entire period of study than is necessary to kill susceptible pathogenic bacteria present in these fluids.

Cefamandole is a relatively new derivative of the cephalosporins. It has been found to be very active against gram-positive cocci and gram-negative bacilli. The in vitro activity against penicillin susceptible and resistant *Staphylococcus aureus* is excellent (1, 6, 7). Cefamandole has also been found to be effective against a significant number of clinical isolates of *Escherichia coli* and *Klebsiella pneumoniae* resistant to other cephalosporins (1). Because of the susceptibility of many of the bacteria causing nosocomial infections, we believe it necessary to determine the character of the excretion and diffusion of the drug from the serum into other body fluids. A comparison of time-serum changes in cefamandole concentration in soft tissue interstitial fluid, bile, and urine was undertaken.

MATERIALS AND METHODS

Multiperforated polypropylene balls measuring 15 mm in diameter were implanted in the tissues of the flank and abdominal wall in six adult mongrel dogs. T-tubes were inserted in the common ducts. After a period of 4 to 6 weeks, sufficient healing had occurred to permit physiological exchange of capsule fluid with the capilliaries. These capsules are identical to those described by Waterman and Kastan (9) for the measurement of antibiotic concentrations in interstitial fluid.

A 20-mg amount of cefamandole nafate per kg of body weight was given intravenously to each animal. Serial blood specimens were obtained by venipuncture. Interstitial fluid from the abdominal wall was withdrawn from the implanted capsule with a 23-gauge needle, and bile was obtained from the T-tube. All specimens were obtained hourly for 4 h. Microbiological assays of antibiotic concentrations in serum, interstitial fluids, and bile were performed by the agar diffusion method described by Sabath and co-workers, using *Bacillus subtilis* as the assay organism (8). Antibiotic standards for the serum level determinations were prepared in pooled canine serum, those for bile concentrations were prepared in pooled canine bile, and those for interstitial fluid levels were prepared in M/15 phosphate buffer (pH 6.0). The concentrations of antibiotics in serum, bile, and interstitial fluids of the liver and abdominal wall soft tissue at varying times were then compared among animals by an analysis of variance.

Multiperforated polypropylene balls measuring 20 mm in diameter were implanted in the flank and abdomen of six adult mongrel dogs. Two 10-mm multiperforated balls connected by polyethelene tubing inserted in the central portion of the capsule were implanted in the renal parenchyma, and a T-tube was inserted in the ipsilateral ureter. The occluded ends of the polyethelene tubes and long limb of the T-tube were sutured beneath the flank skin. After 4 weeks, healing was sufficient to permit physiological fluid exchange between renal interstitium and capsules. The dogs were anesthetized with thiopental sodium and given 20 mg of cefamandole per kg intravenously. Serial samples of blood were drawn from peripheral veins, renal interstitial fluid was extracted from the polyethelene tubing, and soft tissue interstitial fluid was obtained from the capsules with 23-gauge hypodermic needles. The urine was allowed to drip from the T-tube with samples taken at hourly intervals for 4 h. This method of study has been described by Eickenberg and colleagues (4, 5) for determining the concentration of cephalothin in renal interstitial fluid. Completed studies to be published show that in the creatinine, blood urea nitrogen, and *para*-amino hippuric acid clearance test measurements and radio-opaque dye injection X-ray studies there is no communication between the renal capsules and the excretory system. The time concentrations of the cephalosporins in serum, renal interstitial fluid, soft tissue interstitial fluid, and urine were compared by an analysis of variance.

RESULTS

Figure 1 shows the average and the variation in the time concentration changes of serum to interstitial fluid. The serum level remained greater than the interstitial fluid for more than

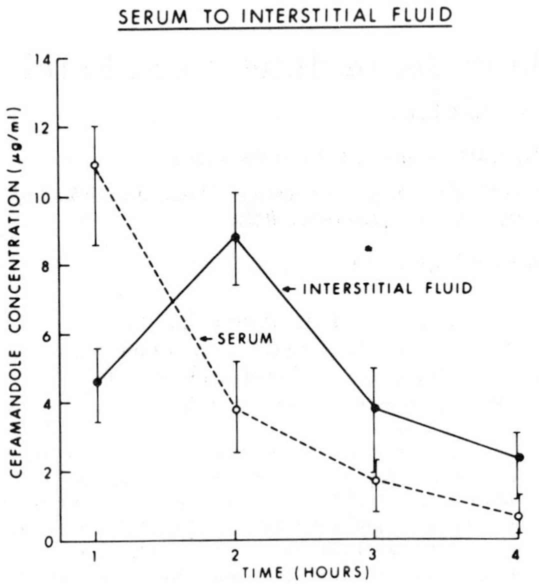

FIG. 1. *Comparison of the concentrations of cefamandole in serum and interstitial fluid at 1 to 4 h after a 20-mg/kg intravenous dose.*

1 h. By 2 h, the antibiotic concentration was greater in the interstitial fluid. As a result of excretion, secretion, and metabolism, the serum concentration became less and the antibiotic began to diffuse back into the vascular compartment. Figure 2 graphically illustrates the average and variation in serum-to-bile concentrations. The bile concentration was 360 μg at 1 h and decreased to 120 μg at 4 h and to 40 μg at 6 h. The analysis of variance showed the relationship during the times of measurement to be significant ($P < 0.01$).

Figure 3 shows that the average and variation in the urine and renal interstitial fluid concentrations, measured as described by Eickenberg and associates (4, 5), are quite high and greatly exceed the concentrations in the serum and in the extrarenal soft tissue interstitial fluid. Cefamandole had an initial peak concentration in the urine of 8,200 μg/ml within 60 min of the single intravenous injection. The greatest quantity appearing in the serum within an hour was 11 μg/ml. After 1 h, the antibiotic concentration in the renal interstitial fluid was 42.6 μg/ml and was greater than both the simultaneously measured serum level (11 μg/ml), and the control soft tissue interstitial fluid concentration (4.6 μg/ml). After 2 h, the serum level (3.9 μg/ml) was less than that in the renal interstitial fluid (38 μg/ml) and soft tissue interstitial fluid (8.8 μg/ml). After 4 h, only a very low concentration was found in

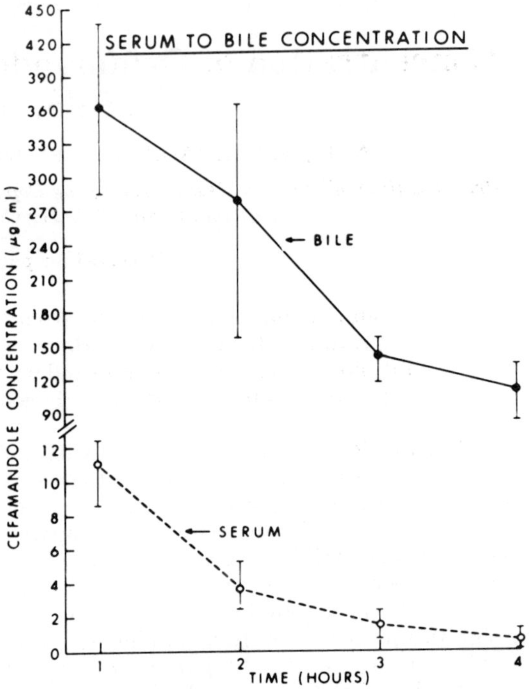

FIG. 2. *Comparison of the serum and bile concentrations at 1 to 4 h after intravenous injection of 20 mg/kg.*

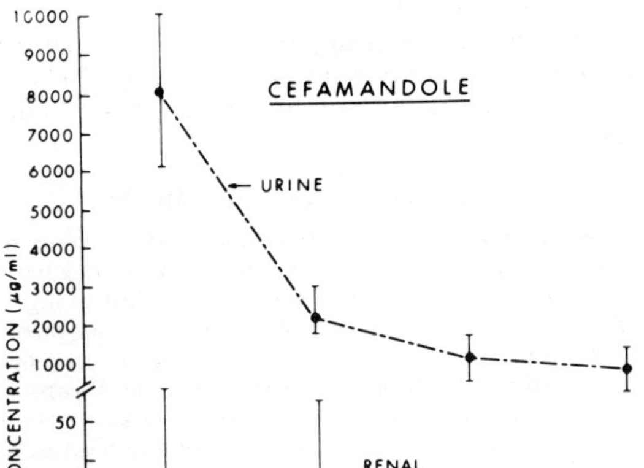

FIG. 3. *Concentrations of cefamandole in serum, soft tissue interstitial fluid, renal interstitial fluid, and urine after intravenous injection of 20 mg/kg.*

serum. The concentration in renal interstitial fluid was 12.6 μg/ml and remained higher than in the soft tissue interstitial fluid (2.4 μg/ml). The analysis of variance showed the relationships to be significant ($P < 0.01$).

DISCUSSION

Cefamandole readily diffuses into body soft tissue interstitial fluid. The rate of diffusion differs little from that of cephalothin (9). Both antibiotic agents increase to satisfactory tissue fluid concentrations in less than 1 h, and the serum and tissue fluids are nearly the same between 90 min and 2 h. The protein binding of cefamandole in pooled dog sera measured by the ultrafiltration method is 40% and is similar to cephalothin (10), and it is consistent with other cephalosporin dog sera protein-binding studies (12). The quantity excreted or secreted into bile is excellent. A comparison with concentrations of other antibiotics in bile previously measured in this laboratory (11) shows the concentration of cefamandole to be greater than that of cephalothin, tetracycline, and ampicillin when each was injected intravenously in the same dosage. Cefazolin was the only antimicrobial agent measured that showed a greater concentration than cefamandole.

The concentrations of cefamandole in urine and renal interstitial fluid were greater than those with cephalothin. Both drugs were measured in the same laboratory animals used by Eickenberg and colleagues (5) to determine renal interstitial fluid antibiotic concentrations.

The concentrations of cefamandole diffusing into interstitial fluid and excreted in bile and urine are greater than those obtained with cephalothin. The graphic patterns of the time concentration changes are very similar. The quantities measured during the period of study were sufficient to be active against most susceptible pathogenic bacteria present in the studied fluids.

ACKNOWLEDGMENT

This work was sponsored by a grant from Eli Lilly & Co.

LITERATURE CITED

1. **Bodey, G. P., and S. Weaver.** 1976. In vitro studies of cefamandole. Antimicrob. Agents Chemother. 9:452-457.
2. **Calnan, J. S., J. J. Pflug, G. D. Chisholm, and L. M. Taylor.** 1972. Pathophysiology of tissue fluid. Proc. R. Soc. Med. 65:715-719.
3. **Chisholm, G. D., P. M. Waterworth, J. S. Calnan, and L. Garrod.** 1973. Concentration of antibacterial agents in interstitial tissue fluid. Br. Med. J. 1:569-573.
4. **Eickenberg, H. U., N. G. Waterman, and L. Scharfenberger.** 1975. Renal interstitial fluid, urine, and serum antibiotic concentration. Surg. Forum 26:589-591.
5. **Eickenberg, H. U., N. G. Waterman, and L. Scharfenberger.** 1975. Concentration of antibiotics in renal interstitial fluid. An experimental model. Urol. Res. 3:165-167.
6. **Eykyn, S., C. Jenkins, A. King, and I. Phillips.** 1973. Antibacterial activity of cefamandole, a new cephalosporin antibiotic, compared with that of cephaloridine, cephalothin, and cephalexin. Antimicrob. Agents Chemother. 3:657-661.
7. **Neu, H. C.** 1974. Cefamandole, a cephalosporin antibiotic with an unusually wide spectrum of activity. Antimicrob. Agents Chemother. 6:177-182.
8. **Sabath, L. D., J. I. Casey, P. A. Ruch, L. L. Stumpf, and M. Finland.** 1976. Rapid microassay for circulating nephrotoxic antibiotics. Antimicrob. Agents Chemother. 10:83-90.
9. **Waterman, N. G., and L. B. Kastan.** 1972. Interstitial fluid and serum antibiotic concentrations. Arch. Surg. 105:192-196.
10. **Waterman, N. G., L. Scharfenberger, and M. Raff.** 1974. Rate of binding of antibiotics to canine serum protein. Antimicrob. Agents Chemother. 5:294-295.
11. **Waterman, N. G., M. J. Raff, L. Scharfenberger, and P. A. Barnwell.** 1976. Antibiotic concentrations in hepatic interstitial and wound fluid. Surg. Gynecol. Obstet. 142:235-238.
12. **Waterman, N. G., M. J. Raff, L. Scharfenberger, and P. A. Barnwell.** 1976. Protein binding and concentrations of cephaloridine and cefazolin in serum and interstitial fluid of dogs. J. Infect. Dis. 133:642-647.

ANTIMICROBIAL AGENTS AND CHEMOTHERAPY, Oct. 1976, p. 736-752
Vol. 10, No. 4

Susceptibility of Anaerobic Bacteria to 23 Antimicrobial Agents

VERA L. SUTTER* AND SYDNEY M. FINEGOLD

Research and Medical Services, Veterans Administration Wadsworth Hospital Center, Los Angeles, California 90073, and Department of Medicine, UCLA School of Medicine, Los Angeles, California 90024*

Received for publication 23 June 1976

The antimicrobial susceptibility of 492 anaerobic bacteria, the majority of which were recent clinical isolates, was determined by the agar dilution technique. Penicillin G was active against most of the strains tested at 32 U or less/ml, but only 72% of *Bacteroides fragilis* strains were susceptible at this level and 9% required 256 U or more/ml. Ampicillin was effective against most of the strains except *B. fragilis* at 16 μg or less/ml. Amoxicillin was active against only 31% of *B. fragilis*, 76% of other *Bacteroides* species, and 67% of *Fusobacterium* species at 8 μg/ml. Two new penicillins, mezlocillin and azlocillin, were similar to ampicillin in their activity. Carbenicillin and ticarcillin inhibited all but a few strains at 128 μg or less/ml. BLP 1654 was somewhat more active than penicillin G against *B. fragilis* but had similar activity against other anaerobes. Cephalothin was inactive against *B. fragilis*, and only 65% of other *Bacteroides* species were inhibited by 32 μg or less/ml. It was effective against all other anaerobes at that level. Cefamandole showed somewhat greater activity than cephalothin against *B. fragilis* but generally less activity against gram-positive organisms. Cefazaflur (SKF 59962) was comparable to cephalothin against *B. fragilis*. Cefoxitin was distinctly more active than cephalothin against *B. fragilis*. These latter two agents were less active than cephalothin against the gram-positive anaerobes. Chloramphenicol remains active against anaerobic bacteria at 16 μg or less/ml, with rare exceptions. Thiamphenicol was similar to chloramphenicol in its activity. Clindamycin was very active against most of the anaerobes at 8 μg or less/ml. Erythromycin and josamycin were also tested, with josamycin showing greater activity against *B. fragilis* than either erythromycin or clindamycin. A new oligosaccharide, everninomicin B, was less active than clindamycin against *B. fragilis* but more active against clostridia and some of the other strains tested. Most of the groups of bacteria tested demonstrated a trend toward resistance to tetracycline. Doxycyline and minocycline were somewhat more active than was tetracycline. Metronidazole was active against the majority of the anaerobes tested; resistance ws demonstrated by some of the gram-positive cocci and gram-positive, non-sporeforming bacilli.

It has been generally accepted by investigators and clinicians knowledgeable in the diagnosis and therapy of anaerobic infections that rapid, routine susceptibility testing of individual isolates of anaerobic bacteria is impractical. Anaerobic infections are frequently polymicrobic and cultures require relatively long periods of time for growth and isolation, so that timely results of susceptibility tests are not feasible. It has been suggested that centers with the capability for testing on a survey basis do so periodically to monitor changing patterns of resistance to commonly recommended agents and to determine the possible effectiveness of newer agents.

The purpose of the present study was to assay the in vitro effect of several drugs currently in use for therapy of anaerobic infections and to determine the activity of several newer agents against anaerobic bacteria recently isolated from clinical material.

MATERIALS AND METHODS

Bacterial strains. A total of 492 strains of anaerobic bacteria was used throughout the study. All but a few were isolated from a variety of clinical specimens received by the Wadsworth Anaerobic Bacteriology Research Laboratory from patients on special studies and from patients seen in consultation by the Infectious Disease Section during the period of September 1972 to June 1975. Exceptions were 21 strains of *Bacteroides melaninogenicus*, 5 of which were reference strains and 16 of which were normal oral or fecal isolates. Table 1 gives the specific iden-

TABLE 1. *Identity of bacterial strains tested*

Organism	No. of strains tested in studies		
	Part I	Part II	Total
Bacteroides fragilis[a]	42	34	76
subsp. *distasonis*	8	3	11
subsp. *fragilis*	18	12	30
subsp. *ovatus*	1	2	3
subsp. *thetaiotaomicron*	9	12	21
subsp. *vulgatus*	4	4	8
Other	2	1	3
Bacteroides melaninogenicus	60	11	71
subsp. *asaccharolyticus*	21	1	22
subsp. *intermedius*	29	6	35
subsp. *melaninogenicus*	10	2	12
Other	0	2	2
Other *Bacteroides* and *Selenomonas*	21	51	72
B. capillosus	0	3	3
B. clostridiiformis subsp. *clostridiiformis*[b]	0	2	2
B. clostridiiformis subsp. *girans*[b]	0	1	1
B. corrodens	2	0	2
B. oralis	4	6	10
B. pneumosintes	2	3	5
B. putredinis	1	1	2
B. ruminicola subsp. *ruminicola*	0	1	1
B. ruminicola subsp. *brevis*	1	3	4
B. splanchnicus[c]	1	0	1
Bacteroides group I	0	6	6
Bacteroides group PS	0	8	8
Bacteroides sp.	10	16	26
Selenomonas sp.	0	1	1
Fusobacterium nucleatum	8	10	18
Other *Fusobacterium*	12	4	16
F. gonidiaformans	2	2	4
F. mortiferum	2	0	2
F. naviforme	1	1	2
F. necrophorum	1	0	1
F. russii	1	0	1
Fusobacterium sp.	5	1	6
Peptococcus and *Gaffkya*	17	42	59
P. asaccharolyticus	2	21	23
P. magnus	4	6	10
P. prevotii	6	8	14
P. saccharolyticus	0	2	2
P. variabilis	4	4	8
Peptococcus sp.	1	0	1
Gaffkya anaerobius	0	1	1
Peptostreptococcus	15	14	29
P. anaerobius	9	9	18
P. micros	5	4	9
Peptostreptococcus sp.	1	1	2
Microaerophilic and anaerobic *Streptococcus*	6	4	10
S. constellatus	0	2	2
S. intermedius	4	2	6
S. morbillorum	2	0	2
Gram-negative cocci	7	19	26
Acidaminococcus fermentans	2	1	3
Veillonella alcalescens	2	6	8
V. parvula	3	12	15
Eubacterium	8	9	17
E. aerofaciens	0	1	1
E. contortum	0	1	1
E. lentum	4	4	8
E. limosum	2	0	2
E. moniliforme	1	0	1
Eubacterium sp.	1	3	4
Arachnia propionica	2	1	3
Propionibacterium	4	8	12
P. acnes	4	5	9
P. avidum	0	2	2
Propionibacterium sp.	0	1	1
Actinomyces	16	0	16
A. israelii	1	0	1
A. naeslundii	5	0	5
A. viscosus	1	0	1
Actinomyces sp.	9	0	9
Bifidobacterium	0	5	5
B. adolescentis var. B	0	2	2
B. infantis	0	1	1
Bifidobacterium sp.	0	2	2
Lactobacillus	10	9	19
L. acidophilus	0	2	2
L. catenaforme	2	1	3
L. fermentum	0	1	1
L. minutis	1	2	3
L. plantarum	2	1	3
Lactobacillus sp.	5	2	7
Clostridium perfringens	8	1	9
Other *Clostridium*	27	7	34
C. bifermentans	2	0	2
C. butyricum	1	0	1
C. difficile	2	0	2
C. glycolicum	1	0	1
C. innocuum	5	3	8
C. paraperfringens	1	0	1
C. plagarum	1	0	1
C. putrificum	1	0	1
C. ramosum	7	3	10
C. sphenoides	1	0	1
C sporogenes	0	1	1
C. tertium	1	0	1
Clostridium sp.	4	0	4

[a] It has recently been proposed that organisms recognized as subspecies of *B. fragilis* be reinstated to species rank (7).

[b] Strains having phenotypic characteristics similar to these have recently been found to have spores and to be genetically similar to *Clostridium*. It has been proposed that they be considered as *C. clostridiiformis* (15) or *C. clostridiiforme* (8). Spores have not been demonstrated in the strains in the present study.

[c] A new *Bacteroides* species described by Werner et al. (48).

tification of the bacteria used in each part of the study. These bacteria were identified according to the criteria of the *Wadsworth Anaerobic Bacteriology Manual* (40) and the Virginia Polytechnic Institute *Anaerobe Laboratory Manual* (13). It has recently been proposed that organisms recognized as subspecies of *Bacteroides fragilis* be given species status (7). We are in agreement with this, but since little or no difference has been found in the susceptibility of these organisms to the antimicrobial agents in the present study and in reports of others (2, 14), we will refer to *B. fragilis* as a group including the five species. The subspecies of *B. melaninogenicus* are also referred to as a group, because no differences were observed in their susceptibility to antimicrobial agents. Six strains had the characteristics of *Bacteroides* group 1 and eight strains had the characteristics of *Bacteroides* group PS. These latter two groups have recently been recognized as distinct from other *Bacteroides* species (L. V. Holdeman, personal communication).

Antimicrobial agents. Laboratory-standard powders were kindly supplied as follows: penicillin G, cephalothin, cefamandole lithium, and erythromycin from Eli Lilly & Co., Indianapolis, Ind.; ampicillin trihydrate and BLP 1654 from Bristol Laboratories, Syracuse, N.Y.; carbenicillin from Roerig, New York, N.Y.; amoxicillin trihydrate and ticarcillin sodium from Beecham-Massengill Pharmaceuticals, Bristol, Tenn.; mezlocillin and azlocillin from Delbay Pharmaceuticals, Inc., Bloomfield, N.J.; sodium cefoxitin from Merck, Sharp and Dohme, Rahway, N.J.; cefazaflur (SKF 59962) from Smith, Kline and French Laboratories, Philadelphia, Pa.; chloramphenicol from Parke-Davis & Co., Detroit, Mich.; thiamphenicol and thiamphenicol glycinate from Zambon, S.p.A., Bresso, Milano, Italy; clindamycin from The Upjohn Co., Kalamazoo, Mich.; everninomicin B from Schering Corp., Bloomfield, N.J.; josamycin from E. I. Dupont de Nemours & Co., Newark, Del.; tetracycline and doxycycline from Pfizer Laboratories, New York, N.Y.; minocycline from Lederle Laboratories, Pearl River, N.Y.; and metronidazole from G. D. Searle & Co., Chicago, Ill.

Procedures. Antimicrobial susceptibility testing was performed by the agar dilution technique as previously described (40). Sets of three laked blood agar plates containing no antibiotic were inoculated before each series of antibiotic-containing plates and incubated anaerobically, in 10% CO_2 in air, and aerobically, to serve as growth and contamination controls. Data were deleted if poor or no growth occurred on the anaerobic growth control plate or if contamination was evident.

Throughout the study, the following antimicrobial agents were included: penicillin G, carbenicillin, BLP 1654, chloramphenicol, clindamycin, tetracycline, doxycycline, minocycline, and metronidazole. During the first part of the study, amoxicillin, ticarcillin, cefoxitin, cefazaflur, thiamphenicol, thiamphenicol glycinate, and everninomicin B were included to determine their possible effectiveness against anaerobes or for comparison of their activity with other drugs. During the second part of the study, the following agents were included: ampicillin, mezlocillin, azlocillin, cephalothin, cefamandole, erythromycin, and josamycin.

RESULTS AND DISCUSSION

Penicillins. The activity of penicillin G against the anaerobes tested is shown in Table 2. An inhibitory concentration of 32 U/ml is considered an acceptable level of susceptibility

TABLE 2. *Activity of penicillin G against anaerobic bacteria*

Bacteria	No. of strains tested	Cumulative % susceptible to indicated concn (U/ml)										
		≤0.1	0.5	1.0	2.0	4.0	8.0	16.0	32.0	64.0	128.0	≥256
Bacteroides fragilis[a]	76	1	3		5	7	13	42	72	91		100
Bacteroides melaninogenicus	66	68	79	83	86	89	94	97	100			
Other *Bacteroides* and *Selenomonas*	72	24	49	51	56	63	71	75	82	93	96	100
Fusobacterium nucleatum	18	72	83	94		100						
Other *Fusobacterium*	16	50	75		88						94	100
Peptococcus and *Gaffkya*	59	49	100									
Peptostreptococcus	29	55	86	90			97		100			
Anaerobic and microaerophilic streptococci	10	50	90					100				
Gram-negative cocci	26	15	69	85	89	92	100					
Eubacterium	17	18	47	59	77	94	100					
Arachnia propionica	3		67	100								
Propionibacterium	12	75	92		100							
Actinomyces	16	69	100									
Bifidobacterium	5	20	100									
Lactobacillus	18	28	89		100							
Clostridium perfringens	9	33	100									
Other *Clostridium*	34	3	53	71	82	97	100					

[a] Includes all strains identified as subspecies of *B. fragilis*.

if a high parenteral dosage is given. Most of the bacteria were inhibited by this concentration or less. However, only 72% of *B. fragilis* strains, 82% of *Bacteroides* species other than *B. fragilis* and *B. melaninogenicus*, and 88% of *Fusobacterium* species other than *Fusobacterium nucleatum* were inhibited by 32 U/ml. Nine percent, or seven of the strains in the *B. fragilis* group (six *B. fragilis* and one *Bacteroides vulgatus*), 4% or three strains of other *Bacteroides* species, and one *Fusobacterium* species required 256 U or more/ml for inhibition. The *B. fragilis* strains included in this study appear to have about the same susceptibility as those tested in a prior study in which strains had been isolated from a variety of sources, including human feces, over a period of several years (39). There was no difference in susceptibility of strains tested in the two parts of the study, with approximately equal proportions of the resistant strains appearing in each segment. The present results with *B. fragilis* and other anaerobes tested are also similar to those reported by others (2, 14, 16, 21, 34, 43, 51), and greater resistance to penicillin does not appear to be emerging.

The activity of ampicillin against the strains tested in the second part of the study is shown in Table 3. With parenteral dosage, levels of at least 16 μg/ml are achievable. Ampicillin inhibited most of the anaerobes tested at concentrations of 16 μg or less/ml but was effective against only 56% of *B. fragilis* strains at this level. The results with *B. fragilis* are similar to those reported by Kislak (16) and overall results show higher minimum inhibitory concentrations (MICs) than those reported by Rotilie et al. (32), who used a microdilution technique for determination of susceptibility.

Amoxicillin, an oral, broad-spectrum penicillin, achieves serum levels of up to 8 μg/ml (24). The activity of this antibiotic against anaerobes was determined during the first part of the study. Amoxicillin was active against many of the strains tested (Table 4), but only 31% of *B. fragilis*, 76% of other *Bacteroides* species, and 67% of *Fusobacterium* species were inhibited by 8 μg or less/ml. One strain each of *Peptostreptococcus anaerobius* and *Streptococcus intermedius* required 16 μg/ml and one strain of *Clostridium perfringens* required 32 μg/ml for inhibition. These studies would indicate that amoxicillin would be less useful in serious anaerobic infections than either penicillin G or ampicillin.

In the second part of the study two new semisynthetic acylureido penicillins, mezlocillin and azlocillin, were tested. Results are shown in Tables 5 and 6. These compounds have similar in vitro effectiveness against the anaerobes tested and, on the basis of weight, are similar to ampicillin in their activity. Pharmacological data on these two compounds are not yet available.

The susceptibility of anaerobes to carbenicillin was tested throughout the study, and results are shown in Table 7. Carbenicillin inhibited all anaerobes tested at a level of 128 μg/

TABLE 3. *Activity of ampicillin against anaerobic bacteria*

Bacteria	No. of strains tested	Cumulative % susceptible to indicated concn (μg/ml)										
		≤0.1	0.5	1.0	2.0	4.0	8.0	16.0	32.0	64.0	128.0	≥256
Bacteroides fragilis[a]	34					6	15	56	82	91		100
Bacteroides melaninogenicus	9	22	67		78	100						
Other *Bacteroides* and *Selenomonas*	50	26	44	48	54	60	72	92	94	98		100
Fusobacterium nucleatum	10	70	80					90	100			
Other *Fusobacterium*	4	25	50				75					100
Peptococcus and *Gaffkya*	41	39	93	100								
Peptostreptococcus	13	23	85				92	100				
Anaerobic and microaerophilic streptococci	4	25	100									
Gram-negative cocci	19	16	79		90	95						100
Eubacterium	9	22	67	78	100							
Arachnia propionica	1			100								
Propionibacterium	7	29	100									
Bifidobacterium	5		100									
Lactobacillus	8	13	75	88					100			
Clostridium perfringens	1	100										
Other *Clostridium*	7	14	71	86	100							

[a] Includes all strains identified as subspecies of *B. fragilis*.

TABLE 4. *Activity of amoxicillin against anaerobic bacteria*

Bacteria	No. of strains tested	Cumulative % susceptible to indicated concn (μg/ml)										
		≤0.1	0.5	1.0	2.0	4.0	8.0	16.0	32.0	64.0	128.0	≥256
Bacteroides fragilis[a]	42	2	5	10	17	26	31	52	83	91	93	100
Bacteroides melaninogenicus	59	71	83	86	90	95	100					
Other *Bacteroides* and *Selenomonas*	21	43	57	62	67	76		86		95	100	
Fusobacterium nucleatum	8	63	88		100							
Other *Fusobacterium*	12	42	67					75		83	92	100
Peptococcus and *Gaffkya*	19	42	90	95	100							
Peptostreptococcus	15	53	87	93				100				
Anaerobic and microaerophilic streptococci	6	67	83					100				
Gram-negative cocci	7	57	86				100					
Eubacterium	7	57	100									
Arachnia propionica	2		100									
Propionibacterium	4	25	75	100								
Actinomyces	16	63	100									
Lactobacillus	10	60	90		100							
Clostridium perfringens	8	75	88						100			
Other *Clostridium*	26	8	77	92	96		100					

[a] Includes all strains identified as subspecies of *B. fragilis*.

TABLE 5. *Activity of mezlocillin against anaerobic bacteria*

Bacteria	No. of strains tested	Cumulative % susceptible to indicated concn (μg/ml)											
		≤0.1	0.5	1.0	2.0	4.0	8.0	16.0	32.0	64.0	128.0	256.0	≥512
Bacteroides fragilis[a]	34						6	27	62	82	91		100
Bacteroides melaninogenicus	9		67		78	89		100					
Other *Bacteroides* and *Selenomonas*	50	10	28	40	50	62	80	88	94	98			100
Fusobacterium nucleatum	10	60	90								100		
Other *Fusobacterium*	4	25	50	75			100						
Peptococcus and *Gaffkya*	42	48	95		100								
Peptostreptococcus	13		70		77	85		100					
Anaerobic and microaerophilic streptococci	4	50	75	100									
Gram-negative cocci	19			11	26	47	68	74	84			90	100
Eubacterium	9		22	44	78				100				
Arachnia propionica	1					100							
Propionibacterium	7	29	86	100									
Bifidobacterium	5	20	80	100									
Lactobacillus	8	13	63	88			100						
Clostridium perfringens	1		100										
Other *Clostridium*	7		29	43	86	100							

[a] Includes all strains identified as subspecies of *B. fragilis*.

ml, with the exception of four strains of *B. fragilis*, a *Bacteroides* species, a *Bacteroides corrodens*, a *Bacteroides clostridiiformis* subsp. *clostridiiformis*, and a *Fusobacterium* species. The MICs of strains in the present study are similar to those of our previous studies (36) and to those of Kislak (16), Staneck and Washington (34), and Zabransky and co-workers (51) but are appreciably lower than those of Blazevic and Matsen (3) and Tally et al. (43). Both of the latter studies utilized prereduced media containing cysteine in determining susceptibility; this might account for some loss of carbenicillin activity.

The activity of ticarcillin against the strains tested in the second part of the study is shown

TABLE 6. *Activity of azlocillin against anaerobic bacteria*

Bacteria	No. of strains tested	Cumulative % susceptible to indicated concn (μg/ml)											
		≤0.1	0.5	1.0	2.0	4.0	8.0	16.0	32.0	64.0	128.0	256.0	≥512
Bacteroides fragilis[a]	34						6	32	65	91		97	100
Bacteroides melaninogenicus	9	11	56		67	89	100						
Other *Bacteroides* and *Selenomonas*	50	12	38	42	50	54	70	80	88	94	98		100
Fusobacterium nucleatum	10	60	90							100			
Other *Fusobacterium*	4	25	50		75	100							
Peptococcus and *Gaffkya*	42	33	95	100									
Peptostreptococcus	13		69	77	85				100				
Anaerobic and microaerophilic streptococci	4	25	100										
Gram-negative cocci	19			5	37	63	79	84			95		100
Eubacterium	9	11	33	44	78				100				
Arachnia propionica	1					100							
Propionibacterium	7	29	100										
Bifidobacterium	5		80	100									
Lactobacillus	8		63	88		100							
Clostridium perfringens	1	100											
Other *Clostridium*	7		57	86	100								

[a] Includes all strains identified as subspecies of *B. fragilis*.

TABLE 7. *Activity of carbenicillin against anaerobic bacteria*

Bacteria	No. of strains tested	Cumulative % susceptible to indicated concn (μg/ml)											
		≤0.1	0.5	1.0	2.0	4.0	8.0	16.0	32.0	64.0	128.0	256.0	≥512
Bacteroides fragilis[a]	76	1	3	5	8	21	25	38	47	80	95		100
Bacteroides melaninogenicus	67	42	85	90	94	97	100						
Other *Bacteroides* and *Selenomonas*	72	7	47	53	68	76	81	88	92	96			100
Fusobacterium nucleatum	18	39	83			94	100						
Other *Fusobacterium*	16	25	44	50	81	88		94					100
Peptococcus and *Gaffkya*	59	25	73	88	98	100							
Peptostreptococcus	29	10	45	69	83	90		93		97	100		
Anaerobic and microaerophilic streptococci	10	20	40	50	80	90					100		
Gram-negative cocci	26		23	42	65	81	89	92	96		100		
Eubacterium	17	12	18	24	47	53	65	88	100				
Arachnia propionica	3				67		100						
Propionibacterium	12	17	83	92					100				
Actinomyces	16	69	100										
Bifidobacterium	5	20		40	60	100							
Lactobacillus	18	17	33	50	89	94		100					
Clostridium perfringens	9		100										
Other *Clostridium*	33		9	21	36	49	61	76	94	100			

[a] Includes all strains identified as subspecies of *B. fragilis*.

in Table 8. With high parenteral dosage schedules, blood levels of ticarcillin are similar to those of carbenicillin (26). The in vitro activity against anaerobes is also quite similar. It was effective against all strains tested at 128 μg or less/ml, with the exception of two strains of *B. fragilis* and one strain each of *Fusobacterium* species and *Fusobacterium gonidiaformans*.

Table 9 indicates the activity of BLP 1654 against the anaerobic bacteria tested throughout the study. Organisms with MICs of 32 μg or less/ml are considered susceptible to this agent (4). Unfortunately, because of its nephrotoxicity, further evaluation of BLP 1654 has been discontinued.

Cephalosporins and similar drugs. The susceptibility of the anaerobic bacteria from the second part of the study to cephalothin is shown in Table 10. All strains of *B. fragilis* were resistant to cephalothin, requiring at least 64 μg/ml for inhibition. Only 65% of other *Bacteroides* species were inhibited by 32 μg/ml. Previous studies indicated 6 to 11% of *B. fragilis* and all strains of other *Bacteroides* species to be inhibited by this concentration (36, 42). All other groups tested in the present study were inhibited by 32 μg or less/ml. Most of the gram-positive anaerobes were inhibited by 8 μg or

TABLE 8. *Activity of ticarcillin against anaerobic bacteria*

Bacteria	No. of strains tested	Cumulative % susceptible to indicated concn (μg/ml)										
		≤0.1	0.5	1.0	2.0	4.0	8.0	16.0	32.0	64.0	128.0	≥256
Bacteroides fragilis[a]	42	2		5	12	14	24	33	50	76	95	100
Bacteroides melaninogenicus	59	41	85	87	90	95	98	100				
Other *Bacteroides* and *Selenomonas*	21	24	48	62	67	71		86	95		100	
Fusobacterium nucleatum	8	38	88			100						
Other *Fusobacterium*	12	25	42	50	58	67	75	83				100
Peptococcus and *Gaffkya*	15	20	60	93	100							
Peptostreptococcus	15	13	53	80	93						100	
Anaerobic and microaerophilic streptococci	6		50			83			100			
Gram-negative cocci	7			29	57	71	86		100			
Eubacterium	7		14	29	43		57	86	100			
Arachnia propionica	2			50	100							
Propionibacterium	4		75						100			
Actinomyces	16	13	81	100								
Lactobacillus	10	10	60	70		80	90	100				
Clostridium perfringens	8		88	100								
Other *Clostridium*	26		8	15	31	54		85	96	100		

[a] Includes all strains identified as subspecies of *B. fragilis*.

TABLE 9. *Activity of BLP 1654 against anaerobic bacteria*

Bacteria	No. of strains tested	Cumulative % susceptible to indicated concn (μg/ml)										
		≤0.1	0.5	1.0	2.0	4.0	8.0	16.0	32.0	64.0	128.0	≥256
Bacteroides fragilis[a]	76	1	3	4	5	8	32	63	90	91	93	100
Bacteroides melaninogenicus	68	50	81	85	87	93	99	100				
Other *Bacteroides* and *Selenomonas*	70	20	46	51	53	56	64	79	93	94	96	100
Fusobacterium nucleatum	18	72	78		83		89		100			
Other *Fusobacterium*	16	31	56			81				88		100
Peptococcus and *Gaffkya*	59	39	95	100								
Peptostreptococcus	28	54	89		93		96	100				
Anaerobic and microaerophilic streptococci	10	30	70	90				100				
Gram-negative cocci	26	8	39	58	73	89			92	96		100
Eubacterium	16	19	50	63	75		100					
Arachnia propionica	3		67		100							
Propionibacterium	11	46	91				100					
Actinomyces	16	25	100									
Bifidobacterium	5		100									
Lactobacillus	18	39	83	94					100			
Clostridium perfringens	9	22	100									
Other *Clostridium*	33		33	70	82	94	100					

[a] Includes all strains identified as subspecies of *B. fragilis*.

TABLE 10. *Activity of cephalothin against anaerobic bacteria*

Bacteria	No. of strains tested	Cumulative % susceptible to indicated concn (μg/ml)											
		≤0.1	0.5	1.0	2.0	4.0	8.0	16.0	32.0	64.0	128.0	256.0	≥512
Bacteroides fragilis[a]	34									15	50	53	100
Bacteroides melaninogenicus	9	44	56			67		78	100				
Other *Bacteroides* and *Selenomonas*	51	2	24	39	41	43	45	51	65	78	92	100	
Fusobacterium nucleatum	10	60	90	100									
Other *Fusobacterium*	4	50	100										
Peptococcus and *Gaffkya*	42	14	74	95	98		100						
Peptostreptococcus	14	14	79		93		100						
Anaerobic and microaerophilic streptococci	4	25	100										
Gram-negative cocci	19		68	84	90	100							
Eubacterium	9	11	33	44	67				100				
Arachnia propionica	1				100								
Propionibacterium	8		88	100									
Bifidobacterium	5		20		40	60	100						
Lactobacillus	8	13	100										
Clostridium perfringens	1			100									
Other *Clostridium*	7		14			29	100						

[a] Includes all strains identified as subspecies of *B. fragilis*.

less/ml. These data are in agreement with those of our earlier study, except that resistant clostridia have not been found as yet.

The activity of cefamandole (7-D-mandelamido-3-[1-methyl-1H-tetrazol-5-ylthiomethyl]-3-cephem-4-carboxylic acid) was compared with that of cephalothin. Cefamandole is a new cephalosporin which has been shown to have a broad spectrum of activity against facultative bacteria (5, 22, 25). It has been shown to be resistant to penicillinase and cephalosporinases derived from facultative bacteria (25, 49). The results of the studies on the activity of cefamandole are shown in Table 11. Since cefamandole is resistant to β-lactamases, the strains of *B. fragilis* tested were more resistant to this agent than would be expected, with only 9% of the strains susceptible to 32 μg/ml. *B. fragilis* β-lactamases have been shown to be different from those produced by *Enterobacteriaceae* (29). It is possible that cefamandole is not resistant to the cephalosporinase produced by these strains. Our results with *B. fragilis* are in disagreement with those recently published by Ernst et al. (12), who found that 57% of their strains were inhibited by 32 μg of cefamandole per ml. This discrepancy could be due to an inoculum effect, since our inoculum is at least 10-fold greater than that used by Ernst and co-workers, or it could be due to carryover of a larger amount of cephalosporinase with the inoculum. The studies of Olsson and co-workers (29) showed that the amount of β-lactamase produced by their strains of *B. fragilis* was medium dependent, and it is possible that greater amounts of the enzyme are produced in the thioglycolate medium used in our studies. Further investigation is necessary to determine the significance of this phenomenon. Cefamandole was more active against *B. melaninogenicus* and other *Bacteroides* species than was cephalothin, had similar activity against *Fusobacterium* species, and was less active against the gram-positive anaerobes. Prior studies with cefazolin indicated that it may be slightly more active than cefamandole against *B. fragilis*, the anaerobic cocci, and clostridia (36).

The activities of cefazaflur (7-trifluoromethylthioacetamido-3-[1-methyl-1H-tetrazol-5-ylthiomethyl]-3-cephem-4-carboxylic acid) and sodium cefoxitin were compared. Cefoxitin is a cephamycin, a class of compounds closely related to the cephalosporins. Results are shown in Tables 12 and 13. Cefazaflur was less active than cefoxitin against *B. fragilis* and other gram-negative anaerobes, was similar in activity against gram-positive, non-sporeforming anaerobes, and was somewhat more active against *Clostridium* species other than *C. perfringens*. Pharmacological studies with animals indicate that serum levels with cefazaflur are similar to those obtained with cephalothin

TABLE 11. *Activity of cefamandole against anaerobic bacteria*

Bacteria	No. of strains tested	Cumulative % susceptible to indicated concn (μg/ml)											
		≤0.1	0.5	1.0	2.0	4.0	8.0	16.0	32.0	64.0	128.0	256.0	≥512
Bacteroides fragilis[a]	34								9	29	56	71	100
Bacteroides melaninogenicus	9	11	56	67		89	100						
Other *Bacteroides* and *Selenomonas*	51	8	24	35	51	55	67	76	90	94	98	100	
Fusobacterium nucleatum	10	80	100										
Other *Fusobacterium*	4	75	100										
Peptococcus and *Gaffkya*	42	17	57	83	88	93	98			100			
Peptostreptococcus	14	7	71	79			86	93	100				
Anaerobic and microaerophilic streptococci	4	25	100										
Gram-negative cocci	19	11		84	95			100					
Eubacterium	9	11	56	78				89	100				
Arachnia propionica	1				100								
Propionibacterium	8	13	100										
Bifidobacterium	5	20	60		100								
Lactobacillus	8	13	75	88		100							
Clostridium perfringens	1				100								
Other *Clostridium*	7		14		57	71	86				100		

[a] Includes all strains identified as subspecies of *B. fragilis*.

TABLE 12. *Activity of cefazaflur against anaerobic bacteria*

Bacteria	No. of strains tested	Cumulative % susceptible to indicated concn (μg/ml)										
		≤0.1	0.5	1.0	2.0	4.0	8.0	16.0	32.0	64.0	128.0	≥256
Bacteroides fragilis[a]	41	2			5				10	12	42	100
Bacteroides melaninogenicus	59	46	81	85	88		93	95	98	100		
Other *Bacteroides* and *Selenomonas*	21	14	43		52	62	67		76	86	91	100
Fusobacterium nucleatum	8	75	100									
Other *Fusobacterium*	12	25	42	50			58		67		75	100
Peptococcus and *Gaffkya*	17	24	94	100								
Peptostreptococcus	15	27	87		93		100					
Anaerobic and microaerophilic streptococci	6	17	67	83								100
Gram-negative cocci	7		86						100			
Eubacterium	7	14	43				57	71	86	100		
Arachnia propionica	2		100									
Propionibacterium	4		75							100		
Actinomyces	16	31	100									
Lactobacillus	10	50	80				90			100		
Clostridium perfringens	8			38		50	88			100		
Other *Clostridium*	26	4	8	15	23	65	73	85	92	100		

[a] Includes all strains identified as subspecies of *B. fragilis*.

(1); therefore, organisms with MICs of 64 μg or more/ml would be considered resistant. Results with cefoxitin against the anaerobes indicate that the majority of strains are inhibited at an achievable level of 32 μg/ml. However, some of the groups of bacteria appear to be more resistant than those reported in a previous study (36). At that time, all *B. fragilis* strains were inhibited by 32 μg/ml, whereas only 85% of recent isolates are susceptible to that level.

Nonetheless, cefoxitin is distinctly more active than any of the cephalosporins against *B. fragilis*. Other *Fusobacterium* species, gram-positive cocci, and gram-positive, non-sporeforming bacilli also are demonstrating higher inhibitory end points. The *B. fragilis* strains in the current study appear to be less susceptible to cefoxitin than those reported by others (6, 28, 42), but the remainder of anaerobes other than *Clostridium* species appear slightly more susceptible than those reported by Tally et al. (42).

Chloramphenicol. The activity of chloramphenicol against the anaerobes tested is shown in Table 14. A level of 16 μg/ml is readily achievable, and all but two of the bacteria were inhibited at this concentration. Only one strain in the *B. fragilis* group (*B. fragilis* subsp. *thetaiotaomicron* or *Bacteroides thetaiotaomicron*)

TABLE 13. *Activity of sodium cefoxitin against anaerobic bacteria*

Bacteria	No. of strains tested	Cumulative % susceptible to indicated concn (μg/ml)										
		≤0.1	0.5	1.0	2.0	4.0	8.0	16.0	32.0	64.0	128.0	≥256
Bacteroides fragilis[a]	40		3	5	8	15	40	65	85	98		100
Bacteroides melaninogenicus	55	20	89	93	98		100					
Other *Bacteroides* and *Selenomonas*	21		43	48	62	71	81		86		91	100
Fusobacterium nucleatum	8	25	75		88	100						
Other *Fusobacterium*	12	8	33	42	50		75	83				100
Peptococcus and *Gaffkya*	17	29	82	88	94			100				
Peptostreptococcus	15		60	73	87	93		100				
Anaerobic and microaerophilic streptococci	6		33	50	83			100				
Gram-negative cocci	7	14	43	100								
Eubacterium	7		14	43	57	71	86		100			
Arachnia propionica	2			100								
Propionibacterium	4		75					100				
Actinomyces	16	38	88	94	100							
Lactobacillus	10		40		60	70	80	90				100
Clostridium perfringens	8		13	50	75			100				
Other *Clostridium*	26		4		19	46	54	58	62	77	100	

[a] Includes all strains identified as subspecies of *B. fragilis*.

TABLE 14. *Activity of chloramphenicol against anaerobic bacteria*

Bacteria	No. of strains tested	Cumulative % susceptible to indicated concn (μg/ml)									
		≤0.1	0.5	1.0	2.0	4.0	8.0	16.0	32.0	64.0	128.0
Bacteroides fragilis[a]	76		1		5	30	86	99	100		
Bacteroides melaninogenicus	68	10	25	56	91	100					
Other *Bacteroides* and *Selenomonas*	72	1	8	38	65	86	96	99			100
Fusobacterium nucleatum	18		72	94	100						
Other *Fusobacterium*	16		50	88	100						
Peptococcus and *Gaffkya*	59	2	3	42	88	98	100				
Peptostreptococcus	29	3	21	66	97		100				
Anaerobic and microaerophilic streptococci	10				40	80	100				
Gram-negative cocci	25		32	68	96	100					
Eubacterium	17		6	24	65	100					
Arachnia propionica	3			33	67	100					
Propionibacterium	12		50	75	92		100				
Actinomyces	16		19	81	88	94	100				
Bifidobacterium	5		20		60	100					
Lactobacillus	18		17	44	83	94		100			
Clostridium perfringens	9				22	100					
Other *Clostridium*	34		3	6	27	68	91	100			

[a] Includes all strains identified as subspecies of *B. fragilis*.

required 32 μg/ml for inhibition, and one strain of *B. clostridiiformis* subsp. *clostridiiformis* was inhibited by 128 μg/ml. These results are similar to previous reports from this laboratory and to those of others (2, 16, 18, 21, 32, 33, 39, 41, 46, 51).

Thiamphenicol, an analogue of chloramphenicol, with substitution of the *p*-nitro group by a methylsulfonyl moiety, and its parenteral form, thiamphenicol glycinate, were tested during the first part of this study. These compounds produce serum levels equivalent to those of chloramphenicol and have been found to produce less serious side effects than does chloramphenicol (46). Results obtained with thiamphenicol are given in Table 15. Thiamphenicol glycinate was equivalent to thiamphenicol in activity. Thiamphenicol was similar in activity to chloramphenicol, with most of the strains tested inhibited by 16 μg or less/ml. The organisms that required 32 μg or more/ml for inhibition were one strain each of *Bacteroides* species, *B. corrodens*, *Lactobacillus plantarum*, and *Clostridium difficile*.

Macrolides and similar drugs. Clindamycin was very active against most of the anaerobes at 8 μg or less/ml (Table 16). All *B. fragilis* strains were inhibited at this level. Strains that required 16 μg or more/ml for inhibition were three of the *Bacteroides* species, nine of the *Peptococcus* species, a *Lactobacillus catenaforme*, and four of the *Clostridium* species.

For most of the groups of anaerobes tested, results are in agreement with previously published studies (2, 17, 18, 21, 32–34, 39, 41, 47, 50, 51). With regard to resistance among the *Peptococcus*, it was not observed by Werner and Böhm (47) but was observed by Martin et al. (21) and in our own earlier studies (18). This may be an important consideration in anaerobic pleuropulmonary infections and in certain other anaerobic infections where clindamycin may be recommended when penicillin cannot be used. Resistance among *Clostridium* species other than *C. perfringens* has been noted previously (34, 41, 50). However, despite the widespread use of this compound over the past few years, resistance does not appear to be emerging among anaerobes previously susceptible to it.

The activity of erythromycin against the anaerobes tested in the second part of the study is indicated in Table 17. These results show that the *B. fragilis* strains, and the anaerobic and microaerophilic streptococci, showed more resistance to erythromycin, whereas the fusobacteria and *Clostridium* species were more susceptible than strains used in the first part of the study. These results were the subject of a previous publication (37). These disparities were not observed with clindamycin in the two parts of the study. Erythromycin was much less active than clindamycin against *B. fragilis*, the fusobacteria, and the gram-negative cocci. It showed greater activity against the anaerobic streptococci and clostridia and had similar activity against the remainder of the strains tested.

Josamycin, a macrolide structurally similar to erythromycin and with similar in vitro activity against facultative bacteria, does not induce

TABLE 15. *Activity of thiamphenicol against anaerobic bacteria*

Bacteria	No. of strains tested	Cumulative % susceptible to indicated concn (μg/ml)									
		≤0.1	0.5	1.0	2.0	4.0	8.0	16.0	32.0	64.0	128.0
Bacteroides fragilis[a]	42				5	21	71	100			
Bacteroides melaninogenicus	59	9	24	51	90	100					
Other *Bacteroides* and *Selenomonas*	21		19	24	57	76	86	91	95		100
Fusobacterium nucleatum	8		100								
Other *Fusobacterium*	12		42	92	100						
Peptococcus and *Gaffkya*	17			35	71	100					
Peptostreptococcus	15		33	47	93	100					
Anaerobic and microaerophilic streptococci	6				50	83		100			
Gram-negative cocci	7		43	86	100						
Eubacterium	7				43	57	100				
Arachnia propionica	2			50	100						
Propionibacterium	4		50	75			100				
Actinomyces	16		25	56	94			100			
Lactobacillus	10		10	30	50	90			100		
Clostridium perfringens	8					100					
Other *Clostridium*	27			4	22	63	78	96		100	

[a] Includes all strains identified as subspecies of *B. fragilis*.

TABLE 16. *Activity of clindamycin against anaerobic bacteria*

Bacteria	No. of strains tested	Cumulative % susceptible to indicated concn (μg/ml)										
		≤0.1	0.5	1.0	2.0	4.0	8.0	16.0	32.0	64.0	128.0	≥256
Bacteroides fragilis[a]	76	17	46	67	84	96	100					
Bacteroides melaninogenicus	64	97	100									
Other *Bacteroides* and *Selenomonas*	72	76	90	93	94		96	99				100
Fusobacterium nucleatum	18	94	100									
Other *Fusobacterium*	16	81	100									
Peptococcus and *Gaffkya*	59	41	76	80	81	83				86	93	100
Peptostreptococcus	29	52	97	100								
Anaerobic and microaerophilic streptococci	10	40	70	80	90		100					
Gram-negative cocci	25	88	100									
Eubacterium	17	41	77	88	100							
Arachnia propionica	3	33	100									
Propionibacterium	12	67	100									
Actinomyces	16	56	100									
Bifidobacterium	5	80		100								
Lactobacillus	18	56	83	89		94				100		
Clostridium perfringens	9	33	57	89	100							
Other *Clostridium*	34	9	41	53	62	79	88	91				100

[a] Includes all strains identified as subspecies of *B. fragilis*.

TABLE 17. *Activity of erythromycin against anaerobic bacteria*

Bacteria	No. of strains tested	Cumulative % susceptible to indicated concn (μg/ml)										
		≤0.1	0.5	1.0	2.0	4.0	8.0	16.0	32.0	64.0	128.0	≥256
Bacteroides fragilis[a]	34	3	6	15	24	47	71	88	94	100		
Bacteroides melaninogenicus	9	44	89	100								
Other *Bacteroides* and *Selenomonas*	51	10	45	78	86	96		98				100
Fusobacterium nucleatum	10					30	70	90		100		
Other *Fusobacterium*	4				25	50	75		100			
Peptococcus and *Gaffkya*	42		5	36	71	83						100
Peptostreptococcus	13	77	85	92	100							
Anaerobic and microaerophilic streptococci	4		100									
Gram-negative cocci	19		5	32	58	79	90	100				
Eubacterium	9	44	100									
Arachnia propionica	1			100								
Propionibacterium	8	88		100								
Bifidobacterium	5	60	100									
Lactobacillus	8	63	88									100
Clostridium perfringens	1			100								
Other *Clostridium*	7	14	71	100								

[a] Includes all strains identified as subspecies of *B. fragilis*.

macrolide resistance among staphylococci (30). It has been shown to be active against *B. fragilis* and other anaerobic bacteria (17, 20, 27, 35). The susceptibility of the anaerobes from the second part of the study is given in Table 18. On a weight basis, josamycin was more active than erythromycin or clindamycin against *B. fragilis* and showed activity similar to that of erythromycin with the remainder of the anaerobes. It, like erythromycin, was more active than clindamycin against the clostridia but was less active than clindamycin against the fusobacteria. It appears to be as active as rosamicin against *B. fragilis* (37) and other anaerobes. However, a direct comparison with the same strains was not made.

A new oligosaccharide, everninomicin B, was tested and the results are shown in Table 19. Pharmacological data are not yet available, but on a weight basis everninomicin is less active

TABLE 18. *Activity of josamycin against anaerobic bacteria*

Bacteria	No. of strains tested	Cumulative % susceptible to indicated concn (μg/ml)										
		≤0.1	0.5	1.0	2.0	4.0	8.0	16.0	32.0	64.0	128.0	≥256
Bacteroides fragilis[a]	34		29	53	77	100						
Bacteroides melaninogenicus	9	56	100									
Other *Bacteroides* and *Selenomonas*	51	12	90	92	98							100
Fusobacterium nucleatum	10					30	80	100				
Other *Fusobacterium*	4				25			50	75	100		
Peptococcus and *Gaffkya*	44		43	82	84		87		93	98	100	
Peptostreptococcus	13	31	85	92								100
Anaerobic and microaerophilic streptococci	4		50	75	100							
Gram-negative cocci	19		5	32	42	68	84	95			100	
Eubacterium	9	33	78	100								
Arachnia propionica	1			100								
Propionibacterium	8	38	100									
Bifidobacterium	5		100									
Lactobacillus	8	38	75	88					100			
Clostridium perfringens	1				100							
Other *Clostridium*	7	14	71	100								

[a] Includes all strains identified as subspecies of *B. fragilis*.

TABLE 19. *Activity of everninomicin B against anaerobic bacteria*

Bacteria	No. of strains tested	Cumulative % susceptible to indicated concn (μg/ml)										
		≤0.1	0.5	1.0	2.0	4.0	8.0	16.0	32.0	64.0	128.0	≥256
Bacteroides fragilis[a]	36			3	6	14	25	42	69	94	97	100
Bacteroides melaninogenicus	58	9	64	78	85	97	100					
Other *Bacteroides* and *Selenomonas*	20			15	40	45	55	65	70	95	100	
Fusobacterium nucleatum	8						50	88		100		
Other *Fusobacterium*	10							40	50			100
Peptococcus and *Gaffkya*	13	69	92									100
Peptostreptococcus	12	50	100									
Anaerobic and microaerophilic streptococci	5	80	100									
Gram-negative cocci	6						33	67	83	100		
Eubacterium	7	43	86	100								
Arachnia propionica	2										50	100
Propionibacterium	4		25									100
Actinomyces	16	69	94	100								
Lactobacillus	7	86	100									
Clostridium perfringens	7	43	71		86	100						
Other *Clostridium*	23	13	83	91	100							

[a] Includes all strains identified as subspecies of *B. fragilis*.

than clindamycin against *B. fragilis* and other gram-negative anaerobes and more active against the clostridia, including strains resistant to clindamycin. It was also more active than was clindamycin against gram-positive, non-sporeforming bacteria, with the exception of the few strains of *Arachnia*, *Propionibacterium*, and *Actinomyces* tested.

Tetracyclines. The activities of tetracycline, doxycycline, and minocycline were determined throughout the study. Results are shown in Tables 20 through 22. Only 42% of strains in the *B. fragilis* group remain susceptible to tetracycline at 4 μg or less/ml and 46% at 8 μg or less/ml. Other groups of anaerobes also exhibited less suceptibility to tetracycline than in prior reports (16, 33, 38). The current results are similar to other recently published data (2, 9, 21, 32, 41, 51). Doxycycline remains more active than tetracycline against anaerobes but is

TABLE 20. *Activity of tetracycline against anaerobic bacteria*

Bacteria	No. of strains tested	Cumulative % susceptible to indicated concn (μg/ml)									
		≤0.1	0.5	1.0	2.0	4.0	8.0	16.0	32.0	64.0	128.0
Bacteroides fragilis[a]	76		25	40		42	46	68	93	99	100
Bacteroides melaninogenicus	67	51	75	76	79	87	94	96	99	100	
Other *Bacteroides* and *Selenomonas*	72	8	33	35	43	50	60	75	93	99	100
Fusobacterium nucleatum	18	33	100								
Other *Fusobacterium*	16	19	88	94				100			
Peptococcus and *Gaffkya*	59	2	25	29	36		37	61	92	100	
Peptostreptococcus	29	28	38	41	48	52	72	86	97	100	
Anaerobic and microaerophilic streptococci	10		50	60	70	90			100		
Gram-negative cocci	26	8	54	69	73			85	92	100	
Eubacterium	17	6	24	59	65		77	82	94	100	
Arachnia propionica	3		67							100	
Propionibacterium	12		58	75	83				100		
Actinomyces	16		56	69	94			100			
Bifidobacterium	5				60				100		
Lactobacillus	17	6	24	53	59	65	77	82	100		
Clostridium perfringens	9	11	22		56	67		78		100	
Other *Clostridium*	33	6	36	46	49	52	61	67	76	91	100

[a] Includes all strains identified as subspecies of *B. fragilis*.

TABLE 21. *Activity of doxycycline against anaerobic bacteria*

Bacteria	No. of strains tested	Cumulative % susceptible to indicated concn (μg/ml)									
		≤0.1	0.5	1.0	2.0	4.0	8.0	16.0	32.0	64.0	128.0
Bacteroides fragilis[a]	76	5	41	42	50	75	88	97	100		
Bacteroides melaninogenicus	67	66	75	78	90	96	97	99		100	
Other *Bacteroides* and *Selenomonas*	72	15	40	43	53	68	79	85	96	99	100
Fusobacterium nucleatum	18	44	100								
Other *Fusobacterium*	16	38	88				100				
Peptococcus and *Gaffkya*	60	8	28	35	40	70	93	98	100		
Peptostreptococcus	29	31	45		66	79	97	100			
Anaerobic and microaerophilic streptococci	10	20	70	90			100				
Gram-negative cocci	26	4	58	69	73	81	96	100			
Eubacterium	17	12	59	65	77	82	88	100			
Arachnia propionica	3		67				100				
Propionibacterium	12	17	75	83		92			100		
Actinomyces	16		63	69	94	100					
Bifidobacterium	5			20	40	60		100			
Lactobacillus	17	12	35	59	71	82	94	100			
Clostridium perfringens	9	11	67			78	89	100			
Other *Clostridium*	33	21	49	52	61	68	82	97		100	

[a] Includes all strains identified as subspecies of *Bacteroides fragilis*.

slightly less active than minocycline against the same strains, except for *C. perfringens*.

Metronidazole. The susceptibility of the anaerobes to metronidazole is shown in Table 23. With the exception of the gram-positive, nonsporeforming bacilli, the majority of strains were inhibited by 16 μg or less/ml. Bacteria requiring MICs of 32 μg or more/ml were two strains of *Bacteroides pneumosintes*, one *Peptococcus saccharolyticus*, one *Peptostreptococcus* species, three *Streptococcus intermedius*, two *Eubacterium* species, two *Arachnia propionica*, eight *Propionibacterium acnes*, two *Propionibacterium avidum*, eight *Actinomyces* species, one *Actinomyces israelii*, one *Actinomyces viscosus*, and one each of *Bifidobacterium* species, *Bifidobacterium adolescentis* var. B, and *Bifidobacterium infantis*. These results generally agree with those in previous publications (11, 19, 23, 31, 34, 41, 44, 45). We did not observe

TABLE 22. *Activity of minocycline against anaerobic bacteria*

Bacteria	No. of strains tested	Cumulative % susceptible to indicated concn (μg/ml)							
		≤0.1	0.5	1.0	2.0	4.0	8.0	16.0	32.0
Bacteroides fragilis[a]	76	29	49	57	70	82	97	100	
Bacteroides melaninogenicus	65	71	74	82	89	97	99	100	
Other *Bacteroides* and *Selenomonas*	70	29	49	56	70	79	90	96	100
Fusobacterium nucleatum	18	67	100						
Other *Fusobacterium*	16	69	94			100			
Peptococcus and *Gaffkya*	58	19	43	59	74	93	97	100	
Peptostreptococcus	28	39	54	75	82	93	100		
Anaerobic and microaerophilic streptococci	10	40	90			100			
Gram-negative cocci	25	12	68	72		92	100		
Eubacterium	16	25	69		81		94	100	
Arachnia propionica	3	33	100						
Propionibacterium	12	42	83		92			100	
Actinomyces	16		88		94	100			
Bifidobacterium	5	40	80		100				
Lactobacillus	17	24	59	71	82	88	100		
Clostridium perfringens	9	22	67					78	100
Other *Clostridium*	33	27	58	61	73	76	97		100

[a] Includes all strains identified as subspecies of *B. fragilis*.

TABLE 23. *Activity of metronidazole against anaerobic bacteria*

Bacteria	No. of strains tested	Cumulative % susceptible to indicated concn (μg/ml)										
		≤0.1	0.5	1.0	2.0	4.0	8.0	16.0	32.0	64.0	128.0	≥256
Bacteroides fragilis[a]	76	1	12	28	57	86	99	100				
Bacteroides melaninogenicus	69	15	81	93	99	100						
Other *Bacteroides* and *Selenomonas*	71	6	42	69	86	94	97		99			100
Fusobacterium nucleatum	18	56	94			100						
Other *Fusobacterium*	16	38	94	100								
Peptococcus and *Gaffkya*	58	3	72	88	98						100	
Peptostreptococcus	29	21	69	76	83	86	93	97				100
Anaerobic and microaerophilic streptococci	10		30			40					50	100
Gram-negative cocci	25	4	60	92	96	100						
Eubacterium	16	6	44	81	88							100
Arachnia propionica	3		33									100
Propionibacterium	12		8			17						100
Actinomyces	16					13		19	50	56	63	100
Bifidobacterium	5					20		40	60	80		100
Lactobacillus	19	11	37	58		68	79			84	90	100
Clostridium perfringens	9		33	78	100							
Other *Clostridium*	32	9	53	81	97	100						

[a] Includes all strains identified as subspecies of *B. fragilis*.

resistant strains of *B. fragilis, Fusobacterium* species, or *Clostridium* species, as was reported by Chow et al. (10).

Although all of the strains in the current study were defined as anaerobes because on initial isolation they grew poorly or not at all in the presence of air, some became more aerotolerant through subsequent in vitro cultivation. For the most part, these were the strains showing the greatest resistance to metronidazole. They belonged in the genus *Streptococcus* and in the various genera of gram-positive, non-sporeforming bacilli. However, the majority of anaerobic bacteria most frequently encountered in infections remain susceptible to achievable levels of metronidazole.

ACKNOWLEDGMENTS

We gratefully acknowledge the contribution of Godfrey K. M. Harding for his studies on identification of subspecies of the *B. melaninogenicus* strains. We thank Lubna Afzal Kureshi and Y. Y. Kwok for their excellent technical assistance and Edward O. Warburton and others at the Biomedical Engineering and Computer Center, Sepulveda VA Hospital, for their excellent assistance in compiling the data.

These studies were supported by grants from Beecham-Massengill Pharmaceuticals, Bristol, Tenn., Bristol Laboratories, Syracuse, N.Y., Delbay Pharmaceuticals, Inc., Bloomfield, N.J., E. I. Dupont de Nemours and Co., Newark, Del., Lederle Laboratories, Pearl River, N.Y., Eli Lilly and Co., Indianapolis, Ind., Pfizer Laboratories, New York, N.Y., Schering Corp., Bloomfield, N.J., G. D. Searle and Co., Chicago, Ill., Smith, Kline and French Laboratories, Philadelphia, Pa., and Zambon, S.p.A., Bresso, Milano, Italy.

LITERATURE CITED

1. **Actor, P., J. V. Uri, J. R. Guarini, I. Zajac, L. Phillips, C. S. Sachs, R. M. De Marinis, J. R. E. Hoover, and J. A. Weisbach.** 1975. A new parenteral cephalosporin. SK&F 59962: *in vitro* and *in vivo* antibacterial activity and serum levels in experimental animals. J. Antibiot. 28:471–476.
2. **Blazevic, D. J.** 1976. Antibiotic susceptibility of the subspecies of *Bacteroides fragilis*. Antimicrob. Agents Chemother. 9:481–484.
3. **Blazevic, D. J., and J. M. Matsen.** 1974. Susceptibility of anaerobic bacteria to carbenicillin. Antimicrob. Agents Chemother. 5:462–465.
4. **Bodey, G. P., V. Rodriguez, N. Horikoshi, and M. Valdivieso.** 1973. New antibiotics of potential importance for immunosuppressed patients. Transplant. Proc. 5(Suppl.):1227–1231.
5. **Bodey, G. P., and S. Weaver.** 1976. In vitro studies of cefamandole. Antimicrob. Agents Chemother. 9:452–457.
6. **Brumfitt, W., J. Kosmides, J. M. T. Hamilton-Miller, and J. N. G. Gilchrist.** 1974. Cefoxitin and cephalothin: antimicrobial activity, human pharmacokinetics, and toxicology. Antimicrob. Agents Chemother. 6:290–299.
7. **Cato, E. P., and J. L. Johnson.** 1976. Reinstatement of species rank for *Bacteroides fragilis, B. ovatus, B. distasonis, B. thetaiotaomicron,* and *B. vulgatus:* designation of neotype strains for *Bacteroides fragilis* (Veillon and Zuber) Castellani and Chalmers and *Bacteroides thetaiotaomicron* (Distaso) Castellani and Chalmers. Int. J. Syst. Bacteriol. 26:230–237.
8. **Cato, E. P., and C. W. Salmon.** 1976. Transfer of *Bacteroides clostridiiformis* subsp. *clostridiiformis* (Burri and Ankersmit) Holdeman and Moore and *Bacteroides clostridiiformis* subsp. *girans* (Prévot) Holdeman and Moore to the genus *Clostridium* as *Clostridium clostridiiforme* (Burri and Ankersmit) comb. nov.: emendation of description and designation of neotype strain. Int. J. Syst. Bacteriol. 26:205–211.
9. **Chow, A. W., V. Patten, and L. B. Guze.** 1975. Comparative susceptibility of anaerobic bacteria to minocycline, doxycycline, and tetracycline. Antimicrob. Agents Chemother. 7:46–49.
10. **Chow, A. W., V. Patten, and L. B. Guze.** 1975. Susceptibility of anaerobic bacteria to metronidazole: relative resistance of non-spore-forming gram-positive bacilli. J. Infect. Dis. 131:182–185.
11. **Dornbusch, K., and C. E. Nord.** 1974. *In vitro* effect of metronidazole and tinidazole on anaerobic bacteria. Med. Microbiol. Immunol. 160:265–267.
12. **Ernst, E. C., S. Berger, M. Barza, N. V. Jacobus, and F. P. Tally.** 1976. Activity of cefamandole and other cephalosporins against aerobic and anaerobic bacteria. Antimicrob. Agents Chemother. 9:852–855.
13. **Holdeman, L. V., and W. E. C. Moore (ed).** 1972. Anaerobe laboratory manual. Virginia Polytechnic Institute and State University, Blacksburg.
14. **Jones, R. N., and P. C. Fuchs.** 1976. Identification and antimicrobial susceptibility of 250 *Bacteroides fragilis* subspecies tested by broth microdilution methods. Antimicrob. Agents Chemother. 9:719–721.
15. **Kaneuchi, C., K. Watanabe, A. Terada, Y. Benno, and T. Mitsuoka.** 1976. Taxonomic study of *Bacteroides clostridiiformis* subsp. *clostridiiformis* (Burri and Ankersmit) Holdeman and Moore and of related organisms: proposal of *Clostridium clostridiiformis* (Burri and Ankersmit) comb. nov. and *Clostridium symbiosum* (Stevens) comb. nov. Int. J. Syst. Bacteriol. 26:195–204.
16. **Kislak, J. W.** 1972. The susceptibility of *Bacteroides fragilis* to 24 antibotics. J. Infect. Dis. 125:295–299.
17. **Kosakai, N., J. Igari, and T. Oguri.** 1969. Susceptibility of recently isolated pathogens to josamycin, erythromycin and lincomycin. Chemotherapy (Tokyo) 17:572–575.
18. **Kwok, Y. Y., F. P. Tally, V. L. Sutter, and S. M. Finegold.** 1975. Disk susceptibility testing of slow-growing anaerobic bacteria. Antimicrob. Agents Chemother. 7:1–7.
19. **Lerner, P. I.** 1974. Susceptibility of pathogenic actinomycetes to antimicrobial compounds. Antimicrob. Agents Chemother. 5:302–309.
20. **Long, S. S., S. Mueller, and R. M. Swenson.** 1976. In vitro susceptibilities of anaerobic bacteria to josamycin. Antimicrob. Agents Chemother. 9:859–860.
21. **Martin, W. J., M. Gardner, and J. A. Washington II.** 1972. In vitro antimicrobial susceptibility of anaerobic bacteria isolated from clinical specimens. Antimicrob. Agents Chemother. 1:148–158.
22. **Meyers, B. R., B. Leng, and S. Z. Hirshman.** 1975. Cefamandole: antimicrobial activity in vitro of a new cephalosoporin. Antimicrob. Agents Chemother. 8:737–741.
23. **Nastro, L. J., and S. M. Finegold.** 1972. Bactericidal activity of five antimicrobial agents against *Bacteroides fragilis*. J. Infect. Dis. 126:104–107.
24. **Neu, H. C.** 1974. Antimicrobial activity and human pharmacology of amoxicillin. J. Infect. Dis. 129(Suppl.):S123–S131.
25. **Neu, H. C.** 1974. Cefamandole, a cephalosporin antibiotic with an unusually wide spectrum of activity. Antimicrob. Agents Chemother. 6:177–182.
26. **Neu, H. C., and G. J. Garvey.** 1975. Comparative in vitro activity and clinical pharmacology of ticarcillin and carbenicillin. Antimicrob. Agents Chemother. 8:457–462.
27. **Ninomiya, K., K. Watanabe, K. Ueno, S. Suzuki, I. Mochizuki, Y. Simizu, T. Isogai, and T. Nisiura.** 1974. Susceptibility of anaerobic bacteria to SF 837. Chemotherapy (Tokyo) 22:1058–1064.
28. **Norrby, R., J. E. Brorsson, and S. Seeberg.** 1976. Comparative study of the in vitro antibacterial activity of cefoxitin, cefuroxime, and cephaloridine. Antimicrob. Agents Chemother. 9:506–510.
29. **Olsson, B., C. E. Nord, and T. Wadström.** 1976. Formation of beta-lactamase in *Bacteroides fragilis:* cell bound and extracellular activity. Antimicrob. Agents Chemother. 9:727–735.
30. **Osono, T., and H. Umezawa.** 1971. Josamycin, a new macrolide antibiotic of resistance non-inducing type, p. 41–120. *In* S. Mitsuhashi (ed.), Drug action and drug resistance in bacteria. University Park Press, Baltimore.
31. **Reynolds, A. V., J. M. T. Hamilton-Miller, and W. Brumfitt.** 1975. A comparison of the *in vitro* activity of metronidazole, tinidazole, and nimorazole against gram-negative anaerobic bacteria. J. Clin. Pathol. 28:775–778.
32. **Rotilie, C. A., R. J. Fass, R. B. Prior, and R. L. Perkins.** 1975. Microdilution technique for antimicrobial susceptibility testing of anaerobic bacteria. Antimicrob. Agents Chemother. 7:311–315.
33. **Sapico, F. L., Y. Y. Kwok, V. L. Sutter, and S. M. Finegold.** 1972. Standardized antimicrobial disc susceptibility testing of anaerobic bacteria: in vitro sus-

ceptibility of *Clostridium perfringens* to nine antibiotics. Antimicrob. Agents Chemother. 2:320–325.

34. **Staneck, J. L., and J. A. Washington II.** 1974. Antimicrobial susceptibilities of anaerobic bacteria: recent clinical isolates. Antimicrob. Agents Chemother. 6:311–315.
35. **Strausbaugh, L. J., J. A. Dilworth, J. M. Gwaltney, Jr., and M. A. Sande.** 1976. In vitro susceptibility studies with josamycin and erythromycin. Antimicrob. Agents Chemother. 9:546–548.
36. **Sutter, V. L., and S. M. Finegold.** 1975. Susceptibility of anaerobic bacteria to carbenicillin, cefoxitin and related drugs. J. Infect. Dis. 131:417–422.
37. **Sutter, V. L., and S. M. Finegold.** 1976. Rosamicin: in vitro activity against anaerobes and comparison with erythromycin. Antimicrob. Agents Chemother. 9:350–351.
38. **Sutter, V. L., Y. Y. Kwok, and S. M. Finegold.** 1972. Standardized antimicrobial disc susceptibility testing of anaerobic bacteria. I. Susceptibility of *Bacteroides fragilis* to tetracycline. Appl. Microbiol. 23:268–275.
39. **Sutter, V. L., Y. Y. Kwok, and S. M. Finegold.** 1973. Susceptibility of *Bacteroides fragilis* to six antibiotics determined by standardized antimicrobial disc susceptibility testing. Antimicrob. Agents Chemother. 3:188–193.
40. **Sutter, V. L., V. L. Vargo, and S. M. Finegold.** 1975. Wadsworth anaerobic bacteriology manual, 2nd ed. University of California, Los Angeles Extension Division, Los Angeles.
41. **Tally, F. P., A. Y. Armfield, V. R. Dowell, Jr., Y. Y. Kwok, V. L. Sutter, and S. M. Finegold.** 1974. Susceptibility of *Clostridium ramosum* to antimicrobial agents. Antimicrob. Agents Chemother. 5:589–593.
42. **Tally, F. P., N. V. Jacobus, J. G. Bartlett, and S. L. Gorbach.** 1975. Susceptibility of anaerobes to cefoxitin and other cephalosporins. Antimicrob. Agents Chemother. 7:128–132.
43. **Tally, F. P., N. V. Jacobus, J. G. Bartlett, and S. L. Gorbach.** 1975. In vitro activity of penicillins against anaerobes. Antimicrob. Agents Chemother. 7:413–414.
44. **Tally, F. P., V. L. Sutter, and S. M. Finegold.** 1972. Metronidazole versus anaerobes. In vitro data and initial clinical observations. Calif. Med. 117:22–26.
45. **Ueno, K., K. Ninomiya, and S. Suzuki.** 1971. Antibacterial activity of metronidazole against anaerobic bacteria. Chemotherapy (Tokyo) 19:111–114.
46. **Van Beers, D., E. Schoutens, M. P. Vanderlinden, and E. Yourassowsky.** 1975. Comparative in vitro activity of chloramphenicol and thiamphenicol on common aerobic and anaerobic Gram-negative bacilli (Salmonella and Shigella excluded). Chemotherapy (Basel) 21:73–81.
47. **Werner, H., and G. Böhm.** 1974. Susceptibility of nonsporing anaerobes of the genera *Bacteroides, Fusobacterium, Sphaerophorus, Peptococcus* and *Peptostreptococcus* to clindamycin. Zentralbl. Bakteriol. Parasitenkd. Infektionskr. Hyg. Abt. 1 Orig. Reihe A 229:401–408.
48. **Werner, H., G. Rintelen, and H. Kunstek-Santos.** 1975. A new butyric acid-producing *Bacteroides* species: *B. splanchnicus* n. sp. Zentralbl. Bakteriol. Parasitenkd. Infektionskr. Hyg. Abt. 1 Orig. Reihe A 231:133–144.
49. **Wick, W. E., and D. A. Preston.** 1972. Biological properties of three 3-heterocyclic-thiomethyl cephalosporin antibiotics. Antimicrob. Agents Chemother. 1:221–234.
50. **Wilkins, T. D., and T. Thiel.** 1973. Resistance of some species of *Clostridium* to clindamycin. Antimicrob. Agents Chemother. 3:136–137.
51. **Zabransky, R. J., J. A. Johnston, and K. J. Hauser.** 1973. Bacteriostatic and bactericidal activities of various antibiotics against *Bacteroides fragilis*. Antimicrob. Agents Chemother. 3:152–156.

Antimicrobial Agents and Chemotherapy, Oct. 1976, p. 753-761
Vol. 10, No. 4

R-Plasmid Transfer In Vivo in the Absence of Antibiotic Selection Pressure

V. PETROCHEILOU, J. GRINSTED, and M. H. RICHMOND*

Department of Bacteriology, University of Bristol, Bristol, BS8 1TD, England

Received for publication 6 April 1976

The persistence of an O18 *Escherichia coli* strain resistant to tetracycline, streptomycin, and sulfonamide has been followed in the fecal flora of a single individual over a period of 9 months. The strain in question carrying an R plasmid was detectable from the beginning of the survey, but it was only after a 10-day period of tetracycline therapy that it reached an all but permanent dominance in the fecal flora. No transfer of the R plasmid carried by the strain to any other coliform could be detected for 202 days after the end of tetracycline treatment. At this point, however, an O88 *E. coli* carrying the same plasmid as the O18 strain appeared briefly as a predominant component of the flora. The two plasmids isolated from the O18 and the O88 *E. coli* strains have been characterized in molecular terms and found to be similar. This suggests that R-plasmid transfer between two *E. coli* strains occurred in an individual who was living a normal daily life and who was not receiving antibiotics.

Previous claims that R-plasmid transfer occurs in man under natural conditions have either been based on experiments in which appropriate marker strains have been fed to volunteers (4, 24) or have been inferred from epidemiological data (10, 18). In all cases, antibiotics have been present at or near the time of transfer, either given deliberately for experimental purposes or administered therapeutically.

In this study we have examined the fecal flora of a single individual for a period of over 9 months. Towards the beginning of this period, tetracycline was administered for a period of 10 days at therapeutic levels, but thereafter antibiotics were not knowingly present. The tetracycline therapy led to the establishment of an O18 *Escherichia coli* line carrying an R plasmid with the marker pattern Tc Sm Su. (Abbreviations of antibiotics are as follows: Tc, tetracycline; Su, sulfonamide; Sm, streptomycin; Ap, ampicillin; Cm, chloramphenicol.) This strain has been detected as a majority component of the fecal flora on two occasions (30 and 9 days) before the beginning of tetracycline treatment, and as a minority strain on four other occasions [36, 12, 2, and 1 day(s) before treatment]. After the end of tetracycline therapy, this strain remained prevalent in the same person for at least 7 months. Twice during this period (202 and 242 days), an O88 *E. coli* expressing a similar marker pattern also appeared briefly as a majority strain.

Molecular examination of the R plasmids carried by the O18 *E. coli* throughout the study and the plasmid present in the O88 *E. coli* on day 202 suggests that they form part of the same plasmid clone and that R plasmid transfer was therefore likely to have occurred between two distinct *E. coli* strains in the alimentary tract of a person not receiving antibiotics.

MATERIALS AND METHODS

Bacterial strains, plasmids, and bacteriophages. *E. coli* UB1139, a nalidixic acid-resistant derivative of *E. coli* K-12, was used as a host for the plasmids under examination. The characteristics of this strain together with those of UB281 (the strain used as recipient in the transduction experiments) and of UB1180 and UB1181 (the strains used for examination of the presence of the *fi* character) are listed in Table 1.

UB1180 was constructed from JC3272 (1) by transferring the F'*lac* factor JCFLO to it (1). UB1181 is a nalidixic acid-resistant derivative of the *E. coli* K-12 multiple auxotroph JN200, provided by M. Jones-Mortimer (Department of Genetics, University of Birmingham, England).

The plasmids used for compatibility tests together with their sources are listed in Table 2.

Bacteriophages MS2 (25), P1*kc* (16), and λC1857 *int-2* (29) were from laboratory stocks.

Media. Nutrient broth consisted of 1.6% (wt/vol) nutrient broth base (Difco) containing 0.5% (wt/vol) NaCl. Nutrient agar was prepared from heart infusion agar (Difco), with the addition, where necessary, of appropriate antibiotics. Lysed blood agar was prepared from blood agar base (Difco) supplemented with 5% (vol/vol) saponin-lysed oxalated horse blood. Minimal salts agar was prepared as described by Grinsted et al. (12).

TABLE 1. *Characteristics of standard E. coli K-12 strains used*

Strain	Genotype	Origin	Reference
UB1139	F^- *lac*$^+$ *leu*$^-$ *met*$^-$ *thy*$^-$ *nal*^{r}		(5)
UB1180	F'*lac*$^+$ *his*$^-$ *trp*$^-$ *lys*$^-$ *str*^{r}	F'*lac*$^+$ derivative of JC3272	(1)
UB1181	F^-*lac*$^-$ *pro*$^-$ *trp*$^-$ *his*$^-$ *arg*$^-$ *ile*$^-$ *met*$^-$ *nal*^{r}	(See text)	
UB281	F^- *pro*$^-$ *met*$^-$ *nal*^{r}		(5)
JC6310	*trp*$^-$ *his*$^-$ *lys*$^-$ *str*^{r} *recA56*	Dr. J. C. Clark	(5)

Drug resistance. Resistance to antibiotics was determined on lysed blood agar by conventional disk tests using "multodisks," unless otherwise stated. The multodisks (type U1, Oxoid Ltd., London) contained tetracycline (50 μg), streptomycin (25 μg), ampicillin (25 μg), sulphafurazole (500 μg), nalidixic acid (30 μg), nitrofurantoin (200 μg), colistin sulfate (10 μg), and chloramphenicol (50 μg).

In certain experiments the minimal inhibitory concentration (MIC) values for strains was determined by plating single colony-forming units on nutrient agar plates containing a range of concentrations of the antibiotic under test. The MIC was recorded as the lowest concentration that did not allow growth.

Conjugation experiments. Exponentially growing donor and recipient broth cultures (containing about 10^8 bacteria/ml) were mixed (0.5 ml of donor plus 1.5 ml of recipient) and incubated for 2 h at 37°C. Samples (0.1 ml) from these mating mixtures and from a series of 10-fold dilutions prepared from them were then plated on appropriate antibiotic agar. Individual colonies obtained on these plates were then purified by subculture on agar containing the same antibiotics.

In experiments to measure the frequency of transfer, samples were taken for plating on selective agar 30 min after mixing.

Transduction experiments. Phage P1*kc* was propagated on *E. coli* UB1139 carrying one of the plasmids under examination using the soft-agar method described by Adams (2). The transduction procedure used was essentially as described by Lennox (16).

Test for the presence of F-pili. The presence of F-pili was determined by following the multiplication of phage MS2 on *E. coli* UB1139 carrying one of the plasmids under examination in liquid medium by the method of Grindley and Anderson (11).

Test for fertility inhibition. The presence of the *fi* character was detected either by observing the inhibition of plaque formation by MS2 on *E. coli* K-12 F^+ when a test plasmid was present in the host strain as well as the F factor (22) or by measuring the extent to which F'*lac* transfer was reduced by the presence of a test plasmid in the same donor cell (7).

Studies on incompatibility. Plasmids were allocated to an incompatibility group by their ability to coexist with plasmids of known compatibility characteristics. *E. coli* UB1139 containing the plasmid under test was mated for 2 h under standard conditions with *E. coli* JC6310 containing one of the standard plasmids listed in Table 2. The mating mixture was plated on minimal agar plates containing either spectinomycin (40 μg/ml) and kanamycin (30 μg/ml), or spectinomycin and carbenicillin (500 μg/ml), thus selecting for JC6310, and thereafter observing the presence and stability of the two plasmids in this strain by testing for the appropriate resistance markers in the two plasmids.

Colonies obtained in this way were purified by restreaking on agar containing the same pair of antibiotics. Isolates that had retained both the plasmids involved in the test were then passed through three successive overnight subcultures in 10 ml of nutrient broth in the absence of antibiotics, and a loopful of the final culture was then streaked on nutrient agar to obtain single colonies. Four clones arising in this way were tested from each mating and at least 100 colonies from each of these clones were scored for the persistence of the two plasmids by patching on agar containing each of the antibiotics used.

Isolation of plasmid DNA. Cleared lysates were prepared essentially as described by Thompson et al. (27). Deoxyribonucleic acid (DNA) was precipitated from these using polyethyleneglycol 6000 (10% wt/vol) and 0.5 M NaCl as described by Humphreys et al. (15). The precipitates were resuspended in SSC buffer (0.15 M NaCl plus 0.015 sodium citrate), extracted twice with chloroform, and then centrifuged in conventional ethidium bromide-CsCl gradients (23).

Radioactive plasmid DNA was prepared and measured as described previously (5, 12).

***Eco*RI endonucleolytic digestion of DNA.** The reaction was carried out in 0.1 M tris(hydroxymethyl)aminomethane buffer, pH 7.5, containing 0.01 M $MgSO_4$. Usually, 2 μl of *Eco*RI endonuclease preparation and either 20 μl of plasmid DNA or 2 μl of λ DNA were used, and the reaction mixture was made up to a total of 40 μl with buffer. Such preparations normally contained about 10 μg of DNA. Mixtures were incubated at 37°C for about 1 h, and the reaction was stopped by the addition of 10 μl of a solution of sucrose (40% wt/vol) and bromophenol blue (0.1% wt/vol) in 0.1 M ethylenediaminetetraacetate, pH 8.0. The effectiveness of the *Eco*RI endonuclease preparation was always cal-

TABLE 2. *Characteristics of plasmid-containing host strains used for compatibility tests*

Plasmid[a]	Source	Incompatibility group	Plasmid resistance pattern	Reference
R1-19K	This lab	FII	Kn	(5)
RP1	This lab	P	Ap Kn Tc	(12)
R144	N. Datta	Ia	Kn	(20)
R388 Cb	This lab	W	Ap Tp Su	(5)
R825	R. Hedges	N	Ap	(17)
R64G[s]	Y. Chabbert	C	Ap Cm Su	(28)

[a] All plasmids were carried in *E. coli* JC6310 (see reference 5 and Table 1).

ibrated against phage λ DNA to ensure complete digestion in a preliminary experiment.

The samples were analyzed in vertical agarose slab gels (0.7% wt/vol). The agarose was dissolved in tris(hydroxymethyl)aminomethane-borate buffer (21), containing ethidium bromide (0.5 μg/ml), and electrophoresis was carried out with the same buffer at a constant current of 60 mA for about 2 h.

The DNA bands were photographed by using illumination from a long-wavelength ultraviolet lamp (UVL 56, Blak-Ray Inc., Calif.).

The *Eco*RI endonuclease was prepared from *E. coli* JK29 essentially as described by Thomas and Davis (26). The strain JK29 was kindly provided by K. Murray (University of Edinburgh, Scotland). Lambda DNA was prepared from λCI857 *int-2* phage by phenol extraction. The particles were obtained by one-step growth in *E. coli* C600 growing in nutrient broth.

RESULTS

Sequence of strains. Table 3 shows the various O-antigen types and the antibiotic resistance patterns of the *E. coli* present as majority strains in the fecal flora of a single individual during the 303 days of the study. These strains were isolated as described previously (13). A therapeutic course of tetracycline (250 mg, twice daily) was administered for 10 days, but thereafter no antibiotic was given. By far the most persistent strain was *E. coli* O18 Tc Sm Su. An O18 *E. coli* strain with the same marker pattern was also present before the onset of tetracycline therapy (Table 3). On days −30 and −9, it was present as one of the majority strains in the flora, whereas on days −36, −12, −2, and −1 it could only be detected by plating fecal suspensions on agar containing tetracycline.

Towards the end of the survey, O18 *E. coli* strains were encountered with the marker pattern Sm Su, and on two occasions (days 202 and 242) a Tc Sm Su pattern was found in an O88 *E. coli*. The other resistant *E. coli* strains encountered in the fecal flora after the end of tetracycline therapy were an O86 Ap Sm Su Cm strain present as a majority component on days 12 to 14 and an O11 Tc Su strain which formed part of the majority flora at the end of the period of therapy and for 9 days afterwards. Before therapy began, an O81 Tc-resistant *E. coli* strain was predominant on day −6, and a small number of colonies of O17 Tc Ap Sm Su were detected, on selective agar only, on day −27.

Resistance patterns of the O18 and O88 *E. coli*. A more detailed examination of the resistance patterns of the O18 and O88 strains isolated in this study showed that all were cross-resistant to streptomycin and to spectinomycin. It seems probable therefore that the R plasmid carried in these strains specified the streptomycin-spectinomycin adenylylating enzyme (6).

E. coli O18 isolates that gave a resistance pattern of Sm Su with standard disks (see Materials and Methods) appeared on days 74, 87, and 130, and thereafter with increasing frequency until this phenotype seemed to displace the O18 Tc Sm Su strains from about day 223 onwards. A more careful comparison of the O18 strains expressing resistance to Tc Sm Su with those that were resistant to Sm and Su alone showed that the tetracycline resistance of the latter type was reduced, but not completely lost. Thus, strains with the pattern Tc Sm Su gave MIC values of 60 μg/ml against tetracycline when measured as single colony-forming units on tetracycline agar, whereas the strains that had the pattern Sm Su when tested with disks gave MIC values against tetracycline of about 10 μg/ml. A variant of this particular O18 *E. coli* that had lost its plasmid gave an MIC against tetracycline of about 1 μg/ml. These results suggest, therefore, either that a new plasmid became prevalent in the O18 strains in this survey around day 130 or that a mutation occurred in the plasmid specifying the high levels of tetracycline resistance to give rise to strains which were more susceptible to this antibiotic without being fully susceptible. This point has been investigated further and will be discussed elsewhere.

Tests for R plasmids and their incompatibility relationships. A total of 30 O18 *E. coli* strains from the series shown in Table 3 (those isolated on days −36, −30, −2, T3, T9, 14, 29, 39, 42, 68, 69, 72, 96, 97, 103, 122, 143, 147, 151, 153, 168, 175, 188, 228, 230, 235, 240, 246, 249, 257) were mated with *E. coli* UB1139 in a standard cross (see Materials and Methods) to see whether the resistance patterns were R plasmid mediated. One isolate of the O88 *E. coli*, isolated on day 202, was treated in the same way as were those of O11 (days 5, 9), O17 (day −27), O81 (day −6), and O86 (day 14). In all cases except the O81 *E. coli* strain, the resistance pattern of the donor was R factor mediated, since in all cases the full pattern could be transferred to UB1139 in a standard cross.

Transduction experiments with phage P1*kc* were then carried out to test whether the resistance markers Tc Sm Su were located on the same plasmid or not. All the antibiotic resistance markers of these plasmids were cotransducible.

Further investigation of the low-level tetracycline resistance phenotype (as, for example, in the O18 Sm Su isolates from days 147, 153, 168, 175, 228, 230, 235, 240, 246, 249, and 257) showed that UB 1139 Spc^R exconjugants (ob-

TABLE 3. *Sequence of E. coli strains in one patient before, during, and after treatment with tetracycline*

No. of isolates (out of 10 colonies from non-selective agar) exhibiting given reaction at stated no. of days[b]

O type	Resistance pattern[a] / Days before therapy	−36	−33	−30	−27	−22	−20	−16	−12	−9	−6	−2	−1
O1						2			10				
O8						1		2		1			
O10											1		
O15													3
O17	Tc Ap Sm Su												
O18		10	6	9	†[c]	2							
O18	Tc Sm Su	†		1					†	1		†	†
O27											1		
O50										1			
O57					7								
O68					3					5	1		
O75											5		
O81	Tc										2		
O107/149						5	10	8		2		10	7

O type	Days of therapy	T1	T2	T3	T5	T6	T7	T8	T9	T10
O18	Tc Sm Su	†	†	10	10	10	10	10	10	8
O11	Tc Su									2

O type	Days after therapy	1	2	3	4	5	6	7	8	9	11	12	13	14	17	18	20	21	22	27	29	31	32	33	35	37
O11	Tc Su	4	2			4	4	4	2	3																
O18	Tc Sm Su	6	8	10	9	6	5	6	6	3	2	†	†	3	7	7	2	10	6	8	4	6	5	10	4	1
O86	Ap Sm Su Cm											3	8	7												
O108											3															
NT[a]												2	2													

O type	Days after therapy	39	41	42	43	45	46	64	65	67	68	69	72	74	76	78	80	81	82	84	87	88	89	90	94	95
O9								5	1																	
O11																		1	1							
O15					3														1				1			
O17																		4								
O18	Tc Sm Su	10	6	6	6	5	6	†	9	10	3	4	1	5	6	10	10	1	3	†	9	10	9	10	4	10
O18	Sm Su													1							1					
O21								2	1																	
O24						1																				

	Days after therapy	96	97	100	103	105	112	115	117	118	122	123	125	129	130	132	137	138
O11																		1
O15		1	1															
O18	Tc Sm Su	9	9		2	3	10	8	†	†	5	10	6	†	1	6	10	†
O18	Sm Su														1			
O20									1	4								
O24									4	4								
O27									2									
O50									3	1				9	6			

	Days after therapy	140	143	147	150	151	153	168	171	175	183	186	188	189	193	197	200	202
O15			2										3	6	10	10		
O18	Tc Sm Su		5	†	†	†	†	†	†	†	2	1	4	4	†	†	10	2
O18	Sm Su			2		10	6	10	5	8	4							
O88	Tc Sm Su																	8

	Days after therapy	208	209	210	216	223	228	230	235	237	240	242	244	246	249	256	257
O9							1										
O15						8											
O18	Tc Sm Su	†	2	†	†	†											
O18	Sm Su		1				3	2	10	1	5	1		10	10	5	5
O21		1					2						1				
O24													3				
O40					3												
O75					1												
O86			5														
O88	Tc Sm Su											5					
O101						2											
O128					4												
NT					2						1	1	4				

[a] Abbreviations: Tc, tetracycline; Su, sulfonamide; Sm, streptomycin; Ap, ampicillin; Cm, chloramphenicol; NT, not typable with available sera.

[b] In instances where number is under 10, the remaining isolates proved not to be *E. coli*.

[c] Culture on selective agar showed presence of strain as a substantial minority component of flora.

tained when low-level resistance O18 strains were used as donors) also showed low-level tetracycline resistance. This variant of the Tet^R phenotype therefore seems to be plasmid coded.

A preliminary experiment carried out on one of the *E. coli* O18 Tc Sm Su strains from this series showed that it would propagate MS2 phage, and this suggested that the plasmid concerned was probably of the F incompatibility group. Accordingly, all the plasmids that had been transferred to strain UB1139 (see above) were tested for their incompatibility with R1-19K (see Materials and Methods). All the plasmids with either a Tc Sm Su or a Sm Su pattern showed a degree of incompatibility with R1-19K, but segregation of the two plasmids after growing for 6 h in broth free of antibiotics was very low; about 80 to 90% of the tested colonies retained both plasmids. For this reason, growth in antibiotic-free broth was extended to three successive overnight subcultures. After that period segregation had occurred in 50 to 95% of the tested colonies. However, individual clones carrying R1-19K and the test plasmid segregated at different rates after release of selection pressure even when they were isolated from the same mating experiment.

The plasmids conferring resistance to the O18 strains in this survey certainly therefore show a degree of incompatibility with R1-19K, but the results are not clear-cut and immediate. This partial incompatibility was also found with all the plasmids whether they specified high- or low-level tetracycline resistance. In contrast, plasmids showing full incompatibility with R1-19K normally segregated completely after growth for 6 h in the absence of selection pressure.

Examination of the Tc Sm Su plasmid from the O88 *E. coli* strain isolated on day 202 also showed this partial incompatibility with R1-19K, and this suggested that this plasmid from the O88 strain may be related to those found in the O18 series.

The *E. coli* O11, O17, O86 isolated on days 9, −27, and 14, respectively, were also tested for incompatibility with R1-19K. All were compatible, and therefore carried plasmids that were different from those in the O18 and O88 strains.

Representative plasmids from the O18 and from one of the O88 strains were also tested for incompatibility with standard plasmids of compatibility groups N, W, C, Ia, and P. No incompatibility was observed in any case.

Fertility inhibition and propagation of phage MS2. All the plasmids that had been transferred to strain UB1139 from the O18 series and from the single O88 strain tested were examined for their ability to propagate the F-pilus specific phage MS2 and also to inhibit the transfer of F′*lac* in a standard test for fertility inhibition (see Materials and Methods). All the plasmids examined in this series with the marker pattern Tc Sm Su, or Sm Su, whether derived from O18 or O88 *E. coli*, propagated MS2 to give an increase in phage number of at least 1,000-fold, inhibited the frequency of transfer of F′*lac* by at least a factor of 100, and also inhibited the lysis of these strains by phage MS2 when transferred into *E. coli* K-12 F$^+$. The combination of MS2 susceptibility, *fi*$^+$ character, and partial incompatibility with R1-19K suggests that the plasmid specifying resistance of Tc Sm Su in both the O18 and O88 *E. coli* isolates examined in this study were very similar in properties to a classical FII class plasmid, and the same was true of the plasmids specifying low-level tetracycline resistance.

R-plasmid isolation from *E. coli* O18 and O88. The R plasmids derived from the O18 strains isolated on days −36, −30, 14, 143, and 249 and from the O88 strain occurring on day 202 were isolated as covalently closed, circular DNA after transfer to UB1139. The isolates from days −36, −30, 14, and 143 showed a Tc Sm Su phenotype, whereas that from day 249 had a Sm Su pattern. Circular molecules were detected in all samples examined after isolation in CsCl-ethidium bromide centrifugation (23) and were sized by electron microscopy (5). Measurement of the contour lengths gave values close to 66×10^6 daltons in all cases. Thus, the plasmids from the O18 and O88 *E. coli* strains all carry plasmids of very similar size.

Cleavage of R plasmids with *Eco*RI restriction endonuclease. Plasmid DNA isolated from those strains examined by electron microscopy (see above) was digested with *Eco*RI restriction endonuclease, and the fragments were separated by electrophoresis in agarose gels. A digest of lambda DNA prepared with the same enzyme at the same time was used as a standard to obtain an approximate size of the fragments. Each plasmid examined gave nine bands ranging in molecular weight from about 15×10^6 to less than 10^6. Figure 1 shows the patterns obtained from the Tc Sm Su plasmids from the O18 strain isolated on day −36 with that found in the O88 *E. coli* isolated 248 days later. All nine bands in the two digests are in similar positions, and this argues that the two plasmids examined in this experiment are extremely similar. Cleavage studies on the plasmids obtained from the *E. coli* O18 strains isolated on days −30, 14, 143, and 249 also show nine bands in identical positions to those shown in Fig. 1.

Plasmid DNA isolated from strains O11, O86,

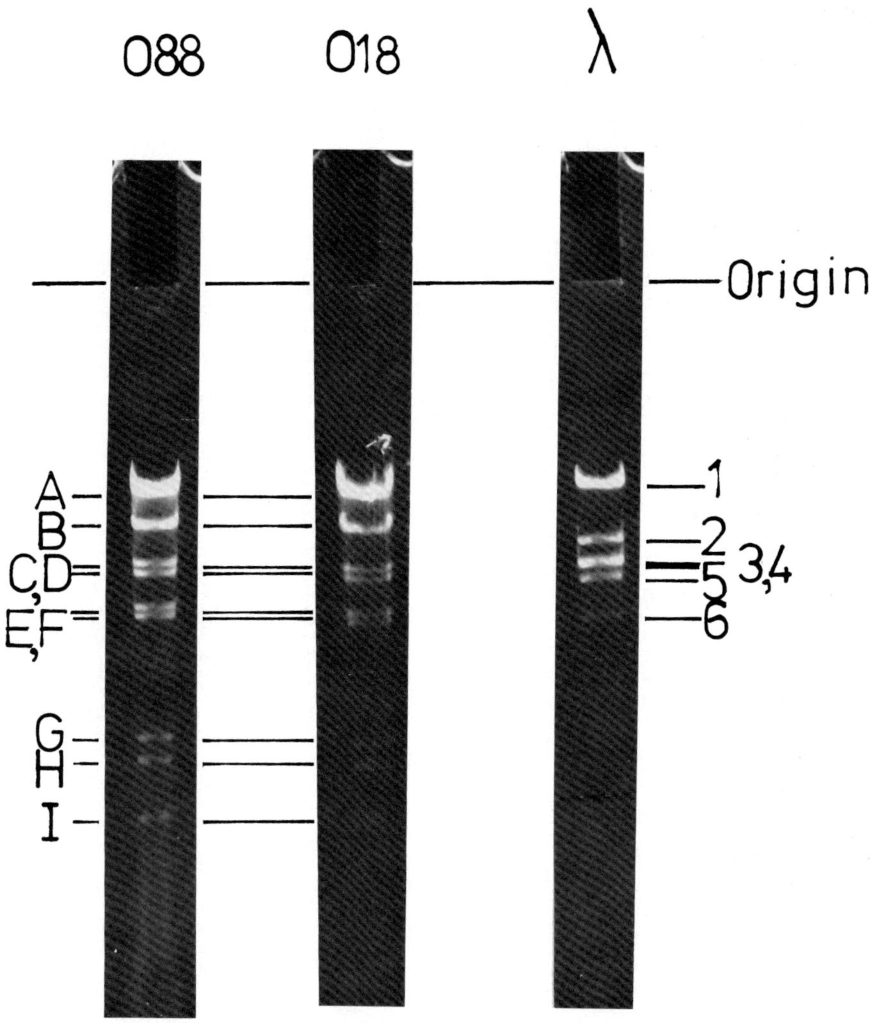

FIG. 1. *EcoRI restriction endonuclease hydrolysis patterns obtained from phage λ DNA and from the plasmids isolated from O18 and O88 E. coli studied in this survey. The six bands (numbers 1–6) obtained from phage λ DNA have molecular weights (× 10^6 d) of 13.7, 4.74, 3.74, 3.48, 3.02, and 2.13 (reference 26). Prolonged separation of the digest from the O18 and O88 plasmids shows that band B is double (data has shown). Electrophoresis was carried out in 0.7% (wt/vol) agarose gels as described. The photographs represent different sections of the same slab gel.*

and O17 (days 9, 14, −27, respectively) gave a completely different pattern when hydrolyzed with *Eco*RI when compared with the one obtained from the O18 and O88 Tc Sm Su plasmids.

DISCUSSION

The pattern of events in this survey of a single individual shows that antibiotic use can lead to the establishment of a resistant *E. coli* strain as a predominant complement of the fecal flora for long periods after the direct selective effect of the antibiotic has ceased (see also reference 14). A strain that had appeared sporadically before treatment became an all but permanent component of the flora afterwards, and it is difficult to escape the conclusion that the tetracycline treatment eliminated all susceptible competitors. The failure of the O17 Tc Ap Sm Su (day −27) and O81 Tc (day −6) strains to emerge at this time presumably means either that they were no longer present in the person's gut flora when therapy commenced or that the O18 strain had an additional selective advantage over the other two tetracycline-resistant *E. coli*. Thus, the survival of resistant *E. coli* in the gut of man seems to be subject to two main influences: the resistance of the strain in the presence of antibiotics and its competitive ability with respect to other bacteria (susceptible or resistant) once the pressure has been removed (14). Thus, antibiotic use is only one of the pressures that leads to the emergence of resistant strains as majority components of mixed populations, and there is no evidence that the carriage of an R plasmid is necessarily a disadvantage, as has been claimed by some (3, 8).

The similarity of marker phenotype, *fi* character, production of F-pili, partial incompatibility with R1-19, and the *Eco*RI endonucleolytic digestion patterns suggests that plasmid transfer may have occurred between the resident O18 *E. coli* followed in this survey and an O88 strain. The alternative possibility is that the serotype O18 strain was converted to O88. This seems improbable since the change would involve the loss of all rhamnose and the gain of mannose and 6-deoxytalose in the lipopolysaccharide, that is, a change from chemotype VII to chemotype XXVI (19). The possibility that the O88 Tc Sm Su plasmid might have appeared exogenously rather than by transfer is also improbable, since it is unlikely that the only Tc Sm Su plasmid to appear in the flora of the individual over a 9-month period should be identical in so many properties with that of the plasmid present throughout. Other studies on Tc Sm Su plasmids of FII compatibility group, isolated elsewhere, have never shown the same banding pattern with *Eco*RI endonuclease as the Tc Sm Su plasmid studied here in the *E. coli* O18 and O88 strains. Nor have any of these other plasmids ever shown partial incompatibility with R1-19K.

Perhaps the most surprising fact to emerge from this survey, and one of great importance for our understanding of the ecology of antibiotic resistance in *E. coli,* is that transfer of the plasmid in question to other *E. coli* could not be detected during a period of nearly 7 months after the strain became established. If transfer did occur the progeny did not survive well enough to become majority components of the fecal flora. So, although plasmid transfer seems to occur in the human gut, these observations, which were a survey of natural events, certainly did not suggest that the phenomenon occurred widely. Whether the process does occur more commonly, but the resulting strains are unable to survive well enough to become majority components of the flora, is unclear. Certainly, there was no evidence that any such transfer had occurred from examination of the samples plated on selective agar during this survey.

ACKNOWLEDGMENTS

We would like to thank P. M. Bennett for carrying out the electron microscopy associated with this study.

This work was supported by a Fellowship from the British Council to V.P., and by a Grant from the Medical Research Council to M.H.R. for epidemiological and molecular studies on R factors and other plasmids.

LITERATURE CITED

1. **Achtman, M., N. Willets, and A. J. Clark.** 1971. Beginning a genetic analysis of conjugational transfer determined by the F factor in *Escherichia coli* by isolation of transfer-deficient mutants. J. Bacteriol. **106:**529–538.
2. **Adams, M. H.** 1959. Bacteriophages, p. 454–456. Interscience Publishers Inc., London.
3. **Anderson, J. D.** 1973. The effect of resistance-transfer (R) factor carriage upon the survival of *E. coli* in vitro and experimentally in man. J. Med. Microbiol. **6:**xix.
4. **Anderson, J. D., W. A. Gillespie, and M. H. Richmond.** 1974. Chemotherapy and antibiotic resistance transfer between Enterobacteria in the human gastrointestinal tract. J. Med. Microbiol. **6:**461–473.
5. **Bennett, P. M., and M. H. Richmond.** 1976. Translocation of a discrete piece of deoxyribonucleic acid carrying an *amp* gene between replicons in *Escherichia coli*. J. Bacteriol. **126:**1–6.
6. **Benveniste, R., and J. Davies.** 1973. Mechanisms of antibiotic resistance in bacteria. Annu. Rev. Biochem. **42:**471–506.
7. **Clowes, R. C., and W. Hayes (ed.).** 1968. Experiments in microbial genetics, p. 134–138. Blackwell Scientific Publications, Oxford.
8. **Cooke, E. M.** 1974. *Escherichia coli* and man, p. 70. Churchill Livingstone, Edinburgh.
9. **Datta, N., and R. W. Hedges.** 1972. R-factors from *Proteus rettgeri*. J. Gen. Microbiol. **72:**349–356.
10. **Farrar, W. E., Jr., M. Eidson, P. Guerry, S. Falkow, L. M. Drusin, and R. B. Roberts.** 1972. Interbacterial transfer of R-factors in the human intestine. *In vivo* aquisition of R-factor-mediated kanamycin resistance by a multi-resistant strain of *Shigella sonnei*. J. Infect. Dis. **126:**22–33.
11. **Grindley, J. N., and E. S. Anderson.** 1971. I-like resistance factors with the fi^+ character. Genet. Res. **17:**267–271.
12. **Grinsted, J., J. R. Saunders, L. C. Ingram, R. B. Sykes, and M. H. Richmond.** 1972. Properties of an R factor which originated in *Pseudomonas aeruginosa* 1822. J. Bacteriol. **110:**529–537.
13. **Hartley, C. L., K. Howe, A. H. Linton, K. B. Linton and M. H. Richmond.** 1972. Distribution of R plasmids among the O-antigen types of *Escherichia coli* isolated from human and animal sources. Antimicrob. Agents Chemother. **8:**122–131.
14. **Hartley, C. L., and M. H. Richmond.** 1975. Antibiotic resistance and survival of *E. coli* in the alimentary tract. Br. Med. J. **4:**71–74.
15. **Humphreys, G. O., G. A. Willshaw, and E. S. Anderson.** 1975. A simple method for the preparation of large quantities of pure plasmid DNA. Biochim. Biophys. Acta **383:**457–463.
16. **Lennox, E. S.** 1955. Transduction of linked genetic characters by bacteriophage P1. Virology **1:**190–206.
17. **Matthew, M., and R. W. Hedges.** 1976. Analytical isoelectric focusing of R factor-determined β-lactamases: correlation with plasmid compatibility. J. Bacteriol. **125:**713–718.
18. **Lowbury, E. J. L., and J. R. Babb.** 1972. Clearance

from a hospital of gram-negative bacilli that transfer carbenicillin-resistance to *Pseudomonas aeruginosa*. Lancet 2:941–945.

19. **Lüderitz, O., K. Jann, and R. Wheat.** 1968. Somatic and capsular antigens of Gram-negative bacteria, p. 105–228. *In* M. Florkin and E. M. Stotz (ed.), Comprehensive biochemistry, vol. 26a. Elsevier Scientific Publishing Co., Amsterdam.
20. **Meynell, E., and N. Datta.** 1967. Mutant drug resistant factors of high transmissibility. Nature (London) 214:885–887.
21. **Peacock, A. C., and C. W. Dingman.** 1968. Molecular weight estimation and separation of ribonucleic acid by electrophoresis in agarose-acrylamide composite gels. Biochemistry 7:668–674.
22. **Pitton, J. S., and E. S. Anderson.** 1970. The inhibition action of transfer factors on lysis of *Escherichia coli* K12 by phage μ2 and ϕ2. Genet. Res. 16:215–224.
23. **Radloff, R., W. Bauer, and J. Vinograd.** 1967. A dye-buoyant-density method for the detection and isolation of closed circular DNA: the closed circular DNA of HeLa cells. Proc. Natl. Acad. Sci. U.S.A. 57:1514–1521.
24. **Smith, H. W.** 1969. Transfer of antibiotic resistance from farm animals and human strains of *E. coli* to resident *E. coli* in the alimentary tract in man. Lancet i:1174–1176.
25. **Strauss, J. H., Jr., and R. L. Sinsheimer.** 1963. Purification and properties of bacteriophage MS2 and of its ribonucleic acid. J. Mol. Biol. 7:43–54.
26. **Thomas, M., and R. W. Davis.** 1975. Studies on the cleavage of bacteriophage lambda DNA with EcoR1 restriction endonuclease. J. Mol. Biol. 91:315–328.
27. **Thompson, R. S., G. Hughes, and P. Broda.** 1974. Plasmid identification using specific endonucleases. Mol. Gen. Genet. 133:141–149.
28. **Witchitz, J. L., and Y. Chabbert.** 1971. Résistance transferable à la gentamicine. I. Expression du charactère de résistance. Ann. Inst. Pasteur Paris 121:733–743.
29. **Zissler, J.** 1967. Integration-negative (*int*) mutants of phage λ. Virology 31:189.

ANTIMICROBIAL AGENTS AND CHEMOTHERAPY, Oct. 1976, p. 762-764 Vol. 10, No. 4

Printed in U.S.A.

NOTES

Inhibition of Bacteriophage Lambda, T1, and T7 Development by R Plasmids of the H Incompatibility Group

DIANE E. TAYLOR* AND ROBERT B. GRANT

Research Institute and Department of Bacteriology, The Hospital for Sick Children, Toronto, Ontario, Canada M5G 1X8

Received for publication 7 June 1976

R plasmids from chloramphenicol-resistant salmonella from Ontario are shown to belong to the H_2 incompatibility subgroup and to mediate a broad-spectrum, phage inhibition function.

In the Mexican typhoid epidemic of 1972 to 1973 and in typhoid outbreaks in India and Vietnam, many isolates of the causative organism were found to be resistant to chloramphenicol (3, 7, 8). This fact has obvious medical significance in view of the previous, long-standing position of chloramphenicol as the drug of choice for the treatment of typhoid fever. The resistance was mediated by transmissible drug resistance factors, which were found to belong to a new incompatibility group, designated "H" (6). Subsequently, two subgroups of H plasmids were identified: H_1 plasmids, which are incompatible with F factors in the autonomous state, and H_2 plasmids, which are compatible with F (10). Both H_1 and H_2 plasmids are *fi*$^-$ and exhibit thermosensitive transfer (10, 11). Both types have been found to have a wide distribution, occurring in various salmonella isolates throughout the world (1).

Recent studies in our laboratory of antibiotic resistance in nontyphoid salmonella from the province of Ontario in Canada have revealed a high incidence of drug resistance plasmids. In Ontario during the summer 1974, 12% of 589 human salmonella and 37% of 204 animal salmonella isolates were resistant to chloramphenicol; the majority of the resistance was transferable to *Escherichia coli* and mediated by a plasmid that also coded for resistance to kanamycin, streptomycin, and tetracycline (Tc), although a few plasmids had determinants for chloramphenicol and Tc only (Grant and Dimambro, unpublished data). In this communication, we demonstrate that these plasmids from Ontario salmonella belong to the H_2 subgroup and that they mediate an unusual phenotype of phage inhibition; they inhibit the growth of a number of bacteriophages in a manner phenotypically similar to the way plasmid F inhibits phage T7.

The plasmids employed in this study are listed in Table 1. The thermosensitive transfer phenotype of each plasmid was demonstrated by simultaneous overnight matings at 26 and 37°C with an *E. coli* donor and an *E. coli* recipient strain by a method described previously (4). In each case the frequency of recombinants expressed as a fraction of total recipient cells was 500- to 50,000-fold greater at 26°C (10^{-1} to 10^{-4}) than at 37°C (10^{-5} to 10^{-8}). This kind of thermosensitive transfer is characteristic of H plasmids (6).

Since the chloramphenicol resistance plasmids from Ontario all exhibit a similar thermosensitivity of transfer, incompatibility experiments were performed between a single member of the Ontario sample, a Tc-sensitive segregant of pAS251-2, pAS251-2Tc$^-$, obtained by mutagenesis with ethyl methane sulfonate, and a standard H plasmid, R27 (Tc$^+$) (5). Transfers were performed in both directions, and the segregation of plasmids from doubly R$^+$ clones was monitored during the growth of the recombinants in nonselective medium. The H_1 standard plasmid and pAS251-2Tc$^-$ were found to be incompatible. The absence of incompatibility with plasmid F places the Ontario H plasmid in the H_2 subgroup.

We have screened for the phage inhibition phenotype with nine different bacteriophages (Table 2). Titrations were performed concurrently with R$^+$ and R$^-$ cells, using three different hosts, namely, two *E. coli* K-12 derivatives and one *E. coli* C strain. All of the H_2 but none of the H_1 subgroup plasmids express the "phage reduction" phenotype. The lambdoid phages $\phi80$ and $\phi21$ show the greatest reduction in the

TABLE 1. *H plasmids employed in this study*

Plasmid designation	Resistance pattern[a]	Subgroup	Original host	Place and data of origin	Source[b]
pSD12	Cm Tc	H_2	*Salmonella typhimurium*	Canada, 1974	OPHL
pSD50	Cm Tc	H_2	*S. typhimurium*	Canada, 1974	OPHL
pSD32	Cm Ka Sm Tc	H_2	*S. typhimurium*	Canada, 1974	OPHL
pSD62	Cm Ka Sm Tc	H_2	*S. typhimurium*	Canada, 1974	OPHL
pSD88	Cm Ka Sm Tc	H_2	*S. typhimurium*	Canada, 1974	OPHL
pSD114	Cm Ka Sm Tc	H_2	*S. anatum*	Canada, 1974	OPHL
pAS251-2	Cm Ka Sm Tc	H_2	*S. typhimurium*	Canada, 1974	HSC
pRG1241	Cm Sm Sp Su Tc	H_1	*S. typhi*	Mexico, 1972	H.W.S.
pRG1252	Cm Sm Sp Su Tc	H_1	*S. typhi*	Vietnam, 1972	H.W.S.
R27	Tc	H_1	*S. typhimurium*	England, 1961	N.D.

[a] Cm, Chloramphenicol; Ka, kanamycin; Sm, streptomycin; Sp, spectinomycin; Su, sulfonamide; Tc, tetracycline.

[b] OPHL, Ontario Public Health Laboratory; HSC, The Hospital for Sick Children, Toronto; H.W.S., H. Williams Smith; N.D., N. Datta.

TABLE 2. *Effect of H_2 plasmids on bacteriophage infection of host*

Phage	Relative EOP (R^+/R^-)	Plaque morphology
λ[a]	10^{-4}	Pinpoint
φ80	10^{-5}	Pinpoint
21	10^{-5}	Pinpoint
P2	10^{-1}–10^{-4}[b]	Pinpoint
T1	10^{-1}	Small center, small halo
T7	10^{-1}	Small, no halo
T4	1	Normal
P1	1	Normal

[a] λ*vir*; λ*cI*.

[b] Varies with host strain.

efficiency of plating (EOP), whereas phages T4 and P1 are unaffected. The phage reduction effect, however, is not the usual restriction and modification phenomenon encountered in plasmids of both *fi*$^+$ and *fi*$^-$ specificities (9), since lysates of the inhibited phages prepared from confluent lysis plates of R^+ cells do not overcome the restriction. The phages do not become modified or adapted to the R^+ host.

When λ infection in R^+ and R^- hosts was compared, adsorption was normal in both hosts, 65 to 80% after 5 min starting with 10^6 phage and 5×10^7 cells/ml, the unadsorbed particles being measured after centrifugation of the infected cells. One-step growth experiments with anti-λ serum showed that abortive infection occurred in 90 to 95% of phage-infected R^+ cells, whereas 5 to 10% had a normal latent period (45 min) and burst size (about 100 plaque-forming units). To investigate the possibility that the cells that had a normal burst of phage had lost their plasmid before being infected, MacConkey plates were inoculated with R^+ cells immediately prior to phage infection. The colonies were subsequently replica plated to a medium that contained 16 μg of chloramphenicol per ml, and it was determined that none of the 1,000 colonies tested had lost the plasmid.

The H_2 plasmids reduce the EOP of T7 by 10-fold and change the plaque size, producing an effect resembling that of a particular mutant of the F factor (2). In addition, unlike the F factor, they markedly reduce the EOP of lambdoid phages. The defect is not in adsorption, but in some other stage of infection. One *fi*$^-$ R factor has been described that inhibits the growth of T1 and λ by a mechanism thought to be restriction without modification (12, 13). Further studies are required to determine whether the H_2 phage reduction phenomenon depends on the restriction of phage deoxyribonucleic acid without modification, permeability effects, or some other unrelated mechanism. Whatever the mechanism, the phage reduction function provides a valuable genetic marker for H_2 plasmids. Together with thermosensitivity of transfer it serves to identify preliminarily this important group of resistance plasmids found in salmonella.

We thank Aina Shapley for technical assistance, S. Toma and H. Lior of the Ontario Public Health Laboratory for salmonella strains, C. Fuerst for anti-λ serum and phage 21, and H. Williams Smith and N. Datta for plasmids.

Diane E. Taylor is a recipient of a postdoctoral fellowship from the Medical Research Council of Canada.

LITERATURE CITED

1. **Anderson, E. S.** 1975. The problem and implications of chloramphenicol resistance in the typhoid bacillus. J. Hyg. 74:289–299.
2. **Blumberg, D. D., C. T. Mabie, and M. H. Malamy.** 1976. T7 protein synthesis in F-factor-containing

cells: evidence for an episomally induced impairment of translation and its relation to an alteration in membrane permeability. J. Virol. 17:94-105.
3. **Butler, T., N. N. Linh, K. Arnold, and M. Pollack.** 1973. Chloramphenicol-resistant typhoid fever in Vietnam associated with R factor. Lancet ii:983-985.
4. **Coetzee, J. N., N. Datta, and R. W. Hedges.** 1972. R factors from *Proteus rettgeri*. J. Gen. Microbiol. 72:543-552.
5. **Datta, N.** 1975. Epidemiology and classification of plasmids, p. 9-15. *In* D. Schlessinger (ed.), Microbiology—1974. American Society for Microbiology, Washington, D.C.
6. **Grindley, N. D. F., J. N. Grindley, and E. S. Anderson.** 1972. R factor compatibility groups. Mol. Gen. Genet. 119:287-297.
7. **Olarte, J., and E. Galindo.** 1973. *Salmonella typhi* resistant to chloramphenicol, ampicillin, and other antimicrobial agents: strains isolated during an extensive typhoid fever epidemic in Mexico. Antimicrob. Agents Chemother. 4:597-601.
8. **Paniker, C. K. J., and K. N. Vimala.** 1972. Transferable chloramphenicol resistance in *Salmonella typhi*. Nature (London) 239:109-110.
9. **Roulland-Dussois, D., R. Yoshimori, P. Greene, and M. Betlach, H. M. Goodman, and H. W. Boyer.** 1975. F factor-controlled restriction and modification of deoxyribonucleic acid, p. 187-198. *In* D. Schlessinger (ed.), Microbiology—1974. American Society for Microbiology, Washington, D.C.
10. **Smith, H. R., N. D. F. Grindley, G. W. Humphreys, and E. S. Anderson.** 1973. Interaction of group H resistance factors with the F factor. J. Bacteriol. 115:623-628.
11. **Smith, H. W.** 1974. Thermosensitive transfer factors in chloramphenicol-resistant strains of *Salmonella typhi*. Lancet ii:281-282.
12. **Watanabe, T., H. Nishida, C. Ogata, T. Arai, and S. Sato.** 1964. Episome-mediated transfer of drug resistance in Enterobacteriaceae. VII. Two types of naturally occurring R factors. J. Bacteriol. 88:716-726.
13. **Watanabe, T., T. Takano, T. Arai, H. Nishida, and S. Sato.** 1966. Episome-mediated transfer of drug resistance in *Enterobacteriaceae*. X. Restriction and modification of phages by *fi*$^-$ R factors. J. Bacteriol. 92:477-486.

ANTIMICROBIAL AGENTS AND CHEMOTHERAPY, Oct. 1976, p. 765-767
Copyright © 1976 American Society for Microbiology
Vol. 10, No. 4
Printed in U.S.A.

Correlation of Resistance to Proflavine and Penicillin in *Escherichia coli*

ROBIN C. McKELLAR, COLIN N. McKENZIE, AND DONN J. KUSHNER*
Department of Biology, University of Ottawa, Ottawa, Ontario, Canada K1N 6N5

Received for publication 6 April 1976

A number of proflavine (PF)-resistant mutants of *Escherichia coli* B were also resistant to penicillin and cephalothin. Mutants resistant to 1.0 mM PF were 10 times more penicillin resistant than were the PF-susceptible, wild-type cells. Single-step mutants selected for resistance to either PF or penicillin were also resistant to the other drug. None of the resistant mutants tested possessed β-lactamase activity. These results suggest that resistance to PF and penicillin in *E. coli* B may be due to permeability changes in the cell envelope.

The role of permeability in bacterial resistance to acridine dyes is uncertain. Earlier reports associated resistance of different strains of *Escherichia coli* to proflavine (PF) and acriflavine (AF) with decreased dye uptake (1, 5, 6, 14, 20, 21, 25). The fact, however, that resistant cells can actively expel acridines has complicated interpretations of experiments based on uptake alone (7, 14).

Work in our laboratory previously suggested that resistance occurred at the metabolic level, since glucose metabolism was inhibited by PF in susceptible but not in resistant *E. coli* (10). It was since found that pyruvate kinase I may be the site of inhibition of glycolysis by PF in sensitive cells. However, purified pyruvate kinase I from susceptible and resistant cells was equally susceptible to PF (unpublished data). These results suggest again that permeability is involved in PF resistance, at least in the sense that some PF-sensitive site(s) may be shielded from the drug by cell structures.

Permeability changes have been implicated as the basis of cross-resistance between unrelated inhibitors. AF resistance due to permeability barriers has been associated with resistance to methanol and thiabendazole in *Dictyostelium discoideum* (24) as well as with resistance to phenethyl alcohol and sodium dodecyl sulfate in *E. coli* (12).

Acridine orange resistance was associated with resistance to penicillin, erythromycin, chloramphenicol, rifampin, and ethidium bromide in *Neisseria gonorrhoeae* (8).

We report here a study of the relation between resistance to PF and penicillin in a number of strains of *E. coli*.

Strains resistant to 1.0 mM PF were isolated from *E. coli* B after growth in Trypticase soy broth (TSB; Baltimore Biological Laboratory [BBL], Cockeysville, Md.) containing successively 0.02, 0.10, 0.20, 0.50, and 1.0 mM PF as previously described (7). Strains resistant to 0.1 mM PF were isolated from Trypticase soy agar (TSA [TSB plus 1.5% agar]; Difco Laboratories, Detroit, Mich.) containing 0.1 mM PF that had been heavily inoculated with *E. coli* B. For these and other experiments, inocula consisted of overnight cultures grown in TSB at 37°C.

Several 1.0 mM PF-resistant strains were exposed to a variety of antibiotics (obtained from BBL and Difco) on TSA plates containing 4 to 5 antibiotic disks/plate. After incubation, susceptibility or resistance was measured as the width of the clear zone surrounding the disk.

All PF-resistant strains exhibited increased resistance to penicillin, cephalothin, and, to a lesser extent, ampicillin (Table 1). PF-susceptible and -resistant strains were equally susceptible to most of the other antibiotics.

To determine the level of PF-associated penicillin resistance, individual strains were inoculated into tubes containing 10 ml of TSB and different concentrations of penicillin. After incubation, growth was measured as absorbance at 660 nm in a Coleman Jr. spectrophotometer. After 24 h, strains resistant to 1.0 mM PF displayed a 10-fold increase in the minimal inhibitory concentration (that is, the lowest concentration completely preventing growth) of penicillin (from 15 to 150 U/ml), whereas those resistant to 0.1 mM PF possessed intermediate levels of penicillin resistance (Fig. 1). These measurements do not distinguish between killing and growth inhibition by penicillin. After 44 h, further growth had taken place in some tubes, but the same pattern still held (minimal inhibitory concentrations, 25 U of penicillin per

TABLE 1. *Susceptibility of PF-resistant strains of E. coli B to antibiotics*[a]

Antibiotic (amt/disk)	Width of clear zone (mm)				
	B[b]	B/Pr	PrA	PrB	PrC
Penicillin, 10 U	2.33 ± 0.11 (6)	0 (7)	0 (4)	0 (4)	0 (4)
Cephalothin, 30 μg	6.58 ± 0.08 (3)	1.00 ± 0.14 (3)	0 (5)	1.20 ± 0.09 (5)	1.50 ± 0.35 (4)
Ampicillin 10 μg	8.33 ± 0.17 (3)	3.63 ± 0.13 (2)	3.0 ± 0.20 (4)	4.90 ± 0.19 (5)	4.75 ± 0.14 (4)
Carbenicillin, 100 μg	10.83 ± 0.17 (3)	4.25 ± 0.10 (4)	7.25 ± 0.14 (4)	6.70 ± 0.12 (5)	6.91 ± 0.15 (6)
Chloramphenicol, 5 μg	2.95 ± 0.10 (6)	0 (6)	2.25 ± 0.14 (4)	1.50 ± 0 (4)	2.63 ± 0.24 (4)
Tetracycline, 30 μg	3.19 ± 0.18 (9)	2.63 ± 0.25 (9)	2.25 ± 0.14 (4)	1.10 ± 0.16 (4)	1.00 ± 0 (4)
Streptomycin, 10 μg	1.60 ± 0.10 (5)	1.75 ± 0.30 (4)	2.00 ± 0.35 (4)	0.67 ± 0.17 (3)	2.63 ± 0.13 (5)
Rifampin, 10 μg	2.50 ± 0 (2)	0.88 ± 0.13 (2)	1.60 ± 0.10 (5)	1.62 ± 0.13 (4)	1.38 ± 0.24 (4)
Gentamicin, 10 μg	1.58 ± 0.08 (3)	1.80 ± 0.17 (3)	NT	NT	NT
Nitrofurodantin, 30 μg	5.80 ± 0.08 (3)	6.00 ± 0.22 (3)	NT	NT	NT
Neomycin, 10 μg	1.50 ± 0 (5)	2.20 ± 0.17 (3)	NT	NT	NT
Septra, 10 μg	4.83 ± 0.17 (3)	3.17 ± 0.73 (3)	NT	NT	NT
Nalidixic acid, 30 μg	4.25 ± 0.14 (3)	4.83 ± 0.17 (3)	NT	NT	NT
Colistin, 10 μg	2.50 ± 0 (3)	3.30 ± 0.08 (3)	NT	NT	NT

[a] Strain B is PF susceptible, and the others are resistant to 1.0 mM PF. Values are presented with standard errors. Bracketed figures represent the number of determinations. NT, Not tested.
[b] Strain.

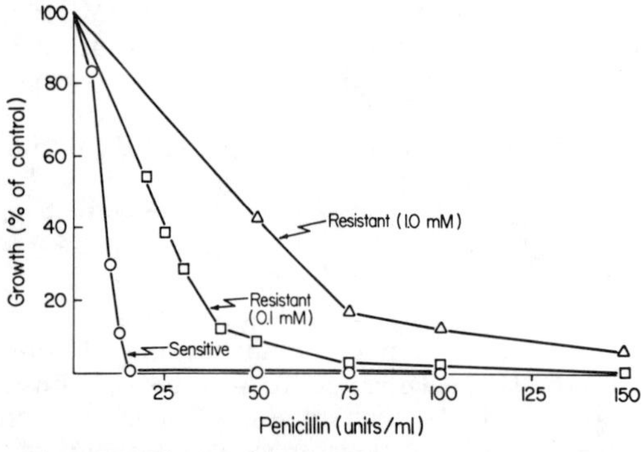

FIG. 1. *Effect of penicillin concentration on growth of PF-susceptible and -resistant E. coli B. Cells were grown in 10 ml of TSB at 37°C for 24 h. Growth was determined as absorbance at 660 nm. One hundred percent growth corresponded to an absorbance of 0.80 at 660 nm.*

ml for the PF-susceptible strain and 300 U/ml for the strain resistant to 1.0 mM PF).

Correlation between PF and penicillin resistance was also studied by replica plating. When 55 colonies of *E. coli* B on TSA not previously exposed to either drug were transferred to a TSA plate containing 25 U of penicillin per ml, no colonies appeared. A similar transfer to TSA containing 0.1 mM PF produced two colonies. Thirteen penicillin-resistant colonies were obtained by spreading 0.5 ml of an overnight culture of *E. coli* B on plates containing 25 U of penicillin per ml and incubating a further 24 h. Twelve of the 13 penicillin-resistant colonies were PF resistant. In a separate experiment 64 PF (0.1 mM)-resistant colonies were obtained in a similar fashion; 54 of these were also resistant to penicillin.

Penicillin resistance is often due to the production of β-lactamase enzymes by resistant bacteria (3, 9, 18); however, in some cases, resistance may result from changes in cell envelope permeability associated with modifications of the lipopolysaccharide layer of the cell wall (2, 11, 15, 16, 19, 22, 23). Such "intrinsic" resistance (29) may occur in cells that lack β-lactamase activity (3).

Three strains resistant to 1.0 mM PF were tested for β-lactamase activity (17). Cells were grown to early log phase in 0.5% glucose mineral salts media (7) at 37°C. In some experiments, penicillin was added to a final concentration of 25 U/ml, and growth was allowed to continue for a further 3 h. PF-susceptible cells lysed within 30 min of penicillin addition, whereas the growth of PF-resistant cells was unaffected by the antibiotic. None of the PF-resistant strains possessed β-lactamase activity, as measured in whole cultures, either untreated or broken by ultrasonic treatment, after growth in the presence or absence of penicillin.

It seems likely from these results that penicillin resistance in *E. coli* B is intrinsic. Since penicillin resistance seems well correlated with PF resistance, we suggest that both phenomena may be caused by permeability changes in the cell envelope.

The study of PF resistance in *E. coli* B/Pr has been complicated by the diversity of binding sites available to PF (4) as well as by the energy-dependent release of bound dye (7, 14). Gross permeability differences to PF do not exist between PF-susceptible and -resistant strains of *E. coli* B (4, 7). It is possible, however, that subtle permeability changes have taken place that are not detectable in PF-binding studies. Nakamura has shown that AF-susceptible and -resistant *E. coli* K-12 bind similar amounts of PF (13), in spite of the fact that AF-resistant cell membranes lack a specific structural protein involved in AF uptake and binding (14).

It now seems possible that *E. coli* mutants selected for resistance to either PF or penicillin have undergone changes in an envelope component(s) that make them resistant to both drugs.

This work was supported by a grant to D. J. Kushner from the National Research Council of Canada.

LITERATURE CITED

1. **Barabas, G., B. M. Mehta, and D. J. Kushner.** 1970. Proflavine binding and release by sensitive and resistant *Bacillus subtilis*. Can. J. Microbiol. **16**:973–981.
2. **Barrett, E., and A. W. Asscher.** 1972. Action of ethylenediamine tetraacetic acid (EDTA) on carbenicillin-resistant strains of *Pseudomonas aeruginosa*. J. Med. Microbiol. 5:355–359.
3. **Citri, N.** 1971. Penicillinase and other β-lactamases, p. 23–46. *In* P. D. Boyer (ed.), The enzymes, vol. 4. Academic Press Inc., New York.
4. **Gravelle, M. J., B. M. Mehta, and D. J. Kushner.** 1972. The elusive permeability barriers and binding sites for proflavine in *Escherichia coli*. Antimicrob. Agents Chemother. **1**:470–475.
5. **Hessler, A. Y.** 1965. Acridine resistance in bacteriophage T2H as a function of dye penetration measured by mutagenesis and photoinactivation. Genetics **52**:711–722.
6. **Kohno, T., and J. R. Roth.** 1974. Proflavine mutagenesis of bacteria. J. Mol. Biol. **89**:17–32.
7. **Kushner, D. J., and S. R. Khan.** 1968. Proflavine uptake and release in sensitive and resistant *Escherichia coli*. J. Bacteriol. **96**:1103–1114.
8. **Maness, M. J., and P. F. Sparling.** 1973. Multiple antibiotic resistance due to a single mutation in *Neisseria gonorrhoeae*. J. Infect. Dis. **128**:321–330.
9. **Massari, S., P. Dell' Antone, R. Colonna, and G. F. Azzone.** Mechanism of atebrin fluorescence changes in energized submitochondrial particles. Biochemistry **13**:1038–1043.
10. **Mehta, B. M., M. J. Gravelle, and D. J. Kushner.** 1973. Effects of energy metabolism on the release of bound proflavine from sensitive and resistant *Escherichia coli*. Antimicrob. Agents Chemother. **4**:332–336.
11. **Monner, D. A., S. Jonsson, and H. G. Boman.** 1971. Ampicillin-resistant mutants of *Escherichia coli* K-12 with lipopolysaccharide alterations affecting mating ability and susceptibility to sex-specific bacteriophages. J. Bacteriol. **107**:420–432.
12. **Nakamura, H.** 1968. Genetic determination of resistance to acriflavine, phenethyl alcohol, and sodium dodecyl sulfate in *Escherichia coli*. J. Bacteriol. **96**:987–996.
13. **Nakamura, H.** 1974. Plasmid-instability in Acr A mutants of *Escherichia coli* K-12. J. Gen. Microbiol. **84**:85–93.
14. **Nakamura, H., and A. Suganuma.** 1972. Membrane mutation associated with sensitivity to acriflavine in *Escherichia coli*. J. Bacteriol. **110**:329–335.
15. **Nelson, B. W., and R. J. Roantree.** 1967. Analysis of lipopolysaccharides extracted from penicillin-resistant, serum-sensitive *Salmonella* mutants. J. Gen. Microbiol. **48**:179–188.
16. **Nordström, K., L. G. Burman, and K. G. Eriksson-Grennberg.** 1970. Resistance of *Escherichia coli* to penicillins. VIII. Physiology of a class II ampicillin-resistant mutant. J. Bacteriol. **101**:659–668.
17. **Novick, R. P.** 1962. Micro-iodometric assay for penicillinase. Biochem. J. **83**:236–240.
18. **Richmond, M. H., G. W. Jack, and R. B. Sykes.** 1971. The β-lactamases of gram-negative bacteria including *Pseudomonads*. Ann. N.Y. Acad. Sci. **182**:243–257.
19. **Richmond, M. H., and R. B. Sykes.** 1973. The β-lactamases of gram negative bacteria and their possible physiological role. Adv. Microb. Physiol. **9**:31–88.
20. **Silver, S.** 1965. Acriflavine resistance: a bacteriophage mutation affecting the uptake of dye by the infected bacterial cells. Proc. Natl. Acad. Sci. U.S.A. **53**:24–30.
21. **Silver, S., E. Levine, and P. M. Spielman.** 1968. Acridine binding by *Escherichia coli*: pH dependency and strain differences. J. Bacteriol. **95**:333–339.
22. **Suginaka, H., A. Ichikawa, and S. Kotani.** 1974. Penicillin-resistant mechanisms in *Pseudomonas aeruginosa:* effects of penicillin G and carbenicillin on transpeptidase and D-alanine carboxypeptidase activities. Antimicrob. Agents Chemother. **6**:672–675.
23. **Weiser, R., A. W. Asscher, and J. Wimpenny.** 1968. In vitro reversal of antibiotic resistance by ethylenediamine tetraacetic acid. Nature (London) **219**:1365–1366.
24. **Williams, K. L., R. H. Kessin, and P. C. Newell.** 1974. Parasexual genetics in *Dictyostelium discoideum*: mitotic analysis of acriflavine resistance and growth in axenic medium. J. Gen. Biol. **84**:59–69.
25. **Woods, D. R., V. R. Schauder, and P. B. Waddington.** 1973. Acriflavine uptake and resistance in *Serratia marcescens* cells and spheroplasts. J. Bacteriol. **114**:59–64.

ANTIMICROBIAL AGENTS AND CHEMOTHERAPY, Oct. 1976, p. 768-769
Vol. 10, No. 4

In Vitro Comparison of Gentamicin, Tobramycin, Sisomicin, and Netilmicin

K. N. BROWN,* J. BENEDICTSON, AND S. SWANBY

Department of Laboratories, Foothills Hospital, Calgary, Alberta, T2N 2T9 Canada

Received for publication 6 July 1976

The antimicrobial activity of gentamicin, tobramycin, sisomicin, and netilmicin (Sch 20569) was compared against 150 strains of organisms. Netilmicin was shown to be the least effective against *Pseudomonas* strains but to have slightly better activity against *Staphylococcus aureus* and *Escherichia coli* than the other agents. The effect of calcium and magnesium in enhancing the differences in activity of these aminoglycosides against *Pseudomonas* strains was also demonstrated.

This study was carried out to compare the in vitro antibacterial activity of four aminoglycoside antibiotics, gentamicin, tobramycin, sisomicin, and netilmicin (Sch 20569), against 148 clinical isolates and two control strains. There were 50 strains each of *Pseudomonas aeruginosa*, *Staphylococcus aureus*, and *Escherichia coli*. The control organisms used were *P. aeruginosa* ATCC 27853 and *E. coli* ATCC 25922.

Minimum inhibitory concentrations (MICs) were determined in the conventional manner in three types of broth: (i) brain heart infusion broth (BHI; BBL 11063) with added calcium and magnesium to provide levels of 75 and 20 mg/liter, respectively; (ii) BHI broth (BBL 11063) unmodified (calcium and magnesium levels were 36 and 14 mg/liter, respectively); and (iii) tryptone broth (Oxord L42). A medium control with no antibiotic added was provided for each organism tested to assure viability, and medium controls with no antibiotic and no organism were also used to assure sterility of the medium. Type (i) broth was used for *Pseudomonas* strains, type (ii) was used for *E. coli* strains, and type (iii) was used for *S. aureus* strains.

Each tube, other than the medium controls, was inoculated with approximately 10^4 colony-forming units of the organism under test.

The results of the MICs of the four antibiotics against these groups of organisms are shown in Fig. 1 (*P. aeruginosa*), Fig. 2 (*S. aureus*), and Fig. 3 (*E. coli*). These illustrate the relationship between MICs and cumulative percentages of strains inhibited.

The most pronounced differences are shown with regard to *P. aeruginosa* (Fig. 1). At the concentration inhibiting 50% of the strains, the MIC of tobramycin was 0.48 μg/ml and that of netilmicin (Sch 20569) was 3.6 μg/ml, whereas gentamicin and sisomicin were almost inseparable at 1.35 and 1.45 μg/ml, respectively. In effect, therefore, a sevenfold difference in activity between tobramycin and netilmicin was demonstrable against this group of *Pseudomonas* strains isolated using BHI broth with added calcium and magnesium.

Figure 2, however, illustrates the converse, in that for the group of staphylococcal isolates tested, the 50% inhibition level was 0.01 μg of netilmicin (Sch 20569) and 0.03 μg of tobramicin per ml, indicating a threefold difference in activity, but in this instance with netilmicin showing the advantage. Gentamicin and sisomicin occupied intermediate positions in their activity.

Netilmicin (Sch 20569) also showed an increase in activity compared with the other aminoglycosides tested against the group of *E. coli* strains, although this difference was less marked. This is shown in Fig. 3. The MICs of netilmicin (Sch 20569) and gentamicin at the 50% inhibition level were 3 and 5 μg/ml, respectively, with tobramycin and sisomicin occupying intermediate positions. These results obtained with gentamicin, tobramycin, and sisomicin are in accord with the work of other investigators who have evaluated these aminoglycosides (1, 2, 5, 6).

Sixteen strains of *P. aeruginosa* were selected from a group of 50. These represented eight gentamicin-susceptible strains and eight gentamicin-resistant strains. These were tested for their MICs to gentamicin, tobramycin, sisomycin, and netilmicin as before, but without added calcium and magnesium in the BHI broth. Therefore, the calcium and magnesium levels were 36 and 14 mg/liter, respectively. For the 16 strains tested, it was demonstrated that

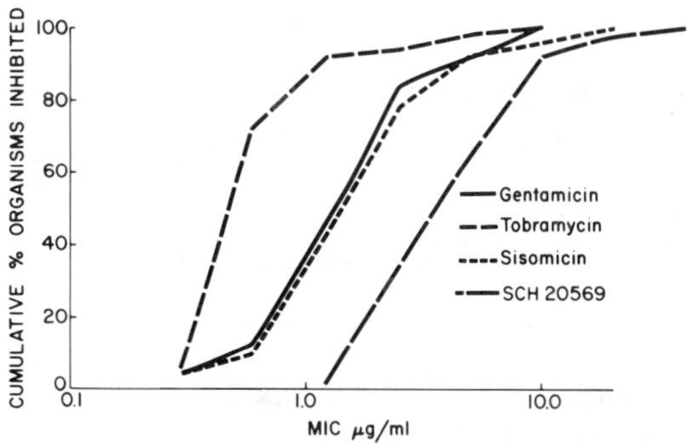

FIG. 1. *MICs of the four antibiotics against P. aeruginosa strains.*

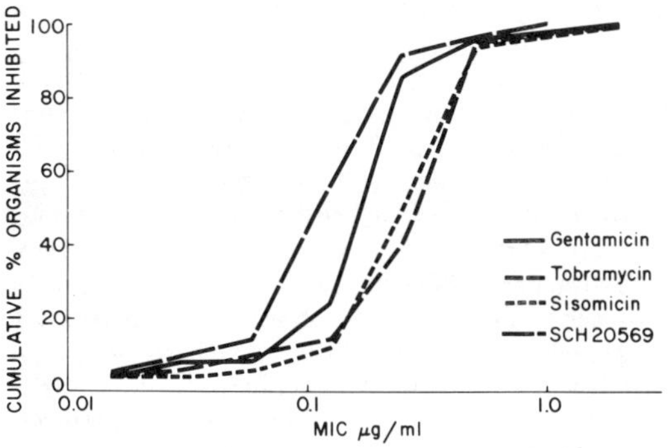

FIG. 2. *MICs of the four antibiotics against S. aureus strains.*

at the 50% inhibition level the MIC range of tobramycin and netilmicin was increased from 0.42 to 1.5 μg/ml without calcium and magnesium to 0.42 to 5.8 μg/ml with added calcium and magnesium. Therefore, the addition of calcium and magnesium apparently increased the differences in activity between tobramycin and netilmicin from three- to sevenfold.

Differences in MICs of gentamicin against *P. aeruginosa* strains have been related to calcium and magnesium concentrations by other workers (3, 4). Our work demonstrates that the addition of calcium and magnesium to BHI broth increased the apparent differences in activity of the antimicrobials tested.

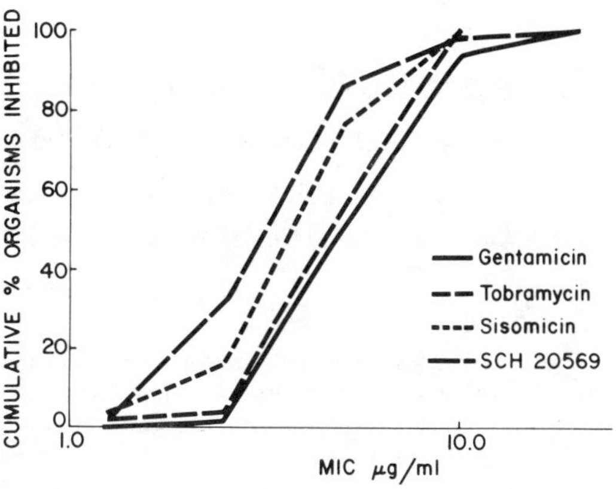

FIG. 3. *MICs of the four antibiotics against E. coli.*

We would like to thank Schering Corporation Limited for their help in furnishing us with quantities of netilmicin (Sch 20569).

LITERATURE CITED

1. **Crowe, C. C., and E. Sanders.** 1973. Sisomicin: evaluation in vitro and comparison with gentamicin and tobramycin. Antimicrob. Agents Chemother. 3:24–38.
2. **Duncan, I. B. R., and J. L. Penner.** 1975. Comparative activity of tobramycin and gentamicin against Pseudomonas, Proteus and Providencia species. Can. Med. Assoc. J. 113:29–31.
3. **Garrod, L. P., and P. M. Waterworth.** 1969. Effect of medium composition on the apparent sensitivity of P. aeruginosa to gentamicin. J. Clin. Pathol. 22:534–538.
4. **Gilbert, D. N., E. Kutscher, P. Ireland, J. A. Barnett, and J. P. Sanford.** 1971. Effect of concentrations of magnesium and calcium on the in-vitro susceptibility of P. aeruginosa to gentamicin. J. Infect. Dis. 124 (Suppl):37–45.
5. **Ries, K., M. E. Levison, and D. Kaye.** 1973. In vitro evaluation of a new aminoglycoside derivative of kanamycin: a comparison with tobramycin and gentamicin. Antimicrob. Agents Chemother. 3:532–533.
6. **Waitz, J. A., E. L. Moss, Jr., C. G. Drabe, and M. J. Weinstein.** 1972. Comparative activity of sisomicin, gentamicin, kanamycin, and tobramycin. Antimicrob. Agents Chemother. 2:431–437.

ANTIMICROBIAL AGENTS AND CHEMOTHERAPY, Oct. 1976, p. 770–772 Vol. 10, No. 4

Therapeutic Effects of Small-Particle Aerosols of Ribavirin on Parainfluenza (Sendai) Virus Infections of Mice

E. W. LARSON,* E. L. STEPHEN, AND J. S. WALKER[1]

United States Army Medical Research Institute of Infectious Diseases, Frederick, Maryland 21701

Received for publication 26 April 1976

Small-particle aerosol administration of ribavirin (1-β-D-ribofuranosyl-1,2,4-triazole-3-carboxamide) increased survival rates, extended the time to death, delayed lung pathology, and reduced pulmonary virus levels in Sendai virus-infected mice.

Infections with the parainfluenza viruses have been reported as a frequent cause of laryngotracheobronchitis in humans, with evidence that these infections account for at least one-third of the cases of croup in children (4). Parainfluenza viruses, types 1 and 2, have been identified most frequently in croup. Parainfluenza virus, type 1 (Sendai), is associated with naturally occurring respiratory infections of mice (5). The pathogenesis of these infections has been described (1, 6, 11). The disease process of Sendai virus infections in rodents closely parallels that seen with parainfluenza in children, and the rodent-Sendai system has been suggested as a suitable animal model for the study of the acute respiratory infections caused by parainfluenza in humans (3, 10).

Ribavirin (1-β-D-ribofuranosyl-1-2,4-triazole-3-carboxamide) has been shown to exhibit antiviral properties against parainfluenza virus types 1 and 3 in vitro (2, 7) and to be therapeutically effective in the treatment of type 1 (Sendai) infections in mice when the drug was administered intraperitoneally (7). In recent work, ribavirin was highly effective for the treatment of influenza type A infections in animals when administered therapeutically as small-particle aerosols (SPAs) (8, 9, 12). This report describes the therapeutic efficacy of ribavirin given as a SPA to mice infected with a lethal respiratory dose of Sendai virus.

Sendai virus, strain D/Sendai/52, was obtained from the American Type Culture Collection. Ten serial intranasal passages of the virus in mice yielded a virus isolate which, when propagated in the allantoic cavity of embryonated chicken eggs, was uniformly lethal for 5- to 7-week-old AKR/J mice after SPA challenge. Mice were exposed to aerosols of the mouse-adapted virus in each of three experiments. In each of the first two studies, one-half of the mice served as untreated, infected controls, whereas the remaining mice were treated continuously with ribavirin administered as SPA during the period from 24 through 72 h after virus challenge. The ribavirin was obtained from Nucleic Acid Research Institute of ICN Pharmaceuticals, Inc., Irvine, Calif. With only one continuous aerosol therapy apparatus, it was necessary to perform the third study to provide for an additional control. Again, one-half of the mice were infected and untreated, but the remaining mice were treated from 24 through 72 h with aerosolized, distilled water (the ribavirin diluent) in the continuous therapy apparatus.

The methods used for challenging mice with infectious virus and the procedures for continuous aerosol therapy have been described previously (8, 9). In the ribavirin studies, the concentration of drug in the spray suspension was adjusted to yield an effective, retained aerosol dose of 50 mg of ribavirin per kg (mouse weight) per day or 100 mg/kg in 48 h of treatment.

Three mice from each of the infected, untreated control and treatment groups were necropsied periodically through 10 days postchallenge in each experiment. The Sendai virus concentrations in lung, tracheobronchial and nasopharyngeal tissues were determined for each mouse and the extent of lung consolidation was scored. The methods used to quantitate virus concentrations in mouse respiratory tissues have been described (8). Virus assays were performed in embryonated chicken eggs; tissue virus levels were measured in terms of median egg infectious doses/whole tissue. In one ribavirin experiment, 40 infected controls and 40 treated mice were challenged for observation of death patterns and time-to-death determinations. The same observations were

[1] Present address; Plum Island Animal Disease Center, P. O. Box 948, Greenport, Long Island, NY 11944.

made on groups of 25 mice in the distilled water control study. All survivor mice were observed for a period of 21 days postinfection.

The mean Sendai virus levels in the respective mouse respiratory tissues from both ribavirin experiments are depicted in Fig. 1. The lung virus concentrations in the mice treated with ribavirin were significantly ($P < 0.05$) lower than those in the infected controls for at least 120 h after treatment was discontinued (72 to 192 h). In contrast, virus levels in the tracheobronchial tissues of treated mice were significantly ($P < 0.05$) below those in the infected controls only at 48 and 72 h. In this tissue, therefore, the effect of treatment did not persist, and the virus concentrations of treated mice approached control levels within 24 h after the termination of treatment. Somewhat lower virus concentrations in nasopharyngeal tissues of ribavirin treated mice were not significantly different from those in the infected, untreated control mice at all periods.

Table 1 summarizes the incidence of lung lesions among the treated and control mice as well as the survival and mean time-to-death properties among the mice which were caged separately for those purposes. Because lung lesions were not observed before 6 days and because in neither experiment did any of the untreated mice, which were designated for necropsy, survive beyond 8 days, statistical comparisons of the lung lesion data were not performed. The evidence suggested, however, that lung pathology developed later in the mice that received ribavirin than in the infected controls. Also, the results in Table 1 show the markedly better survival among the treated mice than among the untreated mice and show that the MTD of the mice that died after treatment was nearly 2 days greater than the MTD of those that died without treatment.

Table 2 presents the mean virus concentrations measured in the respiratory tissues of mice in the distilled water control study. Virus levels were very similar between the untreated and water-treated mice regardless of the respiratory tissue or postinfection period considered. Virus titers at 10 days postchallenge were not measured due to a lack of surviving mice. No lung consolidation was seen in the mice which were necropsied through 96 h (4 days) postinfection, but all of the mice in both groups showed 50 to 75% involvement at 168 h (7 days). All of the 25 mice from each group which were held to determine survival properties died. The geometric MTD were 10.1 days and 9.6 days for the with and without water treatments, respec-

TABLE 1. *Lung lesion scores, survival, and mean time-to-death (MTD) properties of AKR mice after small-particle aerosol challenge with lethal doses of Sendai virus*

Parameter	No. of mice with lesions/ total (mean score[a]) Untreated	Treated[b]	P
Lung lesions			
6 days	2/6(2.5)	0/6	ND[c]
8 days	5/5(3.4)	3/6(2.7)	ND
10 days	–[d]	6/6(3.7)	ND
Survivors (21 days), no./total (%)	0/40 (0)	25/39(64)	<0.005[e]
Geometric MTD (days)	8.1	9.8	<0.005[f]

[a] Mice showing lesions/total examined (mean lesion score of positives) based on a scale of 0 to 4 from negative to total consolidation.

[b] Treated continuously with ribavirin as small-particle aerosol from 24 through 72 h.

[c] No statistical test performed.

[d] No surviving mice.

[e] Chi-square test with Yates correction factor.

[f] Unpaired t test.

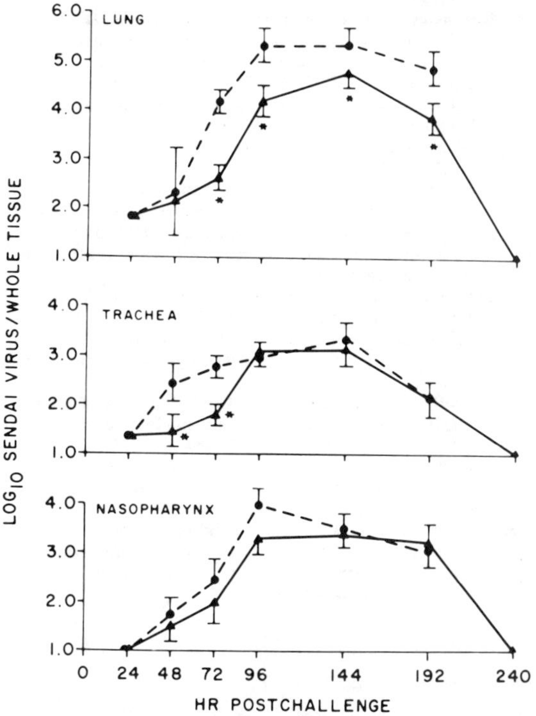

FIG. 1. *Effect of ribavirin continuous aerosol treatment (24 to 72 h) on Sendai virus levels (means and standard errors) in mouse respiratory tissues after lethal small-particle aerosol challenges with mouse-adapted virus. Symbols: ●, untreated; ▲, treated. *, Virus concentration with treatment significantly less than without treatment ($P \leq 0.05$).*

TABLE 2. *Whole tissue concentrations of Sendai virus in the respiratory tract of infected mice with and without distilled water aerosol treatment*

Treatment	Hours postchallenge	Log EID_{50}[a]/whole tissue		
		Lung	Trachea	Nasopharynx
Water[b] treated	48	4.44 (±0.24)[c]	2.76 (±0.36)	3.45 (±0.33)
	96	5.87 (±0.46)	3.77 (±0.04)	4.88 (±0.21)
	168	4.80 (±0.17)	3.22 (±0.08)	4.23 (±0.06)
Untreated	48	3.85 (±0.33)	3.27 (±0.33)	3.27 (±0.43)
	96	5.32 (±0.41)	3.62 (±0.29)	4.10 (±0.32)
	168	4.17 (±0.29)	3.18 (±0.32)	4.06 (±0.41)

[a] EID_{50}, Median egg infectious dose.
[b] Treated continuously with distilled water aerosol from 24 through 72 h.
[c] ± Standard error (n = 3).

tively. These similarities between the control groups were taken as evidence that the results with untreated infected mice in the ribavirin experiments were adequate for control purposes.

In summary, these studies have indicated that ribavirin, when administered as SPA, was therapeutically effective for treating Sendai virus infections of mice. Therapeutic efficacy was demonstrated by increased survival rates, extended times to death, later development of gross lung pathology, and reduction of pulmonary virus concentrations. The effects of ribavirin were similar to those observed in the treatment of type A influenza virus infections (8, 12). Our results suggest that the lung and not the upper respiratory tract may be the important tissue in determining the outcome of Sendai infections in mice. These relatively brief studies have supported the continually accumulating evidence that the aerosol administration of ribavirin represents effective therapy for the management of viral respiratory infections.

LITERATURE CITED

1. **Appell, L. H., R. M. Kovatch, J. M. Reddecliff, and P. J. Gerone.** 1971. Pathogenesis of Sendai virus infection in mice. Am. J. Vet. Res. 32:1835–1841.
2. **Huffman, J. H., R. W. Sidwell, G. P. Khare, J. T. Witkowski, L. B. Allen, and R. K. Robins.** 1973. In vitro effect of 1-β-D-ribofuranosyl-1,2,4-triazole-3-carboxamide (Virazole, ICN 1229) on deoxyribonucleic acid and ribonucleic acid viruses. Antimicrob. Agents Chemother. 3:235–241.
3. **Jakab, G. J., and E. C. Dick.** 1973. Synergistic effect in viral-bacterial infection: combined infection of the murine respiratory tract with Sendai virus and *Pasteurella pneumotropica*. Infect. Immun. 8:762–768.
4. **Knight, V.** 1973. Parainfluenza viruses, p. 125–130. *In* V. Knight (ed.), Viral and mycoplasmal infections of the respiratory tract. Lea and Febiger, Philadelphia.
5. **Parker, J. C., and R. K. Reynolds.** 1968. Natural history of Sendai virus infection in mice. Am. J. Epidemiol. 88:112–125.
6. **Robinson, T. W. E., R. J. R. Cureton, and R. B. Heath.** 1968. The pathogenesis of Sendai virus infection in the mouse lung. J. Med. Microbiol. 1:89–95.
7. **Sidwell, R. W., J. H. Huffman, G. P. Khare, L. B. Allen, J. T. Witkowski, and R. K. Robins.** 1972. Broad-spectrum antiviral activity of Virazole: 1-β-D-ribofuranosyl-1,2,4-triazole-3-carboxamide. Science 177:705–706.
8. **Stephen, E. L., J. W. Dominik, J. B. Moe, R. O. Spertzel, and J. S. Walker.** 1975. Treatment of influenza infection of mice by using rimantadine hydrochlorides by the aerosol and intraperitoneal routes. Antimicrob. Agents Chemother. 8:154–158.
9. **Stephen, E. L., J. S. Walker, J. W. Dominik, H. W. Young, and R. F. Berendt.** 1976. Aerosol therapy of influenza infections of mice and primates with rimantadine, ribavirin and related compounds. Ann. N. Y. Acad. Sci., in press.
10. **Tyrrell, D. A. J., and C. R. Coid.** 1970. Sendai virus infection of rats as a convenient model of acute respiratory infection. Vet. Rec. 86:164–165.
11. **van Nunen, M. C. J., and J. van der Veen.** 1968. Experimental infection with Sendai virus in mice. Arch. Gesamte Virusforsch. 22:388–397.
12. **Walker, J. S., E. L. Stephen, and R. O. Spertzel.** 1976. Small-particle aerosols of antiviral compounds in treatment of type A influenza pneumonia in mice. J. Infect. Dis. 133:A140–A144.

Antimicrobial Agents and Chemotherapy, Oct. 1976, p. 773-775 Vol. 10, No. 4

Printed in U.S.A.

Josamycin and Rosamicin: In Vitro Comparisons with Erythromycin and Clindamycin

SMITH SHADOMY,* MARGARET TIPPLE, and LARRY PAXTON

Department of Medicine, Medical College of Virginia, Virginia Commonwealth University, Richmond, Virginia 23298

Received for publication 10 May 1976

The macrolide antibiotics josamycin and rosamicin were compared in vitro with erythromycin for activity against *Staphylococcus aureus*, *S. epidermidis*, and enterococci and with clindamycin for activity against a variety of anaerobic organisms. Rosamicin and erythromycin were similar in activity and superior to josamycin against aerobic cocci. Most isolates of *S. aureus* (96%), *S. epidermidis* (79%), and the enterococci (87%) were inhibited by 1.56 μg of either of the new macrolide compounds per ml. Clindamycin was the most active compound against the anaerobic organisms.

Josamycin and rosamicin are macrolide antibiotics presently under clinical investigation in this country. Both compounds reportedly are effective in vitro, at physiological pH's, against most gram-positive aerobic cocci, including some resistant to erythromycin. Additionally, both have demonstrated in vitro activity against a variety of anaerobic species (7).

These studies were undertaken to test the in vitro activities of josamycin and rosamicin against a variety of clinical isolates of aerobic gram-positive cocci and to compare these activities with those of another currently available macrolide antibiotic, erythromycin. Studies also were conducted in which these two macrolides were tested against a number of isolates of anaerobic organisms. In these latter studies, josamycin and rosamicin were compared with clindamycin.

Aerobic gram-positive cocci were obtained from specimens submitted to the Clinical Laboratories, Medical College of Virginia Hospitals, during 1975. Identifications were verified by using standard techniques (5). Aerobic gram-positive cocci included: *Staphylococcus aureus*, 48 isolates; *S. epidermidis*, 34 isolates; and enterococci, 39 isolates.

A variety of anaerobes were tested. These included: *Bacteroides fragilis*, 42 isolates; other gram-negative rods including *Bacteroides* spp. and *Fusobacterium* spp., 7 isolates; and 15 isolates of gram-positive organisms including *Peptococcus* spp., *Propionobacter* spp., *Clostridium* spp., and *Actinomyces* spp. Some of the anaerobic organisms were obtained from the American Type Culture Collection, Rockville, Md. Others came from the laboratories of Virginia Polytechnic Institute and State University of Blacksburg, Va., and the Wilmington Medical Center, Wilmington, Del.

Drug minimal inhibitory concentrations (MICs) for all organisms were determined by using the ICS agar dilution technique (2), unmodified for testing with aerobes and modified for anaerobic incubation to permit testing with anaerobes.

Aerobes were tested against josamycin (EN-141, Endo Laboratories lot no. JC526), rosamicin (drug number 14,947, Schering Laboratories, batch no. 5533-122 IIIA), and erythromycin (Eli Lilly & Co., lot no. P-86211). Each drug was dissolved in 95% ethanol with further dilution in sterile 0.1 M phosphate buffer, pH 8.0, to provide stock solutions of 1,000 μg of active drug per ml. These were kept at −20°C until the day of use, at which time they were thawed and diluted to 10 times the desired final concentration in sterile water. The dilutions, 1 volume, then were added to 9 volumes of molten Mueller-Hinton agar (pH 7.2) supplemented with 5% sheep's blood, to provide final drug concentrations ranging from 25 to 0.01 μg/ml. Organisms to be tested were grown overnight in brain heart infusion broth, diluted in broth to contain approximately 10^7 colony-forming units/ml as determined photometrically, and then inoculated onto the prepared plates using a Steers replicator. Plates were incubated for 18 to 24 h at 35 to 37°C. The MIC was taken as the lowest concentration of drug at which complete inhibition of bacterial growth occurred.

Anaerobic organisms were tested against josamycin, rosamicin, and clindamycin (clindamycin HCI hydrate, lot no. 624 DC, Upjohn Co.). Josamycin and rosamicin were prepared as above; clindamycin first was dissolved in and then diluted with water but otherwise was handled identically. Drugs were diluted to 10 times the desired concentrations and then added to molten Brucella agar with 5% sheep's blood to give final concentrations of 128 to 0.05 μg/ml. Plates were stored in a reduced anaerobic jar for 24 h before use. Organisms to be tested were grown for 48 to 72 h in thioglycolate medium without indicator and enriched with hemin (5 μg/ml). The cultures were diluted to contain 10^7 colony-forming units/ml and inoculated onto prepared plates using a Steers replicator. Diluting and plating operations were carried out aerobically, with the time of exposure of the inocula to nonreducing atmosphere kept to a minimum; less than 30 min transpired from the opening of broth cultures to the placement of the inoculated plates in anaerobic containers. The inoculated plates were incubated at 35 to 37°C for 48 to 72 h in GasPak (BBL) jars (GasPak 100[tm] anaerobic system, Becton-Dickinson & Co.).

Cumulative percentages of inhibition were calculated, and individual data pairs for josamycin and rosamicin and for josamycin and erythromycin (or clindamycin) were compared using the *t* test.

Cumulative percent inhibitions for the three macrolides and gram-positive cocci are compared in Table 1. Rosamicin and erythromycin are shown to have inhibited the growth of most strains of *S. aureus* and *S. epidermidis* at lower concentrations than josamicin, whereas rosamicin was more active at lower concentrations than either josamycin or erythromycin when tested against enterococci. If an MIC of 1.56 μg/ml is accepted as the upper limit of probable clinical susceptibility, then 92% of *S. aureus* isolates, 77% of *S. epidermidis,* and 85% of the enterococci were susceptible to this, or lesser, concentrations of all three drugs. A total of 4% of *S. aureus,* 21% of *S. epidermidis,* and 13% of the enterococci were resistant at drug concentrations equal to or greater than 12.5 μg/ml. In this study, there were no isolates showing intermediate levels of susceptibility, and, with one exception, each resistant organism was resistant to all three drugs.

Table 2 compares the cumulative percentage of inhibition of the three drugs for the anaerobic organisms. The responses of the 42 isolates of *B. fragilis* to josamycin and clindamycin were similar at all but the lowest concentrations tested; clindamycin was the most active compound at concentrations of 0.06 and 0.13 μg/ml. Responses to rosamicin did not approximate josamycin and clindamycin at concentrations lower than 4 μg/ml. In contrast, rosamicin and josamycin were most similar in activity against gram-positive anaerobes, although 60% were inhibited at 0.06 μg of clindamycin per ml as compared with an inhibition of 7% by rosamicin and josamycin. The seven isolates of *Bacteroides* sp. and *Fusobacterium* sp. tested were all susceptible to clindamycin at a concentration of 0.06 μg/ml. Responses to rosamicin and josamycin again were similar, with all but one isolate being susceptible to concentrations of 1 μg/ml of less. One isolate of *F. nucleatum* required 16 μg of josamycin per ml for inhibition. When performances of the three drugs against the various groups of anaerobic organisms were compared, significant differences were demonstrated only for josamycin and rosamicin ($P < 0.001$) and for clindamycin and rosamicin ($P < 0.01$) when tested against *B. fragilis*.

Serious infections with aerobic gram-positive cocci such as *S. aureus* and enterococci remain a common clinical problem and, with the increasing use of intravascular prosthetic de-

TABLE 1. *Comparative activities (at MIC levels) of josamycin, rosamicin, and erythromycin against various aerobic gram-positive cocci*[a]

Organism (no. of strains tested)	Antibiotic	Cumulative % of strains inhibited at an MIC (μg/ml) of:								
		0.10	0.20	0.39	0.78	1.56	3.13	6.25	12.5	≥25.0
S. aureus (48)	Josamycin			12.5	83.3	95.8				100
	Rosamicin	2.1	91.7	95.8						100
	Erythromycin	31.3	91.7				95.8			100
S. epidermidis (34)	Josamycin			2.9	41.2	79.4				100
	Rosamicin	2.9	55.9	76.5	79.4					100
	Erythromycin	2.9	70.6	73.5		76.5				100
Enterococci (39)	Josamycin			23.1	79.5	87.2			89.7	100
	Rosamicin		33.3	87.2						100
	Erythromycin	12.8	20.5	33.3	59.0	84.6	87.2			100

[a] As determined by using the ICS agar dilution procedure.

TABLE 2. *Comparative activities (at MIC levels) of josamycin, rosamicin, and clindamycin against various anaerobic organisms*[a]

Organism (no. of strains tested)	Antibiotic	Cumulative % of strains inhibited at an MIC (μg/ml) of:								
		≤0.06	0.125	0.25	0.5	1.0	2.0	4.0	8.0	16.0
B. fragilis (42)	Josamycin		4.8	35.7	57.1	83.3	97.6	100		
	Rosamicin		2.4	9.5	42.9	52.4	83.3	92.9	100	
	Clindamycin	14.3	19.1	31.0	61.9	78.6	95.2	100		
Miscellaneous gram positive (15)	Josamycin	6.7	13.3	20	60	86.7	100			
	Rosamicin	6.7	26.7	60	80	100				
	Clindamycin	60	66.7	80				86.7	100	
Miscellaneous gram negative (7)	Josamycin	14.3	28.6	42.9	71.4	85.7				100
	Rosamicin	14.3	28.6		57.1	100				
	Clindamycin	100								

[a] As determined by using the ICS agar dilution procedure.

vices, *S. epidermidis* now is emerging as a significant pathogen (6). The patient who has such an infection and who for one reason or another is unable to tolerate a penicillin derivative may represent a significant problem in management with other currently available antibiotic agents. A better understanding of the role of anaerobic organisms in serious infections has led to the widespread use of such agents as chloramphenicol and clindamycin in the treatment of infections caused by these organisms (4). Although both are effective drugs, each has the potential for serious side effects. Thus, the search for new antibiotics or chemotherapeutic agents with activity against many of these organisms continues.

Data presented here suggest that, in vitro, josamycin and rosamicin are comparable in activity to erythromycin against several groups of pathogenic, gram-positive aerobic cocci. This is in agreement with previous results with rosamicin reported by Crowe and Sanders (1) and with available data regarding josamycin (3). If subsequent in vitro studies can show that the development of resistance to these agents is not a problem, as it has been with erythromycin, and if in vivo studies can show that these drugs are effective as well as safe and well tolerated, then either or both of these drugs deserve careful attention.

This study was supported by a grant from Schering Corp.

LITERATURE CITED

1. **Crowe, C. C., and W. E. Sanders.** 1974. Rosamicin: evaluation in vitro and comparison with erythromycin and lincomycin. Antimicrob. Agents Chemother. 5:272–275.
2. **Ericsson, H. M., and J. C. Sherris.** 1971. Antibiotic sensitivity testing. Report of an international collaborative study. Acta Pathol. Microbiol. Scand. Sect. B Suppl. 217.
3. **Gomi, J., T. Aoyagi, H. Tomioka, M. Oana, Y. Yoshimura, Y. Mitsuno, K. Kawai, Y. Yamada, Y. Yamada, and T. Takeshita.** 1969. Laboratory and clinical assessment of josamycin. Chemotherapy (Tokyo) 17:618–620.
4. **Gorbach, S. I., and J. G. Bartlett.** 1973. Anaerobic infections. New Engl. J. Med. 920:1289–1294.
5. **Ivler, D.** 1974. Staphylococcus, p. 91–95. *In* E. H. Lennette, E. H. Spaulding, and J. P. Truant (ed.), Manual of clinical microbiology, 2nd ed. American Society for Microbiology, Washington, D.C.
6. **Slaughter, l., J. E. Morris, and A. Starr.** 1973. Prosthetic valvular endocarditis, a 12 year review. Circulation 47:1319–1326.
7. **Sutter, V., and S. M. Finegold.** 1976. Rosamicin: in vitro activity against anaerobes and comparison with erythromycin. Antimicrob. Agents Chemother. 9:350–351.

ANTIMICROBIAL AGENTS AND CHEMOTHERAPY, Oct. 1976, p. 776-777 Vol. 10, No. 4

New Medium for In Vitro Susceptibility Studies with Amphotericin B

C. J. UTZ, S. WHITE, AND S. SHADOMY*

Division of Infectious Diseases, Department of Medicine, Medical College of Virginia, Virginia Commonwealth University, Richmond, Virginia 23298

Received for publication 1 July 1976

Antibiotic medium 20 FDA and antibiotic medium 3 FDA were compared to determine if antibiotic medium 3 would be suitable for in vitro susceptibility testing with amphotericin B.

Many of our previous in vitro studies involving susceptibility testing of amphotericin B against clinical isolates of pathogenic fungi were performed using a broth medium originally recommended by Groves and Randall for use in microbiological assay of this drug (1). This medium, known as antibiotic medium 20 FDA (M-20), more recently has been recommended for routine use in susceptibility testing with both amphotericin B and nystatin (3). Unfortunately, commercial production of M-20 has been discontinued.

With the nonavailability of M-20, it became necessary to choose another medium that would yield diagnostically similar results in in vitro susceptibility tests. A somewhat similar medium, antibiotic medium 3 FDA (Difco Laboratories, M-3) was selected. The main differences between these two media are in the total amounts of yeast extract, dextrose, and tryptone. M-3 contains 5 g of yeast extract per liter less and 10 g of dextrose per liter less than does M-20, whereas M-20 contains 10 g of tryptone per liter. All other constituents of the two media are similar (Table 1).

A brief study was undertaken to compare the two media and to determine if M-3 would be suitable for in vitro susceptibility testing with amphotericin B. Minimal inhibitory (MIC) and minimal fungicidal (MFC) concentrations were determined in both media for a variety of pathogenic yeasts in parallel using a previously described broth dilution method (3). Concentrations of amphotericin B ranged from 50 to 0.05 μg/ml. The drug was initially dissolved in 100% $(CH_3)_2SO$, and a stock concentration of 100 μg/ml was then prepared in 5% $(CH_3)_2SO$ and maintained at −20°C. Five clinical isolates each of *Cryptococcus neoformans* and *Candida albicans* and four of *Candida parapsilosis* were tested. *Saccharomyces cerevisiae* ATCC 9763 was tested along with each isolate as a control. MIC end points were determined after 48 h of incubation at 30°C. The MIC was defined as the

TABLE 1. *Compositions of antibiotic media M-3 and M-20*

Component	M-3 (g/liter)	M-20 (g/liter)
Beef extract	1.5	1.5
Yeast extract	1.5	6.5
Peptone	5.0	5.0
Tryptone		10.0
Dextrose	1.0	11.0
NaCl	3.5	3.5
K_2PO_4	3.68	3.68
$NaHPO_4$	1.32	1.32
Final pH	7.0	6.6

TABLE 2. *In vitro susceptibility tests with amphotericin B in two nonsynthetic media*

Isolate	Antibiotic medium: M-20 MIC[a] (μg/ml)	M-20 MFC[a] (μg/ml)	M-3 MIC (μg/ml)	M-3 MFC (μg/ml)
Cryptococcus neoformans				
9.1	0.05	0.10	0.05	0.05
9.7	0.39	0.39	0.20	0.20
9.17	0.39	0.39	0.05	0.05
9.18	0.05	0.20	0.05	0.05
9.49	0.20	0.20	0.05	0.05
Candida albicans				
7.2	0.39	1.56	0.20	0.20
7.7	0.39	0.78	0.20	0.20
7.18	0.78	1.56	0.20	0.39
7.31	0.39	0.78	0.20	0.20
7.66	0.78	1.56	0.20	0.39
Candida parapsilosis				
7.1	0.39	0.39	0.05	12.5
7.3	0.20	0.39	0.05	0.20
7.6	0.39	6.25	0.20	12.5
7.21	0.10	0.39	0.05	0.05
Saccharomyces cerevisiae				
14 tests	0.39-0.78	0.39-0.78	0.05	0.05

[a] MIC, Minimal inhibitory concentration; MFC, minimal fungicidal concentration.

lowest concentration of drug that inhibited growth as measured by the absence of a visible "button" at the bottom of each tube. MFC were determined by subculturing, on Sabouraud agar, all negative tubes.

Results with this study indicate that M-3 can be used for susceptibility testing with yeast-like organisms and amphotericin B (Table 2). The MIC and MFC results in all 14 individual tests with the control organism *S. cerevisiae* were constant, 0.05 μg/ml, indicating uniformity of results. Most MIC and MFC values measured for the clinical isolates in M-3 were somewhat lower than those measured in M-20. Differences between MIC values measured in the two media were significant (*t* test, $P < 0.001$), but differences in MFC values were not. With only two isolates, *Candida parapsilosis* 7.1 and *C. parapsilosis* 7.6, was a higher MFC measured in M-3 than in M-20. These differences were not critical in determination of clinical susceptibility. Differences between inhibitory and fungicidal end points measured in the two media most likely could be attributed to a lesser production of acid in M-3, with a subsequent reduction in decay of active drug, because of the lower carbohydrate content of this medium. The adverse effect of an acidic pH on the activity of amphotericin B is the primary reason why unbuffered synthetic media, such as yeast nitrogen base, are unsuitable for in vitro testing with polyene compounds (2).

LITERATURE CITED

1. **Grove, D. C. and W. A. Randall.** 1955. Assay methods of antibiotics. Medical Encyclopedia, Inc., New York.
2. **Shadomy, S.** 1974. Laboratory evaluation of antifungal agents, p. 27-36a. *In* 14th National Medicinal Chemistry Symposium. Division of Medicinal Chemistry, American Chemical Society, University of New Hampshire, Durham, N. H.
3. **Shadomy, S., and A. Espinel-Ingroff.** 1974. Susceptibility testing of antifungal agents, p. 569-574. *In* E. H. Lennette, E. H. Spaulding, and J. P. Truant (ed.), Manual of clinical microbiology, 2nd ed. American Society for Microbiology, Washington, D.C.

ERRATA

Gentamicin- and Cephalothin-Associated Rises in Blood Urea Nitrogen

W. LEE FANNING, DIETER GUMP, AND HERSHEL JICK*

Infectious Disease Unit, Medical College of Vermont, Burlington, Vermont 05401, and Boston University School of Medicine, Waltham, Massachusetts 02154

Volume 10, no. 1, p. 81, column 1, Discussion, lines 19–21 should read: ". . . 6.5% of 77 courses of gentamicin after other causes of nephrotoxicity were eliminated (14). A similar estimate for cephalothin given alone . . ."

Acute Diffuse Interstitial Nephritis Related to Chemotherapy of Tuberculosis

WILLIAM J. STONE,* JAMES A. WALDRON, JOHN H. DIXON, JR., R. KIRBY PRIMM, AND ROBERT G. HORN

Departments of Medicine and Pathology, Veterans Administration Hospital, and Vanderbilt University School of Medicine, Nashville, Tennessee 37203*

Volume 10, no. 1, p. 169, column 2, Discussion, line 5: "urethral" should read "ureteral."

ANTIMICROBIAL AGENTS AND CHEMOTHERAPY, Nov. p. 779-785 Vol. 10, No. 5

Printed in U.S.A.

Inhibition of Conjugal Transfer of R Plasmids by Pipemidic Acid and Related Compounds

SHINICHI NAKAMURA,* SATORU INOUE, MASANAO SHIMIZU, SHIZUKO IYOBE, AND SUSUMU MITSUHASHI

Research and Development Division, Dainippon Pharmaceutical Co., Ltd., Suita, Osaka, and Department of Microbiology, School of Medicine, Gunma University, Maebashi, Japan*

Received for publication 5 May 1976

It was found that pipemidic acid and related compounds have the common property of inhibiting the conjugal transfer of R plasmids carried by *Escherichia coli* and *Pseudomonas aeruginosa*. This inhibition was not due to bactericidal activity of the compounds against donors, recipients, or R^+ transconjugants. However, it was correlated inversely with their minimal inhibitory concentrations, depending especially upon sensitivity of donors to the compounds. The inhibition was generally observed in mating systems using various combinations of 14 R plasmids and 9 bacterial strains. The pretreatment of a donor or a recipient strain with pipemidic acid showed only a small inhibitory effect on the transfer of an R plasmid, whereas the presence of the compound during an active mating caused a marked inhibitory effect.

R-mediated drug resistance in bacteria is a serious problem in clinical medicine. In studies thus far made for anti-R plasmid agents, nalidixic acid was found to inhibit the conjugal transfer of R plasmids (10). Pipemidic acid, a new synthetic antibacterial agent active against gram-negative bacteria including *Pseudomonas aeruginosa* (14), is structurally related to nalidixic acid and shows a marked inhibition of the conjugal transfer of R_{100-1} between strains of *Escherichia coli*. This finding raised the questions of whether such inhibition is a common property of this group of compounds and whether it is generally observed in various systems of R plasmid transfer. The present study was carried out to clarify these points.

MATERIALS AND METHODS

R plasmids and bacterial strains. The R plasmids and bacterial strains used in this study are listed in Tables 1 and 2, respectively. Pipemidic acid-resistant strains were made in vitro by 10 serial passages in nutrient broth containing the agent.

Drugs. The chemical structures of the pipemidic acid-related compounds tested are shown in Fig. 1. These were all prepared in the Research Laboratories of Dainippon Pharmaceutical Co., Ltd., according to procedures described previously (6–9; Japanese Patent Publ. 48-37279; Japanese Patent Application Disclosures 49-82670 and 49-126697). Appropriate amounts of 0.1 N sodium hydroxide were added to them when dissolved. Chloramphenicol was purchased from Sankyo Co., Ltd., and tetracycline hydrochloride was purchased from Takeda Chemical Industries, Ltd.

Media. Nutrient broth and SS agar were purchased from Eiken Co., Ltd. ALGa, AGGa, and AMGa broths or agars consisted of medium A (2), 0.5% L-glutamic acid, and 1% lactose, glucose, and maltose, respectively. Appropriate nutrients were added, if necessary, at a concentration of 30 μg/ml unless otherwise described.

Kinetics of R plasmid transfer. In the R plasmid transfer between strains of *E. coli*, donor (W4861 $R_{100-1}{}^+$ or $R_{10}{}^+$) and recipient (58-161) cells grown exponentially in nutrient broth (about 7×10^8 cells/ml each) were mixed at a volume ratio of 1:9 and

TABLE 1. *R plasmids used*

R plasmid	Incompatibility group	Resistance pattern[a]
R_{100-1}	FII	Tc Cm Sm Sa
R_{100}	FII	Tc Cm Sm Sa
R_{10}	FII	Tc Cm Sm Sa
R386	FI	Tc
R144	Iα	Tc Km
R387	K	Sm Cm
N3	N	Tc Sm Sa
RP4	P-1	Apc Tc Km
S-a	W	Sm Sa Cm Km
R446	M	Tc Sm
R14	O	Apc Tc Sm Sa
Rms139	P-2	Tc Cm Sm Sa Cpc
Rms159	P-2	Tc Cm Sm Hg
Rms163	P-5	Tc Cm Sa
RP4	P-1	Tc Km Cpc

[a] Abbreviations: Tc, tetracycline; Cm, chloramphenicol; Sm, streptomycin; Sa, sulfonamides; Km, kanamycin; Apc, ampicillin; Cpc, carbenicillin; Hg, mercuric chloride.

TABLE 2. *Bacterial strains used*

Strain	Genotype
Escherichia coli K-12 W4861	F⁻ *lac⁻ pur⁻*
E. coli K-12 58-161	F⁻ *met⁻*
E. coli K-12 W3630	F⁻ *mal⁻*
E. coli K-12 W3630	F⁻ *mal⁻ ppa*[a]
E. coli K-12 W4354	F⁻ *met⁻*
E. coli K-12 W4354	F⁻ *met⁻ ppa*[b]
Shigella flexneri 2a EW10	
Pseudomonas aeruginosa M243	*trp⁻ his⁻ ilv⁻ met⁻*
P. aeruginosa ML4600	*trp⁻ his⁻*

[a] Resistance to pipemidic acid (*ppa*); MIC, 200 μg/ml.

[b] Resistance to pipemidic acid (*ppa*); MIC, 50 μg/ml.

incubated at 37°C under static conditions. At various times after incubation, a 0.5-ml sample was taken, diluted 100 times with ice-chilled ALGa broth containing L-methionine (10 μg/ml), and divided into two aliquots; one was treated with a blender (Nippon Seiki Co.) at 15,000 rpm for 30 s, and the other was left untreated. Both aliquots were incubated at 37°C for 10 min and diluted appropriately with the same broth. A 1.5-ml amount of each dilution was mixed with an equal volume of ALGa agar plus L-methionine (10 μg/ml) and chloramphenicol (50 μg/ml) and overlaid on the same agar containing chloramphenicol (25 μg/ml). After incubation at 37°C for 48 h, the colonies of R^+ transconjugants were counted.

In the R plasmid transfer between strains of *P. aeruginosa*, donor (M243 $RP4^+$) and recipient

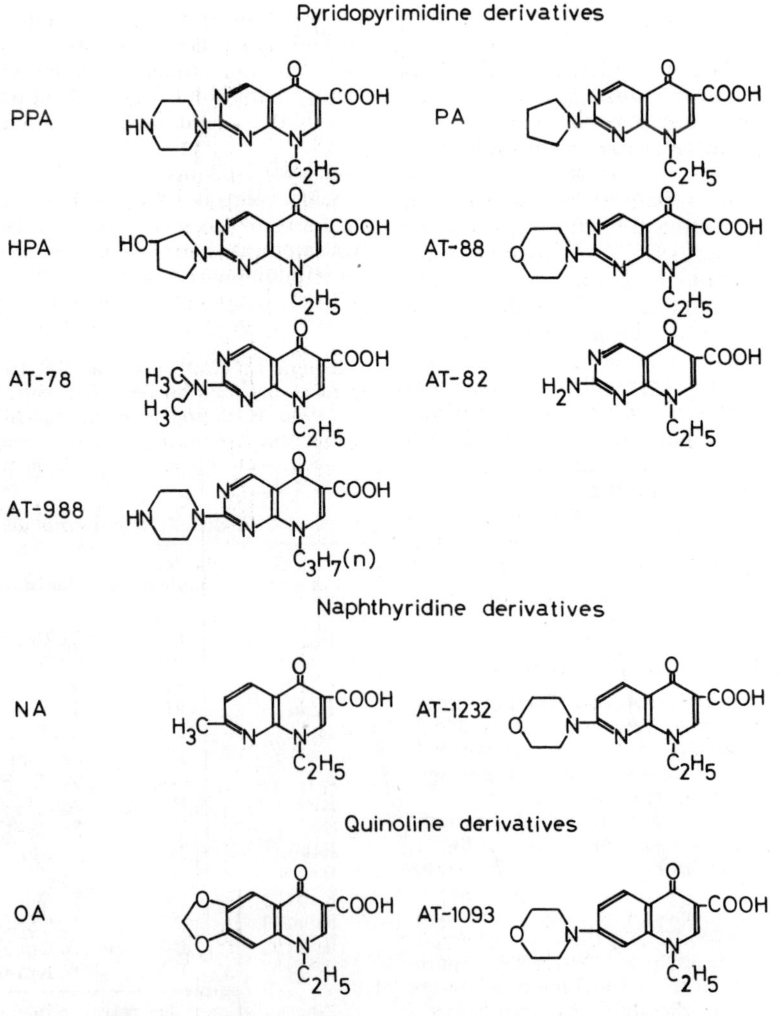

FIG. 1. *Chemical structures of pipemidic acid-related compounds tested. Abbreviations: PPA, pipemidic acid; PA, piromidic acid; HPA, hydroxypiromidic acid; NA, nalidixic acid; OA, oxolinic acid; AT-78, AT-82, AT-88, AT-988, AT-1093, and AT-1232, code numbers of Dainippon Pharmaceutical Co., Ltd.*

(ML4600) cells exponentially grown in nutrient broth containing 0.4% KNO_3 (about 4 × 10^8 cells/ml each) were mated in the same manner as *E. coli*. Samples taken were diluted with AGGa broth containing L-tryptophan and L-histidine followed by the same treatment as *E. coli* except that R^+ transconjugants were selected on AGGa agar containing KNO_3 (0.4%), L-tryptophan, L-histidine, and tetracycline (75 μg/ml).

MIC. The minimal inhibitory concentration (MIC) was determined by the twofold agar dilution method (14).

Inhibition of R plasmid transfer. The procedure of mating was the same as that described for the kinetics experiment except that an appropriate amount of a compound was added to the conjugation mixture. Samples were taken 20 min after mating in *E. coli* and *Shigella flexneri* and 50 min after mating in *P. aeruginosa*, followed by treatment with the blender. The colonies of donors, recipients, and R^+ transconjugants were counted on appropriate agars (ALGa, AGGa, and AMGa agars for *E. coli*, SS agar for *S. flexneri*, and AGGa agar for *P. aeruginosa*) with or without required nutrients and a selective agent. Chloramphenicol (25 μg/ml) was used as a selective agent for bacteria carrying R_{100-1}, R_{100}, R_{10}, R387, and S-a, and tetracycline (25 μg/ml for *E. coli* and 75 μg/ml for *P. aeruginosa*) was used for bacteria carrying one of the other R plasmids. The transfer rate was calculated according to the formula: transfer rate = 100 × (number of R^+ transconjugants of a test group/number of R^+ transconjugants of a control).

Pipemidic acid treatment before and during mating. Donor (W3630 $R_{100-1}{}^+$) and recipient (W4354) cells of *E. coli* grown exponentially in nutrient broth were harvested on membrane filters (Millipore Corp.), resuspended in 1/10 volume of the same broth (about 7 × 10^9 cells/ml), and divided into two aliquots each; one received pipemidic acid (3.13 μg/ml), and the other received distilled water. After incubation at 37°C for 30 min under static conditions, one of the donor cultures and one of the recipient cultures were mixed for mating and incubated for 20 min in the presence or absence of pipemidic acid. Mating mixtures consisted of 0.1 ml of a donor culture, 0.8 ml of a recipient culture, 0.1 ml of a pipemidic acid solution (313 μg/ml) or distilled water, and 9 ml of nutrient broth. Other procedures were as described above.

RESULTS

Kinetics of R plasmid transfer. The time course of R plasmid transfer was investigated in three mating systems. The number of R^+ transconjugants increased exponentially until about 20 min after mixing of donor and recipient cells in the mating systems of *E. coli*, and until about 50 min in the mating system of *P. aeruginosa* (Fig. 2). Sensitivity to the blender treatment disappeared about 20 min (or 50 min) after mixing in both systems. This result indicates that the transfer of the R plasmids was completed in both mating systems 20 min (or 50 min) after mixing.

Inhibition of R plasmid transfer by pipemidic acid-related compounds. The effect of pipemidic acid-related compounds on R plasmid transfer was examined by using two mating systems (Fig. 3). In the mating of *E. coli* W4861

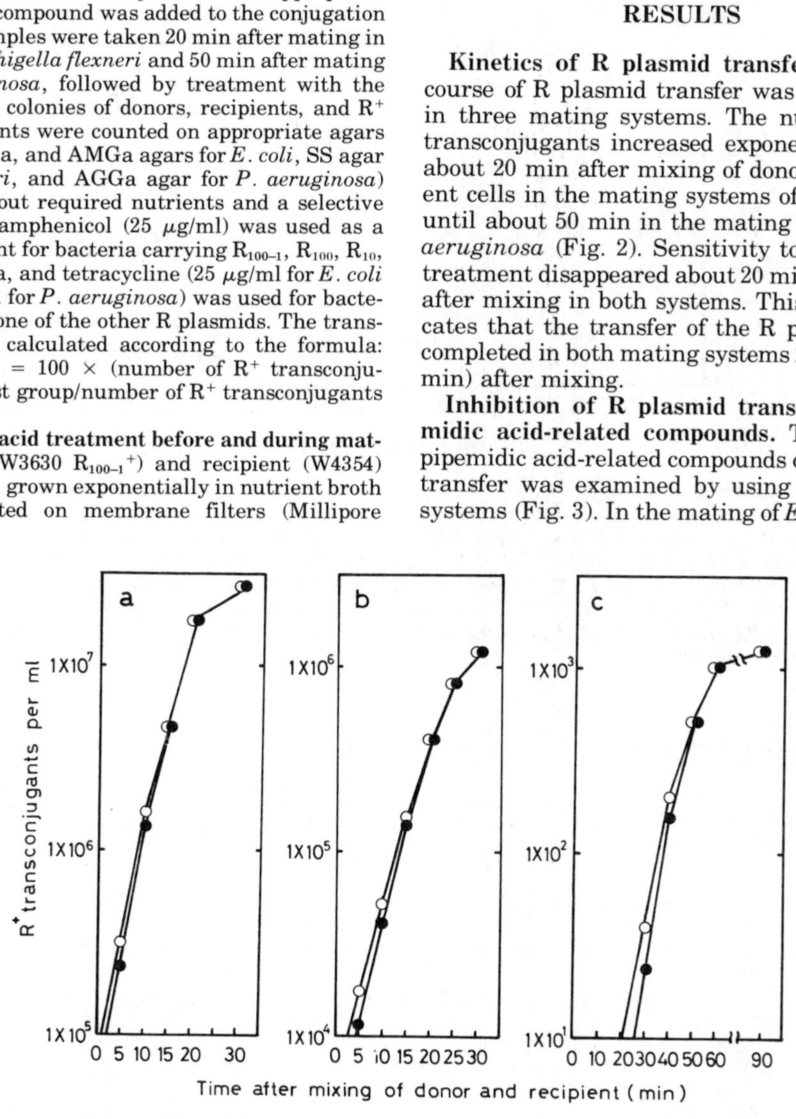

FIG. 2. *Kinetics of R plasmid transfer. (a) Donor, E. coli W4861* $R_{100-1}{}^+$*; recipient, E. coli 58-161. (b) Donor, E. coli W4861* $R_{10}{}^+$*; recipient, E. coli 58-161. (c) Donor, P. aeruginosa M243 RP4*$^+$*; recipient, P. aeruginosa ML4600. Blender treated (●) and untreated (○).*

R_{100-1}^{+} and *E. coli* 58-161 (system A), compounds showing low MICs (such as oxolinic, nalidixic, and pipemidic acids) exhibited significant inhibition of transfer, whereas those showing high MICs (such as AT-82 and AT-1232) were less active. There was a clear inverse correlation between MIC and inhibition of transfer. A similar result was obtained with the mating of *P. aeruginosa* M243 RP4$^+$ and *P. aeruginosa* ML4600 (system B), where pipemidic acid, which showed the lowest MIC, markedly inhibited the transfer of the R plasmid. The inhibition of R plasmid transfer by pipemidic acid-related compounds was not due to a bactericidal activity against donor, recipient, or R$^+$ transconjugant cells (Table 3).

Influence of pipemidic acid resistance of donor and recipient on transfer inhibition. The inhibition of R plasmid transfer by pipemidic acid depended on its antibacterial activity, especially that against the donor. Transfer inhibition was markedly diminished when the

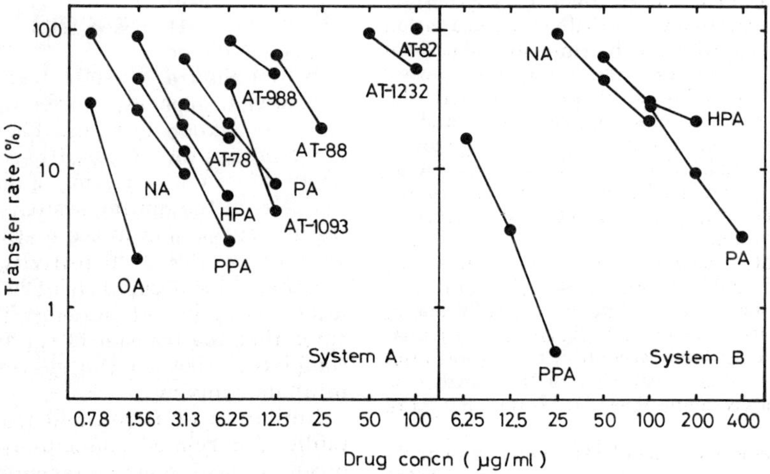

FIG. 3. *Inhibition of R plasmid transfer by pipemidic acid-related compounds. Transfer rate = 100 × (number of R$^+$ transconjugants of a test group/number of R$^+$ transconjugants of a control). System A: Donor, E. coli W4861 R_{100-1}^{+}; recipient, E. coli 58-161. MICs (µg/ml) for the donor and recipient: OA, 1.56 and 0.78; NA, 3.13 and 12.5; PPA, 3.13 and 3.13; HPA, 6.25 and 12.5; AT-78, 6.25 and 50; AT-1093, 12.5 and 50; PA, 12.5 and 50; AT-988, 12.5 and 12.5; AT-88, 25 and 50; AT-1232, 100 and 100; AT-82, >100 and >100. System B: Donor, P. aeruginosa M243 RP4$^+$; recipient, P. aeruginosa ML4600. MICs (µg/ml) for the donor and recipient: PPA, 12.5 and 12.5; NA, 100 and 100; PA, 400 and 400; HPA, 200 and 200. See Fig. 1 for compound abbreviations.*

TABLE 3. *Bactericidal activity of pipemidic, piromidic, hydroxypiromidic, and nalidixic acids*

Drug[a]	Concn (µg/ml)	Colony-forming units/ml					
		E. coli[b]			*P. aeruginosa*[c]		
		W4861R_{100-1}^{+}	58–161	58–161R_{100-1}^{+}	M243RP4$^+$	ML4600	ML4600RP4$^+$
Control	0	8.7×10^7	5.7×10^8	2.4×10^7	5.7×10^7	2.3×10^8	3.7×10^7
PPA	3.13	9.2×10^7	5.5×10^8	2.7×10^7			
	12.5	9.1×10^7	5.3×10^8	2.7×10^7	5.8×10^7	2.2×10^8	3.6×10^7
	25				4.8×10^7	2.4×10^8	3.7×10^7
PA	25	1.0×10^8	4.6×10^8	2.6×10^7			
	400				5.6×10^7	2.4×10^8	2.8×10^7
HPA	6.25	9.6×10^7	5.2×10^8	2.5×10^7			
	200				5.6×10^7	2.2×10^8	2.5×10^7
NA	3.13	1.0×10^8	5.0×10^8	2.7×10^7			
	100				4.7×10^7	2.3×10^8	2.8×10^7

[a] See Fig. 1 for abbreviations.
[b] Contact of cells with drugs for 20 min.
[c] Contact of cells with drugs for 50 min.

donor was resistant to pipemidic acid and less markedly so when the recipient was resistant to it (Fig. 4).

Influence of bacterial strains used as donor or recipient on the transfer inhibition. Transfer inhibition was observed when bacterial strains used as donor or recipient were changed. Pipemidic, piromidic, hydroxypiromidic, and nalidixic acids inhibited the transfer of R_{100-1} at their MIC values against donor cells in four mating systems, using donor strains sensitive to the acids (Table 4). Fluctuation in the degree of inhibition between the four systems could not be ascribed to differences in drug sensitivity of the donors, because the MICs of the compounds against the four donors were the same except for piromidic acid.

Influence of R plasmids on transfer inhibition. Using eleven R plasmids in *E. coli* W4861 and four R plasmids in *P. aeruginosa* M243, we tested the transfer inhibition of these R plasmids by pipemidic, piromidic, hydroxypiromidic, and nalidixic acids. Transfer of the R plasmids was inhibited by these acids at their MIC values against the donors, although the degree of inhibition varied depending on the plasmids used (Table 5). This variance was not due to differences in the MIC values of the compounds toward the donors carrying the R plasmids.

Influence of the time of drug treatment on transfer inhibition. Donor (W3630 $R_{100-1}{}^{+}$) and recipient (W4354) cells of *E. coli* were treated with pipemidic acid before and during mating (Table 6). The transfer rate was markedly decreased when pipemidic acid was present during mating (groups B, D, F, and H), whereas its inhibition was lower when the compound was

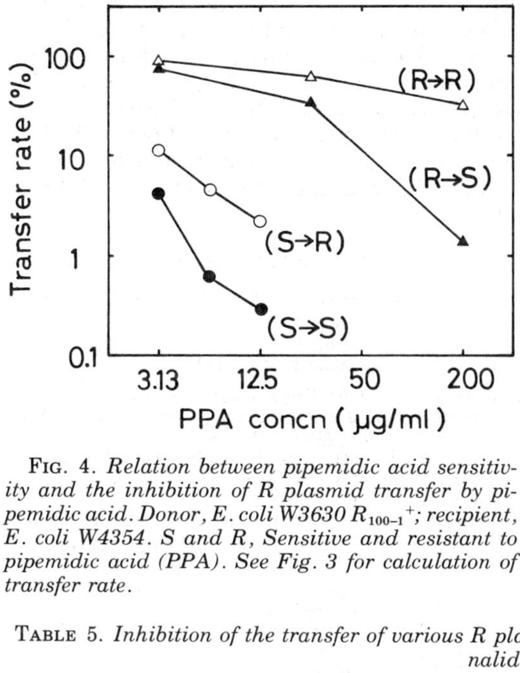

FIG. 4. *Relation between pipemidic acid sensitivity and the inhibition of R plasmid transfer by pipemidic acid. Donor, E. coli W3630 $R_{100-1}{}^{+}$; recipient, E. coli W4354. S and R, Sensitive and resistant to pipemidic acid (PPA). See Fig. 3 for calculation of transfer rate.*

TABLE 4. *Inhibition of R plasmid transfer by pipemidic, piromidic, hydroxypiromidic, and nalidixic acids in various mating systems*

Drug[a]	Concn[b] (μg/ml)	Transfer rate (%)[c] in mating system: I[d]	II[e]	III[f]	IV[g]
PPA	3.13	13.1	3.0	1.0	13.3
PA	25	7.7[h]	21.0	12.9	28.7
HPA	6.25	6.0	10.0	2.6	14.0
NA	3.13	8.9	15.0	4.7	19.3

[a] See Fig. 1 for abbreviations.
[b] MIC for donors.
[c] See Fig. 3 for calculation.
[d] Donor, *E. coli* W4861 $R_{100-1}{}^{+}$; recipient, *E. coli* 58–161.
[e] Donor, *E. coli* W3630 $R_{100-1}{}^{+}$; recipient, *E. coli* W4354.
[f] Donor, *E. coli* W3630 $R_{100-1}{}^{+}$; recipient, *S. flexneri* 2a EW10.
[g] Donor, *E. coli* W4354 $R_{100-1}{}^{+}$; recipient, *E. coli* W3630.
[h] Concentration used was 12.5 μg/ml, which is the MIC against *E. coli* W4861 $R_{100-1}{}^{+}$.

TABLE 5. *Inhibition of the transfer of various R plasmids by pipemidic, piromidic, hydroxypiromidic, and nalidixic acids*

Drug[a]	Concn[b] (μg/ml)	Transfer rate (%)[c] in *E. coli*[d]: R_{100-1}	R_{100}	R_{10}[f]	R386	R144	R387	N3	RP4	S-a	R446	R14	Concn (μg/ml)	Transfer rate (%)[c] in *P. aeruginosa*[e]: Rms 139	Rms 163	RP4	Rms 159
PPA	3.13	13.1	27.3	7.5	15.6	11.3	60.2	50.1	10.3	50.8	38.0	44.2	12.5	1.5	8.5	3.5	0.5
PA	12.5	7.7	9.5	11.6	2.8	0.6	3.8	19.6	3.9	49.2	12.2	28.4	400	0.3	0.5	3.2	0.2
HPA	6.25	5.9	14.4	14.4	3.2	0.5	4.9	24.3	8.4	29.2	12.8	28.4	200	3.9	5.4	21.4	0.9
NA	3.13	8.9	13.7	14.2	6.2	7.8	29.0	23.7	3.5	39.3	22.0	36.8	100	0.5	1.5	21.4	1.4

[a–c] See Table 4.
[d] Donor, *E. coli* W4861 R^{+}; recipient, *E. coli* 58–161.
[e] Donor, *P. aeruginosa* M243 R^{+}; recipient, *P. aeruginosa* ML4600.
[f] The concentrations of PPA, PA, HPA, and NA used were 12.5, 50, 12.5, and 12.5 μg/ml, respectively, because these were the MICs against *E. coli* W4861 $R_{10}{}^{+}$.

TABLE 6. *Relation between the time of pipemidic acid treatment and the inhibition of R plasmid transfer*

Group	Treatment with PPA[a] for:			Transfer rate (%)[d]
	30 min of premixing		20 min of postmixing	
	Donor[b]	Recipient[c]		
A	−	−	−	100
B	−	−	+	4.9
C	+	−	−	37.7
D	+	−	+	2.3
E	−	+	−	42.2
F	−	+	+	5.2
G	+	+	−	34.5
H	+	+	+	2.0

[a] Treated (+) or untreated (−) with pipemidic acid (PPA) at a concentration of 3.13 μg/ml.

[b] *E. coli* W3630 R_{100-1}^+.

[c] *E. coli* W4354.

[d] See Fig. 3 for calculation.

absent during that period (groups A, C, E, and G). Pretreatment of the donor and recipient with pipemidic acid, followed by removal of the compound during mating (groups C, E, and G), caused only a small inhibitory effect on the transfer rate. This result suggests that the inhibition of R plasmid transfer by pipemidic acid is not due to irreversible damage of either donor or recipient, but rather to the interruption of the mating process itself.

DISCUSSION

The present study demonstrated that pipemidic acid-related compounds inhibited the conjugal transfer of R plasmids. Such inhibition was inversely correlated with the antibacterial activity of the compounds against donor cells. However, there is no relationship between their bactericidal activity and the inhibition of R plasmid transfer, because none of the donors, recipients, or R^+ transconjugants were killed during mating under the experimental conditions used. The inhibition was observed in mating systems of a number of bacterial strains carrying various R plasmids. Sensitivity of donors to the compound test and the presence of the compound during mating determined the degree of inhibition of R plasmid transfer. These results appear to be related to those of the pipemidic acid-related compound nalidixic acid, which inhibits the conjugal transfer of F'*lac* only when the donor is sensitive to the drug (1), with the inhibitory effect of the drug lost by dilution of the mating mixture with drug-free medium (5). Pipemidic acid-related compounds inhibit bacterial deoxyribonucleic acid (DNA) synthesis (4, 11, 12). Fenwick and Curtiss (3) demonstrated that nalidixic acid inhibited conjugal DNA replication of R64-11. It is likely that there is a common mechanism for the inhibition of R plasmid transfer via the inhibition of plasmid DNA synthesis by this group of compounds.

It is important from a practical viewpoint that these compounds can exert their action in vivo in humans. The toxicity of pipemidic acid-related compounds is rather low, and some of them, i.e., pipemidic, piromidic, nalidixic, and oxolinic acids, have been applied to human diseases. Roe and Jones (13) found that carbenicillin was ineffective against a mixed infection with a carbenicillin-resistant, avirulent strain of *Klebsiella aerogenes* and a carbenicillin-sensitive, virulent strain of *P. aeruginosa* in burned mice because of the emergence of carbenicillin-resistant *P. aeruginosa* by the transfer of an R plasmid determining carbenicillin resistance. The combined use of nalidixic acid and carbenicillin was effective due to the inhibition of R plasmid transfer by nalidixic acid. This result suggests that the other members of this group of compounds might also be effective in inhibiting in vivo transfer of R plasmids, for some of them are known to be more effective on bacterial infections in vivo than is nalidixic acid (6, 15).

ACKNOWLEDGMENT

We are indebted to H. Hattori for his collaboration in a part of this study.

LITERATURE CITED

1. **Barbour, S. D.** 1967. Effect of nalidixic acid on conjugal transfer and expression of episomal lac in *Escherichia coli* K12. J. Mol. Biol. **28**:373–376.
2. **Davis, B. D., and E. S. Mingioli.** 1950. Mutants of *Escherichia coli* requiring methionine or vitamin B_{12}. J. Bacteriol. **60**:17–28.
3. **Fenwick, R. G., Jr., and R. Curtiss III.** 1973. Conjugal deoxyribonucleic acid replication by *Escherichia coli* K-12: effect of nalidixic acid. J. Bacteriol. **116**:1236–1246.
4. **Goss, W. A., W. H. Deitz, and J. M. Cook.** 1965. Mechanism of action of nalidixic acid on *Escherichia coli*. II. Inhibition of deoxyribonucleic acid synthesis. J. Bacteriol. **89**:1068–1074.
5. **Hollom, S., and R. H. Pritchard.** 1965. Effect of inhibition of DNA synthesis on mating in *E. coli* K-12. Genet. Res. **6**:479–483.
6. **Kaminsky, D., and R. I. Meltzer.** 1968. Quinolone antibacterial agents. Oxolinic acid and related compounds. J. Med. Chem. **11**:160–163.
7. **Lesher, G. Y., E. J. Froelich, M. D. Gruett, J. H. Bailey, and R. P. Brundage.** 1962. 1,8-Naphthyridine derivatives. A new class of chemotherapeutic agents. J. Med. Pharm. Chem. **5**:1063–1065.
8. **Matsumoto, J., and S. Minami.** 1975. Pyrido[2,3-*d*]pyrimidine antibacterial agents. 3. 8-Alkyl- and 8-vinyl-5,8-dihydro-5-oxo-2-(1-piperazinyl)pyrido[2,3-*d*]pyrimidine-6-carboxylic acids and their derivatives. J. Med. Chem. **18**:74–79.

9. **Minami, S., T. Shono, and J. Matsumoto.** 1971. Pyrido[2,3-*d*]pyrimidine antibacterial agents. II. Piromidic acid and related compounds. Chem. Pharm. Bull. 19:1426–1432.
10. Mitsuhashi, S. 1965. Transmissible drug-resistance factor R. Gunma J. Med. Sci. 14:169–209.
11. **Nakamura, S., M. Ishiyama, and M. Shimizu.** 1974. The mechanism of action of piromidic acid and 3′-hydroxypiromidic acid, p. 432–435. *In* G. K. Daikos (ed.), Progress in chemotherapy, Proceedings of the 8th international congress of chemotherapy, vol. 1. Hellenic Society of Chemotherapy, Athens, Greece.
12. **Pianotti, R. S., R. R. Mohan, and B. S. Schwartz.** 1968. Biochemical effects of oxolinic acid on *Proteus vulgaris*. J. Bacteriol. 95:1622–1626.
13. **Roe, E., and R. J. Jones.** 1972. Effects of topical chemoprophylaxis on transferable antibiotic resistance in burns. Lancet ii:109–111.
14. **Shimizu, M., Y. Takase, S. Nakamura, H. Katae, A. Minami, K. Nakata, S. Inoue, M. Ishiyama, and Y. Kubo.** 1975. Pipemidic acid, a new antibacterial agent active against *Pseudomonas aeruginosa*: in vitro properties. Antimicrob. Agents Chemother. 8:132–138.
15. **Shimizu, M., Y. Takase, S. Nakamura, H. Katae, A. Minami, K. Nakata, and N. Kurobe.** 1976. Pipemidic acid: its activities against various experimental infections. Antimicrob. Agents Chemother 9:569–574.

ANTIMICROBIAL AGENTS AND CHEMOTHERAPY, Nov. 1976, p. 786-794 Vol. 10, No. 5

Printed in U.S.A.

Effects of Antibiotics on Metabolism of Peptidoglycan, Protein, and Lipids in *Bifidobacterium bifidum* subsp. *pennsylvanicus*

G. C. MOLENKAMP AND J. H. VEERKAMP*

Department of Biochemistry, University of Nijmegen, Nijmegen, The Netherlands

Received for publication 25 June 1976

The formation of cell envelope components of *Bifidobacterium bifidum* subsp. *pennsylvanicus* was studied by measuring the incorporation of [^{3}H]glycine, ^{14}C-labeled fatty acids, and *N*-benzoyl-[^{14}C]glucosamine into the membrane protein, membrane lipids, and cell wall peptidoglycan, respectively. Inhibition of peptidoglycan synthesis by antibiotics (penicillin G, vancomycin, D-cycloserine, and bacitracin) and by the omission of glucosamine-containing growth factors caused a marked decrease in glycine incorporation into cellular as well as membrane protein, which was accompanied by a considerable enhancement of fatty acid incorporation. The uncoupling of protein and lipid synthesis led to the release of marked amounts of lipids from the cell under these conditions. Arrestment of protein synthesis by antibiotics (chloramphenicol, tetracycline, and actinomycin D) decreased peptidoglycan and lipid synthesis only partially, but did not lead to lipid release. Mg^{2+} deficiency of the medium caused about 60% inhibition of growth and lipid synthesis, but protein synthesis and especially peptidoglycan synthesis were much less inhibited. Staphylococcin 1580 arrested the growth and also the synthesis of protein and peptidoglycan. However, the synthesis and turnover of lipids were considerably increased and a release of large amounts of lipids was observed. Peptidoglycan and cellular protein did not show any turnover either during normal growth or after the inhibition of cell wall and protein synthesis.

Although much information has been gathered about the biosynthesis of bacterial membranes and that of cell walls, relatively little is known about the interaction of these processes during growth (24, 28, 42, 45, 54, 58). Cell wall thickening by antibiotics that inhibit protein synthesis and by amino acid starvation in *Streptococcus faecalis* and other bacteria suggested an interrelationship (28, 58). *Biofidobacterium bifidum* subsp. *pennsylvanicus* is a suitable organism with which to study this relationship because it requires human milk (22) or certain D-glucosamine derivatives (40, 41) as a substrate for cell wall synthesis. Much information was obtained on the composition of its cell wall (65) and cytoplasmic membrane (14, 16). Earlier (14, 15, 63) we observed marked changes in the lipid composition after inhibition of cell wall synthesis.

We report in this paper a study of the incorporation of ^{14}C-labeled fatty acids into cellular and membrane lipids and of [^{3}H]glycine into cellular and membrane protein under normal growth conditions and under conditions in which cell wall synthesis and/or protein synthesis were inhibited. These conditions were effected by various antibiotics, Mg^{2+} deficiency, the omission of glucosamine-containing growth factors, or staphylococcin 1580. Peptidoglycan synthesis was measured by the incorporation of [^{14}C]glucosamine from the synthetic growth factor *N*-benzoyl-[^{14}C]glucosamine. Previously we have shown that a high amount of radioactivity from this compound is incorporated into the amino sugars of the cell wall peptidoglycan (40). Since changes in incorporation may be due to alterations in turnover and/or net synthesis, the turnover of peptidoglycan, protein, and lipids was also studied to arrive at an adequate interpretation. The effect of staphylococcin 1580 on the macromolecular syntheses was included in these investigations because this bacteriocin was bactericidal for many gram-positive bacteria (30) and considerably affected protein synthesis (31, 32).

A disbalance of lipid and protein synthesis was observed under all inhibitory conditions, but only specific inhibitors of peptidoglycan synthesis and staphylococcin 1580 cause a marked release of lipids to the culture medium.

MATERIALS AND METHODS

Organism and cultivation. *B. bifidum* subsp. *pennsylvanicus*, originally called *Lactobacillus bifidus* subsp. *pennsylvanicus* (22), was cultivated at 37°C in a complex medium previously described (13), to which 2% skimmed human milk was added. The gas phase consisted of 90% N_2 and 10% CO_2.

Chemicals. Lysozyme and deoxyribonuclease were obtained from Boehringer Mannheim Corp. Sodium-penicillin G was purchased from Mycofarm, Delft, Netherlands; bacitracin from Farmachemie, Delft, Netherlands; vancomycin HCl from Eli Lilly & Co., Indianapolis, Ind.; D-cycloserine from Sigma Chemical Co., St. Louis, Mo.; chloramphenicol from Mycofarm, Delft, Netherlands; tetracycline from R.I.T., Rijswijk, Netherlands; and actinomycin D from Merck & Co., Rahway, N.J. Staphylococcin 1580 was kindly provided by G. D. Vogels, Department of Microbiology, University of Nijmegen, Netherlands. The preparation was produced by *Staphylococcus epidermis* 1580 and isolated from the culture medium by $(NH_4)_2SO_4$ precipitation and dialysis (33). The activity of each preparation was empirically determined (33).

Instagel and Omnifluor were obtained from Packard Instruments Co., Brussels, Belgium, and New England Nuclear Corp., Dreieichenhain, West Germany, respectively. Radioactive compounds were purchased from the Radiochemical Centre, Amersham, England. *N*-benzoylglucosamine and *N*-benzoyl-[^{14}C]glucosamine were prepared by the method of Konstas et al. (39). The radioactive preparation had a specific activity of 21 μCi/mmol.

Incorporation experiments. Cells from 10-h cultures (exponential phase) were suspended in fresh culture medium (pH 6.8) without human milk. The absorbance at 550 nm of the suspension was approximately set to 1.00. *N*-benzoyl-D-glucosamine was added in an optimal concentration for growth (25 μg/ml). Preincubation was performed for 1 h at 37°C with and without antibiotics. The final concentrations of the antibiotics were: penicillin G, 10 μg/ml; vancomycin, 20 μg/ml; bacitracin, 160 μg/ml (3.24 U/ml); D-cycloserine, 80 μg/ml; chloramphenicol, 60 μg/ml; tetracycline, 50 μg/ml; actinomycin D, 10 μg/ml; and staphylococcin 1580, 50 arbitrary units/ml. After preincubation one normal and one inhibited culture suspension were tested at the same initial absorbance. Radioactive precursors were added in the following amounts per ml: 50 nCi of *N*-benzoyl-[1-^{14}C]glucosamine together with 15 nCi of [2-^{3}H]glycine or separately 5 nCi of [1-^{14}C]oleic acid or 3 nCi of [1-^{14}C]palmitic acid. Incubation was carried out at 37°C under an atmosphere of 90% N_2-10% CO_2.

Incorporation of [^{3}H]glycine and [^{14}C]glucosamine. Samples of 2.5 ml of culture were mixed with 2.5 ml of 10% trichloroacetic acid at 0°C. After centrifugation the precipitate was suspended in 5 ml of 5% trichloroacetic acid and heat for 30 min at 95°C. The trichloroacetic acid-insoluble residue was suspended in 5 ml of 0.01 M NaOH. After mixing with 10 ml of Instagel, the radioactivity was determined.

Incorporation of ^{14}C-labeled fatty acids. Samples of 2.5 ml of culture were mixed with 2.5 ml of medium at 0°C. Cells were isolated, washed twice with cold culture medium, and suspended in 5 ml of 0.01 M NaOH. After mixing with 10 ml of Instagel, the radioactivity was determined.

Isolation of the cytoplasmic membrane fraction. Samples of 2.5 ml of culture were added to 5 ml of medium at 0°C and centrifuged. The cells were suspended in 5 ml of 0.1 M phosphate buffer (pH 6.8), which contained 10 mM Mg^{2+} and 5 mg of lysozyme (EC 3.2.1.17). Protoplast formation was effected by incubation at 37°C for 40 min. Protoplasts were sonically treated four times for 15 s with a Branson sonifier model B12. After 5 min of incubation with deoxyribonuclease (EC 3.1.4.5; 12 μg/ml) the membrane fraction was collected by centrifugation for 30 min at 100,000 × *g*. The preparation was washed twice with 5 ml of phosphate buffer (pH 6.8, 10 mM Mg^{2+}) and taken up in 3 ml of 1% sodium dodecyl sulfate in water. For liquid scintillation counting 2 ml of the membrane suspension was adjusted to 5 ml with water and mixed with 10 ml of Instagel. The rest of the suspension was used for the protein assay.

Turnover experiments. Cells from 10-h cultures were incubated with radioactive precursors (concentrations as described above) during 60 min in fresh culture medium at 37°C. The labeled cells were isolated, washed twice with medium, and reincubated in fresh nonradioactive medium containing *N*-benzoylglucosamine (25 μg/ml). Antibiotics were then added in the same concentration as during the incorporation studies. The turbidity (550 nm) of the culture was about 1.0 at the start. The radioactivity was measured in the cells and in the medium, isolated from samples of 2.5 ml after different periods of incubation at 37°C. The same precipitation procedures were used as during the incorporation studies. Lipids were extracted from the culture medium by the procedure of Bligh and Dyer (3).

Analytical methods. The turbidity of the cultures was assayed at 550 nm. An absorbance of 1.00 corresponds to a dry weight of 0.04 mg/ml of culture. The protein content of membrane suspensions was assayed by the method of Lowry et al. (43). Lipids were extracted from cells as previously described (63) and from the extracellular fluid by the procedure of Bligh and Dyer (3). Silicic acid column and thin-layer chromatography were described previously (14). The amount of radioactivity incorporated from [^{14}C]glycine or *N*-benzoyl-[^{14}C]glucosamine into fatty acyl chains was determined by the method of Cronan (8).

For identification of the labeled amino acids, the hot trichloroacetic acid-insoluble fraction of [^{14}C]-glycine-labeled cells was hydrolyzed with 6 N HCl for 16 h at 100°C. After thin-layer chromatography on cellulose, amino acid detection was performed by autoradiography. The plates were developed with *n*-butanol–pyridine–water (1:1:1, by volume) and n-butanol–acetone–water (4:1:5, by volume).

Samples were assayed for radioactivity in a Tri-Carb liquid scintillation spectrometer model 3380 with an absolute activity analyzer model 544 (Packard Instruments Co., Inc.). The scintillation fluid was a solution of 4 g of Omnifluor in 1 liter of toluene. Aqueous samples were mixed with 2 volumes of Instagel.

RESULTS

The glucosamine unit from *N*-benzoylglucosamine appears to be readily incorporated into the hot trichloroacetic acid-insoluble fraction of the cell. This fraction contains the cell wall peptidoglycan but no teichoic acids (53). Only 1.4% of the total radioactivity was not solubilized after lysozome digestion. About 1.9% of the radioactivity incorporated from *N*-benzoylglucosamine was found in the fatty acyl chains. Thus, the ^{14}C activity of the fraction represented predominantly incorporation into peptidoglycan. Glycine was chosen as a precursor for protein synthesis because this amino acid is very effectively incorporated into the cellular protein without structural modification. Since glycine is not a component of the cell wall peptidoglycan (52), a single precipitation procedure could be used for protein and peptidoglycan. By the use of [^{3}H]glycine and *N*-benzoyl-[^{14}C]- glucosamine it was possible to measure the incorporation of both precursors by one assay in the same sample.

Since glycerol and fatty acids are common components of all lipids, both were investigated as possible precursors for incorporation into the lipid fraction. Glycerol did not appear to be a suitable precursor because it was not incorporated under all experimental conditions. ^{14}C-labeled fatty acids appeared to be good precursors for the lipids. They were not used for the synthesis of other cellular components because 99% of the incorporated radioactivity could be extracted with chloroform-methanol. Oleic and palmitic acids were used because they amounted to about 40 and 25%, respectively, of the total fatty acids (64). These acids were not converted to other fatty acids, as was proved by radio-gas chromatography.

Incorporation studies. Incorporation in control cells varied somewhat, despite the use of completely standardized procedures. These variations are probably due to differences in culture, age, and growth. The problem was overcome by comparing the inhibited cells always with control cells from the same original culture. Since an extended period of growth inhibition may cause widespread damage to the cell, only data for relatively short labeling periods were considered. The data for membrane components were expressed on the basis of the protein content of the membrane preparation, according to Kahane and Razin (34), since the amount of membrane material obtained varied between identical experiments.

When cells from a 10-h culture were suspended in fresh medium containing *N*-benzoylglucosamine, the absorbance doubled after about 90 min (Fig. 1). The increase in incorporation of [^{3}H]glycine, *N*-benzoyl-[^{14}C]glucosamine, and [^{14}C]oleic acid into cellular components was nearly linear for 60 min (Fig. 1 and 2). After this period the incorporation rate of oleic acid decreased. The incorporation of glycine and oleic acid into the membrane fraction rapidly increased in the early part of the incubation period. Since incorporation is expressed per milligram of membrane protein, it tends to become constant, as the increasing incorporation equilibrates with the increase in the membrane protein mass.

Inhibition of cell wall synthesis. Penicillin, vancomycin, and bacitracin appear to be effective inhibitors of growth and *N*-benzoylglucosamine incorporation. Figure 1 shows the results of one representative experiment. Table 1 contains the relative incorporation data for the inhibited cells after 50 and 90 min. These values are fairly representative for all incorporation studies. D-Cycloserine inhibited somewhat less than the former three antibiotics. The incorporation of glycine into cellular and membrane protein was markedly depressed under all conditions of cell wall inhibition, with cycloserine again showing less effect. The apparent incorporation may be due to the net synthesis of cell components and/or turnover. The turnover of glucosamine in peptidoglycan and of glycine in protein was studied in cells labeled for 60 min. The glucosamine and glycine labels were preserved in the macromolecules of the normal cell during the chase period of 90 min, equal to one generation time. The inhibition of cell wall synthesis did not cause a decrease of these labels either.

The amount of [^{3}H]glycine incorporated per milligram of membrane protein decreased to about 74% of the value at the start of the chase period in normal cells. The increase of turbidity (46%) suggests a similar increase in membrane mass, explaining the 30% decrease of the ^{3}H activity. The agreement of the observed and calculated values for isotope dilution indicates an absence of turnover of glycine in the membrane protein during the 90-min chase period. Inhibition of cell wall synthesis caused a slight decrease in the amount of [^{3}H]glycine per milligram of membrane protein, which may be due to isotope dilution and increased turnover.

The addition of penicillin caused a marked increase in the [^{14}C]oleic acid incorporation (Fig. 2), despite a strong inhibition of growth. In this case, and also with vancomycin, the incorporation into cellular lipids reached a

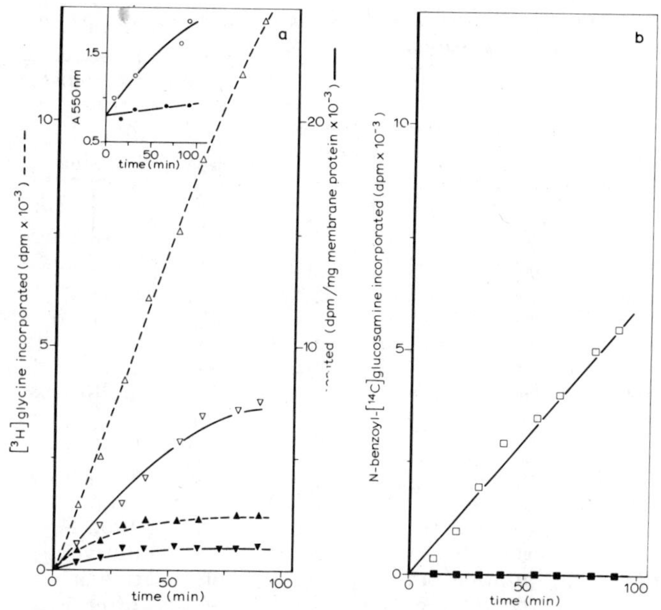

FIG. 1. *Incorporation of [^{3}H]glycine and N-benzoyl-[^{14}C]-D-glucosamine during normal growth (open symbols) and during inhibition with penicillin G (closed symbols). (a) Incorporation of glycine into the hot trichloroacetic acid-insoluble fraction (△) and incorporation of glycine into the membrane fraction per milligram of membrane protein (▽). Insertion, Absorbance of the cultures at 550 nm (A_{550}). (b) Incorporation of N-benzoylglucosamine into the hot trichloroacetic acid-insoluble fraction.*

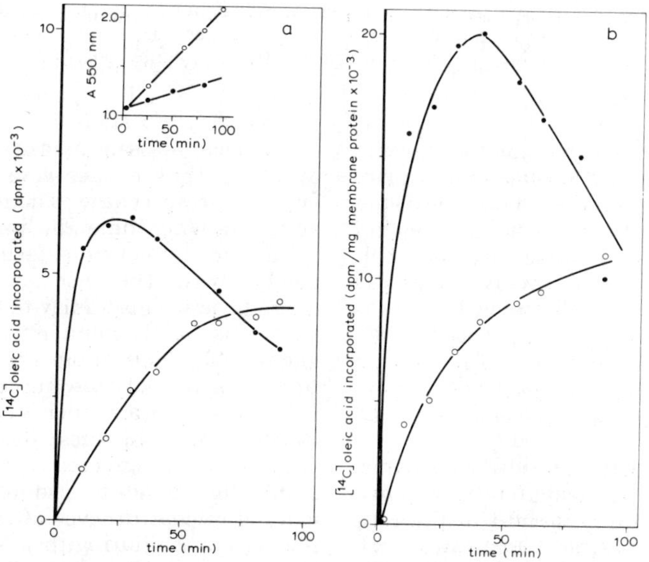

FIG. 2. *Incorporation of [^{14}C]oleic acid during normal growth (open symbols) and during inhibition with penicillin G (closed symbols). (a) Incorporation into the cellular lipids. Insertion, Absorbance of the cultures at 550 nm (A_{550}). (b) Incorporation into the membrane fraction.*

maximum after about 40 min and decreased thereafter. In other cases of inhibition of peptidoglycan synthesis the incorporation was also increased, but did not show a maximal value (Table 1). The increase of oleic acid incorporation was also apparent in the membrane fraction (Table 1). Chromatography of extracted ^{14}C-labeled lipids demonstrated that the in-

TABLE 1. *Influence of inhibition of cell wall synthesis and protein synthesis on the incorporation of N-benzoylglucosamine, glycine, and oleic acid*[a]

Condition	Time (min)	Relative incorporation: Growth	Relative incorporation: N-benzoyl-glucosamine	Glycine: Cells	Glycine: Membrane	Oleic acid: Cells	Oleic acid: Membrane
Penicillin G	50	11	1	13	18	129	209
	90	6	1	11	14	92	95
Vancomycin	50	4	1	5	18	270	420
	90	3	1	5	16	105	165
Bacitracin	50	13	2	16	14	122	155
	90	10	4	18	17	170	215
D-Cycloserine	50	45	13	63	75	147	133
	90	25	24	55	78	144	128
Without N-benzoylglucosamine	50	18		51	48	131	141
	90	15		45	50	127	193
Chloramphenicol	50	27	50	5	1	32	14
	90	30	48	5	1	46	20
Tetracycline	50	23	47	2	2	65	79
	90	25	51	3	1	60	80
Actinomycin D	50	11	24	3	3	93	83
	90	10	20	1	2	128	122
Without additional Mg^{2+}	50	42	90	62	66	38	32
	90	40	95	56	73	53	49
Staphylococcin 1580	50	11	7	15	20	100	144
	90	20	6	17	25	68	131

[a] Cells in the exponential phase were suspended in fresh culture medium containing N-benzoylglucosamine (25 μg/ml). Radioactive precursors were added after preincubation for 1 h with and without antibiotic. The incorporation of N-benzoyl-[^{14}C]glucosamine into peptidoglycan, of [^{3}H]glycine into cellular and membrane protein, and of [^{14}C]oleic acid into cellular and membrane lipids was determined. Growth was measured as the increase in turbidity at 550 nm. Values were calculated as the percentage of those of the control cells. Values for the membrane fraction were calculated per milligram of membrane protein and subsequently expressed as the percentage of those of the control cell membranes. Data are the means of two to four experiments.

creased incorporation was not due to a specific increase in free cellular [^{14}C]oleic acid or glycerides. The glycolipid fraction showed the same relative increase and the phospholipid fraction showed an even larger enhancement of labeling. Inhibition of peptidoglycan synthesis caused similar effects on [^{14}C]palmitic acid incorporation. Its incorporation increased by 80, 135, 30, 17, and 43% after 50 min of incubation with penicillin, vancomycin, bacitracin, and D-cycloserine and without N-benzoylglucosamine, respectively.

During normal growth in nonradioactive medium all of the [^{14}C]oleic acid and [^{14}C]palmitic acid incorporated were conserved in the cells (Fig. 3). Under all conditions that caused cell wall inhibition we observed a considerable decline in the ^{14}C activity of the cellular lipids with a concomitant increase in the radioactivity of the lipids in the culture medium (Fig. 3). Penicillin caused a loss of 76% of the initial cellular [^{14}C]oleic acid activity and of 65% of the [^{14}C]palmitic acid activity after 90 min. With vancomycin and the omission of N-benzoylglucosamine, these values were 75 and 50, and 36 and 37%, respectively. The distribution of ^{14}C activity among the main lipid fractions of the culture medium was determined after a 3-h incubation of [^{14}C]oleic acid-labeled cells in nonradioactive medium with penicillin. The activity was mainly found in the glycolipids (30%) and phospholipids (65%). The detailed composition of the lipids in the culture medium will be reported separately (J. H. Veerkamp, Biochim. Biophys. Acta, in press). The membrane fractions of the inhibited cells also showed a considerable loss of oleic acid-labeled lipids. The marked release of lipids after cell wall inhibition is not coupled with a significant loss of labeled protein or peptidoglycan from [^{3}H]glycine- or [^{14}C]glucosamine-labeled cells.

Inhibition of protein synthesis. Chloramphenicol, tetracycline, and actinomycin D appeared to inhibit [^{3}H]glycine incorporation into total cellular and membrane protein effectively, although growth was not completely arrested (Table 1). Despite the inhibition of glycine incorporation, the incorporation of *N*-benzoyl-[^{14}C]glucosamine continued, although at a decreased rate. The incorporated [^{14}C]glucosamine activity was nearly completely soluble after lysozyme digestion.

The omission of Mg^{2+} from the medium reduced its concentration from 1.0 to 0.14 mM (contamination by other chemicals). The Mg^{2+} deficiency resulted in a decrease in growth and glycine incorporation (Table 1). The incorporation of *N*-benzoylglucosamine was about the same for normal and Mg^{2+}-deficient cultures, despite the lower increase in turbidity in the latter case. The glucosamine activity incorporated after Mg^{2+} omission was again nearly completely digestible by lysozyme.

During the inhibition of protein synthesis the incorporation of [^{14}C]oleic acid continues to a considerable extent, especially in the presence of tetracycline and actinomycin (Table 1). After 60 min the incorporation was higher in the presence of actinomycin than in normal cells. Mg^{2+} deficiency caused a markedly lower incorporation of [^{14}C]oleic acid (Table 1). The distribution of the incorporated activity of oleic acid over the glycerides, the free fatty acid fraction, and the polar lipids was not changed by inhibitors of protein synthesis and by Mg^{2+} deficiency.

Protein and peptidoglycan, prelabeled for 60 min and incubated for 90 min, showed no significant decrease in radioactivity upon inhibition of protein synthesis. The [^{14}C]oleic acid label of cellular lipids was retained during the inhibition of protein synthesis with chloramphenicol and tetracycline and during Mg^{2+} deficiency in nonradioactive medium. Actinomycin caused a 20% decrease in the initial radioactivity after 90 min of incubation. The amount of [^{3}H]glycine per milligram of membrane protein remained constant during incubation with inhibitors of protein synthesis in nonradioactive medium for 90 min, whereas Mg^{2+} omission caused some turnover. In all of these cases the amount of [^{14}C]oleic acid per milligram of membrane protein remained unchanged. No significant release of lipids was detected after the inhibition of protein synthesis by chloramphenicol and tetracycline and during Mg^{2+} deficiency.

Effect of staphylococcin 1580. Staphylococcin 1580 inhibited the growth and incorporation of glycine and *N*-benzoylglucosamine about equally. The incorporation into staphylococcin-inhibited cells was increased for 40 min after the addition of [^{14}C]oleic acid, whereupon it declined as it did after the addition of penicillin and vancomycin. The incorporation of [^{14}C]-palmitic acid showed the same results as for oleic acid. The cellular lipids lost 60% of the [^{14}C]oleic acid label after 90 min of incubation of the cells in nonradioactive medium with staphylococcin. The amount of [^{14}C]oleic acid per milligram of membrane protein decreased by 50% after 90 min. As in the case of inhibitors of cell wall synthesis, staphylococcin 1580 caused a considerable release of lipids to the culture medium (Fig. 3). No significant loss of cellular

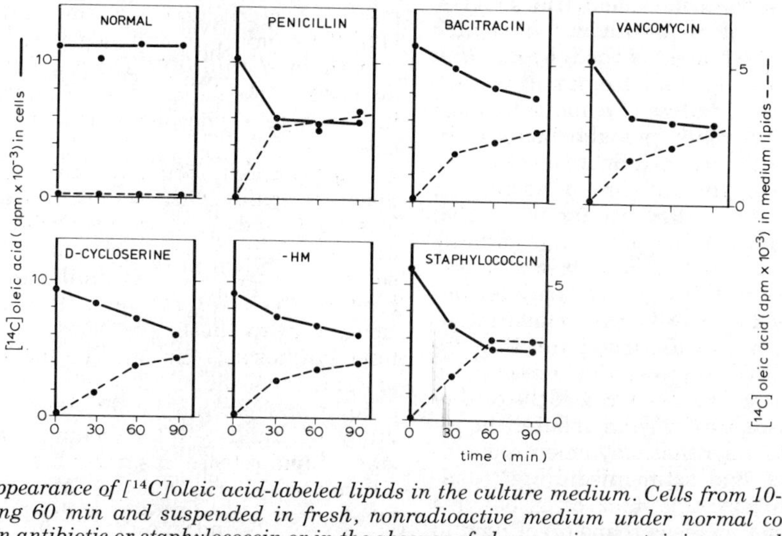

FIG. 3. *Appearance of [^{14}C]oleic acid-labeled lipids in the culture medium. Cells from 10-h cultures were labeled during 60 min and suspended in fresh, nonradioactive medium under normal conditions in the presence of an antibiotic or staphylococcin or in the absence of glucosamine-containing growth factors (-HM). The radioactivity of lipids was determined in the cells (●——●) and in the culture fluid (●– –●).*

labeled peptidoglycan or protein appeared under this condition.

DISCUSSION

Although they are acting at different levels of peptidoglycan synthesis (4, 59, 61), the effects of penicillin, vancomycin, bacitracin, and D-cycloserine on the metabolism of protein and lipids are qualitatively similar and similar to those of omission of human milk. Protein synthesis decreases strongly, but a marked increase in lipid synthesis appears together with a release of fatty acid-labeled lipids. A considerable amount of lipid-^{32}P activity was also found in the culture medium when ^{32}P-labeled cells were incubated under conditions causing inhibition of cell wall synthesis (data not shown). The release of lipids may be due to the uncoupling of protein and lipid synthesis under these conditions. Lipid release after the inhibition of cell wall synthesis has previously been found only for *Corynebacterium alkanolyticum* and *Brevibacterium thiogenitalis* (36, 49). Among the antibiotics that inhibit cell wall synthesis, only penicillin and cephalosporidine induced the release of lipids by these organisms.

The inhibition of protein synthesis by antibiotics did not affect lipid synthesis in some organisms (2, 34, 52) and merely reduced it in others (6, 9, 10, 25, 47, 50). No release of lipids occurred under these conditions of unbalanced synthesis, which may result in an enhanced lipid-to-protein ratio of the membrane (34, 47). Different modes of inhibition of protein synthesis appeared only to promote the release of complexes of lipids with lipopolysaccharides and/or protein by different *Escherichia coli* strains (10, 11, 38, 55). The release of lipids by *Bacillus amyloliquefaciens*, on the other hand, was diminished after the addition of chloramphenicol (20). Under these conditions the increase in lipid content is not corrected by lipid release in our organism. Higgins and Daneo-Moore (25), Higgins et al. (26), and Shockman et al. (58) reported that the inhibition of protein synthesis by amino acid starvation and antibiotics causes an increase in the thickness of the electron-transparent middle layer of the membrane in *S. faecalis*, which they ascribed to an increase in the ratio of lipid to protein. We observed a similar phenomenon in about 20% of the cells of *B. bifidum* subsp. *pennsylvanicus* after the inhibition of protein synthesis by chloramphenicol, tetracycline, and actinomycin. Mg^{2+} deficiency does not cause this thickening, but this condition does not increase the ratio of lipid to protein in our organism either.

The treatment of various gram-positive bacteria with antibiotics inhibitory to protein synthesis resulted in the thickening of the cell wall by continued peptidoglycan synthesis (5, 7, 17, 19, 23, 26, 27, 29, 48, 57). Although the inhibition of protein synthesis caused only a partial inhibition in peptidoglycan synthesis in *B. bifidum* subsp. *pennsylvanicus*, we could not establish an increase in cell wall thickness. However, this organism has a rather thin cell wall (10 to 15 nm), which makes the detection of small increases rather difficult.

The absence of a detectable turnover of cellular proteins was also found in *S. aureus* (66). The membrane proteins appear metabolically stable, in contrast to those of *Mycoplasma laidlawii* (34). Chloramphenicol, tetracycline, and actinomycin equally inhibited glycine incorporation into the total cellular and membrane proteins of *B. bifidum* subsp. *pennsylvanicus*, as they do in *E. coli* (67). A differential inhibitory effect was observed upon the incorporation of glycine into proteins of *Micrococcus lysodeikticus* (18, 62). During the arrest of protein synthesis by chloramphenicol, no turnover of membrane proteins was observed in *E. coli* (2), as was the case in our organism. The rate of membrane protein turnover was decreased by this antibiotic in *M. laidlawii* (34).

Growth of bacteria in a Mg^{2+}-deficient medium causes a loss of ribosomes (35, 44), but only partial inhibition of protein synthesis (46). In our organism protein and peptidoglycan synthesis are less affected than growth during Mg^{2+} deficiency. This may be due to an accumulation of Mg^{2+}, as was found in *Bacillus cereus* T (56). Mg^{2+} limitation affected the cell wall content and composition of various gram-positive bacteria grown in chemostat cultures (12). The synthesis of lipids runs parallel to growth in *B. bifidum* subsp. *pennsylvanicus* during Mg^{2+} depletion of the medium, whereas in *E. coli* total phospholipids increased in this case (21).

Staphylococcin 1580 causes inhibition of some macromolecular syntheses and transport of various compounds in *S. aureus* Oxford 209 P (30–32). The effect of this compound on *B. bifidum* subsp. *pennsylvanicus* is similar to that of inhibitors of cell wall synthesis. Protein and peptidoglycan synthesis are nearly arrested, but lipid synthesis continues. The marked release of lipids is not the result of cell lysis because no protein and peptidoglycan appear in the medium and their cellular amount remains constant. Lipid release has never been reported as a result of bacteriocin action. Most bacteriocins cause a reduction of lipid synthesis (51).

ACKNOWLEDGMENTS

The excellent technical assistance of A. Plas is gratefully acknowledged.

This investigation was supported by the Netherlands Organization for Basic Research.

LITERATURE CITED

1. **Bacchus, A. N., and G. T. Javor.** 1975. Stability of *Escherichia coli* membrane proteins during chloramphenicol treatment. Antimicrob. Agents Chemother. 8:387–389.
2. **Ballesta, J. P. G., and M. Schaechter.** 1971. Effect of shift-down and growth inhibition on phospholipid metabolism of *Escherichia coli*. J. Bacteriol. 107:251–258.
3. **Bligh, E. G., and W. J. Dyer.** 1959. A rapid method of total lipid extraction and purification. Can. J. Biochem. Physiol. 37:911–917.
4. **Blumberg, P. M., and J. L. Strominger.** 1974. Interaction of penicillin with the bacterial cell: penicillin-binding proteins and penicillin-sensitive enzymes. Bacteriol. Rev. 38:291–335.
5. **Cadieux, G., J. R. Coté, and L. G. Mathieu.** 1970. Microscopic observation of cell wall modifications in *Staphylococcus aureus* cells treated with chloramphenicol or phenethyl alcohol. Rev. Can. Biol. 29:219–225.
6. **Card, G. L.** 1973. Metabolism of phosphatidylglycerol, phosphatidylethanolamine, and cardiolipin of *Bacillus stearothermophilus*. J. Bacteriol. 114:1125–1137.
7. **Chung, K. L.** 1971. Thickened cell walls of *Bacillus cereus* grown in the presence of chloramphenicol: their fate during cell growth. Can. J. Microbiol. 17:1561–1565.
8. **Cronan, J. E.** 1967. A rapid method for the estimation of bacterial fatty acid biosynthesis. Anal. Biochem. 21:293–297.
9. **Cronan, J. E., and P. R. Vagelos.** 1972. Metabolism and function of the membrane phospholipids of *Escherichia coli*. Biochim. Biophys. Acta 265:25–60.
10. **Crowfoot, P. D., M. Esfahani, and S. J. Wakil.** 1972. Relation between protein synthesis and phospholipid synthesis and turnover in *Escherichia coli*. J. Bacteriol. 112:1408–1415.
11. **Crowfoot, P. D., T. Oka, M. Esfahani, and S. J. Wakil.** 1972. Turnover of phospholipids in an unsaturated fatty acid auxotroph of *Escherichia coli*. J. Bacteriol. 112:1396–1407.
12. **Ellwood, D. C., and D. W. Tempest.** 1972. Effects of environment on bacterial wall content and composition, p. 83–117. *In* A. H. Rose and D. W. Tempest (ed.), Advances in microbial physiology, vol. 7. Academic Press Inc., London.
13. **Exterkate, F. A., B. J. Otten, H. W. Wassenberg, and J. H. Veerkamp.** 1971. Comparison of the phospholipid composition of *Bifidobacterium* and *Lactobacillus* strains. J. Bacteriol. 106:824–829.
14. **Exterkate, F. A., and J. H. Veerkamp.** 1969. Biochemical changes in *Bifidobacterium bifidum* var. *pennsylvanicus* after cell wall inhibition. I. Composition of lipids. Biochim. Biophys. Acta 176:65–77.
15. **Exterkate, F. A., and J. H. Veerkamp.** 1971. Biochemical changes in *Bifidobacterium bifidum* var. *pennsylvanicus* after cell wall inhibition. IV. Galactolipid composition. Biochim. Biophys. Acta 231:545–549.
16. **Exterkate, F. A., G. F. J. Vrensen, and J. H. Veerkamp.** 1970. Biochemical changes in *Bifidobacterium bifidum* var. *pennsylvanicus* after cell wall inhibition. III. Morphological structure and osmotic properties of the protoplasts and membrane composition. Biochim. Biophys. Acta 219:141–154.
17. **Frehel, C., A. Beaufilo, and A. Ryter.** 1971. Etude au microscope électronique de la croissance de la paroi chez *B. subtilis* et *B. megaterium*. Ann. Inst. Pasteur Paris 121:139–148.
18. **Garcia Mendoza, C., and M. Novaes Ledieu.** 1975. Membrane protein synthesis in *Micrococcus lysodeikticus* and selective effect of chloramphenicol. Can. J. Biochem. 53:615–622.
19. **Giesbrecht, P., and H. Ruska.** 1968. Uber Veranderungen der Feinstrukturen von Bakterien unter der Einwirkung von Chloramphenicol. Klin. Wochenschr. 46:575–582.
20. **Glenn, A. R., and A. R. Gould.** 1973. Inhibition of lipid synthesis in *Bacillus amyloliquefaciens* by inhibitors of protein synthesis. Biochem. Biophys. Res. Commun. 52:356–364.
21. **Günther, T., L. Richter, and J. Schmalbeck.** 1975. Phospholipids of *Escherichia coli* in magnesium deficiency. J. Gen. Microbiol. 86:191–193.
22. **György, P., R. F. Norris, and C. S. Rose.** 1954. Bifidus factor. I. A variant of *Lactobacillus bifidus* requiring a special growth factor. Arch. Biochem. Biophys. 48:193–201.
23. **Hash, J. H., and M. C. Davies.** 1962. Electron microscopy of *Staphylococcus aureus* treated with tetracycline. Science 138:828–829.
24. **Henning, U.** 1975. Determination of cell shape. Annu. Rev. Microbiol. 29:45–60.
25. **Higgins, M. L., and L. Daneo-Moore.** 1972. Morphokinetic reaction of cells of *Streptococcus faecalis* (ATCC 9790) to specific inhibition of macromolecular synthesis: dependence of mesosome growth on deoxyribonucleic acid synthesis. J. Bacteriol. 109:1221–1231.
26. **Higgins, M. L., L. Daneo-Moore, D. Boothby, and G. D. Shockman.** 1974. Effect of inhibition of deoxyribonucleic acid and protein synthesis on the direction of cell wall growth in *Streptococcus faecalis*. J. Bacteriol. 118:681–692.
27. **Higgins, M. L., and G. D. Shockman.** 1970. Early changes in the ultrastructure of *Streptococcus faecalis* after amino acid starvation. J. Bacteriol. 103:244–254.
28. **Higgins, M. L., and G. D. Shockman.** 1971. Procaryotic cell division with respect to wall and membranes. Crit. Rev. Microbiol. 1:29–72.
29. **Hughes, R. C., P. J. Tanner, and E. Stokes.** 1970. Cell wall thickening in *Bacillus subtilis*. Biochem. J. 120:159–170.
30. **Jetten, A. M., and G. D. Vogels.** 1972. Nature and properties of a *Staphylococcus epidermis* bacteriocin. J. Bacteriol. 112:243–250.
31. **Jetten, A. M., and G. D. Vogels.** 1972. Mode of action of a *Staphylococcus epidermis* bacteriocin. Antimicrob. Agents Chemother. 2:456–463.
32. **Jetten, A. M., and G. D. Vogels.** 1973. Effects of colicin A and staphylococcin 1580 on amino acid uptake into membrane vesicles of *Escherichia coli* and *Staphylococcus aureus*. Biochim. Biophys. Acta 311:483–495.
33. **Jetten, A. M., G. D. Vogels, and F. de Windt.** 1972. Production and purification of a *Staphylococcus epidermis* bacteriocin. J. Bacteriol. 112:235–242.
34. **Kahane, I., and S. Razin.** 1969. Synthesis of membrane protein and lipid in *Mycoplasma laidlawii*. Biochim. Biophys. Acta 183:79–89.
35. **Kennell, D., and A. Kotoulas.** 1967. Magnesium starvation of *Aerobacter aerogenes*. I. Changes in nucleic acid composition. J. Bacteriol. 93:334–344.
36. **Kikuchi, M., T. Kanamaru, and Y. Nakao.** 1973. Relation between the extracellular accumulation of L-glutamic acid and the excretion of phospholipids by penicillin-treated *Corynebacterium alkanolyticum*. Agric. Biol. Chem. 37:2405–2408.
37. **Kitanaka, E., K. Ochiai, G. Hamasu, M. Nakao, and J. Nakazawa.** 1972. Cell wall synthesis by *Staphylococcus aureus* in the presence of protein synthesis inhibitory agents. J. Antibiot. 25:679–680.
38. **Knox, K. W., J. Cullen, and E. Work.** 1967. An extracellular lipopolysaccharide-phospholipid-protein complex produced by *Escherichia coli* grown under lysine-limiting conditions. Biochem. J. 103:192–201.
39. **Konstas, S., J. Photaki, and L. Zervas.** 1959. Überführ-

ung von D-Glucosamin in Oxazolon- und Oxazolinderivate. Chem. Ber. 92:1288–1292.

40. **Lambert, R., Y. Saito, and J. H. Veerkamp.** 1965. Incorporation of labeled derivatives of 2-deoxy-2-amino-D-glucose into the cell walls of *Lactobacillus bifidus* var. *pennsylvanicus*. Arch. Biochem. Biophys. **110:**341–344.
41. **Lambert, R., and F. Zilliken.** 1965. Novel growth factors for *Lactobacillus bifidus* var. *pennsylvanicus*. Arch. Biochem. Biophys. **110:**544–550.
42. **Leive, L. (ed.).** 1973. Membranes and walls of bacteria. Marcel Dekker, New York.
43. **Lowry, O. H., N. J. Rosebrough, A. L. Farr, and R. J. Randall.** 1951. Protein measurement with the Folin phenol reagent. J. Biol. Chem. **193:**265–275.
44. **Lutsch, G., and P. Venker.** 1969. Intracytoplasmatische Membranen in *E. coli* nach magnesium- bzw phosphat-Mangel. Naturwissenschaften **56:**568.
45. **Machtiger, N. A., and C. F. Fox.** 1973. Biochemistry of bacterial membranes. Annu. Rev. Biochem. **42:**575–600.
46. **Marchesi, S. L., and D. Kennell.** 1967. Magnesium starvation of *Aerobacter aerogenes*. III. Protein metabolism. J. Bacteriol. **93:**357–366.
47. **Mindich, L.** 1970. Membrane synthesis in *Bacillus subtilis*. II. Integration of membrane proteins in the absence of lipid synthesis. J. Mol. Biol. **49:**433–439.
48. **Nakao, M., E. Kitanaka, K. Ochiai, and J. Nakazawa.** 1972. Cell wall synthesis in *Staphylococcus aureus* in the presence of protein synthesis inhibitory agents. I. Lincomycin, clindamycin and macrolide antibiotics. Jpn. J. Microbiol. **16:**403–413.
49. **Nakao, Y., T. Kanamaru, M. Kikuchi, and S. Yamatodani.** 1973. Extracellular accumulation of phospholipids, UDP-N-acetylhexosamine derivatives and L-glutamic acid by penicillin-treated *Corynebacterium alkanolyticum*. Agric. Biol. Chem. **37:**2399–2404.
50. **Nunn, W. D., and B. E. Tropp.** 1972. Effects of phenethyl alcohol on phospholipid metabolism in *Escherichia coli*. J. Bacteriol. **109:**162–168.
51. **Ohkawa, J., B. Maruo, and M. Kageyama.** 1975. Preferential inhibition of lipid synthesis by the bacteriocin pyocin S_2. J. Biochem. **78:**213–223.
52. **Ono, Y., and D. C. White.** 1971. Consequences of the inhibition of cardiolipin metabolism in *Haemophilus parainfluenzae*. J. Bacteriol. **108:**1065–1071.
53. **Park, J. T., and R. Hancock.** 1960. A fractionation procedure for studies of the synthesis of cell wall mucopeptide and of other polymers in cells of *Staphylococcus aureus*. J. Gen. Microbiol. **22:**249–258.
54. **Rogers, H. J.** 1970. Bacterial growth and the cell envelope. Bacteriol. Rev. **34:**194–214.
55. **Rothfield, L., and M. Pearlman-Kothencz.** 1969. Synthesis and assembly of bacterial membrane components. J. Mol. Biol. **44:**477–492.
56. **Schmidt, G. B., C. L. Rosano, and C. Hurwitz.** 1971. Evidence for a magnesium pump in *Bacillus cereus* T. J. Bacteriol. **105:**150–155.
57. **Shockman, G. D.** 1965. Symposium on the fine structure and replication of bacteria and their parts. IV. Unbalanced cell-wall synthesis: autolysis and cell-wall thickening. Bacteriol. Rev. **29:**345–358.
58. **Shockman, G. D., L. Daneo-Moore, and M. L. Higgins.** 1974. Problems of cell wall and membrane growth, enlargement, and division. Ann. N.Y. Acad. Sci. **235:**161–197.
59. **Siewert, G., and J. L. Strominger.** 1967. Bacitracin, an inhibitor of the dephosphorylation of lipid pyrophosphate, an intermediate in biosynthesis of the peptidoglycan of bacterial cell walls. Proc. Natl. Acad. Sci. U.S.A. **57:**767–773.
60. **Sokawa, Y., E. Nakao, and Y. Kaziro.** 1968. On the nature of the control by RC gene in *E. coli*: amino acid-dependent control of lipid synthesis. Biochem. Biophys. Res. Commun. **33:**108–112.
61. **Strominger, J. L.** 1973. The actions of penicillin and other antibiotics on bacterial cell wall synthesis. Johns Hopkins Med. J. **133:**63–81.
62. **Vambutas, V. K., and M. R. J. Salton.** 1970. Incorporation of [^{14}C]glycine into *Micrococcus lysodeikticus* membrane protein and effects of protein synthesis inhibitors. Biochim. Biophys. Acta **203:**83–93.
63. **Van Schaik, F. W., and J. H. Veerkamp.** 1975. Biochemical changes in *Bifidobacterium bifidum* var. *pennsylvanicus* after cell wall inhibition. VIII. Composition and metabolism of phospholipids at different stages and conditions of growth. Biochim. Biophys. Acta **388:**213–225.
64. **Veerkamp, J. H.** 1970. Biochemical changes in *Bifidobacterium bifidum* var. *pennsylvanicus* after cell wall inhibition. II. Fatty acid composition. Biochim. Biophys. Acta **210:**267–275.
65. **Veerkamp, J. H.** 1971. The structure of the cell wall peptidoglycan of *Bifidobacterium bifidum* var. *pennsylvanicus*. Arch. Biochem. Biophys. **148:**204–211.
66. **Wong, W., F. E. Young, and A. N. Chatterjee.** 1974. Regulation of bacterial cell walls: turnover of cell wall in *Staphylococcus aureus*. J. Bacteriol. **120:**837–843.
67. **Zusman, D. R.** 1973. Membrane protein synthesis in *Escherichia coli*: sensitivity to chloramphenicol. Arch. Biochem. Biophys. **159:**336–341.

ANTIMICROBIAL AGENTS AND CHEMOTHERAPY, Nov. 1976, p. 795-801
Vol. 10, No. 5

Printed in U.S.A.

R Plasmids in *Streptococcus agalactiae* (Group B)

THEA HORODNICEANU,* D. H. BOUANCHAUD, G. BIETH, AND Y. A. CHABBERT

Service de Bactériologie Médicale, Institut Pasteur, 75015 Paris, France

Received for publication 23 April 1976

Two plasmids determining resistance to tetracycline (RIP500) and to chloramphenicol, erythromycin, lincomycin, and pristinamycin I (RIP501) were isolated from a strain of *Streptococcus agalactiae*. The frequency-of-resistance loss is very low for RIP500 (<3 × 10^{4}) but higher for RIP501 (the efficiency was dependent upon the curing agents and incubation temperature and varied between 0.5 and 96%). Derivatives susceptible to all drugs were also obtained. RIP500 and RIP501 have similar molecular weights (17.9 × 10^{6} and 20 × 10^{6}, respectively) and represent different percentages of total deoxyribonucleic acid (0.4 and 4%, respectively). The number of copies of RIP500 and RIP501 per cell is different, and these plasmids are likely replicated under different kinds of control (stringent and/or relaxed). No plasmid deoxyribonucleic acid was found in a derivative of strain B96 susceptible to all drugs.

Increased frequency of the appearance of drug resistance strains in Lancefield group A (12, 27), B (16), and D (29) streptococci has been reported in the last years, especially for erythromycin, lincomycin, and tetracycline antibiotics. Since the initial report of Courvalin et al. of two R plasmids in a group D *Streptococcus faecalis* (8), the existence of plasmids in other strains of streptococci has been demonstrated in *S. mutans* (13), *S. pyogenes* (3, 23), group N (7, 22), and *S. faecium* (6). In all these strains, cryptic (7, 13), metabolic (6, 7, 22), and R plasmids (3, 4, 21) were described. Jacob et al. (20) and Dunny and Clewell (14) reported more recently the capacity of plasmids to promote transfer during mixed incubation in broth in *S. faecalis*.

Evidence of R plasmids in group B streptococci has not yet been reported. This study deals with the genetic and physical properties of two R plasmids (designated RIP500 and RIP501) carried by *S. agalactiae* strain B-49813/75, referred to as strain B96 in this study.

MATERIALS AND METHODS

Bacteria and plasmids. *S. agalactiae* strain B-49813 (designated here as B96), isolated from a clinical sputum specimen, was used in this investigation. The identification on horse blood agar was verified by Fuller's serological test (18). This strain is resistant to tetracycline (T), chloramphenicol (C), macrolide antibiotics (including erythromycin [E], oleandomycin [O], and spiramycin [Sr]), lincomycin (L), and pristinamycin I (PI), a streptogramin B-type antibiotic similar to vernamycin Bα (3). The R plasmids described in this study are: RIP500, mediating resistance to T; and RIP501, resistant to C, E, L, and PI. The wild strain is referred to as B96 (RIP500 + RIP501) (see Table 1). T169, a tetracycline resistance plasmid from *Staphylococcus aureus* strain RN1304 (26), was used as the control in this study.

Media and materials. Brain heart infusion broth (Difco) was used as nutrient broth; tryptic soy agar (Difco) with 5% horse serum and Mueller-Hinton agar (Institut Pasteur) with 5% horse blood were used as nutrient agar. Davis minimal broth (11) supplemented with 2% protease peptone no. 3 (Difco) was used as the semisynthetic medium. Drugs used were as follows: tetracycline (Rhône-Poulenc, France), chloramphenicol (Roussel, France), erythromycin (Abbott, England), lincomycin (The Upjohn Co), and rifampin (Lepetit, France). Reagents used were: acridine orange (ESBE, France), acriflavine (Serlabo, France), ethidium bromide (Boots Drug Co), cesium chloride (ultrapur 2039, Merck), [^{3}H]-thymidine (44 Ci/mmol) and [^{14}C]thymidine (57 mCi/mmol) (Commissariat à l'Energie Atomique, France), Sarkosyl (NL97, Geigy Chemical Corp.), and lysozyme (Sigma).

MICs. The minimum inhibitory concentrations (MICs) were determined by the spot technique (10), using a Steers multiple inoculator apparatus (28). Eighty to 100 colony-forming units were plated onto nutrient agar plates containing doubling concentrations of an antibiotic, starting from 0.015 μg/ml. Antibiotics used and their MICs are listed in Table 1. The MIC was recorded as the lowest concentration of antibiotic preventing colony formation after 18 h of incubation. Resistance to O, S, clindamycin (Cl), virginiamycin, and PI and PII was determined with susceptibility disks.

Curing procedures. Curing by high temperature was as follows. An 18-h broth culture was diluted 1:10 in broth and incubated without aeration for 18 h at 42°C. Control cultures were grown at 37°C. For curing by chemical agents (acridine orange, acriflavine, or ethidium bromide), 1 to 3 mg of the chemicals was placed on nutrient agar (tryptic soy agar plus 5% horse serum) inoculated with a diluted (1:200) 6-h broth culture. After 18 h of incubation at 37°C, three zones were observed: (i) total inhibition, (ii) partial inhibition, and (iii) noninhibition. A loopful from the border of the second zone was subcultured in nutrient broth for 18 h. Master plates were prepared from this broth, as well as from those incubated either at 42 or 37°C and replica-plated for loss of T, C, E, or L resistance. Curing by rifampin was obtained by using nutrient agar plates containing 10, 25, 50, and 100 μg of rifampin per ml, and the plates were inoculated with a 6-h broth culture, 20-fold concentrated by centrifugation. After 18 to 36 h of incubation at 37°C, they were directly replica-plated as described above.

Plasmid deoxyribonucleic acid (DNA) isolation and sedimentation analysis. Streptococci were grown in 20 ml of semisynthetic broth containing 4% (wt/vol) glucose (optical density = 25 Klett units) at 37°C. Bacteria were labeled at optical density = 50 Klett units with 5 μCi of [*methyl*-^{3}H]thymidine or 100 μCi of [*methyl*-^{14}C]thymidine per ml. At optical density = 110 Klett units the cells were harvested and washed in cold tris(hydroxymethyl)aminomethane (0.05 M), ethylenediaminetetraacetic acid (0.001 M), pH 8 (TES buffer). The cells were treated for 1 h at 37°C with lysozyme (final concentration, 400 μg/ml in TES buffer) and for 30 min at 37°C with Sarkosyl (final concentration, 0.5%). These crude lysates (8 ml) were then centrifuged in the presence of cesium chloride (8 g) and ethidium bromide (0.4 ml of a stock solution containing 10 mg/ml). After 48 h at 42,000 rpm (20°C) in a 50 Ti rotor (L2-65 B Beckman ultracentrifuge), gradients were fractionatated by drop collection and counted. Plasmid T169 from *Staphylococcus* strain RN1304 was isolated as described by Novick and Bouanchaud (26). Sedimentation analysis in a neutral sucrose grdient of plasmid molecules was carried out as described recently (19).

RESULTS

Antibiotic resistance of *S. agalactiae* strains. The resistance pattern of 856 group B streptococci isolated from separate patients in the last 5 months of 1975 in Louis Pasteur Hospital, Strasbourg (France), was determined by using the routine susceptibility disk method. A total of 852 strains had the usual susceptibility spectrum of *S. agalactiae*, but four strains were resistant to T, C, E, Sr, O, L, Cl, and PI. One of these resistant strains, referred to as B96, was chosen for further studies. The MICs of different antibiotics are shown in Table 1.

Stability of drug resistance in strain B96. Spontaneous loss of drug resistance after 6 months of storage in nutrient broth at 4°C, or after lyophilization of the strain, was tested by the replica-plating technique (Table 2). As can be seen, no loss of drug resistance was observed, except in a lyophilized sample, in which only C, E, L, and PI markers were lost at low frequency (<0.5%). The results of several "curing" experiments using different agents are summarized in Table 2. One important feature is the detection of a rather large number of clones resistant to T and one clone (from a total of 3,376 clones examined) resistant only to C, E, L, and PI. The lack of loss of T was recently reported by Clewell et al. (4) and was in contrast to the efficiency of curing (31%) obtained by Courvalin et al. (8). Thus, to obtain susceptible clones of B96, the C E L PI-resistant strain was treated by different curing procedures. We obtained an efficiency of 1% with rifampin (25 μg/ml) and 1.2% at the elevated incubation temperature (42°C; Table 2). These results suggested that the resistance markers in B96 strain were plasmid borne and that this strain carried two plasmids, referred to as RIP500 and RIP501, coding for T and C E L PI, respectively. When the wild strain B96 (RIP500 + RIP501) was grown at 42°C, the frequency of colony-forming units of plasmid RIP501 (C E L PI) "cured" was 0.5, 48.5, and 96% in three independent experiments. The RIP500 (T) plasmid was never cured at high temperature. No loss of any resistance markers was obtained with acriflavine or ethidium bromide.

The MICs of antibiotics for all derivatives are shown in Table 1. The same pattern of susceptibility for C, E, L, and T was obtained for another strain of *S. agalactiae* (B19) used as the reference strain in this study. One of the cured cells of strain B96 was further examined for

TABLE 1. *MICs of antibiotics used*

Bacterial strain[a]	Plasmids	Resistance markers	MIC (μg/ml) for:				
			T	C	E	L	PI[b]
B96	RIP500 + RIP501	T C E L PI	64	16	4,000	256	R
B96	RIP500	T	64	2	0.03	0.03	S
B96	RIP501	C E L PI	0.25	32	4,000	256	R
B96		Cured	0.25	2	0.03	0.03	S
B19			0.25	2	0.03	0.03	S

[a] B19 is a susceptible, reference group B strain.

[b] Tested with sensitivity disks. S, Sensitive; R, resistant.

TABLE 2. *Curing of RIP500 and RIP501 by different agents*

Plasmids	Treatment[a]	No. of colonies tested	No. of resistant colonies				Efficiency of curing (%)
			T	C	E	L	
RIP500 + RIP501 (T C E L PI)	37°C	180[b]	180	180	180	180	0
		420[c]	420	418	418	418	0.5
		200[d]	200	199	199	199	0.5
	42°C	64[d]	64	33	33	33	48.5
		340[d]	340	14	14	14	96
	AO	67	66	62	62	62	1.5 for T[e] 7.4 for C E L PI
RIP500 (T)	37°C	133	133				0
	42°C	163	163				0
	AO	460	460				0
	Rif	33	33				0
RIP501 (C E L PI)	37°C	200		200	200	200	0
	42°C	98		97	97	97	1
	AO	250		250	250	250	0
	Rif	78		77	77	77	1.2

[a] AO, Acridine orange; Rif, rifampin.
[b] After 6 months of storage at 4°C.
[c] After lyophilization of the wild strain B96.
[d] Three independent experiments.
[e] A single tetracycline-susceptible clone was obtained from a total of 3,376 clones screened.

spontaneous reversion to high-level resistance on plates containing 8 μg of C and 25 μg of E, L, or T per ml. An inoculum of about 2.2×10^9 cells was spread on the plates; no reversion to C, E, L, or T resistance was observed. From the data shown in Table 2 we could conclude that resistance markers were stable in strain B96, and that curing agents have poor activity (if any) on plasmids RIP500 and RIP501. The same stability has been reported by Jacob and Hobbs in an *S. faecalis* strain (21) and by Clewell and Franke in an *S. pyogenes* strain (3).

Determination of chloramphenicol inactivation. Inactivation of chloramphenicol was demonstrated by using the satellitism test as described by Chabbert and Debruge (2) in *Staphylococcus* strains. Spots of B96 (RIP501) and of B96 (RIP500) were inoculated on nutritive agar containing spores of *Bacillus subtilis* strain ATCC 6633 and 2 μg of C per ml. After 18 h of incubation at 37°C, a dense halo of *B. subtilis* is visible around the spot of B96 (RIP501) but not around that of B96 (RIP500). This observation suggests that an inhibitor of chloramphenicol diffused in the agar from the B96 (RIP501) spot, presumably a chloramphenicol acetyltransferase, which will be described elsewhere.

Isolation of plasmid DNA. Figure 1 shows the results of dye buoyant density centrifugation of the DNA of strain B96 (wild type) and of different variants obtained in curing procedures. Double-label experiments were carried out with mixtures of a lysate of B96 resistant to C E L PI T, and labeled with [^{3}H]thymidine, and a lysate of a derivative susceptible to all drugs of B96 labeled with [^{14}C]thymidine. The percentage of plasmid DNA was, respectively, 4 and 0% of the total bulk DNA (Fig 1a). In another experiment, lysates of B96 resistant to C E L PI T ([^{3}H]thymidine labeled) and of B96 resistant only to T ([^{14}C]thymidine labeled) were analyzed. The results are illustrated in Fig. 1b. The percentage of plasmid DNA was, respectively, 3.8 and 0.4% of the total DNA. In a third experiment (data not shown), it was observed that plasmid DNA represented 3.5% of the total DNA in a variant of B96 resistant to C E L PI but susceptible to T. These findings indicate the presence of plasmids in this strain. The loss of plasmid DNA associated with the loss of resistance provides evidence that the determinants of resistance are plasmid borne. RIP500 (T) and RIP501 (C E L PI) represent approximately 15 and 85% of the total plasmid DNA, respectively.

Determination of molecular weight and size of RIP500 and RIP501. Samples of pure plasmid DNA, obtained from B96 (RIP500) and B96 (RIP501) and labeled, respectively, with [^{14}C]thymidine and [^{3}H]thymidine, were sedimented in sucrose gradients as described in Materials and Methods. Figure 2a shows the results of band sedimentation of RIP501 and

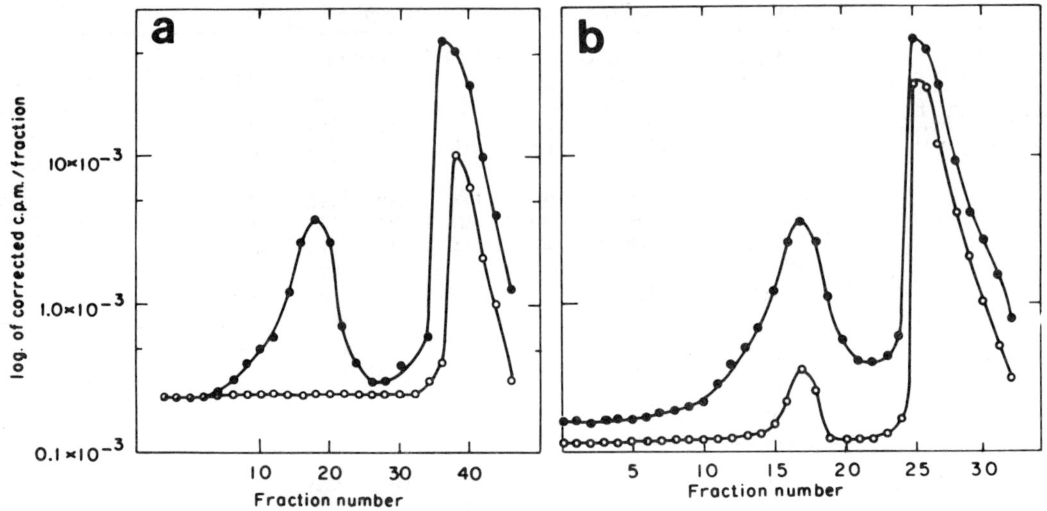

FIG. 1. *Isolation of plasmid DNA in dye buoyant density gradients. (a) Lysate of a mixture of wild strain B96 (RIP500 + RIP501) ([³H]thymidine, ●) and of a susceptible derivative of B96 ([¹⁴C]thymidine, ○). (b) Lysate of a mixture of B96 (RIP500 + RIP501) ([³H]thymidine, ●) and of B96 (RIP500) ([¹⁴C]thymidine, ○). Counts were corrected for double labeling and plotted on a log scale.*

T169 (used as a standard). The two peaks in fractions 24 and 32 represent form I (covalently closed circles of DNA) and form II (open circles) of RIP501 (C E L PI) plasmid. Using the value of $S = 19.55$ for T169 (26), the S value for RIP501 (form I) can be estimated to be 45.13, which corresponds to a molecular weight of 20×10^6, equivalent to 10 nm. The result of band sedimentation of RIP501 (^{3}H-labeled) and RIP500 (^{14}C-labeled) can be seen in Fig. 2b. The S value for RIP500 was calculated to be 43.3, which corresponds to a molecular weight of 17.9×10^6, or 9.07 nm. RIP500 (T) does not give rise to form II molecules, as was found for some plasmids of *S. aureus* (Bouanchaud and Novick, unpublished data) and from this point of view is strikingly different from RIP501 (C E L PI).

Estimation of the number of copies of each plasmid. Assuming that plasmid and chromosomal DNA have the same radioactive specific activity and that the molecular weight of the *S. faecalis* chromosome is 1.47×10^9 (1), the relative number of copies of RIP500 and RIP501 per chromosomal genome equivalent (CGE) can be estimated from the molecular weight and the relative amount of each plasmid. The apparent number of copies is 0.3/CGE for RIP500 (T) and 3/CGE for RIP501 (C E L PI). A summary of the most important physical properties of RIP500 and RIP501, described above, is given in Table 3.

DISCUSSION

There is increasing interest in group B streptococci in the medical literature of the past decade, due to the multiple clinical infections caused by this organism: perinatal-puerperal infections, neonatal sepsis (with or without meningitis), pneumonia, empyema, peritonitis, urinary tract infections, arthritis, and endocarditis (15). Moreover, group B streptococci are usually very susceptible to several antibiotics and especially to penicillin G, which is the drug of choice in the treatment of *S. agalactiae* diseases. However, in penicillin-allergic patients, for whom penicillin is contraindicated, E or L is usually a satisfactory alternative. The appearance of strains resistant to E and L, reported by Eickhoff et al. (16) and Minck (unpublished data) in group B streptococci, and also the high frequency of T-resistant strains (approximately 80% of our recent *S. agalactiae* isolates) could make it difficult to provide an appropriate therapy.

Multiple-drug-resistant plasmids have recently been demonstrated only in group D (4, 8, 21) and A streptococci (3, 23), and at least two R plasmids carried by one strain were generally reported. The *S. agalactiae* strain (B96) described in this study also carries two R plasmids: RIP500 (T) and RIP501 (C E L PI). From this point of view, streptococci seem to be very different from staphylococci, in which the most plasmids described so far encode only for one resistance marker, with the exception of the penicillin erythromycin plasmids reported by Novick (25).

It might be pointed out that an interesting feature of RIP501 is that it also carries the C-resistant marker, which was found only in a few strains of *S. pyogenes* (24).

The molecular weights of *Streptococcus* plasmids are very variable: from 10^6 for a cryptic plasmid in *S. lactis* (22) to 64.5×10^6 for a tetracycline resistance plasmid isolated from an *S. faecalis* strain (9). The molecular weights (and sizes) of RIP500 (T) and RIP501 (C E L PI) are very close, 17.9×10^6 (9.07 nm) and 20×10^6 (10 nm), respectively, but RIP500 (T) represents 0.4% and RIP501 (C E L PI) represents 4% of total DNA. The number of copies of *Streptococcus* plasmids is not easy to define, because of the uncertainty of the size of the bacterial genome. As observed in *Enterobacteriaceae,* smaller plasmids seem to be replicated under relaxed control, and larger plasmids under stringent control (5). The apparent number of copies is 0.3/CGE for RIP500 (T) and 3/CGE for RIP501 (C E L PI). These are minimum estimates, because a variable and, very likely, important proportion of plasmid DNA is lost in the assay procedures. For instance, the number of copies of RIP500 cannot be smaller than 1 to

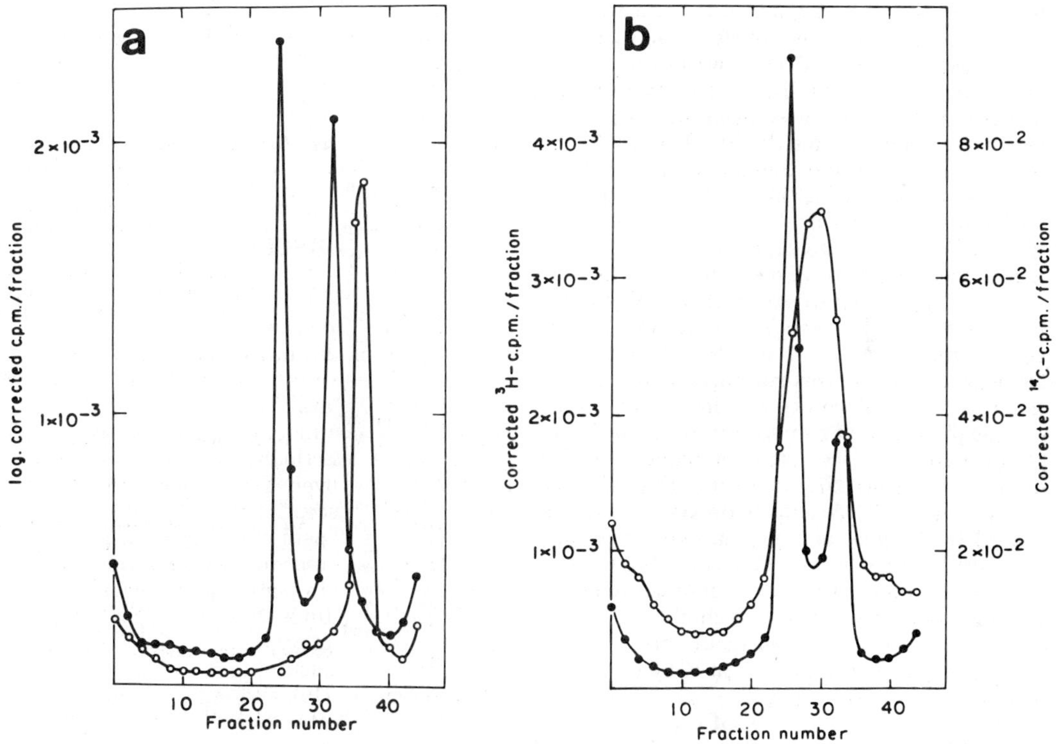

FIG. 2. *Sedimentation analysis of plasmid DNA in a neutral sucrose gradient. (a) RIP501 DNA ([³H]thymidine, ●) and T169 DNA ([¹⁴C]thymidine, ○). (b) RIP501 DNA ([³H]thymidine, ●) and RIP500 DNA ([¹⁴C]thymidine, ○). Note change in scale.*

TABLE 3. *Summary of the most important physical properties of RIP500 and RIP501*

Plasmids	Resistance marker	Mol. wt ($\times 10^{-6}$)	Size (nm)	% of total DNA	Minimum no. of copies per CGE	Form I (CCC) or II (OC)[a]
RIP500	T	17.9	9.07	0.4	0.3 (≥1)	CCC only
RIP501	C E L PI	20	10	3.8–4	≥3	CCC and OC

[a] CCC, Covalently closed circular; OC, open circular.

2/CGE, but a maximum of 1/3 (and often less) of RIP500 plasmid DNA is recovered in the density gradient. The molecular weight of RIP500 (T) is 17.9 × 10^6. Replicating plasmids of the same size have been found to be under stringent control in *S. faecalis* (4) and *S. pyogenes* (3). The DNA of RIP501 (C E L PI) represents 4% of the total DNA, but the data available so far do not allow a decision as to whether the number of copies of this plasmid is 9 to 10 times the number of copies of RIP500 or if the recovery of RIP501 DNA is better than the recovery of RIP500 DNA. However, the fact that RIP500 (T) seems to have less copies per CGE than RIP501 (C E L PI) does not agree with the difficulty in curing of the tetracycline plasmid. Clewell et al. (4) recently reported the same lack of success in curing a tetracycline plasmid, but the number of copies per CGE was larger.

The rather wide RIP500 band in the sucrose gradient is an unexplained but not uncommon feature of this type of experiment, as already shown by Freifelder for the F plasmid (17) and by Horodniceanu and Bouanchaud for the recombinant plasmid pIP218 (19). This fact contrasts with the sharp plasmid bands obtained with RIP501 DNA molecules.

Previous reports have demonstrated the presence of R plasmids in group A and D streptococci (3, 8); in the present study we demonstrate the presence of two R plasmids in group B streptococci. These reports suggest that the existence of R plasmids in other serological groups of human or animal origin is likely and is, perhaps, a more usual phenomenon. The similarity in these *Streptococcus* plasmids merits studies by DNA homology (as recently reported by Yagi et al. [30] for two E-resistant plasmids), to determine their possible interrelationships and define any genetic exchanges among these organisms.

ACKNOWLEDGMENTS

We are greatly indebted to S. Levy for his helpful criticism. We thank Françoise Delbos for expert technical assistance.

This work was partially supported by grants from the Institut National de la Santé et de la Recherche Médicale (T.H.) and the Fondation de l'Industrie Pharmaceutique pour la Recherche (D.H.B.). Strain B49813/75 was a gift from R. Minck (Université Louis Pasteur, Strasbourg, France).

LITERATURE CITED

1. **Bak, A. L., C. Christiansen, and A. Stenderup.** 1970. Bacterial genome sizes determined by DNA renaturation studies. J. Gen. Microbiol. **64:**377–380.
2. **Chabbert, Y. A., and J. Debruge.** 1956. La résistance naturelle des staphylocoques au chloramphénicol. Fréquence des variants sensibles producteurs d'une substance antagoniste au chloramphénicol. Ann. Inst. Pasteur Paris **91:**225–230.
3. **Clewell, D. B., and A. E. Franke.** 1974. Characterization of a plasmid determining resistance to erythromycin, lincomycin, and vernamycin Bα in a strain of *Streptococcus pyogenes*. Antimicrob. Agents Chemother. **5:**534–537.
4. **Clewell, D. B., Y. Yagi, G. M. Dunny, and S. K. Schultz.** 1974. Characterization of three plasmid deoxyribonucleic acid molecules in a strain of *Streptococcus faecalis:* identification of a plasmid determining erythromycin resistance. J. Bacteriol. **117:**283–289.
5. **Clowes, R. C.** 1972. Molecular structure of bacterial plasmids. Bacteriol. Rev. **36:**361–405.
6. **Cook, A. R.** 1976. The elimination of urease activity in *Streptococcus faecium* as evidence for plasmid-coded urease. J. Gen. Microbiol. **92:**49–58.
7. **Cords, B. R., L. L. McKay, and P. Guerry.** 1974. Extrachromosomal elements in group N streptococci. J. Bacteriol. **117:**1149–1152.
8. **Courvalin, P. M., C. Carlier, and Y. A. Chabbert.** 1972. Plasmid-linked tetracycline and erythromycin resistance in group D "*Streptococcus*." Ann. Inst. Pasteur Paris **123:**755–759.
9. **Courvalin, P. M., C. Carlier, O. Croissant, and D. Blangy.** 1974. Identification of two plasmids determining resistance to tetracycline and to erythromycin in group D *Streptococcus*. Mol. Gen. Genet. **132:**181–192.
10. **Daguet, G. L., and Y. A. Chabbert.** 1972. Les antibiotiques en bactériologie médicale, p. 155–156. *In* Techniques en bactériologie. Flammarion, Paris.
11. **Davis, B. D., and E. S. Mingioli.** 1950. Mutants of *Escherichia coli* requiring methionine or vitamin B12. J. Bacteriol. **60:**17–28.
12. **Dixon, J. M. S., and A. E. Lipinski.** 1972. Resistance of group A beta-hemolytic streptococci to lincomycin and erythromycin. Antimicrob. Agents Chemother. **1:**333–339.
13. **Dunny, G. M., N. Birch, G. Hascall, and D. B. Clewell.** 1973. Isolation and characterization of plasmid deoxyribonucleic acid from *Streptococcus mutans*. J. Bacteriol. **114:**1362–1364.
14. **Dunny, G. M., and D. B. Clewell.** 1975. Transmissible toxin (hemolysin) plasmid in *Streptococcus faecalis* and its mobilization of a noninfectious drug resistance plasmid. J. Bacteriol. **124:**784–790.
15. **Eickhoff, T. C.** 1972. Group B streptococci in human infection, p. 533–543. *In* L. W. Wannamaker and J. M. Matsen (ed.), Streptococci and streptococcal diseases. Academic Press Inc., New York.
16. **Eickhoff, T. C., J. O. Klein, A. K. Daly, D. Ingall, and M. Finland.** 1964. Neonatal sepsis and other infectious due to group B beta-hemolytic streptococci. N. Engl. J. Med. **271:**1221–1228.
17. **Freifelder, D.** 1968. Studies with *Escherichia coli* sex factors. Cold Spring Harbor Symp. Quant. Biol. **33:**425–434.
18. **Fuller, A. T.** 1938. The formamide method for the extraction of polysaccharides from hemolytic streptococci. Br. J. Exp. Pathol. **19:**130–139.
19. **Horodniceanu, T., and D. H. Bouanchaud.** 1976. Genetic and physical studies of recombinant plasmids formed between an R plasmid of compatibility group FI and sex factor F of HfrH. J. Bacteriol. **125:**58–67.
20. **Jacob, A. E., G. J. Douglas, and S. J. Hobbs.** 1975. Self-transferable plasmids determining the hemolysin and bacteriocin of *Streptococcus faecalis* var. *zymogenes*. J. Bacteriol. **121:**863–872.
21. **Jacob, A. E., and S. J. Hobbs.** 1974. Conjugal transfer of plasmid-borne multiple antibiotic resistance in *Streptococcus faecalis* var. *zymogenes*. J. Bacteriol. **117:**360–372.

22. **McKay, L. L., and K. A. Baldwin.** 1975. Plasmid distribution and evidence for a proteinase plasmid in *Streptoccus lactis* C2. Appl. Microbiol. 29:546–548.
23. **Malke, H.** 1974. Genetics of resistance to macrolide antibiotics and lincomycin in natural isolates of *Streptococcus pyogenes*. Mol. Gen. Genet. 135:349–367.
24. **Nakae, M., M. Inoue, and S. Mitsuhashi.** 1975. Artificial elimination of drug resistance from group A beta-hemolytic streptococci. Antimicrob. Agents Chemother. 7:719–720.
25. **Novick, R. P.** 1969. Extrachromosomal inheritance in bacteria. Bacteriol. Rev. 33:210–235.
26. **Novick, R. P., and D. H. Bouanchaud.** 1971. Extrachromosomal nature of drug resistance in *Staphylococcus aureus*. Ann. N.Y. Acad. Sci. 182:279–294.
27. **Sanders, E., M. T. Foster, and D. Scott.** 1968. Group A beta-hemolytic streptococci resistant to erythromycin and lincomycin. N. Engl. J. Med. 278:538–540.
28. **Steers, E., E. L. Foltz, and B. S. Graves.** 1959. An inocula replicating apparatus for routine testing of bacterial susceptibility to antibiotics. Antibiot. Chemother. 9:307–311.
29. **Toala, P., A. McDonald, C. Wilcox, and M. Finland.** 1969. Susceptibility of group D *Streptococcus* (Enterococcus) to 21 antibiotics in vitro, with special reference to species differences. Am. J. Med. Sci. 258:416–430.
30. **Yagi, Y., A. E. Franke, and D. B. Clewell.** 1975. Plasmid-determined resistance to erythromycin: comparison of strains of *Streptococcus faecalis* and *Streptococcus pyogenes* with regard to plasmid homology and resistance inducibility. Antimicrob. Agents Chemother. 7:871–873.

ANTIMICROBIAL AGENTS AND CHEMOTHERAPY, Nov. 1976, p. 802–808 Vol. 10, No. 5

Combination of Bacteriostatic and Bactericidal Drugs: Lack of Significant In Vitro Antagonism Between Penicillin, Cephalothin, and Rolitetracycline

FRANZ D. DASCHNER[1]

Children Hospital, Division of Antimicrobial Therapy, University of Munich, 8 Munich 2, Germany

Received for publication 16 April 1976

Although it is generally believed that bactericidal and bacteriostatic drugs should not be combined in vivo, in vitro experiments using the checkerboard dilution technique revealed no antagonism between penicillin/cephalothin and rolitetracycline but rather additive or synergistic activity of either drug combination in 40 to 50% of 20 *Escherichia coli* and 14 *Staphylococcus aureus* strains. Slight antagonism occurred only between 3 and 8 h after combining penicillin/cephalothin and rolitetracycline in either bacteriostatic or bactericidal concentrations, but not after 24 h of incubation, nor was antagonism found with combinations of these drugs in bacteriostatic concentrations. Neither bacteriostatic nor bactericidal activity of penicillin/cephalothin and rolitetracycline was inhibited by pretreatment of one *E. coli* strain with bacteriostatic rolitetracycline or bacteriostatic penicillin/cephalothin concentrations. Penicillin and cephalothin could exert a bactericidal effect after 2-h exposure of the *E. coli* strain to bacteriostatic rolitetracycline concentrations. Combined action of subinhibitory penicillin and rolitetracycline concentrations resulted in more pronounced inhibition of growth than either drug alone. The higher activity of penicillin/cephalothin in combination with rolitetracycline on some *E. coli* and *S. aureus* strains might be due to a better access of rolitetracycline into bacterial cells whose cell walls have been weakened by cell wall-active, bactericidal drugs. Thus, growth of penicillin-induced spheroplasts of *E. coli* and stable staphylococcal L-forms was inhibited by much lower concentrations of rolitetracycline than were the corresponding parent cells with intact cell walls.

According to Jawetz and Gunnison, the antibiotic and chemotherapeutic drugs can be divided into substances the effect of which is mainly bactericidal (e.g., penicillin, cephalosporins) and substances that generally have only bacteriostatic effects (e.g., tetracyclines) (11). They noted that whereas two bactericidal drugs were often synergistic, a combination of bactericidal and bacteriostatic antibiotics often resulted in antagonism in vitro. Several exceptions, however, to this chemotherapeutic rule have been found. The bacteriostatic sulfonamides may act synergistically with the bactericidal polymyxins against *Proteus* species and *Pseudomonas aeruginosa* (20, 22). Antagonism has been described between two penicillins, ampicillin and carbenicillin, when tested against *Enterobacter cloacae* (2). Although increased killing of penicillin-susceptible *Streptococcus viridans* by penicillin plus streptomycin can be demonstrated in vitro, the addition of streptomycin is not needed for effective treatment of patients with *S. viridans* endocarditis (2). Furthermore, it has long been known from in vitro studies that decreasing or increasing the concentration of primarily bactericidal and bacteriostatic drugs results in either bacteriostatic or bactericidal activity (19). None of these studies, however, considered the original finding of Jawetz that even within a given test system, the results of drug combinations may depend on drug concentrations, time of interaction, inoculum size, and other laboratory variables (10). I therefore investigated some of these variables, especially subinhibitory, bacteriostatic, and bactericidal drug concentrations and time of interaction, combining bactericidal (penicillin G, cephalothin) and bacteriostatic (rolitetracycline [RTC]) drugs in vitro. In further experiments with cell wall-defective bacteria (L-forms, spheroplasts), I examined why the combination of bactericidal and bacteriostatic drugs may lead to synergism instead of antagonism (16). RTC was used because with this drug very high serum levels can be obtained in pa-

[1] Present address: Wissenschaftlicher Rat und Professor, Leiter der Klinikhygiene in der Universitäts-Fraunklinik, 7800 Freiburg, West Germany.

tients after intravenous application, levels that exceed the concentrations found to be bactericidal in this study (7, 15).

MATERIAL AND METHODS

Test organisms. All *Escherichia coli* and *Staphylococcus aureus* strains used in this study were isolated from children with nosocomial diseases, mostly urinary tract infections and septicemia. One *E. coli* strain isolated from urine was used throughout the study for the growth and killing curves. The four strains of stable staphylococcal L-forms (L-36, L-65, L-68, L-101) and the corresponding bacterial forms were obtained from B. M. Kagan, Cedars Sinai Medical Center, Los Angeles, Calif., and subcultured weekly as described previously (5).

Antibiotics. Potassium penicillin G was supplied by Bayer (Leverkusen), cephalothin by Eli Lilly & Co. (Bad Homburg), and RTC by Hoechst AG (Frankfurt), each as standard powder. Laboratory standard solutions were prepared by dissolving the antibiotic in Mueller-Hinton broth; they were stored at −22°C and thawed immediately before use. Further dilution was done in Mueller-Hinton broth (Merck AG, Darmstadt).

Media. Mueller-Hinton broth adjusted to pH 7.4 or brain heart infusion broth (Difco) supplemented with 10% sucrose for osmotic stabilization was used for the growth and killing curves. All synergy studies using the checkerboard dilution technique were done in freshly prepared Mueller-Hinton broth, adjusted to pH 7.4 and supplemented with phenol red as indicator to facilitate reading the end points, as described previously (4). Salt serum agar was prepared according to Kagan (12) using gamma globulin-free horse serum (Grand Island Lab., N.J.) instead of human serum.

Synergy studies. The effect of RTC on the inhibitory activity of penicillin G or cephalothin was observed using a microtiter variation of the checkerboard dilution technique, as described previously (4). Briefly, twofold dilutions of RTC in 0.025 ml were made in one direction with a microtiter dilutor. Twofold dilutions of penicillin or cephalothin were added in the same volume manually in the perpendicular direction, using a disposable pipette delivering 0.025 ml/drop. Where each of the antibiotics was used alone, 0.025 ml of broth was added to achieve a volume of 0.05 ml. The inoculum of 0.05 ml from an overnight culture, adjusted to contain approximately 10^6 organisms/ml with a Coleman Junior spectrophotometer, was added by delivering 1 drop from a 0.05-ml disposable drop pipette. The final concentrations of RTC for *E. coli* (*S. aureus*) ranged from 0.09 to 12.5 μg/ml (0.02 to 3.12 μg/ml), those for cephalothin ranged from 0.9 to 125 μg/ml (0.006 to 0.9 μg/ml), and those for penicillin ranged from 117 to 15,000 μg/ml (6 to 768 μg/ml). Inhibitory end points were determined after overnight incubation at 37°C by noting the lowest concentration of antibiotics, alone and in combination, that allowed no visible growth. This was greatly facilitated by change of the indicator from red to yellow. Isobolograms for each strain were constructed by plotting the inhibitory end points on an arithmetic scale in the usual manner. The isobole defining additive effects of the two antibiotics was obtained by drawing a straight line between the minimal inhibitory concentrations (MICs) of each drug acting alone. Synergism would be evident if the line representing combined action of both drugs at various concentrations fell below the additive isobole (21). Since one-tube variations in MICs are commonly observed with serial dilution tests, which have a marked effect on the shape of the isobole, synergism was considered present only when there was, with the combination, at least a fourfold reduction in the MICs of both antibiotics (e.g., a twofold reduction with one antibiotic and a fourfold with the other one, causing only a slight concave bowing of the isobole was not accepted as evidence of synergistic activity). A twofold reduction of the MICs of both or either was considered additive, and no lowering of the end points was regarded as indifference.

Growth curves. Growth curves (Fig. 4) of one *E. coli* strain in Mueller-Hinton broth or osmotically stabilized brain heart infusion broth were obtained by measuring optical density, as described previously (5, 6). Subinhibitory penicillin (150 μg/ml) or RTC concentrations (0.9 μg/ml) were added alone, in combination, or following pretreatment with one of these antibiotics after 3 h of incubation.

Killing curves. Serial colony counts were performed with broth cultures of one *E. coli* strain to determine the time-related bactericidal or bacteriostatic effects of penicillin or cephalothin alone or in combination with RTC. Broth with one or both antibiotics was inoculated with bacteria from an overnight culture and adjusted photometrically to contain an average final inoculum of 0.4×10^6 organisms/ml. At 0, 1, 2, 3, 4, 5, 6, and 24 h, 0.1 ml from each tube was transferred undiluted or in 10-fold dilutions in broth to petri dishes with Endo agar (Difco). Colony-forming units per milliliter were counted after overnight incubation. Typical experiments are shown in Fig. 1 through 3.

Antibiotic susceptibility testing of L-forms. Antibiotic susceptibility testing was done by using the agar dilution technique. From salt serum agar with equal growth of single L-form colonies, 0.5- by 0.5-cm agar blocks were cut out and inversely moved to one-half of the salt serum agar plates containing twofold dilutions of RTC (range, 0.45 to 1,000 μg/ml). The other halves of the plates were inoculated with 0.005 ml of a standardized inoculum (approximately 5×10^5 organisms) of the corresponding parent forms, which resulted in growth of single colonies. One plate was used to test all four L-forms and parent forms; one plate without antibiotics served as growth control. Plates were read after 24 h and again after 48 and 72 h. Antibiotic concentrations that inhibited visible growth of L-forms and parent forms of staphylococci were taken as the MICs.

Incubation. All experiments were done at least in triplicate under aerobic conditions at 37°C.

RESULTS

Synergy studies. Table 1 summarizes the effects of penicillin and cephalothin in combination with RTC on 20 *E. coli* and 14 *S. aureus*

TABLE 1. *Effect of combinations of penicillin (Pen)/cephalothin (Ceph) and RTC on 20 E. coli and 14 S. aureus strains as determined by using the checkerboard dilution technique*

Effect of antibiotic combination	No. of strains			
	E. coli		*S. aureus*	
	Pen/RTC	Ceph/RTC	Pen/RTC	Ceph/RTC
Indifferent	10	10	8	10
Additive	10	7	6	3
Synergistic	0	3	0	1

strains. Three *E. coli* and one *S. aureus* strain were inhibited synergistically by the cephalothin/RTC combination; penicillin/RTC or cephalothin/RTC combinations were found to be additive on at least one-half of the strains tested. More important, however, was the lack of true antagonism of combinations of any of the so-called bactericidal and bacteriostatic antibiotics used in this study. The mean MIC of RTC for the *E. coli* (*S. aureus*) strains was 1.61 (0.69) μg/ml, and that of penicillin was 1,374 (161) μg/ml; the MIC of cephalothin was 15.6 (0.28) μg/ml.

Effect of bacteriostatic/bactericidal penicillin or RTC concentrations alone and in combination (killing curves). Figure 1 shows that significant growth over 24 h of the *E. coli* strain used in this study could be inhibited by certain penicillin (300 μg/ml) or RTC (7.8 μg/ml) concentrations (bacteriostatic concentrations). Increasing the concentrations resulted in immediate and marked bactericidal activity of both drugs. Only slight regrowth occurred beyond 8 h and up to 24 h. Figure 2 summarizes the findings if bacteriostatic/bactericidal penicillin/RTC concentrations or one drug in a bactericidal and the other in bacteriostatic concentration were combined at the beginning of the experiment. Control curves without antibiotics were similar to the one shown in Fig. 1. No antagonism could be found with penicillin/RTC combined in bacteriostatic concentrations (7.8 μg of RTC and 300 μg of penicillin per ml). Slight antagonism occurred between 3 and 8 h after combining RTC or penicillin in either bacteriostatic or bactericidal concentrations. No antagonism, however, could be found after 24 h of incubation.

It is well known that penicillin can destroy bacteria only when they are in the growing stage, so that drugs causing bacteriostasis might render penicillin ineffective if administered simultaneously. In experimental infections in mice, antagonism tended to occur especially if therapy with chlortetracycline was started before therapy with penicillin (14). I therefore studied the effect of penicillin and RTC on *E. coli* cells that had been pretreated with either drug in bactericidal or bacteriostatic concentrations. Neither bacteriostatic nor bactericidal activity of penicillin and RTC was inhibited by pretreatment with bacteriostatic RTC or penicillin concentrations (Fig. 3). In this type of experiment penicillin could exert a prompt bactericidal effect even after 2 h of exposure of the *E. coli* strain to bacteriostatic RTC concentrations (7.8 μg/ml). Killing curves almost identical to those shown in Fig. 1, 2, and 3 were obtained if cephalothin instead of penicillin was used in bactericidal (15.0 μg/ml) or bacteriostatic (5.0 μg/ml) concentrations. Control tubes without antibiotics were assayed in all experiments to be sure that bacteria studied were always in the logarithmic growth phase. All control curves were almost identical to the one shown in Fig. 1.

Growth curves of *E. coli* and antibiotic susceptibility testing of staphylococcal L-forms. The effect of subinhibitory RTC (0.9 μg/ml) and

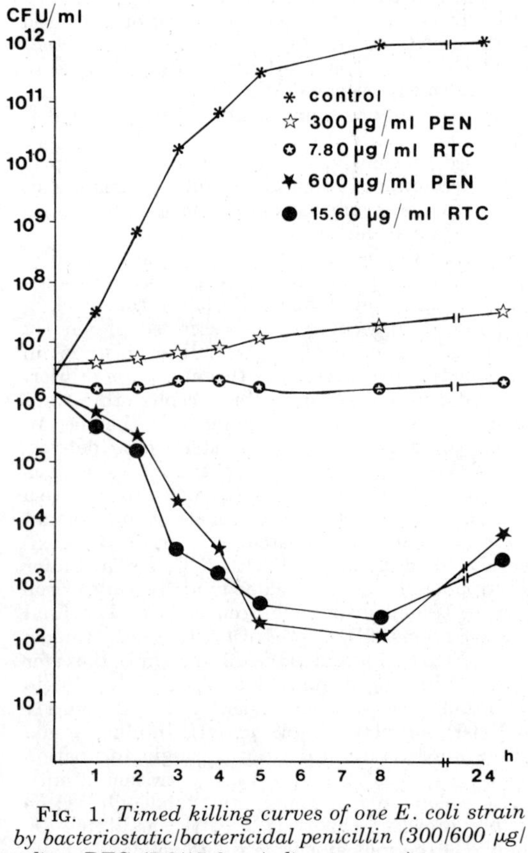

FIG. 1. *Timed killing curves of one E. coli strain by bacteriostatic/bactericidal penicillin (300/600 μg/ml) or RTC (7.8/15.6 μg/ml) concentrations as compared to a control curve without antibiotic.*

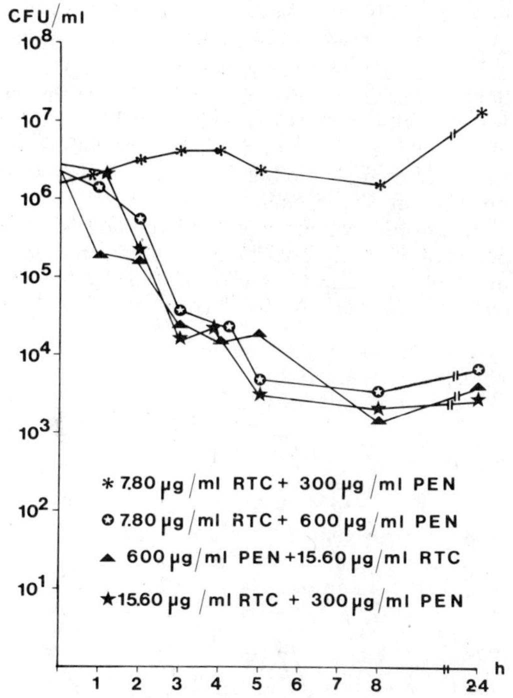

FIG. 2. *Timed killing curves of E. coli by penicillin/RTC combinations in either bacteriostatic or bactericidal concentrations.*

penicillin (150 μg/ml) concentrations on the growth of *E. coli* was studied by measuring optical density at hourly intervals. The curves obtained for growth in Mueller-Hinton broth are shown in Fig. 4, and those obtained for growth in osmotically stabilized brain heart infusion broth are shown in Fig. 5. Combined action of subinhibitory penicillin and RTC concentrations invariably resulted in more pronounced inhibition of growth than with either drug alone. Addition of penicillin or RTC 3 h after pretreatment with the other drug, each in a subinhibitory concentration, led to growth retardation; the growth curves were parallel, approaching the rate of growth inhibition of *E. coli* by penicillin and RTC when both drugs were added at the beginning of the experiment (Fig. 4).

The better activity of both drugs in combination, at least within 3 h of incubation, than either component alone was less obvious when hypertonic osmotically stabilized brain heart infusion broth instead of Mueller-Hinton broth was used for the growth curves (Fig. 5). Addition of RTC in a subinhibitory concentration 3 h after pretreatment with penicillin, however, significantly decreased optical density, suggesting bactericidal activity of RTC. At this time 99.9% of all bacteria were transformed to spheroplasts by penicillin, which has been demonstrated previously (6) as well as in this study by phase-contrast microscopy. This suggested that cell wall alterations induced by penicillin, especially in hypertonic medium, might permit greater access of RTC into the bacterial cell, which thus better reaches its site of action. This assumption could be supported by my finding that growth of four different strains of stable staphylococcal L-forms (cell wall-deficient bacterial forms) was inhibited by significantly lower concentrations of RTC than was that of the corresponding parent forms with intact cell walls (Table 2).

DISCUSSION

Despite the theoretical problems posed by the use of antibiotic combinations, there are five possible justifications for their use in clinical practice (2): (i) the concept of proven clinical synergy; (ii) to broaden the spectrum; (iii) to treat mixed or potentially mixed infections; (iv) to prevent the emergence of resistant organisms; and (v) the use of two potentially toxic drugs in lower dosage to possibly reduce the

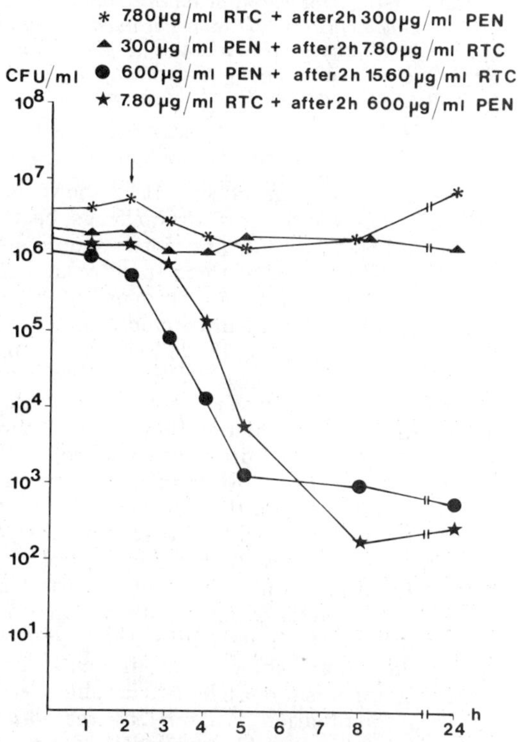

FIG. 3. *Timed killing curves of E. coli by penicillin or RTC added 2 h after pretreatment (arrow) of the bacteria with bacteriostatic RTC or bacteriostatic/bactericidal penicillin concentrations.*

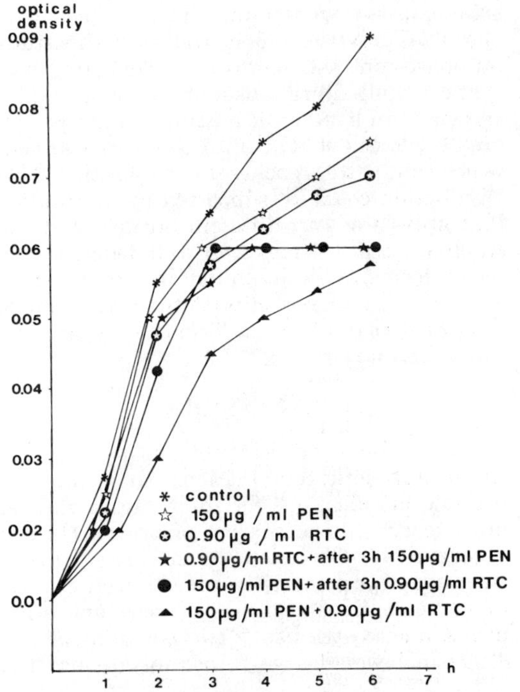

FIG. 4. *Growth of E. coli at subinhibitory concentrations of penicillin or RTC alone or in combination in Mueller-Hinton broth. Addition of penicillin or RTC both in subinhibitory concentrations to cells pretreated with the other drug led to prompt bacteriostasis.*

danger of severe side effects. It is, however, generally believed that, using two drugs, bactericidal and bacteriostatic antibiotics should not be combined because of their in vitro and in vivo antagonism. Antibiotic antagonism, especially between the penicillins chloramphenicol and tetracycline (13, 17, 18, 23), could be demonstrated in various clinical studies. Similarly designed studies, however, failed to show any untoward effect of combinations of bacteriostatic and bactericidal drugs as compared with using only one drug. Finland et al. (9) observed no difference in the antibacterial activity of human plasma when either penicillin or penicillin combined with chloramphenicol was administered to human subjects. Ahern and Kirby (1) treated 25 patients with pneumococcal pneumonia with penicillin alone and 25 with penicillin and chlortetracycline and found neither antagonism nor a beneficial effect from the drug combination. Walker (25) treated patients with streptococcal pharyngitis with penicillin alone or with penicillin and chloramphenicol; duration of fever, frequency of relapses, or other symptoms were not influenced by using penicillin alone or in combination with chloramphenicol. Some recent experimental studies also question the concept of general antagonism between bacteriostatic and bactericidal drugs. Luboshitzky et al. (16) found striking examples of synergism between tetracyclines/cephaloridine on *Serratia* and between tetracycline/kanamycin on *Enterobacter*. The combination of chloramphenicol and cephalothin resulted in an additive effect against four out of six multiple-antibiotic-resistant strains of *Staphylococcus epidermidis* (24). None of these studies, how-

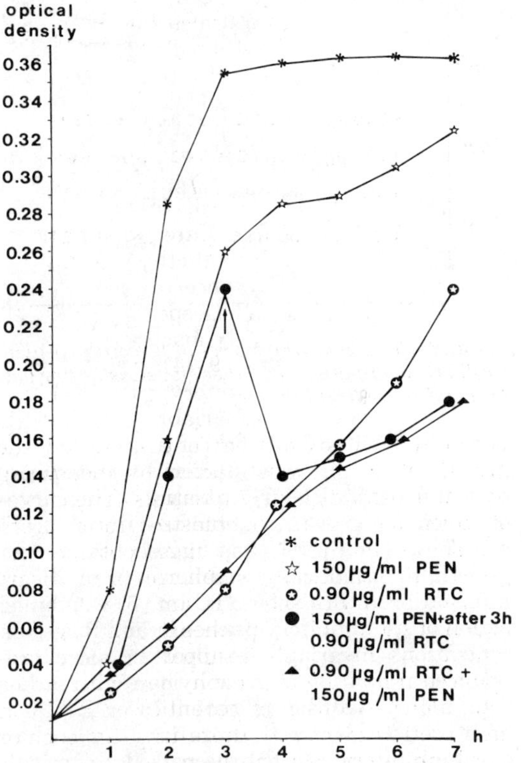

FIG. 5. *Growth of E. coli at subinhibitory penicillin or RTC concentrations alone or in combination in osmotically stabilized brain heart infusion broth. Addition of RTC in subinhibitory concentrations to penicillin-induced spheroplasts resulted in bactericidal activity (arrow).*

TABLE 2. *Susceptibility (MIC) of four staphylococcal L-form and parent strains to RTC*

Strain	MIC (µg/ml)	
	Parent form	L-form
36	125	1.9
65	500	3.9
68	1.9	0.9
101	125	0.45

ever, considered the original finding of Jawetz (10) that results of drug combinations may depend on the bacterial strains, drug concentrations, time of interaction, and other laboratory variables. I therefore investigated some of these variables and found not antagonistic, but additive, indifferent, or synergistic activity between cephalothin/penicillin and tetracycline on various strains of *S. aureus* and *E. coli* when tested by using the checkerboard dilution technique. Slight antagonism between penicillin/cephalothin and RTC, each combined in bactericidal and bacteriostatic concentrations, occurred only between 3 and 8 h, but not at 24 h, of incubation. There was also no antagonism when the drugs were combined in bacteriostatic concentrations. This was also true if penicillin/cephalothin or RTC was added to *E. coli* cells pretreated with either bacteriostatic RTC or penicillin concentrations. Penicillin as well as cephalothin could exert a bactericidal effect after a 2-h exposure of *E. coli* to bacteriostatic RTC concentrations. The latter findings may account for some of the conflicting results of in vitro and in vivo studies concerning the effect of various drug combinations, especially those between so-called primarily bacteriostatic and bactericidal antibiotics (1, 9, 14). Even the combined action of subinhibitory penicillin and RTC concentrations invariably resulted in more pronounced inhibition of growth than did using either drug alone. Bactericidal activity of subinhibitory RTC concentrations on penicillin-induced *E. coli* spheroplasts in osmotically stabilized fluid medium suggested that cell wall-defective bacteria (spheroplasts) might permit greater access of RTC into the bacterial cell, which thus better reaches its site of action. This hypothesis could be supported by comparing the RTC MICs of staphylococcal L-forms and their corresponding parent forms with intact cell walls. L-forms were invariably more susceptible to RTC than the parent forms.

My data confirm those of Mouton and Koelman (19) and Jawetz (10), who found that drug interaction patterns between bactericidal and bacteriostatic drugs are highly dependent on bacterial species, strains, and drug concentrations used. Better activity of tetracyclines on cell wall-defective bacteria as compared with bacterial cells with intact cell walls has been demonstrated previously by Kagan (12). Whether this may account, at least in part, for the additive or synergistic action of penicillin in combination with RTC on certain strains remains to be studied. Combinations of bactericidal drugs with tetracyclines may be necessary to broaden the spectrum in the treatment of certain mixed infections, e.g., with anaerobes, where tetracyclines were shown to be effective in vitro (3). Further clinical studies are necessary to prove the effectiveness of these drug combinations. One of these studies is currently being done in our hospital. At present, however, I would not recommend the use of combinations of bactericidal and bacteriostatic drugs unless antagonism has been excluded, preferably by methods using bactericidal end points.

ACKNOWLEDGMENTS

The enthusiastic technical assistance of Ingrid Emriccson is appreciated.

This work was supported in part by a grant from Hoechst AG, Frankfurt, Germany.

LITERATURE CITED

1. **Ahern, J. J., and W. M. M. Kirby.** 1953. Lack of interference of aureomycin with penicillin in treatment of pneumococcic pneumonia. Arch. Intern. Med. **91**:197–203.
2. **Brumfitt, W.** 1971. Antibiotic combinations. Lancet **ii**:387–389.
3. **Chow, A. W., V. Patten, and L. B. Guze.** 1975. Comparative susceptibility of anaerobic bacteria to minocycline, doxycycline, and tetracycline. Antimicrob. Agents Chemother. **7**:46–49.
4. **Daschner, F.** 1975. Synergismus von Cefazolin und Tobramycin bei Klebsiella pneumoniae als Erreger nosokomialer Infektionen. Infection **3**(Suppl. 1):31–34.
5. **Daschner, F.** 1976. Inhibition of cell wall synthesis by sulfonamides and trimethoprim. Chemotherapy **22**:12–18.
6. **Daschner, F. D., R. Hövel, and W. Marget.** 1973. Action of gentamicin on penicillin G-induced Proteus spherosplasts. Chemotherapy **18**:235–241.
7. **Dimmling, T.** 1972. Vergleichsstudie über drei derzeit gebräuchliche Tetracyclinederivate zur intravenösen Anwendung (Serum- und Urinspiegel). Med. Klin. **67**:1632–1637.
8. **Dowling, H. F.** 1960. The conditions under which the use of combinations of antibiotics is undesirable. Antibiot. Chemother. **8**:114–125.
9. **Finland, M., C. V., Pryles, and W. F. Jones.** 1958. Antibiotic combinations. Antibacterial action of plasma of human subjects after ingestion of penicillin V or chloramphenicol or both. N. Engl. J. Med. **258**:817–824.
10. **Jawetz, E.** 1968. Combined antibiotic action: some definitions and correlations between laboratory and clinical results, p. 203–209. Antimicrob. Agents Chemother. 1967.
11. **Jawetz, E., and J. B. Gunnison.** 1952. Studies on antibiotic synergism and antagonism: a scheme of combined antibiotic action. Antibiot. Chemother. **2**:243–248.
12. **Kagan, B. M.** 1968. Antibiotic sensitivities of staphylococcal L-forms, p. 314–318. *In* L. B. Guze (ed.), Microbial protoplasts, spheroplasts and L-forms. The Williams & Wilkins Co., Baltimore.
13. **Lepper, M. H., and H. F. Dowling.** 1951. Treatment of pneumococcal meningitis with penicillin compared with penicillin plus aureomycin. Arch. Intern. Med. **88**:489–494.
14. **Lepper, M. H., G. G. Jackson, H. F. Dowling, and J. Seto.** 1953. Comparison of results of treatment of pneumococcic infection in mice with multiple doses of aureomycin and penicillin combined with each drug alone. Am. J. Med. Sci. **225**:648–656.

15. **Limson, M. B., and R. B. Guevara, Jr.** 1962. Efficacy of a single intravenous injection of pyrrolidinomethyltetracycline in pneumococcal pneumonia: report of 20 cases with assays of 24 hour antibiotic activity in serum. Antibiot. Chemother. 12:85–90.
16. **Luboshitzky, R., T. Sacks, and J. Michel.** 1973. Bactericidal effect of combinations of antibiotics on Klebsiella-Enterobacter-Serratia. Chemotherapy 19:354–366.
17. **McCabe, W. R., and G. G. Jackson.** 1965. The treatment of pyelonephritis. Bacterial, drug and host factors in success or failure among 252 patients. N. Engl. J. Med. 272:1037–1044.
18. **Mathies, A. W., Jr., J. M. Leedom, D. Ivler, P. F. Wehrle, and B. Portnoy.** 1968. Antibiotic antagonism in bacterial meningitis, p. 218–224. Antimicrob. Agents Chemother. 1967.
19. **Mouton, R. P., and A. Koelman.** 1966. The interaction patterns of combined antibacterial agents. Experiments with two agar diffusion methods. Chemotherapy 11:10–26.
20. **Russell, F. E.** 1962. Synergism between sulfonamide drugs and antibiotics of the polymyxin group against Proteus species in vitro. J. Clin. Pathol. 16:362–366.
21. **Sabath, L. D.** 1968. Synergy of antibacterial substances by apparently known mechanisms, p. 210–217. Antimicrob. Agents Chemother. 1967.
22. **Simmons, N. A.** 1969. Potentiation of inhibitory activity of colistin on Pseudomonas aeruginosa by sulfamethoxazole and sulfamethiazole. Br. Med. J. 3:693–696.
23. **Strohm, J.** 1955. The question of antagonism between penicillin and chlortetracycline, illustrated by therapeutical experiments in scarlatina. Antibiot. Med. 1:6–12.
24. **Traub, W. H.** 1970. In vitro activity of chloramphenicol combined with cephalothin against DNase-positive, multiple-antibiotic resistant strains of Staphylococcus epidermidis. Chemotherapy 15:234–241.
25. **Walker, S. H.** 1953. A study of the possible interference of chloramphenicol with penicillin in acute streptococcal pharyngitis. Antibiot. Chemother. 3:677–680.

ANTIMICROBIAL AGENTS AND CHEMOTHERAPY, Nov. 1976, p. 809-813
Vol. 10, No. 5

Effect of Ribavirin on Murine Cytomegalovirus Infection

JOHN N. DOWLING, BOSKO POSTIC, AND LUCILLE O. GUEVARRA

Department of Medicine, University of Pittsburgh School of Medicine, Pittsburgh, Pennsylvania 15261

Received for publication 1 July 1976

Ribavirin (1-β-D-ribofuranosyl-1,2,4-triazole-3-carboxamide), a new synthetic nucleoside, inhibited murine cytomegalovirus in cell culture. This was shown by the inhibition of viral cytopathic effect and plaque formation, as well as reduction in the yield of virus. Despite this in vitro antiviral effect, ribavirin did not protect mice from mortality produced by a high inoculum of cytomegalovirus. When a lower inoculum was used to initiate a chronic infection, the administration of ribavirin for 9 days had no effect on the titer of cytomegalovirus in the salivary gland, kidney, liver, and spleen. Thus, ribavirin was ineffective in the treatment of both acute and chronic murine cytomegalovirus infections.

Cytomegalovirus causes a broad spectrum of clinical illnesses including congenital infection, the mononucleosis syndrome, and involvement of various organs in immunosuppressed hosts (18). Human cytomegaloviruses (HCMV) are inhibited by the nucleoside analogues adenine arabinoside, cytosine arabinoside, and 5-iodo-2′-deoxyuridine in cell culture (4). In clinical trials, these antiviral agents may transiently suppress urinary excretion of HCMV, but generally fail to eradicate the virus or alter the natural course of disease (2, 3, 8, 9, 13). The search for antiviral agents capable of inhibiting HCMV should therefore be continued.

Rivavirin (1-β-D-ribofuranosyl-1,2,4-triazole-3-carboxamide) is a new synthetic nucleoside which is active in cell culture against numerous deoxyribonucleic acid and ribonucleic acid viruses (5). The in vitro inhibition of herpesviruses, including murine cytomegalovirus (MCMV), by ribavirin has compared favorably with other antiviral compounds (5, 14, 19). In animal systems, ribavirin demonstrated activity against influenza A and B (7), vaccinia (15), and herpes simplex (15) infections. The infection in mice produced by MCMV is well characterized (10, 11, 20) and has been used as a model to evaluate the effectiveness of chemotherapeutic agents (6). This work examines the activity of ribavirin against MCMV in cell culture and in mice. The antiviral effect in cultured cells was first determined by three methods. Then, ribavirin was evaluated in both acute, lethal and chronic, subclinical murine infections.

MATERIALS AND METHODS

Animals. Swiss-Webster CD-1 mice were obtained from Charles River Breeding Laboratories, Wilmington, Mass.

Virus. MCMV of the Smith strain was maintained by animal passage. Weanling mice were inoculated intraperitoneally (i.p.) with approximately 10^5 plaque-forming units (PFU) of MCMV. Four to five weeks later, the mice were sacrificed and their salivary glands were removed. Stock virus consisted of a 10% (wt/vol) salivary gland homogenate in medium 199 containing 25% sorbitol.

Cell culture. MCMV was grown in secondary mouse embryo tissue culture (METC) maintained with medium 199 supplemented with 2% newborn calf serum, 0.2% $NaHCO_3$, penicillin (100 U/ml), streptomycin (100 μg/ml), and nystatin (50 U/ml). Titration was carried out in METC by the plaquing method using tragacanth overlay (12). After 7 days, the tragacanth was removed and the cell sheets were stained with a dye-fixer solution containing 0.5% methylrosaniline chloride, 5% formalin (vol/vol), 50% ethanol (vol/vol), and 0.85% NaCl in distilled water (1). Plaques were enumerated with the aid of a dissecting microscope.

Ribavirin. Ribavirin was kindly supplied by Robert W. Sidwell (ICN Nucleic Acid Research Institute, Irvine, Calif.).

CPE inhibition. MCMV was added to METC in tube cultures. After virus adsorption, ribavirin was added in the appropriate concentration in the maintenance medium. Controls consisted of tubes to which medium without drug was added. Maintenance medium was not changed during the course of an experiment. Tubes were examined daily and scored for cytopathic effect (CPE) on a scale of 0 to 4+. Protection was defined as less than 1+ (<25%) CPE in the test cell sheet at the time when virus control monolayers first showed 4+ (100%) CPE.

Yield reduction. MCMV was grown in tube cultures with or without drug in the maintenance medium, as for the examination of CPE inhibition. At intervals, the medium was removed and titered for MCMV (supernatant virus). After addition of 2.0 ml of fresh medium, the cell cultures were frozen and thawed three times and clarified by low-speed centrifugation, and the infectivity of the supernatant was determined by the plaque method (cell virus).

Plaque reduction. After adsorption of virus onto

METC, varying concentrations of ribavirin were added to the tragacanth overlay. Control cultures received overlay without drug. Plaques were stained and counted as for MCMV titration. The counts on treated and untreated monolayers were contrasted. In addition, plaque sizes were measured using a calibrated ocular in a microscope at ×10 magnification. Ten randomly chosen plaques at each drug concentration were measured, the largest and smallest diameters of a plaque were averaged, and the area was calculated.

Acute MCMV infection. The MCMV suspension was inoculated i.p. with 0.2 ml of medium 199 as carrier. Control animals received medium alone. Ribavirin was administered for a total of 9 days, beginning the day preceding virus inoculation. The total daily drug dose was calculated for a particular group of mice based on their mean weight and given as twice-daily i.p. injections of ribavirin in 0.2 to 0.3 ml of physiological saline. Control animals received saline only.

Chronic MCMV infection. Four-week-old mice were given approximately 10^6 PFU of MCMV, i.p. After 5 weeks, surviving animals were divided into three groups of 17 mice. Two groups were given ribavirin, 50 mg/kg per day and 100 mg/kg per day, i.p. in twice-daily injections for 9 days. The control group received saline twice daily. On the day after the last drug dose, the mice were killed by cervical dislocation, and the organs of each mouse were dissected out. The spleens, kidneys, livers, and salivary glands from each treatment group were pooled, weighed, and ground in a mortar and pestle with sterile sand, and medium 199 was added to make a final 10% organ concentration. These suspensions were centrifuged, and the supernatant was titered for MCMV.

RESULTS

To examine the ability of ribavirin to inhibit CPE, tube cultures of METC were inoculated with 10-fold dilutions of MCMV from 3×10^6 to 3×10^3 PFU. After virus adsorption, between 1 and 1,000 μg of ribavirin per ml was added in the maintenance medium. At each virus concentration tested, 25 μg of ribavirin per ml protected the cell sheet from CPE when control monolayers showed evidence of diffuse CPE. In these experiments, no visible cytotoxicity was produced by 50 μg of ribavirin per ml; concentrations of 100 μg/ml or more regularly produced cell destruction.

Yield reduction was examined in cells infected with 3×10^5 PFU of MCMV and with 25 μg of ribavirin per ml in the medium. Cells and supernatant were harvested from drug and control tubes at intervals from 1 to 96 h and then were titered. The results are shown in Fig. 1. The titer of MCMV in control cells and supernatant began to rise by 31 h after infection and reached 1.4×10^5 and 1.3×10^6 PFU/0.1 ml, respectively, at 96 h. In contrast, ribavirin inhibited productive infection through 72 h. At 96 h, the cell suspension contained only 6.2×10^1 PFU/0.1 ml and the supernatant contained 6.5×10^2 PFU/0.1 ml.

To examine the effect of ribavirin on plaque production, the drug was incorporated into the overlay at varying concentrations after inoculation of cell cultures with 10-fold dilutions of the virus suspension. The effect was measured by the MCMV titer (Table 1). At a concentration of 10 μg/ml, ribavirin reduced the number of plaques 9-fold, and at 25 μg/ml, 19-fold. In addition, there was a marked reduction noted in the size of the plaques that formed with increasing concentrations of ribavirin in the overlay. This obvious difference in plaque size was quantitated by measuring 10 randomly chosen plaques at each drug concentration and calculating their average area (Table 1). The difference in plaque size between 0 and 10 μg/ml is highly significant ($t = 9.98, P < 0.001$), as is the difference between 10 and 25 μg/ml ($t = 5.92, P < 0.001$). The plaques at 50 and 100 μg of ribavirin per ml were so tiny that they could not be accurately enumerated. Therefore, it was not possible to measure titer reduction at drug concentrations above 25 μg/ml.

The reduction in plaque counts was examined further with a lower inoculum of virus,

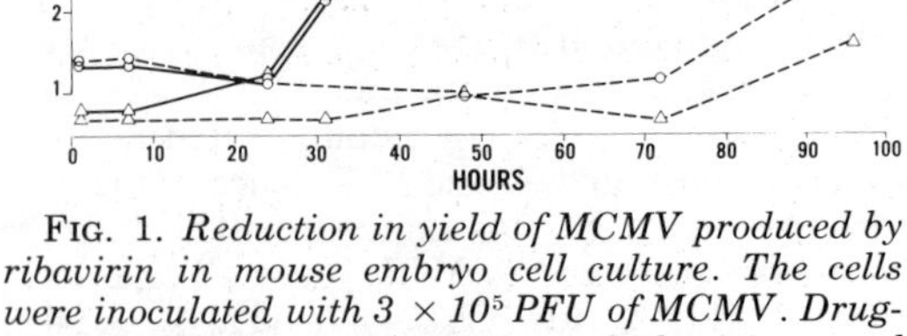

FIG. 1. *Reduction in yield of MCMV produced by ribavirin in mouse embryo cell culture. The cells were inoculated with 3×10^5 PFU of MCMV. Drug-treated cultures contained 25 μg of ribavirin per ml in the maintenance medium.*

TABLE 1. *Inhibition of MCMV plaque formation by ribavirin*

Ribavirin (μg/ml)	Titer (PFU)	Plaque size[a] (mm²)
0	3.3×10^8	0.90
10	3.7×10^7	0.33
25	1.7×10^7	0.13

[a] Average area of 10 plaques measured at 10^{-5} dilution.

approximately 100 PFU, at ribavirin concentrations ranging from 1.0 to 100 μg/ml. For each experiment, a dose-response curve was constructed on a probit graph from which the ribavirin concentration required to inhibit plaque number by 50% was determined. The results are summarized in Table 2. Some variation between experiments, especially in the drug concentration required to completely inhibit plaque formation, is apparent. Nevertheless, concentrations of ribavirin between 9 and 23 μg/ml reduced the plaque number by 50%. Between 25 and 100 μg of ribavirin per ml was required to completely inhibit plaque production.

The effect of ribavirin on acute, lethal MCMV infection was assessed in adult mice weighing about 30 g. In the first experiment, the two inocula of virus chosen, 1.7×10^6 and 2.5×10^6 PFU, killed 25 and 58% of mice, respectively (Table 3). The administration of ribavirin, 50 or 100 mg/kg per day for 9 days, did not protect the animals from death at either virus level. There was no mortality among mice treated with these dosages of ribavirin alone, but the mice were observed to have mild diarrhea. This drug toxicity was reflected in the failure of mice receiving ribavirin to gain weight at the rate of saline-treated controls during the course of the experiment.

Drug toxicity, as manifested by weight loss and mortality, was more striking at higher doses (Table 3, experiment 2). The administration of 150 and 200 mg of ribavirin/kg per day alone for 9 days killed 17 and 45% of mice, respectively. These doses did not protect against mortality due to MCMV. In fact, the toxicity of ribavirin appeared to be additive with the effects of the infection, so that, at each level of virus, mortality increased with increasing drug dose.

To evaluate the effect of ribavirin on chronic, clinically latent MCMV infection, mice infected 5 weeks previously were treated with the drug for 9 days. The titers found in the pooled spleens, livers, kidneys, and salivary glands of these animals are given in Table 4. Some variation in titer between groups is apparent, but there was no consistent reduction in titer related to the dose of ribavirin received.

TABLE 2. *Ribavirin concentration required for 50 and 100% reduction of plaques produced by a small inoculum of MCMV*[a]

Expt	Ribavirin (μg/ml)	
	ED_{50}	ED_{100}
1	8.9	50
2	11.5	>25
3	12.3	25
4	23.0	100

[a] Approximately 100 PFU of MCMV per monolayer.

DISCUSSION

The evaluation of the in vitro activity of antiviral agents is not standardized. Three techniques were used to assess the effect of ribavi-

TABLE 3. *Effect of ribavirin on acute MCMV infection in mice*

Expt	MCMV (PFU/mouse)	Ribavirin (mg/kg per day)	No.	Mortality		Maximum Δ weight (%)
				No.	%	
1		None	6	0	0	+9.8
	None	50	13	0	0	+5.5
		100	14	0	0	−1.8
		None	12	3	25	−14.4
	1.7×10^6	50	11	5	45	−11.3
		100	12	6	50	−18.7
		None	12	7	58	−22.0
	2.5×10^6	50	12	10	83	−20.9
		100	10	4	40	−20.1
2		None	9	0	0	0.0
	None	150	12	2	17	−17.3
		200	12	5	45	−20.8
		None	12	1	8	−9.4
	1.7×10^6	150	12	4	33	−25.8
		200	12	11	92	−29.3
		None	10	5	50	−17.3
	2.5×10^6	150	12	8	67	−23.6
		200	12	12	100	−30.0

TABLE 4. *Effect of ribavirin on chronic MCMV infection in mice*

Ribavirin (mg/kg per day)	MCMV titer (log PFU/0.1 g)			
	Spleen	Liver	Kidney	Salivary gland
None	4.90	0.85	1.84	6.58
50	4.18	1.43	0.59	6.86
100	3.48	1.53	2.58	6.93

rin against MCMV. Ribavirin demonstrated considerable activity whether measured by protection from CPE, reduction in yield, or inhibition of plaque formation. The drug was effective in cell culture against levels of virus equivalent to and exceeding those used to produce lethal infections in mice. The approximate mean lethal dose (LD_{50}) of MCMV in adult animals was 2.5×10^6 PFU (Table 3). Ribavirin at a concentration of 25 μg/ml protected against CPE in cells inoculated with 3×10^6 PFU, or 1.2 LD_{50}, of MCMV and reduced by 19-fold the number of plaques produced by 3.3×10^8 PFU (132 LD_{50}) of MCMV (Table 1).

Despite this activity in cell culture, ribavirin appeared to have little antiviral effect on either acute or chronic MCMV infections in the intact animal. There are a number of considerations that might account for this failure. It is possible that combinations using younger mice or other dosage schedules would have yielded different results. Since resistance to the lethal effects of MCMV infection increases with the age of the animal (12), adult mice were used in these studies in an attempt to maximize any impact of ribavirin. For the same reason, the drug was given for a day preceding the administration of virus. The dosage schedules originally chosen to treat acute MCMV infection were similar to those that appeared to be effective against influenza infection in mice (7). When the given doses produced no protection, larger amounts were tried, but resulted in excessive toxicity. Administration of 200 mg of ribavirin/kg per day for 9 days produced 42% mortality, a figure consistent with the LD_{50} observed in mice by others (7).

Ribavirin had no effect on the titer of MCMV in the organs of chronically infected mice. This suggests that mortality was not favorably influenced because ribavirin failed to exert significant antiviral activity in vivo. Perhaps the drug failed to reach the sites of virus multiplication, or inhibitory concentrations of ribavirin-5′-phosphate, the active form of the drug (17), were not achieved in infected cells. Huffman et al. (5) showed that the activity of ribavirin in cell culture against a particular virus can vary markedly, depending on the cell type used. The efficacy of ribavirin in treating influenza infections (7) indicates that antiviral concentrations are achieved in the lung. The failure of parenterally administered ribavirin to influence the outcome of encephalitis due to herpes simplex or vaccinia virus in mice suggested that the compound did not cross the blood-brain barrier (15). No attempt was made in the present investigation to determine if biologically active drug accumulated in the spleen, liver, kidney, and salivary gland, the target organs of MCMV infection.

The possibility that ribavirin exerted an immunosuppressive effect in mice which interfered with virus elimination must be considered. In a controlled, double-blind study of cytosine arabinoside in patients with disseminated herpes zoster, Stevens et al. (16) found that the duration of disseminated disease was prolonged by drug therapy, especially in patients with stage III and IV lymphoma. This adverse effect was ascribed to depression of host response to zoster produced by cytosine arabinoside.

Recently, Kelsey et al. (6) examined the effects of cytosine arabinoside and 5-iodo-2′-deoxyuridine on MCMV. Both drugs inhibited MCMV in cell culture, but neither affected the lethal outcome of disseminated MCMV infection in suckling mice, even at doses that were lethal for a proportion of drug-treated controls. It is not surprising that nucleoside analogues, which interfere with both host cell and viral nucleic acid synthesis, might fail to have significant antiviral activity at subtoxic doses. Although it would be hazardous to extrapolate our results with MCMV to HCMV infections, it may prove difficult to achieve therapeutic activity with ribavirin in man without incurring unreasonable toxicity.

ACKNOWLEDGMENTS

This study was supported by a special grant from the Monsour Medical Foundation, Jeannette, Pa., and in part by the Veterans Administration.

LITERATURE CITED

1. **Armstrong, J. A.** 1971. Semi-micro, dye-binding assay for rabbit interferon. Appl. Microbiol. 21:723–725.
2. **Barton, B. E., and J. O'H. Tobin.** 1970. The effect of iodoxuridine on the excretion of cytomegalovirus in congenital infection. Ann. N.Y. Acad. Sci. 172:90–95.
3. **Ch'ien, L. T., N. J. Cannon, R. J. Whitley, A. G. Diethelm, W. E. Dismukes, C. W. Scott, R. A. Buchanan, and C. A. Alford, Jr.** 1974. Effect of adenine arabinoside on cytomegalovirus infections. J. Infect. Dis. 130:32–39.
4. **Fiala, M., A. W. Chow, K. Miyasaki, and L. B. Guze.** 1974. Susceptibility of herpesviruses to three nucleoside analogues and their combinations and enhancement of the antiviral effect at acid pH. J. Infect. Dis. 129:82–85.

5. **Huffman, J. H., R. W. Sidwell, G. P. Khare, J. T. Witkowski, L. B. Allen, and R. K. Robins.** 1973. In vitro effect of 1-β-D-ribofuranosyl-1,2,4-triazole-3-carboxamide (Virazole, ICN 1229) on deoxyribonucleic acid and ribonucleic acid viruses. Antimicrob. Agents Chemother. 3:235–241.
6. **Kelsey, D. K., E. R. Kern, J. C. Overall, and L. A. Glasgow.** 1976. Effect of cytosine arabinoside and 5-iodo-2′-deoxyuridine on a cytomegalovirus infection in newborn mice. Antimicrob. Agents Chemother. 9:458–464.
7. **Khare, G. P., R. W. Sidwell, J. T. Witkowski, L. N. Simon, and R. K. Robins.** 1973. Suppression by 1-β-D-ribofuranosyl-1,2,4-triazole-3-carboxamide (Virazole, ICN 1229) of influenza virus-induced infections in mice. Antimicrob. Agents Chemother. 3:517–522.
8. **Kraybill, E. N., J. L. Sever, G. B. Avery, and N. Movassaghi.** 1972. Experimental use of cytosine arabinoside in congenital cytomegalovirus infection. J. Pediatr. 80:485–487.
9. **McCracken, G. H., and J. P. Luby.** 1972. Cytosine arabinoside in the treatment of congenital cytomegalic inclusion disease. J. Pediatr. 80:488–495.
10. **Mannini, A., and D. N. Medearis, Jr.** 1961. Mouse salivary gland virus infections. Am. J. Hyg. 73:329–343.
11. **Medearis, D. N., Jr.** 1964. Mouse cytomegalovirus infection. II. Observations during prolonged infections. Am. J. Hyg. 80:103–112.
12. **Osborn, J. E., and D. L. Walker.** 1970. Virulence and attenuation of murine cytomegalovirus. Infect. Immun. 3:228–236.
13. **Rytel, M. W., and H. M. Kauffman.** 1976. Clinical efficacy of adenine arabinoside in therapy of cytomegalovirus infections in renal allograft recipients. J. Infect. Dis. 133:202–205.
14. **Sidwell, R. W., J. H. Huffman, G. P. Khare, L. B. Allen, J. T. Witkowski, and R. K. Robins.** 1972. Broad-spectrum antiviral activity of Virazole: 1-β-D-ribofuranosyl-1,2,4-triazole-3-carboxamide. Science 177:705–706.
15. **Sidwell, R. W., L. B. Allen, G. P. Khare, J. H. Huffman, J. T. Witkowski, L. N. Simon, and R. K. Robins.** 1973. Effect of 1-β-D-ribofuranosyl-1,2,4-triazole-3-carboxamide (Virazole, ICN 1229) on herpes and vaccinia keratitis and encephalitis in laboratory animals. Antimicrob. Agents Chemother. 3:242–246.
16. **Stevens, D. A., G. W. Jordan, T. F. Waddell, and T. C. Merigan.** 1973. Adverse effect of cytosine arabinoside on disseminated zoster in a controlled trial. N. Engl. J. Med. 289:873–878.
17. **Streeter, D. G., J. T. Witkowski, G. P. Khare, R. W. Sidwell, R. J. Bauer, R. K. Robins, and L. N. Simon.** 1973. Mechanism of action of 1-β-D-ribofuranosyl-1,2,4-triazole-3-carboxamide (Virazole), a new broad-spectrum antiviral agent. Proc. Natl. Acad. Sci. U.S.A. 70:1174–1178.
18. **Weller, T. H.** 1971. The cytomegaloviruses: ubiquitous agents with protean clinical manifestations. N. Engl. J. Med. 285:203–214, 267–274.
19. **Witkowski, J. T., R. K. Robins, R. W. Sidwell, and L. N. Simon.** 1972. Design, synthesis, and broad-spectrum antiviral activity of 1-β-D-ribofuranosyl-1,2,4-triazole-3-carboxamide and related nucleosides. J. Med. Chem. 15:1150–1154.
20. **Wu, B. C., J. N. Dowling, J. A. Armstrong, and M. Ho.** 1975. Enhancement of mouse cytomegalovirus infection during host-versus-graft reaction. Science 190:56–58.

ANTIMICROBIAL AGENTS AND CHEMOTHERAPY, Nov. 1976, p. 814-823 Vol. 10, No. 5
 Printed in U.S.A.

Cefamandole: In Vitro and Clinical Pharmacokinetics

R. S. GRIFFITH* H. R. BLACK, G. L. BRIER, AND J. D. WOLNY

Lilly Laboratory for Clinical Research, Wishard Memorial Hospital, and Indiana University School of Medicine, Indianapolis, Indiana 46202*

Received for publication 7 June 1976

Cefamandole has a broader spectrum and greater potency than the other cephalosporins. It includes *Haemophilus influenzae,* most strains of *Enterobacter,* and many strains of indole-positive *Proteus* and *Bacteroides,* with a lower minimal inhibitory concentration for *Escherichia coli, Klebsiella,* etc. Concentrations of drug in the serum after the parenteral injection of cefamandole exceed manyfold the minimal inhibitory concentrations of over 82% of the bacteria studied. Approximately 65 to 85% is excreted in a biologically active form in the urine. This antibiotic offers advantages of antibacterial effectiveness and at the same time retains the safety of penicillin G and cephalothin in animals.

The clinical efficacy of the cephalosporin antibiotics has been well established (10, 11). Cephalothin, because of pain with intramuscular injection of greater than 0.5- to 1-g doses, is usually administered intravenously. Cephaloridine, virtually painless with intramuscular injection, has been associated with nephrotoxicity. Cefazolin produces high and prolonged serum concentrations, but has relatively high protein binding with slow dissociation, resulting in a low volume of distribution. As a result of molecular manipulation (Fig. 1), cefamandole offers advantages of antibacterial effectiveness and at the same time retains the safety of penicillin G and cephalothin in animals.

MATERIALS AND METHODS

Antibiotic. The lithium salt of cefamandole for in vitro studies was supplied in 20-mg ampoules by Eli Lilly & Co. The cefamandole for clinical use, CT-2883-4F, was cefamandole nafate furnished as 1 g of cefamandole activity per ampoule.

Bacterial strains. A total of 1,152 strains of bacteria were isolated from clinical material at Wishard Memorial and University Hospitals, Indianapolis, Ind.

Susceptibility testing. A serial twofold broth dilution procedure with a Canalco Autotiter IV (Canalco, Inc., Rockville, Md.) was used to establish the minimal inhibitory concentration (MIC) for all strains of bacteria except the *Bacteroides*. These were tested in an anerobic atmosphere with a manually operated Canalco Autotiter.

Mueller-Hinton broth was the medium employed for all of the aerobes and facultative anaerobes. When strains of streptococci and pneumococci were tested, 5% sheep blood was added to the broth. *Haemophilus influenzae* was tested by adding Filtes supplement. The inoculum for these procedures was 10^5 bacteria/ml of media. The MIC was recorded after 18 h of incubation at 37°C. Susceptibility of the *Neisseria* species was evaluated by using solid chocolate agar and a Steers replicator. The inoculum for the Steers replicator was prepared as for the International Collaborative Study agar dilution method.

Protein binding. The percentage of inactivation by human serum (protein binding) was estimated by comparing serum and urine standard curves obtained during the blood and urine assays.

Subjects. Volunteers were ambulatory adult males and females between the ages of 25 and 55 years with no overt physical or laboratory abnormalities. Diet was not restricted.

Injection of antibiotic. For intramuscular injection 3 ml of distilled water was added to each 1-g ampoule of cefamandole. Proportionate amounts of the resulting solution were used to achieve the 250-mg, 500-mg, or 1-g intramuscular dose. The injection was given in the gluteal muscle through a 1.5 inch (ca. 3.8-cm) 20-gauge needle.

For intravenous administration, the 1-g ampoules were placed in solution using 3 ml of distilled water. The dose to be given was then added to 50 ml of 5% glucose and infused rapidly into the antecubital vein over a 10-min period.

Serum assays. Blood samples were drawn before and at intervals after the administration of single doses of cefamandole (see Tables 3 and 5). The blood samples were centrifuged and the sera were frozen until assayed. Serum concentrations were measured using the *Bacillus subtilis* cup plate method (4).

Urine assays. Urine was collected at the intervals shown in Tables 4 and 6. These were assayed using an Elanco Autoturb (Elanco Products Co., Indianapolis, Ind.) with a *Klebsiella* strain as the indicator organism.

RESULTS

Susceptibility studies. Table 1 lists the number of bacterial strains in each species studied and their susceptibility to a given concentration of cefamandole. For ease of interpretation, the cumulative percentage of the susceptible strains is shown in Table 2.

A total of 90 to 100% of the methicillin-susceptible *Staphylococcus aureus*, group A and B streptococci, pneumococci, and gonococci required 2 μg or less of cefamandole per ml for inhibition. A concentration of 64 μg/ml (readily achieved in the urine after a 250-mg dose of cefamandole intramuscularly) inhibited the 19 strains of enterococci studied. Seventy percent of the *Escherichia coli* and indole-negative *Proteus* were inhibited by 4 μg of cefamandole per ml. Eighty percent of the *Bacteroides fragilis* subsp. *fragilis* were inhibited by 32 μg/ml, a concentration achieved by the administration of 1 g or greater doses intravenously.

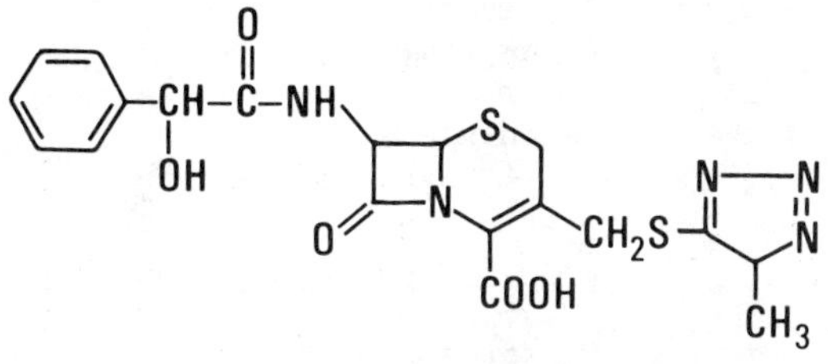

CEFAMANDOLE

FIG. 1. *Structure of cefamandole.*

All 42 strains of *H. influenzae* and the two strains of *Salmonella typhosa* were inhibited by 2 μg of cefamandole per ml.

Sixty-five percent of the 20 strains of *Serratia* were inhibited by 64 μg of cefamandole per ml. A concentration of 8 μg/ml inhibited 82% of the 55 strains of *Proteus mirabilis,* whereas this same concentration inhibited 59% of the 65 indole-positive *Proteus* strains studied. Seventy-one percent of the 24 *Citrobacter* strains were susceptible to 8 μg of cefamandole per ml. Of the 98 strains of *Enterobacter,* 28% were susceptible to 8 μg, 37% to 16 μg, and 46% to 32 μg or less of cefamandole per ml. Therapy of systemic infections due to these organisms and the enterococci obviously would require relatively high intravenous doses daily.

Protein binding. Using a cup plate method, 5 μg of cefamandole per ml in urine produced a

TABLE 1. *Number of isolates susceptible to cefamandole*

Organism	No. of isolates	No. susceptible at an MIC (μg/ml) of:										
		0.12	0.25	0.5	1	2	4	8	16	32	64	>64
Gram-positive cocci												
S. aureus	63	23	9	30	50	60	62	62	62	62	63	
S. aureus[a]	38						22	36	38	38	38	
β-hemolytic streptococci												
Lancefield group A	27	25	26	26	27	27	27	27	27	27	27	
Lancefield group B	13	7	7	9	11	13	13	13	13	13	13	
Lancefield other[b]	7	6	7	7	7	7	7	7	7	7	7	
Group D enterococcus	19									8	19	
Group D non-enterococcus	4	4	4	4	4	4	4	4	4	4	4	
Streptococcus pneumoniae	15	12	15	15	15	15	15	15	15	15	15	
Gram-negative cocci												
Neisseria gonorrhoeae	90	42	63	71	77	80	85	88	90	90	90	
Gram-negative rods												
E. coli	358		6	19	69	168	262	312	312	346	348	10
Klebsiella sp.	114	2		10	53	88	104	106	108	108	113	1
H. influenzae	42			13	40	42	42	42	42	42	42	
P. mirabilis	55		2	6	31	39	42	45	49	51	54	1
Proteus sp. (indole positive)	64			2	16	25	30	38	40	42	43	21
Enterobacter sp.	98				7	11	20	27	36	45	54	44
Serratia	20						1	1	3	5	13	7
Salmonella sp.	20			2	11	15	19	20	20	20	20	
S. typhosa	2		1	1	2	2	2	2	2	2	2	
Shigella sp.	3				1	1	1	2	3			
Citrobacter sp.	24				5	11	16	17	19	20	20	4
Acinetobacter	4									1	2	2
B. fragilis subsp. *fragilis*	72						4	19	44	58	62	10
Cumulative total	1,152	121	140	215	426	608	778	883	934	1,007	1,052	100

[a] Methicillin resistant.

[b] Not class A, B, C, or G.

TABLE 2. *Percentage of isolates susceptible to cefamandole*

Organism	No. of isolates	Isolates (%) susceptible at an MIC (μg/ml) of:										
		0.125	0.25	0.5	1	2	4	8	16	32	64	>64
Gram-positive cocci												
S. aureus	63	5	14	46	94	95	98	98	98	98	100	
S. aureus[a]	38						58	95	100			
β-hemolytic streptococci												
Lancefield group A	27	93	96	96	100							
Lancefield group B	13	54	54	69	85	100						
Lancefield other[b]	7	86	100									
Group D enterococcus	19									42	100	
Group D non-enterococcus	4	100										
S. pneumoniae	15	80	100									
Gram-negative cocci												
N. gonorrhoeae	90	47	70	79	86	89	94	98	100			
Gram-negative rods												
E. coli	358	1	2	5	19	47	73	87	87	97	97	3
Klebsiella sp.	114			9	46	77	91	93	95	95	99	1
H. influenzae	42			31	95	100						
P. mirabilis	55		4	11	56	71	76	82	89	93	98	2
Proteus sp. (indole positive)	65			3	25	29	47	59	63	66	67	33
Enterobacter sp.	98				7	11	20	28	37	46	55	45
Serratia	20						5	5	15	25	65	35
Salmonella sp.	20			10	55	75	95	100				
S. typhosa	2				100							
Shigella sp.	3								100			
Citrobacter sp.	24				21	46	67	71	79	83	83	17
Acinetobacter	4										50	50
B. fragilis subsp. *fragilis*	72						6	26	61	80	86	14
Total	1,152											
Cumulative Susceptible (%)		11	12	19	37	53	68	77	81	87	91	9

[a] Methicillin resistant.
[b] Not class A, B, C, or G.

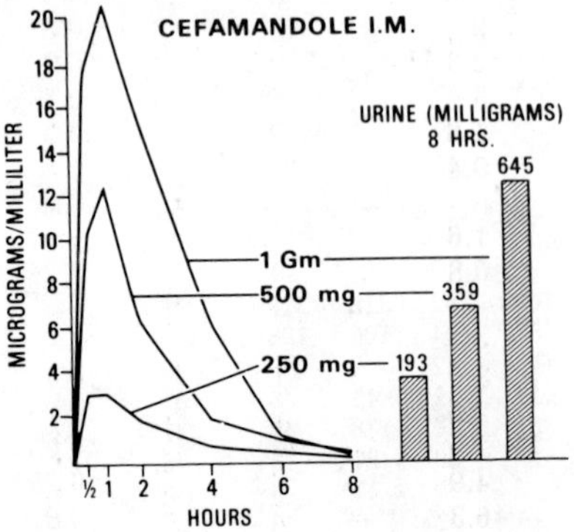

FIG. 2. *Average cefamandole levels in blood and urine excretion after the intramuscular (I.M.) injection of 250, 500, and 1,000 mg.*

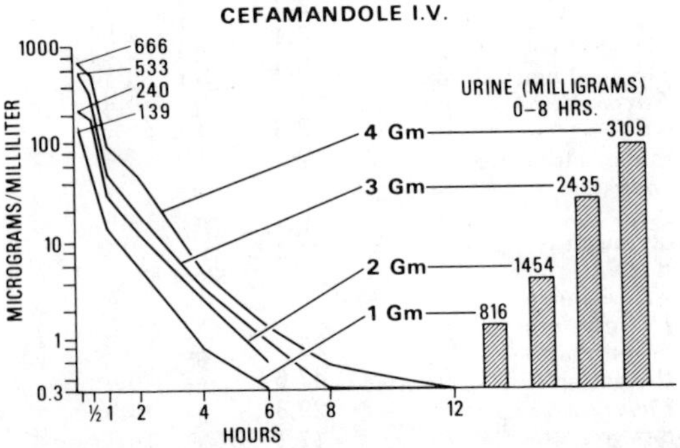

FIG. 3. *Average cefamandole levels in blood and urine excretion after the intravenous (I.V.) injection of 1, 2, 3, and 4 g.*

zone size of 37.4 mm. This was reduced to 30.7 mm when the same concentration in serum was studied. Thus, serum reduced the zone size by 18%. From the standard curve, it was apparent that an 18% reduction of zone size was the same as lowering the concentration of cefamandole from 5 to 1.0 μg/ml, or 80% binding by serum proteins.

When an ultracentrifuge was used to determine protein binding, 70% of the cefamandole went with the protein fraction. These values are similar to those reported for cephalothin by Kirby and Regamey, using the ultrafiltration method (5).

Pharmacology. Figure 2 shows the average levels of cefamandole in the blood and urine excretion after the intramuscular injection of 250, 500, and 1,000 mg. Levels with each dose at 1 h were 2.7, 12.2, and 20.6 μg/ml, respectively. Assayable amounts were still present at 4 h after the 250-mg dose and at 6 to 8 h after the 500-mg and 1-g doses.

The total amount of cefamandole excreted over the 8-h collection period was approximately 65 to 85% after the intramuscular injection. The average concentration in the urine for the 8-h period was 210 μg/ml after the 250-mg dose, 254 μg/ml after the 500-mg dose, and 1,357 μg/ml after the 1-g dose.

Figure 3 compares the average levels of cefamandole in blood and urine excretion after the

TABLE 3. *Concentration of cefamandole in serum after intramuscular administration*

Patient	Concn in serum at h:						
	0	0.5	1	2	4	6	8
250-mg dose							
AB	0	2.8	2.6	1.9	0.8	0.3	
RD	0	3.4	2.8	1.0	<0.3	<0.3	
ME	0	4.8	3.1	1.0	0.3	<0.3	
AF	0	4.5	3.5	1.9	0.6	<0.3	
HG	0	2.2	2.4	1.3	0.5	<0.3	
JH	0	2.6	2.7	1.8	0.6	<0.3	
TH	0	1.7	2.5	1.8	0.7	<0.3	
RM	0	1.5	1.9	1.8	0.8	0.3	
AP	0	3.8	3.0	1.6	0.4	<0.3	
DW	0	2.7	2.2	0.9	<0.3	<0.3	
Mean	0	3.0	2.7	1.5	0.5		
SD[a]	0	1.1	0.5	0.4			
500-mg dose							
AB	0	12.2	20.3	4.4	1.1	0.8	<0.3
RD	0	15.8	15.8	4.4	0.7	<0.3	<0.3
ME	0	16.2	15.7	5.6	1.6	<0.3	<0.3
AF	0	12.2	15.8	9	2	0.4	<0.3
HG	0	12.2	5.7	5.4	1.6	0.3	<0.3
JH	0	3.4	7.5	5.7	2	0.4	<0.3
TH	0	3.4	7.7	7.3	2.3	0.3	<0.3
RM	0	1	3.9	5	3	0.8	<0.3
AP	0	8.3	15.7	8.3	1.8	0.3	<0.3
DW	0	12	13.9	7.3	0.4	<0.3	<0.3
Mean	0	9.7	12.2	6.2	1.6	0.5	
SD	0	5.4	5.5	1.6	0.8	0.2	
1-g dose							
AB	0	25	16	10.8	3.5	1.2	0.4
RD	0	47.6	26.6	14.3	2.5	0.5	<0.25
ME	0	29.3	43.5	21.4	2.5	0.4	<0.25
HG	0	17.1	16.7	17.6	4.9	0.8	<0.25
JH	0	9	9	9.7	6.3	2.2	0.6
TH	0	4.4	12.3	14.4	2.9	0.8	<0.25
RM	0	5.8	14	15.1	6.2	2.2	1.1
AP	0	22.4	40.2	20.4	6.2	1.6	1.2
DW	0	19.5	20.1	13.1	4.0	0.7	<0.25
RB	0	4.1	7.1	20.1	6.0	0.9	0.3
Mean	0	18.4	20.6	15.7	4.5	1.1	0.4
SD	0	13.7	12.5	4.1	1.6	0.7	

[a] SD, Standard deviation.

TABLE 4. *Concentrations of cefamandole in urine after intramuscular administration*

Patient	0–2 h			6–8 h		
	μg/ml	Total volume (ml)	Total mg	μg/ml	Total volume (ml)	Total mg
250-mg dose						
AB	165	480	79	880	130	114
RD	250	474	118	235	405	95
ME	120	1,000	120	185	350	64
AF	400	450	182	625	50	31
HG	205	600	123	340	350	119
JH	95	550	52	240	450	108
TH	80	460	37	340	180	61
RM	90	800	72	290	450	130
AP	190	500	95	150	850	127
DW	270	450	121	445	180	80
Mean	186	576	100	373	339	93
SD[a]	100	183	42	225	22	34
500-mg dose						
AB	300	1,030	309	820	100	82
RD	100	1,120	112	320	850	272
ME	380	890	338	265	450	119
AF	130	1,160	150	350	540	189
HG	210	700	147	500	550	275
JH	120	960	115	300	600	180
TH	160	900	144	350	550	192
RM	150	700	105	230	550	126
AP	320	560	179	390	450	175
DW	220	890	195	350	550	192
Mean	209	891	179	388	519	180
SD	95	192	81	160	184	62
1-g dose						
AB	1,365	230	324	4,875	640	312
RD	2,973	160	476	1,043	255	266
ME	4,800	80	384	1,352	170	230
HG	1,037	100	104	1,997	310	619
JH	750	190	143	1,495	380	568
TH	3,857	95	366	1,295	220	285
RM	1,780	115	205	1,059	340	360
AP	797	240	191	833	420	350
DW	1,520	210	319	1,320	200	264
RB	1,185	100	119	2,178	270	588
Mean	2,006	156	262	1,745	320	384
SD	1,395	62	127	1,176	137	149

[a] SD, Standard deviation.

intravenous injection of 1, 2, 3, and 4 g. Average peak levels at 10 min after the completion of the 10-min intravenous infusion of cefamandole were 139 μg/ml for the 1-g dose and 240, 524, and 666 μg/ml for the 2-, 3-, and 4-g doses, respectively. After equilibration, the corresponding 30-min levels were 54, 196, 279, and 428 μg/ml. Each increase in the amount given prolonged the duration of measurable levels. The antibiotic level was less than 0.3 μg/ml at 8 h after the 2-g dose and was not assayable at 12 h after the 3- and 4-g doses.

A total of 75 to 85% of the intravenous dose was recovered in the urine during the 8-h postinjection period. The average concentration for the 8-h period was 750 μg/ml after the 1-g dose, 1,380 μg/ml after the 2-g dose, 2,110 after the 3-g dose, and 2,550 after the 4-g dose. For closer scrutiny, the actual blood levels and urine excretion for each individual receiving cefamandole are shown in Tables 3 through 6. The average values for the blood levels and urine excretion used for preparing Fig. 2 and 3 are shown in Table 7.

DISCUSSION

The bacteria most frequently isolated from nonhospitalized patients with infection are streptococci, pneumococci, staphylococci, and *E. coli*. Infections caused by these organisms are usually treated with relatively low doses of antibiotics administered orally. Patients with serious infections are usually admitted to a hospital. At the Wishard Memorial Hospital in Indianapolis, 12% of the admissions are related to bacterial infections. An additional 7% are from nosocomial sources (Committee on Infection Control, Wishard Memorial Hospital). This incidence is similar to that reported by others (1). The distribution of the bacteria tested for antibiotic susceptibility (other than group A streptococci and pneumococci) are

TABLE 5. *Concentrations of cefamandole in serum after intravenous administration*

Patient	Concn in serum at h:								
	0	0.17	0.5	1	2	4	6	8	12
1-g dose									
RB	0	214.2	106.1	13.5	5.9	0.8	<0.3		
AF	0	128.5	68.7	24	8.6	1.3	<0.3		
GL	0	92.3	22.2	13.3	5.2	0.7	<0.3		
HL	0	198.5	31.4	13.3	1.6	0.3	<0.3		
BO	0	145.1	78.9	14	3.3	0.3	<0.3		
CK	0	85.1	40.1	14	5.5	1.1	<0.3		
GM	0	100	33.2	14.2	4.0	1.4	0.4		
Mean	0	139.1	54.4	15.2	4.9	0.8			
SD[a]	0	54.1	30.8	3.9	2.2	0.4			
2-g dose									
RB	0	313.8	278	24.5	2.4	1.7	0.5	<0.3	
AF	0	228.1	198.5	38.4	10	4.5	0.8	<0.3	
GL	0	137.7	88.6	22.8	4.5	1.8	0.3	<0.3	
HL	0	109.8	64.1	15	4.4	0.6	0.3	<0.3	
BO	0	301.3	195	23.3	6.4	1	0.3	<0.3	
CK	0	308.5	274.7	49.1	22.5	2.4	0.5	<0.3	
GM	0	284	274.7	40.2	27	3.6	1.1	0	
Mean	0	240.5	196.2	30.5	11	2.2	0.5		
SD	0	85	89.5	12.2	9.7	1.4	0.3		
3-g dose									
CK	0	644.6	318	66.2	26	3.5	1.1	0.3	<0.3
GM	0	526	249.6	54.8	30.9	4.3	1.5	0.6	<0.3
BO	0	370	151.8	63.6	34.6	1.9	0.4	0.3	<0.3
RM	0	588	288.7	68.2	16.2	1.9	0.5	<0.3	<0.3
CS	0	540	389.2	86	27.9	2.7	1	0.3	<0.3
Mean	0	533.7	279.5	67.8	27.1	2.9	0.9	0.3	
SD	0	102.6	87.8	11.4	6.9	1	0.5		
4-g dose									
CK	0	747	675.2	65.2	55.4	4.8	1.6	0.5	<0.3
GM	0	684.4	486	92.7	38.7	6_{e6}	2.6	1	<0.3
BO	0	413.6	326.7	68.9	31.6	2.5	0.6	0.3	<0.3
RM	0	654.4	376.8	67.7	41.1	1.8	1	0.3	<0.3
CS	0	833.1	777.6	100.7	39	4	0.8	0.3	<0.3
Mean	0	666.3	528.5	79	41.2	3.9	1.3	0.5	
SD	0	156.9	193.1	16.4	8.7	1.9	0.8	0.3	

[a] SD, Standard deviation.

shown in Table 8 (Committee on Infection Control, Wishard Memorial Hospital).

All of the group A streptococci and pneumococci and 95% of the methicillin-susceptible *S. aureus* in this study were shown to be susceptible to concentrations of 2 μg or less per ml, easily achieved by doses of 250 mg of cefamandole intramuscularly. Eighty-two percent of the bacterial isolates were inhibited by serum concentrations of 8 μg or less per ml, an amount exceeded after the 500-mg and 1-g doses intramuscularly. Intravenous doses of greater than 1 g gave serum concentrations manyfold higher than the susceptibility of most of the bacterial strains studied. Relatively low therapeutic doses of cefamandole, 0.5 to 1 g intramuscularly or 1 to 2 g intravenously every 6 h, should be clinically effective in infections that would include virtually all of the commonly encountered bacterial organisms, i.e., beta-hemolytic strep-

TABLE 6. *Urine concentration and excretion of cefamandole after intravenous administration*

Patient	0–2 h			2–4 h			4–6 h			6–8 h		
	μg/ml	Volume (ml)	Total mg	μg/ml	Volume (ml)	Total mg	μg/ml	Volume (ml)	Total mg	μg/ml	Volume (ml)	Total mg
1-g dose												
RB	1,780	390	694	510	380	194	29	390	11	16	630	10
AF	1,550	420	651	400	310	124	29	80	2	12	305	4
GL	3,100	150	465	600	140	84	16	190	3	14	210	3
HL	1,800	320	576	490	330	162	30	130	4	11	200	2
BO	1,000	700	700	500	320	160	45	140	6	30	230	7
CK	2,700	220	594	450	350	158	220	120	26	33	130	4
GM	1,600	590	944	1,225	70	86	329	95	31	36	64	2
Mean	1,933	399	661	596	271	138	100	164	12	22	252	5
SD[a]	721	195	149	284	118	42	124	106	12	11	183	3
2-g dose												
RB	3,460	520	1,799	1,110	85	94	45	400	18	18	290	5
AF	1,900	530	1,007	1,675	190	318	50	230	12	38	380	14
GL	3,740	360	1,346	455	485	221	33	450	15	30	150	5
HL	2,800	460	1,288	770	280	216	36	220	8	20	170	3
BO	2,300	615	1,415	1,550	120	186	40	100	4	31	130	4
CK	4,170	120	500	1,375	275	378	40	250	10	35	110	4
GM	6,000	170	1,020	2,420	120	290	34	50	2	32	100	3
Mean	3,481	396	1,196	1,336	222	243	40	243	10	29	190	5
SD	1,369	189	407	643	139	94	6	145	6	8	105	4
3-g dose												
CK	6,950	275	1,911	780	290	226	110	150	17	37	125	5
GM	5,600	410	2,296	800	200	160	380	50	19	104	20	2
BO	2,200	1,040	2,288	840	420	353	112	150	17	38	105	4
RM	3,950	515	2,034	960	250	240	410	150	62	38	170	7
CS	3,750	520	1,950	1,235	400	494	400	190	76	47	330	16
Mean	4,490	552	2,095	923	312	295	282	138	38	53	150	7
SD	1,828	290	185	188	95	131	157	52	29	29	114	5
4-g dose												
CK	7,500	310	2,325	1,710	250	428	640	120	77	38	155	6
GM	5,000	420	2,100	7,600	50	380	780	30	23	108	75	8
BO	4,500	800	3,600	1,000	450	450	500	120	60	92	420	39
RM	9,500	250	2,375	1,740	235	409	175	450	79	120	395	47
CS	6,750	380	2,565	1,200	415	498	275	255	70	26	265	7
Mean	6,650	432	2,593	2,650	280	433	474	195	62	77	262	21
SD	2,013	216	537	2,786	160	45	250	164	23	42	149	20

[a] SD, Standard deviation.

TABLE 7. *Serum concentrations and urine excretion of cefamandole after intramuscular and intravenous administration*

Dose	No. of subjects	Concn in serum at h: 0.17	0.5	1	2	4	6	8	12	Urine excretion at 0–8 h: Avg (μg/ml)	Total (mg)	%
Intramuscular												
250 mg	10		3	2.7	1.5	0.5	<0.3			210	193	77
500 mg	10		9.7	12.2	6.2	1.6	0.5	<0.3		254	359	72
1 g	10		18.4	20.6	15.7	4.5	1.1	0.4		1,357	646	65
Intravenous												
1 g	7	139	54	15	5	0.8	<0.3			750	816	82
2 g	7	240	196	30	11	2.2	0.5	<0.3		1,383	1,454	73
3 g	5	533	279	68	27	2.9	0.9	0.3	<0.3	2,114	2,435	81
4 g	5	666	528	79	41	3.9	1.3	0.5	<0.3	2,660	3,109	78

TABLE 8. *Incidence of bacteria isolated for susceptibility testing at Wishard Memorial Hospital, Indianapolis, Ind.*

Determination	Isolates (%)/mo in: 1968 (707)[a]	1969 (1,419)	1970 (1,646)	1973 (1,712)	1974 (1,026)
S. aureus	20	16	17	17	17
S. epidermis	5	15	21	24	5
E. coli	25	22	21	19	26
Citrobacter	8	9	8	1	1
Proteus sp.	11	10	10	8	9
Klebsiella-Enterobacter	22	14	11	13	19
Pseudomonas	7	7	7	10	9
Serratia		4	1	1	2

[a] Numbers in parentheses indicate the total number of isolates.

TABLE 9. *Mean MIC of isolates susceptible to 64 μg or less of cefamandole per ml*

Organism	Mean MIC	%
Gram-positive cocci		
S. aureus	1.83	100
S. aureus (methicillin resistant)	6.11	100
β-hemolytic streptococci		
Group A	0.16	100
Group B	1.6	100
Other	0.14	100
Group D enterococcus	50.5	100
Group D non-enterococcus	0.1	100
S. pneumoniae	0.14	100
Gram-negative cocci		
N. gonorrhoeae	1.14	100
Gram-negative rods		
E. coli	4.7	97
Klebsiella	4.6	99
P. mirabilis	1	98
Indole-positive *Proteus* sp.	6.5	67
Enterobacter sp.	20.4	55
Salmonella sp.	2.1	100
H. influenzae	0.9	100
Citrobacter sp.	5.5	83
B. fragilis subsp. *fragilis*	21.9	86

tococci, pneumococci, staphylococci, *E. coli*, *Klebsiella*, etc. (Table 9).

Young and Hewitt have used an inhibitory index to illustrate the relative potency of an antibiotic (12). This method has been used to compare the effect of increasing doses of cefamandole (Table 10). Presumably, protein binding would not appreciably affect the antibacterial activity of cefamandole and, therefore, has not been included in the calculations in Table 10. Like penicillin G and cephalothin, cefamandole is rapidly dissociated from the serum proteins, as evidenced by the relatively short half-life and rapid appearance in the urine.

It is obvious that as the dose is increased the number of bacterial species that can be included in the spectrum of cefamandole is also increased. If one utilizes somewhat less stringent criteria (corresponding to an MIC of 32 μg or less per ml, levels that can readily be achieved with parenteral therapy), 80% of the *Bacteroides* strains tested would be susceptible to cefamandole therapy. These results are similar to the median of 32 μg/ml reported by Ernst et al. (2). A similar observation has been made by Moellering et al. for cefoxitin (6).

Although most of the *P. mirabilis* indole-negative strains are susceptible to the cephalosporins, including cefamandole, Eykyn and coworkers called attention to the promising results observed with cefamandole against other enterobacteriaceae (3). However, they found *P. vulgaris* strains were consistently resistant to cefamandole. These findings are in accord with our data. *P. mirabilis* strains required only 8

TABLE 10. *Inhibitory index[a] for cefamandole*

Organism	Mean MIC	Inhibitory index after dose (g) of:						
		Intramuscular			Intravenous			
		0.25 (3.0)[b]	0.5 (12.2)	1 (20.6)	1 (54)	2 (196)	3 (270)	4 (528)
Gram-positive cocci								
S. aureus	1.83	2	7	11	30	107	152	288
S. aureus (methicillin resistant)	6.11		2	3	9	32	46	86
β-hemolytic streptococci								
Group A	0.16	19	76	128	338	1,225	1,744	3,300
Group B	1.6	2	8	13	34	122	174	330
Other	0.14	21	87	147	385	1,400	1,993	3,771
Group D enterococcus	50.4				1	4	6	10
Group D non-enterococcus	0.1	30	122	206	540	1,960	2,790	5,280
S. pneumoniae	0.14	21	87	147	385	1,400	1,993	3,771
Gram-negative cocci								
N. gonorrhoeae	1.14	3	11	18	47	172	245	463
Gram-negative rods								
E. coli	4.7		3	4	11	42	59	112
Klebsiella	4.6		3	4	12	43	61	115
P. mirabilis	1	3	12	20	54	196	279	528
Indole-positive *Proteus* sp.	6.5		2	3	8	30	43	81
Enterobacter sp.	20.4			1	3	10	14	26
Salmonella sp.	2.1	1	6	10	26	93	133	251
H. influenzae	0.9	3	14	23	60	217	310	587
Citrobacter sp.	5.5		2	4	10	36	51	96
B. fragilis subsp. *fragilis*	21.9			1	2	9	13	24

[a] Ratio between the mean peak serum levels and the mean MIC of the isolates susceptible to 64 μg or less per ml.
[b] Numbers in parentheses indicate mean peak blood level in micrograms per milliliter.

μg/ml to inhibit 82%, whereas 59% of the indole-producing strains of *Proteus* were inhibited by this concentration.

We found that 46% of the 98 strains of *Enterobacter* were susceptible to 32 μg of cefamandole per ml, whereas Washington reported 73% of 30 strains of *E. aerogenes* and 67% of 51 strains of *E. cloacae* were inhibited by 8 μg/ml (9). Eykyn emphasized that there is often a striking inoculum effect among organisms with moderate to high MIC values, with only partial inhibition of large inocula by concentrations of cefamandole (3). Inoculum effect has been observed with other cephalosporins and penicillins (8).

In addition to the inoculum effect, the discrepancies in the cefamandole MICs of *Enterobacter* reported by other workers are apparently associated with whether the susceptibility tests were performed in broth or agar (3, 7, 9).

The higher cefamandole MICs in broth (as used in our study) may reflect an emergence of resistant variants from the heterogenous composition of the culture, not detected by lower inocula or by the end-point criteria usually used in agar dilution methods (C. M. Findell and J. C. Sherris, Abstr. Annu. Meet. Am. Soc. Microbiol. 1976, A14, p. 3).

Since the strains of *Enterobacter*, indole-positive *Proteus*, and enterococci vary in susceptibility, laboratory tests should be used as a guide to selection of antibiotic therapy. *Pseudomonas* strains are universally resistant to cefamandole.

In conclusion the majority (82%) of the bacterial strains isolated from hospitalized patients with infection were susceptible to the peak serum concentrations (8 to 16 μg/ml) obtained after 500-mg to 1-g doses of cefamandole administered intramuscularly.

A total of 65 to 85% of the parenterally injected cefamandole appeared as the biologically active form in urine over an 8-h collection period.

Very high serum concentrations of 270 and 528 μg/ml were obtained 0.5 h after a 10-min infusion of 3 and 4 g of cefamandole intravenously. As has been shown with other antibiotics, higher doses would be needed only for the treatment of infections due to less susceptible organisms or in those patients with severe or overwhelming infections.

LITERATURE CITED

1. **Bennett, J. V., W. E. Scheckler, D. G. Maki, and P. S. Brachman.** 1970. Current national patterns–United States. *In* Proceedings of the International Conference on Nosocomial Infections, 3–6 August, p. 42–49. American Hospital Association, Chicago.
2. **Ernst, E. C., S. Berger, M. Barza, N. V. Jacobus, and F. P. Tally.** 1976. Activity of cefamandole and other cephalosporins against aerobic and anaerobic bacteria. Antimicrob. Agents Chemother. 9:852–855.
3. **Eykyn, S., C. Jenkins, A. King, and I. Phillips.** 1973. Antibacterial activity of cefamandole, a new cephalosporin antibiotic, compared with that of cephaloridine, cephalothin, and cephalexin. Antimicrob. Agents Chemother. 3:657–661.
4. **Grove, D., and W. A. Randall.** 1955. Assay methods for antibiotics. *In* Antibiotic monogr. no. 2. Medical Encyclopedia, Inc., New York.
5. **Kirby, W. M. M., and C. Regamey.** 1973. Pharmacokinetics of cefazolin compared with four other cephalosporins. J. Infect. Dis. 128(Suppl.):S341–S347.
6. **Moellering, R. C., Jr., M. Dray, and L. J. Kung.** 1974. Susceptibility of clinical isolates of bacteria to cefoxitin and cephalothin. Antimicrob. Agents Chemother. 6:320–323.
7. **Neu, H. C.** 1974. Cefamandole, a cephalosporin antibiotic with an unusually wide spectrum of activity. Antimicrob. Agents Chemother. 6:177–182.
8. **Sabath, L. D., C. Garner, C. Wilcox, and M. Finland.** 1975. Effect of inoculum and of beta-lactamase on the anti-staphylococcal activity of thirteen penicillins and cephalosporins. Antimicrob. Agents Chemother. 8:344–349.
9. **Washington, J. A., II.** 1976. The in vitro spectrum of the cephalosporins. Mayo Clin. Proc. 51:237–250.
10. **Weinstein, L.** 1975. Chemotherapy of microbial diseases, p. 1158–1166. *In* L. S. Goodman and A. Gilman (ed.), Pharmacological basis of therapeutics, 5th ed. Macmillan Co., New York.
11. **Weinstein, L., and K. Kaplan.** 1970. The cephalosporins. Microbiological, chemical, and pharmacological properties and use in chemotherapy of infection. Ann. Intern. Med. 72:729–739.
12. **Young, L. S., and S. L. Hewitt.** 1973. Activity of five aminoglycoside antibiotics in vitro against gram-negative bacilli and *Staphylococcus aureus*. Antimicrob. Agents Chemother. 4:617–625.

ANTIMICROBIAL AGENTS AND CHEMOTHERAPY, Nov. 1976, p. 824–826
Copyright © 1976 American Society for Microbiology

Vol. 10, No. 5
Printed in U.S.A.

Effect of Osmolality on the Response of *Escherichia coli* to Mecillinam

DAVID GREENWOOD

Department of Microbiology, University of Nottingham, City Hospital, Nottingham, NG5 1PH, England

Received for publication 29 June 1976

The influence of osmolality on the effect of the novel β-lactam antibiotic, mecillinam, on *Escherichia coli* was examined in a turbidimetric system. Both sucrose and sodium chloride were able to protect *E. coli* from the effects of mecillinam during the stage of conversion to morphologically abnormal forms, and the additional presence of small amounts of magnesium sulfate protected the spherical forms from subsequent lysis. More phenotypically "resistant" survivors were recovered in osmotically protective media than in broth of low osmolality. Sucrose appeared a better protective agent than sodium chloride, but growth of the phenotypically resistant population was much slower in the sucrose-containing than in sodium chloride-containing medium.

Mecillinam, previously known by its manufacturer's code, FL 1060, is an anomalous β-lactam antibiotic whose behavior differs in several important respects from that of other penicillins and cephalosporins (4, 5, 10, 12). Among the unusual properties of mecillinam is its ability to convert susceptible gram-negative bacilli to spherical forms by a generalized effect on the cell wall (4, 6), whereas sufficient concentrations of most other β-lactam agents induce the formation of osmotically sensitive spheroplasts at discrete sites typically associated with incipient points of cell division (7, 9). It has been claimed that conversion of gram-negative bacilli to spherical forms by mecillinam is independent of sucrose concentration (10), implying that such forms are not osmotically sensitive, but our own studies (4, 8), using sodium chloride to vary the osmolality, have indicated that the formation and fate of spherical forms is very dependent on the osmotic environment. Recently, Tybring and Melchior (13) have suggested that NaCl, but not sucrose, is active in protecting the spherical forms and that the effect is related not to osmolality, but to specific conductivity of the medium.

The question of the fate of mecillinam-treated bacteria may be of some importance because, in contrast to the situation with other β-lactam agents, abnormal forms surviving the destructive effect of the drug are able to grow and divide in its presence and this may influence its therapeutic efficacy.

MATERIALS AND METHODS

A strain of *Escherichia coli* (laboratory code ECSA 2), originally isolated from infected urine, was used throughout. *E. coli* ECSA 2 was chosen because in a previous study of the response of several *E. coli* strains to mecillinam (4) this strain showed an intermediate type of response to changes in the osmolality of the growth medium.

Mecillinam was a gift from Leo Laboratories Ltd. Suitable concentrations were freshly prepared as required in sterile distilled water.

Cultures were grown from small inocula in complete broth (7) containing the required amount of NaCl or sucrose, in the light path of a simple photometric device (14) connected to a potentiometric recorder. In this way the turbidity of the cultures could be continuously monitored. The cultures were mixed by using a magnetic stirrer. Mecillinam was added at a standard point in the logarithmic growth phase when the turbidity of the culture reached 12% of maximum.

Osmolality measurements were made by the cryostatic method using an advanced osmometer (Advanced Instruments Inc.).

Morphological observations were made on untreated wet preparations by interference contrast microscopy.

RESULTS

The osmolality of complete medium without supplements was found to be about 170 mOsm/kg; the addition of 10% (wt/vol) sucrose increased the osmolality to about 455 mOsm/kg; the addition of 1% (wt/vol) NaCl increased the osmolality to about 470 mOsm/kg.

Continuous turbidimetric monitoring was used in order to follow the kinetics of bacterial response to mecillinam. The relationship of turbidimetric changes to alterations in morphology and viability of *E. coli* has been discussed elsewhere (4).

Continuous turbidimetric records of *E. coli*

ECSA 2 exposed to mecillinam (10 μg/ml; 80 times the minimum inhibitory concentration) are shown in Fig. 1. In complete medium alone a small increase in opacity occurred after the addition of mecillinam over a period of about 90 min, corresponding to the period during which morphological changes develop (4), after which the opacity again declined. A fresh increase in opacity, shown by microscopy to be due to the growth of morphologically abnormal cells (4), occurred about 20 h after the addition of mecillinam. In the presence of 1% NaCl or 10% sucrose, the opacity of the culture continued to follow the normal growth curve for at least 90 min after the addition of mecillinam, after which a marked fall in opacity occurred. This fall in opacity occurred sooner and was more profound in the presence of NaCl than in the presence of sucrose. A fresh, progressive increase in opacity due to morphologically abnormal forms occurred as the lytic phase came to an end, but the increase was much slower in the presence of sucrose (Fig. 1C) than in the presence of NaCl (Fig. 1D).

The influence of 0.1% magnesium sulfate ($MgSO_4 \cdot 7H_2O$) on the response of *E. coli* ECSA 2 to mecillinam is shown in Fig. 2. Alone, it had little effect on the response curve, except that regrowth due to morphologically abnormal forms occurred somewhat sooner (16 h rather than 20 h after antibiotic addition). In medium containing 1% NaCl, the additional presence of $MgSO_4$ modified the rate of fall in opacity and allowed recovery to occur sooner, whereas in medium containing 10% sucrose, the additional presence of $MgSO_4$ totally abolished the lytic phase.

DISCUSSION

The death of gram-negative bacilli, after exposure to β-lactam antibiotics, is generally due to osmotic lysis (3, 7). However, two fractions of the bacterial population may survive exposure to β-lactam agents; morphologically normal persisters (1, 2) and those cells having an intracellular osmolality below that of the environment, which survive as spheroplasts (3, 7). Mecillinam converts sensitive gram-negative bacilli to forms resembling spheroplasts, but, because it lacks the ability of other β-lactam agents to inhibit division, cells surviving exposure to mecillinam are (unlike conventional spheroplasts) able to grow and divide in a morphologically abnormal form (4).

The reliance of mecillinam on low environmental osmolality to achieve its lethal effect (4, 8) has been questioned by Tybring and Melchior (13) who relate protection to the specific conductivity of the medium. Results obtained in the present study, however, indicate that both sucrose and NaCl are active in protecting *E. coli* from the early effects of mecillinam, although lysis of part of the population subsequently occurred in the presence of both substances, when cell wall damage was sufficiently advanced (4); this delayed lysis occurred sooner and was more profound in the presence of NaCl. The additional presence of $MgSO_4$, which has a stabilizing effect on cell wall-deficient *E. coli* (11), modified the lytic response in the presence of NaCl and abolished it in the presence of sucrose. The inferior protective ability of NaCl, which is also found in ampicillin-induced spheroplasts (3), is probably related to the flow of ions into the cell, whereas sucrose, a nonfermentable substrate for *E. coli*, is likely to be excluded.

Although sucrose appeared better able than NaCl to protect cells from the early effects of mecillinam, it was also found to allow growth of the surviving, phenotypically resistant fraction of the population at a much reduced rate compared with NaCl. This may explain the findings of Tybring and Melchior (13) that NaCl, but not sucrose, had a protective effect on me-

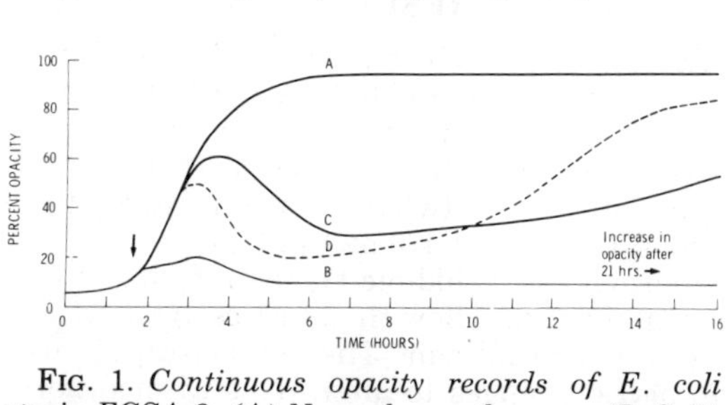

FIG. 1. *Continuous opacity records of E. coli strain ECSA 2. (A) Normal growth curve; (B,C,D) mecillinam was added (arrow) to achieve a concentration of 10 μg/ml. Medium contained (A,B) no addition; (C) 10% sucrose; (D) 1% NaCl.*

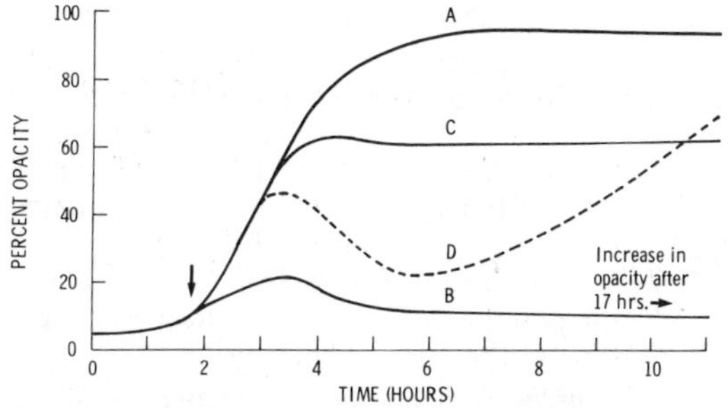

FIG. 2. *Continuous opacity records of E. coli strain ECSA 2. (A) Normal growth curve; (B,C,D) mecillinam was added (arrow) to achieve a concentration of 10 μg/ml. Medium contained 0.1% $MgSO_4 \cdot 7H_2O$ and (A,B) no further addition; (C) 10% sucrose; (D) 1% NaCl.*

cillinam-treated gram-negative bacilli. In their experiments results were expressed as the minimal inhibitory concentration estimated in the presence of various osmotically active agents. Minimal inhibitory concentration tests read at a fixed point in time after overnight incubation may clearly be influenced by differences in growth rates of the surviving cells as a slow growing population may not achieve a visible turbidity by the time of inspection.

The question of whether the ready emergence of phenotypically resistant forms reduces the therapeutic efficacy of mecillinam has not yet been resolved. However, the markedly enhanced effect obtained when *E. coli* is exposed to mecillinam in conditions of relatively low osmolality suggests that it may be advisable to reduce the osmolality when practicable (for example, by increased fluid intake in urinary tract infection) in treatment with this antibiotic.

ACKNOWLEDGMENT

I am grateful to George Sharp for the osmolality measurements.

LITERATURE CITED

1. **Greenwood, D.** 1972. Mucopeptide hydrolases and bacterial "Persisters." Lancet **ii**:465–466.
2. **Greenwood, D., and F. O'Grady.** 1970. Trimodal response of *Escherichia coli* and *Proteus mirabilis* to penicillins. Nature (London) **228**:457–458.
3. **Greenwood, D., and F. O'Grady.** 1972. The effect of osmolality on the response of *Escherichia coli* and *Proteus mirabilis* to pencillins. Br. J. Exp. Pathol. **53**:457–464.
4. **Greenwood, D., and F. O'Grady.** 1973. FL 1060: a new β-lactam antibiotic with novel properties. J. Clin. Pathol. **26**:1–6.
5. **Greenwood, D., and F. O'Grady.** 1973. The two sites of penicillin action in *Escherichia coli*. J. Infect. Dis. **128**:791–794.
6. **Greenwood, D., and F. O'Grady.** 1973. Penicillin and the site of wall growth in gram-negative bacilli. Naturwissenschaften **60**:435–436.
7. **Greenwood, D., and F. O'Grady.** 1973. Comparison of the responses of *Escherichia coli* and *Proteus mirabilis* to seven β-lactam antibiotics. J. Infect. Dis. **128**:211–222.
8. **Greenwood, D., H. L. Brooks, R. Gargan, and F. O'Grady.** 1974. Activity of FL 1060, a new β-lactam antibiotic, against urinary tract pathogens. J. Clin. Pathol. **27**:192–197.
9. **Lederberg, J.** 1956. Bacterial protoplasts induced by penicillin. Proc. Natl. Acad. Sci. U.S.A. **42**:574–577.
10. **Lund, F., and L. Tybring.** 1972. 6β-amidinopenicillanic acids—a new group of antibiotics. Nature (London) New Biol. **236**:135–137.
11. **McQuillen, K.** 1960. Bacterial protoplasts, p. 249–359. *In* I. C. Gunsalus and R. Y. Stanier (ed.), The bacteria, vol. I. Academic Press Inc., New York.
12. **Park, J. T., and L. Burman.** 1973. FL 1060, a new penicillin with a unique mode of action. Biochem. Biophys. Res. Commun. **51**:863–868.
13. **Tybring, L., and N. H. Melchior.** 1975. Mecillinam (FL 1060), a 6β-amidinopenicillanic acid derivative: bactericidal action and synergy in vitro. Antimicrob. Agents Chemother. **8**:271–276.
14. **Watson, B. W., C. L. Gauci, L. Blache, and F. O'Grady.** 1969. A simple turbidity cell for continuously monitoring the growth of bacteria. Phys. Med. Biol. **14**:555–558.

Antimicrobial Agents and Chemotherapy, Nov. 1976, p. 827–836
Vol. 10, No. 5

Biological Activity of Netilmicin, a Broad-Spectrum Semisynthetic Aminoglycoside Antibiotic

GEORGE H. MILLER,* GEORGE ARCIERI, MARVIN J. WEINSTEIN, AND J. ALLAN WAITZ

Chemotherapy Department and Antibiotic Clinical Research, Schering Corporation, Bloomfield, New Jersey 07003*

Received for publication 19 July 1976

Netilmicin (Sch 20569) is a new broad-spectrum semisynthetic aminoglycoside derived from sisomicin. Netilmicin was compared to gentamicin, tobramycin, and amikacin in a variety of in vitro test systems as well as in mouse protection tests. Netilmicin was found to be similar in activity to gentamicin against aminoglycoside-susceptible strains in both in vitro and in vivo tests. Netilmicin was also active against many aminoglycoside-resistant strains of gram-negative bacteria, particularly those known to possess adenylating enzymes (ANT 2′) or those with a similar resistance pattern. Netilmicin was found to be markedly less toxic than gentamicin in chronic studies in cats, although gentamicin appeared less toxic in acute toxicity tests in mice. The concentrations of netilmicin and gentamicin in serum were compared in dogs after intramuscular dosing, and the pharmacokinetics including peak concentrations in serum were found to be similar.

In recent years, many new semisynthetic antibiotics that have improved chemotherapeutic properties have been prepared. Semisynthetic penicillins that are active against penicillinase-producing strains of staphylococci or against gram-negative bacteria are the most common examples. Another example of this approach is amikacin, a semisynthetic aminoglycoside which is currently undergoing clinical evaluation. Amikacin is active against many aminoglycoside-resistant gram-negative strains (5); however, strains resistant to it have been reported (5, 8, 10), and the investigation of other semisynthetic aminoglycosides would seem worthwhile. Recently, it was reported from our laboratories (14) that the 1-*N*-alkylation of certain aminoglycosides leads to a group of semisynthetic aminoglycosides which possess activity against many aminoglycoside-resistant bacteria. These compounds appear to have a unique spectrum against aminoglycoside-resistant gram-negative strains, which is different from other clinically used aminoglycosides. This report presents the results of microbiological investigations of one of these antibiotics, netilmicin (Sch 20569), which is the 1-*N*-ethyl derivative of sisomicin. In addition to its activity against aminoglycoside-resistant strains, netilmicin has a pharmacokinetic profile which is similar to that of gentamicin and, when compared to gentamicin, appears to have greatly reduced chronic toxicity.

MATERIALS AND METHODS

Netilmicin and gentamicin were used as sulfate salts, and all results are expressed in terms of base activity, as determined by bioassay. Tobramycin, provided by Eli Lilly & Co., and amikacin, provided by Bristol Laboratories, were used as the bases. Methods used were generally similar to those reported earlier (10, 11).

In vitro activity. In vitro activity was studied using an agar dilution method on Mueller-Hinton agar. An inoculum of approximately 10^3 to 10^4 organisms was delivered onto the agar surface from an overnight culture in Mueller-Hinton broth using the inocula replicating apparatus of Steers et al. (9). The minimal inhibitory concentration (MIC) was defined as the lowest concentration at which less than six discrete colonies were visible. In vitro activity was also studied by means of conventional broth dilution tests with Mueller-Hinton broth as the medium. The inoculum used was 0.05 ml of a 1:1000 dilution of an overnight culture; the volume of medium in each tube was 3 ml. The MIC was defined as the lowest concentration that prevented visible growth. In vitro bactericidal activity was assessed in a manner similar to the broth MIC determinations. After a 48-h incubation, the tubes containing the lowest concentration of antibiotic allowing growth and the three next highest concentrations of antibiotic were streaked onto the surface of Mueller-Hinton agar. After a 24-h incubation, the minimum bactericidal concentration (MBC) was read as the lowest concentration preventing visible growth on the plates.

In vivo tests. Mouse protection tests and acute toxicity tests were performed with groups of seven male CF1 mice weighing approximately 20 g each. In the protection tests, mice were dosed once subcutaneously 1 h after intraperitoneal infection with approximately 10^7 organisms/mouse. Usually, five to seven dose levels were used in each test, and mean protective dose (PD_{50}) values were calculated by probit procedures. Comparative studies were always carried out simultaneously using the same inoculum (10). Cats used in the ataxia tests were mongrel males weighing between 2.5 and 4 kg each. The antibiotics were administered subcutaneously. Ataxia studies were similar to those described earlier (12, 13). Dogs were male beagle-type mongrels weighing approximately 10 kg each. Antibiotics were administered intramuscularly.

RESULTS

The results of agar dilution tests are shown comparing netilmicin with gentamicin in Fig. 1 and with gentamicin, tobramycin, and amikacin in Tables 1 and 2. Netilmicin was found to have the same potency as gentamicin against aminoglycoside-sensitive strains of gram-negative bacteria other than *Pseudomonas*. It is approximately one to two dilutions less active than gentamicin against aminoglycoside-sensitive strains of *Pseudomonas* (Table 1). Netilmicin is active against aminoglycoside-resistant strains (Table 2) that possess the following aminoglycoside-inactivating enzymes: (i) either type of aminoglycoside-phosphorylating enzyme APH (3′)-I or APH (3′)-II and (ii) aminoglycoside-adenylating enzymes, ANT (2″). It is also active against many but not all strains that possess the acetylating enzymes AAC (3)-I and AAC (3)-III. In particular, it was found to

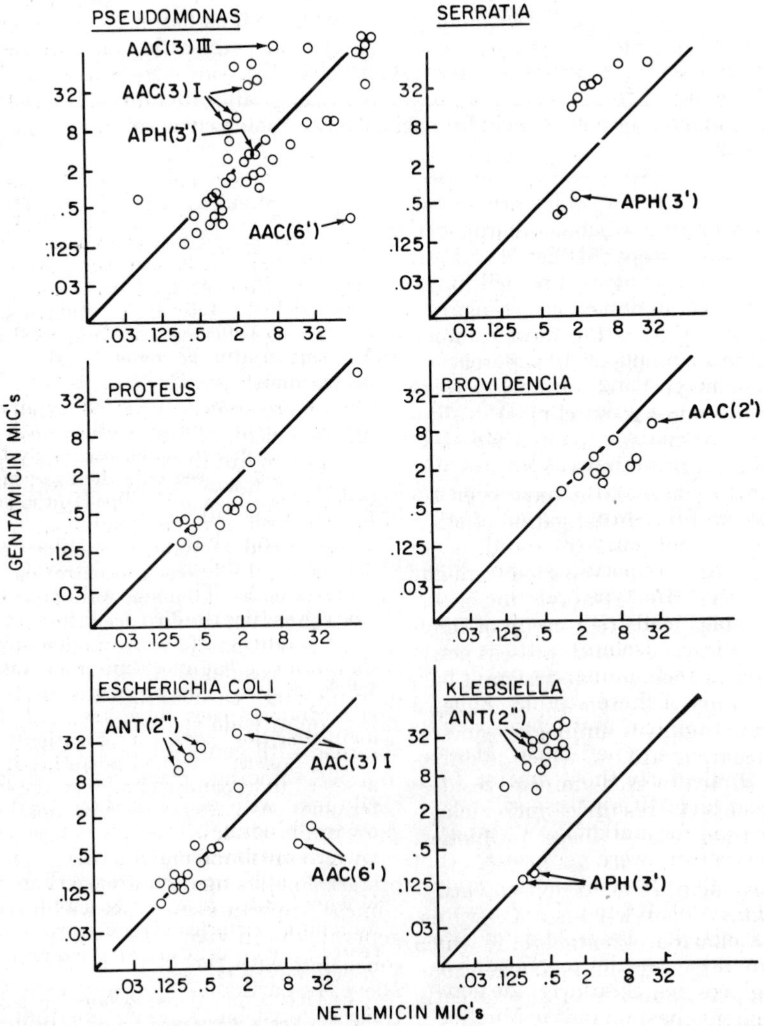

FIG. 1. *In vitro activity of netilmicin compared to gentamicin. MICs (μg/ml, 24 h, Mueller-Hinton agar) of gentamicin versus those of netilmicin.*

TABLE 1. *In vitro activity against susceptible strains*

Organism	No. of strains[a]	Median MIC (μg/ml)			
		Netilmicin	Gentamicin	Tobramycin	Amikacin
Staphylococcus aureus	13	0.125 (0.015–0.25)[b]	0.125 (0.03–0.25)	0.125 (0.03–0.25)	0.5 (0.125–2)
Streptococcus	4	8 (4–8)	16 (4–16)	16 (16)	128 (64–128)
Enterobacter	6	0.25 (0.25–4)	0.25 (0.25–1)	0.5 (0.25–2)	1 (1–4)
Escherichia coli	11	0.25 (0.015–1)	0.25 (0.015–1)	0.25 (0.015–0.5)	1 (0.015–2)
Providencia	8	4 (2–16)	2 (2–8)	2 (1–4)	0.5 (0.25–1)
Proteus mirabilis	3	0.25 (0.25–0.5)	0.5 (0.25–0.5)	0.25 (0.25–0.5)	1 (0.5–1)
Proteus morganii	3	0.5 (0.25–1)	0.5 (0.5)	0.5 (0.5)	1 (0.125–1)
Proteus rettgeri	4	2 (2–4)	1 (1–4)	1 (1–4)	1 (0.5–1)
Proteus vulgaris	3	0.5 (0.25–4)	0.25 (0.25–1)	0.5 (0.25–2)	1 (1)
Pseudomonas aeruginosa	24	1 (0.06–8)	1 (0.25–8)	0.5 (0.06–2)	2 (0.25–8)
Serratia species	2	1	0.5	1	2

[a] MICs were determined by agar dilutions methods on Mueller-Hinton agar.
[b] Range.

be active against *Escherichia coli* which possess these enzymes but to have variable activity against *Pseudomonas* which possess these enzymes. Netilmicin is not active against strains that possess the acetylating enzyme AAC (2′), and like amikacin it is not active against strains having the acetylating enzyme AAC (6′). Thus, netilmicin has a unique spectrum of activity against resistant gram-negative strains that is different from that of both tobramycin and amikacin. Its activity against the gentamicin-tobramycin-resistant strains that produce the adenylating enzyme ANT (2″) would seem to be very important, since the appearance of strains of this type has increased recently (5). We specifically studied a large number of recent clinical isolates with as yet undefined mechanisms of aminoglycoside resistance (Fig. 2). Many of these strains, which were resistant to gentamicin and tobramycin, were found to be sensitive to netilmicin. Many of these strains, particularly those among the *Enterobacteriaceae*, had MICs with netilmicin severalfold lower than for amikacin. A variety of additional in vitro tests were performed.

Studies in which the pH of Mueller-Hinton broth was varied from pH 6.6 to pH 8.2 showed that netilmicin's activity is greater at the higher pH in a manner parallel to gentamicin and other aminoglycosides. Similarly, the addition of calcium and magnesium ions to Mueller-Hinton broth decreases the activity of netilmicin against *Pseudomonas* but not against other gram-negative strains in a manner similar to gentamicin, sisomicin, tobramycin, and amikacin. The results of a study comparing the broth and agar dilution MICs with the bactericidal levels (minimum bactericidal concentrations) of netilmicin, gentamicin, tobramycin, and amikacin are shown in Fig. 3. Generally, minimum bactericidal concentrations were equal to or one to two dilutions higher than MICs. The addition of horse serum to Mueller-Hinton broth caused small changes in netilmicin activity, indicating that protein binding is not a large factor in determining the activity of this aminoglycoside. There is considerable uncertainty regarding the choice of the proper experimental conditions for studying serum binding of aminoglycosides (7; D. R. Myers, W. M. Bennett, and G. D. Olsen, Clin. Res. 24:133A, 1976), and a wide variety of results have been obtained with gentamicin (1, 2) ranging from 0 to >50% binding. Details of such tests with netilmicin will be published elsewhere and show low binding comparable to gentamicin.

In vivo antibacterial activity. The results of protection tests against a variety of bacteria of clinical importance are shown in Table 3. In general, the in vivo activity of netilmicin was consistent with the in vitro activity described above. In particular, netilmicin shows good activity against bacterial strains that are resistant to gentamicin and tobramycin and possess

TABLE 2. *In vitro activity against aminoglycoside-resistant strains*[a]

Strain	Mechanism[b]	Median MIC (μg/ml)			
		Netilmicin	Gentamicin	Tobramycin	Amikacin
Escherichia coli					
St. Michael 589	APH (3′)-I	1	1	1	2
Baker 2	APH (3′)-I	0.5	1	1	2
W677/R55	ANT (2″)	0.5	32	32	1
JR66	ANT (2″), APH (3′)	0.5	32	32	2
LA290/R55	ANT (2″)	0.25	16	16	0.5
JR88	AAC (3)-I	4	128	1	4
JR90	AAC (3)-I	2	64	1	4
R5/W677	AAC (6′)	32	1	32	32
HL97/W677	AAC (6′)	16	0.5	16	16
Swidinsky 4195	Unknown	2	8	32	8
Klebsiella					
18 strains	ANT (2″)[c]	0.5 (0.25–1)[d]	32 (8–64)	32 (8–128)	1 (0.5–4)
AD17	APH (3′)-II	0.25	0.25	0.5	1
AD18	APH (3′)-II	0.25	0.25	0.25	1
Georgetown 3694	ANT (2″)	0.5	16	16	1
Georgetown 3020	ANT (2″)	0.125	8	4	0.5
Providencia					
164	AAC (2′)	32	16	8	4
Proteus rettgeri					
Anderson	AAC (3)-II[c]	128	128	32	1
Pseudomonas aeruginosa					
D-2	APH (3′)	4	4	1	4
Stone 130	AAC (3)-I	2	16	0.25	2
Stone 138	AAC (3)-I	4	64	0.25	2
Capetown 18	AAC (3)-I	2	16	0.25	2
71PD	AAC (3)-I[c]	4	64	0.5	2
630PD	AAC (3)-I[c]	4	128	0.5	4
G 64PD	AAC (3)-I[c]	8	>128	0.5	4
Travers 1	AAC (3)-III	2	128	128	2
4184	Unknown	32	>128	32	2
Delaware (3 strains)	Unknown	>128	>128	64	4
Delaware 5	Unknown	>128	64	32	4
Delaware 7	Unknown	16	8	2	32
Delaware 8	Unknown	64	16	8	2
Delaware 9	Unknown	>128	>128	64	8
Shriners 10099	Unknown	64	16	2	32
Shriners 10006	Unknown	32	16	2	32
GN315	AAC (6′)-I	128	0.5	16	16
Shreveport 3796	Unknown	>128	>128	64	4
Serratia species					
Dalton	APH (3′)-I	2	1	2	2
1484	Unknown	32	128	16	2
6 strains	ANT (2″)[c]	4 (2–8)	64 (32–128)	32 (32–128)	4 (4–8)

[a] MICs were determined by agar dilution techniques on Mueller-Hinton agar.
[b] The resistance pattern has been determined by enzymatic inactivation studies.
[c] The resistance pattern has been determined by an aminoglycoside sensitivity pattern (5).
[d] Numbers in parentheses represent the range.

the adenylating enzyme ANT (2″). The activity of netilmicin against strains of *Pseudomonas aeruginosa* possessing acetylating enzymes or a pattern of antibiotic susceptibilities similar to strains possessing acetylating enzymes is variable and may be related to the virulence of the strain.

Acute toxicity in mice. The acute toxicity of

netilmicin was equal to that of sisomicin and approximately twice that of gentamicin (Table 4) when they were given intravenously. When given intraperitoneally or subcutaneously, the acute toxicity was approximately three to four times that of gentamicin. These latter values suggest that the absorption of netilmicin from the injection site may be somewhat more rapid than that of gentamicin. Observation of the animals at the time of death suggests that the mechanism of the acute toxicity is a neuromuscular blockade similar to that of other aminoglycosides. Detailed pharmacological studies with netilmicin will be published separately.

Ataxia studies in cats. Netilmicin was compared to gentamicin with respect to causing ataxia in cats after daily subcutaneous administration of a large dose (40 mg/kg) of either drug. This dose level produces peak serum levels in the range of 80 to 100 μg/ml. Cats were dosed 7 days a week with the antibiotics dissolved in water and contained in a volume of 0.5 ml/kg. Each day, the cats were observed for impairment of righting reflex and the appearance of ataxia. The results of these tests are shown in Table 5, in terms of the number of days for each cat to become ataxic. Earlier data for gentamicin are included. It is apparent from these data that netilmicin is substantially less toxic than gentamicin. Gentamicin, as has been reported for sisomicin (12), produced diminution of righting reflexes in 10 to 15 days, with ataxia appearing several days later. Animals were sacrificed in a moribund condition on the days shown. In this same study netilmicin was given daily for a period of 3 months, and no

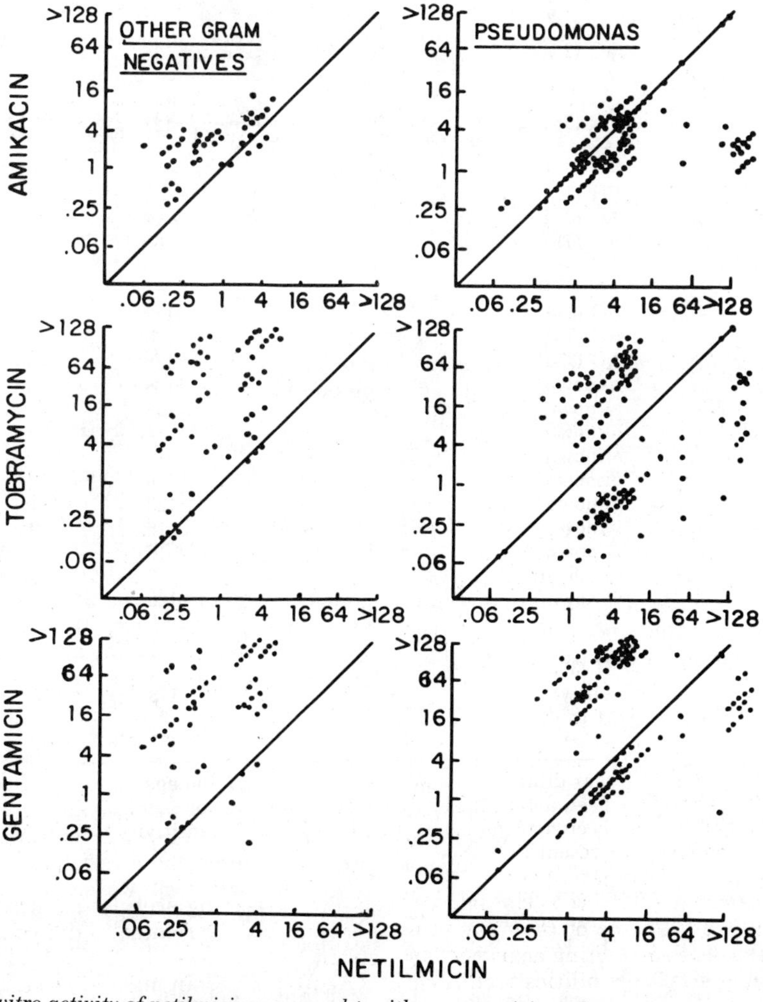

FIG. 2. *In vitro activity of netilmicin compared to either gentamicin, tobramycin, or amikacin. MICs (μg/ml, 24 h, Mueller-Hinton agar) of either gentamicin, tobramycin, or amikacin versus those of netilmicin.*

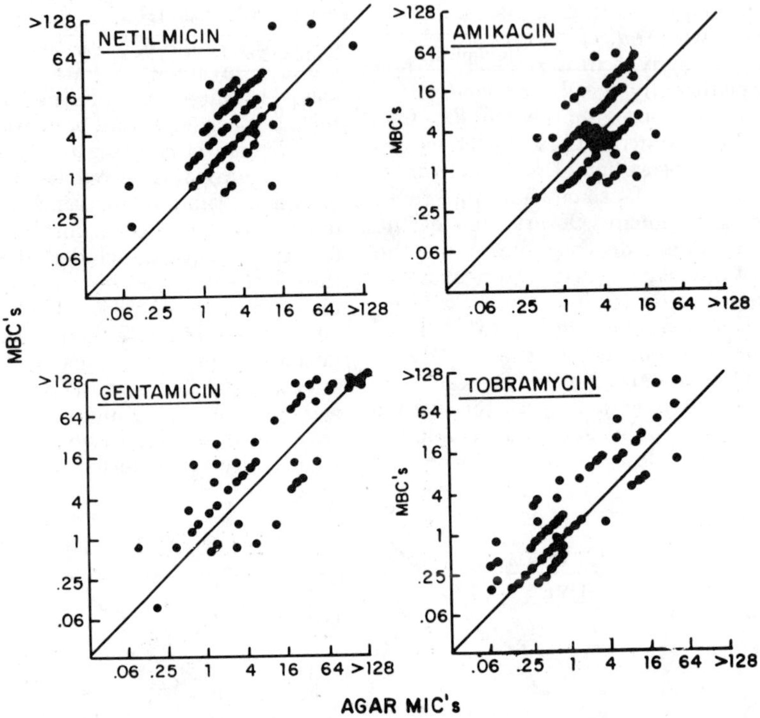

FIG. 3. *Relationship of minimum bactericidal concentrations (MBCs) to agar MICs for netilmicin, gentamicin, tobramycin, and amikacin. MBCs (μg/ml, Mueller-Hinton broth and agar) versus MICs (μg/ml, 24 h, Mueller-Hinton agar).*

impairment of righting reflexes was seen nor was any ataxia observed in the five cats dosed. One cat died on day 89 of treatment from unknown causes, while the other four cats were sacrificed after the 92nd dose in apparently normal condition. At this time, animals were killed, and tissues were submitted for histopathological examination. Mild renal tubular cell changes were noted in these cats; however, renal tubular necrosis was not seen in any animal. It appears from this study that netilmicin is markedly less toxic in cats than is gentamicin. Other studies on rats and dogs to be described elsewhere confirm the markedly reduced chronic toxicity of netilmicin.

Absorption in dogs. The concentrations of netilmicin in the serum of dogs were, in general, similar to those seen with gentamicin or sisomicin when comparable doses were administered (12). Serum levels obtained in a study of male beagle dogs in which netilmicin was compared to gentamicin in a crossover design are shown in Table 6. It can be seen that peak serum levels and serum half-lives are similar for both compounds. Detailed pharmacokinetic studies of netilmicin in mice, rats, and dogs will be published separately.

DISCUSSION

Netilmicin is a new semisynthetic aminoglycoside that appears to have a different spectrum of activity in vitro against resistant gram-negative strains than either gentamicin, tobramycin, or amikacin. Netilmicin was similar in potency to gentamicin against sensitive strains of the family *Enterobacteriaceae* and was active against all the tested clinical isolates of *Enterobacteriaceae* that were resistant to gentamicin and tobramycin. Against these isolates, netilmicin was substantially more potent than amikacin. Against sensitive strains of *P. aeruginosa,* netilmicin was about twofold less active than gentamicin but was active against many of the gentamicin- or tobramycin-resistant strains. Against these resistant *P. aeruginosa* organisms netilmicin was equipotent with amikacin. Many of the gentamicin-resistant strains of *P. aeruginosa* that apparently possess various AAC (3) acetylating enzymes are resistant to netilmicin. All of these isolates ap-

TABLE 3. *In vivo antibacterial activity in mice*

Infecting organism	PD_{50} (mg/kg)			
	Netilmicin	Gentamicin	Tobramycin	Amikacin
Staphylococcus aureus				
Grey	4.0	20.0	15.0	45.0
306	0.5	0.3	3.0	0.4
Enterobacter				
Casey	1.0	3.0	5.0	10.0
Escherichia coli				
St. Michael 589	<0.25	<0.25	<0.25	1.0
F14 Bk	<0.25	0.25	<0.25	1.0
ATCC 10536	<0.25	0.25	0.5	1.0
Klebsiella species				
Georgetown 3020	0.3	>50.0	15.0	<0.25
Oklahoma 6	<0.5	>50.0	>50.0	2.0
Rahal 1	<0.25	40.0	30.0	1.0
Rahal 3	4.0	>50.0	60.0	15.0
Rahal 5	1.0	40.0	>50.0	<0.5
Rahal 13	<0.5	25.0	50.0	<0.5
Rahal 14	<0.5	50.0	>50.0	3.0
Rahal 18	<0.5	50.0	>50.0	2.0
Rahal Nixon	<0.5	1.5	4.0	20.0
Rahal Fortenza 1	1.0	1.5	<0.5	1.0
Rahal Fortenza 2	2.5	3.0	20.0	20.0
Proteus mirabilis				
Allen	0.4	0.5	15.0	5.0
Pseudomonas aeruginosa				
Travers 1	<0.5	≥50.0	5.0	2.0
Stone 130	0.25	4.0	2.5	25.0
Stone 138	0.25	35.0	1.0	15.0
Capetown 18	<0.5	≥50.0	1.5	10.0
Shriners 10999	>50.0	>50.0	>50.0	>50.0
Delaware 1	40.0	>50.0	>50.0	>50.0
Delaware 9	>50.0	25.0	>50.0	>50.0
G 64PD	40.0	>50.0	2.5	5.0
4148 PD	50.0	>50.0	15.0	2.0
630 PD	>50.0	>50.0	25.0	>50.0
Cohen				
Ming	>50.0	>50.0	>50.0	>50.0
Rube	>50.0	>50.0	35.0	>50.0
Davi	60.0	>50.0	50.0	15.0
Van T.	>50.0	>50.0	40.0	>50.0
Simo	2.5	30.0	4.0	5.0
Robi C.	2.5	25.0	40.0	35.0
Harr C.	20.0	15.0	10.0	20.0
Hous	2.0	3.0	<0.5	15.0
Hine	1.0	1.0	1.0	4.0
Pittsburgh				
10	>50.0	40.0	50.0	>50.0
16	35.0	40.0	3.0	40.0
4	40.0	20.0	3.0	>50.0
13	30.0	15.0	20.0	>50.0
Rahal				
Bro	>50.0	>50.0	40.0	>50.0
Oxe	>50.0	60.0	20.0	>50.0
Loe	50.0	35.0	20.0	40.0
324	<0.5	2.0	2.5	<0.5
Let	<0.25	1.5	0.25	2.0

TABLE 3. *Continued*

Infecting organism	PD_{50} (mg/kg)			
	Netilmicin	Gentamicin	Tobramycin	Amikacin
Pseudomonas aeruginosa—Cont.				
Washington				
Nas	>50.0	>50.0	35.0	>50.0
Glott	>50.0	40.0	20.0	50.0
Stern	>50.0	35.0	10.0	>50.0
Walker	50.0	35.0	10.0	50.0
Tab	25.0	15.0	10.0	35.0
Blise	2.0	4.0	3.0	30.0
Artem	4.0	4.0	10.0	4.0
Mot	15.0	2.0	3.0	35.0
Watanakunakorn				
P200	>50.0	20.0	35.0	4.0
P81	20.0	15.0	2.0	20.0
P192	60.0	15.0	>50.0	40.0
P183	40.0	15.0	15.0	50.0
Serratia species				
4	30.0	10.0	>50.0	35.0
5	4.0	5.0	25.0	15.0
Univ. of Texas 153	3.0	>50.0	>50.0	>50.0
Univ. of Texas 168	0.3	50.0	>50.0	50.0

TABLE 4. *Acute toxicity in mice*

Route of administration	LD_{50} (mg/kg)[a]		
	Netilmicin	Gentamicin[b]	Sisomicin[c]
Intravenous	40	75	34
Intraperitoneal	125	430	221
Subcutaneous	175	485	288

[a] LD_{50}, Mean lethal dose.
[b] Data from reference 9.
[c] Data from reference 12.

pear to be sensitive to amikacin, whereas those with the type I enzyme (AAC (3)-I) also appear sensitive to tobramycin. The observed in vivo activity of netilmicin appears to be consistent with its in vitro spectrum and potency.

Although the acute toxicity of netilmicin is greater than that of gentamicin, its chronic toxicity in cats and other species is substantially less than that of gentamicin. The calculation of therapeutic indices from antibiotic sensitivity data and animal toxicity test results is

TABLE 5. *Chronic toxicity of netilmicin and gentamicin in cats*

Antibiotic	Cat no.	Daily dose (mg/kg)	Day of impaired reflexes	Day ataxic	Day of death
Netilmicin	8814	40	>92	>92	>92[a]
	8815	40	>92	>92	>92[a]
	8589	40	>89	>89	89
	8763	40	>92	>92	>92[a]
	8630	40	>92	>92	>92[a]
Gentamicin	8643	40	9	–	10[b]
	8811	40	13	–	13[b]
	8793	40	15	18	18[b]
	8764	40	15	18	18[b]
	8694	40	11	–	12
Earlier gentamicin results[c]	5[d]	20	31.2	31.4	>63
	21[d]	40	17.2	17.5	24
	8[d]	60	12.9	12.8	17.6

[a] On day 92 the study was terminated, and the remaining cats were sacrificed in an apparently normal condition.
[b] The cats were in a moribund condition and sacrificed on the day indicated.
[c] One of the cats receiving a daily dose of 40 mg/kg lived for 70 days (reference 11).
[d] Number of cats used in study.

TABLE 6. *Serum levels in dogs after a single intramuscular dose (10 mg/kg)*

Compound[a]	Avg serum levels (μg/ml) at time (h) after dosing											Pharmacokinetic constants[b]			
	0.166	0.333	0.5	1	2	3	4	5	6	7	8	K_a (min^{-1})	K_{el} (min^{-1})	$t_{1/2}$ (nin)	AUC (μg/min per ml)
Netilmicin	16.1 (3.9)[c]	21.6 (4.1)	23.4 (4.3)	19.2 (2.7)	10.5 (1.1)	7.2 (0.6)	3.3 (1.8)	2.4 (1.3)	1.2 (0.4)	0.8 (0.3)	0.5 (0.23)	0.95	0.0090	77	3300
Gentamicin	14.9 (2.5)	22.3 (4.0)	28.2 (2.0)	20.2 (2.9)	13.7 (6.8)	6.3 (0.8)	3.3 (1.5)	2.4 (0.4)	1.4 (0.4)	0.9 (0.4)	1.0 (0.5)	0.92	0.0096	72	3500

[a] Serum levels of netilmicin were evaluated during week 1 and those of gentamicin were determined in the same dogs during week 2.

[b] The data were fitted to a single-compartment open model by a regression analysis technique to obtain the absorption rate constant (K_a) and the serum elimination rate constant (K_{el}) as well as the serum half-lives ($t_{1/2}$) and the area under the curve (AUC) values.

[c] The values in parentheses are the observed standard deviations obtained with the three dogs.

difficult, but on the basis of its similarity in potency to gentamicin and its reduced chronic toxicity, it seems clear that netilmicin has a potentially greater therapeutic index than gentamicin. Serum levels in dogs, as well as in other species (unreported data), indicate that netilmicin is well absorbed and tolerated after parenteral administration. The pharmacokinetics of netilmicin are similar to those seen with gentamicin. Compared to gentamicin, netilmicin appears to possess the combination of an improved therapeutic index, a broader spectrum of activity against resistant strains, as well as similar pharmacokinetics. Netilmicin appears to have sufficient advantages and promise for clinical usefulness. Since this report was prepared, two in vitro studies with netilmicin have been published (3, 6). These studies are in agreement with the in vitro results reported here.

ACKNOWLEDGMENTS

The studies reported here were performed by E. L. Moss, Jr., F. Menzel, and F. Sabatelli.

We thank S. Cohen, J. J. Rahal, Jr., J. Washington, and C. Watanakunakorn for providing some of the strains used in our studies.

LITERATURE CITED

1. **Black, J., B. Calesnick, D. Williams, and M. J. Weinstein.** 1964. Pharmacology of gentamicin, a new broad-spectrum antibiotic, p. 138–146. Antimicrob. Agents Chemother. 1963.
2. **Gordon, R. C., C. Regamey, and W. M. M. Kirby.** 1972. Serum protein binding of aminoglycoside antibiotics. Antimicrob. Agents Chemother. 2:214–216.
3. **Kabins, S. A., C. Nathans, and S. Cohen.** 1976. In vitro comparison of netilmicin, a semisynthetic derivative of sisomicin, and four other aminoglycoside antibiotics. Antimicrob. Agents Chemother. **10**:139–145.
4. **Noriega, E. R., R. E. Leibowitz, A. S. Richmond, E. Rubinstein, S. Schaeffer, M. S. Simberkoff, and J. J. Rahal, Jr.** 1975. Nosocomial infection caused by gentamicin-resistant, streptomycin-sensitive *Klebsiella*. J. Infect. Dis. **131**:S45–S50.
5. **Price, K. E., T. A. Pursiano, M. D. DeFuria, and G. E. Wright.** 1974. Activity of BBK-8 (amikacin) against clinical isolates resistant to one or more aminoglycoside antibiotics. Antimicrob. Agents Chemother. **5**:143–152.
6. **Rahal, J. J., Jr., M. S. Simberkoff, K. Kagan, and N. H. Moldover.** 1976. Bactericidal efficacy of Sch 20569 and amikacin against gentamicin-sensitive and -resistant organisms. Antimicrob. Agents Chemother. **9**:595–599.
7. **Ramirez-Ronda, C. H., R. K. Holmes, and J. P. Sanford.** 1975. Effects of divalent cations on binding of aminoglycoside antibiotics to human serum proteins and to bacteria. Antimicrob. Agents Chemother. **7**:239–245.
8. **Shimada, K., T. Inamatsu, M. Kanno, K. Ubukata, A. Kobayashi, S. Kubo, A. Saito, Y. Ueda, K. Shimizu, and K. Okuzumi.** 1975. Bacteria resistant to gentamicin. Chemotherapy (Tokyo) 23:2599–2604.
9. **Steers, E., E. L. Foltz, and B. S. Graves.** 1959. An inocula replicating apparatus for routine testing of bacterial susceptibility to antibiotics. Antibiot.

Chemother. 9:307–311.
10. **Waitz, J. A.** 1975. Laboratory evaluation of aminoglycoside antibiotics. Dev. Ind. Microbiol. **16**:161–174.
11. **Waitz, J. A., E. L. Moss, Jr., E. M. Oden, G. H. Wagman, and M. J. Weinstein.** 1972. Biological activity of Sch 14342, an aminoglycoside coproduced in the gentamicin fermentation. Antimicrob. Agents Chemother. **2**:464–469.
12. **Waitz, J. A., E. L. Moss, Jr., E. M. Oden, and M. J. Weinstein.** 1970. Biological studies with Antibiotic 6640, a new broad spectrum aminoglycoside antibiotic. J. Antibiot. **23**:559–565.
13. **Waitz, J. A., E. L. Moss, Jr., and M. J. Weinstein.** 1971. Aspects of the chronic toxicity of gentamicin sulfate in cats. J. Infect. Dis. **124**:S125–S129.
14. **Wright, J. J.** 1975. Synthesis of 1-N-ethyl-sisomicin: a broad-spectrum semi-synthetic aminoglycoside antibiotic. J. Chem. Soc. Chem. Commun. **6**:206–208.

ANTIMICROBIAL AGENTS AND CHEMOTHERAPY, Nov. 1976, p. 837-844
Vol. 10, No. 5

Ticarcillin in Combination with Cephalothin or Gentamicin as Empiric Antibiotic Therapy in Granulocytopenic Cancer Patients

STEPHEN C. SCHIMPFF,* SHELDON LANDESMAN, DAVIS M. HAHN, HAROLD C. STANDIFORD, CLARENCE L. FORTNER, VIOLA MAE YOUNG, AND PETER H. WIERNIK

Baltimore Cancer Research Center, National Cancer Institute at the University of Maryland Hospital, Baltimore, Maryland 21201, and Department of Medicine, Baltimore Veterans Administration Hospital, Baltimore, Maryland 21218*

Received for publication 1 June 1976

Ticarcillin was used in combination with either cephalothin or gentamicin as initial empiric antibiotic therapy for 127 patient trials of suspected infection in granulocytopenic cancer patients. Bacteremia was present in 20%, nonbacteremic microbiologically documented infections in 21%, clinically documented infections in 23%, and possible infections in 5%; infection was doubtful in 31%. Although *Staphylococcus aureus* was the most common single organism isolated (23%), gram-negative bacilli accounted for 54% of all pathogens. Both antibiotic regimens were highly efficacious, with complete resolution in 46% of bacteremias, 88% of nonbacteremic microbiologically documented infections, and 95% of clinically documented infections. Among bacteremias, 8 of 9 caused by *S. aureus* but only 4 of 15 (27%) caused by gram-negative bacilli were completely resolved with these antibiotic combinations. Reasons for nonresponse in bacteremias were persistent granulocytopenia, mixed infection and, in two patients, antibiotic-resistant organisms. Toxicities other than hypokalemia were minimal. Although the rate of further infections was high overall (18/127), only one occurred among the 39 patients with <4 days of antibiotic therapy. Ticarcillin in combination with either cephalothin or gentamicin was effective as initial empiric therapy of suspected infection in granulocytopenic cancer patients.

Despite advances in preventive technique (23), serious infections continue to occur in granulocytopenic cancer patients (6, 13). Prompt empiric use of broad-spectrum bactericidal antibiotics in recent years has substantially reduced the morbidity and mortality of infection in this patient population (5–7, 10, 13–17, 24–26, 29; W. H. Greene, S. C. Schimpff, V. M. Young, and P. H. Wiernik, Ann. Intern. Med. 78:825–826, 1973). Various combinations of carbenicillin, gentamicin, and cephalothin have been utilized with encouraging results, especially for *Pseudomonas aeruginosa* (5–7, 10, 13–15, 17, 24–26, 29; Greene et al., Ann. Intern. Med. 78:825–826). A new semisynthetic penicillin, ticarcillin (α-carboxyl-3-thienylmethyl penicillin), has been introduced for investigational use (1). Ticarcillin is quite similar to carbenicillin in structure and activity; it is more active than carbenicillin on a milligram-per-milligram basis against most strains of *P. aeruginosa* (15, 18, 20, 28). Like carbenicillin, ticarcillin demonstrates in vitro synergy against most strains of *P. aeruginosa* combined with gentamicin (28). Because of the increased in vitro efficacy of ticarcillin as compared with carbenicillin against *P. aeruginosa*, ticarcillin can be given in approximately one-half the dosage of carbenicillin, thereby lessening the possibility of dose-related side effects (circulatory congestion, hypokalemia, and coagulation dysfunction). Like carbenicillin, however, ticarcillin has little activity against *Klebsiella* spp. and is inactivated by the beta-lactamase of penicillin-resistant strains of *Staphylococcus aureus*.

The increased in vitro activity of ticarcillin against *P. aeruginosa* combined with its potential for less toxicity suggested its use as part of an empiric antibiotic approach for suspected infection in febrile granulocytopenic cancer patients. Ticarcillin was therefore studied in combination with either cephalothin or gentamicin because these two combinations will cover most bacterial infections that occur in this patient population (12, 22). The 127 patient trials reported here represent the largest single institution series utilizing ticarcillin for neutropenic patients with suspected infections.

MATERIALS AND METHODS

The patients were hospitalized at the Baltimore Cancer Research Center (BCRC) and were part of a prospective, randomized evaluation of the International Antimicrobial Therapy Project Group under the sponsorship of the European Organization for Research on Treatment of Cancer; the complete protocol and initial Group results have been published (11, 12).

Patients were eligible for the present study if their absolute granulocyte count was $<1,000/\mu l$ and they had an oral temperature of 38.3°C (101°F) or greater in the absence of an obvious noninfective cause of fever (e.g., blood products or cytotoxic drugs).

Before beginning antibiotic therapy, all patients at the BCRC had, at a minimum, the following evaluation (12): (i) complete history and physical examination emphasizing subtle findings of inflammation (22); (ii) chest radiograph; (iii) two separate blood cultures; (iv) cultures of clinically relevant sites; (v) urinalysis (usually performed by the attending physician); (vi) surveillance cultures (nose, gingiva, axilla, and perianum) (24); and (vii) serum electrolytes, blood urea nitrogen, creatinine, glucose, and a complete blood count including differential. In cases of pneumonia, recognized at fever onset, where sputum samples are of minimal value in these granulocytopenic patients, transtracheal aspiration was performed (depending on bleeding parameters), and if this was unrewarding, the patient underwent transtracheal selective bronchial brushing (2).

Patients were then randomized to receive one of the following two-drug regimens: ticarcillin-cephalothin, ticarcillin-gentamicin, or cephalothin-gentamicin. As this paper relates to the use of ticarcillin, only those 127 patient trials at the BCRC in which ticarcillin was utilized are reported here. The complete 19-institution Group study will be reported separately.

Each antibiotic was dissolved in 50 ml of 5% dextrose and water and infused separately over approximately 10 to 20 min for each antibiotic. The dosages were: ticarcillin (kindly supplied by Robert L. Vann, Beecham Laboratories, Bristol, Tenn.), 12 g/m^2 per day (average, 5 g every 6 h); cephalothin, 7 g/m^2 per day (average, 3 g every 6 h); and gentamicin, 180 mg/m^2 per day (average, 80 mg every 6 h or 4.5 mg/kg per day). Antibiotic dosage was adjusted accordingly for renal dysfunction.

Follow-up laboratory evaluations included complete blood count and platelet count four to five times per week. Electrolytes, blood urea nitrogen, creatinine, and SMA-12 were usually performed two to three times per week.

Based on the clinical course and microbiological data, each febrile episode was classified as to whether the infection was: (i) microbiologically documented, (ii) clinically documented, (iii) possible, or (iv) doubtful. The definitions used were substantially the same as those used at this institution since 1969 (25). Antibiotic response was defined as: (i) improvement (a return of temperature to normal or to the preinfectious state with complete disappearance of all signs and symptoms of infection); (ii) temporary improvement (a return of temperature to normal and resolution of signs and symptoms of infection lasting at least 5 days but followed by a relapse of the same infection either while the patient was still receiving antibiotics or within 1 week after antibiotic discontinuation); (iii) failure (no or poor response to antibiotic therapy); a change of antibiotics or the addition of granulocyte transfusions (21) resulted in the trial being classified as an antibiotic failure regardless of the patient's ultimate clinical course (such changes were made in consultation with the investigators); or (iv) nonevaluable (improvement or no change without any specific relationship to antibiotics). Most patients in this category had febrile episodes that were classified as doubtful. When a patient had a documented viral or fungal infection, the infection was classified as microbiologically documented but nonevaluable in terms of response to the antibiotic regimens (12, 25).

Antibiotic alteration and changes. The patients with microbiologically documented *P. aeruginosa*, *Klebsiella* spp., *Enterobacter* spp., or *Escherichia coli* infections were given only the original combination unless the trial was deemed a failure. Nonactive antibiotics were discontinued from the combination once antibiotic susceptibility testing was completed (e.g., cephalothin would be discontinued in a *P. aeruginosa* infection) (12). The physician was allowed to substitute methicillin once culture results indicated *S. aureus*. The infection was considered improved based on the above definitions, provided a response was obvious by the time methicillin was substituted.

If, at the end of 96 h, the patient remained febrile without significant change in the fever pattern, without a site of infection by complete reevaluation, and without positive findings from cultures, then both antibiotics were discontinued and the patient was recultured and observed closely (12).

Antibiotic susceptibility testing and antibiotic serum levels. Antibiotic susceptibility testing of all isolates was performed by the method of Bauer et al. (3) as recommended by the Food and Drug Administration (9). Ticarcillin disk-resistant gram-negative bacilli were further evaluated by a microtiter technique to determine minimal inhibitory concentrations. Serum levels of ticarcillin and gentamicin were determined for some patients at 1 and 5 h after completion of antibiotic infusion by a modified agar well diffusion method described by Bennett et al. (4). For ticarcillin, the assay organism was *P. aeruginosa* NTCC 10701, which was resistant to gentamicin and cephalothin. For the gentamicin assay, beta-lactamase was added to the serum to destroy the ticarcillin. Thereafter the aminoglycoside concentration was determined by using *Bacillus subtilis* as the assay organism.

RESULTS

Patient characteristics. There were 62 patient trials with ticarcillin-cephalothin and 65 with ticarcillin-gentamicin (Table 1). Both groups were equivalent with regard to age, sex ratio, tumor type (>75% of patients had acute leukemia), and numbers of patients receiving oral nonabsorbable antibiotics or treated in reverse isolation rooms for infection prophylaxis.

Classification, site, and etiology of infection. Of the 127 patient trials, there were 26 (20%) bacteremias, 27 (21%) nonbacteremic microbiologically documented infections, 29 (23%) clinically documented infections, 6 (5%) possible infections, and 39 (31%) episodes where infection was doubtful.

The most common sites of infection were skin and soft tissue (20), oral lesions (18), perianal lesions (12), urinary tract (8), colon (8), lower respiratory tract (7), and nose and sinuses (5).

The organisms that caused most infections were *S. aureus* (15), *Klebsiella* spp. (12), *P. aeruginosa* (10), *E. coli* (9), *Candida* spp. (6), *Serratia marcescens* (6), group D *Streptococcus* sp. (3), and *Proteus mirabilis* (2).

Response to therapy. Responses are tabulated in Table 2. The 39 doubtful infections, 12 infections caused in whole or part by fungi or viruses, and 8 nonevaluable patient trials (five patients for whom antibiotics were added or changed against protocol, one afebrile patient, two invalid randomizations) were excluded from analysis of response but were analyzed for side effects. The response rate (Table 2; only improvement [complete resolution] is tabulated) was essentially the same for the two antibiotic regimens (ticarcillin-cephalothin and ticarcillin-gentamicin). Overall, 46% of the bacteremias, 88% of the nonbacteremic microbiologically documented infections, and 95% of the clinically documented infections improved. By definition, the six patients with possible infection improved.

S. aureus (Table 2) was the most common organism isolated and caused most of the bac-

TABLE 1. *Patient population*

Determination	Ticarcillin + cephalothin	Ticarcillin + gentamicin	Total
Patient trials	62	65	127
Mean age (yr)	40	41	41
Male/female	38/24	37/28	75/52
Tumor type			
Acute nonlymphocytic leukemia	39	35	74
Acute lymphocytic leukemia	4	8	12
Lymphoma	11	11	22
Carcinoma/sarcoma	8	10	18
Oral nonabsorbable antibiotics	37	36	73
Reverse isolation	9	4	13

TABLE 2. *Responses to antibiotic combinations*[a]

Infection or organism	Ticarcillin + cephalothin	Ticarcillin + gentamicin	Total
Classification of infection			
Bacteremia	8/14[b] (57)[c]	3/10 (30)	11/24 (46)
Microbiologically documented	4/5 (80)	10/11 (91)	14/16 (88)
Clinically documented	13/14 (93)	8/8 (100)	21/22 (95)
Possible	5/5 (100)	1/1 (100)	6/6 (100)
Total	29/37 (78)	22/30 (73)	51/67 (76)
Pathogen			
Staphylococcus aureus	8/8 (100)	5/6 (83)	13/14 (93)
Klebsiella spp.	1/2 (50)	5/8 (62)	6/10 (60)
Escherichia coli	1/4 (25)	2/3 (67)	3/7 (43)
Pseudomonas aeruginosa	3/4 (75)	1/3 (33)	4/7 (57)
Serratia marcescens	0/2 (0)	0/3 (0)	0/5 (0)
Other bacteria	1/2 (50)	4/4 (100)	5/6 (83)
Total	14/22 (64)	17/27 (63)	31/49 (63)

[a] Total pathogens exceeds total microbiologically documented infections because of multiple pathogens in some infections.

[b] Improved/total.

[c] Percentage.

TABLE 3. *Response to antibiotic regimens with bacteremia*

Organism	Ticarcillin + cephalothin	Ticarcillin + gentamicin	Total (%)
Staphylococcus aureus	6/6[a]	2/3	8/9 (89)
Klebsiella spp.	1/3	1/4	2/7 (29)
Escherichia coli	0/3	0/1	0/4 (0)
Serratia marcescens	0/2	0/3	0/5 (0)
Group D *Streptococcus* sp.	1/1		1/1
Enterobacter cloacae		1/1	1/1
Pseudomonas aeruginosa	1/1		1/1
Total (%)[b]	8/14 (57)	3/10 (30)	11/24 (46)

[a] Improved/total.
[b] Total bacteremias is less than total pathogens because of mixed bacteremias.

teremias. Thirteen of 14 (93%) of the *S. aureus* infections improved. It is noteworthy that the ticarcillin-gentamicin combination appeared about as efficacious as the cephalothin-ticarcillin combination as initial empiric antibiotic therapy for *S. aureus* infections. The response rate for gram-negative bacillary infections was considerably less than that for *S. aureus*.

Twenty-eight organisms caused 24 bacteremias (Table 3). Eight of nine (89%) *S. aureus* bacteremias improved. The one patient listed as not responding had an *S. aureus* endometritis susceptible to both ticarcillin and gentamicin; the patient improved slowly with the addition of granulocyte transfusions. The patients with gram-negative bacteremias, as a group, did poorly, with only 4 of 15 (27%) showing a complete response without the need for other antibiotics or granulocyte transfusions. Three additional patients had a definite temporary improvement but relapsed shortly thereafter; the remaining eight patients did not respond to initial therapy.

Failure to respond to initial antibiotic therapy usually depended on the type of infection and the patient's current status rather than the specific antibiotic combination. The presence of gram-negative bacteremia was a major adverse prognostic finding (27% improvement rate for gram-negative bacteremia compared with improvement in 89% for *S. aureus* bacteremias, 88% for nonbacteremic microbiologically documented infections, and 95% for clinically documented infections). Among the 12 antibiotic failures in all categories, poor prognostic indicators included gram-negative bacteremias in eight, mixed organism infections in three, and clinical shock at presentation in two. Only two patients had organisms ultimately found to be resistant to both antibiotics administered. These 12 patients each had a granulocyte count below 500/μl (median, 100/μl; range, 1 to 450); 10 of the 12 had been granulocytopenic for over 30 days, and all 12 patients had aplastic bone marrows at the onset of infection (such that peripheral granulocytes did not begin to return to normal for at least 10 days in any patient). Seven of the 12 patients had progressive neoplasia unresponsive to therapy.

Granulocyte transfusions were given to six of these patients who failed to respond adequately to initial antibiotic therapy. Two died shortly; one began to improve but died of a *Torulopsis glabrata* pneumonia with sepsis. Two patients had bacteremias caused by resistant organisms (*E. coli* and *S. marcescens*, each resistant to ticarcillin, cephalothin, and gentamicin) which improved upon the addition of granulocyte transfusions and institution of polymyxin B. Finally, one patient with progressive *S. aureus* endometritis (susceptible to the antibiotic combination that she was receiving) slowly improved after the addition of granulocyte transfusions.

Clinical shock was present in three patients at the time of randomization. One patient had an *S. aureus* and *P. aeruginosa* bacteremia associated with a subclavian catheter and died while receiving the first dose of antibiotics (excluded from analysis as nonevaluable). The second patient had an *E. coli* bacteremia from a perianal lesion caused by both *E. coli* and *P. aeruginosa;* he died within 3 days. A third patient with *Klebsiella pneumoniae* bacteremia from an oral lesion had a temporary improvement to initial intensive measures including empiric ticarcillin plus cephalothin, but ultimately succumbed despite addition of gentamicin and granulocyte transfusions.

Antibiotic susceptibility was not of major importance provided the bacteremia was caused by an organism(s) susceptible to at least one of the two antibiotics in the combination. Among the 15 patients with gram-negative bacteremia, only 2 were infected by an organism resistant to ticarcillin, cephalothin, and gentamicin and hence to the combination administered empirically. Both had progressive infection until switched to polymyxin B and granulocyte transfusions; with this therapy they each made full recoveries as their own peripheral granulocytes returned. Seven of the 15 had bacteremias susceptible to only one of the two drugs given; three improved, but the other four died of infection. Five patients had gram-negative bacteremias susceptible to both antibiotics administered. None improved fully, although three patients had a temporary improvement and two with progressive infection improved once granulocyte transfusions were added.

Granulocyte counts over the first few days of therapy were critical in determining responses to antibiotic therapy (Table 4). For patients with gram-negative bacteremias, the antibiotic failure rate was 78% (seven of nine) for those patients who had either no rise or a minimal rise in granulocytes during therapy of $<100/\mu l$. However, only one of six (17%) patients with an *S. aureus* bacteremia and minimal rise in granulocytes failed to respond to initial antibiotic therapy. Finally, none of 7 (0%) and one of 17 (6%) patients with nonbacteremia microbiologically documented or clinically documented infections and minimal rise failed to respond to antibiotic therapy. Thus patients with a gram-negative bacteremia and lack of a prompt rise in their peripheral granulocyte level had a very poor prognosis, whereas other patients usually responded to antibiotic therapy alone despite persistent granulocytopenia.

The 15 patients with gram-negative bacteremia, which tended to occur in the patients with the most severe and prolonged depression in their granulocyte count before infection, represented a minority of the total infections in this series. These same patients were among those in whom the granulocyte count did not rise during therapy. Review of these patients' records suggests that the lack of a granulocyte rise during infection was related to the preinfectious state of the patient (advanced acute leukemia or lymphoma refractory to therapy) and probably not the bacteremia per se. It therefore appears that antibiotic failure or response was dictated in this series as much or more by patient status than by the type of infecting organism.

TABLE 4. *Granulocyte rise and failure to respond to antibiotics*

Granulocyte rise	Bacteremia[a]		Microbiologically documented[a]	Clinically documented
	Gram-negative	*S. aureus*		
0–99	7/9[b]	1/6	0/7	1/17
100–499	1/2		1/3	0/2
500–999			0/3	0/1
>1000	1/1	0/1	0/3	0/5
Total	9/12	1/7	1/16	1/25

[a] Bacterial infections only.
[b] Antibiotic failures/evaluable patients.

Side effects. Two patients receiving ticarcillin plus cephalothin and two receiving ticarcillin plus gentamicin developed a rash that was believed related to one of the antibiotics; however, other drugs, notably allopurinol, could not be discounted as either a cause or a potentiator. Two patients receiving ticarcillin plus cephalothin but none receiving ticarcillin plus gentamicin developed a rise in serum creatinine from a normal baseline value (<1.5 mg/100 ml) to >1.5 mg/100 ml without any potential cause other than antibiotic administration. Hypokalemia (serum potassium <3.5 meq/liter) occurred in 23% of patients receiving ticarcillin plus cephalothin and 20% receiving ticarcillin plus gentamicin. Serious fluid overload, apparently related to the disodium salt of ticarcillin, occurred only once. One patient, who had preexisting renal dysfunction secondary to multiple myeloma, inadvertently received a full dosage of ticarcillin with subsequent development of a bleeding diathesis characterized by petechiae, ecchymoses, and epistaxis in association with reduced fibrinogen and prolongation of partial thromboplastin and prothrombin times. The serum level of ticarcillin 9 h after the final dose was 1,050 $\mu g/ml$; ticarcillin was discontinued and the bleeding diathesis was resolved.

Further infections. Further infections (any infection occurring during antibiotic administration or within 7 days after their discontinuation) occurred in 5 of 62 (8%) ticarcillin-plus-cephalothin trials and 13 of 65 (20%) ticarcillin-plus-gentamicin trials (Table 5). The further infections with the former regimen included two bacterial and three fungal infections with three deaths; with the latter regimen there were nine bacterial and three fungal infections with four deaths.

Seventeen of the further infections occurred in the patients with documented infections (i.e., prolonged antibiotic therapy), whereas only one of the 39 infection-doubted patients (i.e., 4 days or less of antibiotics) developed a further infection. The median days on antibiotics before a further infection was 11.5. All patients were still granulocytopenic at the onset of further infection.

Infection doubted. Thirty-nine patients (31%) of the entire group were classified as having infection doubted. In some patients the cause of fever was rapidly apparent (blood products or chemotherapy), but in many others fever persisted without change during antibiotic administration. In such patients, after com-

TABLE 5. *Further infections*

Ticarcillin + cephalothin		Ticarcillin + gentamicin	
Infection	Course[a]	Infection	Course
Staphylococcus aureus conjunctivitis	Day 4, improved	Mucositis	Day 12, improved
Pseudomonas aeruginosa perianal lesion	Day 20, died	*S. aureus* pneumonia	Day 11, improved
Aspergillus pneumonia	Day 7, improved	*Escherichia coli* cellulitis	Day 7, improved
Torulopsis glabrata pneumonia	Day 7, died	*Klebsiella pneumoniae* pharyngitis	Day 12, improved
Candida albicans pneumonia	Day 7, died	*E. coli* cellulitis	Day 30, improved
		Serratia marcescens bacteremia	Day 10, improved
		S. marcescens bacteremia	Day 15, died
		E. coli + *K. pneumoniae* bacteremia	Day 14, died
		K. pneumoniae bacteremia	Day 17, improved
		S. aureus + *S. faecalis* bacteremia	Day 8, improved
		Aspergillus pneumonia	Day 13, improved
		C. albicans pneumonia	Day 8, died
		Disseminated candidiasis	Day 18, died

[a] Day indicates day after start of antibiotics that further infection was clinically recognized. Improved, cured with appropriate therapy; died, died of this further infection.

plete reassessment (history, examination, chest radiograph, and repeat cultures), all antibiotics were discontinued at 96 h and the patient was observed. In this series, only one patient was subsequently proven to have had an infection "masked" by the antibiotic regimen, thus suggesting that it is quite safe to discontinue empiric antibiotics after 96 h provided that a thorough reevaluation fails to disclose infection. This approach can substantially reduce the risk of further infection.

Blood levels. Serum samples were obtained for antibiotic determinations (Table 6) at 1 and 5 h after completion of antibiotic infusion. In all cases, ticarcillin was the second of the two antibiotics given. Infusions frequently took more than the planned 20 min per antibiotic. The mean serum level of ticarcillin was 180 μg/ml at 1 h and 35 μg/ml at 5 h. The mean gentamicin serum level was 2.3 μg/ml at 1 h and 0.8 μg/ml at 5 h. Cephalothin was not assayed.

TABLE 6. *Antibiotic serum levels*

Serum levels	Mean	Median	Range	Samples[a]
Ticarcillin				
1 h	180	146	19–530	44
5 h	35	21	0–220	21
Gentamicin				
1 h[b]	2.3	2.1	0.9–4.8	24
5 h	0.8	0.6	0.4–2.4	10

[a] Each 1-h sample represents a separate patient; 5-h samples were taken from same patient (minus some not collected).

[b] One-hour samples for gentamicin represent approximately 1.25 to 1.5 h because gentamicin administration preceded ticarcillin administration.

DISCUSSION

Ticarcillin was utilized in these combinations because of its promise based on in vitro studies of being a suitable alternative to carbenicillin for the treatment of organisms such as *P. aeruginosa, E. coli, Enterobacter* spp., and some strains of *Proteus* spp. Multiple laboratory evaluations have shown that ticarcillin is more effective on a weight basis than carbenicillin against *P. aeruginosa* (17, 20). This allows for use of a lower dosage with potential for fewer dose-related side effects of sodium overload, hypokalemia, and coagulation abnormalities. In addition, synergism frequently occurs between ticarcillin and gentamicin when tested against *P. aeruginosa* (8). The combinations chosen in this study included ticarcillin plus gentamicin because of the activity of ticarcillin and gentamicin together against *P. aeruginosa* and because gentamicin could be expected to have broad coverage against most of the other organisms, including *S. aureus,* that might be expected to infect this patient population. The other combination, ticarcillin plus cephalothin, includes ticarcillin for its activity against *P. aeruginosa, Enterobacter* spp., and many strains of *E. coli* and *Proteus* spp. and has cephalothin for activity against *Klebsiella* spp., some strains of *E. coli,* and *S. aureus.*

Rodriguez et al. (19) used ticarcillin as a single agent for empiric therapy of similar types of patients and observed improvement in 16 of 20 infections, including some bacteremias, caused by *Pseudomonas* spp. This drug was not effective therapy, however, for organisms such as *Klebsiella* spp., which would not be expected to respond based on in vitro evaluations. Klastersky and colleagues (15) used the combinations of ticarcillin plus tobramycin and ticarcillin plus cephalothin in a program similar to the present study (although only 33% of the patients were granulocytopenic) and achieved overall improvement in 11 of 15 (73%) *P. aeruginosa* infections.

The present investigation indicates that these two antibiotic combinations, which included ticarcillin, were efficacious against susceptible strains of gram-negative bacilli provided the peripheral granulocyte count began to rise during therapy. Failure to respond to either of these antibiotic combinations was usually associated with the combination of gram-negative bacteremia and persistent granulocytopenia during antibiotic therapy. Although most failures occurred in patients with persistent granulocytopenia, either antibiotic combination usually produced a good response despite granulocytopenia if the patient did not have a gram-negative bacteremia.

There was a lower rate of gram-negative bacteremia in this series than in previous investigations of empiric antibiotic therapy at this center (25; Greene et al., Ann. Intern. Med. **78**:825–826, 1973), probably because of improved preventive techniques (24) and earlier institution of the empiric antibiotic regimen. The few patients who nevertheless developed a gram-negative bacteremia were among the patients with the most prolonged and persistent granulocytopenia and hence the worst prognosis. The paradoxical result has been a reduced incidence but an increased mortality from gram-negative bacteremia. For similar reasons, only three patients presented with bacteremic shock, but each died rapidly.

For those patients not in shock, early institution of granulocyte transfusions were often lifesaving until bone marrow function could recover (21). It would appear that granulocyte transfusions are both indicated and essential in patients with gram-negative bacteremia and hypoplastic bone marrows.

The patients with *S. aureus* infections, including those with bacteremias, fared well on both empiric antibiotic regimens. It must be noted that patients receiving ticarcillin-gentamicin were switched to methicillin alone once the culture results indicated *S. aureus* as a single infecting organism. This conversion generally occurred on days 3 to 5 of therapy, i.e., at a time when initial response to the initial therapy was apparent. This suggests that even in these high-risk patients, an aminoglycoside such as gentamicin is sufficient early coverage for *S. aureus*.

Immediate institution of empiric antibiotics is undoubtedly useful in this patient setting, but overuse may lead to further infection. The median time on antibiotics before further infection was 11.5 days. Seventeen of 18 occurred among the patients with documented infection, i.e., those patients who required prolonged antibiotic therapy. Only one of 39 patients with infection doubted (i.e., antibiotics discontinued within 96 h) developed a further infection, emphasizing the importance of limiting unnecessary prolongation of antibiotic therapy.

Side effects from either combination were relatively few in number and included hypokalemia in an equivalent percentage (20 to 23%) with either antibiotic combination. Circulatory congestion occurred once, rash thought possibly to be due to ticarcillin occurred four times, and a coagulation abnormality related to an excessively high blood level of ticarcillin in a patient with azotemia occurred once (8). These side effects were minimal and suggest that ticarcillin in either combination was relatively safe. Unfortunately, this was not a comparative study with carbenicillin, so no specific comments can be made as to relative degrees of hypokalemia or circulatory overload between ticarcillin and carbenicillin.

Ticarcillin in combination with either cephalothin or gentamicin appears to be safe and efficacious when used in a program of prompt empiric antibiotic therapy for febrile granulocytopenic cancer patients.

ACKNOWLEDGMENTS

We wish to thank Robert Good and the staff of Hazelton Laboratories, and Paula Salvatore, Norman Friedman, W. R. Robinson, and the clinical staff of the Baltimore Cancer Research Center for their assistance with this investigation. Beverly Tatem performed the antibiotic serum assays; Charles Schiffer and Joseph Aisner kindly supplied data on granulocyte transfusions and carefully reviewed the manuscript.

LITERATURE CITED

1. **Acred, P., P. A. Hunter, L. Mizen, and G. N. Rolinson.** 1971. α-Carboxyl-3-thienylmethylpenicillin (BRL 2288), a new semisynthetic penicillin: in vivo evaluation, p. 396–401. Antimicrob. Agents Chemother. 1970.
2. **Aisner, J., L. K. Kvols, E. A. Sickles, S. C. Schimpff, and P. H. Wiernik.** 1976. Transtracheal selective bronchial brushing for pulmonary infiltrates in patients with cancer. Chest **69**:367–371.
3. **Bauer, A. W., W. M. M. Kirby, J. C. Sherris, and M. Turck.** 1966. Antibiotic susceptibility testing by a standardized single disk method. Am. J. Clin. Pathol. **43**:493–496.

4. **Bennett, J. V., E. J. Brodie, and W. M. M. Kirby.** 1966. Simplified accurate method for antibiotic assay of clinical specimens. Appl. Microbiol. **14**:170–177.
5. **Bloomfield, C. D., and B. J. Kennedy.** 1974. Cephalothin, carbenicillin, and gentamicin combination therapy for febrile patients with acute nonlymphocytic leukemia. Cancer **34**:431–437.
6. **Bodey, G. P.** 1975. Infections in cancer patients. Cancer Treatment Rev. **2**:89–128.
7. **Bodey, G. P., V. Rodriguez, and J. K. Luce.** 1969. Carbenicillin therapy of gram-negative bacilli infections. Am. J. Med. Sci. **275**:408–414.
8. **Brown, C. H., III, E. A. Natelson, W. Bradshaw, C. P. Alfrey, Jr., and T. W. Williams, Jr.** 1975. Study of the effects of ticarcillin on blood coagulation and platelet function. Antimicrob. Agents Chemother. **7**:652–675.
9. **Food and Drug Administration.** 1971. Antibiotic susceptibility discs, drug efficacy study implementation. Fed. Reg. **36**:6899–6902.
10. **Gaya, H.** 1975. Antimicrobial therapy in neutropenic patients with malignant disease, p. 117–125. *In* J. Klastersky (ed.), Clinical use of combinations of antibiotics. Hodder and Stoughton, London.
11. **Gaya, H., J. Klastersky, S. C. Schimpff, D. Fiere, S. Widmaier, and G. Nagel.** 1975. Prospective randomly-controlled trial of three antibiotic combinations for empirical therapy of suspected sepsis in neutropenic cancer patients. Eur. J. Cancer **11**(Suppl.):S5–S8.
12. **Gaya, H., J. Klastersky, S. C. Schimpff, and M. H. N. Tattersall.** 1975. Protocol for an international prospective trial of initial therapy regimens in neutropenic patients with malignant disease. Eur. J. Cancer **11**(Suppl.):S1–S4.
13. **Levine, A. S., S. C. Schimpff, R. G. Graw, Jr., and R. C. Young.** 1974. Hematologic malignancies and other marrow failure states: progress in the managment of complicating infections. Semin. Hematol. **11**:141–202.
14. **Klastersky, J.** 1975. The clinical use of combinations of antibiotics in patients predisposed to severe infection, p. 11–23. *In* J. Klastersky (ed.), Clinical use of combinations of antibiotics. Hodder and Stoughton, London.
15. **Klastersky, J., A. Henri, C. Hensgens, and D. Daneau.** 1974. Gram negative infections in cancer. Study of empiric therapy comparing carbenicillin-cephalothin with and without gentamicin. J. Am. Med. Assoc. **227**:45–48.
16. **Klastersky, J., C. Hensgens, and L. Debusscher.** 1975. Empiric therapy for cancer patients: comparative study of ticarcillin-tobramycin, ticarcillin-cephalothin, and cephalothin-tobramycin. Antimicrob. Agents Chemother. **7**:640–645.
17. **Middleman, E. A., A. Watanabe, H. Kaizer, and G. P. Bodey.** 1972. Antibiotic combinations for infections in neutropenic patients. Evaluation of carbenicillin plus either cephalothin or kanamycin. Cancer **30**:573–579.
18. **Neu, H. C., and G. J. Garvey.** 1975. Comparative in vitro activity and clinical pharmacology of ticarcillin and carbenicillin. Antimicrob. Agents Chemother. **8**:457–462.
19. **Rodriguez, V., G. P. Bodey, N. Horikoshi, J. Inagaki, and K. B. McCredie.** 1973. Ticarcillin therapy of infections. Antimicrob. Agents Chemother. **4**:427–431.
20. **Rodriguez, V., J. Inagaki, and G. P. Bodey.** 1973. Clinical pharmacology of ticarcillin (α-carboxyl-3-thienylmethyl penicillin, BRL-2288). Antimicrob. Agents Chemother. **4**:31–36.
21. **Schiffer, C. A., J. Aisner, S. W. Betts, and P. H. Wiernik.** 1975. Clinical experience with transfusion of granulocytes obtained by continuous flow filtration leukopheresis. Am. J. Med. **58**:373–381.
22. **Schimpff, S. C.** 1975. Diagnosis of infection in patients with cancer. Eur. J. Cancer **11**(Suppl.):S29–S38.
23. **Schimpff, S. C.** 1976. Laminar air flow room reverse isolation and microbial suppression to prevent infection in patients with cancer. Cancer Chemother. Rep. **59**:1055–1060.
24. **Schimpff, S. C., W. H. Greene, V. M. Young, and P. H. Wiernik.** 1974. Significance of *Pseudomonas aeruginosa* in the patient with leukemia or lymphoma. J. Infect. Dis. **130**(Suppl):S24–S31.
25. **Schimpff, S. C., W. Satterlee, V. M. Young, and A. Serpick.** 1971. Empiric therapy with carbenicillin and gentamicin for febrile patients with cancer and granulocytopenia. N. Engl. J. Med. **284**:1061–1065.
26. **Tattersall, M. H. N., A. S. D. Spiers, and J. H. Darrell.** 1972. Initial therapy with combination of five antibiotics in febrile patients with leukaemia and neutropenia. Lancet **i**:162–166.
27. **Viola, M. V.** 1967. Acute leukemia and infection. J. Am. Med. Assoc. **201**:923–926.
28. **Wald, E. R., H. C. Standiford, B. A. Tatem, F. M. Calia, and R. B. Hornick.** 1975. BL-P1654, ticarcillin, and carbenicillin: in vitro comparison alone and in combination with gentamicin against *Pseudomonas aeruginosa*. Antimicrob. Agents Chemother. **7**:336–340.
29. **Zinner, S. H., and W. R. McCabe.** 1975. Gram-negative rod bacteremia in cancer patients. A review with emphasis on the antibody response. Eur. J. Cancer **11**(Suppl.):S39–S47.

ANTIMICROBIAL AGENTS AND CHEMOTHERAPY, Nov. 1976, p. 845-849
Vol. 10, No. 5

Comparative Nephrotoxicities of Netilmicin and Gentamicin in Rats

FRIEDRICH C. LUFT, MOO NAHM YUM, AND STUART A. KLEIT

Departments of Medicine and Pathology, Indiana University School of Medicine, Indianapolis, Indiana 46202*

Received for publication 10 June 1976

The relative nephrotoxicities of netilmicin (Sch 20569) and gentamicin were compared in rats at doses of 30, 60, 90, and 120 mg/kg per day for 15 days. Both drugs caused proteinuria and a decrease in urine osmolality; however, netilmicin produced significantly less changes at all doses than gentamicin. Whereas gentamicin resulted in a decline in creatinine clearance at all doses, netilmicin failed to cause a decline in creatinine clearance. Renal-cortical concentrations of antibiotic at sacrifice were similar in animals receiving either drug. Light-microscopic changes were less severe with netilmicin than gentamicin. Cytosegresomes with myeloid bodies were identified electron microscopically in the kidneys of animals receiving either netilmicin or gentamicin at all doses. Electron-microscopic manifestations were similar. The data indicate that in the rat, netilmicin is distinctly less nephrotoxic than gentamicin.

Netilmicin (Sch 20569) is a new semisynthetic aminoglycoside which has in vitro bactericidal efficacy against both gentamicin-sensitive and gentamicin-resistant microorganisms (11). In vitro studies have shown that the spectrum of activity of netilmicin is similar to that of gentamicin against most gram-negative bacteria and *Staphylococcus aureus*. Although it has been shown to be active against many gentamicin-resistant organisms, it is somewhat less active than gentamicin against strains of *Pseudomonas aeruginosa* (12). In molecular structure, it closely resembles gentamicin C_{1a}, a component of the gentamicin complex. Fourteen-day and ninety-day chronic studies in rats, dogs, and cats have suggested that netilmicin has significantly less oto- and nephrotoxicity than gentamicin (12). To compare their relative toxicities in greater detail and to define the ultrastructural morphological changes rendered by netilmicin in kidney, we studied the effects of repetitive injections of both drugs at several different doses in rats. Parameters of renal function and concentrations of drug in renal cortex at sacrifice, as well as light- and electron-microscopic changes were monitored.

(This paper was presented in part at the 16th Interscience Conference on Antimicrobial Agents and Chemotherapy, Chicago, Ill., 29 October 1976.)

MATERIALS AND METHODS

Adult, male Sprague-Dawley rats weighing 200 to 225 g were selected, housed singly in metabolic cages, allowed free access to water, and fed a standard Purina rat diet ad libitum. The metabolic cages were equipped with screens below the animals' living space to avoid contamination of the urine specimens with feces or other debris. The design of the cages was such that the animals were unable to contaminate the specimens with drinking water. The 24-h urine samples were collected under mineral oil to preclude evaporation.

Four groups of 24 rats each, half of which received netilmicin and half of which received gentamicin, were studied. Eight control animals which received saline diluent accompanied each of the four experimental groups. Groups 1, 2, 3, and 4 received the drugs subcutaneously in 1 ml of saline diluent at doses of 30, 60, 90, and 120 mg/kg per day, respectively. Urine specimens were collected on days 3, 5, 8, 10, 12, and 15, at which time urine volume, urine protein excretion, and urine osmolality were measured.

Eight animals from each group, four receiving netilmicin and four receiving gentamicin, were sacrificed 24 h after a previous injection of antibiotic on days 5, 10, and 15. Four control animals for each group were sacrificed on days 5 and 15. Serum was collected for the measurement of urea nitrogen and creatinine clearance. The kidneys were removed and were examined by light and electron microscopy. In addition, homogenates were prepared for the measurement of antibiotic concentrations in renal tissue. These were compared to antibiotic concentrations in urine obtained on those same days. Urine specimens for antibiotic assay were obtained by direct needle puncture of the bladder.

The kidneys were halved through the hilus along the long axis to obtain a maximum area of light microscopy, fixed in buffered 10% formalin, embedded in paraffin, and stained with hematoxylin and eosin or by the periodic acid Schiff reaction. The histological sections were coded and read blind by one of us (M.N.Y.). To assess the extent of the tubular necrosis, the entire cortical area was systematically examined using a mechanical stage at low magnification. Additional small samples of the kidneys were fixed in cold 4% glutaraldehyde solution in 0.1 M phosphate buffer (pH 7.4), postfixed in cold 1% phosphate-buffered osmium tetroxide solution, and embedded in Epon 812 epoxy resin. Ultrathin sections were stained with urnayl acetate and lead citrate and viewed under a Philips 300 electron microscope.

Antibiotic concentrations in urine and renal tissue were measured by an agar well diffusion method (1). *Bacillus subtilis* served as the marker organism. Renal tissue was weighed, homogenized, and diluted as necessary with phosphate buffer (pH 8). Those kidneys acquired on day 15 were further divided into cortex and medulla. The fractions were homogenized and similarly analyzed. Urine concentrations were measured after dilution in pH 8 phosphate buffer. Concentrations in renal tissue are expressed as micrograms per gram of tissue, whereas urine concentrations are expressed as micrograms per milliliter.

Urine protein was determined by a biuret method; serum urea nitrogen and creatinine were measured by standard autoanalyzer techniques (9). Osmolality was determined by freezing-point depression. A statistical analysis of variance was used to compare animals receiving netilmicin to those receiving gentamicin and to controls.

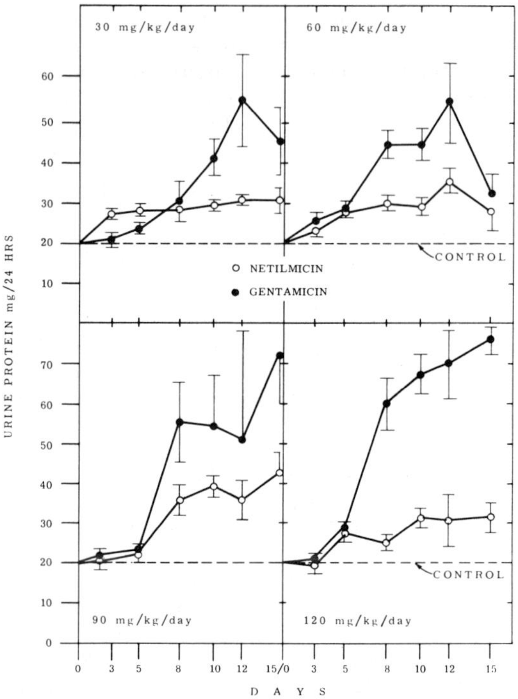

FIG. 1. *Mean values of controls are represented by a broken line. Bars represent standard error. Both drugs caused proteinuria at all doses tested, but netilmicin did so at a lesser degree.*

RESULTS

The administration of both drugs caused moderate increases in urine volume which are not graphically displayed. Significant differences between netilmicin and gentamicin were apparent only at the 30-mg/kg per day dose after 10 days of treatment. Proteinuria (Fig. 1) uniformily occurred with both regimens and was significantly increased above controls by day 5 at all doses ($P < 0.05$). The protein excretion of animals receiving gentamicin exceeded those receiving netilmicin by day 10 at 30 mg/kg per day ($P < 0.01$) and by day 8 at 60, 90, and 120 mg/kg per day, respectively ($P < 0.01$).

Urine osmolality (Fig. 2) decreased with both regimens at all doses. Gentamicin resulted in significant depression of urine osmolality compared with controls by day 8 at 30 and 60 mg/kg per day, by day 3 at 90 mg/kg per day, and by day 5 at 120 mg/kg per day ($P < 0.01$). Significant differences were observed between netilmicin and gentamicin by day 8 at 30, 60, and 120 mg/kg per day ($P < 0.05$) and by day 5 at 90 mg/kg per day ($P < 0.01$).

The serum urea nitrogen and creatinine clearance data are displayed in Tables 1 and 2. Significant serum urea nitrogen elevations compared to controls and to animals receiving netilmicin were observed in those receiving gentamicin at the 60-, 90-, and 120-mg/kg doses ($P < 0.05$). Netilmicin failed to cause a significant decrease in creatinine clearance at any of the doses tested ($P > 0.05$). Gentamicin resulted in a significant decrease by day 15 at 30 mg/kg per day, by day 10 at 60 and 90 mg/kg per day, and by day 5 at 120 mg/kg per day ($P < 0.05$). There was no mortality in netilmicin-treated animals, whereas three animals died with gentamicin treatment at 90 mg/kg per day and one animal died at 120 mg/kg per day.

Antibiotic concentrations in bladder urine at sacrifice ranged from 30 to 90 μg/ml and were similar with both regimens. Antibiotic concentrations in renal cortex at sacrifice are displayed in Fig. 3. Both drugs achieved high concentrations in renal cortex that exceeded those found in medulla fivefold or greater. There was no apparent differences among the regimens ($P > 0.05$).

Dose-related tubular damage involving primarily the convoluted portion of the proximal tubule was observed by light microscopy. In general, the changes with netilmicin were milder and occurred after a longer duration of treatment. At the 30-mg/kg per day dose, cloudy swelling was seen in animals receiving netilmicin, whereas those receiving gentamicin exhibited, in addition, patchy areas of tubular necrosis. At the higher doses, tubular necrosis developed after 10 days of treatment with either drug, but was more extensive in animals receiving gentamicin (Table 3).

Electron-microscopic changes noted with both drugs at all doses were the formation of large numbers of cytosegresomes containing myeloid bodies within the proximal tubular cells. These bodies were also found within the lumina of the proximal tubules. Mild mitochondrial swelling and dilation of the cisternae of the rough endoplasmic reticulum were noted as well.

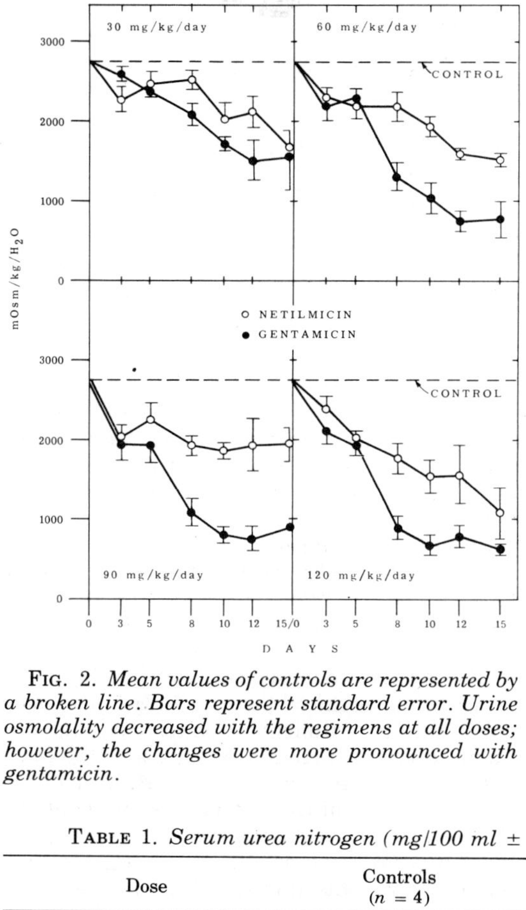

FIG. 2. *Mean values of controls are represented by a broken line. Bars represent standard error. Urine osmolality decreased with the regimens at all doses; however, the changes were more pronounced with gentamicin.*

DISCUSSION

Netilmicin appeared less toxic than gentamicin by all parameters of renal function measured. The drug resulted in less proteinuria, less depression in urine osmolality, and no decline in creatinine clearance at the doses studied. Increases in serum urea nitrogen observed with netilmicin were significantly less than those with gentamicin. These mild increases, not accompanied by significant decreases in creatinine clearance, may reflect "pre-renal" azotemia on the basis of mild dehydration since the animals were polyuric; however, no specific measurements of plasma volume or renal blood flow were done so the point remains conjectural. Serum urea nitrogen concentrations with netilmicin were significantly different from controls only on days 10 and 15 at the 90-mg/kg per day dose, a time at which the serum urea nitrogen concentrations of the controls were lower than generally seen. No consistent proteinuria occurred with netilmicin treatment.

The manifestations of netilmicin nephrotoxicity were similar to those ascribed to gentami-

TABLE 1. *Serum urea nitrogen (mg/100 ml ± standard error) determined at time of sacrifice.*

Dose	Controls (n = 4)	Netilmicin (n = 4)	Gentamicin (n = 4)
30 mg/kg per day			
5 days	15 ± 0.48	14 ± 0.48	16 ± 2.26
10 days		13 ± 0.7	15 ± 0.25
15 days	16 ± 1.56	15 ± 0.25	7 ± 0.85
60 mg/kg per day			
5 days	20 ± 0.65	26 ± 2.06	21 ± 0.61
10 days		23 ± 1.25	41 ± 12[a, b]
15 days	19 ± 0.48	23 ± 1.75	63 ± 11.7[a, b]
90 mg/kg per day			
5 days	13 ± 0.43	13 ± 0.78	13 ± 0.25
10 days		20 ± 0.75[c]	137 ± 16[a, b]
15 days	12 ± 0.29	18 ± 0.65[c]	240[a, b] (n = 1)
120 mg/kg per day			
5 days	20 ± 0.65	23 ± 0.48	22 ± 1
10 days		24 ± 1.7	138 ± 8[a, b]
15 days	19 ± 0.78	20 ± 1.47	194 ± 33[a, b] (n = 3)

[a] $P \leq 0.05$, gentamicin versus controls.
[b] $P \leq 0.05$, gentamicin versus netilmicin.
[c] $P \leq 0.05$, netilmicin versus controls.

TABLE 2. *Creatinine clearance (ml/min ± standard error) determined at time of sacrifice*

Dose	Controls (n = 4)	Netilmicin (n = 4)	Gentamicin (n = 4)
30 mg/kg per day			
5 days	1.47 ± 0.20	1.37 ± 0.07	1.41 ± 0.06
10 days		1.45 ± 0.24	1.07 ± 0.03
15 days	1.24 ±0.03	1.22 ± 0.06	0.84 ± 0.09[a, b]
60 mg/kg per day			
5 days	1.74 ± 0.09	1.42 ± 0.07	1.66 ± 0.09
10 days		1.37 ± 0.09	0.34 ± 0.04[a, b]
15 days	1.72 ± 0.08	1.50 ± 0.1	0.21 ± 0.03[a, b]
90 mg/kg per day			
5 days	1.62 ± 0.12	1.26 ± 0.17	1.56 ± 0.29
10 days		1.31 ± 0.35	0.45 ± 0.11[a, b]
15 days	1.78 ± 0.20	1.68 ± 0.11	0.1[a, b] (n = 1)
120 mg/kg per day			
5 days	1.60 ± 0.13	1.55 ± 0.04	1.07 ± 0.06[a, b]
10 days		1.29 ± 0.05	0.26 ± 0.025[a, b]
15 days	1.69 ± 0.16	1.62 ± 0.13	0.20 ± 0.02[a, b] (n = 3)

[a] $P \leq 0.05$, gentamicin versus controls.
[b] $P \leq 0.05$, gentamicin versus netilmicin.

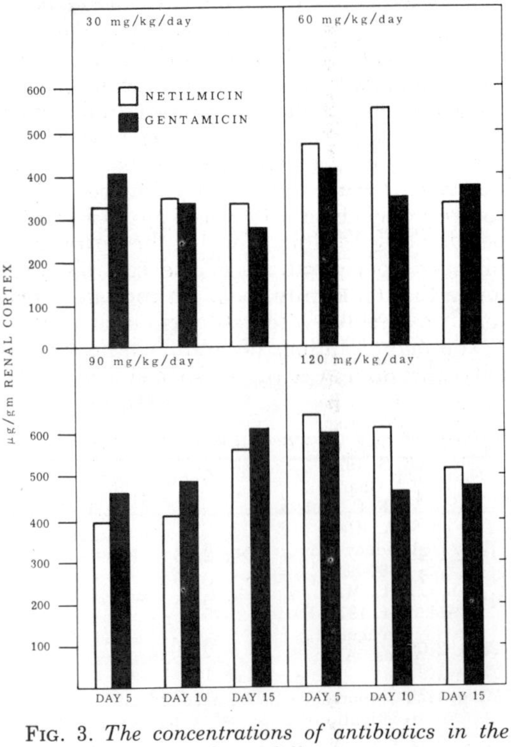

FIG. 3. *The concentrations of antibiotics in the renal cortex. No significant differences were apparent between the regimens.*

cin and other aminoglycosides (10). Proteinuria and a decrease in urine osmolality were early manifestations of toxicity, whereas alterations in glomerular filtration, observed only with gentamicin in the present study, occurred later. Histological changes observed with light microscopy were similar to those reported previously with gentamicin and other aminoglycosides (8, 10). This proved to be the case for the electron-microscopic changes as well. The formation of cytosegresomes with myeloid bodies was first described in the English literature by Kosek et al., who noted these changes in Fischer 344 rats with doses of gentamicin as low as 1 mg/kg per day after 48 h (6). Houghton et al. have recently published an elaborate series of photomicrographs which displayed the electron-microscopic changes seen with gentamicin at 40 mg/kg per day in Fischer 344 rats (5). Their observations are very similar to the findings in the present study. The origin and the significance of the electron-microscopic changes observed in proximal tubular epithelium remain unknown. Houghton et al. suggest that the cell may isolate and subsequently eject gentamicin-injured or possibly gentamicin-bound cytoplasmic structures in the form of myeloid bodies (5). Aminoglycosides are known to accumulate in renal cortex in which they have long half-lives (7). Since they impair protein synthesis in susceptible bacteria (4), it is conceivable that they impair protein or lipid synthetic processes in mammalian cells as well.

Whether or not renal-cortical concentrations of aminoglycosides correlate with the degree of nephrotoxicity is not established with certainty. In a previous publication, we reported that the renal-cortical concentrations achieved with an experimental aminoglycoside which proved to be most nephrotoxic were greater than a number of less toxic aminoglycosides (8). Dellinger et al. noted a protective effect of cephalothin against gentamicin nephrotoxicity (2)

TABLE 3. *Extent of tubular necrosis at 10 days of treatment (four rats in each group)*

Symptom	No. of rats receiving antibiotic[a]							
	Net (30 mg/kg)	Gen (30 mg/kg)	Net (60 mg/kg)	Gen (60 mg/kg)	Net (90 mg/kg)	Gen (90 mg/kg)	Net (120 mg/kg)	Gen (120 mg/kg)
Cloudy swelling without necrosis	4	4	4		2			
Necrosis involving 25% of total cortical area				1	2		4	
Necrosis involving 25–50% of total cortical area				3				
Necrosis involving 50–75% of total cortical area						1		
Necrosis involving 75–100% of total cortical area						3		4

[a] Net, Netilmicin; Gen, gentamicin.

and were able to demonstrate renal cortical concentrations of gentamicin that were significantly lower in rats given gentamicin and cephalothin simultaneously as compared with animals given gentamicin alone (3). In the present study, the renal cortical concentrations of netilmicin were not significantly different from those of gentamicin. Furthermore, the concentrations found with both drugs did not appear related to the dose. It is possible that the doses at which the drugs were given saturated all available binding sites and that with a lower dose, such as that used by Dellinger et al., a difference would have been apparent. Also, present bioassay techniques of aminoglycosides in homogenates of renal tissue are relatively crude. More sensitive assay systems may demonstrate a correlation between degree of toxicity and the renal-cortical concentration of aminoglycosides.

In summary, the present study presents evidence that netilmicin was significantly less nephrotoxic than gentamicin in the rat. The morphological changes engendered in proximal tubular epithelium by both drugs were similar in character, but less severe with netilmicin. The nephrotoxicity of the drugs could not be correlated with concentrations of the drugs in homogenates of renal cortex at sacrifice.

ACKNOWLEDGMENT

F. Luft is the recepient of grants-in-aid from the Schering Corp., Bloomfield, N.J., and the Kidney Foundation of Indiana.

LITERATURE CITED

1. **Brier, G. L., J. Wolny, and J. W. Smith.** 1975. Serum bioassay for antimicrobial agents, p. 57–71. *In* Technical improvement service number 21, American Society of Clinical Pathologists, Chicago.
2. **Dellinger, P., T. Murphy, V. Pinn, M. Barza, and L. Weinstein.** 1976. Protective effect of cephalothin against gentamicin-induced nephrotoxicity in rats. Antimicrob. Agents Chemother. 9:172–178.
3. **Dellinger, P., T. Murphy, M. Barza, V. Pinn, and L. Weinstein.** 1976. Effect of cephalothin on renal cortical concentration of gentamicin in rats. Antimicrob. Agents Chemother. 9:587–588.
4. **Hahn, F. E., and S. G. Sarre.** 1969. Mechanism of action of gentamicin. J. Infect. Dis. 119:364–369.
5. **Houghton, D. C., M. Hartnett, M. Campbell-Boswell, G. Porter, and W. Bennett.** 1976. A light and electron microscopic analysis of gentamicin nephrotoxicity in rats. Am. J. Pathol. 82:589–600.
6. **Kosek, J. C., R. I. Mazze, and M. J. Cousins.** 1974. Nephrotoxicity of gentamicin. Lab. Invest. 30:48–57.
7. **Luft, F. C., and S. A. Kleit.** 1974. Renal parenchymal accumulation of aminoglycoside antibiotics in rats. J. Infect. Dis. 130:656–659.
8. **Luft, F. C., V. Patel, M. N. Yum, B. Patel, and S. A. Kleit.** 1975. Experimental aminoglycoside nephrotoxicity. J. Lab. Clin. Med. 86:213–220.
9. **Natelson, S.** 1971. Techniques of clinical chemistry, p. 606–612. Charles C Thomas Co., Springfield, Ill.
10. **Patel, V., F. C. Luft, M. N. Yum, B. Patel, W. Zeman, and S. A. Kleit.** 1975. Enzymuria in gentamicin-induced kidney damage. Antimicrob. Agents Chemother. 7:364–369.
11. **Rahal, J. J., M. S. Simberkoff, K. Kagan, and N. H. Moldover.** 1976. Bacterial efficacy of Sch 20569 and amikacin against gentamicin-sensitive and -resistant organisms. Antimicrob. Agents Chemother. 9:595–599.
12. **Schering Corporation.** 1975. Informational material for the investigational drug Sch 20569. Schering Corp., Bloomfield, N.J.

ANTIMICROBIAL AGENTS AND CHEMOTHERAPY, Nov. 1976, p. 850-855
Vol. 10, No. 5

Antibiotic Penetrance of Ascitic Fluid in Dogs

DALE N. GERDING,* JAMES P. KROMHOUT, JOHN J. SULLIVAN, AND WENDELL H. HALL

Infectious Disease Section, Department of Medicine, Veterans Administration Hospital, and The University of Minnesota Medical School, Minneapolis, Minnesota 55417*

Received for publication 17 June 1976

Antibiotic concentrations in ascitic fluid after parenteral therapy may be important in the treatment of peritonitis. We have created ascites in dogs by partial ligation of the inferior vena cava. Ascitic fluid volume was measured at the time each antibiotic was administered. Nine antibiotics were studied in the same three dogs. Antibiotic concentration in ascitic fluid was found to vary inversely with ascites volume. Percentage of penetration (ratio of ascites peak to serum peak ×100) ranged from 5.8 to 65% among the drugs studied. Only metronidazole showed a statistically significant higher percentage of penetration than other antimicrobials. Concentrations in ascitic fluid after single doses of cephalothin (15 mg/kg) and the aminoglycosides (2 mg/kg, gentamicin and tobramycin; 7.5 mg/kg, amikacin and kanamycin) did not exceed the minimum inhibitory concentration of many gram-negative rods and may justify the use of higher than usual initial parenteral doses, or possibly initial intraperitoneal administration in seriously ill patients.

Patients with hepatic cirrhosis and ascites are at increased risk of developing spontaneous bacterial peritonitis (2, 3). Successful antibiotic therapy of this highly fatal disease is likely to depend upon both the antimicrobial spectrum of the drugs selected and their ability to penetrate into ascitic fluid. Previous studies of peritoneal transport of antibiotics in man have been performed during peritoneal dialysis (6, 17, 18). Such studies, utilizing a protein-free fluid that is rapidly exchanged, may not accurately reflect the kinetics of antibiotics in ascitic fluid arising as a result of cirrhosis. Furthermore, patients with cirrhosis frequently have low serum albumin levels, which may alter the serum binding of certain antibiotics and change their pharmacokinetics. There is little information on ascitic fluid penetration of newer antibiotics, particularly those of the cephalosporin and aminoglycoside groups. The only paper directly addressing this topic suggested that cephalothin should be administered by both the intravenous and intraperitoneal routes in the initial treatment of peritonitis in cirrhotics with ascites (24).

Because the literature data concerning antibiotic penetration of ascitic fluid does not seem to be adequate, we elected to study this problem utilizing a previously described model (13) for the creation of ascites in dogs. In this paper we report the ascitic fluid penetrance of single doses of nine antibiotics in this dog model. In addition, ascitic fluid volume was measured and compared with ascites concentrations for several of the antibiotics studied.

(Presented in part at the 15th Interscience Conference on Antimicrobial Agents and Chemotherapy, Washington, D.C., 1975.)

MATERIALS AND METHODS

Creation of ascites in dogs. Mongrel dogs weighing 18 to 22 kg were anesthetized with intravenous pentobarbital, and the inferior vena cava was ligated through a right thoracotomy according to the technique of McKee et al. (13). An umbilical tape was used to ligate the vena cava by tying down loosely on a 1.5-mm-diameter rigid tube that was then removed. Three of the first seven dogs prepared in this manner developed ascites and were used for the antibiotic studies. Two of the three dogs required 15 g of sodium chloride daily in their diets periodically to maintain the ascites. All dogs were housed in separate pens, fed commercial dry dog food, and given free access to water.

Large collateral veins developed on the abdomen and thoracic wall, and the animals showed obvious loss of muscle mass after the procedure. Previous microscopic studies by McKee et al. (13) have shown that the procedure results in passive congestion of the liver with marked dilation of subcapsular lymphatics and venous sinusoids. Ascites formation occurs primarily by means of fluid escape from the capsular surface of the liver (7).

Ascitic fluid volume and characteristics. The volume of ascitic fluid was measured before each antibiotic administration according to the method of Luttwak (11) using ^{125}I-labeled human serum albumin. Five microcuries of ^{125}I-labeled albumin was injected into the peritoneal cavity, and the volume of fluid was determined by counting a 10-ml sample of ascitic fluid obtained 30 min after injection. Stability of the volume determination at 10, 20, and 30 min as shown by Luttwak (11) was confirmed.

Cell counts were determined on a Coulter counter (Coulter Electronics, Inc., Hialeah, Fla.). Differentials were hand counted. Total protein, albumin, creatinine, blood urea nitrogen, bilirubin, serum glutamic-oxalacetic transaminase, and alkaline phosphatase were determined using the Auto Analyzer (Technicon, Terrytown, N.Y.).

Antibiotic administration. Antibiotics were administered intramuscularly in the gluteus muscle, except for metronidazole, which was given orally. Each antibiotic was administered to the same three dogs. Dosages are given in Table 2 and are based on the dry weight of each dog before the creation of ascites. Serum and ascites specimens were obtained at zero time, 0.5, 1 through 6, and 24 h after antibiotic administration. Blood was obtained from the jugular vein and ascites fluid was obtained by midline abdominal wall aspiration. Dogs were fasting 12 h at the onset of each study and were allowed water ad libitum but no food for the 24 h of an experiment.

Antibiotic assays. Antibiotic assays were performed in triplicate using a microbiological disk-plate method with a 24-h incubation at 37°C (10, 16). *Bacillus subtilis* ATCC 6633 was used for the assay of cephalothin and all the aminoglycosides. *Sarcina lutea* was the indicator organism for cephaloridine and clindamycin. *Staphylococcus aureus* 6538P was used for cefazolin. Metronidazole was assayed by the method of Levison (9), modified by using a strain of *Clostridium perfringens* obtained from the University of Minnesota. One molar phosphate buffer (pH 8.0) was added to the clindamycin specimens immediately after drawing to interrupt further hydrolysis from ester to active clindamycin. Specimens were placed on 6.35-mm paper disks (Schleicher and Schuell, Inc., Keene, N.H.) using disposable 20-μl pipettes (Unopette, Becton-Dickinson and Co., Rutherford, N.J.). For each antibiotic, the initial standard curves were prepared in both pooled dog ascitic fluid and serum. No differences were noted between standard curves obtained from serum or ascitic fluid for any of the antibiotics, and subsequent assays were done with dog serum only for the standard curve. All antibiotics were supplied as sterile dry powders or solutions. Tobramycin was furnished through the courtesy of Eli Lilly and Co., Indianapolis, Ind., and amikacin was supplied by Bristol Laboratories, Syracuse, N.Y.

Statistical analysis. Standard error of the mean was determined by the method of Mantel (12). Antibiotic serum half-life ($t_{1/2}$) was calculated from the standard formula using the slope of the regression line determined by the method of least squares (5). The nonparametric Mann-Whitney U test was used to determine statistical significance (1).

RESULTS

Serum and ascitic fluid characteristics. Ascitic fluid chemical and cellular characteristics are shown in Table 1 for the three dogs studied and six additional dogs. Leukocyte and erythrocyte counts tended to be slightly higher for specimens obtained after repeated paracenteses during the course of an antibiotic study. Maximum hematocrit was 1.2%.

Serum total protein and albumin were reduced in these animals, ranging from 3.7 to 4.8 g/100 ml (mean, 4.5) for protein and from 1.5 to 2.7 g/100 ml (mean, 2.2) for albumin. Blood urea nitrogen, serum creatinine, bilirubin, serum glutamic-oxalacetic transaminase, and alkaline phosphatase were normal. Protein electrophoresis in two animals revealed qualitatively similar patterns for ascitic fluid and serum, but quantitatively both globulins and albumin were lower in ascites.

Ascites volume and antibiotic concentration in ascitic fluid. Ascitic fluid volume ranged from 2.2 to 10.8 liters in the three dogs during the course of the study (Table 2). Volumes for an individual dog changed slowly and did not vary by more than a liter from week to week unless sodium chloride was withheld or added to the diet. The variation of ascitic fluid antibiotic concentration with ascites volume for cefazolin is shown in Fig. 1. Peak concentrations of cefazolin in serum were similar for the three dogs (22, 24, and 29 μg/ml). Other antibiotics showed a similar variation of ascites concentration with volume, but ascitic fluid volumes often were more closely grouped and the range of ascites antibiotic concentrations was not as wide as with cefazolin. During the first few hours after administration, the relationship of ascitic fluid antibiotic level to ascitic fluid volume is linear when plotted on a semilogarithmic graph, as shown in Fig. 2 for amikacin and cefazolin. After 2 to 3 h, ascitic fluid peak concentrations begin to occur and the relationship becomes nonlinear.

Ascitic fluid levels of antibiotics. Mean peak levels and ranges of antibiotic concentrations and percentage of penetration (ratio of ascites peak to serum peak ×100) are shown in Table 2. Typical pharmacokinetic curves for the study are shown for cefazolin and cephalothin (Fig. 3) and for metronidazole and clindamycin (Fig. 4). Kinetic curves for cephaloridine and

TABLE 1. *Characteristics of ascitic fluid from nine dogs*

Determination	Mean	Range
Leukocyte count	975	110–2,000
% Polymorphonuclears (%)	50	16–77
Erythrocyte count	7,500	300–20,000
Total protein (g/100 ml)	3.1	1.9–3.8
Albumin (g/100 ml)	1.7	1.2–1.9
pH	7.62	7.5–7.7

TABLE 2. *Mean and range of ascites volume, peak serum level, peak ascites level and percentage of penetration (ratio of ascites peak to serum peak ×100) for nine antibiotics administered to the same three dogs*

Antibiotic	Dose (mg/kg)	Ascites volume (liters)		Serum peak (μg/ml)		Ascites peak (μg/ml)		% Penetration	
		Mean	Range	Mean	Range	Mean	Range	Mean	Range
Cephaloridine	15	6.2	3.7–9.4	27.7	23–35	5.3	3.5–6.8	19.1	15.2–24.3
Cefazolin	15	5.8	2.2–10.8	24.0	22–29	6.2	2.7–9.0	25.8	11.3–32.7
Cephalothin	15	5.1	3.3–8.3	14.5	10–18	3.1	1.3–5.4	21.4	8.4–30.0
Kanamycin	7.5	4.6	3.2–6.4	21.3	19–25	2.4	1.1–4.3	11.3	5.8–21.5
Amikacin	7.5	5.6	3.3–9.1	19.4	17–23	3.3	1.9–4.6	17.0	8.6–25.0
Gentamicin	2	3.5	3.0–3.8	8.9	5.4–15	1.7	0.6–3.7	19.1	11.1–24.7
Tobramycin	2	4.6	2.3–7.5	6.4	4–8.2	1.1	0.6–1.5	17.2	13.4–21.5
Clindamycin	8.6	5.8	2.8–10.5	7.8	4.8–10.5	2.1	1.4–3.3	26.9	13.3–39.3
Metronidazole	250[a]	5.9	4.2–9.1	12.1	9.8–15.5	5.7	4.2–6.7	47.0	38.2–65.0

[a] Dose in milligrams.

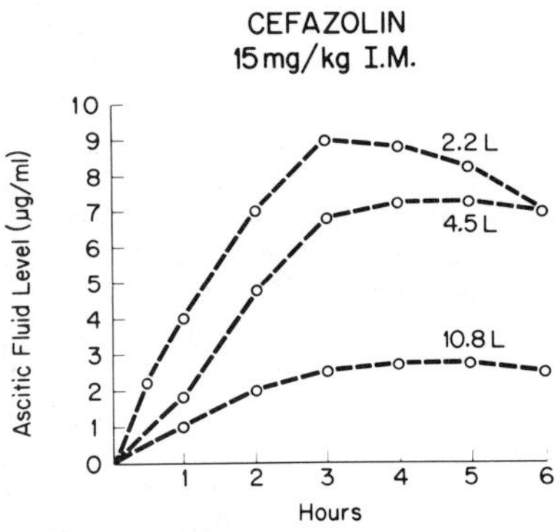

FIG. 1. *Ascitic fluid level of cefazolin in three dogs with different ascites volumes given the same dose of cefazolin based on dry weight. Peak serum concentrations were similar in the three animals.*

all the aminoglycosides were similar to those in Fig. 3. The kinetics of metronidazole (oral administration) showed a later serum peak and a longer $t_{1/2}$ than the other drugs tested. Clindamycin, administered as the phosphate, requires hydrolysis to the active form of the drug, resulting in later serum and ascites peaks. There were no statistical differences in percentage of penetration among the cephalosporins, aminoglycosides, and clindamycin. Metronidazole percentage of penetration was significantly higher ($P < 0.05$) than all cephalosporins and aminoglycosides, but was not statistically higher ($P < 0.10$) than clindamycin. Peak concentration of antibiotic in ascitic fluid occurred 4 h after administration for all drugs, except cephalothin (2 h), kanamycin (3 h), and clindamycin (5 h). Detectable concentrations of antibiotic were present in ascitic fluid at 24 h for clindamycin, metronidazole, amikacin, cefazolin, and cephaloridine. Ascitic fluid clindamycin mean concentration at 24 h was 1.1 μg/ml (range, 0.9 to 1.3) and was the highest of the nine drugs tested.

Serum $t_{1/2}$ for the aminoglycosides was 0.9 h for kanamycin, 1.3 h for amikacin and tobramycin, and 1.7 h for gentamicin. Percentage of penetration (Table 2) closely paralleled serum $t_{1/2}$ for the aminoglycosides. Cefazolin had the longest $t_{1/2}$ of the cephalosporins (1.5 h); this compared with 1.1 and 1.2 h for cephalothin and cephaloridine, respectively. Clindamycin (3.3 h) and metronidazole (4.2 h) had a considerably longer serum $t_{1/2}$ than the other drugs tested. In general, the percentage of penetration of the antibiotics (Table 2) paralleled the serum $t_{1/2}$.

DISCUSSION

Two physiological factors are believed to be responsible for ascites formation in cirrhosis: obstruction to hepatic venous outflow and prehepatic portal venous obstruction (8, 25). The model chosen for this study produces ascites largely by means of the former mechanism, and results in a somewhat higher ascites protein content than in cirrhosis, largely because fluid "weeps" from the liver surface (7). Secondary factors contributing to ascites formation in cirrhosis (reduced serum albumin, and salt and water retention) are also present in this model (13). Thus, the model approximates the physiological situation in cirrhosis except for the absence of portal vein obstruction.

The study was deliberately performed with single doses of each antibiotic to determine the ascites penetration of initial systemic administrations, possibly a critical factor in seriously ill patients with peritonitis. No attempt was made to establish equilibrium conditions. Previous studies of antibiotic concentrations in perito-

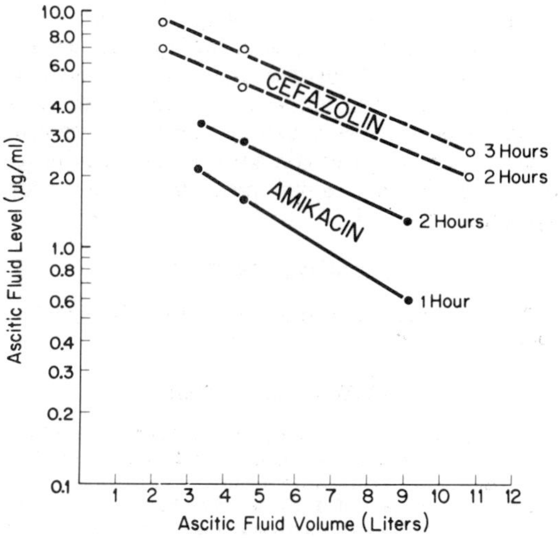

FIG. 2. *Semilogarithmic plot of cefazolin (broken line) and amikacin (solid line) ascitic fluid concentrations as a function of ascitic fluid volume for the first 3 h after intramuscular injection.*

neal dialysis fluid in humans have indicated that therapeutically adequate concentrations of methicillin and tetracycline can be expected after 1 to 2 h after systemic administration (17). In similar studies, tobramycin and gentamicin concentrations have been therapeutically inadequate (18, 23). Renal function was abnormal in all the patients studied, resulting in longer than normal serum $t_{1/2}$. Cephalothin penetrance of ascitic fluid in uninfected cirrhotic patients was studied by Wilson and associates (24). Mean peak ascites concentration was 3.22 µg/ml 1 h after a 1-g intravenous administration. Ascites volume ranged from 4 to 12 liters.

The results of the present study show that ascitic fluid concentrations of antibiotics are inversely proportional to the volume of ascites present. Percentage of penetration (ratio of ascites peak to serum peak ×100) can be expected to range from 8.4 to 32.7% for the cephalosporins, from 5.8 to 25% for the aminoglycosides, from 13.3 to 39.3% for clindamycin, and from 38.2 to 65% for metronidazole, depending upon the ascites volume present (Table 2). Among the cephalosporins and aminoglycosides studied, no single antibiotic was found to penetrate peritoneal fluid preferentially. The mean peak ascitic fluid cephalothin concentration achieved in this study (3.1 µg/ml) is virtually identical to the level achieved in the only comparable human study (24). Metronidazole was the only drug studied that showed a statistically higher percentage of penetration than the others. Metronidazole was also the only drug administered

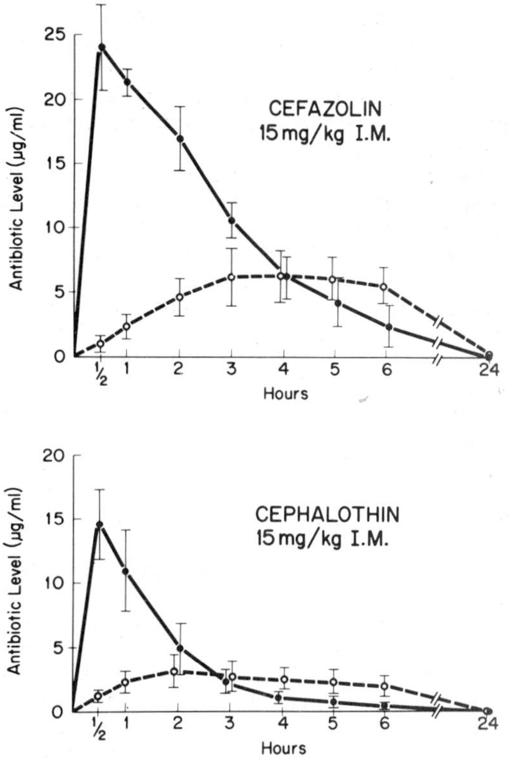

FIG. 3. *Cefazolin and cephalothin levels in serum (solid line) and ascitic fluid (broken line) in the same three dogs. Vertical bars indicate standard error of the mean.*

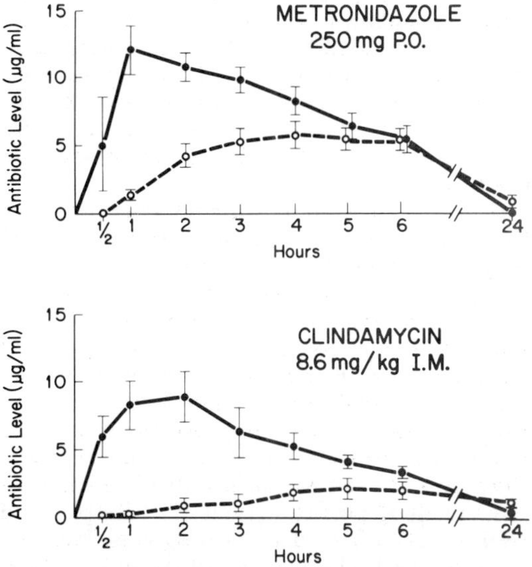

FIG. 4. *Metronidazole and clindamycin levels in serum (solid line) and ascitic fluid (broken line) in the same three dogs. Vertical bars indicate standard error of the mean.*

orally, and it had the longest serum $t_{1/2}$. Levels of metronidazole, as measured by bioassay, reflect activity of both parent drug and biologically active metabolites (19), which may account in part for the long $t_{1/2}$ and high percentage of penetration.

We find it interesting that the differences in serum protein binding of the cephalosporins in dogs (22) appear to have no affect on the concentrations achieved in ascitic fluid. It has been shown that cefazolin is 80% serum protein bound, cephalothin is 40% bound, and cephaloridine is only 10% bound; but the time required for maximum binding in vitro has been shown to be up to 50 min for cefazolin (22). A similar delay in in vivo binding of cefazolin could account for its high percentage of penetration. Since serum albumin was low in these dogs, cefazolin serum binding may have been lower than in normal canine serum. In addition, bound as well as unbound drug may diffuse from serum to peritoneal cavity from the liver surface.

The concentrations of clindamycin and metronidazole in ascitic fluid after a single dose exceed the minimum inhibitory concentration (MIC) of most anaerobic and gram-positive aerobic organisms toward which they might be directed (14, 20). In comparison to the in vitro MIC of gram-negative bacilli (15, 26), the ascitic fluid concentrations of the aminoglycosides appear to be marginal at best. This may be due to the short serum $t_{1/2}$ observed in the dog, in comparison with observations in humans. Similarly, cephalothin ascitic fluid concentrations appear to be inadequate for most susceptible gram-negative bacilli (21), at the dosage used in this study (1 g human equivalent). Concentrations of cephaloridine and cefazolin compare well with the in vitro MIC of gram-negative bacilli (21).

In the presence of peritoneal inflammation, the penetrance of antibiotics into ascitic fluid may be increased, as observed by Smithivas and associates (18) for gentamicin. Early experimental observations by David (4), however, indicate that in severe peritonitis, peritoneal absorption may be markedly inhibited.

Based on our observations in dogs, we believe that the ascitic fluid concentrations of some antibiotics (cephalothin and the aminoglycosides) may be somewhat low after a single administration, particularly if the ascitic fluid volume is large, disregarding possible enhanced penetration due to inflammation. Antibiotic kinetics in ascitic fluid suggest that accumulation will occur with subsequent doses (Fig. 3 and 4). Because initial peritoneal concentrations may be marginal, we suggest maximizing the initial systemic dose or intraperitoneal installation of the first dose of aminoglycosides or cephalothin if the patient is critically ill. Because of possible respiratory paralysis and ototoxicity, aminoglycoside dosages intraperitoneally should not exceed recommendations for systemic therapy.

ACKNOWLEDGMENT

This work was supported by a grant from Eli Lilly & Co., Indianapolis, Ind.

LITERATURE CITED

1. **Auble, D.** 1952. Extended tables for the Mann-Whitney statistic. Institute of Educational Research, School of Education, Indiana University, Bloomington, Ind.
2. **Conn, H. O., and M. J. Fessel.** 1971. Spontaneous bacterial peritonitis in cirrhosis. Variations on a theme. Medicine 50:161–197.
3. **Curry, N., R. W. McCallum, and P. H. Guth.** 1974. Spontaneous peritonitis in cirrhotic ascites. Am. J. Dig. Dis. 19:685–692.
4. **David, V. C.** 1925. Peritonitis. An experimental study. Surg. Gynecol. Obstet. 45:287–293.
5. **Goldstein, A., L. Aronow, and S. Kolman.** 1974. The time course of drug action, p. 301–355. *In* Principles of drug action. Harper & Row, Publishers, New York.
6. **Greenberg, P. A., and J. P. Sanford.** 1967. Removal and absorption of antibiotics in patients with renal failure undergoing peritoneal dialysis. Ann. Intern. Med. 66:465–479.
7. **Hyatt, R. E., G. H. Lawrence, and J. R. Smith.** 1955. Observations on the origin of ascites from experimental hepatic congestion. J. Lab. Clin. Med. 45:274–280.
8. **Hyatt, R. E., and J. R. Smith.** 1954. The mechanism of ascites. A physiological appraisal. Am. J. Med. 16:434–448.
9. **Levison, M. E.** 1974. Microbiological agar diffusion assay for metronidazole concentrations in serum. Antimicrob. Agents Chemother. 5:466–468.
10. **Lilly Research Laboratories.** 1970. Paper disc or cup plate antibiotic assay procedures. Eli Lilly & Co., Indianapolis, Ind.
11. **Luttwak, E. M.** 1973. Quantitative studies of ascitic fluid. Surg. Gynecol. Obstet. 136:269–272.
12. **Mantel, N.** 1951. Rapid estimation of standard errors of means for small samples. Am. Stat. 5:26–27.
13. **McKee, F. W., J. A. Schwing, G. H. Tishkoff, and R. E. Hyatt.** 1949. Experimental ascites. Effects of sodium chloride and protein intake on protein metabolism of dogs with constricted inferior vena cava. Surg. Gynecol. Obstet. 89:529–540.
14. **Oppenheimer, S., and M. Turck.** 1968. Laboratory and clinical evaluation of 7-chloro-7-deoxylincomycin. Am. J. Med. Sci. 256:314–321.
15. **Reynolds, A. V., J. M. T. Hamilton-Miller, and W. Brumfit.** 1974. Newer aminoglycosides—amikacin and tobramycin. An *in vitro* comparison with kanamycin and gentamicin. Br. Med. J. 3:778–780.
16. **Sabath, L. D., J. I. Casey, P. A. Ruch, L. L. Stumpf, and M. Finland.** 1971. Rapid microassay for circulating nephrotoxic antibiotics, p. 83–89. Antimicrob. Agents Chemother. 1970.
17. **Shear, L., J. H. Shinaberger, and K. G. Barry.** 1965. Peritoneal transport of antibiotics in man. N. Engl. J. Med. 272:666–669.
18. **Smithivas, T., P. J. Hyams, R. Matalon, M. S. Simber-**

koff, and J. J. Rahal, Jr. 1971. The use of gentamicin in peritoneal dialysis. I. Pharmacologic results. J. Infect. Dis. **124**:S77–S83.
19. **Speck, W. T., A. B. Stein, and H. S. Rosenkranz.** 1976. Metronidazole bioassay. Antimicrob. Agents Chemother. **9**:260–261.
20. **Staneck, J. L., and J. A. Washington II.** 1974. Antimicrobial susceptibilities of anaerobic bacteria: recent clinical isolates. Antimicrob. Agents Chemother. **6**:311–315.
21. **Washington, J. A., II.** 1976. The *in vitro* spectrum of the cephalosporins. Mayo Clin. Proc. **51**:237–250.
22. **Waterman, N., L. Scharfenberger, and M. J. Raff.** 1974. Rate of binding of antibiotics to canine serum protein. Antimicrob. Agents Chemother. **5**:294–295.
23. **Weinstein, A. J., A. W. Karchmer, and R. C. Møellering, Jr.** 1973. Tobramycin concentrations during peritoneal dialysis. Antimicrob. Agents Chemother. **4**:432–434.
24. **Wilson, D. E., T. C. Chalmers, and M. A. Madoff.** 1967. The passage of cephalothin into and out of ascitic fluid. Am. J. Med. Sci. **253**:449–452.
25. **Witte, M. H., C. L. Witte, and A. E. Dumont.** 1971. Progress in liver disease: physiological factors involved in the causation of cirrhotic ascites. Gastroenterology **61**:742–750.
26. **Young, L. S., and W. H. Hewitt.** 1973. Activity of five aminoglycoside antibiotics in vitro against gram-negative bacilli and *Staphylococcus aureus*. Antimicrob. Agents Chemother. **4**:617–625.

ANTIMICROBIAL AGENTS AND CHEMOTHERAPY, Nov. 1976, p. 856-860
Vol. 10, No. 5
Printed in U.S.A.

Antifungal Properties of Electrically Generated Metallic Ions

T. J. BERGER,* J. A. SPADARO, RICHARD BIERMAN, S. E. CHAPIN, AND R. O. BECKER

Veterans Administration Hospital, Syracuse, New York 13210, and Department of Orthopedics, State University of New York, Upstate Medical Center, Syracuse, New York 13210*

Received for publication 15 July 1976

A qualitative and quantitative investigation was undertaken to study the susceptibility of unicellular eucaryotic organisms (yeasts) to metallic cations generated by low levels of direct current. Results were characteristic of effects obtained previously using clinical and standard bacteria test organisms. The present study demonstrated that anodic silver (Ag^+) at low direct currents had inhibitory and fungicidal properties. Broth dilution susceptibility tests were made on several species of *Candida* and one species of *Torulopsis*. Growth in all isolates was inhibited by concentrations of electrically generated silver ions between 0.5 and 4.7 μg/ml, and silver exhibited fungicidal properties at concentrations as low as 1.9 μg/ml. The inhibitory and fungicidal concentrations of electrically generated silver ions are lower than those reported for other silver compounds.

We have previously examined the bactericidal activities of a variety of metallic ions generated from pure metallic anodes by direct currents. We reported (3, 4, 11) that the silver ion was an effective antibacterial agent when liberated by low levels of direct current. Quantitatively it was more effective against both gram-positive and gram-negative organisms than silver sulfadiazine. All other metals tested lacked bactericidal properties except when associated with high levels of direct current (400 μA) and the accompanying major pH changes.

Lukens (6) reviewed the work of S. E. A. McCallan and F. Wilcoxon, who examined the fungitoxicity of the elements in relation to their position in the periodic table. Generally, toxicity within a group increased with atomic weight. Silver and osmium were the most toxic elements. Data from J. G. Horsfall have been summarized (7) and show that metals are arranged in the following descending order of fungitoxicity: Ag > Hg > Cu > Cd > Cr > Ni > Pb > Co > Zn > Fe > Ca. Practically all work has involved the fungitoxicity of the metals as salts in combination with various anions. Since the electrically generated silver ion appeared to be superior to the silver compounds in antibacterial activity, we have attempted to determine the antifungal properties of several electrically generated metallic ions including silver. This article reports the results of this study.

MATERIALS AND METHODS

Qualitative studies. A 0.5-ml portion of nutrient broth (Gibco, T1859) or fluid Sabouraud medium (Gibco, 1401500) containing exponential-phase yeast (optical density at 500 nm, 0.1 to 0.3) was spread with a glass rod onto brain heart infusion agar (BHI; Gibco, T1904) or Sabouraud agar (Gibco, 1402240). Electrode culture plates (60 by 15 mm) were prepared as previously described (3). Silver, copper, zinc, and titanium wires that were at least 99.9% pure were used. Battery-operated constant-current generators (11) were applied to all electrodes (except controls) after yeast inoculation and throughout incubation in the dark (37°C, 24 h). The current levels employed were 0.4, 4.0, and 40.0 μA.

The following parameters were recorded for all control and experimental culture plates: (i) currents and applied potentials were taken at 0 and 24 h; (ii) subcultures, after 24 h, were taken aseptically at three points along each electrode and at 3-mm intervals out from each electrode (+ and −); (iii) pH measurements were made using pH test paper (Hydrion) at the same points as above; (iv) general observations such as zone size (radius), gas production, medium discoloration, and tarnishing of metal electrode were recorded, and photographs were taken.

The experimental organisms employed were *Candida albicans* I and *C. krusei*; both were derived from the VA hospital (Syracuse, N.Y.) and the Upstate Medical Center (Syracuse, N.Y.). *C. albicans* was maintained on BHI agar at 4°C, and *C. krusei* was maintained on Sabouraud dextrose agar (Gibco, 1402240) at 4°C, and both were transferred onto fresh media every 2 months.

Quantitative studies. The broth dilution susceptibility test (2) was employed to determine minimum inhibitory concentrations (MIC) and minimum fungicidal concentrations (MFC) of electrically generated silver in nutrient broth. The silver ions used in the yeast susceptibility test were liberated in nutrient broth from pure silver wire anodes via battery-operated constant-current generators at 75 μA for 4 h. The current and voltage levels were monitored at the beginning and end of silver generation. The chamber used to generate silver and the determination of the silver concentrations via emission spectroscopy have been previously described (3). The organisms used in the quantitative studies were *C. albicans* I, *C. albicans* II, *C. parapsilosis*, *C. pseudotropicalis*, *C. tropicalis*, and *Torulopsis glabrata*. These yeasts were obtained from the Upstate Medical Center and maintained on BHI as above. The final concentrations for all organisms used in the susceptibility test were between 10^4 and 10^6 cells/ml. All organisms were incubated in the dark at 37°C for 24 h. All inoculations and testing in the quantitative studies were performed in nutrient broth.

RESULTS

Qualitative studies at low current levels. Initially the four metals (silver, copper, zinc, and titanium) were tested against *C. albicans* using BHI plate cultures. When silver was shown to be the most reactive, experiments were then repeated using silver against *C. krusei*. The results presented in Table 1 were based on the sterility of stab tests from three points along each electrode. The extent of sterility depended on the number of points that demonstrated a lack of viable organisms. All data are the average of at least two separate experiments with the following two exceptions: the copper electrode experiment and the *C. krusei* inoculated in nutrient broth, which were performed only once. The yeasts were grown in an initial inoculating medium of nutrient broth with subsequent plating on BHI agar plates.

At 0.4 and 4.0 μA, copper and zinc showed no effect on *C. albicans* at either electrode, whereas 1/3 of the test points at the titanium cathode (negative) were sterile. However, all test points were sterile at the silver anode (positive) for both *C. albicans* and *C. krusei* in the same current ranges. There were also clear zones present, having a 6-mm radius from the wire (see Fig. 1a and b). Interestingly, in one of two experiments with *C. albicans*, the Ag cathode also showed clearing zones of 1.5-mm radius at 0.4 μA and 5.5-mm radius at 4 μA. These clearing zones had spots of yeast growth randomly throughout, and these zones proved to be nonsterile (Table 1). We had previously

TABLE 1. *Sterility near metal electrodes with weak direct currents*

Inoculating medium[a]	Current (A)	Electrode	Potential[b] (V)	No. of sterile subcultures near electrode[c]			
				C. albicans I		*C. krusei*	
				Pos.	Neg.	Pos.	Neg.
NB	0.4	Silver	0.47	+++	0		
		Silver	0.46			+++	0
		Copper	0.04	0	0		
		Zinc	0.03	0	0		
		Titanium	2.15	0	+		
NB	4.0	Silver	0.91	+++	0		
		Silver	0.58			+++	0
		Copper	0.54	0	0		
		Zinc	0.35	0	0		
		Titanium	3.12	0	+		
NB	40.0	Silver	1.65	+++	0		
		Silver	1.20			+++	0
		Copper	1.10	0	0		
		Zinc	0.50	0	0		
		Titanium	8.0+	+	+		
Sabouraud	0.4	Silver	0.53			0	0
Sabouraud	4.0	Silver	0.84			+++	0
Sabouraud	40.0	Silver	2.05			+++	++

[a] NB, Nutrient broth; Sabouraud, fluid Sabouraud medium. The yeasts were initially grown in either of these two media with subsequent plating on BHI agar or Sabouraud agar, respectively.

[b] Potential at 24 h.

[c] Sterility of the region near the electrode was measured by subculturing tests, which were taken at three points along each electrode (+ and −). The degree of sterility was categorized as follows: 0, lack of sterility at all three points along the electrode with no stab tests sterile; +, 1/3 of stab tests sterile; ++, 2/3 of stab tests sterile; +++, all stab tests sterile. Pos., positive; Neg., negative.

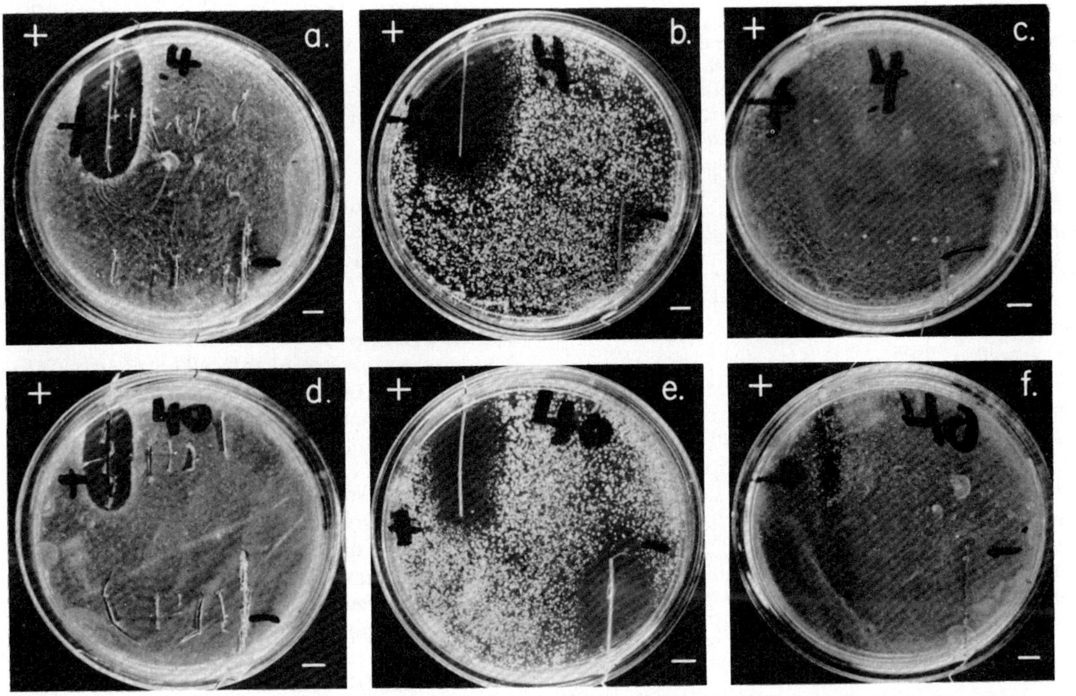

FIG. 1. *(a and d) Culture plates of C. albicans with Ag electrode at 0.4 and 40 μA after 24 h of incubation; (b and e) C. krusei with Ag at 0.4 and 40 μA; (c and f) C. albicans with titanium at 0.4 and 40 μA. Note the presence of clear sterile zones at all Ag anodes (+). C. krusei also has a nonsterile clear zone at the Ag cathode. Titanium has a small clear zone at both 40 μA positive and negative.*

seen similar clearing zones at the Ag cathode (only at the 4-μA level) with some bacteria (11). *C. krusei* at the Ag cathode exhibited no clear zones at 0.4 μA but also had a partially clear zone of 3-mm radius at 4 μA. This also proved to be nonsterile (Table 1). The control electrode (no current) generally had no clear zones, but occasionally a small clear zone of 1-mm radius or less was observed around the control Ag wire. These small zones proved to be nonsterile but do indicate some diffusion of Ag ions away from the Ag wire.

The silver, copper, and zinc electrode pairs at these current levels had potentials of less than 1 V. There were no pH shifts, gas formation, or agar discoloration seen for any of these metals at either current. However, at 4 μA a very slight tarnishing of the metal electrode was noticed for all three metals.

The titanium electrodes appeared slightly tarnished relative to the control and had an interelectrode potential greater than 2.0 V at 0.4 and 4 μA. Other than the appearance of a slight gas formation at the titanium anode in the 4.0-μA plate, there were no other changes observed (see Fig. 1c).

Qualitative studies at higher current. At 40 μA, all metals except zinc had a final interelectrode potential greater than 1 V. Silver again had a clear zone at the anode with a 4-mm radius for *C. albicans* and a 6-mm radius for *C. krusei*. The Ag wire appeared tarnished, and the zones proved to be sterile in both cases (Table 1). At the Ag cathode there was no clear zone produced with *C. albicans*, but with *C. krusei* there was a 6-mm-radius clear zone present that on subculture proved to be nonsterile. Both culture plates of the above had gas bubbles present at the cathode (see Fig. 1d and e). There were no substantial pH shifts except at the points directly adjacent to the cathode, where the pH shifted about +0.5 units as compared to the control.

The copper anode at 40 μA produced a 3-mm clear zone that proved to be nonsterile. A bluish discoloration appeared at the anode, along with gas formation at the cathode. A pH shift of +1.0 unit was observed at the cathode relative to the control.

Zinc at 40 μA had no zones, and no other changes were noted. Titanium at 40 μA exhibited 1/3 of the test points sterile at the anode and cathode with slight tarnishing, and no pH shift or discoloration of the medium was observed. At both positive and negative electrodes gas formation was evident (see Fig. 1f).

Fluid Sabouraud medium was also used to grow the inoculum of *C. krusei*. Once turbid growth was achieved, the inoculum was plated onto Sabouraud agar and treated with silver electrodes. The potentials increased with increasing currents, as seen with *C. krusei* grown from an inoculum in nutrient broth. However, no test points were sterile until the 4.0-μA level, and at 40 μA 2/3 of the test points were sterile at the cathode. There was a brownish discoloration of the medium around the anode at all three current levels, with the greatest discoloration at 40 μA. At 40 μA there was a pH shift of +2.5 units at both positive and negative poles, with gas formation evident only at the negative. Thus *C. krusei* was inhibited at a higher current level at the Ag anode when the inoculum was prepared in Sabouraud medium.

Quantitative studies. Since copper, zinc, and titanium showed no significant killing at the current levels used, attention was focused primarily on the inhibitory and fungicidal properties of the anodically released silver. The quantitative studies confirm the results obtained in the qualitative experiments using electrically generated silver ions.

The MIC and MFC of silver for six yeasts are summarized in Table 2. All data are averages of two or three experiments. All organisms were inhibited by a silver concentration of 4.7 μg/ml or less, and the fungicidal concentration of silver was as low as 1.9 μg/ml. These values were generally lower than the values reported for other silver compounds against *Candida* (1, 5, 12).

TABLE 2. *MICs and MFCs of electrically generated silver for some yeasts in nutrient broth*

Organism	Anodic Ag (μg/ml)	
	MIC[a]	MFC[b]
Candida parapsilosis	4.7	—[c]
C. pseudotropicalis	2.4	4.0
Torulopsis glabrata	1.6	2.6
C. tropicalis	1.0	—[c]
C. albicans I	0.5	1.9
C. albicans II	3.5	13.8

[a] A 0.5-ml portion (10^4 to 10^6 organisms) was added to the twofold serial dilution of silver-treated broth. The MIC was interpreted as the lowest concentration of Ag not associated with turbidity after the control tube appeared turbid at 37°C (between 4 and 50 h).

[b] A 0.5-ml portion was removed from the nonturbid tubes and mixed with a tube of agar. The MFC was defined as the minimum concentration of Ag at which all yeast cells were killed.

[c] Silver concentration greater than 15 μg/ml.

DISCUSSION

Golubovich completely interrupted the growth of *C. utilis* (10^6 cells/ml) with 4.7 μg of $AgNO_3$ per ml (5). Our findings show that electrically produced silver not only stops growth at concentrations below that used by Golubovich but also kills some species of *Candida* in the same range and without nitrate.

Avakyan (1) reported that silver (in the form of $AgNO_3$), in comparison to other heavy metals, was the most toxic to yeasts and bacteria. But overall the yeasts were less sensitive to the action of the heavy metals than the bacteria. Our results with yeasts show that their MIC and some MFC values are in the same range as those reported for 16 bacterial species (4). Thus, electrically released silver-ion therapy seems to be just as effective against some unicellular eucaryotic organisms as with procaryotic ones. Wlodkowski (12), using *C. albicans* isolates, reported an MIC of 100 μg/ml with Ag-sulfadiazine, and only 2% of the isolates had an MIC lower than 3.12 μg/ml. With the method reported here the MIC has been found to be 4.7 μg/ml or less for all six organisms tested so far in nutrient broth.

The data reported here illustrate that the use of silver wire in conjunction with low electrical current is more effective for inhibiting and killing yeasts than other contemporary silver compounds in use. The effectiveness of anodic silver against *Candida* even compares favorably with its inhibition of relatively resistant bacterial organisms. We have tested, for example, two strains of *Enterobacter cloacae* (7779 and 7780, gifts of H. S. Rosenkranz) that were isolated from a burn ward in which Ag-sulfadiazine was used. These two organisms had an MIC of 400 μg/ml with Ag-sulfadiazine (10). In tests with anodic Ag, the MICs obtained for the same two organisms were less than 3.0 μg of Ag per ml.

There is now strong evidence in the literature that the active component of any silver compound is the silver itself (5, 8, 9, 11). Our results confirm these findings, since they show the action of killing yeast residues specifically at the anode (+) where silver ions are produced. Whether we are dealing with just free silver ions or some electrochemical silver complex has yet to be determined. The data show that electrically generated silver cations are more effective than silver sulfadiazine or silver nitrate.

ACKNOWLEDGMENTS

We are grateful to Jack TerBeek and his staff at the Ritter Co., Rochester, N.Y., for support of this work and for supplying the constant current generators. We also thank the Clinical Laboratory, Upstate Medical Center, Syracuse, N.Y., for providing the yeast cultures.

This work was supported by Veterans Administration research grant no. 0865-01 and by a grant from the Ritter Co., Division of Sybron Corp.

LITERATURE CITED

1. **Avakyan, Z. A.** 1967. Comparative toxicity of heavy metals for certain microorganisms. Microbiology 36:366–369.
2. **Bailey, W. R., and E. G. Scott.** 1974. Determination of susceptibility of bacteria to antimicrobial agents, p. 316–317. *In* Diagnostic microbiology. The C.V. Mosby Co., St. Louis.
3. **Barranco, S. D., J. A. Spadaro, T. J. Berger, and R. O. Becker.** 1974. *In vitro* effect of weak direct current on *Staphylococcus aureus*. Clin. Orthop. Relat. Res. 100:250–255.
4. **Berger, T. J., J. A. Spadaro, S. E. Chapin, and R. O. Becker.** 1976. Electrically generated silver ions: quantitative effects on bacterial and mammalian cells. Antimicrob. Agents Chemother. 9:357–358.
5. **Golubovich, V. W., and I. L. Rabotnova.** 1974. Kinetics of growth inhibition in *Candida utilis* by silver ions. Microbiology 43:948–950.
6. **Lukens, R. J.** 1971. Structure-activity relationship, p. 76–90. *In* A. Kleinzellar, G. F. Springer, and H. G. Wittmann (ed.), Molecular biology, biochemistry and biophysics, vol. 10. Chemistry of fungicidal action. Springer-Verlag, New York.
7. **Martin, H.** 1969. The distribution of fungicidal activity over the periodic system, p. 101–107. *In* D. C. Torgeson (ed.), Fungicides, vol. 11. Chemistry and physiology. Academic Press Inc., New York.
8. **Modak, S. M., and C. L. Fox, Jr.** 1973. Binding of silver sulfadiazine to the cellular components of *Pseudomonas aeruginosa*. Biochem. Pharmacol. 22:2391–2404.
9. **Rosenkranz, H. S., and H. S. Carr.** 1972. Silver sulfadiazine: effect on the growth and metabolism of bacteria. Antimicrob. Agents Chemother. 2:367–372.
10. **Rosenkranz, H. S., J. E. Coward, T. J. Wlodkowski, and H. S. Carr.** 1974. Properties of silver sulfadiazine-resistant *Enterobacter cloacae*. Antimicrob. Agents Chemother. 5:199–201.
11. **Spadaro, J. A., T. J. Berger, S. D. Barranco, S. E. Chapin, and R. O. Becker.** 1974. Antibacterial effects of silver electrodes with weak direct current. Antimicrob. Agents Chemother. 6:637–642.
12. **Wlodkowski, T. J., and H. S. Rosenkranz.** 1973. Antifungal activity of silver sulfadiazine. Lancet ii:739–740.

ANTIMICROBIAL AGENTS AND CHEMOTHERAPY, Nov. 1976, p. 861-863 Vol. 10, No. 5

Printed in U.S.A.

NOTES

Preparation of Isolated Intestinal Villi Useful for Studying Hydrolysis Rates of Penicillin and Cephalosporin Esters

WALTER E. WRIGHT* AND VERLE D. LINE

The Lilly Research Laboratories, Indianapolis, Indiana 46206

Received for publication 27 July 1976

A method for the preparation of freeze-dried intestinal villi from hamsters and mice is described. The villi, consisting largely of epithelial cells rich in esterase activity, are useful for hydrolysis studies of penicillin and cephalosporin esters.

Esterification of the carboxyl group of certain cephalosporins and penicillins often results in increases in oral absorption of the parent drug (1, 3). Almost complete hydrolysis of the ester function can occur during oral absorption in vivo, especially during passage through the intestinal wall (1). Since the intact ester does not possess antibacterial activity, it is often neces-

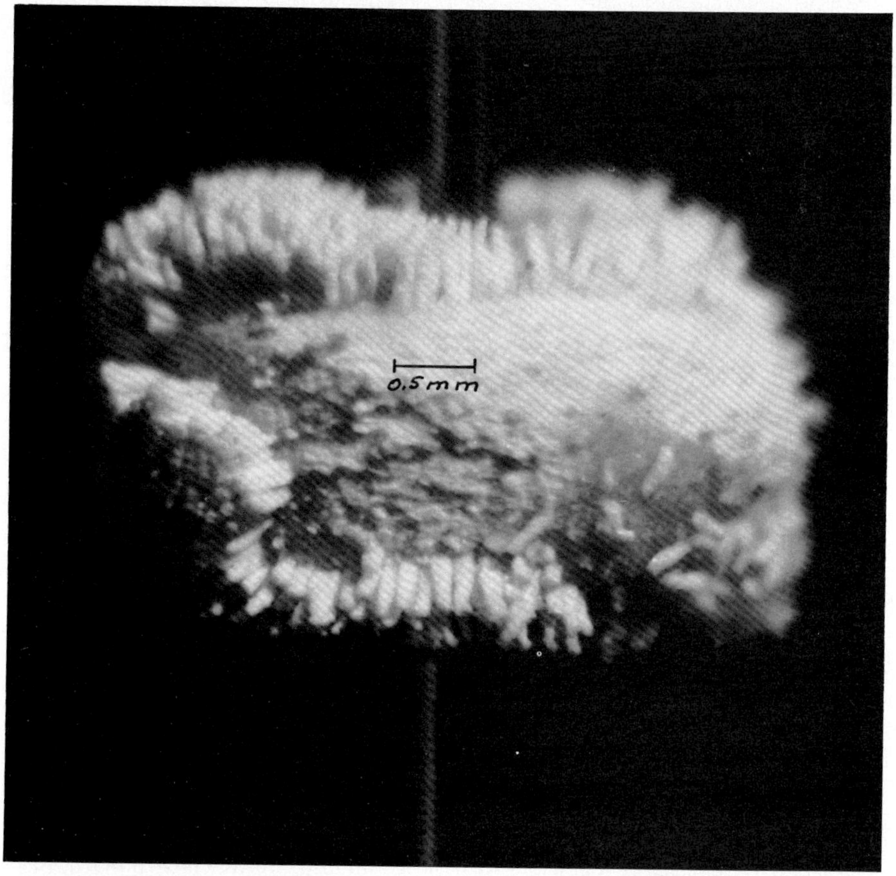

FIG. 1. *Freeze-dried intestinal tissue from a hamster, showing both an area brushed free of villi and areas with villi still attached. Note the uniform manner in which the villi break free from the underlying nonvillus tissue.*

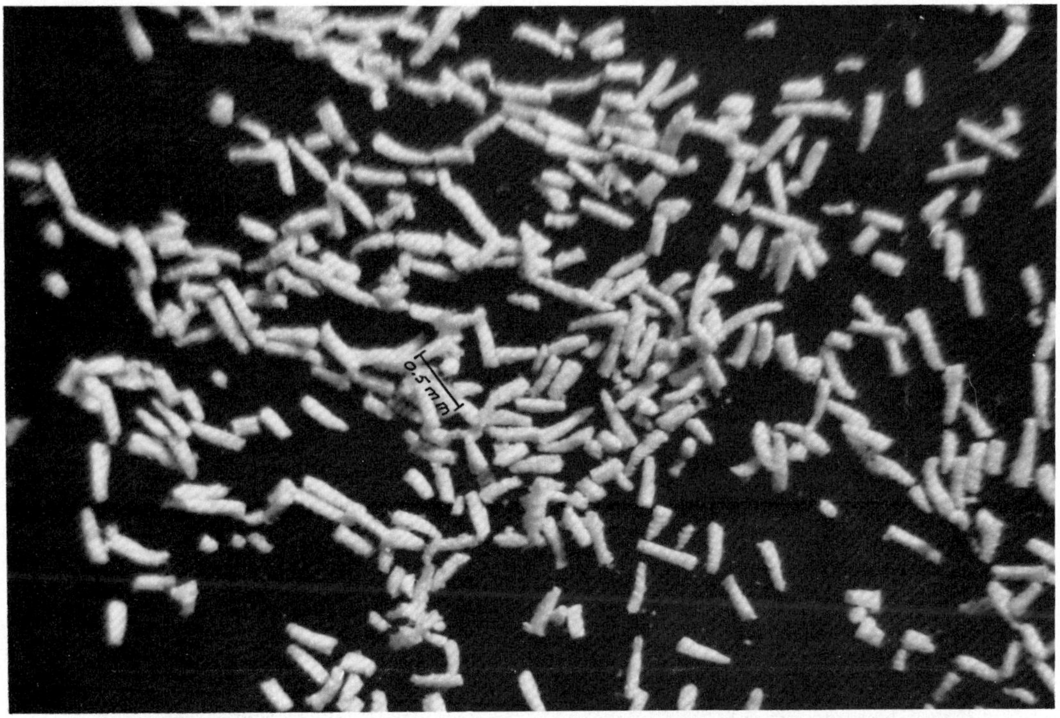

FIG. 2. *Freeze-dried villi removed from the piece of hamster intestinal tissue shown in Fig. 1.*

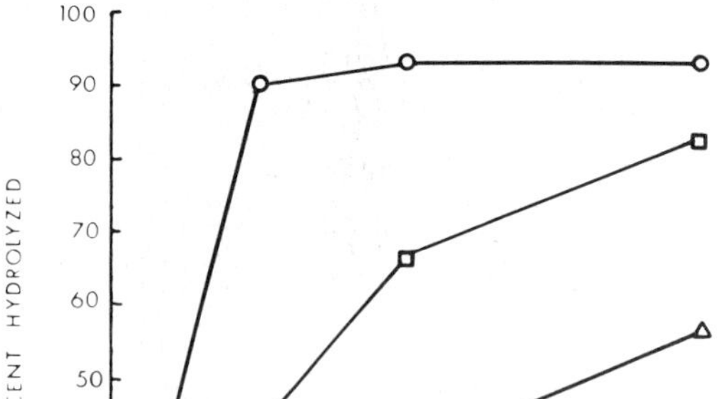

FIG. 3. *Hydrolysis of pivampicillin by freeze-dried hamster intestinal villi. Conditions: 0.1 M sodium phosphate buffer, pH 6.0, 37.5°C, pivampicillin, 20 μg/ml, with dried hamster villi at 0.05 (△), 0.1 (□), or 1.0 (○) mg/ml of incubation solution. One-hour control incubations showed less than 6% hydrolysis in the absence of villi.*

sary to hydrolyze the ester group in vitro for purposes of bioassay or purity determination. In addition, it would be useful to have an esterase preparation with some degree of stability and reproducibility for comparing in vitro hydrolysis rates within a series of esters. The epithelial layer of the small intestine is rich in esterase activity. The following describes the preparation of isolated intestinal villi containing a high fraction of epithelial cells and having utility for the hydrolysis of esters in vitro.

Unfasted male hamsters [Eng:ELS(SYR)] ranging from 120 to 140 g were anesthetized with ether, and the entire small intestine was removed by cutting along the mesentery next to the serosal wall. The distal one-fifth of the intestine was discarded. The contents were removed from the remaining four-fifths of the intestine by washing through with several volumes of iced Krebs-Ringer bicarbonate buffer previously gassed with 95% O_2-5% CO_2 (2). The washed intestine was placed under fresh buffer in a shallow tray and everted (4) on a glass rod. While keeping the intestine under the buffer, the intestine was cut in sections about 0.5 mm long and immediately pooled in a sintered-glass funnel containing iced buffer aerated through the funnel stem from below with the gas mixture. The spontaneous contraction of the serosal musculature causes the sections to form round or oval shapes with the villi extended. These intestinal pieces were immersed and frozen without delay in Krebs-Ringer bicarbonate buffer and freeze dried under vacuum. The dried tissue pieces were transferred to clean vials. Gentle tapping of the vials on a solid surface removed the light, powdery buffer from the dried tissue pieces. The pieces were again transferred to clean vials for the separation of the villi. Under a low-power dissecting microscope, the dry brittle villi were brushed off the surface of the piece with a microspatula or a flattened wire (Fig. 1). It was sometimes helpful to impale the pieces on a fine stiff wire to steady them during villi removal. The denuded nonvillus portions, which consisted of the crypt region, submucosa, vascular tissue, muscular layers, serosa, and mesentery, were discarded. A single hamster intestine usually yielded from 100 to 150 mg of dried villi (Fig. 2), representing about one-third of the total weight of the intact dried intestine. The yield of villi depends on the weight of the animal and the thoroughness of removal of the villi from the underlying tissue. Depending on the anatomical site from which it is removed, the mass of a single villus will consist of between 50 and 75% epithelial cells. This estimate was made by separate histological studies of normal intestinal tissue sections.

Mice can also serve as a source of intestinal villi but, because of their small size relative to hamsters, are not as convenient to use and the yield of villi is smaller. Although rats could be used as a source of epithelial tissue, the short, blunt shape of the villi makes them difficult to separate from the rest of the intestinal tissue. Krebs-Ringer bicarbonate buffer is the buffer of choice because, when dry, it is powdery and falls free from the tissue. Many other buffers dry as a glass and adhere to the tissue.

The ability of freeze-dried hamster villi to hydrolyze an ampicillin ester is shown in Fig. 3. Pivampicillin (3) was incubated in the presence of varying concentrations of the villi. Periodic samples were removed, and the enzymatic reaction was quenched with 39 volumes of anhydrous methanol. The methanol solutions with the partially hydrolyzed ester were assayed for free ampicillin by a disk plate method against *Sarcina lutea* ATCC 9341, using conventional techniques. The ability of the quench procedure to satisfactorily block further enzymatic hydrolysis is apparent from the minimal hydrolysis of the zero-time samples. These samples show that by proper selection of enzyme (villi) and substrate concentrations, one can either gather data suitable for enzyme-substrate kinetic studies or effect complete hydrolysis for assay purposes.

Preparations of hamster and mouse intestinal villi are currently being used to study the hydrolysis of a series of cephalosporin esters in an attempt to correlate such behavior with oral absorption performance. Whereas these isolated villi are useful as an enzyme source, they are not suitable as a preparation for studying intestinal absorption directly since freeze drying disrupts the structural integrity of the epithelial cell layer.

LITERATURE CITED

1. **Binderup, E., W. O. Godtfredsen, and K. Roholt.** 1971. Orally active cephalosporin esters. J. Antibiot. **24**:767–773.
2. **Umbreit, W. W., R. H. Burris, and J. F. Stauffer.** 1972. Manometric and biochemical techniques, 5th ed., p. 146. Burgess Publishing Co., Minneapolis.
3. **von Daehne, W., W. O. Godtfredsen, K. Roholt, and L. Tybring.** 1971. Pivampicillin, a new orally active ampicillin ester, p. 431–437. Antimicrob. Agents Chemother. 1970.
4. **Wilson, T. H., and G. Wiseman.** 1954. The use of sacs of everted small intestine for the study of the transference of substances from the mucosal to the serosal surface. J. Physiol. **123**:116–125.

ANTIMICROBIAL AGENTS AND CHEMOTHERAPY, Nov. 1976, p. 864-865 Vol. 10, No. 5

Sisomicin Versus Netilmicin: In Vitro Susceptibility Testing

D. J. FLOURNOY

Laboratory Service, Clinical Microbiology Section, Veterans Administration Hospital, Oklahoma City, Oklahoma 73104

Received for publication 2 July 1976

Antimicrobial susceptibility to sisomicin and netilmicin (Sch 20569) was determined on 164 clinical isolates using a broth microdilution method. Sisomicin was active against 86.1%, and netilmicin against 96.4%, of the isolates. In addition, netilmicin was active against 93.7% of the strains that were resistant to gentamicin, kanamycin, tobramycin, and sisomicin.

Gentamicin is used often in the treatment of bacterial infections. Two significant factors can be associated with gentamicin usage: the increased occurrence of resistant strains and toxicity. These factors have stimulated studies on new drugs that could potentially replace gentamicin or be used whenever gentamicin cannot. This study compared the susceptibility of clinical isolates to two new aminoglycosides, sisomicin and netilmicin. Netilmicin is a semisynthetic derivative of sisomicin, which is produced by *Micromonospora inyoensis*. Netilmicin and sisomicin closely resemble gentamicin in molecular structure.

The organisms studied were initial clinical isolates identified by conventional methods in the clinical microbiology section of the Oklahoma City Veterans Administration Hospital.

Antibiotic powders of sisomicin and netilmicin were donated by the Schering Corp. Antimicrobial disks, used for agar diffusion testing, were obtained commercially.

Minimal inhibitory concentrations (MICs) were determined by a broth microdilution method. Mueller-Hinton broth (Difco) was used as the diluent. The final volume in each microtiter plate well was 0.1 ml. Microtiter plates were incubated for 16 to 18 h at 35°C after inoculation. The MIC was taken as the highest dilution of antimicrobial in which no visible growth appeared. MICs of 4 μg or less per ml were considered as indicative of susceptibility for sisomicin and netilmicin. Disk agar diffusion studies were performed by the method of Bauer et al. (1).

Table 1 notes the MICs performed on 156 isolates. The median MICs for sisomicin and netilmicin were similar for most isolates except *Serratia marcescens* and *Proteus* sp. other than *Proteus mirabilis*. Netilmicin was significantly more active in the former group. The following isolates were not mentioned in Table 1: two strains of *Micrococcus* sp., two *Pseudomonas* sp., one *Citrobacter freundii*, one *Providencia* sp., and two *Acinetobacter calcoaceticus*. Their range of susceptibility was from 4 to $\leq$0.125 μg/ml.

Disk diffusion susceptibility studies on 164 isolates showed: gentamicin (88.5% susceptible), kanamycin (58.8%), tobramycin (86.7%), and sisomicin (89.1%). Susceptibility testing results to gentamicin and sisomicin were identical in 161 (97.5%) of the isolates. Sixteen isolates were resistant to gentamicin, kanamycin, tobramycin, and sisomicin. Fifteen of these strains were resistant to sisomicin and susceptible to netilmicin as determined by MIC studies (Table 2). One isolate, *Proteus rettgeri* F21, was resistant to both sisomicin and netilmicin. This isolate was susceptible to amikacin as determined by disk agar diffusion testing. Twelve of the sixteen strains were isolated from urinary tract sources.

The similarity of gentamicin and sisomicin has been previously mentioned (2, 5, 8, 9). However, netilmicin has been reported to be significantly more active than gentamicin against clinical isolates of *Enterobacteriaceae*, *Staphylococcus aureus*, and *Pseudomonas aeruginosa* (6). Another study (4) showed netilmicin to be effective against gentamicin-resistant *Enterobacteriaceae*. This report discloses netilmicin to be significantly more active than sisomicin. These differences in activity appear to be the result of distinct enzymes. Kabins et al. (4) found that gentamicin-resistant organisms possess an aminoglycoside-adenylating enzyme, whereas netilmicin resistance was associated with an acetylating enzyme. They also reported that *Proteus* sp. have an acetylating enzyme, which may explain (Table 2) higher MICs for two aminoglycoside-resistant *Proteus rettgeri* in this study. Since the MICs for *Proteus mirabilis* were lower than those for other *Proteus* sp. (Table 1), the presence of acetylating enzymes may differ in the two groups.

This investigation shows *P. aeruginosa* to be susceptible to netilmicin, as determined by

TABLE 1. *Comparison of in vitro activity of sisomicin (S) and netilmicin (N)*

Organism	No. of strains	Drug	MIC, μg/ml	
			Range	Median
Staphylococcus aureus	25	S	≤0.125–0.5	≤0.125
		N	≤0.125–0.5	≤0.125
Staphylococcus epidermidis	6	S	All≤0.125	≤0.125
		N	All≤0.125	≤0.125
Group D enterococcus	8	S	1–8	8
		N	2–8	4
Pseudomonas aeruginosa	29	S	≤0.125–1	≤0.125
		N	≤0.125–2	0.25
Escherichia coli	30	S	≤0.125–128	0.25
		N	≤0.125–2	0.25
Klebsiella pneumoniae	16	S	All≤0.125	≤0.125
		N	≤0.125–0.25	≤0.125
Enterobacter	14[a]	S	≤0.125–32	≤0.125
		N	≤0.125–1	≤0.125
Serratia marcescens	7	S	≤0.125–>128	32
		N	≤0.125–2	0.25
Proteus mirabilis	14	S	≤0.125–4	0.25
		N	≤0.125–2	0.50
Proteus, other	7[b]	S	≤0.125–64	0.50
		N	≤0.125–16	4

[a] Includes nine *Enterobacter aerogenes*, two *E. agglomerans*, and three *E. cloacae* isolates.
[b] Includes one *Proteus morganii*, four *P. rettgeri*, and two *P. vulgaris* isolates.

TABLE 2. *MICs of aminoglycoside-resistant isolates*

Isolate	MIC, μg/ml	
	Sisomicin	Netilmicin
Escherichia coli H4	16.0	0.5
Enterobacter aerogenes D6	32.0	1.0
Serratia marcescens B8	128.0	2.0
E. coli C9	16.0	1.0
S. marcescens E9	128.0	1.0
Proteus rettgeri F9	32.0	4.0
Enterobacter agglomerans		0.5
A10	16.0	0
E. coli E12	16.0	≤0.125
S. marcescens C14	32.0	0.25
S. marcescens F15	32.0	0.25
E. agglomerans A17	16.0	≤0.125
E. coli C17	32.0	0.5
E. cloacae A20	16.0	0.5
P. rettgeri F21	64.0	16.0
S. marcescens A24	>128.0	2.0
E. coli G24	128.0	1.0

broth dilution studies. Kabins et al. (4) noted a higher degree of *P. aeruginosa* susceptibility when MICs were done in broth than agar. Which is the most representative method relating to in vivo activity? Is *P. aeruginosa* generally susceptible or resistant to netilmicin in vivo? Two reports (3, 7) have suggested that MICs performed in agar are more clinically significant due to the greater similarity of cation concentration between agar and serum than broth and serum. In vivo studies involving *P. aeruginosa* infections would help to answer these questions.

This investigation was supported by a grant from the Schering Corp.

LITERATURE CITED

1. **Bauer, A. W., W. M. M. Kirby, J. C. Sherris, and M. Turck.** 1966. Antibiotic susceptibility testing by a standardized single disc method. Am. J. Clin. Pathol. 45:493–496.
2. **Crowe, C. C., and E. Sanders.** 1973. Sisomicin: evaluation in vitro and comparison with gentamicin and tobramycin. Antimicrob. Agents Chemother. 3:24–28.
3. **Gilbert, D. N., E. Kutscher, P. Ireland, J. A. Barnett, and J. P. Sanford.** 1971. Effect of the concentrations of magnesium and calcium on the *in vitro* susceptibility of *Pseudomonas aeruginosa* to gentamicin. J. Infect. Dis. 124(Suppl.):S37–S45.
4. **Kabins, S. A., C. Nathan, and S. Cohen.** 1976. In vitro comparison of netilmicin, a semisynthetic derivative of sisomicin, and four other aminoglycoside antibiotics. Antimicrob. Agents Chemother. 10: 139–145.
5. **Levison, M. E., and D. Kaye.** 1974. In vitro comparison of four aminoglycoside antibiotics: sisomicin, gentamicin, tobramycin, and BB-K8. Antimicrob. Agents Chemother. 5:667–669.
6. **Rahal, J. J., M. S. Simberkoff, K. Kagan, and N. H. Moldover.** 1976. Bactericidal efficacy of Sch 20569 and amikacin against gentamicin-sensitive and -resistant organisms. Antimicrob. Agents Chemother. 9:595–599.
7. **Reller, L. B., F. D. Schoenknecht, M. A. Kenny, and J. C. Sherris.** 1974. Antibiotic susceptibility testing of *Pseudomonas aeruginosa*: selection of a control strain and criteria for magnesium and calcium content in media. J. Infect. Dis. 130:454–463.
8. **Waitz, J. A., E. L. Moss, C. G. Drube, and M. J. Weinstein.** 1972. Comparative activity of sisomicin, gentamicin, kanamycin, and tobramycin. Antimicrob. Agents Chemother. 2:431–436.
9. **Young, L. S., and W. L. Hewitt.** 1973. Activity of five aminoglycoside antibiotics in vitro against gram-negative bacilli and *Staphylococcus aureus*. Antimicrob. Agents Chemother. 4:617–625.

ANTIMICROBIAL AGENTS AND CHEMOTHERAPY, Nov. 1976, p. 866-867 Vol. 10, No. 5

Printed in U.S.A.

Stability of Gentamicin in Serum

SUE M. JONES, DONNA J. BLAZEVIC, AND HENRY H. BALFOUR, JR.*

Department of Laboratory Medicine and Pathology and Department of Pediatrics, University of Minnesota, Minneapolis, Minnesota 55455

Received for publication 1 July 1976

Patients' sera were divided into three portions when the initial gentamicin level was determined and were stored at −20, 4, and 25°C in plastic or glass tubes. Gentamicin levels were repeated after 1 and 2 days of storage at the respective temperatures. There was no significant difference in gentamicin levels among portions, except those from a patient in renal failure with high serum concentrations of carbenicillin.

Because of practical problems our laboratory has been concerned with the stability of gentamicin in serum samples during storage. It is not always possible in a clinical laboratory to perform a gentamicin level determination on a serum sample at the time it is received. This study was undertaken to determine whether storage of serum samples at various temperatures in either glass or plastic vials would affect the gentamicin level.

Serum samples for gentamicin determinations were tested shortly after receipt in the laboratory and then were divided into three portions. The portions were placed at random in either glass (Kimble) or plastic (Falcon) tubes and were stored at −20, 4, and 25°C. The gentamicin determinations were repeated on these samples 1 and 2 days after collection. Thus, seven determinations were done on each specimen: a level of fresh serum and levels after 1 and 2 days of storage at −20, 4, and 25°C. The levels were measured by a rapid gentamicin disk diffusion bioassay using a multiple-antibiotic-resistant strain of *Klebsiella pneumoniae* (ATCC 27799) (2).

Forty-four specimens from 33 patients were tested. Seven of the 44 specimens were exhausted before all seven separate determinations could be performed. Eight of the patients (14 samples) were receiving only gentamicin, whereas the other patients were receiving multiple antibiotics (Table 1).

The gentamicin levels at 0, 1, and 2 days were compared using the statistical paired comparisons method (1). In this method the individual differences of the paired samples were determined for each group (e.g., all values obtained after storage of the sera for 1 day at 4°C in glass tubes were compared with the values obtained on those same fresh sera).

No significant change in the concentration of gentamicin in the groups of paired sera stored at the three temperatures in either glass or plastic containers was found, with one exception. Two separate samples of serum from a patient with renal failure who had carbenicillin levels >500 μg/ml showed a decrease in gentamicin level after 1 day of storage at room temperature and a decrease at all temperatures after 2 days of storage (Table 2).

It has been previously reported by McLaughlin and Reeves (3) and Riff and Jackson

TABLE 1. *Antibiotics administered to patients in study*

Antibiotics	Patients	Samples
Gentamicin only	8	14
Gentamicin +		
Carbenicillin	1	2
Chloramphenicol, cephalothin, nystatin	1	2
Methicillin, nystatin, sulfisoxazole	1	1
Ampicillin	3	3
Clindamycin	5	7
Cephalothin	10	11
Methicillin	1	1
Nystatin	1	1
Neomycin	1	1
Penicillin G	1	1

TABLE 2. *Gentamicin levels in sera of renal failure patient receiving gentamicin and carbenicillin*

Original gentamicin result[a]	Day 1			Day 2		
	−20°C	4°C	25°C	−20°C	4°C	25°C
5.8	4.8	5.8	<2	3.8	2.5	<2
6.6	7.0	5.3	2.0	4.9	4.0	<2

[a] Concentration of gentamicin expressed in micrograms per milliliter.

(4) that large doses of carbenicillin in patients with normal renal function or moderate doses in patients in renal failure can significantly inactivate gentamicin. Riff and Jackson found that the rate of inactivation is influenced by the relative concentration of the two drugs, the fluid into which they are placed, and the temperature. In serum, they found the half-life of gentamicin with carbenicillin to be 24 h.

The presence of other antibiotics did not affect the results of gentamicin determinations.

In conclusion, sera for gentamicin levels may be stored for 1 to 2 days in either glass or plastic tubes with no significant change in the levels, except those from patients expected to have high serum levels of carbenicillin. In such cases, the sera for gentamicin levels either should be tested immediately or be stored at −20°C for no longer than 1 day. It may also be possible to inactivate the carbenicillin by addition of beta-lactamase; however, that was not evaluated in the present study.

We want to thank A. L. Fox who originally suggested that this study be performed. This study was supported in part by Public Health Service grant HL06314 from the National Heart and Lung Institute.

LITERATURE CITED

1. **Daniel, W. W.** 1974. Biostatistics – a foundation for analysis in the health sciences, p. 163–166. John Wiley & Sons, New York.
2. **Lund, M. E., D. J. Blazevic, and J. M. Matsen.** 1974. Rapid gentamicin bioassay using a multiple-antibiotic-resistant strain of *Klebsiella pneumoniae*. Antimicrob. Agents Chemother. 4:569–573.
3. **McLaughlin, J. E., and D. S. Reeves.** 1971. Clinical and laboratory evidence for inactivation of gentamicin by carbenicillin. Lancet i:261–264.
4. **Riff, L. J., and G. G. Jackson.** 1972. Laboratory and clinical conditions for gentamicin inactivation by carbenicillin. Arch. Intern. Med. 130:887–891.

ANTIMICROBIAL AGENTS AND CHEMOTHERAPY, Dec. 1976, p. 869–871 Vol. 10, No. 6

Printed in U.S.A.

Reevaluation of the Disk Diffusion Method for Sulfonamide Susceptibility Testing of *Neisseria meningitidis*

SUSAN HAMMERBERG, MELVIN I. MARKS,* AND GERRY WEINMASTER

Departments of Pediatrics (Infectious Diseases) and Microbiology, McGill University-Montreal Children's Hospital Research Institute, Montreal, Quebec H3H 1P3, Canada

Received for publication 30 June 1976

Lack of correlation between quantitative minimal inhibitory concentration (MIC) determinations and disk diffusion susceptibility tests in our laboratory prompted a study to reevaluate the use of the disk diffusion test for sulfonamide susceptibility testing of *Neisseria meningitidis*. One hundred and sixty-three recent clinical isolates of *N. meningitidis* were examined for sulfonamide susceptibility by the agar dilution and disk diffusion methods. Optimal inocula for each of the tests were determined, and thereafter all disk diffusion tests were compared with quantitative MICs as determined by the agar dilution method using sulfadiazine and an inoculum of 10^6 colony-forming units (CFU)/ml. The clearest and most reproducible zone diameters were obtained with a 10^7-CFU/ml inoculum in the disk diffusion test. There was complete correlation between the disk zone diameters for 300-μg disks of sulfadiazine and sulfathiazole and the agar dilution test MICs. All isolates with a zone diameter of <20 mm were resistant to sulfadiazine, whereas those with zone diameters of ≥30 mm were susceptible. False susceptible and false resistant readings were obtained with 300-μg sulfisoxazole disks. These data suggest that inocula and type of sulfonamide are critical factors in the disk diffusion test for meningococcal susceptibility testing. Sulfonamide disks are not interchangeable for susceptibility testing of meningococci.

Disagreements between quantitative minimal inhibitory concentrations (MICs) and disk diffusion susceptibilities for sulfonamide testing of *Neisseria meningitidis* were noted on several occasions in our laboratory. This prompted the present study to reevaluate selected technical aspects of the disk diffusion method for estimation of sulfonamide susceptibility of *N. meningitidis*. Inaccuracies in these results may be reflected clinically by inappropriate use of chemoprophylactic agents in meningococcal carriers and occasionally by therapeutic errors, and may influence certain epidemiological observations.

MATERIALS AND METHODS

Bacteria. One hundred and sixty-three recent clinical isolates of *N. meningitidis* were tested for sulfonamide susceptibility by agar dilution and disk diffusion methods. These bacteria were isolated from contacts and index cases of meningococcal meningitis and/or bacteremia and stored in sheep blood at −70°C. Serogroups were as follows: group A, 25; group B, 58; group C, 42; group Y, 9; group 29e, 6; group X, 3; and 20 were not typed.

Media. Mueller-Hinton agar (Difco) (Ca^{2+}, 7.0 mg/100 ml; Mg^{2+}, 3.6 mg/100 ml) and Mueller-Hinton broth (Difco) were used for all agar dilution and disk diffusion tests. Sheep blood agar plates were used for subculture of isolates from frozen sheep blood.

Antimicrobial agents. Disks (300 μg) of sulfadiazine, sulfathiazole, and sulfisoxazole (Difco) were tested. Sulfadiazine was provided in powder form by May and Baker Canada Ltd. A stock solution of 800 mg/100 ml was prepared and used immediately for preparation of the agar dilution plates.

Agar dilution tests. Square petri dishes (100 by 15 mm; Falcon) were prepared within 48 h of testing by combining twofold dilutions of sulfadiazine (0.5 ml) with 9.5 ml of Mueller-Hinton agar, yielding test combinations of 40 to 0.009 mg of sulfadiazine per 100 ml. The inoculum was prepared by swabbing sufficient growth from a pure blood agar culture into 10 ml of Mueller-Hinton broth to produce an optical density of 0.13 to 0.15 at 625 nm in a Coleman Junior spectrophotometer. This standard, and suspensions prepared by eye comparison, yielded viable bacterial counts of approximately 10^8 colony-forming units (CFU)/ml (MacFarland no. 1 turbidity standard can be used as an alternative to the spectrophotometric standard providing it is prepared on a biyearly basis or when clumping is noted). A 10^{-2} dilution of this inoculum was placed in a Steers replicator, and the plates were inoculated and dried at room temperature (3). Plates were read after incubation in 5% CO_2 at 37°C for 16 to 20 h. MIC was defined as the lowest concentration of drug giving an 80% (or sudden) reduction in surface growth of bacteria.

Disk diffusion test. Round petri dishes (100 by 15

mm; Fisher) were prepared with a uniform agar depth of 4 mm and placed in the incubator for 30 min before inoculation. The plates were inoculated with a swab dipped into a 10^{-1} dilution of the standard inoculum (described above), giving a colony count of approximately 10^7 CFU/ml. The swab was squeezed on the side of the tube to remove excess fluid and then streaked on the plate in four directions. After drying for 3 to 5 min, disks were applied and the plates were inverted and incubated in 5% CO_2 at 37°C for 16 to 20 h. The zone diameter was measured with a ruler from the back of the plate, ignoring any haze within the definite margin of inhibition.

RESULTS

Preliminary experiments were carried out to determine suitable inocula for the disk diffusion and agar dilution tests. An inoculum of 10^6 CFU/ml gave the clearest results for the agar dilution test. When an inoculum of 10^7 CFU/ml was used for both the agar dilution and disk diffusion tests, trailing end points occurred, making the interpretation of the exact MIC difficult; several false susceptible disk readings resulted. When 10^6 CFU/ml was used for the disk diffusion test, however, false susceptible results were also encountered. An inoculum of 10^7 CFU/ml produced a preconfluent growth on the surface of the agar as well as two clearly distinguishable populations. Therefore, an inoculum of 10^6 CFU/ml was used for the agar dilution studies, and 10^7 CFU/ml was used for disk diffusion.

Several other parameters were also examined. Incubation of plates in 9% CO_2, 5% CO_2, and a candle jar (approximately 2% CO_2) did not alter the disk or agar dilution test results. Similarly, agar depth (10 ml versus 25 ml) had no effect on agar dilution MICs, and each isolate had the same MIC to sulfadiazine, sulfathiazole, and sulfisoxazole.

A total of 163 recent clinical isolates of *N. meningitidis* were tested for susceptibility with sulfathiazole disks, and the results were correlated with the MIC to sulfadiazine determined by the agar dilution method (Fig. 1). All 45 isolates with a disk zone diameter of <20 mm were resistant (MIC ≥ 1 mg/100 ml), whereas all 118 isolates with a zone diameter of ≥30 mm were susceptible.

Sixty-nine of these isolates were also tested with 300-μg disks of sulfadiazine and sulfisoxazole, and the arithmetic mean of three determinations was correlated with the sulfadiazine agar dilution MICs (Fig. 2 and 3). Although <20- and >30-mm zone diameters with sulfathiazole and sulfadiazine disks clearly separated the populations into resistant and susceptible, respectively, comparable criteria for sulfisoxazole were <33 and >40 (Fig. 3).

Although zone diameter variations for a single isolate as great as 12 mm were recorded when tests were repeated in triplicate, there was no cross-over from resistant to susceptible populations, or vice versa, with sulfathiazole

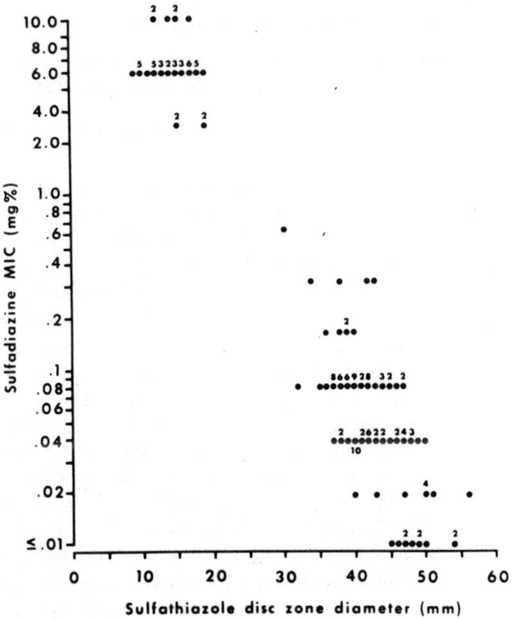

FIG. 1. *Relationship between agar dilution susceptibility to sulfadiazine and zone of inhibition around a 300-μg sulfathiazole disk for 163 recent clinical isolates of N. meningitidis.*

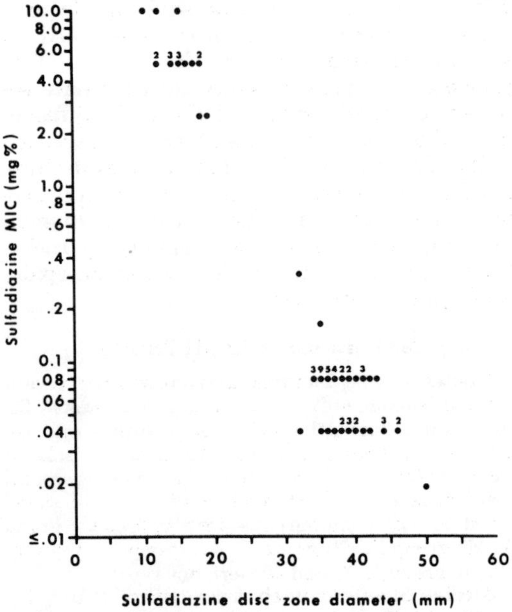

FIG. 2. *Relationship between agar dilution susceptibility to sulfadiazine and inhibition zone around a 300-μg sulfadiazine disk.*

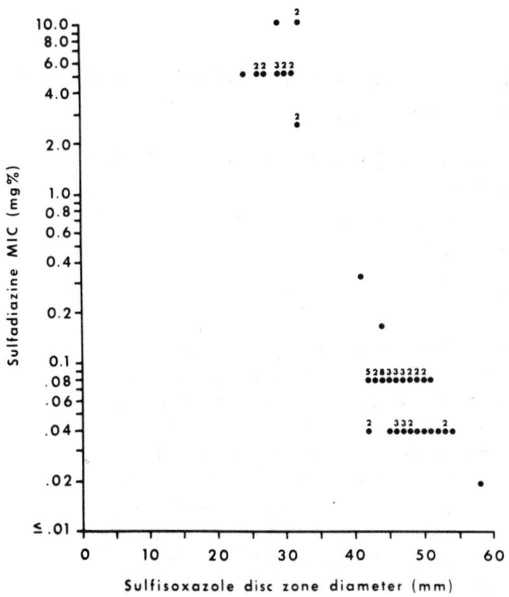

FIG. 3. *Relationship between sulfadiazine agar dilution MIC and 300-μg sulfisoxazole disk zone diameter.*

and sulfadiazine disks. However, several false susceptible and resistant results were noted with repeated sulfisoxazole disk diffusion tests. This is not reflected in Fig. 3 since only the mean zone diameters of three separate experiments are illustrated. Zone diameter variations increased in direct proportion to the size of the zone of inhibition.

DISCUSSION

Our studies confirm the accuracy and reproducibility of the disk diffusion test in predicting resistance and susceptibility of *N. meningitidis* to sulfonamides. The method we used for disk diffusion testing is the same as described by Bennett et al. (1) without the modifications subsequently used by Wiggins et al. (4). A critical difference in our results, however, is the different disk zone criteria for susceptibility and resistance. The disk zone diameters that we found useful in predicting agar dilution MICs for *N. meningitidis* are ≥30 mm = susceptible and <20 mm = resistant, using sulfadiazine and sulfathiazole 300-μg disks and the inocula and other test characteristics described above. Previous publications recommended disk zone diameters of >40 and <30 mm, respectively (1, 4).

The inoculum used in our agar dilution studies was smaller than that described by Bennett et al. (1). We were only able to accurately reproduce clear end points for MIC determinations of *N. meningitidis* with an inoculum of 10^6 CFU/ml. Bennett et al. (1), however, were able to do this with an inoculum of 5×10^7 CFU/ml, whereas Wiggins et al. (4) used a different method of standardizing their inoculum to a McFarland no. 5 tube. These differences are small ones and do not appear to account for the difference in disk zone diameter readings mentioned above. Nevertheless, these results, and those obtained in the disk diffusion studies, illustrate the importance of carefully standardizing the inoculum for use in determining susceptibilities of *N. meningitidis* to sulfonamides.

It has been stated that different sulfonamide preparations are interchangeable for disk susceptibility testing, although this was not specifically tested for *N. meningitidis* (2). In our studies, sulfathiazole and sulfadiazine gave almost identical results; however, sulfisoxazole was less useful, and its use was associated with false readings. There is no ready explanation for this difference in disk activity. Differences in antibacterial activity of the three sulfonamide preparations were ruled out, but diffusion was not evaluated.

As stated by Bennett et al. (1) and Wiggins et al. (4), *N. meningitidis* with zone diameters in the intermediate zone of susceptibility (20 to 30 mm in the test described above) should have their susceptibilities to sulfonamide confirmed by a quantitative method, if clinically indicated. It is clear that certain technical aspects of meningococcal susceptibility testing are critical, and any changes in inocula, type of sulfonamide, disk concentration, media, etc., should be evaluated in a careful comparative manner with a quantitative test before introduction into the clinical diagnostic laboratory.

ACKNOWLEDGMENT

Meningococcal typing antisera were kindly provided by Paul Kenny, National Communicable Disease Center, Ottawa. Theodore Eickhoff provided invaluable advice throughout this study.

This work was supported in part by grant 604-7-863, Department of Health and Welfare, Canada.

LITERATURE CITED

1. **Bennett, J. V., H. M. Camp, and T. C. Eickhoff.** 1968. Rapid sulfonamide disc sensitivity test for meningococci. Appl. Microbiol. **16**:1056–1060.
2. **Petersdorf, R. G., and J. C. Sherris.** 1965. Methods and significance of *in vitro* testing of bacterial sensitivity to drugs. Am. J. Med. **39**:766–779.
3. **Steers, E., E. L. Foltz, and B. S. Graves.** 1959. An inocula replicating apparatus for routine testing of bacterial sensitivity testing to antibiotics. Antibiot. Chemother. **9**:307–311.
4. **Wiggins, G. L., J. V. McLaughlin, S. T. Bickman, W. L. Jones, and A. Balows.** 1970. Susceptibility of *Neisseria meningitidis* strains from the civilian population to sulfadiazine, penicillin, and rifampin. Appl. Microbiol. **20**:893–898.

ANTIMICROBIAL AGENTS AND CHEMOTHERAPY, Dec. 1976, p. 872–877 Vol. 10, No. 6

Printed in U.S.A.

Comparison of the Epidemiology of Bacterial Resistance to Mecillinam and Ampicillin

J. D. ANDERSON,* MONICA A. ADAMS, JANE C. BARRINGTON, W. N. SPENCE, AND C. A. SHEPHERD

Infection Control Laboratory, Clifton Hospital, and Department of Biology, University of York, York, YO3 6RD, England*

Received for publication 26 July 1976

Mecillinam is a new type of β-lactam antibiotic (an amidinopenicillanic acid) that is particularly active against *Enterobacteriaceae* and is taken orally as in the form of an ester, pivmecillinam. Assessment of any new antibiotic should include a survey of levels of bacterial resistance and investigation of its capacity to select resistant organisms or harm the commensal flora. Antibiotic resistance patterns of 2,000 *Enterobacteriaceae* isolated from the urine of patients with significant urinary tract infections were therefore determined. Mecillinam-resistant *Enterobacteriaceae* were found to be much less common than ampicillin-amoxycillin-resistant organisms both in the community and in hospital patients. Most ampicillin-resistant *Enterobacteriaceae* from infected urines were susceptible to mecillinam, but the relatively rare mecillinam-resistant organisms were usually resistant to ampicillin and cephaloridine. The fecal flora of 26 healthy volunteers who served as controls or were given repeated courses of therapeutic doses of either ampicillin or pivmecillinam was studied. Pivmecillinam had only a transient effect on the aerobic fecal flora and in contrast to ampicillin did not increase populations of resistant *Enterobacteriaceae,* which would be a potential hazard to the patient and contaminate the environment.

Although the development of bacterial resistance has often reduced the benefits of chemotherapy (1, 11), relatively little information is available for clinicians on the effect of specific antibiotics or regimens on the selection of resistant commensals or pathogens. Gram-negative bacteria in the gut are of great importance, since they form a large reservoir from which resistant organisms arising by cross-infection, mutation, or antibiotic resistance (R) factor transfer may be disseminated. Resistant gut bacteria may be selected every time a patient is treated with an antibiotic. These resistant populations present a potential hazard to the patient and increase levels of resistance in the environment. The ideal antibiotic, while effective in curing infection, should not select resistant organisms or harm the commensal flora. There is, therefore, a need to identify effective antibiotics and antibiotic regimens which are least likely to do harm. We have studied the epidemiology of bacterial resistance to a novel antibiotic that may well be used widely in treating urinary tract infections (6, 7, 30, 31) employing antibiotic regimens suitable for these infections.

This drug (mecillinam, a 6β-amidinopenicillanic acid derivative) is a penicillin analogue that is particularly active against gram-negative bacteria and differs from other penicillins and the cephalosporins in that the β-lactam nucleus is linked to the side chain by an amidino instead of an amido group (17). For oral therapy it must be given as its pivavoyloxymethyl ester (pivmecillinam), which is well absorbed and, although lacking antibacterial activity, is rapidly hydrolyzed to mecillinam by blood esterases (23). Although mecillinam has not yet been introduced into general use, its structural resemblance to the cephalosporins and penicillins raises the possibility that these β-lactam antibiotics may have already selected a high level of resistance to mecillinam in bacteria. Furthermore, slow growing, mecillinam-resistant phenotypic variants may arise in vitro when *Enterobacteriaceae* are grown under certain conditions in the presence of mecillinam (12, 17, 18, 29). These variants lose their antibiotic resistance when subcultured in the absence of mecillinam but could be a potential cause of treatment failure in vivo.

MATERIALS AND METHODS

Determination of MICs of antibiotics. Cephaloridine was obtained in the anhydrous form from vials of Ceporin injection (Glaxo Laboratories Ltd.). Ampicillin (as the trihydrate) was a gift from Beecham Research Laboratories Ltd. Mecillinam (as the hydrochloride dihydrate) was a gift from Leo Laboratories Ltd. Oxoid (Oxoid Ltd., Basingstoke, Hants) diagnostic susceptibility test agar (CM 261) was supplemented with 5% saponin-lysed oxalated horse blood for minimal inhibitory concentration (MIC) determinations.

Doubling dilutions of the antibiotics in lysed blood agar (2 to 1,024 μg/ml) were prepared by adding suitable volumes of stock solutions to agar cooled to 45°C. Plates were allowed to dry in a laminar air flow cabinet for 15 min and then inoculated with small volumes (0.002 ml) of a range of dilutions of saline suspensions of bacteria prepared from colonies taken from 18-h agar plate cultures. Bacterial suspensions that were sufficiently dense to form discrete colonies on antibiotic-free control media after incubation at 37°C for 18 h were selected for estimation of MICs.

Survey of urinary *Enterobacteriaceae*. Populations of viable bacteria in all urines submitted to the hospital laboratory with a request for bacteriologic examination were determined by the "calibrated loop" technique on MacConkey agar (CM 7, Oxoid Ltd.). Organisms isolated from infected urines were generally classified by their colonial appearance and by simple biochemical reactions. All mecillinam-resistant organisms and a random selection of 100 other isolates were identified in greater detail (8).

Antibiotic susceptibility patterns of all organisms from significant urinary infections, i.e., catheter specimens containing $\geq 10^3$ organisms per ml and all other specimens containing $\geq 10^5$ cells per ml of a single organism, were determined by the antibiotic paper disk test (method A, reference 28) on Welcotest agar (Wellcombe Foundation Ltd., Beckenham, Kent). Susceptibility to mecillinam was determined with disks provided by Leo Laboratories Ltd. and to other antibiotics with a suitable "polydisc" (Scientific Hospital Supplies Ltd., Liverpool 7). An amoxycillin disk on the polydisc used in our routine laboratory was, for convenience, used to determine the susceptibility of organisms to ampicillin. Beecham Pharmaceuticals Research Division, Brockham Park, Surrey (R. Sutherland, Senior Research Bacteriologist, private communication) recommends that amoxycillin 25-μg disks may be used in routine laboratories to determine the susceptibility of urinary pathogens to both amoxycillin and ampicillin. Furthermore, in an independent survey, susceptibility test results with ampicillin and amoxycillin were the same for 56 out of 57 urinary *Enterobacteriaceae* (5).

Investigation of the aerobic fecal flora. Eight healthy volunteers who served as controls were given no antibiotics. Thirteen others were given 400 mg of pivmecillinam four times daily for 5 days (as pivmecillinam hydrochloride capsules, 200 mg, equivalent to 68% anhydrous mecillinam; Leo Laboratories Ltd.). The majority of these individuals were given a second course of antibiotic and some a third course. Five more volunteers were each given two courses of 250 mg of ampicillin (as Penbritin capsules, Beecham Research Laboratories) four times daily for 5 days.

The aerobic fecal flora for of all volunteers were studied quantitively on MacConkey agar and on MacConkey agar containing either 10 μg of mecillinam per ml or 10 μg of ampicillin per ml (2). Coliforms (lactose-fermenting, bile-tolerant, gram-negative bacilli), non-lactose-fermenting *Enterobacteriaceae, Pseudomonas* spp., and fecal streptococci were enumerated separately. The antibiotic susceptibility patterns of a representative selection of resistant *Enterobacteriaceae* from each plate were confirmed by the antibiotic disk susceptibility test method (28) on Welcotest agar. The ability of the fecal strains of *Proteus* to transfer resistance was determined by a method similar to that used with other antibiotics (2).

RESULTS

Survey of urinary *Enterobacteriaceae*. Antibiotic disk susceptibility tests showed that mecillinam resistance was much less common than ampicillin-amoxycillin resistance both in the community and in hospital patients. Ampicillin-amoxycillin-resistant organisms were usually susceptible to mecillinam, but mecillinam-resistant organisms were usually resistant to these antibiotics and cephaloridine and frequently to other antibiotics (Table 1). Out of a random sample of 100 of the urinary *Enterobacteriaceae,* 85% were *Escherichia coli,* 7% were *Proteus* sp., 5% were *Klebsiella* sp., 3% were *Citrobacter* sp., and 2% were *Enterobacter* sp. In contrast, of the 37 mecillinam-resistant organisms, 59% were *Klebsiella* sp. (all but two isolates were a single serotype of *Klebsiella pneumoniae*), 28% were *Proteus* sp., and 16% were *E. coli*. The majority of mecillinam-resistant organisms had MICs of mecillinam and ampicillin on lysed blood agar medium of >1,024 μg/ml and of between 128 and 256 μg/ml for cephaloridine. The MICs of mecillinam-resistant urinary *Proteus* isolates varied widely on other media.

Effect of therapeutic doses of pivmecillinam upon the fecal flora. Out of 34 specimens of feces obtained from 13 healthy individuals over a period of 9 days, mecillinam-resistant *Enterobacteriaceae* were only found in two samples from a single individual. The fecal flora of these individuals was then monitored during and after a 5-day course of pivmecillinam. There was no significant increase in a mecillinam-resistant *Proteus rettgeri* which had been present before chemotherapy (about 3×10^5/g) in the feces of the single individual, and this organism disappeared within a week after completion of the course. No mecillinam-resistant coliforms or *Proteus* were detected in the feces of any of the remaining 12 individuals who had been treated with this antibiotic.

TABLE 1. *Antibiotic resistance pattern of 2,000 Enterobacteriaceae isolated from patients with significant[a] urinary tract infections in the York Health District*

Source of urine specimens	No. of organisms examined	% Organisms susceptible to all antibiotics tested	% Organisms resistant by the disk antibiotic susceptibility test with disks containing:							
			Mecillinam (10 µg)	Amoxycillin (for ampicillin, 25 µg)	Cephaloridine (25 µg)	Sulphatriad (300 µg)	Trimethoprim (2.5 µg)	Nitrofurantoin (200 µg)	Colistin (10 µg)	Gentamicin (10 µg)
General practice and antenatal patients	705	63.0	0.4	17.7	–	17.3	9.9	5.2	–	0.1
Hospital outpatients	227	53.3	0.4	26.9	–	26.0	9.7	4.0	–	0
Hospital inpatients	1,068	38.4	3.1	37.5	–	27.9	23.9	13.7	–	0.2
All mecillinam-resistant isolates	37	0	100	91.9	78.4	70.3	67.6	35.1	29.7	0

[a] See Materials and Methods for definition of significance.

Eleven of the 13 persons, including the one who had harbored the resistant *Proteus*, were given a second course of pivmecillinam about 3 weeks after completion of the first course, and two were given a third course. Repeated courses of pivmecillinam were given to increase the chances of detecting resistant organisms arising during antibiotic treatment with a regimen intended for urinary infections. No mecillinam-resistant *Enterobacteriaceae* were found in any of the individuals given two or more courses of pivmecillinam. Thus, out of a total of 206 fecal samples from individuals who had received no antibiotics, 100 samples from individuals given ampicillin in the trial described below, and 254 samples from 13 persons given one or more courses of pivmecillinam, the only mecillinam-resistant enterobacteria found was the *P. rettgeri* previously discussed. This organism was sensitive to the common urinary antibiotics other than colistin, and its mecillinam resistance could not be transferred in vitro to a laboratory strain of *E. coli*.

In some individuals, fecal coliform populations fell during treatment with pivmecillinam and then returned to normal levels (Table 2, columns 3 to 5). Although large individual variations in the fecal flora preclude a firm conclusion, pivmecillinam did not appear to select ampicillin-resistant coliforms (Table 2, column 6), *Proteus* sp. or *Pseudomonas* sp., but did transiently increase populations of fecal streptococci, which were resistant to mecillinam (MIC $\geq$ 256 µg/ml).

Changes in the fecal flora in 33 specimens obtained from two individuals given a third course of pivmecillinam resembled the pattern found during the first two courses of treatment with this antibiotic.

Effect of therapeutic doses of ampicillin upon the fecal flora. Small numbers of ampicillin-resistant organisms were found in the feces of five individuals prior to treatment with this agent (Table 2, column 8). The fecal flora of these individuals was then monitored during and after two separate courses of ampicillin in therapeutic amounts. In contrast to pivmecillinam, this antibiotic exerted a strong selection pressure for ampicillin-resistant organisms. These two courses of ampicillin did not appear to have any marked effect upon total populations of coliforms, *Pseudomonas* sp., *Proteus* sp., or fecal streptococci.

Side effects of antibiotics. No adverse effects were noted in any of the five individuals given ampicillin. One individual receiving pivmecillinam complained of persistent mild dyspepsia and declined to take a second course of treatment. A second person complained of

TABLE 2. *Effect of two courses of therapeutic doses of pivmecillinam or ampicillin upon the fecal flora of healthy volunteers*

Time of sampling	Volunteers given pivmecillinam: No. of specimens of feces examined	% of specimens with counts of *Enterobacteriaceae* (per g of feces) of: $<10^4$	10^4–10^6	$>10^6$	Mean % of ampicillin-resistant *Enterobacteriaceae*	Volunteers given ampicillin: No. of specimens of feces examined	Mean % of ampicillin-resistant *Enterobacteriaceae*
Days 1–9	34	0	9	91	<0.1	12	<0.1
During first 5-day course of treatment	37	16	51	32	<0.1	16	55
Days 15–19	32	9	28	63	<0.1	5	56
Days 20–24	20	0	30	70	<0.1	11	12
Days 25–29	16	0	13	87	<0.1	6	0.2
Days 30–34	22	0	9	91	<0.1	8	<0.1
During second 5-day course of treatment	30	43	17	40	<0.1	15	51
Days 40–44	20	40	45	15	2.3	16	72
Days 45–49	19	10	16	74	<0.1	5	0.2
Days 50–54	15	0	20	80	<0.1	6	0.7
Days 55–59	10	0	20	80	<0.1	12	2.5

occasional slight dyspepsia during the first course of treatment but discontinued treatment on day 1 of the second course because of dyspepsia and nausea. A third individual who had suffered with dyspepsia during previous treatment with ampicillin or tetracycline complained of mild occasional dyspepsia during the first course of treatment, but none during the second course when the tablets had been taken with milk or food. Alcoholic drinks may have exacerbated or caused some of the incidents of dyspepsia. No other side effects were noted, and all individuals were questioned to ensure that they had not suffered from rashes or diarrhea and had taken the capsules as directed.

DISCUSSION

Levels of antibiotic resistance in the community and in hospitals influence the primary choice of antibiotic and may determine the outcome of treatment. Populations of resistant organisms tend to increase with antibiotic use (1, 11, 15) and to fall when antibiotics are withdrawn (3, 15, 16, 20, 25). Available evidence indicates that antibiotics differ in their capacity to select resistant organisms, e.g., ampicillin (2, 9, 13, 25) and tetracycline (2, 9, 10, 13, 24, 25), which tend to increase numbers of resistant organisms in the feces, while co-trimoxazole (19, 21, 27) or amoxycillin (25) do not.

In contrast to ampicillin and some other antibiotics, mecillinam resistance was uncommon in fecal and urinary *Enterobacteriaceae* in the present study. Mecillinam-resistant phenotypic variants of susceptible organisms which may be formed under certain conditions in the laboratory (12, 17, 18, 29) were not found in this or in another (14) study of the fecal flora. However, other regimens might have a different effect upon the gut flora, and mecillinam-resistant *Enterobacteriaceae* were found in the feces of 7 out of 12 chronic salmonella carriers who had been given one or more 28-day courses of pivmecillinam. Some of this resistance was multiple and some was R-factor mediated, but all mecillinam-resistant organisms disappeared from the feces within 1 to 4 weeks of completion of treatment (14). Similarly, mecillinam-resistant *Enterobacteriaceae* were found during and after treatment in two out of six patients with acute salmonellosis who had been given pivmecillinam for 14 days (14). These studies with salmonella infections may not be representative of conditions found in the treatment of other infections, and no resistant organisms were found in the urine when pivmecillinam was used in four clinical trials of the treatment of urinary tract infections (6, 7, 30, 31).

The broad spectrum of mecillinam is consistent with experimental evidence that it has a different mode of action (18, 29) and greater resistance to β-lactamases then ampicillin (22, 29).

Although the outcome of therapy depends on factors other than the results of laboratory susceptibility tests, the survey summarized in Table 1 suggests that one may expect pivmecillinam to be effective against the majority of urinary tract infections caused by *Enterobacteriaceae*. Results of these disk susceptibility tests with urinary pathogens are in general agreement with a recent detailed survey of MIC and cidal concentrations of mecillinam for *En-*

terobacteriaceae isolated from hospital patients (22). All mecillinam-resistant *Klebsiella* infections occurred in hospital patients and most took place over a short period of time in catheterized patients in two surgical wards. Most of the resistant organisms had the same antibiogram, and there was other evidence that this relatively high level of resistance in a small number of patients was due to cross-infection by a single strain. As with many other hospital infections, control of cross-infection would appear to be more relevant than chemotherapy.

Therapeutic doses of pivmecillinam appeared to have only a transient effect upon the aerobic fecal flora, which generally returned to normal levels within a week of stopping treatment. No attempts were made to monitor the effect of pivmecillinam upon the anaerobic fecal flora. Although *Bacteroides fragilis* may inhibit antibiotic resistance transfer between coliforms in the laboratory (4), there is no evidence that anaerobes play a direct role in such transfer in the gut. Furthermore, *B. fragilis* has been shown to be resistant to mecillinam (22).

Upper gastrointestinal tract symptoms noted in three individuals in this relatively small investigation have only been reported in one other trial (6) but obviously deserve further consideration.

One cannot exclude the possibility that there will be a slow buildup of resistance when pivmecillinam is used on a larger scale. However, the evidence available so far indicates that if pivmecillinam is used for treating urinary infection, it would be unlikely to produce long-term changes in the fecal flora or promote the development of resistant organisms which might effect the patient or the environment.

ACKNOWLEDGMENTS

We are grateful to R. Warr of York University for his interest. This work was supported by a grant for locally organized clinical research to J.D.A. from the North Yorkshire Area Health Authority and a grant for apparatus from Leo Laboratories Ltd.

LITERATURE CITED

1. **Anderson, E. S.** 1968. The ecology of transferable drug resistance in the enterobacteria. Annu. Rev. Microbiol. 22:131–180.
2. **Anderson, J. D., W. A. Gillespie, and M. H. Richmond.** 1973. Chemotherapy and antibiotic-resistance transfer between enterobacteria in the human gastro-intestinal tract. J. Med. Microbiol. 6:461–473.
3. **Anderson, J. D.** 1974. The effect of R-factor carriage on the survival of *Escherichia coli* in the human intestine. J. Med. Microbiol. 7:85–90.
4. **Anderson, J. D.** 1975. Factors that may prevent transfer of antibiotic resistance between gram-negative bacteria in the gut. J. Med. Microbiol. 8:83–88.
5. **Anderson, J. D., M. Warner, and H. L. Forshaw.** 1975. Studies on the effect of amoxycillin and ampicillin on *Enterobacteriaceae* in an experimental model of urinary infection. J. Antimicrob. Chemother. 1:197–204.
6. **Bentzen, A. J., R. Vejlsgaard, J. Jacobsen, and L. Tybring.** 1975. Clinical evaluation of a novel β-lactam antibiotic: pivmecillinam (FL 1039). Infection 3:154–160.
7. **Christoffersen, J. C., H. G. Iversen, J. Jacobsen, B. Korner, H. K. Petersen, F. Rasmussen, and L. Tybring.** 1974. FL 1039 in bacteriuria following prostatectomy. A double blind comparison with pivampicillin and placebo. Scand. J. Urol. Nephrol. 8:185–192.
8. **Cowan, S. T.** 1974. Cowan and Steel's manual for the identification of medical bacteria, 2nd ed. Cambridge University Press, London.
9. **Datta, N.** 1971. R factors in *Escherichia coli*. Ann. N.Y. Acad. Sci. 182:59–64.
10. **Datta, N., M. C. Faiers, D. S. Reeves, W. Brumfitt, F. Ørskov, and I. Ørskov.** 1971. R factors in *Escherichia coli* in faeces after oral chemotherapy in general practice. Lancet 1:312–315.
11. **Finland, M.** 1971. Changes in susceptibility of selected pathogenic bacteria to widely used antibiotics. Ann. N.Y. Acad. Sci. 182:5–20.
12. **Greenwood, D., H. L. Brooks, R. Gargan, and F. O'Grady.** 1974. Activity of FL 1060, a new β-lactam antibiotic, against urinary tract pathogens. J. Clin. Pathol. 27:192–197.
13. **Jonsson, M.** 1973. Antibiotic resistance and R-factors in gram-negative bacteria isolated in a hospital for infectious diseases. Scand. J. Infect. Dis. 5:41–47.
14. **Jonsson, M., and G. Tunevall.** 1975. FL 1039: a new β-lactam derivative for the treatment of infections with gram-negative bacteria. A clinical evaluation in salmonella patients. Infection 3:31–36.
15. **Lacey, R. W.** 1975. A critical appraisal of the importance of R-factors in the *Enterobacteriaceae in vivo*. J. Antimicrob. Chemother. 1:25–37.
16. **Lowbury, E. J. L., J. R. Babb, and E. Roe.** 1972. Clearance from a hospital of gram-negative bacilli that transfer carbenicillin-resistance to *Pseudomonas aeruginosa*. Lancet 2:941–945.
17. **Lund, F., and L. Tybring.** 1972. 6-β-Amidinopenicillanic acids–a new group of antibiotics. Nature (London) New Biol. 236:135–137.
18. **Matsuhashi, S., T. Kamiryo, P. M. Blumberg, P. Linnett, E. Willoughby, and J. L. Strominger.** 1974. Mechanism of action and development of resistance to a new amidino penicillin. J. Bacteriol. 117:578–587.
19. **Moorehouse, E. C., and W. Farrell.** 1973. Effect of co-trimoxazole on faecal enterobacteria: no emergence of resistant strains. J. Med. Microbiol. 6:249–252.
20. **Price, D. J. E., and J. D. Sleigh.** 1970. Control of infection due to *Klebsiella aerogenes* in a neurosurgical unit by withdrawal of all antibiotics. Lancet 2:1213–1215.
21. **Näff, H.** 1971. Über die Veränderungen der normalen Darmflora des Menschem durch Bactrim. Pathol. Microbiol. 37:1–22.
22. **Neu, H. C.** 1976. Mecillinam, a novel penicillanic acid derivative with unusual activity against gram-negative bacteria. Antimicrob. Agents Chemother. 9:793–799.
23. **Roholt, K., B. Nielsen, and E. Kristensen.** 1975. Pharmacokinetic studies with mecillinam and pivmecillinam. Chemotherapy 21:146–166.
24. **Schmidt, H., E. From, and G. Heydenreich.** 1973. Bacteriological examination of rectal specimens during long-term oxytetracycline treatment for acne vulgaris. Acta Dermatovener (Stockholm). 53:153–156.
25. **Shaw, E. J., N. Datta, G. Jones, F. M. Marr, and W. J.**

B. Froud. 1973. Effect of stay in hospital and oral chemotherapy on the antibiotic sensitivity of bowel coliforms. J. Hyg. 71:529–534.

26. **Søgaard, H., C. Zimmerman-Nielsen, and K. Siboni.** 1974. Antibiotic-resistant gram-negative bacilli in a urological ward for male patients during a nine-year period: relationship to antibiotic consumption. J. Infect. Dis. 130:646–650.
27. **Speller, D. C. E., and D. M. Bruten.** 1972. Faecal flora after prolonged co-trimoxazole treatment. Br. Med. J. 3:416.
28. **Stokes, E. J., and P. M. Waterworth.** 1972. Antibiotic disk sensitivity tests by diffusion methods. Association of Clinical Pathologists Broadsheet 55 (Revised).
29. **Tybring, L.** 1975. Mecillinam (FL 1060), a 6β-amidinopenicillanic acid derivative: in vitro evaluation. Antimicrob. Agents Chemother. 8:266–270.
30. **Verrier-Jones, E. R., and A. W. Asscher.** 1975. Treatment of recurrent bacteriuria with pivmecillinam (FL 1039). J. Antimicrob. Chemother. 1:193–196
31. **Wise, R., D. S. Reeves, J. M. Symonds, and P. J. Wilkinson.** 1976. A clinical investigation of pivmecillinam, a novel β-lactam antibiotic, in the treatment of urinary tract infection. Chemotherapy 22:335–339.

ANTIMICROBIAL AGENTS AND CHEMOTHERAPY, Dec. 1976, p. 878-884
Vol. 10, No. 6

In Vitro Activity of Gentamicin, Amikacin, and Netilmicin Alone and in Combination with Carbenicillin Against *Serratia marcescens*

STEVEN M. POGWIZD AND STEPHEN A. LERNER*

Departments of Medicine, Biophysics and Theoretical Biology, and Microbiology, University of Chicago Pritzker School of Medicine, Chicago, Illinois 60637

Received for publication 6 April 1976

The inhibitory and bactericidal effects of gentamicin, amikacin, netilmicin (Sch 20569), and carbenicillin were tested against 55 clinical isolates of *Serratia marcescens* that had been subtyped into 26 strains by biotyping and serotyping. Three major patterns of resistance to gentamicin, netilmicin, and carbenicillin were recognized among these isolates. (i) Most of the 27 isolates that were susceptible to gentamicin (minimal bactericidal concentration [MBC] ≤6.25 μg/ml) were susceptible to carbenicillin (MBC ≤125 μg/ml) and resistant to netilmicin (MBC ≥12.5 μg/ml). (ii) Most of the 11 isolates with moderate resistance to gentamicin (MBC of 12.5 to 25 μg/ml) were also susceptible to carbenicillin and resistant to netilmicin. (iii) The 17 isolates with high-level resistance to gentamicin (MBC ≥ 50 μg/ml) were all highly resistant to carbenicillin (MBC ≥8,000 μg/ml) but susceptible to netilmicin (MBC ≤6.25 μg/ml). The susceptibility to amikacin was unpredictable among these groups of isolates but, overall, 80% of the isolates were killed by 25 μg of amikacin/ml, which is within the range of peak serum concentrations used therapeutically. Clinically attainable subinhibitory concentrations of carbenicillin enhanced the activity of the three aminoglycosides against all isolates with MBCs of carbenicillin ≤2,000 μg/ml. The 17 isolates with high-level resistance to carbenicillin and gentamicin, as well as the four isolates with high-level resistance to carbenicillin but not to gentamicin, were not susceptible to such enhancement of aminoglycoside activity by carbenicillin.

Serratia marcescens has been isolated with increasing frequency from patients who are hospitalized or subject to intravenous drug abuse (18, 21, 22, 37, 43, 44). At the University of Chicago Hospitals and Clinics, approximately 600 isolates of *S. marcescens* have been recovered from clinical specimens annually. Although most of these isolates were from sites of colonization, some were implicated in a variety of serious infections.

Antibiotic therapy of serious *Serratia* infections has been difficult. The advent of gentamicin improved inhibition of many *Serratia* strains in vitro over results achieved with other agents such as kanamycin, chloramphenicol, and nalidixic acid (8, 30, 39, 41, 43, 44). This made possible more effective treatment of some clinical infections (44). However, treatment of infections in relatively inaccessible sites, such as cardiac valvular vegetations, may be limited by a requirement for higher serum levels of gentamicin, which may potentiate the risk of toxicity. Furthermore, gentamicin resistance has lately become an increasingly serious problem for the treatment of *Serratia* infections. At this institution, in particular, disk susceptibility testing of *S. marcescens* isolates showed a dramatic increase in the incidence of resistance to gentamicin during successive 6-month periods from January 1973 through June 1975 (0, 5, 17, 30, and 50%, respectively).

The addition of sublethal concentrations of carbenicillin has been shown to produce a synergistic bactericidal effect with gentamicin and other aminoglycoside antibiotics against some strains of *Pseudomonas* and other gram-negative bacilli, both in vitro (1, 2, 12, 14–16, 24, 33, 35, 40) and in animal-model infections (2). By reducing the effective bactericidal concentration of gentamicin, synergistic enhancement of gentamicin activity may increase its clinical effectiveness in the treatment of infections caused by marginally susceptible strains as well as those caused by resistant strains. Also, the risks of toxicity may be reduced by the use of lower concentrations of gentamicin in serum. For these reasons, carbenicillin has been used with gentamicin in the treatment of infections due to *Serratia* (6, 7, 9, 21, 27) as well as other gram-negative organisms (2, 13, 23, 32, 34), although synergism against *Serratia* has only rarely been examined in vitro (7, 42).

Newer aminoglycoside antibiotics, such as tobramycin and amikacin, have exhibited greater in vitro activity than gentamicin against some strains of *Pseudomonas* and other gram-negative bacilli (4, 5, 11, 15, 17, 25, 45). Amikacin, in particular, has been shown to be effective against *S. marcescens* both in vitro (4, 25, 35, 44) and in clinical infections (10, 19, 36). Although most strains of *Serratia* that have been tested with amikacin were very susceptible to gentamicin, there have been occasional reports of its effectiveness against gentamicin-resistant strains (25, 35). In a recent report, netilmicin (Sch 20569), a new semisynthetic aminoglycoside, was shown to have activity against many gentamicin-resistant gram-negative bacilli, although it was less active than gentamicin against some of the 20 *Serratia* strains tested (26). Synergism with carbenicillin may enhance the bactericidal activity of these two aminoglycosides.

The present in vitro study was undertaken to examine the effects of two therapeutic alternatives to the use of gentamicin alone against each of a series of 55 recent clinical isolates of *S. marcescens*. (i) The activities of amikacin and netilmicin were compared with that of gentamicin. (ii) The activity of each of the three aminoglycosides in combination with sublethal concentrations of carbenicillin was compared with the activity of each aminoglycoside alone.

MATERIALS AND METHODS

Bacterial strains. Fifty-five clinical isolates of *S. marcescens* were obtained for this study from the Clinical Microbiology Laboratory of the University of Chicago Hospitals and Clinics. Isolates were chosen to include approximately 50% resistant to gentamicin by disk susceptibility testing. These isolates were grouped into 26 strains by biotype and serotype testing (28) carried out by F. Kocka and E. Roemisch of the Clinical Microbiology Laboratory. One strain included seven isolates, two had six, and the other thirty-six isolates were distributed among the remaining twenty-three strains, with fifteen strains (58%) each having only one isolate. The subtyping of this collection of *Serratia* isolates assured the diversity of this population in which the response to various antibiotics was studied. Subtyping also indicated that colonization and infection with this organism were not limited to a predominant hospital strain.

Antibiotics. Gentamicin and netilmicin were gifts of Schering Corp.; amikacin was a gift of Bristol Laboratories; and carbenicillin was a gift of Beecham, Inc. Stock solutions of the aminoglycoside antibiotics were made up in water according to concentrations of their bases and were kept at −20°C. These solutions were diluted in Trypticase soy broth (TSB) (BBL) for use in susceptibility testing. Carbenicillin solutions were prepared fresh before each experiment by dissolving disodium carbenicillin in water and diluting further in TSB.

Antibiotic susceptibility testing. The susceptibility of the *Serratia* isolates to the aminoglycosides and to carbenicillin was determined by a broth dilution method in a single experiment. A culture of each isolate grown overnight in TSB at 37°C was diluted to 10^{-4} with TSB for inoculation. Portions of 0.5 ml were added to sets of tubes, each of which contained 0.5 ml of a twofold dilution of one of the antibiotics in TSB. The minimal inhibitory concentration (MIC) was the lowest concentration that prevented the development of visible turbidity during incubation at 37°C for 18 h. Cultures without visible growth were subcultured by streaking with a 0.01-ml calibrated loop onto Columbia sheep blood agar plates (BBL), which were then incubated at 37°C for 18 h. The minimal bactericidal concentration (MBC) of an antibiotic was the lowest concentration in a culture from which fewer than 10 colonies grew. In the majority of cases, MICs were within two dilutions of the MBCs.

Testing of synergism. The effects of sublethal concentrations of carbenicillin on the bactericidal activities of the aminoglycosides for each *S. marcescens* isolate was determined by a variation of the checkerboard technique (29). Twofold serial dilutions of carbenicillin in TSB (0.25 ml) were mixed with 0.25 ml of twofold serial dilutions of each aminoglycoside in TSB. Each tube was inoculated with 0.5 ml of a 10^4-fold TSB dilution of a culture that had grown in TSB for 18 h at 37°C. All tubes that remained clear after incubation at 37°C for 18 h after inoculation were subcultured with a 0.01-ml calibrated loop onto blood agar plates. For all isolates with MBC of carbenicillin ≤500 μg/ml, the MBC of an aminoglycoside alone was compared with its MBC in the presence of one-fourth of the MBC of carbenicillin. For isolates with MBC of carbenicillin >500 μg/ml, the reduction of the aminoglycoside MBCs was scored in the presence of carbenicillin at the clinically attainable concentration of 125 μg/ml (and also at 500 μg/ml). Synergism was defined as a fourfold or greater reduction of the aminoglycoside MBC in the presence of these subinhibitory concentrations of carbenicillin. For each isolate, the MBCs of each drug in the synergism tests were within one tube dilution of the MBCs obtained previously.

RESULTS

Susceptibility to gentamicin, amikacin, netilmicin, and carbenicillin. No isolates were killed at concentrations of gentamicin <3.12 μg/ml (Fig. 1). Only 27 isolates (49%) were killed, and 32 (58%) were inhibited by 6.25 μg of gentamicin per ml, which is within the range of peak serum concentrations used to treat patients with this drug. Eleven isolates (20%) were moderately resistant to the antibiotic, re-

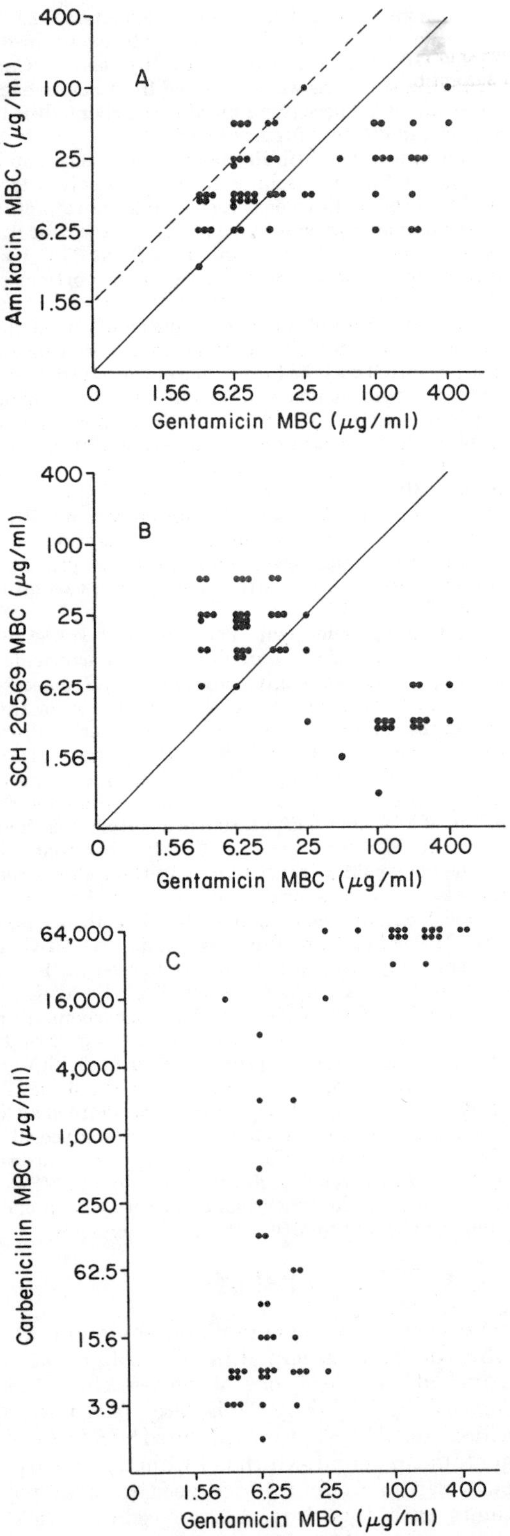

quiring 12.5 to 25 μg/ml for bactericidal effect. Seventeen (31%) were highly resistant to gentamicin, with MBCs of 50 to 400 μg/ml.

In comparison, 44 *Serratia* isolates (80%) were killed and 52 (94%) were inhibited by 25 μg of amikacin per ml (Fig. 1A), a peak concentration in serum that has been used in the treatment of patients (3, 10, 19, 36). The remaining 11 isolates all had MBCs of 50 to 100 μg/ml.

Netilmicin showed a greater difference between MICs and MBCs. At a concentration of 6.25 μg/ml, 40 isolates (73%) were inhibited, but only 20 (36%) were killed (Fig. 1B). All isolates were killed at 50 μg/ml.

There was little difference between MICs and MBCs of carbenicillin for this series of isolates. Carbenicillin was able to inhibit and kill 30 (54%) at a concentration of 125 μg/ml (Fig. 1C), which is clinically attainable in serum. Even at only 15.6 μg/ml, carbenicillin was bactericidal to 44% of the isolates. Although only four isolates had MBCs in the range of 250 to 2,000 μg/ml, 21 (38%) were found to be highly resistant, with MBCs greater than 2,000 μg/ml (8,000 to 64,000 μg/ml).

Figures 1A and 1B compare the MBCs of amikacin and of netilmicin with the MBC of gentamicin for each *Serratia* isolate. Amikacin is compared at four times the concentration of gentamicin, since the clinically achievable peak serum levels of amikacin are approximately four times higher than those of gentamicin (3, 36, 41). For all but three isolates, the MBCs of amikacin were at or less than four times the comparable MBCs of gentamicin. Furthermore, 8 of 11 isolates with MBCs of gentamicin at 12.5 to 25 μg/ml, as well as 12 of 17 with higher MBCs of gentamicin, were shown to be susceptible to amikacin (MBC ≤25 μg/ml). There was, however, no correlation between the levels of susceptibility to these two drugs.

In contrast, there was an inverse correlation between the susceptibility to gentamicin and to netilmicin for most isolates. All isolates that were highly resistant to gentamicin (MBC ≥ 50 μg/ml) were susceptible to netilmicin (MBC ≤6.25 μg/ml). On the other hand, 35 of the 38

FIG. 1. *Comparison of MBCs of gentamicin with MBCs of amikacin (A), netilmicin (Sch 20569) (B), and carbenicillin (C) for each of the 55 isolates of S. marcescens. The solid line indicates equal susceptibility to the aminoglycosides on a weight basis. The dashed line in (A) compares the susceptibility to gentamicin with the susceptibility to amikacin at an equivalent fourfold higher MBC (see text).*

strains that were either susceptible or moderately resistant to gentamicin (MBC ≤25 μg/ml) were resistant to netilmicin (MBC ≥12.5 μg/ml).

An analysis of the MBCs of gentamicin and carbenicillin for each isolate (Fig. 1C) indicated that all 17 isolates (from at least six different strains) that were highly resistant to gentamicin (MBC ≥50 μg/ml) were also highly resistant to carbenicillin (MBC ≥8,000 μg/ml). Of the four additional isolates that were highly resistant to carbenicillin, two had MBCs of gentamicin at 25 μg/ml and the other two were susceptible (MBC ≤6.25 μg/ml). Of this total of 21 isolates with MBCs of carbenicillin ≥8,000 μg/ml (represented by closed circles in Fig. 2A–C), 18 had MBCs of netilmicin ≤6.25 μg/ml, whereas 15 had MBCs of amikacin ≤25 μg/ml. Of the remaining 34 isolates that were more susceptible to carbenicillin, 33 had MBCs of gentamicin ≤12.5 μg/ml, and 31 MBCs of amikacin ≤25 μg/ml. On the other hand, only 2 of these 34 isolates showed MBCs of netilmicin ≤12.5 μg/ml.

Synergism studies. Figure 2 compares the aminoglycoside MBCs of each *S. marcescens* isolate with its MBCs in the presence of sublethal concentrations of carbenicillin. All 34 isolates (from at least 17 strains) with MBCs of carbenicillin ≤2,000 μg/ml were susceptible to enhancement of the bactericidal effect of these aminoglycosides by the addition of carbenicillin at one-fourth of its MBC (or at 125 μg/ml for the two isolates whose MBC of carbencillin was 2,000 μg/ml). In particular, the MBCs of the three aminoglycosides for these 34 isolates were reduced synergistically in all but eight instances. (In these marginal cases, which involved seven of the isolates, there was reduction of an aminoglycoside MBC to one-half rather than one-fourth.) With the addition of carbenicillin at concentrations used to test for synergism, 33 of these 34 isolates with MBCs of carbenicillin ≤2,000 μg/ml were killed by only 1.56 μg of gentamicin per ml, whereas only four were killed by this concentration of gentamicin alone. Thirty-three of these thirty-four isolates were killed by 6.25 μg of amikacin per ml in combination with carbenicillin; six were killed by this concentration of amikacin alone. Netilmicin at 3.12 μg/ml killed 31 of these isolates in the presence of the sublethal concentrations of carbenicillin, whereas none was killed by this concentration of netilmicin without the addition of carbenicillin.

For the remaining 21 isolates (from at least nine different strains), there was no reduction of MBCs of any of the three aminoglycosides in the presence of carbenicillin at either 125 μg/ml or 500 μg/ml (Fig. 2A–C). These were all the isolates which were not killed, or even inhibited, by 2,000 μg of carbenicillin per ml; their MBCs were all ≥8,000 μg/ml.

DISCUSSION

The range of susceptibility to gentamicin in this series of isolates (Fig. 1) appeared to be shifted toward greater levels of resistance than has usually been seen for *S. marcescens* (4, 8, 11, 20, 38, 45–47), with MBCs up to 400 μg/ml and none less than 3.12 μg/ml. Clinically important resistance of gentamicin (MBC ≥12.5 μg/ml) was present in 51% of the isolates in the series, in agreement with disk susceptibility testing. Such a high incidence of gentamicin resistance as was shown among recent isolates of *S. marcescens* in our hospital has not been reported (4, 8, 11, 20, 38, 45–47) until very recently (37). This decrease in susceptibility to gentamicin exhibited by the diverse strains in this series provided an opportunity to test alternative antibiotic regimens in vitro.

Amikacin was more active than gentamicin against a majority of isolates when its MBCs were compared with those of gentamicin in a therapeutically equivalent ratio of 4:1. Although there was an absence of high-level resistance to amikacin, some gentamicin-resistant isolates, as well as some susceptible isolates, exhibited low-level resistance to amikacin.

While Rahal et al. (26) have reported that netilmicin has activity against many gentamicin-resistant gram-negative bacilli, they found that all of their six gentamicin-resistant *Serratia* isolates were resistant to netilmicin. However, all isolates in our series that were highly resistant to gentamicin showed susceptibility to netilmicin. Since blood levels of netilmicin used in animals were comparable to those of gentamicin (31), netilmicin may be a useful antibiotic for infections caused by gentamicin-resistant *Serratia*.

The results of the studies on synergism against this series showed that the addition of subinhibitory concentrations of carbenicillin yielded synergistic killing with aminoglycosides for all isolates with MBCs of carbenicillin ≤2,000 μg/ml. Although most of these isolates exhibited MBCs of carbenicillin well within the range of concentrations that are achievable clinically in the serum, it is likely that the addition of relatively low levels of aminoglycosides would ensure more rapid bactericidal effect than the use of carbenicillin alone (1, 40).

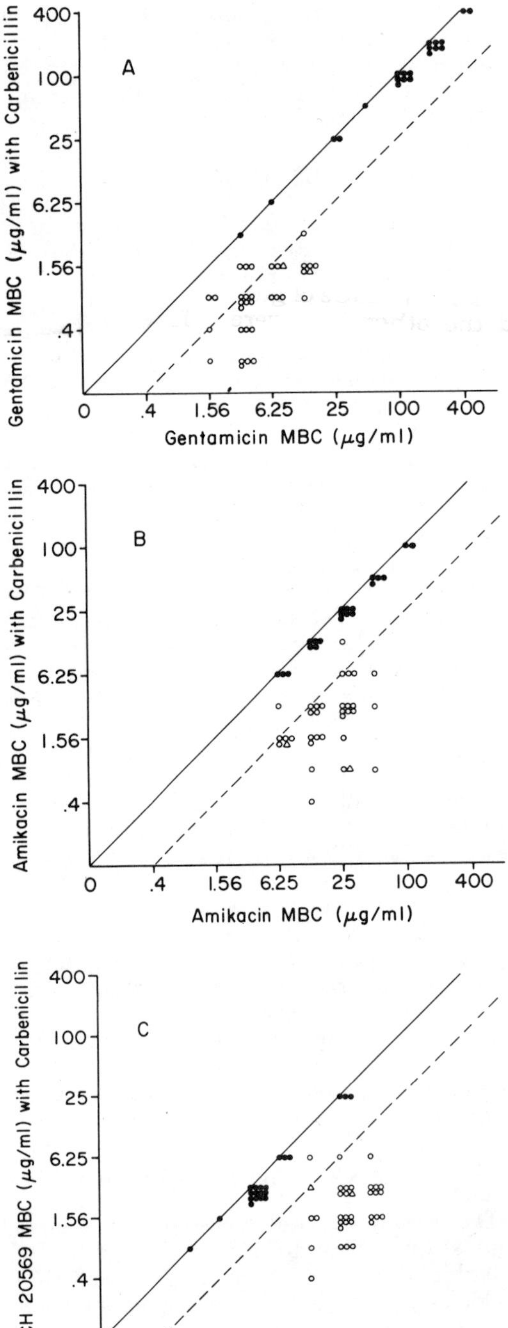

FIG. 2. *Killing of each of the 55 S. marcescens isolates by the combination of carbenicillin with gentamicin (A), amikacin (B), and netilmicin (Sch 20569) (C). For each isolate, the MBC of the aminoglycoside alone is compared with the MBC of the aminoglycoside in the presence of carbenicillin at the following concentrations: at one-fourth the MBC of carbenicillin for isolates with MBCs ≤500 μg/ml (○), at 125 μg/ml for isolates with MBCs at 2,000 μg/ml (△), and at 500 μg/ml for isolates with MBCs >2,000 μg/ml (●). The solid line indicates equal susceptibility to the aminoglycoside with and without carbenicillin. The dashed line indicates a synergistic reduction of the MBC of the aminoglycoside to one-fourth by the addition of carbenicillin.*

The only isolates that were not susceptible to synergistic lowering of aminoglycoside MBCs in the presence of carbenicillin at 125 μg/ml (or even at 500 μg/ml) were those with MBCs of carbenicillin ≥8,000 μg/ml. This group of isolates included two that were susceptible to gentamicin and many that were susceptible to amikacin and/or netilmicin. Therefore, in our series of isolates, lack of susceptibility to synergism with concentrations of carbenicillin that are clinically attainable in serum seems to correlate with high-level resistance to carbenicillin.

It thus appears that a synergistic combination of amikacin or gentamicin with carbenicillin may provide a more effective treatment regimen than the use of gentamicin alone for infections caused by *Serratia* isolates that are susceptible or only moderately resistant to gentamicin (especially if they are susceptible to killing by ≤2,000 μg of carbenicillin per ml). For isolates which are highly resistant to gentamicin (and generally highly resistant to carbenicillin as well), netilmicin or, in some cases, amikacin may be adequately bactericidal alone. Further clinical evaluation of amikacin, netilmicin, and combinations of carbenicillin with aminoglycosides are needed for the treatment of *Serratia* infections.

ACKNOWLEDGMENTS

This study was supported by a grant from the Schering Corporation.

We are indebted to Frank Kocka and Elinor Roemisch for providing and typing the *S. marcescens* isolates used. We also thank Frank Kocka for his constructive criticism of the manuscript.

LITERATURE CITED

1. **Anderson, E. L., P. K. Gramling, P. R. Vestal, and W. E. Farrar, Jr.** 1975. Susceptibility of *Pseudomonas aeruginosa* to tobramycin or gentamicin alone and combined with carbenicillin. Antimicrob. Agents Chemother. 8:300–304.
2. **Andriole, V. T.** 1974. Antibiotic synergy in experimental infection with *Pseudomonas*. II. The effect of carbenicillin, cephalothin, or cephanone combined with tobramycin or gentamicin. J. Infect. Dis. 129:124–133.
3. **Black, R. E., W. K. Lau, R. J. Weinstein, L. S. Young, and W. L. Hewitt.** 1976. Ototoxicity of amikacin. Antimicrob. Agents Chemother. 9:956–961.

4. **Bodey, G. P., and D. Stewart.** 1973. In vitro studies of BB-K8, a new aminoglycoside antibiotic. Antimicrob. Agents Chemother. 4:186–192.
5. **Britt, M. R., R. A. Garibaldi, J. N. Wilfert, and C. B. Smith.** 1972. In vitro activity of tobramycin and gentamicin. Antimicrob. Agents Chemother. 2:236–241.
6. **Bryan, C. S., S. R. Marney, Jr., R. H. Alford, and R. E. Bryant.** 1975. Gram-negative bacillary endocarditis: interpretation of the serum bactericidal test. Am. J. Med. 58:209–215.
7. **Farhoudi, H. O., T. Banks, and N. Ali.** 1974. A case report of *Serratia* endocarditis with review of the literature. Med. Ann. D.C. 43:401–406.
8. **Greenup, P., and D. J. Blazevic.** 1971. Antibiotic susceptibilities of *Serratia marcescens* and *Enterobacter liquefaciens*. Appl. Microbiol. 22:309–314.
9. **Harris, J. A., and C. G. Cobbs.** 1973. *Serratia* endocarditis in patients with a Starr-Edwards valve: report of a case of bacteriologic cure with antimicrobial therapy. South. Med. J. 66:1117–1120.
10. **Howard, J. B., and G. H. McCracken, Jr.** 1975. Pharmacological evaluation of amikacin in neonates. Antimicrob. Agents Chemother. 8:86–90.
11. **Hyams, P. J., M. S. Simberkoff, and J. J. Rahal, Jr.** 1973. In vitro bactericidal effectiveness of four aminoglycoside antibiotics. Antimicrob. Agents Chemother. 3:87–94.
12. **Klastersky, J., R. Cappel, and D. Daneau.** 1972. Clinical significance of in vitro synergism between antibiotics in gram-negative infections. Antimicrob. Agents Chemother. 2:470–475.
13. **Klastersky, J., R. Cappel, and D. Daneau.** 1973. Therapy with carbenicillin and gentamicin for patients with cancer and severe infections caused by gram-negative rods. Cancer 31:331–336.
14. **Klastersky, J., G. Swings, and D. Daneau.** 1970. Antimicrobial activity of the carbenicillin/gentamicin combination against gram-negative bacilli. Am. J. Med. Sci. 260:373–380.
15. **Kluge, R. M., H. C. Standiford, B. Tatem, V. M. Young, W. H. Greene, S. C. Schimpff, F. M. Calia, and R. B. Hornick.** 1974. Comparative activity of tobramycin, amikacin, and gentamicin alone and with carbenicillin against *Pseudomonas aeruginosa*. Antimicrob. Agents Chemother. 6:442–446.
16. **Kluge, R. M., H. C. Standiford, B. Tatem, V. M. Young, S. C. Schimpff, W. H. Greene, F. M. Calia, and R. B. Hornick.** 1974. The carbenicillin-gentamicin combination against *Pseudomonas aeruginosa*: correlation of effect with gentamicin sensitivity. Ann. Intern. Med. 81:584–587.
17. **Levison, M. E., and D. Kaye.** 1974. In vitro comparison of four aminoglycoside antibiotics: sisomycin, gentamicin, tobramycin, and BB-K8. Antimicrob. Agents Chemother. 5:667–669.
18. **Maki, D. G., C. G. Hennekens, C. W. Phillips, W. V. Shaw, and J. V. Bennett.** 1973. Nosocomial urinary tract infection with *Serratia marcescens*: an epidemiologic study. J. Infect. Dis. 128:579–587.
19. **Meyer, R. D., R. P. Lewis, E. D. Carmalt, and S. M. Finegold.** 1975. Amikacin therapy for serious gram-negative bacillary infections. Ann. Intern. Med. 83:790–800.
20. **Meyers, B. R., B. Leng, and S. Z. Hirschman.** 1975. Comparison of the antibacterial activities of sisomicin and gentamicin against gram-negative bacteria. Antimicrob. Agents Chemother. 8:757–758.
21. **Mills, J., and D. Drew.** 1976. *Serratia marcescens* endocarditis: a regional illness associated with intravenous drug abuse. Ann. Intern. Med. 84:29–35.
22. **Myerowitz, R. L., A. A. Medeiros, and T. F. O'Brien.** 1971. Recent experience with bacillemia due to gram-negative organisms. J. Infect. Dis. 124:239–246.
23. **Nunnery, A. W., W. D. Hamilton, and H. D. Riley, Jr.** 1970. Carbenicillin: *in vivo* synergism and combined therapy. J. Infect. Dis. 122(Suppl.):78–83.
24. **Phair, J. P., C. Watanakunakorn, and T. Bannister.** 1969. In vitro susceptibility of *Pseudomonas aeruginosa* to carbenicillin and the combination of carbenicillin and gentamicin. Appl. Microbiol. 18:303–306.
25. **Price, K. E., T. A. Pursiano, M. D. DeFuria, and G. E. Wright.** 1974. Activity of BB-K8 (amikacin) against clinical isolates resistant to one or more aminoglycoside antibiotics. Antimicrob. Agents Chemother. 5:143–152.
26. **Rahal, J. J. Jr., M. S. Simberkoff, K. Kagan, and N. H. Moldover.** 1976. Bactericidal efficacy of Sch 20569 and amikacin against gentamicin-sensitive and -resistant organisms. Antimicrob. Agents Chemother. 9:595–599.
27. **Rodriguez, V., J. P. Whitecar, Jr., and G. P. Bodey.** 1970. Therapy of infections with the combination of carbenicillin and gentamicin, p. 386–390. Antimicrob. Agents Chemother. 1969.
28. **Roemisch, E., and F. E. Kocka.** 1976. Comparison of methods for differentiating among *Serratia marcescens* isolated from clinical specimens. Am. J. Clin. Pathol. 66:96–100.
29. **Sabath, L. D.** 1968. Synergy of antibacterial substances by apparently known mechanisms, p. 210–217. Antimicrob. Agents Chemother. 1967.
30. **Sanford, J. P.** 1967. Sensitivity tests of *Klebsiella, Enterobacter,* and *Serratia*. J. Infect. Dis. 119:388–390.
31. **Schering Corporation.** 1975. Informational material for the investigational drug SCH 20569. Schering Corp., Bloomfield, N.J.
32. **Schimpff, S., W. Satterlee, V. M. Young, and A. Serpick.** 1971. Empiric therapy with carbenicillin and gentamicin for febrile patients with cancer and granulocytopenia. N. Engl. J. Med. 284:1061–1065.
33. **Smith, C. B., P. E. Dans, J. N. Wilfert, and M. Finland.** 1969. Use of gentamicin in combination with other antibiotics. J. Infect. Dis. 119:370–377.
34. **Smith, C. B., J. N. Wilfert, P. E. Dans, T. A. Kurrus, and M. Finland.** 1970. *In vitro* activity of carbenicillin and results of treatment of infections due to *Pseudomonas* with carbenicillin singly and in combination with gentamicin. J. Infect. Dis. 122(Suppl).:14–25.
35. **Sonne, M., and E. Jawetz.** 1969. Combined action of carbenicillin and gentamicin on *Pseudomonas aeruginosa* in vitro. Appl. Microbiol. 17:893–896.
36. **Tally, F. P., T. J. Louie, W. M. Weinstein, J. G. Bartlett, and S. L. Gorbach.** 1975. Amikacin therapy for severe gram-negative sepsis: emphasis on infections with gentamicin-resistant organisms. Ann. Intern. Med. 83:484–488.
37. **Thomas, F. E., Jr., J. M. Leonard, and R. H. Alford.** 1976. Sulfamethoxazole-trimethoprim-polymixin therapy of serious multiply drug-resistant *Serratia* infections. Antimicrob. Agents Chemother. 9:201–207.
38. **Thornton, G. F., and V. T. Andriole.** 1969. Antibiotic sensitivities of nonpigmented *Serratia marcescens* to gentamicin and carbenicillin. J. Infect. Dis. 119:393–394.
39. **Thornton, G. F., and J. A. Cramer.** 1971. Antibiotic susceptibility of nonpigmented *Serratia marcescens,* p. 514–516. Antimicrob. Agents Chemother. 1970.
40. **Wald, E. R., H. C. Standiford, B. A. Tatem, F. M. Calia, and R. B. Hornick.** 1975. BL-P1654, ticarcillin, and carbenicillin: in vitro comparison alone and in combination with gentamicin against *Pseudomonas aeruginosa*. Antimicrob. Agents Chemother. 7:336–340.
41. **Weinstein, R. J., L. S. Young, and W. L. Hewitt.** 1975. Activity of three aminoglycosides and two penicillins

against four species of gram-negative bacilli. Antimicrob. Agents Chemother. 7:172–178.

42. **Weinstein, R. J., L. S. Young, and W. L. Hewitt.** 1975. Comparison of methods for assessing in vitro antibiotic synergism against *Pseudomonas* and *Serratia*. J. Lab. Clin. Med. 86:853–862.
43. **Wilfert, J. N., F. F. Barrett, W. H. Ewing, M. Finland, and E. H. Kass.** 1970. *Serratia marcescens*: biochemical, serological, and epidemiological characteristics and antibiotic susceptibility of strains isolated at Boston City Hospital. Appl. Microbiol. 19:345–352.
44. **Wilfert, J. N., F. F. Barrett, and E. H. Kass.** 1968. Bacteremia due to *Serratia marcescens*. N. Engl. J. Med. 279:286–289.
45. **Young, L. S., and W. L. Hewitt.** 1973. Activity of five aminoglycoside antibiotics in vitro against gram-negative bacilli and *Staphylococcus aureus*. Antimicrob. Agents Chemother. 4:617–625.
46. **Yu, P. K., and J. A. Washington II.** 1973. Comparative in vitro activity of three aminoglycoside antibiotics: BB-K8, kanamycin, and gentamicin. Antimicrob. Agents Chemother. 4:133–139.
47. **Yu, P. K., and J. A. Washington II.** 1974. Comparison of in vitro antibacterial activities of gentamicin and verdamicin. Antimicrob. Agents Chemother. 6:526–528.

ANTIMICROBIAL AGENTS AND CHEMOTHERAPY, Dec. 1976, p. 885-888
Vol. 10, No. 6
Printed in U.S.A.

Effect of 9-β-D-Arabinofuranosyladenine 5′-Monophosphate and 9-β-D-Arabinofuranosylhypoxanthine 5′-Monophosphate on Experimental Herpes Simplex Keratitis

HERBERT E. KAUFMAN AND EMILY D. VARNELL*

Department of Ophthalmology, College of Medicine, University of Florida, Gainesville, Florida 32610

Received for publication 13 August 1976

Treatment of established experimental keratitis caused by herpes simplex virus with 9-β-D-arabinofuranosyladenine 5′-monophosphate (Ara-AMP) or 9-β-D-arabinofuranosylhypoxanthine 5′-monophosphate (Ara-HxMP) showed that the Ara-AMP, in a concentration of 2 or 20%, had a significant effect on the keratitis but that 0.4% Ara-HxMP showed only minimal activity. Ara-AMP was also effective in the treatment of idoxuridine-resistant keratitis. No local toxicity with a high concentration (20%) of Ara-AMP was seen, but the duration of therapy was brief.

Idoxuridine (IDU) has been used for the treatment of herpes simplex keratitis for approximately 13 years (10). Although it is an extremely useful drug, a more potent drug with less potential side effects would be desirable. In the study of drugs active against herpes simplex keratitis in humans, experimental herpes simplex keratitis in rabbits has been found to be extremely predictive. The previous technique of analysis (1) using multiple parameters that are weighted in an arbitrary way (the Draize score) was abandoned, but the corneal ulcer, the most important clinical parameter, was scored using a blind rating of severity. The score of the ulcers in experimental keratitis, when treatment of the eye was delayed until the disease was well established and the treated group was compared to the control, has been found to be extremely accurate in the prediction of the effect in humans. This has been validated with a number of separate drugs in both animals and humans (4, 7, 8, 11, 12, 15).

In this experimental keratitis system, cytosine arabinoside has been found to be approximately as active as, but more toxic than (6), IDU (9). Adenine arabinoside (Ara-A) is approximately as active as IDU (7) and, in large-scale double-blind studies in humans (4, 11, 12), it is approximately as effective as IDU, with no significant differences between them. Trifluorothymidine is more effective than IDU both in experimental keratitis in rabbits (8) and in humans (15).

The monophosphates of Ara-A and adenine hypoxanthine (Ara-Hx) are much more soluble than the nucleosides. Much hope has been raised that the increased solubility might enable the attainment of more effective antiviral levels. Because of the high degree of predictability of these systems for humans, and because some studies with modified keratitis systems have shown an effect both of Ara-AMP and of Ara-HxMP (14) (Fig. 1), it seemed important to document the effects of these drugs and, where possible, their dose response relationships, in a system known to be an effective predictor for humans.

MATERIALS AND METHODS

New Zealand white rabbits weighing 2 to 4 lb (ca. 0.92 to 1.8 kg) were used in these studies. Keratitis was produced by traumatizing the corneas in a standard manner, instilling the virus suspension, and gently rubbing the lids over the cornea (10). The virus utilized was either the McKrae strain of herpes simplex virus type 1 prepared in human embryonic kidney cells or an IDU-resistant virus prepared by repeatedly growing the McKrae virus in the presence of increasing concentrations of IDU in the medium (5). Corneal ulcers were graded on a scale of 0 to 4+, where 0 indicated no lesions, and 1+, 2+, 3+, and 4+ indicated 25, 50, 75, and 100% ulceration, respectively. Grading was done in a blind manner, using a slit lamp after fluorescein staining. Both eyes of each rabbit were infected and treated identically. Only keratitis was evaluated in this study because of the close correlation it has to the benefits seen in human disease.

The Ara-AMP, supplied as a lyophilized powder (Parke, Davis & Co.), was diluted in aqueous solutions. The Ara-HxMP (supplied by R.W. Sidwell, ICN Pharmaceuticals, Inc.) was also prepared in an aqueous solution of pH 6 to 6.5. The 3.3% Ara-A (Parke, Davis & Co.) and 0.5% Stoxil (Smith Kline & French Laboratories, IDU) were both ointment preparations. Treatment was started 3 days after

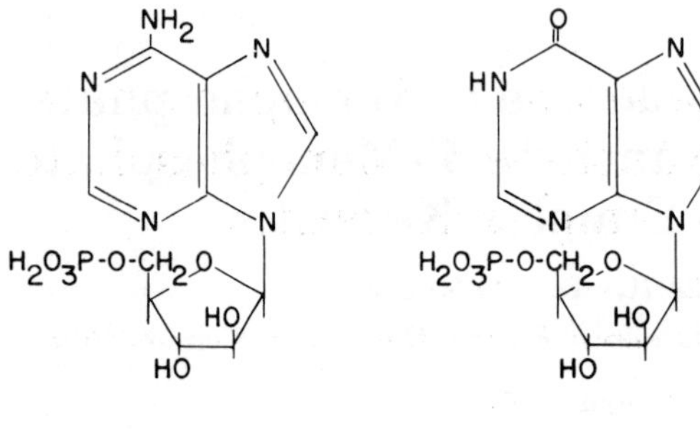

FIG. 1. *Structures of Ara-AMP and Ara-HxMP.*

infection, at a time when dendritic ulcers were present in all eyes, and was continued for 5 days. All medications were given six times a day at approximately 4, 8, and 11 a.m. and 2, 5, and 11 p.m.

The severity levels of keratitis in the treatment groups were compared against one another each day with the Kruskal-Wallis one-way analysis of variance (3). If the test statistic was significant at the 5% level of significance, multiple comparisons were then made by the Dunn technique (2) and were run at the 1% level of significance.

RESULTS

The data (Table 1) indicate that the 3.3% Ara-A- and the 0.4% Ara-AMP-treated groups both gave better results than the control group and the 0.4% Ara-HxMP-treated group. In this study, therefore, Ara-A and Ara-AMP appeared to be active and potent antivirals, whereas the Ara-HxMP showed minimal activity.

Similarly, the expected therapeutic effect of Ara-A was significantly better than the control; however, no difference was seen between the Ara-Hx, Ara-HxMP, and control groups (Table 2).

There is a good dose response effect of Ara-AMP (Table 3). Toxicity was not seen either in infected or noninfected traumatized eyes with the higher concentration of Ara-AMP, but the total duration of therapy was very brief, compared with many clinical situations.

Trifluorothymidine, Ara-AMP, and Ara-A are all highly active against IDU-resistant virus (Table 4).

DISCUSSION

Ara-AMP is known to enter some tissue culture cell systems apparently unchanged and without dephosphorylization (13). Its effect on keratitis is similar to that expected for the parent compound, Ara-A, except that it is significantly more soluble than Ara-A and may be deaminated more slowly. When higher concentrations of Ara-AMP are used, an increased therapeutic effect is apparent. In these experiments no toxicity was seen, although the duration of therapy was brief. The great solubility of this drug may not only make it more usable for superficial herpes keratitis, but it might also increase penetration of the drug into the corneal stroma. Preliminary experiments in our laboratory suggest that this is the case. One of the drawbacks of the parent compound, Ara-A, in systemic use is its lack of solubility and its need to be administered with very large volumes of fluid. The administration of the great volumes (more than 2 liters a day to a typical patient) makes intravenous administration sometimes hazardous for ill patients. A more soluble and equally effective compound such as Ara-AMP might be used either as intravenous push or as an intramuscular injection with no loss in activity, but with much greater therapeutic convenience and safety due to the re-

TABLE 1. *Effect of Ara-AMP and Ara-HxMP on herpes keratitis*

Treatment[a] (%)	No. of eyes	Severity of keratitis[b] on treatment day: 4	5
Ara-AMP, 0.4	22	0.70[c, d]	0.54[c, d]
Ara-HxMP, 0.4	24	1.41	1.08
Ara-A, 3.3	22	0.60[c, d]	0.63[d]
Saline control	18	1.58	1.19

[a] All treatments were given six times daily. Treatment started 3 days after infection and continued for 5 days.

[b] 0, Normal cornea; 4, complete corneal ulceration.

[c] Significantly better than control, at the 1% level.

[d] Significantly better than Ara-HxMP, at the 1% level.

TABLE 2. *Comparison of Ara-Hx and Ara-HxMP on herpes keratitis*

Treatment[a] (%)	Severity of keratitis[b] on treatment day: 4	5
Ara-A, 3.3	0.05[c]	0[c]
Ara-Hx, 0.3	1.28	1.00
Ara-HxMP, 0.5	1.82	1.60
Saline control	2.50	2.00

[a] All treatments were given six times daily; 20 eyes were tested with each treatment. Treatment started 3 days after infection and continued for 5 days.

[b] 0, Normal cornea; 4, complete corneal ulceration.

[c] Significantly better than control, at the 1% level.

TABLE 3. *Dose-response of Ara-AMP in treatment of herpetic keratitis*

Treatment[a] (%)	Severity of keratitis[b] on treatment day:	
	4	5
Ara-AMP, 20	0.40[c, d]	0.35[c, d]
Ara-AMP, 2	0.82	0.83
Ara-AMP, 0.2	1.06	0.95
Stoxil, 0.5	0.11[c, d, e]	0.03[c, d, e]
Saline control	1.61	1.98

[a] All treatments were given six times daily; 24 eyes were tested with each treatment. Treatment started 3 days after infection and continued for 5 days.

[b] 0, Normal cornea; 4, complete corneal ulceration.

[c] Significantly better than control, at the 1% level.

[d] Significantly better than 0.2% Ara-AMP, at the 1% level.

[e] Significantly better than 20% and 2% Ara-AMP, at the 1% level.

TABLE 4. *Effect of Ara-AMP on IDU-resistant herpetic keratitis*

Treatment[a] (%)	No. of eyes	Severity of keratitis[b] on treatment day:	
		3	5
Trifluorothymidine, 1	24	0.12[c]	0.06[c]
Ara-AMP, 20	24	0.07[c]	0.04[c]
Ara-A, 3.3	20	0.20[c]	0.25[c]
Saline control	24	1.01	1.10

[a] All treatments were given six times daily. Treatment started 3 days after infection and continued for 5 days.

[b] 0, Normal cornea; 4, complete ulceration.

[c] Significantly better than control, at the 1% level.

duced amounts of fluid required for its administration.

Ara-HxMP may well penetrate the cell intact under some circumstances, as does Ara-AMP, but this is not certain. Previous studies of this drug were done with experimental herpetic keratitis (14), but they were undertaken with systems that had not been shown to be valid predictors in humans. Multiple criteria (e.g., corneal opacity, lesion size, erythema, conjunctival swelling, and discharge) were combined to evaluate effectiveness, although many of them may have nothing to do with the primary effect of the drug used for treating corneal ulcers. These therapeutic entities are also arbitrarily weighted in a statistically unvalidated manner. In the experiments described above, treatment was begun 24 h after infection, a time usually considered too early for the appearance of lesions that can clearly be identified as herpes. In addition, there is no indication that grading of these ulcers was done on a blind basis.

The system used in the present study has been shown to be an extremely accurate predictor of the drug effect in humans, and it suggests that Ara-HxMP is not likely to be useful for the treatment of herpetic keratitis in humans. Higher concentrations of Ara-HxMP might have significant activity, but Ara-HxMP is clearly less effective than Ara-AMP. Ara-AMP, on the other hand, has an activity comparable to that of Ara-A. At higher concentrations, which are possible because of increased solubility, Ara-AMP appears to have significant advantages over the parent compound.

ACKNOWLEDGMENTS

This study was supported by Public Health Service grants EY-00007 and Ey-00446 from the National Eye Institute.

LITERATURE CITED

1. **Draize, J. H., G. Woodard, and H. O. Calverty.** 1944. Methods for the study of irritation and toxicity of substances applied topically to the skin and mucous membranes. J. Pharmacol. Exp. Ther. 82:377–390.
2. **Dunn, O. J.** 1964. Multiple comparisons using rank sums. Technometrics 6:241–252.
3. **Hollander, M., and D. A. Wolf.** 1973. Nonparametric statistical methods, p. 129–130. John Wiley and Sons, Inc., New York.
4. **Hyndiuk, R. A., R. O. Schultz, and D. S. Hull.** 1975. Herpetic keratitis-clinical evaluation of adenine arabinoside and idoxuridine, p. 331–335. *In* D. Pavan-Langston, R. A. Buchanan, and C. A. Alford, Jr., (ed.), Adenine arabinoside: an antiviral agent. Raven Press, New York.
5. **Kaufman, H. E.** 1965. In vivo studies with antiviral agents. Ann. N.Y. Acad. Sci. 130:168–180.
6. **Kaufman, H. E., J. A. Capella, E. D. Maloney, J. E. Robbins, G. M. Cooper, and M. H. Uotila.** 1964. Corneal toxicity of cytosine arabinoside. Arch. Ophthalmol. 72:535–540.
7. **Kaufman, H. E., E. D. Ellison, and W. M. Townsend.** 1970. The chemotherapy of herpes iritis with adenine arabinoside and cytarabine. Arch. Ophthalmol. 84:783–787.
8. **Kaufman, H. E., and C. Heidelberger.** 1964. Therapeutic antiviral action of 5-trifluoromethyl-2′-deoxyuridine. Science 145:585–586.
9. **Kaufman, H. E., and E. D. Maloney.** 1963. IDU and cytosine arabinoside in experimental herpetic keratitis. Arch. Ophthalmol. 69:626–629.
10. **Kaufman, H. E., A. B. Nesburn, and E. D. Maloney.** 1962. IDU therapy of herpes simplex. Arch. Ophthalmol. 67:583–591.
11. **Laibson, P. R., and J. H. Krachmer.** 1975. Controlled comparison of adenine arabinoside and idoxuridine therapy of human superficial dendritic keratitis, p. 323–330. *In* D. Pavan-Langston, R. A. Buchanan, and C. A. Alford, Jr. (ed.), Adenine arabinoside: an antiviral agent. Raven Press, New York.
12. **Pavan-Langston, D., and C. H. Dohlman.** 1972. A dou-

ble blind clinical study of adenine arabinoside therapy of viral keratoconjunctivitis. Am. J. Ophthalmol. 74:81–88.

13. **Plunkett, W., L. Lapi, P. J. Ortiz, and S. S. Cohen.** 1974. Penetration of mouse fibroblasts by the 5′-phosphate of 9-β-D-arabinofuranosyladenine and incorporation of the nucleotide into DNA. Proc. Natl. Acad. Sci. U.S.A. 71:73–77.
14. **Sidwell, R. W., L. B. Allen, J. H. Huffman, G. V. Revankar, R. K. Robins, and R. L. Tolman.** 1975. Viral keratitis-inhibitory effect of 9-β-D-arabinofuranosylhypoxanthine 5′-monophosphate. Antimicrob. Agents Chemother. 8:463–467.
15. **Wellings, P. C., P. N. Awdry, F. H. Bors, B. R. Jones, D. C. Brown, and H. E. Kaufman.** 1972. Clinical evaluation of trifluorothymidine in the treatment of herpes simplex corneal ulcers. Am. J. Ophthalmol. 73:932–942.

ANTIMICROBIAL AGENTS AND CHEMOTHERAPY, Dec. 1976, p. 889-892
Vol. 10, No. 6
Printed in U.S.A.

Antibiotic Synergy and Antagonism Against Clinical Isolates of *Klebsiella* Species

ROBERT M. D'ALESSANDRI, DAVID J. McNEELY, AND RONICA M. KLUGE*

Division of Infectious Diseases, Department of Medicine, College of Medicine, University of Florida, Gainesville, Florida 32610

Received for publication 7 July 1976

Minimal inhibitory concentrations of kanamycin, gentamicin, amikacin, cephalothin, and chloramphenicol were determined in Trypticase soy broth for 70 clinical isolates of *Klebsiella* species. Gentamicin and amikacin were the most active on a weight basis. Chloramphenicol was more active than kanamycin, and cephalothin was the least active of all. Studies using a microtiter modification of the checkerboard technique were performed to evaluate the comparative activity of the three aminoglycosides in combination with either chloramphenicol or cephalothin. The cephalothin-aminoglycoside combinations demonstrated synergy in >80% of the isolates tested. No antagonism was noted. The chloramphenicol-aminoglycoside combinations showed antagonism in 35 to 45% of the isolates tested. The data suggest that the chloramphenicol-aminoglycoside combinations be used with caution when treating serious infections where *Klebsiella* is a potential pathogen.

The combination of a cephalosporin and an aminoglycoside antibiotic is considered the treatment of choice for serious *Klebsiella* infections (3, 11). This is based on the finding of antimicrobial synergy in vitro and the suggestion that combined antibiotic therapy retards the development of resistance to either antibiotic (2).

In patients allergic to the cephalosporins, or in patients with polymicrobial bacteremia in whom both *Enterobacteriaceae* and anaerobes are potential pathogens, the combination of chloramphenicol and an aminoglycoside antibiotic is often recommended. There is some in vitro evidence to indicate that such a combination may have an antagonistic effect (2, 4, 8).

Kanamycin and gentamicin are the most commonly used aminoglycosides in clinical practice today. Amikacin, an investigational aminoglycoside, is pharmacologically related to kanamycin. In a recent report (H. Standiford, B. Tatum, and F. Calia, Prog. Abstr. Intersci. Conf. Antimicrob. Agents Chemother., 15th, Washington, D.C., Abstr. 263, 1975), amikacin in clinically achievable levels was found to be more active in vitro against *Klebsiella* strains than gentamicin. In the present study the comparative activity of kanamycin, gentamicin, amikacin, chloramphenicol, and cephalothin against *Klebsiella* isolates was evaluated. In addition, the activity of each aminoglycoside in combination with either chloramphenicol or cephalothin was determined.

MATERIALS AND METHODS

Seventy clinical isolates of *Klebsiella* species were obtained from the Veterans Administration Hospital and the Shands Teaching Hospital, Gainesville, Fla. Isolates were maintained on tryptic soy agar at 4°C until studied.

Solutions of each antibiotic were prepared in concentrations of 80 μg/ml. The solutions were divided into 4-ml portions and stored at −20°C. Fresh solutions were prepared monthly. All susceptibility testing was performed in tryptic soy broth (TSB). The concentration of calcium in the TSB ranged between 3.4 and 4.1 mg/100 ml; the magnesium concentration was between 1.2 and 1.3 mg/100 ml.

The minimal inhibitory concentration (MIC) of each drug alone was measured by the standard twofold tube dilution method. The MICs of the combination of each aminoglycoside with chloramphenicol and each aminoglycoside with cephalothin were measured using a microtiter modification of the checkerboard technique (7). The final concentration of antibiotic ranged from 40 to 0.5 μg/ml, and the inoculum consisted of a 10^{-3} dilution of a 4-h culture. Pour plates were made to determine the exact inoculum. MIC results were considered valid when the inoculum fell between 10^5 and 5×10^5 colony-forming units.

The character of the antibiotic interaction was determined by plotting an isobologram (Fig. 1) for each microtiter plate (10). The concentration of aminoglycoside formed the ordinate, and the concentration of either cephalothin or chloramphenicol formed the abscissa. The MICs of each drug alone and of the combinations as read from the microtiter plate were plotted on the isobologram. If the points fell on a straight line joining the aminoglycoside

MIC to the cephalothin or chloramphenicol MIC, an additive interaction was recorded. If the curve bowed upward, antagonism was recorded, whereas if the curve bowed downward toward the coordinates, synergy was recorded.

RESULTS

A comparison of the MICs of kanamycin, gentamicin, and amikacin against 70 *Klebsiella* isolates is seen in Table 1. Fifty-six isolates were sensitive to 10 μg or less of kanamycin per ml, a clinically achievable level. Twelve isolates were moderately resistant, requiring 20 μg/ml. Only two isolates were resistant to more than 40 μg of kanamycin per ml. All 70 isolates were sensitive to 5 μg or less of gentamicin per ml. Sixty-eight of the 70 isolates were sensitive to 10 μg or less of amikacin per ml. One isolate was moderately resistant, with an MIC of 20 μg/ml, and one isolate was resistant with an MIC of 40 μg of amikacin per ml. On a weight basis gentamicin was the most active of the three aminoglycosides and kanamycin was the least active. Sixty-eight of the isolates were sensitive to 20 μg or less of chloramphenicol per ml, an easily achieved serum level. Only two isolates were resistant to more than 40 μg/ml. Only 49 isolates were sensitive to 20 μg or less of cephalothin per ml, a clinically achievable level. However, 15 isolates were resistant to more than 40 μg/ml, and 6 isolates with an MIC of 40 μg/ml were moderately resistant.

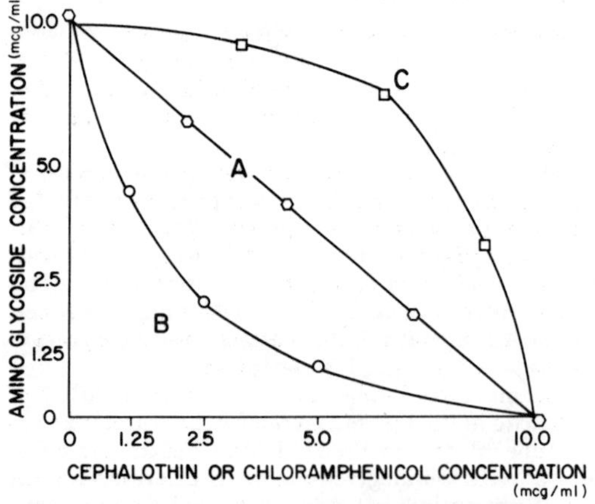

FIG. 1. *Isobologram with three isobols representing additive effect (A), synergy (B), and antagonism (C).*

The results of combining cephalothin with each of the three aminoglycosides are seen in Table 2. The combination of cephalothin and kanamycin was synergistic in 32 of 35 isolates (92%). For the remainder of the isolates an additive effect was noted. Cephalothin with gentamicin was synergistic in 36 of 38 isolates (95%). Cephalothin and amikacin showed synergy in 26 of 38 isolates (68%). The cephalothin-gentamicin combination was synergistic for a statistically greater number of isolates than was the cephalothin-amikacin combination ($P < 0.01$). The statistical significance was similar when comparing the cephalothin-kanamicin and cephalothin-amikacin combinations. None of the cephalothin-aminoglycoside combinations were antagonistic.

In Table 3 are the results of testing the combination of chloramphenicol with each of the three aminoglycosides against *Klebsiella* isolates. Chloramphenicol with kanamycin and chloramphenicol with amikacin were synergistic in 14 of 39 and 13 of 40 isolates, respectively. Chloramphenicol with gentamicin was synergistic in 20 of 39 isolates. This difference in synergy between chloramphenicol with kanamycin or amikacin and chloramphenicol with gentamicin was not statistically significant ($P > 0.10$). It is important to note that each combination was antagonistic against 35 to 45% of the isolates tested. Synergy was demonstrated for 47 of 118 combinations using the aminoglycosides with chloramphenicol; another 47 of these 118 combinations showed antagonism. In the aminoglycosides with cephalothin group, synergy was noted with 94 of 111 combinations and no antagonism was shown. The difference in synergy between the two groups was statistically significant ($P < 0.001$). The difference in

TABLE 1. *MICs of aminoglycosides, chloramphenicol, and cephalothin against 70 clinical isolates of Klebsiella pneumoniae*

Antimicrobial agent	No. of strains inhibited							
	<1.25[a]	1.25	2.5	5.0	10.0	20.0	40.0	>40.0
Gentamicin	3 (4)[b]	21 (30)	38 (88)	8 (100)				
Amikacin	1 (1)	13 (19)	30 (62)	17 (87)	7 (97)	1 (99)	1 (100)	
Kanamycin	0 (0)	4 (6)	6 (14)	31 (59)	15 (80)	12 (97)	0 (99)	2 (100)
Chloramphenicol	0 (0)	3 (4)	16 (27)	29 (68)	16 (91)	4 (97)	0 (97)	2 (100)
Cephalothin	0 (0)	0 (0)	16 (23)	14 (43)	15 (64)	4 (70)	6 (79)	15 (100)

[a] MIC (micrograms per milliliter).
[b] Numbers in parentheses represent the cumulative percentage of strains inhibited.

TABLE 2. *Cephalothin-aminoglycoside combination*

Cephalothin with:	No. of isolates tested			
	Additive (%)	Synergistic (%)	Antagonistic (%)	Total
Kanamycin	3 (8.5)	32 (91.5)	0	35
Gentamicin	2 (5.2)	36 (94.8)	0	38
Amikacin	12 (31.5)	26 (68.5)	0	38
Total	17 (15.3)	94 (84.7)	0	111

TABLE 3. *Chloramphenicol-aminoglycoside combination*

Chloramphenicol with:	No. of isolates tested			
	Additive (%)	Synergistic (%)	Antagonistic (%)	Total
Kanamycin	10 (25.6)	14 (35.9)	15 (38.4)	39
Gentamicin	5 (12.8)	20 (51.4)	14 (35.8)	39
Amikacin	9 (22.5)	13 (32.5)	18 (45.0)	40
Total	24 (20.2)	47 (39.9)	47 (39.9)	118

TABLE 4. *Comparison of MIC of five antibiotics against Klebsiella isolates in TSB and MHB*

Organism	MIC (μg/ml)									
	Gentamicin		Amikacin		Kanamycin		Chloramphenicol		Cephalothin	
	TSB	MHB	TSB	MHB	TSB	MHB	TSB	MHB	TSB	MHB
STH 14	0.625	0.156	1.25	0.313	5.00	0.156	2.50	1.25	5.00	1.25
STH 32	1.25	0.156	1.25	0.313	5.00	1.25	5.00	2.50	10.0	2.50
VAH 44	2.50	0.625	2.50	0.625	20.0	10.0	5.00	5.00	40.0	40.0
VAH 49	5.00	0.313	10.0	1.25	20.0	2.5	2.50	2.50	10.0	5.00
STH 68	0.625	0.313	5.00	0.313	5.00	0.313	2.50	1.25	40.0	40.0

antagonism was also statistically significant at the same level.

DISCUSSION

Gentamicin was the most active aminoglycoside in this system, followed by amikacin and kanamycin against 70 clinical isolates of *Klebsiella* species. This hierarchy of in vitro activity against *Klebsiella* has been reported previously (1). In terms of clinically achievable serum antimicrobial levels, gentamicin, amikacin, and chloramphenicol have greater in vitro activity than kanamycin or cephalothin. Cephalothin was the least active, with only 68% of isolates sensitive to 20 μg/ml or less.

A partial explanation for the relatively high MICs of kanamycin and amikacin in this system may be the use of TSB as the test medium. It has been shown that aminoglycoside MICs against different *Enterobacteriaceae,* including *Klebsiella,* are four- to sixfold higher in TSB than in nutrient broth or Mueller-Hinton broth (MHB) (1, 2). The exact mechanism for this is only partially understood. Two parameters that have been shown to affect aminoglycoside activity in various media are the pH of the growth medium and the electrolyte content. TSB contains added dextrose (250 mg/ml), and this is, of course, fermentable by the *Klebsiella* with a resultant fall in pH during growth. The net result is a diminution in the aminoglycoside effectiveness (1). TSB has a generally higher cation content than MHB or brain heart infusion broth (12), and this increased cation content (particularly calcium and magnesium) has been shown to adversely affect in vitro aminoglycoside activity (13).

To determine if our *Klebsiella* isolates followed this pattern, we performed simultaneous twofold tube dilution MICs of gentamicin, amikacin, kanamycin, chloramphenicol, and cephalothin in TSB and MHB for 5 of our 70 *Klebsiella* isolates (see Table 4). There was an average fourfold drop in the aminoglycoside MIC when MHB was used for susceptibility testing, but the relative order of activity against *Klebsiella* was similar to that determined in TSB (i.e., gentamicin > amikacin > kanamycin). No difference in chloramphenicol MIC was apparent, but a trend to a lower MIC of cephalothin in MHB was demonstrated.

To further delineate the media effect, if any, on the synergy results, microtiter synergy studies were repeated in MHB for two of the five organisms surveyed in Table 4 (STH 32 and VAH 49). Whereas the absolute values for the combination MICs were reduced two- to fourfold, the isobologram curves denoting synergy or antagonism were superimposable in 11 of the 12 plates when compared to the corresponding TSB synergy plate results.

In summary, synergy was demonstrated most commonly with the cephalothin-gentamicin and cephalothin-kanamycin combinations. Cephalothin-amikacin also exhibited synergy that was significantly greater than the respective aminoglycoside-chloramphenicol combination. None of the cephalothin-aminoglycoside combinations showed antagonism as opposed to 35 to 45% of the chloramphenicol-aminoglycoside combinations. In comparing the MIC data with the checkerboard results, there was no consistent sensitivity pattern with which one could predict whether or not the combinations of antibiotics would be synergistic or antagonistic.

The clinical importance of in vitro synergy or antagonism is uncertain in the absence of an in vivo model or a clinical trial. Until such data are available, the finding of significant antagonism using the chloramphenicol-aminoglycoside combinations mitigates against the indiscriminate use of this antibiotic combination in situations in which *Klebsiella* is a potential pathogen. The finding of synergy in over 80% of the cephalothin-aminoglycoside combinations tested suggests that this combination be used in therapy of serious *Klebsiella* infections. In addition, there is some clinical evidence to support the use of these combinations in serious gram-negative infections (5, 6, 9).

LITERATURE CITED

1. **Bodey, G. P., and D. Stewart.** 1973. In vitro effectiveness of BB-K8, a new aminoglycoside antibiotic. Antimicrob. Agents Chemother. 4:182–192.
2. **Bulger, R. J.** 1967. *In vitro* effectiveness of kanamycin and kanamycin/cephalothin against klebsiella. Ann. Intern. Med. 67:523–532.
3. **Holloway, W. J., and W. A. Taylor.** 1973. Gram-negative rods, p. 104–106. *In* Sepsis. Futura Publishing Co., Mt. Kisco, N.Y.
4. **Jawetz, E., and J. B. Gunnison.** 1952. Studies on antibiotic synergism and antagonism: a scheme of combined antibiotic action. Antibiot. Chemother. 2:243–248.
5. **Klastersky, J., R. Cappel, and D. Daneau.** 1972. Clinical significance of in vitro synergism between antibiotics in gram-negative infections. Antimicrob. Agents Chemother. 2:470–475.
6. **Klastersky, J., R. Cappel, G. Swings, and L. Vandenborre.** 1971. Bacteriological and clinical activity of the ampicillin/gentamicin and cephalothin/gentamicin combinations. Am. J. Med. Sci. 262:283-290.
7. **Kluge, R. M., H. C. Standiford, B. Tatum, V. M. Young, W. H. Greene, S. C. Schimpff, F. M. Calia, and R. B. Hornick.** 1974. Comparative activity of tobramycin, amikacin, and gentamicin alone and with carbenicillin against *Pseudomonas aeruginosa*. Antimicrob. Agents Chemother. 6:442–446.
8. **Luboshitzky, R., T. Sacks, and J. Michel.** 1973. Bactericidal effect of combinations of antibiotics on klebsiella-enterobacter-serratia. Chemotherapy 19:354–366.
9. **Martin, C. M., A. J. Cuomo, M. J. Geraghty, J. R. Zager, and T. C. Mandes.** 1969. Gram negative rod bacteremia. J. Infect. Dis. 119:506–517.
10. **Sabath, L. D.** 1968. Synergy of antibacterial substances by apparently known mechanisms, p. 210–217. Antimicrob. Agents Chemother. 1967.
11. **Sanford, J. P.** 1975. Klebsiella and other gram-negative bacterial pneumonias, p. 286–288. *In* P. B. Beeson and W. McDermott (ed.), Textbook of medicine, W. B. Saunders Co., Philadelphia.
12. **Warren, E., R. J. Snyder, and J. A. Washington, II.** 1972. Four-hour microbiological assay of gentamicin in serum. Antimicrob. Agents Chemother. 1:46–48.
13. **Washington, J. A., II, R. E. Ritts, Jr., and W. J. Martin.** 1970. In vitro susceptibility of gram-negative bacilli to gentamicin. Mayo Clin. Proc. 45:146–149.

ANTIMICROBIAL AGENTS AND CHEMOTHERAPY, Dec. 1976, p. 893–898 Vol. 10, No. 6

Effect of Clindamycin on Aminoglycoside Activity in a Murine Model of Invasive *Escherichia coli* Infection

EDEM EKWO[1] AND GEORGES PETER[2]

Departments of Pediatrics and Medicine, Roger Williams General Hospital, Providence, Rhode Island 02908; Department of Pediatrics, Rhode Island Hospital, Providence, Rhode Island 02902; and Sections of Reproductive and Developmental Medicine and Medicine, Brown University Program in Medicine, Providence, Rhode Island 02908

Received for publication 28 June 1976

Previous studies have demonstrated that the early in vitro bactericidal activity of gentamicin and amikacin is inhibited by clindamycin. To investigate the possible clinical implications of these findings, the effect of clindamycin in combination with gentamicin or amikacin was compared with that of the aminoglycoside alone in the treatment of normal and neutropenic mice with *Escherichia coli* peritonitis and bacteremia. Mice treated with saline or clindamycin alone experienced rapid multiplication of bacteria in the peritoneal cavity, bacteremia, and subsequent death. Gentamicin or amikacin given 2 h after *E. coli* inoculation significantly reduced the mortality and peritoneal bacterial counts in normal and neutropenic mice in comparison with untreated controls. Prior or simultaneous administration of clindamycin with either aminoglycoside did not inhibit survival or bacterial clearance from the peritoneum. The only clindamycin effect was slight enhancement of survival of neutropenic mice treated with multiple doses of amikacin and clindamycin in comparison to those treated with amikacin alone.

Increased awareness of the significance of anaerobic bacteria (4, 7) has resulted in the addition of clindamycin to antibiotic regimens for the critically ill patient with suspected infection (2, 16). The use of multiple antibiotics concurrently in the same patient, however, necessitates consideration of possible antimicrobial synergy or antagonism. Two recent studies have demonstrated that clindamycin inhibits the in vitro killing of *Escherichia coli* and *Klebsiella pneumoniae* by gentamicin (16; L. Riff and D. Matulionis, Prog. Abstr. Intersci. Conf. Antimicrob. Agents Chemother., 14th, San Francisco, Calif., Abstr. 291, 1974). In the study from this laboratory by Zinner et al., antagonism of either gentamicin or amikacin was observed after 4 h of incubation with clindamycin concentrations frequently achieved in patients (16).

To investigate the possible clinical importance of these findings, the effect of clindamycin on the in vivo therapeutic efficacy of gentamicin and amikacin was evaluated in a murine model of lethal *E. coli* infection. Since antibiotic antagonism, especially of early killing, may be clinically significant only in the host with diminished phagocytic function (13), these studies were performed in both normal and neutropenic mice.

(This paper was presented in part at the 15th Interscience Conference on Antimicrobial Agents and Chemotherapy, 24–26 September 1975, Washington, D.C.)

MATERIALS AND METHODS

Animals. White, male, pathogen-free, Swiss-Webster mice, strain SW/1CR (Ancare Corp., Manhasset, N.Y.), weighing 18 to 20 g, were used.

Induction of neutropenia. Cyclophosphamide (kindly supplied by Mead Johnson Laboratories, Evansville, Ind.) (Cytoxan), diluted in sterile saline immediately before use, was administered intraperitoneally (i.p.) in three divided doses (days 0, 1, and 3) totaling 350 mg/kg. Daily leukocyte and differential counts on tail vein blood were performed on five mice on days 2 through 9. As shown in Fig. 1, diminished circulating leukocytes (mean, 5,400 ± 591/mm^3) and neutropenia of less than 100/mm^3 on day 4, and persistence of less than 1,000 neutrophils per mm^3 through day 8 in both infected and noninfected mice occurred in the cyclophosphamide-treated mice. Nontreated mice (injected i.p. with sterile saline) demonstrated mean leukocyte and neutrophil counts of 10,700 ± 2,936/mm^3 and 3,210 ± 600/mm^3, respectively.

[1] Present address: Department of Pediatrics, University of Iowa Hospitals and Clinics, Iowa City, IA 52242.

[2] Address reprint requests to: Dr. Georges Peter, Division of Infectious Diseases, Rhode Island Hospital, Providence, RI 02902.

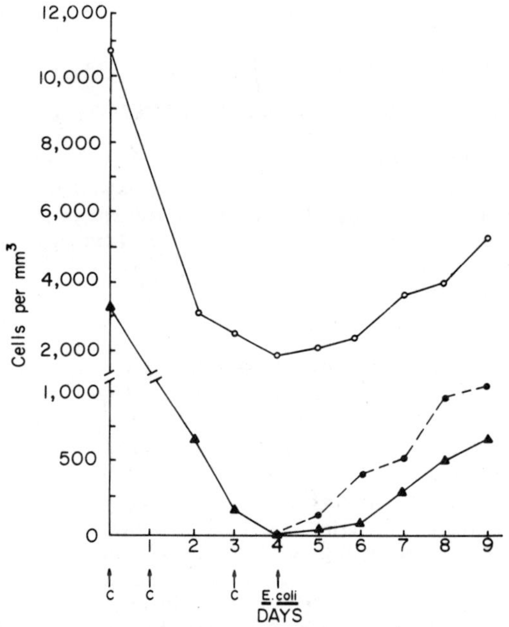

FIG. 1. *Mean circulating leukocytes and neutrophils in mice treated with cyclophosphamide (C). Verticle arrows below the X-axis indicate cyclophosphamide and, for later experiments, E. coli injections. Symbols:* ○, *leukocytes in noninfected mice;* ●, *neutrophils in infected mice;* ▲, *neutrophils in noninfected mice.*

Bacteria. One representative strain of *E. coli* was selected for the animal experiments from the 20 strains previously studied in vitro in this laboratory, whose early killing by gentamicin and amikacin was antagonized by clindamycin at 15 μg/ml (16). The definition of antagonism for this paper is that of Sabath (10). The minimal inhibitory concentrations of gentamicin and amikacin at 18 h of incubation for this strain were 1.8 μg/ml and 2.5 μg/ml, respectively. Clindamycin alone at concentrations up to 100 μg/ml did not inhibit its growth. The test strain was stored on corked Trypticase soy agar slants until use.

For injection into mice, this *E. coli* strain was grown overnight in Mueller-Hinton broth at 37°C, diluted 1:10, and then shaken for 1 h in a 37°C water bath to reach log-phase growth. This suspension was standardized against a known concentration of bacteria by optical density (transmission at 45%; wavelength, 610 nm; didymicin filter on the Coleman Jr. II) to give 10^8 colony-forming units (CFU)/ml (as determined by a standard pour-plate technique) and subsequently diluted in Mueller-Hinton broth to obtain the desired concentration.

Antibiotics. Gentamicin sulfate (Schering Corp., Bloomfield, N.J.), amikacin sulfate (Bristol Laboratories, Syracuse, N. Y.), and clindamycin hydrochloride (Upjohn Co., Kalamazoo, Mich.) were dissolved and diluted in sterile distilled water and stored at −40°C until use. All products were kindly supplied by the respective manufacturer.

Infection of mice. Groups of 18 mice were injected i.p. with 0.3 ml of different concentrations of *E. coli* ranging from 10^2 to 10^8 CFU/ml. Cyclophosphamide-treated mice were infected at the time of maximum neutropenia (day 4, as shown on Fig. 1). Cumulative mortality was determined by survival at least 5 days after infection. The mean lethal dose (LD_{50}) was calculated by the method of Reed-Muench (9). In addition, blood was obtained aseptically from the aorta of mice sacrificed 2 h after infection and quantitively cultured by pour-plate dilution to assess bacteremia.

Antibiotic treatment. Normal and neutropenic mice infected with 10 times their respective LD_{50} inoculum of *E. coli* were treated 2 h later with one of the following regimens: gentamicin, amikacin, clindamycin, clindamycin and gentamicin, clindamycin and amikacin, or sterile saline (control group). Multiple antibiotics were administered at separate sites. Antibiotic doses were given in 0.2-ml volumes i.p. and included the following: gentamicin, 3 and 5 mg/kg; amikacin, 10 and 15 mg/kg; and clindamycin, 15, 30, 50, and 100 mg/kg. Multiple-dose therapy with these drugs was given from 2 to 48 h after infection with the following dosages: gentamicin, 3 and 5 mg/kg; amikacin, 10 and 15 mg/kg; clindamycin, 30 mg/kg.

Serum gentamicin concentrations were determined by the method of Sabath et al. (11). Groups of 10 noninfected, normal mice given a single dose of gentamicin (1, 5, and 7 mg/kg) were bled 30 or 60 min later from the tail vein.

Peritoneal lavage. Neutropenic mice challenged with 0.3 ml of an approximate LD_{50} *E. coli* inoculum (5×10^4 CFU/ml) were given gentamicin (3 and 5 mg/kg), amikacin (10 and 15 mg/kg), clindamycin (30 mg/kg), or clindamycin and an aminoglycoside, or sterile saline (control) 2 h later. The bacterial content of the peritoneal cavity was quantitated by the method of Cohn (2) on mice (three to five in each group) sacrificed at 2, 3, 4, 6, and 8 h after infection.

Chi-square with Yates correction where applicable and the paired *t* tests were used for statistical analyses.

RESULTS

Cumulative mortality of normal and neutropenic mice infected with 0.3 ml of different concentrations of *E. coli* is shown in Fig. 2. Deaths occurred within the first 36 h after infection. The differing mortality curves for normal and neutropenic mice demonstrate the increased susceptibility of the neutropenic mice to bacterial challenge. The LD_{50} (absolute number of bacteria) of 3×10^3 CFU for neutropenic mice was significantly less ($P < 0.001$) than that of 3×10^6 CFU for the non-immunosuppressed mice. Blood cultures obtained 2 h after infection with 5×10^4 CFU demonstrated a

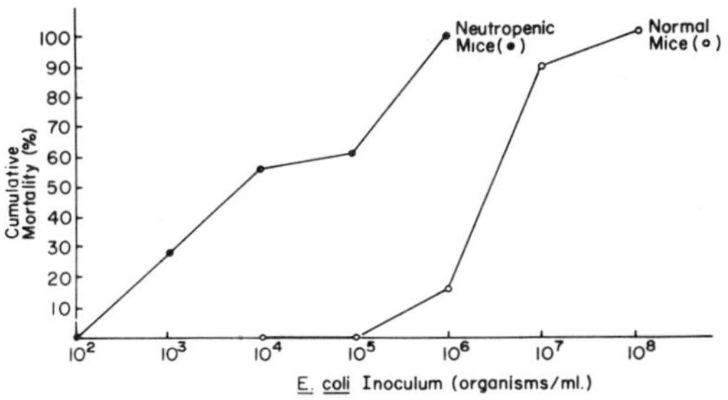

FIG. 2. *Cumulative mortality of normal and neutropenic mice infected with differing inocula of E. coli in groups of 18. Mice were injected i.p. with 0.3 ml of the bacterial concentration (X-axis) and mortality was determined by 5-day survival. The calculated mean lethal doses in the text are expressed in the absolute number of bacteria.*

mean of 2.14 (± 0.62) × 10^2 CFU/ml in five normal mice and 2.28 (±0.187) × 10^3 CFU/ml in five neutropenic mice.

Quantitation of serum gentamicin concentrations 30 and 60 min postdose in normal, uninfected mice demonstrated dose-related peak serum concentrations of <1.5 μg/ml and of 3.0 μg/ml and 5.0 μg/ml for 1-mg/kg, 5-mg/kg, and 7-mg/kg doses, respectively. These concentrations for the two higher doses exceeded the minimal inhibitory concentration of the test strain.

Treatment of normal mice infected with 3 × 10^7 organisms with either gentamicin (5 mg/kg) or amikacin (15 mg/kg) 2 h later significantly reduced mortality. Twenty-four percent (6 out of 25) of gentamicin-treated and 28% (7 out of 25) of amikacin-treated mice died in comparison to 95% (38 out of 40) of both control and clindamycin-treated (30 mg/kg) animals ($P < 0.001$). Clindamycin at 15, 30, or 50 mg/kg administered simultaneously at 30 or 60 min before either aminoglycoside did not affect aminoglycoside-induced survival.

Similar experiments with neutropenic mice infected with 3 × 10^4 organisms and treated 2 h later demonstrated similar antibiotic effects (Fig. 3). The cumulative mortality of 45% (9 out of 20) for the mice receiving gentamicin (5 mg/kg) was significantly different ($P < 0.05$) from that for control or clindamycin-treated mice. Survival was not appreciably affected by clindamycin (30 mg/kg) in conjunction with 5 mg of gentamicin per kg. Gentamicin at 3 mg/kg and amikacin at 10 mg/kg resulted in 58% (14 out of 24) and 64% (16 out of 25) cumulative mortality, respectively; concomitant clindamycin at either 30 or 50 mg/kg did not alter these survival curves (data not shown). Clindamycin in very high doses (100 mg/kg) gave similar results with or without an aminoglycoside.

Treatment with multiple 3- and 5-mg/kg doses of gentamicin also reduced mortality significantly ($P < 0.005$). This effect was dose related; 90% (18 out of 20) of mice treated with 5 mg/kg survived in comparison to 60% (12 out of 20) given 3 mg/kg (Fig. 4A). The efficacy of gentamicin was not inhibited by concomitant clindamycin therapy at either 30-mg/kg (Fig. 4A) or 50-mg/kg doses (not shown).

Figure 4B demonstrates the results with multiple-dose amikacin and clindamycin treatment. Amikacin alone at the 10-mg/kg dose resulted in 40% (8 out of 20) and 45% (9 out of 20) survival at 48 and 96 h, respectively. The addition of clindamycin (30-mg/kg per dose) to amikacin further reduced the mortality to 7% (2 out of 30) at both 48 and 96 h. This difference achieved statistical significance ($P < 0.001$). However, similar experiments with amikacin

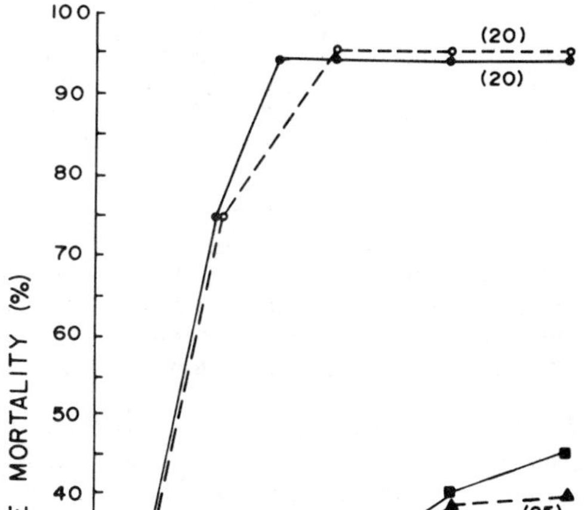

FIG. 3. *Cumulative mortality of infected neutropenic mice infected with 3 × 10^4 E. coli and treated with single doses of gentamicin and/or clindamycin 2 h after infection. Control mice received sterile saline (●). Clindamycin (30 mg/kg) (○); gentamicin (5 mg/kg) (■); gentamicin (5 mg/kg) plus clindamycin (30 mg/kg) (▲).*

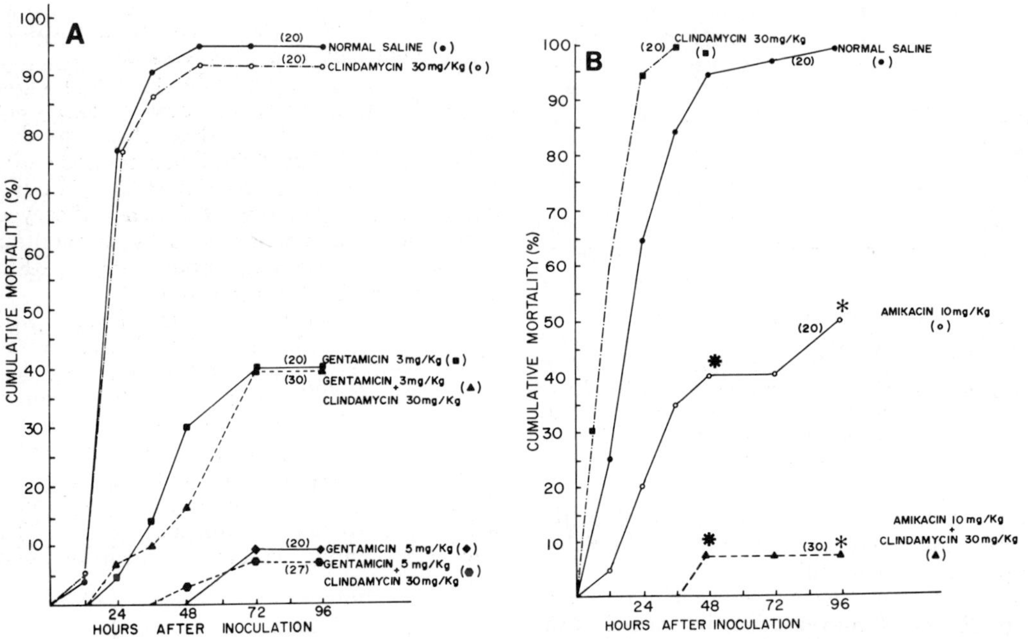

FIG. 4. *Cumulative mortality of infected neutropenic mice treated with multiple doses of an aminoglycoside and/or clindamycin. (A) Gentamicin and/or clindamycin were given at 2, 10, 32, 40, and 48 h after infection. (B) Amikacin was given at 2, 14, 26, and 38 h and clindamycin was given at 2, 8, 14, 26, 32, and 38 h. Control mice received sterile saline. Significant differences in mortality ($P < 0.001$) are denoted by matching symbols.*

at the 15-mg/kg per dose did not demonstrate any effect from the addition of clindamycin (data not shown). Amikacin at this higher dose resulted in 75% (15 out of 20) survival at 96 h; with clindamycin, survival was 80% (16 out of 20).

Peritoneal lavage of infected neutropenic mice demonstrated that both aminoglycosides (gentamicin, 3 and 5 mg/kg; amikacin, 10 and 15 mg/kg) resulted in 90 to 95% reduction in the quantitative recovery of bacteria from the peritoneal cavity from 2 to 6 h after antibiotic administration. Figure 5 shows that the bacterial clearance with gentamicin was not altered by clindamycin. No inhibition could be demonstrated at either gentamicin dose, even if clindamycin was administered 30 to 60 min before. Results with amikacin and clindamycin were nearly identical to those with gentamicin and are not shown here.

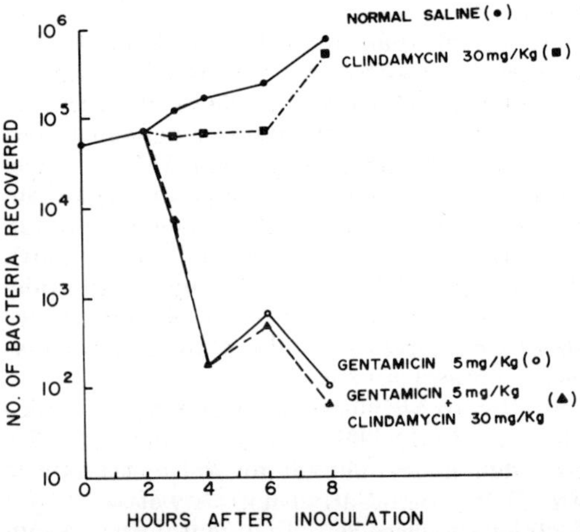

FIG. 5. *Recovery of E. coli from the peritoneal cavity of neutropenic mice inoculated i.p. with 5 × 10^4 organisms at zero time and given gentamicin and/or clindamycin 2 h later. Three to five mice in each treatment group were sacrificed at 0, 2, 3, 4, 6, and 8 h.*

DISCUSSION

In this study, clindamycin did not inhibit the therapeutic effect of either gentamicin or amikacin in an otherwise lethal *E. coli* infection. In vivo antagonism could not be demonstrated with differing doses and schedules of clindamycin and the aminoglycosides, even in neutropenic mice. This was true when clindamycin was administered 30 and 60 min before the injection of gentamicin. The lack of correlation between these in vivo findings and those demonstrating in vitro inhibition by clindamycin of the early antibacterial activity of two aminoglycosides contrasts with those with chloramphenicol and gentamicin reported by Sande and Overton (13). These investigators found that chloramphenicol inhibition of early in vitro bactericidal activity of gentamicin appeared significant in neutropenic, but not normal, mice infected with *Proteus mirabilis*. In their work, neutropenia was induced by irradiation. The markedly increased susceptibility to *E. coli* bacteremia and death of mice treated with cyclophosphamide reported here and by Grogan (5) indicates that the lack of clindamycin antagonism probably cannot be explained by inadequate immunosuppression. Since serum concentrations of clindamycin were not determined, the lack of clindamycin antagonism might be explained by insufficient serum clindamycin activity. The wide range of doses, 15 to 100 mg/kg, at which clindamycin was tested lessens the likelihood of this possibility, however.

A possible explanation for the lack of clindamycin antagonism is that the degree of inhibition of aminoglycoside activity by clindamycin was insufficient to cause in vivo antagonism in this murine model. In the study by Sande and Overton, the addition of chloramphenicol to gentamicin resulted in an approximate three-log difference in the number of viable organisms (13) in comparison with a less than 100-fold difference in our in vitro studies with clindamycin and an aminoglycoside (16).

The in vitro findings that prompted this series of experiments did demonstrate that at 18 h of incubation (in contrast to findings at 4 h), high concentrations of clindamycin (20 to 25 μg/ml) did reduce the minimal inhibitory concentration and minimal bactericidal concentration of gentamicin and amikacin for the same strains of *E. coli* (16). In neutropenic mice, multiple doses of amikacin and clindamycin did result in slightly enhanced survival in comparison to mice receiving multiple doses of amikacin alone. These findings might be interpreted to give clinical signficance to in vitro antibiotic interactions noted after 18 to 24 h of incubation, rather than after 2 to 4 h. However, similar experiments with gentamicin and clindamycin did not demonstrate this correlation between "late" in vitro findings and therapeutic results.

The discrepancy between in vivo and in vitro results has also been noted in the treatment of an experimental *Staphylococcus aureus* infection with antibiotic combinations (14). These findings support the conclusion of Jawetz that "antagonism between antimicrobial drugs undoubtedly occurs . . . , but with the exception of special situations, the effect is not of sufficient magnitude to interfere with a successful outcome of treatment" (6). Results of in vitro tests are dependent upon several laboratory variables, including drug concentrations, time of interaction, and inoculum size. For example, clindamycin combined with gentamicin against gram-negative organisms has been reported in different test systems to be antagonistic (16; Riff and Matulionis, Prog. Abstr. Intersci. Conf. Antimicrob. Agents Chemother., Abstr. 291, 1974), indifferent (3, 12), or synergistic (13). Studies of antibiotic combinations in human and experimental infections are affected by additional immunological and pharmacological considerations, including phagocytic function (13), interval between infection and treatment (11), and drug distribution. Antagonism can be obscured by a large excess of one drug at the site of infection (16), as well as by adequate local phagocytic factors. Any of these factors may help to explain the lack of correlation of these in vivo findings with in vitro results.

ACKNOWLEDGMENTS

We thank Katherine S. Elias and Richard B. Provonchee for their technical assistance, and Stephen H. Zinner for his advice and encouragement during the study and in the preparation of the manuscript.

This study was supported by the Cancer Research Center Public Health Service grant no. CA 13943 from the National Cancer Institute.

LITERATURE CITED

1. **Andriole, V. T.** 1971. Synergy of carbenicillin and gentamicin in experimental infection with Pseudomonas. J. Infect. Dis. 124:S46–S55.
2. **Cohn, Z. A.** 1962. Determinants of infection in the peritoneal cavity. I. Response to and the fate of *Staphylococcus aureus* and *Staphylococcus albus* in the mouse. Yale J. Biol. Med. 35:12–28.
3. **Fass, R. J., C. A. Rotile, and R. B. Prior.** 1974. Interaction of clindamycin and gentamicin in vitro. Antimicrob. Agents Chemother. 6:582–587.
4. **Finegold, S. M., J. G. Bartlett, A. W. Chow, D. J. Flora, S. L. Gorbach, E. J. Harder, and F. P. Tally.** 1975. Management of anaerobic infections. Ann. Intern. Med. 83:275–389.
5. **Grogan, J. B.** 1975. Pseudomonas aeruginosa infection in mice after treatment with cyclophosphamide. Arch. Surg. 110:1473–1476.
6. **Jawetz, E.** 1968. The use of combinations of antimicrobial drugs. Annu. Rev. Pharm. 8:151–170.
7. **Kagnoff, M. F., D. Armstrong, and A. Blevins.** 1972. Bacteroides bacteremia. Cancer 29:245–251.
8. **Ledger, W., T. J. K. Focog, L. S. Richard, and F. R. Fekety.** 1974. The use of clindamycin in treatment of obstetrics-gynecology patients with severe infection. Obstet. Gynecol. 43:490–497.
9. **Reed, L. J., and H. Muench.** 1938. A simple method of estimating fifty percent end-point. Am. J. Hyg. 27:493–497.
10. **Sabath, L. D.** 1968. Synergy of antibacterial substances by apparently known mechanisms, p. 210–217. Antimicrob. Agents Chemother. 1967.
11. **Sabath, L. D., J. I. Casey, P. A. Ruch, L. L. Stumpf, and M. Finland.** 1971. Rapid microassay of gentami-

cin, kanamycin, neomycin, streptomycin and vancomycin in serum or plasma. J. Lab. Clin. Med. 78:457–463.

12. **Sabath, L. D., and I. Toftegaard.** 1974. Rapid microassays for clindamycin and gentamicin when present together and the effect of pH and of each on the antibacterial activity of the other. Antimicrob. Agents Chemother. 6:54–59.
13. **Sande, M. A., and J. W. Overton.** 1973. In vivo antagonism between gentamicin and chloramphenicol in neutropenic mice. J. Infect. Dis. 128:247–250.
14. **Steigbigel, R. T., R. L. Greenman, and J. S. Remington.** 1975. Antibiotic combinations in the treatment of experimental *Staphylococcus aureus* infection. J. Infect. Dis. 131:245–251.
15. **Tattersall, M. H. N., A. S. D. Spiers, and J. H. Darrell.** 1972. Initial therapy with combination of five antibiotics in febrile patients with leukemia and neutropenia. Lancet i:162–165.
16. **Zinner, S. H., R. B. Provonchee, K. S. Elia, and G. Peter.** 1976. Effect of clindamycin on the in vitro activity of amikacin and gentamicin against gram-negative bacilli. Antimicrob. Agents Chemother. 9:661–664.

ANTIMICROBIAL AGENTS AND CHEMOTHERAPY, Dec. 1976, p. 899-901 Vol. 10, No. 6

Printed in U.S.A.

Comparison of Josamycin and Erythromycin in the Therapy of *Mycoplasma pneumoniae* Pneumonia

RICHARD P. WENZEL,* J. OWEN HENDLEY, WENDELL K. DODD, AND JACK M. GWALTNEY, JR.

Departments of Internal Medicine and Pediatrics, University of Virginia School of Medicine, Charlottesville, Virginia 22901*

Received for publication 7 June 1976

A controlled, double-blind study was performed to compare the efficacy of two macrolide antibiotics, erythromycin and josamycin, in the therapy of *Mycoplasma pneumoniae* pneumonia. Marine Corps recruit volunteers received one of the two antibiotics in a dosage of 2 g daily for 7 days. Twelve of 21 men treated with josamycin and 9 of 25 men treated with erythromycin had confirmed *M. pneumoniae* pneumonia. The josamycin-treated group remained hospitalized for 5.4 ± 1.2 days compared to 5.1 ± 2.0 days for the erythromycin-treated group ($0.60 > P > 0.50$). Fever days were similar for the josamycin-treated (1.4 ± 0.4) and erythromycin-treated (1.2 ± 0.3) groups ($P = 0.95$). There was no difference in resolution of signs and symptoms of illness in the two study populations. Thus, josamycin is as efficacious as erythromycin in the therapy of *M. pneumoniae* pneumonia.

Mycoplasma pneumoniae is an important cause of bronchitis and pneumonia in older children and young adults (1, 3, 6, 12, 15). Two antibiotics, erythromycin and tetracycline, have been shown to be efficacious in reducing hospitalization time, days of fever, cough, and resolution of chest film infiltrates in patients with *M. pneumoniae* pneumonia (5, 8, 10, 11). Recently a new investigational macrolide antibiotic, josamycin (9), was shown to have activity in vitro against *M. pneumoniae* and was demonstrated to have few gastrointestinal side effects (13). Josamycin has been suggested as an alternative antibiotic for therapy of *M. pneumoniae* pneumonia. The purpose of this study was to compare the relative efficacy of josamycin and erythromycin in the therapy of naturally occurring *M. pneumoniae* pneumonia.

MATERIALS AND METHODS

Time and location of study. The study period began on July 1, 1975, and continued to October 15, 1975, at the Marine Corps Recruit Depot, Parris Island, S.C.

Volunteers. Forty-six Marine Corps recruits at Parris Island, S.C., with pneumonia, who had been informed of the nature of the study and its possible hazards and who had signed the consent form, comprised the study group. Pneumonia was considered present if there was a consistent clinical picture and either an infiltrate on chest X ray or the presence of rales on admission. All but three patients had an infiltrate, and all confirmed *M. pneumoniae* pneumonia cases had the presence of both infiltrate and rales. No volunteer had a known allergy to erythromycin. Twenty-one men received josamycin, and 25 received erythromycin double-blind and randomized fashion.

Antibiotics. Either josamycin (2 g/day; Endo Laboratories, Inc., Garden City, N.Y.) or erythromycin base (2 g/day) in four 6-h doses was administered to volunteers for 7 days or until it was no longer tolerated. Both antibiotics were administered by Navy Corpsmen during the day at 6 a.m., 12 a.m., 6 p.m., and 12 p.m., thus in close relationship to meals or the evening snack.

Blood levels of josamycin and erythromycin obtained at 10:00 a.m. on hospital day 3 were determined by a standard bioassay method employing *Sarcina lutea* ATCC 9341 grown overnight in brain heart infusion broth. Tests were kindly performed by Joe W. McGahen, Stine Laboratories, Wilmington, Del. Sixteen determinations were performed for josamycin and 17 for erythromycin.

Surveillance and sampling. All patients hospitalized with pneumonia who volunteered for the study received one of the two antibiotics and were observed daily. On admission and on day 7, throat swabs for *M. pneumoniae* culture were obtained. Paired sera (admission and day 21) for antibody testing were collected. A clinical sheet was completed daily to evaluate acceptability. Fever days and hospital days were counted to compare efficacy of the two antibiotics.

Serum antibody. The metabolic inhibition test of Taylor-Robinson et al. (14) was employed using four to 16 CCU of organisms per well to assess antibody response to the vaccine (12).

***M. pneumoniae* cultures.** Throat swabs were placed in Hayflick's pleuropneumonia-like organism (mycoplasmas) collecting media and, on return to a central facility, portions were incubated before being sent (within 3 days) in insulated and cooled containers to Charlottesville. In Charlottesville, portions were placed in pleuropneumonia-like organism diphasic media with a color indicator for growth. All presumed isolates were confirmed by disk inhibition (anti-*M. pneumoniae* antibody) on pleuropneumonia-like organism agar (4).

Clinical evaluation. A daily scoring system for each volunteer was used to test the efficacy of antibiotics: rales and wheezes if present were arbitrarily scored two (2); malaise, cough, and headache were scored as one (1), two (2), or three (3) if present and considered mild, moderate, or severe, respectively. Separate scoring for gastrointestinal symptoms were calculated daily. Nausea, vomiting, diarrhea, abdominal pain, and anorexia were each graded as one (1), two (2), or three (3) if present and considered mild, moderate, or severe, respectively, by the volunteers.

Analysis of data. Any volunteer with a positive pharyngeal culture or fourfold serum antibody rise to *M. pneumoniae* was considered ill with that agent. Student's *t* test analyses were performed in the comparison of hospital days and fever days in the two antibiotic-treated groups. To test the difference in resolution of signs and symptoms, the mean scoring system was determined for each antibiotic study group and plotted by day.

RESULTS

Seventy-two-hour mean (standard deviation) antibiotic levels were 1.15 μg/ml (0.58) and 2.95 μg/ml (2.12) for patients receiving josamycin or erythromycin, respectively. Twelve of 21 men who were treated with josamycin and 9 of 25 who were treated with erythromycin had confirmed *M. pneumoniae* pneumonia. Pneumonia was similar in degree of infiltrate in all *M. pneumoniae* confirmed cases, and in every patient was confined to a single lobe. There was no significant difference in the number of hospital days or fever days between the josamycin and erythromycin groups (Table 1). The josamycin-treated groups remained hospitalized for a mean of 5.4 days compared to a mean of 5.1 days for the erythromycin-treated group. Fever was present for a mean of 1.4 days in the josamycin-treated group and a mean of 1.2 days for the erythromycin-treated group. When the mean scoring system for efficacy was employed there was no difference in the resolution of signs or symptoms of *M. pneumoniae* pneumonia (malaise, cough, headache, rales, and wheezes) in the josamycin- and erythromycin-treated groups (Fig. 1).

Since gastrointestinal symptoms were considered possible side effects, mean scores for each antibiotic group were compared (Fig. 2).

TABLE 1. *Antibiotic efficacy against M. pneumoniae pneumonia*[a]

Study group	Hospital days[b]	Fever days[c]
Josamycin (n = 12)	5.4 ± 1.2	1.4 ± 0.4
Erythromycin (n = 9)	5.1 ± 2.0	1.2 ± 0.3

[a] Student's t test.
[b] $0.60 > P > 0.50$.
[c] $P = 0.95$.

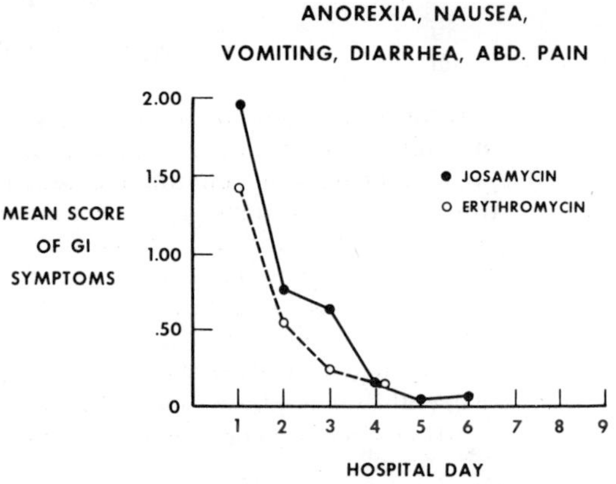

FIG. 1. *Mean daily scores for symptoms and signs of M. pneumoniae pneumonia in josamycin- and erythromycin-treated groups. There were 12 volunteers in the josamycin-treated group on admission and nine in the erythromycin-treated group.*

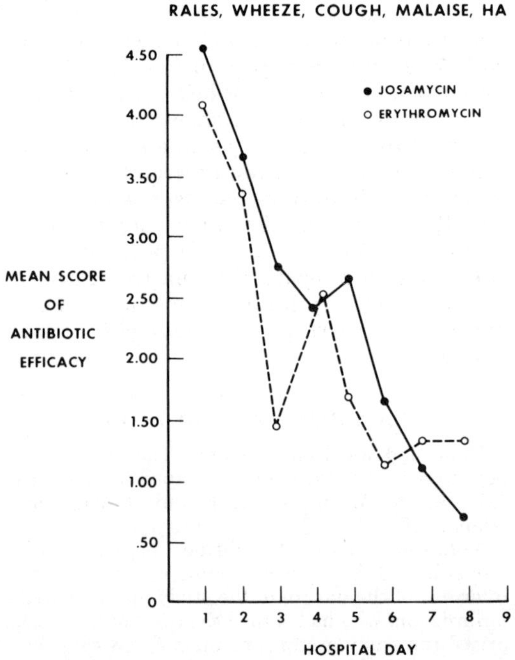

FIG. 2. *Mean daily scores for gastrointestinal symptoms in the patients treated with josamycin or erythromycin. There were 21 volunteers in the josamycin-treated group and 25 in the erythromycin-treated group on admission.*

There was continued resolution of symptoms with time in both antibiotic-treated groups, suggesting that these were not side effects but perhaps coincident symptoms. Furthermore, there was no difference in the rate of resolution of these symptoms.

DISCUSSION

In the evaluation of josamycin and erythromycin for treatment of *M. pneumoniae* pneumonia in Marine Corps recruits, both antibiotics were well tolerated at doses of 2 g daily. Blood levels were ≥100 times the reported median mycoplasmacidal drug levels for josamycin (0.015 μg/ml) and erythromycin (0.007 μg/ml) (13). It should be pointed out, however, that our subjects (highly motivated Marine Corps recruits) were quite anxious to leave the hospital to return to their original platoons; therefore, their minor complaints might not have been voiced. We conclude that josamycin is as efficacious as erythromycin in the therapy of *M. pneumoniae* pneumonia, and that in Marine Corps recruits gastrointestinal symptoms were similar in patients treated with josamycin or erythromycin.

ACKNOWLEDGMENTS

We acknowledge the invaluable assistance of Walter R. Stephenson of the Marine Corps Recruit Depot, Parris Island, S.C., John H. Gannon of the United States Navy, and Joe W. McGahen of Stine Laboratories, Newark, Del.

This research was jointly supported by E. I. du Pont de Nemours & Co., Inc., Wilmington, Del., and by its subsidiary, Endo Laboratories, Inc., Garden City, N.Y.

LITERATURE CITED

1. **Alexander, E.R., H.M. Foy, G.E. Kenny, R.A. Kronmal, R. McMahn, E.R. Clarke, W.A. MacColl, and J.T. Grayston.** 1966. Pneumonia due to *Mycoplasma pneumoniae*. N. Engl. J. Med. 275:131-136.
2. **Brown, R.C., J.O. Hendley, and J.M. Gwaltney, Jr.** 1972. *Mycoplasma pneumoniae* vaccine: antigenicity of buffered antigens in volunteers. Infect. Immun. 5:657-661.
3. **Chanock, R.M.** 1965. Mycoplasma infections of man. N. Engl. J. Med. 273:1199-1206.
4. **Clyde, W.A.** 1964. Mycoplasma species identification based upon growth inhibition by specific antisera. J. Immunol. 92:958-965.
5. **Foy, H.J., G.E. Kenny, R. McMahan, A.M. Mansy, and J.T. Grayston.** 1970. *Mycoplasma pneumoniae* pneumonia in an urban area. J. Am. Med. Assoc. 214:1666-1672.
6. **Grayston, J.T., E.R. Alexander, G.E. Kenny, E.R. Clarke, J.C. Fremont, and W.A. MacColl.** 1965. *Mycoplasma pneumoniae* infections. J. Am. Med. Assoc. 191:369-374.
7. **Hayflick, L.** 1965. Cell cultures and mycoplasmas. Tex. Rep. Biol. Med. 23:285.
8. **Kingston, J.R., R.M. Chanock, M.C. Mufson, L.P. Hellman et al.** 1961. Eaton agent pneumonia. J. Am. Med. Assoc. 176:118-123.
9. **Nakazawa, S.**, S. Oka, K. Ishitiara, H. Sato, and Y. Hirasawa. 1969. Laboratory and clinical evaluation of josamycin in pediatrics. Chemotherapy (Nihon Kagaku Ryoho Gakkai) 17:664-672.
10. **Rasch, J.R., and W. J. Mogabgab.** 1966. Therapeutic effect of erythromycin on *Mycoplasma pneumoniae* pneumonia, p. 693-699. Antimicrob. Agents Chemother. 1965.
11. **Shames, J.M., R.B. George, W.B. Holliday, J.R. Rasch, and W.J. Mogabgab.** 1970. Comparison of antibiotics in the treatment of mycoplasma pneumonia, Arch. Int. Med. 125:680-684.
12. **Steinberg, P., R.J. White, S.L. Fuld, R.R. Gutekunst, R.M. Chanock, and L.B. Senterfit.** 1969. Ecology of *Mycoplasma pneumoniae* infections in Marine recruits at Parris Island, South Carolina. Am. J. Epidemiol. 89:62-73.
13. **Strausbaugh, L.J., J.A. Dilworth, J.M. Gwaltney, Jr., and M.A. Sande.** 1976. In vitro susceptibility studies with josamycin and erythromycin. Antimicrob. Agents Chemother. 9:546-548.
14. **Taylor-Robinson, D., R.H. Purcell, D.C. Wong, and R.M. Chanock.** 1973. A colour test for the measurement of antibody to certain mycoplasma species based upon the inhibition of acid production, J. Hyg. 64:91-104.
15. **Wenzel, R.P., D.P. McCormick, E.P. Smith, D.L. Clark, and W.E. Beam, Jr.** 1971. Acute respiratory disease: clinical and epidemiologic observations of military trainees. Mil. Med. 136:873-880.

ANTIMICROBIAL AGENTS AND CHEMOTHERAPY, Dec. 1976, p. 902–911
Copyright © 1976 American Society for Microbiology
Vol. 10, No. 6
Printed in U.S.A.

Cephalosporin and Aminoglycoside Concentrations in Peritoneal Capsular Fluid in Rabbits

DALE N. GERDING,* WENDELL H. HALL, ELIZABETH A. SCHIERL, AND ROBERT E. MANION

Infectious Disease Section, Department of Medicine, Veterans Administration Hospital, and University of Minnesota Medical School, Minneapolis, Minnesota 55417*

Received for publication 1 July 1976

To study the penetration of antibiotics into peritoneal tissue fluid, a subcutaneous tissue capsule model was modified by implanting multiple, perforated spherical capsules in the peritoneal cavity of rabbits. Capsules became vascularized, encased in connective tissue, and filled with fluid having a mean protein concentration of 3.6 g/100 ml. Capsular fluid was obtained by percutaneous needle aspiration and assayed for antibiotic by the disk plate bioassay technique. Cephalosporins were administered intramuscularly at a dose of 30 mg/kg. Mean peak concentrations of cephaloridine and cefazolin were significantly higher than cephalothin and cephapirin in capsular fluids, but the percent penetration (ratio of capsular mean peak to serum mean peak) ranged from 8.7 to 16.9% and was not significantly different among the cephalosporins. At 24 h the capsular concentration of cefazolin was significantly greater than for the other cephalosporins ($P < 0.001$). Lower rabbit serum protein binding observed at high in vivo concentrations may have enabled cefazolin to penetrate capsular fluid, but in vitro protein binding studies did not confirm a decrease in serum protein binding at high concentrations within the clinical range. Kanamycin and amikacin showed comparable capsular fluid peak concentrations as did gentamicin and tobramycin. The percent penetration ranged from 15.2 to 34.5% for the aminoglycosides. The only statistical difference was that amikacin penetration was significantly higher than that for tobramycin. Mean capsular concentrations of amikacin, cefazolin, and cephaloridine compared most favorably with the minimum inhibitory concentration of gram-negative bacilli at the dosages used in this study.

Among the factors determining successful antibiotic therapy, the ability of the antibiotic to reach an extravascular site of infection seems particularly important. Intra-abdominal infections (abscesses and peritonitis) are commonly caused by a mixed bacterial flora and are often treated with antibiotics administered both parenterally and locally. If parenteral administration alone fails to achieve adequate levels in peritoneal tissues, intraperitoneal therapy may be required. In addition, members of certain classes of antibiotics, such as the cephalosporins and aminoglycosides, may differ in their penetration of extravascular tissue. A perforated tissue capsule model (14) was adapted for use intraperitoneally in rabbits (11) to determine the penetration of antibiotics into peritoneal capsular fluid.

The purpose of this paper is: (i) to describe the peritoneal tissue capsule model used in rabbits and (ii) to evaluate the capsular penetration of single doses of four cephalosporin and four aminoglycoside drugs in this model. A limited comparison of the penetration of subcutaneous capsules and intraperitoneal capsules was also performed.

(This paper was presented in part at the 14th Interscience Conference on Antimicrobial Agents and Chemotherapy, 11–13 September 1974, San Francisco, Calif., and the Symposium on Antibiotics, Section on Medicine of the New York Academy of Medicine, 20 November 1974, New York, N.Y.)

MATERIALS AND METHODS

Capsules. Various tissue capsules used in the study are shown in Fig. 1. Fabricated stainless-steel mesh cylinders and 5-ml plastic syringe barrels drilled with 60 to 70 holes (1.6 mm) were implanted subcutaneously. Ordinary table tennis balls were drilled with 200 to 250 holes and implanted in the peritoneal cavity.

Implantation. Albino rabbits (2.5 to 5.25 kg) were anesthetized with 50 to 75 mg of intravenous sodium pentobarbital. For subcutaneous implantations the

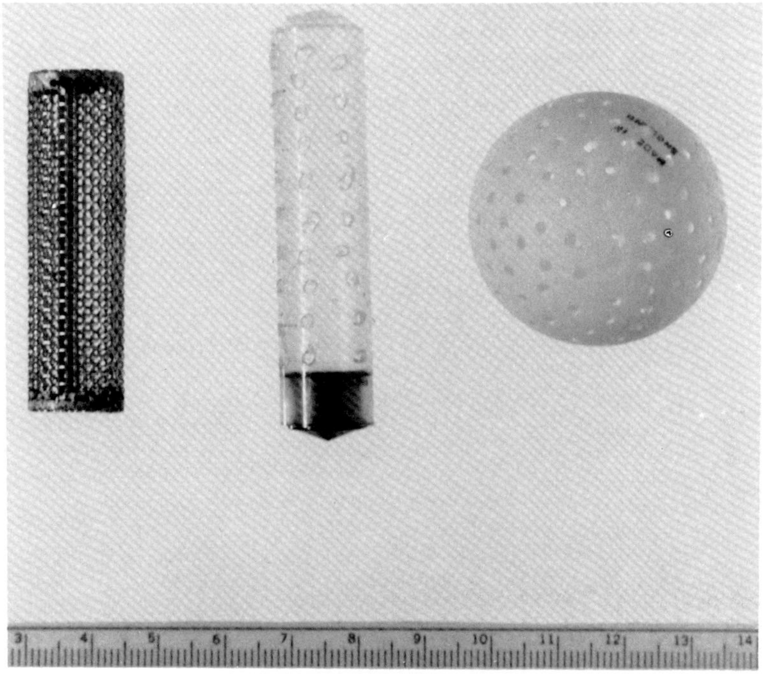

FIG. 1. *Subcutaneous (stainless-steel mesh and perforated syringe barrel) and peritoneal (perforated table tennis ball) capsules. Mesh cylinders are 5.2 cm long by 1.5 cm in diameter. Syringe barrels are 6.1 cm long and 1.4 cm in diameter.*

flanks were shaved and the skin was swabbed with povidone-iodine followed by absolute alcohol. A 5-cm incision was made and the subcutaneous space was dissected bluntly. One to three ethylene oxide-sterilized cylinders were implanted in each flank and positioned 2 to 3 cm apart. The skin was closed with metal clips. For intraperitoneal implantation the abdomen was cleansed in the same manner as were the flanks. A 5-cm midline incision was made just below the xiphoid and the peritoneum was opened with scissors. Two to five sterile peritoneal capsules were inserted and manually maneuvered under the abdominal wall into well-separated positions. No attempt was made to fix the capsules in place. The abdominal wall was closed with interrupted silk sutures and the skin was closed with metal clips.

Antibiotics. Tobramycin and cephaloridine were furnished through the courtesy of Eli Lilly & Co., Indianapolis, Ind., and amikacin and cephapirin were furnished by Bristol Laboratories, Syracuse, N.Y. All antibiotics were supplied as sterile dry powders or solutions.

Antibiotics were administered intramuscularly in the quadriceps muscle or intravenously in the marginal ear vein over 25 min with a Harvard pump (Harvard Apparatus Co., Dover, Mass.). Blood for antibiotic levels was obtained from ear or mammary veins and occasionally by cardiac puncture. Capsular fluid was obtained by percutaneous puncture with a 22-gauge needle through one of the capsular perforations. No capsules were studied until a minimum of 30 days after implantation. Blood and capsular fluid were obtained for antibiotic assay immediately prior to antibiotic administration, at 30 min after intramuscular injection, and 5 min after intravenous infusion and then hourly for 6 h and again at 24 h after administration. Occasional capsular specimens showing evidence of gross bleeding were rejected. All of the cephalosporins (cefazolin, cephaloridine, cephalothin, and cephapirin) and the aminoglycosides (gentamicin, tobramycin, kanamycin, and amikacin) were studied in three to six rabbits each. Capsular antibiotic levels were determined in 10 capsules for each of the antibiotics.

Assays. Antibiotic assays were performed in triplicate by using a microbiological disk plate method with 24 h of incubation at 37°C (20, 26). Aminoglycosides were assayed using *Bacillus subtilis* ATCC 6633 as the indicator organism in antibiotic medium 5 at pH 8.0 (Difco Laboratories, Detroit, Mich.). *B. subtilis* ATCC 6633 was also used for the assay of cephalothin, using 75% synthetic agar and 25% biochemical medium 6 at pH 8.0 (20). Biochemical medium 6 is similar to antibiotic medium 5 (Difco), but contains 6 g of yeast extract per liter and 17.5 g of agar per liter. Cephapirin and cephaloridine were assayed with *Sarcina lutea* ATCC 9341, using either antibiotic medium one (Difco) or biochemical medium 6, respectively. Cefazolin was assayed with *Staphylococcus aureus* ATCC 6538P on antibiotic medium 11 (Difco) at pH 6.0. All fluid specimens were placed on 6.35-mm paper disks (Schleicher and Schuell, Inc., Keene, N.H.), using disposable 20-μl capillary pipettes (Unopette, Becton, Dickinson &

Co., Rutherford, N.J.). Initially, standard curves for capsular fluids were determined using both pooled rabbit serum and pooled capsular fluid. No differences were noted between standard curves using serum or capsular fluid for any of the eight antibiotics assayed, and therefore subsequent assays were performed using only rabbit serum as a standard.

Protein binding. Binding of cefazolin to rabbit serum was measured by an ultracentrifugation method (22). Specimens were centrifuged at 295,000 × *g* for 3 h at a temperature of 33 to 35°C with pH maintained in the range of 7.2 to 7.6. The concentration of cefazolin was measured in the uppermost 0.5 ml of a total serum volume of 8 ml. Binding studies were performed on serum specimens obtained from rabbits 30 min after intramuscular injection with cefazolin at doses of 30 and 15 mg/kg and on rabbit serum in vitro at concentrations of 22, 88, and 300 μg/ml.

Pressures. Capsular hydrostatic fluid pressures were measured using a water manometer while the rabbit was secured on its back on a holding board at 45°. Pressures were measured 8 to 9 weeks after implantation. Freshly drawn iced capsular fluid specimens unexposed to air were used for pH measurements.

Statistics. Serum antibiotic half-life ($t_{1/2}$) was calculated by the standard formula, using the slope of the regression line determined by the method of least squares (12) from the arithmetic means of three to six experiments. Each serum antibiotic $t_{1/2}$ was calculated over the period extending from 2 to 5 h after administration, except that for cephalothin the 1- to 4-h period was used because of the short $t_{1/2}$ in serum. Capsular fluid $t_{1/2}$ was determined over the period from 4 to 6 h after injection, using the mean of 10 capsules for each antibiotic. The standard error of the mean was determined by the method of Mantel (21). All statistical analysis was done by the nonparametric Mann-Whitney U Test (3). A probability value of less than 0.05 was used for statistical significance. The area under the curve (AUC) was calculated in triplicate using a planimeter.

RESULTS

Capsule characteristics. Peritoneal capsules adhered to omental or bowel surfaces and became encased in a thin layer of connective tissue that covered both their internal and external surfaces (Fig. 2). Vascularization occurred through perforations in the capsule wall and was most prominent at the point of attachment to the bowel or omentum. Sagittal microscopic sections showed connective tissue fibroblasts and mononuclear cell infiltrates, with occasional areas of fat within the capsules. Large blood vessels were seen only in areas of omental attachment (Fig. 3).

Capsular fluid characteristics are given in Table 1. Specimens were obtained from 3 weeks to 8 months after implantation. There was a trend toward lower leukocyte and erythrocyte counts and higher pH in older capsules, and differential counts showed fewer polymorphonuclears with an increasing duration of implantation. The total protein and albumin remained relatively high but stable.

Capsular pressures ranged from −0.7 to +2.2 cm of water in a series of 20 measurements within five capsules. The mean capsular pressure was +0.9 cm of water. Immediately after the aspiration of 0.4 to 0.6 ml of fluid, the

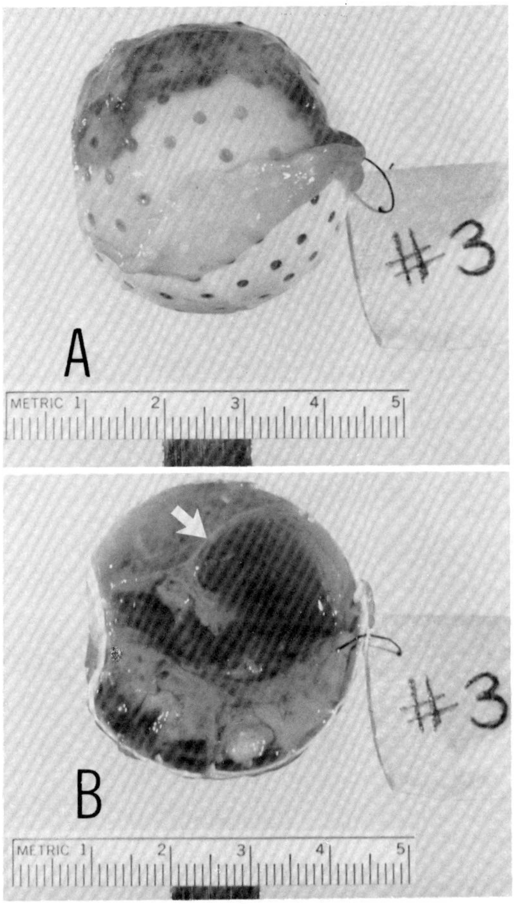

FIG. 2. *Gross appearance of a capsule removed 6 months after implantation. (A) External surface showing dark vascularized area at the upper pole that was dissected free from omental attachment. The thin layer of connective tissue has been reflected at the lower pole to show nodules of tissue that had penetrated the capsule perforations. (B) Sectioned capsule showing thick connective tissue lining at the inferior pole (region of omental attachment). Thin connective tissue layer at the upper pole has separated from the capsule wall during sectioning (arrow). The central dark area was filled with capsule fluid.*

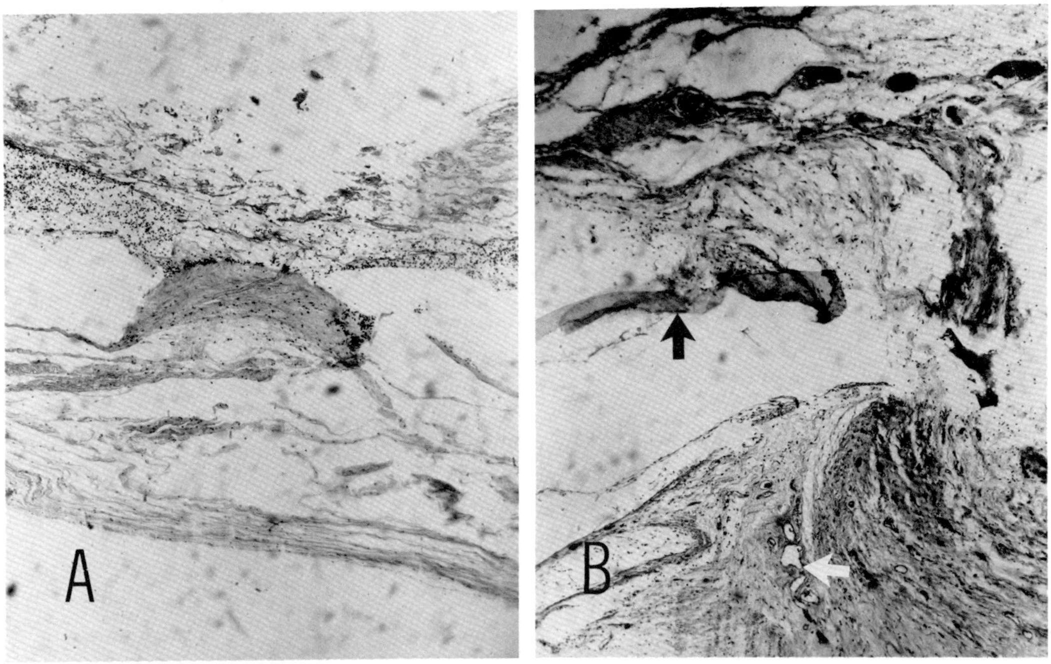

FIG. 3. *Microscopic appearance of capsule tissue (×30). (A) Area of thin connective tissue extending through a chamber perforation, showing fibroblasts and mononuclear cells. The capsule wall has been destroyed by the fixative. (B) Section through area of omental attachment, showing remnant of capsule wall (black arrow) and vascular channels (white arrow) near a capsule perforation.*

TABLE 1. *Capsule fluid characteristics (5 to 10 specimens examined)*

Determination	Mean	Range
Leukocyte count/mm^3	1,006	70–2,600
Polymorphonuclears (%)	36	19–60
Erythrocyte count/mm^3	493	196–5,250
pH	7.54	7.49–7.61
Total protein (g/100 ml)	3.6	2.9–4.1
Albumin (g/100 ml)	2.6	2.1–3.0

pressure decreased by a mean of 8.1 cm of water (range, 6.4 to 11.1 cm). Pressures returned to base line levels within 1 h, often rising to previous levels within 15 min after aspiration.

Cephalosporins. Serum and capsular pharmacokinetics are shown in Fig. 4. The cephalosporins were all administered intramuscularly at a dose of 30 mg/kg. Mean peak serum levels were highest for cefazolin and lowest for cephalothin, but there was considerable variability among the rabbits in serum levels, particularly with cephalothin. Capsular levels also showed considerable variability, even for capsules implanted in the same rabbit. For both cephaloridine and cephalothin, peak capsular levels occurred 2 h after administration, whereas capsular peaks for cephapirin and cefazolin occurred 3 and 4 h, respectively, after administration.

Peak serum and capsular levels (mean and range) are shown in Table 2. The peak serum concentration for cefazolin was significantly higher than for the other three cephalosporins (P range, <0.02 to <0.005). Peak serum levels were not significantly different for the other three cephalosporins when compared with each other. Mean peak capsular levels of both cefazolin and cephloridine were significantly higher than for cephapirin and cephlothin ($P < 0.005$, cefazolin versus cephapirin; $P < 0.025$, cefazolin versus cephalothin; $P < 0.025$, cephaloridine versus cephapirin; $P < 0.04$, cephaloridine versus cephalothin). Peak levels for cefazolin versus cephaloridine and cephapirin versus cephalothin were not significantly different.

When the ratio of mean capsular peak to mean serum peak was used to determine the percent penetration, it was found to range from 8.7 to 16.9% for the cephalosporins (Table 2). There was no statistically significant difference in percent penetration among the four cephalosporins.

The ratio of mean capsular peak to serum AUC was also calculated. For cefazolin, cephaloridine, and cephapirin there were no statistically significant differences. However, cephalothin, which showed the lowest serum AUC, showed significantly higher ratios of capsular

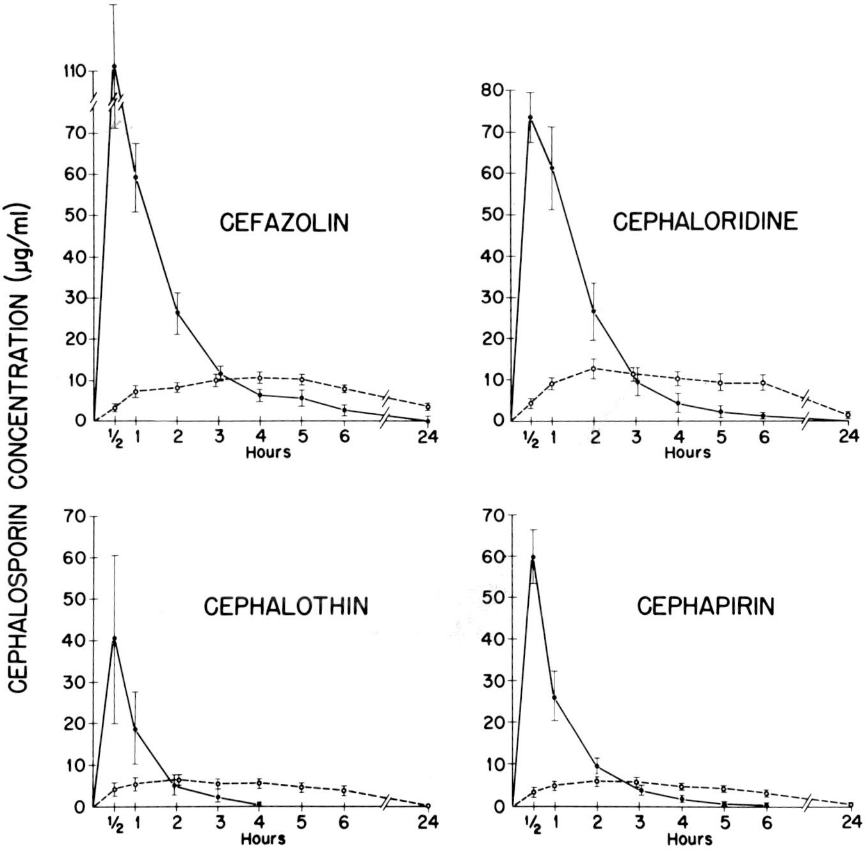

FIG. 4. *Concentrations of four cephalosporins in serum (solid line) and peritoneal capsular fluid (broken line). Administration was intramuscular at a dose of 30 mg/kg. Each point on the serum curve is a mean of 3 to 6 determinations, and each point on the capsular curve is a mean of 10 determinations. Vertical bars indicate standard errors of the mean.*

TABLE 2. *Serum and capsular mean peak concentrations and ranges (micrograms per milliliter), percent penetration (ratio of mean capsule peak to mean serum peak × 100), and mean capsular concentration and range at 24 h (micrograms per milliliter) for four cephalosporins and four aminoglycosides*[a]

Antibiotic	Serum peak		Capsule peak		% Penetration	Capsule concn at 24 h	
	Mean	Range	Mean	Range		Mean	Range
Cefazolin (6)	111.3	76–165	10.5	4.6–17	9.5	3.1	1.1–3.9
Cephaloridine (3)	73.7	66–84	12.4	3.1–27	16.9	1.3	0.8–2.3
Cephapirin (4)	60.0	50–76	5.2	4.0–9.2	8.7	0.2	0–0.8
Cephalothin (3)	40.2	16.5–78	6.1	1.0–12.5	15.1	0	0
Kanamycin (3)	21.4	18.6–27	4.7	1.0–12.5	22.0	0.6	0–1.7
Amikacin (3)	19.7	17.4–28.8	6.8	1.4–13	34.5	1.2	0–2.7
Tobramycin (5)	6.5	3.5–8.2	1.0	0.4–1.8	15.2	0.3	0–0.7
Gentamicin (5)	4.7	5.1–7.8	1.4	0.3–2.3	29.8	0.4	0.1–0.9

[a] Ten capsules were studied with each antibiotic. The number of animals studied is in parentheses.

peak to AUC than was the case for cefazolin or cephapirin ($P < 0.04$). Cephalothin was not significantly different from cephaloridine in this regard. A comparison of capsular AUC to serum AUC was not performed because total capsular AUC could not accurately be determined from the available data (Fig. 4).

Capsular levels at 24 h (Table 2) were significantly higher for cefazolin than for the other three cephalosporins ($P < 0.001$). At 24 h the cephaloridine capsular level was significantly higher than for cephapirin ($P > 0.01$) and cephalothin ($P > 0.001$). Cephapirin and cephalothin levels were not significantly different from each other at 24 h.

Because cefazolin has been reported to be highly bound to human serum protein (18), we determined the binding of cefazolin to rabbit serum protein at two different in vivo serum cefazolin concentrations. Binding was 86% at a cefazolin concentration of 30 μg/ml, but dropped to 61% at the higher concentration of 82 μg/ml. However, in vitro rabbit serum binding determinations at 22, 88, and 300 μg/ml showed bindings of 95, 95, and 74%, respectively, much higher than the binding observed on in vivo specimens.

Serum and capsular $t_{1/2}$ is shown in Table 3. For the cephalosporins $t_{1/2}$ was 3.5 to 6.5 times longer in capsules than in serum. Cefazolin had the longest serum $t_{1/2}$ and cephaloridine had the longest capsular $t_{1/2}$. The $t_{1/2}$ in serum and capsules was similar for cephalothin and cephapirin.

Aminoglycosides. Kanamycin and amikacin were administered intramuscularly at a dose of 7.5 mg/kg. Gentamicin and tobramycin were administered either intramuscularly or by a 25-min intravenous infusion at a dose of 2 mg/kg. Data using intramuscular and intravenous administration routes were pooled for both tobramycin and gentamicin because similar serum peaks and serum $t_{1/2}$ were observed. Serum and capsular kinetics for the four aminoglycosides are shown in Fig. 5. As expected, peak levels of amikacin and kanamycin were similar, but the peak serum level of gentamicin (± standard error) was lower (4.7 ± 1.3 μg/ml) than the peak for tobramycin (6.5 ± 0.9 μg/ml). This difference was largely artifactual, resulting from a distribution of serum peaks between the 30-min and 1-h specimens for gentamicin, whereas tobramycin peaks occurred consistently at 30 min. When the mean of the serum peak concentration for gentamicin was calculated, disregarding the time of occurrence, it was 6.1 ± 0.7 μg/ml, a value in close agreement with the tobramycin peak.

TABLE 3. *Serum and capsule $t_{1/2}$*

Antibiotic	Serum $t_{1/2}$	Capsule $t_{1/2}$ (h)
Cefazolin	1.4	4.9
Cephaloridine	0.9	5.9
Cephapirin	0.6	3.9
Cephalothin	0.8	3.9
Kanamycin	1.1	5.1
Amikacin	2.0	12.6
Tobramycin	1.3	3.9
Gentamicin	1.3	5.8

Peak capsular concentrations occurred at 3 h for kanamycin, amikacin, and tobramycin and at 4 h for gentamicin, possibly a reflection of the later serum peaks with gentamicin. Peak capsular concentrations of amikacin versus kanamycin were not significantly different nor were peak capsular concentrations of tobramycin versus gentamicin (Table 2). The ratio of mean peak capsule concentration to mean peak serum concentration (percent penetration) ranged from 15.2% for tobramycin to 34.5% for amikacin (Table 2). The only significant difference in percent penetration was for amikacin versus tobramycin ($P < 0.01$). Although the value for gentamicin was nearly twice that of tobramycin, this was largely an artifact due to slurring of the gentamicin serum peak. When the actual mean serum gentamicin peak of 6.1 μg/ml was used for calculation, the percent penetration of gentamicin was 23%, which was not significantly different from the value for tobramycin.

The ratio of mean capsular peak concentration to serum AUC was not significantly different for any of the aminoglycosides. Although the capsular concentration of amikacin was twice as high as that of kanamycin at 24 h (Table 2), this was not a significant difference. Similarly, gentamicin and tobramycin concentrations at 24 h were not significantly different.

Serum and capsular $t_{1/2}$ for the aminoglycosides is given in Table 3. The $t_{1/2}$ in capsules was 3 to 6.3 times as long as in serum. For amikacin, capsular $t_{1/2}$ was the longest of all antibiotics tested (12.6 h) and correlated fairly well with the concentration of the drug measured at 24 h (1.2 μg/ml).

Additional capsular antibiotic studies. An extensive comparison of peritoneal to subcutaneous capsular antibiotic concentrations was abandoned when subcutaneous cylinders were found unsatisfactory for chronic use because fluids were frequently contaminated with blood or easily infected or the cylinders quickly filled with connective tissue. However, cefazolin was studied successfully with five subcutaneous cylinders in two rabbits. The mean peak serum concentration (± standard error) was 98.5 ± 1.5 μg/ml. The mean peak subcutaneous cylinder level was 11.0 ± 2.0 μg/ml and occurred at 4 h. The percent penetration was 11.2%. In similar rabbits with peritoneal capsules the serum mean peak was 111.3 ± 14.8 μg/ml and the peritoneal capsular mean peak was 10.5 ± 1.2

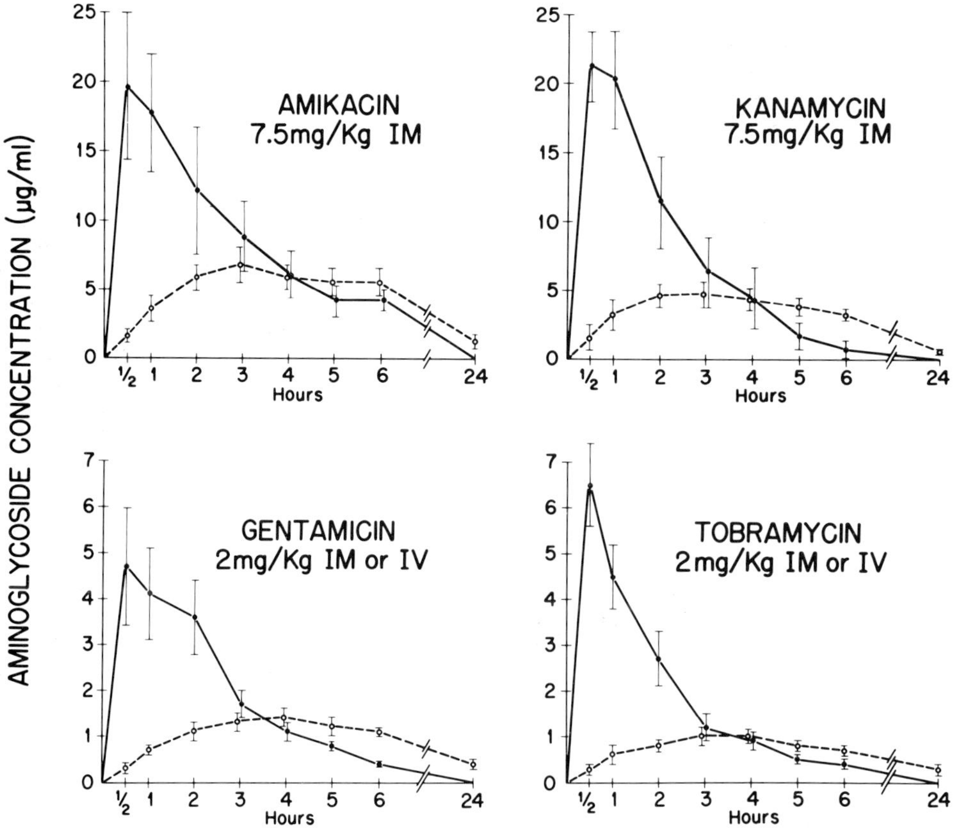

FIG. 5. *Concentrations of four aminoglycosides in serum (solid line) and peritoneal capsular fluid (broken line). Each point on the serum curve is a mean of 3 to 5 determinations, and each point on the capsular curve is a mean of 10 determinations. Vertical bars indicate standard error of the mean.*

μg/ml, with a percent penetration of 9.5%. Therefore, serum and capsular peak levels and percent penetration for cefazolin were not significantly different in the two types of capsules.

Anecdotally, during preparation of one of the rabbits for surgery, ascites was noted and on exploration the liver surface was observed to be nodular. Capsules were implanted and the animal was studied to determine the concentration of amikacin in ascitic fluid for comparison with peritoneal capsular fluid. The peak ascitic level of amikacin was 7.8 μg/ml, as compared with a mean peak capsular fluid level of 6.8 ± 1.2 μg/ml. Unfortunately this animal expired before concentrations of other antibiotics in ascitic fluid could be measured.

Because of a concern that the aspiration of intraperitoneal capsular fluid might artifactually induce the penetration of capsules by serum containing high concentrations of antibiotics (particularly in the first 2 h after administration), a series of experiments was performed to investigate this possibility. Some capsular aspirations were delayed until 3 to 4 h after the administration of antibiotics (when the serum antibiotic concentration was considerably lower) for a comparison with the levels achieved in capsules aspirated beginning at 30 min after administration. Tobramycin, cephalothin, and cefazolin were studied sequentially in the same animal. No increase in antibiotic levels was observed in capsules repeatedly aspirated beginning at 30 min as compared with those aspirated only at 3 to 4 h. However, in the course of these experiments it was noted that certain capsules consistently yielded higher antibiotic concentrations than others, regardless of the antibiotic used. At autopsy those capsules showing the higher antibiotic concentrations appeared to have larger areas of vascular attachment than those exhibiting somewhat lower levels. Thus, consistent variation in achievable capsular antibiotic concentrations could be demonstrated between capsules, but artifactual induction of consistently increased concentrations by repeated aspiration was not seen.

DISCUSSION

The use of perforated capsules as a means of measuring interstitial tissue fluid pressure in dogs was first described by Guyton (14). He implanted capsules both subcutaneously and intramuscularly, and pressures within were found to range from −2.6 mm of Hg in muscle to −7.1 mm of Hg in subcutaneous tissue. Mean capsular fluid protein was only 1.96 g/100 ml. Additional studies were done in dogs by Calnan et al. to further characterize subcutaneous capsular fluid and its dynamics (7). The total protein in capsular fluid averaged 2.54 g/100 ml (30 to 45% of serum proteins). Sodium was found to be freely diffusible from blood to capsular fluid and back. Albumin was also readily diffusible from blood to tissue fluid, but over a longer period of time, requiring 48 h to equilibrate. Other studies have shown a diffusion rate for albumin one-third that expected for pure water (15). We are unaware of reports of the characteristics of fluid in intraperitoneally implanted capsules, other than our own preliminary results (11). Our mean capsular protein concentration was 3.6 g/100 ml (55% of the serum protein level) in rabbits, nearly twice as high as values reported for subcutaneous capsules in dogs and slightly higher than for subcutaneous capsules in rabbits (29). The majority of peritoneal capsular protein was albumin (mean, 2.6 g/100 ml). Hydrostatic fluid pressures in peritoneal capsules were slightly positive, disagreeing with the subcutaneous capsule observations of Guyton. However, intra-abdominal pressure measurements are influenced by several factors, including the position of the animal, abdominal muscle tension, and gastrointestinal contents; the latter two factors were uncontrolled in the measurement of pressures in this study (17).

Several authors have employed subcutaneously implanted capsules in the study of antibiotic penetration into tissue fluid (1, 4, 8, 10, 29, 31). Using capsules implanted for 1 h to 14 days, Alexander et al. showed high concentrations of cefazolin, cephaloridine, penicillin, and ampicillin in tissue fluid in dogs (1). Concentrations of oxacillin, nafcillin, clindamycin, cephalothin, and gentamicin were considerably lower. In capsules implanted for a minimum of 4 weeks, Chisholm et al. (8) demonstrated peak concentrations of ampicillin that were about 25% of the serum peak concentrations. The peak concentration of gentamicin in tissue fluid exceeded 50% of the serum peak concentration, whereas the tobramycin tissue fluid concentration did not appear to reach 10% of the peak serum concentration. The dosage of gentamicin was 80 mg intramuscular, but for tobramycin it was only 50 mg intramuscular. Ehrlich and coworkers measured cephaloridine concentrations in fluid collected in 10-day-old subcutaneous mesh cylinders in rabbits and found them to be similar to the intraperitoneal capsular levels obtained in this study (10). Their maximum tissue fluid cephaloridine levels were reached 1½ h after intravenous bolus infusion, in close agreement with the peak concentration time of 2 h observed after an intramuscular injection in the present study. Waterman and Kastan (31) found that the cephalothin concentration reached a peak of 12 μg/ml in interstitial fluid from 4-week-old subcutaneous capsules in dogs after a 40-mg/kg intravenous dose. This appeared to be approximately 10% of the peak serum concentration, again in agreement with the observations made here.

The extravascular concentration of an antibiotic is thought to depend upon a number of factors, including: (i) the concentration gradient from serum to extravascular fluid, (ii) the degree of binding to protein and tissues, (iii) the lipid solubility, and (iv) the ionization state or pKa. The binding of antibiotics to serum proteins is felt to be an important factor limiting penetration into interstitial fluid (19). Somewhat surprisingly, the known degree of binding of the various cephalosporins to human serum proteins did not appear to correlate with the peritoneal capsular fluid concentrations in the rabbit model. Cefazolin, which is 86% bound to human serum (18), achieved particularly high capsular concentrations. Our protein binding determinations in rabbit serum obtained in vivo confirmed the high binding of cefazolin at low concentrations (86% at 30 μg/ml), but binding dropped to only 61% at a concentration of 82 μg/ml. Diminished protein binding at drug concentrations in excess of 100 μg/ml has previously been described by Rolinson and Sutherland (25). A decrease in serum protein binding at high clinical serum concentrations would provide an attractive explanation for the extravascular penetration of cefazolin, but we were unable to confirm the decrease in binding on in vitro studies and, in fact, found binding to be 95% in rabbit serum at drug concentrations in the clinical range. Waterman et al. (32) have also observed high capsular fluid concentrations of cefazolin in dogs, despite high serum protein binding, and have attributed this to the slow rate of binding of cefazolin to serum proteins (33).

In contrast to the cephalosporins, the aminoglycosides used in this study have little or no detectable binding to human serum protein (9, 13). Although the percent penetration of amikacin was the highest among the aminoglycosides, this was statistically significant only when compared with tobramycin. This difference could possibly be due to the higher dose of amikacin (7.5 versus 2 mg/kg). Kanamycin and amikacin are pharmacologically very similar (9). With the same large dose of kanamycin and amikacin, capsular fluid concentrations of amikacin were slightly higher (Table 2), although this was not significant statistically. Gentamicin and tobramycin also have similar pharmacokinetics (16, 27). Serum and capsular peak concentrations were similar for the two drugs (Table 2). Although the percent penetration of gentamicin appeared to be almost twice as great as for tobramycin (Table 2), this difference could be misleading, due to the lower serum peak of gentamicin resulting from a distribution of peak concentrations between 30 min and 1 h. When the actual serum peak concentration of 6.1 μg/ml was used, there were no statistical differences between tobramycin and gentamicin.

The general pattern of slow accumulation and elimination of drugs from peritoneal capsular fluids has also been seen in subcutaneous tissue capsule models (1, 4, 8, 10, 31), as well as in other models of extravascular antibiotic penetration (5, 6, 28). Our calculations of capsular fluid $t_{1/2}$ (Table 3) are based on only three determinations in each capsule over a 2-h period and should not be construed as highly precise measures, but rather as representative figures for capsular fluid kinetics after the administration of a single parenteral dose. Nevertheless, all capsular $t_{1/2}$ values were in the range of 3.9 to 5.9 h, with the exception of amikacin (12.6 h). From capsule fluid concentrations calculated at 24 h (Table 2), the calculated capsular $t_{1/2}$ of amikacin appears to be somewhat long, whereas the $t_{1/2}$ of cefazolin seems too short. Both of these discrepancies are likely due to the short time period used in the calculation of the $t_{1/2}$. Finally, slow capsular fluid kinetics suggest the probable accumulation of antibiotic in capsules with repeated doses. The exact degree of accumulation is likely to be greatest for those drugs with the longest capsular $t_{1/2}$, but this will also depend upon the frequency of systemic administration.

The basic question of the need for local antibiotic instillation in peritoneal infection cannot be answered from the results of the single-dose studies performed here. Concentrations of cephalosporins and aminoglycosides in capsular fluid, although substantial, are not in excess of the minimum inhibitory concentration of some relevant organisms, particularly gram-negative bacilli (24, 30).

At the dosage used in this study, capsular concentrations of cefazolin and cephaloridine compare favorably with the minimum inhibitory concentration of the majority of *Enterobacteriaceae*, whereas cephapirin and cephalothin levels are somewhat low (30). Furthermore, the assay method employed in this study also measured the desacetyl metabolites of cephalothin and cephapirin, which are biologically active, but to a lesser degree than the parent compounds (34, 35). Among the aminoglycosides, only amikacin capsular concentrations are consistently in excess of the minimum inhibitory concentration of the *Enterobacteriaceae* (24). Although kinetics suggest that accumulation probably occurs with repeated systemic doses, this remains to be proven, and we emphasize that no attempt has been made in this study to achieve equilibrium conditions. Furthermore, the effect of inflammation in altering tissue penetration might be expected to raise capsular fluid concentrations (paralleling the situation in meningitis), but this is also an unproven hypothesis.

Intraperitoneal implantation of tissue capsules has circumvented several of the technical difficulties we have encountered with subcutaneous implants (bleeding, infection, rapid tissue growth). If the similar penetration shown for cefazolin in the two models is confirmed with other antibiotics, this would suggest that either model can provide equivalent results representative of interstitial tissue fluid penetrance in general. However, peritoneal capsular concentrations of antibiotics are variable, even in the same animal, probably as a result of the inconstant degree of vascularity of capsules. Future studies comparing antibiotic penetrance should either be done with large numbers of capsules (as in this study) or by paired cross-over studies in the same capsules in the same animals. The potential of the tissue capsule model for in vivo study of the interaction of microorganisms with antimicrobials has already been emphasized (2, 23, 29). Experimental infections in intraperitoneal capsules and the effect of antibiotic treatment on those infections warrant further investigation.

ACKNOWLEDGMENTS

This work was supported by a grant from Eli Lilly & Co., Indianapolis.

We wish to thank Horace H. Zinneman and Lance R. Peterson for the determination of protein concentrations and protein binding.

LITERATURE CITED

1. **Alexander, J. W., N. S. Sykes, M. M. Mitchell, and M.V. Fisher.** 1973. Concentration of selected intravenously administered antibiotics in experimental surgical wounds. J. Trauma 13:423–434.
2. **Arko, R. J.** 1972. *Neisseria gonorrhea*: experimental infection of laboratory animals. Science 77:1200–1201.
3. **Auble, D.** 1952. Extended tables for the Mann-Whitney Statistic. Institute of Educational Research, School of Education, Indiana University, Bloomington.
4. **Baker, G., and T. K. Hunt.** 1968. Penicillin concentrations in experimental wounds. Am. J. Surg. 115:531–534.
5. **Barza, M., T. Samuelson, and L. Weinstein.** 1974. Penetration of antibiotics into fibrin loci *in vivo*. II. Comparison of nine antibiotics: effect of dose and degree of protein binding. J. Infect. Dis. 129:66–72.
6. **Barza, M., and L. Weinstein.** 1974. Penetration of antibiotics into fibrin loci *in vivo*. I. Comparison of penetration of ampicillin into fibrin clots, abscesses, and "interstitial fluid." J. Infect. Dis. 129:59–65.
7. **Calnan, J. S., J. J. Pflug, G. D. Chisholm, and L. M. Taylor.** 1972. Pathophysiology of tissue fluid. Proc. R. Soc. Med. 65:715–719.
8. **Chisholm, G. D., P. M. Waterworth, J. S. Calnan, and L. P. Garrod.** 1973. Concentration of antibacterial agents in interstitial tissue fluid. Br. Med. J. 1:569–573.
9. **Clarke, J. T., R. D. Libke, C. Regamey, and W. M. M. Kirby.** 1974. Comparative pharmacokinetics of amikacin and kanamycin. Clin. Pharmacol. Ther. 15:610–616.
10. **Ehrlich, H. P., V. Licko, and T. K. Hunt.** 1973. Kinetics of cephaloridine in experimental wounds. Am. J. Med. Sci. 265:33–44.
11. **Gerding, D. N., and W. H. Hall.** 1975. The penetration of antibiotics into peritoneal fluid. Bull. N.Y. Acad. Med. 51:1016–1019.
12. **Goldstein, A., L. Aronow, and S. Kolman.** 1968. Principles of drug action, p. 196, 287, 295. Harper and Row, New York.
13. **Gordon, R. C., C. Regamey, and W. M. M. Kirby.** 1972. Serum protein binding of the aminoglycoside antibiotics. Antimicrob. Agents Chemother. 2:214–216.
14. **Guyton, A. C.** 1963. A concept of negative interstitial pressure based on pressures in implanted perforated capsules. Circ. Res. 12:399–414.
15. **Guyton, A. C., H. J. Granger, and A. E. Taylor.** 1971. Interstitial fluid pressure. Physiol. Rev. 51:527–563.
16. **Harikoshi, N., M. Valdivieso, and G. P. Bodey.** 1974. Clinical pharmacology of tobramycin. Am. J. Med. Sci. 266:453–458.
17. **Hartman, W.** 1973. Intra-abdominal pressure in small ruminants. Zentralbl. Veterinaermed. Reihe A 20:498–502.
18. **Kirby, W. M. M., and C. Regamey.** 1973. Pharmacokinetics of cefazolin compared with four other cephalosporins. J. Infect. Dis. 128(Suppl.):S341–346.
19. **Kunin, C. M.** 1974. Blood level measurements and antimicrobial agents. Clin. Pharmacol. Ther. 16:251–256.
20. **Lilly Reasearch Laboratories.** 1970. Paper disc or cup plate antibiotic assay procedures. Eli Lilly & Co., Indianapolis.
21. **Mantel, N.** 1951. Rapid estimation of standard errors of means for small samples. Am. Stat. 5:26–27.
22. **Mattie, H., W. R. O. Goslings, and E. L. Noach.** 1973. Cloxacillin and nafcillin: serum binding and its relationship to antibacterial effect in mice. J. Infect. Dis. 128:170–177.
23. **Rathleu, T.** 1973. Cultivation of pathogenic *Treponema pallidum* in chambers surgically implanted in experimental animals. Acta Pathol. Microbiol. Scand. 81: 269–271.
24. **Reynolds, A. V., J. M. T. Hamilton-Miller, and W. Brumfit.** 1974. Newer aminoglycosides—amikacin and tobramycin: an *in vitro* comparison with kanamycin and gentamicin. Br. Med. J. 3:778–780.
25. **Rolinson, G. N., and R. Sutherland.** 1965. The binding of antibiotics to serum proteins. Br. J. Pharmacol. 25:638–650.
26. **Sabath, L. D., J. I. Casey, P. A. Ruch, L. L. Stumpf, and M. Finland.** 1971. Rapid microassay for circulating nephrotoxic antibiotics, p. 83–89. Antimicrob. Agents Chemother. 1970.
27. **Stratford, B. C., and S. Dixson.** 1974. Serum levels of gentamicin and tobramycin after slow intravenous bolus injection. Lancet i:378–379.
28. **Tan, J. S., A. Trott, J. P. Phair, and C. Watanakunakorn.** 1972. A method for measurement of antibiotics in human interstitial fluid. J. Infect. Dis. 126:492–497.
29. **Tight, R. R., R. B. Prior, R. L. Perkins, and C. A. Rotilie.** 1975. Fluid and penicillin G. dynamics in polyethylene chambers implanted subcutaneously in rabbits. Antimicrob. Agents Chemother. 8:495–497.
30. **Washington, J. A., II.** 1976. The *in vitro* spectrum of the cephalosporins. Mayo Clin. Proc. 51:237–250.
31. **Waterman, N. G., and L. B. Kastan.** 1972. Interstitial fluid and serum antibiotic concentrations. Arch. Surg. 105:192–196.
32. **Waterman, N. G., M. J. Raff, L. Scharfenberger, and P. A. Barnwell.** 1976. Protein binding and concentrations of cephaloridine and cefazolin in serum and interstitial fluid of dogs. J. Infect. Dis. 133:642–647.
33. **Waterman, N. G., L. Scharfenberger, and M. J. Raff.** 1974. Rate of binding of antibiotics to canine serum protein. Antimicrob. Agents Chemother. 5:294–295.
34. **Wick, W. E.** 1966. In vitro and in vivo laboratory comparison of cephalothin and desacetylcephalothin, p. 870–875. Antimicrob. Agents Chemother. 1965.
35. **Yamanaka, Y., S. Kono, H. Tateishi, and H. Aratani.** 1974. Pharmacologic studies of cephapirin. Second report. Distribution, fate, and excretion. Chemotherapy 22:1208–1218.

ANTIMICROBIAL AGENTS AND CHEMOTHERAPY, Dec. 1976, p. 912-914 Vol. 10, No. 6

Printed in U.S.A.

NOTES

Bacteriocin Production by Group A Streptococcal L-Forms

WALERIA HRYNIEWICZ[1]* AND JOHN R. TAGG[2]

Departments of Pediatrics and Microbiology, University of Minnesota Medical School, Minneapolis, Minnesota 55455

Received for publication 26 May 1976

L-forms induced from a bacteriocin-producing strain of group A streptococcus retained both the ability to produce the streptococcin and producer strain immunity to the homologous bacteriocin. L-forms of a spontaneously cured (bacteriocin negative) derivative of this same strain failed to produce streptococcin but were sensitive to its action.

Streptococcin A-FF22 (SA) is a bacteriocin produced by group A streptococcus strain FF22 (M type 52). Characterization and partial purification of this bacteriocin have been described previously (7, 8). Recent results (Tagg, unpublished observations) indicate that SA may exist in two forms: firmly bound to the cell envelope or as an extracellular product. Studies of bacteriocin production by L-forms have been few in number, and none of these have related to group A streptococcal L-forms (1). Among gram-negative bacteria, the effect of cell wall loss on susceptibility to colicins is a controversial subject, with some studies indicating that the cell wall is necessary for attachment of these bacteriocins (4) and others indicating that the cell membrane carries the specific receptors (5).

It was of interest to determine whether L-forms of group A streptococcus strain FF22 are capable of bacteriocin production and also whether loss of cell wall results in increased sensitivity to SA.

Group A streptococcus L-forms of strain FF22 (SA^+) and of strain SPON1 (SA^-), a non-SA-producing spontaneously cured derivative, were induced with group C streptococcal phage-associated lysin (muralysin), using the method described by Maxted (3). The induction medium was composed of brain heart infusion (Difco) supplemented with 10% horse serum, 25% sucrose, and 1.2% agar (Difco). L-form induction and the first few passages were in the presence of penicillin (10 IU/ml), but subsequent propagation was on penicillin-free medium to eliminate this possible source of non-bacteriocin inhibition.

After 3 to 5 days of incubation at 37°C, morphologically typical L-forms developed and were maintained by the technique of agar block transfers. After 10 to 15 passages, stable L-forms were established as evidenced by their failure to revert to bacterial forms on penicillin-free L-form medium and on blood agar medium. Occasional spontaneous reversion was observed during the first few passages on penicillin-free medium or blood agar. The revertants were characterized as identical to the parent form by morphology on blood agar, staining, and serological grouping and typing. Tests (7, 8) of the bacteriocin produced in tryptic soy broth cultures by the revertant and by the parent strain indicated a similar titers and activity spectra.

Four agar blocks containing stable L-forms from two independent inductions of the SA^+ strain and of its SA^- derivative were placed on penicillin-free L-form agar medium and incubated for 48 h. The blocks were removed, and L-form growth in the absence of bacterial forms was confirmed. The plate was exposed to chloroform vapors to kill surface colonies (8) and then overlayered with an indicator layer of soft agar containing *Staphylococcus aureus* strain CIT (6). After overnight incubation at 37°C, a wide zone of inhibition was observed around the L-form colonies derived from the SA^+ strain (Fig. 1). The SA^- L-form colonies were not inhibitory. To eliminate inhibitory effects due to residual penicillin, which might have been present in the agar block, penicillinase (Bacto Penase, Difco) was included in the L-form me-

[1] Present address: Department of Bacteriology, National Institute of Hygiene, 00-791 Warsaw, Poland.

[2] Present address: Department of Microbiology, University of Otago, Dunedin, New Zealand.

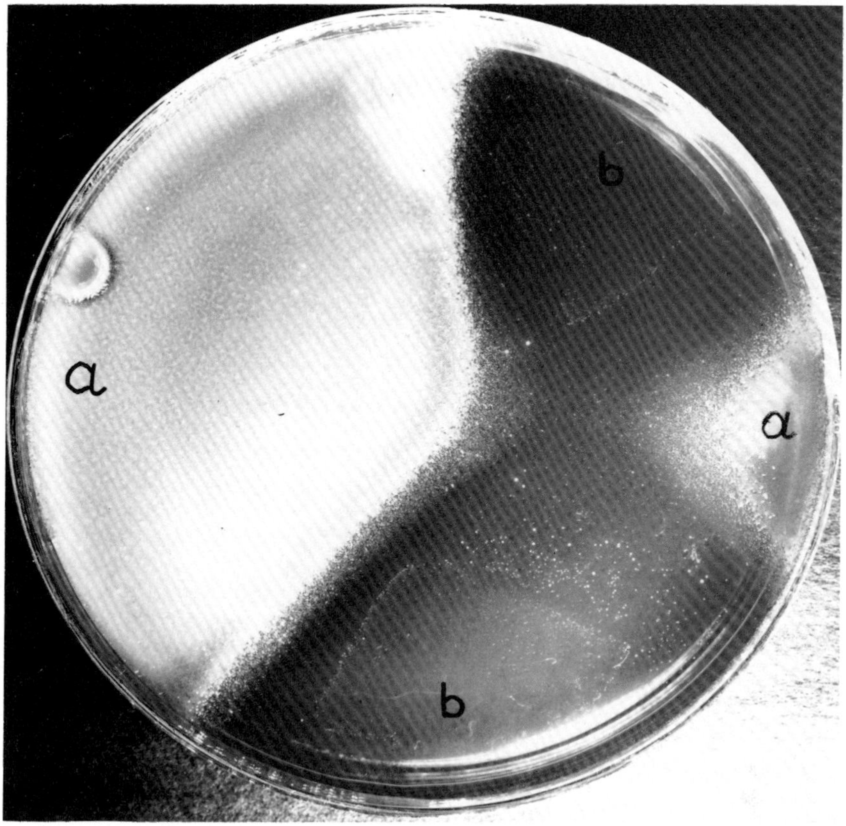

FIG. 1. *Inhibition of Staphylococcus aureus CIT by bacteriocin-producing streptococcal group A L-forms. (a) S. aureus CIT; (b) streptococcal L-forms (SA+).*

dium. No reduction in inhibitory effect was observed with the inclusion of penicillinase.

The bacteriocin sensitivity of SA^+ and SA^- L-forms was tested by incorporating partially purified streptococcin (8) into L-form medium in the concentrations indicated in the table. L-forms were allowed to grow on bacteriocin-containing agar medium for 48 h, and then the parent bacterial strains were spread onto adjacent areas of the same plate. No loss of bacteriocin activity occurred under the test conditions. Group A streptococcus strain FF22 (SA^+) and its L-form derivative appeared resistant to the bacteriocin (Table 1). By comparison, both the cured strain and its L-form were considerably more sensitive to the streptococcin. Application of studies in liquid medium should provide more precise information.

From these data we conclude that L-forms induced from an SA^+ group A streptococcus retain the ability to produce bacteriocin. Other reported studies (2) have shown that group A streptococcal L-forms still produce M protein and various other extracellular products that are elaborated by the parent streptococcus. It is apparent that retention of an intact cell wall is not essential for SA production. Moreover, producer strain immunity to the homologous bacteriocin seems to be preserved in the L-form phase of group A streptococcus strain FF22.

TABLE 1. *Effect of streptococcin A-FF22 (SA) on growth of SA^+ and SA^- streptococci and L-forms*

Organism	Growth at SA concn (U/ml of medium)[a] of:		
	64	32	16
Strain FF22 (SA^+)	+++[b]	+++	+++
L-form derivative (SA^+)	+++	+++	+++
Strain SPON1 (SA^-)	+	±	−
L-form derivative (SA^-)	++	−	−

[a] Streptococcin units are as defined previously (8).
[b] Symbols: ±, 1 to 5 colonies; +, 6 to 10 colonies; ++, 11 to 50 colonies; +++, over 50 colonies.

The SA$^-$ derivative L-forms seem to retain the sensitivity of the parent bacterial form to the bacteriocin, the implication being that the cell wall may not be necessary to effect the bactericidal action of SA.

We are grateful to Lewis W. Wannamaker for helpful advice and criticism and to S. Skjold for a sample of phage-associated lysin.

This research was done by one of the authors (W.H.) on leave of absence from the National Institute of Hygiene, Warsaw, and was supported by Public Health Service research grant 05-327-2. Support was also provided by Public Health Service research grant AI08724 from the National Institute of Allergy and Infectious Diseases. J.R.T. had a Career Investigator Fellowship from the American Heart Association.

LITERATURE CITED

1. **Harwick, H. J., J. Z. Montgomerie, G. M. Kalamanson, E. G. Hubert, C. S. Potter, and L. B. Guze.** 1971. Differential action of a streptococcal bacteriocin on mycoplasmas and microbial L-forms. Infect. Immun. 4:194–198.
2. **Maxted, W. R.** 1964. Streptococcal bacteriophages, p. 25–44. *In* J. W. Uhr (ed.), The streptococcus, rheumatic fever and glomerulonephritis. The Williams & Wilkins Co., Baltimore.
3. **Maxted, W. R.** 1972. Specific procedures and requirements for the isolation, growth and maintenance of the L-phase of some microbial groups, p. 423–449. *In* J. R. Norris and D. W. Ribbons (ed.), Methods in microbiology, vol. 7A. Academic Press Inc., New York.
4. **Sabet, S. F., and C. A. Schnaitman.** 1971. Localization and solubilization of colicin receptors. J. Bacteriol. 108:422–430.
5. **Smarda, J., and U. Taubeneck.** 1968. Situation of colicin receptors in surface layers of bacterial cells. J. Gen. Microbiol. 52:161–172.
6. **Tagg, J. R., A. S. Dajani, and L. W. Wannamaker.** 1975. Bacteriocin of a group B streptococcus: partial purification and characterization. Antimicrob. Agents Chemother. 7:764–772.
7. **Tagg, J. R., A. S. Dajani, L. W. Wannamaker, and E. D. Gray.** 1973. Group A streptococcal bacteriocin. Production, purification and mode of action. J. Exp. Med. 138:1168–1183.
8. **Tagg, J. R., R. S. D. Read, and A. R. McGiven.** 1973. Bacteriocin of group A streptococcus: partial purification and properties. Antimicrob. Agents Chemother. 4:214–221.

ANTIMICROBIAL AGENTS AND CHEMOTHERAPY, Dec. 1976, p. 915-917
Vol. 10, No. 6

Cultivation of *Staphylococcus aureus* in a Synthetic Medium of Low Ultraviolet Absorptivity

B. G. CHARLES AND B. D. RAWAL*

Department of Pharmacy, University of Queensland, St. Lucia, Queensland 4067, Australia

Received for publication 3 May 1976

A new synthetic medium having negligible ultraviolet absorbance is described for growing staphylococci in experiments requiring ultraviolet spectrophotometry of cell-free portions of the culture.

In studying the mechanisms of action of antimicrobial agents acting on bacteria, tests for leakage of cellular contents are widely used. The detection of large amounts of 260-nm-absorbing substances in the filtrate of a culture exposed to the antimicrobial agent under study provides adequate evidence of damage to the cell envelope. Obviously neither the antimicrobial agent nor the culture medium should exhibit a high degree of ultraviolet absorptivity. Although interference due to residual drug may be eliminated by its physical removal, absorptivity due to the medium itself cannot be easily differentiated from that of leaked cell contents. A simple synthetic medium with negligible ultraviolet absorptivity of its own is indeed the obvious answer. Morris and Russell (3) used a simple glucose phosphate medium for measuring cellular leakage from *Escherichia coli* by novobiocin. Staphylococci, however, need more complex media; both Difco AOAC synthetic broth and the liquid medium of Laue and MacDonald (2) supported the growth of staphylococci but exhibited a high degree of ultraviolet absorptivity (Fig. 1). Presently attempts were made to obtain adequate growth of staphylococci in a synthetic medium having minimal ultraviolet absorptivity at wavelengths between 350 and 250 nm.

In developing the synthetic medium, the minimal medium of Davis and Mingioli (1) was supplemented with several amino acids and growth factors as listed in Table 1. Solutions of each of these compounds were scanned for light absorbance between 350 and 250 nm on a Hitachi-Perkin Elmer double-beam spectrophotometer with glass-distilled water as the blank. The concentration of each compound that gave an absorbance of 0.02 or less in the 350- to 250-nm range was chosen for inclusion in the medium.

The ultraviolet light absorptivity of the SM4 medium was compared with that of the synthetic medium of Laue and MacDonald (2) and Difco AOAC synthetic broth, using distilled water as the blank. The ultraviolet spectra of these three media (Fig. 1) revealed that medium SM4 had the lowest and negligible absorbance in the ultraviolet region.

A collection of 20 strains of *Staphylococcus aureus* having diverse antimicrobial resistance profiles (Table 2) was used for determining the growth-promoting ability of this medium. These 20 strains were individually subcultured daily for 3 successive days in 10.0 ml of tryptone soya broth (Oxoid). After the third passage, the cultures were centrifuged at 4,000 rpm for 30 min. The cell pellets were resuspended in 5.0 ml of sterile physiological saline. Varying inocula (0.05, 0.1, 0.2 and 0.5 ml) from these "unwashed" suspensions were each added to 5.0 ml of membrane-filtered SM4 medium in duplicate. One set was used for measuring the initial absorbance at 450 nm (Abs_0), and the other was incubated at 37°C for 18 h, at which time the absorbance (Abs_{18}) was measured again at 450 nm.

To subject the absorbance readings to statistical analysis, Abs_0 was subtracted from Abs_{18} for each culture. These corrected absorbance values for each culture are shown in Table 2. An analysis of variance of these absorbance readings for each culture with respect to inoculum size and antimicrobial resistance (Table 3) showed that the growth of *S. aureus* in the SM4 medium was inoculum dependent but independent of the antibiotic resistance.

Further confirmation of the growth-promoting ability was determined by comparing the doubling time of a multiply antibiotic-resistant strain (PS84) with that of an antibiotic-sensitive strain (62) in a growth curve study. Two milliliters of inoculum, prepared as above, was added to 50.0 ml of SM4 medium. Samples (3.0

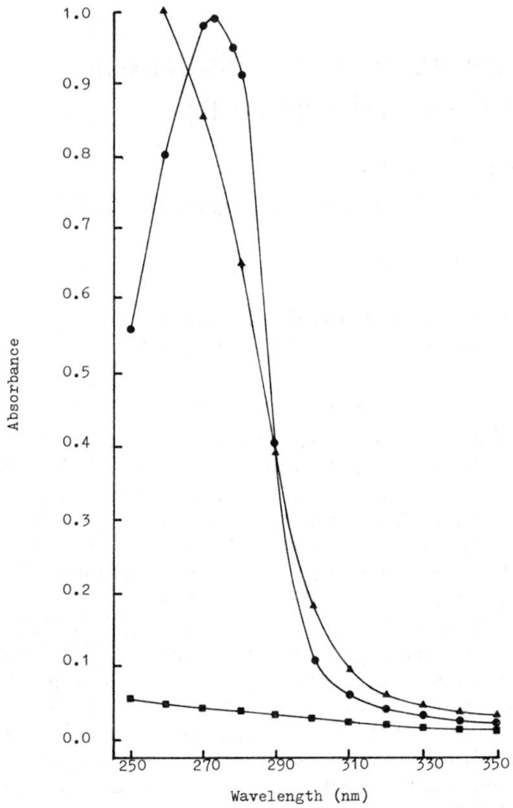

FIG. 1. *Spectral comparison of SM4 medium with other synthetic media. Symbols: (■) SM4 medium; (▲) Laue and MacDonald (2) medium (1:2 dilution); (●) AOAC medium (Difco) (1:3 dilution).*

ml) were removed at 3-h intervals up to 18 h of incubation in a shaking water bath at 37°C. Viable cell numbers were determined in each sample by using the surface plate method. Both strains exhibited a doubling time of 77 min; this confirmed the above observation that the growth of staphylococci in the SM4 medium was independent of the antibiotic resistance of the strain. It may, however, be argued that the method of preparing inocula, which did not involve washing, failed to exclude growth due to the carry-over from the nonsynthetic broth. The possible role of traces of tryptone soya broth, via the unwashed inoculum, in promoting the growth in SM4 medium was studied by measuring the duration of the lag phase and doubling time of parallel cultures inoculated with unwashed and washed suspensions; the latter were prepared by further centrifugations (thrice) of the unwashed suspensions before resuspension in saline. Strain PS84 was used in this experiment. The ratio of inoculum to the

TABLE 1. *Formula of SM4 synthetic medium*

Component	Amt (g/liter)
DL-Aspartic acid	0.180
L-Valine	0.170
L-sodium glutamate	0.090
DL-β-Phenylalanine	0.010
L-Proline	0.070
L-Arginine monohydrochloride	0.025
L-Histidine monohydrochloride	0.050
Glycine	0.050
DL-Leucine	0.050
L-Cystine	0.005
L-α-Alanine	0.080
Nicotinic acid	0.0002
Thiamine hydrochloride	0.00001
Sodium citrate	0.5
Ammonium sulfate	1.0
Magnesium sulfate	0.1
D-Glucose	2.0
Potassium dihydrogen orthophosphate	3.0
Dipotassium hydrogen orthophosphate	7.0

SM4 medium was 1:26. The cultures were observed for 28 h under stationary incubation at 37°C to obtain accurate measurements of the lag-phase duration. Viable counts of three hourly samples were performed by the surface plate method. Lag phase in cultures inoculated with unwashed and washed suspensions lasted for 10 and 21 h, respectively. Doubling time, however, for both cultures was 80 min. These results indicate that traces of tryptone soya broth introduced with the unwashed inoculum, if at all, did not enhance the doubling time. The observed growth was therefore attributable to the SM4 medium itself. Increased lag phase in the culture inoculated with the washed suspension is possibly due to the handling of the cells during washing.

The role of the carry-over of the nonsynthetic medium during the experiments with unwashed inocula was investigated in yet another way. It was hypothesized that if the nonsynthetic medium was carried over, then the unwashed inoculum must significantly increase the immediate ultraviolet absorptivity of the SM4 medium; the nonsynthetic medium has very high absorptivity. To test this, washed and unwashed inocula from strain PS84 were introduced into the SM4 medium; the ratio of the inoculum to the medium was 1:26, same as used in the growth curve experiment above. Immediately after the inoculation, the suspensions were membrane filtered to determine the absorbance at 260 nm. The filtrates from uninoculated SM4 medium, SM4 medium inoculated with unwashed suspension, and SM4 medium inoculated with washed suspension had absorb-

TABLE 2. *Growth of Staphylococcus aureus in SM4 medium using four inocula (absorbance at 450 nm)*

Antibiotic sensitivity profile no.[a]	Strain no.	$Abs_{18} - Abs_0$			
		0.5	0.2	0.1	0.05
1	8	0.30	0.45	0.30	0.20
	56	0.43	0.56	0.63	0.31
	66	0.35	0.50	0.43	0.18
	89	0.36	0.53	0.48	0.52
	91	0.36	0.19	0.17	0.02
	PS84	0.51	0.58	0.65	0.30
2	32	0.13	0.12	0.04	0.00
	79	0.35	0.45	0.40	0.34
3	9	0.26	0.16	0.23	0.12
4	50	0.30	0.41	0.34	0.03
5	12	0.36	0.29	0.03	0.00
6	38	0.36	0.46	0.48	0.57
7	12	0.36	0.29	0.03	0.00
	42	0.36	0.28	0.11	0.04
	54	0.44	0.35	0.67	0.18
	62	0.46	0.55	0.32	0.52
	84	0.34	0.58	0.64	0.54
	86	0.00	0.03	0.04	0.03
	Oxford	0.48	0.57	0.65	0.29
	NCTC 4163	0.44	0.31	0.09	0.00

[a] 1, Resistant to benzylpenicillin, erythromycin, streptomycin, and tetracycline; 2, resistant to chloramphenicol, benzlpenicillin, streptomycin, and oleandomycin; 3, resistant to benzylpenicillin, streptomycin, and oleandomycin; 4, resistant to tetracycline and oleandomycin; 5, resistant to oleandomycin; 6, resistant to benzylpenicillin; 7, sensitive to the above antibiotics.
[b] Milliliters of inoculum per 5.0 ml of medium.

TABLE 3. *Analysis of variance: cultivation of Staphylococcus aureus in SM4 medium with respect to inoculum size and antibiotic sensitivity*

Source of variation	Sums of squares	Degrees of freedom	Variance		
			Mean squares	Ratio	*P*
Inoculum size	0.3539	3	0.1180	3.3	0.02–0.05
Antibiotic sensitivities	0.0039	1	0.0039	0.1	0.7–0.8
Interaction	0.0184	3	0.0061	0.2	NS[a]
Error	2.5464	72	0.0354		
Total	2.9226	79			

[a] Not significant.

ances of 0.068, 0.12, and 0.09, respectively; the carry-over of the nonsynthetic medium, under our experimental conditions, was not significant. The observed growth is therefore attributed to the SM4 medium. The medium is considered suitable for growing staphylococci in experiments demanding minimal ultraviolet absorptivity of the culture medium.

LITERATURE CITED

1. **Cruickshank, R.** 1968. Medical microbiology. E. Livingstone Ltd., London.
2. **Laue, P., and R. E. MacDonald.** 1968. Growth stimulation of *Staphylococcus aureus* by L-cystine or L-djenkolic acid. J. Bacteriol. 95:2420–2421.
3. **Morris, A., and A. D. Russell.** 1970. Novobiocin-induced leakage of intracellular substances form *Escherichia coli* Microbios 5:35–41.

ANTIMICROBIAL AGENTS AND CHEMOTHERAPY, Dec. 1976, p. 918–920
Vol. 10, No. 6

Comparative In Vitro Studies of Cinoxacin, Nalidixic Acid, and Oxolinic Acid

RALPH C. GORDON,[1]* LYNNE I. STEVENS, CHARLES E. EDMISTON, JR., AND KANWAL MOHAN

Departments of Human Development, Medicine, and Microbiology and Public Health, Michigan State University, East Lansing, Michigan 48824

Received for publication 23 July 1976

Cinoxacin and nalidixic acid were found to be similar in in vitro activity against 138 *Shigella* isolates and somewhat less active than oxolinic acid on a weight basis. Cross-resistance developed when 10 shigellae were transferred on increasing amounts of the respective agent contained in Mueller-Hinton agar. Plate dilution studies of the effect of changes in agar pH on the minimum inhibitory concentration revealed that the antibacterial activity increased with decreasing pH. Protein binding investigations revealed a high degree of binding, with nalidixic acid > oxolinic acid > cinoxacin.

Cinoxacin, nalidixic acid, and oxolinic acid are synthetic organic acids that are similar in their in vitro activity against gram-negative bacteria (1, 2, 7, 8, 12). These agents are currently reserved for treatment of urinary tract infections, and cinoxacin has not yet been approved for clinical use. The present laboratory studies were carried out to compare their activity against shigellae and to investigate influence of pH on antibacterial activity, development of resistance in vitro, and the degree of binding by human serum proteins.

Antimicrobial susceptibility testing was carried out on 138 isolates of *Shigella* (25 *S. flexneri* and 113 *S. sonnei*) using the Steers replicator (11) and incorporation of the agents into Mueller-Hinton agar (6), with a final inoculum of 10^4 to 10^5 organisms delivered to the plates. The minimum inhibitory concentration (MIC) was the lowest concentration of antimicrobial allowing growth of five or fewer colonies after 24 h at 37°C.

The influence of adjustment of agar pH on MIC by the addition of 1 N NaOH or 1 N HCl was evaluated for five isolates each of *S. flexneri* and *S. sonnei*. The pH values of 7.0, 7.3, and 8.0 were measured using a pH meter at 25°C and checking a portion before adding the antimicrobial.

The development of bacterial resistance was investigated by transferring five isolates each of the two species on gradually increasing concentrations of the agents in agar three times per week for 6 weeks beginning with subinhibitory concentrations. MIC determinations were then carried out on the original organisms (fresh clinical isolates) and on isolates that had been transferred on the three series of plates, looking for resistance and cross-resistance. These strains were then transferred twice a week for 3 weeks on drug-free agar, looking for loss of resistance on repeat MIC determinations.

Binding by human serum was estimated using broth dilution (9) and centrifugation (5) methods with paper disk assay (10) and an antimicrobial concentration of 14 μg/ml of 98% serum.

Results of plate dilution susceptibility studies are presented in Fig. 1. On a weight basis,

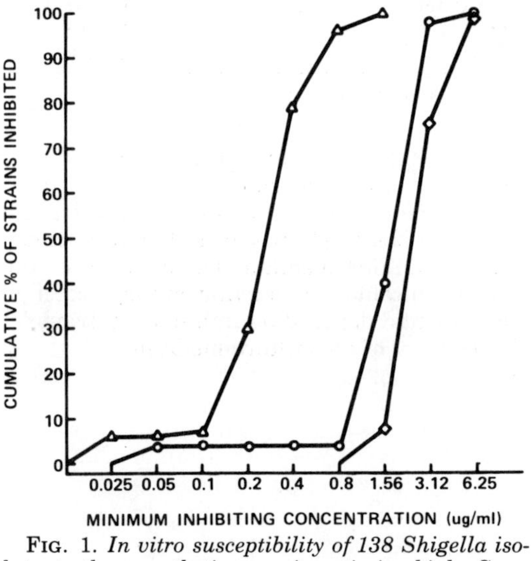

FIG. 1. *In vitro susceptibility of 138 Shigella isolates to three synthetic organic antimicrobials. Symbols: △, oxolinic acid; ○, cinoxacin; ◇, nalidixic acid.*

[1] Present address: Infectious Disease Research Laboratory, A. P. Beutel Health Center, Texas A & M University, College Station, TX 77843.

TABLE 1. *Effect of varying pH of Mueller-Hinton agar on MIC*

Strain	MIC (μg/ml) of:								
	Oxolinic acid			Nalidixic acid			Cinoxacin		
	7.0[a]	7.3	8.0	7.0	7.3	8.0	7.0	7.3	8.0
S. sonnei 1	0.39	0.39	3.12	1.56	6.25	12.5	0.78	1.56	12.5
S. sonnei 2	0.39	0.2	3.12	1.56	6.25	12.5	0.78	1.56	12.5
S. sonnei 3	0.39	0.2	0.39	1.56	6.25	12.5	0.78	1.56	25.0
S. sonnei 6	0.78	0.2	0.78	1.56	6.25	12.5	0.78	1.56	25.0
S. sonnei 10	0.39	0.2	3.12	1.56	6.25	6.25	3.12	1.56	6.25
S. flexneri 99	0.39	0.2	3.12	1.56	6.25	12.5	0.78	1.56	12.5
S. flexneri 113	0.39	0.2	0.39	1.56	6.25	12.5	0.78	1.56	25.0
S. flexneri 117	0.78	0.2	0.78	1.56	6.25	>25.0	1.56	1.56	25.0
S. flexneri 124	0.39	0.2	0.78	1.56	6.25	25.0	1.56	1.56	25.0
S. flexneri 130	0.78	0.2	0.78	1.56	6.25	25.0	1.56	1.56	>25.0

[a] pH of agar.

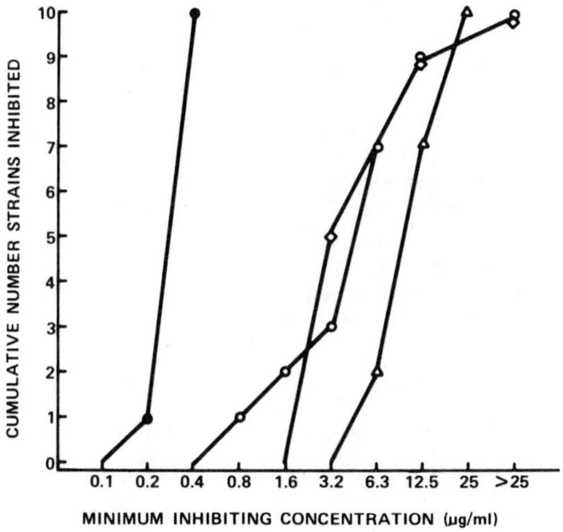

FIG. 2. *In vitro susceptibility of 10 Shigella isolates to oxolinic acid before and after 18 passages on agar plates containing oxolinic acid, nalidixic acid, and cinoxacin. Symbols: ●, fresh clinical isolates; ◇, nalidixic acid transfers; ○, cinoxacin transfers; △, oxolinic acid transfers.*

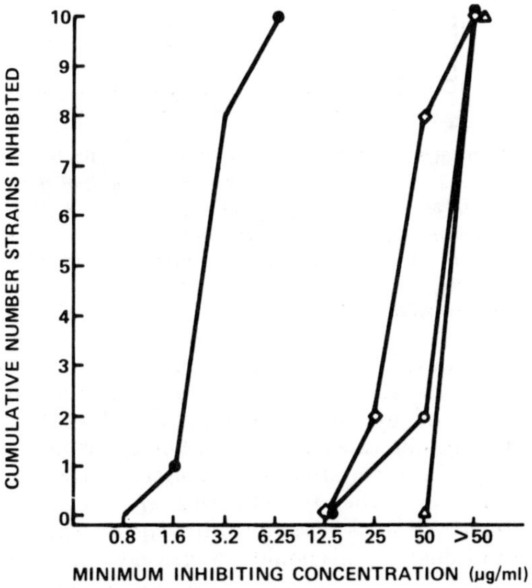

FIG. 3. *In vitro susceptibility of 10 Shigella isolates to nalidixic acid after passage on agar plates containing nalidixic acid, cinoxacin, or oxolinic acid. Symbols: ●, fresh clinical isolates; ◇ nalidixic acid transfers; ○, cinoxacin transfers; △, oxolinic acid transfers.*

oxolinic acid was most active; all isolates were inhibited by 1.56 μg or less per ml. Cinoxacin was somewhat more active than nalidixic acid; 40% as opposed to 8% was inhibited by 1.56 μg/ml. However, all isolates were inhibited at a concentration of 6.25 μg of either agent per ml. An increase in agar pH resulted in a raised MIC of all three agents, but this increase in MIC was less apparent with oxolinic acid (Table 1). Figures 2 through 4 illustrate that 18 passages on agar containing the single agent resulted in the development of resistance and cross-resistance of the 10 isolates. Seven of the ten strains were inhibited by 12.5 μg or less of oxolinic acid per ml after passage. No loss of resistance was noted after six transfers on antimicrobial-free agar. Evaluation of the susceptibility of these *Shigella* isolates to other antimicrobials was not carried out in the current work; however, previous studies (3, 6) have demonstrated that nalidixic acid and oxolinic acid are active against organisms resistant to multiple other agents. The degree of serum protein binding was greater with nalidixic acid (89 to 91%) than with oxolinic acid (80 to 85%) or cinoxacin (77 to 83%). Results for nalidixic acid are in agreement with those of Buchbinder and colleagues (2) and higher than the 66% for

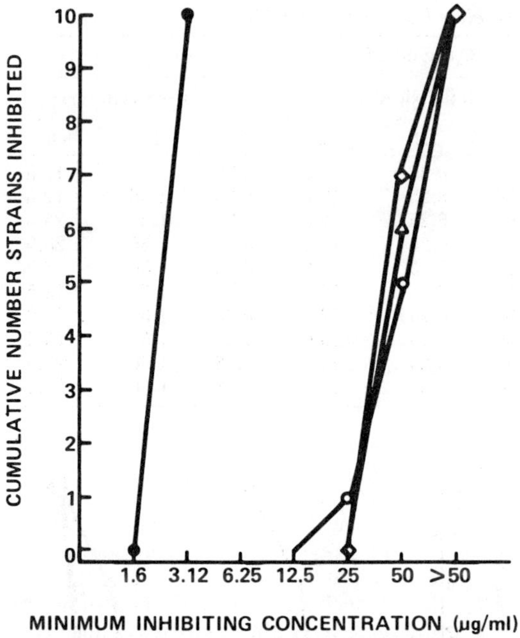

FIG. 4. *In vitro susceptibility of 10 Shigella isolates to cinoxacin after 18 passages on agar plates containing cinoxacin, nalidixic acid, or oxolinic acid. Symbols: ●, fresh clinical isolates; ○, cinoxacin transfers; ◇, nalidixic acid transfers; △, oxolinic acid transfers.*

nalidixic acid and 16% for cinoxacin reported by Wick and associates (12). A recent study by Giamarellou and Jackson (4) found that increasing the concentration of horse serum in a broth dilution system had no effect on the MIC of cinoxacin when tested with *Escherichia coli*, *Proteus*, and *Klebsiella-Enterobacter* species. Additional work should be carried out using several methods of determination of protein binding, taking into consideration the effects of pH on antibacterial activity, to further determine the binding characteristics of these agents.

This research was supported by Public Health Service General Research Support grant RR 05656-05 from the National Institutes of Health and by a grant from Eli Lilly & Co., Indianapolis, Ind. H. R. Black of the Lilly Research Laboratories furnished cinoxacin. F. C. Nachod of Sterling-Winthrop Research Institute and F. J. Turner of the Warner-Lambert Research Institute kindly supplied nalidixic acid and oxolinic acid, respectively. We thank Maria Patterson for critically reviewing the manuscript.

LITERATURE CITED

1. **Atlas, E., H. Clark, F. Silverblatt, and M. Turck.** 1969. Nalidixic acid and oxolinic acid in the treatment of chronic bacteriuria. Ann. Intern. Med. **70**:713–721.
2. **Buchbinder, M., J. C. Webb, L. Anderson, and W. R. McCabe.** 1963. Laboratory studies and clinical pharmacology of nalidixic acid (WIN 18,320), p. 308–317. Antimicrob. Agents Chemother. 1962.
3. **Byers, P. A., H. L. DuPont, and M. C. Goldschmidt.** 1976. Antimicrobial susceptibilities of shigellae isolated in Houston, Texas, in 1974. Antimicrob. Agents Chemother. **9**:288–291.
4. **Giamarellou, H., and G. G. Jackson.** 1975. Antibacterial activity of cinoxacin in vitro. Antimicrob. Agents Chemother. **7**:688–692.
5. **Gordon, R. C., C. Regamey, and W. M. M. Kirby.** 1973. Serum protein binding of erythromycin, lincomycin and clindamycin. J. Pharm. Sci. **62**:1074–1077.
6. **Gordon, R. C., T. R. Thompson, W. Carlson, J. W. Dyke, and L. I. Stevens.** 1975. Antimicrobial resistance of shigellae isolated in Michigan. J. Am. Med. Assoc. **231**:1159–1161.
7. **Kurtz, S., and M. Turck.** 1975. In vitro activity of cinoxacin, an organic acid antibacterial. Antimicrob. Agents Chemother. **7**:370–373.
8. **Lumish, R. M., and C. W. Norden.** 1975. Cinoxacin: in vitro antibacterial studies of a new organic acid. Antimicrob. Agents Chemother. **7**:159–163.
9. **Rolinson, G. N.** 1967. The significance of protein binding of antibiotics in vitro and in vivo, p. 254–283. *In* A. P. Waterson (ed.), Recent advances in medical microbiology. Little, Brown & Co., Boston.
10. **Simon, H. J., and E. J. Yin.** 1970. Microbioassay of antimicrobial agents. Appl. Microbiol. **19**:573–579.
11. **Steers, E., E. L. Foltz, and B. S. Graves.** 1959. Inocula replicating apparatus for routine testing of bacterial susceptibility to antibiotics. Antibiot. Chemother. (Washington, D.C.) **9**:307–311.
12. **Wick, W. E., D. A. Preston, W. A. White, and R. S. Gordee.** 1973. Compound 64716, a new synthetic antibacterial agent. Antimicrob. Agents Chemother. **4**:415–420.

ANTIMICROBIAL AGENTS AND CHEMOTHERAPY, Dec. 1976, p. 921-922
Vol. 10, No. 6

Procedure for Expediting Determinations of Antibiotic Susceptibility of Gram-Negative, Urinary Tract Pathogens

DENNIS L. WEGNER[1]* AND THOMAS R. NEBLETT

Division of Bacteriology and Serology, Department of Pathology, Henry Ford Hospital, Detroit, Michigan 48202

Received for publication 30 July 1976

Standardized direct disk diffusion antibiotic susceptibility testing on monomicrobial urine specimens is compared with the Food and Drug Administration method. The direct procedure yields acceptable data and may conserve 24 h in reporting results.

Disk diffusion antibiograms of bacterial urinary tract pathogens are most appropriately determined by the Food and Drug Administration (FDA) recommended procedure (3, 5, 6, 7), which requires a single isolate to prepare inocula for susceptibility testing. The necessity to await pure cultures causes 36 to 48 h to elapse before antibiotic susceptibility data become available. This period has been shortened in clinically urgent situations by using the urine specimen itself as inoculum for disk diffusion testing (1, 4). Because the urine sometimes contains inhibitory factors and varying quantities of organisms, sensitivity data so obtained may differ from information collected by the accepted method.

Previous studies in this laboratory (9) showed that when bacteremia is caused by a single, rapidly growing pathogen, 24 h may be conserved by inoculating a small volume of blood culture fluid into a relatively large volume of nutrient broth and growing it to standard density. This results in an inoculum for disk diffusion testing that is standardized and in which toxic factors are eliminated by dilution. The present study shows that the principle is also applicable to the susceptibility testing of urine specimens containing a single gram-negative organism.

Urine specimens from patients with suspected urinary tract infection were inoculated onto MacConkey agar plates, colistin-nalidixic acid sheep blood agar, and 10% sheep blood agar plates. One drop of each urine specimen (ca. 0.01 ml) was inoculated into 2 ml of Columbia broth with a Pasteur capillary pipette.

The Columbia broth suspensions were incubated for 4 to 6 h at 35°C. Those showing turbidity were Gram stained and subsequently adjusted with 0.9% NaCl to match a 0.5 McFarland $BaSO_4$ standard. Mueller-Hinton agar plates were inoculated evenly, and antibiotic disks (BBL) were applied. After 18 to 24 h of incubation at 35°C, inhibition zone diameters were measured to the nearest whole millimeter with a linear scale. Urine specimens shown to be polymicrobic by stain or culture, those containing gram-positive organisms, and specimens containing slow-growing organisms were not considered.

Isolated colonies from the blood agar plates were used to prepare inocula for the FDA standardized Bauer-Kirby procedure. Zone sizes for each isolate and drug tested by the direct and standard procedure were recorded and compared to interpretive standards established by the FDA method (5).

Seventy-two urine specimens, containing single, rapidly growing, gram-negative pathogens, were evaluated. Bacterial titers of the specimens ranged from 30,000 organisms per ml to greater than 500,000 organisms per ml. Antibiograms of 26 *Escherichia coli*, 12 *Proteus mirabilis*, 11 *Klebsiella pneumoniae*, 9 *Serratia marcescens*, 9 *Enterobacter cloacae*, 3 *Enterobacter aerogenes*, and 2 *Proteus vulgaris* were obtained by both methods.

Data ((Table 1) for the *E. coli* isolates are representative of the group of organisms. For each urine isolate and each antibiotic tested, discrepancies between zones obtained by both methods averaged less than 2 mm. Results obtained by the two methods necessitated a change in interpretive susceptibility category in only seven unrelated instances (1.0%).

Since polymicrobic suspensions yield unreliable antibiotic susceptibility data (8), this technique is only applicable to the testing of monomicrobic urine specimens. Fortunately, the majority of bacterial urinary tract infections are caused by single gram-negative organisms

[1] Present address: Department of Pathology, Mercy Hospital, Des Moines, IA 50314.

TABLE 1. *Comparison of experimental direct and indirect methods for obtaining antibiograms of E. coli isolates[a] from urine specimens*

Antibiotic (concn)	Mean difference (mm)[b]	Range (mm)
Ampicillin (10 μg)	1.2	0–3
Tetracycline (30 μg)	1.5	0–3
Cephalothin (30 μg)	1.6	0–4
Colistin (10 μg)	0.2	0–1
Gentamicin (10 μg)	1.2	0–2
Carbenicillin (100 μg)	1.0	0–3
Nalidixic acid (30 μg)	1.0	0–3
Furadantin (300 μg)	1.1	0–3
Gantrisin (2 μg)	1.1	0–4

[a] Twenty-six urine specimens containing *E. coli* as the sole bacterial pathogen were evaluated.

[b] For each urine isolate, the antibiotic zones of inhibition were obtained by both the experimental direct and indirect Bauer-Kirby methods. Averages and ranges of the individual differences were then computed.

(2). Because of the mixed flora at the terminal end of the urinary tract, extreme care must be exercised in specimen collection.

Bacteria from a few urine specimens from patients receiving antibiotics grew on solid isolation media but did not grow in direct susceptibility nutrient broth. Therefore, if clinically feasible, it is also recommended that urine specimens for direct susceptibility testing be collected before initiation of antimicrobial therapy.

Because of the chance of polymicrobic urinary tract infection or infection by slow-growing organisms, direct susceptibility testing on all urine specimens is not recommended as a replacement for the FDA procedure. However, in clinically urgent situations, such as bacteremia secondary to bacteriuria, it is felt that this technique is a valid means to conserve 24 h.

LITERATURE CITED

1. **Barry, A. L., L. J. Joyce, A. P. Adams, and E. J. Benner.** 1973. Rapid determination of antimicrobial susceptibility for urgent clinical situations. Am. J. Clin. Pathol. 59:693–699.
2. **Barry, A. L., P. B. Smith, M. Turck, and T. L. Gavan, (ed.).** 1975. Laboratory diagnosis of urinary tract infections. Cumitech 2. American Society for Microbiology, Washington, D. C.
3. **Bauer, A. W., W. M. M. Kirby, J. C. Sherris, and M. Turck.** 1966. Antibiotic sensitivity testing by a standardized single disk method. Am. J. Clin. Pathol. 45:493–496.
4. **Kunin, C. M.** 1972. Detection, prevention, and management of urinary tract infections, p. 99. Lea and Febiger, Philadelphia.
5. **National Committee for Clinical Laboratory Standards.** 1975. Performance standards for antimicrobial disc susceptibility tests. Villanova, Pa.
6. **Rules and Regulations.** 1972. Antibiotic susceptibility discs. Fed. Regist. 37:20525–25029.
7. **Rules and Regulations.** 1973. Antibiotic susceptibility discs: correction. Fed. Regist. 38:2576.
8. **Shahidi, A., and P. C. Ellner.** 1969. Effect of mixed cultures on antibiotic susceptibility testing. Appl. Microbiol. 18:776–780.
9. **Wegner, D. L., C. R. Mathis, and T. R. Neblett.** 1976. Direct method to determine the antibiotic susceptibility of rapidly growing blood pathogens. Antimicrob. Agents Chemother. 9:861–862.

ANTIMICROBIAL AGENTS AND CHEMOTHERAPY, Dec. 1976, p. 923-925
Vol. 10, No. 6

Chemically Defined Medium for Susceptibility Testing of Antimicrobial Agents

PAULA F. DOUGHERTY,* DAVID W. YOTTER, AND THOMAS R. MATTHEWS

Nucleic Acid Research Institute, ICN Pharmaceuticals, Inc., Irvine, California 92715

Received for publication 11 June 1976

A defined medium was developed that supports growth of many of the bacterial and fungal pathogens frequently isolated in clinics.

The problem of medium interference with susceptibility testing of antimicrobial agents has been recognized for some time (4, 7, 9). In our laboratory, in vitro evaluation of potential chemotherapeutic agents that may act as metabolic inhibitors required a chemically defined medium (1, 11, 13, 14). This medium needed to be simple and inexpensive to prepare. It was also desirable that the medium support the growth of both bacteria and fungi.

Defined medium (DM) is an extensive modification of synthetic amino acid medium (SAAM) and synthetic amino acid medium, fungal (SAAMF) (6, 8). DM contains no purines or pyrimidines. Amino acid concentrations are reduced. Folic acid is replaced by folic acid precursors that can be modified for sulfonamide studies. One liter of DM contains 75 mg of Ca^{2+} and 27 mg of Mg^{2+} (12). Vitamins are provided at 10^{-7} M (2).

DM retains the buffer system of MOPS [2-(*N*-morpholino)propane sulfonic acid] and tris [2-amino-2(hydroxymethyl)-1,3-propanediol] (5) at the concentration used in SAAM (0.04 M). This gives the medium a higher buffering capacity than is found in commonly used media (6).

Some components of SAAM and SAAMF are present in lower concentration in DM. This reduces the cost of DM to one-third that of SAAM.

DM has the advantage of supporting both bacterial and fungal growth. Some fastidious organisms may require enrichment, as can be the case with media such as Mueller-Hinton (15).

To prepare 1 liter of DM, place in a large beaker: distilled water (500.0 ml); minimum essential medium amino acids (50×) without glutamine (GIBCO) (50.0 ml); L-glutamine (625 ml); L-asparagine, L-proline, L-cysteine, and glycine (250.0 mg each); sodium pyruvate (375.0 mg); K_2HPO_4 (870.0 mg); MOPS (8.25 g); tris(hydroxymethyl)aminomethane (Tris) (6.25 g); fumaric acid (375.0 mg); and dextrose (5.0 g). Stir while warming to 45°C. Add 1.0 ml of a solution containing the following: distilled water (250.0 ml); biotin (6.1 mg); thiamine hydrochloride (8.5 mg); choline chloride (3.5 mg); riboflavin (9.5 mg); nicotinamide (3.0 mg); pyri-

TABLE 1. *Component concentration per liter of defined medium*

Component	Amt/liter
L-Arginine	262.5 mg
L-Cystine	60.0 mg
L-Hystidine	77.5 mg
L-Isoleucine	131.25 mg
L-Leucine	131.0 mg
L-Lysine	145.0 mg
L-Methionine	37.5 mg
L-Phenylalanine	80.0 mg
L-Threonine	120.0 mg
L-Tryptophan	25.0 mg
L-Tyrosine	90.0 mg
L-Valine	115.0 mg
L-Glutamine	625.0 mg
L-Asparagine	250.0 mg
L-Proline	250.0 mg
L-Cysteine	250.0 mg
Glycine	250.0 mg
Sodium pyruvate	375.0 mg
K_2HPO_4	870.0 mg
MOPS	8.25 g
Tris	6.25 g
Fumaric acid	375.0 mg
Dextrose	5.0 g
Biotin	0.0244 mg
Thiamine hydrochloride	0.034 mg
Choline chloride	0.014 mg
Riboflavin	0.038 mg
Nicotinamide	0.012 mg
Pyridoxal hydrochloride	0.02 mg
Pyridoxamin · 2HCl	0.024 mg
Pyridoxine hydrochloride	0.021 mg
Calcium pantothenate	0.022 mg
Inositol	0.018 mg
p-Aminobenzoic acid (optional)	0.014 mg
$CaCl_2 \cdot 2H_2O$	270.0 mg
$MgCl_2 \cdot 6H_2O$	228.0 mg
$FeCl_2 \cdot 6H_2O$	30.0 mg
$ZnSO_4 \cdot 7H_2O$	7.0 mg
$MnCl_2 \cdot 4H_2O$	5.0 mg

doxal hydrochloride (5.0 mg); pyridoxamin·2HCl (6.0 mg); pyridoxine hydrochloride (5.3 mg); pantothenic acid (5.5 mg); inositol (4.5 mg); and *para*-aminobenzoic acid (3.5 mg) (added as an optional enrichment; omit for sulfonamide testing. Add distilled water to bring the volume to 1,000 ml. Adjust the pH to 7.3 by adding Tris. Filter sterilize into a sterile flask containing 0.5 ml of each of the following mineral solutions. Solution A contains: distilled water (5.0 ml); $CaCl_2 \cdot 2H_2O$ (2.7 g); and $MgCl_2 \cdot 6H_2O$ (2.28 g). Solution B contains: distilled water (5.0 ml); $FeCl_3 \cdot 6H_2O$ (300.0 mg); $ZnSO_4 \cdot 7H_2O$ (70.0 mg); and $MnCl_2 \cdot 4H_2O$ (50.0 mg).

We have found it convenient to prepare DM as a 10× concentrate and store it frozen in 100-ml aliquots in screw-capped bottles. Fluid DM is prepared by adding 100 ml of the thawed 10× concentrate to 900 ml of sterile distilled water and mixing thoroughly. DM agar is prepared by adding 100 ml of the thawed 10× concentrate to 900 ml of sterile, molten 1.6% purified agar (Difco) that has been cooled to 45°C. The vitamin solution may also be prepared in quantity and stored frozen for up to 6 months.

Final concentration of all components is given in Table 1. Genera of organisms that we have used for susceptibility testing in DM are given in Table 2.

All organisms used were clinical isolates received from many sources. Selection of gram-negative bacteria was based on uniqueness of biochemical profile, determined by the API 20E system (Analytab Products Inc., Carle Place, N.Y.), and antibiogram, determined by the disk diffusion method.

DM has been used in our laboratory for 38 months. This medium is usually prepared in 4-liter volumes of a 10× concentrate and frozen for use during a 3-month interval. During initial modification studies, growth of bacteria and *Candida albicans* in DM broth was compared with growth in SAAM broth using optical density readings (660 nm). Final readings after 18 h of incubation were uniform.

Standard drugs such as gentamicin, ampicillin, cephalexin, tolnaftate, and 5-fluorocytosine as well as potential chemotherapeutic agents were tested in DM using disk diffusion, broth dilution, and agar dilution methods (3, 10, 15). Quantitative and qualitative in vitro inhibitory

TABLE 2. *Growth of genera on defined medium*

Genus	No. of strains showing growth	No. of strains showing no growth	Genus	No. of isolates showing growth	No. of isolates showing no growth
Bacteria			Fungi		
Aeromonas	3	0	*Allescheria*	1	0
Acinetobacter	13	0	*Alternaria*	1	0
Alcaligenes	4	0	*Aspergillus*	6	0
Arizona	2	0	*Blastomyces*	2	0
Brucella	7	14	*Candida*	77	0
Citrobacter	8	0	*Cephalosporium*	1	0
Enterobacter	28	0	*Cryptococcus*	8	0
Enterococcus	8	0	*Epidermophyton*	2	0
Escherichia	78	0	*Eupenicillium*	1	0
Flavobacterium	1	0	*Fonsecaea*	2	0
Klebsiella	33	0	*Fusarium*	1	0
Listeria	2	0	*Geotrichum*	2	0
Proteus	56	0	*Histoplasma*	3	0
Providence	8	0	*Keratinomyces*	1	0
Pseudomonas	73	0	*Microsporum*	9	0
Salmonella	22	0	*Mucor*	2	0
Serratia	15	0	*Neurospora*	1	0
Shigella	6	0	*Nocardia*	3	0
Staphylococcus	39	44	*Penicillium*	1	0
Streptococcus	5	15	*Phialophora*	2	0
			Rhizopus	1	0
			Rhodotorula	1	0
			Scopulariopsis	2	0
			Sepedonium	1	0
			Sporotrichum	1	0
			Torulopsis	7	0
			Trichophyton	22	0
			Trichosporon	1	0
			Ustilago	1	0

values for these drugs have remained consistent during the 3- to 4-month use period of a single batch. More importantly, these values have remained consistent from one batch of DM to the next.

Organisms that have not grown well on DM include isolates of *Brucella*, *Enterococcus*, *Staphylococcus*, and *Streptococcus*. Attempts were made to enhance the growth of these organisms by the addition of 25 mg of uracil, uridine, and cytidine per liter and elimination of dextrose from the medium. No growth enhancement was achieved by these alterations.

DM has the advantages of being totally defined, simple to prepare, relatively low in cost, and reproducible from batch to batch. DM can be easily modified for special studies; for example, purines or pyrimidines can be added for activity reversal studies. Mg^{2+} and Ca^{2+} concentrations are suitable for aminoglycoside testing against *Pseudomonas* (12). The ability of DM to support both bacterial and fungal growth is particularly useful. Although DM may not be practical for general use in susceptibility testing, we have found DM to be very useful for routine in vitro evaluation of potential chemotherapeutic agents that may act as metabolic inhibitors.

LITERATURE CITED

1. **Bartholomew, D. G., J. H. Huffmon, T. R. Matthews, R. K. Robins, and G. R. Revanbar.** 1976. Imidazo-[1,2-*c*]pyrimidine nucleosides. Synthesis and biological evaluation of certain 1-β-D-arabinofuranosyl)-imidazol[1,2-*c*]pyrimidines. J. Med. Chem. **19**:814–816.
2. **Burrows, W.** 1968. Textbook of microbiology. W. B. Saunders Co., Philadelphia.
3. **Ericsson, H. M., and J. C. Sherris.** 1971. Antibiotic sensitivity testing. Report of an international collaborative study. Acta Pathol. Microbiol. Scand. Suppl. 217, p. 12.
4. **Garrod, L. P., and P. M. Waterworth.** 1969. Effect of medium composition on the apparent sensitivity of *Pseudomonas aeruginosa* to gentamicin. J. Clin. Pathol. **22**:534–538.
5. **Good, N. E., G. D. Winget, W. Winter, T. N. Connolly, S. Izawa, and R. M. Singh.** 1966. Hydrogen ion buffers for biological research. Biochemistry **5**:467–477.
6. **Hoeprich, P. D., A. L. Barry, and G. D. Fay.** 1971. Synthetic medium for susceptibility testing, p. 494–497. Antimicrob. Agents Chemother. 1970.
7. **Hoeprich, P. D., and P. D. Finn.** 1971. Influence of culture media on the antistaphylococcal activity of fosfomycin. Appl. Microbiol. **22**:781–783.
8. **Hoeprich, P. D., and P. D. Finn.** 1972. Obfuscation of the activity of antifungal antibiotics by culture media. J. Infect. Dis. **126**:353–361.
9. **Koch, A. E., and J. J. Burchall.** 1971. Reversal of the antimicrobial activity of trimethoprim by thymidine in commercially prepared media. Appl. Microbiol. **22**:812–817.
10. **Marymount, J. H., and R. M. Wentz.** 1966. Serial dilution antibiotic sensitivity testing with the microtitrator system. Am. J. Clin. Pathol. **45**:548–551.
11. **Novinson, T., T. Okabe, R. K. Robins, and T. R. Matthews.** 1976. Synthesis and antimicrobial activity of some novel heterocycles: the azolo-*as*-triazines. J. Med. Chem. **19**:517–520.
12. **Reller, B. L., F. D. Shoenknecht, M. A. Kenny, and J. C. Sherris.** 1974. Antibiotic susceptibility testing of *Pseudomonas aeruginosa*: selection of a control strain and criteria for magnesium and calcium content in media. J. Infect. Dis. **130**:454–463.
13. **Revankar, G. R., T. R. Matthews, and R. K. Robins.** 1975. Synthesis and antimicrobial activity of certain imidazo[1,2-*a*]-pyrimidines. J. Med. Chem. **18**:1253–1255.
14. **Srivastava, P. C., A. R. Newman, T. R. Matthews, and R. K. Robins.** 1975. Synthesis of 5-amino-1-(5-deoxy-β-D-ribofuranosyl)imidazole-4-carboxamide and related 5′-deoxyimidazole ribonucleosides. J. Med. Chem. **18**:1237–1240.
15. **Washington, J. A., II, and A. L. Barry.** 1974. Dilution test procedures, p. 410–417. *In* E. H. Lennette, E. H. Spaulding, and J. P. Truant (ed.), Manual of clinical microbiology, 2nd ed. American Society for Microbiology, Washington, D.C.

ANTIMICROBIAL AGENTS AND CHEMOTHERAPY, Dec. 1976, p. 926-928
Vol. 10, No. 6

Medium for Use in Antibiotic Susceptibility Testing of Anaerobic Bacteria

TRACY D. WILKINS* AND SARAH CHALGREN

Anaerobe Laboratory, Virginia Polytechnic Institute and State University, Blacksburg, Virginia 24061

Received for publication 3 August 1976

A medium is described which was designed for use in testing the minimal inhibitory concentration of antibiotics for anaerobic bacteria by agar dilution. It contains: Trypticase (1%), Gelysate (1%), yeast extract (0.5%), glucose (0.1%), pyruvate (0.1%), arginine (0.1%), NaCl (0.5%), hemin (5 μg/ml), vitamin K_1 (0.5 μg/ml), agar (1.5%). The medium does not require the addition of blood to support growth of most clinical isolates of anaerobic bacteria.

At present there is no standard medium for use in testing the antibiotic susceptibility of anaerobic bacteria. Mueller-Hinton agar has been used as a standard medium for susceptibility testing of facultative bacteria for many years, but it will not support the growth of most species of anaerobic bacteria (10). A collaborative group has been working for 2 years on the development of a standard anaerobic method for determination of minimal inhibitory concentrations (MICs) of antibiotics by agar dilution. This working group consists of: V. L. Sutter (Wadsworth V.A. Hospital), W. J. Martin (UCLA), C. Thornsberry (Center for Disease Control), V. R. Dowell (Center for Disease Control), J. E. Rosenblatt (Mayo Clinic), R. J. Zabransky (Mt. Sinai, Milwaukee), and ourselves. Brucella Agar (Difco) with 5% sheep blood was suggested as a standard medium, but the group was concerned with the possible variation the blood might introduce into the test. Sheep blood varies from different suppliers, changes with age, and is easily contaminated. Brucella Agar without blood does not support growth of many anaerobes (10). We therefore undertook the development of a suitable medium that would not require the addition of blood. The medium described in Table 1 supports the growth of the anaerobes commonly isolated in clinical laboratories. The reasons for inclusion of each ingredient are given below.

Trypticase (BBL) is the best peptone that we have found for growth of anaerobes. This has also been found by others; Trypticase is the peptone component of both Schaedler medium (7) and Lombard-Dowell broth (9). We also used Trypticase because it is derived from a pure protein, casein, and should be a more consistent product than meat peptones. We also used Gelysate (BBL) peptone, which is from another pure protein, gelatin. In addition to its derivation from a pure protein, we used Gelysate because it complemented the amino acid composition of Trypticase and, in particular, was high in glycine. Glycine is fermented by some anaerobic cocci (1). Both Trypticase and Gelysate were used in 1% concentration to ensure adequate amounts of amino acids and peptides and to provide some buffering capacity.

Yeast extract was added to supply vitamins and other growth factors such as purines and pyrimidines. Several anaerobes tested, including strains of *Peptostreptococcus anaerobius* and *Bacteroides melaninogenicus*, required 0.5% and did not grow as well with 0.25%. IsoVitaleX (B-D) could not replace yeast extract; however, it may be possible to replace yeast extract at some future date with a known mixture of vitamins, purines, pyrimidines, etc.

Glucose (0.1%) was added to allow growth of the obligately saccharolytic organisms and to stimulate faster growth of most strains. We obtained faster growth of saccharolytic organisms with higher concentrations of glucose, but this resulted in a drastic drop in the pH. This was not desirable, since some antibiotics vary greatly in activity at different pH values and this could affect any slower-growing organisms on the same plate.

Arginine was added to make certain that enough would be available for *Eubacterium lentum*, which uses the arginine dihydrolase pathway (8) for energy production.

Pyruvate was added for two reasons. First, many asaccharolytic cocci, such as the *Veillonella*, utilize pyruvate as an energy source (2, 6). Second, pyruvate degrades hydrogen peroxide, forming acetate, CO_2, and H_2O. This is not nearly as fast as the reaction catalyzed by catalase, but it is more convenient to use, since pyruvate can be autoclaved with the medium.

Hemin was added to satisfy the requirements

TABLE 1. *Preparation of Wilkins-Chalgren medium*

1. Dispense the following ingredients and dissolve in 1,000 ml of water—the pH should be 7.0 to 7.2.

	Catalog no.	Company	Amt (g)
Trypticase (pancreatic digest of casein)	11921	BBL	10
Gelysate (pancreatic digest of gelatin)	11870	BBL	10
Yeast extract	0127-01	Difco	5
Glucose	D-16 73412	Fisher	1
NaCl	S-271 78440 or 78443	Fisher	5
L-Arginine—free base	A-5006	Sigma	1
Pyruvic acid—sodium salt	P-2256	Sigma	1
Agar	0140-01	Difco	15

2. Add heme and vitamin K_1 solutions to yield final concentrations of 5 μg/ml for hemin and 0.5 μg/ml for K_1 (Table 2)
3. Boil for 1 min (until agar dissolves)
4. Autoclave at 121°C for 15 min on slow exhaust aerobically
5. Cool in water bath to 50 to 55°C
6. Add antibiotic solution and dispense into petri plates

TABLE 2. *Preparation of hemin and vitamin K_1 solutions*

Vitamin K_1 stock—Add 0.2 ml of stock per liter = 0.5 μg/ml, final concentration
- Sigma Chemical Co., St. Louis, catalog no. V-3501
- Stock = 0.05 ml of vitamin K_1 solution + 20 ml of 95% ethanol
- Filter sterilize (membrane filter)
- Keep stock solution in dark bottle in refrigerator for 1 month and then discard

Hemin stock—Add 10 ml of stock per liter = 5.0 μg/ml, final concentration
- Sigma Chemical Co., St. Louis, catalog no. H-2375 hemin equine type III
- 0.5 g of hemin + 10 ml of 1 N NaOH + 990 ml of water
- Autoclave at 121°C for 12 min on fast exhaust = 500 μg/ml
- Stock solution kept at room temperature under N_2 atmosphere

of *Bacteroides fragilis* (M. D. Appleman, J. J. Johnson, and T. D. Wilkins, Abstr. Annu. Meet. Am. Soc. Microbiol. 1976, I128, p. 132; 11) and other species of *Bacteroides* (5). In a commercial formulation, this could be mixed well with the other ingredients, but for making small batches we added both hemin and vitamin K_1 as a solution (Table 2) before autoclave sterilization (4). Vitamin K_1 was added, since some strains of *B. melanogenicus* require it (3). NaCl was added to make the medium isotonic so that blood could be added for use as an isolation medium when hemolysis reactions need to be detected.

Antibiotics were added (1 ml per 50 ml of medium) when the medium had been cooled to 50°C. Plates were poured immediately after addition of the antibiotic solution. The plates could be used as soon as they were dry or after storage for 1 day in either an anaerobic chamber or GasPak (BBL) type jar. Storage for a longer time would risk decay of the antibiotic in the agar, but we have not noticed any effect on growth of anaerobic bacteria.

The medium given in Table 1 has been used by seven separate laboratories to determine the MIC of 5 antibiotics on 10 standard strains of anaerobic bacteria (V. L. Sutter, A. L. Barry, W. J. Martin, J. E. Rosenblatt, V. R. Dowell, Jr., C. Thornsberry, T. D. Wilkins, and R. J. Zabransky, Prog. Abstr. Intersci. Conf. Antimicrob. Agents Chemother., 16th, Chicago, Ill., Abstr. 453, 1976). The results have been reproducible, even though the seven laboratories made the medium from the separate components and used different lots of these components.

Except for Trypticase and Gelysate peptones, the ingredients should not have to be obtained from the sources listed in Table 1, as long as good-quality products are used. However, some batches of agar from other suppliers would not remain as a liquid at 50°C, which is the temperature at which the antibiotic solution is added. Standard strains will be made available by the working group which can be used to quality control the medium composition.

The medium has been in use in our laboratory for a year and has consistently grown anaerobes as well or better than media such as Brucella Agar or Schaedler blood agar. It has the advantage of being made from relatively reproducible components and does not contain meat infusions, etc., that can vary greatly in composition.

This work was supported by Public Health Service grant GM-14604 from the National Institute of General Medical Sciences and by grants from the Upjohn Co. and Pfizer Co.

LITERATURE CITED

1. **Douglas, H. C.** 1951. Glycine fermentation by nongas forming anaerobic micrococci. J. Bacteriol. 62:517–518.
2. **Foubert, E. I., Jr., and H. C. Douglas.** 1948. Studies on the anaerobic micrococci. I. Taxonomic consideration. J. Bacteriol. 56:25–34.
3. **Gibbons, R. J., and J. B. MacDonald.** 1960. Hemin and vitamin K compounds as required factors for the cultivation of certain strains of *Bacteroides melaninogenicus*. J. Bacteriol. 80:164–170.
4. **Holdeman, L. V., and W. E. C. Moore (ed.).** 1975. Anaerobe laboratory manual, 3rd ed. Virginia Polytechnic Institute and State University, Blacksburg, Va.
5. **Quinto, G., and M. Sebald.** 1964. Identification of three hemin-requiring *Bacteroides* strains. Am. J. Med. Technol. 30:381–384.
6. **Rogosa, M.** 1964. The genus *Veillonella*. 1. General cultural, ecological, and biochemical consideration. J. Bacteriol. 87:162–170.
7. **Schaedler, R. W., R. Dubos, and R. Costello.** 1965. The development of the bacterial flora in the gastrointestinal tract of mice. J. Exp. Med. 122:59–66.
8. **Sperry, J. F., and T. D. Wilkins.** 1976. Arginine, a growth limiting factor for *Eubacterium lentum*. J. Bacteriol. 127:780–784.
9. **Stargel, M. D., F. S. Thompson, S. E. Phillips, G. L. Lombard, and V. R. Dowell, Jr.** 1976. Modification of the Miniteck miniaturized differentiation system for characterization of anaerobic bacteria. J. Clin. Microbiol. 3:291–301.
10. **Sutter, V. L., Y-Y. Kwok, and S. M. Finegold.** 1973. Susceptibility of *Bacteroides fragilis* to six antibiotics determined by standardized antimicrobial disc susceptibility testing. Antimicrob. Agents Chemother. 3:188–193.
11. **Varel, V. H., and M. P. Bryant.** 1974. Nutritional features of *Bacteroides fragilis* subsp. *fragilis*. Appl. Microbiol. 18:251–257.

U.S. POSTAL SERVICE

STATEMENT OF OWNERSHIP, MANAGEMENT AND CIRCULATION

(Required by 39 U.S.C. 3685)

1. TITLE OF PUBLICATION: ANTIMICROBIAL AGENTS AND CHEMOTHERAPY

2. DATE OF FILING: 10/1/76

3. FREQUENCY OF ISSUE: MONTHLY

A. NO. OF ISSUES PUBLISHED ANNUALLY: 12

B. ANNUAL SUBSCRIPTION PRICE: mem.$13, non-mem.$50

4. LOCATION OF KNOWN OFFICE OF PUBLICATION *(Street, City, County, State and ZIP Code) (Not printers)*: 1913 EYE STREET, N.W. WASHINGTON, D.C. 20006

5. LOCATION OF THE HEADQUARTERS OR GENERAL BUSINESS OFFICES OF THE PUBLISHERS *(Not printers)*: 1913 EYE STREET, N.W. WASHINGTON, D.C. 20006

6. NAMES AND COMPLETE ADDRESSES OF PUBLISHER, EDITOR, AND MANAGING EDITOR

PUBLISHER *(Name and Address)*: AMERICAN SOCIETY FOR MICROBIOLOGY, 1913 EYE STREET, N.W. WASHINGTON, D.C. 20006

EDITOR *(Name and Address)*: DR. GLADYS L. HOBBY,INF.DISEASE RESEARCH INST. P.O.BOX 495, EAST ORANGE, NJ. 07019

MANAGING EDITOR *(Name and Address)*: ROBERT A. DAY, 1913 EYE STREET, N.W. WASHINGTON, D.C. 20006

7. OWNER *(If owned by a corporation, its name and address must be stated and also immediately thereunder the names and addresses of stockholders owning or holding 1 percent or more of total amount of stock. If not owned by a corporation, the names and addresses of the individual owners must be given. If owned by a partnership or other unincorporated firm, its name and address, as well as that of each individual must be given.)*

NAME	ADDRESS
American Society for Microbiology	1913 Eye Street, N.W. Wash., D.C. 20006

8. KNOWN BONDHOLDERS, MORTGAGEES, AND OTHER SECURITY HOLDERS OWNING OR HOLDING 1 PERCENT OR MORE OF TOTAL AMOUNT OF BONDS, MORTGAGES OR OTHER SECURITIES *(If there are none, so state)*

NAME	ADDRESS
NONE	

9. FOR COMPLETION BY NONPROFIT ORGANIZATIONS AUTHORIZED TO MAIL AT SPECIAL RATES *(Section 132.122, PSM)*
The purpose, function, and nonprofit status of this organization and the exempt status for Federal income tax purposes *(Check one)*

[XX] HAVE NOT CHANGED DURING PRECEDING 12 MONTHS [ ] HAVE CHANGED DURING PRECEDING 12 MONTHS *(If changed, publisher must submit explanation of change with this statement.)*

10. EXTENT AND NATURE OF CIRCULATION	AVERAGE NO. COPIES EACH ISSUE DURING PRECEDING 12 MONTHS	ACTUAL NO. COPIES OF SINGLE ISSUE PUBLISHED NEAREST TO FILING DATE
A. TOTAL NO. COPIES PRINTED *(Net Press Run)*	2582	2,438
B. PAID CIRCULATION 1. SALES THROUGH DEALERS AND CARRIERS, STREET VENDORS AND COUNTER SALES	None	None
2. MAIL SUBSCRIPTIONS	1,683	1,874
C. TOTAL PAID CIRCULATION *(Sum of 10B1 and 10B2)*	1,683	1,874
D. FREE DISTRIBUTION BY MAIL, CARRIER OR OTHER MEANS SAMPLES, COMPLIMENTARY, AND OTHER FREE COPIES	3	3
E. TOTAL DISTRIBUTION *(Sum of C and D)*	1,686	1,877
F. COPIES NOT DISTRIBUTED 1. OFFICE USE, LEFT OVER, UNACCOUNTED, SPOILED, AFTER PRINTING	1,896	1,561
2. RETURNS FROM NEWS AGENTS	None	None
G. TOTAL *(Sum of E, F1 and 2—should equal net press run shown in A)*	2,582	2,438

11. I certify that the statements made by me above are correct and complete.
SIGNATURE AND TITLE OF EDITOR, PUBLISHER, BUSINESS MANAGER, OR OWNER: Robert A. Day, Managing Editor

12. FOR COMPLETION BY PUBLISHERS MAILING AT THE REGULAR RATES *(Section 132.121, Postal Service Manual)*

39 U. S. C. 3626 provides in pertinent part: "No person who would have been entitled to mail matter under former section 4359 of this title shall mail such matter at the rates provided under this subsection unless he files annually with the Postal Service a written request for permission to mail matter at such rates."

In accordance with the provisions of this statute, I hereby request permission to mail the publication named in Item 1 at the phased postage rates presently authorized by 39 U. S. C. 3626.

SIGNATURE AND TITLE OF EDITOR, PUBLISHER, BUSINESS MANAGER, OR OWNER

PS Form 3526 *(Page 1)* Apr. 1976 (See instructions on reverse)

ERRATUM

Mutanolysin, Bacteriolytic Agent for Cariogenic Streptococci: Partial Purification and Properties

KANAE YOKOGAWA, SHIGEO KAWATA, SHINZO NISHIMURA, YASUHIKO IKEDA, AND YOSHIO YOSHIMURA

Research and Development Division, Dainippon Pharmaceutical Co. Ltd., Osaka, Japan

Volume 6, no. 2, p. 156–165: The figure legends should read as follows.

FIG. 1. *Results of mutanolysin subjected to electrofocusing. Symbols: ——, pH; – – –, proteolytic activity; . . ., OD at 280 nm; –·–, lytic activity.*

FIG. 2. *Activities of lytic and proteolytic enzymes in mutanolysin at different pH values. In all cases, 0.01 M buffers (final concentration) and 10 μg of mutanolysin were used. Symbols: ○, lytic activity; ●, proteolytic activity. Buffers used were glycine-HCl (pH 3 to 4), citrate (pH 5 to 6), phosphate (pH 7 to 9), Tris-hydrochloride (pH 10), glycine-NaOH (pH 11), Ringer (pH 12), and Sörensen (pH 13).*

FIG. 3. *Lytic and proteolytic activities as determined by change in incubation temperature. Symbols: ○, lytic activity; ●, proteolytic activity.*

FIG. 4. *Effect of heat on lytic and proteolytic activities. Mutanolysin was dissolved in distilled water at a concentration of 1 mg/ml and heated at various temperatures for 10 min prior to the assay. Symbols: ○, lytic activity; ●, proteolytic activity.*

FIG. 5. *Effect of pH on the stability of lytic and proteolytic enzymes. The incubation mixture containing 500 μg of mutanolysin in 1 ml of buffer was incubated at 37 C. After 24 h, the residual lytic (○) and proteolytic (●) activities were assayed.*

FIG. 6. *Time course curves of lysis and viable cell counts by mutanolysin on S. mutans. Streptococci were incubated with 80 μg of mutanolysin per 4 ml of reaction mixture, and the optical density at 600 nm (– – –) and the viable cell counts (——) at various times during incubation were measured. Symbols: ●, S. mutans AHT; ○, S. mutans BHT.*

FIG. 7. *Lysis of S. mutans by mutanolysin in human and hamster saliva. The reactions were carried out at 37 C with 100 μg of mutanolysin in 4 ml of human saliva (○), hamster's saliva (●), or phosphate buffer (▲). Solid line, natural saliva; broken line, neutral saliva.*

FIG. 8. *Time course of cell lysis. The incubation time with mutanolysin and the magnifications were as follows: (a) 0 min, ×26,000; (b) 5 min, ×35,000; (c) 5 min, ×11,000; (d) 5 min, ×8,750; (e) 20 min, ×33,000; (f) 30 min, ×29,000; (g) 60 min, ×7,500; (h) 60 min, ×28,000.*

FIG. 9. *Analysis of cell wall digests for amino groups and reducing groups. A suspension of 250 mg of cell walls in 0.02 M phosphate buffer, pH 6.5, containing 10^{-3} M $MgSO_4$, 400 mg of NaN_3, and 1,100 units of mutanolysin was incubated and assayed for free amino groups (□), reducing sugars (■), and optical density at 600 nm (▲).*

AUTHOR INDEX

VOLUME 10

Adams, Monica A., 872
Ahern, Mary Jean, 457
Aitken, Connie L., 436
Ajello, Libero, 75
Alam, A. K. M. Jamiul, 610
Anderson, J. D., 872
Andersson, Karl-Erik, 604
Andriole, Vincent T., 457
Appel, Gerald B., 623
Arcieri, George, 827

Baca, B., 258
Badal, R. E., 83
Baird, Ian M., 626
Baker, Carol J., 128
Balfour, Henry H., Jr., 866
Bardos, T. J., 682
Barrett, Fred F., 128
Barrington, Jane C., 872
Barry, A. L., 83
Bartholomew, Luanna, 507
Barza, Michael, 421, 569
Baum, Jules, 569
Becker, Jeffrey M., 483
Becker, R. O., 856
Beebe, J. L., 179
Bellinger, Mary Ann, 417
Benedictson, J., 768
Berger, Stephen, 421
Berger, T. J., 856
Bernardo, Peter D., 283
Berquist, Kenneth R., 571
Betts, Robert F., 253
Bhathena, Dinyar, 555
Bierman, Richard, 856
Bieth, G., 795
Black, H. R., 814
Blackman, Jane, 234
Blackwell, C. Caroline, 288
Blazevic, Donna J., 866
Bobek, Miroslav, 119
Bodey, Gerald P., 652
Bolton, W. Kline, 450
Bond, John H., 639
Bouanchaud, D. H., 258, 795
Bourque, Michael, 157
Bradshaw, M. W., 467
Breinig, Mary K., 28
Briedis, Dalius J., 592
Brier, G. L., 814
Brotherton, Thomas, 322
Broughton, Alan, 652
Brown, Arthur, 277
Brown, K. N., 768
Bruckner, H. W., 185
Bryan, L. E., 573
Buck, R. E., 426
Bullock, Ward E., 555

Burch, K., 464
Burt, Sharon J., 567
Busch, David F., 713

Cabana, B. E., 307
Capmau, M. L., 258
Chabbert, Y. A., 795
Chadha, K. C., 682
Chalgren, Sarah, 926
Chapin, S. E., 856
Chappell, W. Adrian, 344
Chardon, H., 258
Charles, B. G., 915
Chello, P., L., 185
Cheng, Yung-Chi, 119
Chisholm, D. R., 426
Chiu, Peter J. S., 277
Chow, A. W., 102
Clark, D. C., 215
Cohen, S., 139
Collins, M. S., 318
Condon, R. G., 363
Cooksey, Robert C., 123
Cox, F., 464
Coyle, Marie B., 436
Cupp, James, 96

D'Alessandri, Robert M., 889
Daschner, Franz D., 802
Del Bene, Victor E., 106
Demain, A. L., 265
Denes, Alexander E., 436
DeRegis, R. G., 426
Desser, Kenneth B., 447
Dilworth, John A., 450
Dixon, John H., Jr., 164
Dodd, Wendell K., 899
Domin, Barbara A., 119
Dominik, J. W., 549
Dougherty, Paula F., 923
Douglas, R. Gordon, 253
Dowling, John N., 809
Drach, John C., 64
Due, Susan L., 630
Duma, Richard J., 370
Duval, J., 258

Earhart, C. F., 150
Ebert, James W., 571
Edmiston, Charles E., Jr., 918
Effinger, L. J., 83
Ehret, Josephine M., 241
Eickenberg, H. U., 733
Eickhoff, Theodore C., 241
Ekwo, Edem, 893
English, Arthur R., 89, 132, 491
Ernst, E. Chaim, 421

Esparza, Jose, 176
Evangelisti, D. G., 89

Fanning, W. Lee, 80
Farrar, W. Edmund, Jr., 123
Fass, Robert J., 34
Feigin, Ralph D., 322
Feigl, Polly, 436
Ferretti, Joseph J., 274
Field, Charles R., 727
Finegold, Sydney M., 713, 736
Finkelstein, Frederic O., 457
Finley, Ruth, 370
Fisher, E., 464
Flournoy, D. J., 864
Fortner, Clarence L., 837
Freimer, Earl H., 288
Frey, C. A., 543
Fu, Kwung P., 511, 526
Fuchs, P. C., 146
Fukada, Shigemi, 1

Gaafar, Hassan A., 417
Galgiani, John N., 721
Gerding, Dale N., 850, 902
Gerster, J. F., 20
Girard, A. E., 89
Girard, Dennis, 491
Glasgow, Lowell A., 668, 691
Goebel, P., 258
Goedde, Lola W., 253
Goldberger, Mark J., 623
Gordon, Ralph C., 918
Grant, Robert B., 762
Greenstone, G., 399
Greenwood, D., 249
Greenwood, David, 824
Griffith, R. S., 814
Grinsted, J., 753
Guerrant, Richard L., 450
Guevarra, Lucille O., 809
Gump, Dieter, 80
Guze, L. B., 102, 462
Gwaltney, Jack M., Jr., 899

Hahn, Davis M., 837
Hall, Henrietta E., 344
Hall, Wendell H., 850, 902
Hamilton, John R., 691
Hammerberg, S., 399
Hammerberg, Susan, 869
Hardi, Robert, 682
Hasilik, Andrej, 402
Hasuda, K., 573
Heifetz, C. L., 543
Helstad, Arlan G., 727
Heman-Ackah, Samuel M., 223
Hendley, J. Owen, 899

Hirschman, Shalom Z., 25, 384
Ho, Y. K., 682
Hoeffler, U., 387
Holloway, B. W., 411, 573
Horn, Robert G., 164
Horodniceanu, Thea, 795
Hottendorf, G. H., 307
Howard, Jorge B., 205
Hryniewicz, Waleria, 912
Hughes, R. G., Jr., 682

Iglewski, Barbara H., 354
Inoue, Satoru, 779
Inuzuka, Manabu, 325, 333
Ishida, Nakao, 14
Islam, M. Rafiqul, 610
Iyobe, S., 573, 799

Jackson, Jean, 234
Jacob, Ginette B., 623
Jick, Hershel, 80
Johnson, Deanne, 354
Johnson, James E., 211
Jones, R. N., 146
Jones, Sue M., 866

Kabins, S. A., 139
Kaminura, Toshiaki, 1
Kane, Anne, 569
Kau, Donald L. K., 630
Kauffman, Carol A., 626
Kaufman, Herbert E., 885
Kaye, Donald, 188
Kayser, F. H., 664
Keim, G. R., Jr., 687
Keith, Alec, 96
Kelleher, J. J., 229
Kern, Earl R., 668, 691
Kisch, Alexander L., 507
Klastersky, J., 395
Kleit, Stuart A., 845
Kluge, Ronica M., 889
Ko, H. L., 387
Komarmy, Louis, 564
Koppel, G. A., 470
Kraus, Linda L., 677
Kromhout, James P., 850
Kulesza, J. S., 687
Kumagai, Katsuo, 57
Kunin, Calvin M., 503
Kureshi, Lubna Afzal, 713
Kurzynski, Terrence A., 727
Kushner, Donn J., 765
Kvam, D. C., 20

Lambe, D. W., Jr., 112
Lampe, Mary F., 436
Landesman, Sheldon, 837
Larson, E. W., 770
Laslie, W. W., 112
Lawton, William D., 417
Lee, B. K., 363
Lee, Wie-Shing, 564
Lees, Tracy, 322

Le Goffic, F., 258
Leitner, F., 426
Lerner, Stephen A., 878
Levin, N., 464
Levinson, Warren, 234
Levison, Matthew E., 188
Lichliter, Wayne D., 483
Lietman, Paul S., 347
Ligeti, P., 179
Lilly, Ralph B., 447
Lindmark, Donald G., 476
Line, Verle D., 861
Long, James F., 277
Lopez, Ruben, 697
Luft, Friedrich C., 845
Luke, Robert G., 555
Lynch, John E., 89, 132

McCardell, Barbara A., 498
McCord, Ronald S., 28
McCracken, George H., Jr., 205
McKellar, Robin C., 765
McKenzie, Colin N., 765
McNeely, David J., 889
McRipley, R. J., 38, 45
Madhavan, T., 464
Mahoney, David F., 470
Majid, M. A., 610
Mallette, M. F., 613
Manion, Robert E., 902
Mårdh, Per-Anders, 604
Marks, Melvin I., 399, 869
Marmion, LeRoy C., 447
Marr, J. J., 707
Martel, A., 258
Matthews, Thomas R., 923
Mattie, H., 441
Mayhall, C. G., 707
Maynard, James E., 571
Medoff, G., 707
Melethil, Srikumaran, 421
Meyer, Richard D., 677
Meyers, Burt R., 25, 384
Mikelens, Peter, 234
Miki, Kazuyo, 1
Miller, George, 277
Miller, George H., 827
Miller, M. M., 687
Miller, Warren M., 630
Mills, B. J., 411
Misiek, M., 426
Mitsuhashi, S., 573, 779
Miyano, Hiroshi, 325, 333
Moe, J. B., 549
Mohan Kanwal, 918
Mohs, Edgar, 205
Molenkamp, G. C., 786
Montgomerie, J. Z., 102
Morahan, Page S., 28
Morioka, Kayoko, 191
Morse, Stephen A., 354
Müller, Miklós, 476
Murakawa, Takeo, 1
Murphy, Bert L., 571

Naider, Fred, 483
Nakamoto, Shoji, 1
Nakamura, Shinichi, 779
Nathan, C., 139
Neblett, Thomas R., 921
Neu, Harold C., 511, 526, 535, 623
Nishida, Minoru, 1
Novo, Ernesto, 176
Nuttall, Charles E., 555

O'Callaghan, Cynthia H., 245
Ogawa, Mayumi, 191
O'Grady, F., 249
Oka, Tetsuo, 579
Okada, Naohiko, 1
Olsen, Gregg A., 668
Overall, James C., Jr., 668, 691

Padhye, Arvind A., 75
Pappagianis, D., 318
Parry, Michael F., 623
Pasiecznik, Karen A., 677
Paxton, Larry, 773
Pearson, I. A., 543
Perkins, Robert L., 34
Peter, Georges, 893
Petrocheilou, V., 753
Phair, John P., 626
Pickering, Larry K., 652
Pickett, M. J., 102
Piña, Carmen I., 176
Pogwizd, Steven M., 878
Pohlod, D., 464
Polish, Louis, 96
Pootjes, C. F., 498
Postic, Bosko, 809
Poutsiaka, J. W., 687
Powell, James T., 639
Prasad, S. S. S. V., 293
Price, K. E., 426
Primm, R. Kirby, 164
Prior, Richard B., 34
Pulverer, G., 387
Purdy, Michael A., 182
Pursiano, T. A., 426

Quay, John F., 630
Quinn, E. L., 464
Quintiliani, Richard, 157

Rahaman, M. Mujibur, 610
Rattie, Elisabeth S., 283
Ravin, Louis J., 283
Rawal, B. D., 915
Reese, Richard E., 253
Retsema, James A., 132, 491
Reusser, Fritz, 618
Ribner, Bruce, 25
Richmond, M. H., 215, 219, 753
Ripa, Torvald, 604
Robson, Hugh G., 592, 646
Rohde, Wolfgang, 234
Rohlfing, S. R., 20

Ronda-Lain, Conchita, 697
Rozgonyi, Ferenc, 377
Ruckinsky, Tom, 96
Ruiz, Daniel E., 34

Sagai, H., 573
Saito, Noriyuki, 14
Sakamoto, Hiroshi, 1
Sande, Merle A., 450
Sanders, Christine C., 519
Sandham, H. J., 196, 200
Sands, Jeffrey, 96
Santanam, P., 664
Santoro, Jerome, 188
Sasaki, Kenji, 14
Sawai, Tetsuo, 191
Scharfenberger, L., 733
Schierl, Elizabeth, A., 902
Schimpff, Stephen C., 87
Schling, Marion, 417
Schwartz, Pauline M., 64
Scott, Rita E., 646
Segal, Ester, 75
Sesnie, J. C., 543
Severin, M. J., 380
Shadomy, Smith, 733, 776
Sharma, Ram A., 119
Shaw, William V., 347
Shepherd, C. A., 872
Sherris, John C., 436
Shethna, Y. I., 293
Shimizu, Fumio, 57
Shimizu, Masanao, 779
Shimizu, Yoshinobu, 57
Shipman, Charles, Jr., 64
Shive, Karen, 150
Sibley, P. L., 687
Siebert, W. T., 467
Silver, Barry, 399
Slepack, Jerry M., 626
Smilack, J. D., 467
Snipes, Wallace, 96
Solomons, I. A., 89
Soussy, C. J., 258
Spadaro, J. A., 856
Spence, W. N., 872
Standiford, Harold C., 837
Staniforth, Susan E., 245
Stephen, E. L., 549, 770
Stevens, David A., 447, 721
Stevens, Lynne I., 918
Stone, William J., 164
Strausbaugh, Larry J., 450
Strong, James E., 652
Sullivan, Hugh R., 630
Sullivan, John J., 850
Sutter, Vera L., 713, 736
Suzuki, Fujio, 14
Swanby, S., 768
Sykes, R. B., 245

Tagg, John R., 299, 912
Tanner, Widmar, 402
Tapia, Alfonso, 697
Taylor, Diane E., 762
Taylor, Richard L., 613
Thijssen, H. H. W., 441
Thorne, Grace M., 123
Thys, J. P., 395
Tilton, Richard C., 157
Tipple, Margaret, 773
Tomasz, Alexander, 697
Tomoeda, Munemitsu 325, 333
Toyama, Hiromi, 333
Trujillo, Hugo, 205
Trust, T. J., 598
Tsai, Y. H., 426
Tuke, Gregory C., 288
Turner, J. R., 470
Tzianabos, T., 344

Utz, C. J., 776
Uwaydah, Marwan, 52

Vandamme, E. J., 265
Vanderkelen, B., 395
Van Harken, D. R., 307
Varani, J., 229
Varnell, Emily D., 885
Vaughan, Patrick, 354
Veerkamp, J. H., 786
Verbist, L., 173, 657

Wadsö, Ingemar, 604
Wagman, G. H., 363
Waitz, J. Allan, 827
Waks, Susan B., 697
Waldron, James A., 164
Walker, J. S., 549, 770
Wanda, Paul, 96
Wannamaker, L. W., 299
Ward, Margie, 274
Washington, John A., II, 211
Watanakunakorn, Chatrchai, 382
Waterman, N. G., 733
Webb, Bette J., 128
Wegner, Dennis L., 921
Weinmaster, Gerry, 869
Weinrich, A. Elise, 106
Weinstein, M. J., 363, 827
Weld, H. G., 196, 200
Wenzel, Richard P., 899
Westerman, E. L., 467
Whitby, J. L., 598
Whitcher, Jack, 234
White, Lendell A., 344
White, S., 776
White, Thomas J., 347
Whitney, R. R., 38, 45
Wiernik, Peter H., 837
Wiley, J. L., 380
Wilkins, Tracy D., 926
Williams, T. W., Jr., 467
Wilson, Stephen G., 519
Wlodkowski, T. J., 179
Wolny, J. D., 814
Woods, D. R., 567
Wotton, Sandra, 215, 219
Wright, Walter E., 861

Yamagishi, Saburo, 191
Yancovitz, Stanley, 25
Yaremchuk, K., 464
Yielding, K. Lemone, 182
Yokota, Yoshiko, 1
Yoon, Y. H., 687
Yoshikawa, Thomas T., 462
Yoshimori, R. N., 102
Yotter, David W., 923
Young, Viola Mae, 837
Yrios, John W., 727
Yum, Moo Nahm, 845

Zaidi, I. H., 687

SUBJECT INDEX

VOLUME 10

Acanthamoeba species
susceptibility to a variety of therapeutic agents, 370
Acinetobacter calcoaceticus var. *anitratus*
susceptibility to minocycline, 102
2″-Adenylyltransferase
enzymatic adenylylation as a means of determining aminoglycoside antibiotic concentrations in serum, 664
4′-Adenylyltransferase
enzymatic adenylylation as a means of determining aminoglycoside antibiotic concentrations in serum, 664
Aeromonas hydrophila
inducible oxacillin-hydrolyzing penicillinase isolated from fish, 191
Agrobacterium tumefaciens
chemical nature of agrocin 84 and its effect on a virulent strain, 498
Agrocin 84
chemical nature, 498
effect on a virulent strain of *A. tumefaciens*, 498
5-Allyl-2′-deoxyuridine
antiviral action and cellular toxicity, 119
Amikacin
activity against *P. aeruginosa* and *Enterobacteriaceae*, 592
activity alone and in combination with carbenicillin against *S. marcescens*, 878
comparative pharmacology with kanamycin in 45 neonates, 205
effect of renal failure and dialysis on serum concentration, 464
5″-Amino-5″-deoxybutirosin
antibacterial activity in vitro in mice, 543
Aminoglycoside
concentrations in peritoneal capsular fluid in rabbits, 902
effect of clindamycin on activity in a murine model of *E. coli* infection, 893
Aminoglycoside antibiotics
new plasmid-mediated nucleotidylation in *S. aureus*, 258
Aminoglycosides
activity against gentamicin-resistant *P. aeruginosa*, 399
enzymatic adenylylation by 4′-adenylyltransferase and 2″-adenylyltransferase for determining concentrations, 664
mutants of *P. aeruginosa* that show specific hypersensitivity, 411
S. aureus strains displaying unusual resistance, 519
susceptibility of gentamicin-resistant *Enterobacteriaceae* and *P. aeruginosa*, 677
Amoxycillin
triple crossover study on absorption and excretion, 173
Amphotericin B
nephrotoxicity, 555
new medium for in vitro susceptibility studies, 776
toxicological studies in mice, rats, and dogs, 687
Amphotericin B methyl ester
toxicological studies in mice, rats, and dogs, 687
Ampicillin
epidemiology of bacterial resistance, 872
short-term storage in microdilution trays for antimicrobial susceptibility tests, 83
susceptibility of *H. influenzae* type b, 322
triple crossover study on absorption and excretion, 173
9-β-D-Arabinofuranosyladenine 5′-monophosphate
effect on experimental herpes simplex keratitis, 885
9-β-D-Arabinofuranosylhypoxanthine 5′-monophosphate
effect on experimental herpes simplex keratitis, 885
Arabinosyladenine
antiviral activity in herpes simplex virus-infected KB cells, 64
Arabinosylhypoxanthine
antiviral activity in herpes simplex virus-infected KB cells, 64
Ascitic fluid
antibiotic penetrance in dogs, 850

Bacillus brevis ATCC 9999
nutrition, 265
Bacillus megaterium
mode of action of penicillins, 579
Bacillus thuringiensis subsp. *thuringiensis*
mode of action of an antitumor protein on Yoshida ascites sarcoma cells, 293
Bacteriocin
production by group A streptococcal L-forms, 912
production by *N. gonorrhoeae*, 417
Bacteriophage φ6
inactivation by butylated hydroxytoluene and butylated hydroxyanisole, 96
Bacteriophage lambda
inhibition of development by R plasmids of the H incompatibility group, 762
Bacteriophage T1
inhibition of development by R plasmids of the H incompatibility group, 762
Bacteriophage T7
inhibition of development by R plasmids of the H incompatibility group, 762
Benzylpenicillin
short-term storage in microdilution trays for antimicrobial susceptibility tests, 83
Beta-lactam antibiotics
synergy of mecillinam in combination, 535
Beta-lactamase
activity in anaerobic bacteria, 106
Beta-lactamases
substrate inhibition, 470
susceptibility of seven cephalosporins, 219
Bifidobacterium bifidum subsp. *pennsylvanicus*
effects of antibiotics on metabolism of peptidoglycan, protein, and lipids, 786

BL-3849A
antiviral activity, 691
BL-P1654
activity in vitro as compared with ticarcillin and carbenicillin, 241
BL-S786
laboratory evaluation, 426
Butylated hydroxyanisole
inactivation of bacteriophage ϕ6, 96
Butylated hydroxytoluene
inactivation of bacteriophage ϕ6, 96

Candida albicans
basis for the design of anticandidal agents from studies of peptide utilization, 483
Carbenicillin
activity against gentamicin-resistant *P. aeruginosa*, 399
activity in combination with gentamicin, amikacin, and netilmicin against *S. marcescens*, 878
activity in vitro as compared with ticarcillin and BL-P1654, 241
short-term storage in microdilution trays for antimicrobial susceptibility tests, 83
susceptibility testing with 100-μg disks, 112
synergistic activity in combination with gentamicin in experimental *Pseudomonas* bacteremia in neutropenic rats, 646
Carboxypeptidase Y
inhibition of synthesis rate by tunicamycin in *S. cerevisiae*, 402
[^{14}C]cefaclor
metabolism in three species of laboratory animals, 630
Cefamandole
comparison of thrombophlebitis associated with cephalothin and cephapirin, 467
concentration in serum interstitial fluid, bile, and urine, 733
in vitro and clinical pharmacokinetics, 814
pharmacokinetics, 421
pharmacokinetics in patients undergoing hemodialysis and peritoneal dialysis, 457
pharmacokinetics in the presence of renal failure and in patients undergoing hemodialysis, 623
Cefatrizine
evaluation in vitro as compared with other cephalosporins, 288
susceptibility of *H. influenzae* type b, 322
Cefazolin
pharmacological study during intermittent and continous infusion, 395
treatment of acute enteric fever, 52
Cefazolin-gentamicin
synergism against enterococci, 157
Ceftezole
in vitro and in vivo evaluation, 1
Cell wall-inhibitory antibiotics
suppression of lytic and bactericidal effects, 697
Cephalosporin
concentrations in peritoneal capsular fluid in rabbits, 902
derivative, ceftezole, 1
dual-action, 249
dual mode of action, 245
preparation of intestinal villi useful for studying hydrolysis rates of esters, 861
Cephalosporins
ability to penetrate the surface layers of *E. coli*, 219
antibacterial activity against *Enterobacteriaceae* and nonfermentative gram-negative bacilli, 657
comparative study of seven, 219
comparison of in vitro activity against gram-negative and -positive bacteria resistant to cephaloridine, 507
comparison of thrombophlebitis associated with three antibiotics, 467
penetration in *E. coli* of beta-lactamase-nonsusceptible, 215
substrate inhibition of beta-lactamases, a method for predicting enzymatic stability, 470
susceptibility of respiratory tract anaerobes, 713
susceptibility to beta-lactamases, 219
Cephalothin
association in rises in blood urea nitrogen, 80
combined with ticarcillin as therapy in granulocytopenic cancer patients, 837
comparison of thrombophlebitis associated with cephapirin and cefamandole, 467
lack of significant in vitro antagonism with penicillin and rolitetracycline, 802
pharmacokinetics, 421
short-term storage in microdilution trays for antimicrobial susceptibility tests, 83
susceptibility of *S. aureus* strains, 707
Cephapirin
comparative pharmacokinetics and metabolism in laboratory animals and humans, 307
comparison of thrombophlebitis associated with cephalothin and cefamandole, 467
pharmacokinetics, 421
Cephradine
pharmacokinetic interpretation of levels in serum, 283
Chloramphenicol
enzymological microassay, 347
susceptibility of *H. influenzae* type b, 322
Cholera
effects of doxycycline in actively purging patients, 610
Cinoxacin
antimicrobial activity against 2,968 clinical bacterial isolates, 146
compared in vitro with nalidixic acid and oxolinic acid, 918
Citrobacter freundii
antibiotic resistance in water containing ornamental fishes, 598
Clindamycin
compared with josamycin and rosamicin, 773
comparison with josamycin and rosamicin against *B. fragilis*, 188
effect on aminoglycoside activity in a murine model of *E. coli* infection, 893
Coliform bacteria
evolution of transferable antibiotic resistance, 567
Cytomegalovirus
effect of ribavirin on infection, 809

Doxycycline
effects in actively purging cholera patients, 610

Encephalomyocarditis virus
treatment with exogenous interferon, polyinosinic acid-polycytidylic acid, or polyinosinic acid-polycytidylic acid-poly-L-lysine complex on infections in mice, 668
Enteric fever
cefazolin treatment, 52
Enterobacteriaceae
antibacterial activity of nine cephalosporins, 657
comparative activity of netilmicin, gentamicin, amikacin, and tobramycin, 592
susceptibility to netilmicin and aminoglycoside antibiotics, 677
Erythromycin
compared with josamycin and rosamicin, 773
comparison with josamycin and rosamicin against *B. fragilis*, 188
comparison with josamycin in the therapy of *M. pneumoniae* pneumonia, 899
Erythromycin stearate
pharmacology compared with josamycin, 450
Escherichia coli
ability of seven cephalosporins to penetrate the surface layers, 219
actions of tetracyclines as studied by microcalorimetry, 604
correlation of resistance to proflavine and penicillin, 765
effect of clindamycin on aminoglycoside activity in a murine model of infection, 893
effect of osmolality on the response to mecillinam, 824
penetration of beta-lactamase-nonsusceptible penicillins and cephalosporins, 215
tetracycline action, 223
Escherichia coli B
phleomycin-induced solubilization of deoxyribonucleic acid in uninfected and T-bacteriophage-infected, 150
Escherichia coli K-12
nalidixic acid inhibition of post-ultraviolet recovery, 182
specific action of 4-nitropyridine 1-oxide on Pro^+ strains, 325, 333
5-Ethyl-deoxyuridine
antiviral action and cellular toxicity, 119
Experimental surgical-wound infections
characterization and quantitation in evaluating topical antibacterial agents, 38
responsiveness to topical chemotherapy, 45

Flumequine
bioevaluation for urinary tract use, 20

Gentamicin
activity against bacteria associated with intra-abdominal sepsis, 34
activity against *P. aeruginosa* and *Enterobacteriaceae*, 592
activity alone and in combination with carbenicillin against *S. marcescens*, 878
activity as compared with sisomicin in mouse protection tests with gram-negative bacilli, 384
activity in vitro as compared with Sch 20656, netilmicin, and tobramycin, 382
association in rises in blood urea nitrogen, 80
combined with ticarcillin as therapy in granulocytopenic cancer patients, 837
effect on growth of viral, chlamydial, and rickettsial agents in mice and embryonated eggs, 344
in vitro comparison with tobramycin, sisomicin, and netilmicin, 768
nephrotoxicity as compared with netilmicin, 845
renal extraction in anesthetized dogs, 277
stability in serum, 866
susceptibility of *S. aureus* strains, 707
synergistic activity in combination with gentamicin in experimental *Pseudomonas* bacteremia in neutropenic rats, 646
Gentamicin-carbenicillin
nosocomial infection with resistant *P. aeruginosa*, 626
Glutarimide
new antibiotic, 9-methylstreptimidone, 14
Gramicidin S
nutrition of *B. brevis* ATCC 9999, the producer of, 265

Haemophilus influenzae
new method for detecting inactivation of penicillins, 564
Haemophilus influenzae type b
susceptibility to cefatrizine, ampicillin, and chloramphenicol, 322
Herpes simplex keratitis
effect of 9-β-D-arabinofuranosyladenine 5′-monophosphate and 9-β-D-arabinofuranosylhypoxanthine 5′-monophosphate, 885
Herpes simplex virus
antiviral activity of arabinosyladenine and arabinosylhypoxanthine in infected KB cells, 64
inactivation by hydroxyquinolines, 234
photoinactivation in rabbit kidney cells, 229
specific inactivation by silver nitrate, 57
Herpes simplex virus type 1
differential effects of 5-methylmercapto-2′-deoxyuridine on replication, 682
Herpes simplex virus type 2
antiviral effect of pyran against infection in mice, 28
Hydroxyquinolines
inhibition of ribonucleic acid-dependent deoxyribonucleic acid polymerase and inactivation of Rous sarcoma virus and herpes simplex virus, 234

Influenza virus
therapeutic effects of ribavirin in mice, 549
Interferon
effect of treatment on encephalomyocarditis virus infections in mice, 668
Isoxazolylpenicillins
active metabolites in humans, 441

Josamycin
activity against *B. fragilis*, in vitro, 188
compared with erythromycin and clindamycin, 773
comparison with erythromycin in the therapy of

M. pneumoniae pneumonia, 899
pharmacology compared with erythromycin stearate, 450
susceptibility of common clinical isolates, 253

Kanamycin
comparative pharmacology with amikacin in 45 neonates, 205
Klebsiella species
antibiotic synergy and antagonism against clinical isolates, 889

L5178Y cells
inhibition by methotrexate and antibiotics, 185
Lactobacilli
effect of long-term therapies with penicillin and sulfadiazine in dental plaque, 200

Mannitol
inability in reducing amphotericin B nephrotoxicity, 555
Mecillinam
effect of osmolality on the response of *E. coli*, 824
epidemiology of bacterial resistance, 872
synergy combined with beta-lactam antibiotics, 535
Melanin
inhibition of antibiotic activity, 569
Metallic ions
antifungal properties, 856
Methicillin
genotypic stability of resistance in *S. aureus* at supraoptimal temperature, 377
short-term storage in microdilution trays for antimicrobial susceptibility tests, 83
Methotrexate
inhibition of L5178Y cells in culture, 185
5-Methylmercapto-2′-deoxyuridine
differential effects on replication of herpes simplex virus type 1, 682
9-Methylstreptimidone
antiviral and interferon-inducing activity, 14
Metronidazole
antitrichomonad action, mutagenicity, and reduction, 476
comparison with josamycin and rosamicin against *B. fragilis*, 188
Miconazole
therapy of thrombocytosis and anemia, 447
Minocycline
activity against bacteria associated with intra-abdominal sepsis, 34
susceptibility of *A. calcoaceticus* var. *antitratus*, 102
Murine coccidioidomycosis
treatment with polymyxin B, 318
Mycoplasma pneumoniae
comparison of josamycin and erythromycin in the therapy of pneumonia, 899

Naegleria species
susceptibility to a variety of therapeutic agents, 370
Nafcillin
short-term storage in microdilution trays for antimicrobial susceptibility tests, 83
Nalidixic acid
compared in vitro with cinoxacin and oxolinic acid, 918
inhibition of post-ultraviolet recovery in *E. coli* K-12, 182
Neisseria gonorrhoeae
absence of penicillin-degrading enzymes in penicillin-resistant strains, 179
bacteriocin production, 417
inhibition by a bacteriocin from *P. aeruginosa*, 354
multiple antibiotic resistance in clinical strains isolated in South Carolina, 639
Neisseria meningitidis
reevaluation of the disk diffusion method for sulfonamide susceptibility testing, 869
Neomycin
influence when combined with oxytetracycline on *S. typhimurium*, 89
Nephritis
related to tuberculosis chemotherapy, 164
Netilmicin
activity against *P. aeruginosa* and *Enterobacteriaceae*, 592
activity alone and in combination with carbenicillin against *S. marcescens*, 878
activity in vitro as compared with Sch 20656, gentamicin, and tobramycin, 382
biological activity, 827
compared with sisomicin in susceptibility testing, 864
in vitro comparison with four other aminoglycoside antibiotics, 139
in vitro comparison with gentamicin, tobramycin, and sisomicin, 768
in vitro study compared with other aminoglycosides, 526
nephrotoxicity as compared with gentamicin in rats, 845
susceptibility of gentamicin-resistant *Enterobacteriaceae* and *P. aeruginosa*, 677
synergistic effect, 511
Nitroimidazoles
antitrichomonad action, mutagenicity, and reduction, 476
4-Nitropyridine 1-oxide
mechanism of action, 333
specific action on *E. coli* K-12 Pro^+ strains, 325, 333

Oxacillin
short-term storage in microdilution trays for antimicrobial susceptibility tests, 83
susceptibility of *S. aureus* strains, 707
Oxolinic acid
compared in vitro with cinoxacin and nalidixic acid, 918
Oxytetracycline
influence when combined with neomycin on *S. typhimurium*, 89

Parainfluenza (Sendai) virus
therapeutic effects of small-particle aerosols of ribavirin on infections of mice, 770
Penicillin
absence of degrading enzymes in resistant *N. gon-*

orrhoeae strains, 179
correlation of resistance in *E. coli*, 765
effect of long-term therapy on *S. mutans* and lactobacilli in dental plaque, 200
effects of low concentrations on *S. mutans*, 196
lack of significant in vitro antagonism with cephalothin and rolitetracycline, 802
preparation of intestinal villi useful for studying hydrolysis rates of esters, 861
Penicillinase
inducible oxacillin-hydrolyzing, 191
Penicillin G
change in susceptibility of group B streptococci from 1968 through 1975, 380
Penicillins
mode of action in *B. megaterium*, 579
new method for detecting inactivation by *H. influenzae* and *S. aureus*, 564
penetration in *E. coli* of beta-lactamase-nonsusceptible, 215
susceptibility of respiratory tract anaerobes, 713
Phleomycin
solubilization of deoxyribonucleic acid in *E. coli* B, 150
Physarum gyrosum
growth on agar plates and in liquid culture, 613
Pipemidic acid
inhibition of conjugal transfer of R plasmids, 779
Pirbenicillin
pharmacokinetic parameters in mice, 491
Polyinosinic acid-polycytidylic acid
effect of treatment on encephalomyocarditis virus infections in mice, 668
Polyinosinic acid-polycytidylic acid–poly-L-lysine complex
effect of treatment on encephalomyocarditis virus infections in mice, 668
Polymyxin B
treatment of murine coccidioidomycosis, 318
Proflavine
correlation of resistance in *E. coli*, 765
Propionibacterium acnes
antimicrobial susceptibility, 387
5-Propyl-deoxyuridine
antiviral action and cellular toxicity, 119
Proteus
effect of organic mercurials and sulfhydryl compounds on urease activity, 503
Prototheca species
susceptibility to antifungal agents, 75
Pseudomonas
synergistic activity of carbenicillin and gentamicin in bacteremia in neutropenic rats, 646
Pseudomonas aeruginosa
activity of newer aminoglycosides and carbenicillin against gentamicin-resistant, 399
classification of R plasmids by incompatibility, 573
comparative activity of netilmicin, gentamicin, amikacin, and tobramycin, 592
inhibition of *N. gonorrhoeae* by a bacteriocin, 354
mutants that show specific hypersensitivity to aminoglycosides, 411
nosocomial infection with gentamicin-carbenicillin-resistant, 626
susceptibility to netilmicin and aminoglycoside antibiotics, 677
Pyran
antiviral effect against herpes simplex virus type 2 infection in mice, 28

recBC
nalidixic acid inhibition requirement for function, 182
Resistance
C. freundii to antibiotics, 598
R factor
mediation of antibiotic resistance in *S. marcescens*, 123
Ribavirin
effect on murine cytomegalovirus infection, 809
therapeutic effects against influenza virus infections in mice, 549
therapeutic effects of small-particle aerosols on parainfluenza (Sendai) virus infections of mice, 770
Ribonucleic acid-dependent deoxyribonucleic acid polymerase
inhibition by hydroxyquinolines, 234
Ribonucleic acid polymerase
inhibition by tirandamycin, 618
Rolitetracycline
lack of significant in vitro antagonism with penicillin and cephalothin, 802
Rosamicin
activity against *B. fragilis*, in vitro, 188
compared with erythromycin and clindamycin, 773
Rous sarcoma virus
inactivation by hydroxyquinolines, 234
R-plasmid
transfer in vivo in the absence of antibiotic selection pressure, 753
R plasmids
classification by incompatibility in *P. aeruginosa*, 573
inhibition of bacteriophage lambda, T1, and T7 development, 762
inhibition of conjugal transfer by pipemidic acid and related compounds, 779
S. agalactiae (group B), 795

Saccharomyces cerevisiae
inhibition of synthesis rate of carboxypeptidase Y by tunicamycin, 402
Salmonella typhimurium
influence of a combination of neomycin and oxytetracycline, 89
Sch 20656
activity in vitro as compared with netilmicin, gentamicin, and tobramycin, 382
Serratia marcescens
activity of gentamicin, amikacin, and netilmicin alone and in combination, 878
R factor-mediated antibiotic resistance, 123
Sisomicin
activity as compared with gentamicin in mouse protection tests with gram-negative bacilli, 384

compared with netilmicin in susceptibility testing, 864
in vitro comparison of netilmicin, a semisynthetic derivative, 139
in vitro comparison with gentamicin, tobramycin, and netilmicin, 768
pharmacokinetic parameters, 25
Staphylococcus aureus
cultivation in a synthetic medium of low ultraviolet absorptivity, 915
genotypic stability of methicillin resistance at supraoptimal temperature, 377
new method for detecting inactivation of penicillins, 564
nucleotidylation of aminoglycoside antibiotics, 258
strains displaying unusual resistance to aminoglycosides, 519
susceptibility of strains to oxacillin, cephalothin, and gentamicin, 707
tetracycline action, 223
Streptococcal L-forms
bacteriocin production by group A, 912
Streptococci
antimicrobial susceptibility of group B, 128
change in susceptibility of group B to penicillin G from 1968 through 1975, 380
Streptococcin A-FF22
genetic basis of production, 299
Streptococcus agalactiae (group B)
R plasmids, 795
Streptococcus mutans
effect of long-term therapies with penicillin and sulfadiazine, 200
effects of low concentrations of penicillin and sulfadiazine, 196
susceptibility to antimicrobial agents, 274
Sulfadiazine
effect of long-term therapy on *S. mutans* and lactobacilli in dental plaque, 200
effects of low concentrations on *S. mutans*, 196
Sulfonamide
reevaluation of the disk diffusion method for susceptibility testing of *N. meningitidis*, 869
Susceptibility
anaerobic bacteria to 23 antimicrobial agents, 736
procedure for expediting determinations in gram-negative, urinary tract pathogens, 921
Susceptibility testing
chemically defined medium, 923
comparison of direct and standardized antimicrobial tests, 211
medium for use with anaerobic bacteria, 926
of anaerobic bacteria with 100-μg carbenicillin disks, 112
reproducibility of control strains, 436
sisomicin versus netilmicin, 864
turbidimetric technique for yeasts, 721

Talampicillin
triple crossover study on absorption and excretion, 173
Tetracycline
comparison of action on *S. aureus* and *E. coli* by microbial kinetics, 223
Tetracyclines
actions on *E. coli* as studied by microcalorimetry, 604
mediation of photoinactivation of Venezuelan equine encephalitis virus, 176
3-(5-Tetrazolyl)penam
laboratory evaluation, 132
Thioglycolate broth disk method
antibiotic susceptibility testing of anaerobes, 727
Thrombocytosis
reversibility due to miconazole therapy, 447
Thrombophlebitis
comparison associated with three cephalosporin antibiotics, 467
Ticarcillin
activity in vitro as compared with BL-P1654 and carbenicillin, 241
combined with cephalothin or gentamicin as therapy in granulocytopenic cancer patients, 837
Tirandamycin
inhibition of bacterial ribonucleic acid polymerase, 618
Tobramycin
activity against *P. aeruginosa* and *Enterobacteriaceae*, 592
activity in vitro as compared with Sch 20656, netilmicin, and gentamicin, 382
in vitro comparison with gentamicin, sisomicin, and netilmicin, 768
radioimmunoassay of iodinated, 652
Trimethoprim-sulfamethoxazole
concentrations in blood after a single, large oral dose, 462
Tunicamycin
inhibition of synthesis rate of carboxypeptidase Y in *S. cerevisiae*, 402

Venezuelan equine encephalitis virus
photoinactivation mediated by tetracyclines, 176
Verdamicin
formation of methylated and phosphorylated metabolites during the fermentation process, 363
5-Vinyl-deoxyuridine
antiviral action and cellular toxicity, 119
Virazole
antiviral effects in chronic hepatitis B surface antigen-seropositive chimpanzees, 571

Yoshida ascites sarcoma cells
mode of action of a purified antitumor protein from the proteinaceous crystal of *B. thuringiensis* subsp. *thuringiensis*, 293

INDEX TO DATE OF ISSUE

Month	Date of Issue	Pages
July	22 July 1976	1–190
August	23 August 1976	191–386
September	23 September 1976	387–572
October	19 October 1976	573–778
November	16 November 1976	779–867
December	14 December 1976	869–929